Textbook of
Interventional Cardiology

Textbook of Interventional Cardiology

sixth edition

ERIC J. TOPOL, MD
Director, Scripps Translational Science Institute
Chief Academic Officer, Scripps Health
Sr. Consultant, Division of Cardiology, Scripps Clinic
Professor of Genomics, The Scripps Research Institute
La Jolla, California

PAUL S. TEIRSTEIN, MD
Chief of Cardiology
Director, Interventional Cardiology
Scripps Clinic
Director, Scripps Prebys Cardiovascular Institute
Scripps Health
La Jolla, California

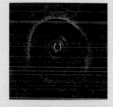
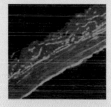
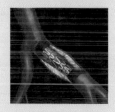
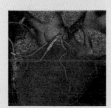

ELSEVIER
SAUNDERS

1600 John F. Kennedy Blvd.
Ste 1800
Philadelphia, PA 19103-2899

Notices

Knowledge and best practice in this field are constantly changing. As new research and experience broaden our understanding, changes in research methods, professional practices, or medical treatment may become necessary.

Practitioners and researchers must always rely on their own experience and knowledge in evaluating and using any information, methods, compounds, or experiments described herein. In using such information or methods they should be mindful of their own safety and the safety of others, including parties for whom they have a professional responsibility.

With respect to any drug or pharmaceutical products identified, readers are advised to check the most current information provided (i) on procedures featured or (ii) by the manufacturer of each product to be administered, to verify the recommended dose or formula, the method and duration of administration, and contraindications. It is the responsibility of practitioners, relying on their own experience and knowledge of their patients, to make diagnoses, to determine dosages and the best treatment for each individual patient, and to take all appropriate safety precautions.

To the fullest extent of the law, neither the Publisher nor the authors, contributors, or editors, assume any liability for any injury and/or damage to persons or property as a matter of products liability, negligence or otherwise, or from any use or operation of any methods, products, instructions, or ideas contained in the material herein.

Acquisitions Editor: Dolores Meloni
Developmental Editor: Taylor Ball
Editorial Assistant: Brad McIlwain
Publishing Services Manager: Catherine Jackson
Project Manager: Sara Alsup
Design Direction: Ellen Zanolle
Illustrations manager: Karen Giacomucci
Marketing Manager: Helena Mutak

Printed in Canada

Last digit is the print number: 9 8 7 6 5 4 3 2 1

This book is dedicated to Alvin S. Teirstein, MD (1927–2011). Forever a student, in his final year he introduced himself as PGY 58. He was a clinician, a teacher, a father, and a giant.

And to our wives, Susan and Jacki, who have given us loving support throughout our careers.

Takashi Akasaka, MD, PhD
Professor, Department of Cardiovascular Medicine
Wakayama Medical University
Wakayama, Japan

Ibrahim Akin, MD
Universitätsklinikum Hamburg-Eppendorf
Abteilung Kardiologie
Hamburg, Germany

Jorge R. Alegria, MD
Assistant Professor
Co-Medical Director of Adult Congenital Heart Disease Clinic
Department of Medicine
Saha Cardiovascular Research Center
University of Kentucky
Lexington, Kentucky

Alexandra Almonacid, MD
Brigham and Women's Hospital
Boston, Massachusetts

Carlos L. Alviar, MD
Post Doctoral Residency Fellow
Department of Medicine
St. Luke's-Roosevelt Hospital Center
Columbia University College of Physicians and Surgeons
New York, New York

Dominick J. Angiollilo, MD, PhD
Associate Professor of Medicine
Director of Cardiovascular Research
University of Florida College of Medicine Jacksonville
Jacksonville, Florida

Gary M. Ansel, MD
MidOhio Cardiology and Vascular Consultants
Columbus, Ohio

Saif Anwaruddin, MD
Assistant Professor of Medicine
Penn Heart and Vascular Center
University of Pennsylvania
Philadelphia, Pennsylvania

David T. Balzer, MD
Professor, Pediatrics
Division of Pediatric Cardiology
Washington University School of Medicine at St. Louis
Director, Cardiac Catheterization Laboratory
St. Louis Children's Hospital
St. Louis, Missouri

Amr T. Bannan, MD
Director, Cardiac Catheterization Laboratories
Hospital of the University of Pennsylvania
Philadelphia, Pennsylvania

Gregory W. Barsness, MD
Assistant Professor of Medicine
Departments of Cardiovascular Diseases and Radiology
Mayo Clinic
Rochester, Minnesota

Robert H. Beekman III, MD
Professor of Pediatric Cardiology
Cincinnati Children's Hospital Medical Center
Cincinnati, Ohio

Farzin Beygui, MD, PhD
Pitié-Salpêtrière University Hospital
Institut de Cardiologie
Paris, France

John A. Bittl, MD
Ocala Heart Institute
Munroe Regional Medical Center
Ocala, Florida (JAB)

Philipp Bonhoeffer, MD
Professor and Chief of Cardiology
Director of the Cardiac Catheterisation Laboratory
Great Ormond Street Hospital for Children, NHS Trust
London, United Kingdom

Michael Braendle, MD, MS
Associate Professor of Endocrinology
Zurich School of Medicine
Zurich, Switzerland
Division Chief, Division of Endocrinology and Diabetes
Department of Internal Medicine
Kantonsspital St. Gallen
St. Gallen, Switzerland

J. Matthew Brennan, MD
Assistant Professor of Medicine
Division of Cardiology
Duke University School of Medicine
Durham, North Carolina

Ralph Brindis, MD, MPH
Clinical Professor of Medicine
University of California, San Francisco
San Francisco, California
Regional Senior Advisor for Cardiovascular Diseases
Kaiser Permanente
Oakland, California

Eric Brochet, MD
Cardiology Department
Hopital Bichat
Paris, France

David Burke, MD
Clinical Assistant Professor of Medicine
Michigan State University/Kalamazoo Center for Medical Studies
Clinical Cardiologist
Heart Center for Excellence
Kalamazoo, Michigan

Heinz Joachim Büttner, MD
Chief of Interventional Cardiology, Herz-Zentrum Bad Krozingen
Universitäres Herz- und Kreislaufzentrum Freiburg—Bad Krozingen
Germany

Robert Byrne, MB
Interventional Cardiologist
Deutsches Herzzentrum and 1. Medizinische Klinik rechts der Isar
Technische Universität
Munich, Germany

Christopher P. Cannon, MD
Associate Professor of Medicine
Harvard Medical School
Associate Physician, Cardiovascular Division,
Brigham and Women's Hospital
Boston, Massachusetts

Ivan P. Casserly, MB, BCh
Assistant Professor of Medicine, University of Colorado
University of Colorado—Denver
Anschutz Medical Campus
Denver, Colorado

Matthews Chacko, MD
Assistant Professor of Medicine
The Johns Hopkins University
Director, Peripheral Vascular Interventions
Faculty, Interventional Cardiology, CCU & the Thayer Firm
The Johns Hopkins Hospital
Baltimore, Maryland

Derek P. Chew, MBBS, MPH
Professor of Cardiology
Department of Cardiovascular Medicine
Flinders University
Regional Director of Cardiology
Department of Cardiovascular Medicine
Southern Adelaide Health Service
Adelaide, South Australia
Australia

Leslie Cho, MD
Director, Cleveland Clinic's Women's Cardiovascular Center
Section Head, Preventive Cardiology and Rehabilitation
Robert and Suzanne Tomsich Department of Cardiovascular
   Medicine
Cleveland Clinic
Cleveland, Ohio

Louise Coats, PhD
Director of Cardiology
Freeman Hospital
Newcastle upon Tyne, United Kingdom

Antonio Colombo, MD
EMO-GVM Centro Cuore Columbus and San Raffaele Scientific
   Institute
Milan, Italy

Marco A. Costa, MD, PhD
University Hospitals Harrington-McLaughlin Heart & Vascular
   Institute
Case Western Reserve University School of Medicine
Cleveland, Ohio

Alain Cribier, MD
Professor of Cardiology
Rouen University
Chief of Cardiology
Hospital Charles Nicolle
Rouen, France

Kevin J. Croce, MD, PhD
Instructor in Medicine
Harvard Medical School
Associate Physician
Cardiovascular Division
Brigham and Women's Hospital
Boston, Massachusetts

Fernando Cura, MD, PhD
Sub-Director of Interventional Cardiology and Endovascular
   Therapies
Instituto Cardiovascular de Buenos Aires
Buenos Aires, Argentina

Gregory J. Dehmer, MD
Professor of Medicine
Texas A&M Health Science Center College of Medicine
Director, Cardiology Division
Scott & White Healthcare
Temple, Texas

Robert S. Dieter, MD
Department of Cardiology
Edward Hines, Jr. VA Hospital
Hines, Illinois

John S. Douglas, Jr., MD
Professor of Medicine
Director, Interventional Cardiology
Emory University School of Medicine
Director, Cardiac Catheterization Laboratories
Emory University Hospital
Atlanta, Georgia

Helene Eltchaninoff, MD
Professor of Cardiology
Rouen University
Chief, Cardiac Catheterization Laboratory
Hospital Charles Nicolle
Rouen, France

Marvin H. Eng, MD
Assistant Profressor of Medicine
University of Texas Health Sciences Center San Antonio
San Antonio, Texas

Peter J. Fitzgerald, MD, PhD
Director, Center for Cardiovascular Technology
Director, Cardiovascular Core Analysis Laboratory (CCAL)
Stanford University Medical School
Stanford, California

Valentin Fuster, MD
Professor of Medicine
Department of Cardiology
Mount Sinai School of Medicine
Director, Zena and Michael A. Wiener Cardiovascular Institute
New York, New York

Mario J. Garcia, MD
Professor, Department of Medicine (Cardiology)
Professor, Department of Radiology
The Pauline Levitt Endowed Chair in Medicine
Chief, Division of Cardiology, Department of Medicine
Co-Director of the Montefiore-Einstein Heart Center
Montefiore Medical Center
Bronx, New York

Scot Garg, MB ChB, MRCP
Department of Interventional Cardiology
Erasmus Medical Center
Rotterdam, Netherlands

Jeffrey Goldstein, MD
Assistant Professor of Medicine
Southern Illinois School of Medicine
Cardiologist
Prairie Heart Institute
Springfield, Illinois

Nilesh J. Goswani, MD
Director, Coronary Care Unit and Chest Pain Center
Prairie Heart Institute
Springfield, Illinois

William A. Gray, MD
Assistant Professor of Clinical Medicine
Columbia University College of Physicians and Surgeons
Director, Endovascular Services
Columbia University Medical Center / New York-Presbyterian
    Hospital
New York, New York

Giulio Guagliumi, MD
Cardiovascular Department
Ospedali Riuniti di Bergamo
Bergamo, Italy

Hidehiko Hara, MD
Minneapolis Heart Institute Foundation
Minneapolis, Minnesota

Rani Hasan, MD
Fellow, Department of Cardiology
The Johns Hopkins University School of Medicine
Baltimore, Maryland

Timothy D. Henry, MD
Director of Research
Minneapolis Heart Institute Foundation
Professor of Medicine—University of Minnesota
Minneapolis, Minnesota

Howard C. Herrmann, MD
Professor of Medicine
University of Pennsylvania School of Medicine
Director, Interventional Cardiology Program and Cardiac
    Catheterization Laboratories
Hospital of the University of Pennsylvania
Philadelphia, Pennsylvania

Dominique Himbert, MD
Cardiology Department
Hopital Bichat
Paris, France

Russel Hirsch, MD
Assistant Professor
University of Cincinnati College of Medicine
Director, Cardiac Catheterization Laboratory
Cincinnati Children's Hospital
Cincinnati, Ohio

David R. Holmes, Jr., MD
Scripps Professor of Medicine
Mayo Clinic College of Medicine
Consultant
Mayo Clinic
Rochester, Minnesota

Yasuhiro Honda, MD
Clinical Associate Professor of Medicine
Division of Cardiovascular Medicine
Stanford University School of Medicine
Co-Director, Cardiovascular Core Analysis Laboratory
Center for Cardiovascular Technology
Stanford University Medical Center
Stanford, California

Hüseyin Ince, MD
Universitätsklinikum Hamburg-Eppendorf
Hamburg, Germany

Bernard Iung, MD
Professor of Cardiology
University of Paris VII
Hospital Doctor
Service de Cariologie
Hopital Bichat
Paris, France

Hani Jneid, MD
Assistant Professor of Medicine
Baylor College of Medicine
Houston, Texas

Samuel L. Johnston, MD
Cardiologist/Cardiac Electrophysiologist
Cascade Heart, PS
Southwest Washington Medical Center
Vancouver, Washington

James G. Jollis, MD
Professor of Medicine and Radiology
Departments of Medicine
Division of Cardiology
Duke University School of Medicine
Durham, North Carolina

David Kandzari, MD
Director, Interventional Cardiology and
Interventional Cardiology Research
Piedmont Heart Institute
Atlanta, Georgia

Samir R. Kapadia, MD
Professor of Medicine
Director, Sones Cardiac Catheterization Laboratories
Director, Interventional Cardiology Fellowship
Department of Cardiovascular Medicine
Cleveland Clinic
Cleveland, Ohio

Adnan Kastrati, MD
Professor of Cardiology
Deutsches Herzzentrum and 1. Medizinische Klinik rechts der Isar
Technische Universität
Munich, Germany

Dean J. Kereiakes, MD
Medical Director
The Christ Hospital Heart and Vascular Center and The Lindner
  Research Center
Professor of Clinical Medicine
Ohio State University
Cincinnati, Ohio

Morton J. Kern, MD
Professor of Medicine
Departments of Medicine and Cardiology
Associate Chief, Cardiology
University of California Irvine
Orange, California

Ahmed A. Khattab, MD
Associate Professor of Cardiology
University Hospital Bern
Bern, Switzerland

Young-Hak Kim, MD, PhD
Heart Institute, Asan Medical Center
University of Ulsan College of Medicine
Seoul, Korea

Ajay J. Kirtane, MD, SM
Chief Academic Officer
Director, Interventional Cardiology Fellowship Program
Columbia University Medical Center
New York—Presbyterian Hospital
New York, New York

Raghu Kolluri, MD
Director of Vascular Medicine
Prairie Heart Institute
Springfield, Illinois

Amar Krishnaswamy, MD
Fellow, Interventional Cardiology
Cleveland Clinic
Cleveland, Ohio

Takashi Kubo, MD, PhD
Assistant Professor, Department of Cardiovascular Medicine
Wakayama Medical University
Wakayama, Japan

Roger Laham, MD
Angiogenesis Research Center
Department of Medicine
Harvard Medical School
Beth Israel Deaconess Medical Center
Boston, Massachusetts

John Lasala, MD, PhD
Associate Professor, Medicine
Director, Interventional Cardiology
Medical Director, Cardiac Catheterization Lab
Washington University School of Medicine
St. Louis, Missouri

Michael J. Lim, MD
Interim Director and Associate Professor of Medicine
Cardiology Division
Saint Louis University
St. Louis, Missouri

Thomas R. Lloyd, MD
Professor, Pediatric Cardiology
Department of Pediatrics and Communicable Diseases
University of Michigan Health System
Ann Arbor, Michigan

Daniel Mark, MD, MPH
Professor of Medicine
Duke University Medical Center
Director, Outcomes Research
Duke Clinical Research Institute
Durham, North Carolina

Bernhard Meier, MD
Professor of Cardiology
Faculty of Medicine
University of Bern
Director of Cardiology
University Hospital
Bern, Switzerland

Gilles Montalescot, MD, PhD
Professor of Cardiology
Pitié-Salpêtrière University Hospital
Institut de Cardiologie
Paris, France

Pedro R. Moreno, MD
Professor of Cardiology
Department of Medicine
The Mount Sinai Medical Center
New York, New York

Jeffrey W. Moses, MD
Professor of Medicine
Columbia University Medical Center
Director, Center for Interventional Vascular Therapy
New York Presbyterian Hospital
New York, New York

Arashk Motiei, MD
Assistant Professor of Medicine
Department of Cardiovascular Disease
Mayo Clinic
Rochester, Minnesota

Debabrata Mukherjee, MD
Chief, Cardiovascular Medicine
Professor of Internal Medicine
Vice Chairman, Department of Internal Medicine
Texas Tech University
El Paso, Texas

Srihari S. Naidu, MD
Assistant Professor of Medicine
SUNY—Stony Brook School of Medicine
Director, Cardiac Catheterization Laboratories
Winthrop University Hospital
Mineola, New York

Brahmajee K. Nallamothu, MD, MPH
Associate Professor of Cardiovascular Medicine
Department of Internal Medicine
University of Michigan Medical School
Ann Arbor, Michigan

Craig R. Narins, MD
Associate Professor of Medicine and Surgery
Divisions of Cardiology and Vascular Surgery
University of Rochester Medical Center
Rochester, New York

Gjin Ndrepepa, MD
Associate Professor of Cardiology
Deutsches Herzzentrum
Technische Universität
Munich, Germany

Franz-Josef Neumann, MD, PhD
Honorary Professor of Cardiology
Albert Ludwigs-Universitat, Frieburg
Medical Director and Chairman
Herz-Zentrum Bad Krozingen
Bad Krozingen, Germany

Christoph A. Nienaber, MD
Professor of Internal Medicine and Cardiology
University of Rostock School of Medicine
Head, Division of Cardiology and Vascular Medicine
University Hospital Rostock
Rostock, Germany

Masakiyo Nobuyoshi, MD
Division of Cardiology
Kokura Memorial Hospital
Kokura, Japan

Igor Palacios, MD
Director of Interventional Cardiology
Division of Cardiology
Massachusetts General Hospital
Harvard Medical School
Boston, Massachusetts

Seung-Jung Park, MD, PhD
Heart Institute, Asan Medical Center
University of Ulsan College of Medicine
Seoul, Korea

Uptal D. Patel, MD
Assistant Professor of Medicine and Pediatrics
Department of Pediatrics
Duke University School of Medicine
Durham, North Carolina

Marc S. Penn, MD, PhD
Director of Research
Summa Cardiovascular Institute
Summa Health System
Akron, Ohio
Professor of Medicine and Integrative Medical Sciences
Northeast Ohio Medical University
Rootstown, Ohio

Jeffrey Popma, MD
Associate Professor of Medicine
Harvard Medical School
Director, Interventional Cardiology Clinical Services
Department of Medicine (Cardiovascular Division)
Beth Israel Deaconess Medical Center
Boston, Massachusetts

Matthew J. Price, MD
Director, Cardiac Catheterization Laboratory
Scripps Clinic
Assistant Professor, Scripps Translational Science Institute
La Jolla, California

Vivek Rajagopal, MD
Staff Cardiologist
Piedmont Heart Institute
Atlanta, Georgia

Kausik K. Ray, MBChB, MRCP, MD, MPhil
Professor of Cardiovascular Disease Prevention
Department of Clinical Services
St. George's University of London
Consultant Cardiologist
Department of Cardiology
St. George's Hospital NHS Trust
London, United Kingdom

G. Russell Reiss, MD
Fellow, Interventional Cardiology, Center for Interventional
 Vascular Therapy
Attending Surgeon, Department of Cardiothoracic Surgery
New York-Presbyterian Hospital
Columbia University
New York, New York

Krishna Rocha-Singh, MD
Medical Director, Prairie Vascular Institute
Prairie Cardiovascular Consultants
Medical Director, Prairie Education and Research Cooperative
Springfield, Illinois

Marco Roffi, MD
Director, Interventional Cardiology Unit
Division of Cardiology, University Hospital
Geneva, Switzerland

R. Kevin Rogers, MD, MSc
Vascular Medicine and Interventional Fellow
Massachusetts General Hospital
Boston, Massachusetts

Javier Sanz, MD
Assistant Professor Medicine/Cardiology
Cardiac MR/CT Program
Cardiovascular Institute
Mount Sinai School of Medicine
New York, NY

Bruno Scheller, MD
Department of Cardiology
Division of Internal Medicine III
University of Saarland
Homburg/Saar, Germany

Albert Schömig, MD
Professor of Medicine
Deutsches Herzzentrum and 1. Medizinische Klinik rechts der Isar
Technische Universität
Munich, Germany

Robert S. Schwartz, MD
Minneapolis Heart Institute and Foundation
Minneapolis, Minnesota

Patrick Serruys, MD, PhD
Professor and Head, Department of Interventional Cardiology
Erasmus University
Director, Clinical Research Program of the Catheterization
　Laboratory
Rotterdam, Netherlands

Shinichi Shirai, MD
Division of Cardiology
Kokura Memorial Hospital
Kokura, Japan

Mehdi H. Shishehbor, DO, MPH
Staff, Interventional Cardiology & Vascular Medicine
Associate Director, Interventional Cardiology Fellowship
Department of Cardiovascular Medicine
Cleveland Clinic
Cleveland, Ohio

Mitchell J. Silver, DO
MidOhio Cardiology and Vascular Consultants
Columbus, Ohio

Daniel I. Simon, MD
University Hospitals Harrington-McLaughlin Heart & Vascular
　Institute
Case Western Reserve University School of Medicine
Cleveland, Ohio

Vasile Sirbu, MD
Director, Cardiovascular Department
Ospedali Riuniti di Bergamo
Bergamo, Italy

Goran Stankovic, MD
Clinic for Cardiology, Department for Diagnostic and
　Catheterization Laboratories
Clinical Center of Serbia
Medical School of Belgrade
Belgrade, Serbia

Curtiss Stinis, MD
Director of Peripheral Interventions
Division of Cardiology
Scripps Clinic and Research Foundation
La Jolla, California

Gregg W. Stone, MD
Director of Cardiovascular Research and Education
Columbia University Medical Center
New York—Presbyterian Hospital
New York, New York

Gus Theodos, MD
Department of Cardiovascular Medicine
Cleveland Clinic
Cleveland, Ohio

On Topaz, MD
Professor of Medicine and Pathology
Chief, Division of Cardiology
Charles George Veterans Affairs Medical Center
Asheville, North Carolina

Christophe Tron, MD
Cardiology Department
Hopital Bichat
Paris, France

Alec Vahanian, MD
Professor of Cardiology
University of Paris VII
Head, Cardiology Department
Hoptial Bichat
Paris, France

Robert A. Van Tassel, MD
Minneapolis Heart Institute and Foundation
Minneapolis, Minnesota

Christopher J. White, MD
Chairman, Department of Cardiovascular Diseases
The John Ochsner Heart & Vascular Institute
Ochsner Clinic Foundation
New Orleans, Louisiana

Matthew R. Williams, MD
Surgical Director, Cardiovascular Transcatheter Therapies
Assistant Professor, Department of Cardiothoracic Surgery
Interventional Cardiologist, Center for Interventional Vascular
　Therapy
New York-Presbyterian Hospital
Columbia University
New York, New York

Paul Yock, MD
The Martha Meier Weiland Professor, School of Medicine
Professor of Bioengineering and, by courtesy, of Mechanical
　Engineering and at the GSB
Stanford University
Stanford, California

Hiroyoshi Yokoi, MD
Deartment of Cardiology
Kokura Memorial Hospital
Fukuoka, Japan

Alan Zajarias, MD
Assistant Professor of Medicine
Cardiovascular Division
Washington University School of Medicine
St. Louis, Missouri

Khaled Ziada, MD
Associate Professor of Medicine
Director, Cardiac Catheterization Laboratories
Director, Cardiovascular Interventional Fellowship
Gill Heart Institute, University of Kentucky
Lexington, Kentucky

Andrew A. Ziskind, MD
Senior Executive, Accenture
Chicago, Illinois

Matthew Zussman, MD
Fellow, Pediatric Cardiology
Cincinnati Children's Hospital
Cincinnati, Ohio

The 6th Edition of the *Textbook of Interventional Cardiology* has been more extensively revamped than any other previous edition, starting with the addition of a co-editor which we refer to as T + T and what will hopefully be viewed as T^2 with respect to the product transcending the sum of the editors input and perspective. We have tried to fully capture the excitement in the field of interventional cardiology, highlighting such breakthroughs as transcatheter aortic valve implantation (TAVI). In this procedure, the sense at the moment the stent valve is deployed is a combination of exhilaration and anxiety, reminiscent of the early pioneering days of balloon angioplasty, and new device development. Over the years, coronary intervention became increasingly predictable and, in many ways, routine, with the progressive maturation of stents and leaps forward in our adjunct pharmacologic therapies. In some ways, the field of interventional cardiology lost a bit of its pioneering spark that had so characterized this discipline from its inception in the 1980s. In those heady times, performing balloon angioplasty in the coronary artery was unpredictable. The predictability provided by stents was replaced with the upredictability of stent thrombosis. Interventional cardiologists, and scientests, had to not only rise to the challenge for each individual patient, but also discover the vital innovations that would perpetuate the prominence and importance of the specialty.

Today, the challenges continue, but they have morphed considerably. The profile of patients who undergo coronary intervention has dramatically increased in complexity including patients wth advanced age, those with left main stem lesions, chronic occlusions, and what would formerly have been considered prohibitive complexity. Whatever happened to patients with Type A lesions? How can we break the maximal SYNTAX score barrier for PCI? At the same time, the crisis in health care economics has placed an undue burden on interventional cardiologists with respect to time, constraints in equipment selection, and fulfilling the responsibility of 24/7 coverage for such emergencics as acute myocardial infarction. There is also the incremental pressure from scorecarding initiatives and challenges to the appropriateness of procedures. But, hopefully, all of these challenges are outweighed by the immense gratification of helping a symptomatic patient with limitations in the quality of life get back to his or her baseline.

This book is intended to serve as a resource for the interventional cardiology community, which not only includes practicing cardiologists, but also the team involved in procedures, referring physicians, and those training or who have aspiration to train in this awe inspiring field. We have changed authors of several chapters to provide a sense of newness and a fresh perspective, and have added several chapters that reflect how the field has changed such as left mainstem disease, thrombus containing lesions, transradial intervention, complications of procedures, the role of cardiac surgeons, and optical coherence tomography. In every chapter, we have sought the authors who are widely regarded as the true expert(s) in the field. Going forward, we fully recognize that there needs to be increased cooperativity with cardiac surgeons—the rising popularity of hybrid and collaborative valve procedures that capitalize on the best parts of percutaneous and surgical approaches is clearly indicative of that collaboration.

We want to express our genuine and deep appreciation to all 130 authors from all over the world who have graciously contributed to this new edition. The old line "it takes a village" needs to be replaced by "it takes a world" to comprehensively and authentically present the ever-burgeoning field of interventional cardiology. We thank Taylor Ball and Natasha Andjelkovic both at Elsevier, for their first rate, professional support of this endeavor. And we are especially grateful to the interventional community of readers of this book who have supported it as the primary reference textbook source for over 25 years. That represents a large sense of responsibility for us to maintain and we hope to have lived up to that, and perhaps exceeded expectations with the 6th edition.

Paul S. Teirstein and Eric J. Topol
La Jolla, California, 2011

CONTENTS

Patient Selection

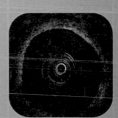

Individualized Assessment for Percutaneous or Surgical Revascularization

SCOT GARG | PATRICK W. SERRUYS

KEY POINTS

- Changes in the demographics of patients presenting in need of revascularization, advances in percutaneous and surgical revascularization techniques, and results from contemporary studies of percutaneous versus surgical revascularization have all made it imperative that patients be assessed as individuals prior to the selection of a treatment strategy.

- Coronary revascularization must be appropriately tailored, taking into account a patient's comorbidities, coronary anatomy, and personal preferences.

- Risk stratification plays an important role in the individualized assessment of patients undergoing revascularization.

- Risk models can be used to assist physicians in risk-stratifying these patients. Broadly speaking, there are three groups of such models: those assessing patients on the basis of their clinical comorbidities, their coronary anatomy, or a combination of the two.

- The increasingly active involvement of patients in the decision-making process has ensured that the final verdict regarding the modality of revascularization is made only after appropriate discussions have taken place among all interested parties.

Introduction

The revascularization of patients with coronary artery disease (CAD) has progressed exponentially since Andreas Grüntzig performed the first balloon angioplasty in 1977.[1] These developments, which have been fueled by new technology, have blurred the boundary between what is considered exclusively surgical disease and what can be treated percutaneously. Consequently there is a greater need than ever to tailor revascularization appropriately, taking into consideration a patient's comorbidities, coronary anatomy, and personal preferences. This chapter first explores the increasing requirement for a more individualized assessment of patients undergoing revascularization; then it reviews the risk models currently available to assist in this stratification process. Finally, risk stratification from the individual patient's perspective is discussed.

The Need for Individualized Patient Assessment

Three major confounding factors have made it imperative that patients be assessed as individuals prior to the selection of a revascularization strategy.

PATIENT COMORBIDITIES

The demographics of patients in need of revascularization who present to tertiary care services are changing. This has largely been the consequence of increased longevity of the general population, a lower threshold to investigate patients presenting with symptoms suggestive of obstructive coronary disease, and increased resources, making revascularization by percutaneous coronary intervention (PCI) or coronary artery bypass grafting (CABG) more accessible. Owing to their generally older age, patients in need of revascularization are now more likely to have comorbidities, such as diabetes, hypertension, and hyperlipidemia.[2,3] These factors are all implicated in accelerating the progression of CAD; consequently patients are more likely to present with more extensive disease. The Arterial Revascularization Therapies Studies (ARTS) Parts I and II were separated by a period of 5 years and, although both studies had the same inclusion criteria, patients in ARTS II had a significantly greater incidence of risk factors and overall increased disease complexity (Table 1-1).[4]

Comorbidities must be taken into consideration in assessing patients for revascularization, as these have the potential to significantly influence outcomes; moreover, the impact of treatment may depend on the underlying revascularization strategy selected. Of note, Legrand et al.[5] demonstrated that patient age was a significant independent predictor of major adverse cardiovascular and cerebrovascular events (MACCE) in patients enrolled in the ARTS I and II studies who were treated with CABG but not in those who received PCI. In a collaborative patient-level analysis of 10 randomized trials of patients with multivessel disease (MVD) treated with PCI using bare metal stents (BMS) and CABG, Hlatky et al.[6] demonstrated comparable 5-year mortality rates among both the PCI and CABG treatment groups in patients without diabetes. Importantly, among those with diabetes, mortality was significantly higher in patients treated with PCI even after multivariate adjustment (Figure 1-1). The clear importance of patient comorbidities is highlighted by their central presence in the risk models now used to assist in decision making. This topic is discussed at greater length further on in this chapter.

TECHNOLOGICAL ADVANCES

The introduction in 2002 of the drug-eluting stent (DES) revolutionized the practice of interventional cardiology, primarily owing to the dramatic reduction in rates of repeat revascularization resulting from its use.[7] The impressive results seen with the use of the DES promptly led to an expansion in the indications for PCI, such that bifurcation lesions, chronic total occlusions, and MVD were increasingly treated with PCI. Previously, these lesion subsets had been deemed more appropriate for surgical revascularization. Evidence of this expansion can be seen in the changing baseline lesion characteristics of patients enrolled in "all comers" PCI studies such as SIRTAX (sirolimus-eluting and paclitaxel-eluting stents for coronary revascularization trial),[8] LEADERS (Limus Eluted from A Durable versus ERodable Stent coating study)[9] and studies of complex (triple-vessel disease [3VD], and/or left main [LM]) CAD such as ARTS I,[10] ARTS II,[11] and the SYNTAX study (SYNergy between percutaneous coronary intervention with TAXus and cardiac surgery) (Table 1-1).[12] Further evidence in support of this change come from assessments of "real world" clinical practice, which indicate that approximately one-third of patients

TABLE 1-1 The Changing Baseline Demographics of Patients Enrolled in Trials of Drug-Eluting Stents

	"All Comers" Studies		Complex Disease Studies		
	SIRTAX[8]	LEADERS[9]	ARTS I[10]	ARTS II[11]	SYNTAX[12]
Year(s) of enrollment	2003–2004	2006–2007	1997–1998	2003	2005–2007
Stent type	DES	DES	BMS	DES	DES
Demographics					
Age, years (mean ± SD)	62 ± 11	65 ± 11	61 ± 10	63 ± 10	65 ± 10
Diabetes, %	20	24	19	26	26
Hypertension, %	61	73	45	67	69
Hypercholesterolemia, %	59	67	58	74	78
Previous myocardial infarction, %	29	33	44	34	32
Left ventricular function, % (mean ± SD)	57 ± 12	56 ± 12	61 ± 12	60 ± 12	59 ± 13
Lesion characteristics (per patient)					
Multivessel disease, %	59	23	96	100	92
Bifurcation lesions, %	8	22	35	34	72
Total occlusions, %	19	12	3	17	24
SYNTAX score (mean ± SD)	12 ± 7	14 ± 9	—	21 ± 10	28 ± 12
Mean number of diseased lesions	1.4	1.5	2.8	3.6	3.6*
Procedural characteristics (per patient)					
Mean number of stents	1.2 ± 0.5	1.3 ± 0.7†	2.8 ± 1.3	3.7 ± 1.5	4.6 ± 2.3
Total stent length, mm (mean±SD)	25.9 ± 15.5	24.7 ± 15.5†	47.6 ± 21.7	72.5 ± 32.1	86.1 ± 47.9

*Treated lesions.
†Per lesion.
SD, standard deviation; DES, drug-eluting stent; BMS, bare metal stent.

with complex disease are now treated with PCI.[13] Coupled with this expanding use of PCI, driven largely through the beneficial effects of DES, the new lower-profile balloons and guidewires are among other advances; these also include new adjunctive pharmacological therapies and the increasing availability of percutaneous extracorporeal circulatory support (Figure 1-2).[14,15] From a technical point of view, therefore, the majority of coronary lesions can now be addressed with PCI; however, this approach may not always be appropriate, necessitating the careful selection of individual patients.

CLINICAL TRIAL RESULTS

Randomized trials comparing CABG and PCI have centered on two major patient groups: those with isolated lesions of the proximal left anterior descending artery and those with complex disease, namely 3VD and/or LM disease. Taking the results of these studies at face value and irrespective of which patient group has been assessed, results at short- and long-term follow-up suggest that there are no differences in the hard clinical outcomes of death and myocardial infarction (MI) between patients treated with PCI or CABG (Table 1-2).[6,16–20] Undisputedly CABG has been associated with a clear, consistent, and significant reduction in rates of repeat revascularization. Importantly, all of these studies have several notable limitations that restrict the ability to extrapolate their results to routine clinical practice. This, consequently, reinforces the need to assess patients individually before a revascularization therapy is selected.

1. The inclusion criteria have commonly excluded (through patient assessment) patients with impaired left ventricular function, LM disease, and multiple comorbidities. Moreover, although these studies have been assessing patients with MVD, this extent of CAD was actually seen in only about one-third of patients. Overall, only approximately 5 to 10% of all potential patients were enrolled; therefore the comparable outcomes observed in these studies and subsequent metanalyses can be applied to only a fraction of those in need of revascularization. It must be appreciated, however, that this step of patient selection was necessary to enable ethical randomization (i.e., to ensure that patients were suitable for both PCI and CABG). Yet paradoxically and unsurprisingly, by eliminating those patients at highest risk, the subsequent mortality was comparable. Of note, clinical outcomes of the sizable proportion of patients with complex disease who were screened but not enrolled in the randomized arm of the study have rarely been reported other than in the BARI (Bypass Angioplasty Revascularization Investigation)[21,22] and SYNTAX studies.[12]

Number of patients*									
CABG no diabetes	3263	3169	3089	2877	2677	2267	1592	1380	1274
CABG diabetes	615	587	575	532	498	421	257	225	200
PCI no diabetes	3298	3217	3148	2918	2725	2281	1608	1393	1288
PCI diabetes	618	574	555	508	475	373	218	179	160

Figure 1-1 Cumulative survival curve of long-term mortality stratified according to diabetic status among patients with multivessel disease who were randomized to treatment with either percutaneous coronary intervention or coronary artery bypass graft surgery. The influence of diabetic status on outcome is highlighted not only by the higher mortality among diabetics versus nondiabetic patients but also by the greater impact diabetic status had on patients treated with PCI compared with CABG. (Reprinted with permission from Hlatky MA, Boothroyd DB, Bravata DM, et al. Coronary artery bypass surgery compared with percutaneous coronary interventions for multivessel disease: a collaborative analysis of individual patient data from ten randomised trials. Lancet. 2009;373(9670):1190–1197.)

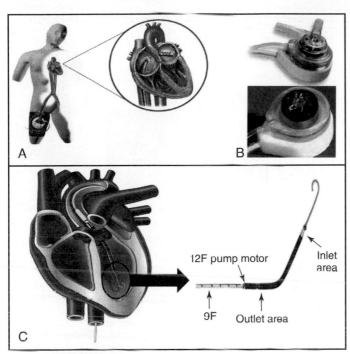

Figure 1-2 Devices that are increasingly available to provide assistance during high-risk PCI include those providing percutaneous extracorporeal circulatory support, such as the TandemHeart (A, B) and the Impella device (C). The TandemHeart (A) removes oxygenated blood from the left atrium and returns it to the peripheral arterial circulation with the aid of a centrifugal pump (B). *(Reprinted with permission from Vranckx P, Meliga E, De Jaegere PP, et al: The TandemHeart, percutaneous transseptal left ventricular assist device: a safeguard in high-risk percutaneous coronary interventions. The six-year-Rotterdam experience. EuroIntervention 2008;4(3):331–337.)* The Impella left ventricular assist device (C) is a miniaturized rotary blood pump, which is placed retrograde across the aortic valve and aspirates (inlet area) up to 2.5 L/min of blood from the left ventricular cavity and subsequently expels (outlet area) this blood into the ascending aorta. *(Reprinted with permission from Valgimigli M, Steendijk P, Serruys PW, et al: Use of Impella Recover LP 2.5 left ventricular assist device during high-risk percutaneous coronary interventions: clinical, haemodynamic and biochemical findings. EuroIntervention. 2006;2(1):91–100.)*

2. Clinical results have been presented for all patients en masse irrespective of the severity of their disease. There is wide variation in the complexity of disease and not all 3VD disease is the same, as highlighted by the important results of the SYNTAX study,[12] discussed below. Overall, considering these limitations, these early randomized trials of PCI versus CABG indicate, somewhat paradoxically, that if patients are selected appropriately, comparable outcomes are achievable irrespective of the modality of revascularization selected. Moreover, in this group of patients with comparable outcomes, patient choice plays an important role in determining the overall treatment strategy, as discussed further in the last part of this chapter.

The SYNTAX Trial

The SYNTAX trial, which to date has been the largest assessment of treatment with PCI or CABG in patients with complex disease, represents an important study that clearly indicates the importance and potential benefits of evaluating patients at an individual level.

This study aimed to supply evidence to support the already established, but not evidence-based practice of performing PCI in patients with complex disease[13]; it also sought to identify which patients should be treated only with CABG. The study design attempted to address the limitations of the earlier trials described above; in doing so, it was anticipated that the results would be more relevant to clinicians' everyday practice. Specifically, it was intended to do the following:

- To ensure that the results would be applicable to routine practice, the study was designed as "an all comers" trial such that there were no specific inclusion criteria other than the need to have 3VD or LM disease (in isolation or with CAD). Exclusion criteria were minimal and limited to prior revascularization, recent MI, or the requirement for concomitant cardiac surgery.[23] In contrast to the earlier studies, 70.9% of eligible patients were enrolled.
- The previously indicated problem of reporting outcomes from all patients with complex CAD together, irrespective of disease severity, was addressed in the SYNTAX study through the utilization of the newly developed SYNTAX score (SXscore) (Table 1-3), which enabled CAD complexity to be quantified.
- To ensure the assessment of patients on an individual level, all patients eligible for enrollment were discussed at a "Heart Team" conference at which an interventional cardiologist and cardiac surgeon carried out a careful, through review of each patient in

TABLE 1-2	A Summary of Metanalyses Reporting Long-Term Outcomes in Patients with Isolated Proximal LAD Disease or Multi-Vessel Disease Randomized to Percutaneous or Surgical Revascularization							
Study	*No. of Patients (PCI/CABG)*	*POBA/BMS/ DES (%)*	*Follow-up (months)*	*Death (PCI vs. CABG)*	*MI (PCI vs. CABG)*	*Stroke (PCI vs. CABG)*	*Repeat Revascularization (PCI vs. CABG)*	*MACCE (PCI vs. CABG)*
Isolated proximal LAD								
Aziz et al.[16]	1952 (1300/652)	0/91/9	34	2.9% vs. 3.4%	2% vs. 1.1%	2.4% vs. 3.5%	14.3% vs. 4.4%*	21.4% vs. 11.1%*
Kapoor et al.[17]	1210 (633/577)	22/59/19	60	9.4% vs. 7.2%	NA	NA	33.5% vs. 7.3%*	NA
Multivessel disease								
Bravata et al.[20]	9963 (5019/4944)	56/42/2	60	9.3% vs. 11.3%	0.6% vs. 1.2%*	11.9% vs. 10.9%	46.1% vs. 40.1% vs. 9.8%*‡	—
Daemen et al.[19]	3051 (1518/1533)	4/96/0	60	8.5% vs. 8.2%	2.5% vs. 2.9%	6.6% vs. 6.1%	25.0% vs. 6.3%*	34.2% vs. 19.6%*
Hlatky et al.[6]	7812 (3923/3889)	63/37/0	5.9	10.0% vs. 8.4%	16.7% vs. 15.4%†	—	24.5% vs. 9.9%*†	36.4% vs. 20.1%*

*P < 0.001.
†Composite with death.
‡Balloon angioplasty vs. PCI vs. CABG.

PCI, percutaneous coronary intervention; CABG, coronary artery bypass grafting; MI, myocardial infarction; NA, not available; MACCE, major adverse cardiovascular and cerebrovascular events (a composite of death, stroke, MI, and repeat revascularization); POBA, balloon angioplasty; BMS, bare metal stent; DES, drug-eluting stent.

TABLE 1-3	The SYNTAX Score Algorithm[38]*
1. Arterial dominance	
2. Arterial segments involved per lesion	
3. Diameter of stenosis	
i. Total occlusion	
ii. Significant lesions (50–99%)	
Adverse lesion characteristics	
4. Total occlusion	
i. Number of segments involved	
ii. Age of the total occlusion (>3 months)	
iii. Blunt stump	
iv. Bridging collaterals	
v. First segment beyond the occlusion visible by antegrade or retrograde filling	
vi. Side branch involvement	
5. Trifurcation	
i. Number of segments diseased	
6. Bifurcation	
i. Medina type	
ii. Angulation between the distal main vessel and the side branch < 70 degrees	
7. Aorto-ostial lesion	
8. Severe tortuosity	
9. Length > 20 mm	
10. Heavy calcification	
11. Thrombus	
12. Diffuse disease/small vessels	
i. Number of segments with diffuse disease/small vessels	

*The angiographic components of the SYNTAX score. Each component is assigned a specific weight according to its contribution to procedural risk. The characteristics above are scored for each lesion with a greater than 50% diameter stenosis; these are added together to provide the total SYNTAX score. Full definitions of all variables are published[38,39] and available online (www.syntaxscore.com).

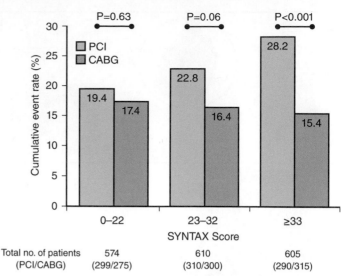

Figure 1-3 Two-year rates of major adverse cardiovascular and cerebrovascular events (a composite of death, stroke, myocardial infarction, and repeat revascularization) among the 1,800 patients randomized to PCI or CABG in the SYNTAX study, stratified according to SYNTAX score. Of note, clinical outcomes were comparable between PCI and CABG in those with an SXscore of 0 to 22, trended in favor of CABG in those with an SXscore of 23 to 32, and were significantly lower with CABG in those with an SXscore ≥ 33.[25]

terms of his or her anginal status, comorbidities, and coronary anatomy using the respective Braunwald score, euroSCORE, and SXscore (discussed later in this chapter). The consensus reached from this meeting was then used to allocate the patient to one of the three arms of the trial. In total, 3,075 patients were enrolled into the following groups:

1. Randomized group (1,800 patients [58.5%]: 897 CABG, 903 PCI): these patients had CAD suitable for treatment with PCI or CABG. The mean SXscores in this group were 26.1 and 28.8, respectively, in patients treated with CABG and PCI.
2. CABG registry (1,077 patients [35.0%]): these patients had CAD unsuitable for PCI, as clearly reflected in the high mean SXscore for this group of 37.8.
3. PCI registry (198 patients [6.4%]): these patients were deemed unsuitable for CABG. The most common reason for this decision was the presence of multiple comorbidities[24] as reflected in the mean euroSCORE of patients in this group, which was 2 points higher than the mean in the randomized group (5.8 vs. 3.8).

Overall the study failed to meet the prespecified primary endpoint of noninferiority in terms of 12-month major adverse cardio- and cerebrovascular events (MACCE), a composite of death, stroke, MI, and repeat revascularization (17.8% vs. 12.4%, $P = 0.002$). This was driven by significantly lower rates of repeat revascularization with CABG (13.5% vs. 5.9%, $P < 0.0001$). Moreover, consistent with prior studies of MVD, there were no significant differences in the overall safety endpoints of death, MI, or death/stroke/MI out to 12 months of follow-up. Results at the 2-year follow-up, which are considered hypothesis-generating in view of the failure to reach the primary endpoint, are somewhat similar to earlier results, with comparable rates of death (PCI 6.2% vs. CABG 4.9%, $P = 0.24$) and the composite of death/stroke and MI (10.8% vs. 9.6%, $P = 0.44$), while significantly higher rates of repeat revascularization (17.4% vs. 8.6%, $P < 0.001$) and

overall MACCE (23.4% vs. 16.3%, $P < 0.001$) were seen with PCI.[25] As indicated earlier, the analysis of all patients irrespective of disease severity does not provide adequate information for clinicians, who daily see patients with wide variations in CAD complexity. To address this limitation of earlier studies, patient outcomes in the SYNTAX study were stratified according to terciles of the SXscore. As shown in Figure 1-3, clinical outcomes between patients treated with PCI and CABG were similar in those with low SXscores, trended in favor of CABG in the intermediate group, and were significantly lower in the CABG group among patients with high SXscores. The intermediate group was further subdivided into a 3VD cohort, where outcomes were lower with CABG, and into an LM cohort, where outcomes were comparable between PCI and CABG (Figure 1-4).[26,27] These results reiterate the importance of assessing patients when a revascularization strategy is being selected. The SYNTAX study was able to identify those patients in whom either PCI or CABG was appropriate and, perhaps more importantly, the group of patients in whom CABG was the optimal treatment. Considering the distribution of CAD in the SYNTAX study, overall one-third of patients with 3VD/LM disease were deemed to have CAD that could be treated safely and effectively with PCI or CABG; in the remaining two-thirds, CABG remained the standard of care. Although these results were consistent with what was already practiced,[13] validation of the SXscore importantly facilitates a more objective assessment of patients, as discussed in the following pages.

Individual Assessment—From a Physician's Perspective

There is no disputing the need and potential benefit of selecting a revascularization strategy only after an individualized patient assessment or risk stratification. Risk stratification is performed routinely and subconsciously by physicians in everyday clinical practice and is in essence behind all clinical decisions that are made. Stratification of risk is vital in assessing patients for revascularization, as this treatment is considered appropriate only when *"the expected benefits, in terms of survival or health outcomes (symptoms, functional status, and/or quality of life) exceed the expected negative consequences of the procedure."*[28] The

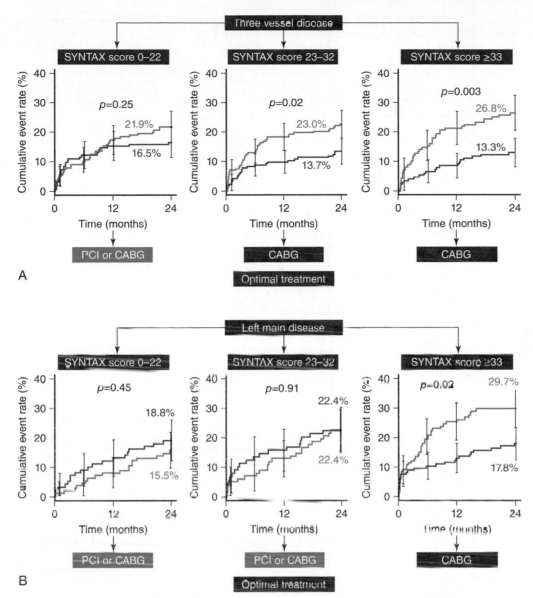

Figure 1-4 The evidence supporting the use of the SYNTAX score as a tool to assist in revascularization decisions. A. In patients with three-vessel disease, the rate of major adverse cardiovascular and cerebrovascular events (MACCE, a composite of death, stroke, myocardial infarction, and repeat revascularization) at 2-year follow-up was comparable only between patients treated with PCI and CABG for SYNTAX scores of 0 to 22; for all other SYNTAX scores, outcomes were significantly better following CABG.[26] B. In patients with left main disease, clinical outcomes were comparable between patients treated by PCI or CABG for all SYNTAX scores, apart from those above 32, when outcomes were significantly better with CABG (CABG: purple line; PCI: green line).[27]

factors that have increased the importance of risk stratification in contemporary practice have already been discussed. The currently available methods of stratifying patients for risk are described in the following paragraphs.

QUALITATIVE VERSUS QUANTITATIVE RISK ASSESSMENT

Qualitative risk stratification is subjective and relies on the clinician's experience. This assessment is advantageous from an individual's perspective because it possesses the greatest sensitivity. In qualitative risk stratification, all factors relevant to assessing risk in a particular individual are considered; in the risk model, only the select list of variables involved are considered. Moreover, this subjective qualitative assessment also allows risk to be calculated and tailored to the expertise of the physician performing the procedure, as opposed to a clinician in

another region who may use different techniques and have different equipment available. Finally, this assessment does not require a calculator or computer and can be "computed" subconsciously very quickly. The major disadvantages of this method of risk assessment are its dependence on an operator's prior experience and its high interobserver variability.

Quantitative risk stratification can be performed using a variety of risk models that incorporate clinical variables sourced from large patient databases.[29-36] These risk models largely incorporate objective variables, thus ensuring adequate reproducibility of the score. However, models such as the American College of Cardiology/American Heart Association (ACC/AHA) lesion score[37] or the SYNTAX score,[38] which include angiographic variables, continue to have documented intra- and interobserver variability.[39,40] In addition to their role in the risk stratification of individual patients, these quantitative risk models have increasing use in the wider context of overall healthcare. They can provide a vital measure of overall patient care and can help to identify future directions to further improve outcomes. Clinical governance and the increasing requirement to report clinical performance (and complications) publicly have also propelled the need to risk stratify patients, thereby allowing useful comparisons of performance to be made between clinicians (and institutions) and the standards dictated by regulatory authorities.[41] In addition, the calculation of risk using accepted risk models can aid clinicians who are faced with an increasing need to justify their clinical decisions to peers, regulatory bodies, and patients. In comparison to the qualitative risk models, the use of a finite number of variables makes these model less sensitive and therefore less able to accurately predict risk in an individual, such that they are more effective in predicting risk for a population of patients with similar comorbidities. The number of variables included in the model must strike a balance between sufficient numbers to enable the calculation of a meaningful prediction of risk; however, the number must not be so excessive as to prevent the use of the model in routine practice. In addition, a minimal number of variables reduces the chances of colinearity between independent variables, which can result in the collection of redundant information[34] while also increasing the chances of "overfitting" the model and thereby reducing the overall accuracy of the results.[42] The applicability of a risk model to contemporary practice must also take into consideration the time at which the model was developed. Risk models rely on large patient databases to derive appropriate weighting factors for variables in the model and thus to enable the final calculation of risk. It follows that they are developed using retrospective information, which may no longer be relevant in the era when the model is being used. The euroSCORE (European System for Cardiac Operative Risk Evaluation), for example, was developed in 1999; however, there have been calls for its recalibration, since repeated evaluations indicate that it overestimates risk by a factor of 2 to 3, which has largely been attributed to improvements in surgical techniques and lower perioperative mortality in the decade following its construction.[43,44] The Society of Thoracic Surgeons (STS) score is also derived from a large patient database; however, unlike the euroSCORE, the STS calculator is periodically recalibrated to ensure the applicability of its results to contemporary practice.[45]

■ Risk Models in Contemporary Practice

Numerous risk models are available to assist clinicians in stratifying risk among patients undergoing revascularization. Some models are appropriate for patients prior to the selection of a revascularization strategy while others have been validated only in patients undergoing a particular form of treatment. Nevertheless, the various models can largely be categorized according to the variables (clinical, angiographic, or a combination of both) used in the overall estimation of risk. Table 1-4 summarizes the different risk models used in contemporary practice; they are described in more detail below.

CLINICALLY BASED SCORES

These risk scores incorporate only clinical variables and do not require any data from angiography. They offer the advantage that they can be computed relatively quickly, usually at the bedside, and that they principally include variables that are not subject to user interpretation, thereby ensuring excellent reproducibility.

euroSCORE

The additive euroSCORE[30] is a clinical risk score that is calculated from 17 different clinical variables (Table 1-5); it has been used since 1999 to predict in-hospital and long-term mortality in patients undergoing cardiac surgery.[30,46,47] Early validation studies, however, suggested that it underestimated risk in those at highest risk, resulting in the development of the logistic euroSCORE, which uses the same clinical

	Summary of Contemporary and Newly Developed Risk Models for Assessment of Risk in Patients Undergoing Revascularization			
TABLE 1-4				
	Number of Variables Used to Calculate Score		**Validated in PCI/CABG**	
Risk Model	CLINICAL	ANGIOGRAPHIC	PCI	CABG
euroSCORE[12,29–31,46–53]	17	0	+	+
Mayo Clinic Risk Score[32,54,65]	17	0	+	+
ACEF[34]	3	0	−	+
National Cardiovascular Database Registry risk model[35]	8	0	+	−
AHA/ACC Lesion classification[37,55–58]	0	11*	+	−
SYNTAX score[4,12,26,27,38,39,48,53,57–64]	0	11*	+	+
Society of Thoracic Surgery score[36,45,54,66]	40	2	−	+
Global Risk Classification[67]	17	11*	+	+
Clinical SYNTAX score[68]	3	11*	+	−

*Per lesion.
PCI, percutaneous coronary intervention; CABG, coronary artery bypass grafting surgery; ACEF, age, creatinine and ejection fraction;
AHA/ACC, American Heart Association/American College of Cardiology.

variables but requires the use of an online calculator (available at www.euroscore.org) to quantify risk.[31]

In addition to its assessment and validation in patients undergoing surgical revascularization, the euroSCORE has also been evaluated in numerous studies of patients undergoing PCI,[12,48–52] the majority of which specifically enrolled patients with LM disease.[12,48–51] Of note, all studies, irrespective of disease severity, have demonstrated the euroSCORE to be an independent predictor of mortality[49,52] and/or MACCE at follow-up ranging from 1- to 3-years.[12,48–51] Importantly those studies which also included a surgical control group, such as the SYNTAX study, the MAIN-COMPARE study, and the registry by Rodés-Cabau et al., also demonstrated that the euroSCORE was an independent predictor of MACCE in surgical patients.[48,50,53] Specifically in the SYNTAX study, which represents the only randomized study assessing the euroSCORE, the additive euroSCORE was shown to be an independent predictor of MACCE at 1-year follow-up irrespective of the method of revascularization (OR: 1.21; 95% CI [1.12–1.32], p < 0.001) in 705 patients undergoing LM revascularization.[48] Similarly at intermediate follow-up of 23-months, Rodés-Cabau et al., identified a euroSCORE ≥ 9 as the best predictor of MACCE after PCI and CABG amongst 249 octogenarians with LM disease.[50] In the MAIN-COMPARE registry which enrolled over 1500 patients with LM disease followed up for a median of 3.1 years, the euroSCORE has been identified as an independent predictor of death/MI/stroke irrespective of revascularization strategy.[53] In addition in the same registry a euroSCORE ≥ 6 has been shown to be an independent predictor of mortality following either PCI or CABG.[49]

The ability of the euroSCORE to identify patients at high risk for adverse events is not confined to those with LM disease. Romagnoli et al. have previously reported that the euroSCORE was an independent predictor of in-hospital mortality among over 1,100 patients, 70% of whom had single-vessel disease. Moreover, the C-statistic for the prediction of in-hospital mortality using the euroSCORE in this population was 0.91.[52] In summary, while acknowledging that most of these studies have been nonrandomized observational studies, the findings do suggest that the euroSCORE is a valuable tool in the individual assessment of risk prior to the selection of a revascularization strategy. Furthermore, these data indicate that the euroSCORE has little utility in helping to determine treatment strategy, as the risk for adverse events from a high euroSCORE is similar following either PCI or CABG.

TABLE 1-5	The Components of the euroSCORE and Relevant Weighting Factors of the Additive and Logistic euroSCOREs[30,31]*		Logistic β Coefficient
Patient Characteristics Additive			
Age	Per 5 years or part thereof over the age of 60 years	1	0.07
Gender	Female	1	0.33
Chronic pulmonary disease	Long-term use of bronchodilators or steroids for respiratory disease	1	0.49
Peripheral arteriopathy	*Claudication, carotid stenosis >50%, previous or planned intervention on the abdominal aorta, limb arteries or carotids	2	0.66
Neurological dysfunction	Severely affected mobility or day to day function	2	0.84
Previous cardiac surgery	Previous opening of the pericardium	3	1.00
Serum creatinine	Preoperatively greater than 200micromol/L	2	0.65
Active endocarditis	Antibiotic therapy at time of surgery	3	1.10
Critical preoperative state	†Preoperative cardiac arrest, ventilation, renal failure, inotropic support, intra-aortic balloon pump use, ventricular arrhythmia	3	0.91
Cardiac-Related Factors			
Unstable angina	Rest pain requiring iv nitrates	2	0.57
Left ventricular function	Moderate (30–50%)	1	0.42
	Poor (<30%)	3	1.09
Recent MI	Within 90 days	2	0.55
Pulmonary hypertension	Systolic pulmonary pressure >60 mmHg	2	0.77
Operation-Related Factors			
Emergency	Operation performed before the start of the next working day	2	0.71
Other than isolated CABG	Major cardiac procedure other than or in addition to CABG	2	0.54
Surgery on thoracic aorta		3	1.16
Postinfarct septal rupture		4	1.46
Constant β₀			−4.79

*The logistic euroSCORE can be calculated at www.euroscore.org.
†Any of the following.

Mayo Clinic Risk Score

The Mayo Clinic Risk Score (MCR) is a clinically based risk score incorporating seven variables (Table 1-6); it was initially developed to predict in-hospital mortality in patients undergoing PCI; however, subsequent validation has also been performed in patients undergoing CABG.[32,54] The score was initially validated in 7,457 PCI patients from the Mayo Clinic database, with resulting C-statistics of 0.74 and 0.89 for the prediction of MACCE and procedural death, respectively.[32] A subsequent larger external validation performed in over 300,000 patients from the National Cardiovascular Data Registry demonstrated good predictive ability for the MCRS, with a C-statistic of 0.885 for

the prediction of in-hospital mortality.[33] In patients undergoing CABG, a strong association has been demonstrated between the MCRS and mortality; however, the MCRS's overall performance has been shown to be inferior to the STS score.[54] These results suggest that the MCRS can be used to assess risk in patients undergoing revascularization; however, validated outcomes are limited to in-hospital mortality only. Additional studies assessing the impact of the MCRS in patients randomized to PCI and CABG remain outstanding.

Age, Creatinine, Ejection Fraction Score

The Age, Creatinine, Ejection Fraction (ACEF) score represents a newly developed risk model that uses just three clinical variables: patient age,

TABLE 1-6	The Mayo Clinic Risk Score[32]	
Variable		**Points**
Age, years		See below
Creatinine, mg/dL		See below
Left ventricular ejection fraction, %		See below
Preprocedural shock		9
Myocardial infarction < 24 hours		4
Congestive heart failure on presentation (without acute MI or shock)		3
Peripheral vascular disease		2
Mayo Clinic Risk Score*		Sum of the above

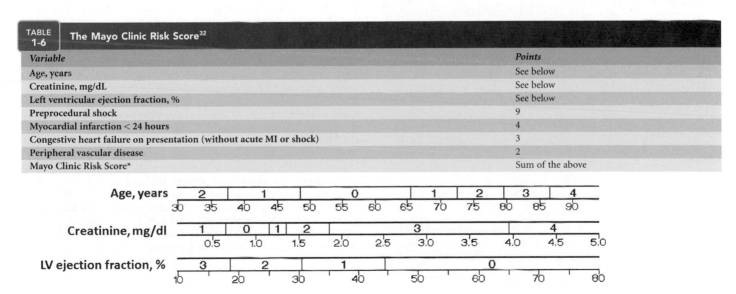

*The Mayo Clinic Risk Score[32] Congestive heart failure (CHF) is not entered in patients presenting with MI or shock. If creatinine is unavailable: 1 point is added if the patient is male or has CHF. If ejection fraction is unavailable: 1 point is added if the patient has CHF. For all other variables, if a risk factor is unknown, no points are added.

ejection fraction (%), and serum creatinine to predict in-hospital mortality in patients undergoing elective CABG.[34] These three variables are combined using a simple formula: (patient age/ejection fraction [%]) + (1 if creatinine >2mg/dL). The only published data thus far come from a single institution and include the initial data set of 4557 patients, and a subsequent validation series of 4091 patients. Nevertheless results demonstrated a similar accuracy and calibration for the prediction of in-hospital mortality with the ACEF score when compared with other more complicated surgical risk scores such as the euroSCORE and the Cleveland Clinic Score. The current data, although limited to a single center, indicates a role for the ACEF score in the assessment of risk in patients undergoing CABG; however the precise role of the ACEF score in assessing patients undergoing revascularization (PCI or CABG) will only be defined following its evaluation in patients undergoing PCI.

National Cardiovascular Database Registry CathPCI Risk Prediction Score

The National Cardiovascular Database Registry (NCDR) CathPCI risk-prediction score is the most contemporary clinically based risk model currently available. It incorporates information from eight clinical variables (Table 1-7), each of which is assigned an appropriate weighted value. These are then added together to give a final score, which can be translated into a risk of in-hospital mortality (Figure 1-5).[35] This score was developed using data from over 180,000 patients from the voluntary U.S. NCDR database and validated in over 400,000 patients from the same database who underwent PCI between March 2006 and March 2007. Of note, the C-statistic for the prediction of in-hospital mortality was consistently above 0.90 for in-hospital mortality, while a lower but nevertheless adequate C-statistic of 0.83 was seen for 30-day mortality. There are as yet no data on the use of this model in patients undergoing CABG; however, it is worth acknowledging that a number of variables used in the NCDR model are also used in the euroSCORE. Moreover, the large numbers of patients which have been used to validate the NCDR model and its high discriminatory ability certainly indicate that it may, in due course, become an important risk-stratification tool for patients undergoing revascularization.

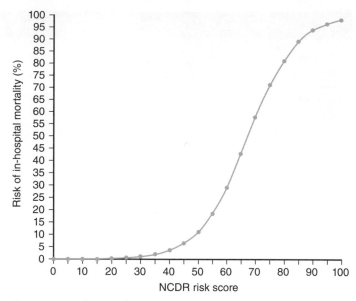

Figure 1-5 The predicted risk of in-hospital mortality using the National Cardiovascular Database Registry risk score described in Table 1-7.[35]

ANGIOGRAPHY-BASED SCORES

Two major angiography-based scores have been developed, both independent of patient clinical variables, since they are calculated using only angiographic data. As alluded to earlier, this introduces a subjective element to the assessment of risk[39,40] and consequently also a degree of intra- and interobserver variability, which is notably absent from the clinical scores described above. Finally, these scores can be computed only after diagnostic coronary angiography has been performed, thereby moving assessment further down the treatment pathway.

ACC/AHA Lesion Classification

The ACC/AHA lesion classification, which was initially devised in 1986 and modified in 1990, uses 11 angiographic variables to categorize lesions into four groups: types A, B1, B2, and C. Historical studies prior to the arrival of DES indicated that ACC/AHA lesion classification did have a prognostic impact on early and late outcomes.[37,55] In contemporary practice, evaluation of the ACC/AHA lesion classification is limited to retrospective registries, the largest of which is the German Cypher registry, which enrolled over 6,700 patients with approximately 8,000 lesions. At 6-month follow-up, no definite relationship was identified between clinical outcomes and ACC/AHA lesion class.[56] These results are at variance with the positive relationship identified between ACC/AHA lesion class and clinical outcomes in smaller studies of patients with more complex disease.[57,58] Specifically Valgimigli et al. reported that a higher ACC/AHA lesion score (derived by assigning 1, 2, 3, and 4 points to type A, B1, B2, and C lesions respectively) correlated with poor clinical outcomes among 306 patients with three-vessel disease undergoing PCI with DES.[57] More recently Capodanno et al. demonstrated that the ACC/AHA lesion score predicted both cardiac death ($P = 0.001$) and MACCE ($P = 0.02$) at 1-year follow-up among 255 patients with LM undergoing PCI with DES.[57] Of note, in this study the ACC/AHA lesion score was also found to be an independent predictor of cardiac death but not MACCE.

Syntax Score

The SXscore represents a comprehensive angiographic scoring system that allows the complexity of CAD to be quantified.[38,39] Both lesion

TABLE 1-7	The National Cardiovascular Database Registry Risk Model*			
Variable	*Scoring Response Categories*			
Age	<60	≥60, <70	≥70, <80	≥80
Weighted score	0	4	8	14
Cardiogenic shock	No	Yes		
Weighted score	0	25		
Prior CHF	No	Yes		
Weighted score	0	5		
Peripheral vascular disease	No	Yes		
Weighted score	0	5		
Chronic lung disease	No	Yes		
Weighted score	0	4		
GFR (mL/min)	<30	30–60	60–90	>90
Weighted score	18	10	6	0
NYHA Class IV	No	Yes		
Weighted score	0	4		
PCI Status (STEMI)	Elective	Urgent	Emergent	Salvage
Weighted score	12	15	20	38
PCI Status (no STEMI)	Elective	Urgent	Emergent	Salvage
Weighted score	0	8	20	42

*The risk of in-hospital mortality is derived using Figure 1-5.
CHF, congestive cardiac failure; GFR, glomerular filtration rate; NYHA, New York Heart Association; PCI, percutaneous coronary intervention; STEMI, ST-elevation myocardial infarction.

| TABLE 1-8 | A Summary of the Results of the Most Prominent Studies Which Have Assessed the Impact of the SYNTAX Score on Clinical Outcomes in Patients Undergoing PCI | | | | | | |

Study Name	No. of Patients (FUP, mo)	MACE, % (Tercile 1 vs. 2 vs. 3)	Death, % (Tercile 1 vs. 2 vs. 3)	MI, % (Tercile 1 vs. 2 vs. 3)	Repeat Revascularization, % (Tercile 1 vs. 2 vs. 3)	Independent Predictor MORTALITY	Independent Predictor MACE
All-Comers Population							
LEADERS[60]	1397 (12)	7.8 vs. 8.9 vs. 15.4*	1.5 vs. 2.1 vs. 5.6*	4.3 vs. 4.9 vs. 5.9	4.7 vs. 6.1 vs. 8.7[†¶]	+	+
SIRTAX[62]	848 (60)	12.5 vs. 21.2 vs. 24.2*	6.3 vs. 8.1 vs. 11.8	3.1 vs. 8.7 vs. 8.1[†]	9.4 vs. 15.7 vs. 15.7[†¶]	−	+
Complex Disease							
ARTS-II[4]	607 (60)	19.9 vs. 29.9 vs. 32.9*	2.4 vs. 7.5 vs. 6.5	3.3 vs. 7.0 vs. 7.0	13.9 vs. 22.6 vs. 24.6[†‡]	NA	+
SYNTAX[12]	903 (12)	13.6 vs. 16.7 vs. 23.4*	2.0 vs. 3.3 vs. 8.0*	2.7 vs. 4.9 vs. 7.0	11.5 vs. 12.1 vs. 16.8	NA	NA
Left Main Disease							
SYNTAX LM cohort[48]	357 (12)	7.7 vs. 12.6 vs. 25.4*	0.9 vs. 1.0 vs. 9.7*	1.7 vs. 2.9 vs. 7.5	7.7 vs. 9.7 vs. 17.2[†]	NA	+
CUSTOMIZE registry[58]	255 (12)	7.4 vs. 21.4 vs. 20.4	2.5 vs. 1.1 vs. 13.1[§]	NA	NA	+	+
MAIN-COMPARE[53]	819 (36)	4.6 vs. 9.4 vs. 11.4[†‖]	NA	NA	NA	−	−
Rotterdam registry[61]	148 (48)	46.2 vs. 55.1 vs. 69.6[†]	NA	NA	NA	+	−

*<0.01
[†]<0.05
[¶]Clinically indicate-target lesion revascularization.
[‡]All revascularization
[§]Cardiac death
[‖]MACE defined as death/M/stroke
NA, not reported
FUP, follow-up
Mo, months

location and adverse lesion characteristics are used in the calculation, which can be performed using either a downloadable calculator or the SXscore website (www.syntaxscore.com)(Table 1-3). The score, which uses several historical anatomical scores as its base, was initially devised specifically for the SYNTAX trial as a means to "force" the cardiologist and cardiac surgeon to study the coronary angiogram in detail. At that time, it was also hypothesized that the SXscore might also correlate with clinical outcome.[38] The score was first used prospectively in the SYNTAX trial and has since been calculated in a number of different clinical trials both in elective and acute PCI patients, with simple or complex disease followed up for between 1 to 5 years.[4,12,48,53,57–62] The main results from these studies at maximum follow-up are shown in Table 1-8. In all studies irrespective of follow-up duration, a higher SXscore tercile has consistently been associated with the poorest outcomes.[4,12,48,53,57–62] Moreover, several studies have also identified the SXscore as an independent predicting MACCE[4,48,57–60] and/or mortality[58,60,61] in patients undergoing PCI. Overall, these results support the role of the SXscore in risk stratifying patients following diagnostic coronary angiography.

Importantly prospective data from the SYNTAX trial, and retrospective analysis of the CUSTOMIZE registry, both of which included a surgical control arm, have also provided evidence which supports the use of the SXscore in helping determine revascularization strategy. This expanded role stems from the identification of the SXscore as an independent predictor of MACCE for patients undergoing PCI, whilst no similar relationship has been demonstrated in patients treated with CABG. In the SYNTAX study the rate of MACCE among patients with 3VD/LM disease undergoing PCI was 19.4%, 22.8%, and 28.2% for SXscore terciles low, intermediate, and high, which contrasts with respective rates amongst CABG patients of 17.4%, 16.4%, and 15.4%. This flat relationship amongst CABG patients is somewhat expected as bypass anastomoses are inserted distal to underlying complex disease. In practice these results suggest patients with a high SXscore have significantly better outcomes, and a lower risk of events following CABG compared to those having PCI. In patients with a low SXscore both treatment modalities offer comparable outcomes, whilst in the intermediate group, CABG offers superior outcomes in patients with 3VD, whilst comparable outcomes are seen in LM patients (Figures 1-3

and 1-4).[26,77] A similar relationship was seen in the CUSTOMIZE registry where rates of MACCE amongst LM patients treated with PCI and CABG for those with an SXscore ≤ 34 were 8.1% and 6.2% (P = 0.46) respectively, compared to 32.7% and 8.5% (P < 0.001) for those with SXscores greater than 34.

The absence of any relationship between the SXscore and events rates among surgical patients is further supported by Lemesle et al., who reported on outcomes of 320 patients undergoing CABG stratified according to SXscore tercile. At 1-year follow-up, rates of death/stroke/MI were 9.4%, 7.5%, and 10.4%, respectively, in patients in the low, intermediate, and high SXscore terciles (P = 0.75).[63] In contrast, Birim et al. identified the SXscore as an independent predictor of 1-year MACCE among a cohort of 148 patients undergoing CABG.[64] The small sample size and retrospective design may have influenced these results, which have not yet been repeated or fully explained. A positive correlation has been reported between the SXscore and the ACC/AHA lesion score; however more detailed analysis indicates that the SXscore has a superior discriminative ability for both cardiac death (SX score 0.83 vs. 0.76 ACC/AHA)[58] and MACCE (SXscore 0.73 vs. ACC/AHA 0.56).[57]

In summary, in the short period of time since its introduction, the SXscore has been evaluated in a number of different studies, all of which suggest that it has a role to play in risk stratifying patients undergoing revascularization. In addition, results from those studies including a surgical treatment arm offer evidence that the SXscore also has utility in assisting in important revascularization decisions in patients with CAD.

COMBINED RISK SCORES

The previous discussion has reviewed risk models that rely on either clinical or angiographic variables. There is no disputing that for a complete individualized patient assessment, both factors must be taken into consideration. Moreover, current evidence indicates that clinically and angiographically based risk models may be better suited to predicting different patient outcomes. Clinically based scores appear to be better at predicting clinical endpoints such as death or MI, while angiographically based scores appear to be superior for the prediction of angiographic success and the risk of repeat revascularization. Of note, Peterson et al. observed only a minimal improvement in the ability of the NCDR CathPCI risk score to predict in-hospital mortality following the inclusion of angiographic variables.[35] These findings are in line with previous reports demonstrating that the MCRS was superior to the ACC/AHA lesion classification in the prediction of death/stroke/MI/emergent CABG but inferior for the prediction of angiographic failure.[65] These differential outcomes, according to the variables assessed in the risk model, have raised interest in combined risk models, which assess risk by considering both clinical and angiographic variables. In view of this, several combined clinical and angiographic risk scores have been developed. Other than the STS score, the newer combined scores have yet to be validated in large patient populations, such that outcome data are currently confined to small, retrospective studies with limited follow-up. The most prominent combined risk scores include the following.

Society of Thoracic Surgery Score

The Society of Thoracic Surgery (STS) score predicts the risk of operative mortality and morbidity after cardiac surgery and is calculated by means of an online calculator that requests information on 40 clinical and 2 angiographic variables (presence of LM lesion and number of vessels diseased).[36,45] As alluded to earlier and unlike the euroSCORE, the STS score undergoes periodic recalibration, which is vital to ensure that its results remain applicable to contemporary practice. In comparison with other clinically based models in patients undergoing CABG, the STS score has been shown to be superior to both the MCRS[54] and the euroSCORE.[66] Importantly, however, there has been no evaluation of the STS score in patients undergoing PCI or any comparison between the STS score and angiographically based scores. Consequently the role of the STS score in the assessment of patients undergoing revascularization is confined to those in whom surgical revascularization has already been selected.

euroSCORE-SYNTAX

The euroSCORE and the SXscore are the most extensively studied risk models in patients undergoing revascularization. Moreover, the combination of both scores should offer the potential to harness the positive aspects of each—namely, the ability of the euroSCORE to identify patients at high risk of adverse events irrespective of treatment modality and the ability of the SXscore to assist in establishing the optimal revascularization strategy. Although the principal behind combining both scores is simple, the method of actually combining both into an effective risk model has been harder to establish. In the SYNTAX study, simply subdividing patients in SXscore tertiles by a euroSCORE above or below the median failed to demonstrate a consistent and understandable relationship. This may in part have been due to the small numbers of patients in each subgroup. A more recent suggestion, which appears to hold promise, has been described by Capodanno et al., who developed a Global Risk Classification (GRC). The GRC categorizes patients into low-, medium-, and high-risk groups using a matrix that incorporates a patient's euroSCORE, which is subdivided into the historically defined groups of low (0–2), intermediate (3–5), and high risk (≥6) and their SXscore, which is divided into low, intermediate, and high terciles (Figure 1-6).[67] The GRC has so far been applied only to a population of 255 patients undergoing LM revascularization, for which SXscores were calculated retrospectively. At 2-year follow-up the rates of cardiac death in patients in the low, intermediate, and high SXscore terciles were 3.9%, 5.4%, and 21.9%, respectively, while rates of 1.6%, 16.0%, and 31.4%, respectively, were seen in the low, intermediate, and high GRC groups. Additional results indicate that the GRC had a greater discriminatory ability when it was compared with other risk scores, including the euroSCORE and the SXscore for the prediction of in-hospital and 2-year mortality. Overall the study reiterated the importance of considering both clinical and angiographic variables in the assessment of overall risk, and it provided a combined scoring system that requires additional validation in a large patient group.

		SYNTAX Score Tercile		
		Low	Intermediate	High
euroSCORE	Low	Low	Low	Intermediate
	Medium	Low	Low	Intermediate
	High	Intermediate	Intermediate	High

- Global Risk Classification (GRC) is derived using the above matrix
- The GRC divides patients into Low, Intermediate, and High risk groups as shown.

Figure 1-6 The Global Risk Classification matrix.[67]

Clinical Syntax Score

The Clinical SYNTAX score (CSS) was born out of the need to include a clinical component to the angiographic SXscore.[68] The CSS score incorporates as its clinical component the ACEF score,[34] which has been modified by replacing serum creatinine (which originally received 1 point if it was >2 mg/dL) with a weighted score linked to the creatinine clearance. This modification was implemented to improve the discrimination of risk, which was previously observed when a similar modification was incorporated into the euroSCORE.[69] The CSS is calculated by multiplying the SXscore with this modified ACEF score (Figure 1-7). Currently the CSS has been evaluated only in patients enrolled with complex disease who were enrolled in the ARTS II study. Nevertheless, at 5-year follow-up among patients with triple-vessel disease, the CSS was shown to have a superior discriminative ability compared to the SXscore and ACEF in the prediction of both mortality (CSS 0.80 vs. SXscore 0.70 vs. ACEF 0.73) and MACCE (CSS 0.67 vs. SXscore 0.64 vs. ACEF 0.59).[68] Further evaluation is necessary to validate this score in a larger, more diverse patient population.

Individual Assessment—From a Patient's Perspective

The above discussion has focused entirely on the factors physicians must take into account in making revascularization decisions. Importantly, however, in the era of increased patient choice and transparency and greater patient involvement in decision making, it is vital also to consider these issues from the patient's perspective through the assessment of health-related quality of life (QoL). This patient-oriented approach is all the more important given the comparable rates of mortality and MI that have been reported among patients with complex disease treated with PCI or CABG at both short- and long-term follow-up (Table 1-2).[4,6,12,19,25,70] Unfortunately data on this key topic are limited to only the handful of studies that have assessed PCI in patients receiving DES. Of note, early studies comparing PCI (with BMS) and CABG indicated a trend toward improved QoL outcomes with CABG; however, these results have largely been driven by higher

$$\text{Clinical SYNTAX Score} = \text{SYNTAX Score} \times \left(\frac{\text{Age}}{\text{LV ejection fraction (\%)}} + \text{1 point for each 10ml creatinine clearance}^{*} < 60\text{ml/min/1.73m}^2 \right)$$

*Calculated using the Cockcroft/Gault equation

Figure 1-7 The Clinical SYNTAX score formula.[68]

rates of repeat revascularization with BMS, a phenomenon addressed following the introduction of DES.[7] For example the Stent or Surgery (SoS) study reported a favorable health related QoL with CABG compared with PCI in terms of reduced anginal frequency and physical limitation at 6 months, with the superior reduction in anginal frequency maintained as long as 12 months.[71] Similarly at 12-month follow-up in the Medicine, Angioplasty or Surgery Study (MASS II), patients treated with CABG had a greater improvement in health-related QoL compared with those who were treated with PCI and medical therapy.[72] Data on QoL from patients treated with DES and CABG are limited to the 12-month results from the SYNTAX study and 3-year results from the ARTS II study.[73,74] Encouragingly, results from the SYNTAX study indicate that despite recruitment of a very complex patient population, treatment with PCI or CABG does lead to a significant improvement in QoL compared with baseline. Moreover, consistent with earlier studies, a greater improvement in QoL is seen in those treated with CABG as opposed to PCI. It is noteworthy that the difference in anginal frequency between both groups according to the Seattle Angina Questionnaire, which was 1.7 when administered at 6 and 12 months, is less than that deemed to be clinically relevant and also less than that observed in other studies such as SoS (a 3-point difference at 12 months), and COURAGE (a 3- to 6-point difference) (Figure 1-8).[75] Similarly, data from the ARTS II study indicate the absence of any significant difference in anginal status between patients treated with DES as opposed to those treated with CABG from as early as 1 month after the index procedure through to 3-year follow-up. Of note, treatment with BMS led to consistently higher rates of angina.[74] Although these results appear to indicate that QoL after revascularization with PCI or CABG is largely comparable, it must be stressed that these results are based on study populations, and as with the risk models discussed previously, individual patients may have different concerns that are not captured in these evaluations. For example, some patients may be more willing to accept the increased chances of a repeat procedure with PCI, as this option allows them to return to normal activity promptly after the procedure; conversely, others may be content with the longer convalesce from CABG, as this offers a suitable trade-off with the subsequently lower risk of repeat revascularization.[76] Interestingly, in the SYNTAX study, physical

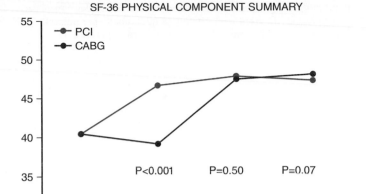

SF-36 PHYSICAL COMPONENT SUMMARY

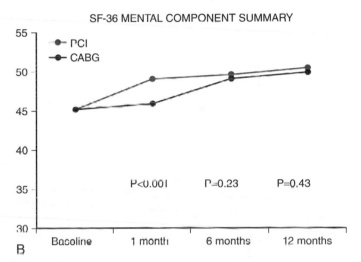

SF-36 MENTAL COMPONENT SUMMARY

Figure 1-9 The temporal change in the Short Form (36) Health Survey (SF-36) physical and mental component during follow-up after revascularization with either PCI or CABG in the SYNTAX study. Importantly at 1 month, a significantly better outcome for both parameters was noted in those treated with PCI; however by 12 months, this difference had eroded such that both treatments were comparable.[73]

limitations, QoL, and treatment satisfaction were all significantly better with PCI than with CABG at 1 month; however, by 6 months, these differences were comparable (Figure 1-9).

Clearly an individual patient's views on these issues cannot be captured in a questionnaire but only through a frank discussion between the patient, cardiologist, and cardiac surgeon. Therefore in patients where PCI or CABG is an equally valid revascularization technique, the thoughts and concerns of individual patients must also be considered before deciding on the optimal revascularization strategy.

Conclusions

The face of revascularization is changing because greater numbers of patients who require revascularization are presenting with comorbidities and more extensive CAD. Concurrent with this have been the advances in PCI and surgical technology, which has lead to a blurring of the classic divisions grouping those patients and coronary lesions that are suitable exclusively for PCI or CABG. This welcome change has increased the importance of assessing patients as individuals, taking into consideration their comorbidities, angiographic findings, and ultimately, where appropriate, their personal preferences prior to the establishment of a treatment strategy. To aid physicians in

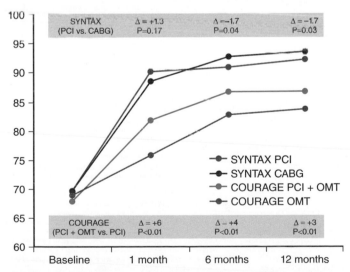

Figure 1-8 The change in Seattle Angina Questionnaire anginal frequency during follow-up of the SYNTAX study and the COURAGE study.[73,75] All therapies led to a reduction in anginal frequency; however, the improvement was greatest following surgical revascularization. Importantly, the difference between PCI and CABG in the SYNTAX study is not considered clinically significant; moreover, it is considerably less than the difference between PCI and optimal medical therapy (OMT) and OMT alone in the COURAGE study.

quantifying this risk, numerous risk models have been developed, each incorporating different clinical and angiographic parameters. The importance of these models in contemporary practice is in part emphasized by their inclusion, for the first time, in society guidelines on myocardial revascularization.[77,78] Unfortunately, however, no validation has been performed of all models in the same patient population and thus no one model can be recommended above another. Nevertheless, the evidence indicates that risk stratification, irrespective of how it is performed, plays an important role in the assessment of patients undergoing revascularization.

REFERENCES

1. Grüntzig A: Transluminal dilatation of coronary-artery stenosis. *Lancet* 1(8058):263, 1978.
2. Hilliard AA, From AM, Lennon RJ, et al: Percutaneous revascularization for stable coronary artery disease temporal trends and impact of drug-eluting stents. *JACC Cardiovasc Interv* 3(2):172–179, 2010.
3. Vranckx P, Boersma E, Garg S, et al: Cardiovascularr profile of patients included in stent trials: a meta-analysis of individual patient data from randomized clinical trials. Insights from 33 prospective stent trials in Europe. *EuroIntervention*. In press.
4. Serruys PW, Onuma Y, Garg S, et al: 5-Year Clinical outcomes of the ARTS II (Arterial Revascularization Therapies Study II) of the sirolimus-eluting stent in the treatment of patients with multivessel de novo coronary artery lesions. *J Am Coll Cardiol* 55:1093–1101, 2010.
5. LeGrand V, Garg S, Serruys PW, et al: Influence of age on the clinical outcomes of coronary revascularization for the treatment of patients with multivessel de novo coronary artery lesions. Sirolimus-eluting stent vs. coronary artery bypass surgery and bare metal stent: insight from the Multicenter Randomized Arterial Revascularization Therapy Study Part I (ARTS-I) and Part II (ARTS-II). *Eurointervention* 6(7):838–845, 2011.
6. Hlatky MA, Boothroyd DB, Bravata DM, et al: Coronary artery bypass surgery compared with percutaneous coronary interventions for multivessel disease: a collaborative analysis of individual patient data from ten randomised trials. *Lancet* 373(9670):1190–1197, 2009.
7. Garg S, Serruys PW: Coronary stents: current status. *J Am Coll Cardiol* 56(10 Suppl):S1–S42, 2010.
8. Windecker S, Remondino A, Eberli FR, et al: Sirolimus-eluting and paclitaxel-eluting stents for coronary revascularization. *N Engl J Med* 353(7):653–662, 2005.
9. Windecker S, Serruys PW, Wandel S, et al: Biolimus-eluting stent with biodegradable polymer versus sirolimus-eluting stent with durable polymer for coronary revascularisation (LEADERS): a randomised non-inferiority trial. *Lancet* 372(9644):1163–1173, 2008.
10. Serruys PW, Unger F, Sousa JE, et al: Comparison of coronary-artery bypass surgery and stenting for the treatment of multivessel disease. *N Engl J Med* 344(15):1117–1124, 2001.
11. Serruys PW, Ong ATL, Morice M-C, et al: Arterial Revascularisation Therapies Study Part II: sirolimus-eluting stents for the treatment of patients with multivessel de novo coronary artery lesions. *EuroIntervention* 1(2):147–156, 2005.
12. Serruys PW, Morice MC, Kappetein AP, et al: Percutaneous coronary intervention versus coronary-artery bypass grafting for severe coronary artery disease. *N Engl J Med* 360(10):961–972, 2009.
13. Kappetein AP, Dawkins KD, Mohr FW, et al: Current percutaneous coronary intervention and coronary artery bypass grafting practices for three-vessel and left main coronary artery disease. Insights from the SYNTAX run-in phase. *Eur J Cardiothorac Surg* 29(4):486–491, 2006.
14. Sjauw KD, Konorza T, Erbel R, et al: Supported high-risk percutaneous coronary intervention with the Impella 2.5 device the Europella registry. *J Am Coll Cardiol* 54(25):2430–2434, 2009.
15. Vranckx P, Schultz CJ, Valgimigli M, et al: Assisted circulation using the TandemHeart during very high-risk PCI of the unprotected left main coronary artery in patients declined for CABG. *Catheter Cardiovasc Interv* 74(2):302–310, 2009.
16. Aziz O, Rao C, Panesar SS, et al: Meta-analysis of minimally invasive internal thoracic artery bypass versus percutaneous revascularisation for isolated lesions of the left anterior descending artery. *BMJ* 334(7594):617–625, 2007.
17. Kapoor JR, Gienger AL, Ardehali R, et al: Isolated disease of the proximal left anterior descending artery: comparing the effectiveness of percutaneous coronary interventions and coronary artery bypass surgery. *J Am Coll Cardiol Intervent* 1(5):483–491, 2008.
18. Thiele H, Neumann-Schniedewind P, Jacobs S, et al: Randomized comparison of minimally invasive direct coronary artery bypass surgery versus sirolimus-eluting stenting in isolated proximal left anterior descending coronary artery stenosis. *J Am Coll Cardiol* 53(25):2324–2331, 2009.
19. Daemen J, Boersma E, Flather M, et al: Long-term safety and efficacy of percutaneous coronary intervention with stenting and coronary artery bypass surgery for multivessel coronary artery disease: a meta-analysis with 5-year patient-level data from the ARTS, ERACI-II, MASS-II, and SoS trials. *Circulation* 118(11):1146–1154, 2008.
20. Bravata DM, Gienger AL, McDonald KM, et al: Systematic review: the comparative effectiveness of percutaneous coronary interventions and coronary artery bypass graft surgery. *Annals of Internal Medicine* 147(10):703, 2007.
21. Comparison of coronary bypass surgery with angioplasty in patients with multivessel disease. The Bypass Angioplasty Revascularization Investigation (BARI) investigators. *N Engl J Med* 335(4):217–225, 1996.
22. The final 10-year follow-up results from the BARI randomized trial. *J Am Coll Cardiol* 49(15):1600–1606, 2007.
23. Ong AT, Serruys PW, Mohr FW, et al: The SYNergy between percutaneous coronary intervention with TAXus and cardiac surgery (SYNTAX) study: design, rationale, and run-in phase. *Am Heart J* 151(6):1194–1204, 2006.
24. Serruys PW, Morice MC, Kappetein AP, et al: Supplementary appendix: percutaneous coronary intervention versus coronary-artery bypass grafting for severe coronary artery disease *N Engl J Med* 360(10):961–972, 2009. DOI: 910.1056/NEJMoa0804626.
25. Kappetein AP: Optimal revascularization strategy in patients with three-vessel disease and/or left main disease. The 2-year outcomes of the SYNTAX trial. Presentation at the ESC Congress, Barcelona, September 2, 2009. Available online www.syntaxscore.com.
26. Morice MC: Multivessel disease lessons from SYNTAX (early results and 2 year follow-up): interventional perspectives. Presentation at Transcatheter Cardiovascular Therapeutics, San Francisco, September 21, 2009.
27. Serruys PW: Left main lessons from SYNTAX (early results and 2 year follow-up): interventional perspectives. Presentation Transcatheter Cardiovascular Therapeutics, 21st September 2009. [Available online: www.tctmd.com/txshow.aspx?tid=939076&id=83938&trid=938634.]
28. Patel MR, Dehmer GJ, Hirshfeld JW, et al: ACCF/SCAI/STS/AATS/AHA/ASNC 2009 appropriateness criteria for coronary revascularization: a report by the American College of Cardiology Foundation Appropriateness Criteria Task Force, Society for Cardiovascular Angiography and Interventions, Society of Thoracic Surgeons, American Association for Thoracic Surgery, American Heart Association, and the American Society of Nuclear Cardiology Endorsed by the American Society of Echocardiography, the Heart Failure Society of America, and the Society of Cardiovascular Computed Tomography. *J Am Coll Cardiol* 53(6):530–553, 2009.
29. Roques F, Nashef SA, Michel P, et al: Risk factors and outcome in European cardiac surgery: analysis of the euroSCORE multinational database of 19030 patients. *Eur J Cardiothorac Surg* 15(6):816–822; discussion 822–813, 1999.
30. Nashef SA, Roques F, Michel P, et al: European system for cardiac operative risk evaluation (euroSCORE). *Eur J Cardiothorac Surg* 16(1):9–13, 1999.
31. Roques F, Michel P, Goldstone AR, et al: The logistic euroSCORE. *Eur Heart J* 24(9):881–882, 2003.
32. Singh M, Rihal CS, Lennon RJ, et al: Bedside estimation of risk from percutaneous coronary intervention: the New Mayo Clinic risk scores. *Mayo Clin Proc* 82(6):701–708, 2007.
33. Singh M, Peterson ED, Milford-Beland S, et al: Validation of the Mayo Clinic risk score for in-hospital mortality after percutaneous coronary interventions using the national cardiovascular data registry. *Circ Cardiovasc Intervent* 1(1):36–44, 2008.
34. Ranucci M, Castelvecchio S, Menicanti L, et al: Risk of assessing mortality risk in elective cardiac operations: age, creatinine, ejection fraction, and the law of parsimony. *Circulation* 119(24):3053–3061, 2009.
35. Peterson ED, Dai D, DeLong ER, et al: Contemporary mortality risk prediction for percutaneous coronary intervention: results from 588,398 procedures in the National Cardiovascular Data Registry. *J Am Coll Cardiol* 55(18):1923–1932, 2010.
36. Shroyer AL, Coombs LP, Peterson ED, et al: The Society of Thoracic Surgeons: 30-day operative mortality and morbidity risk models. *Ann Thorac Surg* 75(6):1856–1864; discussion 1864–1855, 2003.
37. Ryan TJ, Bauman WB, Kennedy JW, et al: Guidelines for percutaneous transluminal coronary angioplasty. A report of the American Heart Association/American College of Cardiology Task Force on Assessment of Diagnostic and Therapeutic Cardiovascular Procedures (Committee on Percutaneous Transluminal Coronary Angioplasty). *Circulation* 88(6):2987–3007, 1993.
38. Sianos G, Morel MA, Kappetein AP, et al: The SYNTAX Score: an angiographic tool grading the complexity of coronary artery disease. *EuroIntervention* 1(2):219–227, 2005.
39. Serruys PW, Onuma Y, Garg S, et al: Assessment of the SYNTAX score in the Syntax study. *Eurointervention* 5(1):50–56, 2009.
40. Garg S, Girasis C, Sarno G, et al: The SYNTAX score revisited: a reassessment of the SYNTAX score reproducibility. *Catheter Cardiovasc Intervent* 75(6):946–952, 2010.
41. Califf RM, Peterson ED, Gibbons RJ, et al: Integrating quality into the cycle of therapeutic development. *J Am Coll Cardiol* 40(11):1895–1901, 2002.
42. Concato J, Feinstein AR, Holford TR: The risk of determining risk with multivariable models. *Ann Intern Med* 118(3):201–210, 1993.
43. Choong CK, Sergeant P, Nashef SA, et al: The euroSCORE risk stratification system in the current era: how accurate is it and what should be done if it is inaccurate? *Eur J Cardiothorac Surg* 35(1):59–61, 2009.
44. Bhatti F, Grayson AD, Grotte G, et al: The logistic euroSCORE in cardiac surgery: how well does it predict operative risk? *Heart* 92(12):1817–1820, 2006.
45. Shahian DM, O'Brien SM, Filardo G, et al: The Society of Thoracic Surgeons 2008 cardiac surgery risk models: part 1. Coronary artery bypass grafting surgery. *Ann Thorac Surg* 88(1 Suppl):S2–22, 2009.
46. Toumpoulis IK, Anagnostopoulos CE, DeRose JJ, et al: European system for cardiac operative risk evaluation predicts long-term survival in patients with coronary artery bypass grafting. *Eur J Cardiothorac Surg* 25(1):51–58, 2004.
47. De Maria R, Mazzoni M, Parolini M, et al: Predictive value of euroSCORE on long term outcome in cardiac surgery patients: a single institution study. *Heart* 91(6):779–784, 2005.
48. Morice MC, Serruys PW, Kappetein AP, et al: Outcomes in patients with de novo left main disease treated with either percutaneous coronary intervention using TAXUS Express2 paclitaxel-eluting stent or coronary artery bypass graft treatment in the SYNTAX trial. *Circulation* 121(24):2645–2653, 2010.
49. Min SY, Park DW, Yun SC, et al: Major predictors of long-term clinical outcomes after coronary revascularization in patients with unprotected left main coronary disease: analysis from the MAIN-COMPARE study. *Circ Cardiovasc Interv* 3(2):127–133, 2010.
50. Rodes-Cabau J, Deblois J, Bertrand OF, et al: Nonrandomized comparison of coronary artery bypass surgery and percutaneous coronary intervention for the treatment of unprotected left main coronary artery disease in octogenarians. *Circulation* 118(23):2374–2381, 2008.
51. Kim YH, Ahn JM, Park DW, et al: EuroSCORE as a predictor of death and myocardial infarction after unprotected left main coronary stenting. *Am J Cardiol* 98(12):1567–1570, 2006.
52. Romagnoli E, Burzotta F, Trani C, et al: EuroSCORE as predictor of in-hospital mortality after percutaneous coronary intervention. *Heart* 95(1):43–48, 2009.
53. Kim Y-H, Park D-W, Kim W-J, et al: Validation of SYNTAX (Synergy between PCI with Taxus and Cardiac Surgery) score for prediction of outcomes after unprotected left main coronary revascularization. *J Am Coll Cardiol Intv* 3(6):612–623, 2010.
54. Singh M, Gersh BJ, Li S, et al: Mayo Clinic risk score for percutaneous coronary intervention predicts in-hospital mortality in patients undergoing coronary artery bypass graft surgery. *Circulation* 117(3):356–362, 2008.
55. Kastrati A, Schomig A, Elezi S, et al: Prognostic value of the modified American College of Cardiology/American Heart Association stenosis morphology classification for long-term angiographic and clinical outcome after coronary stent placement. *Circulation* 100(12):1285–1290, 1999.
56. Khattab AA, Hamm CW, Senges J, et al: Prognostic value of the modified American College of Cardiology/American Heart Association lesion morphology classification for clinical outcome after sirolimus-eluting stent placement (results of the prospective multicenter German Cypher Registry). *Am J Cardiol* 101(4):477–482, 2008.
57. Valgimigli M, Serruys PW, Tsuchida K, et al: Cyphering the complexity of coronary artery disease using the syntax score to predict clinical outcome in patients with three-vessel lumen obstruction undergoing percutaneous coronary intervention. *Am J Cardiol* 99(8):1072–1081, 2007.
58. Capodanno D, Di Salvo ME, Cincotta G, et al: Usefulness of the SYNTAX Score for Predicting Clinical Outcome After Percutaneous Coronary Intervention of Unprotected Left Main Coronary Artery Disease. *Circ Cardiovasc Intervent* 2(4):302–308, 2009.
59. Capodanno D, Capranzano P, Di Salvo ME, et al: Usefulness of SYNTAX score to select patients with left main coronary artery disease to be treated with coronary artery bypass graft. *JACC Cardiovasc Interv* 2(8):731–738, 2009.
60. Wykrzykowska J, Garg S, Girasis C, et al: Value of the Syntax Score (SX) for Risk Assessment in the "All-comers" Population of the Randomized Multicenter Leaders Trial. *J Am Coll Cardiol* 56(4):272–277, 2010.
61. Onuma Y, Girasis C, Piazza N, et al: Long-term clinical results following stenting of the Left Main Stem—Insights from RESEARCH and T-SEARCH Registries. *J Am Coll Cardiol Intv* 3(6):584–594, 2010.
62. Girasis C, Garg S, Raber L, et al: Prediction of 5-year clinical outcomes using the SYNTAX score in patients undergoing PCI

from the Sirolimus eluting stent compared with paclitaxel eluting stent for coronary revascularisation (SIRTAX) trial. Abstract at American College of Cardiology meeting, March 14–16th 2010, Atlanta GA.

63. Lemesle G, Bonello L, de Labriolle A, et al: Prognostic value of the Syntax score in patients undergoing coronary artery bypass grafting for three-vessel coronary artery disease. *Catheter Cardiovasc Interv* 73(5):612–617, 2009.

64. Birim O, van Gameren M, Bogers AJ, et al: Complexity of coronary vasculature predicts outcome of surgery for left main disease. *The Annals of thoracic surgery* 87(4):1097–1104; discussion 1104–1095, 2009.

65. Singh M, Rihal CS, Lennon RJ, et al: Comparison of Mayo Clinic risk score and American College of Cardiology/American Heart Association lesion classification in the prediction of adverse cardiovascular outcome following percutaneous coronary interventions. *J Am Coll Cardiol* 44(2):357–361, 2004.

66. Ad N, Barnett SD, Speir AM: The performance of the euroSCORE and the Society of Thoracic Surgeons mortality risk score: the gender factor. *Interact Cardiovasc Thorac Surg* 6(2):192–195, 2007.

67. Capodanno D, Miano M, Cincotta G, et al: EuroSCORE refines the predictive ability of SYNTAX score in patients undergoing left main percutaneous coronary intervention. *Am Heart J* 159(1):103–109, 2010.

68. Garg S, Sarno G, Garcia Garcia HM, et al: A new tool for the risk stratification of patients with complex coronary artery disease: the clinical SYNTAX score. *Circ Cardiovasc Interv* 3(4):317–326, 2010.

69. Walter J, Mortasawi A, Arnrich B, et al: Creatinine clearance versus serum creatinine as a risk factor in cardiac surgery. *BMC Surg* 3:4, 2003.

70. Serruys PW, Ong AT, van Herwerden LA, et al: Five-year outcomes after coronary stenting versus bypass surgery for the treatment of multivessel disease: the final analysis of the Arterial Revascularization Therapies Study (ARTS) randomized trial. *J Am Coll Cardiol* 46(4):575–581, 2005.

71. Zhang Z, Mahoney EM, Stables RH, et al: Disease-specific health status after stent-assisted percutaneous coronary intervention and coronary artery bypass surgery: one-year results from the Stent or Surgery Trial. *Circulation* 108(14):1694–1700, 2003.

72. Favarato ME, Hueb W, Boden WE, et al: Quality of life in patients with symptomatic multivessel coronary artery disease: a comparative post hoc analyses of medical, angioplasty or surgical strategies-MASS II trial. *Int J Cardiol* 116(3):364–370, 2007.

73. Cohen DJ, Van Hout B, Serruys PW, et al: Synergy between PCI with Taxus and Cardiac Surgery Investigators. Quality of life after PCI with drug-eluting stents or coronary-artery bypass surgery. *N Engl J Med* 364(11):1016–1026, 2011.

74. van Domburg R, Daemen J, Morice M, et al: Short- and long-term health related quality-of-life and anginal status of the Arterial Revascularisation Therapies Study part II, ARTS-II; sirolimus-eluting stents for the treatment of patients with multivessel coronary artery disease. *EuroIntervention* 5:962–967, 2010.

75. Weintraub WS, Spertus JA, Kolm P, et al: Effect of PCI on quality of life in patients with stable coronary disease. *N Engl J Med* 359(7):677–687, 2008.

76. Federspiel J, Stearns S, Van Domburg R, et al: Risk-benefit trade-offs in revascularization choices. *EuroIntervention* 6(8):936–941, 2011.

77. Wijns W, Kolh P, Danchin N, et al: Guidelines on myocardial revascularization: The Task Force on Myocardial Revascularization of the European Society of Cardiology (ESC) and the European Association for Cardio-Thoracic Surgery (EACTS). *Eur Heart J* 31:2501–2555, 2010.

78. Guidelines on myocardial revascularization. *Eur J Cardiothorac Surg* 38(Suppl):S1–S52, 2010.

Evidence-Based Interventional Practice

FRANZ-JOSEF NEUMANN | HEINZ JOACHIM BÜTTNER

KEY POINTS

- When coronary revascularization is considered, prognostic and symptomatic indications must be distinguished.

- In general, percutaneous coronary intervention (PCI) for single-vessel disease is justified only if an improvement of symptoms can be anticipated, or ischemia comprising >10% of the left ventricle can be relieved.

- With multi-vessel disease or left main stenosis, the decision for PCI versus coronary artery bypass grafting (CABG) depends on the complexity of coronary artery involvement, which can be gauged by the SYNTAX-score.

- In patients with left main stenosis and a SYNTAX score <33 or with multi-vessel disease and a SYNTAX score <22 in the absence of left main stenosis, the 3-year outcome of PCI is similar to that after CABG, provided that complete revascularization can be achieved. Thus, PCI is an acceptable alternative to bypass surgery in many cases with multi-vessel disease or left main stenosis.

- In patients with diabetes mellitus, the threshold for recommending PCI instead of CABG should be higher than in non-diabetic patients. Depending on SYNTAX-score and risk for surgery, multi-vessel PCI may offer a reasonable option in diabetic patients.

- In most instances, individualized decisions must be taken jointly by the cardiac surgeon and the interventional cardiologist.

Introduction

CHANGING PARADIGMS OF CORONARY REVASCULARIZATION

When the era of interventional cardiology began, with the pioneering work of Andreas Grüntzig on plain balloon angioplasty, percutaneous coronary intervention, PCI (for list of abbreviations and acronyms see Table 2-1), was a treatment option only for isolated proximal coronary lesions not involving the ostium or the left main stem. In the late 1980s, coronary stents were developed with the goal of reducing the risk of restenosis and achieving a more predictable acute result of angioplasty, thus avoiding the dreaded abrupt closure due to dissection. As shown subsequently, stents were successful in achieving this goal. Nevertheless, they created a new problem: subacute stent thrombosis. After intense research on peri- and postinterventional antithrombotic treatment, the concept of dual or triple antiplatelet therapy emerged, which significantly reduced the incidence of this complication. The use of coronary stents in conjunction with optimized antithrombotic treatment extended the spectrum of coronary lesions for which PCI was considered a reasonable treatment option and thereby led to a substantial expansion of interventional techniques. Because of the large number of patients who were now being treated with coronary stents, restenosis due to neointima formation became a serious problem. Although various studies demonstrated that stents, compared with plain balloon angioplasty, reduced the need for reintervention, restenosis rates continued to be relevant, ranging from just above 10% in the simplest lesions to more than 50% with diffuse disease in patients with diabetes.

Thus it is not surprising that the community of interventional cardiologists celebrated the advent of the new drug-eluting stents as a major breakthrough, given that the initial studies suggested zero restenosis rates. In the meantime, it has become clear that drug-eluting stents compared with bare metal stents reduce the need for target-vessel reintervention by around 80%, thus largely reducing but not eliminating the problem of restenosis. Subsequently, drug-eluting stents led to another massive expansion of the proportion of patients treated with PCI. With the widespread use of these stents for PCI, reports appeared pointing to a new problem that had not been seen with bare metal stents: that is, late stent thrombosis. Yet a thorough reevaluation of the data from randomized studies—with uniform application of definitions for definite, probable, and possible stent thrombosis—failed to confirm these alarming initial reports.[1] Nevertheless, there may be a slight increase in the risk of very late (>1 year) stent thrombosis after the placement of drug-eluting stents as compared with bare metal stents.[2] It is, however, reassuring that the risk of serious late complications such as death and myocardial infarction (MI) has never been shown to be higher with drug-eluting stents than with bare metal stents.[2] In some high-risk instances, drug-eluting stents may even improve survival.[3] Despite the remaining problems of PCI, its use has increased exponentially over the past decades. Initially, this increase has come at the expense of lone medical therapy. More recently, however, with the advent of drug-eluting stents, there has been a shift of patients with multivessel disease and other complex coronary anatomies from CABG to PCI. This shift has been facilitated by both physician and patient preference for the supposedly easier approach to coronary revascularization, given the idea that the problem of restenosis has been largely solved. There is, however, reasonable concern that this shift has led to the overuse of PCI and that, in some patients, it may not yield the same outcome as CABG, which for a number of indications is an established treatment option with a well-documented survival benefit compared with medical therapy.

THE SCOPE OF THIS CHAPTER

In comparing PCI with lone medical treatment or with bypass surgery, it is important to scrutinize the available evidence that PCI offers at least as great a benefit as CABG, on the one hand, or a greater benefit than lone medical treatment, on the other. This review summarizes and discusses the currently available evidence so as to present a rationale for clinical decision making.

Pharmacological therapy and coronary revascularization—by either CABG or PCI—are the mainstays of treatment for coronary artery disease. The prime objective of such treatment is improved survival (prognostic indication); other reasonable treatment goals are relief of symptoms and improved quality of life (symptomatic indication). In pursuing these goals, the prevention of MI is a key issue pertaining to both survival and quality of life. In deciding on the optimal revascularization strategy in a patient with coronary artery disease, it is necessary to determine first whether there is a prognostic or symptomatic indication for coronary revascularization and then to choose the most appropriate revascularization modality. This chapter presents criteria for both these elements in clinical decision making, focusing primarily on the prognostic indication for coronary revascularization. Based on a review of the general criteria for revascularization, the efficacy and safety of PCI as compared with CABG are discussed. Thereafter, the role of PCI in symptomatic indications for coronary revascularization is addressed, predominantly in comparison with lone medical therapy. The focus is on stable coronary disease. Acute coronary syndromes including MI are touched only briefly because these are discussed in depth in other chapters.

TABLE 2-1	List of Abbreviations Acronyms

ACIP: Asymptomatic Cardiac Ischemia Pilot study

ACME: Angioplasty Compared to Medicine

APPROACH: Alberta Provincial Project for Outcome Assessment in Coronary Heart Disease

ARTS: Arterial Revascularization Therapies Study

AVERT: Atorvastatin Versus Revascularization Treatments

AWESOME: Angina With Extremely Serious Operative Mortality Evaluation

BARI: Bypass Angioplasty Revascularization Investigation

BARI 2D: Bypass Angioplasty Revascularization Investigation in Type 2 Diabetes

CABG: Coronary Artery Bypass Grafting

CABRI: Coronary Angioplasty versus Bypass Revascularization Investigation

CARDia: Coronary Artery Revascularization in Diabetes

CASS: Coronary Artery Surgery Study

COMBAT: Randomized Comparison of Bypass Surgery versus Angioplasty Using Sirolimus-Eluting Stent in Patients With Left Main Coronary Artery Disease

COURAGE: Clinical Outcomes Utilizing Revascularization and Aggressive Drug Evaluation

EAST: Emory Angioplasty versus Surgery Trial

ECSS: European Coronary Surgery Study

ERACI: Argentine Randomized Trial of Percutaneous Transluminal Coronary Angioplasty Versus Coronary Artery Bypass Surgery in Multivessel Disease

FINESSE: Facilitated Intervention with Enhanced Reperfusion Speed to Stop Events

FRISC: Fragmin and Revascularization during Instability in Coronary Artery Disease

GABI: German Angioplasty Bypass Surgery Investigation

ICTUS: Invasive versus Conservative Treatment in Unstable Coronary Syndromes

ISAR-SWEET: Intracoronary Stenting and Antithrombotic Regimen: Is Abciximab a Superior Way to Eliminate Elevated Thrombotic Risk in Diabetics?

ISAR-LEFT-MAIN: Intracoronary Stenting and Antithrombotic Regimen: Drug-Eluting Stents for Unprotected Left Main Stem Disease

LAD: left anterior descending coronary artery

LV: left ventricular

MACCE: major adverse cardiac and cerebrovascular event, comprising death from any cause, stroke, myocardial infarction, or repeat revascularization

MAIN-COMPARE: Revascularization for Unprotected Left Main Coronary Artery Stenosis: Comparison of Percutaneous Coronary Angioplasty Versus Surgical Revascularization registry

MASS: Medicine, Angioplasty, or Surgery Study

PCI: percutaneous coronary intervention

RITA: Randomized Intervention Treatment of Angina

SIMA: Stenting versus Internal Mammary Artery

SoS: Stent or Surgery Trial

SYNTAX: Synergy Between PCI with Taxus Drug-Eluting Stent and Cardiac Surgery

TACTICS: Treat Angina with Aggrastat and Determine Cost of Therapy with an Invasive or Conservative Strategy

TIMI: Thrombolysis in Myocardial Infarction

VA Study: Veterans Administration Cooperative Study

Prognostic Indications for Coronary Revascularization

CLINICAL PRESENTATION

Myocardial Infarction with ST-Segment Elevation

In acute MI, as shown by a metanalysis of the randomized trials in this setting, fibrinolysis reduces mortality by 18% as compared with conservative treatment.[4] On top of this benefit, coronary reperfusion by primary PCI reduces in-hospital mortality by an additional 37%.[5] In addition to its effect on survival, PCI compared with fibrinolysis reduces the risk of reinfarction and stroke, particularly that of hemorrhagic stroke,[6] and the initial benefit is maintained during long-term follow-up.[6] The largest survival benefit by PCI is obtained when the delay conferred by PCI compared with fibrinolysis is shorter than 35 minutes.[5] Nevertheless, even with delays by PCI compared with fibrinolysis ranging between 35 and 120 minutes, there is a significant survival benefit by PCI ranging around 24% on average.[5] Prespecified subgroup analyses of the FINESSE study suggest that even with delays as long as 2.55 to 4 hours, direct PCI is the preferred strategy in terms of safety and efficacy.[7] Although fibrinolysis is more effective within the first 1 to 3 hours after the onset of pain than after larger delays, the benefit from PCI as compared with fibrinolysis is largely independent of the time from onset of pain to intervention.[5] CABG in the setting of MI, although it can be performed, delays reperfusion compared with PCI and is associated with a high perioperative risk. Hence CABG has only a niche indication in this setting. In summary, acute MI is an accepted and well-documented prognostic indication for PCI.

Acute Coronary Syndromes without ST-Segment Elevation

There has been a long-standing debate about two competing treatment strategies for acute coronary syndromes without ST-segment elevation.[8] The conservative strategy reserves coronary angiography and revascularization to those patients who continue to have a spontaneous or inducible myocardial ischemia despite maximal medical therapy. On the other hand, the invasive strategy suggests coronary angiography and revascularization irrespective of the primary success of medical treatment. Various studies have addressed this issue. A metanalysis published in 2005 concluded that the invasive strategy, while increasing the risk of in-hospital death and MI (early hazard), significantly reduced death and MI during the entire follow-up—ranging from 6 months to 2 years in various studies—by 18% (95% confidence interval, 2% to 42%).[9] Supporting this analysis, the 5-year follow-up of RITA-3 revealed that, as compared with the conservative strategy, the benefit of the invasive strategy with respect to death and MI continued to increase with time.[10] At 5 years after intervention, the incidence of death and MI was 20.0% in the conservative arm but 16.6% in the interventional arm ($P = 0.04$). Moreover, there was an increased survival benefit of the invasive strategy as compared with the conservative strategy during the 5-year follow-up (88% vs. 85%), which almost reached statistical significance ($P = 0.054$). The 5-year follow-up of FRISC-II also demonstrated a significant reduction in the long-term incidence of death and MI by the invasive strategy as compared with the conservative strategy (5-year incidence 19.9% vs. 24.5%, $P = 0.009$).[11] The benefit from the invasive strategy compared with the conservative one is not uniform across the spectrum of acute coronary syndromes. The pivotal studies—FRISC-II, TACTICS-TIMI 18, and RITA-3[12-14]—consistently show that the benefit from the invasive strategy is linked to various markers of risk, whereas patients without these risk markers may be treated according to the same principles as patients with stable angina. The risk factors that could be established in previous studies include elevated myocardial marker proteins, dynamic ST-segment changes, ongoing myocardial ischemia, hemodynamic instability, and diabetes mellitus.[15] This concept of a routine invasive strategy has recently been challenged by the ICTUS trial.[16] It accepts the need for coronary revascularization in the majority of patients but challenges troponin levels as the sole criterion for revascularization. It randomized 1,200 patients to a routine invasive versus a selective invasive strategy. To be included, patients had to have unstable angina with elevated cardiac troponin levels. During a 1-year follow-up, 54% of the patients in the selectively invasive arm and 76% of those in the routine invasive arm underwent coronary revascularization. It is noteworthy that the rate of coronary revascularization in the conservative arm of ICTUS was as high as that in the invasive arm of RITA-3. During 1-year follow-up, the primary endpoint of ICTUS—which was death or MI and hospital readmission for unplanned coronary revascularization—was not significantly different between the two treatment arms. Secondary analyses, however, revealed a significant increase in MIs in the invasive arm (15% vs. 10%), which could be attributed to an early hazard of the intervention. The ICTUS trial is consistent with other

TABLE 2-2	Poor Prognosis in Stable Angina (Average Annual Mortality Risk > 3%)
High-risk treadmill score	
Stress-induced large or moderate-sized nuclear perfusion defect (particularly if in the anterior wall)	
Stress-induced multiple perfusion defects with LV dilation or increased lung parenchymal uptake of thallium-201 isotope	
Echocardiographic wall-motion abnormality involving >2 segments developing at a low dose of dobutamine (≤10 mcg/kg/min) or at a low heart rate (120 bpm)	
Stress-induced echocardiographic evidence of extensive ischemia	

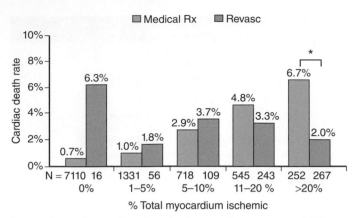

Figure 2-1 Observed cardiac death rates during a mean follow-up of 1.9 years in patients undergoing revascularization (Revasc) versus medical therapy (Medical Rx) as a function of the amount of inducible ischemia. Increase in cardiac death frequency as a function of inducible ischemia. *P < 0.001. (From Hachamavitch R, Hayes SW, Friedman JD, et al: Comparison of the short-term survival benefit associated with revascularization compared with medical therapy in patients with no prior coronary artery disease undergoing stress myocardial perfusion single photon emission computed tomography. Circulation. 2003;107:2900–2907.)

previous trials suggesting that there is a need for revascularization in the majority of patients presenting with high-risk acute coronary syndromes. As a new aspect, ICTUS suggests that even among patients with positive troponins, there is a low-risk subset in whom the long-term benefit from revascularization cannot compensate for the incidence of peri-interventional complications. In this respect, ICTUS challenges the elevation of myocardial marker proteins as the only criterion for recommending revascularization. As published recently, the increased incidence of peri-interventional MI with routine invasive as compared with selective invasive strategy had no significant impact on 5-year survival or survival free of MI.[17] Hence there does not appear to be a long-term down side to the routine invasive strategy. Therefore taking advantage of the other benefits of the routine invasive strategy—such as a shorter hospital stay and lower need for unplanned revascularization—may be justified.

In summary, the majority of patients with high-risk acute coronary syndromes benefit from coronary revascularization with respect to the possibility of imminent MI or death.

Stable Angina—Severe Angina or Large Ischemic Area

Among patients with chronic stable angina, those with severe angina, large or multiple perfusion defects on functional testing, or a low threshold for the induction of ischemia (Table 2-2) have a poor prognosis with an annual mortality risk >3%. If these high-risk features are associated with double- or triple-vessel disease, patients benefit from revascularization irrespective of left ventricular function. In an analysis of 5,303 patients in the CASS registry, surgical benefit was greatest in patients who exhibited at least 1 mm of ST-segment depression and could exercise only into stage 1 or less. In the surgical group with triple-vessel disease and severe exercise-induced ischemia, 7-year survival was 81%, whereas it was 58% in the corresponding medical group.[18] Likewise, in another registry including 2,023 patients with severe angina and two-vessel disease, 6-year survival was 76% in patients treated medically and 89% in patients treated surgically (P < 0.001).[19] Cox multivariate analyses showed that surgical treatment was a beneficial independent predictor of survival for patients with two-vessel coronary disease and Canadian Cardiovascular Society class 3 or 4 angina. ACIP is a more recent trial that was designed to compare the efficacy of medical therapy versus revascularization.[20] In ACIP, 558 patients with angiographically documented coronary artery disease, mostly multivessel disease, and stable coronary artery disease were randomly assigned to medical therapy, adjusted either to suppress angina or both angina and evidence of ischemia during ambulatory ECG monitoring or revascularization with either PCI or CABG. Revascularization was significantly more effective in relieving ischemia than either of the medical strategies. During 1-year follow-up, the ACIP trial appeared to show better outcome in patients treated with revascularization. Mortality was 4.4% and 1.6% in the two conservative groups, whereas none of the patients in the revascularization group had died during the 1-year follow-up period. The apparent benefit of revascularization was largely confined to patients with double- or triple-vessel disease. A registry of 10,627 consecutive patients who underwent exercise or adenosine myocardial perfusion single photon emission computed tomography (SPECT) demonstrated that patients with large ischemic areas on functional testing benefit from revascularization.

The patients included in this retrospective analysis had no prior MI or revascularization and were followed for a mean of 1.9 years. The treatment received within 60 days of stress testing was revascularization by either CAGB or PCI in 671 patients and medical therapy in 9,956 patients. To adjust for nonrandomization of treatment, a propensity score was developed. On the basis of the Cox proportional hazards model predicting cardiac death, patients undergoing medical therapy demonstrated a survival advantage over patients undergoing revascularization in the setting of no or mild ischemia, whereas those undergoing revascularization had an increasing survival benefit over patients undergoing medical therapy when moderate to severe ischemia was present (Figure 2-1).[21] Consistent results were obtained in a nuclear substudy on 314 patients of the COURAGE study.[22] In this substudy, the extent of residual posttreatment ischemia—assessed as percentage of the left ventricle by myocardial perfusion SPECT—was a predictor of outcome: rates of death or MI ranged from 0% to 39% for patients with no residual ischemia to ≥10% residual ischemia despite treatment, (P = 0.002 [risk-adjusted P = 0.09]) (Figure 2-2). With respect to treatment, a ≥5% reduction in ischemic myocardium lowered the risk of death or MI (P = 0.037 [risk-adjusted P = 0.26]), particularly if baseline ischemia was ≥10% (P = 0.001 [risk-adjusted P = 0.08]). PCI on top of optimal medical therapy increased the likelihood of achieving this goal. The findings of this substudy suggest that revascularization is indicated if, in addition to optimal medical therapy, it affords at least a 5% reduction in myocardial ischemia.

Thus, although adequately powered randomized trials addressing the impact of severe angina or large perfusion defects on outcome in patients with chronic stable angina are lacking, the bulk of the currently available evidence suggests that these patients benefit from revascularization, particularly if more than one vessel is affected.

CORONARY ANATOMY

Until now our understanding of the anatomical conditions that constitute a survival benefit from coronary revascularization as compared with lone medical therapy is largely based on milestone studies performed during the 1970s. Soon after CABG was introduced in 1969, three randomized trials compared surgical revascularization with lone medical therapy: the VA Study, ECSS, and CASS. Although these studies are outdated in many respects, including a low use of arterial conduits and limited means of pharmacological risk factor

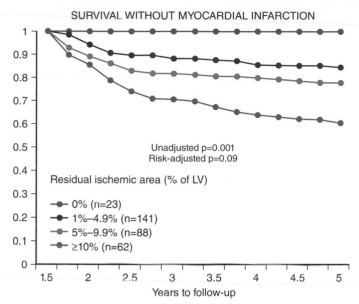

SURVIVAL WITHOUT MYOCARDIAL INFARCTION

Unadjusted p=0.001
Risk-adjusted p=0.09

Residual ischemic area (% of LV)

- 0% (n=23)
- 1%–4.9% (n=141)
- 5%–9.9% (n=88)
- ≥10% (n=62)

Figure 2-2 Survival without myocardial infarction depending on residual ischemic area. *(Reproduced with permission from Shaw LJ, Berman DS, Maron DJ, et al: Optimal medical therapy with or without percutaneous coronary intervention to reduce ischemic burden: results from the Clinical Outcomes Utilizing Revascularization and Aggressive Drug Evaluation (COURAGE) trial nuclear substudy. Circulation 117(10): 1283–1291,2008.)*

modification and platelet inhibition, it is unlikely that they will ever be replicated. In concert with analyses of large registry databases, the early studies established the conditions in which CABG improves survival as compared with medical therapy (Table 2-3). A metanalysis of all published randomized trials of CABG versus lone medical treatment for coronary artery disease identified left main disease (diameter of stenosis ≥ 50%), multivessel disease, and involvement of the proximal left anterior descending coronary artery (LAD) as significant predictors of a survival benefit from CABG.[23] In the cumulative experience of seven studies, the VA study being the first, surgical revascularization for left main disease was associated with a 65% relative reduction in mortality as compared with lone medical therapy.[23] Notably, in left main disease there was a survival benefit of surgery irrespective of the presence or absence of spontaneous or inducible symptoms or signs of ischemia or reduced left ventricular function. The same is also true for triple- or double-vessel disease involving the proximal LAD.[24]

In all other conditions, the indication for surgical coronary revascularization depends on a combination of anatomical and clinical criteria. If triple-vessel disease is associated with impaired LV function (LV ejection fraction < 50%), surgical revascularization improves survival irrespective of LAD involvement.[25,26] In the presence of severe angina or large areas of ischemia on functional testing, surgical revascularization of triple- or double-vessel disease is also indicated for both symptomatic and prognostic reasons even in the absence of LV dysfunction.[18,19] Coronary revascularization has never been shown to confer a survival benefit in patients with single-vessel disease. This is also true for isolated proximal LAD stenoses. Yusuf's metanalysis[23] showing a survival benefit from surgery in patients with LAD involvement must be interpreted with the notion that this result was obtained

TABLE 2-3	Conditions in Which CABG Improves Survival as Compared with Medical Therapy
Left main disease	
Triple- or double-vessel disease involving the proximal LAD	
Triple- or double-vessel disease in the presence of severe angina or large areas of ischemia on functional testing	
Triple-vessel disease associated with impaired LV function	

in a cohort having predominantly multivessel disease. More recently, the randomized MASS (Medicine, Angioplasty or Surgery Study) trial compared lone medical treatment with plain balloon angioplasty or CABG in 214 patients with symptomatic, isolated, high-grade stenosis of the LAD.[27] During a 5-year follow-up, there was no appreciable difference between the three treatment arms with regard to either death or MI. Although the power to detect small differences in event rates was low in MASS, its results are consistent with the current judgment that there is no prognostic indication for coronary revascularization in stable single-vessel disease. No study ever demonstrated that, in patients with stable angina, the risk of subsequent MI can be reduced by either bypass surgery or PCI. The degree of stenosis is a notoriously poor predictor of subsequent events. Although the risk of subsequent MI is higher with high-grade stenoses than with low-grade stenoses, the latter are far more frequent than the former. Thus the majority of infarctions are triggered by low-grade stenoses. Despite recent advances,[28,29] our current means of identifying vulnerable plaques are limited.

TECHNICAL FEASIBILITY

Apart from the extent and distribution of coronary artery disease, the probability of achieving complete revascularization is an important criterion for the choice of the most appropriate revascularization strategy. In CABG, a number of studies have demonstrated that patients who are completely revascularized have better long-term outcomes than those with incomplete revascularization.[30] The same is also true for PCI. Several studies from the pre-stent era have confirmed better long-term outcomes after complete revascularization than after an incomplete procedure.[31,32] The reasons for not treating all diseased vessels may include technical obstacles such as heavy calcification, tortuous vessels or chronic total occlusions, the presence of serious concomitant disease, or the intention to treat only the "culprit lesion" thought to be responsible for the patient's symptoms. A recent analysis of a total of 21,945 stent patients from New York State's Percutaneous Coronary Interventions Reporting System assessed the issue of incomplete revascularization with current practices of coronary revascularization. A follow-up period of 3 years was reported.[33] In this registry, 68.9% of the stent patients were incompletely revascularized. After adjustment for comorbidities and other baseline characteristics associated with increased risk, incompletely revascularized patients were significantly more likely to die at any time than completely revascularized patients (adjusted hazard ratio – 1.15; 95% confidence interval, 1.01 to 1.30). The risk associated with incomplete revascularization increased with the number of vessels that were not revascularized and was higher with nonrevascularized chronic total occlusions than in nonrevascularized nonocclusive lesions. Incompletely revascularized patients with total occlusions and ≥2 nonrevascularized vessels were at the highest risk compared with completely revascularized patients (hazard ratio = 1.36; 95% confidence interval, 1.12 to 1.66) (Figure 2-3). Given the major impact of the extent of revascularization on long-term survival, consideration must be given to the likelihood of achieving complete revascularization. When PCI is unlikely to achieve

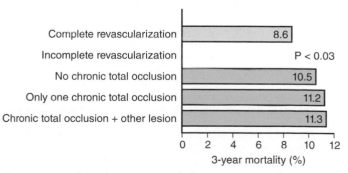

Figure 2-3 Adjusted 3-year survival after complete revascularization versus incomplete revascularization.

complete revascularization, surgery may offer better prospects. Yet this may not always be the case. In some instances, poor target vessels for CABG may be treated by PCI with higher chances of success.

Prognostic Indication for Revascularization: PCI Versus CABG

MULTIVESSEL DISEASE

From the late 1980s to the early 1990s, several studies compared plain balloon angioplasty with CABG. Among them were three larger trials—RITA (n = 1011), CABRI (n = 1154), and BARI (n = 1829)—and three smaller trials—GABI (n = 358), EAST (n = 392), and the Toulouse monocentric study (n = 152). In each of these trials survival after PCI versus CABG was similar, as was the incidence of Q-wave MI, but repeat revascularization was more frequently needed after PCI. However, Hoffmann et al., in a metanalysis based on data extracted from the literature, showed a significant survival benefit from surgery as compared with PCI of 3% absolute at 5 years and of 4% absolute at 8 years.[34] The results of the early studies antedating the stent era are, of course, not reflective of the current practice of coronary revascularization. Since the early studies, major advances have been achieved in PCI, CABG, and medical treatment, including coronary stents, effective antiplatelet therapy, the use of arterial conduits up to complete arterial revascularization, and vigorous pharmacological risk-factor modification. For these reasons, the results of randomized trials performed in the pre-stent era cannot be transferred to current practice.

Lessons from Studies with Bare Metal Stents

Randomized Studies. Five randomized trials compared stenting with CABG for multivessel disease: ARTS,[35,36] SoS,[37] ERACI-2,[38,39] MASS-2,[40] and AWESOME.[41] Four major studies were incorporated in a metanalysis based on individual patient data, which confirmed the results of the majority of the individual studies.[42] This metanalysis comprised ARTS, SoS, ERACI-2, and MASS-2 but excluded AWESOME, because the high-risk characteristics of the patients in this last trial were clearly different from those of the patient population of the four other trials. This metanalysis confirmed that PCI with stent placement was associated with a similar 1-year incidence of death, MI, or stroke as CABG (Figure 2-4). Nevertheless, the need for repeat revascularization was considerably higher after PCI, although the observed gap with CABG surgery has narrowed from the approximately 30% reported in the pre-stent era to approximately 14% (Figure 2-4). As compared with PCI, CABG was associated with a slightly lower frequency of recurrent angina (77% vs. 82%; P = 0.002). Another metanalysis based on aggregate data from ARTS, SoS, ERACI-2, and SIMA, a study on isolated proximal LAD stenosis, extended the analysis to a follow-up of 3 years.[34] The point estimates for both the 3-year incidence of death and nonfatal MI were lower after PCI than after CABG. However, a significant difference was found only for nonfatal MI (Figure 2-5). Moreover, this metanalysis confirmed that the 1-year incidence of repeat intervention was 15% absolute higher after PCI than after CABG but did not demonstrate any significant further changes from 1 to 3 years. For ARTS, the largest trial comparing PCI with CABG for the treatment of multivessel disease,[35,36] 5-year results are available. ARTS included a total of 1,205 patients with at least two de novo lesions located in different vessels and territories not including the left main coronary artery. In this study, 600 patients were randomly assigned to stenting and 605 to bypass surgery; 67% of the patients had a double-vessel disease and 32% triple-vessel disease. At 5 years, the incidence of death was 8% in the stent group versus 7.6% in the CABG group (relative risk 1.05 [95% confidence interval, 0.71 to 1.55], P = 0.83). Likewise, there was no significant difference in cerebrovascular accident (3.8% vs. 3.5%, relative risk 1.10 [95% confidence interval, 0.62 to 1.97], P = 0.76), Q-wave MI (6.7% vs. 5.6%, relative risk 1.19 [95% confidence interval, 0.76 to 1.85], P = 0.47), non-Q-wave MI (1.8% vs. 0.8%, relative risk 2.22 [95% confidence interval, 0.78 to 6.35], P = 0.14), or the composite thereof (18.2% vs. 14.9%, relative risk 1.22 [95% confidence

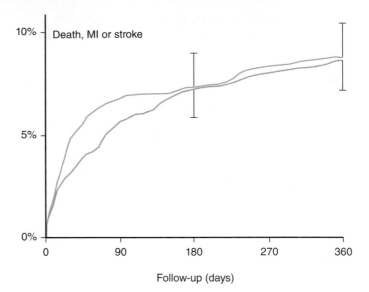

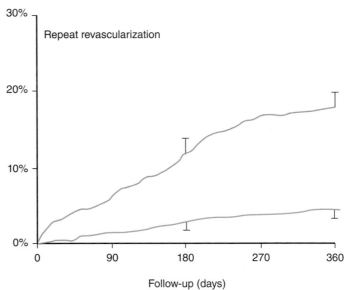

Figure 2-4 Metaanalysis of ARTS, SoS, ERACI-2 and MASS-2. Incidence of adverse cardiovascular events and repeat revascularization procedures during 1-year follow-up in patients allocated to PCI with multiple stenting (blue line) or CABG surgery (green line). *(From Mercado N, Wijns W, Serruys PW, et al: One-year outcomes of coronary artery bypass graft surgery versus percutaneous coronary intervention with multiple stenting for multisystem disease: A meta-analysis of individual patient data from randomized clinical trials. J Thorac Cardiovasc Surg. 2005;130:512–519.)*

interval 0.95 to 1.58], P = 0.14). There was, however, a significant difference in the incidence of repeat revascularization (30.3% vs. 8.8%, relative risk 3.46 [95% confidence interval, 2.61 to 4.60], P < 0.001). In the stent group, 10.5% of the revascularizations involved CABG, whereas it was 1.2% in the CABG group. In summary, the 5-year outcome with respect to the serious endpoints death, MI, and cerebrovascular accident with the surgical and nonsurgical approaches was similar. With the primarily catheter-based approach, there was a 90% chance of avoiding CABG during the subsequent 5 years, with a similar outcome with respect to death, cerebrovascular accident, and MI as with the surgical approach but at the expense of a 20% higher incidence of repeat catheter interventions. Consistent with the long-term results of ARTS, the recently published 10-year results of MASS-2 showed no significant survival benefit of CABG over PCI (hazard ratio

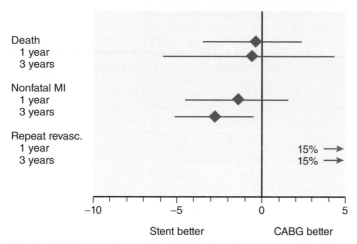

% Difference in risk stent vs. CABG

Death
1 year
3 years

Nonfatal MI
1 year
3 years

Repeat revasc.
1 year 15% →
3 years 15% →

−10   −5   0   5

Stent better   CABG better

Figure 2-5 Metaanalysis of randomized studies comparing stenting with CABG. Risk difference for various events at 1 year and at 3 years. The lines represent the 95% confidence interval. MI, myocardial infarction; revasc., revascularization.

[95%-confidence limit]: 1.03 [0.69–1.53], $P = 0.88$), but a substantially increased need for repeat interventions with PCI versus CABG (hazard ratio [95%-confidence limit]: 3.71 [1.82–7.52], $P < 0.0001$).[43]

The studies described so far compared PCI with CABG in cohorts that were well suited for both procedures. The important question of whether patients at high risk for CABG surgery and refractory myocardial ischemia should undergo PCI as an alternative procedure was addressed in AWESOME.[41] This multicenter study included patients with myocardial ischemia refractory to medical management and the presence of one or more risk factors for adverse outcome with CABG, including prior open heart surgery, age > 70 years, LV ejection fraction <35%, MI within 7 days, or the need for intra-aortic balloon pumping. Over a 5-year period, 2,431 patients met the entry criteria. By physician consensus, 1,650 patients formed a physician-directed registry assigned to CABG ($n = 692$), PCI ($n = 651$) or further medical therapy ($n = 307$) and 781 were angiographically eligible for random allocation. Of the patients who were angiographically acceptable, 454 consented to randomized assignment between CABG and PCI; the remaining 327 constituted a patient choice registry. At all time points during the 5-year follow-up of the randomized study there was a nonsignificant survival benefit of PCI over CABG (97% vs. 95% at 30 days and 75% vs. 70% at 5 years).[44] Within the first 3 years after randomization, more patients randomized to PCI received a subsequent revascularization (37% vs. 18%, $P < 0.001$), whereas between 3 and 5 years of follow-up repeat revascularization was similarly frequent in both the PCI group and the CABG group (6% vs. 4%). In the physician-directed subgroup, the 3-year survival rate was 76% for both CABG and PCI. In the patient-choice subgroup, the 3-year survival was 80% with CABG but 98% with PCI. The findings of the AWESOME Registry[45] therefore support the findings of the main study. The AWESOME investigators specifically addressed the issue of whether, in patients with previous CABG, PCI is the preferred option for repeat intervention.[46] In the subgroup with previous CABG, 3-year survival rates were 73% and 76% with CABG or PCI respectively in the randomized patients, 71% versus 77% in the physician-directed registry, and 65% versus 86% ($P = 0.001$) in the patient-choice registry. The authors concluded that PCI is preferable to CABG for many post-CABG patients.

Registries. It has been argued that the randomized studies comparing PCI with CABG in multivessel disease comprised only a small proportion of the patients presenting at dedicated high-volume centers.[47]

Therefore, it is claimed, the results of these trials may not be applicable to the vast majority of patients in need for coronary revascularization. It is thus an important question whether the absence of a substantial difference in survival between PCI and CABG can also be verified in large registries. Contrary to the randomized studies comparing PCI bare metal stents to CABG, several large registry analyses from the Cleveland, New York, and Rotterdam databases found a significant difference in risk-adjusted survival favoring CABG over PCI.[48–50] Despite these statistically clear-cut results, the implications of the findings in these registries must be interpreted cautiously, as several limitations derive from the nonrandomized nature of these comparisons. Adjustment by proportional hazard models cannot fully substitute for randomization, as comprehensive inclusion of all confounders is impossible. One important confounder that was not included in any of the risk adjustment was subsequently published by the New York group—that is, incomplete revascularization. These investigators noted that in their registry 69% of the patients receiving a stent had incomplete revascularization. In the same registry, incomplete revascularization after PCI had a statistically significant and clinically relevant impact on outcome, as discussed above. Between patients completely revascularized and those incompletely revascularized there was a 2.1% survival disadvantage in 3 years in the absence of a total occlusion and a 2.7% difference in the presence of a nonrecanalized total occlusion.[33] The difference between complete and incomplete revascularization within the stent group of the New York registry was on the same order of magnitude as the difference between the stent group and the CABG group in the entire registry. The comprehensive analysis from the Duke registry gives additional insight.[51] This registry comprised 18,481 patients with significant coronary artery disease between 1986 and 2000 who were assigned by physician preference to medical therapy ($n = 6,862$), PCI ($n = 6,292$), or CABG ($n = 5,327$). Each group was categorized into three subgroups according to the baseline severity of coronary artery disease: low severity (predominantly single-vessel), intermediate severity (predominantly two-vessel), and high severity (all three-vessel). Mortality was evaluated by Cox models adjusted for cardiac risk, comorbidity, and propensity for selection of a specific treatment. In all three anatomical subgroups, revascularization conferred a significant survival benefit as compared with medical therapy (Figure 2-6). The extent of this survival benefit varied with the degree of coronary artery disease, ranging from an additional 8 months gained during 15 years in the low-severity group to 24 months gained in the high-severity group. In the low- and intermediate-severity groups, the benefit from revascularization was independent of the treatment modality, with similar results by CABG and PCI. In the high-severity subgroup, however, CABG was associated with a small but significant survival benefit of 8 months during 15 years. It is noteworthy that the impact of revascularization versus medical treatment is substantially larger than the impact of the choice of revascularization modality. In summary, registry data comparing PCI with bare metal stents to CABG suggest a small survival benefit of surgery versus PCI in patients with multivessel disease. A large proportion of this survival benefit appears to be attributed to patients with the most complex anatomy and to those who do not achieve complete revascularization with PCI.

Lessons from Studies with Drug-Eluting Stents

Registries. The New York cardiac registry was also interrogated for the comparison of CABG with drug-eluting stents.[52] In an analysis based on 7,437 patients with CABG and 9,963 patients with drug-eluting stents, CABG continued to be associated with lower mortality rates than did treatment with drug-eluting stents; it was also associated with lower rates of death or MI and repeat revascularization. Among patients with three- or two-vessel disease who underwent CABG compared with those who received a drug-eluting stent, the adjusted hazard ratio for death was 0.80 (95% confidence interval [CI], 0.65 to 0.97) and 0.71 (95% CI, 0.57 to 0.89), respectively.[52] Yet the same limitations apply as for the bare-metal-stent analysis of the same database (see above). Specifically, the issue of completeness of revascularization was

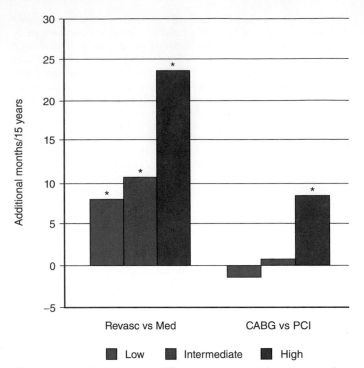

Figure 2-6 Adjusted survival differences versus initial treatment selection. Results are shown according to the severity of coronary artery disease: low (blue bar), intermediate (orange bar), and high (purple bar). *$P < 0.5$; CABG, coronary artery bypass grafting; PCI, percutaneous coronary intervention; Revasc, revascularization. *(From Smith PK, Califf RM, Tuttle RH, et al: Selection of surgical or percutaneous coronary intervention provides differential longevity benefit. Ann Thorac Surg. 2006;82:1420–1428.)*

not addressed. ARTS II, a 45-center, 607-patient registry, intended to compare 1-year outcomes of the sirolimus-eluting stent against the historical results of the two arms of ARTS I.[53] To achieve the number of treatable lesions per patient comparable to ARTS I, patients were stratified to ensure that at least one-third had three-vessel disease.

Compared with ARTS I, ARTS II comprised a higher-risk cohort: 53.5% had three-vessel disease, and diabetes was present in 26.2%. Mean stented length was 72.5 mm, with 3.7 stents implanted per patient. The 5-year incidence[54] of death/stroke/MI was 12.9% in ARTS II versus 14% in the CABG arm of ARTS I ($P = 0.1$) and 18.1% in the bare-metal-stent arm of ARTS I ($P = 0.007$). The 5-year rate of MACCE (of major adverse cardiovascular and cerebrovascular events) in ARTS II of 27.5% was significantly higher than that among patients in ARTS I who received CABG (21.1%, $P = 0.02$) and lower than among ARTS I patients who received bare metal stents (41.5%, $P < 0.001$). The authors concluded that at 5 years, the sirolimus-eluting stent had a safety record comparable to that of CABG and superior to the placement of bare metal stents. Nevertheless, surgery still afforded a lower need for repeat revascularization, although overall event rates in ARTS II approached the surgical results in ARTS I.

Randomized Studies. The promising results of ARTS II had to be interpreted cautiously because this study does not account for advances in surgical technique that may have occurred since the days of ARTS I. Thus, randomized studies were needed to clarify the role of drug-eluting stents compared with CABG for multivessel disease. This issue was the objective of the SYNTAX trial.[55] This randomized trial compared PCI with paclitaxel-eluting stents and CABG for treating patients with previously untreated three-vessel or left main coronary artery disease or both. The study enrolled 1,800 patients, in whom the local cardiac surgeon and interventional cardiologist determined that equivalent anatomical revascularization could be achieved with either treatment. The primary endpoint, MACCE, at 1 year was significantly higher in the PCI group (17.8% vs. 12.4% for CABG; $P = 0.002$), in large part because of an increased rate of repeat revascularization (13.5% vs. 5.9%, $P < 0.001$). Apart from reintervention, there were no significant differences in any of the components of the primary endpoint or a combination thereof except for stroke, which was significantly more likely to occur with CABG (2.2% vs. 0.6% with PCI; $P = 0.003$). Three-year results of SYNTAX have been reported (Table 2-4).[56] By 3 years, the primary endpoint, MACCE, was reached in 28.0% of the PCI group and in 20.2% of the CABG group ($P < 0.001$). This difference was largely caused by a difference in the need for reintervention (19.7% vs. 10.7%, $P < 0.001$). The composite risk of death, MI, and stroke, however, was similar between the two groups (14.1% vs.

TABLE 2-4	Three-Year Outcomes in SYNTAX Stratified to Coronary Involvement and SYNTAX Score											
	Any			**<22**			**22 to 32**			**>32**		
Syntax Scores	PCI	CABG	P	PCI	CABG	P	PCI	CABG	P	PCI	CABG	P
Entire cohort, number of patients	903	897		299	275		310	300		290	315	
First endpoint: MACCE	20.2%	28.0%	<0.001	22.7%	22.5%	0.098	27.4%	18.9%	0.02	34.1%	19.5%	<0.001
Death	8.6%	6.7%	0.13	5.4%	6.5%	0.66*	8.5%	7.8%	0.85*	6.0%	12.2%	0.01*
Death, MI, stroke	14.1%	12.0%	0.21	9.5%	11.8%	0.37*	14.3%	12.6%	0.58*	18.8%	11.8%	0.01*
Repeat revasc.	19.7%	10.7%	<0.001	17.5%	12.3%	0.09*	17.4%	10.1%	0.008*	24.4%	9.9%	<0.001
Three-vessel subset, number of patients	546	549		1981	171		207	208		155	166	
First endpoint: MACCE	28.8%	18.8%	<0.001	25.8%	22.2%	0.45	29.4%	16.8%	0.008	31.4%	17.9%	0.004
Death	9.5%	5.7%	0.02	7.3%	6.8%	0.86	10.3%	5.7%	0.09	11.1%	4.5%	0.03
Death, MI, stroke	14.8%	10.6%	0.04	11.2%	12.3%	0.75	16.1%	11.3%	0.16	17.7%	8.3%	0.01
Repeat revasc.	19.4%	10.0%	<0.001	18.8%	11.6%	0.06	18.2%	8.4%	0.04	21.5%	10.5%	0.006
Left-main subset, number of patients	357	348		118	104		103	92		135	149	
First endpoint: MACCE	22.3%	26.8%	0.20	18.0%	23.0%	0.33	23.4%	23.3%	0.90	37.3%	21.2%	0.003
Death	7.3%	8.4%	0.64	2.6%	6.0%	0.21	4.9%	12.4%	0.06	13.4%	7.6%	0.10
Death, MI, stroke	13.0%	14.3%	0.60	6.9%	11.0%	0.26	10.8%	15.6%	0.29	20.1%	15.7%	0.034
Repeat revasc.	20.0%	11.7%	0.004	15.4%	13.4%	0.69	15.9%	14.0%	0.75	27.7%	9.2%	<0.001

*P values by chi-square test, incidences calculated from reported incidences in the left-main and three-vessel subsets.
MACCE, major adverse cardiac and cardiovascular events; MI, myocardial infarction; revasc., revascularization.

12.6%, $P = 0.21$). Considering individual components, there was a trend toward higher 3-year mortality (8.6% vs. 6.7%, $P = 0.13$) and a significantly higher 3-year rate of MI (7.1% vs. 3.6%, $P = 0.002$) in the PCI group, whereas in the CABG group a trend toward more frequent strokes prevailed (3.4% vs. 2.0%, $P = 0.07$). In SYNTAX, randomization was stratified according to left main involvement. In the 1,095 patients who belonged to the subset defined by three-vessel disease without left main stenosis, PCI compared with CABG performed less well than in the entire SYNTAX study (Table 2-4).[57] Three-year mortality after PCI in the three-vessel-disease stratum was significantly higher than after CABG (6.2% vs. 2.9%, $P = 0.01$), as was the incidence of MI (7.1% vs. 3.3%, $P = 0.005$), while there was no significant difference in stroke rate (2.6% vs. 2.9%, $P = 0.64$). Thus both the 3-year composite of death, MI, and stroke as well as 3-year MACCE after PCI were significantly inferior to those after CABG (14.8% vs. 10.6%, $P = 0.04$; and 28.0% vs. 20.2%, $P < 0.001$, respectively). The authors of the SYNTAX trial also stratified the study patients to tertiles of the SYNTAX score (Table 2-4). This score was developed prospectively to gauge the extent and complexity of coronary artery disease. In the lowest tertile of SYNTAX scores (those below 22), 3-year mortality in the three-vessel-disease subset after PCI was similar to that after CABG (7.3% vs. 6.8%, $P = 0.86$). Likewise, there was only a statistically insignificant and clinically irrelevant numerical increase in MACCE with PCI as compared with CABG (25.8% vs. 22.2%, $P = 0.45$). These results in the lowest tertile of SYNTAX scores in the three-vessel-disease subset were consistent with the results in the corresponding subset of the entire study (5.4% vs. 6.5%, $P = 0.66$ for death; and 22.7% vs. 22.5%, $P = 0.98$, for MACCE). In the highest tertile of SYNTAX scores (>32), PCI was associated with excess 3-year mortality compared with CABG both in the three-vessel-disease subset and in the entire study cohort (5.4% vs. 6.5%, $P = 0.66$; and 11.1% vs. 4.5%, $P = 0.03$, respectively). Similar to the finding in the entire subset with three-vessel disease, mortality in the middle tertile was also higher at 3 years after PCI than after CABG (10.3% vs. 5.7%, $P = 0.09$). In the two highest tertiles of SYNTAX scores in the three-vessel disease subset, there were also major differences in 3-year MACCE, favoring CABG over PCI. In the majority of patients suffering from three-vessel disease without left main involvement, the SYNTAX study suggests CABG as the preferred revascularization strategy because it improves survival and reduces the risk of MI as well as the need for reintervention. In patients with SYNTAX scores <22, however, PCI afforded similar outcomes with respect to survival and major cardiovascular and cerebrovascular events, a finding that was independent of left main involvement. In this setting, PCI will be the treatment of choice because it is associated with less discomfort to the patient and less resource consumption.

SPECIAL CONSIDERATIONS IN DIABETIC PATIENTS

Compared with nondiabetic patients, patients with diabetes often have a more advanced type of coronary atherosclerosis, with diffuse disease in small-lumen vessels. With any treatment modality for coronary revascularization, diabetic patients have an inferior outcome compared with nondiabetics. This was first shown for CABG. In patients with diabetes mellitus as compared with nondiabetics, CABG is associated with a more rapid progression of atherosclerosis in both grafted and nongrafted vessels as well as an accelerated degeneration of venous bypass grafts. Nevertheless, CASS demonstrated that in older diabetic patients, coronary revascularization confers a substantial benefit as compared with lone medical therapy.[58] Likewise, PCI in patients with diabetes is associated with a substantially increased risk of adverse short- and long-term outcome as compared with PCI in nondiabetics. In particular, it has been shown that the risk of restenosis after any type of PCI is substantially increased in diabetics as compared with nondiabetics.[59,60] Moreover, whereas restenosis has little impact on survival in patients without diabetes, Bertrand and coworkers demonstrated that restenosis after plain balloon angioplasty in diabetics has a major impact on 10-year mortality, with a 45% relative increase

for nonocclusive stenosis and more than a twofold increase with occlusive stenosis.[61] The risk of peri-interventional death and MI is also increased by about twofold after plain balloon angioplasty in diabetics as compared with nondiabetics.[62] Comparing coronary bypass surgery with plain balloon angioplasty for multivessel disease, BARI reported 5- and 7-year mortalities in diabetics of 34.5% and 44.3%, whereas after bypass surgery the respective mortalities were 19.4% and 23.6% ($P = 0.03$ and 0.01, respectively).[63] The findings in BARI that were subsequently confirmed by the 8-year analysis of EAST[64] led to a clinical alert from the National Heart, Lung and Blood Institute for the abandonment of plain balloon angioplasty as a treatment option for multivessel coronary artery disease. Studies done in the era of plain balloon angioplasty, however, are not transferable to current practice. As first demonstrated by the studies on abciximab, the increased risk of thrombotic complications during early and longer-term follow-up can be abrogated by intense antiplatelet therapy.[65,66] More recently, the ISAR-SWEET study suggested that a similar effect can be achieved by effective pretreatment with clopidogrel.[67] In addition, it has been shown by various studies that stents as compared with plain balloon angioplasty reduce the subsequent incidence of restenosis, although this incidence continues to be higher in diabetics than in nondiabetics.[60,68,69] Given the major impact of restenosis on survival, it is plausible that stents as compared with plain balloon angioplasty may improve the long-term outcome of PCI substantially. Finally, the recently improved means of achieving tight metabolic control can further improve outcome after catheter intervention.[70,71]

Because coronary revascularization in diabetics differs in many respects from that in nondiabetics, the indication for PCI in diabetics deserves special attention.

Studies with Bare Metal Stents

Of the studies comparing bare metal stents with CABG, ARTS, AWESOME, and ERACI-2 reported subgroup analyses for diabetics. Of the 1,205 patients included in ARTS, 112 diabetics were randomly assigned to stent implantation and 69 to bypass surgery.[72] Mortality during 1-year follow-up, however, was higher in the stent group (6.3%) than in the surgical group (3.1%), although statistical significance was missed ($P = 0.294$). Notably, in the PCI group there was a significant difference in event-free survival between diabetics and nondiabetics (63.4% vs. 76.2%), which was not present in the surgical group. During 1-year follow-up, the incidence of MIs also trended higher in the PCI group than in the surgical group (6.3% vs. 3.1%, $P = 0.294$) whereas the incidence of stroke was higher by trend in the surgical group (6.3 vs. 1.8%, $P = 0.10$). As in the entire ARTS cohort, the need for repeat intervention (mostly catheter intervention) was significantly higher in the stent group than in the surgical group. In the aggregate, ARTS suggested bypass surgery as the preferred treatment for multivessel disease in diabetics. Nevertheless, the number of diabetics included in ARTS was too low to allow for definite conclusions. Analysis of the 90 diabetics in ERACI (without stent) and ERACI-2 (with stent), on the other hand, did not reveal any advantage of CABG over PCI with bare metal stents. The AWESOME study addressed patients with a high risk for CABG (see above). The number of diabetics included in AWESOME was 144 in the randomized study, 89 in the patient-choice registry, and 525 in the physician-choice registry.[73] In the randomized study, the 4-year mortality of diabetics after catheter intervention was not significantly different from that after bypass surgery, with the point estimates favoring catheter intervention (19% vs. 28%, $P = 0.27$). Similar results were obtained in the patient-choice registry (11% vs. 15%, $P = 0.73$) and the physician-choice registry (29% vs. 27%, $P = 0.77$). The results of AWESOME, therefore, suggest that in patients with multivessel disease and refractory angina who have an increased risk for CABG, coronary implantation of bare metal stents is a safe alternative to surgical revascularization. APPROACH, the only large registry that addressed stent-supported PCI with bypass surgery in patients with diabetes, did not reveal any benefit of CABG as compared with PCI.[74]

Studies with Drug-Eluting Stents

Drug-eluting stents are particularly appealing in diabetics because they offer a solution to the most crucial problem of PCI in this patient subset—that is, restenosis. A metanalysis of the diabetic patients in randomized studies comparing drug-eluting stents with bare metal stents confirmed that in diabetes mellitus, drug-eluting stents confer a similar relative reduction in restenosis as do bare metal stents in non-diabetics.[75] Nevertheless, the excess risk of restenosis in diabetics as compared with nondiabetics prevailed even with drug-eluting stents.[75] There were no safety issues with respect to the 1-year incidence of death or of the composite of death and nonfatal MI when drug-eluting stents were compared with bare metal stents in diabetics. Based on the older studies for PCI in diabetes, it may be anticipated that the reduction in restenosis by drug-eluting stents as compared with bare metal stents may confer a survival benefit during longer-term follow-up in diabetics.[61] Hence the role of PCI as compared with CABG in the treatment of multivessel disease must be reassessed in the era of drug-eluting stents. FREEDOM, a large NIH-sponsored trial addressing this issue, has just finished recruitment after inclusion of 1,800 patients, but results are still pending. Currently, decision making must be based on the prespecified diabetic subgroup analysis of SYNTAX[76] and on the drug-eluting-stent subgroup analysis of CARDia.[77]

In SYNTAX, randomization was stratified for diabetes. Among 452 patients with medically treated diabetes, 221 were assigned to CABG and 231 to PCI.[76] Concerning the primary endpoint of SYNTAX, the 1-year incidence of MACCE, CABG was superior to PCI (14.2% vs. 26.0%; $P = 0.003$).[76] To a large extent, this was due to a lower need for repeat revascularization (6.4% vs. 20.3%; $P < 0.001$). There were, however, no significant differences in the 1-year composite of death, MI, and stroke (10.3% vs. 10.1%; $P = 0.98$) or 1-year death (6.4% vs. 8.4%; $P = 0.43$). There appeared to be a trend toward lower mortality with CABG as compared with PCI (5.7% vs. 12.5%; $P = 0.12$) only in the small group of insulin-treated diabetics; this was not observed in diabetics on oral agents only (6.8% vs. 5.8%; $P = 0.72$). For death as well as for the composite of death, MI, and stroke, the relative risks for major outcome variables comparing PCI with CABG were similar in diabetics and nondiabetics (Figure 2-7). With interaction P values close to the level of statistical significance, the surplus of repeat revascularization with PCI and thus the surplus in MACCE were more prominent in diabetics (Figure 2-7). Stratifying the diabetic subgroup of SYNTAX to anatomic complexity as judged by tertiles of SYNTAX scores reveals that, similar to the findings in the entire study, PCI in

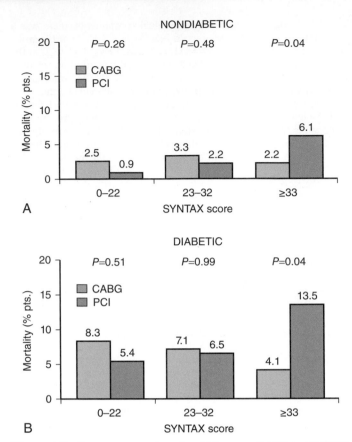

Figure 2-8 One-year mortality after PCI versus CABG in SYNTAX, stratified to diabetic status and tertiles of SYNTAX score.

the highest tertile of SYNTAX scores was associated with a significant excess in 1-year mortality as compared with CABG (Figure 2-8). Although the risk ratios for mortality were similar in diabetics and nondiabetics, the absolute difference in survival between CABG and PCI was higher in diabetics than in nondiabetics owing to the higher overall risk in diabetes (Figure 2-8). Three-year outcomes in the diabetic cohort have been reported.[78] The combined 3-years incidence in death, MI, and stroke is still not significantly different between PCI and CABG (16.3% vs. 14.0%; $P = 0.53$). Likewise, the difference in repeat revascularization seen at 1 year was largely maintained during follow-up, although additional repeat revascularization had to be performed in both groups during years 2 and 3 (7.7% after PCI vs. 6.5% after CABG, not significant). MACCE in the lowest tertile of SYNTAX scores was not significantly different between PCI and CABG (29.8% vs. 30.5%; $P = 0.98$), whereas in the middle and upper tertiles of SYNTAX scores, PCI resulted in a higher 3-year incidence of MACCE than CABG (36.2% vs. 21.0%, $P = 0.04$; 45.9% vs. 18.5%, $P < 0.001$; respectively). In summary, the overall level of risk in the diabetic cohort of SYNTAX is higher than in the entire cohort, but on the whole, the findings are largely consistent with those in the entire study except for a higher risk of restenosis. Specifically, the subgroup analysis of diabetics suggests that the noninferiority of PCI compared with CABG in patients with SYNTAX scores <22, as found in the entire study, also applies to diabetics. The CARDia trial was designed to compare PCI against CABG in patients with diabetes.[77] A total of 510 diabetic patients with multivessel or complex single-vessel coronary disease were randomized to CABG or PCI with bare metal stents in the first 30% of the patients and subsequently with sirolimus-eluting stents. The primary endpoint, the 1-year composite incidence of all-cause mortality, MI, was 10.5% in the CABG group and 13.0% in the PCI group ($P = 0.39$), all-cause mortality rates were 3.2% and 3.2%,

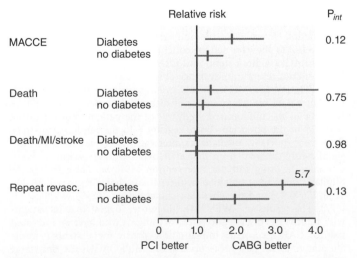

Figure 2-7 Relative risks for various events comparing PCI to CABG in the diabetic and the nondiabetic subset of SYNTAX. P_{int}, interaction P value; MACCE, major adverse cardiac and cerebrovascular events.

and the rates of repeat intervention were 2.0% and 11.8% ($P < 0.001$), respectively. Thus the 1-year rate of MACCE after CABG was significantly lower than that after PCI (11.3% vs. 19.3%, hazard ratio: 1.77, 95% confidence interval: 1.11 to 2.82; $P = 0.02$). With respect to the primary endpoint as well as MACCE, there were interactions with the stent type, favoring drug-eluting stents over bare metal stents ($P = 0.076$ and $P = 0.131$, respectively). Nevertheless, the observed 1-year rate of MACCE in the subgroup with sirolimus-eluting stents was 18.0% after PCI as compared with 12.9% after CABG. Owing to the reduced power of the subgroup analysis, no conclusions can be drawn from the lack of statistical significance for this finding. Comparing CARDia with SYNTAX, it is conspicuous that the 1-year incidences of MACCE as well as the corresponding hazard ratio for PCI versus CABG are lower in the drug-eluting-stent subgroup of CARDia than in the diabetic subgroup of SYNTAX. This may be explained by a lower risk profile in CARDia compared with the diabetic subgroup for SYNTAX. For example, three-vessel disease accounted for 63% of patients in CARDia as compared with 71% in SYNTAX. On average, 3.6 stents per patient were implanted in CARDia at a total stent length of 71 mm. The respective figures for the SYNTAX trial were 4.6 and 86 mm, respectively, in the study as a whole. Moreover, only 1% of the lesions treated by PCI in CARDia were bifurcations, compared with 73% of the lesions in SYNTAX. Given the SYNTAX finding that increased lesion complexity has a disproportionately adverse effect on the outcome of PCI compared with CABG, the findings in the DES-subgroup of CARDia and those in the diabetic subgroup of SYNTAX are remarkably consistent. Taken together, the DES subset of CARDia and the diabetic subset of SYNTAX suggest that PCI with drug-eluting stents is a reasonable alternative to CABG in patients with multivessel disease and low lesion complexity. Nevertheless, owing to the inherent limitations of subgroup analyses and the limited number of patients, these studies cannot definitely clarify the issue of PCI in multivessel disease in diabetics. The FREEDOM trial will provide the statistical power and duration of follow-up to clarify the efficacy of PCI versus CABG in general as well as in specific subsets defined by clinical variables and/or lesion complexity.

LEFT MAIN DISEASE

Since the early days of A. Grüntzig, plain balloon angioplasty has been considered contraindicated in unprotected left main stem lesions because of the almost inevitable fatality when the procedure fails and because CABG had been established as a therapy that reduced mortality compared with lone medical treatment. With the advent of coronary stents, however, the verdict against catheter treatment of left main stenosis was challenged. Stents are particularly attractive for percutaneous treatment of left main disease because they reduce acute complications and restenosis, especially in large-diameter vessels. Moreover, stents overcome the elastic recoil within the aortic wall, which represents a major problem with left main percutaneous transluminal coronary angioplasty (PTCA). It was thus not surprising that several groups reported favorable results of registries on bare metal stenting of unprotected left main stenosis.[79–84]

Registries with Drug-Eluting Stents

Several registries have addressed the efficacy and safety of drug-eluting stents in the treatment of left main disease. In 2005, three key studies were published that comprised cohorts of 85 to 102 patients treated with drug-eluting stents for unprotected left main disease and historic control groups with bare metal stents of 64 to 121 patients.[85–87] These studies suggested that drug-eluting stents as compared with bare metal stents may improve outcome—an assumption that was subsequently confirmed by nonrandomized comparisons and a small randomized study.[88–91] In ISAR-LEFT-MAIN, comprising 607 patients treated with a drug-eluting stent, 2-year mortality was 9.7 and angiographic restenosis 17.7%, with no significant difference between sirolimus- and paclitaxel-eluting stents.[92] Consistent results were reported from a multicenter registry.[93]

In 2006, the first two nonrandomized studies comparing implantation of drug-eluting stents for unprotected left main disease with CABG were published. The study by Lee et al.[94] compared 50 patients who underwent PCI with drug-eluting stents for unprotected left main disease with 123 patients at the same institutions who underwent CABG. At 6 months, freedom from death, MI, cerebrovascular events, and target-vessel revascularization was 83% after CABG and 89% after PCI ($P = 0.20$). Freedom from death, MI, and cerebrovascular events at 6 months, however, was significantly higher after PCI (95.6%) than after CABG (82.9%) ($P = 0.03$). By multivariable Cox regression analysis, CABG was an independent predictor of major adverse cardiovascular and cerebrovascular events. Similar results were obtained in the study by Chieffo et al.,[95] which compared 107 patients with unprotected left main disease who were treated with PCI and drug-eluting stent implantation with 142 patients undergoing CABG. At 1 year, the rate of death, MI, and cerebrovascular events was significantly lower in PCI-treated patients as compared with CABG-treated patients (3.7% vs. 8.5%, $P < 0.001$). This difference prevailed after adjustment by propensity analysis with respect to baseline differences between the two cohorts (adjusted odds ratio 0.39, 95% confidence interval, 0.18 to 0.82, $P = 0.01$). On the other hand, there was a significant increase in target-vessel revascularization in the PCI-treated patients (19.6% vs. 3.6%). Subsequently, several nonrandomized studies comparing PCI with drug-eluting stents versus CABG reported consistent results.[96–102] The largest of these studies is the MAIN-COMPARE registry, for which 5-year results have been reported.[100] The MAIN-COMPARE registry evaluated 2,240 patients with unprotected left main coronary artery disease who received coronary stents ($n = 1,102$) or underwent CABG ($n = 1,138$). Among the PCI-treated patients, 318 received bare metal stents and 784 drug-eluting stents. Median follow-up was 5.2 years. The 5-year incidences after PCI versus CABG were 11.8% and 13.6% ($P = 0.06$) for death, 12.2% and 14.7% ($P = 0.03$) for the composite of death, Q-wave MI, or stroke, and 16.0% versus 4.0% ($P < 0.001$) for target-vessel revascularization. After adjustment for differences in baseline risk factors, the corresponding hazard ratios were 1.13 (95% confidence interval: 0.88 to 1.44, $P = 0.35$) for death; 1.07 (95% confidence interval: 0.84 to 1.37, $P = 0.59$) for the composite of death, Q-wave MI or stroke; and 5.11 (95% confidence interval: 3.52 to 7.42, $P < 0.001$) for target-vessel revascularization. Comparisons of bare metal stents with concurrent CABG and of drug-eluting stents with concurrent CABG yielded similar results. Hence with respect to clinically important endpoints, CABG for unprotected left main disease did not afford a superior 5-year outcome as compared with PCI. Yet a higher need for reintervention had to be faced when therapy was primarily based on PCI instead of CABG.

The registry data and nonrandomized studies thus do not support the concept that every left main stenosis should be treated surgically.

Randomized Studies with Drug-Eluting Stents

In SYNTAX, 705 patients belonged to the prespecified subset with left main disease (Table 2-4).[103,104] During 3-year follow-up,[103] the incidence of MACCE did not differ significantly between PCI and CABG (22.3% vs. 26.8%, $P = 0.20$) (Table 2-4). The composite of death, MI, and stroke to 3 years was also similar between the two groups (13.0% vs. 14.3%, $P = 0.60$), as were mortality (7.3% vs. 8.4%, $P = 0.64$) and rate of MI (6.9% vs. 4.1%, $P = 0.14$). At 3 years, reintervention was significantly more frequent in the PCI group (20.0% vs. 11.7%, $P = 0.004$), whereas stroke was significantly more frequent in the CABG group (1.2% vs. 4.0%, $P = 0.02$). The extent of coronary artery disease outside the left main had a major impact on outcome after PCI versus CABG. As in the entire study, there was excess 3-year mortality and excess 3-year MACCE after PCI compared with CABG in the tertile with SYNTAX scores >32 (13.4% vs. 7.6%, $P = 0.10$; and 37.3% vs. 21.2%, $P = 0.003$, respectively) (Table 2-4). On the other hand, in the two lower tertiles of SYNTAX scores, there were trends toward lower mortality with PCI (2.6% vs. 6.0%, $P = 0.21$, for SYNTAX score <22; 4.9% vs. 12.4%, $P = 0.06$, for SYNTAX score 22–32) and there was no increase in MACCE with PCI as compared with CABG (18.0% vs.

23.0%, $P = 0.21$, for SYNTAX score <22; 23.4% vs. 23.3%, $P = 0.90$, for SYNTAX score 22–32) (Table 2-4). Thus the results of the SYNTAX study suggest that PCI is the treatment of choice for left main disease unless there is extensive coronary artery disease, as judged by SYNTAX scores >32. The key results of SYNTAX left main are corroborated by another multicenter trial that randomized 201 patients with unprotected left main to undergo sirolimus-eluting stenting ($n = 100$) or CABG using predominantly arterial grafts ($n = 101$).[105] At 1 year, the primary clinical endpoint of major adverse cardiac events—comprising cardiac death, MI, and the need for target vessel revascularization—was reached in 13.9% of patients after surgery as opposed to 19.0% after PCI ($P = 0.19$ for noninferiority). The combined rates for death and MI were comparable (surgery 7.9% vs. stenting 5.0%, noninferiority $P < 0.001$), but stenting was inferior to surgery for repeat revascularization (5.9% vs. 14.0%, noninferiority $P = 0.35$). Perioperative complications were higher after surgery (4% vs. 30%; $P < 0.001$). Like SYNTAX, this trial suggests equipoise between PCI and CABG with respect to prognostically relevant endpoints. The two randomized trials comparing CABG to PCI with drug-eluting stents for left main disease have been included in a metanalysis together with six nonrandomized studies.[106] Consistently, this metanalysis suggests that the risk of death as well as that of death, MI, or stroke is insignificantly higher with CABG as compared with drug-eluting stents (odds ratio [95% confidence interval]: 1.12 [0.80 to 1.56] and 1.25 [0.86 to 1.82], respectively), whereas the risk for target vessel revascularization is significantly lower (odds ratio [95% confidence interval]: 0.44 [0.32 to 0.59]).[106] In summary, based on currently available evidence, PCI with drug-eluting stents is a reasonable treatment option for many patients with unprotected left main disease. In general, survival and freedom from MI and stroke are at least as good as after surgery and patients may thus decide whether they want to exchange the discomfort of surgery for the potential inconvenience of repeat revascularization procedures. Concerning specific subsets, SYNTAX has taught us that the differential outcome of the two treatment strategies critically depends on the extent of concomitant coronary artery disease outside the left main. With widespread, diffuse disease outside the left main, CABG is more beneficial (including a survival benefit), whereas with no or minor disease outside the left main PCI leads to better outcomes.

▣ Symptomatic Indication for Revascularization: PCI Versus Medical Therapy Alone

Several studies of the pre-stent era compared PCI with lone medical therapy in single- or double-vessel disease without a prognostic indication for bypass surgery. A metanalysis that—apart from ACME, RITA-2, and AVERT—also included MASS and one smaller German trial demonstrated a significant 30% reduction in angina but a significant increase in the need for CABG with PCI as compared with medical treatment and trends toward increased risk of death, MI, and nonscheduled PCI.[107] This metanalysis supports the concept that compared with lone medical therapy, PCI in patients with stable angina reduces symptoms but may be associated with a higher incidence of serious complications such as death and MI. It must be considered, however, that none of the studies included in this metanalysis used contemporary interventional techniques, including the systematic use of stents with vigorous peri- and postinterventional antiplatelet treatment or strict risk-factor modification, in particular the administration of statins, after PCI. Modern peri- and postinterventional drug therapy would have reduced the risk of death and MI, and each of the three elements of modern interventional treatment—stents, statins, and antiplatelet drugs—would have reduced the need for subsequent unplanned revascularization procedures. Hence it may be anticipated that, with modern interventional approaches, the complications of catheter intervention would have been substantially lower without corrupting the beneficial effect of this treatment of angina as compared

with lone medical therapy. The role of PCI compared with lone medical therapy in patients without an established prognostic indication for coronary revascularization therefore needed reassessment in the light of contemporary interventional techniques and optimal peri- and postinterventional treatment. This was the goal of the randomized COURAGE trial.[107] COURAGE involved 2,287 patients who had objective evidence of myocardial ischemia and significant coronary artery disease; 1,149 patients were assigned to undergo PCI with optimal medical therapy (PCI group) and 1,138 to receive optimal medical therapy alone (medical therapy group). Patients with persistent Canadian Cardiovascular Society class IV angina, a markedly positive stress test, unprotected left main disease, or hazardous PCI, as in ostial stenosis of the LAD, were not eligible for the study. COURAGE was highly successful in applying state-of-the-art preventive and antiischemic pharmacological treatment. Drug-eluting stents, however, were not available except for the last 6 months of the study. Thus only 2.7% of the COURAGE trial PCI patients received drug-eluting stents. Among patients randomized to PCI, 6.4% did not have the procedure. On the other hand, 32% of the patients assigned to the medical therapy group crossed over to PCI during follow-up. Repeat PCI was also performed in 21% of the patients in the PCI group. During a median follow-up of 4.6 years, the cumulative primary event rates, the composite of death from any cause and nonfatal MI, were 19.0% in the PCI group and 18.5% in the medical therapy group (hazard ratio for the PCI group, 1.05; 95% confidence interval, 0.87 to 1.27; $P = 0.62$).[108] Considering components of the primary endpoint, numbers of death were 85 in the PCI group and 95 in the medical therapy group, those of spontaneous MI 108 and 109, and those of peri-PCI MI 35 and 9, respectively. At 1 year and at 3 years but not at 5 years, a significantly higher proportion of patients in the PCI group as compared with the medical therapy group were free of angina (66% vs. 58%, $P < 0.001$; 72% vs. 67%, $P = 0.02$; and 74% vs. 72%, $P = 0.35$; respectively). The striking 72% angina-free status at 5 years in the medical therapy group may be attributed to the fact that 43% of these patients began the trial with minimal (Canadian Cardiovascular Society class I) or no angina and 32% went on to subsequent revascularization for relief of symptoms. Given the failure to reduce the risk of death and MI and the marginal symptomatic benefit of PCI plus optimal medical therapy over optimal medical therapy alone, it was concluded that an initial recommendation of PCI on top of optimal medical therapy offers no important advantage over an initial recommendation of optimal medical therapy alone.

More recently, results consistent with the COURAGE trial were reported from the BARI 2D trial.[109] BARI 2D included 2,368 patients with both type 2 diabetes and coronary artery disease. These patients were stratified as potential candidates for CABG ($n = 763$) or for PCI ($n = 1,605$) and then randomly assigned to prompt revascularization or intense medical therapy. There also was a subrandomization to insulin sensitization or insulin provision therapy. At 5 years, rates of survival did not differ significantly between the revascularization group (88.3%) and the medical therapy group (87.8%, $P = 0.97$). The rates of freedom from major cardiovascular events also did not differ significantly among the groups: 77.2% in the revascularization group and 75.9% in the medical treatment group ($P = 0.70$). Taken together, COURAGE and BARI-2D suggest that with optimal medical treatment, a conservative approach that reserves revascularization to patients with progression of angina, the development of an acute coronary syndrome, or severe ischemia is preferred over a strategy of prompt revascularization. Some caveats against an uncritical generalization of this concept need to be considered. The first comes from the authors of the COURAGE trial themselves. In their nuclear substudy of COURAGE, they demonstrated that the beneficial effect of therapy on prognosis is linked to a substantial reduction in stress-induced ischemia to a low residual level.[22] In their substudy, a reduction of the area of stress-induced ischemia of ≥5% and to ≤10% of the left ventricle was needed for a prognostic effect, especially if baseline ischemia was >10%. Although this was achieved more frequently after PCI than after medical therapy alone, a substantial number of PCI patients fell short of this goal. This may not be considered an inherent limitation of PCI but rather a consequence of a PCI strategy that focused on the culprit lesion. Despite the fact that 69% of patients assigned to PCI had multivessel disease and 65% had multiple reversible perfusion defects on nuclear imaging, only 36% of the patients received more than one stent. Thus, in a substantial proportion of patients, PCI resulted in incomplete revascularization. With respect to the overall outcome of the study, this will have diluted the beneficial effect of complete revascularization in some of the patients, as demonstrated in the nuclear substudy of COURAGE.[22] The findings of the BARI 2D trial also support the concept that revascularization will improve prognosis if a relevant area of the left ventricle can be relieved from ischemia. In this trial, the low-risk patients stratified as PCI candidates derived no benefit from revascularization as compared with primarily medical treatment, whereas patients stratified as CABG candidates fared better with revascularization (major adverse events 22.4% vs. 30.5%, $P = 0.01$; $P = 0.002$ for interaction between stratum and study group). Compared with PCI candidates, CABG candidates more often had three-vessel disease and a jeopardy score >50% (odds ratios 4.4 and 4.1, respectively). Thus, in BARI 2D, the larger reduction in ischemia in the CABG group as compared with that in the PCI group resulted in a prognostic benefit. The second caveat comes from the observation of a 13% relative reduction in mortality by PCI plus optimal medical therapy compared with optimal medical therapy alone in COURAGE. COURAGE, however, was not powered to establish the statistical significance of this finding. Yet when all the information derived from 17 randomized trials comparing PCI-based invasive treatment strategy with medical treatment is considered, the metanalysis suggests that the PCI-based invasive strategy improves long-term survival compared with a strategy of medical treatment only (odds ratio for all-cause death: 0.80; 95% confidence interval: 0.64 to 0.99, $P = 0.263$ for heterogeneity across the trials).[110] This inference is further supported by analysis of the large Duke University Medical Center registry, which included 18,481 patients (Figure 2-6).[51] As detailed above, this study demonstrated that even in patients with a low severity of coronary artery disease (one or two vessels ≥75%, none ≥95%), the initial revascularization by PCI conferred a significant survival benefit of 8 months in 7 years (adjusted for pertinent covariables) over conservative treatment alone. In summary, currently available evidence suggests that stable patients who are free of symptoms under antianginal medication and free of relevant residual inducible ischemia should be managed conservatively. PCI in stable angina should be reserved for those patients who are not free of symptoms or have an area of stress-induced ischemia of >10% of the left ventricle under the tolerated medical therapy.

Summary

When coronary revascularization is considered, prognostic and symptomatic indications must be distinguished. With prognostic indications, PCI offers an alternative to CABG; with symptomatic indications, PCI competes with medical treatment. In the absence of an acute coronary syndrome, PCI for single-vessel disease is justified only if an improvement in symptoms can be anticipated or if there is a large area (>10% of left ventricle) of inducible ischemia.

In patients with multivessel disease with or without left main stenosis, the choice of revascularization therapy will depend on the complexity of coronary artery involvement. With low complexity, such as a SYNTAX score <22, there is currently no evidence that CABG offers a relevant benefit over PCI with drug-eluting stents. In patients with a high complexity (e.g., SYNTAX score >32), however, current evidence demonstrates a survival benefit of CABG over PCI; PCI in such patients is therefore discouraged. With an intermediate complexity of coronary artery involvement and three-vessel disease, there also is a preference for surgery. The risks of death, myocardial infarction, or stroke appear to be lower after CABG than after PCI. Patients also must be informed about the higher need for repeat procedures after PCI, which has to be weighed against the discomfort of surgery. Left main stenosis is not a contraindication to PCI. In fact, for a given range of SYNTAX scores, the outcome after PCI with left main involvement is superior to that without left main involvement. Hence, PCI is still preferable at an intermediate range of SYNTAX scores. In patients with diabetes mellitus, however, it is unclear whether multivessel PCI can achieve a prognostic benefit similar to that of CABG. Despite drug-eluting stents, vigorous antiplatelet treatment, and tight metabolic control, diabetic patients continue to be at increased risk of death and reintervention. Thus, for a given range of coronary lesion complexity, the threshold for CABG should be lower in diabetic than in nondiabetic patients. Individualized decisions have to be taken that consider the likelihood of complete revascularization and the risk associated with either approach, the patient's life expectancy based on age and comorbidities, as well as the patient's preference after thorough counseling. Such decisions must be reached jointly by the cardiac surgeon and the interventional cardiologist.

REFERENCES

1. Mauri L, Hsieh WH, Massaro JM, et al: Stent thrombosis in randomized clinical trials of drug-eluting stents. *N Engl J Med* 356(10):1020–1029, 2007.
2. Roukoz H, Bavry AA, Sarkees ML, et al: Comprehensive meta-analysis on drug-eluting stents versus bare-metal stents during extended follow-up. *Am J Med* 122(6):581 e581–510, 2009.
3. Marroquin OC, Selzer F, Mulukutla SR, et al: A comparison of bare-metal and drug-eluting stents for off-label indications. *N Engl J Med* 358(4):342–352, 2008.
4. Fibrinolytic Therapy Trialists' (FTT) Collaborative Group: Indications for fibrinolytic therapy in suspected acute myocardial infarction: collaborative overview of early mortality and major morbidity results from all randomised trials of more than 1000 patients. *Lancet* 343(8893):311–322, 1994.
5. Boersma E: The Primary Coronary Angioplasty vs. Thrombolysis Group. Does time matter? A pooled analysis of randomized clinical trials comparing primary percutaneous coronary intervention and in-hospital fibrinolysis in acute myocardial infarction patients. *Eur Heart J* 27:779–788, 2006.
6. Keeley EC, Boura JA, Grines CL: Primary angioplasty versus intravenous thrombolytic therapy for acute myocardial infarction: a quantitative review of 23 randomised trials. *Lancet* 361:13–20, 2003.
7. Ellis SG, Tendera M, de Belder MA, et al: Facilitated PCI in patients with ST-elevation myocardial infarction. *N Engl J Med* 358(21):2205–2217, 2008.
8. Hillis LD, Lange RA: Optimal management of acute coronary syndromes. *N Engl J Med* 360(21):2237–2240, 2009.
9. Mehta SR, Cannon CP, Fox KA, et al: Routine vs. selective invasive strategies in patients with acute coronary syndromes: a collaborative meta-analysis of randomized trials. *JAMA* 293:2908–2917, 2005.
10. Fox KA, Poole-Wilson P, Clayton TC, et al: 5-year outcome of an interventional strategy in non-ST-elevation acute coronary syndrome: the British Heart Foundation RITA 3 randomised trial. *Lancet* 366(9489):914–920, 2005.
11. Lagerqvist B, Husted S, Kontny F, et al: 5-year outcomes in the FRISC-II randomised trial of an invasive versus a non-invasive strategy in non-ST-elevation acute coronary syndrome: a follow-up study. *Lancet* 368(9540):998–1004, 2006.
12. Cannon CP, Weintraub WS, Demopoulos LA, et al: Comparison of early invasive and conservative strategies in patients with unstable coronary syndromes treated with the glycoprotein IIb/IIIa inhibitor tirofiban. *N Engl J Med* 344(25):1879–1887, 2001.
13. Fox KA, Poole-Wilson PA, Henderson RA, et al: Interventional versus conservative treatment for patients with unstable angina or non-ST-elevation myocardial infarction: the British Heart Foundation RITA 3 randomised trial. Randomized Intervention Trial of unstable Angina. *Lancet* 360(9335):743–751, 2002.
14. FRISCII, Investigators. Invasive compared with non-invasive treatment in unstable coronary-artery disease: FRISC II prospective randomised multicentre study. *Lancet* 354:708–715, 1999.
15. Bertrand ME, Simoons ML, Fox KA, et al: Task Force on the Management of Acute Coronary Syndromes of the European Society of Cardiology. Management of acute coronary syndromes in patients presenting without persistent ST-segment elevation. *Eur Heart J* 23:1809–1840, 2002.
16. de Winter RJ, Windhausen F, Cornel JH, et al: Invasive versus Conservative Treatment in Unstable Coronary Syndromes (ICTUS) Investigators. Early invasive versus selectively invasive management for acute coronary syndromes. *N Engl J Med* 353:1095–1104, 2005.
17. Damman P, Hirsch A, Windhausen F, et al: 5-year clinical outcomes in the ICTUS (Invasive versus Conservative Treatment in Unstable coronary Syndromes) trial a randomized comparison of an early invasive versus selective invasive management in patients with non-ST-segment elevation acute coronary syndrome. *J Am Coll Cardiol* 55(9):858–864, 2010.
18. Weiner DA, Ryan TJ, McCabe CH, et al: The role of exercise testing in identifying patients with improved survival after coronary artery bypass surgery. *J Am Coll Cardiol* 8(4):741–748, 1986.
19. Mock MB, Fisher LD, Holmes DR, Jr, et al: Comparison of effects of medical and surgical therapy on survival in severe angina pectoris and two-vessel coronary artery disease with and without left ventricular dysfunction: a Coronary Artery Surgery Study Registry Study. *Am J Cardiol* 61(15):1198–1203, 1988.
20. Pepine CJ, Geller NL, Knatterud GL, et al: The Asymptomatic Cardiac Ischemia Pilot (ACIP) study: design of a randomized clinical trial, baseline data and implications for a long term outcome trial. *J Am Coll Cardiol* 24(1):1–10, 1994.
21. Hachamovitch R, Hayes SW, Friedman JD, et al: Comparison of the short-term survival benefit associated with revascularization compared with medical therapy in patients with no prior coronary artery disease undergoing stress myocardial perfusion single photon emission computed tomography. *Circulation* 107(23):2900–2907, 2003.
22. Shaw LJ, Berman DS, Maron DJ, et al: Optimal medical therapy with or without percutaneous coronary intervention to reduce ischemic burden: results from the Clinical Outcomes Utilizing Revascularization and Aggressive Drug Evaluation (COURAGE) trial nuclear substudy. *Circulation* 117(10):1283–1291, 2008.

23. Yusuf S, Zucker D, Peduzzi P, et al: Effect of coronary artery bypass graft surgery on survival: overview of 10-year results from randomised trials by the Coronary Artery Bypass Graft Surgery Trialists Collaboration. *Lancet* 344(8922):563–570, 1994.
24. ECSS, Group: Long-term results of prospective randomised study of coronary artery bypass surgery in stable angina pectoris. European Coronary Surgery Study Group. *Lancet* 2(8309):1173–1180, 1982.
25. Passamani E, Davis KB, Gillespie MJ, et al: A randomized trial of coronary artery bypass surgery. Survival of patients with a low ejection fraction. *N Engl J Med* 312(26):1665–1671, 1985.
26. Peduzzi P, Hultgren HN: Effect of medical vs. surgical treatment on symptoms in stable angina pectoris. The Veterans Administration Cooperative Study of surgery for coronary arterial occlusive disease. *Circulation* 60(4):888–900, 1979.
27. Hueb WA, Bellotti G, de Oliveira SA, et al: The Medicine, Angioplasty or Surgery Study (MASS): a prospective, randomized trial of medical therapy, balloon angioplasty or bypass surgery for single proximal left anterior descending artery stenoses. *J Am Coll Cardiol* 26(7):1600–1605, 1995.
28. Kubo T, Maehara A, Mintz GS, et al: The dynamic nature of coronary artery lesion morphology assessed by serial virtual histology intravascular ultrasound tissue characterization. *J Am Coll Cardiol* 55(15):1590–1597, 2010.
29. Barlis P, Serruys PW, Gonzalo N, et al: Assessment of culprit and remote coronary narrowings using optical coherence tomography with long-term outcomes. *Am J Cardiol* 102(4):391–395, 2008.
30. Bell MR, Gersh BJ, Schaff HV, et al: Effect of completeness of revascularization on long-term outcome of patients with three-vessel disease undergoing coronary artery bypass surgery. A report from the Coronary Artery Surgery Study (CASS) Registry. *Circulation* 86(2):446–457, 1992.
31. Bourassa MG, Kip KE, Jacobs AK, et al: Is a strategy of intended incomplete percutaneous transluminal coronary angioplasty revascularization acceptable in nondiabetic patients who are candidates for coronary artery bypass graft surgery? The Bypass Angioplasty Revascularization Investigation (BARI). *J Am Coll Cardiol* 33(6):1627–1636, 1999.
32. Cowley MJ, Vandermael M, Topol EJ, et al: Is traditionally defined complete revascularization needed for patients with multivessel disease treated by elective coronary angioplasty? Multivessel Angioplasty Prognosis Study (MAPS) Group. *J Am Coll Cardiol* 22(5):1289–1297, 1993.
33. Hannan EL, Racz M, Holmes DR, et al: Impact of completeness of percutaneous coronary intervention revascularization on long-term outcomes in the stent era. *Circulation* 113(20):2406–2412, 2006.
34. Hoffman SN, TenBrook JA, Wolf MP, et al: A meta-analysis of randomized controlled trials comparing coronary artery bypass graft with percutaneous transluminal coronary angioplasty: one- to eight-year outcomes. *J Am Coll Cardiol* 41(8):1293–1304, 2003.
35. Serruys PW, Ong AT, van Herwerden LA, et al: Five-year outcomes after coronary stenting versus bypass surgery for the treatment of multivessel disease: the final analysis of the Arterial Revascularization Therapies Study (ARTS) randomized trial. *J Am Coll Cardiol* 46(4):575–581, 2005.
36. Serruys PW, Unger F, Sousa JE, et al: Comparison of coronary-artery bypass surgery and stenting for the treatment of multivessel disease. *N Engl J Med* 344(15):1117–1124, 2001.
37. SoS, Investigators: Coronary artery bypass surgery versus percutaneous coronary intervention with stent implantation in patients with multivessel coronary artery disease (the Stent or Surgery trial): a randomised controlled trial. *Lancet* 360(9338):965–970, 2002.
38. Rodriguez A, Bernardi V, Navia J, et al: Argentine Randomized Study: Coronary Angioplasty with Stenting versus Coronary Bypass Surgery in patients with Multiple-Vessel Disease (ERACI II): 30-day and one-year follow-up results. ERACI II Investigators. *J Am Coll Cardiol* 37(1):51–58, 2001.
39. Rodriguez AE, Baldi J, Fernandez Pereira C, et al: Five-year follow-up of the Argentine randomized trial of coronary angioplasty with stenting versus coronary bypass surgery in patients with multiple vessel disease (ERACI II). *J Am Coll Cardiol* 46(4):582–588, 2005.
40. Hueb W, Soares PR, Gersh BJ, et al: The medicine, angioplasty, or surgery study (MASS-II): a randomized, controlled clinical trial of three therapeutic strategies for multivessel coronary artery disease: one-year results. *J Am Coll Cardiol* 43(10):1743–1751, 2004.
41. Morrison DA, Sethi G, Sacks J, et al: Percutaneous coronary intervention versus coronary artery bypass graft surgery for patients with medically refractory myocardial ischemia and risk factors for adverse outcomes with bypass: a multicenter, randomized trial. Investigators of the Department of Veterans Affairs Cooperative Study #385, the Angina With Extremely Serious Operative Mortality Evaluation (AWESOME). *J Am Coll Cardiol* 38(1):143–149, 2001.
42. Mercado N, Wijns W, Serruys PW, et al: One-year outcomes of coronary artery bypass graft surgery versus percutaneous coronary intervention with multiple stenting for multisystem disease: a meta-analysis of individual patient data from randomized clinical trials. *J Thorac Cardiovasc Surg* 130(2):512–519, 2005.
43. Hueb W, Lopes N, Gersh BJ, et al: Ten-year follow-up survival of the medicine, angioplasty, or surgery study (mass ii): A randomized controlled clinical trial of 3 therapeutic strategies for multivessel coronary artery disease. *Circulation* 122:949–957, 2010.
44. Stroupe KT, Morrison DA, Hlatky MA, et al: Cost-effectiveness of coronary artery bypass grafts versus percutaneous coronary intervention for revascularization of high-risk patients. *Circulation* 114(12):1251–1257, 2006.
45. Morrison DA, Sethi G, Sacks J, et al: Percutaneous coronary intervention versus coronary bypass graft surgery for patients with medically refractory myocardial ischemia and risk factors for adverse outcomes with bypass: The VA AWESOME multicenter registry: comparison with the randomized clinical trial. *J Am Coll Cardiol* 39(2):266–273, 2002.
46. Morrison DA, Sethi G, Sacks J, et al: Percutaneous coronary intervention versus repeat bypass surgery for patients with medically refractory myocardial ischemia: AWESOME randomized trial and registry experience with post-CABG patients. *J Am Coll Cardiol* 40(11):1951–1954, 2002.
47. Grapow MT, von Wattenwyl R, Guller U, et al: Randomized controlled trials do not reflect reality: real-world analyses are critical for treatment guidelines! *J Thorac Cardiovasc Surg* 132(1):5–7, 2006.
48. Brener SJ, Lytle BW, Casserly IP, et al: Propensity analysis of long-term survival after surgical or percutaneous revascularization in patients with multivessel coronary artery disease and high-risk features. *Circulation* 109(19):2290–2295, 2004.
49. Hannan EL, Racz MJ, Walford G, et al: Long-term outcomes of coronary-artery bypass grafting versus stent implantation. *N Engl J Med* 352(21):2174–2183, 2005.
50. van Domburg RT, Takkenberg JJ, Noordzij LJ, et al: Late outcome after stenting or coronary artery bypass surgery for the treatment of multivessel disease: a single-center matched-propensity controlled cohort study. *Ann Thorac Surg* 79(5):1563–1569, 2005.
51. Smith PK, Califf RM, Tuttle RH, et al: Selection of surgical or percutaneous coronary intervention provides differential longevity benefit. *Ann Thorac Surg* 82(4):1420–1428; discussion 1428–1429, 2006.
52. Hannan EL, Wu C, Walford G, et al: Drug-eluting stents vs. coronary-artery bypass grafting in multivessel coronary disease. *N Engl J Med* 358(4):331–341, 2008.
53. Serruys PW, Ong ATL, Morice MC, et al: Arterial Revascularisation Therapies Study Part II—Sirolimus-eluting stents for the treatment of patients with multivessel de novo coronary artery lesions. *EuroIntervention* 1:147–156, 2005.
54. Serruys PW, Onuma Y, Garg S, et al: 5-year clinical outcomes of the ARTS II (Arterial Revascularization Therapies Study II) of the sirolimus-eluting stent in the treatment of patients with multivessel de novo coronary artery lesions. *J Am Coll Cardiol* 55(11):1093–1101, 2010.
55. Serruys PW, Morice MC, Kappetein AP, et al: Percutaneous coronary intervention versus coronary-artery bypass grafting for severe coronary artery disease. *N Engl J Med* 360(10):961–972, 2009.
56. Kappetein AP: The 3-year outcomes of the SYNTAX trial. *24 EACTS Annual Meeting* Geneva, Switzerland; 2010.
57. Mohr FW: The 3-year outcomes of the SYNTAX trial in the subset of pateints with three-vessel disease. *Transcath Ther* Washington, DC; 2010.
58. Barzilay JI, Kronmal RA, Bittner V, et al: Coronary artery disease and coronary artery bypass grafting in diabetic patients aged > or = 65 years (report from the Coronary Artery Surgery Study [CASS]Registry). *Am J Cardiol* 74:334–339, 1994.
59. Van Belle E, Abolmaali K, Bauters C, et al: Restenosis, late vessel occlusion and left ventricular function six months after balloon angioplasty in diabetic patients. *J Am Coll Cardiol* 34(2):476–485, 1999.
60. Elezi S, Kastrati A, Pache J, et al: Diabetes mellitus and the clinical and angiographic outcome after coronary stent placement. *J Am Coll Cardiol* 32(7):1866–1873, 1998.
61. Van Belle E, Ketelers R, Bauters C, et al: Patency of percutaneous transluminal coronary angioplasty sites at 6-month angiographic follow-up: A key determinant of survival in diabetics after coronary balloon angioplasty. *Circulation* 103(9):1218–1224, 2001.
62. Kip KE, Faxon DP, Detre KM, et al: Coronary angioplasty in diabetic patients. The National Heart, Lung, and Blood Institute Percutaneous Transluminal Coronary Angioplasty Registry. *Circulation* 94(8):1818–1825, 1996.
63. BARI I: Seven-year outcome in the Bypass Angioplasty Revascularization Investigation BARI) by treatment and diabetic status. *J Am Coll Cardiol* 35(5):1122–1129, 2000.
64. King SBr, Kosinski AS, Guyton RA, et al: Eight-year mortality in the Emory Angioplasty versus Surgery Trial (EAST). *J Am Coll Cardiol* 35(5):1116–1121, 2000.
65. Marso SP, Lincoff AM, Ellis SG, et al: Optimizing the percutaneous interventional outcomes for patients with diabetes mellitus: results of the EPISTENT diabetic substudy. *Circulation* 100(25):2477–2484, 1999.
66. Bhatt DL, Marso SP, Lincoff AM, et al: Abciximab reduces mortality in diabetics following percutaneous coronary intervention. *J Am Coll Cardiol* 35:922–928, 2000.
67. Mehilli J, Kastrati A, Schühlen H, et al: Randomized clinical trial of abciximab in diabetic patients undergoing elective percutaneous coronary interventions after treatment with a high loading dose of clopidogrel. *Circulation* 110:3627–3635, 2004.
68. Van Belle E, Bauters C, Hubert E, et al: Restenosis rates in diabetic patients: a comparison of coronary stenting and balloon angioplasty in native coronary vessels. *Circulation* 96(5):1454–1460, 1997.
69. Van Belle E, Perie M, Braune D, et al: Effects of coronary stenting on vessel patency and long-term clinical outcome after percutaneous coronary revascularization in diabetic patients. *J Am Coll Cardiol* 40(3):410–417, 2002.
70. Otsuka Y, Myazaki S, Okumara H: Abnormal glucose tolerance, not small vessel diameter, is a determinant of long-term prognosis in patients treated with balloon coronary angioplasty. *Eur Heart J* 21:1790–1796, 2000.
71. Takagi T, Akasaka T, Yamamuro A, et al: Troglitazone reduces neointimal tissue proliferation after coronary stent implantation in patients with non-insulin dependent diabetes mellitus: a serial intravascular ultrasound study. *J Am Coll Cardiol* 36(5):1529–1535, 2000.
72. Abizaid A, Costa MA, Centemero M, et al: Clinical and economic impact of diabetes mellitus on percutaneous and surgical treatment of multivessel coronary disease patients: insights from the Arterial Revascularization Therapy Study (ARTS) trial. *Circulation* 104(5):533–538, 2001.
73. Sedlis SP, Morrison DA, Lorin JD, et al: Percutaneous coronary intervention versus coronary bypass graft surgery for diabetic patients with unstable angina and risk factors for adverse outcomes with bypass: outcome of diabetic patients in the AWESOME randomized trial and registry. *J Am Coll Cardiol* 40(9):1555–1566, 2002.
74. Dzavik V, Ghali WA, Norris C: Long-term survival in 11,661 patients with multivessel coronary artery disease in the era of stenting: a report from the Alberta Provincial Project for Outcome Assessment in Coronary Heart Disease (APPROACH) Investigators. *Am Heart J* 142:119–126, 2001.
75. Scheen AJ, Warzee F, Legrand VM: Drug-eluting stents: meta-analysis in diabetic patients. *Eur Heart J* 25(23):2167–2168; author reply 2168–2169, 2004.
76. Banning AP, Westaby S, Morice MC, et al: Diabetic and nondiabetic patients with left main and/or 3-vessel coronary artery disease: comparison of outcomes with cardiac surgery and paclitaxel-eluting stents. *J Am Coll Cardiol* 55(11):1067–1075, 2010.
77. Kapur A, Hall RJ, Malik IS, et al: Randomized comparison of percutaneous coronary intervention with coronary artery bypass grafting in diabetic patients. 1-year results of the CARDia (Coronary Artery Revascularization in Diabetes) trial. *J Am Coll Cardiol* 55(5):432–440, 2010.
78. Kappetein AP: Three-year outcomes of the SYNTAX trial: Focus on diabetes. *Transcath Ther* Washington, DC; 2010.
79. Ellis SG, Tamai H, Nobuyoshi M, et al: Contemporary percutaneous treatment of unprotected left main coronary stenoses: initial results from a multicenter registry analysis 1994–1996. *Circulation* 96(11):3867–3872, 1997.
80. Silvestri M, Barragan P, Sainsous J, et al: Unprotected left main coronary artery stenting: immediate and medium-term outcomes of 140 elective procedures. *J Am Coll Cardiol* 35(6):1543–1550, 2000.
81. Park SJ, Park SW, Hong MK, et al: Stenting of unprotected left main coronary artery stenoses: immediate and late outcomes. *J Am Coll Cardiol* 31(1):37–42, 1998.
82. Park SJ, Hong MK, Lee CW, et al: Elective stenting of unprotected left main coronary artery stenosis: effect of debulking before stenting and intravascular ultrasound guidance. *J Am Coll Cardiol* 38(4):1054–1060, 2001.
83. Lee BK, Hong MK, Lee CW, et al: Five-year outcomes after stenting of unprotected left main coronary artery stenosis in patients with normal left ventricular function. *Int J Cardiol* 2006.
84. Park SJ, Park SW, Hong MK, et al: Long-term (three-year) outcomes after stenting of unprotected left main coronary artery stenosis in patients with normal left ventricular function. *Am J Cardiol* 91(1):12–16, 2003.
85. Park SJ, Kim YH, Lee BK, et al: Sirolimus-eluting stent implantation for unprotected left main coronary artery stenosis: comparison with bare metal stent implantation. *J Am Coll Cardiol* 45(3):351–356, 2005.
86. Chieffo A, Stankovic G, Bonizzoni E, et al: Early and mid-term results of drug-eluting stent implantation in unprotected left main. *Circulation* 111(6):791–795, 2005.
87. Valgimigli M, van Mieghem CA, Ong AT, et al: Short- and long-term clinical outcome after drug-eluting stent implantation for the percutaneous treatment of left main coronary artery disease: insights from the Rapamycin-Eluting and Taxus Stent Evaluated At Rotterdam Cardiology Hospital registries (RESEARCH and T-SEARCH). *Circulation* 111(11):1383–1389, 2005.
88. Buszman PE, Buszman PP, Kiesz RS, et al: Early and long-term results of unprotected left main coronary artery stenting: the LE MANS (Left Main Coronary Artery Stenting) registry. *J Am Coll Cardiol* 54(16):1500–1511, 2009.
89. Palmerini T, Marzocchi A, Tamburino C, et al: Two-year clinical outcome with drug-eluting stents versus bare-metal stents in a real-world registry of unprotected left main coronary artery stenosis from the Italian Society of Invasive Cardiology. *Am J Cardiol* 102(11):1463–1468, 2008.
90. Biondi-Zoccai GG, Lotrionte M, Moretti C, et al: A collaborative systematic review and meta-analysis on 1278 patients undergoing percutaneous drug-eluting stenting for unprotected left main coronary artery disease. *Am Heart J* 155(2):274–283, 2008.

91. Erglis A, Narbute I, Kumsars I, et al: A randomized comparison of paclitaxel-eluting stents versus bare-metal stents for treatment of unprotected left main coronary artery stenosis. *J Am Coll Cardiol* 50(6):491–497, 2007.

92. Mehilli J, Kastrati A, Byrne RA, et al: Paclitaxel- versus sirolimus-eluting stents for unprotected left main coronary artery disease. *J Am Coll Cardiol* 53(19):1760–1768, 2009.

93. Khattab AA, Hamm CW, Senges J, et al: Sirolimus-eluting stent treatment for unprotected versus protected left main coronary artery disease in widespread clinical routine: 6-month and 3-year clinical follow-up results from the prospective multicentre German Cypher Registry. *Heart* 93(10):1251–1255, 2007.

94. Lee MS, Kapoor N, Jamal F, et al: Comparison of coronary artery bypass surgery with percutaneous coronary intervention with drug-eluting stents for unprotected left main coronary artery disease. *J Am Coll Cardiol* 47(4):864–870, 2006.

95. Chieffo A, Morici N, Maisano F, et al: Percutaneous treatment with drug-eluting stent implantation versus bypass surgery for unprotected left main stenosis: a single-center experience. *Circulation* 113(21):2542–2547, 2006.

96. Palmerini T, Marzocchi A, Marrozzini C, et al: Comparison between coronary angioplasty and coronary artery bypass surgery for the treatment of unprotected left main coronary artery stenosis (the Bologna Registry). *Am J Cardiol* 98(1):54–59, 2006.

97. Chieffo A, Park SJ, Valgimigli M, et al: Favorable long-term outcome after drug-eluting stent implantation in nonbifurcation lesions that involve unprotected left main coronary artery: a multicenter registry. *Circulation* 116(2):158–162, 2007.

98. Kang SJ, Park DW, Mintz GS, et al: Long-term vascular changes after drug-eluting stent implantation assessed by serial volumetric intravascular ultrasound analysis. *Am J Cardiol* 105(10):1402–1408, 2010.

99. Park DW, Kim YH, Yun SC, et al: Long-term outcomes after stenting versus coronary artery bypass grafting for unprotected left main coronary artery disease: 10-year results of bare-metal stents and 5-year results of drug-eluting stents from the ASAN-MAIN (ASAN Medical Center-Left MAIN Revascularization) Registry. *J Am Coll Cardiol* 56(17):1366–1375, 2010.

100. Park DW, Seung KB, Kim YH, et al: Long-term safety and efficacy of stenting versus coronary artery bypass grafting for unprotected left main coronary artery disease: 5-year results from the MAIN-COMPARE (Revascularization for Unprotected Left Main Coronary Artery Stenosis: Comparison of Percutaneous Coronary Angioplasty Versus Surgical Revascularization) registry. *J Am Coll Cardiol* 56(2):117–124, 2010.

101. Cheng CI, Lee FY, Chang JP, et al: Long-term outcomes of intervention for unprotected left main coronary artery stenosis: coronary stenting vs coronary artery bypass grafting. *Circ J* 73(4):705–712, 2009.

102. Sanmartin M, Baz JA, Claro R, et al: Comparison of drug-eluting stents versus surgery for unprotected left main coronary artery disease. *Am J Cardiol* 100(6):970–973, 2007.

103. Serruys PW: Three-year follow-up of the SYNTAX trial: Optimal revascularization strategy in patients with left main disease. *Transcath Ther* Washington, DC; 2010.

104. Morice MC, Serruys PW, Kappetein AP, et al: Outcomes in patients with de novo left main disease treated with either percutaneous coronary intervention using paclitaxel-eluting stents or coronary artery bypass graft treatment in the Synergy Between Percutaneous Coronary Intervention with TAXUS and Cardiac Surgery (SYNTAX) trial. *Circulation* 121(24):2645–2653, 2010.

105. Boudriot E, Walter T, Liebetrau C, et al: Randomized comparison of percutaneous coronary intervention with sirolimus-eluting stents versus coronary artery bypass grafting in unprotected left main stem stenosis. *J Am Coll Cardiol* 57(5):538–545, 2011.

106. Lee MS, Yang T, Dhoot J, et al: Meta-analysis of studies comparing coronary artery bypass grafting with drug-eluting stenting in patients with diabetes mellitus and multivessel coronary artery disease. *Am J Cardiol* 105(11):1540–1544, 2010.

107. Bucher HC, Hengstler P, Schindler C, et al: Percutaneous transluminal coronary angioplasty versus medical treatment for non-acute coronary heart disease: meta-analysis of randomised controlled trials. *BMJ* 321(7253):73–77, 2000.

108. Boden WE, O'Rourke RA, Teo KK, et al: Optimal medical therapy with or without PCI for stable coronary disease. *N Engl J Med* 356(15):1503–1516, 2007.

109. Frye RL, August P, Brooks MM, et al: A randomized trial of therapies for type 2 diabetes and coronary artery disease. *N Engl J Med* 360(24):2503–2515, 2009.

110. Schömig A, Mehilli J, de Waha A, et al: A meta-analysis of 17 randomized trials of a percutaneous coronary intervention-based strategy in patients with stable coronary artery disease. *J Am Coll Cardiol* 52(11):894–904, 2008.

3

Diabetes

MARCO ROFFI | MICHAEL BRAENDLE

KEY POINTS

- Diabetes confers an equivalent cardiovascular risk to aging 15 years.

- Diabetes-associated deaths—two-thirds of them being cardiovascular—are on an exponential rise following the diabetes "epidemics" observed in western countries.

- Although mortality rates from coronary artery disease (CAD) have declined in the western world during the past 30 years and diabetic individuals have also benefited from the decline, a more than twofold higher risk of dying from CAD in men and women with diabetes has persisted over time.

- CAD is more prevalent, more severe, and occurs at younger age among patients with diabetes. Chronic hyperglycemia, dyslipidemia, and insulin resistance have been associated with an accelerated form of atherogenesis, characterized by a prothrombotic state, enhanced inflammation, and endothelial dysfunction.

- Diabetic patients undergoing coronary revascularization have worse outcomes—in the settings of both percutaneous coronary intervention (PCI) and coronary artery bypass grafting (CABG)—than nondiabetic individuals. PCI with first-generation drug-eluting stents (DESs) and CABG appear to have comparable midterm results in diabetic patients with multivessel disease in terms of death, myocardial infarction (MI), or stroke. Conversely, surgery remains superior to PCI for repeat revascularization.

- Diabetic patients with both non-ST-elevation acute coronary syndromes (ACS) and those with ST-elevation myocardial infarction (STEMI) have higher short- and long-term morbidity and mortality rates than their nondiabetic counterparts. However, they derive a greater benefit from aggressive management, including early invasive strategy, potent platelet inhibition, and primary angioplasty.

- The evidence for a cardiovascular benefit of intensive glycemic control primarily rests on the long-term follow-up of study cohorts treated early in the course of type 1 and type 2 diabetes as well as subset analyses of several large interventional trials.

- The risks of aggressive glycemic control may outweigh the benefits in some diabetic patients, such as those with diabetes of very long duration, a known history of severe hypoglycemia, poor glycemic control, advanced atherosclerosis, and advanced age or frailty.

- Aggressive modification of additional risk factors, including the control of blood pressure and cholesterol level, cigarette smoking cessation, weight loss, and exercise remain key to the prevention of cardiovascular complications in diabetic individuals.

Introduction

Diabetes mellitus is a metabolic condition characterized by dysfunction in insulin secretion and/or insulin action resulting in chronic hyperglycemia, which deeply affects the cardiovascular (CV) system. In the last few decades, the increased prevalence of diabetes has assumed epidemic proportion in western countries, and the developing world is expected to follow a similar pattern. In diabetic patients, the CV risk is magnified to a greater extent than would be expected based on the clustering of additional risk factors; that is, it has been estimated that hypertension, dyslipidemia, physical inactivity, and central obesity account for no more than 25% of the CV risk in diabetic patients. While diabetes affects both the macro- and the microvasculature, this chapter focuses just on the macrovascular aspects and specifically on CAD. For the purpose of this chapter, unless otherwise noted, the term *diabetes* refers to type 2 diabetes mellitus, which accounts for over 90% of all cases in western countries.

THE BURDEN OF THE DISEASE

According to the American Diabetes Association (ADA), in 2007 diabetes affected 23.6 million individuals in the United States, corresponding to 11% and 21% of the population over 20 and 60 years of age, respectively.[1] In the same year, 1.6 million new cases of diabetes were diagnosed. While 50% of these individuals were women, the condition remained unrecognized in 25% of those affected. In addition, the U.S. Department of Health and Human Services estimated that in 2004, approximately 40% of American adults aged 40 to 74 years, or 41 million, had prediabetes, a disturbance of glucose metabolism predisposing to overt diabetes, heart disease, and stroke.[2] Also in the United States, the prevalence of diabetes is expected to more than double from 2005 to 2050.[3] The proportional rises are projected to be largest in the elderly, with an expected increase of 220% among those 65 to 74 years of age and 450% ≥75 years of age, respectively. With respect to race, the most affected will be Hispanics, followed by African Americans. As a result, the prevalence of diabetes among African Americans >75 years of age is expected to increase by as much as 600%.[3] One report has estimated that in the year 2010, the worldwide prevalence of diabetes among adults stood at 6.4% (285 million individuals), while it is expected to increase to 7.7% (439 million individuals) by the year 2030.[4] The total estimated cost of diabetes in the United States in 2007 was $172 billion, divided into $116 billion for direct medical costs and $58 billion for indirect medical costs (e.g., disability, work loss).[1] The total healthcare cost associated with this condition is expected to rise to $192 billion by the year 2020.[5] After adjusting for age and gender, the average medical expenditures for individuals with diabetes are more than double those for their nondiabetic counterparts.

Diagnostic Criteria of Diabetes, Prediabetes, and Metabolic Syndrome

The diagnostic criteria of diabetes according to the ADA are reported in Table 3-1. In addition to the long-standing established diagnostic criteria based on fasting plasma glucose or 75-g oral glucose tolerance test, in 2009 an International Expert Committee recommended the assessment of the hemoglobin A_{1C} (HbA_{1c}) to diagnose diabetes, with a threshold of >6.5%.[6] Disturbances of the glucose metabolism, characterized by impaired fasting glucose levels or impaired glucose tolerance, can be detected long before the development of overt diabetes. These two metabolic abnormalities do negatively affect the CV system and were recently grouped under the term *prediabetes* (Table 3-1). Metabolic syndrome comprises a cluster of lipid and nonlipid risk factors of metabolic origin mediated by insulin resistance, such as pathological glucose metabolism, obesity, hypertension, and dyslipidemia. Several organizations have proposed definitions of the metabolic syndrome that may differ not only in the set of criteria included but also in the cut-offs to define the presence or absence of an individual component of the syndrome (Table 3-2). However, both the concept

TABLE 3-1	Diagnosis of Diabetes Mellitus, Impaired Glucose Tolerance, and Impaired Fasting Glucose According to the ADA

Diabetes mellitus

Hb A_{1c} >6.5%[*]

or

Fasting plasma glucose ≥126 mg/dL (7.0 mmol/L)

or

2-hour plasma glucose ≥200 mg/dL (11.1 mmol/L) during an oral glucose tolerance test (OGTT)

or

In a patient with classic symptoms of hyperglycemia or hyperglycemic crisis, a random plasma glucose ≥200 mg/dL (11.1 mmol/L).

Impaired glucose tolerance (IGT)

2-hour plasma glucose ≥140 mg/dL (7.8 mmol/L) and <200 mg/dL (11.1 mmol/L) during OGTT

Impaired fasting glucose (IFG)

Fasting plasma glucose of ≥100 mg/dL) (5.6 mmol/L) and <126 mg/dL (7 mmol/L)

[*]The test should be performed in a certified laboratory.
ADA = American Diabetes Association.
Reprinted with permission from the ADA.[101]

and the clinical utility of the metabolic syndrome have been critically appraised. Accordingly, a case-control study on the incidence of myocardial infarction (MI) performed in 52 countries and involving a total of 26,903 subjects showed that the risk of MI associated with metabolic syndrome was not greater than the sum of the risks associated with the components of this condition.[7]

Pathophysiology of Atherosclerosis in Diabetes

In patients with diabetes, CAD is more prevalent, more advanced, and occurs at a younger age compared with nondiabetic counterparts. Several metabolic abnormalities—including chronic hyperglycemia, dyslipidemia, oxidative stress, and insulin resistance—have been associated with the accelerated atherogenesis observed in diabetes (Fig. 3-1).[8] In addition to metabolic disturbances, diabetes alters the function of multiple cell lines, including endothelial cells, smooth muscle cells, and platelets. Despite the description of several peculiarities characterizing diabetes-associated atherosclerosis, the exact mechanisms underlying the initiation and progression of the atherosclerotic process remain elusive.[9]

INSULIN RESISTANCE

Insulin resistance describes a reduced sensitivity to the action of insulin observed in body tissues, thereby affecting both glucose disposal in muscles and fat and insulin-mediated suppression of hepatic glucose output. As a consequence, in patients with type 2 diabetes, higher concentrations of insulin are needed to stimulate peripheral glucose disposal and suppress hepatic glucose production. On a biologic level, insulin resistance has been associated, among others, with enhanced coagulation, proinflammation, and endothelial dysfunction. In insulin-resistant subjects, endothelium-dependent vasodilatation was found to be reduced and the degree of the impairment correlated with the severity of this metabolic abnormality. Abnormal endothelium-dependent vasodilatation in insulin-resistant states may be explained by alterations in intracellular signaling that reduce the production of endothelium-derived nitric oxide (NO). Finally, insulin resistance is associated with elevations in the levels of free fatty acids, which may also contribute to a decrease in NO synthase activity and reduced production of NO in insulin-resistant states. In addition to diabetes, clinical manifestations of insulin resistance include hypertension, dyslipidemia, and overall an increased CV risk. Even among nondiabetic patients, high fasting plasma insulin was found to be an independent risk factor for long-term mortality in patients with acute MI.

ENDOTHELIAL DYSFUNCTION AND END-OXIDATIVE STRESS

Diabetic vascular disease is characterized by endothelial dysfunction—a biological abnormality that has been related to hyperglycemia, increased production of free fatty acids, decreased bioavailability of NO, increased formation of advanced glycation end products (AGE), altered lipoproteins, hypertension, and, as previously mentioned, insulin resistance. A decreased bioavailability of NO, with subsequent impaired endothelium-dependent vasodilation, has been observed in diabetic individuals even prior to detectable atherosclerosis. Nitric

TABLE 3-2	The Metabolic Syndrome—Definitions		
	WHO (1999)	**NCEP ATP III (2001)**	**IDF (2004)**
	Impaired glucose tolerance, or diabetes and/or insulin resistance[*] together with two or more of the following:	Three or more of the following five risk factors:	Central obesity—ethnicity-specific plus any two of the following criteria:
Fasting plasma glucose		>100 mg/dL (5.6 mmol/L)[†]	≥100 mg/dL (5.6 mmol/L) or previously diagnosed diabetes
Blood pressure	≥140/90 mm Hg	≥130/≥85 mm Hg	≥130 or ≥85 mmHg or treatment of previously diagnosed hypertension
Triglycerides	≥150 mg/dl (1.7 mmol/L)	≥150 mg/dL (1.7 mmol/L)	≥150 mg/dl (1.7 mmol/L) or specific treatment for this abnormality
	and/or		
HDL cholesterol	Men: <35 mg/dl (0.9 mmol/l)	Men: <40 mg/dL (1.03 mmol/L)	<40 mg/dl (1.03 mmol/L) in males
	Women: <39 mg/dL (1.0 mmol/L)	Women: <50 mg/dL (1.29 mmol/L)	<50 mg/dL (1.29 mmol/L) in females
Obesity	Men: waist-hip ratio >0.90	Men: waist circumference >102 cm	Europid[‡] men: waist circumference ≥94 cm
	Women: waist-hip ratio >0.85 and/or BMI > 30 kg/m²	Women: waist circumference >88 cm	Europid[‡] women: waist circumference ≥80 cm
Microalbuminuria	≥20 mcg/min or albumin:creatinine ratio ≥30 mg/g		

[*]Insulin sensitivity measured under hyperinsulinemic euglycemic conditions, glucose uptake below lowest quartile for background population under investigation.
[†]The 2001 definition identified fasting plasma glucose of ≥110 mg/dL (6.1 mmol/L) as elevated. This was modified in 2004 to be ≥100 mg/dL (5.6 mmol/L), in accordance with the American Diabetes Association's updated definition of impaired fasting glucose (IFG)
[‡]The values for other ethnicities are reported in the manuscript.[101]
WHO, World Health Organization; NCEP ATP III, National Cholesterol Education Program Adult Treatment Panel III; IDF, International Diabetes Federation.
Adapted with permission from Alberti et al.[102]

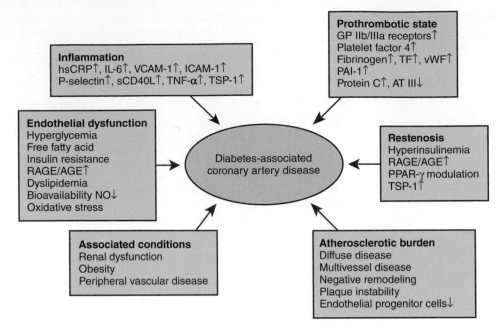

Figure 3-1 Pathophysiology of diabetes mellitus-associated coronary artery disease. hs-CRP = high-sensitivity C-reactive protein; IL-6 = interleukin-6; VCAM-1 = vascular cell adhesion molecule-1; ICAM-1 = intracellular adhesion molecule-1; sCD40L = soluble CD40 ligand; TNF-α = tumor necrosis factor-α; TSP-1 = thrombospondin-1; RAGE = receptor for advanced glycation end-products (AGE); GP = glycoprotein; TF = tissue factor; vWF = von Willebrand factor; PAI-1 = plasminogen activator inhibitor-1; AT = antithrombin; PPAR-γ = peroxisome proliferator-activated receptor-γ. (*Adapted with permission from Roffi M, Topol EJ. Percutaneous coronary intervention in diabetic patients with non-ST-segment elevation acute coronary syndromes. Eur Heart J. 2004;25:190–198.*)

oxide is a potent vasodilator and a key compound of the endothelium-mediated control mechanisms of vascular relaxation. In addition, it inhibits platelet activation, limits inflammation by reducing leukocyte adhesion to endothelium and migration into the vessel wall, and reduces the proliferation and migration of vascular smooth muscle cells. As a consequence, intact NO metabolism in the vessel wall has a protective effect by inhibiting atherogenesis. The impaired vasodilatation observed among diabetic individuals may also be due to an increased production of vasoconstrictors, particularly endothelin-1. Despite the evidence of increased endothelin-1, angiotensin II, and abnormal sympathetic nervous system activity, the mechanisms of vascular smooth muscle cell dysfunction and hypertension in diabetes remain elusive. The formation of AGE is the consequence of the oxidation of amino groups by glucose. Additional processes induced by augmented AGE production include subendothelial cellular proliferation and matrix expression, cytokine release, macrophage activation, and expression of adhesion molecules. Although the underlying mechanisms remain incompletely understood, it has been postulated that oxidative stress due to chronic hyperglycemia plays an important role in the etiology of diabetic complications. Hyperglycemia may induce the production of reactive oxygen species in the mitochondria of the endothelial cells directly via glucose metabolism and auto-oxidation and indirectly through the formation of AGE and their receptor binding, suggesting links between hyperglycemia, AGE, and oxidative stress.

PROTHROMBOTIC STATE

The observation that diabetic patients are characterized by a hypercoagulable state is based on both clinical and laboratory findings. The prothrombotic state seen in diabetes is related to endothelial dysfunction, impaired fibrinolysis, increased levels of coagulation factors, and enhanced platelet reactivity. Manifestations of atherothrombosis include sudden cardiac death, ACS, ischemic stroke, peripheral arterial ischemia (i.e., intermittent claudication and critical limb ischemia), and coronary stent thrombosis. An angioscopic study performed in ACS patients revealed that plaque ulceration and intracoronary thrombus were more frequent among diabetic patients than in nondiabetic individuals. Similarly, the incidence of thrombus was found to be higher in atherectomy specimens from patients with diabetes undergoing PCI than in those from nondiabetic patients. With respect to

laboratory findings, subjects at various stages of diabetes proved to have increased numbers of activated platelets compared with healthy controls. Accordingly, platelets of diabetic individuals have a greater platelet activation and aggregation response to shear stress and platelet-activating agonists. In addition, an increased platelet-surface expression of the glycoprotein (GP) Ib receptor, which mediates binding to von Willebrand factor, and of the GP IIb/IIIa receptor, which mediates platelet-fibrin interaction, has been described. Finally, basal thromboxane B(2) is significantly increased in resting platelets from diabetic patients even in the absence of vascular complications and in cases of well-controlled diabetes. Moreover, both decreased endothelial production of the antiaggregants NO—as previously mentioned—and prostacyclin; increased levels of procoagulant agents such as fibrinogen, tissue factor, von Willebrand factor, platelet factor 4, and factor VII; and decreased concentrations of endogenous anticoagulants such as protein C and antithrombin III have been documented (Fig. 3-1). Finally, elevated levels of plasminogen activator inhibitor-1 (PAI-1) may impair endogenous tissue plasminogen activator-mediated fibrinolysis. Overall, diabetes is characterized by increased intrinsic platelet activation, decreased endogenous inhibition of platelet activity, and increased blood coagulation in the presence of impaired endogenous fibrinolysis.

INFLAMMATORY STATE

Inflammation has been related not only to acute CV events but also to the initiation and progression of atherosclerosis. Several CV risk factors, including diabetes, may trigger an inflammatory state. Although it is plausible that metabolic disturbances associated with diabetes trigger vascular inflammation, the converse may also be true. Accordingly, C-reactive protein (CRP), a key proinflammatory cytokine in patients with atherosclerosis, has been shown to independently predict the risk of developing type 2 diabetes. Inflammatory parameters are elevated in diabetes; in the context of insulin resistance in the absence of overt diabetes, these include high-sensitivity CRP, Il-6, tumor necrosis factor (TNF)-α, and a circulating/soluble form of CD40 ligand (sCD40L) (Fig. 3-1). In addition, an increased expression of adhesion molecules such as endothelial (E)-selectin VCAM-1 and ICAM-1 has been detected. The morphological substrate of increased vascular inflammatory activity can be derived by an analysis of coronary atherectomy specimen of ACS patients, showing that tissue from diabetic patients exhibited a larger content of lipid-rich atheromas and a more pronounced macrophage infiltration compared with specimens from nondiabetic individuals. The receptor for AGE (RAGE) may play an important role in inflammatory processes and endothelial activation, likely accelerating the processes of coronary atherosclerotic development, especially in diabetic patients. It has been demonstrated that CRP upregulates RAGE expression in endothelial cells. These observations reinforce the mechanistic link in diabetes among inflammation, endothelial dysfunction, atherothrombosis, and, as detailed below, accelerated restenosis.

PLAQUE INSTABILITY AND IMPAIRED VASCULAR REPAIR

In addition to promoting atherogenesis, diabetes is associated with plaque instability. Accordingly, it has been shown that atherosclerotic lesions in diabetic patients contain fewer vascular smooth muscle cells compared with lesions in controls. As the source of collagen, vascular smooth muscle cells strengthen the atheroma, making it less likely to rupture and cause thrombosis. In addition, diabetic endothelial cells may produce an excess of cytokines, which decrease the de novo synthesis of collagen by vascular smooth muscle cells. Finally, diabetes enhances the production of matrix metalloproteinases, which lead to the breakdown of collagen, potentially decreasing the mechanical stability of the plaque's fibrous cap. Overall, diabetes alters vascular smooth muscle function in ways that promote the formation of atherosclerotic lesions, plaque instability, and clinical events. In addition, it has been demonstrated that the coronary arteries of diabetic patients, more frequently than those in nondiabetic individuals, have lipid-rich plaques, which are known to be more prone to rupture. Moreover, observations have suggested that human endothelial progenitor cells, which are supposed to be important regulators of vascular repair, exhibit impaired proliferation, adhesion, and incorporation into the vascular structures of diabetic patients. In addition to the dysfunction already described, it has been found that in culture, the number of endothelial progenitor cells obtained from diabetic patients was reduced compared with those obtained from age- and sex-matched control subjects, and that this reduction was inversely related to HbA$_{1c}$ levels. An investigation has documented that the level of endothelial progenitor cells was particularly low among diabetic patients with peripheral arterial disease; the investigators hypothesized that depletion of this cell line may be involved in the pathogenesis of diabetic complications of the peripheral vasculature. Overall, in diabetes mellitus, atherosclerosis develops more aggressively and faster, leading more frequently to thrombotic events through the interaction between a vessel wall prone to plaque rupture and hypercoagulable blood. Finally, a link between macrovascular and microvascular disease in diabetes has been suggested, with hyperglycemia being the driving force for both large- and small-vessel disease. Accordingly, both increased angiogenesis and microangiopathy may contribute to accelerated atherosclerosis and the development of vulnerable plaque through processes such as hypoxia and changes in the vasa vasorum.

Cardiovascular Disease in Diabetes

Adults with diabetes have a CV death rate that is up to fourfold greater than that of nondiabetic individuals. Moreover, among diabetic individuals, CVD accounts for over two-thirds of total mortality.[2] With respect to gender, the adjusted risk of CV death among diabetic men is three times greater than that among their nondiabetic peers. Among diabetic women, the risk may be as high as sixfold as great as it is among those who are not diabetic. A population-based study has estimated that diabetes confers an equivalent CV risk to aging 15 years.[10] Although in the western countries, such as the United States, the age-adjusted mortality rates of other major multifactorial diseases such as CAD, stroke, or cancer have declined or remained stable over the last 20 years, the diabetes "epidemic" has led to a 30% increase of

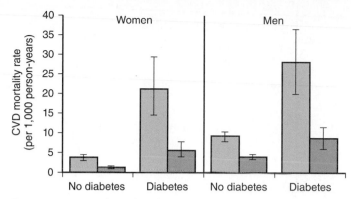

Figure 3-2 Age-adjusted cardiovascular disease (CVD) mortality rates among participants in their Framingham Heart Study with and without diabetes mellitus by sex and time period. Green bars represent earlier time period (1950 to 1975); gray bars represent later time period (1976 to 2001). *(Reproduced with permission from Preis SR, Hwang SJ, Coady S, et al. Trends in all-cause and cardiovascular disease mortality among women and men with and without diabetes mellitus in the Framingham Heart Study, 1950 to 2005. Circulation. 2009;119:1728–1735.)*

diabetes-related deaths in the same time span.[11] Nevertheless, the Framingham Heart Study documented a major reduction in CV mortality in both diabetic (hazard ratio [HR] 0.31) and nondiabetic (HR 0.38) individuals enrolled in the years 1975 to 2001 compared with those enrolled in the years 1950 to 1975 (Fig. 3-2).[12] The absolute benefit was dramatic in the diabetic population, with mortality going from 24.1 to 6.8 per 1,000 person-years. Among nondiabetic individuals, it went from 6.3 to 2.4 per 1,000 person-years. Although mortality rates from CAD have declined in the western world during the past 30 years and people with diabetes have also benefited from this decline, the more than twofold higher risk of dying from CAD in men and women with diabetes has persisted over time.[13] In 2001, the Adult Treatment Panel III of the National Cholesterol Education Program (NCEP ATP III) recommended considering diabetes as a CAD risk equivalent, therefore mandating aggressive CV prevention.[14] This notion has been confirmed by a study including all residents in Denmark at least 30 years of age and following them for 5 years by individual-level linkage of nationwide registers. At baseline, 71,801 (2.2%) had diabetes mellitus and 79,575 (2.4%) had a prior MI. Regardless of age, the age-adjusted Cox proportional HR for cardiovascular death was 2.4 both in men with diabetes mellitus without a prior MI and in nondiabetic men with a prior MI, with nondiabetics without prior MI as the reference (Fig. 3-3).[15]

THE ANATOMICAL PATTERN OF CORONARY ARTERY DISEASE

Autopsy and angiographic studies have shown that patients with diabetes more frequently have left main coronary artery lesions, multivessel disease, and diffuse CAD. An angiographic study on patients with angina has demonstrated that the greater the impairment of glucose metabolism (i.e., normal, impaired glucose tolerance, newly diagnosed diabetes, and known diabetes) the smaller the average vessel diameter and the longer the coronary lesions. It is a common belief that diabetic patients, compared with their nondiabetic counterparts, have an impaired ability to develop coronary collaterals. However, a study measuring coronary collateral flow using intracoronary pressure and Doppler guidewires did not find such differences between diabetic and nondiabetic patients in the setting of stable CAD. Finally, intravascular ultrasound studies have shown that the coronary arteries of diabetic patients are less likely to undergo favorable remodeling—an early compensatory enlargement at atherosclerotic sites—in response to atherosclerosis.

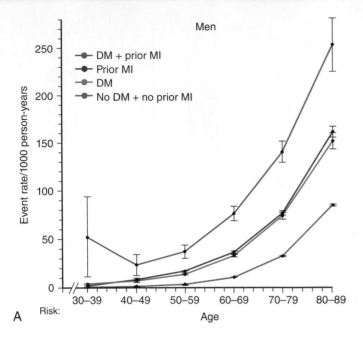

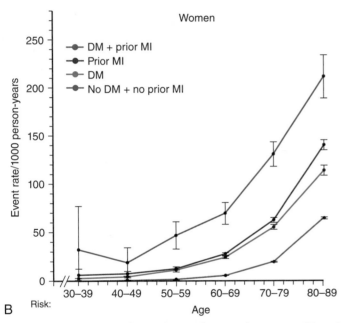

Figure 3-3 Event rates for cardiovascular mortality in men (A) and women (B) stratified by age and sex in relation to diabetes mellitus (DM) and prior myocardial infarction (MI). *(Reproduced with permission from Schramm TK, Gislason GH, Kober L, et al. Diabetes patients requiring glucose-lowering therapy and nondiabetics with a prior myocardial infarction carry the same cardiovascular risk: a population study of 3.3 million people. Circulation. 2008;117:1945–1954.)*

PERIPHERAL ARTERIAL AND CEREBROVASCULAR DISEASE

Epidemiological evidence confirms an association between diabetes and peripheral artery disease, with an incidence estimated to range between twofold and more than fourfold compared with nondiabetic individuals. In the Framingham cohort, the presence of diabetes increased the risk of claudication fourfold in men and ninefold in women. A study addressing the prevalence of peripheral artery disease among patients according to the degree of associated metabolic disturbance found that the rate of abnormal ankle-brachial indices ranged

between 7% in individuals with normal glucose tolerance and 21% in those requiring multiple antidiabetic medications. Diabetes-associated vascular disease of the lower extremities is characterized by extensive vascular calcification and a more frequent infrapopliteal involvement. The lower limb amputation rate among diabetic patients is up to 13-fold compared with that among nondiabetic individuals. In 2004, over 71,000 lower limb amputations were performed in U.S. patients with diabetes, corresponding to over 60% of all nontraumatic lower limb amputations.[16] Similar to what has been observed in the coronary and peripheral arterial circulation, diabetes triggers cerebrovascular disease. Accordingly, patients with diabetes more commonly have more advanced extracranial and intracranial atherosclerosis than do nondiabetic individuals. Case-control stroke studies and prospective epidemiological data have correlated poor glycemic control and stroke risk and have identified diabetes as an independent predictor of ischemic stroke, with an increased risk ranging from 1.8-fold to nearly 6-fold.[2] Particularly ominous is the impact of diabetes in individuals below 55 years of age, with a greater than 10-fold increased risk of stroke. Finally, diabetes increases the risk of stroke-related dementia more than threefold, doubles the risk of recurrence, and increases total and stroke-related mortality.

Cardiovascular Diagnostic Modalities in Diabetic Patients

Diabetic patients have significantly higher rates of silent ischemia than the general population. It has been estimated that in the United States, as many as 12.5 million diabetic patients may have asymptomatic CAD.[17] In the absence of typical symptoms, diabetic patients may suffer from myocardial ischemia more frequently than their nondiabetic counterparts, and most studies investigating the prevalence of silent ischemia have found higher rates in diabetic patients. The FIELD (Fenofibrate Intervention and Event Lowering in Diabetes) study followed 9,795 diabetic patients aged 50 to 75 years with routine ECG for a mean of 5 years.[18] In this study, 37% of all MIs identified were silent. Older age, longer diabetes duration, prior CVD, higher HbA$_{1c}$ levels, and albuminuria independently predicted the risk of silent MI. The diagnostic and prognostic value of stress testing diabetic patients has been extensively investigated (Tables 3-3 and 3-4).[19] Exercise ECG testing is a well-established and inexpensive test to guide the clinician in the diagnosis and risk stratification of diabetic patients with suspected CAD. Sensitivity and specificity for the diagnosis of CAD in diabetic patients presenting with angina and in nondiabetic patients appear comparable. In asymptomatic patients, an abnormal exercise ECG test may be helpful to identify a subgroup of patients with advanced CAD. Patients with a negative stress test in the presence of normal exercise capacity are at low risk of CV events, at least in the short run. Stress nuclear imaging has the most extensive literature among the noninvasive imaging modalities for both diagnostic and prognostic purposes in diabetes. With respect to stress echocardiography, several studies have addressed its prognostic accuracy in diabetes, while the data on its diagnostic value are scarce (Tables 3-3 and 3-4).[19] The assessment of coronary artery calcium is a well-established index of atherosclerosis. Electron beam computed tomography (CT) and multidetector CT make it possible to measure the calcium content of coronary arteries, and a scoring system has been developed to that purpose. Several studies have identified the coronary artery calcium score as a strong predictor for CV events and all-cause mortality in diabetic individuals. The PREDICT (Prospective Evaluation of Diabetic Ischaemic Disease by Computed Tomography) study evaluated prospectively calcium score as a predictor of CV events in 589 asymptomatic individuals with type 2 diabetes.[20] The risk of a CV event rose with an increased calcium score (Fig. 3-4). In addition, calcium score had greater predictive value for events than a broad range of conventional and novel risk factors. Finally, a prospective cohort study in West London found that calcium score was superior to established risk factors in predicting the presence of silent myocardial ischemia on

TABLE 3-3	Summary of Studies Using Stress Testing in the Diagnosis of Suspected CAD in Diabetic Patients							
Type of Test	*Study*	*DM Subjects, n*	*Reference Standard*	*Sensitivity, %*	*Specificity, %*	*PPV, %*	*NPV, %*
ECG	Lee et al.	190	Angiography	47	81	85	41
DSE	Hennessy et al.	52	Angiography	82	54	84	50
Nuclear	Kang et al.	138	Angiography	86	56	NA	NA

CAD, coronary artery disease; PPV, positive predictive value; NPV, negative predictive value; ECG, exercise ECG stress test; DSE, dobutamine stress echocardiography; NA, not available; DM, diabetes mellitus.

Reprinted with permission from Albers et al.,[19] in which the references can be found.

perfusion scans.[21] The introduction of coronary CT angiography has changed the field of noninvasive imaging. In addition to existing functional imaging techniques assessing myocardial perfusion and wall motion, CT angiography allows for the detection of both coronary stenoses and calcified and noncalcified plaques. In asymptomatic diabetic individuals, coronary CT angiography revealed a high prevalence of occult CAD (between 64% and 92%) with a high proportion of significant coronary stenosis.[22] A German study of 140 asymptomatic diabetic individuals suggests that an atherosclerotic burden score based on the number of diseased coronary segments on coronary CT angiography may significantly improve the risk prediction for CV events over and above conventional risk-factor assessment.[23] A study of 313 diabetic patients, mean age 62 years, suggested that the negative predictive value of this imaging modality was excellent, since the mortality was 0% over a mean follow-up of 20 months among those with no evidence of disease.[24] The extent of screening for CAD in asymptomatic diabetic patients is a source of controversy. Cardiac testing should be considered in the presence of features of increased CV risk such as peripheral or cerebrovascular disease, renal disease, albuminuria, abnormal resting ECG, diabetic complications, and both traditional and novel CV risk factors.[25] In the DIAD (Detection of Ischemia in Asymptomatic Diabetics) study, 1,123 diabetic participants with no symptoms of CAD were randomly assigned to adenosine stress radionuclide myocardial perfusion imaging or no screening in addition to optimal medical treatment.[26] At a mean follow-up of 4.8 years, the cumulative cardiac death or MI was 2.9% (0.6% per year), with no difference between the two groups. In the screened group, participants with normal results (N = 409) or small defects (N = 50) had lower event rates than the 33 patients with moderate or large defects on perfusion imaging (0.4% per year vs. 2.4% per year [HR 6.3, P = 0.001]) (Fig. 3-5). Nevertheless, the positive predictive value of having moderate or large defects on perfusion scans was only 12%. The overall rate of coronary revascularization was low in both groups (5.5% in the screened group and 7.8% in the unscreened group). The authors concluded that more aggressive screening for CAD did not improve the outcome of asymptomatic diabetic patients over optimal medical therapy and lifestyle modification. However, because the event rates were lower than estimated, the study was underpowered. In addition, among 33 patients with moderate to large perfusion defects detected by screening, the rate of coronary angiography was only 15%.

Revascularization in Diabetic Patients with Stable Coronary Disease

Nearly 1.5 million coronary revascularization procedures, either CABG or PCI, are performed each year in the United States, and approximately one-quarter of them involve diabetic patients.[27] Despite improvements in the management of diabetic patients undergoing coronary revascularization—both from a pharmacological and medical device standpoint—diabetes remains an independent predictor of CV events following percutaneous and surgical revascularization. Until recently, comparative data between medical management and revascularization for the diabetic population were sparse. Similarly, little data—mainly derived from subgroup analyses of trials initiated in the late 1980s and early 1990s—were available on the safety and efficacy of PCI versus CABG. However, high-quality comparative data are now available on medical management versus revascularization and on PCI with drug-eluting stents (DESs) versus CABG in diabetic patients. For the choice of revascularization in the individual diabetic patient, several parameters should be taken into account, such as clinical presentation (ACS vs. stable CAD), coronary anatomy, left ventricular function, coexisting conditions, and patient preference (Fig. 3-6).

PERCUTANEOUS CORONARY INTERVENTION

While in-hospital and 30-day outcomes after PCI in diabetic patients have frequently been found to be comparable with those in their nondiabetic counterparts, invariably diabetes remained associated with increased target-vessel revascularization (TVR), major adverse cardiovascular and cerebrovascular events (MACCE), and late mortality. Although stenting has definitely improved the outcomes of diabetic patients undergoing PCI compared with balloon angioplasty, in-stent restenosis remained a challenge for PCI. Accordingly, the outcomes of

TABLE 3-4	Summary of Studies Using Stress Testing in the Diagnosis of CAD in Asymptomatic Diabetic Patients							
Type of Test	*Study*	*DM Subjects, n*	*Reference Standard*	*Sensitivity, %*	*Specificity, %*	*PPV, %*	*NPV, %*
ECG	Blandine et al.	98	Angiography	NA	NA	90	NA
ECG	Koistinen et al.	136	Angiography	NA	NA	94	NA
ECG	Bacci et al.	206	Angiography	NA	NA	79	NA
ECG	Penfornis et al.	56	Angiography	NA	NA	60	NA
DSE	Penfornis et al.	56	Angiography	NA	NA	69	NA
Nuclear	Blandine et al.	103	Angiography	NA	NA	63	NA
Nuclear	Wackers et al.	1123	None	NA	NA	NA	NA
Nuclear	Rajagopalan et al.	1427	Angiography	92	68	89	60
Nuclear	Penfornis et al.	56	Angiography	NA	NA	75	NA

CAD, coronary artery disease; PPV, positive predictive value; NPV, negative predictive value; ECG, exercise ECG stress test; DSE, dobutamine stress echocardiography; NA, not available; DM, diabetes mellitus.

Reprinted with permission from Albers et al.,[19] in which the references can be found.

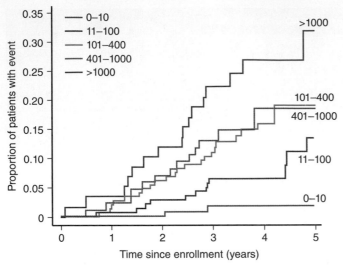

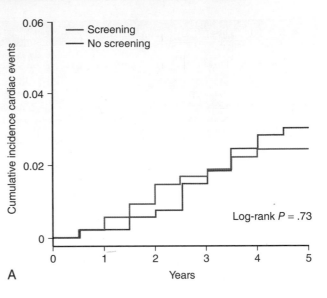

Figure 3-4 Proportions of patients with an event with increasing time since recruitment into the PREDICT study in successive coronary artery calcification score categories (Agatston units). *(Reproduced with permission from Elkeles RS, Godsland IF, Feher MD, et al. Coronary calcium measurement improves prediction of cardiovascular events in asymptomatic patients with type 2 diabetes: the PREDICT study. Eur Heart J. 2008;29:2244–2251.)*

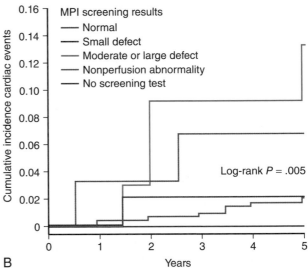

Figure 3-5 A. Cumulative incidence of cardiac events in 561 participants randomized to systematic baseline screening with stress myocardial perfusion imaging (MPI) and 562 participants randomized to receive no screening in the DIAD study. B. Cumulative incidence of cardiac events according to results of systematic screening with stress MPI: normal, small defect, moderate or large defect, and nonperfusion abnormality. *(Data from Young LH, Wackers FJ, Chyun DA, et al. Cardiac outcomes after screening for asymptomatic coronary artery disease in patients with type 2 diabetes: the DIAD study: a randomized controlled trial. JAMA. 2009;301:1547–1555.)*

diabetic patients remained unfavorable in large-scale registries and subgroup analyses of clinical trials compared with those of their nondiabetic counterparts despite a broad use of bare metal stents (BMSs). A metanalysis of six trials with BMSs published up to 2002, including 1,166 diabetic and 5,070 nondiabetic patients, identified diabetes as an independent predictor of restenosis (odds ratio [OR] 1.3), and the restenosis rate in diabetic patients was 37%.[28] Similar observations were made in a restenosis trial including a large diabetic population (N = 2,694) undergoing BMS implantation, the PRESTO (Prevention of REStenosis with Tranilast and its Outcomes) study.[29] No difference in in-hospital events was observed between diabetic and nondiabetic patients. But after adjusting for baseline characteristics, diabetes was identified as independent predictor of death (relative risk [RR] 1.9) and TVR (RR 1.3) at 9 months. Drug-eluting stents have revolutionized the field of interventional cardiology by dramatically reducing the incidence of restenosis and, as a consequence, of the need for TVR. However, even in the DES era, diabetic patients have worse outcomes compared with those who are nondiabetic. The EVASTENT matched multicenter cohort registry enrolled 1,731 patients undergoing DES implantation (sirolimus-eluting stent, Cypher, Cordis). For each diabetic patient enrolled (stratified as single- or multiple-vessel disease), a nondiabetic patient was subsequently included.[30] The median follow-up was 465 days, and 1-year follow-up was available for 98.5% of patients. The worst outcomes were observed among diabetic patients with multivessel disease, while diabetic patients with single-vessel disease had outcomes similar to those of nondiabetic individuals with multivessel disease (Fig. 3-7). Overall, diabetic patients had higher 1-year mortality, stent thrombosis, and TVR rates, and the group at higher risk were diabetic patients treated with insulin. With respect to DES in diabetic patients, an initial subgroup analysis on four DES-versus-BMS trials including 428 patients showed that DES implantation was associated with a statistically significant increase in CV mortality at 4 years (adjusted HR 3.0).[31] However, a harmful effect of DESs in diabetic patients could not be reproduced in subsequent studies that were adequately powered. A network metanalysis of 35 randomized trials comparing DES with BMS and including 3,852 diabetic patients showed that DESs, while not affecting overall mortality or MI rates in diabetic patients, were associated with a sizable reduction in target-lesion revascularization (TLR), with a relative RR of 60%

to 70% (depending on the type of stent used) and absolute RR of ~16% (Fig. 3-8).[32] An analysis of all patients undergoing PCI in nonfederal hospitals in Massachusetts between April 2003 and September 2004 included 5,051 diabetic patients and allowed for a comparison of two propensity-matched diabetic cohorts of 1,476 patients each.[33] While the unadjusted cumulative incidence of mortality at 3 years was 14.4% in the DES group and 22.2% in the BMS group (P < 0.001), the corresponding risk-adjusted mortality, MI, and TVR rates at 3 years in propensity-matched cohorts were 17.5% versus 20.7% (P = 0.02), 13.8% versus 16.9% (P = 0.02), and 18.4% versus 23.7% (P < 0.001), respectively. Despite these encouraging results, concerns persist over the risk of DES thrombosis in diabetic patients. Accordingly some trials and registries, albeit not all, have identified diabetes mellitus and particularly insulin-requiring diabetes as an

CORONARY ANATOMY	CLINICAL SETTING	CO-EXISTING CONDITIONS
SYNTAX score	Stable CAD	EUROSCORE
Targets adequate/not adequate for CABG	Non-ST-ACS	STS score
Lesions can/cannot be treated with PCI	STEMI	Ventricular function
Ischemic burden	Cardiogenic shock	Age
		Valvular heart disease
PATIENT-RELATED FACTORS		Renal insufficiency
Frailty		Pulmonary disease
Preference		Coagulation or bleeding disorders
Compliance to antiplatelet agents		Cerebrovascular disease
Tolerance of dual antiplatelet therapy		Peripheral vascular disease
Scheduled non-cardiac surgery		Previous cardiac surgery
Need for anticoagulation		Limited life expectancy

Figure 3-6 Parameters guiding the choice of revascularization strategy in diabetic patients. STEMI = ST-elevation myocardial infarction; ACS = acute coronary syndromes; CAD = coronary artery disease; CABG = coronary artery bypass grafting; PCI = percutaneous coronary interventions; STS = Society of Thoracic Surgery.

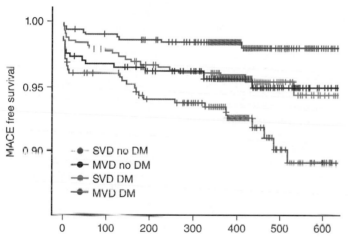

Figure 3-7 Major adverse cardiac and cerebrovascular event (MACCE)-free survival rates according to the presence of diabetes and the number of diseased vessels in the EVASTENT study. MVD = multivessel disease; SVD: single vessel disease; dm = diabetes mellitus. (*Reproduced with permission from Machecourt J, Danchin N, Lablanche JM, et al. Risk factors for stent thrombosis after implantation of sirolimus-eluting stents in diabetic and nondiabetic patients: the EVASTENT Matched-Cohort Registry. J Am Coll Cardiol. 2007;50:501–508.*)

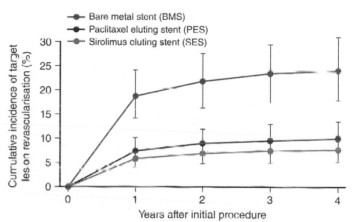

Figure 3-8 Cumulative incidence of target-lesion revascularization and corresponding hazard ratios (95% credibility intervals) for three stent types estimated from a network metanalysis for pairwise comparisons in patients with diabetes. BMS = bare metal stent; SES = sirolimus-eluting stent (Cypher, Cordis); PED = paclitaxel-eluting stent (Taxs, Boston Scientific). (*Reproduced with permission from Stettler C, Allemann S, Wandel S, et al. Drug eluting and bare metal stents in people with and without diabetes: collaborative network meta-analysis. BMJ. 2008;337:a1331.*)

independent predictor of late DES thrombosis. In the previously described EVASTENT matched cohort registry, the 1-year stent thrombosis rate was 3.5% and 1.8% ($P < 0.033$) in diabetic and nondiabetic patients, respectively.[30] Among diabetic individuals, stent thrombosis occurred in 4.3% in the presence of multivessel disease and in 2.3% in single-vessel disease, while in nondiabetic individuals the corresponding rates were 3.0% and 0.8% ($P = 0.03$). Insulin-requiring diabetes was identified as independent predictor of stent thrombosis (OR 2.9, $P = 0.004$). Similarly, in a large trial of patients undergoing PCI for ACS, approximately half were treated with DESs and half with BMSs. At a median follow-up of 14 months, the rate of stent thrombosis was 2.8% and 1.4% (HR 2.0; $P < 0.0001$) respectively in diabetic ($N = 3,146$) and nondiabetic ($N = 10462$) individuals.[34] In the diabetic subgroup, the rates of stent thrombosis for patients treated with insulin ($N = 776$) and those on oral hypoglycemic drugs were 3.7% and 2.5%,

respectively. Sufficient comparative data among DESs for diabetic patients are available only for the first-generation devices, namely the sirolimus-eluting stent Cypher (Cordis) and the paclitaxel-eluting stent Taxus (Boston Scientific). A metanalysis of five head-to-head studies dedicated to a diabetic patient population (total $N = 1,173$) demonstrated that the sirolimus-eluting stent was significantly more effective with respect to TLR (5.1% vs. 11.4%; OR 0.41, $P < 0.001$) and angiographic binary restenosis (5.6% vs. 16.4%; OR 0.30, $P < 0.001$) compared with the paclitaxel-eluting stent. With respect to cardiac death (2.2% vs. 2.9%), MI (1.5% vs. 2.6%), and stent thrombosis (0.6% vs. 1.2%), no statistically significant differences were identified.

With respect to second-generation DESs, a subgroup analysis of the diabetic population ($N = 414$) of the head-to-head trial comparing the biolimus-eluting stent (Bomatrix, Biosensor) and the sirolimus-eluting stent (Cypher) showed no difference in death, MI, or TVR at

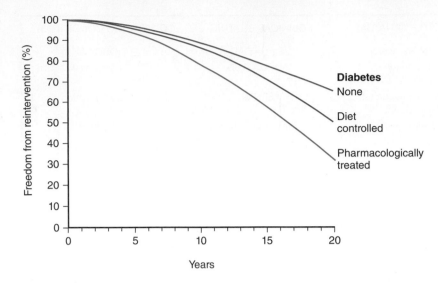

Figure 3-9 Predicted freedom from repeat coronary revascularization after coronary artery bypass surgery stratified by diabetes mellitus and its treatment. *(Reprinted with permission from Sabik JF, Blackstone EH, Gillinov AM, et al. Occurrence and risk factors for reintervention after coronary artery bypass grafting. Circulation. 2006;114(1 Suppl):I454–1460.)*

9 months.[35] Similarly, a subgroup analysis for the diabetic population (*N* = 1,140) of the head-to-head trial allocating patients to the everolimus-eluting stent (Xience, Abbott) and the Taxus stent showed no difference in the target-lesion failure at 1 year (6.4% vs. 6.9%).[36]

CORONARY ARTERY BYPASS SURGERY

Paralleling what was described for PCI, diabetes still negatively affects outcomes following CABG. The impact of diabetes on morbidity and mortality in patients undergoing surgical coronary revascularization was addressed in a retrospective analysis of the Society of Thoracic Surgery database, including 41,663 diabetic patients among a total population of 146,786.[37] At 30 days, the mortality was significantly higher in the diabetes group (3.7% vs. 2.7%). The unadjusted and adjusted mortality OR for diabetes were 1.4 and 1.2, respectively. With respect to diabetes treatments at presentation, the adjusted mortality OR for patients on oral hypoglycemic drugs and on insulin were 1.1 and 1.4, respectively. In addition, the overall morbidity and the infection rates were significantly higher among diabetic patients. Looking into long-term mortality following CABG, a prospective cohort study including 11,186 consecutive diabetic patients and 25,455 nondiabetic patients undergoing CABG from 1992 to 2001 detected a significantly higher annual mortality rate among diabetic patients (5.5%) compared with nondiabetic individuals (3.1%).[38] The annual mortality increased to 8.4%, 16.3%, and 26.3% among diabetic patients with vascular disease, renal failure, or both, respectively. In addition to increased periprocedural morbidity and mortality as well as long-term mortality, diabetic patients must undergo repeat revascularization following CABG more frequently than their nondiabetic counterparts. A prospective single-center analysis on 26,927 patients who were contacted every 5 years up to 25 years following CABG identified diabetes as an independent predictor of subsequent coronary revascularization (Fig. 3-9).[39] As part of the metabolic syndrome, diabetes is frequently associated with obesity, hypertension, and hypertriglyceridemia. Using a single-center database that included 6,428 patients undergoing CABG, the impact of these four factors (the "deadly quartet") on 8-year mortality following CABG was assessed.[40] Compared with individuals with no risk factors, the HR for mortality increased from 1.6 for one risk factor to 3.9 for four risk factors. The yearly mortality ranged from 1% in patients with no risk factors to 3.3% in patients with four risk factors. The use of multiple arterial conduits, including bilateral internal mammary grafts, has been shown to improve the long-term results of CABG and to reduce the need for repeat revascularization. A retrospective analysis of the Montreal Heart Institute of 4,382 patients undergoing CABG compared the outcomes of diabetic and nondiabetic patients according to the use of a single (SIMA) or bilateral internal mammary artery (BIMA). Outcomes of diabetic and nondiabetic patients undergoing grafting with a SIMA (*n* = 419 and 2,079) or BIMA (*n* = 214 and 1,594) were addressed at a mean follow-up of 11 years. Cox regression analysis with interaction term and propensity scoring showed that BIMA grafting significantly decreased the risk of death (HR = 0.72) and coronary reoperation (HR = 0.38) in both diabetic and nondiabetic patients.[41] The Leipzig experience with 1,515 consecutive patients who underwent BIMA grafting included 519 diabetic patients. Multiple regression analysis showed that, in addition to repeat operation (OR 12.7), both non-insulin-dependent (OR 4.6) and insulin-dependent patients with diabetes mellitus (OR 6.9) had a significantly increased risk of sternal infection.[42] The ART (Arterial Revascularisation Trial) randomized 3,102 patients to SIMA or BIMA with a primary outcome of survival at 10 years. A mean of three grafts were applied in both groups and 41% of the procedures were performed off pump. Mortality at 30 days was 1.2% in both groups, while at 1 year it was 2.3% in the SIMA group and 2.5% in the BIMA group (Fig. 3-10).[43] The rates of stroke, MI, and repeat revascularization were

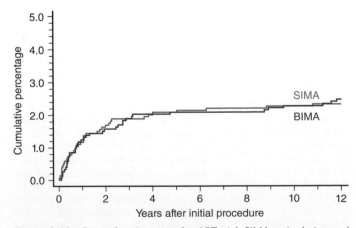

Figure 3-10 Survival to 1 year in the ART trial. SIMA = single internal mammary artery; BIMA = bilateral internal mammary artery. *(Reproduced with permission from Taggart DP, Altman DG, Gray AM, Lees B, Nugara F, Yu LM, Campbell H, Flather M. Randomized trial to compare bilateral vs. single internal mammary coronary artery bypass grafting: 1-year results of the Arterial Revascularisation Trial (ART). Eur Heart J. 2010;31:2470–2481.)*

all ≤2% at 1 year and similar between the two groups. Sternal wound reconstruction for infection was required in 0.6% and 1.9% of the SIMA and BIMA groups, respectively (RR 3.2, 95% CI 1.5–6.8). The results of the ART suggest that the use of BIMA grafts is feasible on a routine basis. The 10-year outcome analysis of the study will show whether BIMA grafting results in lower mortality and the need for repeat intervention. While no outcome data for the diabetes subgroup ($N = 734$) are available, it is notable that diabetic patients suffered half of all sternal wound reconstructions, although they accounted for only 24% of the studied population. At this time it is unknown whether the increased risk of sternal wound infection associated with BIMA grafting in diabetic patients will be counterbalanced by a long-term benefit in terms of MACCE. Despite the overall encouraging results of BIMA grafting, a cross-sectional observational study on over half a million CABG surgeries performed in the United States between 2002 and 2005 showed that this revascularization technique was performed in only 4% of the patient population.[44] With respect to the impact of off-pump surgery, a metanalysis of 10 randomized trials comparing off- and on-pump technique and including 2,018 patients showed no impact on mortality but suggested a benefit of off-pump surgery in terms of stroke and MI at the price of an increased risk of repeat revascularization.[45] No data on off-pump surgery are available for diabetic patients.

REVASCULARIZATION VERSUS MEDICAL MANAGEMENT

The Euro Heart Survey on Diabetes and the Heart recruited patients with CAD at 110 centers in 25 European countries. A total of 3,488 patients (2,063 nondiabetic and 1,425 diabetic) were enrolled and prospectively followed for 1 year.[46] The population consisted of approximately one-third of stable and two-thirds of unstable CAD patients. The study investigated the impact of evidence-based medicine—defined as the combined use of renin-angiotensin-aldosterone system inhibitors, beta blockers, any antiplatelet agent, and statins—and of revascularization (PCI or CABG) on mortality and MACCE. Of the eligible patients, 44% of those with diabetes and 43% of those without diabetes received evidence-based medicine, while 34% and 40%, respectively, were revascularized. A preferential benefit from both evidence-based medicine and revascularization in diabetic patients was identified. Revascularization was associated with a statistically significant reduction in mortality (5.7% vs. 8.6%) and death, MI, or stroke (9.9% vs. 16.9%) in diabetic patients (Fig. 3-11). In addition, a statistically significant interaction between diabetic status and treatment effect was identified for evidence-based medicine with respect to MACCE (HR 0.61, $P = 0.015$ and HR 0.61, $P = 0.025$, respectively).[46] The BARI (Bypass Angioplasty Revascularization Investigation) 2D trial randomly assigned 2,368 diabetic patients with stable CAD in a 2 × 2 design to either prompt revascularization with intensive medical therapy or intensive medical therapy alone and to either insulin-sensitization or insulin-provision therapy.[47] Primary endpoints were the 5-year rate of death and of MACCE defined as a composite of death, MI, or stroke. Randomization was stratified according to the choice of PCI or CABG as the more appropriate intervention. Survival did not differ between the revascularization group (88.3%) and the medical therapy group (87.8%). The rates of freedom from MACCE also did not differ among the groups: they were 77.2% in the revascularization group and 75.9% in the medical treatment group (Fig. 3-12). There was no significant difference in primary endpoints between the revascularization group and the medical therapy group in the PCI stratum; however, in the CABG stratum, the rate of MACCE was significantly lower in the revascularization group (22.4%) than in the medical therapy group (30.5%, $P = 0.01$; $P = 0.002$ for interaction between stratum and treatment assignment).[47] Since BARI 2D did not compare PCI and CABG, no conclusion can be drawn from that trial on the efficacy of these strategies in diabetic patients. Patients randomized in the CABG stratum were at higher risk than those randomized in the PCI stratum. With respect to the factors influencing the choice

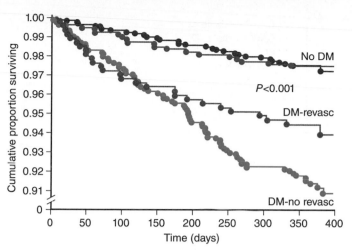

Figure 3-11 Kaplan-Meier curves on survival comparing patients with and without diabetes (DM) who were revascularized or not in the Euro Heart Survey on Diabetes. *(Reproduced with permission from Anselmino M, Malmberg K, Ohrvik J, et al. Evidence-based medication and revascularization: powerful tools in the management of patients with diabetes and coronary artery disease: a report from the Euro Heart Survey on diabetes and the heart. Eur J Cardiovasc Prev Rehabil. 2008;15:216–223.)*

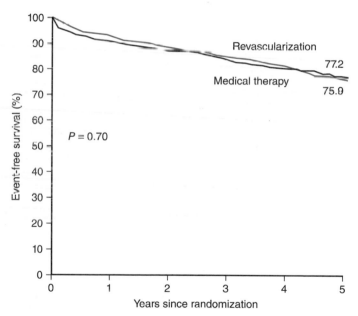

Figure 3-12 Freedom from major cardiovascular events, revascularization vs. medical therapy at 5 years in the BARI 2D trial. *(Reproduced with permission from Frye RL, August P, Brooks MM, et al. A randomized trial of therapies for type 2 diabetes and coronary artery disease. N Engl J Med. 2009;360:2503–2515.)*

of revascularization in BARI 2D, multivariate analysis showed that the selection of CABG over PCI was significantly driven by age >65 years (OR 1.4) and angiographic factors including triple-vessel disease (OR 4.4), left anterior descending (LAD) stenosis ≥70% (OR 2.9), proximal LAD stenosis ≥50% (OR 1.8), total occlusion (OR 2.4), and multiple type C lesions (OR 2.1).[48] How to explain the differential benefit observed in diabetic patients from revascularization in the EHS (Euro Heart Survey on Diabetes and the Heart) and BARI 2D? First, the baseline risk of the populations was different. While in BARI 2D enrollment was limited to patients with stable CAD, in the EHS two-thirds of the patients were admitted for ACS. Accordingly the annual

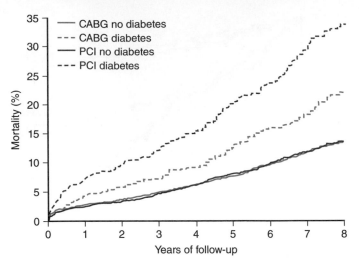

Figure 3-13 Mortality in patients assigned to coronary artery bypass graft (CABG) or percutaneous coronary intervention (PCI) by diabetes status in an analysis of ten randomized trials. *(Reproduced with permission from Hlatky MA, Boothroyd DB, Bravata DM, et al. Coronary artery bypass surgery compared with percutaneous coronary interventions for multivessel disease: a collaborative analysis of individual patient data from ten randomised trials. Lancet. 2009;373:1190–1197.)*

mortality rates in diabetic patients treated conservatively in the EHS were approximately three times greater than those observed in BARI 2D (7.6% at 1 year in EHS vs. 2.4%/year in BARI 2D). Similarly, the rate of mortality, MI, or stroke was 14.5% at 1 year in EHS while the corresponding annual rate was 4.8% in BARI 2D.

PCI VERSUS CABG IN DIABETIC PATIENTS WITH MULTIVESSEL DISEASE

An insight into the comparative results of angioplasty or BMS-based PCI versus CABG in diabetic patients can be obtained by a pooled analysis of individual patient data from 10 randomized trials comparing the effectiveness of CABG with angioplasty (6 trials) or BMS-based PCI (4 trials) in 7,812 patients with multivessel CAD. Over a median follow-up of 5.9 years, no difference in mortality was observed among nondiabetic patients; however, among patients with diabetes (CABG, $N = 615$; PCI, $N = 618$), mortality was substantially lower in the CABG group (23%) than in the PCI group (29%) (HR 0.70, 0.56-0.87) (Fig. 3-13).[49] In the New York cardiac registries, 37,212 patients with multivessel CAD who underwent CABG and 22,102 patients with multivessel disease who underwent BMS-based PCI were identified. Over 12,300 patients in the CABG group and 5,500 patients in the PCI group had diabetes.[50] Among diabetic patients, multivariate analyses showed a significant mortality benefit at 3 years for CABG versus PCI in patients with three-vessel disease with proximal and nonproximal LAD involvement and in those with two-vessel disease with proximal and nonproximal LAD involvement (adjusted HR ranging from 0.59 to 0.71). Only among diabetic patients with two-vessel disease and no LAD involvement did the mortality benefit not reach statistical significance (HR 0.69, 95% CI 0.46–1.03).[50] Several studies are now available to compare DES-based PCI and CABG in diabetic patients. An epidemiological study assessed the clinical outcomes of patients with multivessel disease who underwent revascularization with CABG ($N = 7437$) or DES ($N = 9963$) between 2003 and 2004 in New York State.[51] Patients undergoing CABG were older, more likely to be male and Caucasian, had lower ejection fraction, prior MI, other coexisting conditions, and three-vessel CAD. The outcomes of diabetic patients treated with CABG ($N = 2,844$) did not differ from those undergoing PCI ($N = 3,256$) with respect to the adjusted rate of death (HR = 0.97, $P = 0.75$) and death or MI (HR = 0.84, $P = 0.07$). The CARDia (Coronary Artery Revascularization in

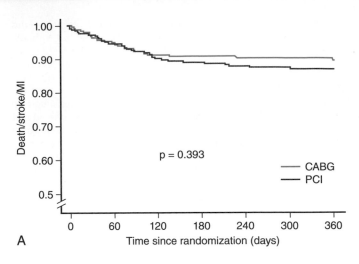

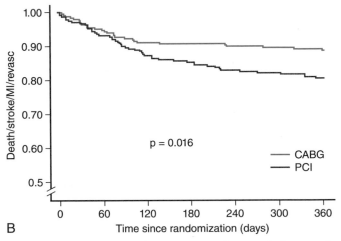

Figure 3-14 One-year Kaplan-Meier event-free survival curves for coronary artery bypass grafting (CABG) and percutaneous coronary intervention (PCI) for the primary outcome of death, myocardial infarction (MI), or stroke (A) and death, MI, stroke, or repeat revascularization (revasc) in the CARDia trial. *(Reproduced with permission from Kapur A, Hall RJ, Malik IS, et al. Randomized comparison of percutaneous coronary intervention with coronary artery bypass grafting in diabetic patients. 1-year results of the CARDia trial. J Am Coll Cardiol. 2010;55:432–440.)*

Diabetes) trial compared PCI and CABG in 510 diabetic patients with symptomatic multivessel CAD. At 1 year of follow-up, the primary endpoint of death, MI, and stroke was 10.5% in the CABG group and 13.0% in the PCI group (HR 1.25, $P = 0.39$). The need of repeat revascularization was 2.0% in the CABG group and 11.8% in the PCI group (HR 6.2, $P < 0.001$). While all-cause mortality rates did not differ (3.2%) the corresponding rates of death, MI, stroke or repeat revascularization were 11.3% and 19.3% (HR 1.77, $P = 0.02$) (Fig. 3-14).[52] In the first phase of the study, patients were randomized to either CABG or BMS implantation; thereafter, patients ($N = 350$) were randomized to CABG or DES implantation. In patients randomized after the introduction of DES, the death, MI, stroke, or repeat revascularization rates in the CABG and PCI groups were 12.9% and 18.0% (HR 1.41, P = NS), respectively. The SYNTAX (SYNergy between percutaneous coronary intervention with TAXus and cardiac surgery) study randomly assigned 1,800 patients (452 with diabetes) to receive paclitaxel (Taxus) DES-based PCI or CABG. The rate of major adverse cardiac and cerebrovascular events (MACCE) at 1 year (the death, stroke, MI, or repeat revascularization rates) were higher among diabetic patients treated with DES (26.0%) than among those

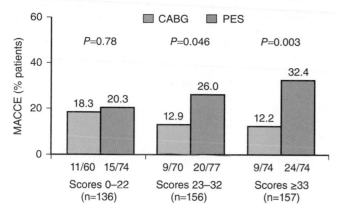

Figure 3-15 One-year major adverse cardiac and cerebrovascular events (MACCE), defined as death, cerebrovascular accident, myocardial infarction or repeat revascularization according to the SYNTAX score in diabetic patients randomized in the SYNTAX trial randomized to coronary artery bypass grafting (CABG) or paclitaxel eluting stenting (PES). *(Reproduced with permission from Banning AP, Westaby S, Morice MC, et al. Diabetic and nondiabetic patients with left main and/or 3-vessel coronary artery disease: comparison of outcomes with cardiac surgery and paclitaxel-eluting stents. J Am Coll Cardiol. 2010;55:1067–1075.)*

who underwent CABG (14.2%) ($P = 0.003$). Conversely, no difference was observed among diabetic patients in the rate of death, stroke, or MI (10.3% for CABG vs. 10.1% for PCI).[53] The presence of diabetes was associated with significantly increased mortality after either revascularization treatment. Mortality was higher after PCI than after CABG (4.1% vs. 13.5%, $P = 0.04$) for diabetic patients with highly complex lesions (i.e., SYNTAX score ≥ 33). Treatment with PCI rather than CABG resulted in higher repeat revascularization rates for diabetic patients (6.4% vs. 20.3%, $P < 0.001$). The more complex the lesions according to the SYNTAX score, the greater the disadvantage of PCI in terms of MACCE, driven by an increased TVR rate (Fig. 3-15). In summary, CABG should be considered superior to angioplasty and BMS-based PCI in diabetic patients with multivessel disease both in terms of MACCE and late mortality. In the era of first-generation DES, based on the results of the CARDia and SYNTAX trials, it can be stated that at one year diabetic patients treated with PCI or CABG have similar mortality rates as well as a similar rate of the composite of death, MI, or stroke. However, the risk of repeat revascularization remains substantially higher for diabetic patients undergoing PCI compared with those undergoing CABG. Finally, diabetic patients undergoing PCI had fewer strokes than those undergoing CABG, though—possibly owing to the sample size—the difference did not reach statistical significance. Important information will come from the follow-up of CARDia and SYNTAX as well as from the ongoing FREEDOM (Future REvascularization Evaluation in patients

with Diabetes mellitus: Optimal management of Multivessel disease) trial, a randomized study of DES-based PCI versus CABG in at least 1,900 diabetic patients with multivessel disease. In the PCI arm, the choice of DES will be left at the discretion of the operator and hopefully newer-generation DESs will be well represented. The primary outcome measure will be the composite of all-cause mortality, nonfatal MI, or stroke at 4 years. The only guideline so far published that incorporates all the mentioned data coming from the European Society of Cardiology and the European Association for Cardio-Thoracic Surgery recommends revascularization in all stable diabetic patients with extensive CAD in order to improve MACCE-free survival (class I, level of evidence A).[54] In addition, it is stated that CABG, rather than PCI, should be considered in diabetic patients when the extent of the CAD justifies a surgical approach (especially in multivessel disease), and the patient's risk profile is acceptable (class IIa, level of evidence B).

Diabetes and Non-ST-Elevation Acute Coronary Syndromes

The high prevalence of abnormal glucose metabolism in patients with CAD, particularly among those with acute manifestations of the disease, has been detected in large-scale surveys in both the United States and Europe. In the American registry CRUSADE (Can Rapid risk stratification of Unstable angina patients Suppress ADverse outcomes with Early implementation of the ACC/AHA guidelines), the prevalence of diabetes was 33% among 46,410 patients with non-ST-elevation ACS.[55] Within the National Registry of Myocardial Infarction, the prevalence of diabetes among patients presenting with ST-elevation MI (STEMI) and non-ST-elevation MI (NSTEMI) was 27% and 34%, respectively.[56] The Euro Heart Survey addressed glucose metabolism in 2,107 patients with unstable CAD.[57] The prevalence of known diabetes in this patient population was 32%. Among patients without known diabetes, an oral glucose tolerance test detected impaired glucose tolerance and diabetes in an additional 36% and 22% of cases, respectively.[57] Diabetic patients more frequently than their nondiabetic counterparts have characteristics and comorbidities that may negatively impact their outcomes in the setting of ACS. Nevertheless, even after accounting for imbalances in baseline characteristics, several studies have shown that diabetes remains an independent predictor of short-term morbidity and mortality in the setting of ACS—an observation reinforced by an analysis of the CRUSADE registry (Table 3-5).[58] In this dataset, the in-hospital mortality rates were 6.8% for diabetic patients on insulin, 5.4% for diabetic patients not treated with insulin, and 4.4% for nondiabetic patients. Similarly, at long-term follow-up, diabetic patients presenting with non-ST-elevation ACS have significantly higher rates of mortality, recurrent MI, stroke, and heart failure compared with their nondiabetic counterparts.[59] The prognostic gap between diabetic and nondiabetic individuals presenting with ACS was confirmed in a large-scale ACS trial mandating an early pharmacoinvasive strategy for non-ST-elevation

TABLE 3-5	In-Hospital Clinical Outcomes in Diabetic Patients with Non-ST-Elevation ACS in the Crusade Registry				
				AOR (95% CI)	
Clinical Outcome	*Nondiabetic*	*NIDDM*	*IDDM*	NIDDM*	IDDM†
N	31,049	9,773	5,588		
Death (%)	4.4	5.4	6.8	1.14 (1.02–1.29)	1.29 (1.12–1.49)
Reinfarction (%)	3.2	3.5	3.8	1.07 (0.96–1.19)	1.07 (0.93–1.24)
Congestive heart failure (%)	8.0	12.4	13.7	1.25 (1.16–1.34)	1.19 (1.09–1.31)
Shock (%)	2.5	3.2	3.5	1.22 (1.05–1.41)	1.18 (0.97–1.44)
Red blood cell transfusion (%)	12.9	17.4	20.8	1.31 (1.23–1.40)	1.51 (1.40–1.63)

ACS, acute coronary syndrome; NIDDM, non-insulin-dependent diabetes; IDDM, insulin-dependent diabetes; AOR, adjusted odds ratio;
*Nondiabetic vs. type 2 diabetic patients.
†Nondiabetic vs. insulin-dependent diabetic patients.
Reprinted with permission from Brogan GX, Peterson ED, Mulgund J, et al: Treatment disparities in the care of patients with and without diabetes presenting with non-ST-segment elevation acute coronary syndromes. *Diabetes Care* 29:9–14, 2006.

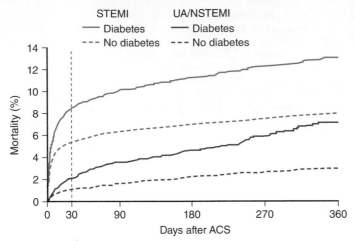

Figure 3-16 Cumulative Incidence of all-cause mortality through 1 year after acute coronary syndromes enrolled in 11 clinical trials. STEMI = ST-segment elevation myocardial infarction; UA = unstable angina; NSTEMI = non-ST-segment elevation myocardial infarction. *(Data from Donahoe SM, Stewart GC, McCabe CH, et al. Diabetes and mortality following acute coronary syndromes. JAMA. 2007; 298:765–775.)*

ACS and primary PCI for STEMI. Within the ACUITY (Acute Catheterization and Urgent Intervention Triage Strategy) trial, a study comparing different antithrombotic regimens in patients with moderate-risk non-ST-elevation ACS undergoing early invasive treatment found that diabetic patients (N = 3,852) had higher rates of 30-day mortality (2.1% vs. 1.3%; P < 0.001) and death, MI, or unplanned revascularization (8.7% vs. 7.2%; P = 0.003) compared with nondiabetic individuals.[60] In addition, diabetic patients had more major bleeding than their nondiabetic counterparts (5.7% vs. 4.2%; P < 0.001). A pooled study of ACS patients enrolled in several randomized clinical trials comprised 46,577 STEMI and 15,459 non-ST-elevation ACS patients. A subgroup analysis of the diabetic population (17% of the total) showed that mortality at 30 days was significantly higher among patients with diabetes than among those without diabetes both in the setting of non-ST-elevation ACS (2.1% vs. 1.1%, P < 0.001) and STEMI (8.5% vs. 5.4%, P < 0.001), with adjusted risks for 30-day mortality in diabetes versus no diabetes of 1.8 for non-ST-elevation ACS and 1.4 for STEMI.[61] Diabetes was also associated with a significantly higher mortality at 1 year for both presentations (HR 1.7 and 1.2, respectively). At 1 year, patients with diabetes presenting with non-ST-elevation ACS had a risk of death that approached that of nondiabetic individuals presenting with STEMI (7.2% vs. 8.1%) (Fig. 3-16).[61] An analysis of the CRUSADE registry addressed the utilization of evidence-based therapy in nondiabetic (N = 31,049), non-insulin-dependent diabetic (N = 9,773), and insulin-treated diabetic (N = 5,588) patients with non-ST ACS.[58] This analysis demonstrated improved treatment utilization among diabetic patients not receiving insulin, comparable with the treatment given to nondiabetic patients. Conversely, insulin-treated diabetic patients were less likely than nondiabetic patients to receive aspirin (adjusted OR 0.83), beta blockers (adjusted OR 0.89), heparin (adjusted OR 0.90), GP IIb/IIIa inhibitors (adjusted OR 0.86), cardiac catheterization within 48 hours of presentation (adjusted OR 0.80) or PCI (adjusted OR 0.87). Compared with nondiabetic patients, insulin-treated and non-insulin-treated diabetic patients were more likely to undergo CABG (adjusted OR 1.34 and 1.35, respectively).[58]

EARLY INVASIVE VERSUS CONSERVATIVE STRATEGY

In diabetic patients with non-ST-elevation ACS, the positive impact of an early invasive strategy can be derived from subgroup analyses of large-scale randomized studies. The FRISCII (Fragmin and Fast

Revascularisation during InStability in Coronary artery disease) study randomized 2,457 patients to an invasive or conservative strategy and detected a significant survival benefit associated with the invasive strategy at 1 year.[62] The reduction in 1-year death or MI associated with early coronary angiography, if needed, followed by revascularization, was marked among diabetic patients (N = 299) in terms of relative and particularly absolute risk reduction (39% and 9.3%, respectively). Among nondiabetic individuals, the effect was less pronounced (28% and 3.1%, respectively). Owing to differences in sample size, the benefit observed in diabetic patients barely missed statistical significance, while such significance was achieved in nondiabetic individuals. In addition, diabetic patients undergoing early invasive therapy had a 38% reduction in the relative risk of 1-year death (7.7% vs. 12.5%), again not reaching statistical significance because of the small sample size.[62] In the TACTICS (Treat Angina with Aggrastat and Determine Cost of Therapy with an Invasive or Conservative Strategy)-TIMI 18 trial, an early invasive strategy was associated with a significant 22% reduction in the relative risk of death, MI, or rehospitalization for ACS at 6 months compared with an early conservative strategy.[63] All patients were treated with aspirin, clopidogrel, and tirofiban. Diabetic patients derived a greater benefit than individuals not affected by diabetes from an early invasive strategy both in terms of absolute (7.6% and 1.8%, respectively) and relative (27% and 13%, respectively) 6-month event reduction. While the 2007 European ACS guidelines recommend an early invasive strategy for all diabetic patients presenting with ACS, the 2011 ACC/AHA recommendations state that decisions on whether to perform stress testing, angiography, and revascularization should be similar in patients with and without diabetes.[64,65]

DIABETES AND ST-ELEVATION MYOCARDIAL INFARCTION

Paralleling the observations for non-ST-elevation ACS, also in the setting of STEMI, diabetes is an independent predictor of morbidity and mortality. A large retrospective study evaluating admission glucose of 141,680 patients presenting with acute MI demonstrated a linear correlation between glucose levels and mortality (Fig. 3-17).[66] Compared with individuals with admission glucose ≤110 mg/dL, for individuals with glucose >140 to 170, >170 to 240, and >40 mg/dL, the HRs for mortality were 1.1, 1.3, 1.5, and 1.8 at 30 days, respectively, and 1.1, 1.2, 1.3, and 1.5 at 1 year, respectively. The impact of diabetes on outcomes following the acute MI phase was addressed in the VALIANT (VALsartan In Acute myocardial iNfarcTion) trial, a contemporary large-scale study.[67] It enrolled 3,400 patients with known diabetes, 580 with newly diagnosed diabetes and 10,719 with no diabetes. At 1 year, patients with previously known and newly diagnosed diabetes had a similar increased risk of mortality (adjusted HRs of 1.4 and 1.5, respectively) and of CV events (adjusted HRs of 1.4 and 1.3, respectively) compared with those without diabetes. As observed in the setting of non-ST-elevation ACS, also in the management of acute MI, diabetic patients are less frequently exposed to evidence-based therapy. According to the RIKS-HIA (Swedish Register of Information and Knowledge about Swedish Heart Intensive care Admissions), after adjustments for differences in baseline characteristics between the diabetic and nondiabetic patients, patients with diabetes were significantly less likely to be treated with reperfusion therapy, heparins, or statins or to be revascularized, while the use of angiotensin converting enzyme (ACE) inhibitors was more prevalent among diabetic than nondiabetic patients.[68] This was the case despite the fact that the same analysis documented a mortality benefit associated with the administration of several of these therapies in the diabetic population.[68]

REPERFUSION THERAPY

With respect to fibrinolytic therapy, the metanalysis of the Fibrinolytic Therapy Trialists' Collaborative Group, involving all the large randomized trials of fibrinolytic therapy versus placebo in STEMI, demonstrated a greater than twofold survival benefit at 35 days among

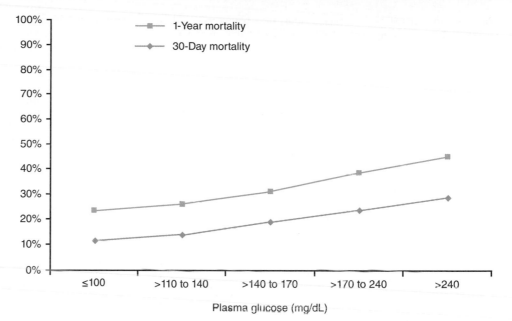

Figure 3-17 Relationship between admission plasma glucose values and 30-day and 1-year mortality rates among patients presenting with acute myocardial infarction. *(Reprinted with permission from Kosiborod M, Rathore SS, Inzucchi SE, et al. Admission glucose and mortality in elderly patients hospitalized with acute myocardial infarction: implications for patients with and without recognized diabetes. Circulation. 2005;111:3078–3086.)*

diabetic patients ($N = 2,236$) compared with nondiabetic individuals ($N = 19,423$), corresponding to 3.7 lives and 1.5 lives saved per 100 patients treated, respectively. While CABG in the setting of STEMI is typically reserved for failed PCI and for MI-related mechanical complications, primary PCI may be preferred over thrombolytic therapy in diabetic patients. However, the data to support this notion are limited. A pooled analysis of individual patient data from 19 randomized trials comparing primary PCI with fibrinolysis for the treatment of STEMI included 6,315 patients, 877 (14%) of whom had diabetes. The 30-day mortality rate (9.4% vs. 5.9%; $P < 0.001$) was higher in patients with diabetes. Mortality was significantly lower after primary PCI compared with fibrinolysis in both patients with diabetes (unadjusted OR 0.49; $P = 0.004$) and those without diabetes (unadjusted OR 0.69; $P = 0.001$). After multivariate analysis, primary PCI was associated with a significant decrease in 30-day mortality in patients with and without diabetes, with a point estimate of greater benefit in diabetic patients (OR 0.50 in diabetic patients and 0.68 in nondiabetic patients).[69]

GLUCOSE-LOWERING THERAPY

The DIGAMI (Diabetes mellitus, Insulin Glucose infusion in Acute Myocardial Infarction) study was designed to test the hypothesis that intensive glucose-lowering therapy in patients with diabetes and acute MI improved outcomes. A total of 620 patients were randomized to standard treatment plus insulin-glucose infusion titrated according to glucose levels for at least 24 hours, followed by subcutaneous insulin treatment for 3 months after discharge or standard treatment. Active treatment was associated with a statistically significant mortality reduction at 3.5 years (33% vs. 44%; relative risk reduction [RRR] 0.72). This translated into an impressive number needed to treat of 9 to save one life. In addition, insulin infusion was associated with a reduction in recurrent MI and heart failure rates at follow-up. In the DIGAMI 2 study, three glucose-lowering strategies were compared among 1,253 diabetic patients with suspected acute MI: group 1, acute insulin-glucose infusion titrated to glucose levels for 24 hours, followed by insulin-based long-term glucose control; group 2, insulin-glucose infusion for 24 hours, followed by standard glucose control; and group 3, routine metabolic management according to local practice.[70] At 2 years, the mortality rates between the three groups were comparable and no significant differences in non-fatal MI or stroke were detected. However, the achieved blood glucose

levels during the study period were identical in the three groups. Therefore, in the presence of tight glycemic control, insulin is not to be considered superior to oral hypoglycemic drugs in terms of CV outcomes

Antithrombotic Therapy in Diabetes

ASPIRIN

While the value of aspirin among diabetic patients in *secondary* prevention in a dose ranging from 75 to 162 mg/day is well established, until recently only one prospective trial was available to address the efficacy of aspirin in *primary* prevention for these patients. The ETDRS (Early Treatment Diabetic Retinopathy Study) enrolled 3,711 diabetic patients in the 1980s and randomized them to aspirin 650 mg/day or placebo.[71] The administration of aspirin over 5 years was associated with a nonsignificant reduction in all-cause mortality and fatal or nonfatal MI (RR 0.91 and 0.83, respectively). Two recent trials failed to demonstrate a significant reduction in CV events with aspirin compared with placebo in the primary prevention setting of diabetic individuals. In the JPAD (Japanese Primary Prevention of Atherosclerosis with Aspirin for Diabetes), 2,539 patients with type 2 diabetes without a history of atherosclerotic disease were assigned to low-dose aspirin (81 or 100 mg/day) or no aspirin and were followed for a median of 4.4 years.[72] Primary endpoints were atherosclerotic events, including fatal or nonfatal ischemic heart disease, fatal or nonfatal stroke, and peripheral artery disease. The occurrence of the primary endpoint did not differ between the two groups (1.4%/year in the aspirin group and 1.7%/year in the placebo group). Similarly, no difference was observed in all-cause mortality. However, the combined endpoint of fatal coronary events and fatal cerebrovascular events was significantly reduced with aspirin (HR, 0.10; 95% CI, 0.01-0.79; $P = 0.0037$). In the POPADAD (Prevention of Progression of Arterial Disease and Diabetes) study, 1,276 adults received 100 mg aspirin or placebo for a median follow-up of 6.7 years.[73] The primary endpoints of death from coronary heart disease or stroke, nonfatal MI or stroke, or amputation above the ankle for critical limb ischemia did not differ between patients treated with aspirin (18.2% vs. 18.3%). Similarly, no difference was observed in the rates of death from coronary heart disease or stroke (6.7% vs. 5.5%). In the 2010 update, the ADA recommended aspirin therapy (75–162 mg/day) as a primary prevention strategy in diabetic patients at increased cardiovascular risk (i.e., 10-year risk >10%), such as most men >50 years of age or women >60 years of age who have at least one additional major risk factor (family history of CVD, hypertension, smoking, dyslipidemia, or albuminuria).[74]

CLOPIDOGREL

The CHARISMA (Clopidogrel for High Atherothrombotic Risk and Ischemic Stabilization, Management, and Avoidance) trial investigated the safety and efficacy of long-term administration of aspirin (75–162 mg/day) and clopidogrel (75 mg/day) in comparison with aspirin alone in patients with established atherosclerotic disease or with multiple CV risk factors.[75] In the large diabetic population enrolled ($N = 6,556$)—mainly a primary prevention cohort—no benefit of the combination therapy was observed after a median follow-up of 28 months, while the bleeding rate increased. The CURE (Clopidogrel in Unstable angina to prevent Recurrent Events) trial randomized patients with ACS primarily medically managed to aspirin or aspirin and clopidogrel for 9 to 12 months. Diabetic patients ($N = 2840$) did not derive a significant benefit from the combined treatment.[76] The CURRENT-OASIS 7 (Clopidogrel Optimal Loading Dose Usage to Reduce Recurrent Events/Optimal Antiplatelet Strategy for Interventions) study randomized 25,087 ACS patients in a 2×2 factorial design to a clopidogrel high-dose regimen (600-mg loading dose on day 1 followed by 150 mg once daily on days 2–7, followed by 75 mg once daily on days 8–30) versus a clopidogrel low-dose regimen (300-mg loading dose on day 1, followed by 75 mg once daily on days 2–30). Patients in each clopidogrel-dose group were further randomized in an open-label fashion to high-dose ASA (300–325 mg daily) or low-dose ASA (75–100 mg daily).[77] Approximately 70% of patients had a non-ST-elevation ACS and the remaining 30% had STEMI. Angiography was performed in 99% of the patients, of whom 70% were suitable for PCI and 30% were not. The primary efficacy composite endpoint—specifically the first occurrence of death from CV causes, MI, or stroke up to day 30—was not met in either randomized cohort. In the subgroup of patients undergoing PCI, there was a 15% statistically significant reduction in the primary composite endpoint with double-dose clopidogrel compared with the standard dose (HR 0.85, $P = 0.036$). In addition, there was a 42% relative risk reduction in stent thrombosis in those who received the double dose (HR 0.58, $P = 0.001$). However, major and severe bleeding was significantly higher in patients receiving double-dose clopidogrel, although this was not associated with an increase in intracerebral hemorrhage or fatal bleeding. In patients who did not undergo PCI, there was no clinical benefit of high-dose clopidogrel. Comparisons between the two ASA dosages showed no significant differences in efficacy or safety. Although no data are yet available on diabetic patients in this cohort, these results encourage using a high dose of clopidogrel for diabetic patients, since the rate of early stent thrombosis is increased in this population.

ANTIPLATELET RESISTANCE

As mentioned earlier in this chapter, patients with diabetes mellitus are characterized by enhanced platelet reactivity, which exposes them to an increased risk of atherothrombotic events. Although aspirin and clopidogrel, used either solely or in combination, are associated with improved clinical outcomes in high-risk patients, diabetic patients treated with antiplatelet agents remain at higher risk of recurrent ischemic events in the setting of ACS and PCI. Recent investigations link this observation to a reduced responsiveness or "resistance," defined as the failure of an antiplatelet agent to adequately block its specific target on the platelet—that is, the COX-1 receptor for aspirin and the $P2Y_{12}$ receptor for clopidogrel. While the data on the prevalence of aspirin resistance and its impact on CV outcomes in diabetic patients are sparse, a bulk of evidence supports the notion that an inadequate response to clopidogrel is more prevalent in diabetic than in nondiabetic individuals. Accordingly, clopidogrel nonresponsiveness is

approximately four times more frequently observed among diabetic than nondiabetic patients undergoing elective PCI at 24 hours following a standard 300-mg loading dose.[78] In addition, platelet reactivity remains persistently elevated in diabetic patients even in the clopidogrel maintenance phase, especially among the individuals treated with insulin.[79] These findings may relate to the high rate of atherothrombotic events observed in diabetic patients, particularly in those at the most advanced stage of the disease (i.e., insulin-requiring). This may also explain why DES studies have repeatedly identified diabetes—and especially its insulin-requiring form—as a predictor of stent thrombosis.

PRASUGREL AND TICAGRELOR

Prasugrel is a third-generation thienopyridine that inhibits the $P2Y_{12}$ receptor more rapidly and more consistently (i.e., with smaller individual variation) than standard and higher doses of clopidogrel in healthy volunteers and in patients with CAD, including those undergoing PCI. These properties may be particularly important for diabetic patients, based on frequently encountered resistance to clopidogrel. TRITON-TIMI 38 (The Trial to Assess Improvement in Therapeutic Outcomes by Optimizing Platelet Inhibition With Prasugrel-Thrombolysis in Myocardial Infarction 38) randomized 13,608 subjects with ACS (both STEMI and non-ST-elevation ACS) to clopidogrel or prasugrel for 6 to 15 months. Among these, 3,146 subjects had diabetes and 776 were treated with insulin on admission. The primary endpoint (death from cardiovascular causes, MI, or stroke) was significantly reduced with prasugrel compared with clopidogrel among subjects without diabetes as well as those with diabetes (9.2% vs. 10.6%; HR 0.86; $P = 0.02$ for nondiabetic patients and 12.2% vs. 17.0%; HR 0.70; $P < 0.001$ for their diabetic counterparts, respectively) (Fig. 3-18).[34] The beneficial effect of prasugrel was observed among diabetic subjects treated with insulin (14.3% vs. 22.2%; HR 0.63; $P = 0.009$) as well as those on oral hypoglycaemic drugs (11.5% vs. 15.3%; HR 0.74; $P = 0.009$). Myocardial infarction was reduced by 18% with prasugrel among subjects without diabetes (7.2% vs. 8.7%; $P = 0.006$) and by 40% among subjects with diabetes (8.2% vs. 13.2%; $P < 0.001$). In the interaction analyses for treatment benefit, diabetic status showed a trend ($P = 0.09$) for the primary endpoint and was significant ($P = 0.02$) for MI, suggesting a preferential benefit of prasugrel in the diabetic population. Although TIMI major bleeds were increased among subjects without diabetes on prasugrel (1.6% vs. 2.4%; HR 1.43; $P = 0.02$), the rates were similar among subjects with diabetes for clopidogrel and prasugrel (2.6% vs. 2.5%). Net clinical benefit with prasugrel was greater for diabetic patients (14.6% vs. 19.2%; HR 0.74; $P = 0.001$) than for nondiabetic individuals (11.5% versus 12.3%; HR 0.92; $P = 0.16$, $P_{interaction} = 0.05$). Finally, the rate of stent thrombosis both in the overall population and in the diabetic population was significantly reduced by the allocation to prasugrel (0.9% vs. 2.0% and 2.0% vs. 3.5%, respectively). In the PLATO (PLATelet inhibition and patient Outcomes) trial, ticagrelor reduced the primary composite endpoint of cardiovascular death, MI, or stroke, but with similar rates of major bleeding compared with clopidogrel in 18,624 patients with ACS (both STEMI and non-ST-elevation ACS). In diabetic patients ($N = 4662$), including 1,036 patients on insulin, the reduction in the primary composite endpoint (HR: 0.88, 95% CI: 0.76–1.03) (Fig. 3-19), all-cause mortality (HR: 0.82, 95% CI: 0.66–1.01), and stent thrombosis (HR: 0.65, 95% CI: 0.36–1.17) with ticagrelor was consistent with the overall cohort and without significant diabetes status-by-treatment interactions.[80] There was no heterogeneity in treatment efficacy between patients with or without ongoing insulin treatment. Owing to the differences in protocols and populations enrolled in the TRITON and PLATO studies, no comparisons with respect to safety or efficacy of the two molecules in diabetic patients can be made at this time. While prasugrel has been approved by the FDA in the United States as well as in many European countries. As of June 1, 2011, ticagrelor has been approved in some European countries, but not in the United States.

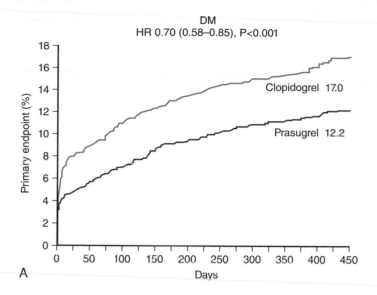

DM
HR 0.70 (0.58–0.85), P<0.001

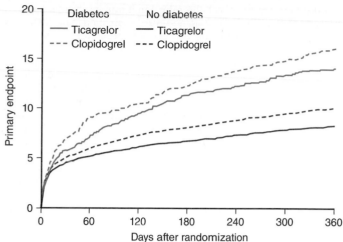

Figure 3-19 Cumulative incidence of the primary composite of cardiovascular death, myocardial infarction and stroke in the PLATO trial according to the randomization to ticagrelor (solid lines) or clopidogrel (dotted lines) and the presence (blue lines) or absence (red lines) of diabetes. *(Reproduced with permission from James S, Angiolillo DJ, Cornel JH, et al. Ticagrelor vs. clopidogrel in patients with acute coronary syndromes and diabetes: a substudy from the PLATelet inhibition and patient Outcomes (PLATO) trial. Eur Heart J. 2010;31:3006–3016.)*

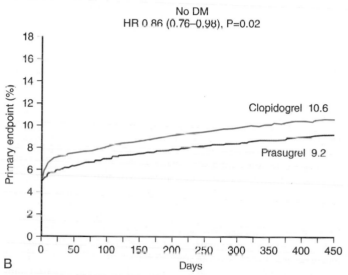

No DM
HR 0.86 (0.76–0.98), P=0.02

Figure 3-18 Kaplan-Meier event-free survival curves. Primary efficacy end point (cardiovascular death/nonfatal myocardial infarction/nonfatal stroke) stratified by diabetic status in the TRITON-TIMI 38 study. DM = diabetes mellitus. *(Reproduced with permission from Wiviott SD, Braunwald E, Angiolillo DJ, et al. Greater clinical benefit of more intensive oral antiplatelet therapy with prasugrel in patients with diabetes mellitus in the trial to assess improvement in therapeutic outcomes by optimizing platelet inhibition with prasugrel-Thrombolysis in Myocardial Infarction 38. Circulation. 2008;118:1626–1636.)*

GLYCOPROTEIN IIB/IIIA RECEPTOR ANTAGONISTS

In the era before clopidogrel loading, the use of intravenous platelet GP IIb/IIIa receptor inhibitors markedly reduced both the early hazard and the 1-year mortality in diabetic patients undergoing PCI.[81] Subsequently, the ISAR-SWEET (Intracoronary Stenting and Antithrombotic Regimen) study—although underpowered—suggested that, in diabetic patients with stable CAD who were not treated with insulin but pretreated with 600 mg of clopidogrel, GP IIb/IIIa inhibitors did not confer additional benefit.[82] In the setting of non-ST elevation ACS, however, a mortality benefit of GP IIb/IIIa inhibitors has been detected among diabetic patients. Accordingly, a metanalysis of the diabetic populations (N = 6,458) enrolled in the six large-scale GP IIb/IIIa inhibitor ACS trials detected a highly significant 26% mortality

reduction associated with the use of these agents compared with placebo at 30 days.[83] These findings were reinforced by a statistically significant interaction between treatment and diabetic status. The use of these potent platelet inhibitors was associated with a similar proportionate reduction in mortality for patients treated with insulin and those on a hypoglycemic diet or oral hypoglycemic drugs. Even more striking was the mortality reduction (70%) associated with the use of GP IIb/IIIa inhibitors among those diabetic patients who underwent PCI. However, the patients included in the trials were not pretreated with clopidogrel. The value of GP IIb/IIIa inhibitors in addition to clopidogrel loading for diabetic patients at the time of mechanical revascularization for STEMI cannot be adequately assessed, since little data are available. In a double-blind, randomized, placebo-controlled trial, 984 patients with STEMI undergoing primary PCI were randomly assigned to either high-bolus-dose tirofiban or placebo in addition to aspirin, heparin, and 600 mg of clopidogrel. The primary endpoint was the extent of residual ST-segment deviation 1 hour after PCI, which was significantly reduced in the tirofiban group. Among the 220 diabetic patients enrolled, the benefit of tirofiban was significant and more pronounced than in nondiabetic patients with respect to residual ST deviation and total CK increase; in addition, a trend toward lower mortality in diabetic patients at 1 year was identified (4.6% vs. 11.6%, P = 0.07).[84]

ANTICOAGULANTS

The SYNERGY (Superior Yield of the New Strategy of Enoxaparin, Revascularization, and Glycoprotein IIb/IIIa inhibitors) trial compared the low-molecular weight heparin (LMWH) enoxaparin with unfractionated heparin (UFH) in 9,978 ACS patients undergoing an early invasive strategy and found no difference in outcomes at 30 days and 6 months in the overall study population as well as in the diabetic cohort (N = 2,926).[85] The A-to-Z (Aggrastat-to Zocor) trial randomized 3,987 ACS patients to enoxaparin or UFH in addition to aspirin and tirofiban and found no benefit of enoxaparin. Among diabetic patients (N = 751), the composite of death, MI, or refractory ischemia at 30 days was nonsignificantly lowered with enoxaparin (8.4% vs. 10.7%).[86] Therefore heparin and LMWH should be seen as equivalent alternatives for diabetic patients in the setting of ACS and PCI.

Investigation of the direct thrombin inhibitor bivalirudin for PCI started with the REPLACE-2 (Randomized Evaluation in percutaneous coronary intervention Linking Angiomax to reduced Clinical Events) trial. This study showed the noninferiority of bivalirudin plus provisional GP IIb/IIIa inhibition compared with routine GP IIb/IIIa inhibition in addition to aspirin and clopidogrel in terms of 30-day death, MI, urgent revascularization, or in-hospital major bleeding. The outcomes up to 1 year with the two strategies were also comparable among the 1,624 diabetic patients enrolled.[87] Subsequent data became available also on the use of bivalirudin in diabetic patients with ACS undergoing PCI. Accordingly, the diabetes subgroup analysis ($N = 3,852$) of the ACUITY (Acute Catheterization and Urgent Intervention Triage Strategy) trial showed comparable results in terms of 30-day ischemic endpoints (8.9% vs. 7.9%) and less major bleeding (7.1% vs. 3.7%, $P < 0.001$), between heparin plus GP IIb/IIIa inhibitors and bivalirudin monotherapy in this moderate-risk non-ST-elevation ACS population. Finally, the use of bivalirudin in the setting of primary PCI for STEMI has been addressed in the HORIZONS-AMI (Harmonizing Outcomes with Revascularization and Stents in Acute Myocardial Infarction) study. While in the overall study population ($N = 3,602$) anticoagulation with bivalirudin alone, as compared with heparin plus glycoprotein IIb/IIIa inhibitors, resulted in significantly reduced 30-day rates of major bleeding and net adverse clinical events, no specific data are available for the diabetic patient population.[88] The OASIS 5 (Fifth Organization to Assess Strategies in Acute Ischemic Syndromes) study randomly assigned 20,078 patients with non-ST-elevation ACS to receive either fondaparinux (2.5 mg daily) or enoxaparin (1 mg/kg of body weight twice daily) for a mean of 6 days.[89] The study met the noninferiority criteria for the efficacy primary endpoint—combined death, MI, or refractory ischemia at 9 days—of fondaparinux compared with enoxaparin (5.8% vs. 5.7%), while the rate of major bleeding at 9 days was markedly lower with fondaparinux than with enoxaparin (2.2% vs. 4.1%; HR 0.52; $P < 0.001$). During the trial, a significant increase in coronary- and catheter-related thrombosis at the time of PCI in the group on fondaparinux was reported, and the safety committee allowed for the additional use of UFH for patients undergoing PCI. So far no specific data are available on the efficacy and safety of fondaparinux in diabetic patients with non-ST-elevation ACS. The influence of fondaparinux on the outcome of STEMI patients was investigated in the OASIS 6 trial.[90] This trial exhibited an advantage of adjunctive fondaparinux use over placebo/unfractionated heparin in patients referred for conservative treatment only and for pharmacological reperfusion, but fondaparinux was inferior to unfractionated heparin in STEMI patients referred for primary PCI. Again, no specific data for the diabetic population in this trial were reported. Therefore, the role of fondaparinux in diabetic patients with ACS undergoing PCI still awaits definition.

Diabetes Management and Treatment Goals

GLYCEMIC CONTROL

An adequate glycemic control remains of paramount importance in the management of the diabetic patients. Several studies have demonstrated the link between elevated HbA$_{1c}$ plasma levels and CV risk. A multivariate analysis of the UKPDS (United Kingdom Prospective Diabetes Study) involving 2,693 diabetic patients without known CV disease demonstrated that, for each increment of 1% in HbA$_{1c}$ at baseline, the CV risk increased independently by approximately 10% over a median follow-up of 8 years. The EPIC (European Prospective Investigation into Cancer) study carefully analyzed the relationship of HbA$_{1c}$ measurement to incident cardiovascular events in a 6-year cohort study of 10,232 diabetic and nondiabetic men and women between ages 45 and 79 years. After adjustment for several cardiovascular risk factors, there was a 21% increase in cardiovascular events for every 1% increase in HbA$_{1c}$ level above 5%.[91] Although hyperglycemia has been associated with CVD and epidemiological evidence links lower blood

glucose levels to a decrease in CV events, the impact of good glycemic control on macrovascular events initially appeared less marked with the exception of patients presenting with acute MI[70] or undergoing CABG.[92] However, 10-year follow-up data from the UKPDS has shown that prior intensive glucose control will have positive effects lasting beyond the period of intense glycemic control.[93] Accordingly, the participants originally randomized to intensive glycemic control benefited from a statistically significant long-term reduction in MI (15% with sulfonylurea or insulin as initial pharmacotherapy, 33% with metformin as initial pharmacotherapy) and in all-cause mortality (13% and 27%, respectively) compared with those assigned to conventional glycemic control. Because of ongoing uncertainty regarding whether intensive glycemic control can reduce the increased risk of CVD events in individuals with type 2 diabetes, several large long-term trials were launched in the past decade to compare the effects of intensive versus standard glycemic control on CVD outcomes in patients with established type 2 diabetes and a relatively high risk for CV events. In 2008, the findings of three large, long-term clinical studies of glucose control and macrovascular disease in patients with type 2 diabetes were reported: ACCORD (the Action to Control CardiOvascular Risk in Diabetes,[94] ADVANCE (the Action in Diabetes and Vascular disease: preterax and diamicron modified release Controlled Evaluation),[95] and VADT (the Veterans Affairs Diabetes Trial).[96] Details of these three studies are shown in Table 3-6. Overall, they suggested no significant reduction in CVD outcomes with intensive glycemic control in these populations. However, in the ACCORD study, an unexplained increased all-cause mortality in the intensive glycemic control group was detected. Hypothesized mechanisms include hypoglycemia, weight gain, rapid lowering of HbA$_{1c}$ level, and medication interactions.[97] All three trials were carried out in participants with established diabetes (mean duration 8-11 years) and either known CVD or multiple risk factors (i.e., high likelihood of established atherosclerosis) suggesting the presence of established atherosclerosis. Subset analysis suggests that a benefit from intensive glycemic control on CV outcomes may be observed in patients with a shorter duration of diabetes, better glucose control, younger age, no previous CV event, or fewer CV risk factors at the time of initiation of the intensified glucose control regiment. PROACTIVE (PROspective piogliAzone Clinical Trial in macroVascular Events) was another large scale outcome study to investigate prospectively the effect of an oral glucose-lowering drug (pioglitazone) on macrovascular outcomes. The study enrolled 5,238 patients with type 2 diabetes and evidence of macrovascular disease. Patients were randomly allocated to receive either pioglitazone or placebo in addition to their usual treatment regimen. At 36 months of follow up, HbA$_{1c}$ was reduced by 0.9% (versus 0.3% with placebo), HDL cholesterol increased by 0.54 mmol/L (versus 0.3 mmol/L), and triglycerides decreased by 0.064 mmol/L (vs. an increase of 0.07 mmol/L for placebo) with pioglitazone treatment. There was a nonsignificant 10% relative risk reduction (RRR) with pioglitazone in the primary endpoint ($P = 0.09$), which was a composite of all-cause mortality, nonfatal MI (including silent MI), stroke, ACS, endovascular or surgical intervention in the coronary or leg arteries, and amputation above the ankle. Pioglitazone was also associated with a significant RRR of 16% ($P = 0.02$) in the principal secondary endpoint of time to first event of death from any cause, MI (excluding silent MI), and stroke. Taken together, these findings suggest that improved glycemic and lipid control associated with pioglitazone treatment lead to a reduced incidence of macrovascular events. In type 1 diabetes, optimization of glycemic control is effective in preventing or delaying retinopathy, nephropathy, and neuropathy. Within the DCCT (Diabetes Control and Complications Trial), fewer CV events occurred in the intensive treatment group than in the conventional treatment group, but the small number of CV events in the relatively young cohort precluded a determination of whether the use of intensive diabetes therapy affected the CV risk. Long-term follow-up data on EDIC (the DCCT/Epidemiology of Diabetes Interventions and Complications) study cohort showed that intensive insulin therapy significantly reduced the risk of nonfatal MI, stroke, and CV death by 57% among 1,182

TABLE 3-6	Comparison of the Three Trials of Intensive Glycemic Control and Cardiovascular Outcomes		
	Accord	Advance	Vadt
Participant characteristics			
n	10,251	11,140	1,791
Mean age (years)	62	66	60
Duration of diabetes (years)	10	8	11.5
History of CVD (%)	35	32	40
Median baseline A1C (%)	8.1	7.2	9.4
On insulin at baseline (%)	35	1.5	52
Protocol characteristics			
A1C goals (%) (I vs. S)*	<6.0 vs. 7.0-7.9	≤6.5 vs. "based on local guidelines"	<6.0 (action if >6.5) vs. planned separation of 1.5
Protocol for glycemic control (I vs. S)*	Multiple drugs in both arms	Multiple drugs added to gliclazide vs. multiple drugs with no gliclazide	Multiple drugs in both arms
Management of other risk factors	Embedded blood pressure and lipid trials	Embedded blood pressure trial	Protocol for intensive treatment in both arms
On-study characteristics			
Achieved median A1C (%) (I vs. S)	6.4 vs. 7.5	6.3 vs. 7.0	6.9 vs. 8.5
On insulin at study end (%) (I vs. S)*	77 vs. 55*	40 vs. 24	89 vs. 0.74
Weight changes (kg)			
Intensive glycemic control arm	+3.5	−0.1	+7.8
Standard glycemic control arm	+0.4	−1.0	13.4
Severe hypoglycemia (participants with one or more episodes during study) (%)			
Intensive glycemic control arm	16.2	2.7	21.2
Standard glycemic control arm	5.1	1.5	9.9
Outcomes			
Definition of primary outcome	Nonfatal MI, nonfatal stroke, CVD death	Microvascular plus macrovascular (nonfatal MI, nonfatal stroke, CVD death) outcomes	Nonfatal MI, nonfatal stroke, CVD death, hospitalization for heart failure, revascularization
HR for primary outcome (95% CI)	0.90 (0.78–1.04)	0.9 (0.82–0.98); macrovascular 0.94 (0.84–1.06)	0.88 (0.74–1.05)
HR for mortality findings (95% CI)	1.22 (1.01–1.46)	0.93 (0.83–1.06)	1.07 (0.81–1.42)

*Insulin rates for ACCORD are for any use during the study.
I, intensive glycemic control; S, standard glycemic control.

TABLE 3-7	Summary of Glycemic Recommendations for Nonpregnant Adults with Diabetes	
A1C		<7.0%*
Preprandial capillary plasma glucose		70–130 mg/dL (3.9–7.2 mmol/L)
Peak postprandial capillary plasma glucose†		<180 mg/dL (<10.0 mmol/L)
Key concepts in setting glycemic goals:		
A1C is the primary target for glycemic control		
Goals should be individualized based on:		
Duration of diabetes		
Age/life expectancy		
Comorbid conditions		
Known CVD or advanced microvascular complications		
Hypoglycemia unawareness		
Individual patient considerations		
More or less stringent glycemic goals may be appropriate for individual patients		
Postprandial glucose may be targeted if A1C goals are not met despite reaching preprandial glucose goals		

*Referenced to a nondiabetic range of 4.0% to 6.0% using a DCCT-based assay.
†Postprandial glucose measurements should be made 1 to 2 hours after the beginning of the meal, generally peak levels in patients with diabetes.
Adapted with permission from the American Diabetes Association.[74]

advanced disease and should not aggressively attempt to achieve near normal HbA$_{1C}$ levels in patients in whom such a target cannot be reasonably easily and safely achieved.[74] The recommendations of the ADA glycemic goals for patients with diabetes are shown in Table 3-7.

MULTIFACTORIAL INTERVENTION

Aggressive CV risk-factor modification—including optimal glycemic control, cigarette smoking cessation, control of blood pressure and cholesterol levels, as well as weight reduction and exercise, is an essential part of diabetes care. In fact, CV morbidity and mortality rates increase more steeply in diabetic subjects than in nondiabetic ones in the presence of additional risk factors. Dietary intervention, increased physical activity, and moderate weight loss not only improve glycemic control but also lower blood pressure and favorably affect lipid metabolism. Regular physical activity may reduce HbA$_{1c}$ levels by 10% to 20%, both systolic and diastolic blood pressure by 5 to 12 mm Hg, triglyceride levels by 20%, and may increase HDL cholesterol levels. Large cohort studies have documented that higher levels of habitual aerobic fitness and physical activity are associated with significantly lower cardiovascular and overall mortality among diabetic individuals. In order to achieve and maintain an effective lifestyle modification, diabetic subjects should receive multidisciplinary counseling by dietitians, diabetes educators, exercise trainers, and physicians. The Steno-2 study compared the efficacy of a targeted, intensified, multifactorial intervention with that of conventional treatment on modifiable risk factors for CV disease in 160 patients with diabetes and microalbuminuria.[99] The primary endpoint was a composite of CV death, nonfatal MI, stroke, revascularization, and amputation. Intensive treatment was characterized by a stepwise implementation of behavior modification and pharmacological therapy that targeted hyperglycemia, hypertension, dyslipidemia, and microalbuminuria, along with secondary CV prevention with aspirin. Conventional treatment was in accordance with national guidelines. After a mean follow-up of 8 years, patients receiving intensive therapy had a significantly lower risk of CVD (HR 0.47), nephropathy (HR 0.39), retinopathy (HR 0.42), and autonomic neuropathy (HR 0.37). The authors concluded that a target-driven, long-term, intensified intervention aimed at multiple risk factors in patients with type 2 diabetes and microalbuminuria halves the risk of cardiovascular and microvascular events. In 2008, the Steno-2 study reported the results of an additional 5.5 years of follow-up.[100] Even though few patients achieved all the treatment goals during

patients followed up for 17 years.[98] Thus, intensive diabetes therapy has long-term beneficial effects on the risk of CVD in patients with type 1 diabetes. In summary, the evidence for a cardiovascular benefit of intensive glycemic control primarily rests on the long-term follow-up of study cohorts treated early in the course of type 1 and type 2 diabetes as well as subset analyses of ACCORD, ADVANCE, and VADT. However, the mortality findings in ACCORD and subgroup analyses of VADT suggest that the risks of very aggressive glycemic control may outweigh its benefits in some patients, such as those with a long duration of diabetes, known history of severe hypoglycemia, advanced atherosclerosis, and advanced age or frailty. Certainly care providers should be vigilant in preventing severe hypoglycemia in patients with the intervention phase and several parameters of metabolic control were no different between the intensive treatment and conventional treatment groups at the end of the follow-up period, intensive intervention with multiple drug combinations and behavior modification had sustained beneficial effects with respect to vascular events and overall as well as CV mortality. Thus, in addition to glycemic control, intensification of cholesterol and blood pressure-lowering therapies remain a mainstay of diabetes management. The recommended treatment goals according to the ADA are summarized in Table 3-8.[74]

TABLE 3-8 Treatment Goals for Diabetic Patients According to the ADA

Glycemic control	Hb A_{1c} < 7.0 %*
Blood pressure	<130/80 mm Hg
Lipids	LDL < 100 mg/dL (<2.6 mmol/L)†

*Referenced to a nondiabetic range of 4.0% to 6.0% using a DCCT-based assay.
†In individuals with overt CVD, a lower LDL cholesterol goal of <70 mg/dL (1.8 mmol/L), using a high dose of a statin, is an option.
Adapted with permission from the American Diabetes Association.[74]

REFERENCES

1. American Diabetes Association: National Diabetes Fact Sheet, Diabetes Statistics. Available at: http://www.diabetes.org/diabetes-basics/diabetes-statistics/Accessed May 2, 2010.
2. Lloyd-Jones D, Adams RJ, Brown TM, et al: Heart disease and stroke statistics—2010 update: a report from the American Heart Association. *Circulation* 121:e46–e215, 2010.
3. Narayan KM, Boyle JP, Geiss LS, et al: Impact of recent increase in incidence on future diabetes burden: U.S., 2005–2050. *Diabetes Care* 29:2114–2116, 2006.
4. Shaw JE, Sicree RA, Zimmet PZ: Global estimates of the prevalence of diabetes for 2010 and 2030. *Diabetes Res Clin Pract* 87:4–14, 2010.
5. Hogan P, Dall T, Nikolov P: Economic costs of diabetes in the U.S. in 2002. *Diabetes Care* 26:917–932, 2003.
6. International Expert Committee report on the role of the A1C assay in the diagnosis of diabetes. *Diabetes Care* 32:1327–1334, 2009.
7. Mente A, Yusuf S, Islam S, et al: Metabolic syndrome and risk of acute myocardial infarction: a case-control study of 26,903 subjects from 52 countries. *J Am Coll Cardiol* 55:2390–2398, 2010.
8. Roffi M, Topol EJ: Percutaneous coronary intervention in diabetic patients with non-ST-segment elevation acute coronary syndromes. *Eur Heart J* 25:190–198, 2004.
9. Creager MA, Luscher TF, Cosentino F, et al: Diabetes and vascular disease: pathophysiology, clinical consequences, and medical therapy: Part I. *Circulation* 108:1527–1532, 2003.
10. Booth GL, Kapral MK, Fung K, et al: Relation between age and cardiovascular disease in men and women with diabetes compared with non-diabetic people: a population-based retrospective cohort study. *Lancet* 368:29–36, 2006.
11. McKinlay J, Marceau L: U.S. public health and the 21st century: diabetes mellitus. *Lancet* 356:757–761, 2000.
12. Preis SR, Hwang SJ, Coady S, et al: Trends in all-cause and cardiovascular disease mortality among women and men with and without diabetes mellitus in the Framingham Heart Study, 1950 to 2005. *Circulation* 119:1728–1735, 2009.
13. Dale AC, Vatten LJ, Nilsen TI, et al: Secular decline in mortality from coronary heart disease in adults with diabetes mellitus: cohort study. *BMJ* 337:a236, 2008.
14. Executive Summary of The Third Report of The National Cholesterol Education Program (NCEP) Expert Panel on Detection, Evaluation, And Treatment of High Blood Cholesterol In Adults (Adult Treatment Panel III). *JAMA* 285:2486–2497, 2001.
15. Schramm TK, Gislason GH, Kober L, et al: Diabetes patients requiring glucose-lowering therapy and nondiabetics with a prior myocardial infarction carry the same cardiovascular risk: a population study of 3.3 million people. *Circulation* 117:1945–1954, 2008.
16. Center of Disease Control and Prevention: National Diabetes Fact Sheet, 2007. Accessed at http://www.cdc.gov/diabetes/pubs/pdf/ndfs_2007.pdf on May 15, 2010.
17. Wackers FJ, Zaret BL: Detection of myocardial ischemia in patients with diabetes mellitus. *Circulation* 105:5–7, 2002.
18. Burgess DC, Hunt D, Li L, et al: Incidence and predictors of silent myocardial infarction in type 2 diabetes and the effect of fenofibrate: an analysis from the Fenofibrate Intervention and Event Lowering in Diabetes (FIELD) study. *Eur Heart J* 31:92–99, 2010.
19. Albers AR, Krichavsky MZ, Balady GJ. Stress testing in patients with diabetes mellitus: diagnostic and prognostic value. *Circulation* 2006;113:583–592.
20. Elkeles RS, Godsland IF, Feher MD, et al: Coronary calcium measurement improves prediction of cardiovascular events in asymptomatic patients with type 2 diabetes: the PREDICT study. *Eur Heart J* 29:2244–2251, 2008.
21. Anand DV, Lim E, Hopkins D, et al: Risk stratification in uncomplicated type 2 diabetes: prospective evaluation of the combined use of coronary artery calcium imaging and selective myocardial perfusion scintigraphy. *Eur Heart J* 27:713–721, 2006.
22. Rivera JJ, Nasir K, Choi EK, et al: Detection of occult coronary artery disease in asymptomatic individuals with diabetes mellitus using non-invasive cardiac angiography. *Atherosclerosis* 203:442–448, 2009.
23. Hadamitzky M, Hein F, Meyer T, et al: Prognostic value of coronary computed tomographic angiography in diabetic patients without known coronary artery disease. *Diabetes Care* 33:1358–1363, 2010.
24. Van Werkhoven JM, Cademartiri F, Seitun S, et al: Diabetes: prognostic value of CT coronary angiography—comparison with a nondiabetic population. *Radiology* 256:83–92, 2010.
25. Bax JJ, Young LH, Frye RL, et al: Screening for coronary artery disease in patients with diabetes. *Diabetes Care* 30:2729–2736, 2007.
26. Young LH, Wackers FJ, Chyun DA, et al: Cardiac outcomes after screening for asymptomatic coronary artery disease in patients with type 2 diabetes: the DIAD study: a randomized controlled trial. *JAMA* 301:1547–1555, 2009.
27. Smith SC, Jr, Faxon D, Cascio W, et al: Prevention Conference VI: Diabetes and Cardiovascular Disease: Writing Group VI: revascularization in diabetic patients. *Circulation* 105:e165–e169, 2002.
28. Gilbert J, Raboud J, Zinman B: Meta-analysis of the effect of diabetes on restenosis rates among patients receiving coronary angioplasty stenting. *Diabetes Care* 27:990–994, 2004.
29. Mathew V, Gersh BJ, Williams BA, et al: Outcomes in patients with diabetes mellitus undergoing percutaneous coronary intervention in the current era: a report from the Prevention of REStenosis with Tranilast and its Outcomes (PRESTO) trial. *Circulation* 109:476–480, 2004.
30. Machecourt J, Danchin N, Lablanche JM, et al: Risk factors for stent thrombosis after implantation of sirolimus-eluting stents in diabetic and nondiabetic patients: the EVASTENT Matched-Cohort Registry. *J Am Coll Cardiol* 50:501–508, 2007.
31. Spaulding C, Daemen J, Boersma E, et al: A pooled analysis of data comparing sirolimus-eluting stents with bare-metal stents. *N Engl J Med* 356:989–997, 2007.
32. Stettler C, Allemann S, Wandel S, et al: Drug eluting and bare metal stents in people with and without diabetes: collaborative network meta-analysis. *BMJ* 337:a1331, 2008.
33. Garg P, Normand SL, Silbaugh TS, et al: Drug-eluting or bare-metal stenting in patients with diabetes mellitus: results from the Massachusetts Data Analysis Center Registry. *Circulation* 118:2277–2285, 2008.
34. Wiviott SD, Braunwald E, Angiolillo DJ, et al: Greater clinical benefit of more intensive oral antiplatelet therapy with prasugrel in patients with diabetes mellitus in the trial to assess improvement in therapeutic outcomes by optimizing platelet inhibition with prasugrel-Thrombolysis in Myocardial Infarction 38. *Circulation* 118:1626–1636, 2008.
35. Windecker S, Serruys PW, Wandel S, et al: Biolimus-eluting stent with biodegradable polymer versus sirolimus-eluting stent with durable polymer for coronary revascularisation (LEADERS): a randomised non-inferiority trial. *Lancet* 372:1163–1173, 2008.
36. Stone GW, Rizvi A, Newman W, et al: Everolimus-eluting versus paclitaxel-eluting stents in coronary artery disease. *N Engl J Med* 362:1663–1674, 2010.
37. Carson JL, Scholz PM, Chen AY, et al: Diabetes mellitus increases short-term mortality and morbidity in patients undergoing coronary artery bypass graft surgery. *J Am Coll Cardiol* 40:418–423, 2002.
38. Leavitt BJ, Sheppard L, Maloney C, et al: Effect of diabetes and associated conditions on long-term survival after coronary artery bypass graft surgery. *Circulation* 110(11 Suppl 1):II41–II44, 2004.
39. Sabik JF, Blackstone EH, Gillinov AM, et al: Occurrence and risk factors for reintervention after coronary artery bypass grafting. *Circulation* 114(1 Suppl):I454–I460, 2006.
40. Sprecher DL, Pearce GL: How deadly is the "deadly quartet"? A post-CABG evaluation. *J Am Coll Cardiol* 36:1159–1165, 2000.
41. Stevens LM, Carrier M, Perrault LP, et al: Influence of diabetes and bilateral internal thoracic artery grafts on long-term outcome for multivessel coronary artery bypass grafting. *Eur J Cardiothorac Surg* 27:281–288, 2005.
42. Pevni D, Uretzky G, Mohr A, et al: Routine use of bilateral skeletonized internal thoracic artery grafting: long-term results. *Circulation* 118:705–712, 2008.
43. Taggart DP, Altman DG, Gray AM, et al: Randomized trial to compare bilateral vs. single internal mammary coronary artery bypass grafting: 1-year results of the Arterial Revascularisation Trial (ART). *Eur Heart J* 31:2470–2481, 2010.
44. Tabata M, Grab JD, Khalpey Z, et al: Prevalence and variability of internal mammary artery graft use in contemporary multivessel coronary artery bypass graft surgery: analysis of the Society of Thoracic Surgeons National Cardiac Database. *Circulation* 120:935–940, 2009.
45. Feng ZZ, Shi J, Zhao XW, et al: Meta-analysis of on-pump and off-pump coronary arterial revascularization. *Ann Thorac Surg* 87:757–765, 2009.
46. Anselmino M, Malmberg K, Ohrvik J, et al: Evidence-based medication and revascularization: powerful tools in the management of patients with diabetes and coronary artery disease: a report from the Euro Heart Survey on diabetes and the heart. *Eur J Cardiovasc Prev Rehabil* 15:216–223, 2008.
47. Frye RL, August P, Brooks MM, et al: A randomized trial of therapies for type 2 diabetes and coronary artery disease. *N Engl J Med* 360:2503–2515, 2009.
48. Kim LJ, King SB, Kent K, et al: Factors related to the selection of surgical versus percutaneous revascularization in diabetic patients with multivessel coronary artery disease in the BARI 2D trial. *JACC Cardiovasc Intervent.* 2:384–392, 2009.
49. Hlatky MA, Boothroyd DB, Bravata DM, et al: Coronary artery bypass surgery compared with percutaneous coronary interventions for multivessel disease: a collaborative analysis of individual patient data from ten randomised trials. *Lancet* 373: 1190–1197, 2009.
50. Hannan EL, Racz MJ, Walford G, et al: Long-term outcomes of coronary-artery bypass grafting versus stent implantation. *N Engl J Med* 352:2174–2183, 2005.
51. Hannan EL, Wu C, Walford G, et al: Drug-eluting stents vs. coronary-artery bypass grafting in multivessel coronary disease. *N Engl J Med* 358:331–341, 2008.
52. Kapur A, Hall RJ, Malik IS, et al: Randomized comparison of percutaneous coronary intervention with coronary artery bypass grafting in diabetic patients. 1-year results of the CARDia trial. *J Am Coll Cardiol* 55:432–440, 2010.
53. Banning AP, Westaby S, Morice MC, et al: Diabetic and nondiabetic patients with left main and/or 3-vessel coronary artery disease: comparison of outcomes with cardiac surgery and paclitaxel-eluting stents. *J Am Coll Cardiol* 55:1067–1075, 2010.
54. Lockowandt U, Sarris G, Vouhe P, et al: Guidelines on myocardial revascularization: The Task Force on Myocardial Revascularization of the European Society of Cardiology (ESC) and the European Association for Cardio-Thoracic Surgery (EACTS). *Eur Heart J* 31:2501–2555, 2010.
55. Bhatt DL, Roe MT, Peterson ED, et al: Utilization of early invasive management strategies for high-risk patients with non-ST-segment elevation acute coronary syndromes: results from the CRUSADE Quality Improvement Initiative. *JAMA* 292:2096–2104, 2004.
56. Roe MT, Parsons LS, Pollack CV, et al: Quality of care by classification of myocardial infarction: treatment patterns for ST-segment elevation vs. non-ST-segment elevation myocardial infarction. *Arch Intern Med* 165:1630–1636, 2005.
57. Bartnik M, Ryden L, Ferrari R, et al: The prevalence of abnormal glucose regulation in patients with coronary artery disease across Europe. The Euro Heart Survey on diabetes and the heart. *Eur Heart J* 25:1880–1890, 2004.
58. Brogan GX, Peterson ED, Mulgund J, et al: Treatment disparities in the care of patients with and without diabetes presenting with non-ST-segment elevation acute coronary syndromes. *Diabetes Care* 29:9–14, 2006.
59. Malmberg K, Yusuf S, Gerstein HC, et al: Impact of diabetes on long-term prognosis in patients with unstable angina and non-Q-wave myocardial infarction: results of the OASIS Registry. *Circulation* 102:1014–1019, 2000.
60. Feit F, Manoukian SV, Ebrahimi R, et al: Safety and efficacy of bivalirudin monotherapy in patients with diabetes mellitus and acute coronary syndromes: a report from the ACUITY trial. *J Am Coll Cardiol* 51:1645–1652, 2008.
61. Donahoe SM, Stewart GC, McCabe CH, et al: Diabetes and mortality following acute coronary syndromes. *JAMA* 298:765–775, 2007.
62. Wallentin L, Lagerqvist B, Husted S, et al: Outcome at 1 year after an invasive compared with a non-invasive strategy in unstable coronary-artery disease: the FRISC II invasive randomised trial. FRISC II Investigators. Fast Revascularisation during Instability in Coronary artery disease. *Lancet* 356:9–16, 2000.
63. Cannon CP, Weintraub WS, Demopoulos LA, et al: Comparison of early invasive and conservative strategies in patients with unstable coronary syndromes treated with the glycoprotein IIb/IIIa inhibitor tirofiban. *N Engl J Med* 344:1879–1887, 2001.
64. Bassand JP, Hamm CW, Ardissino D, et al: Guidelines for the diagnosis and treatment of non-ST-segment elevation acute coronary syndromes. The Task Force for the Diagnosis and Treatment of Non-ST-Segment Elevation Acute Coronary Syndromes of the European Society of Cardiology. *Eur Heart J* 28:1598–1660, 2007.

65. Wright RS, Anderson JL, Adams CD, et al: 2011 ACCF/AHA Focused Update of the Guidelines for the Management of Patients with Unstable Angina/Non-ST-Elevation Myocardial Infarction (Updating the 2007 Guideline). A Report of the American College of Cardiology Foundation/American Heart Association Task Force on Practice Guidelines. *Circulation* 123:2022–2060, 2011.

66. Kosiborod M, Rathore SS, Inzucchi SE, et al: Admission glucose and mortality in elderly patients hospitalized with acute myocardial infarction: implications for patients with and without recognized diabetes. *Circulation* 111:3078–3086, 2005.

67. Aguilar D, Solomon SD, Kober L, et al: Newly diagnosed and previously known diabetes mellitus and 1-year outcomes of acute myocardial infarction: the VALsartan In Acute myocardial iNfarcTion (VALIANT) trial. *Circulation* 110:1572–1578, 2004.

68. Norhammar A, Malmberg K, Ryden L, et al: Under utilisation of evidence-based treatment partially explains for the unfavourable prognosis in diabetic patients with acute myocardial infarction. *Eur Heart J* 24:838–844, 2003.

69. Timmer JR, Ottervanger JP, de Boer MJ, et al: Primary percutaneous coronary intervention compared with fibrinolysis for myocardial infarction in diabetes mellitus: results from the Primary Coronary Angioplasty vs Thrombolysis-2 trial. *Arch Intern Med* 167:1353–1359, 2007.

70. Malmberg K, Ryden L, Wedel H, et al: Intense metabolic control by means of insulin in patients with diabetes mellitus and acute myocardial infarction (DIGAMI 2): effects on mortality and morbidity. *Eur Heart J* 26:650–661, 2005.

71. ETDRS Investigators: Aspirin effects on mortality and morbidity in patients with diabetes mellitus. Early Treatment Diabetic Retinopathy Study report 14. *JAMA* 268:1292–1300, 1992.

72. Ogawa H, Nakayama M, Morimoto T, et al: Low-dose aspirin for primary prevention of atherosclerotic events in patients with type 2 diabetes: a randomized controlled trial. *JAMA* 300:2134–2141, 2008.

73. Belch J, MacCuish A, Campbell I, et al: The prevention of progression of arterial disease and diabetes (POPADAD) trial: factorial randomised placebo controlled trial of aspirin and antioxidants in patients with diabetes and asymptomatic peripheral arterial disease. *BMJ* 337:a1840, 2008.

74. Standards of medical care in diabetes—2010. *Diabetes Care* 33(Suppl 1):S11–S61, 2010.

75. Bhatt DL, Fox KA, Hacke W, et al: Clopidogrel and aspirin versus aspirin alone for the prevention of atherothrombotic events. *N Engl J Med* 354:1706–1717, 2006.

76. Yusuf S, Zhao F, Mehta SR, et al: Effects of clopidogrel in addition to aspirin in patients with acute coronary syndromes without ST-segment elevation. *N Engl J Med* 345:494–502, 2001.

77. Mehta SR, Tanguay JF, Eikelboom JW, et al: Double-dose versus standard-dose clopidogrel and high-dose versus low-dose aspirin in individuals undergoing percutaneous coronary intervention for acute coronary syndromes (CURRENT-OASIS 7): a randomised factorial trial. *Lancet* 376:1233–1243, 2010.

78. Angiolillo DJ, Fernandez-Ortiz A, Bernardo E, et al: Platelet function profiles in patients with type 2 diabetes and coronary artery disease on combined aspirin and clopidogrel treatment. *Diabetes* 54:2430–2435, 2005.

79. Angiolillo DJ, Bernardo E, Ramirez C, et al: Insulin therapy is associated with platelet dysfunction in patients with type 2 diabetes mellitus on dual oral antiplatelet treatment. *J Am Coll Cardiol* 48:298–304, 2006.

80. James S, Angiolillo DJ, Cornel JH, et al: Ticagrelor vs. clopidogrel in patients with acute coronary syndromes and diabetes: a substudy from the PLATelet inhibition and patient Outcomes (PLATO) trial. *Eur Heart J* 31:3006–3016, 2010.

81. Bhatt DL, Marso SP, Lincoff AM, et al: Abciximab reduces mortality in diabetics following percutaneous coronary intervention. *J Am Coll Cardiol* 35:922–928, 2000.

82. Mehilli J, Kastrati A, Schuhlen H, et al: Randomized clinical trial of abciximab in diabetic patients undergoing elective percutaneous coronary interventions after treatment with a high loading dose of clopidogrel. *Circulation* 110:3627–3635, 2004.

83. Roffi M, Chew DP, Mukherjee D, et al: Platelet glycoprotein IIb/IIIa inhibitors reduce mortality in diabetic patients with non-ST-segment-elevation acute coronary syndromes. *Circulation* 104:2767–2771, 2001.

84. Timmer JR, Ten Berg J, Heestermans AA: Pre-hospital administration of tirofiban in diabetic patients with ST-elevation myocardial infarction: a sub-analysis of the on Time 2 trial. *Eurointervention* 6:336–342, 2010.

85. Mahaffey KW, Cohen M, Garg J, et al: High-risk patients with acute coronary syndromes treated with low-molecular weight or unfractionated heparin: outcomes at 6 months and 1 year in the SYNERGY trial. *JAMA* 294:2594–2600, 2005.

86. Blazing MA, de Lemos JA, White HD, et al: Safety and efficacy of enoxaparin vs unfractionated heparin in patients with non-ST-segment elevation acute coronary syndromes who receive tirofiban and aspirin: a randomized controlled trial. *JAMA* 292:55–64, 2004.

87. Gurm HS, Sarembock IJ, Kereiakes DJ, et al: Use of bivalirudin during percutaneous coronary intervention in patients with diabetes mellitus: an analysis from the randomized evaluation in percutaneous coronary intervention linking angiomax to reduced clinical events (REPLACE)-2 trial. *J Am Coll Cardiol* 45:1932–1938, 2005.

88. Stone GW, Witzenbichler B, Guagliumi G, et al: Bivalirudin during primary PCI in acute myocardial infarction. *N Engl J Med* 358:2218–2230, 2008.

89. Yusuf S, Mehta SR, Chrolavicius S, et al: Comparison of fondaparinux and enoxaparin in acute coronary syndromes. *N Engl J Med* 354:1464–1476, 2006.

90. Yusuf S, Mehta SR, Chrolavicius S, et al: Effects of fondaparinux on mortality and reinfarction in patients with acute ST-segment elevation myocardial infarction: the OASIS-6 randomized trial. *JAMA* 295:1519–1530, 2006.

91. Khaw KT, Wareham N, Bingham S, et al: Association of hemoglobin A1c with cardiovascular disease and mortality in adults: the European prospective investigation into cancer in Norfolk. *Ann Intern Med* 141:413–420, 2004.

92. Furnary AP, Gao G, Grunkemeier GL, et al: Continuous insulin infusion reduces mortality in patients with diabetes undergoing coronary artery bypass grafting. *J Thorac Cardiovasc Surg* 125:1007–1021, 2003.

93. Holman RR, Paul SK, Bethel MA, et al: 10-year follow-up of intensive glucose control in type 2 diabetes. *N Engl J Med* 359:1577–1589, 2008.

94. Gerstein HC, Miller ME, Byington RP, et al: Effects of intensive glucose lowering in type 2 diabetes. *N Engl J Med* 358:2545–2559, 2008.

95. Patel A, MacMahon S, Chalmers J, et al: Intensive blood glucose control and vascular outcomes in patients with type 2 diabetes. *N Engl J Med* 358:2560–2572, 2008.

96. Duckworth W, Abraira C, Moritz T, et al: Glucose control and vascular complications in veterans with type 2 diabetes. *N Engl J Med* 360:129–139, 2009.

97. Kahn SE: Glucose control in type 2 diabetes: still worthwhile and worth pursuing. *JAMA* 301:1590–1592, 2009.

98. Nathan DM, Cleary PA, Backlund JY, et al: Intensive diabetes treatment and cardiovascular disease in patients with type 1 diabetes. *N Engl J Med* 353:2643–2653, 2005.

99. Gaede P, Vedel P, Larsen N, et al: Multifactorial intervention and cardiovascular disease in patients with type 2 diabetes. *N Engl J Med* 348:383–393, 2003.

100. Gaede P, Lund-Andersen H, Parving HH, et al: Effect of a multifactorial intervention on mortality in type 2 diabetes. *N Engl J Med* 358:580–591, 2008.

101. Diagnosis and classification of diabetes mellitus. *Diabetes Care* 33 Suppl 1:S62–S69, 2010.

102. Alberti KG, Zimmet P, Shaw J: Metabolic syndrome—a new world-wide definition. A Consensus Statement from the International Diabetes Federation. *Diabet Med* 23:469–480, 2006.

Prior Evaluation: Functional Testing, Multidetector CT

MARIO J. GARCIA

Introduction

Noninvasive testing in patients with known or suspected CAD is conducted to establish the diagnosis of coronary atherosclerosis as the cause of symptoms and/or to determine whether a patient would benefit from medical therapy and/or myocardial revascularization. Functional tests such as stress electrocardiography, stress echocardiography, and stress scintigraphic myocardial perfusion imaging (MPI) attempt to quantify the presence of ischemia based on electrical, mechanical, and perfusion abnormalities. Over the last decade, cardiac computed tomographic angiography (CCTA) has evolved as a noninvasive alternative to invasive catheterization for the evaluation of coronary anatomy. In general, anatomical tests such as CCTA have greater sensitivity for the detection of CAD, whereas functional tests have greater ability to predict benefit from revascularization. This chapter provides an overview of the methodology and interpretation of these tests with the objectives of providing guidelines for appropiate test selection and treatment.

Stress Testing

Anginal symptoms in patients with obstructive CAD are caused by an imbalance between myocardial oxygen supply and oxygen demand. Asymptomatic patients with CAD have normal resting blood flow even in the presence of epicardial coronary artery stenosis. Myocardial perfusion pressure and blood flow are maintained by compensatory dilation of the coronary arterioles. During stress, myocardial oxygen demand increases but myocardial blood flow cannot increase proportionally, thus leading to the development of ischemia. Myocardial ischemia results in progressive metabolic and functional alterations including electrical repolarization abnormalities and abnormal regional diastolic and systolic myocardial function. On these principles, different stress testing modalities attempt to quantify the burden of obstructive CAD based on the extent of myocardial hypoperfusion, ST depression, and wall motion abnormalities. Stress may be accomplished by a number of methods, including exercise, pharmacological maneuvers, and even mental tests. Whenever possible, exercise is the preferred modality, since the information obtained may be more easily related to functional limitations. The choice between electrocardiography (ECG) versus echocardiography or MPI is often determined by local availability, costs, and patient characteristics. In general, specificity has been reported to be higher with stress echocardiography and sensitivity higher with MPI. Accordingly, many clinicians prefer stress echocardiography for individuals with a lower pretest probability of obstructive CAD and MPI for those with a higher probability. Although exercise ECG has lower sensitivity and specificity than stress imaging modalities, it is cost-effective and provides comparable prognostic information in patients who have a normal resting ECG and are able to exercise. One disadvantage of exercise ECG is that it cannot localize the ischemic region, rendering it less useful as a guide for targeting revascularization. Stress cardiac magnetic resonance (CMR) can provide both perfusion and wall motion information with accuracy comparable to stress MPI; however, both of these modalities are currently limited to pharmacologic stress in selected reference centers. Over the last two decades, the prognostic utility of stress testing has been increasingly recognized. Exercise capacity, heart rate response, and the extent of ST depression as well as wall motion and perfusion abnormalities are powerful predictors of outcome. Patients with decreased exercise tolerance and chronotropic incompetence during exercise stress testing have been shown to have increased adverse events independently of other factors. Chronotropic incompetence may be a marker of impaired autonomic dysfunction, which has been associated with cardiac events. Chronotropic response may be defined as the proportion of age-predicted maximal heart rate achieved or the proportion of heart rate reserve used. The latter is defined as follows:

$$(\text{Peak heart rate} - \text{resting heart rate})/(220 - \text{age} - \text{resting heart rate})$$

It is the preferred method as it has been shown to be largely independent of age, functional capacity, or exercise protocol. It is defined as failure to use at least 80% of the heart rate reserve. Chronotropic incompetence has been shown to be associated with the angiographic severity of CAD and increased mortality.

Heart rate recovery is another index that appears to be related to autonomic tone. Most evidence suggests that a rapid reactivation of vagal tone is the major determinant of a decline in heart rate during the first 30 seconds to 1 minute after exercise. Unlike chronotropic incompetence, heart rate recovery is not significantly affected by the administration of beta blockers. Heart rate recovery is calculated as the difference in heart rate at peak versus 1 minute after exercise. A value <12 beats per minute is considered abnormal. Patients evaluated for suspected or known CAD with an abnormal heart rate recovery have a markedly increased mortality rate that is independent of other risk factors.[1] Although both impaired chronotropic response and heart rate recovery are powerful predictors of outcomes, it is unknown whether these are modifiable. Moreover, their association with mortality may be independent of the presence or severity of CAD. Therefore they may have limited value in guiding therapeutic interventions.

ECG STRESS TESTING

Detection of ischemia by ECG stress testing relies on the development of abnormal repolarization, manifesting as ST-segment depression during and/or immediately after exercise. This is achieved by serial or continuous recordings of a 12-lead ECG, which is often aided by computer analysis. Exercise ECG testing has modest diagnostic accuracy; it is most useful when performed in patients with an intermediate pretest probability of obstructive CAD. It is now recognized that the early reported sensitivities of exercise ECG testing were affected by a verification bias (positive studies are more likely to be referred for catheterization). This bias leads to overestimation of sensitivity and underestimation of specificity. Recent data suggest that the true sensitivity of exercise testing may be as low as 50%. Despite this limitation, exercise ECG testing remains a useful prognostic test. An index derived from the exercise ECG test that incorporates exercise time, magnitude of ST-segment deviation, and angina—also known as the Duke treadmill score—has proven to be a powerful prognosticator of events. The Duke Treadmill score index is calculated as follows:

$$\text{Exercise time} - (5 \times \text{maximum net ST-segment deviation}) - (4 \times \text{angina index})$$

Maximum net ST-segment deviation is defined as the maximum deviation (elevation or depression) noted in any of the 12 ECG leads as compared with baseline. The treadmill anginal index is defined as having a value of 0 if no angina occurs, 1 if angina occurs during exercise but is not test-limiting, or 2 if test-limiting angina occurs. Exercise time is measured based on the Bruce protocol and appears to be the most important determinant of prognosis.[4] Using the Duke treadmill score, patients may be divided into categories of low (score ≥ +5), intermediate (score < 5 but ≥ −10), and high risk (score < −10). The 5-year survival rates among patients categorized as low, intermediate, and high risk were initially reported at 97%, 91%, and 72%, respectively. The prognostic information derived from the Duke treadmill score is independent of coronary angiography findings. The predictive utility of the Duke score has been validated in many different subpopulations, including women. A low score is associated with a very low risk for cardiac death (0.3%–1.2% per year).

STRESS ECHOCARDIOGRAPHY

The interpretation of stress echocardiography is based on the identification of regional wall motion abnormalities induced by ischemia in the presence of obstructive CAD. The test has gained increasing acceptance following the introduction of digital acquisition, harmonic imaging, and contrast agents, all of which have incrementally contributed to increased image quality, reproducibility, and accuracy. The performance and interpretation of stress echocardiography require close supervision and attention to detail. Accordingly, accuracy varies significantly between experienced and inexperienced centers. Real time three-dimensional echocardiography facilitates faster data acquisition and better image segmentation and has been shown to improve diagnostic accuracy.[3] Strain imaging has also been shown to improve the accuracy for detecting stress-induced ischemia and/or viability in dysfunctional segments.[4] In stress echocardiography, regional wall motion is assessed from parasternal long, parasternal short, and apical images using a 17-segment model of the LV.[5] Each segment is described as either normal, hypokinetic, akinetic, or dyskinetic, and the results of the individual segments are averaged to calculate a global wall motion score. The diagnosis of CAD is based on the detection of either resting or stress-induced regional wall motion abnormalities (Figs. 4-1, 4-2, and 4-3). In most cases, resting regional wall motion abnormality implies a prior myocardial infarction while a stress-induced regional wall motion abnormality implies ischemia caused by obstructive CAD. Stress echocardiography may also be used to evaluate the severity of ischemic mitral insufficiency.

Exercise Echocardiography

Exercise stress may be performed with a treadmill, supine or prone bicycle, and even arm ergometry. Treadmill stress echocardiography is by far the most commonly used modality in the United States. With treadmill exercise, only pre- and postexercise images are obtained. This is done while the patient lies in a supine lateral position. Postexercise images must be obtained within 1 minute of termination of exercise. Any delay can result in resolution of regional wall motion abnormalities, thus reducing the sensitivity of the test. Bicycle ergometry allows the operator to obtain images while the patient is still exercising; thus, in theory, it is capable of detecting more subtle wall motion abnormalities caused by transient ischemia. Both treadmill and bicycle ergometry allow evaluation of important functional data such as exercise capacity, blood pressure response, hemodynamic responses to exercise including the assessment of cardiac output and pulmonary pressures, as well as standard ECG ST-segment analysis. The complete interpretation of the test takes into account all of these variables. Several studies have reported sensitivities ranging from 71% to 97% and specificities ranging from 64% to over 90%. The differences in results often relate to the definition of wall motion abnormalities. If hypo- or akinesis is required, sensitivity tends to be lower and specificity higher. On the other hand, if tardokinesis (delayed contraction or postsystolic shortening) or lack of hyperkinesis is the accepted definition, sensitivity is higher and specificity tends to be lower. Reported accuracy parameters also vary according to whether obstructive CAD is defined as a >50% or >70% reduction in diameter. The sensitivity of exercise echocardiography is lower for the detection of single-vessel CAD, in particular in the circumflex coronary artery distribution. Quite often, ischemia is only detected in the territory supplied by the most stenotic vessel in those patients with multivessel disease, especially if the test is discontinued at a submaximal workload.

Resting and/or exercise-induced wall motion abnormalities may occur in patients with cardiomyopathies, microvascular disease, severe hypertension (increased afterload), or valvular disease; they are often a cause of false-positive interpretations. Several stress echocardiographic variables have been shown to have important prognostic value in patients with known or suspected CAD. A low exercise wall motion score index or a fall in exercise ejection fraction is highly predictive of an increased risk of adverse cardiac events. This prognostic value is equivalent to that of an MPI perfusion defect of >15%. Echocardiographic variables have incremental independent prognostic utility over other variables, such as the Duke Treadmill score.[6] The rate of cardiac events in individuals with a normal exercise echocardiogram has been reported in several studies to be <1% per year.

Pharmacological Stress Echocardiography

Intravenous dobutamine, dipyridamole, or adenosine may be used as pharmacological stressors with echocardiography. Dobutamine is the most commonly used stressor in the United States. It is administered by continuous infusion at incremental rates starting from 5 and up to 50 mcg/kg per minute. It is often complemented by handgrip exercise and/or intravenous atropine (0.5–2.0 mg) to increase heart rate. Dobutamine increases myocardial oxygen demand by increasing contractility and heart rate. Adenosine and dipyridamole are used in many centers in Europe and South America. These agents induce ischemia by coronary steal. In order to induce regional wall motion abnormalities, the required doses are typically much higher than those used to provoke vasodilation during pharmacological MPI studies. The reported

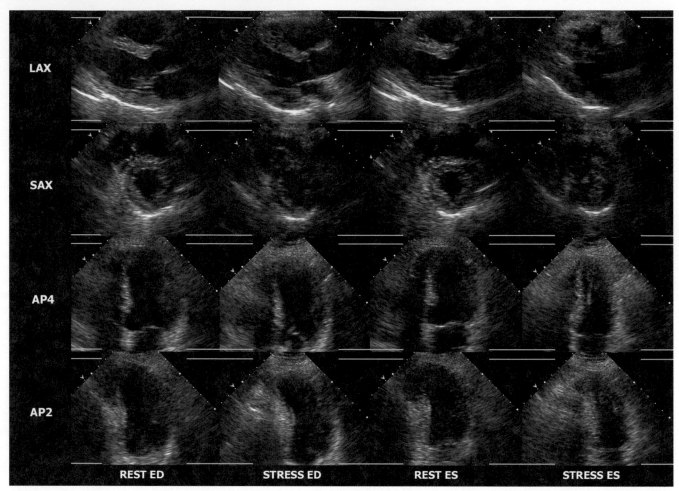

Figure 4-1 Normal stress echo response. Images obtained at end-diastole (ED) and end-systole (ES) at rest and immediately after exercise stress from the parasternal long axis (LAX), short axis (SAX), and apical four-chamber (AP4) and two-chamber (AP2) windows. Notice the decrease in end-systolic LV cavity size after stress.

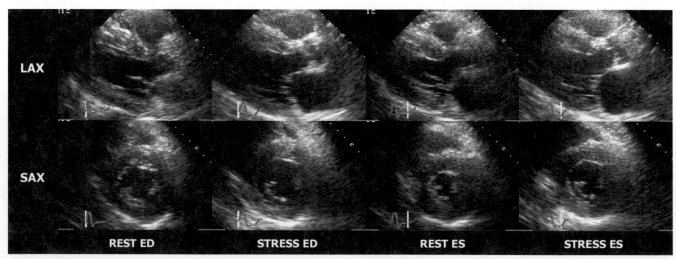

Figure 4-2 Abnormal stress echo response in a patient with severe multivessel CAD. Images obtained at end-diastole (ED) and end-systole (ES) at rest and immediately after exercise stress from the parasternal long axis (LAX) and short axis (SAX) windows. Notice the end-systolic dilatation of LV cavity.

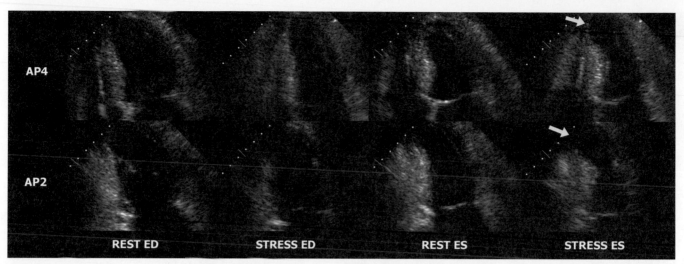

Figure 4-3 Abnormal stress echo response in a patient with severe stenosis of the mid-left anterior descending coronary artery. Images obtained at end-diastole (ED) and end-systole (ES) at rest and immediately after exercise stress from the apical four-chamber (AP4) and two-chamber (AP2) windows. Notice the relative end-systolic dilatation of the LV apical segments (arrows).

sensitivity and specificity of dobutamine echocardiography for the detection of obstructive CAD are equivalent to those reported for exercise echocardiography. The sensitivity is reduced in patients with concentric hypertrophy who experience cavity obliteration early during the test as well as in those who do not reach the target heart rate. Echocardiographic variables obtained during pharmacological stress have also been shown to have significant prognostic value.[7] A normal dobutamine stress echocardiogram is associated with a low cardiac event rate in patients with suspected CAD and in those at clinically determined intermediate or high cardiac risk undergoing noncardiac surgery. The presence of stress-induced regional wall motion abnormalities, particularly when detected at low heart rates, is a strong predictor of cardiac events. Dobutamine stress echocardiography allows further risk stratification even in patients at intermediate or high risk who are receiving perioperative beta blockers.[8] Dobutamine echocardiography may be performed for risk assessment in patients after myocardial infarction. In this setting, extensive resting regional wall motion abnormalities, stress-induced ischemia, absence of viability, and worsening left ventricular (LV) function with stress are associated with an increased risk of adverse events. In patients with ischemic heart disease and chronic LV dysfunction, dobutamine echocardiography is useful to identify myocardial viability. Improvement in regional contractility at lower rates of dobutamine (5–10 mcg/kg per minute) in segments that are akinetic or hypokinetic at rest predicts functional recovery after revascularization, particularly when those same segments exhibit a reduction in contractility at high dobutamine rates (biphasic response). Patients with ischemic LV dysfunction and viable myocardium who undergo revascularization have better outcomes than those who are not revascularized or have no evidence of viability regardless of revascularization. The sensitivity with which dobutamine echocardiography predicts recovery of function ranges between 74% and 88%; the specificity is between 73% and 87%. Compared with MPI, dobutamine stress echocardiography has higher specificity but lower sensitivity and overall similar accuracy for predicting functional recovery.[9]

Contrast Perfusion Imaging

Echocardiographic contrast agents consist of inert perfluorocarbon gases encapsulated in a biodegradable shell. Contrast microbubbles have a small diameter (<10 microns) that allows them to cross the pulmonary capillary bed. These agents are commercially available and approved for endocardial border definition in patients with suboptimal echocardiographic images. When they are exposed to ultrasound, these microbubbles act as strong reflectors owing to their liquid-gas interface. Contrast echocardiography may be used to evaluate myocardial perfusion. Since the LV myocardium has a dense capillary bed, the injection of contrast microbubbles results in myocardial enhancement proportional to the myocardial blood volume. During vasodilator stress in the presence of a flow-limiting stenosis, there is a reduction in capillary blood flow and myocardial blood volume in the segments supplied by the stenotic vessel. This may be detected as either a delay in myocardial enhancement following contrast injection or a relative reduction in enhancement in ischemic compared with normal segments (Fig. 4-4). Studies have shown relatively good agreement between myocardial contrast echocardiography and MPI for the detection of ischemia.[10,11] An earlier study performed in high-risk patients but with normal wall motion at rest reported a sensitivity of 85% by myocardial contrast echocardiography versus 74% by MPI for the detection of obstructive CAD.[12] The high spatial and temporal resolution of myocardial contrast echocardiography makes it suitable for the detection of nontransmural ischemia and milder ischemia where blood flow may be reduced but blood volume is preserved (late enhancement). However, data have been limited to a few reports and, in some studies where the sensitivity has been reported to be high, the specificity has been low. A previously published multicenter trial performed in 123 patients reported a sensitivity of 84% but a specificity of only 56%.[13] Protocols for image acquisition and interpretation are considerably more technically demanding than those required for scintigraphic MPI. Thus, at present the use of contrast echocardiography for myocardial perfusion assessment is not an approved clinical indication in the United States.

STRESS SCINTIGRAPHIC MYOCARDIAL PERFUSION IMAGING

The assessment of myocardial perfusion imaging (MPI) by nuclear scintigraphic methods relies on the administration of a radionuclide isotope that is accumulated by the myocardium in proportion to blood flow. MPI is performed with either single-photon-emitting or dual-photon-emitting isotopes using single photon emission computed tomography (SPECT) or positron emission tomography (PET) imaging systems, respectively. Thallium-201, technetium-99m sestamibi, and technetium-99m tetrofosmin are isotopes commercially available for SPECT imaging. Currently, technetium-99m-based isotopes are preferred for their higher photon energy, which results in higher image quality, and their shorter half-life, which results in lower radiation exposure. These isotopes emit single photons that travel through tissues and must be detected on a photon-sensitive detector. The direction of the traveling photon is determined by adding a lead collimator, which

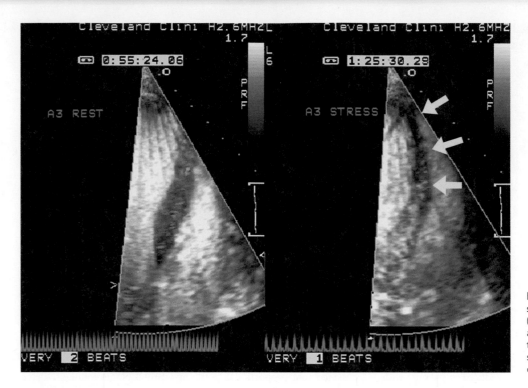

Figure 4-4 Myocardial contrast perfusion study showing a stress-induced (adenosine) perfusion defect not present at rest in the mid- and apical anteroseptal region (arrows) in a patient with severe stenosis of the mid-left anterior descending coronary artery.

acts as an x-ray filter between the source and the detector. This collimator rejects most of the photons not traveling along certain directions; therefore only a percentage of the emitted photons are used for imaging. Spatial resolution is given by the space between the bars in the collimator. Increasing spatial resolution improves image quality but requires higher rejection of photons, thus reducing efficiency and increasing radiation exposure to the patient. Most dual-photon-emitting isotopes are produced using a cyclotron and have a very short half-life. These isotopes decay with the emission of a positron; after a series of collisions with atomic electrons from the tissues, it annihilates with a nearby electron and produces two high-energy photons emitted in opposite directions. A PET system relies on the simultaneous detection of the photons. These photons travel toward detectors positioned around the subject, where they interact, becoming absorbed and producing an electrical signal. The detector signals are processed by specialized coincidence circuitry. If the difference in the time of arrival of these photons is smaller than a predetermined value (typically <10 ns) a signal is recorded. Unlike SPECT imaging, PET does not require collimation, since the position of the emitting target is determined by the simultaneous registration of the two photons traveling at 180 degrees. Thus, the efficiency of PET is several magnitudes greater, providing higher resolution, lower noise, and lower radiation exposure. The signals recorded are used to reconstruct a three-dimensional image. The spatial resolution of PET images is closely related to the physical size of the detector elements and has dramatically increased in recent times with the introduction of time-of-flight (TOF) technology (Fig. 4-5). With either SPECT or PET cardiac perfusion studies, images are obtained after stress and at rest. For segmentation of the LV, a 17-segment model is applied. Images are interpreted visually or by using automated quantification based on normalized data. Myocardial scar is determined by the presence of a relative perfusion defect (compared with the segment with highest counts), which persists on both stress and resting images. Ischemia is determined by the presence of a perfusion defect on stress images that improves or resolves on the resting images (Figs. 4-6, 4-7, 4-8, and 4-9).

Exercise Scintigraphic MPI

Exercise stress is well suited for SPECT MPI. At peak exercise, either on a treadmill or bicycle ergometer, patients are injected with the radioisotope. Acquisition of the stress images is performed after a few minutes to up to 1 hour after exercise, depending on the radioisotope used. Resting images are obtained before or after the exercise images following the administration of a separate dose of the isotope at rest. Different isotopes may be used for resting and for stress imaging—for example, thallium-201 injected at rest and technetium-99m sestamibi injected at peak stress.

The mean reported sensitivity and specificity for exercise SPECT is 86% and 74%, respectively.[14] Most of the studies reported, however, are potentially subjected to verification bias. Accordingly, true sensitivity may be overestimated and specificity underestimated. In order to estimate the true specificity of the test, the normalcy rate has been studied in populations at low risk of having CAD. The mean normalcy rate in these populations has been reported at 89%. Sensitivity and specificity are higher for the detection of multivessel disease, followed by single-vessel disease in the left anterior descending artery distribution, right coronary artery, and circumflex. False-positive results are often attributed to attenuation artifacts from large breasts in women and the diaphragm in obese individuals. Excessive bowel radioactivity may also result in false-positive or false-negative results. The introduction of ECG gated SPECT imaging has allowed assessment of LV function in addition to perfusion. Studies have shown a good correlation for the assessment of LV ejection fraction between SPECT and other tomographic modalities.[15] However, LV volumes may be underestimated and ejection fraction overestimated in ventricles with a small LV cavity and hypertrophy of the walls because of partial volume effects. The accuracy of SPECT determination of LV volumes and ejection fraction is also limited in patients with extensive perfusion defects and LV aneurysms, where the entire geometry of the LV cavity cannot be defined. However, the additional information derived from regional systolic function in gated studies has improved the diagnostic accuracy of the test. Quite frequently, artifacts caused by soft tissue attenuation may be discriminated from true ischemia or scar by the demonstration of normal regional wall motion. Another recent advancement in SPECT imaging has been the introduction of attenuation correction. Commercially available SPECT attenuation correction systems measure the nonhomogeneous attenuation distribution utilizing external collimated radionuclide sources or x-ray CT (hybrid systems). The application of attenuation correction in patients with excessive

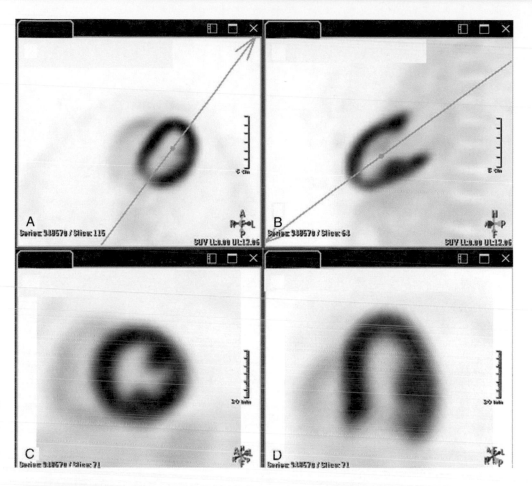

Figure 4-5 Example of a PET-FDG study obtained with time-of-flight (TOF) imaging. The high spatial resolution allows visualization of the papillary muscles in the transverse (A), sagittal oblique (B), short-axis (C), and horizontal long-axis (D) planes.

Figure 4-6 SPECT technetium-99m sestamibi exercise stress study showing normal myocardial perfusion during stress and at rest

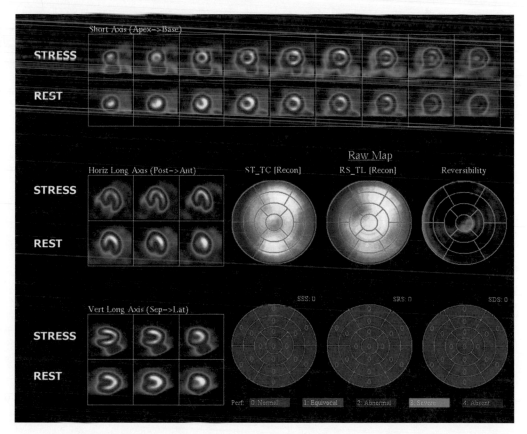

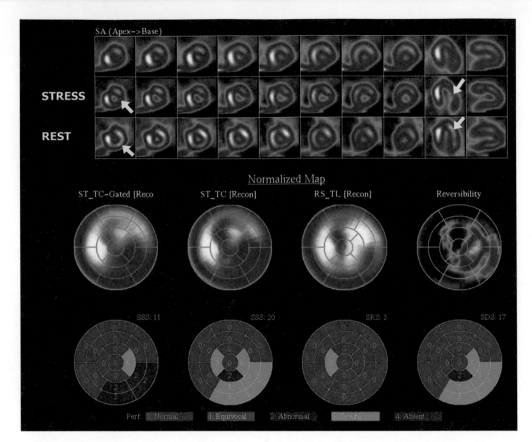

Figure 4-7 SPECT technetium-99m sestamibi exercise stress study showing a large myocardial perfusion defect in the posterolateral walls during stress (white arrows) with complete reversibility on the resting study, indicating ischemia.

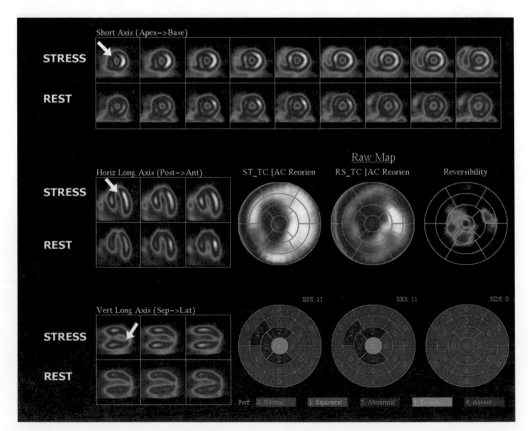

Figure 4-8 SPECT technetium-99m sestamibi exercise stress study showing a mid-size myocardial perfusion defect in the anteroseptal and apical walls during stress (white arrows) without reversibility on the resting study, indicating scar.

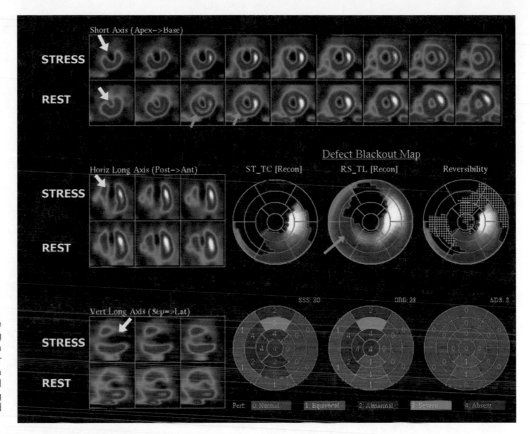

Figure 4-9 SPECT technetium-99m sestamibi exercise stress study showing a large myocardial perfusion defect in the anteroseptal, anterior, and inferior walls during stress (white arrows), with partial reversibility (inferior and septal walls, green arrows) on the resting study, indicating both scar and ischemia.

subdiaphragmatic activity corrects by enhancing the affected regions of the myocardium such as the inferior and posterior LV walls. Several studies have shown significant improvements in specificity and modest improvements in sensitivity with the use of attenuation correction.[16,17] The demonstrated benefits of attenuation correction are greater in patients with increased indexed body mass.[18] More recently, SPECT systems where the traditional Anger camera is replaced with individual cesium iodide (CsI) scintillation crystals coupled to solid-state photodiodes have shown improved efficiency, making it possible to obtain higher counts and improving signal-to-noise ratio and spatial resolution without increasing isotope dose or acquisition time. Several studies have shown that a normal exercise stress SPECT study predicts a very low likelihood (<1%) of adverse events, such as cardiac death or myocardial infarction, for at least 12 months and that this level of risk is independent of gender, age, symptom status, and even the presence of CAD. Therefore in those patients with abnormal scans, baseline clinical characteristics such as diabetes, as well as severe and extensive SPECT perfusion abnormalities it is possible to define incremental levels of risk as well as which populations of patients will benefit most from revascularization.[19]

Pharmacological Scintigraphic MPI

In the United States, many patients who are referred for evaluation of suspected or known CAD are unable to exercise. Both adenosine and dipyridamole are vasodilator agents that, in the absence of epicardial artery stenosis, increase myocardial blood flow three to five times over baseline. In the presence of a stenosis, a relative perfusion defect may be seen, indicating either failure to increase regional blood flow compared with myocardial segments supplied by a normal vessel or reduced myocardial blood flow due to coronary steal. For this reason, in some patients with multivessel disease and balanced ischemia, pharmacological stress SPECT studies may appear normal. The average reported sensitivity and specificity of adenosine SPECT for the detection of CAD are similar to those of exercise SPECT studies, at 90% and 75%,

respectively. With dipyridamole SPECT, sensitivity is similar (89%) but specificity is lower (65%). As previously discussed, verification bias may exaggerate true sensitivity and underestimate specificity. The sensitivities and specificities are also higher for multivessel than for single-vessel disease. Pharmacological stress SPECT studies may also be performed with dobutamine. The mean reported sensitivity and specificity of this test are 82% and 75%, respectively. Unlike dobutamine echocardiography, monitoring of ischemia-induced functional abnormalities is difficult during SPECT MPI. For this reason, dobutamine is not a preferred stressor in most clinical instances. Pharmacological SPECT is a powerful prognosticator in populations of patients with suspected CAD and in those at risk being evaluated prior to noncardiac surgery. The risk of death in patients with normal scans has been reported to be low but higher than in patients with negative exercise SPECT (1%-3% per year). This probably reflects higher comorbidities in selected populations of patients who cannot exercise. In patients undergoing noncardiac surgery, a pharmacological stress test has a significant negative predictive value but a low positive predictive value. For that reason, it has been recommended that this test be used in populations at moderate risk, such as those with anginal symptoms, prior infarction, and/or diabetes. The role of stress MPI is well accepted for the evaluation of symptoms, but has not been clearly established for screening asymptomatic patients at risk. In the DIAD[54] (Detection of Ischemia in Asymptomatic Diabetics) study, a randomized controlled trial in which 1,123 participants with type 2 diabetes and no symptoms of CAD were randomly assigned to be screened with adenosine-stress MPI or not to be screened, the cardiac event rates were low and were not significantly reduced by MPI screening for myocardial ischemia over a follow-up period of 4.8 years.[21] Pharmacological stress imaging may be performed with PET. Its higher spatial resolution, efficiency, and lower attenuation make PET a superior method in certain patient groups, such as the obese. Cardiac PET has also been validated for the quantitative assessment of regional myocardial perfusion, left ventricular function, and viability. Current PET

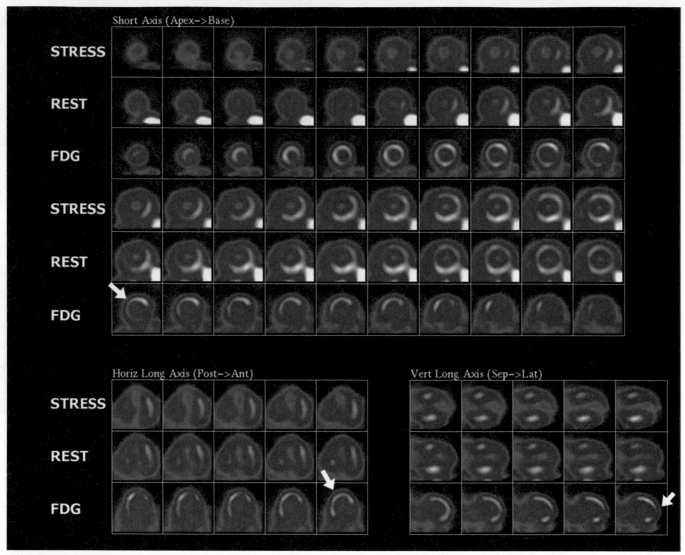

Figure 4-10 PET myocardial viability study obtained in a patient with ischemic LV dysfunction. Both resting and stress rubidium-82 images show an extensive anteroapical perfusion defect (arrows). The fluorine-18-2-fluoro-2-deoxyglucose (FDG) images show matched preserved metabolic activity indicating hypoperfused but viable myocardium (arrows).

stress myocardial perfusion protocols require pharmacological stress because of the short half-life of rubidium-82. Given that it can be produced on-site without a cyclotron from a column generator, this is the preferred radioisotope for the assessment of perfusion in clinical practice. Two other radioisotopes approved for cardiac PET use in the United States are nitrogen-13 ammonia (perfusion) and fluorine-18-2-fluoro-2-deoxyglucose (metabolic viability). In patients with suboptimal SPECT results, follow-up cardiac PET has demonstrated superior accuracy. Most PET studies obtained in patients with a previous equivocal SPECT result are unequivocally classified as normal or mildly positive.[21] PET is one of the most sensitive methods for the identification of myocardial viability in patients with ischemic LV dysfunction. PET defines viable myocardium as the presence of a perfusion/metabolism mismatch. Images are obtained using a perfusion isotope such as rubidium-82 and a metabolic agent such as fluorine-18-2-fluoro-2-deoxyglucose. Scar myocardium exhibits reduced uptake of both tracers, whereas ischemic viable myocardium shows preserved metabolic activity (Fig. 4-10). The extent of viability by PET has been shown in numerous studies as able to predict functional myocardial recovery after revascularization. Patients with viable myocardium by PET who undergo revascularization have improved survival compared with those with viable myocardium on medical therapy or those without viability regardless of treatment.

CARDIAC MAGNETIC RESONANCE

Cardiac magnetic resonance (CMR) is an excellent method for the assessment of global and regional systolic LV function. The most widely used steady-state free precession technique (SSFP) allows clear identification of endocardial borders caused by a high blood-pool signal. In addition, the tomographic approach allows for the measurement of volumes without geometric assumptions, resulting in accurate measurements even in those patients with previous myocardial infarction and distorted LV geometry. Image quality is preserved even in obese patients, making this method ideal for patients with technically difficult echocardiographic images. In addition, in using intravenous paramagnetic contrast agents, CMR can provide an accurate assessment of myocardial perfusion.

Dobutamine CMR

CMR can evaluate global and regional LV function at rest and during bicycle ergometry or pharmacological stress. Dobutamine is the most commonly used stressor for the evaluation of ischemia-induced regional wall motion abnormalities. The average reported sensitivity and specificity for the detection of obstructive CAD are 89% and 84%, respectively. The protocols used are similar to those used in echocardiography for the evaluation of both ischemia and viability. One of the limitations of dobutamine CMR is the inability to obtain accurate ECG monitoring of ST-segment deviation during the test. For this reason many centers have favored the use of vasodilator stress and CMR perfusion imaging.

CMR Perfusion Imaging

An intravenous paramagnetic agent such as gadolinium DTPA may be used to evaluate myocardial perfusion. Gadolinium DTPA is an extracellular agent that, during its first pass, will enhance the intravascular compartment. This is followed by extracellular deposition. Areas of fibrosis and scarring in the LV accumulate gadolinium over time, exhibiting "delayed enhancement." Using a fast imaging protocol with steady-state precession (FISP) based sequence, the first-pass enhancement of the myocardium may be imaged by CMR in near real-time. CMR makes it possible to identify areas of myocardial hypoenhancement at rest in the presence of severely reduced myocardial blood flow (Fig. 4-11). In most circumstances, resting blood flow is normal in segments supplied by stenotic vessels owing to compensatory arteriolar vasodilation. However, adenosine or dipyridamole may induce ischemia in these cases by reducing myocardial perfusion pressure. The high spatial resolution of CMR permits the visualization of nontransmural ischemia or infarction. A study comparing CMR and SPECT MPI for the detection of CAD demonstrated similar sensitivities for both techniques for the detection of transmural ischemia or infarction.[22] On the other hand, SPECT identified only 28% of subendocardial infarcts, whereas CMR correctly identified 92%. In a recent multicenter study of patients undergoing cardiac catheterization for the evaluation of symptoms, perfusion CMR was compared with SPECT MPI. Based on receiver operating characteristic (ROC) analysis, perfusion CMR at the optimal gadolinium-DTPA dose ($n = 42$, 0.1 mmol/kg) performed much like SPECT (area under ROC curve [AUC]: 0.86 ± 0.06 vs. 0.75 ± 0.09 for SPECT, $P = 0.12$).[23] CMR studies have also shown abnormal myocardial perfusion in patients with syndrome X[24] and others with microvascular dysfunction. Quantitative analysis of CMR perfusion images can be performed to determine the ratio of stress/resting blood flow or myocardial perfusion reserve (MPR). Studies have shown that in patients with obstructive CAD, MPR increases following percutaneous intervention.[25] Delayed gadolinium-enhanced CMR is a powerful technique for evaluating the presence of scar in patients with ischemic LV dysfunction. The extent of infarct transmurality as determined by CMR predicts functional recovery in patients referred for revascularization (Fig. 4-12).[26] Coronary imaging may be performed with CMR. Although the method is well established for the evaluation of congenital coronary anomalies, it is less accurate for evaluating CAD. In a recent metanalysis of 20 studies (989 patients) comprising patients with suspected CAD assessed by MRI, mean sensitivity and specificity for the detection of obstructive CAD were 87.1% (CI, 83.0%–90.3%) and 70.3% (CI, 58.8%–79.7%), considerably lower than the respective values found in a metanalysis of 89 studies (7,516 patients) assessed by cardiac computed tomographic angiography (CCTA, 97.2% (95% CI, 96.2%–98.0%) and 87.4% (CI, 84.5%–89.8%).[27]

Cardiac Computed Tomography

Cardiac computed tomography (CCT) has now been extensively validated as an accurate noninvasive method of evaluating the coronary anatomy. Technical advances available in modern scanners now make it possible to obtain adequate image quality in most patients. Image acquisition and interpretation can be performed very rapidly, making this technology suitable for the evaluation of ambulatory patients.

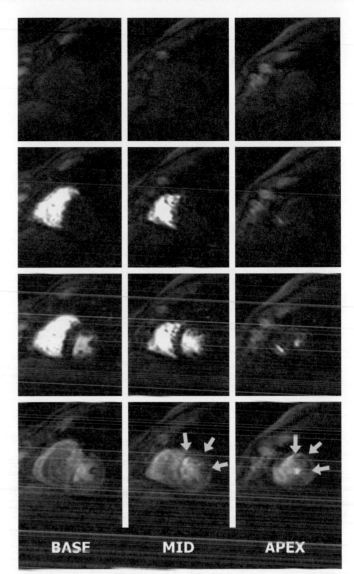

Figure 4-11 First-pass gadolinium DTPA myocardial perfusion study. From top to bottom, sequential cross-sectional images obtained at the base (left), middle, and apex (right panels). The first row of images is acquired before the arrival of contrast. The second row demonstrates the arrival of contrast in the right ventricle. The third row shows its arrival in the left ventricular cavity, and the fourth row shows enhancement of the myocardium. The arrows demonstrate an area of subendocardial hypoenhancement in a patient with severe stenosis of a large marginal branch.

Multidetector CT (MDCT) technology has recently overcome many of its previous limitations, providing ECG-gated acquisition with short acquisition time, submillimeter spatial resolution, and adequate spatial resolution (80–200 msec), thus allowing excellent visualization of the coronary arteries. Moreover, the rate of technological advancement with MDCT has rapidly exceeded that of electron-beam computed tomography (EBCT) and CMR. Image quality is undergoing constant refinement, and the number of un-interpretable coronary studies has gradually decreased from 20% to 40% using four detectors to 15% to 25% using 16 detectors; it is now as low as 3% to 10% with systems using 64, 128, 256, and 320 detectors. CCT can provide an accurate and reproducible assessment of coronary calcification. By adding iodine contrast for intravascular enhancement, one can also use cardiac computed tomographic angiography (CCTA) to provide visualization of noncalcified coronary plaques and assess the severity of stenosis.

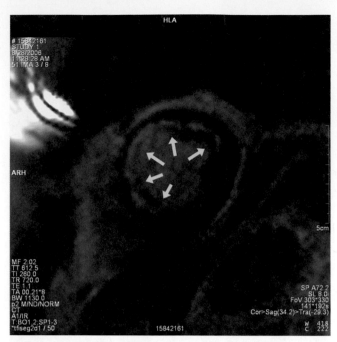

Figure 4-12 Mid-LV cross-sectional image obtained 20 minutes after injection of gadolinium DTPA, demonstrating a large area of subendocardial fibrosis (white rim indicated by arrows) involving 50% of transmural thickness in the septum and anterior walls.

CORONARY ARTERY CALCIUM SCORING

Coronary artery calcium scoring (CAC) quantifies coronary calcification using a radiographic density-weighted volume of high attenuation regions (>130 Hounsfield units). The prognostic value of CAC has been clearly established.[28] Keelan et al. demonstrated that a CAC Agatston score >100 was an independent predictor (OR = 1.88) of cardiovascular outcomes (death and nonfatal myocardial infarction) at 7 years' follow-up. Although very high calcium scores impart an approximately 10-fold increased event risk, they do not always imply a tight coronary stenosis. The role of CAC for screening asymptomatic individuals is controversial, and the routine incorporation of this type of investigation into a comprehensive risk screening with CRP and cholesterol measurements is still under debate. There is some evidence to support the incorporation of CAC into the overall risk stratification of older individuals, using clinical algorithms such as the Framingham Risk Score. In the South Bay Heart Watch study,[29] a CAC > 300 was associated with a significant increase in cardiac event rates compared with that determined by clinical score alone. These data support the belief that CAC can improve risk prediction, especially among patients at intermediate Framingham risk in whom clinical decision making is most difficult. Patients with low Framingham risk derive no significant additional benefit from CAC. Furthermore, it is costly to use CAC to improve cardiovascular risk prediction in populations with no cardiac symptoms who are at low risk. Some even suggest that its wide clinical implementation may in aggregate have a detrimental effect on the quality of life of screened populations.[30] However, in a published study of 6,723 asymptomatic patients, CAC was shown to be the strongest predictor of cardiovascular death, nonfatal myocardial infarction, angina, and revascularization (total events = 162) independent of race. In this study, the risk increased 7.7-fold in patients with a CAC score between 101 and 300 compared with 0 and 9.7 fold in patients with a score > 300.[31] The addition of CAC to MPI provides incremental value over and above myocardial perfusion findings.[32] In patients with normal stress perfusion, adding a CAC score can improve detection of CAD, particularly in patients with a high pretest likelihood, such as those with diabetes.[33] Although evidence of calcified plaque is not specific for obstructive CAD,[34] there is a proportional relationship between the extent of CAC and risk for cardiac events, even in patients with a normal MPI.[35]

CARDIAC COMPUTED TOMOGRAPHIC ANGIOGRAPHY

Although the actual acquisition of a cardiac computed tomographic angiography (CCTA) study takes less than 15 seconds, patient preparation and data interpretation require extensive training and extreme attention to detail. Patient selection is important, since extensive coronary calcification and poor x-ray penetration in obese patients may compromise image quality. The frequency of artifacts related to diaphragmatic and/or cardiac motion has been significantly reduced with the newest wide detector coverage (128-, 256-, and 320-slice) scanners and dual-source imaging. However, most patients still require beta-blocker administration and cooperation with breath-holding during the scan acquisition.

Over the last few years, significant attention has focused on excessive radiation exposure with medical imaging.[36] In response, the industry, in collaboration with medical imaging leaders, has implemented several strategies to reduce radiation dose during CCTA. These include reduction in the volume of coverage, use of lower peak x-ray-tube currents and wider adoption of prospective ECG-gated acquisition. The use of prospective gating is very effective in reducing dose[37] but limits CCTA image acquisition to a predetermined brief phase of the cardiac cycle. Thus, analysis of left ventricular function cannot be performed when this acquisition mode is being used. Patients in whom functional analysis is required, or those with rapid or irregular heart rates who may require reconstruction of multiple cardiac phases for coronary vessel examination, should be imaged using conventional spiral retrospective ECG-gated acquisition, which requires higher overall radiation exposure. CCTA is very useful in assessing the origin and course of congenitally anomalous coronary arteries and the three-dimensional relationship of anomalous coronary arteries with the aorta and pulmonary arterial trunk.[38-40] Myocardial bridges and coronary arteriovenous fistulas can also be well visualized by CCTA.

CCTA Evaluation of Coronary Luminal Stenosis

Figures 4-13 and 4-14 are CCTA studies obtained from a patient with normal coronaries and another with severe multivessel disease. The corresponding invasive angiogram from the latter is shown in Figure 4-15. Several single-center and multicenter studies have examined the accuracy of CCTA for establishing the diagnosis of obstructive CAD. Most of these studies have been performed in patients being referred for diagnostic coronary angiography based on clinical indications. The prevalence of obstructive CAD in patients enrolled in these studies ranged anywhere from 35% to 80%. Accuracy has been defined in these studies based on segment-based, vessel-based, and/or patient-based analysis. Segment-based analysis has been restricted in many of these studies to segments >1.5 or >2 mm in diameter. In most studies, previously stented segments have been excluded. Either a >50% or >70% reduction in luminal diameter on invasive coronary angiography has been used as the reference standard to adjudicate a positive result. On vessel-based analysis, a positive result has been defined as the presence of one or more abnormal segments in the specific vessel's distribution. On patient-based analysis, a positive result has been defined as one or more abnormal segments anywhere in the coronary arterial tree.

In single-center studies performed with the first generation of 16-slice scanners, the sensitivity of MDCT coronary angiography ranged between 72% and 95% in segment-based analysis and 85% and 100% in patient-based analysis. The specificity has been reported as between 86% and 98% in segment-based analysis and between 78% and 86% in patient-based analysis. In a multicenter study[41] that enrolled 187 patients with high or intermediate risk with an Agatston calcium score <600, 71% of segments were deemed evaluable on MDCT. All nonevaluable segments were censored as "positive," since in clinical practice they would also lead to the performance of

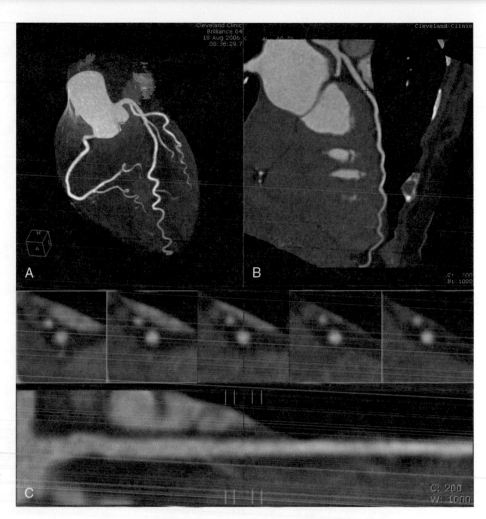

Figure 4-13 MDCT coronary angiography showing normal coronary arteries. A. Volume-rendered maximum-intensity projection of the aortic root and coronary arteries. B. Curved multiplanar reconstruction of the left anterior descending coronary artery (LAD). C. Series of cross-sectional images obtained from the mid-LAD at 1 mm intervals.

angiography. The sensitivity, specificity, and positive/negative predictive values for detecting >50% luminal stenoses in segment-based analysis were 89%, 65%, 13%, and 99%. In patient-based analysis, the sensitivity, specificity, positive/negative predictive values were 98%, 54%, 50%, and 99%. The results of this study suggest that the clinical utility of CCTA, given its high negative predictive value, lies primarily in the exclusion of obstructive CAD.

Prospective multicenter trials have demonstrated improved diagnostic characteristics of 64-slice CCTA in comparison to 16-slice CCTA.[42,43] The ACCURACY trial, a 15-center U.S.-based multicenter study examining 230 patients undergoing CCTA prior to elective diagnostic coronary angiography observed sensitivity, specificity, and positive (PPV) and negative predictive values (NPV) of CCTA to detect a ≥50% or ≥70% stenosis of 95%, 83%, 64%, 99%, respectively and 94%, 83%, 48%, 99% respectively. It is likely that there will always be a discrepancy between CCTA and invasive coronary angiography for the quantitative assessment of luminal stenosis. Unlike angiography, CCTA provides data on both the lumen and vessel wall plaque. Thus the results of CCTA are more comparable with those of intravascular ultrasound (IVUS). In addition, CCTA provides an infinite number of projections because of its three-dimensional nature. Thus, in many cases, a presumed "false positive" CCTA finding may represent a "false negative" coronary angiogram in which adequate projections were not obtained. The prognostic utility of CCTA has been examined in several single-center studies. Among 169 low- to intermediate-risk patients who underwent both exercise treadmill testing and CCTA, the presence of obstructive (≥70%) stenosis was associated with both ST-segment depression (adjusted odds ratio [OR] 3.38 [1.32, 8.64], P = 0.001) and

elevated risk Duke treadmill scores (adjusted OR 4.67 [1.97, 11.03], P < 0.001). In this study, there was a graded relationship between the extent and severity of CAD and the exercise time as well as the likelihood of ST-segment depression.[44] In another study of 163 low- to intermediate-risk patients who underwent both MPI and CCTA, the extent and severity of CAD as measured by a modified Duke coronary artery jeopardy score was independently associated with a severely abnormal MPI result (OR 2.25 [1.12–4.41], P = 0.02) for the highest risk group as compared with those without disease.[45] In a single-center study, a cohort of 1,127 low- to intermediate-risk symptomatic patients underwent 16-slice CCTA for the diagnosis of stable chest pain syndromes, the severity of intraluminal stenosis, left main or proximal LAD stenosis, and the number of coronary segments involved. Their results were associated with increased mortality over an intermediate-term observation period averaging 15 ± 3.9 months.[46] In this study the negative predictive value for death of a normal CCTA was 99.7%. In a multicenter study of 541 intermediate-probability patients referred for symptoms or CAD risk factors who prospectively underwent both CCTA and MPS, the annualized hard event rate was 1.8% in those with no or mild CAD versus 4.8% in those with ≥50% stenosis by CCTA and 1.1% in those with a normal MPS versus 3.8% in those with an abnormal MPS.[47] In multivariate analysis, CCTA-visualized obstructive plaque and abnormal MPS were independent predictors of late events after adjustment for clinical risk factors, with significantly improved prediction by the combined use of CCTA and MPI compared with either modality alone (log-rank test P value < 0.005). Over the study period, those with concordantly normal CCTA and MPS results had an annualized hard event rate of 1%; those with

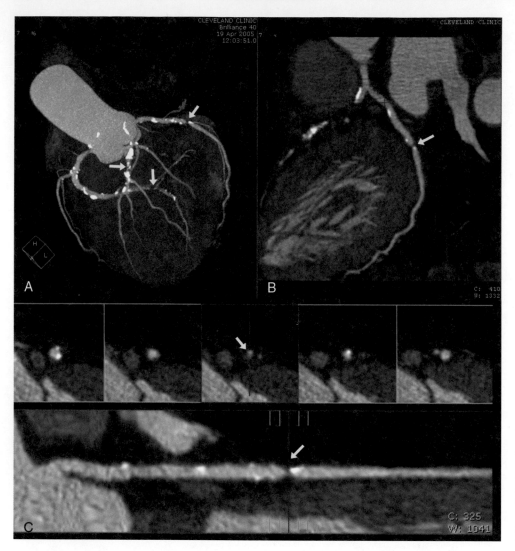

Figure 4-14 MDCT coronary angiography showing obstructive multivessel disease. A. Volume-rendered maximum-intensity projection of the aortic root and coronary arteries. B. Curved multiplanar reconstruction of the left circumflex coronary artery (LCX). C. Series of cross-sectional images obtained from the mid-LCX at 1-mm intervals. Arrows indicate areas of severe stenosis caused predominantly by noncalcified (dark) atherosclerotic plaques.

concordantly abnormal CCTA and MPS results had a hard event rate of 9.0%; and those with discordant CCTA and MPS results with either abnormal CCTA or abnormal MPS had event rates of 3.8% and 3.7% respectively. In a multicenter study of 368 patients presenting to the emergency department for evaluation of acute chest pain who underwent 64-slice CCTA after initially negative troponin measurements and ECGs, none of the 185 patients with no visualized CAD had ACS, while 7 of the 115 with nonobstructive plaque and 24 of the 68 with significant obstructive or nondiagnostic exams had ACS during the index hospitalization.[48] In this study, CCTA incrementally improved prediction of ACS beyond the TIMI risk score, with an area under the curve (AUC) for CCTA-visualized extent of plaque of 0.88 and CCTA-visualized stenotic disease of 0.82 compared with the AUC of the TIMI risk score of 0.63. The current data on CCTA for ACS suggest that in this selected population, a normal CCTA has a very high negative predictive value, allowing for safe early discharge in a large proportion of low-risk suspected ACS patients. Although several studies have demonstrated the predictive value of low-density plaque components and eccentric remodeling, the benefit of CCTA in asymptomatic patients is not yet well established. In one study, 1,000 asymptomatic patients underwent 64-slice CCTA as part of a general health evaluation; those with no plaque had no major adverse cardiac events over an average observation of 17 ± 2 months, while 15 of the 215 individuals with any plaque had later unstable angina or underwent revascularization.[49] However, most events occurred within 90 days of the CCTA and were

driven by revascularization procedures in this open-label trial. Furthermore, most events occurred in patients with an abnormal CAC, indicating that CCTA provided no significant incremental prognostic value in asymptomatic patients. Accurate assessment of previously stented coronary vessels remains an important limitation of CCTA coronary angiography.[50] A noninvasive, accurate test for in-stent restenosis would be invaluable in patients with postinterventional chest pain. This is particularly true because the widespread use of drug-eluting stents reduces the incidence of in-stent restenosis, thus reducing the positive yield from repeated invasive coronary angiography. In a study using 16-slice MDCT, only 126 of 232 stents (54%) could be evaluated.[51] Smaller stents in vessels <3 mm were harder to evaluate accurately. Internal luminal diameter is often underestimated. Studies performed with 64-slice scanners have shown improved sensitivity and specificity.[52] Nevertheless, the ability to evaluate the lumen of stented vessels depends on the type and diameter of the stent. Practical delineation of in-stent stenosis remains difficult in stents with a diameter <3 mm. CCTA is useful in the evaluation of coronary artery bypass grafts (CABG) (Fig. 4-16). The reported sensitivity, specificity, and positive/negative predictive values for detecting total graft occlusion were 96%, 95%, 81%, and 99%, respectively, using 16-slice scanners.[53] In a more recent study using 64-slice scanners,[54] CCTA images of 138 grafts, native vessels, and anastomotic sites were compared with invasive coronary angiograms. The grafts included both venous and arterial bypass conduits. All the grafts were "evaluable" by CCTA, with

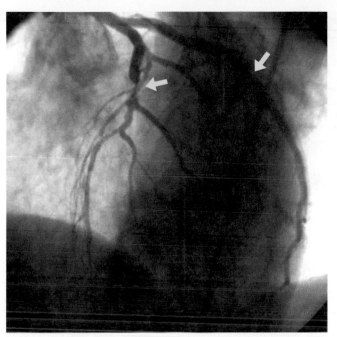

Figure 4-15 Angiographic left anterior projection of the left coronary artery and branches obtained by catheterization in the previous patient in Figure 4-14. Arrows indicate severe stenotic lesions in the LAD and the left circumflex coronary artery.

or in whom a high contrast load should be avoided. MDCT may also be useful in symptomatic patients with recent CABG in whom graft occlusion is suspected. CCTA is useful in defining the three-dimensional location of preexisting coronary grafts in relation to the chest wall in patients undergoing repeated sternotomy.

CCTA Evaluation of Coronary Atherosclerotic Plaque

In contrast to invasive coronary angiography, CCTA is also capable of imaging the vessel wall. Several studies have documented the ability of CCTA to visualize atherosclerotic coronary plaques[55–57] and differentiate calcified from noncalcified lesions based on Hounsfield unit values.[58] Whether MDCT could be used in clinical practice as a screening test remains to be proven, but in selected patients at low to intermediate risk, it could potentially help to justify lifelong aggressive preventive intervention. MDCT plaque characterization could also potentially serve to devise optimal revascularization strategies.

Guiding Interventions with CCTA

Because of its three-dimensional capabilities, CCTA has a great potential as a guide to interventions. In electrophysiology, MDCT has already been adopted, as it provides an anatomical roadmap for complex electrophysiological procedures such as radiofrequency ablation of atrial fibrillation. CCTA can define the anatomical course, calibre, length of a diseased segment, and the extent of calcification in patients with chronic total occlusions (CTO) of a coronary vessel.[59] In addition, MDCT images may be projected side by side with the fluoroscopy images in the catheterization laboratory.

Hybrid Imaging

Until the advent of CCTA, noninvasive imaging for the detection of CAD had mainly relied on functional imaging techniques to assess perfusion or wall motion abnormalities as indirect evidence of CAD. Functional imaging has been proven to be very valuable in determining prognosis and establishing the need for revascularization. However, neither echocardiographic, MPI, nor CMR stress testing can establish the presence of mild to moderate CAD. Moreover, decisions regarding revascularization cannot rely solely on functional imaging without knowledge of the coronary anatomy. CCTA is capable of providing detailed information about the coronary anatomy, including luminal

sensitivity, specificity, and positive/negative predictive values of 100%, 94%, 92%, and 100%, respectively. Evaluation of the distal anastomosis is often limited by surgical clips, constituting artifacts. Analysis of the native vessels is often more difficult in patients with previous CABG owing to poor runoff, more extensive calcification, and smaller lumen size. This can potentially limit the diagnostic utility of CCTA in this setting. In patients with previous CABG, CCTA should be considered as an alternative to invasive angiography in patients in whom direct catheterization carries a risk, such as those with suspected atheroma

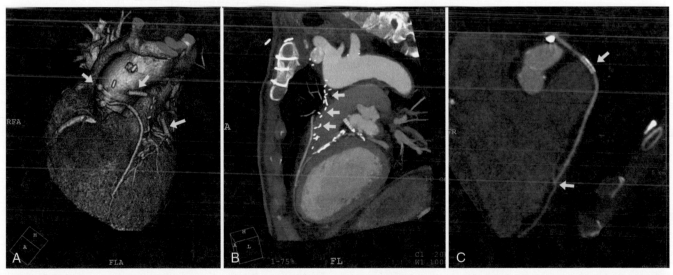

Figure 4-16 MDCT coronary angiography obtained in a patient with previous coronary artery bypass grafts. A. Volume-rendered projection of the heart. Arrows indicate the stump of an occluded bypass to the circumflex and stents previously deployed in this vessel. The graft is not visualized owing to the lack of contrast opacification. B. Oblique sagittal maximum-intensity-projection image showing a series of staples corresponding to an occluded left internal thoracic graft to the LAD. C. Curved multiplanar reconstruction of a saphenous vein bypass graft to the LAD. The arrows indicate a stent in the proximal segment and the location of anastomosis to the distal LAD.

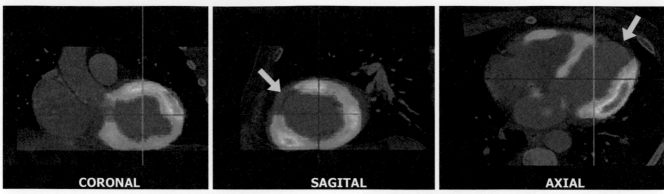

Figure 4-17 Hybrid imaging. Fusion of anatomical (MDCT) and functional images (PET rubidium-82) in a patient with a large apical myocardial infarction (arrows). Notice the thinning of the myocardium, matching the lack of perfusion.

stenosis and wall plaque. Because of the latter, it may establish the presence of atherosclerosis even earlier than invasive coronary angiography. However, the technique is limited in spatial and temporal resolution, making the differentiation between moderate and severe luminal stenosis difficult in most cases. In a study of 114 patients undergoing both MPI and CCTA, 90% of patients with no visualized plaque by CCTA had normal MPI, 45% with any plaque by CCTA had abnormal MPI, and only 50% with any >50% plaque by CCTA had abnormal MPI.[60] The rationale for the development of PET-CT or SPECT-CT hybrid systems is that in many patients, a knowledge of both coronary anatomy and extent of ischemia is needed to make management decisions. Hybrid systems consist of an MDCT and either a SPECT or a PET camera mounted next to each other and sharing the same patient table. This facilitates the registration of functional and anatomical data in three-dimensional space (Fig. 4-17). In oncology, the use of hybrid PET-CT systems has largely replaced the use of either modality alone. The benefit of integrating anatomical and functional data is clear, given the small size and large possible volume of distribution of metastatic tumors. However, in cardiology, the development of the technology has advanced before a clinical need has been clearly established.

Conclusions

The objectives of noninvasive cardiac imaging in patients with known or suspected CAD are to provide (1) confirmatory evidence that CAD has been the cause of symptoms and (2) guidance for the appropriate selection of medical therapy and/or revascularization. In most cases, the extent of anatomic CAD is directly related to the extent and severity of stress-induced myocardial perfusion abnormalities. However, abnormal myocardial perfusion may also be associated with vascular dysfunction in the setting of nonobstructive CAD. Conversely, normal myocardial perfusion may be present in patients with obstructive CAD with increased collateral flow.[61] Hence, since the objective of myocardial revascularization is to reduce myocardial ischemia, one may conclude that the results of functional imaging tests are more important than knowledge of the coronary anatomy to guide therapeutic decisions in patients with known or suspected CAD.

In patients who have been evaluated by both MPI and CCTA, the frequency of inducible ischemia is 0%, 5%, 33%, 54%, and 86% for CCTA stenosis of 0%, 0% to 60%, 60% to 70%, 70% to 80%, and >80%, respectively ($P < 0.0001$).[62] Thus when severe ischemia is present and a false-positive result is unlikely, the likelihood of obstructive CAD is high. The additional information provided by CCTA in such cases is minimal in terms of dictating patient management. On the other hand, real-world experience has shown that a significant proportion of patients who are evaluated by functional tests have inconclusive, false-positive, or false-negative results. Thus anatomical demonstration of CAD by CCTA may play an important role as a less expensive and safer alternative to diagnostic invasive coronary angiography in these cases.

A recent metanalysis of comparative studies performed with 64-multislice CCTA demonstrated diagnostic sensitivities and specificities of 94% (93%-97%) and 85% (80%-90%).[63] From these studies it is clear that the strengths of CCTA are its high sensitivity and high negative predictive value, exceeding 95%.[64] These characteristics suggest that CCTA would be most useful as a first diagnostic test for excluding obstructive CAD in low- to intermediate-risk patients.

In comparison with CCTA, MPI has a lower sensitivity, in the range of 85% to 90%,[65] and even lower for the detection of single-vessel CAD. The rate of false-positive MPI scans has been reduced with the use of technetium-99m radioisotopes, attenuation-correction algorithms, and the incorporation of gated LV ejection fraction and regional wall motion analysis. The result has been improved specificity in the range of 80% to 90%.[66-68] Specificity is also very high with stress echocardiography. Therefore, the strengths of functional stress imaging tests are their higher specificity and positive predictive value. Accordingly, stress imaging would be most useful as a first diagnostic test for confirming obstructive CAD in intermediate- to high-risk patients. Several ongoing prospective multicenter trials are seeking to determine the utility of anatomical versus functional imaging tests in specific clinical scenarios.

REFERENCES

1. Cole CR, Blackstone EH, Pashkow FJ, et al: Heart-rate recovery immediately after exercise as a predictor of mortality. *N Engl J Med* 341:1351–1357, 1999.
2. Nishime EO, Cole CR, Blackstone EH, et al: Heart rate recovery and treadmill exercise score as predictors of mortality in patients referred for exercise ECG. *JAMA* 284:1392–1398, 2000.
3. Ahmad M, Xie T, McCulloch M, et al: Real-time three-dimensional dobutamine stress echocardiography in assessment stress echocardiography in assessment of ischemia. Comparison with two-dimensional dobutamine stress echocardiography. *J Am Coll Cardiol* 37:1303–1309, 2001.
4. Voigt JU, Exner B, Schmiedehausen K, et al: Strain-rate imaging during dobutamine stress echocardiography provides objective evidence of inducible ischemia *Circulation* 107:2120–2126, 2003.
5. Quinones MA, Douglas PS, Foster E, et al: ACC/AHA clinical competence statement on echocardiography: a report of the American College of Cardiology/American Heart Association/American College of Physicians/American Society of Internal Medicine Task Force on Clinical Competence. *J Am Coll Cardiol* 41:687–708, 2003.
6. Marwick TH, Case C, Vasey C, et al: Prediction of mortality by exercise echocardiography: a strategy for combination with the Duke treadmill score. *Circulation* 103:2566–2571, 2001.
7. Sicari R, Pasanisi E, Venneri L, et al: Stress echo results predict mortality. A large-scale multicenter prospective international study. *J Am Coll Cardiol* 41:589–595, 2003.
8. Boersma E, Poldermans D, Bax JJ, et al: Predictors of cardiac events after major vascular surgery. Role of clinical characteristics, dobutamine echocardiography, and beta-blocker therapy. *JAMA* 285:1865–1873, 2001.
9. Bax JJ, Poldermans D, Elhendy A, et al: Sensitivity, specificity, and predictive accuracies of various noninvasive techniques for detecting hibernating myocardium *Curr Probl Cardiol* 26:141–186, 2001.

10. Heinle SK, Noblin Goree-Best P, et al: Assessment of myocardial perfusion by harmonic power Doppler imaging at rest and during adenosine stress: comparison with (99m)Tc-sestamibi SPECT imaging, *Circulation* 102:55–60, 2000.
11. Wei K, Crouse L, Weiss J, et al: Comparison of usefulness of dipyridamole stress myocardial contrast echocardiography to technetium-99m sestamibi single-photon emission computed tomography for detection of coronary disease (PB127 multicenter phase 2 trial results). *Am J Cardiol* 91:1293–1298, 2003.
12. Peltier M, Vancraeynest D, Pasquet A, et al: Assessment of the physiologic significance of coronary disease with dipyridamole real-time myocardial contrast echocardiography. *J Am Coll Cardiol* 43:257–264, 2004.
13. Jeetley P, Hickman M, Kamp O: Myocardial contrast echocardiography for the detection of coronary artery stenosis: a prospective multicenter study in comparison with single-photon emission computed tomography. *J Am Coll Cardiol* 47(1):141–145, 2006.
14. Underwood SR, Anagnostopoulos C, Cerqueira M, et al: Myocardial perfusion scintigraphy: the evidence. *Eur J Nucl Med Mol Imaging* 31:261–291, 2004.
15. Ioannidis JP, Trikalinos TA, Danias PG: Electrocardiogram-gated single-photon emission computed tomography versus cardiac magnetic resonance imaging for the assessment of left ventricular volumes and ejection fraction: a meta-analysis. *J Am Coll Cardiol* 39:2059–2068, 2002.
16. Hendel RC, Berman DS, Cullom SJ, et al: Multicenter clinical trial to evaluate the efficacy of correction for photon attenuation and scatter in SPECT myocardial perfusion imaging. *Circulation* 99:2742–2749, 1999.
17. Links JM, Becker LC, Rigo P, et al: Combined corrections for attenuation, depth-dependent blur, and motion in cardiac SPECT: a multicenter trial. *J Nucl Cardiol* 7:414–425, 2000.
18. Bateman TM, Heller GV, Johnson LL, et al: Relative performance of attenuation-corrected and uncorrected ECG-gated SPECT myocardial perfusion imaging in relation to body mass index. *Circulation* 108:IV–455, 2003.
19. Hachamovitch R, Hayes SW, Friedman JD, et al: Identification of a threshold of inducible ischemia associated with a short-term survival benefit with revascularization compared to medical therapy in patients with no prior CAD undergoing stress myocardial perfusion SPECT. *Circulation* 107:2899–2906, 2003.
20. Young LH, Wackers FJ, Chyun DA, et al: Cardiac outcomes after screening for asymptomatic coronary artery disease in patients with type 2 diabetes: the DIAD study: a randomized controlled trial. *JAMA* 301(15):1547–1555, 2009.
21. Bateman TM, McGhie I, O'Keefe JH, et al: High clinical value of follow-up myocardial perfusion PET in patients with a diagnostically indeterminate myocardial perfusion SPECT study. *Circulation* 108:IV–454, 2003.
22. Wagner A, Mahrholdt H, Holly TA, et al: Contrast-enhanced MRI and routine single photon emission computed tomography (SPECT) perfusion imaging for detection of subendocardial myocardial infarcts: an imaging study. *Lancet* 361:374–379, 2003.
23. Schwitter J, Wacker CM, van Rossum AC, et al: MR IMPACT: comparison of perfusion-cardiac magnetic resonance with single-photon emission computed tomography for the detection of coronary artery disease in a multicentre, multivendor, randomized trial. *Eur Heart J* 29(4):480–489, 2008.
24. Panting JR, Gatehouse PD, Yang GZ, et al: Abnormal subendocardial perfusion in cardiac syndrome X detected by cardiovascular magnetic resonance imaging. *N Engl J Med* 346:1948–1953, 2002.
25. Al-Saadi N, Nagel E, Gross M., et al: Noninvasive detection of myocardial ischemia from perfusion reserve based on cardiovascular magnetic resonance. *Circulation* 101:1379–1383, 2000.
26. Kim RJ, Wu E, Rafael A, et al: The use of contrast-enhanced magnetic resonance imaging to identify reversible myocardial dysfunction. *N Engl J Med* 343(20):1445–1453, 2000.
27. Schuetz GM, Zacharopoulou NM, Schlattmann P, et al: Meta-analysis: noninvasive coronary angiography using computed tomography versus magnetic resonance imaging. *Ann Intern Med* 152(3):167–177, 2010.
28. Keelan PC, Bielak LF, Ashai K, et al: Long-term prognostic value of coronary calcification detected by electron-beam computed tomography in patients undergoing coronary angiography. *Circulation* 104:412–417, 2001.
29. Greenland P, LaBree L, Azen SP, et al: Coronary artery calcium score combined with Framingham score for risk prediction in asymptomatic individuals. *JAMA* 291:210–215, 2004.
30. O'Malley PG, Greenberg BA, Taylor AJ: Cost-effectiveness of using electron beam computed tomography to identify patients at risk for clinical coronary artery disease. *Am Heart J* 148:106–113, 2004.
31. Detrano R, Guerci AD, Carr JJ, et al: Coronary calcium as a predictor of coronary events in four racial or ethnic groups. *N Engl J Med* 358(13):1336–1345, 2008.
32. Schenker MP, Dorbala S, Hong EC, et al: Interrelation of coronary calcification, myocardial ischemia, and outcomes in patients with intermediate likelihood of coronary artery disease: a combined positron emission tomography/computed tomography study. *Circulation* 117(13):1693–1700, 2008.
33. Anand DV, Lim E, Hopkins D, et al: Risk stratification in uncomplicated type 2 diabetes: prospective evaluation of the combined use of coronary artery calcium imaging and selective myocardial perfusion scintigraphy. *Eur Heart J* 27(6):713–721, 2006.
34. Greenland P, Bonow RO, Brundage BH, et al: ACCF/AHA 2007 clinical expert consensus document on coronary artery calcium scoring by computed tomography in global cardiovascular risk assessment and in evaluation of patients with chest pain: a report of the American College of Cardiology Foundation Clinical Expert Consensus Task Force (ACCF/AHA Writing Committee to Update the 2000 Expert Consensus Document on Electron Beam Computed Tomography) developed in collaboration with the Society of Atherosclerosis Imaging and Prevention and the Society of Cardiovascular Computed Tomography. *J Am Coll Cardiol* 49(3):378–402, 2007.
35. Berman DS, Wong ND, Gransar H, et al: Relationship between stress-induced myocardial ischemia and atherosclerosis measured by coronary calcium tomography. *J Am Coll Cardiol* 44(4):923–930, 2004.
36. Hausleiter J, Meyer T, Hermann F, et al: Estimated radiation dose associated with cardiac CT angiography. *JAMA* 301(5):500–507, 2009.
37. Raff GL, Chinnaiyan KM, Share DA, et al: Radiation dose from cardiac computed tomography before and after implementation of radiation dose-reduction techniques. *JAMA* 301(22):2340–2348, 2009.
38. Taylor AJ, Byers JP, Cheitlin MD, et al: Anomalous right or left coronary artery from the contralateral coronary sinus: "high-risk" abnormalities in the initial coronary artery course and heterogeneous clinical outcomes. *Am Heart J* 133:428–435, 1997.
39. Shi H, Aschoff AJ, Brambs HJ, et al: Multislice CT imaging of anomalous coronary arteries. *Eur Radiol* 14:2172–21781, 2004.
40. Memisoglu E, Hobikoglu G, Tepe MS, et al: Congenital coronary anomalies in adults: Comparison of anatomic course visualization by catheter angiography and electron beam CT. *Catheter Cardiovasc Interv* 66:34–42, 2005.
41. Garcia MJ, Lessick J, Hoffmann MHK: Accuracy of 16-row multidetector computed tomography for the assessment of coronary artery stenosis. *JAMA* 296:404–411, 2006.
42. Miller JM, Rochitte CE, Dewey M, et al. Diagnostic performance of coronary angiography by 64-row CT. *N Engl J Med* 359(22):2324–2336, 2008.
43. Meijboom WB, Meijs MF, Schuijt JD, et al: Diagnostic accuracy of 64-slice computed tomography coronary angiography: a prospective, multicenter, multivendor study. *J Am Coll Cardiol* 52(25):2135–2144, 2008.
44. Lin FY, Saba S, Weinsaft JW, et al: Relation of plaque characteristics defined by coronary computed tomographic angiography to ST-segment depression and impaired functional capacity during exercise treadmill testing in patients suspected of having coronary heart disease. *Am J Cardiol* 103(1):50–58, 2009.
45. Lin F, Shaw LJ, Berman DS, et al: Multidetector computed tomography coronary artery plaque predictors of stress-induced myocardial ischemia by SPECT. *Atherosclerosis* 197(2):700–709, 2008.
46. Min JK, Shaw LJ, Devereux RB, et al: Prognostic value of multidetector coronary computed tomographic angiography for prediction of all-cause mortality. *J Am Coll Cardiol* 50(12):1161–1170, 2007.
47. Van Werkhoven JM, Schuijf JD, Gaemperli O, et al: Prognostic value of multislice computed tomography and gated single-photon emission computed tomography in patients with suspected coronary artery disease. *J Am Coll Cardiol* 53(7):623–632, 2009.
48. Hoffmann U. AHA Scientific Sessions, New Orleans, 2008.
49. Choi EK, Choi SI, Rivera JJ, et al: Coronary computed tomography angiography as a screening tool for the detection of occult coronary artery disease in asymptomatic individuals. *J Am Coll Cardiol* 52(5):357–365, 2008.
50. Gilard M, Cornily JC, Rioufol G, et al: Noninvasive assessment of left main coronary stent patency with 16-slice computed tomography. *Am J Cardiol* 95:110–112, 2005.
51. Hong C, Chrysant GS, Woodard PK, et al: Coronary artery stent patency assessed with in-stent contrast enhancement measured at multi-detector row CT angiography: initial experience. *Radiology* 233:286–291, 2004.
52. Leber AW, Knez A, von Ziegler F, et al: Quantification of obstructive and nonobstructive coronary lesions by 64-slice computed tomography: a comparative study with quantitative coronary angiography and intravascular ultrasound. *J Am Coll Cardiol* 46:147–154, 2005.
53. Schlosser T, Konorza T, Hunold P, et al: Noninvasive visualization of coronary artery bypass grafts using 16-detector row computed tomography. *J Am Coll Cardiol* 44:1224–1229, 2004.
54. Ropers D, Pohle FK, Kuettner A, et al: Diagnostic accuracy of noninvasive coronary angiography in patients after bypass surgery using 64-slice spiral computed tomography with 330-ms gantry rotation. *Circulation* 114(22):2334–2341, 2006.
55. Kopp A, Schroeder S, Baumbach A, et al: Non-invasive characterization lesion morphology and composition by multislice: just results in comparison with intracoronary ultrasound. *Euro Radiol* 11(9):1607–1611, 2001.
56. Schoenhagen P, Tuzcu EM, Stillman AE, et al: Non-invasive assessment of plaque morphology and remodeling in mildly stenotic coronary segments: comparison of 16-slice computed tomography and intravascular ultrasound. *Coronary Artery Dis* 14:459–462, 2003.
57. Achenbach S, Moselewski F, Ropers D, et al: Detection of calcified and noncalcified coronary atherosclerotic plaque by contrast-enhanced, submillimeter multidetector spiral computed tomography. A segment-based comparison with intravascular ultrasound. *Circulation* 109:14–17, 2004.
58. Carrascosa PM, Capunay CM, Garcia-Merletti P, et al: Characterization of coronary atherosclerotic plaques by multidetector computed tomography. *Am J Cardiol* 97(5):598–602, 2006.
59. Ehara M, Terashima M, Kawai M, et al: Impact of multislice computed tomography to estimate difficulty in wire crossing in percutaneous coronary intervention for chronic total occlusion. *J Invas Cardiol* 21(11):575–582, 2009.
60. Schuijf JD, Wijns W, Jukema JW, et al: Relationship between noninvasive coronary angiography with multi-slice computed tomography and myocardial perfusion imaging. *J Am Coll Cardiol* 48(12):2508–2514, 2006.
61. Wolak AB, Bax JJ, Marwic TH, et al, editors: *Hurst's The Heart: Manual of Cardiology*, ed 12, New York, 2008, McGraw Hill.
62. Lin FY, Saba S, Weinsaft JW, et al: Relation of plaque characteristics defined by coronary computed tomographic angiography to ST-segment depression and impaired functional capacity during exercise treadmill testing in patients suspected of having coronary heart disease. *Am J Cardiol* 103(1):50–58, 2009.
63. Janne d'Othee B, Siebert U, Cury R, et al: A systematic review on diagnostic accuracy of CT-based detection of significant coronary artery disease. *Eur J Radiol* 65(3):449–461, 2008.
64. Budoff MJ, Achenbach S, Blumenthal RS, et al: Assessment of coronary artery disease by cardiac computed tomography: a scientific statement from the American Heart Association Committee on Cardiovascular Imaging and Intervention, Council on Cardiovascular Radiology and Intervention, and Committee on Cardiac Imaging, Council on Clinical Cardiology. *Circulation* 114(16):1761–1791, 2006.
65. Mieres JH, Shaw LJ, Arai A, et al: Role of noninvasive testing in the clinical evaluation of women with suspected coronary artery disease: Consensus statement from the Cardiac Imaging Committee, Council on Clinical Cardiology, and the Cardiovascular Imaging and Intervention Committee, Council on Cardiovascular Radiology and Intervention, American Heart Association. *Circulation* 111(5):682–696, 2005.
66. Masood Y, Liu YH, Depuey G, et al: Clinical validation of SPECT attenuation correction using x-ray computed tomography-derived attenuation maps: multicenter clinical trial with angiographic correlation. *J Nucl Cardiol* 12(6):676–686, 2005.
67. Fricke E, Fricke H, Weise R, et al: Attenuation correction of myocardial SPECT perfusion images with low-dose CT: evaluation of the method by comparison with perfusion PET. *J Nucl Med* May; 46(5):736–744, 2005.
68. Duvall WL, Croft LB, Corriel JS, et al: SPECT myocardial perfusion imaging in morbidly obese patients: image quality, hemodynamic response to pharmacologic stress, and diagnostic and prognostic value. *J Nucl Cardiol* 13(2):202–209, 2006.

Contrast-Induced Acute Kidney Injury and the Role of Chronic Kidney Disease in PCI

J. MATTHEW BRENNAN | BRAHMAJEE K. NALLAMOTHU |
UPTAL D. PATEL

KEY POINTS

- Acute kidney injury (AKI) after cardiac catheterization and percutaneous coronary intervention (PCI) is common, primarily because of exposure to contrast agents; it is associated with worse clinical outcomes.

- The prevalence of chronic kidney disease (CKD) is rising and it is a key risk factor for AKI after cardiac catheterization and PCI.

- The presence of CKD and end-stage renal disease (ESRD) is associated with worse short- and long-term outcomes even after successful PCI, including higher rates of restenosis and repeat revascularization. The use of coronary stenting and drug-eluting stents may diminish this risk.

- Beyond the use of serum creatinine levels, calculation of the glomerular filtration rates and a simple risk score can help to identify high-risk patients prior to their procedures.

- Established keys to preventing AKI after cardiac catheterization and PCI include periprocedural hydration and the use of low- or iso-osmolar contrast agents.

- Evidence appears to favor the safety and efficacy of antioxidant agents like N-acetylcysteine in high-risk patients, but not all trials are consistent.

- Intraprocedural strategies should consistently be used to minimize the volume of contrast agent exposure as much as possible.

Introduction

Alterations of the kidney are commonly encountered in the interventional cardiology setting. Sudden changes are manifest during AKI that are sustained during procedures, while chronic decreased function is a predisposing risk factor. Contrast-induced AKI, also known as contrast-induced nephropathy, is a widely recognized complication of cardiac catheterization and PCI. A transient rise in serum creatinine levels, a common marker for the development of mild renal dysfunction, occurs in more than 15% of patients undergoing these procedures. Although many of these rises are unlikely to be clinically significant, even mild AKI after cardiac catheterization and PCI has been associated with longer hospital stays and greater inpatient costs as well as worse short- and long-term mortality. Contrast-induced AKI after cardiac catheterization and PCI is believed to be primarily caused by intraprocedural exposure to contrast agents, which are nephrotoxic in high-doses.[1] The single most important risk factor that has been linked to the development of AKI after cardiac catheterization and PCI is the presence of preexisting CKD. Other clinical factors like diabetes mellitus and hemodynamic instability, which are also highly prevalent in this population, may also contribute to and exacerbate its clinical course. In a small proportion of patients, AKI may be related to renal atheroembolic disease from diffuse atherosclerosis of the aorta. In patients without CKD or other risk factors, the development of renal dysfunction after these procedures is rare. Importantly, recent diagnostic and therapeutic advances have improved our ability to identify those patients who are at highest risk for developing contrast-induced AKI and to minimize its occurrence. In this chapter we provide a summary of this data with an additional focus on patients with CKD, given its strong association with AKI as well as subsequent cardiovascular complications. We discuss the role of nonpharmacological and pharmacological strategies for reducing the likelihood that AKI will develop in high-risk patients. Finally, we briefly comment on two groups of patients who represent growing segments of the population undergoing coronary revascularization: those with ESRD and those with heart failure.

Epidemiology of Acute Kidney Injury

DEFINITIONS OF ACUTE KIDNEY INJURY

Several definitions have been used to identify AKI, resulting in wide variation in estimates of its incidence. Within the context of contrast-induced AKI, the interventional cardiology and radiology literature commonly define contrast-induced AKI as a rise in serum creatinine of at least 0.5 mg/dL or a 25% increase from baseline within 48 to 72 hours after the procedure.[2,3] However, these definitions differ from those in the cardiothoracic and nephrology literature, which seeks to evaluate AKI in a variety of settings not limited to contrast exposure.[4] The Society of Thoracic Surgeons defines postoperative renal insufficiency as a twofold or greater elevation of creatinine that must exceed 2.0 mg/dL, whereas renal failure is defined as AKI requiring dialysis.[5] In contrast, definitions from the nephrology community include graded criteria for AKI by the Acute Kidney Injury Network group (AKIN criteria) and the Acute Dialysis Quality Initiative (RIFLE criteria, including stages of Risk, Injury, Failure, Loss, and End stage).[6,7] In an attempt to standardize the definition of AKI across the scientific community, these systems grade AKI on the basis of urine output or change in creatinine from baseline, with the mildest stage of AKI defined as the rapid development (<48 hours) of renal dysfunction, including either a rise in serum creatinine (absolute rise ≥0.3 mg/dL [≥26.4 micromol/L] or relative rise ≥50% from baseline) or a reduction in urine output to less than 0.5 mL/kg per hour for >6 hours. The severity of AKI can be further staged based on the magnitude of increase in serum creatinine or reduction in urine output. Although some studies have sought to determine the relative advantages between these criteria, there remains no clear consensus.[8,9] Greater recognition of this problem has led to several reports based on data from the Contrast-Induced Nephropathy Consensus Working Panel, an international multidisciplinary group that convened to address the challenges of contrast-induced AKI.[10]

INCIDENCE OF ACUTE KIDNEY INJURY

The incidence of AKI depends on both the population studied and the definition used. Using a common definition of contrast-induced nephropathy (a rise in serum creatinine levels of 0.5 mg/dL or a 25% increase from baseline), the reported incidence ranges from 8% to 15% in the general population[11] and up to 28% in those with acute coronary syndromes (ACSs).[12]

PROGNOSIS OF ACUTE KIDNEY INJURY

In most cases, AKI after cardiac catheterization and PCI is completely reversible, with a typical clinical course consistent with acute tubular necrosis and nonoliguric AKI. Abnormalities in serum creatinine levels start within 24 to 48 hours after the procedure, peak at 5 days, and then completely recover within 2 to 4 weeks.[13] The need for renal replacement therapy with hemodialysis or peritoneal dialysis is rare.[14] Among those who do require renal replacement therapy (1%–4%), less than 50% require it permanently.[10] The requirement for renal replacement therapy appears to be more likely in the setting of renal atheroembolic disease, which has a more progressive course than contrast-induced nephropathy and a lower likelihood of recovery.

Importantly, the development of AKI after cardiac catheterization and PCI has been associated with several clinical outcomes unrelated to renal disease, including longer hospital stays and greater inpatient costs.[15] Recent reports also suggest that the development of contrast-induced nephropathy predicts short- and long-term mortality.[16–19] What remains unclear from this literature, however, is whether the development of AKI after PCI is simply a marker of greater disease acuity or additional comorbidities like diabetes mellitus.

PATHOPHYSIOLOGY OF CONTRAST-INDUCED AKI

The most common reason for AKI after cardiac catheterization and PCI is related to the use of intravascular contrast agents. Despite their widespread use in imaging studies, however, the exact mechanisms responsible for the development of contrast-induced nephropathy remain unknown.[1] Most studies suggest that both (1) direct toxic injury to the renal tubules and (2) ischemic injury to the renal medulla from vasomotor changes and decreased perfusion are responsible. The latter appears to be mediated partly by the development of reactive oxygen species like superoxide and has important implications for treatment with scavenging agents.[20] Diabetes mellitus and heart failure may also exacerbate contrast-induced nephropathy, specifically by impeding vasodilatory responses in the renal vasculature (Table 5-1).[21] However, these mechanisms are often insufficient in the absence of reduced renal function. The presence of CKD, or a reduction in

functional renal mass, appears to be necessary for these mechanisms to cause AKI from ischemic injury. In addition, this risk appears to be multiplied in the presence of diabetes.[10] A much less common but well-recognized cause of AKI after cardiac catheterization and PCI is renal atheroembolic disease. This disease process is part of the larger cholesterol embolization syndrome, which can result from the embolism of minor atheromatous debris from the aorta or other large vessels and its movement into small arteries in different vascular beds.[22] The clinical spectrum of renal atheroembolic disease includes blue toe syndrome, livedo reticularis, visual deficits, and abdominal pain from mesenteric ischemia.[22] Laboratory abnormalities include elevated eosinophil counts in the blood and eosinophiluria. AKI is believed to be caused by distal and partial occlusion of the small arteries, leading to ischemic atrophy as opposed to large areas of infarction.[23] Treatment for renal atheroembolic disease is largely supportive. Finally, additional factors may exacerbate the development of AKI after cardiac catheterization and PCI. Many medications may directly contribute to renal toxicity or worsen microvascular changes in the renal medulla, thus extending areas of ischemic injury. Table 5-2 lists several of these agents as well as others that should be monitored closely owing to their potential interactions with contrast agents.[24] For example, metformin can cause lactic acidosis in the setting of renal dysfunction; this has led the Food and Drug Administration to recommend withholding it on the day of exposure to contrast agents and for 48 to 72 hours after. Similarly, volume depletion and hemodynamic changes from heart failure or cardiogenic shock may aggravate contrast-induced nephropathy. In case reports, anticoagulants like warfarin and heparin, given their potential to prevent proper healing of atheromas in the aorta after instrumentation, have been implicated as causative agents in renal atheroembolic disease.[23,25]

Risk Factors for Contrast-Induced AKI

Several bedside tools have been created to predict a patient's risk of developing contrast-induced nephropathy after cardiac catheterization and PCI.[26,27] One model by Mehran and colleagues, developed in 8,357 patients undergoing PCI, uses eight readily available variables to calculate an overall risk score for predicting both the risk of contrast-induced nephropathy and nephropathy requiring dialysis (Fig. 5-1).[77] Variables in this model are scored from 1 to 6 and then summed to generate risks of contrast-induced nephropathy ranging from 7.5% to 57.3% and risks of nephropathy requiring dialysis from 0.04% to 12.6%. The use of models such as these allows clinicians to appropriately discuss the potential benefits and risks of cardiac catheterization with high-risk patients prior to their procedures. They also may help target potential strategies to minimize the risk of developing

TABLE 5-1	Risk Factors for the Development of Contrast-Induced Nephropathy
Clinical factors	
Chronic kidney disease	
Diabetes mellitus	
Advanced age	
Female gender	
Peripheral vascular disease	
Hypertension	
Ejection fraction <40%	
Presenting factors	
Acute coronary syndrome	
Hypotension	
Heart failure	
Volume depletion	
Concomitant nephrotoxic medications	
Anemia	
Procedural factors	
Intra-aortic balloon pump placement	
Multivessel disease	
Contrast amount	
Contrast type	

TABLE 5-2	Concomitant Drugs to Monitor with Exposure to Contrast Agents
Drugs influencing renal hemodynamics	
Nonsteroidal anti-inflammatory drugs (NSAIDs)	
Cyclo-oxygenase-2 inhibitors	
Nesiritide	
ACE inhibitors	
Angiotensin receptor blockers	
Dipyrimadole	
Drugs that cause tubular toxicity	
Diuretics including mannitol	
Antibiotics including aminoglycosides, vancomycin, amphotericin B	
Immunosuppressants including tacrolimus and cyclosporine A	
Drugs with potentially enhanced toxicity after contrast-induced nephropathy	
Metformin	
Statins	

Adapted from Erley C. Concomitant drugs with exposure to contrast media. *Kidney Int.* 2006;100:S20–S24.

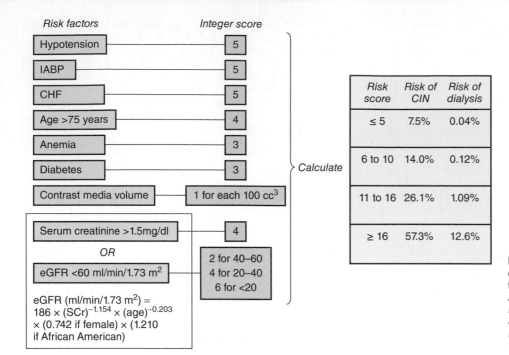

Risk score	Risk of CIN	Risk of dialysis
≤ 5	7.5%	0.04%
6 to 10	14.0%	0.12%
11 to 16	26.1%	1.09%
≥ 16	57.3%	12.6%

Figure 5-1 Risk score for determining risk of contrast-induced nephropathy and dialysis following PCI. (*Adapted from Mehran R et al, A simple risk score for prediction of contrast-induced nephropathy after percutaneous coronary intervention: development and initial validation. J Am Coll Cardiol 2004;44: 1393.*)

contrast-induced AKI. One of the most powerful predictors of AKI following cardiac catheterization is the presence of preexisting CKD; in most cases with long-term complications, patients have preexisting evidence of advanced CKD. The risk of developing AKI following cardiac catheterization increases with increasing severity of CKD, such that patients undergoing PCI with a baseline serum creatinine >1.5 mg/dL or an estimated glomerular filtration rate (eGFR) of <60 mL/min per 1.73 m² have an expected 30% incidence of contrast-induced nephropathy with an adjusted odds ratio of 2.05 (95% CI 1.59-2.66) of developing contrast-induced nephropathy.[27] In addition to CKD, several other risk factors for developing renal dysfunction after cardiac catheterization and PCI have been identified (Table 5-1). Most importantly, these appear to be related to demographics like advanced age, comorbidities like diabetes mellitus, periprocedural factors like hemodynamic instability or heart failure, and evidence of volume depletion.[28] Additional factors include the use of intra-aortic balloon pumps and nephrotoxic medications like nonsteroidal anti-inflammatory drugs (NSAIDs).

CHRONIC KIDNEY DISEASE

The population of patients with CKD worldwide is growing at a tremendous rate. Consequently, these high-risk patients are now encountered much more frequently in the cardiac catheterization laboratory. In one recent registry, for example, 25% of patients undergoing PCI had at least mild CKD.[29] For the interventional cardiologist, identifying these patients is important for two reasons. First, this group represents those patients who are at highest risk for developing renal dysfunction following PCI and require specific preventive therapies prior to their procedures. Second, patients with CKD at baseline are also more likely to have worse cardiovascular outcomes after their procedures. This latter finding is due in part to the well-established relationship between CKD and cardiovascular disease. Until recently, defining patients with CKD was problematic owing to a multitude of nonstandardized definitions and inaccurate assessments of glomerular filtration rates (GFR). The National Kidney Foundation now specifically defines CKD as the presence of sustained abnormalities of renal function, manifest by either a reduced GFR or the presence of kidney damage.[30] Kidney damage is defined by structural or functional abnormalities of the kidney in the presence or absence of decreased GFR manifest by either pathological abnormalities (assessed by renal biopsy) or markers of kidney damage including laboratory abnormalities (in the composition of blood or urine) and radiographic abnormalities (on imaging tests).[30] Once GFR has been assessed, patients with CKD can be stratified into one of five stages (Table 5-3) in order of increasing impairment: stage 1 (GFR ≥90 mL/min per 1.73 m²),

TABLE 5-3	Stages of CKD, Action Recommendations, and Prevalence			
CKD Stages	**Description**	**GFR mL/min per 1.73m²**	**Action Recommendation**	**Prevalence (%)**
1	Kidney damage with normal or increased GFR	≥90	Diagnosis and treatment Treatment of coexisting conditions Slowing progression CVD risk reduction	1.8
2	Kidney damage with mild decrease in GFR	60–89	Estimation of progression	3.2
3	Moderate decrease in GFR	30–59	Evaluation and treatment of complications	7.7
4	Severe decrease in GFR	15–29	Referral to nephrologist Consideration for renal replacement therapy	0.4
5	Kidney failure	<15	Replacement (if uremia present)	0.2

Adapted from National Kidney Foundation Kidney Disease Outcome Quality Initiative Advisory B: K/DOQI clinical practice guidelines for chronic kidney disease: evaluation, classification, and stratification. Kidney Disease Outcome Quality Initiative, *American Journal of Kidney Dis*. 2002;39:S1–S246, and Coresh J et al. Prevalence of chronic kidney disease in the United States; *JAMA*. 2007;298(17):2038–2047.

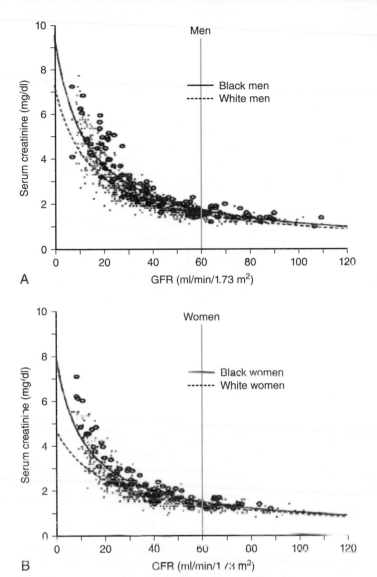

Figure 5-2 Relationship of measured serum creatinine levels to measured glomerular filtration rates in the Modification of Diet in Renal Disease Study, by men (A) and women (B). *(Adapted from Levey AS et al. A more accurate method to estimate glomerular filtration rate from serum creatinine: a new prediction equation. Modification of Diet in Renal Disease Study Group. Ann Intern Med 1999;130:464.)*

stage 2 (GFR 60-89 mL/min), stage 3 (GFR 30-59 mL/min), stage 4 (GFR 15-29 mL/min), and stage 5 (GFR <15 mL/min). Patients with GFRs of ≥60 mL/min are considered to have CKD if they meet additional criteria, demonstrating evidence of kidney damage based on pathological, laboratory, or imaging tests. Such markers of kidney damage include microalbuminuria, proteinuria, abnormalities of the urinary sediment, or abnormal radiological findings. In all cases, CKD requires that kidney disease has persisted for 3 months or longer. Importantly, a normal serum creatinine does not necessarily reflect normal kidney function, and standard reference ranges for normal often misclassify patients with early disease (Fig. 5-2).[31] Such errors result from the fact that serum creatinine alone does not accurately reflect the level of GFR because of nonlinear relationships that vary according to age, gender, race, and lean body mass. Both direct and indirect measures of GFR are available. Direct measurements of GFR may be more accurate, but they are impractical in routine clinical practice. Indirect measurements of GFR are obtained by incorporating serum creatinine values into formulas such as the Cockcroft-Gault equation or the equation of the Modification of Diet in Renal Disease

(MDRD) study.[30] Although the MDRD study equation has generally been purported to have less bias, both formulas have limitations in accuracy, especially for patients with normal kidney function.[32] In addition, these formulas do not perform well for many other individuals who were not well represented in the cohorts from which these equations were developed, including those who have very high or low muscle mass, weight, or age; are severely ill or hospitalized; ingest no or large amounts of meat; or are from minority racial and ethnic groups, such as Asians or Hispanics.[32] Nonetheless in the ACS setting, more conservative estimation of kidney function using the Cockcroft-Gault equation is preferable for drug dosage adjustments so as to minimize overdosing, which may otherwise increase the risk of bleeding in high-risk groups including women and the elderly.[33] In addition to developing AKI, patients with CKD are at particularly high risk for death and adverse cardiovascular events following interventional procedures.[34-36] The risk of adverse outcomes is progressive, with an independent, graded association between reduced GFR and risk of hospitalizations, cardiovascular events, and death.[34,36,37] Consequently, the National Kidney Foundation, American Heart Association, and the Seventh Joint National Committee on Prevention, Detection, Evaluation, and Treatment of High Blood Pressure have classified the presence of CKD as a cardiovascular risk factor.[30,35,38]

Mechanisms by which CKD increases cardiovascular risk are unclear and under investigation. The progressive increase in cardiovascular risk associated with declining kidney function is largely explained by a larger burden of traditional risk factors.[39] However, CKD is also associated with many nontraditional risk factors including renal decline, albuminuria, proteinuria, homocysteinemia, elevated uric acid levels, anemia, dysregulation of mineral metabolism and arterial calcification, oxidative stress, inflammation, malnutrition, endothelial dysfunction, insulin resistance, and conditions promoting coagulation, all of which are associated with accelerated atherosclerosis.[30,35,40] Finally, another contributing factor may be the paradox of lower rates of appropriate therapy with risk-factor modification and intervention among CKD patients than in the general population despite established awareness of their high cardiovascular risk, a concept referred to as "therapeutic nihilism."[41]

Minimizing the Risk of Acute Kidney Injury

Patients with CKD often have existing comorbidities that may complicate their procedure and post-procedure management. As always, developing a systematic approach that reviews the patient's history, physical examination, and laboratory studies is critical (Fig. 5-3). As described earlier, the clinician needs to pay particular attention to accurate assessment of the degree of CKD at baseline as well as several clinical risk factors that have been consistently associated with poor outcomes in patients with CKD, such as diabetes mellitus, concomitant medication use, and volume depletion or hemodynamic instability. Most of the approaches below are designed to minimize the risk of contrast-induced AKI after cardiac catheterization and PCI.

PERIPROCEDURAL STRATEGIES

Most strategies to reduce the risk of procedural complications in patients with CKD must be considered even before cardiac catheterization and PCI begin. These include measures to carefully prepare the patient with adequate hydration and the use of specific drug therapies.

Periprocedural Hydration

Adequate hydration is a particular concern, since most patients are asked to avoid oral intake starting the night before their procedures. They can easily present to the catheterization laboratory in a relatively dehydrated state. It is important to initiate intravenous fluid early in these cases while carefully monitoring patients with heart failure who may be sensitive to rapid volume changes. The best-studied fluid

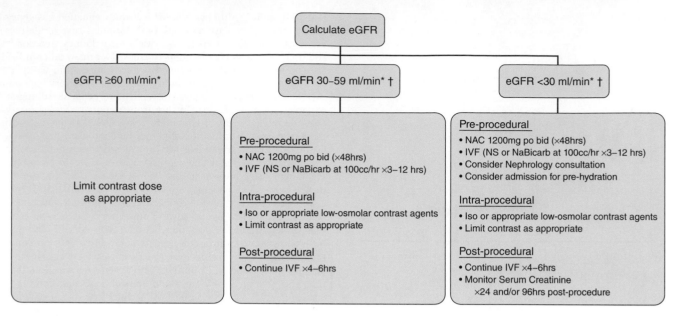

*Discontinue Metformin
†Discontinue NSAIDS and other Nephrotoxic medications

Figure 5-3 Strategies to reduce the risk of contrast-induced AKI in patients undergoing cardiac catheterization. (*Adapted from McCullough PA. Contrast-induced acute kidney injury. J Am Coll Cardiol 2008;51:1419–1428.*)

regimen in clinical trials has been 0.45% normal saline infusions at a rate of 1 mL/kg per minute for 6 to 12 hours prior to the procedure and continuing after the procedure.[42] Data from a large trial suggest that the substitution of isotonic saline for 0.45% normal saline may modestly reduce the incidence of contrast-induced nephropathy, particularly among patients with diabetes mellitus and those receiving large doses of contrast agents.[43] A small clinical trial of 36 patients with serum creatinine levels at baseline ≥1.4 mg/dL demonstrated that 1 L orally followed by 6 hours of intravenous hydration starting at the time of contrast agent exposure was equivalent to preprocedural intravenous hydration.[44] This approach may be more realistic for outpatients who come in on the day of their procedures. From a practical standpoint, a quick assessment of the adequacy of hydration is possible prior to contrast injection by assessing the left ventricular end-diastolic pressure with a pigtail or multipurpose catheter even if a pulmonary capillary wedge pressure is unavailable. If the patient appears to be dehydrated based on his or her hemodynamic parameters, fluid boluses may be given intermittently prior to contrast agent exposure. Recently there has been great interest in the use of sodium bicarbonate infusions to hydrate patients with CKD during the periprocedural time period. Sodium bicarbonate may relieve oxidative stress, which is thought to be a potential mechanism of action by which contrast-induced nephropathy occurs. Although one early clinical trial suggested a benefit of sodium bicarbonate versus sodium chloride infusion,[45] more recent studies have not demonstrated a difference in the incidence of contrast-induced AKI with these agents.[46,47]

Medications

Several medications have also been used to reduce the risk of contrast-induced nephropathy. The most extensively studied of these agents is N-acetylcysteine, which has been evaluated in more than 20 randomized clinical trials.[48] The premise behind the use of N-acetylcysteine is that it acts as a scavenger of reactive oxygen species and promotes vasodilatory effects in the renal medulla. The first of these trials was reported by Tepel and colleagues and evaluated its use in 83 patients receiving intravenous contrast agents for computed tomography.[49] This study found an approximately 90% relative risk reduction in contrast-induced nephropathy with the use of acetylcysteine, but not all studies have shown a consistent benefit. In total, the evidence

suggests that there is a potential benefit with its use. It is certainly very reasonable to consider its use in high-risk patients, given its good safety profile and low cost. The most commonly studied regimen for N-acetylcysteine has been 600 mg orally twice a day starting a day prior to the procedure, but there is evidence that other routes of administration are effective and that higher doses may result in even better clinical outcomes. In one study, intravenous N-acetylcysteine was prepared as 150 mg/kg in a 500-mL bolus infusion and given over 30 minutes starting just prior to contrast agent exposure.[50] This study demonstrated efficacy with the use of N-acetylcysteine and may be an effective alternate regimen when time constraints prevent its oral use. Most recently, in a provocative trial of 354 patients, the use of N-acetylcysteine routinely in all patients undergoing primary PCI for ST-elevation myocardial infarction regardless of serum creatinine levels at baseline also demonstrated benefit.[51] Not only did the use of N-acetylcysteine prevent the development of contrast-induced nephropathy but, remarkably, its use has led to reductions in in-hospital death. In this study, there appeared to be dose-dependent effects, with a higher dose of N-acetylcysteine (1,200 mg bolus intravenously followed by 1,200 mg orally twice a day for 2 days) being superior to standard doses. Most recent studies have reported on an oral regimen of 1200 mg twice daily.[52,53]Another important medication that has been studied extensively in randomized clinical trials is fenoldopam. Fenoldopam works as a dopamine-receptor agonist and is believe to preserve renal blood flow despite insults from contrast agent exposure. A series of small clinical studies had suggested significant benefit in terms of the reduction of contrast-induced nephropathy, particularly in high-risk patients.[54,55] However, enthusiasm for the use of fenoldopam has fallen since publication of the large, multicenter CONTRAST trial in 2003.[56] In this study, no benefit was seen with fenoldopam in 315 patients who had estimated GFRs <60 mL/min and underwent cardiac catheterization. The use of a high-dose statin has been shown to shorten time to recovery from contrast-induced AKI in ACS patients[57]; however, this result has not been consistently replicated.[58] Additional agents that have been studied include probucol, ascorbic acid, captopril, theophylline (or aminophylline), dopamine, atrial natriuretic peptides, calcium channel blockers, and prostaglandin E_1. Most of these agents have either been studied in only a few trials (ascorbic acid[59]) or have yielded largely conflicting results (theophylline[60]). Thus their routine use cannot be recommended. Medications that should be avoided unless otherwise indicated include mannitol or furosemide for forced diuresis (without hemodynamic monitoring), given their potential to result in volume depletion and exacerbate AKI.[42]

Other Strategies

Several other nonpharmacological strategies have been suggested as approaches for minimizing AKI after cardiac catheterization and PCI. However, many of these require intense resources, and their use is limited to the highest-risk patients. The use of forced diuresis with a combination of intravenous hydration, furosemide, dopamine, and mannitol may be valuable, but only if it is implemented after the measurement of right- and left-sided filling pressures with adjustments made according to baseline pressures.[61] In this setting, with a careful protocol to ensure adequate hydration, one clinical trial suggested that the use of forced diuresis led to higher rates of urine flow. However, only modest clinical benefits were noted in regard to serum creatinine levels and the incidence of contrast-induced nephropathy. Another approach that has been suggested is the prophylactic use of hemodialysis or hemofiltration after or during contrast agent exposure. Although contrast agents can be effectively removed from the blood by hemodialysis, clinical studies have not consistently demonstrated a benefit.[62,63] One explanation for this has been that it may result in hemodynamic or inflammatory changes that are nephrotoxic and thus offset the removal of contrast agents. To better address this issue, Marenzi and colleagues studied the use of hemofiltration in 114 patients with severe CKD undergoing PCI.[64] Hemofiltration has the advantage of avoiding hypovolemia and can provide high-volume hydration without concerns of intravascular congestion. In this group, the use of hemofiltration starting at least 4 to 6 hours prior to PCI was associated with improved clinical outcomes including lower rates of renal replacement therapy as well as reduced in-hospital and 1-year mortality. The intensive resources required for this intervention limit its use to tertiary care centers and the highest-risk patients.

INTRAPROCEDURAL STRATEGIES

Intraprocedural strategies for approaching patients with CKD largely depend on (1) the choice of contrast agent, (2) minimizing the volume that is used as much as possible, and (3) avoiding use of potentially nephrotoxic medications. However, this must be done without sacrificing the operator's ability to adequately and safely perform the procedure, which always requires a careful balance. Appropriate visualization of the lesion and adjacent coronary anatomy is essential for success during PCI and should not be sacrificed. General strategies to consider during the case include the use of smaller guiding catheters when possible, since these are associated with lower volumes of contrast agents.[65] It is also important to minimize the use of contrast agents during the diagnostic portion of the case if ad hoc PCI is performed. This can be done by potentially avoiding left ventriculograms and using noninvasive tests like echocardiography to evaluate systolic wall motion and function. The use of biplane coronary angiography, which allows the operator to obtain two simultaneous views with one injection during cineangiography, is another commonly used tool. Other proposed intraprocedural strategies to limit contrast-induced AKI include both coronary sinus cannulation with extracorporeal column filtration and intraprocedural hypothermia. Although the feasibility of the coronary cannulation system has been demonstrated in a swine model and small human studies,[66–68] these results have not been widely validated. Intraprocedural hypothermia has also not been shown to be effective for the prevention of contrast-induced nephropathy.[69]

The Choice and Use of Contrast Agent

The choice of contrast agent is an important intraprocedural consideration and has evolved considerably over the last several years with the development of low- and iso-osmolar contrast agents. Traditional iodine-based contrast agents were hypertonic, including ionic compounds like diatrizoate (Hypaque, Renografin), which frequently caused mild hemodynamic changes in addition to contrast-induced nephropathy. Given substantially lower costs in recent years, most laboratories have switched to the routine use of low-osmolar, nonionic contrast agents, which improve hemodynamic effects and patient comfort. An important effect of low-osmolar agents is believed to be a reduction in contrast-induced nephropathy. In a metanalysis that included data from 25 trials, the risk of contrast-induced nephropathy was 39% lower in patients who received low-osmolar contrast agents as compared with hypertonic contrast agents.[70] This benefit appeared to be even more pronounced in patients with pre-existing renal disease with a 50% risk reduction in that population. The introduction of iodixanol (Visipaque), an iso-osmolar contrast agent, has raised the question of whether the incidence of contrast-induced nephropathy can be further reduced. In a widely cited study of patients with CKD and diabetes mellitus, the use of iso-osmolar contrast agents reduced the incidence of AKI by over 90% when compared with low-osmolar contrast agents.[71] An additional study comparing these two types of contrast agents also suggested a reduction in major adverse cardiovascular events with the use of iso-osmolar contrast in patients undergoing high-risk PCI.[72] However, more recent studies have not replicated these results,[73,74] and the relative benefit of iso-osmolar agents remains unclear. Nonetheless, updated PCI guidelines recommend the use of iso-osmolar contrast agents (level of evidence, A)[75] or low-molecular-weight agents other than ioxaglate or iohexol (level of evidence, B).[76] Finally, some investigators have begun to use alternative, non-iodine-based contrast agents like gadolinium, particularly in peripheral angiography. Although case reports of its use in the coronary circulation do exist, many questions remain regarding the overall safety and feasibility of this approach, particularly given the high serum osmolality of these agents and the risk of nephrogenic systemic fibrosis in patients with severe renal impairment.[77–79] Regardless of the selection of a contrast agent, it is imperative to use the least amount of volume that is required for adequate visualization of the coronary artery and technical success of the procedure. In patients at particularly high risk, the maximum allowable contrast dose [MACD = five times body weight (kg)/serum Cr (mg/dL)] should be calculated before the procedure so that the interventional cardiologist and team can be aware of its use during the procedure. Staging nonurgent procedures is also a potential approach in many settings and will minimize the risk of developing contrast-induced nephropathy. Unfortunately there are few data on the optimal timing between sequential procedures.

Special Populations

END-STAGE RENAL DISEASE

Not all patients with CKD go on to develop ESRD; in fact, most will die of other nonrenal causes, especially from cardiovascular disease. However, patients with ESRD who do undergo cardiac catheterization and PCI represent an important group that may be at risk for intraprocedural as well as short- and long-term complications. Overall, the epidemiology of ESRD is better understood than that of CKD. In the United States, both the incidence and prevalence of ESRD have doubled in the past decade, and they are expected to increase significantly in the future.[26] In 2003, over 450,000 people required dialysis or transplantation for ESRD in the United States; however, by 2030, estimates suggest that this number will increase to more than 2 million.[26] The dramatically increased rates of cardiovascular disease and accelerated atherosclerosis have long been recognized in ESRD.[80] More than 50% of deaths among patients with ESRD are due to cardiovascular events and more than 20% of cardiac deaths can be attributed to acute myocardial infarction.[81] The 2-year mortality rate after myocardial infarction among patients with ESRD is approximately 50%, or twice the mortality rate after myocardial infarction in the general population.[35,81] This excess cardiovascular mortality risk ranges from 500-fold higher in individuals aged 25 to 35 to five-fold higher in individuals aged >85 years.[82] In most patients who are chronically on dialysis, routine dialysis postprocedurally is not needed after exposure to contrast agents.[63,83] But the studies in this area involved only a select group of patients. So although it appears that most patients can be maintained on their routine schedules for dialysis, special care and attention may be needed for specific groups like those with poor cardiac function or evidence of residual renal function, which is more common among patients treated with peritoneal dialysis. Preservation of residual renal function is vital to successful treatment with peritoneal dialysis: once it is lost, patients often require hemodialysis. An additional concern regarding patients with advanced CKD and ESRD is the anatomy of their coronary arteries, which are frequently diffusely diseased.[84] These issues can raise technical challenges in the delivery of coronary devices during routine PCI, particularly for those with ESRD due to extensive coronary calcification. Additional strategies like rotational atherectomy may be required under these circumstances for plaque modification prior to coronary stent delivery. After PCI, the presence of CKD and ESRD has also been associated with higher rates of major adverse cardiovascular events, including restenosis and repeat target vessel revascularization. In the era before routine stenting, restenosis was a substantial problem, with rates as high as 80% in patients with ESRD. Although the likelihood of these complications has diminished with newer devices, there still appears to be an increased risk.[85,86] For example, Rubenstein and colleagues demonstrated that CKD was independently predictive of worse outcomes, including repeat revascularization, in a cohort of 3,334 patients undergoing PCI during a period when coronary stenting and atherectomy were being introduced.[86] Within this study population, there also appeared to be no difference between patients with CKD and ESRD.[86] Although the data are limited, some reports have also suggested that the use of drug-eluting stents may minimize the risk of restenosis even further in patients with CKD and ESRD.[87–90] This area requires further investigation. Another critical issue in these patients is determining the risks and benefits of PCI versus surgical revascularization. This is a controversial area and clinical trials have been unable to directly inform this issue, since most have excluded patients with significant CKD and ESRD. In the absence of adequate clinical trial data, this decision is often individualized and relies upon the goals of treatment, the likelihood of technical success with PCI, and the patient's operative risk with bypass surgery.[91,92] Finally, it is important for the interventional cardiologist to appropriately select and dose adjunctive drug therapy in patients with CKD and ESRD. The risks and benefits of many drugs routinely used as adjunctive therapy in PCI, including glycoprotein IIb/IIIa inhibitors and bivalirudin, need to be carefully weighed in this population owing to the diminished renal clearance of such agents in these patients and potential to increase the risk for bleeding.[93–95]

CONGESTIVE HEART FAILURE AND RISK OF AKI

Patients with advanced heart failure (NYHA classes III-IV) are among the highest-risk populations for the development of contrast-induced AKI, with an incidence of 38.5% and an odds ratio of 2.25 (95% CI 1.68-3.01) compared with those who do not have advanced heart failure.[27] These patients pose a particularly difficult management dilemma as the use of volume-loading strategies is generally discouraged. Gentle diuresis of patients with pulmonary edema is often necessary to allow supine patient positioning for catheterization, and the relief of excess portal pressure in these patients may reduce the risk of contrast-induced nephropathy.[96] The administration of preprocedural N-acetylcysteine is reasonable, and measures to limit contrast volume (e.g., biplane angiography, selective angiographic views, noninvasive left ventricular functional assessment) are encouraged. Finally, in heart failure patients with low left ventricular end-diastolic pressures following cardiac catheterization, limited gentle hydration (i.e., 100 mL/hr for 2 to 4 hours) may be considered.

■ The Future

Serum cystatin C has been suggested as a superior alternative to serum creatinine in quantifying GFR in patients with CKD because cystatin C has a fairly constant rate of production.[32] However, serum levels of cystatin C may also be influenced by age, gender, and muscle mass.[97] Currently, it provides only a marginal improvement in the accuracy of estimating kidney function over methods based on serum creatinine. In addition, many laboratories are not yet equipped to perform this test. Eventually, there may be a role for an estimating equation combining cystatin C and serum creatinine when more accurate GFR estimates are needed, particularly within the normal GFR range. Assessment of AKI using serum markers of renal clearance, including serum creatinine and cystatin C, is inherently problematic and leads to the poor sensitivity and specificity observed when compared with biopsy-proven kidney injury. In fact, measures of structural injury are better markers of AKI and able to detect smaller tubular insults than the current methods of relying upon serum creatinine-based changes in renal clearance. In search of such improved biomarkers for detecting AKI, several new ones have been identified, while those previously known have been evaluated more thoroughly. Despite several dozen unique biomarkers of AKI that have been identified or are under investigation, most of the current interest has focused on a small handful of promising biomarkers: neutrophil gelatinase-associated lipocalin, interleukin-18, and kidney injury molecule-1.[4,98] Although some early results are encouraging, none have been validated for routine clinical use. Once validated in large studies that support their diagnostic and predictive capacities, such biomarkers are likely to replace assessment of AKI by changes in serum creatinine. This evolution of renal assessment moves closer to the paradigm within the field of cardiology in which structural injury is assessed separately from overall function. Sudden changes in these new biomarkers will be used to detect AKI similar to how serum troponin and creatine kinase are used to evaluate acute coronary syndromes. Likewise, overall function will be assessed with estimating equations using serum creatinine (with or without new biomarkers like cystatin C), similar to the way in which ventricular function is evaluated with an ejection fraction and other measurements. In addition to clarifying the role of various alterations of the kidney, this evolution also has the potential to improve clinical outcomes by helping to identify more successful treatments.[4]

REFERENCES

1. Persson PB, Tepel M: Contrast medium-induced nephropathy: the pathophysiology. *Kidney Int Suppl* S8–S10, 2006.
2. Kelly AM, Dwamena B, Cronin P, et al: Meta-analysis: effectiveness of drugs for preventing contrast-induced nephropathy. *Ann Intern Med* 148:284–294, 2008.
3. McCullough PA, Adam A, Becker CR, et al: Epidemiology and prognostic implications of contrast-induced nephropathy. *Am J Cardiol* 98:5K–13K, 2006.
4. Hudson C, Hudson J, Swaminathan M, et al: Emerging concepts in acute kidney injury following cardiac surgery. *Semin Cardiothorac Vasc Anesth* 12:320–330, 2008.
5. Ferguson TB, Jr, Dziuban SW, Jr, Edwards FH, et al: The STS National Database: current changes and challenges for the new millennium. Committee to Establish a National Database in Cardiothoracic Surgery, The Society of Thoracic Surgeons. *Ann Thorac Surg* 69:680–691, 2000.

6. Bellomo R, Ronco C, Kellum JA, et al: Acute renal failure: definition, outcome measures, animal models, fluid therapy and information technology needs: the Second International Consensus Conference of the Acute Dialysis Quality Initiative (ADQI) Group. *Crit Care* 8:R204–R212, 2004.
7. Mehta RL, Kellum JA, Shah SV, et al: Acute Kidney Injury Network: report of an initiative to improve outcomes in acute kidney injury. *Crit Care* 11:R31, 2007.
8. Bagshaw SM, George C, Bellomo R: A comparison of the RIFLE and AKIN criteria for acute kidney injury in critically ill patients. *Nephrol Dial Transplant* 23:1569–1574, 2008.
9. Haase M, Bellomo R, Matalanis G, et al: A comparison of the RIFLE and Acute Kidney Injury Network classifications for cardiac surgery-associated acute kidney injury: a prospective cohort study. *J Thorac Cardiovasc Surg* 138:1370–1376, 2009.

10. McCullough PA: Contrast-induced acute kidney injury. *J Am Coll Cardiol* 51:1419–1428, 2008.
11. Barrett BJ, Parfrey PS: Clinical practice. Preventing nephropathy induced by contrast medium. *N Engl J Med* 354:379–386, 2006.
12. Senoo T, Motohiro M, Kamihata H, et al: Contrast-induced nephropathy in patients undergoing emergency percutaneous coronary intervention for acute coronary syndrome. *Am J Cardiol* 105:624–628, 2010.
13. McCullough PA, Sandberg KR: Epidemiology of contrast-induced nephropathy. *Rev Cardiovasc Med* 4 Suppl 5:S3–S9, 2003.
14. Freeman RV, O'Donnell M, Share D, et al: Nephropathy requiring dialysis after percutaneous coronary intervention and the critical role of an adjusted contrast dose. *Am J Cardiol* 90:1068–1073, 2002.

15. McCullough PA, Wolyn R, Rocher LL, et al: Acute renal failure after coronary intervention: incidence, risk factors, and relationship to mortality. *Am J Med* 103:368–375, 1997.
16. Rihal CS, Textor SC, Grill DE, et al: Incidence and prognostic importance of acute renal failure after percutaneous coronary intervention. *Circulation* 105:2259–2264, 2002.
17. Marenzi G, Lauri G, Assanelli E, et al: Contrast-induced nephropathy in patients undergoing primary angioplasty for acute myocardial infarction. *J Am Coll Cardiol* 44:1780–1785, 2004.
18. Bartholomew BA, Harjai KJ, Dukkipati S, et al: Impact of nephropathy after percutaneous coronary intervention and a method for risk stratification. *Am J Cardiol* 93:1515–1519, 2004.
19. Gupta R, Gurm HS, Bhatt DL, et al: Renal failure after percutaneous coronary intervention is associated with high mortality. *Catheter Cardiovasc Intervent* 64:442–448, 2005.
20. Katholi RE, Woods WT, Jr, Taylor GJ, et al: Oxygen free radicals and contrast nephropathy. *Am J Kidney Dis* 32:64–71, 1998.
21. Toprak O, Cirit M: Risk factors for contrast-induced nephropathy. *Kidney Blood Press Res* 29:84–93, 2006.
22. Fukumoto Y, Tsutsui H, Tsuchihashi M, et al: The incidence and risk factors of cholesterol embolization syndrome, a complication of cardiac catheterization: a prospective study. *J Am Coll Cardiol* 42:211–216, 2003.
23. Mannesse CK, Blankestijn PJ, Man in 't Veld AJ, Schalekamp MA: Renal failure and cholesterol crystal embolization: a report of 4 surviving cases and a review of the literature. *Clin Nephrol* 36:240–245, 1991.
24. Erley C: Concomitant drugs with exposure to contrast media. *Kidney Int Suppl* S20–S24, 2006.
25. Hyman BT, Landas SK, Ashman RF, et al: Warfarin-related purple toes syndrome and cholesterol microembolization. *Am J Med* 82:1233–1237, 1987.
26. Halkin A, Singh M, Nikolsky E, et al: Prediction of mortality after primary percutaneous coronary intervention for acute myocardial infarction: the CADILLAC risk score. *J Am Coll Cardiol* 45:1397–1405, 2005.
27. Mehran R, Aymong ED, Nikolsky E, et al: A simple risk score for prediction of contrast-induced nephropathy after percutaneous coronary intervention: development and initial validation. *J Am Coll Cardiol* 44:1393–1399, 2004.
28. Mehran R, Nikolsky E: Contrast-induced nephropathy: definition, epidemiology, and patients at risk. *Kidney Int Suppl* S11–S15, 2006.
29. Blackman DJ, Pinto R, Ross JR, et al: Impact of renal insufficiency on outcome after contemporary percutaneous coronary intervention. *Am Heart J* 151:146–152, 2006.
30. National Kidney Foundation Kidney Disease Outcome Quality Initiative Advisory B: K/DOQI clinical practice guidelines for chronic kidney disease: evaluation, classification, and stratification. Kidney Disease Outcome Quality Initiative. *Am J Kidney Dis* 39:S1–S246, 2002.
31. Levey AS, Bosch JP, Lewis JB, et al: A more accurate method to estimate glomerular filtration rate from serum creatinine: a new prediction equation. Modification of Diet in Renal Disease Study Group [comment]. *Ann Intern Med* 130:461–470, 1999.
32. Stevens LA, Coresh J, Greene T, Levey AS: Assessing kidney function–measured and estimated glomerular filtration rate. *N Engl J Med* 354:2473–2483, 2006.
33. Melloni C, Peterson ED, Chen AY, et al: Cockcroft-Gault versus modification of diet in renal disease: importance of glomerular filtration rate formula for classification of chronic kidney disease in patients with non-ST-segment elevation acute coronary syndromes. *J Am Coll Cardiol* 51:991–996, 2008.
34. Go AS, Chertow GM, Fan D, et al: Chronic kidney disease and the risks of death, cardiovascular events, and hospitalization. *N Engl J Med* 351:1296–1305, 2004.
35. Sarnak MJ, Levey AS, Schoolwerth AC, et al: Kidney Disease as a Risk Factor for Development of Cardiovascular Disease: A Statement From the American Heart Association Councils on Kidney in Cardiovascular Disease, High Blood Pressure Research, Clinical Cardiology, and Epidemiology and Prevention. *Circulation* 108:2154–2169, 2003.
36. Patel UD, Young EW, Ojo AO, et al: CKD progression and mortality among older patients with diabetes. *Am J Kidney Dis* 46:406–414, 2005.
37. Anavekar NS, Gans DJ, Berl T, et al: Predictors of cardiovascular events in patients with type 2 diabetic nephropathy and hypertension: a case for albuminuria. *Kidney Int Suppl* S50–S55, 2004.
38. Chobanian AV, Bakris GL, Black HR, et al: The Seventh Report of the Joint National Committee on Prevention, Detection, Evaluation, and Treatment of High Blood Pressure: the JNC 7 report. [comment][erratum appears in *JAMA*. 2003;290(2):197]. *JAMA* 289:2560–2572, 2003.
39. Shlipak MG, Fried LF, Cushman M, et al: Cardiovascular mortality risk in chronic kidney disease: comparison of traditional and novel risk factors. *JAMA* 293:1737–1745, 2005.
40. Best PJ, Reddan DN, Berger PB, et al: Cardiovascular disease and chronic kidney disease: insights and an update. *Am Heart J* 148:230–242, 2004.
41. Anavekar NS, McMurray JJ, Velazquez EJ, et al: Relation between renal dysfunction and cardiovascular outcomes after myocardial infarction. *N Engl J Med* 351:1285–1295, 2004.
42. Solomon R, Werner C, Mann D, et al: Effects of saline, mannitol, and furosemide to prevent acute decreases in renal function induced by radiocontrast agents. *N Engl J Med* 331:1416–1420, 1994.
43. Mueller C, Buerkle G, Buettner HJ, et al: Prevention of contrast media-associated nephropathy: randomized comparison of 2 hydration regimens in 1620 patients undergoing coronary angioplasty. *Arch Intern Med* 162:329–336, 2002.
44. Taylor AJ, Hotchkiss D, Morse RW, et al: PREPARED: Preparation for Angiography in Renal Dysfunction: a randomized trial of inpatient vs outpatient hydration protocols for cardiac catheterization in mild-to-moderate renal dysfunction. *Chest* 114:1570–1574, 1998.
45. Merten GJ, Burgess WP, Gray LV, et al: Prevention of contrast-induced nephropathy with sodium bicarbonate: a randomized controlled trial. *JAMA* 291:2328–2334, 2004.
46. Brar SS, Shen AY, Jorgensen MB, et al: Sodium bicarbonate vs sodium chloride for the prevention of contrast medium-induced nephropathy in patients undergoing coronary angiography: a randomized trial. *JAMA* 300:1038–1046, 2008.
47. Maioli M, Toso A, Leoncini M, et al: Sodium bicarbonate versus saline for the prevention of contrast-induced nephropathy in patients with renal dysfunction undergoing coronary angiography or intervention. *J Am Coll Cardiol* 52:599–604, 2008.
48. Nallamothu BK, Shojania KG, Saint S, et al: Is acetylcysteine effective in preventing contrast-related nephropathy? A meta-analysis. *Am J Med* 117:938–947, 2004.
49. Tepel M, van der Giet M, Schwarzfeld C, et al: Prevention of radiographic-contrast-agent-induced reductions in renal function by acetylcysteine. *N Engl J Med* 343:180–184, 2000.
50. Baker CS, Wragg A, Kumar S, et al: A rapid protocol for the prevention of contrast induced renal dysfunction: the RAPPID study. *J Am Coll Cardiol* 41:2114–2118, 2003.
51. Marenzi G, Assanelli E, Marana I, et al: *N*-acetylcysteine and contrast-induced nephropathy in primary angioplasty. *N Engl J Med* 354:2773–2782, 2006.
52. Jo SH, Koo BK, Park JS, et al: N-acetylcysteine versus AScorbic acid for preventing contrast-Induced nephropathy in patients with renal insufficiency undergoing coronary angiography NASPI study-a prospective randomized controlled trial. *Am Heart J* 157:576–583, 2009.
53. Thiele H, Hildebrand L, Schirdewahn C, et al: Impact of high-dose N-acetylcysteine versus placebo on contrast-induced nephropathy and myocardial reperfusion injury in unselected patients with ST-segment elevation myocardial infarction undergoing primary percutaneous coronary intervention. The LIPSIA-N-ACC (Prospective, Single-Blind, Placebo-Controlled, Randomized Leipzig Immediate PercutaneouS Coronary Intervention Acute Myocardial Infarction N-ACC) Trial. *J Am Coll Cardiol* 55:2201–2209, 2010.
54. Madyoon H, Croushore L, Weaver D, et al: Use of fenoldopam to prevent radiocontrast nephropathy in high-risk patients. *Catheter Cardiovasc Intervent* 53:341–345, 2001.
55. Kini AS, Mitre CA, Kamran M, et al: Changing trends in incidence and predictors of radiographic contrast nephropathy after percutaneous coronary intervention with use of fenoldopam. *Am J Cardiol* 89;999–1002, 2002.
56. Stone GW, McCullough PA, Tumlin JA, et al: Fenoldopam mesylate for the prevention of contrast-induced nephropathy: a randomized controlled trial. *JAMA* 290:2284–2291, 2003.
57. Xinwei J, Xianghua F, Jing Z, et al: Comparison of usefulness of simvastatin 20 mg versus 80 mg in preventing contrast-induced nephropathy in patients with acute coronary syndrome undergoing percutaneous coronary intervention. *Am J Cardiol* 104:519–524, 2009.
58. Jo SH, Koo BK, Park JS, et al: Prevention of radiocontrast medium-induced nephropathy using short term high-dose simvastatin in patients with renal insufficiency undergoing coronary angiography (PROMISS) trial—a randomized controlled study. *Am Heart J* 155:499 e1–e8, 2008.
59. Spargias K, Alexopoulos E, Kyrzopoulos S, et al: Ascorbic acid prevents contrast-mediated nephropathy in patients with renal dysfunction undergoing coronary angiography or intervention. *Circulation* 110:2837–2842, 2004.
60. Bagshaw SM, Ghali WA: Theophylline for prevention of contrast-induced nephropathy: a systematic review and meta-analysis. *Arch Intern Med* 165:1087–1093, 2005.
61. Stevens MA, McCullough PA, Tobin KJ, et al: A prospective randomized trial of prevention measures in patients at high risk for contrast nephropathy: results of the PRINCE Study. Prevention of Radiocontrast Induced Nephropathy Clinical Evaluation. *J Am Coll Cardiol* 33:403–411, 1999.
62. Lee PT, Chou KJ, Liu CP, et al: Renal protection for coronary angiography in advanced renal failure patients by prophylactic hemodialysis. A randomized controlled trial. *J Am Coll Cardiol* 50:1015–1020, 2007.
63. Deray G: Dialysis and iodinated contrast media. *Kidney Int Suppl* S25–S29, 2006.
64. Marenzi G, Marana I, Lauri G, et al: The prevention of radiocontrast-agent-induced nephropathy by hemofiltration. *N Engl J Med* 349:1333–1340, 2003.
65. Grossman PM, Gurm HS, McNamara R, et al: Percutaneous coronary intervention complications and guide catheter size: bigger is not better. *JACC Cardiovasc Intervent* 2:636–644, 2009.
66. Michishita I, Fujii Z: A novel contrast removal system from the coronary sinus using an adsorbing column during coronary angiography in a porcine model. *J Am Coll Cardiol* 47:1866–1870, 2006.
67. Danenberg HD, Lotan C, Varshitski B, et al: Removal of contrast medium from the coronary sinus during coronary angiography: feasibility of a simple and available technique for the prevention of nephropathy. *Cardiovasc Revasc Med* 9:9–13, 2008.
68. Duffy SJ, Ruygrok P, Juergens CP, et al: Removal of contrast media from the coronary sinus attenuates renal injury after coronary angiography and intervention. *J Am Coll Cardiol* 56:525–526, 2010.
69. Stone GW, Dixon SR, Foster M, et al: Abstract 3794: Systemic Hypothermia to Prevent Contrast Nephropathy: the COOL RCN Pilot Trial. *Circulation* 114:II_811–II_812, 2006.
70. Barrett BJ, Carlisle EJ: Metaanalysis of the relative nephrotoxicity of high- and low-osmolality iodinated contrast media. *Radiology* 188:171–178, 1993.
71. Aspelin P, Aubry P, Fransson SG, et al: Nephrotoxic effects in high-risk patients undergoing angiography. *N Engl J Med* 348: 491–499, 2003.
72. Davidson CJ, Laskey WK, Hermiller JB, et al: Randomized trial of contrast media utilization in high-risk PTCA: the COURT trial. *Circulation* 101:2172–2177, 2000.
73. Kuhn MJ, Chen N, Sahani DV, et al: The PREDICT study: a randomized double-blind comparison of contrast-induced nephropathy after low- or isoosmolar contrast agent exposure. *AJR Am J Roentgenol* 191:151–157, 2008.
74. Laskey W, Aspelin P, Davidson C, et al: Nephrotoxicity of iodixanol versus iopamidol in patients with chronic kidney disease and diabetes mellitus undergoing coronary angiographic procedures. *Am Heart J* 158:822–828 e3, 2009.
75. King SB, III, Smith SC, Jr, Hirshfeld JW, Jr, et al: 2007 Focused Update of the ACC/AHA/SCAI 2005 Guideline Update for Percutaneous Coronary Intervention: a report of the American College of Cardiology/American Heart Association Task Force on Practice Guidelines: 2007 Writing Group to Review New Evidence and Update the ACC/AHA/SCAI 2005 Guideline Update for Percutaneous Coronary Intervention, Writing on Behalf of the 2005 Writing Committee. *Circulation* 117:261–295, 2008.
76. Kushner FG, Hand M, Smith SC, Jr, et al: 2009 Focused Updates: ACC/AHA Guidelines for the Management of Patients With ST Elevation Myocardial Infarction (updating the 2004 Guideline and 2007 Focused Update) and ACC/AHA/SCAI Guidelines on Percutaneous Coronary Intervention (updating the 2005 Guideline and 2007 Focused Update): a report of the American College of Cardiology Foundation/American Heart Association Task Force on Practice Guidelines. *Circulation* 120:2271–2306, 2009.
77. Sarkis A, Badaoui G, Azar R, et al: Gadolinium-enhanced coronary angiography in patients with impaired renal function. *Am J Cardiol* 91:974–975, A4, 2003.
78. Bokhari SW, Wen YH, Winters RJ: Gadolinium-based percutaneous coronary intervention in a patient with renal insufficiency. *Catheter Cardiovasc Intervent* 58:358–361, 2003.
79. Kribben A, Witzke O, Hillen U, et al: Nephrogenic systemic fibrosis: pathogenesis, diagnosis, and therapy. *J Am Coll Cardiol* 53:1621–1628, 2009.
80. Lindner A, Charra B, Sherrard DJ, et al: Accelerated atherosclerosis in prolonged maintenance hemodialysis. *N Engl J Med* 290:697–701, 1974.
81. Herzog CA, Ma JZ, Collins AJ: Poor long term survival after acute myocardial infarction among patients on long-term dialysis. *N Engl J Med* 339:799–805, 1998.
82. Levey AS, Beto JA, Coronado BE, et al: Controlling the epidemic of cardiovascular disease in chronic renal disease: what do we know? What do we need to learn? Where do we go from here? National Kidney Foundation Task Force on Cardiovascular Disease. *Am J Kidney Dis* 32:853–906, 1998.
83. Hamani A, Petitclerc T, Jacobs C, et al: Is dialysis indicated immediately after administration of iodinated contrast agents in patients on haemodialysis? *Nephrol Dial Transplant* 13:1051–1052, 1998.
84. Bocksch W, Fateh-Moghadam S, Mueller E, et al: Percutaneous coronary intervention in patients with end-stage renal disease. *Kidney Blood Press Res* 28:275–279, 2005.
85. Azar RR, Prpic R, Ho KK, et al: Impact of end-stage renal disease on clinical and angiographic outcomes after coronary stenting. *Am J Cardiol* 86:485–489, 2000.
86. Rubenstein MH, Harrell LC, Sheynberg BV, et al: Are patients with renal failure good candidates for percutaneous coronary revascularization in the new device era? *Circulation* 102:2966–2972, 2000.
87. Daemen J, Lemos P, Aoki J, et al: Treatment of coronary artery disease in dialysis patients with sirolimus-eluting stents: 1-year clinical follow-up of a consecutive series of cases. *J Invas Cardiol* 16:685–687, 2004.
88. Halkin A, Mehran R, Casey CW, et al: Impact of moderate renal insufficiency on restenosis and adverse clinical events after paclitaxel-eluting and bare metal stent implantation: results from the TAXUS-IV Trial. *Am Heart J* 150:1163–1170, 2005.
89. Abdel-Latif A, Mukherjee D, Mesgarzadeh P, et al: Drug-eluting stents in patients with end-stage renal disease: meta-analysis and systematic review of the literature. *Catheter Cardiovasc Intervent* 76:942–948, 2010.
90. Douglas PS, Brennan JM, Anstrom KJ, et al: Clinical effectiveness of coronary stents in elderly persons: results from 262,700 Medicare patients in the American College of Cardiology-National Cardiovascular Data Registry. *J Am Coll Cardiol* 53:1629–1641, 2009.
91. Reddan DN, Szczech LA, Tuttle RH, et al: Chronic kidney disease, mortality, and treatment strategies among patients with clinically significant coronary artery disease. *J Am Soc Nephrol* 14:2373–2380, 2003.

92. Williams M: Coronary revascularization in diabetic chronic kidney disease/end-stage renal disease: a nephrologist's perspective. *Clin J Am Soc Nephrol* 1:209–220, 2006.

93. Freeman RV, Mehta RH, Al Badr W, et al: Influence of concurrent renal dysfunction on outcomes of patients with acute coronary syndromes and implications of the use of glycoprotein IIb/IIIa inhibitors. *J Am Coll Cardiol* 41:718–724, 2003.

94. Alexander KP, Chen AY, Roe MT, et al: Excess dosing of antiplatelet and antithrombin agents in the treatment of non-ST-segment elevation acute coronary syndromes. *JAMA* 294:3108–3116, 2005.

95. Tsai TT, Maddox TM, Roe MT, et al: Contraindicated medication use in dialysis patients undergoing percutaneous coronary intervention. *JAMA* 302:2458–2464, 2009.

96. Damman K, van Deursen VM, Navis G, et al: Increased central venous pressure is associated with impaired renal function and mortality in a broad spectrum of patients with cardiovascular disease. *J Am Coll Cardiol* 53:582–588, 2009.

97. Knight EL, Verhave JC, Spiegelman D, et al: Factors influencing serum cystatin C levels other than renal function and the impact on renal function measurement. *Kidney Int* 65:1416–1421, 2004.

98. Malyszko J, Bachorzewska-Gajewska H, Poniatowski B, et al: Urinary and serum biomarkers after cardiac catheterization in diabetic patients with stable angina and without severe chronic kidney disease. *Renal Failure* 31:910–919, 2009.

6

Preoperative Coronary Intervention

CRAIG R. NARINS

KEY POINTS

- Perioperative myocardial infarction (MI) can result from either coronary plaque rupture or a myocardial oxygen supply-demand mismatch related to a preexisting coronary stenosis; it typically occurs in the first 48 hours following surgery. Even if clinically silent, it is a powerful predictor of future adverse cardiac events.

- Beta-blocker therapy is associated with reduced cardiac event rates among properly selected patients at risk for complications during noncardiac surgery, but it can be harmful if used indiscriminately, especially among lower-risk individuals.

- The indications for performing preoperative coronary angiography and revascularization are the same as in the nonoperative setting.

- When it is undertaken in the preoperative period, percutaneous coronary intervention (PCI) is associated with increased procedural risk, especially among patients requiring vascular surgery.

- Because no prospective trial to date has demonstrated short- or long-term benefits from a strategy of routine preoperative PCI among patients with coronary disease, the indications for preoperative PCI are very limited. The use of PCI to "get a patient through" noncardiac surgery is unproven and potentially harmful.

- Noncardiac surgery performed within 6 weeks of bare metal stent (BMS) implantation or 12 months of drug-eluting stent (DES) placement is associated with elevated rates of stent thrombosis, an often catastrophic event associated with substantial mortality.

- Among patients with previously placed drug-eluting stents who require unanticipated noncardiac surgery, the decision to continue or suspend aspirin and thienopyridine therapy for surgery requires individualized assessment of the risks and implications of bleeding complications versus stent thrombosis and should be made with multidisciplinary input from the cardiologist, surgeon, and other involved subspecialists.

- Novel antiplatelet agents and bedside assays of platelet function offer promise in the management of antiplatelet therapy in the perioperative period.

- While prevention of cardiac complications through proper patient selection and management remains the cornerstone of achieving low surgical mortality rates, prompt recognition and treatment of post-operative complications when they do occur represents an equally important factor in optimizing surgical outcomes.

Introduction

Of the over 30 million surgical procedures requiring the use of general anesthesia performed annually in the United States, approximately one-third involve patients who are at risk for or have known coronary artery disease. Given the physiological stresses that accompany surgery, the perioperative period represents a time of substantially heightened risk for adverse cardiac events. Current evidence suggests that the routine use of coronary revascularization in the preoperative setting is unlikely to reduce the incidence of subsequent cardiac events. Nevertheless, selected patients at particularly increased risk for cardiac complications related to noncardiac surgery may benefit from preoperative PCI. Optimal performance of preoperative PCI requires awareness of several procedural issues that are unique to the preoperative setting. This chapter provides a clinically oriented review of preoperative PCI,

including the indications for coronary angiography and revascularization prior to upcoming surgery, the utility of various medical and interventional strategies to reduce perioperative risk among patients with known or suspected coronary disease, technical approaches to performing angioplasty and stenting prior to noncardiac surgery, and strategies for managing patients with prior DES placement who subsequently require unanticipated noncardiac surgery.

Overview of Perioperative MI

As with MI outside the context of surgery, perioperative MI can result either from the rupture of an atherosclerotic plaque with thrombotic occlusion of the involved coronary artery or from a transient stress-induced mismatch of myocardial oxygen supply and demand, typically in the setting of a fixed coronary artery stenosis or occlusion.[1] Thrombosis of a previously implanted coronary stent represents another potential mechanism of perioperative MI and has been described among patients undergoing noncardiac surgery early following BMS implantation and up to several years after DES placement. In the vast majority of instances, perioperative MI does not occur during the surgical procedure itself but rather within the first 48 hours following surgery. This period is associated with multiple hemodynamic stresses and hematological alterations that can predispose to plaque rupture, myocardial oxygen supply-demand mismatch, and a hypercoagulable state (Fig. 6-1). The incidence of myocardial ischemia and infarction in the period surrounding noncardiac surgery is a function of both the type of surgery and the risk profile of the population being studied. The ACC/AHA guidelines for perioperative assessment classify specific operations as high risk (>5% reported rate of cardiac death and nonfatal MI), intermediate risk (1%–5%), or low risk (<1%) (Table 6-1).[2] Perioperative MI, whether clinically apparent or silent, is associated with increased mortality in both the short and long term. In-hospital survival rates for perioperative MI typically exceed 90%, which is similar to that of MI in the nonoperative setting. As with clinically silent MI detected following PCI, even smaller infarcts detected following noncardiac surgery are associated with up to a two- to fourfold increase in medium- to late-term mortality independent of other clinical factors.[3,4]

DETERMINING OPERATIVE RISK

Concepts

For the process of preoperative evaluation to be a clinically useful exercise, two goals must be met: (1) the evaluation must result in the identification of a subgroup of patients at heightened risk of short- or long-term cardiac complications during or after surgery, and, equally important; (2) once this higher-risk group is identified, there must exist some intervention that can modify that risk, whether the intervention involves canceling surgery, or serves to make surgery safer (for example by prescribing a medication, changing operative approach or route of anesthesia, or intervening to correct an underlying problem, as through coronary revascularization). Several models have been devised that allow prediction of operative risk based on a patient's clinical history and the results of noninvasive testing. In culling findings from a wealth of studies, the ACC/AHA consensus guidelines for preoperative evaluation prior to noncardiac surgery have become a widely used clinical tool not only to identify operative risk but also to serve as a guideline for the appropriateness of further testing and intervention.

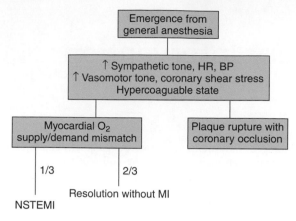

Figure 6-1 Pathophysiological events contributing to the genesis of perioperative MI. BP, blood pressure; HR, heart rate; NSTEMI, non-ST-segment elevation myocardial infarction.

The guidelines recommend a stepwise approach in determining the need for invasive testing prior to noncardiac surgery. First, patient-specific risk is determined through the assessment of clinical risk factors and symptoms, overall functional capacity, and the timing and results of prior coronary evaluation and treatment if applicable. Second, surgery-specific cardiac risk is determined based on the expected incidence of cardiac events associated with the particular surgery the patient is scheduled to undergo, as previously discussed. The decision of whether to perform noninvasive stress testing is then based on assessment of the patient and surgery-specific risks. Despite the comprehensive nature of the ACC/AHA preoperative guidelines, adherence to the guidelines in "real-world" clinical practice is highly variable.[5]

INDICATIONS FOR CORONARY ANGIOGRAPHY

The indications for performing coronary angiography as part of a preoperative assessment are identical to those in the nonoperative setting, and include the following[2,6]:

- Noninvasive test results suggesting a high risk of adverse outcomes, such as extensive (multivessel distribution) myocardial ischemia, prior to high-risk surgery.

TABLE 6-1	Cardiac Risk* for Noncardiac Surgical Procedures
Vascular (reported cardiac risk often greater than 5%)	
Aortic and other major vascular surgery	
Peripheral vascular surgery	
Intermediate (reported cardiac risk generally less than 5%)	
Intraperitoneal and intrathoracic surgery	
Carotid endarterectomy	
Head and neck surgery	
Orthopedic surgery	
Prostate surgery	
Low (reported cardiac risk generally less than 1%)	
Endoscopic procedures	
Superficial procedure	
Cataract surgery	
Breast surgery	
Ambulatory surgery	

*Death and/or MI.
From The ACC/AHA Guidelines on Perioperative Cardiovascular Evaluation and Care for Noncardiac Surgery.[2]

- An equivocal noninvasive test result in a patient with multiple clinical risk factors facing high-risk surgery
- The presence of exertional angina not responsive to appropriate medical therapy, especially when the patient is facing a moderate- or high-risk surgical procedure.
- The presence of unstable angina or recent MI.

It must be emphasized that, given the absence of prospective data indicating that surgical risk can be favorably influenced by preoperative coronary revascularization, the concept that PCI or coronary artery bypass grafting (CABG) should be undertaken to "get the patient through" a subsequent noncardiac surgery is not supported by evidence-based standards; these interventions should be used sparingly if at all for this indication. The ACC/AHA consensus guidelines assert that preoperative coronary revascularization is likely "appropriate for only a small subset of patients at very high risk."

Pharmacological Therapy

Because all individuals with known or suspected coronary disease have the potential to benefit from appropriate pharmacological therapy at the time of surgery regardless of whether preoperative coronary revascularization is undertaken, current principles regarding the use of perioperative beta-blocker and statin therapy are briefly reviewed.

BETA BLOCKERS

Beta blockers are thought to ameliorate cardiac stress in the perioperative setting by a number of mechanisms, including reduction of adrenergic stimulation, improvements in the balance of myocardial oxygen demand and supply, diminution of arrhythmic potential, and potential anti-imflammatory and plaque-stabilizing effects. Based on the results of two relatively small trials published in the 1990s demonstrating significant reductions in mortality associated with perioperative beta-blocker therapy among patients at risk for coronary events, guidelines advocating routine beta-blocker administration for patients at risk for cardiac complications or undergoing higher-risk surgical procedures became widely adopted. Several ensuing trials failed to demonstrate benefit from routine perioperative beta-blocker therapy among higher-risk patients, raising questions regarding therapeutic efficacy (Table 6-2). Publication of the more recent DECREASE-IV (Dutch Echocardiographic Cardiac Risk Evaluation Applying Stress Echo) and POISE (Patients Undergoing Non-Cardiac Surgery) trials has provided new insights while simultaneously raising new questions regarding the role of perioperative beta-blocker therapy.[7,8] The DECREASE-IV trial, which demonstrated a significant reduction in the incidence of cardiac death or nonfatal MI associated with perioperative bisoprolol therapy among patients at intermediate cardiac risk undergoing noncardiac surgery, appeared to settle the controversy in favor of beta-blocker therapy. In DECREASE-IV, bisoprolol was initiated at a low dose 30 days prior to surgery and carefully titrated to a goal heart rate of 50 to 70 beats per minute in 1,066 patients. Conflicting findings from the much larger POISE trial, however, again raised doubts regarding the safety and effectiveness of routine perioperative beta-blocker use. In POISE, 8,351 patients at risk for or with known coronary artery disease were assigned to receive either extended-release metoprolol or placebo beginning 2 to 4 hours before noncardiac surgery and continued for 30 days. At 30-day follow-up, the incidence of the composite primary endpoint of cardiovascular death, nonfatal MI, or nonfatal cardiac arrest was significantly lower among those assigned to metoprolol (5.8% vs. 6.9%), yet this advantage was offset by significantly increased frequencies of both all-cause mortality and stroke among individuals treated with beta blockers rather than placebo.

Many observers believe that the discordant results of trials examining perioperative beta blockade are multifactorial and likely attributable to differences with respect to the baseline cardiac risk of the populations under study, the particular beta blocker used, and whether therapy was begun well in advance of surgery and titrated to effect or simply started at a fixed uniform dose a few hours before the

TABLE 6-2	**Results of Randomized Trials of Beta-Blocker Therapy during Noncardiac Surgery**								
				Composite Cardiac Endpoint (%)		**All-Cause Mortality (%)**		**Nonfatal MI (%)**	
	Drug	N	*Follow-up*	BETA-BLOCKER	PLACEBO	BETA-BLOCKER	PLACEBO	BETA-BLOCKER	PLACEBO
McSPI	Atenolol	200	2 years	17*	32	10*	21	NR	NR
DECREASE-I	Bisoprolol	112	30 days	3*	34	3*	17	0*	17
DIPOM	Metoprolol XL	921	18 months	21	20	16	16	NR	NR
MaVS	Metoprolol	496	30 days	10	12	0	1.6	7.7	8.4
POBBLE	Metoprolol	103	30 days	34	32	5.7	2.3	6	11
POISE	Metoprolol XL	8,351	30 days	5.8*	6.9	3.1*	2.3	4.2*	5.7
DECREASE-IV	Bisoprolol	1,066	30 days	2.1*	6.0	1.9	3.0	2.1*	6.0

NR, not reported.
*P value < 0.05.

operation.[9,10] Based on the latest study data, the ACC/AHA established updated guidelines in 2009 for the use of beta blockers for noncardiac surgery. The guideline statement concludes that while the most recent studies suggest that "beta blockers reduce perioperative ischemia and may reduce the risk of MI and cardiovascular death in high-risk patients, routine administration of higher-dose long-acting metoprolol in beta-blocker naive patients on the day of surgery and in the absence of dose titration is associated with an overall increase in mortality." The lone class-I recommendation for beta blockade in the current guidelines states that "beta blockers should be continued in patients undergoing surgery who are [already] receiving beta blockers" for appropriate indications. Class IIa recommendations support the use of beta blockers *titrated to heart rate and blood pressure* for patients undergoing vascular or intermediate-risk surgery who are at high cardiac risk as a result of either (1) known coronary artery disease, (2) the finding of cardiac ischemia on preoperative testing, or (3) the presence of more than one clinical risk factor for coronary disease. The routine administration of high-dose beta blockers in the absence of dose titration is now contraindicated (class III) for patients undergoing noncardiac surgery who are not currently taking beta blockers.

STATIN THERAPY

Proposed mechanisms by which statins may reduce perioperative cardiac complications relate to the plaque-stabilizing effects of these agents, including their anti-inflammatory and anti-thrombotic properties, and the favorable influences these drugs exert on plaque-related endothelial dysfunction.[11] The withdrawal of statin therapy in the perioperative period has been associated with increased cardiac events.[12] Recent randomized trials have supported earlier observational studies suggesting that statin therapy administered prior to noncardiac surgery may be associated with a reduction in major adverse events. The DECREASE-III trial randomized 497 statin-naive patients scheduled to undergo vascular surgery to receive fluvastatin 80 mg daily or placebo started a median of 37 days preoperatively.[13] All patients also received titrated beta-blocker therapy. Fluvastatin therapy was associated with significant reductions in the incidence of perioperative myocardial ischemia on continuous ECG monitoring (10.8% vs. 19%, hazard ratio [HR] 0.55; 95% confidence interval [CI], 0.34–0.88) and in 30-day cardiovascular death or MI (HR, 0.47; 95% CI, 0.24–0.94) (Fig. 6-2). In the DECREASE-IV trial, which utilized a 2 × 2 factorial design to study the effects of perioperative fluvastatin and bisoprolol therapy, randomization to fluvastatin 80 mg daily was associated with a nonsignificant trend toward reduced 30-day cardiac events (HR, 0.65; 95% CI, 0.35–1.10).[8]

Current ACC/AHA guidelines recommend (with a class I indication) that patients currently taking statins who are scheduled for noncardiac surgery should continue therapy. In addition, the guidelines provide class II support for statin use among patients undergoing vascular surgery with or without clinical risk factors and for patients undergoing intermediate-risk procedures who have at least one clinical risk factor for coronary disease.

Preoperative Coronary Revascularization

As perioperative myocardial infarction is often related to the presence of preexisting coronary stenosis, coronary revascularization prior to surgery was previously looked upon as a potential means to limit the occurrence of ischemic events during and after surgery. Randomized clinical trials, however, have failed to demonstrate clinical benefits from a strategy of routine coronary revascularization prior to noncardiac surgery, and the indications for preoperative coronary artery bypass grafting (CABG) or PCI are now quite limited.

CORONARY ARTERY BYPASS GRAFTING

Noncardiac surgery appears safe for individuals with remote CABG who subsequently require a major noncardiac surgical procedure. Among patients followed in the CASS (Coronary Artery Surgery Study) registry who required high-risk noncardiac surgery during follow-up, prior CABG was associated with reduced postoperative MI and mortality compared with medically managed coronary disease. Other observational reports have indicated that for patients with prior CABG, mortality rates associated with noncardiac surgery are comparable with those observed among patients without evidence of coronary disease. While a history of remote CABG may be protective during future surgical procedures, the role of CABG undertaken as a preemptive measure among patients discovered to have severe

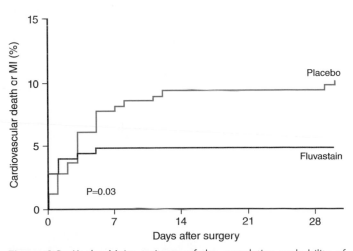

Figure 6-2 Kaplan-Meier estimate of the cumulative probability of cardiovascular death or MI during the 30-day follow-up period after surgery among subjects randomized to fluvastatin (red line) or placebo (blue line) in the DECREASE-III trial (4.8% vs. 10.1%, HR for fluvastatin 0.47; 95% CI, 0.24-0.94). *(From Schouten O, Boersma E, Hoeks SE, et al. Fluvastatin and perioperative events in patients undergoing vascular surgery.* N Engl J Med *2009;361:980–989.)*

coronary artery disease during a preoperative risk assessment remains unproven. Performance of CABG can substantially delay subsequent noncardiac surgery, and prophylactic CABG may not be feasible if the required noncardiac surgical procedure is urgent or semiurgent. Attempts to perform noncardiac surgery very shortly after CABG may be associated with further increased operative risks. For example, in one observational study, patients undergoing vascular surgery within 1 month of CABG demonstrated a fivefold increase in operative mortality compared with matched controls who underwent vascular surgery without preceding CABG (20.6 vs. 3.9%, $P < 0.005$).[14]

PERCUTANEOUS CORONARY INTERVENTION

Risks of Preoperative Percutaneous Coronary Intervention

Decision analyses have suggested that coronary angiography and intervention prior to vascular surgery should be carried out only when the risk of the vascular surgery is relatively high (>5%) and the anticipated risk of angiography and revascularization is relatively low (<3%). Unfortunately, the mere presence of peripheral vascular disease requiring surgical intervention is associated with an increased risk of adverse events during PCI. Among 2,340 patients enrolled in the BARI trail or registry, the presence of peripheral vascular disease was associated with a 50% relative increase in major in-hospital cardiovascular events following PCI (11.7 vs. 7.8%) and a nearly twofold increased likelihood of adverse events following CABG. Within another large registry of 25,114 patients who underwent PCI, the presence of peripheral or cerebral artery disease was independently associated with significantly increased likelihoods of in-hospital death (2.8% vs. 1.3%), MI (3.0% vs. 2.0%), stroke (0.8% vs. 0.3%), nephropathy (3.3% vs. 0.8%), major vascular complications (3.4% vs. 2.2%), and need for blood transfusion (8.2% vs. 4.2%). The significantly elevated risks of performing PCI among individuals with coexisting peripheral vascular disease, as highlighted by these studies, should be kept in mind in deciding whether to undertake PCI prior to planned vascular surgery.

Observational Studies of Preoperative Percutaneous Coronary Intervention

A variety of retrospective analyses extending from the pre-stent era to current practice have addressed the relationship between preoperative PCI and the likelihood of adverse cardiac events during subsequent noncardiac surgery (Tables 6-3, 6-4, and 6-5). Conclusions that can be drawn from these studies are, however, limited. Almost all reports suffer from small size, retrospective design, frequent absence of

TABLE 6-3	Complication Rates of Noncardiac Surgery following Balloon Angioplasty			
Author	**N**	**MI (%)**	**Death (%)**	**Interval between Angioplasty and Surgery**
Allen (1991)	148	0.7	2.7	11 months
Huber (1992)	50	5.6	1.9	9 days
Elmore (1993)	14	0	0	10 days
Jones (1993)	108	3.7	0.9	14 days
Gottlieb (1998)	194	0.5	0.5	11 days
Posner (1999)	686	2.2	2.6	1 year
Hassan (2001)	251	0.8	0.8	21 months
Brilakis (2005)	350	0.6	0.3	<2 months
Leibowitz (2006)	122	2.9	14.7	Early (0-14 days)
		6.8	9.1	Late (14-62 days)

Adapted (and expanded) from the ACC/AHA Guidelines on Perioperative Cardiovascular Evaluation and Care for Noncardiac Surgery.[2]

standardized indications to determine which patients were referred for PCI, a wide variety of noncardiac surgical procedures, variable timing between preoperative PCI and subsequent noncardiac surgery (days to years), and, perhaps most importantly, the lack of control groups. Also, in most reports patients who died following PCI did not go on to noncardiac surgery and thus were not included in follow-up, so the true complication rates from a strategy of preoperative PCI were underreported. Among studies of preoperative balloon angioplasty performed in the pre-stent era, in-hospital mortality following subsequent noncardiac surgery ranged from 0% to 2.7% for patients who underwent surgery following either recent (within 2 weeks) or remote (up to 29 months) preoperative angioplasty. Higher perioperative mortality rates (ranging from 2.9% to 20%) have been reported in more recent studies that examined outcomes following coronary BMS or DES implantation prior to noncardiac surgery.

RANDOMIZED TRIALS OF PREOPERATIVE REVASCULARIZATION

The landmark CARP (Coronary Artery Revascularization Prophylaxis) trial compared the strategies of preoperative coronary revascularization versus stand-alone medical therapy for the reduction of early and late cardiac events following major vascular surgery.[15] The trial enrolled 510 patients scheduled for vascular surgery at one of 18 Veterans Affairs Medical Centers. Patients were eligible if angiographically

TABLE 6-4	Complication Rates of Noncardiac Surgery following Coronary Stent Placement				
Author	**N**	**MI (%)**	**Death (%)**	**Major Bleeding (%)**	**Timing of Stenting and Surgery**
Kaluza (2000)	40	17.5	20	27.5	All deaths and MI occurred when surgery was performed <2 weeks after stenting.
Wilson (2003)	207	1.4	2.9	33	All deaths and MI occurred when surgery was performed <6 weeks after stenting.
Sharma (2004)	47	NR	17.0	25.6	Fivefold increase in mortality when surgery performed early (<3 weeks) vs. late (>3 weeks) after stenting.
Reddy (2005)	56	10.7	7.1	5.4	Death or MI occurred in 38% who had surgery within 2 weeks of stenting, but none who had surgery after 6 weeks.
Leibowitz (2006)	94	7.4	13.8	16	Significantly more adverse events occurred when surgery was performed within 2 weeks of PCI.
Vicenzi (2006)*	103	11.7	4.9	3.9	2.1-fold more events when surgery was performed early (<35 days) rather than late (>90 days) after stenting.
Schouten (2007)*	192	2.6	0	23	MACCE rate 13.3% vs. 0.6% when surgery performed early (<30 days) vs. late (>30 days) after stenting.
Brotman (2007)*	114	1.8	0	NR	Low MACCE rate.
Kim (2008)	101	0	0	NR	No MACCE occurred.
Nuttall (2008)	899	2.0	3.4	4.8	>Threefold greater MACCE rate when surgery performed early (<30 days) rather than late (>30 days) after stenting.
Van Kuijk (2009)	174	0.6	17.4	NR	MACCE rate 50% when surgery performed early (≤30 days) vs. 4% when performed late (>30 days) after stenting.

*Studies marked by an asterisk included patients with BMSs or DESs. Unmarked studies included only patients who received BMSs.
MACCE, major adverse cardiac and cerebrovascular events; NR = not reported.
Adapted (and expanded) from the ACC/AHA Guidelines on Perioperative Cardiovascular Evaluation and Care for Noncardiac Surgery.[2]

Author	N	MI (%)	Death (%)	Major Bleeding (%)	Timing of Stenting and Surgery
Assali (2009)	78	5.1	2.6	16.7	Frequency of MACCE did not differ significantly between those with early (<1 year) vs. late (>1 year) NCS following DES placement.
Rabbitts (2008)	520	2.7	2.7	14.8	Frequency of MACCE was not significantly associated with the time between PCI and NCS.
Rhee (2008)	141	1.4	3.5	NR	Only patients undergoing NCS <1 year post-DES included. Discontinuance of clopidogrel ≥7 days preop was the strongest predictor of MACCE.
Godot (2008)	96	12.5	2.1	0	Frequency of MACCE was not significantly associated with the time between PCI and NCS.
Compton (2006)	38	0	0	NR	No MACE noted in this small series. Clopidogrel was stopped prior to NCS in 60% of patients
Kim (2008)	138	1.4	0.7	NR	The adverse events occurred 6,264 and 367 days after stent placement.
Van Kuijk (2009)	376	9.6	0.5	NR	MACCE rate 18% when surgery performed early (≤1 year) vs. 9% when performed late (>1 year) after stenting.

TABLE 6-5 Complication Rates of Noncardiac Surgery following Placement of Coronary Drug-Eluting Stents

MACCE, major adverse cardiac and cerebrovascular events; NCS, noncardiac surgery; NR, not reported.

proven coronary artery disease with a ≥70% stenosis in at least one major epicardial coronary artery was present and were randomized to either coronary revascularization followed by vascular surgery (N = 258) or to vascular surgery without preceding coronary revascularization (N = 252). Among the group randomized to coronary revascularization, 41% underwent CABG and 59% were treated with PCI. The majority of patients enrolled in the CARP trial were at low to intermediate rather than high risk for perioperative coronary events. The median age was 66 years, and while 42% had suffered a prior MI, only 38% noted the presence of angina at the time of study entry. Most patients had one- or two-vessel coronary disease with preserved left ventricular function; those with left main stenosis of ≥50%, a left ventricular ejection fraction of <20%, or severe aortic stenosis were excluded. The results of the CARP trial indicated that preoperative revascularization was not associated with any apparent benefit over conservative therapy. Whereas patients assigned to coronary revascularization had a significantly longer delay between randomization and vascular surgery (54 vs. 18 days), neither preoperative PCI nor CABG was associated with a reduction in the occurrence of adverse cardiac events following vascular surgery at 30-day or 2.7 year follow-up (Fig. 6-3). One criticism of the CARP trial was that the process of preoperative risk stratification used in the study did not follow the ACC/AHA guidelines, in which coronary angiography is generally considered only after noninvasive testing has demonstrated moderate or severe inducible ischemia. In the CARP study, noninvasive testing was not mandated, and less than 50% of enrolled subjects underwent a stress imaging study that documented moderate or severe ischemia prior to coronary angiography.

The DECREASE-V pilot study was designed to evaluate the effectiveness of prophylactic coronary revascularization prior to major vascular surgery among a higher-risk group of patients than those enrolled in the CARP trial.[16] A total of 101 patients with extensive myocardial ischemia on noninvasive stress imaging were randomized to either revascularization (65% had PCI, 35% had CABG) or no revascularization prior to vascular surgery. Within this relatively small cohort, preoperative coronary revascularization was not associated with significant differences in the occurrence of death or MI either at 30 days or 1 year following noncardiac surgery (Fig. 6-4). The authors calculated that, based on the event rates observed in this pilot study, a sample size of >600 patients would be required for a randomized study to establish definitively that coronary revascularization is superior to medical therapy to improve postoperative outcome in high-risk patients by 20% compared with optimal medical therapy.

Despite their potential shortcomings, the CARP and DECREASE-V results lend strong support to the concept that performing prophylactic coronary revascularization for the purpose of "getting a patient through" noncardiac surgery is generally not appropriate. At present, preoperative PCI should be considered only among patients who have an indication for coronary revascularization unrelated to the

noncardiac surgery, particularly those with medically refractory angina, unstable angina, or recent MI. For these limited patient groups at the highest risk for adverse cardiac events, sufficient data regarding the efficacy and safety of preoperative revascularization is lacking, and the potential risks and benefits of preoperative revascularization need to be carefully weighed on an individual basis. Multidisciplinary communication involving the patient's primary care physician, cardiologist, cardiac surgeon, anesthesiologist, and surgeon intending to perform the noncardiac procedure can be crucial in determining a rational preoperative strategy. Such a discussion can allow consideration of issues such as life expectancy, anticipated risks and benefits of preoperative PCI or CABG, the risks, necessity, and urgency of the planned noncardiac surgical procedure, and the potential risks that antiplatelet agents such as aspirin or thienopyridine therapy may pose during the operation.

Technical Aspects of Preoperative PCI

When the decision has been made to perform preoperative PCI, several important technical considerations exist. Foremost is the length of delay that is permissible between PCI and the subsequent noncardiac

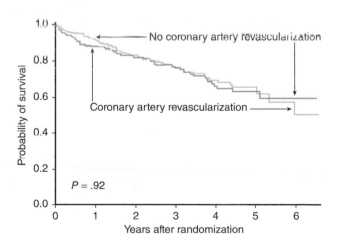

No. at risk

Revascularization	226	175	113	65	18	7
No revascularization	229	172	108	55	17	12

Figure 6-3 Kaplan-Meier survival curve for patients enrolled in the CARP trial. There was no difference in early or late mortality following noncardiac surgery among patients with coronary artery disease who were randomized to undergo preoperative coronary revascularization rather than conservative therapy. (*From McFalls EO, Ward HB, Moritz TE, et al. Coronary-artery revascularization before elective major vascular surgery. N Engl J Med 2004;351:2795–2804.*)

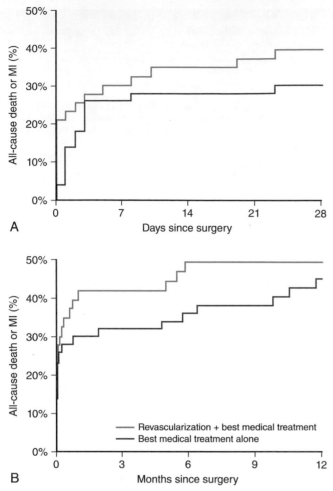

Figure 6-4 Preoperative revascularization was not associated with a significant difference in all-cause death or MI following noncardiac surgery among patients with three or more cardiac risk factors and extensive stress-induced ischemia enrolled in the DECREASE-V pilot study. *(From Poldermans D, Schouten O, Vidakovic R, et al. A clinical randomized trial to evaluate the safety of a noninvasive approach in high-risk patients undergoing major vascular surgery: the DECREASE-V Pilot Study. J Am Coll Cardiol 2007;49:1763–1769.)*

surgical procedure, which often dictates whether stand-alone balloon angioplasty, bare metal stenting, or drug-eluting stent implantation is performed.

Balloon Angioplasty. Because of less reliable short and long-term results, balloon angioplasty without stent placement has become an infrequently used strategy for most patients undergoing PCI. Stand-alone balloon angioplasty may, however, have a role in the preoperative setting as this approach does not introduce the possibility of perioperative stent thrombosis or mandate the use of thienopyridine therapy, and therefore can permit surgery to be performed with little delay following PCI (Table 6-3). Current ACC/AHA guidelines recommend delaying surgery for 2 to 4 weeks following balloon angioplasty to allow for initial healing at the site of vessel injury and to overcome the usual time frame during which acute vessel closure and recoil typically occur. Surgery should not be delayed for more than 8 to 12 weeks following angioplasty because restenosis becomes a potential concern after this interval. Thus, for a patient in whom PCI is deemed necessary prior to surgery, but delaying surgery for more than 2 weeks is undesirable, balloon angioplasty without stenting may represent a reasonable option. It should, however, be kept in mind that abrupt vessel closure

or an inadequate angiographic result can occur in up to 10% to 20% of attempts at stand-alone balloon angioplasty, and that unplanned stenting may become necessary.

Bare Metal Stents. Among patients undergoing PCI, routine stent implantation is associated with improved immediate and late results compared with balloon angioplasty alone. In the face of noncardiac surgery, however, the presence of a recently placed coronary stent introduces the possibility of stent thrombosis during the perioperative period, an event that is associated with substantial morbidity and mortality. Antiplatelet therapy with aspirin and a thienopyridine is typically recommended for at least 4 weeks following placement of a BMS to reduce the likelihood of stent thrombosis while stent endothelialization is occurring. When noncardiac surgery is undertaken soon (within 4 to 6 weeks) after coronary stent implantation, several observational studies have demonstrated an alarmingly high rate of adverse cardiac events, especially when dual antiplatelet therapy is interrupted prior to surgery (Table 6-4). A report by Kaluza et al. was the first to highlight concerns regarding stent placement prior to noncardiac surgery.[17] Among 40 patients who underwent bare metal stenting less than 6 weeks prior to noncardiac surgery, there were 8 deaths, 7 MIs, and 11 major bleeding episodes at the time of surgery. The majority of ischemic cardiac events were the result of stent thrombosis. Within another cohort of 56 individuals who underwent noncardiac surgery after coronary bare metal stenting, perioperative death or MI occurred among 38% of patients who had surgery within 2 weeks of stenting; however no patients in whom surgery was delayed for >6 weeks experienced adverse cardiac sequelae.[18] In a much larger series of 899 patients who underwent a noncardiac surgical procedure at the Mayo Clinic within 1 year of coronary BMS implantation, much lower rates of perioperative death (3.4%) and MI (2.0%) were reported. Consistent with other reports, however, a greater than threefold excess of major adverse cardiac events was observed among individuals who underwent surgery earlier than 30-days post-PCI.[19] The likelihood of stent thrombosis when noncardiac surgery is performed early following stent placement is further amplified when thienopyridine therapy is discontinued prior to the surgical procedure. Within a small group of patients who underwent noncardiac surgery within 3 weeks of bare metal stenting, Sharma noted a dramatic 86% incidence of stent thrombosis among patients in whom thienopyridine therapy was discontinued prior to surgery, compared with a 5% incidence of thrombosis among those whose in whom thienopyridine therapy was not stopped.[20] Similarly, among a separate contingent of 192 patients treated with either BMSs or DESs prior to noncardiac surgery, the perioperative mortality rate was 30.7% for individuals with premature discontinuation of thienopyridine therapy (<30 days after bare metal stenting or <3-6 months after DES placement) prior to surgery), but no deaths occurred among patients who completed the full course of dual antiplatelet therapy.[21] In summary, given the risk of perioperative stent thrombosis when the interval between PCI and surgery is short, noncardiac surgery should be delayed for 6 weeks following BMS implantation. This will permit at least partial endothelialization of the stent as well as completion of a full 4-week course of thienopyridine therapy with additional time after drug discontinuation for return of platelet function prior to surgery.

Drug-Eluting Stents. DESs have further reduced the likelihood of restenosis following PCI compared with BMSs, yet they are poorly suited for use in the preoperative setting. By inhibiting cellular proliferation, drug-eluting stents not only limit the development of fibrointimal hyperplasia but also inhibit the protective process of stent endothelialization. Stent thrombosis therefore remains a concern for months to years (instead of weeks) following DES implantation and mandates a prolonged course of thienopyridine therapy.[22] At present, dual antiplatelet therapy for at least 12 months following DES placement is recommended; however, reports of DES thrombosis beyond 1 year suggest that even longer courses of thienopyridine therapy may be beneficial, particularly for patients with high-risk clinical

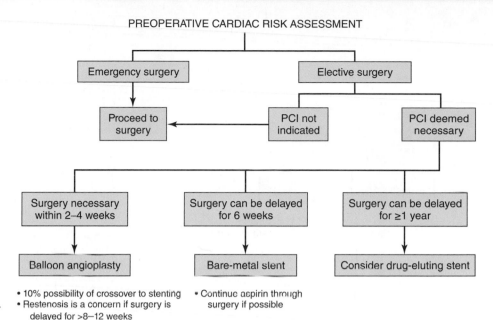

Figure 6-5 Algorithm outlining device selection for preoperative PCI.

PREOPERATIVE CARDIAC RISK ASSESSMENT

Emergency surgery | Elective surgery

Proceed to surgery | PCI not indicated | PCI deemed necessary

Surgery necessary within 2–4 weeks | Surgery can be delayed for 6 weeks | Surgery can be delayed for ≥1 year

Balloon angioplasty | Bare-metal stent | Consider drug-eluting stent

- 10% possibility of crossover to stenting
- Restenosis is a concern if surgery is delayed for >8–12 weeks

- Continue aspirin through surgery if possible

or anatomical features of stent thrombosis.[23] Such features include diabetes mellitus, renal insufficiency, reduced ejection fraction, and DES use for "off-label" indications (including left main, bifurcation, or small vessel stenting and implantation of multiple or overlapping stents). Even when used for "on-label" indications, long-term follow-up studies have demonstrated that DES thrombosis can occur well beyond a year after stent implantation at rates of 0.2% to 0.5% per year. Drawing upon the observation that perioperative stent thrombosis risk following BMS implantation is greatest when surgery is performed prior to completion of the customary 4-week course of theinopyirdine therapy, the current ACC/AHA guidelines for perioperative care recommend delaying surgery when possible for at least 12 months following DES placement. Prior to all PCI procedures, patients should routinely be asked whether any noncardiac surgical procedure is planned or likely within the next 12 months; if so balloon angioplasty or bare metal stenting should be performed in lieu of DES placement.

Recommendations

If PCI is felt to be necessary prior to noncardiac surgery, the primary factors that dictate procedural approach are (1) the amount of time available between PCI and surgery and (2) whether the planned surgical procedure allows for continuation of antiplatelet therapy during the perioperative period (Fig. 6-5). If surgery is urgent for a life-threatening problem, PCI is typically not performed. Stand-alone balloon angioplasty can be considered in instances when surgery can be delayed for at least 1 to 2 weeks, as this approach circumvents the need for thienopyridine therapy and the possibility of perioperative stent thrombosis. As noted, however, the possibility that bailout stent placement may become necessary during attempts at balloon angioplasty should be considered. A strategy of simple balloon angioplasty is also less likely to yield adequate results with certain disease patterns—for example, multivessel or left main disease. BMS placement appears to represent the preferred approach if surgery can be postponed for preferably 6 weeks following stent placement so as to permit stent endothelialization and completion and washout of thienopyridine therapy. If the bleeding risks of the planned surgical procedure are low, such that aspirin and thienopyridine can be continued perioperatively, it may be possible, if necessary, to perform surgery earlier following BMS placement, although the safety of this approach remains uncertain and postponing surgery for a full 6 weeks is strongly recommended. The use of a DES should be avoided if the planned surgical procedure cannot be delayed for at least 12 months.

Management of Patients with Drug-Eluting Stents Who Require Noncardiac Surgery

Even if DES use is avoided among patients with impending surgery, it is inevitable that some individuals with a previously placed DES will need unanticipated noncardiac surgery within or beyond the ensuing year. It has been estimated that approximately 5% of patients who receive a DES require surgery during the first 12 months after stent placement.[24] For these individuals, perioperative management of antiplatelet therapy requires careful attention.[25–27] While studies identifying the ideal waiting period for surgery among DES recipients are lacking at present, current guidelines advise that noncardiac surgery be delayed if possible for at least 1 year following DES implantation to allow completion of a full course of dual antiplatelet therapy. Despite this recommendation, studies to date have reached conflicting conclusions regarding the presence or absence of a significant association between the timing of noncardiac surgery following DES placement and the risk of perioperative cardiac events. In a retrospective analysis by Assali et al. that included 78 patients who underwent noncardiac surgery at least 6 months after DES implantation (median = 414 days), the incidence of perioperative cardiac death or nonfatal MI did not differ significantly between patients who had surgery 6 to 12 months versus more than 12 months following stent placement (9.1% vs. 6.7%, respectively).[28] Event rates in this relatively small population were not influenced by the continuation or cessation of clopidogrel perioperatively, as one-third of adverse events occurred among patients in whom clopidogrel had been continued through surgery. This finding conflicts with that of Rhee et al., who found that discontinuation of clopidogrel ≥7 days before surgery was the strongest predictor of major adverse cardiovascular and cerebrovascular events (MACCE) among a group of 141 patients with prior DES placement.[29] In the largest reported series to date, Rabbitts et al. found that the frequency of MACCE was not significantly associated with the time interval between DES placement and subsequent noncardiac surgery among 520 patients who underwent surgery up to 730 days (median = 203 days) following PCI. Significant univariate risk factors for MACCE

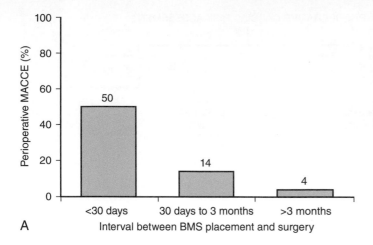

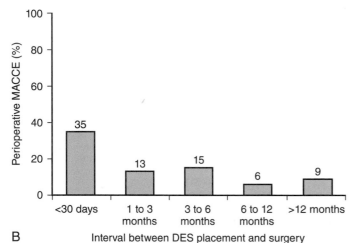

Figure 6-6 Association between the time interval from stent placement and noncardiac surgery and the occurrence of perioperative major adverse cardiovascular and cerebrovascular events (MACCE) following (a) bare-metal stent (BMS) and (b) drug-eluting stent (DES) placement. *(Derived from the results of van Kuijk JP, Flu WJ, Schouten O, et al. Timing of noncardiac surgery after coronary artery stenting with bare metal or drug-eluting stents. Am J Cardiol 2009;104:1229–1234.)*

were older age, shock at the time of PCI, prior MI, and continuation of thienopyridine into the operative period.[30] Conversely, among 376 patients who underwent noncardiac surgery at various intervals following DES placement at another center from 2002 to 2007, MACCE rates fell from 18% when surgery was performed in first year after stenting to 9% when surgery was performed more than 1 year following PCI (Fig. 6-6).[31]

ASPIRIN, THIENOPYRIDINES, AND SURGICAL BLEEDING RISK

Despite conflicting data, most authors believe that continuing dual aspirin and thienopyridine therapy through surgery will probably reduce the likelihood of perioperative DES thrombosis, especially when the surgical procedure must be performed within 12 months of stent placement. While likely providing some protection against potentially catastrophic adverse cardiac events, continuation of dual antiplatelet therapy during surgery involves the trade-off of an increased probability of hemorrhagic complications. The likelihood and consequences of perioperative bleeding events is a function of the surgical procedure being performed. For example, intracranial, spinal, and certain types of retinal surgery represent situations in which even

small amounts bleeding into a closed space can have devastating consequences, and cessation of antiplatelet agents is typically considered mandatory in advance of these procedures. With a few exceptions, continuation of aspirin during most surgical procedures is generally considered safe. In the largest evaluation of aspirin use during noncardiac surgery, aspirin therapy was associated with a 1.5-fold increase in overall bleeding complications among nearly 50,000 patients who underwent a variety of surgical procedures.[32] Despite the increase in overall bleeding, however, there was no increase in fatal bleeding among aspirin users except during intracranial surgery and transurethral prostatectomy. The withdrawal of aspirin prior to surgery, conversely, was associated with an increased incidence of cardiac, cerebral, and peripheral vascular adverse events. Clopidogrel, when continued during cardiac or noncardiac surgery, is associated more consistently than aspirin with hemorrhagic events. Among individuals undergoing on- or off-pump coronary bypass surgery, clopidogrel use is linked to increased incidences of major bleeding, surgical reexploration for bleeding, and the need for blood product transfusions but not with excess mortality.[33–35] Although the implications of continued clopidogrel use during noncardiac surgery are less well defined, increases in nonfatal bleeding complications and transfusion rates have likewise been described.[36] For some vascular procedures, pretreatment aspirin and clopidogrel may produce beneficial effects. For example, in one prospective study of patients undergoing carotid endarterectomy, pretreatment with aspirin and clopidogrel was associated with a reduction in cerebral emboli as detected by intraoperative transcranial Doppler monitoring but no increase in clinical bleeding complications.[37]

SUMMARY AND RECOMMENDATIONS

The decision as to whether to suspend or continue antiplatelet therapy during noncardiac surgery among patients with a preexisting DES should be based on careful consideration of the potential risks and consequences of perioperative stent thrombosis versus bleeding complications. Communication between the surgeon and cardiologist is critical in determining how to properly manage antiplatelet therapy around the time of surgery on a patient-by-patient basis. The ACC/AHA perioperative guidelines admonish that "healthcare providers who perform invasive or surgical procedures and who are concerned about periprocedural and postprocedural bleeding must be made aware of the potentially catastrophic risks of premature discontinuation of thienopyridine therapy."

In considering whether to stop or continue thienopyridine therapy prior to surgery, the following factors should be taken into account:

1. How much time has elapsed since stent was placed? While definitive data are lacking, continuation of dual antiplatelet therapy is especially important when surgery cannot be deferred for 1 year following DES implantation. If theinopyirdine therapy must be stopped, ACC/AHA guidelines urge that "aspirin be continued if at all possible and the thienopyridine be restarted as soon as possible after the procedure." A recent metanalysis of all reported cases of late or very late DES thrombosis supports the concept that short-term discontinuation of thienopyridine may be safer if aspirin is continued.[38]

2. What is the patient-specific risk of stent thrombosis? It should be determined whether the patient possesses any additional risk factors for stent thrombosis, such as diabetes mellitus, renal insufficiency, or use of DES in an "off label" manner, which may increase the propensity for thrombosis. The presence of such risk factors favors the continuation of dual antiplatelet therapy through surgery whenever possible.

3. What are the potential consequences of stent thrombosis for the particular patient? For instance, stent occlusion may be especially devastating for patients with preexisting left ventricular dysfunction or in circumstances when the stent is located in a vessel with a large territory of supply, such as an unprotected left main or a single remaining patent coronary artery or bypass graft.

4. What are the potential risks and consequences of excess surgical bleeding for the proposed operation? For operations involving closed spaces, such as intracerebral, spinal, or retinal surgery, the adverse consequences of bleeding may be so dire that temporary cessation of antiplatelet therapy is mandated. Since clopidogrel results in irreversible inhibition of platelet function, when the decision is made to discontinue therapy in advance of surgery, the drug should be stopped at least 5 days prior to the procedure to allow adequate time for platelet regeneration. Likewise, clopidogrel should be restarted with a 300- or 600-mg bolus as soon as possible following surgery.

EMERGING STRATEGIES

Preoperative "Bridging"

For patients receiving dual antiplatelet therapy who are considered to be at particularly elevated risk for stent thrombosis but for whom antiplatelet agents must be stopped prior to surgery, "bridging" therapy, in which a parenteral glycoprotein IIb/IIIa receptor antagonist is administered during the thienopyadine washout period immediately prior to surgery, has been proposed as a means to shorten the vulnerable period during which platelet function may be inadequately inhibited.[39] The small-molecule IIb/IIIa receptor anagonists eptifibatide and tirofiban both have relatively short physiological half-lives with near complete recovery of platelet function within several hours of drug cessation and may represent suitable bridging agents. Because abciximab, like clopidogrel, results in irreversible inhibition of platelet function, this agent is not appropriate for preoperative bridging. While preoperative bridging is theoretically attractive, published reports of it remain sparse. Broad et al. described their experience with bridging therapy among three patients with paclitaxel-eluting stents who were felt to be at high risk of perioperative stent thrombosis.[40] Clopidogrel was discontinued 5 days before surgery and aspirin was continued. Three days before surgery, patients were hospitalized for initiation of tirofiban and unfractionated heparin infusions that were stopped 6 hours prior to surgery. Clopidogrel was restarted on the first postoperative day with a loading dose of 300 mg. No ischemic or hemorrhagic complications were encountered. While clinical experience with this approach remains anecdotal, bridging therapy with a IIb/IIIa receptor antagonist may represent a reasonable approach for DES patients in whom the risks or consequences of stent thrombosis are felt to be substantial.

New Antiplatelet Agents

The pharmacodynamic properties of several newer antiplatelet agents may render them especially well suited for use in the preoperative setting (Table 6-6). Ticagrelor is an orally administered nonthienopyadine platelet $P2Y_{12}$ receptor antagonist with more potent and consistent platelet inhibition than clopidogrel.[41] Unlike ticlopidine, clopidogrel, and prasugrel, which bind irreversibly to the $P2Y_{12}$ receptor and therefore require several days for the manufacture of new platelets following drug cessation for return of platelet activity, ticagrelor binds reversibly to the $P2Y_{12}$ receptor, permitting a more rapid return of platelet activity. Given its relatively short half-life (6 to 13 hours), cessation of ticagrelor as little as 1 day prior to surgery might be an option. In the DISPERSE-2 (Dose Confirmation Study Assessing Anti-Platelet Effects of AZD6140 vs. Clopidogrel in non-ST segment Elevation Myocardial Infarction-2) trial, 990 patients hospitalized with non-ST-elevation MI were randomized to ticagrelor versus clopidogrel and no significant differences in minor or major bleeding rates were detected between the two agents. Among a small subgroup of 84 patients who required CABG, however, major bleeding events were less common among those randomized to ticagrelor versus clopidogrel when surgery was performed within 5 days of drug cessation (36% vs. 64%), with little difference when surgery was delayed beyond 5 days (50% vs. 60%).[42] In the randomized PLATO (Platelet Inhibition and Patient Outcomes) trial of over 18,000 patients hospitalized with acute MI, ticagrelor was associated with significant reductions in cardiac death and myocardial infarction but no increase in overall bleeding events compared with clopidogrel. Among patients requiring CABG, ticagrelor was not associated with a significant difference in major bleeding complications compared with clopidogrel.[43] Cangrelor, a reversible $P2Y_{12}$ receptor antagonist that is administered intravenously, has a very rapid onset of action and a half-life of only 3 minutes, allowing recovery of platelet function within 60 minutes of its cessation.[44] While cangrelor was not effective in reducing ischemic endpoints among >14,000 patients undergoing PCI in the CHAMPION (Cangrelor versus Standard Therapy to Achieve Optimal Management of Platelet Inhibition) series of trials,[45,46] the drug's remarkably rapid onset and offset of action may render it valuable as a perioperative bridging agent. In the ongoing BRIDGE (Maintenance of Platelet Inhibition with Cangrelor after Discontinuation of Thienopyridines in Patients Undergoing Surgery) trial, the safety and efficacy of cangrelor among hospitalized patients awaiting CABG surgery will be assessed.

Platelet Function Testing

Substantial interindividual variability exists with respect to the degree of platelet inhibition produced by clopidogrel. A variety of assays with the ability to rapidly assess the level of platelet inhibition on a patient-specific basis have recently garnered much interest in the interventional cardiology community and may be of value in the preoperative management of patients at risk for stent thrombosis who require discontinuation of thienopyradine agents prior to surgery.[47-49] While guidelines currently recommend delaying surgery for at least 5 days after discontinuation of clopidogrel, platelet function may recover more rapidly in some individuals, leaving them vulnerable to ischemic events for a longer than desirable period of time. With serial platelet function testing, it may be possible to determine precisely when platelet reactivity has recovered sufficiently to allow the safe performance of surgery while minimizing the window of increased risk for stent thrombosis. Although intuitively attractive, the safety and efficacy of such an approach requires further clinical testing before its widespread use can be recommended.

Postoperative Care

While prevention of operative complications through proper patient selection and management remains the cornerstone of achieving low surgical mortality rates, prompt recognition and treatment of postoperative complications when they do occur represents another critical element in optimizing surgical outcomes. In a provocative study of

TABLE 6-6	Pharmacokinetics of Antiplatelet Agents				
Drug	Route of Administration	Reversible Platelet Inhibition?	Time to Peak Activity after Loading Dose*	Elimination Half-Life*	Time to Platelet Recovery after Discontinuation*
Ticlopidine	Oral	No	3-5 days	4-5 days	5-7 days
Clopidogrel	Oral	No	2–6 hours	8 hours	5-7 days
Prasugrel	Oral	No	1 hour	8 hours	5-7 days
Ticagrelor	Oral	Yes	2 hours	8 hours	<48 hours
Cangrelor	Intravenous	Yes	<10 minutes	3 minutes	<60 minutes

*Times are approximate and demonstrate interindividual variability.

over 84,000 patients included in the American College of Surgeons Quality Improvement Program who underwent inpatient general or vascular surgery from 2005 to 2007, hospitals were divided into quintiles based on overall risk-adjusted mortality rates. While the major surgical complication rates were similar among hospitals in the lowest and highest mortality quintiles (16.2 vs. 18.2%), the ultimate mortality rates among patients with major complications varied dramatically, from 12.5% among hospitals in the lowest mortality quintile to 21.4% among hospitals in the highest mortality quintile.[50] These findings indicate that variations in mortality rates between hospitals can be explained to a substantial degree not by differences in initial surgical complication rates, but by the care that patients receive after complications have occurred.

Because the vast majority of perioperative cardiac events occur within the first 24 to 48 hours following surgery, close surveillance of patients at increased risk for such events is essential during the early postoperative period. Continuous telemetry monitoring and routine assessment of serum troponin levels are recommended for patients at risk of cardiac events during this interval. For patients in whom aspirin and/or thienopyradine therapy was suspended prior to surgery, these agents should be resumed as soon as safely possible, since the prothrombotic milieu engendered by surgery persists into the postoperative period. If an acute ST-segment-elevation MI does occur early postoperatively, primary PCI is the treatment of choice. Thrombolytic therapy is contraindicated after all but the most minor surgical procedures because of the potential for hemorrhagic complications related to the surgical site. For this reason, patients at heightened risk for perioperative MI (including those with prior DES placement or in whom dual antiplatelet therapy must be suspended prior to surgery) should have their surgical procedure performed at an institution with the on-site ability to perform primary PCI on a continuous basis. Following vascular surgery involving the aorta or iliofemoral arteries, the use of an intra-aortic balloon pump may not be possible and the radial artery may represent the preferred approach for coronary angiography and PCI. Among patients requiring emergency PCI in the very early postoperative period, bleeding complications related to the surgical site remain a concern; however, angioplasty can be performed safely in most instances with the use of only aspirin and a single dose of unfractionated heparin or a bolus and brief infusion of bivalirudin. While published outcome data are limited, in one report of 48 patients who underwent PCI for acute MI within 1 week of noncardiac surgery, many of whom presented with cardiogenic shock, the survival rate was 65% and only one individual had significant bleeding at the operative site.

REFERENCES

1. Priebe HJ: Triggers of perioperative myocardial ischaemia and infarction. *Br J Anaesth* 93:9–20, 2004.
2. Fleisher LA, Beckman JA, Brown KA, et al: 2009 ACCF/AHA focused update on perioperative beta blockade incorporated into the ACC/AHA 2007 guidelines on perioperative cardiovascular evaluation and care for noncardiac surgery: a report of the American College of Cardiology Foundation/American Heart Association Task Force on Practice Guidelines. *Circulation* 120:e169–e276, 2009.
3. Bursi F, Babuin L, Barbieri A, et al: Vascular surgery patients: perioperative and long-term risk according to the ACC/AHA guidelines, the additive role of post-operative troponin elevation. *Eur Heart J* 26:2448–2456, 2005.
4. Chong CP, Lam QT, Ryan JE, et al: Incidence of post-operative troponin I rises and 1-year mortality after emergency orthopaedic surgery in older patients. *Age Ageing* 38:168–174, 2009.
5. Hoeks SE, Scholte op Reimer WJ, Lenzen MJ, et al: Guidelines for cardiac management in noncardiac surgery are poorly implemented in clinical practice: results from a peripheral vascular survey in the Netherlands. *Anesthesiology* 107:537–544, 2007.
6. Poldermans D, Bax J, Boersma E, et al: Guidelines for pre-operative cardiac risk assessment and perioperative cardiac management in non-cardiac surgery. The Task Force for Preoperative Cardiac Risk Assessment and Perioperative Cardiac Management in Non-cardiac Surgery of the European Society of Cardiology (ESC) and endorsed by the European Society of Anaesthesiology (ESA). *Eur Heart J* 30:2769–2812, 2009.
7. Devereaux PJ, Yang H, Yusuf S, et al: Effects of extended-release metoprolol succinate in patients undergoing non-cardiac surgery (POISE trial): a randomised controlled trial. *Lancet* 371:1839–1847, 2008.
8. Dunkelgrun M, Boersma E, Schouten O, et al: Bisoprolol and fluvastatin for the reduction of perioperative cardiac mortality and myocardial infarction in intermediate-risk patients undergoing noncardiovascular surgery: a randomized controlled trial (DECREASE-IV). *Ann Surg* 249:921–926, 2009.
9. Chopra V, Eagle KA: Perioperative beta-blockers for cardiac risk reduction: time for clarity. *JAMA* 303:551–552, 2010.
10. Poldermans D, Schouten O, van Lier F, et al: Perioperative strokes and beta-blockade. *Anesthesiology* 111:940–945, 2009.
11. Biccard BM: A peri-operative statin update for non-cardiac surgery. Part I: The effects of statin therapy on atherosclerotic disease and lessons learnt from statin therapy in medical (non-surgical) patients. *Anaesthesia* 63:52–64, 2008.
12. Le Manach Y, Godet G, Coriat P, et al: The impact of postoperative discontinuation or continuation of chronic statin therapy on cardiac outcome after major vascular surgery. *Anesth Analg* 104:1326–1333, 2007.
13. Schouten O, Boersma E, Hoeks SE, et al: Fluvastatin and perioperative events in patients undergoing vascular surgery. *N Engl J Med* 361:980–989, 2009.
14. Breen P, Lee JW, Pomposelli F, et al: Timing of high-risk vascular surgery following coronary artery bypass surgery: a 10-year experience from an academic medical centre. *Anaesthesia* 59:422–427, 2004.
15. McFalls EO, Ward HB, Moritz TE, et al: Coronary-artery revascularization before elective major vascular surgery. *N Engl J Med* 351:2795–2804, 2004.
16. Poldermans D, Schouten O, Vidakovic R, et al: A clinical randomized trial to evaluate the safety of a noninvasive approach in high-risk patients undergoing major vascular surgery: the DECREASE-V Pilot Study. *J Am Coll Cardiol* 49:1763–1769, 2007.
17. Kaluza GL, Joseph J, Lee JR, et al: Catastrophic outcomes of noncardiac surgery soon after coronary stenting. *J Am Coll Cardiol* 35:1288–1294, 2000.
18. Reddy PR, Vaitkus PT: Risks of noncardiac surgery after coronary stenting. *Am J Cardiol* 95:755–757, 2005.
19. Nuttall GA, Brown MJ, Stombaugh JW, et al: Time and cardiac risk of surgery after bare-metal stent percutaneous coronary intervention. *Anesthesiology* 109:588–595, 2008.
20. Sharma AK, Ajani AE, Hamwi SM, et al: Major noncardiac surgery following coronary stenting: when is it safe to operate? *Cath Cardiovasc Intervent* 63:141–145, 2004.
21. Schouten O, van Domburg RT, Bax JJ, et al: Noncardiac surgery after coronary stenting: early surgery and interruption of antiplatelet therapy are associated with an increase in major adverse cardiac events. *J Am Coll Cardiol* 49:122–124, 2007.
22. Luscher TF, Steffel J, Eberli FR, et al: Drug-eluting stent and coronary thrombosis: biological mechanisms and clinical implications. *Circulation* 115:1051–1058, 2007.
23. Grines CL, Bonow RO, Casey DE, Jr, et al: Prevention of premature discontinuation of dual antiplatelet therapy in patients with coronary artery stents: a science advisory from the AHA, ACC, SCAI, ACS, and ADA. *Circulation* 115:813–818, 2007.
24. Vicenzi MN, Meislitzer T, Heitzinger B, et al: Coronary artery stenting and non-cardiac surgery—a prospective outcome study. *Br J Anaesth* 96:686–693, 2006.
25. Practice alert for the perioperative management of patients with coronary artery stents: a report by the American Society of Anesthesiologists Committee on Standards and Practice Parameters. *Anesthesiology* 110:22–23, 2009.
26. Brilakis ES, Banerjee S, Berger PB: Perioperative management of patients with coronary stents. *J Am Coll Cardiol* 49:2145–2150, 2007.
27. Mollmann H, Nef HM, Hamm CW, et al: How to manage patients with need for antiplatelet therapy in the setting of (un-)planned surgery. *Clin Res Cardiol* 98:8–15, 2009.
28. Assali A, Vaknin-Assa H, Lev E, et al: The risk of cardiac complications following noncardiac surgery in patients with drug eluting stents implanted at least six months before surgery. *Cathet Cardiovasc Intervent* 74:837–843, 2009.
29. Rhee SJ, Yun KH, Lee SR, et al: Drug-eluting stent thrombosis during perioperative period. *Int Heart J* 49:135–142, 2008.
30. Rabbitts JA, Nuttall GA, Brown MJ, et al: Cardiac risk of noncardiac surgery after percutaneous coronary intervention with drug-eluting stents. *Anesthesiology* 109:596–604, 2008.
31. van Kuijk JP, Flu WJ, Schouten O, et al: Timing of noncardiac surgery after coronary artery stenting with bare metal or drug-eluting stents. *Am J Cardiol* 104:1229–1234, 2009.
32. Burger W, Chemnitius JM, Kneissl GD, et al: Low-dose aspirin for secondary cardiovascular prevention—cardiovascular risks after its perioperative withdrawal versus bleeding risks with its continuation—review and meta-analysis. *J Int Med* 257:399–414, 2005.
33. Ferraris VA, Ferraris SP, Moliterno DJ, et al: The Society of Thoracic Surgeons practice guideline series: aspirin and other antiplatelet agents during operative coronary revascularization (executive summary). *Ann Thorac Surg* 79:1454–1461, 2005.
34. Fox KA, Mehta SR, Peters R, et al: Benefits and risks of the combination of clopidogrel and aspirin in patients undergoing surgical revascularization for non-ST-elevation acute coronary syndrome: the Clopidogrel in Unstable angina to prevent Recurrent ischemic Events (CURE) Trial. *Circulation* 110:1202–1208, 2004.
35. Kapetanakis EI, Medlam DA, Petro KR, et al: Effect of clopidogrel premedication in off-pump cardiac surgery: are we forfeiting the benefits of reduced hemorrhagic sequelae? *Circulation* 113:1667–1674, 2006.
36. Chassot PG, Delabays A, Spahn DR: Perioperative antiplatelet therapy: the case for continuing therapy in patients at risk of myocardial infarction. *Br J Anaesth* 99:316–328, 2007.
37. Payne DA, Jones CI, Hayes PD, et al: Beneficial effects of clopidogrel combined with aspirin in reducing cerebral emboli in patients undergoing carotid endarterectomy. *Circulation* 109:1476–1481, 2004.
38. Eisenberg MJ, Richard PR, Libersan D, et al: Safety of short-term discontinuation of antiplatelet therapy in patients with drug-eluting stents. *Circulation* 119:1634–1642, 2009.
39. Abualsaud A, Eisenberg M: Peroperative management of patients with drug-eluting stents. *J Am Coll Cardiol Intervent* 131–142, 2010.
40. Broad L, Lee T, Conroy M, et al: Successful management of patients with a drug-eluting coronary stent presenting for elective, non-cardiac surgery. *Br J Anaesth* 98:19–22, 2007.
41. Storey RF, Husted S, Harrington RA, et al: Inhibition of platelet aggregation by AZD6140, a reversible oral P2Y12 receptor antagonist, compared with clopidogrel in patients with acute coronary syndromes. *J Am Coll Cardiol* 50:1852–1856, 2007.
42. Cannon CP, Husted S, Harrington RA, et al: Safety, tolerability, and initial efficacy of AZD6140, the first reversible oral adenosine diphosphate receptor antagonist, compared with clopidogrel, in patients with non-ST-segment elevation acute coronary syndrome: primary results of the DISPERSE-2 trial. *J Am Coll Cardiol* 50:1844–1851, 2007.
43. Wallentin L, Becker RC, Budaj A, et al: Ticagrelor versus clopidogrel in patients with acute coronary syndromes. *N Engl J Med* 361:1045–1057, 2009.
44. Ferreiro JL, Ueno M, Angiolillo DJ: Cangrelor: a review on its mechanism of action and clinical development. *Exp Rev Cardiovasc Ther* 7:1195–1201, 2009.
45. Bhatt DL, Lincoff AM, Gibson CM, et al: Intravenous platelet blockade with cangrelor during PCI. *N Engl J Med* 361:2330–2341, 2009.
46. Harrington RA, Stone GW, McNulty S, et al: Platelet inhibition with cangrelor in patients undergoing PCI. *N Engl J Med* 361:2318–2329, 2009.
47. Jones N, Broomhead R, Kaur J, et al: "To MAP or not to MAP; is that the question?" The role of platelet function tests in the perioperative management of patients on antiplatelet therapy. *Curr Anaesth Crit Care* 21:91–99, 2010.
48. Lippi G, Favaloro EJ, Salvagno GL, et al: Laboratory assessment and perioperative management of patients on antiplatelet therapy: from the bench to the bedside. *Clin Chim Acta* 405:8–16, 2009.
49. Price MJ: Monitoring platelet function to reduce the risk of ischemic and bleeding complications. *Am J Cardiol* 103:35A–39A, 2009.
50. Ghaferi A, Birkmeyer J, Dimick J: Variation in Hospital Mortality Associated with Inpatient Surgery. *New Engl J Med* 361:1368–1375, 2009.

7

Gender and Ethnicity Issues in Percutaneous Coronary Interventions

LESLIE CHO

KEY POINTS

- Women who present for percutaneous coronary interventions (PCIs) are older and have more comorbidities compared with men. Women and men have similar short-term and long-term benefits with bare metal stent (BMS) and drug-eluting stent (DES). Moreover, women and men have similar mortality rate after PCIs. However, women have higher rates of vascular complications and bleeding after PCI.

- Women presenting with unstable angina or non-ST elevation myocardial infarction (NSTEMI) with negative biomarkers are less likely to benefit from an invasive strategy and should have their risk stratified with stress testing.

- Women and men have similar benefit with glycoprotein (GP) IIb/IIIa inhibitor, adenosine diphosphate (ADP) receptor inhibitors, and direct thrombin inhibitors.

- Women derive similar benefit as do men with primary PCI for ST-elevation MI (STEMI).

- Race-specific analyses in PCI are still rare. However, African American patients who present for PCIs are younger, female, more likely to have comorbidities, and present with acute coronary syndrome (ACS) or STEMI.

Introduction

Cardiovascular disease (CVD) remains the leading cause of death regardless of gender and race.[1] Until recently, information has been extrapolated from large studies and registries and has been applied to all population groups irrespective of gender, race, or ethnicity. However, there is a growing body of literature that has shown differences in cardiovascular disease manifestations and treatment effects, depending on gender and race. In this chapter, we will explore gender and racial differences in PCIs, acute myocardial infarction (AMI), acute coronary syndrome (ACS), stable angina, and adjunctive pharmacotherapy.

Gender

CVD is the leading cause of mortality and morbidity among women in the United States. It claims the lives of more women than the next five major causes of death in women combined.[1] CVD in women occurs about 10 years later than in men, and in part, this has contributed to the misconception that cardiovascular disease is predominately a problem of the male gender. There has been much reported gender differences in outcomes between women and men, which may be explained by differences in comorbidities, pathophysiologic differences between genders, and disparities in treatment and outcomes following the cardiovascular event.[1]

PERCUTANEOUS CORONARY INTERVENTIONS

More than 1.3 million PCIs are performed annually in the United States. An estimated 33% of PCIs are performed in women.[1] Compared with men, women undergoing PCIs are 5 years older and have higher prevalences of hypertension, diabetes, and other comorbidities.[2] They are less likely to have had a history of MI, PCIs, or coronary bypass graft surgery (CABG). At the time of PCIs, they have less multi-vessel disease and are more likely to present with unstable angina. Unlike men, they require more urgent procedures and are more likely to have rotational atherectomy. Compared with men, women have similar lesions types, less multi-vessel disease, and more preserved left ventricular (LV) function.[2,3] However, paradoxically, despite better LV function, women tend to have higher incidences of congestive heart failure (CHF), and more functional impairment after revascularization than do men.[4] Early reports of patients undergoing balloon angioplasty found lower procedural success rates in women. In addition, earlier registry studies showed that women had higher in-hospital mortality after PCIs even after adjusting for baseline comorbidites.[5] However, recent studies report similar procedural success rates of 90% in both groups.[3,5] Improved morbidity and mortality outcomes were observed in more recent studies despite older age and more complex lesion types (Tables 7-1 and 7-2),[3,5] Table 7-1 shows the recently published data regarding in-hospital deaths and MI rates by gender. The table also includes large published studies since 2000, which reported odds ratios adjusted for age and risk factors. Even though there are variations in each of the studies, they show no differences in in-hospital mortality and morbidity rates. With newer-generation stents and balloons, smaller sheath sizes and catheters, and advances in adjunctive pharmacotherapies, adjusted long-term mortality and morbidity rates after PCI have become similar between men and women[3,5-7] (see Table 7-2) (Fig. 7-1). There has been much controversy surrounding less frequent use of diagnostic catheterization and delays in PCIs in women compared with men.[6] These issues will be addressed further in the section on ACS and MI later in the chapter.

GENDER AND DEVICES

No gender-based comparisons were made in the earlier randomized clinical trials comparing bare metal stent (BMS) with balloon angioplasty. Re-stenosis and revascularization rates were not well defined for women after BMS because of the small sample of women in prospective trials with systematic angiographic follow-up. Even though women tend to have a smaller vessel size and a higher prevalence of diabetes, initially some intriguing studies reported that women had similar or lower target vessel revascularization (TVR) rates compared with their male counterparts after PCIs.[9] However, systematic angiographic and clinical follow-up have not validated these studies. In the drug-eluting stent (DES) era, both sirolimus and taxus stents have shown favorable outcomes in women. Both the SIRIUS trial and the TAXUS IV trial have demonstrated the superiority of DES with reduction in re-stenosis, TVR, and major adverse cardiac events at 1-year follow-up in women and men.[10,11] In TAXUS IV, 1314 patients with severe coronary artery stenosis were randomized to paclitaxel stent versus BMS. Women comprised 27.9% of the study population. Re-stenosis rates were similar in women and men treated with the TAXUS stent (7.6% vs. 8.6%, $P = 0.80$), as was late loss (0.23 mm vs. 0.22 mm, $P = 0.90$). Compared with BMS stents, women treated with the TAXUS stent had a significant reduction in 9-month re-stenosis (29.2% vs. 8.6%, $P < 0.001$) and 1-year target lesion revascularization rates (TLR) (14.9% vs. 7.6%,

TABLE 7-1	In-Hospital Death and Myocardial Infarction after Percutaneous Coronary Interventions by Gender			
Study	#Women/Men	Women %	Men %	Adjusted OR (95% CI)
Peterson 2001:				
In-hospital death	35,571/74,137	1.8%	1.0%	1.07 (0.9–1.2)
In-hospital MI		1.5%	1.2%	1.25 (1.1–1.4)
Jacobs 2002:				
In-hospital death	895/1,629	2.2%	1.3%	1.6 (0.76–3.35)
In-hospital MI		0.2%	0.7%	
Lansky 2002:				
In-hospital death	2,077/5,295	1.4%	0.7%	2.28 (1.15–4.55)
Watanabe 2001:				
In-hospital death	29,227/53,556	1.2%	0.6%	1.65 (1.33–2.04)
Malenka 2002:				
In-hospital death	3,983/8,057	1.04%	0.79%	1.24 (0.96–1.60)
In-hospital MI		1.71%	1.36%	1.02 (0.85–1.24)

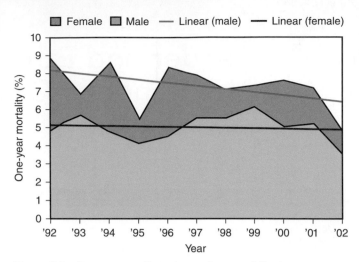

Figure 7-1 One-year unadjusted mortality rates following percutaneous coronary intervention (PCI) in women and men from 1992 to 2002 from The Cleveland Clinic. *(Reproduced with permission from Chiu et al. Impact of female sex on outcome after percutaneous coronary intervention. Am Heart J. 2004;148(6):998–1002.)*

$P = 0.02$). Of note, women had higher unadjusted TLR rates compared with men at 1 year; however, female gender was not an independent predictor of TLR (OR 1.72, 95% CI 0.68–4.37, $P = 0.25$).[12] A patient pooled analysis from four randomized sirolimus vs. BMS trials was done to assess for gender differences.[13] In 1748 patients, of whom 497 were women, sirolimus-coated stents were associated with significant reduction in the rates of in-segment binary re-stenosis in women (6.3% vs. 43.8%) as well as in men (6.4% vs. 35.6%), which resulted in significant reduction in 1-year major adverse cardiac events ($P < 0.0001$). Few gender-based studies on the efficacy of directional atherectomy (DCA) exist. No gender-specific data on rotational atherectomy, cutting balloon angioplasty, extraction atherectomy, or gamma brachytherapy are available. DCA is no longer used, but from a historical perspective, it appears to be associated with lower procedural success and more bleeding complications in women.[14] Likewise, large devices such as the Excimer laser angioplasty also are associated with higher morbidity rates in women with higher coronary perforation rates.[14]

VASCULAR COMPLICATIONS

Women have experienced greater vascular complications such as major hematoma, retroperitoneal bleed, bleeding complications requiring transfusion, and vascular injury requiring surgery after PCI compared with men.[7,15,16] Much of this is likely caused by smaller vessel size and aggressive anticoagulation. With the development of weight-adjusted heparin dosing, introduction of smaller sheath size, and early sheath

removal, vascular complications have decreased.[15,16] However, even in the current era, women continue to have 1.5 to 4 times higher risk of vascular complication compared with men.[7,10,15,16] Table 7-3 shows different vascular complication rates by gender as reported in recently published large studies. Of note, there have been no gender-specific data on arterial vascular puncture closure devices. Since women have higher rates of vascular complications, they might be ideal candidates for radial access. Data are somewhat complicated.[17]

GENDER DIFFERENCES BY CLINICAL SYNDROME

Acute Coronary Syndrome

Women who present with ACS are older and have higher incidences of diabetes and hypertension compared with men. They also have less severe coronary artery disease, with greater absence of critical obstructions and more preserved left ventricular function. In ACS, women are more likely to have elevated cross-reactive (C-reactive) protein (CRP) and brain natriuretic peptide (BNP), whereas men are more likely to have elevated creatine kinase-MB and troponin.[18] Randomized trials have shown the benefit of invasive strategy over conservative treatment in ACS; however, results in women have been confusing. A meta-analysis of eight large ACS trials, in which 3075 subjects were women and 7075 were men, has shed some insight into the confusion.[19] These

TABLE 7-2	Long-Term Outcome of Percutaneous Coronary Interventions in ACS Patients by Gender			
	#Women/Men	Women	Men	Adjusted OR (95% CI)
Jacobs 2002:				
1-yr Death	895/1,629	6.5%	4.3%	1.26 (0.85–1.87)
1-yr Death/ myocardial infarction		11.1%	9.0%	1.14 (0.86–1.50)
Lansky 2002:				No difference between gender noted; however OR was not reported
1-yr death	2,077/5,295	4.4%	3.3%	
1-yr MACE		29.2%	32.7%	
Mehili 2000:				
1-yr death	1,001/3,263	4.0%	4.1%	0.99 (0.54–1.13)
1-yr MACE		6.0%	5.8%	—
Chiu 2004:				
1-year death	5,301/12,738	7%	5%	1.14 (0.93–1.41)
1 year MACE	—			1.05 (0.97–1.13)

TABLE 7-3	Vascular Injury Complication by Gender			
	# Women/Men	Women	Men	P-value
Chiu 2004:				
Blood transfusion	5,301/12,738	12%	4%	<0.001
Major hematoma		5%	2%	<0.001
Pseudoaneurysm		0.6%	0.3%	0.005
Lansky 2002:				
Major hematoma	562/1,520	2.5%	1.5%	0.005
Retroperitoneal bleed		0.5%	0.2%	0.05
Surgical repair		3.8%	2.4%	0.001
Welty 2001:				
Vascular injury	2,101/3,888	1.6%	0.6%	0.001
Peterson 2001:				
Vascular injury	35,571/74,137	5.4%	2.7%	0.001

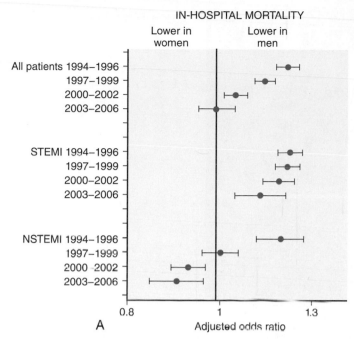

Figure 7-2 In-hospital mortality rates for women and men. (Reprinted with permission from Rogers WJ, Frederick PD, Stoehr E, et al: Trends in presenting characteristics and hospital mortality among patients with ST elevation and non-ST elevation myocardial infarction in the National Registry of Myocardial Infarction from 1990 to 2006. Am Heart J 2008;156:1026–1034.)

studies found that among ACS patients, as it was in men, an invasive strategy was safe and effective in women who had positive biomarkers when the composite endpoints of death, MI, or re-hospitalization (OR 0.67, 95% CI 0.50–0.88) were reduced. However, in women with negative biomarkers, an invasive strategy did not reduce major adverse cardiac events and was associated with a trend toward higher rates for death or MI (OR 1.35; 95% CI 0.78–2.35).[19] A recent study from the National Registry of Myocardial Infarction in which 1.9 million patients were included showed that since 2000, women with NSTEMI had lower adjusted mortality than their male counterparts, which may be attributed to less obstructive CAD at the time of presentation in women (Fig. 7-2).[28] Much has been reported on gender differences in the diagnosis and treatment of ACS, STEMI, and stable angina. Studies have shown delays in diagnosis and in health care–seeking behaviors as well as underutilization of cardiac catheterization and revascularization in women compared with men throughout the spectrum of CAD and treatment. In 2005, the CRUSADE investigators published their registry data on gender differences in patients with NSTEMI–ACS. In this large registry of over 35,000 patients, of which 41% were women, they found that women were less likely to receive guidelines-recommended therapy such as heparin (adjusted OR 0.91, 95% CI 0.86–0.97), angiotensin-converting enzyme inhibitors I (ACE-I) (adjusted OR 0.95, 95% CI 0.90–0.99), and GP IIb/IIIa inhibitors (adjusted OR 0.87, 95% CI 0.81–0.92), compared with men, during acute hospitalization.[20] Even troponin-positive patients were less likely to receive GP IIb/IIIa inhibitors (adjusted OR 0.87, 95% CI 0.81–0.92). Moreover, women were less likely to undergo diagnostic catheterization (adjusted OR 0.86, 95% CI 0.82–0.91) or PCI (adjusted OR 0.91, 95% CI 0.86–0.96) during hospitalization.[20] Women were less likely to receive guidelines-recommended medical therapies such as aspirin (adjusted OR 0.91 95% CI 0.85–0.98), ACE I (adjusted OR 0.93, 95% CI 0.88–0.98), and statin (adjusted OR 0.92, 95% CI 0.88–0.98) at the time of discharge. The CRUSADE registry confirms the unfortunate presence of continued treatment disparities between the groups. Another published study using the ACC-NCDR (American College of

Cardiology–National cardiovascular data registry) registry regarding gender differences among patients with ACS both NSTEMI and STEMI again showed gender disparities in treatment.[21] Of 199,690 patients, the 55,691 women, in spite of having fewer high-risk criteria, had higher rates of in-hospital complications. For example, although the adjusted mortality among women and men was similar (OR 0.97, 95% CI 0.88–1.07, P = 0.52), women had higher rates of complications such as CHF (OR 0.80, 95% CI 0.69–0.92, P = 0.002), bleeding complications (OR 0.55, 95% CI 0.52–0.58, P < 0.01), and cardiogenic shock (OR 0.82, 95% CI 0.75–0.89, P < 0.01). Moreover, they found that women were less likely to receive aspirin (OR 1.16, 95% CI 1.13–1.20, P < 0.01) or GP IIb/IIIa inhibitor (OR 1.10, 95% CI 1.08–1/13, P < 0.01) at admission and were less likely to be discharged on statins (OR 1.10, 95% CI 1.07–1.13, P < 0.01) or aspirin (PR 1.17, 95% CI 1.13–1.21, P < 0.01). These findings call for significant improvements in the care of ACS patients and highlight the importance of continued investigations into barriers that contribute to these differences.

ST Elevation Myocardial Infarction

Women with MI are older and have more comorbidities compared with their male counterparts. Moreover, they are likely to present to hospital later than men with a higher Killip class. At the time of presentation, women have less severe CAD and more preserved left ventricular function. In the majority of cases, the initial presentation of CAD in women is sudden cardiac death (SCD) or acute MI. Surprisingly, there appear to be differences in plaque morphology between women and men with acute MI. Autopsy studies have shown more plaque erosion than plaque rupture in young women after fatal MI compared with men or older women (Fig. 7-3, A and B).[22] Also, women appear to have more distal microvascular embolization compared with men during fatal MI.[23] The overall superiority of primary PCI over fibrinolytic therapy for women has been demonstrated.[24] Because of more comorbidities in women at presentation, the absolute benefit with primary PCI is greater for women than for men. An estimated 56 deaths could be prevented for every 1000 women treated with primary PCI compared with 42 fewer deaths per 1000 men.[24] A study has shown that there are gender-associated differences in the amount of myocardial salvage after primary PCI for STEMI. In this study, myocardial salvage achieved by primary PCI was greater in women than in men.[25] Improved salvage may be attributed to gender-specific hypoxic tolerance. Female cells have a higher baseline expression of the protein Bcl-2, showing a higher inherited hypoxic tolerance than male cells.[25]

Gender-specific data regarding primary stenting versus primary balloon angioplasty in STEMI have been available. Women with STEMI benefitted from primary stenting with less re-infarction, TVR, and TLR. The CADILLAC trial which enrolled 2082 patients, of which 27% were women, to BMS versus primary balloon angioplasty with or without GP IIb/IIIa inhibitor, found superior efficacy and safety with primary stenting with or without abciximab compared with balloon angioplasty (Fig. 7-4).[10] In women, primary stenting resulted in a reduction in the 1-year composite of death, re-infarction, ischemia-driven TVR, or disabling stroke from 28.1% to 19.1% (P = 0.01) compared with percutaneous transluminal coronary angioplasty (PTCA).[10] The addition of abciximab to primary stenting significantly reduced the 30-day ischemic TVR without increasing bleeding or stroke rates for women.[14] Much controversy has surrounded mortality rate differences between women and men after STEMI (see Table 7-4). There appears to be higher in-hospital mortality rates among women undergoing PCI for STEMI compared with men. A large study using Nationwide Inpatient Sample of 11,717 women and 24,028 men found a 5.2% in-hospital mortality rate in women compared with a 2.7% mortality rate in men. Even after adjusting for age, hypertension, institutional volume, and pulmonary disease, women had higher mortality rate (OR 1.47, 95% CI 1.23–1.75).[26] Similarly, the New York State Department of Health database found that women had significantly higher adjusted in-hospital mortality rate (OR 2.69 95% CI 1.4–5.2).[27] The recently published data from the National Registry of Myocardial

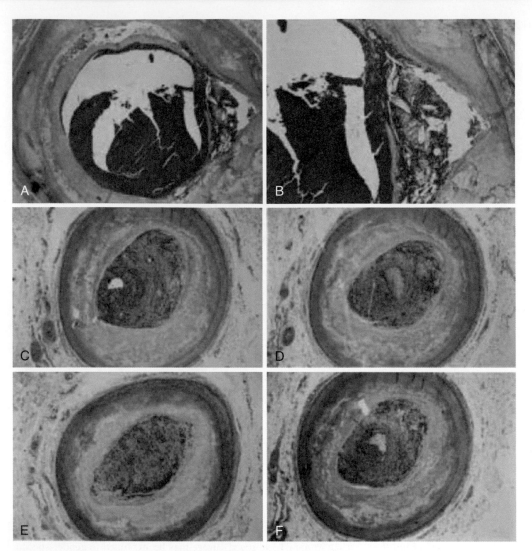

Figure 7-3 **A** and **B,** Plaque ulcer with hemorrhagic core. **C, D, E,** and **F,** Plaque erosion. Note the lack of continuity between thrombus and the plaque. *(Reproduced with permission from Arbustini et al. Plaque erosion is a major substrate for coronary thrombosis in acute myocardial infarction. Heart 1999;82(3):269–272.)*

TABLE 7-4	Short-Term and Long-Term Outcome in Percutaneous Coronary Interventions in Patients with Myocardial Infarction by Gender			
PCI–MI studies	*# Women/ Men*	*Female*	*Men*	*Adjusted rates OR (95% CI)*
Watanabe 2001:				
In-hospital death	11,717/ 24,028	5.2%	2.7%	1.47(1.23–1.75)
Vakili 2001:				
In-hospital death	317/727	7.9%	2.3%	2.69(1.4–5.2)
Mehili 2000:				
30-day death	502/1,435	8.4%	8.5%	—
1-year death		13.8%	12.9%	0.65(0.49–0.87)
Lansky 2005:				
30-day death	562/1,520	4.6%	1.1%	—
1-year death		7.6%	3.0%	1.11(0.53–2.36)
Antonucci 2001:				
6-months death	230/789	12%	7%	1.25(0.63–2.47)

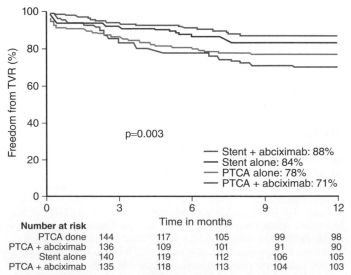

p=0.003

— Stent + abciximab: 88%
— Stent alone: 84%
— PTCA alone: 78%
— PTCA + abciximab: 71%

Number at risk				
PTCA done	144	117	105	99	98
PTCA + abciximab	136	109	101	91	90
Stent alone	140	119	112	106	105
PTCA + abciximab	135	118	113	104	103

Figure 7-4 Target vessel revascularization rate in women enrolled in the CADILLAC trial. *(Reproduced with permission from Lansky et al. Percutaneous coronary intervention and adjunctive pharmacotherapy in women: a statement for healthcare professionals from the American Heart Association. Circulation 2005;111(7):940–953.)*

Infarction showed that women with STEMI have higher in hospital mortality rates compared with men (see Fig. 7-2).[28] However, by 30 days and 1 year, there appears to be no difference in mortality rates between the two groups (see Table 7-4). Of note, female gender is an independent risk factor for the development of cardiogenic shock as a complication of acute MI. However, there is no gender difference in the mortality rates of cardiogenic shock once age is adjusted. Thus, the ACC/AHA guidelines for the treatment of STEMI recommend PCI or CABG for patients age <75 years who are in cardiogenic shock and have lesions amenable to revascularization, regardless of gender.[4] Many studies have shown delay in time to treatment, time to invasive diagnostic test, and time to revascularization in women. Women with STEMI are less likely to undergo primary angioplasty within 2 hours or have accepted pharmacologic treatment on admission. Even at discharge, women are less likely to be on accepted medical treatment.[29] The older age of the female patients, the symptom differences, and the delay in presentation after AMI have been suggested as possible explanations. While these factors may explain initial treatment differences, it does not explain the treatment disparities once the diagnosis has been made. Continued quality improvement in the diagnosis and treatment of women with CAD are needed.

GENDER DIFFERENCES IN ADJUNCTIVE PHARMACOTHERAPY

Anti-platelet Therapy

Aspirin. Aspirin remains the mainstay of anti-platelet therapy in patients with CAD. It acts by irreversibly inactivating cyclo-oxygenase (COX), which leads to the inhibition of platelet thromboxane A2 synthesis; this ultimately leads to the inhibition of thromboxane-mediated platelet aggregation. Aspirin's effectiveness in secondary prevention is well established. However, aspirin's role in primary prevention in women has been controversial. An early prospective prevention cohort study of 87,678 healthy women aged 34 to 65 years found that 325 mg of aspirin once to six times a week was associated with a significant reduction of myocardial infarction (P = 0.005).[30] However, recently, a randomized primary prevention trial of 39,876 women receiving 100 mg aspirin administered every other day found no cardiovascular risk reduction (RR 0.91, 95% CI 0.80–1.15).[31] Aspirin reduced the risk of ischemic stroke by 24% but had no effect on the risk of MI. Of note, there was a consistent cardiovascular risk reduction with aspirin in women age 65 years. A meta-analysis of six randomized controlled trials of primary prevention in 51,342 women and 44,144 men demonstrated gender-specific benefits. In women, aspirin decreased the rate of ischemic stroke (OR 0.76, 95% CI 0.63–0.93, P = 0.0008) but had no benefit in reducing MI. In contrast, men had a reduction in MI (OR 0.68, 95% CI 0.54–0.86, P = 0.001), but there was no significant reduction in the incidence of stroke.[32] The treatment variability has been attributed to baseline clinical differences as well as to unique gender-specific responses to aspirin therapy. After aspirin therapy, both men and women showed similar inhibition of platelets in the COX-1 direct pathway. In aggregation assays that were indirectly dependent on the COX-1 pathway, compared with men, women had a modest increase in platelet reactivity after aspirin therapy.[33]

Aspirin resistance also appears to be more common in women than in men. A recent study of 326 patients with cardiovascular disease assessed the prevalence and clinical significance of aspirin resistance by optical platelet aggregation.[34] Of the 326 patients, 17 patients were aspirin resistant. In this study, aspirin resistance was defined as mean platelet aggregation of ≥70% with 10 μM ADP and a mean aggregation of ≥20% with 0.5 mg/mL arachidonic acid. Women were more likely to be aspirin resistant. A much larger study from the Heart Outcome Prevention Evaluation (HOPE) trial assessed the relationship between aspirin resistance and the risk of adverse cardiovascular outcomes.[35] Patients in the study had a history of CAD, stroke, peripheral vascular disease, or diabetes plus at least one other cardiovascular risk factor. Aspirin resistance was determined by measuring urinary levels of

11-dehydro-thromboxane B2, a stable metabolite of thromboxane A2. Higher baseline urinary levels of 11-dehydro-thromboxane B2 were associated with increased MI, stroke, and CVD mortality rates (P = 0.01).[35] Female gender was independently associated with higher baseline levels of 11-dehydrothromboxane B2 level, indicating that women may be more resistant to aspirin (P = 0.0004).[35] Of greater concern is the lack of aspirin therapy in women with CAD. In a large secondary prevention trial of women, only 83% of those with established CAD or CVD were on aspirin therapy.[36] Even among patients with unstable angina, women were less likely to be on aspirin therapy. This dismal rate is confirmed in other large registries and speaks to the treatment gap that still exists in practice.[36,37] Despite the advances in therapy, proven medical therapy after PCI such as the use of aspirin, ACE inhibitors, beta-blockers, and statin continue to be underutilized in all patients, most specifically in women.[37]

Thienopyridines. Clopidogrel and ticlopidine inhibit platelet aggregation by inhibiting the ADP receptor binding to the platelet receptor. When given in addition to aspirin, these agents reduce the rates of subacute stent thrombosis after stent implantation. The CURE-PCI study enrolled 2658 patients with ACS treated with PCI, of which 30.2% were women, and assigned them to either long-term or short-term clopidogrel plus aspirin. They found that clopidogrel for up to 12 months was superior to aspirin alone.[38] A trend toward benefit was seen in women (RR 0.77, 95% CI 0.52–1.15) compared with the statistically significant benefit seen in men (RR 0.65, 95% CI 0.48, 0.87). In the CREDO trial, 2116 patients were enrolled, of which 29% were women, long-term treatment with clopidogrel for up to 12 months after elective PCI compared with short-term clopidogrel was associated with a 27% relative risk reduction in the primary endpoint of death, MI, or stroke.[39] In women, there was a 32% relative risk reduction in the primary endpoint; however, it did not reach statistical significance (OR 32.1, 95% CI 58.9–12.1).[39] With regard to clopidogrel loading dose, there are no gender-specific data. The optimal timing and loading dose for women at both high risk and low risk have yet to be determined. In the ISAR-REACT trial, which enrolled 2159 patients with low risk for PCI pretreated with 600 mg of clopidogrel, and assigned them to either abciximab or placebo; the study found no additional benefit to GP IIb/IIIa inhibitor.[40] In this study, women comprised 24% of the population. All patients who had a diagnosis of ACS, insulin-dependent diabetes, and other high risk criteria were excluded from this trial. Death, MI, and TVR at 30 days did not differ between the abciximab and placebo groups in either the entire population (4.0% vs. 4.0%, P = NS) or the female subset (3.0% vs. 3.0%, P = NS).[40] For the new thienopyridine, Prasugrel, no gender-specific analysis has been done to date.

Glycoprotein IIb/IIIa Inhibitors. GP IIb/IIIa inhibitors, in addition to unfractionated heparin, are beneficial to women undergoing PCIs and are not associated with an independent risk of major bleeding complications.[16] However, the risk of minor bleeding complications is increased in women.[16] In the pooled analysis of abciximab high-risk PCI trials, abciximab conferred equal benefit to both men and women.[16] The composite incidence of death, MI, or urgent revascularization was reduced from 16.0% to 9.9% at 6 months in women (P < 0.001); at 1 year, there was a significant reduction in mortality (4.0% vs. 2.5%, P = 0.03) in the women treated with abciximab.[16] Although women experienced more major bleeding than men (3.0% vs. 1.3%, P < 0.05), it was unrelated to abciximab. However, abciximab therapy was associated with increased minor bleeding in women (6.7% abciximab vs. 4.7% placebo. P = 0.01).[16] A meta-analysis of six large placebo-controlled trials of mostly small-molecule GP IIb/IIIa inhibitors in ACS patients undergoing PCIs showed a significant reduction in the combined endpoint of death and nonfatal MI after PCI.[41] This benefit extended to 6 months after the index PCI. In this meta-analysis, a highly significant interaction was seen between gender and treatment.[41] In men, there was a 19% reduction in the 30-day death or MI with GP IIb/IIIa inhibitors compared with placebo (OR 0.81, 95% CI

0.75–0.89).[41] In contrast, in women, there was an 11% increased risk of 30-day death or MI with GP IIb/IIIa inhibitor use (OR 1.15, 95% CI 1.01–1.30).[41] Even after adjusting for age and comorbidities, a gender difference in treatment effect was still present. However, once patients were stratified according to troponin concentration, there was no differential treatment effect between women and men.[41] A reduction in the 30-day death or MI with GP IIb/IIIa inhibitors was seen in women (OR 0.93, 95% CI 0.68–1.28) and men (0.82, 95% CI 0.65–1.03) with positive baseline troponin, whereas no risk reduction was seen in patients with negative troponin.[41] Tirofiban and eptifibatide have both been shown to be safe and efficacious in women during PCIs.[42,43] However, abciximab has been shown to be superior to tirofiban in preventing peri-procedural and 30-day ischemic complications, a finding that was consistent and unrelated to gender.[44] Abciximab has never been compared directly with double-bolus eptifibatide. In women undergoing PCIs for STEMI, use of GP IIb/IIIa inhibitors has shown reduction of short-term ischemic events.[14] However, the use of GP IIb/IIIa inhibitors in rescue PCIs after failed thrombolysis has been associated with increased bleeding rates, especially in women and older adults.[45,46]

Anti-thrombin Agents

Unfractionated Heparin. Unfractionated heparin has been used as the main anticoagulation therapy in PCIs. In the early days of PCIs, empiric heparin dosing was used. However, ACT levels after a fixed dose of unfractionated heparin vary substantially because of the differences in body sizes, concomitant use of other medications, and the presence of certain disease states such as ACS that increase heparin resistance. This issue is of particular concern in women, since they tend to have higher rates of bleeding. Thus, the weight-based dosing of heparin is essential for women.[14] In those patients who are not receiving GP IIb/IIIa inhibitors, a weight-adjusted heparin dosing of 70 to 100 U/kg should be given to achieve ACT of 250 to 300 seconds with the HemoTec device and 300 to 350 seconds with the Hemochron device.[47] The unfractionated heparin bolus should be reduced to 50 to 70 U/kg when GP IIb/IIIa inhibitors are given to achieve a target ACT of 200 seconds with either the HemoTec device or the Hemochron device.[47]

Low-Molecular-Weight Heparin. The efficacy and safety of the low-molecular-weight heparin (LMWH) enoxaparin in patients with ACS undergoing PCIs have been studied in two non-inferiority trials.[48,49] The A-to-Z study enrolled 3987 patients (29% women) and the SYNERGY study enrolled 9978 patients (34% women) and found no statistical benefit of enoxaparin over standard UFH in PCI.[48,49] In the A-to-Z trial, 8.6% of the women on enoxaparin reached the primary endpoint of death, MI, or refractory ischemia at 7 days compared with 9.3% of the women on unfractionated heparin. This was not statistically significant.[48] In the SYNERGY trial, patients with ACS who were treated with an early invasive strategy were given either enoxaparin or unfractionated heparin. At 30 days, death or MI occurred in 13.5% of the women on enoxaparin compared with 12.9% of the women on unfractionated heparin ($P = 0.59$).[49] Bleeding rate by gender has not been reported.

Direct Thrombin Inhibitors. The direct thrombin inhibitor bivalirudin has emerged as an alternative antithrombotic therapy during PCIs. The REPLACE-2 trial demonstrated that the bivalirudin with provisional GP IIb/IIIa inhibitors was non-inferior compared with heparin and GP IIb/IIIa inhibition with regard to major adverse cardiac events and was associated with less bleeding among patients undergoing PCIs.[50] This trial enrolled 6010 patients, of which 1537 were women. In a prospectively defined analysis of gender, there were no differences in the individual or composite ischemic endpoints of death, MI, or urgent revascularization at 30 days or 6 months between genders with bivalirudin or heparin and GP IIb/IIIa inhibitors.[15] In women treated with heparin and GP IIb/IIIa inhibitors, the composite of death, MI, and urgent revascularization at 30 days occurred in 7.5% versus 6.7% of the women treated with bivalirudin ($P = 0.58$).[15] In women, major bleeding occurred in 5.9% in the heparin and GP IIb/IIIa inhibitors group compared with 3.7% in the bivalirudin group ($P = 0.04$).[15] Similarly, a decrease occurred in minor bleeding (28.2% vs. 16.0%, $P < 0.001$), and access site bleeding was decreased with bivalirudin (4.1% vs. 1.6%, $P = 0.003$).[15] Thus, for lower-risk female patients undergoing PCIs, bivalirudin appears to provide better protection against ischemic events and lower bleeding events compared with heparin and GP IIb/IIIa inhibitors.

▩ Ethnicity

Currently, African Americans, Hispanic Americans, Asian Americans, and Native Americans comprise 30% of the U.S. population. By 2050, they will comprise 47.5% of the population. Thus, it is important to understand the dissimilarities between the groups and determine whether they are clinically relevant. Discussions on race or ethnicity in medicine are fraught with difficulties, since race is neither scientific nor physiologic. Race can provide information regarding similar environmental factors and some physiologic risk factors such as obesity, diabetes, and hypertension; however, since it is self-reported, it is often prone to inaccuracies. The importance of the environment cannot be overemphasized, since there is only 0.1% genetic variance between the races.

CORONARY ARTERY DISEASE

Heart disease is the leading cause of death for all races in the U.S. population. African Americans have the highest rates of mortality from heart disease.[1] The mortality rate for African Americans is 1.6 times that of whites.[1] The average annual death rate for heart disease by race is shown in Table 7-5. The prevalence of coronary artery disease (CAD) is also higher in African Americans compared with their white counterparts regardless of gender.[1] Furthermore, the onset of disease occurs 5 years earlier in African Americans. Death rates for stroke are also higher in African Americans. Various ethnic minority groups are experiencing increasing rates of ischemic heart disease. Rates of CAD are increasing in Asian Americans, Hispanic Americans, and Native Americans.[1] Despite the increased incidence of CAD among African Americans, the presence of obstructive epicardial CAD on the angiogram is less than in whites.[51] Paradoxically, there is greater prevalence of complications from atherosclerosis in African Americans despite lower

TABLE 7-5	Cardiovascular Disease in US: AHA 2010 Heart and Stroke Statistics[1]						
	Total	White Male	White Female	African American Male	African American Female	Mexican American Male	Mexican American Female
Prevalence	81.1 M	38.1%	34.4%	44.6%	46.9%	28.5%	34.5%
Mortality	831 K	340 K	372 K	47.9 K	50.9 K	—	—

M = Million, K = Thousand.

TABLE 7-6	Short-Term and Long-Term Percutaneous Coronary Interventions Outcome in African Americans	
Study	Total # of Patients (% African Americans)	Adjusted Even Rate Comparing African Americans to Whites (OR, 95% CI)
Maynard 2001:		
In-hospital Death	24,625 (11%)	0.97 (0.83–1.12) Death
2-year Death		1.11 (1.05–1.17) Death
Leborgne 2004:		
1-year death	10,561 (12%)	1.35 (1.06–1.71) Death
Slater 2003:		
1-year Death	4,618 (9.7%)	0.65 (0.36–1.14) Death, MI, or CABG
2-year Death		1.47 (1.06–2.04) Death, MI or CABG
Chen 2005:		
1-year Death	8,832 (8.0%)	1.45 (1.14–1.84) Death or MI

incidence of obstructive CAD. The most likely reasons for the increased prevalence of CAD among African Americans are increased rates of hypertension, diabetes, and smoking, and not inherent differences in the pathophysiology of CAD.[51] Of note, African Americans tend to have higher prevalence of peripheral arterial disease than do their white counterparts (adjusted OR 2.39, 95% CI 1.11–5.12). This was seen in the National Health and Nutrition examination survey in the United States.[52] This finding was confirmed by the GENOA study, which also showed that this difference was not explained by risk factor differences.[53] The study showed that African American men (adjusted OR 4.7, 95% CI 1.4–16.0) and women (adjusted OR 2.2, 95% CI 1.2–4.2) had higher rates of peripheral arterial disease even after adjusting for age and comorbidities than did white Americans.

PERCUTANEOUS CORONARY INTERVENTIONS (Table 7-6)

African American patients undergoing PCIs are younger, more likely to be female, more likely to have hypertension, diabetes, and chronic renal insufficiency than their white counterparts. They are more likely to have urgent rather than elective PCIs. Immediate procedural success rates between African Americans and white Americans appear to be similar.[54] Short-term rates of death or MI after PCIs are also similar between the groups.[55] However, some have reported lower long-term survival rates in African Americans than in their white counterparts.[56] In a large PCI registry, there was an increased adjusted mortality rate among African Americans at 2 years (OR 1.87, 95% CI 1.15–3.04).[57] In another large single-center PCI registry, there was an increased 2-year adjusted mortality rate in African Americans (OR 1.45, 95% CI 1.14–1.84).[54] Differences in long-term outcomes after PCIs are likely to be multi-factorial, potentially because of differences in the access to and quality of health care for African Americans. Studies have shown that African Americans receive fewer preventive health services and less specialist care, and physicians treating them have had less rigorous clinical training.[58] Another possibility is the high prevalence of left ventricular hypertrophy together with increased endothelin-1 levels in African Americans.[59] Endothelin-1, a potent vasoconstrictor, is stimulated by transforming growth factor beta (TGF-β), which is increased in African Americans with hypertension. The combination of left ventricular hypertrophy and endothelial dysfunction in conjunction with CAD may contribute to greater rates of mortality.[51] Despite the recent interest in the field, race-specific analyses of PCIs are still rare.

ACUTE CORONARY SYNDROME

With regard to ACS, African American patients are likely to be younger and have hypertension, diabetes, heart failure, and renal insufficiency. They are also less likely to have insurance coverage or specialist care.[60]

Recently, the investigator of CRUSADE, a large NSTEMI registry, found that African American patients were more likely to receive older ACS treatments such as aspirin, Beta-blockers, or ACE-inhibitors but were significantly less likely to receive newer ACS therapies such as GP IIb/IIIa inhibitors, clopidogrel, and statin therapy.[60] Also, African Americans were less likely to receive cardiac catheterization, revascularization, or smoking cessation counseling. In-hospital death or post-admission MI were similar between African Americans and white patients in CRUSADE (adjusted OR 0.92, 95% CI 0.81–1.05), which was confirmed recently by data from the National Registry of Myocardial Infarction.[28] Several factors may explain the decreased rates of catheterization and revascularization in African Americans. In addition to patient preference and physician recommendations, African Americans with ACS are more likely to be treated in low-volume hospitals.[61] While there are some data regarding race-specific differential antihypertensive medication responses, to our knowledge, there are no race-specific data on adjunctive PCI pharmacotherapy.

ST ELEVATION MYOCARDIAL INFARCTION

At the time of presentation with STEMI, African Americans are younger, are more likely to be female, have more comorbidities, and present in higher Killip class.[67] Because of their younger age, they are less likely to have disease in two or more vessels. In a large fibrinolysis trial, the 30-day survival rates were similar between African Americans and whites. However, African Americans had a higher rate of in-hospital stroke (OR 1.75, 95% CI 1.19–2.59) and more major bleeding events (OR 1.32, 95% CI 1.13–1.55).[62] According to National Registry of Myocardial Infarction data, in-hospital mortality rates for STEMI patients are similar between African Americans and their white counterparts (Fig. 7-5).[28] However, at 5 years, the death rate was significantly higher among African Americans despite their younger age (OR 1.63, 95% CI 1.41–1.90).[67] Studies have demonstrated different practice patterns by racial and ethnic groups in acute MI.[63,64] African Americans are less likely to undergo cardiac catheterization

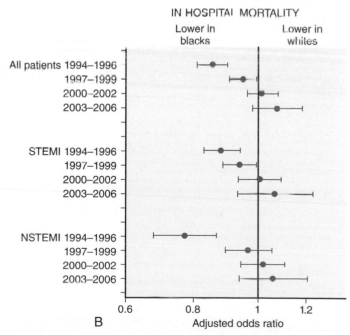

Figure 7-5 In-hospital mortality rate for African Americans and white Americans. *(Reprinted with permission from Rogers WJ, Frederick PD, Stoehr E, et al: Trends in presenting characteristics and hospital mortality among patients with ST elevation and non-ST elevation myocardial infarction in the National Registry of Myocardial Infarction from 1990 to 2006. Am Heart Journal 2008;156:1026–1034.)*

and revascularization following STEMI.[63,64] Recently, a study assessing racial and ethnic differences in time to acute reperfusion for patients with STEMI was reported using the national registry of myocardial infarction (NRMI).[63] The investigators found that whites tended to be older than patients from racial and ethnic minority groups and insurance status differed significantly between these groups.[63] Types of hospital patients also differed markedly by race.[63] They found that door-to-drug time and door-to-balloon time were significantly longer for nonwhite patients. Even after adjusting for age, gender, insurance status, clinical characteristics, time of arrival, time since symptom onset, and hospital characteristics, there was still difference between white and nonwhite patients. In the fully adjusted model, door-to-balloon time was 8.7 minutes longer in African Americans compared with whites ($P < 0.001$) and 3.7 minutes longer for Hispanic patients compared with whites ($P = 0.002$).[63] Similarly, a fully adjusted model of door-to-drug time showed a 5.1-minute increase in African Americans ($P < 0.001$), 1.3-minute increase in Hispanic Americans ($P = 0.006$), and 1.7-minute increase in Asian Americans ($P = 0.01$) compared with their white counterparts.[63] Even though a substantial portion of the racial and ethnic disparities in time-to-treatment is accounted for by the hospital where a patient is admitted, racial and ethnic treatment disparities persist, even after adjusting for hospital and clinical factors.

TREATMENT DIFFERENCES

Because of complex issues of social, political, physiologic, and genetic variances in minority populations, disparities exist in health care. African Americans as well as other ethnic minority groups are less likely to undergo cardiovascular procedures such as catheterization and revascularization either with stent or CABG.[65,66] While it is important to note that patients from ethnic minority groups are more likely to be treated in low-volume hospitals and to refuse invasive procedures than their white counterparts, there still appears to be some amount of treatment disparities.[67] In reviewing over 100 studies, the National Institute of Medicine's 2001 report found that patients from minority groups are less likely to receive the needed services compared with their white counterparts even after accounting for access to health care. The committee considered three sets of factors associated with treatment differences, assuming that each group had similar access to health care. The first set of factors were those related to the operation of health care systems. For instance, because of lack of interpretative services for non–English speaking patients or minorities, these patients were more likely to be enrolled in lower-cost health plans that place greater limits on testing and access to specialists. The second set of factors were related to providers, such as bias against minority patients or greater uncertainty in diagnoses in these patients by health care providers. Lastly, patient preferences were considered.[68] In the report they concluded that even though "myriad sources contribute to these (treatment) disparities, some evidence suggest that bias, prejudice, and stereotyping on the part of the health care providers may contribute to differences in care".[68] Studies have shown that regardless of the physician's race, information about patients' ethnicity, age, and lifestyle was used to make decisions about cardiac intervention.[69] To eliminate disparities in care, the National Institute of Medicine recommended a comprehensive, multi-level strategy, including training and educating health care providers, policy and regulatory strategies that address health plans and health services, to promote better use of clinical practice guidelines.

▥ Conclusion

Much has been learned in the last few years regarding gender and racial differences in coronary artery disease. There is much more to be learned about the differences between these groups in pathophysiology, clinical manifestations, treatments, and outcomes. The pervasive and continuing treatment disparities found among women and patients from minority groups calls all health care providers and researchers to improve their understanding of and quality of care for these patients.

REFERENCES

1. Writing Group M, Lloyd-Jones D, Adams RJ, et al: Heart disease and stroke statistics—2010 update: A report from the American Heart Association. *Circulation* 121(7):e46–e215, 2010.
2. Jacobs AK: Coronary revascularization in women in 2003: Sex revisited. *Circulation* 107(3):375–377, 2003.
3. Malenka DJ, Wennberg DE, Quinton HA, et al: Gender-related changes in the practice and outcomes of percutaneous coronary interventions in Northern New England from 1994 to 1999. *J Am Coll Cardiol* 40(12):2092–2101, 2002.
4. Smith SC, Jr, Feldman TE, Hirshfeld JW, Jr, et al: ACC/AHA/SCAI 2005 guideline update for percutaneous coronary intervention: A report of the American College of Cardiology/American Heart Association Task Force on Practice Guidelines (ACC/AHA/SCAI Writing Committee to Update 2001 Guidelines for Percutaneous Coronary Intervention). *Circulation* 113(7):e166–e286, 2006.
5. Jacobs AK, Johnston JM, Haviland A, et al: Improved outcomes for women undergoing contemporary percutaneous coronary intervention: a report from the National Heart, Lung, and Blood Institute Dynamic registry. *J Am Coll Cardiol* 39(10):1608–1614, 2002.
6. Peterson ED, Roe MT, Mulgund J, et al: Association between hospital process performance and outcomes among patients with acute coronary syndromes. *JAMA* 295(16):1912–1920, 2006.
7. Chiu JH, Bhatt DL, Ziada KM, et al: Impact of female sex on outcome after percutaneous coronary intervention. *Am Heart J* 148(6):998–1002, 2004.
8. Schulman KA, Berlin JA, Harless W, et al: The effect of race and sex on physicians' recommendations for cardiac catheterization. *N Engl J Med* 340(8):618–626, 1999.
9. Mehilli J, Kastrati A, Bollwein H, et al: Gender and restenosis after coronary artery stenting. *Eur Heart J* 24(16):1523–1530, 2003.
10. Lansky AJ, Pietras C, Costa RA, et al: Gender differences in outcomes after primary angioplasty versus primary stenting with and without abciximab for acute myocardial infarction: Results of the Controlled Abciximab and Device Investigation to Lower Late Angioplasty Complications (CADILLAC) trial. *Circulation* 111(13):1611–1618, 2005.
11. Moses JW, Leon MB, Popma JJ, et al: Sirolimus-eluting stents versus standard stents in patients with stenosis in a native coronary artery. *N Engl J Med* 349(14):1315–1323, 2003.
12. Lansky AJ, Costa RA, Mooney M, et al: Gender-based outcomes after paclitaxel-eluting stent implantation in patients with coronary artery disease. *J Am Coll Cardiol* 45(8):1180–1185, 2005.
13. Solinas E, Nikolsky E, Lansky AJ, et al: Gender-specific outcomes after sirolimus-eluting stent implantation. *J Am Coll Cardiol* 50(22):2111–2116, 2007.
14. Lansky AJ, Hochman JS, Ward PA, et al: Percutaneous coronary intervention and adjunctive pharmacotherapy in women: a statement for healthcare professionals from the American Heart Association. *Circulation* 111(7):940–953, 2005.
15. Chacko M, Lincoff AM, Wolski KE, et al: Ischemic and bleeding outcomes in women treated with bivalirudin during percutaneous coronary intervention: A subgroup analysis of the Randomized Evaluation in PCI Linking Angiomax to Reduced Clinical Events (REPLACE)-2 trial. *Am Heart J* 151(5):1031–e1037, 2006.
16. Cho L, Topol EJ, Balog C, et al: Clinical benefit of glycoprotein IIb/IIIa blockade with Abciximab is independent of gender: Pooled analysis from EPIC, EPILOG and EPISTENT trials. Evaluation of 7E3 for the prevention of ischemic complications. Evaluation in percutaneous transluminal coronary angioplasty to improve long-term outcome with abciximab GP IIb/IIIa blockade. Evaluation of platelet IIb/IIIa inhibitor for stent. *J Am Coll Cardiol* 36(2):381–386, 2000.
17. Pristipino C, Pelliccia F, Granatelli A, et al: Comparison of access-related bleeding complications in women versus men undergoing percutaneous coronary catheterization using the radial versus femoral artery. *Am J Cardiol* 100(10):1604, 2007.
18. Wiviott SD, Cannon CP, Morrow DA, et al: Differential expression of cardiac biomarkers by gender in patients with unstable angina/non-ST-elevation myocardial infarction: A TACTICS-TIMI 18 (Treat Angina with Aggrastat and determine Cost of Therapy with an Invasive or Conservative Strategy-Thrombolysis In Myocardial Infarction 18) substudy. *Circulation* 109(5):580–586, 2004.
19. O'Donoghue M, Boden WE, Braunwald E, et al: Early invasive vs conservative treatment strategies in women and men with unstable angina and non-ST-segment elevation myocardial infarction: A meta-analysis. *JAMA* 300(1):71–80, 2008.
20. Blomkalns AL, Chen AY, Hochman JS, et al: Gender disparities in the diagnosis and treatment of non-ST-segment elevation acute coronary syndromes: Large-scale observations from the CRUSADE (Can Rapid Risk Stratification of Unstable Angina Patients Suppress Adverse Outcomes With Early Implementation of the American College of Cardiology/American Heart Association Guidelines) National Quality Improvement Initiative, *J Am Coll Cardiol* 45(6):832–837, 2005.
21. Akhter N, Milford-Beland S, Roe MT, et al: Gender differences among patients with acute coronary syndromes undergoing percutaneous coronary intervention in the American College of Cardiology-National Cardiovascular Data Registry (ACC-NCDR). *Am Heart J* 157(1):141–148, 2009.
22. Arbustini E, Dal Bello B, Morbini P, et al: Plaque erosion is a major substrate for coronary thrombosis in acute myocardial infarction. *Heart* 82(3):269–272, 1999.
23. Kolodgie FD, Burke AP, Wight TN, et al: The accumulation of specific types of proteoglycans in eroded plaques: A role in coronary thrombosis in the absence of rupture. *Curr Opin Lipidol* 15(5):575–582, 2004.
24. Tamis-Holland JE, Palazzo A, Stebbins AL, et al: Benefits of direct angioplasty for women and men with acute myocardial infarction: Results of the Global Use of Strategies to Open Occluded Arteries in Acute Coronary Syndromes Angioplasty (GUSTO II-B) angioplasty substudy. *Am Heart J* 147(1):133–139, 2004.
25. Mehilli J, Ndrepepa G, Kastrati A, et al: Gender and myocardial salvage after reperfusion treatment in acute myocardial infarction. *J Am Coll Cardiol* 45(6):828–831, 2005.
26. Watanabe CT, Maynard C, Ritchie JL: Comparison of short-term outcomes following coronary artery stenting in men versus women. *Am J Cardiol* 88(8):848–852, 2001.
27. Vakili BA, Kaplan RC, Brown DL: Sex-based differences in early mortality of patients undergoing primary angioplasty for first acute myocardial infarction. *Circulation* 104(25):3034–3038, 2001.
28. Rogers WJ, Frederick PD, Stoehr E, et al: Trends in presenting characteristics and hospital mortality among patients with ST elevation and non-ST elevation myocardial infarction in the National Registry of Myocardial Infarction from 1990 to 2006. *Am Heart J* 156(6):1026–1034, 2008.
29. Gan SC, Beaver SK, Houck PM, et al: Treatment of acute myocardial infarction and 30-day mortality among women and men, *N Engl J Med* 343(1):8–15, 2000.

30. Manson JE, Stampfer MJ, Colditz GA, et al: A prospective study of aspirin use and primary prevention of cardiovascular disease in women. *JAMA* 266(4):521–527, 1991.

31. Ridker PM, Cook NR, Lee IM, et al: A randomized trial of low-dose aspirin in the primary prevention of cardiovascular disease in women. *N Engl J Med* 352(13):1293–1304, 2005.

32. Berger JS, Roncaglioni MC, Avanzini F, et al: Aspirin for the primary prevention of cardiovascular events in women and men: a sex-specific meta-analysis of randomized controlled trials. [Erratum appears in *JAMA*, 2006 May 3;295(17):2002]. *JAMA* 295(3):306–313, 2006.

33. Becker DM, Segal J, Vaidya D, et al: Sex differences in platelet reactivity and response to low-dose aspirin therapy. *JAMA* 295(12):1420–1427, 2006.

34. Gum PA, Kottke-Marchant K, Poggio ED, et al: Profile and prevalence of aspirin resistance in patients with cardiovascular disease. *Am J Cardiol* 88(3):230–235, 2001.

35. Eikelboom JW, Hirsh J, Weitz JI, et al: Aspirin-resistant thromboxane biosynthesis and the risk of myocardial infarction, stroke, or cardiovascular death in patients at high risk for cardiovascular events. *Circulation* 105(14):1650–1655, 2002.

36. Vittinghoff E, Shlipak MG, Varosy PD, et al: Risk factors and secondary prevention in women with heart disease: The Heart and Estrogen/progestin Replacement Study.[Summary for patients in Ann Intern Med. 2003 Jan 21;138(2):I10; PMID: 12529114]. *Ann Intern Med* 138(2):81–89, 2003.

37. Jani SM, Montoye C, Mehta R, et al: Sex differences in the application of evidence-based therapies for the treatment of acute myocardial infarction: The American College of Cardiology's Guidelines Applied in Practice projects in Michigan. *Arch Intern Med* 166(11):1164–1170, 2006.

38. Mehta SR, Yusuf S, Peters RJ, et al: Effects of pretreatment with clopidogrel and aspirin followed by long-term therapy in patients undergoing percutaneous coronary intervention: the PCI CURE study. *Lancet* 358(9281):527–533, 2001.

39. Steinhubl SR, Berger PB, Mann JT, 3rd, et al: Early and sustained dual oral antiplatelet therapy following percutaneous coronary intervention: A randomized controlled trial. *JAMA* 288(19):2411–2420, 2002.

40. Kastrati A, Mehilli J, Schuhlen H, et al: A clinical trial of abciximab in elective percutaneous coronary intervention after pretreatment with clopidogrel. *N Engl J Med* 350(3):232–238, 2004.

41. Boersma E, Harrington RA, Moliterno DJ, et al: Platelet glycoprotein IIb/IIIa inhibitors in acute coronary syndromes: a meta-analysis of all major randomised clinical trials.[Erratum appears in Lancet 2002 Jun 15;359(9323):2120]. *Lancet* 359(9302):189–198, 2002.

42. Fernandes LS, Tcheng JE, O'Shea JC, et al: Is glycoprotein IIb/IIIa antagonism as effective in women as in men following percutaneous coronary intervention? Lessons from the ESPRIT study. *J Am Coll Cardiol* 40(6):1085–1091, 2002.

43. Iakovou I, Dangas G, Mehran R, et al: Gender differences in clinical outcome after coronary artery stenting with use of glycoprotein IIb/IIIa inhibitors. *Am J Cardiol* 89(8):976–979, 2002.

44. Topol EJ, Moliterno DJ, Herrmann HC, et al: Comparison of two platelet glycoprotein IIb/IIIa inhibitors, tirofiban and abciximab, for the prevention of ischemic events with percutaneous coronary revascularization. *N Engl J Med* 344(25):1888–1894, 2001.

45. Cantor WJ, Kaplan AL, Velianou JL, et al: Effectiveness and safety of abciximab after failed thrombolytic therapy. *Am J Cardiol* 87(4):439–442, 2001.

46. Jong P, Cohen EA, Batchelor W, et al: Bleeding risks with abciximab after full-dose thrombolysis in rescue or urgent angioplasty for acute myocardial infarction. *Am Heart J* 141(2):218–225, 2001.

47. Chew DP, Bhatt DL, Lincoff AM, et al: Defining the optimal activated clotting time during percutaneous coronary intervention: aggregate results from 6 randomized, controlled trials. *Circulation* 103(7):961–966, 2001.

48. Blazing MA, de Lemos JA, White HD, et al: Safety and efficacy of enoxaparin vs unfractionated heparin in patients with non-ST-segment elevation acute coronary syndromes who receive tirofiban and aspirin: a randomized controlled trial. *JAMA* 292(1):55–64, 2004.

49. Ferguson JJ, Califf RM, Antman EM, et al: Enoxaparin vs unfractionated heparin in high-risk patients with non-ST-segment elevation acute coronary syndromes managed with an intended early invasive strategy: Primary results of the SYNERGY randomized trial. *JAMA* 292(1):45–54, 2004.

50. Lincoff AM, Bittl JA, Harrington RA, et al: Bivalirudin and provisional glycoprotein IIb/IIIa blockade compared with heparin and planned glycoprotein IIb/IIIa blockade during percutaneous coronary intervention: REPLACE-2 randomized trial.[Erratum appears in JAMA, 2003 Apr 2;289(13):1638]. *JAMA* 289(7):853–863, 2003.

51. Yancy C: *Heart disease in varied populations*, Vol 2, ed 7, Philadelphia, 2005, Saunders.

52. Selvin E, Erlinger TP: Prevalence of and risk factors for peripheral arterial disease in the United States: results from the National Health and Nutrition Examination Survey, 1999–2000. *Circulation* 110(6):738–743, 2004.

53. Kullo IJ, Bailey KR, Kardia SL, et al: Ethnic differences in peripheral arterial disease in the NHLBI Genetic Epidemiology Network of Arteriopathy (GENOA) study. *Vasc Med* 8(4):237–242, 2003.

54. Chen MS, Bhatt DL, Chew DP, et al: Outcomes in African Americans and whites after percutaneous coronary intervention. *Am J Med* 118(9):1019–1025, 2005.

55. Iqbal U, Pinnow EE, Lindsay J, Jr: Comparison of six-month outcomes after percutaneous coronary intervention for Whites versus African-Americans. *Am J Cardiol* 88(3):304–305, 2001.

56. Leborgne L, Cheneau E, Wolfram R, et al: Comparison of baseline characteristics and one-year outcomes between African-Americans and Caucasians undergoing percutaneous coronary intervention. *Am J Cardiol* 93(4):389–393, 2004.

57. Slater J, Selzer F, Dorbala S, et al: Ethnic differences in the presentation, treatment strategy, and outcomes of percutaneous coronary intervention (a report from the National Heart, Lung, and Blood Institute Dynamic Registry). *Am J Cardiol* 92(7):773–778, 2003.

58. Lillie-Blanton M, Maddox TM, Rushing O, et al: Disparities in cardiac care: rising to the challenge of Healthy People 2010. *J Am Coll Cardiol* 44(3):503–508, 2004.

59. Schiffrin EL: Role of endothelin-1 in hypertension and vascular disease. *Am J Hypertension* 14(6 Pt 2):83S–89S, 2001.

60. Sonel AF, Good CB, Mulgund J, et al: Racial variations in treatment and outcomes of black and white patients with high-risk non-ST-elevation acute coronary syndromes: Insights from CRUSADE (Can Rapid Risk Stratification of Unstable Angina Patients Suppress Adverse Outcomes With Early Implementation of the ACC/AHA Guidelines?) *Circulation* 111(10):1225–1232, 2005.

61. Trivedi AN, Sequist TD, Ayanian JZ: Impact of hospital volume on racial disparities in cardiovascular procedure mortality. *J Am Coll Cardiol* 47(2):417–424, 2006.

62. Mehta RH, Marks D, Califf RM, et al: Differences in the clinical features and outcomes in African Americans and whites with myocardial infarction. *Am J Med* 119(1):70e–78e, 2006.

63. Bradley EH, Herrin J, Wang Y, et al: Racial and ethnic differences in time to acute reperfusion therapy for patients hospitalized with myocardial infarction. *JAMA* 292(13):1563–1572, 2004.

64. Manhapra A, Canto JG, Vaccarino V, et al: Relation of age and race with hospital death after acute myocardial infarction. *Am Heart J* 148(1):92–98, 2004.

65. Lucas FL, DeLorenzo MA, Siewers AE, et al: Temporal trends in the utilization of diagnostic testing and treatments for cardiovascular disease in the United States, 1993–2001. *Circulation* 113(3):374–379, 2006.

66. Werner RM, Asch DA, Polsky D: Racial profiling: the unintended consequences of coronary artery bypass graft report cards. *Circulation* 111(10):1257–1263, 2005.

67. Rosen AB, Tsai JS, Downs SM: Variations in risk attitude across race, gender, and education. *Med Decision Making* 23(6):511–517, 2003.

68. Smedley B, Stith A, Nelson A: *Unequal treatment: Confronting racial and ethnic disparities in health care*, Washington, D.C., 2001, Institute of Medicine of the National Academies, Board of Health Sciences Policy.

69. Chen J, Rathore SS, Radford MJ, et al: Racial differences in the use of cardiac catheterization after acute myocardial infarction. *N Engl J Med* 344(19):1443–1449, 2001.

Pharmacologic Intervention

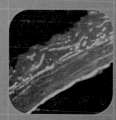

Platelet Inhibitor Agents

MATTHEW J. PRICE | DOMINICK J. ANGIOLLILO

KEY POINTS

- Dual anti-platelet therapy with aspirin and a P2Y12 receptor inhibitor is the cornerstone of therapy after percutaneous coronary intervention (PCI).

- The thienopyridines—ticlopidine, clopidogrel, and prasugrel—are P2Y12 inhibitors that are pro-drugs, and therefore require conversion into an active metabolite to exert their anti-platelet effect. This active metabolite irreversibly binds and antagonizes the P2Y12 receptor for the lifespan of the platelet.

- Prasugrel reduces ischemic events, compared with clopidogrel, in patients undergoing PCI but is associated with a higher risk of bleeding. Net clinical benefit is greatest in patients without a history of stroke or transient ischemic attack, who are <75 years of age, and weigh >60 kg.

- Several genetic polymorphisms reduce the enzymatic activity of CYP2C19, which is critical for the conversion of clopidogrel to its active metabolite. When treated with clopidogrel, carriers of these alleles with reduced function, especially those with two copies (poor metabolizers), are at higher risk of thrombotic events after PCI compared with patients with normal alleles. The CYP2C19 genotype does not influence the clinical effectiveness of prasugrel or ticagrelor.

- Ticagrelor, a non-thienopyridine, is a direct, reversible P2Y12 antagonist. In patients with acute coronary syndrome, including those treated with an invasive strategy, ticagrelor reduced ischemic events and cardiovascular mortality compared with clopidogrel. While overall bleeding was not increased with ticagrelor, there was an increased risk of non–CABG-related bleeding.

- There is substantial inter-individual variability in the anti-platelet effect of clopidogrel. High on-treatment platelet reactivity according to several platelet function tests can identify patients at risk for ischemic events after percutaneous coronary intervention (PCI). The clinical benefit of personalized anti-platelet strategies based on platelet function testing is being tested in several randomized clinical trials.

- The effects of thrombin, the most potent platelet activator, are mediated primarily through the protease-activated receptor 1 (PAR1) receptor. PAR1 antagonists may offer a wide therapeutic window between ischemia reduction and bleeding risk and are currently being examined in clinical trials.

- In the modern era of pretreatment with P2Y12 inhibitors, the benefit of glycoprotein (GP) IIb/IIIa inhibition appears to be restricted to high-risk patients with acute coronary syndrome (ACS) with elevated cardiac biomarkers.

Basic Principles of Anti-Platelet Therapy

Platelets have a key role in normal hemostasis and in the pathogenesis of atherothrombotic disease. Platelets provide an initial hemostatic plug at the site of vascular injury and promote pathophysiologic thrombosis, which, in turn, precipitates myocardial infarction (MI), stroke, and peripheral vascular occlusions. Therefore, anti-platelet agents are key in cardiovascular disease management. In particular, the goal of anti-platelet treatment strategies is to reduce the risk of recurrent atherothrombotic events without excessive bleeding

complications. However, because both pathologic and physiologic functions of platelets are caused by the same mechanism, it is difficult to separate therapeutic benefits from potential harmful effects. Platelet plug formation at sites of vascular injury occurs in three stages: (1) initiation phase, which involves platelet adhesion; (2) extension phase, which includes activation, additional recruitment, and aggregation; (3) perpetuation phase, characterized by platelet stimulation and stabilization of clot.[1] Circulating platelets are quiescent under normal circumstances and do not bind to the intact endothelium. However, endothelial damage leads to the exposure of circulating platelets to the subendothelial extracellular matrix and triggers platelet recruitment and adhesion (Fig. 8-1).[2] In the initial phase of primary hemostasis, the tethering of platelets at sites of vascular injury is mediated by GP Ib-IX-V receptor complex, which binds von Willebrand factor (vWF). Subendothelial collagen exposed by damaged vessel engages platelets via GP VI and GP Ia/IIa receptors. These interactions allow the arrest and activation of adherent platelets. In the extension phase, additional platelets are recruited and activated via soluble agonists. These platelet-activating factors include adenosine diphosphate (ADP), thromboxane A2 (TXA2), epinephrine, serotonin, collagen, and thrombin. Signaling via ADP receptors contributes to platelet activation during both protective hemostasis and pathologic thrombosis. Two ADP receptors are expressed by platelets: P2Y1 which couples to $G\alpha q$ and contributes to initial aggregation, and P2Y12 which couples to $G\alpha_{12}$ and decreases cyclic adenosine monophosphate (cAMP), stabilizing the platelet aggregate.[3] P2Y12 receptor signaling also stimulates surface expression of P-selectin and secretion of TXA2. TXA2 is produced de novo and, like ADP, is released from adherent platelets. It is generated from arachidonic acid through conversion by cyclo-oxygenase 1 (COX-1) and thromboxane synthase. TXA2 binds platelet receptors $TP\alpha$ and $TP\beta$; however, its effects in platelets are mediated primarily through $TP\alpha$. ADP and TXA2 are secreted from adherent platelets and contribute to the recruitment of circulating platelets and promote alterations in platelet shape and granule secretion. Thus platelet activation is amplified and sustained during the extension phase. Thrombin, generated at the site of vascular injury, represents the most potent platelet activator.[4] Thrombin contributes to the formation of the hemostatic plug and platelet thrombus growth. Thrombin also directly activates platelets through stimulation of the protease-activated receptors (PARs). Human platelets express two PARs for thrombin: PAR1 and PAR4. Thrombin facilitates the production of fibrin from fibrinogen, contributing to the formation and stabilization of the hemostatic plug.[4] The final common pathway is activation of the integrin GP IIb/IIIa, which allows platelets to bind fibrinogen with high affinity, leading to platelet aggregates.[5] In the perpetuation phase, the platelet-rich thrombus and coagulation cascades reinforce one another and culminate in the generation of a stable platelet-fibrin–rich plug at the sites of injury.

The mechanisms by which anti-platelet drugs interfere with platelet function involve targeting enzymes or receptors that are critical for the synthesis or action of important mediators of these functional responses. Current and investigational oral anti-platelet therapies target key platelet signaling pathways (Fig. 8-2). This chapter reviews the mechanism of action, efficacy and safety of anti-platelet agents inhibiting key platelet-signaling pathways, including the TXA2 pathway, P2Y12 receptor, PAR1 receptor, phosphodiesterase III, and the GP IIb/IIIa receptor, focusing on their roles in PCI.

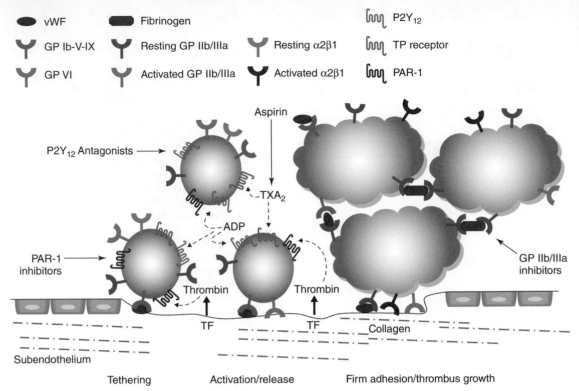

Figure 8-1 Platelet mediated thrombosis. The interaction between von Willebrand factor (vWF) and the platelet receptor glycoprotein (GP) Ib-V-IX mediates platelet tethering to the subendothelium at the sites of injury. GP VI binds collagen with low affinity. This triggers intracellular signals that shift platelet integrins to a high-affinity state and induce the release of the secondary mediators adenosine diphosphate (ADP) and thromboxane A2 (TXA2). In parallel, tissue factor (TF) locally triggers thrombin formation, which also contributes to platelet activation via binding to the platelet protease-activated receptor 1 (PAR1). Ultimately, the integrin GP IIb/IIIa, which is the final common pathway mediating platelet aggregation, transforms from a resting to an activated phase which allows it to bind fibrinogen with high affinity, leading to platelet aggregates. In the perpetuation phase, the platelet-rich thrombus and coagulation cascades reinforce one another contributing to thrombus growth and culminate in the generation of a stable platelet-fibrin–rich plug at the sites of injury. (Adapted from Varga-Szabo D, Pleines I, Nieswandt B: Cell adhesion mechanisms in platelets, Arterioscler Thromb Vasc Biol 28:403–412, 2008.)

Aspirin

MECHANISM OF ACTION

Aspirin irreversibly inactivates the cyclo-oxygenase activity of prostaglandin H (PGH) synthase 1 and 2, also referred to as COX-1 and COX-2. PGH synthase 1 and 2 convert arachidonic acid to PGH2, which acts as a substrate for the generation of several prostanoids, including TXA2 and prostacyclin (PGI2). Aspirin enters the COX channel and acetylates the amino acid serine at position 529 and 516 of COX-1 and COX-2, respectively, thereby preventing arachidonic acid access to the catalytic site of the enzyme through steric hindrance. Mature platelets express only COX-1 and are the primary sources of TXA2. TXA2 is released by the platelet in response to a variety of agonists and induces platelet aggregation through the G-protein–coupled TXA2 receptor, TP. Other cells, including the vascular endothelium, express both COX-1 and COX-2. COX-1 is responsible for the production of cytoprotective prostaglandins PGE2 and PGI2 in the gastric mucosa and COX-2 is the main source of vascular PGI2. Gastric mucosal cells, unlike mature platelets, can synthesize COX-1 and therefore recover the ability to produce prostaglandins within hours after aspirin exposure. Higher levels of aspirin are required to inhibit COX-2 compared with COX-1, and therefore low-dose aspirin is sufficient to inhibit platelet TXA2 production but insufficient to affect the generation of vascular PGI2, which is a platelet inhibitor and vasodilator. In addition to its primary effect on platelet aggregation through inhibition of the PGH synthase COX-1 activity, aspirin may also exert anti-platelet effects via COX-1–independent pathways.

PHARMACOKINETICS AND PHARMACODYNAMICS

Aspirin is rapidly absorbed in the stomach and small intestine, achieving peak plasma levels in 30 to 40 minutes. Esterases in the gastrointestinal (GI) mucosa and liver hydrolyze aspirin into salicylic acid, which then interacts with platelets in the portal circulation. The half-life is short, approximately 20 to 30 minutes, but the pharmacodynamic effect is prolonged, given the permanent inactivation of platelet COX-1 activity. Low-dose aspirin requires several days to effectively suppress TXA2 production. A loading dose is needed to quickly achieve effective platelet inhibition in aspirin-naïve subjects. Loading doses greater than 300 mg do not appear to provide additional pharmacodynamic benefit at 2 hours after ingestion. The American College of Cardiology (ACC)/American Heart Association (AHA)/Society for Cardiovascular Angiography and Interventions (SCAI) 2007 PCI guidelines state that patients not already taking daily long-term aspirin therapy should be given 300 mg to 325 mg of aspirin at least 2 and preferably 24 hours before PCI is performed (Class I, Level of Evidence: C).[6]

ASPIRIN DOSE AFTER PERCUTANEOUS CORONARY INTERVENTION

Maintenance aspirin regimens of as low as 30 mg daily are adequate to completely inhibit serum TXB2 production (a marker of platelet thromboxane production) in healthy individuals. Collaborative meta-analyses of the clinical benefit of long-term aspirin in high-risk patients show that doses greater than 75 to 150 mg are no more effective in reducing ischemic events but are associated with a greater risk of

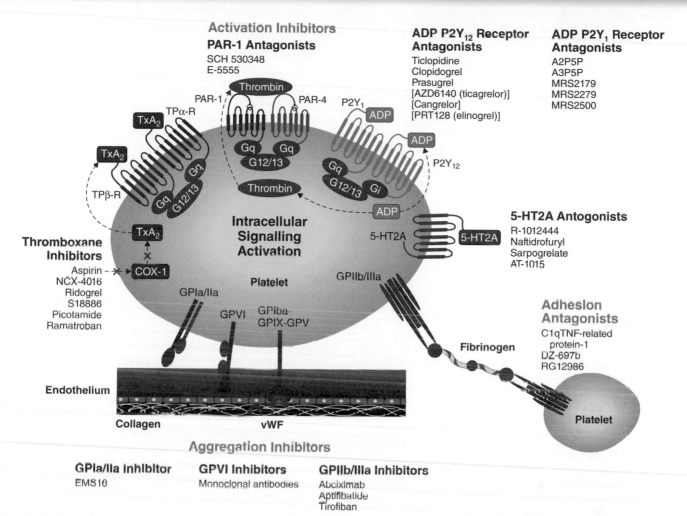

Figure 8-2 Sites of action of current and emerging anti-platelet agents. Platelet adherence to the endothelium occurs at the sites of vascular injury through the binding of glycoprotein (GP) receptors to exposed extracellular matrix proteins (collagen and von Willebrand factor [vWF]). Platelet activation occurs via complex intracellular signaling processes and causes the production and release of multiple agonists, including thromboxane A2 (TXA2) and adenosine diphosphate (ADP), and local production of thrombin. These factors bind to their respective G protein coupled receptors, mediating paracrine and autocrine platelet activation. Further, they potentiate each other's actions (P2Y12 signaling modulates thrombin generation). The major platelet integrin GP IIb/IIIa mediates the final common step of platelet activation by undergoing a conformational shape change and binding fibrinogen and vWF leading to platelet aggregation. The net result of these interactions is thrombus formation mediated by platelet–platelet interactions with fibrin. Current and emerging therapies inhibiting platelet receptors, integrins, and proteins involved in platelet activation include thromboxane inhibitors, ADP receptor antagonists, GP IIb/IIIa inhibitors, and the novel PAR antagonists and adhesion antagonists. *TP*, thromboxane receptor; *5-HT2A*, 5-hydroxy tryptamine 2A receptor. Reversible-acting agents are indicated by brackets. *(Reproduced with permission from Angiolillo DJ, Capodanno D, Goto S: Platelet thrombin receptor antagonism and atherothrombosis, Eur Heart J 31:17–28, 2010.)*

bleeding. However, patients undergoing PCI and receiving stents are not represented in these studies. The ACC/AHA/SCAI 2007 PCI guidelines state that in patients without allergy or risk of bleeding, aspirin 162 mg to 325 mg daily should be given for at least 1 month after bare metal stent (BMS) implantation, 3 months after sirolimus-eluting stent implantation, and 6 months after paclitaxel-eluting stent implantation, after which daily long-term aspirin use should be continued indefinitely at a dose of 75 mg to 162 mg (Class I, Level of Evidence, B).[6] The impact of different aspirin dosages on ischemia and bleeding in stented patients was examined in a post hoc, observational analysis of the PCI cohort of the Clopidogrel in Unstable Angina to Prevent Recurrent Ischemic Events (CURE) trial. This analysis suggested that doses of aspirin <200 mg may be optimal after PCI with BMSs.[7] The study stratified the 2658 patients who underwent PCI for acute coronary syndrome in the CURE trial into three groups: high-dose (≥200 mg), medium-dose (>100 mg to <200 mg), and low-dose aspirin (≤100 mg).[7] There were no differences in the unadjusted or adjusted rates of death, MI, or stroke between groups (high-dose versus

low-dose, adjusted HR 1.00 [95% CI 0.67–1.48]; medium-dose versus low-dose, adjusted HR 1.09 [95% CI 0.73–1.60]). Unadjusted and adjusted rates of major bleeding were significantly greater with high-dose aspirin compared with low-dose aspirin (adjusted HR 2.03 [95% CI 1.15–3.57]). The Clopidogrel and Aspirin Optimal Dose Usage to Reduce Recurrent Events—Seventh Organization to Assess Strategies in Ischemic Syndromes (CURRENT–OASIS 7) examined the safety and efficacy of higher-dose aspirin (300 to 325 mg daily) compared with lower-dose aspirin (75 to 100 mg daily) in 25,086 patients with ACS treated with an invasive strategy. All patients received an aspirin loading dose ≥300 mg the day of randomization, and patients were also randomized in a 2-by-2 factorial design to standard-dose or double-dose clopidogrel. In the overall cohort, the rate of cardiovascular death, MI, or stroke at 30 days was not different between higher-dose or lower-dose aspirin (4.2 versus 4.4%, HR 0.97 [95% CI 0.86–1.09], P = 0.61). The incidence of major bleeding as defined by the trial was not different between groups (2.3% vs. 2.3%, HR 0.99 [95% CI 0.84 to 1.17], P = 0.9). Minor bleeding was more frequent with higher-dose aspirin (5.0% versus 4.4%, HR 1.13 [95% CI 100–1.27], $P = 0.04$), as was GI bleeding (0.4% versus 0.2%, $P = 0.04$). The findings were similar among those patients who underwent PCI, approximately 42% of whom received a drug-eluting stent, and there was no difference in the incidence of stent thrombosis within the PCI cohort. Therefore, a treatment strategy of lower-dose aspirin in invasively managed patients with ACS for 30 days appears to provide similar ischemic outcomes as higher-dose aspirin with less minor bleeding and less GI bleeding. However, longer treatment durations have not been examined in a randomized fashion.

▣ P2Y12 Inhibitors

BASIC PRINCIPLES

The platelet P2Y12 receptor plays a central role in amplifying the effect of various stimuli on platelet activation, promoting thrombus growth and stability. It is an inhibitory G-protein coupled receptor (Gα12) that is activated by ADP. ADP is released from dense granules after platelet activation from a variety of stimuli. ADP binding to the P2Y12 receptor leads to a series of intracellular signaling events that result in further granule release and amplification of platelet activation, conformational changes of the GP IIb/IIIa receptor, and stabilization of the platelet aggregate. P2Y12 activation further amplifies other responses to platelet activation including P-selectin expression, microparticle formation, procoagulant changes in the surface membrane, and potentiation of shear stress–induced platelet aggregation. The intracellular effect of P2Y12 receptor activation is mediated by signal transduction via a secondary messenger system that activates phosphoinositide-3-kinase (PI3K) and inhibits adenylyl cyclase. PI3K activation leads to GP IIb/IIIa receptor activation through activation of a serine-threonine protein kinase B (PKB/Akt) and Rap1b GTP binding protein. Inhibition of adenylyl cyclase decreases intracellular levels of cyclic adenosine monophosphate (cAMP), a key co-factor for the phosphorylation of vasodilator-stimulated phosphoprotein (VASP). De-phosphorylated VASP helps promote the conformational change of the GP IIb/IIIa receptor to its active state. Therefore, P2Y12 activation, through its action on cAMP levels, drives the de-phosphorylation of VASP and, in turn, GP IIb/IIIa activation.

THIENOPYRIDINES

The thienopyridines—ticlopidine, clopidogrel, and prasugrel—are pro-drugs that require biotransformation into an active metabolite to exert their anti-platelet effect. The active metabolite irreversibly binds and antagonizes the P2Y12 receptor for the platelet's lifespan (7 to 10 days). Differences in the rapidity and magnitude of platelet inhibition between the thienopyridines are predominantly the result of differences in pro-drug metabolism that affect the efficiency of active metabolite formation. Since the interaction between the active metabolite and the P2Y12 receptor is irreversible, a substantial waiting period for platelet functional recovery is required after thienopyridine exposure, which appears to be related to the magnitude of the initial inhibition.[8,9]

Ticlopidine

Ticlopidine was the first thienopyridine to be introduced into clinical practice. It has a slow onset of action, is poorly tolerated, and its use is associated with blood dyscrasias. The incidence of neutropenia has been reported to be 2.4%, peaking at 4 to 6 weeks after the start of therapy; the incidence of aplastic anemia is 1 in 4000 to 8000 patients; and the incidence of thrombotic thrombocytopenic purpura is approximately 1 in 2000 to 4000 patients. The onset of hematologic disorders is rare after 3 months of therapy. Therefore, hematologic monitoring is required before initiation and for the first 3 months of exposure. The Stent Anticoagulation Re-stenosis Study (STARS) demonstrated that the combination of aspirin and ticlopidine significantly reduced the rate of death, angiographically evident stent thrombosis, MI, or revascularization at 30 days by 85% compared with aspirin alone and by

80% compared with the combination of aspirin and warfarin.[10] Ticlopidine has been widely replaced by clopidogrel, given its better tolerability and lack of blood monitoring requirements.

Clopidogrel

Metabolism. Clopidogrel is a pro-drug that requires hepatic conversion into an active metabolite to exert its anti-platelet effect (Fig. 8-3). Approximately 85% of absorbed clopidogrel is hydrolyzed by human carboxylesterase[1] in the liver into an inactive carboxylic acid metabolite, so only a fraction of absorbed clopidogrel is available for conversion into the active metabolite by the cytochrome P450 (CYP) system. Hepatic biotransformation of absorbed clopidogrel into the active metabolite is thought to occur through a two-step process. The thiophene ring of clopidogrel is first oxidized to 2-oxo-clopidogrel, which is then hydrolyzed to a highly labile active metabolite (R-130964) that forms a disulfide bond with the P2Y12 receptor as platelets pass through the liver. The first metabolic step involves the isoenzymes CYP2C19, CYP2B6, and CYP1A2, and the second step involves the isoenzymes CYP2C19, CYP2B6, CYP3A4, CYP3A5, and CYP2C9. An alternative pathway for the oxidative biotransformation of clopidogrel that does not involve CYP2C19 has been suggested.[11] In this formulation, CYP-catalyzed oxidation of clopidogrel to 2-oxo-clopidogrel is mediated by CYP3A, CYP2B6, and CYP1A2, and conversion of 2-oxo-clopidogrel to the thiol active metabolite is mediated by the esterase, paraoxonase-1 (PON1). The catalytic activity of PON1 is proposed to be the rate-determining step for the active metabolite formation of clopidogrel.

Pharmacodynamics. A daily dose of clopidogrel 75 mg requires 3 to 7 days to reach steady-state platelet inhibition. A loading dose provides a rapid onset of action. However, the clinical benefit of a 300 mg loading dose may not be seen until 6 hours or as long as 15 hours after administration.[12,13] Larger doses provide higher circulating levels of active metabolite, more rapid onset, and more intense inhibition.[14,15] Peak inhibition after a 600-mg loading dose occurs at 4 to 6 hours after exposure.[14,16] A 900-mg loading dose may or may not provide more rapid and additional suppression of platelet function compared with 600 mg, as the intestinal absorption of clopidogrel may be limited at doses greater than 600 mg.[14,15] A maintenance dose regimen of 150 mg daily is associated with greater inhibition than a dose of 75 mg daily.[17,18] There is wide variability among individuals in the anti-platelet effect of clopidogrel after either a loading dose or a maintenance dose. Higher doses of clopidogrel reduce, but do not eliminate, this variability. The pharmacodynamic response to clopidogrel has been associated with CYP2C19 genotype, age, diabetes mellitus, body mass index, gender, ACS presentation, active smoking, renal dysfunction, pretreatment reactivity, and concomitant therapy with calcium channel blockers or proton pump inhibitors (PPIs).[19–22] However, clinical characteristics and the CYP2C19 genotype only partly explain the variability in on-treatment reactivity.[20,23] The level of ADP-induced platelet reactivity measured by several ex vivo platelet function tests have been associated with clinical outcomes in clopidogrel-treated patients undergoing PCI.[24]

Clinical Studies

Non–ST Elevation Acute Coronary Syndrome. The longer-term ischemic benefit of clopidogrel in patients presenting with ACS was established by the Clopidogrel in the Unstable Angina to Prevent Recurrent Ischemic Events (CURE) Trial. This trial randomized 12,562 patients presenting with non–ST elevation ACS to aspirin and clopidogrel (300 mg loading dose followed by 75 mg daily) or aspirin alone for 3 to 12 months.[25] The composite endpoint of cardiovascular death, nonfatal MI, or stroke occurred in 9.3% of the patients in the clopidogrel group and 11.4% of the patients in the placebo group ($P < 0.001$). Clopidogrel therapy was associated with an increased rate of major bleeding as defined by the trial (3.7 vs. 2.7%, $P = 0.001$). In the population of patients enrolled in CURE that underwent PCI (17% of the overall cohort, 82% of whom received a BMS), pretreatment with clopidogrel for a median of 6 days reduced the rate of cardiovascular

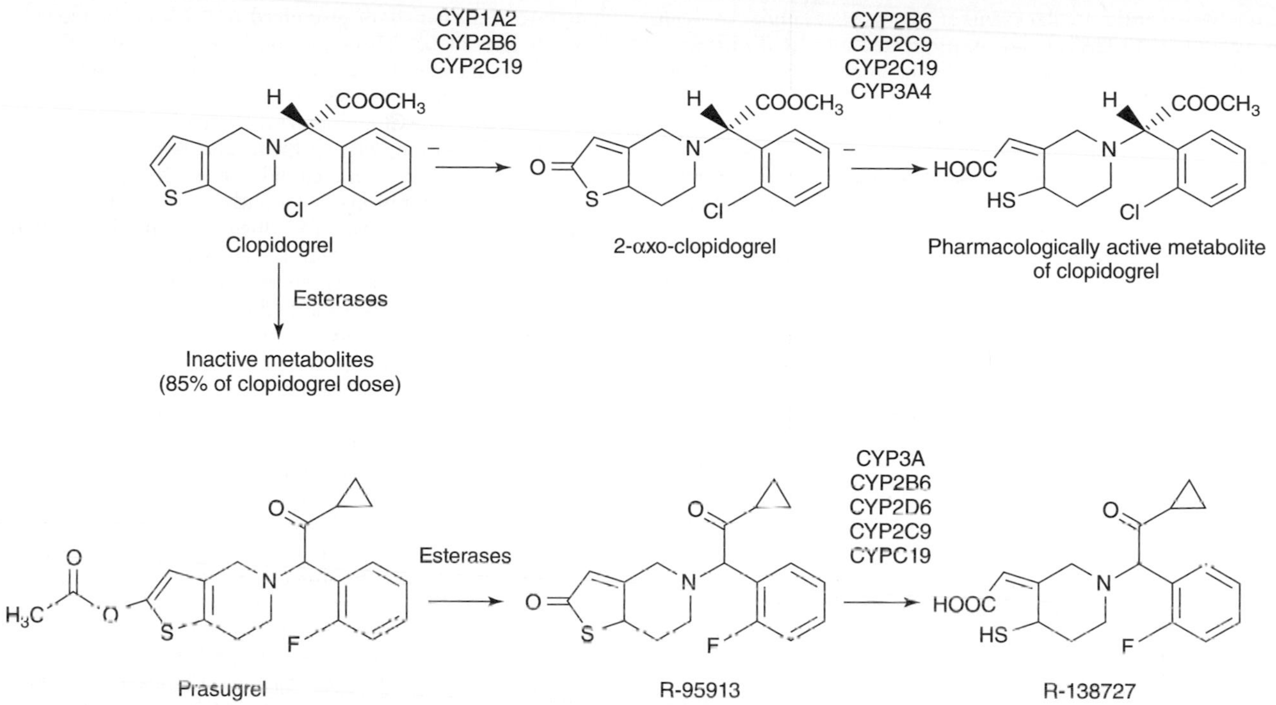

Figure 8-3 Comparative metabolism of clopidogrel and prasugrel. Both clopidogrel and prasugrel are pro-drugs, requiring biotransformation into their respective active metabolites to exert an anti-platelet effect. Clopidogrel undergoes a two-step process mediated by CYP450 isoenzymes with involvement of CYP2C19 and CYP2B6 in both steps. A substantial portion of absorbed clopidogrel is shunted into a dead end pathway by esterases. Prasugrel undergoes a one-step oxidation after the formation of a thiolactone intermediate. The greater inhibitory effect of prasugrel compared with clopidogrel is believed to be attributable to differences in the efficiency of active metabolite formation. (Adapted with permission from Giusti B, Abbate R: Response to antiplatelet treatment: from genes to outcome, Lancet 376:1278–1281, 2010.)

death, MI, or urgent target-vessel revascularization within 30 days from 6.4% to 4.5% ($P = 0.03$).

ST Elevation Myocardial Infarction. The Clopidogrel as Adjunctive Reperfusion Therapy-Thrombolysis in Myocardial Infarction (CLARITY-TIMI)-28 trial randomized 3491 patients ≤75 years of age receiving aspirin and fibrinolytic therapy within 12 hours of an ST elevation myocardial infarction to clopidogrel 300 mg followed by 75 mg daily or placebo. All patients underwent mandated angiography 2 to 8 days later. Clopidogrel significantly reduced the rate of an occluded infarct related artery, death, or recurrent MI before angiography (15.0% vs. 21.7%, $P < 0.001$), without increasing TIMI-defined major bleeding, minor bleeding, or intracranial hemorrhage.[26] A prespecified analysis of patients who underwent PCI demonstrated that clopidogrel significantly reduced ischemic events from randomization through 30 days, from PCI through 30 days, and from randomization to PCI.[27] This trial supports the use of clopidogrel in patients ≤75 years old presenting with ST elevation myocardial infarction (STEMI) and treated with aspirin and fibrinolysis.

Pretreatment for Percutaneous Coronary Intervention. The rationale for clopidogrel pretreatment is based on the slow onset of a substantial pharmacodynamic effect even after a clopidogrel loading dose. The Clopidogrel for the Reduction of Events During Observation (CREDO) trial randomized 2116 patients with stable coronary artery disease (CAD), unstable angina, or recent ACS to a clopidogrel 300 mg loading dose or placebo 3 to 24 hours before PCI. All patients received clopidogrel 75 mg daily for 28 days thereafter; patients in the control arm did not receive a loading dose. Pretreatment did not significantly reduce the primary composite endpoint of death, MI, and urgent target revascularization at 28 days (6.8% vs. 8.3%, $P = 0.23$). Post hoc analysis suggested that longer durations of pretreatment were associated with improved outcomes, but little benefit was achieved when the treatment duration was less than 12 hours.[13] A prospectively planned analysis of the 1863 patients in CLARITY-TIMI 28 undergoing PCI

after mandated angiography showed that pretreatment for a median duration of 3 days in patients with STEMI treated with aspirin and fibrinolysis significantly reduced the incidence of cardiovascular death, MI, or stroke following PCI (3.6% vs. 6.2%, $P = 0.008$) and from randomization through 30 days (7.5% vs. 12.0% $P = 0.001$).[27] Unfortunately, the use of a 300 mg loading dose in CREDO, PCI-CURE, and PCI-CLARITY and the prolonged duration of pretreatment in PCI-CURE and PCI-CLARITY limit their applicability to current practice patterns for both elective and urgent PCIs. The ischemic benefit of a shorter pretreatment duration of high dose clopidogrel before PCI has not been examined in a large, randomized, placebo-controlled trial. Post hoc analysis of the Intracoronary Stenting and Antithrombotic Regimen-Rapid Early Action for Coronary Treatment (ISAR-REACT) trial, which compared abciximab with placebo in elective PCI patients who were treated with clopidogrel 600 mg for at least 2 hours before intervention, showed no incremental benefit from durations of pretreatment >2 to 3 hours.[28] The PRAGUE-8 study randomized 1028 patients undergoing coronary angiography and potential ad hoc PCI for stable angina to either clopidogrel 600 mg >6 hours before angiography or clopidogrel 600 mg in the catheterization laboratory only in the case of PCI.[29] There were no differences in the rate of death, MI, stroke, or re-intervention between groups at 7 days, either in the entire population or the subgroup undergoing PCI (0.8% vs. 1.0%, $P = 0.7$; 1.3% vs. 2.8%, $P = 0.4$, respectively), but bleeding was increased in the pretreatment group (3.5% vs. 1.4%, $P = 0.025$). The findings of this small trial support a strategy of "on the table" clopidogrel loading before ad hoc PCI in elective patients, although the findings must be interpreted within the context of the relatively small sample size and very low event rates. The findings are supported by another smaller trial, Antiplatelet therapy for Reduction of MYocardial Damage during Angioplasty (ARMYDA) PRELOAD, which randomized 409 patients (39 with acute coronary syndrome) to a 600 mg clopidogrel loading dose 4 to 8 hours before PCI or a 600 mg load given in the catheterization laboratory after coronary angiography and before PCI.[30] The rates of major adverse cardiovascular events at 30 days were similar between groups, occurring in 10.8% of patients pretreated compared with 8.8% in the patients receiving clopidogrel in the laboratory ($P = 0.7$). There were no differences in the rates of bleeding.

Dosing Strategies. Pharmacodynamic studies have demonstrated that higher clopidogrel loading doses and maintenance doses provide more rapid onset of action and greater levels of inhibition compared with a 300-mg loading dose and a 75-mg maintenance dose, respectively.[14-16,31] Two large randomized studies, CURRENT-OASIS 7 and The Gauging Responsiveness With A VerifyNow Assay–Impact on Thrombosis And Safety (GRAVITAS), have examined the efficacy and safety of higher dose clopidogrel in patients managed invasively or undergoing PCI.

The CURRENT–OASIS 7 trial examined the ischemic benefit of a higher-dose strategy in 25,086 patients with non–ST elevation ACS and ST elevation ACS undergoing an early invasive strategy, of whom 17,263 underwent PCI.[32] Before angiography, patients were randomized to receive (1) a 600 mg loading dose, followed by 150 mg daily for 6 days and 75 mg daily thereafter or (2) a 300-mg loading dose followed by 75 mg daily thereafter. Patients were also randomized to high-dose aspirin or low-dose aspirin in a 2-by-2 factorial design. The primary endpoint, a composite of cardiovascular death, MI, or stroke at 30 days, was no different with double-dose clopidogrel or standard-dose clopidogrel (4.2% vs. 4.4%, $P = 0.30$). A potential interaction was observed with aspirin dosing, where patients receiving double-dose clopidogrel had better outcomes when treated with higher-dose aspirin. This observation must be taken within the context that the interaction P value was 0.04, which did not meet the trial's prespecified criteria for significance ($P = 0.01$ to adjust for multiple comparisons) and that a mechanism for this potential interaction is unknown. Major bleeding, as defined by the trial, was significantly greater in the patients randomized to double-dose clopidogrel (2.5% vs. 2.0%, HR, 1.24 [95% CI, 1.05–1.46], $P = 0.01$), although there were no differences in fatal bleeding, coronary artery bypass graft (CABG)–related bleeding, or TIMI-criteria major bleeding. Within the subgroup of patients who underwent PCI, high-dose clopidogrel was associated with a 13% relative risk reduction in the primary endpoint (3.9% vs. 4.5%, $P = 0.04$).[33] However, the interaction test between patients who did or did not undergo PCI did not reach the prespecified threshold for statistical significance, and therefore the possibility that the results of the PCI subgroup are a chance finding cannot be excluded.[32] The GRAVITAS trial tested whether an additional clopidogrel loading dose followed by a 6-month course of clopidogrel 150 mg daily would reduce thrombotic events compared with clopidogrel 75 mg daily in patients who had undergone PCI with a drug-eluting stent (DES) and displayed high on-treatment reactivity according to ex vivo platelet function testing 12 to 24 hours after the intervention. Unlike the population examined by the CURRENT-OASIS 7 trial, the predominant indication for PCI in the enrolled population was stable CAD or low-risk unstable angina. There was no difference in the rate of cardiovascular death, nonfatal MI, or stent thrombosis at 6 months between groups (2.3% vs. 2.3%, $P = 0.9$). The incidence of severe or moderate bleeding per the Global Utilization of Streptokinase and t-PA for Occluded Coronary Arteries (GUSTO) criteria was not increased with the high-dose regimen (1.4% vs. 2.3%, $P = 0.10$). The higher-dose clopidogrel regimen had a significant, but only modest, effect on platelet inhibition in patients with high on-treatment reactivity to standard dosing, which may partly explain the similar outcomes of the two groups.

Duration of Therapy. The small but incremental risk of late thrombosis with DESs has raised uncertainty about the optimal duration of dual anti-platelet therapy after PCI. Observational studies have shown that discontinuation of anti-platelet therapy after DES has been associated with late and very late stent thrombosis, but the interpretation of these studies is limited by study design and the presence of potentially unmeasured confounders. Randomized trials from the BMS era

demonstrate the benefit of prolonged aspirin and clopidogrel over the first year after PCI.[12,34] Patients who have undergone PCI could possibly receive benefits from very long-term clopidogrel because of a reduction in atherosclerosis-mediated events, rather than stent-mediated events. The Clopidogrel for High Atherothrombotic Risk and Ischemic Stabilization, Management, and Avoidance (CHARISMA) trial compared aspirin and clopidogrel with aspirin alone over a median treatment duration of 28 months in 15,603 patients with either clinically evident cardiovascular disease or multiple risk factors.[35] While there was no difference in the rate of cardiovascular death, MI, or stroke between treatment groups in the overall cohort, a post hoc analysis showed that aspirin and clopidogrel appeared to provide a significant 17% relative risk reduction in the rate of composite ischemic endpoint in patients with a prior MI, ischemic stroke, or symptomatic peripheral arterial disease (PAD).[36] In contrast, a randomized study of 2701 patients who underwent DES placement and were free of major adverse cardiovascular or cerebrovascular events at 1 year observed no significant ischemic benefit for extended aspirin and clopidogrel therapy compared with aspirin alone.[37] These findings will be confirmed or rebutted by the Dual Antiplatelet Therapy (DAPT) trial (clinicaltrials.gov identifier NCT00977938), which will randomize more than 20,000 patients treated with either a drug-eluting or bare metal stent who are event-free at 12 months post procedure to receive either aspirin and a thienopyridine or aspirin and placebo for an additional 18 months. Current ACC/AHA/SCAI guidelines state that all patients receiving a DES should be given clopidogrel 75 mg daily for at least 12 months if they are not at high risk of bleeding; and for patients receiving a BMS, clopidogrel should be given for a minimum of 1 month, ideally up to 12 months, unless the patient is at increased risk of bleeding, in which case it should be given for a minimum of 2 weeks.[6] In the setting of ACS, for post-PCI patients receiving a stent (BMS or DES), a daily maintenance dose should be given for at least 12 months and for up to 15 months unless the risk of bleeding outweighs the anticipated net benefit afforded by a thienopyridine, and continuation beyond 15 months may be considered in patients undergoing DES placement.[38]

Role of CYP2C19. The anti-platelet effect of clopidogrel is dependent on the generation of an active metabolite through the hepatic CYP450 system. Patients who are carriers for genetic polymorphisms that reduce the catalytic activity of CYP2C19 have lower clopidogrel active metabolite levels and diminished platelet inhibition with treatment. Approximately 5% to 12% of the variability in ADP-induced platelet reactivity appears to be explained by the carriage of the reduced function CYP2C19*2 allele.[20,23] The sensitivity of active metabolite generation to changes in the catalytic activity of CYP2C19 may be attributed to the important contribution of this enzyme to both steps in clopidogrel biotransformation. Decreased CYP2C19 function could lead to a bottleneck at the level of hepatic activation, thereby shunting the pro-drug into the pathway leading to an inactive carboxylic acid metabolite.

Predicted Metabolic Phenotype. Patients can be classified on the basis of the predicted metabolic phenotype of the CYP2C19 genotype. The single nucleotide polymorphisms that affect enzyme activity are described using the established "star allele" nomenclature. The CYP2C19*1 allele denotes the lack of known polymorphisms and therefore is considered to be a wild type. CYP2C19*2 is the most common reduced-function allele, with an allelic frequency of approximately 13% in Caucasians, 18% in African Americans, and 30% in Asians. CYP2C19*3 is the second most common reduced-function allele, with an allelic frequency of approximately 10% in Asians but is rare in other ethnicities. Much less common reduced function alleles include *4, *5, *6, *7, *8, and *10. The *17 variant is associated with increased gene transcription and increased catalytic activity of the enzyme. The combination of two alleles (genotype) can be used to predict the metabolic phenotype of a particular individual (Table 8-2). Metabolic phenotype is associated with the pharmacokinetics and

TABLE 8-1 Key Randomized Clinical Trials of P2Y12 Inhibitors in Patients Undergoing Invasive Management for Acute Coronary Syndrome Percutaneous Coronary Intervention or Both

Drug	Trial Name	N	Population Studied	Intervention	Control	Primary Endpoint	Duration of FU	Treatment Effect
Clopidogrel	PCI-CURE*	2,658	NSTE-ACS	Clopidogrel 300 mg load, 75 mg daily thereafter + ASA	Clopidogrel open-label for 28 d + ASA	CV Death, MI, or Revascularization	9 mo	RR 0.70 [95% CI 0.50–0.97] $P = 0.03$
	CREDO	2,116	Stable CAD and unstable angina	Clopidogrel 300 mg pre-PCI, then 75 mg daily + ASA	Clopidogrel 75/mg day for 28 d + ASA	CV death, MI, or stroke	1 year	RRR 26.9% [95% CI 3.9%–44.4%] $P = 0.02$
	PCI-CLARITY*	1,863	STEMI treated with fibrinolytics; PCI 2–8 days later	Clopidogrel 300 mg pre-PCI, then 75 mg daily + ASA	Open-label clopidogrel starting at time of PCI + ASA	CV death, MI, or stroke	30 d	OR, 0.54 [95% CI, 0.35–0.85] $P = 0.008$
	CURRENT-OASIS 7	25,807	NSTE-ACS and STEMI with intended PCI	Clopidogrel 600 mg before angiography, 150 mg daily for 6 days, then 75 mg daily + ASA	Clopidogrel 300 mg before angiography, then 75 mg daily + ASA	CV death, MI, or stroke	30 d	Overall cohort: HR 0.94 [95% CI 0.83–1.06] $P = 0.30$ PCI cohort:* (N = 17263) HR 0.86 [95% CI 0.74–0.99] $P = 0.04$*
	GRAVITAS	2,214	Patients with high on-treatment reactivity to standard clopidogrel 12 to 24 hours after PCI	Clopidogrel 600 mg, then 150 mg daily + ASA	Clopidogrel 75 mg + ASA	CV death, nonfatal MI, stent thrombosis	6 mo	HR 1.01 [95% CI 0.58–1.76] $P = 0.97$
Prasugrel	TRITON-TIMI 38	13,608	NSTE-ACS and STEMI with planned PCI	Prasugrel 60-mg load, 10 mg thereafter + ASA	Clopidogrel 300 mg load, 75 mg thereafter + ASA	CV death, MI, or stroke	450 d	HR 0.81 [95% CI, 0.73–0.90] $P < 0.001$
Ticagrelor	PLATO Invasive	13,408 (PCI in 77%)	NSTE-ACS and STEMI, intended early invasive management	Ticagrelor 180-mg load, 90 mg bid thereafter + ASA	Clopidogrel 300–600 mg load, 75 mg/d thereafter + ASA	CV death, MI, or stroke	12 m	HR 0.84 [95% CI 0.75–0.94] $P = 0.0025$
Cangrelor	CHAMPION PLATFORM	5,362	Stable CAD or ACS, PCI	Cangrelor + ASA + post-PCI clopidogrel 600-mg	ASA + clopidogrel 600 mg post-PCI	Death, MI, or Revascularization	48 m	OR 0.87 [95% CI 0.71–1.07] $P = 0.17$
	CHAMPION PCI	8,877	Stable CAD or ACS with PCI	Cangrelor + ASA + post-PCI clopidogrel 600-mg	ASA + clopidogrel 600 mg pre-PCI	Death, MI, or Revascularization	48 m	OR 1.05 [95% CI 0.88–1.24] $P = 0.59$

*Post-randomization analysis of larger clinical trial.

NSTE-ACS, non–ST elevation acute coronary syndrome; *STEMI*, ST elevation myocardial infarction; *ASA*, aspirin; *MI*, myocardial infarction; *ACS*, acute coronary syndrome; *PCI*, percutaneous coronary intervention; *RR*, risk reduction; *RRR*, relative risk reduction; *OR*, odds ratio; *HR*, hazard ratio; *CI*, confidence interval. *CURE*, Clopidogrel in Unstable Angina to Prevent Recurrent Ischemic Events (CURE); *CREDO*, Clopidogrel for the Reduction of Events During Observation; *CLARITY*, Clopidogrel as Adjunctive Reperfusion Therapy–Thrombolysis in Myocardial Infarction; *CURRENT-OASIS 7*, Clopidogrel and Aspirin Optimal Dose Usage to Reduce Recurrent Events–Seventh Organization to Assess Strategies in Ischemic Syndromes; *GRAVITAS*, Gauging Responsiveness with A VerifyNow assay–Impact on Thrombosis And Safety; *TRITON-TIMI 38*, Therapeutic Outcomes by Optimizing Platelet Inhibition with Prasugrel–Thrombolysis in Myocardial Infarction 38; *PLATO*, Platelet Inhibition and Patient Outcomes; *CHAMPION*, Cangrelor versus Standard Therapy to Achieve Optimal Management of Platelet Inhibition.

TABLE 8-2 Classification of Predicted Metabolic Phenotype According to CYP2C19 Genotype

CYP2C19 Genotype	Predicted Phenotype
*17/*17	Ultra-rapid metabolizer
*1/*17	Ultra-rapid metabolizer
*1/*1	Extensive metabolizer
*1/*2–*8	Intermediate metabolizer
*17/*2–*8	Intermediate metabolizer/unknown
*2–*8/*2–*8	Poor metabolizer

pharmacodynamics of clopidogrel. In a study of healthy volunteers, ultra-rapid metabolizers had the highest exposure to active metabolite and the greatest platelet inhibition, and poor metabolizers had the lowest exposure and least platelet inhibition with both loading and maintenance doses.[39] The frequency of poor metabolizers is approximately 2% in the Caucasian population.

CYP2C19 and Clinical Outcomes. A collaborative meta-analysis of nine studies involving 9685 patients of whom 91% had a PCI reported a significantly increased risk of the composite endpoint of cardiovascular death, MI, or ischemic stroke in carriers of at least one reduced-function CYP2C19 allele (HR 1.57 [95% CI 1.13–2.16], $P = 0.006$) and in patients with two reduced-function CYP2C19 alleles (HR 1.76 [95% CI, 1.24–2.50], $P = 0.002$). Carriers of at least one reduced-function CYP2C19 allele had an increased risk of stent thrombosis (HR, 2.81 [95% CI, 1.81–4.37], $P < 0.0001$); the risk of stent thrombosis was especially strong in patients with two reduced-function alleles (HR 3.97; 95% CI, 1.75–9.02; $P = 0.001$). The influence of CYP2C19 genotype on outcomes is less apparent in populations treated with clopidogrel for indications other than PCI. In the genetic substudy of the Atrial Fibrillation Clopidogrel Trial with Irbesartan for Prevention of Vascular Events (ACTIVE)-A, which was a randomized comparison of aspirin and clopidogrel compared with aspirin alone for the prevention of thromboembolic events in atrial fibrillation (AF), the primary outcome was similar in carriers and noncarriers of the CYP2C19*2 reduced-function alleles. Similarly, in the CURE trial, in which only 14% of patients presenting with ACS underwent PCI, there was no difference in ischemic outcomes according to CYP2C19 genotype.[40]

U.S. Food and Drug Administration's Boxed Warning. The U.S. Food and Drug Administration (FDA) mandated a warning in the Plavix package insert in the fall of 2009 that highlights the impact of CYP2C19 on the exposure to clopidogrel active metabolite, platelet inhibition, and clinical outcomes. This warning emphasizes that the effectiveness of clopidogrel is dependent on bioactivation by CYP2C19 and that poor metabolizers generate less active metabolite and have less platelet inhibition with the recommended dosage of clopidogrel (i.e., 300-mg load and 75-mg daily maintenance dose). Furthermore, the warning states that compared with patients with normal CYP2C19 function, cardiovascular event rates are higher in poor metabolizers with ACS or those who are undergoing PCI when treated with recommended doses of clopidogrel. The warning goes on to state that tests are available to identify a patient's CYP2C19 genotype; that these tests can be used as an aid in determining therapeutic strategy and that alternative treatment or treatment strategies should be considered in patients identified as poor metabolizers of CYP2C19. A subsequent ACCF/AHA Clopidogrel Clinical Alert stated that the evidence base was insufficient to recommend routine genetic testing, but testing to determine if a patient is a poor metabolizer may be considered before starting clopidogrel therapy in patients believed to be at moderate or high risk for poor outcomes, for example, those undergoing elective high-risk PCI. The alert also noted that if genotyping identifies a poor metabolizer, other anti-platelet therapies, particularly prasugrel for coronary patients, should be considered, taking into account the balance of potential ischemic benefit with the known increased risk of bleeding.[41]

Other Genetic Polymorphisms

PON1. An alternative model for the bioactivation of clopidogrel posits a central role for the paraoxonase-1 enzyme (PON1) in hydrolyzing 2-oxo-clopidogrel into the thiol active metabolite. A genetic variant that lowers the activity of PON1 (Q192R) and may reduce the efficiency of clopidogrel bioactivation has been identified. Carriage of two PON1 loss-of-function alleles was associated with definite stent thrombosis in a prospective cohort of 1982 patients with ACS (HR 10.20 [95% CI, 4.39–71.43], $P < 0.001$).[11]

ABCB1. P-glycoprotein is an adenosine triphosphate (ATP)—dependent efflux pump encoded by the *ABCB1* gene. It is expressed in the intestinal epithelial cells; increased expression or function can influence the bioavailability of drugs that are its substrate. Healthy subjects homozygous for the 3435 C->T polymorphism have decreased pharmacodynamic effect of clopidogrel.[42] The results of clinical outcomes studies are inconsistent. A genetic substudy of the TRial to assess Improvement in the Therapeutic outcomes by Optimizing platelet INhibition with prasugrel–Thrombolysis in Myocardial Infarction (TRITON–TIMI) 38 study reported that ABCB1 3435 TT homozygotes had a significantly increased risk of adverse cardiovascular events during treatment with clopidogrel after PCI for ACS, whereas event rates were highest in ABCB1 3435 CC homozygotes in the genetic

substudy of the Platelet Inhibition and Patient Outcomes (PLATO) trial.[42,43]

Proton Pump Inhibitors

PPIs are extensively metabolized by CYP2C19 and CYP3A4. The different PPIs inhibit CYP2C19 activity to varying degrees. Omeprazole, lansoprazole, and esomeprazole demonstrate more potent inhibition by ex vivo assays, and lesser inhibition is observed with pantoprazole and rabeprazole. PPIs interfere with the pharmacodynamic effect of clopidogrel. In the Omeprazole Clopidogrel Aspirin (OCLA) study, 124 patients who had undergone coronary stent implantation received aspirin and clopidogrel (300 mg loading dose followed by 75 mg daily) and were randomized to either omeprazole 20 mg daily or placebo for 7 days.[44] Omeprazole significantly decreased the inhibitory effect of clopidogrel as assessed by VASP phosphorylation analysis. Administering the two drugs 12 hours apart does not mitigate the clopidogrel–PPI interaction.[45] A pharmacodynamic interaction does not appear to occur with pantoprazole.[45,46] Large retrospective cohort and population-based studies have reported an association between concomitant PPI and clopidogrel use with an increased risk of recurrent cardiovascular events, including MI.[47,48] Although these analyses adjust for baseline differences among treatment groups, unmeasured confounders may, in part, explain these observations, as patients treated with PPIs after PCI have substantially more comorbidities than those patients not treated with PPIs. Post hoc analysis of the TRITON-TIMI 38 randomized trial found no association between PPI use and the risk of cardiovascular death, MI, or stroke in patients treated with clopidogrel.[49] The Clopidogrel and the Optimization of Gastrointestinal Events Trial (COGENT) was a multi-center, randomized, phase III study of the safety and efficacy of a fixed-dose combination of clopidogrel 75 mg or omeprazole 20 mg in patients at high risk for GI bleeding who required aspirin and clopidogrel therapy for at least 12 months.[50] The primary endpoint was the time to first occurrence of an upper GI clinical event; the primary cardiovascular endpoint was a composite of cardiovascular death, nonfatal MI, coronary revascularization, or ischemic stroke. The study was not powered a priori for the cardiovascular endpoint; it was halted prematurely for lack of funding. A total of 3873 patients were randomized, of whom approximately 42% had a history of ACS. At 180 days, the rate of the composite GI endpoint was significantly lower in the combination clopidogrel–omeprazole group compared with clopidogrel alone (1.1% vs. 2.9%, HR 0.34 [95% CI, 0.18–0.63], $P < 0.001$), and there appeared to be no difference in the incidence of cardiovascular events (4.9% vs. 5.7%, HR 0.99 [95% CI, 0.68–1.44], $P = 0.96$). The cardiovascular endpoint was driven predominantly by the need for coronary revascularization (generally not a platelet-driven phenomenon); cardiovascular death or MI occurred in only 23 patients in the omeprazole group and in 20 patients in the placebo group. Given the possibility of a 44% increased hazard for cardiovascular events in the low-risk group that was studied, the COGENT results may not rule out a clinically meaningful difference in cardiovascular events with the use of omeprazole in patients administered clopidogrel for its labeled indications.[51] The findings of a meta-analysis of 13 studies involving 48,674 clopidogrel-treated patients suggested that the clinical impact of concomitant PPI use might be significant only in patients with high baseline cardiovascular risk.[52] An ACC Foundation/American College of Gastroenterology/AHA 2010 Expert Consensus Document on the Concomitant Use of Proton Pump Inhibitors and Thienopyridines states that clinical decisions regarding concomitant use of PPIs and thienopyridines must balance overall risks and benefits, considering both cardiovascular and GI complications.[53] Patients with ACS and prior upper GI bleeding are at substantial cardiovascular risk, so dual anti-platelet therapy with concomitant use of a PPI may provide the optimal balance of risk and benefit. Among stable patients undergoing coronary revascularization, a history of GI bleeding should inform the choice of revascularization method; if a coronary stent is selected to treat such patients, the risk–benefit trade-off may favor concomitant use of dual anti-platelet therapy plus a PPI.

PRASUGREL

Metabolism

Prasugrel is a thienopyridine, like ticlopidine and clopidogrel, but its biotransformation into the active metabolite is substantially more efficient (see Fig. 8-3). Hydrolysis by human carboxylesterase 2 during absorption forms a thiolactone precursor, which is then oxidized in a single CYP-dependent step to the active metabolite. CYP3A4/5 and CYP2B6 are major contributors to this process, whereas CYP2C19 and CYP2C9 play a minor role; oxidation by intestinal CYP3A also occurs.[54] The biotransformation of prasugrel is more efficient than that of clopidogrel, since there is no competing metabolic pathway to an inactive metabolite. The greater magnitude of inhibition of platelet aggregation achieved by prasugrel 60-mg compared with clopidogrel 600 mg is caused by differences in active metabolite exposure.[55] The area under the concentration-time curve of prasugrel active metabolite is dose proportionate between 10 mg and 60 mg. Genetic polymorphisms that reduce the catalytic activity of CYP2C19 have no effect on active metabolite formation, the achieved level of platelet inhibition, or clinical outcomes in patients with ACS treated with PCI.[54,56]

Pharmacodynamics

Compared with clopidogrel, a prasugrel 60-mg loading dose followed by 10 mg daily provides a more rapid onset of action, significantly greater P2Y12 inhibition, and less inter-individual variability in the extent of inhibition. Prasugrel 60 mg achieves greater than twice the mean inhibition of platelet aggregation (IPA) at 4 hours after administration compared with a clopidogrel 300-mg loading dose in patients with stable coronary artery disease (ADP 5 mmol/L, 74% vs. 37%; ADP 20 mmol/L, 68% vs. 30%), and the stronger effect on IPA can be detected as early as 15 to 30 minutes after administration.[57] Prasugrel 10 mg daily provides a greater level of IPA compared with clopidogrel 75 mg daily (ADP 5 mmol/L, 59% vs. 31%; ADP 20 mmol/L, 58% vs. 31%).[57] A randomized pharmacodynamic study demonstrated that a prasugrel 60-mg load followed by 10 mg daily also provides a greater level of platelet inhibition than clopidogrel 600 mg followed by 150 mg daily.[58] The variability in inhibition among individuals is substantially less with prasugrel 60 mg or 10 mg compared with clopidogrel. However, prasugrel maintenance doses of less than 10 mg daily are associated with greater degrees of inter-individual variability in the extent of inhibition.[57]

Clinical Studies

The clinical efficacy and safety of prasugrel in ACS were examined in TRITON–TIMI 38.[59] In this phase III, randomized, active-control, time-to-event trial, 13,608 patients with moderate- to high-risk ACS undergoing treatment with PCI were assigned a prasugrel 60-mg loading dose followed by 10 mg daily or a clopidogrel 300-mg loading dose followed by 75 mg daily for 6 to 15 months. The primary efficacy endpoint was a composite of death from cardiovascular causes, nonfatal MI, or stroke. To be eligible, patients were required to be naïve to thienopyridine therapy. Randomization to the study drug occurred after diagnostic coronary angiography and the determination that PCI was to be performed except in the case of STEMI, when randomization was allowed before the assessment of coronary anatomy. Over a median duration of therapy of 14.5 months, the primary composite endpoint occurred in 12.1% of the patients receiving clopidogrel and 9.9% of patients receiving prasugrel ($P < 0.001$). The treatment effect of prasugrel was driven primarily by a reduction in the rate of nonfatal MI. The benefit of prasugrel was similar in patients with non–ST elevation ACS (HR, 0.82 [95% CI, 0.73–0.93], $P = 0.002$) or STEMI (HR 0.79 [95% CI, 0.65–0.97], $P = 0.02$). The rate of definite or probable stent thrombosis was also significantly reduced with prasugrel (1.13% vs. 2.35%, HR 0.48 [95% CI, 0.36–0.64], $P < 0.001$). Key elements of the TRITON-TIMI 38 study design that may have impacted the findings

were the timing of study drug administration and the clopidogrel dosing strategy to which prasugrel was compared (clopidogrel 300-mg loading dose at the time of PCI). Prespecified landmark analyses for efficacy were performed from randomization to day 3 and from day 3 to the end of the trial to separate the events that could be attributed to the loading dose of the study drug. These analyses demonstrated that in addition to an early benefit, prasugrel provided a significant reduction in the rates of MI and stent thrombosis after 3 days, supporting the hypothesis that prasugrel is superior to clopidogrel during the chronic phase of management after PCI (nonfatal MI: HR 0.69 [95% CI, 0.58–0.83], $P < 0.001$; stent thrombosis: HR 0.45 [95% CI, 0.32–0.64], $P < 0.001$).[60] Further landmark analyses also showed that prasugrel reduced stent thrombosis both early (≤30 days, 0.64% vs. 1.56%, $P < 0.001$) and late (>30 days, 0.49% vs. 0.82%, $P = 0.03$).[61] Although prasugrel provided a significant benefit with regard to ischemic outcomes, a significant hazard for major bleeding was also observed (HR 1.32, [95% CI, 1.03–1.68], $P = 0.03$), including fatal bleeding. A determination of net clinical outcome (combination of ischemic and bleeding events) may be helpful to assess the overall benefit of prasugrel for a particular patient, assuming that the components of this composite (death from any cause, nonfatal MI, stroke, and major non–CABG-related bleeding) can be considered of equivalent importance to the physician and the patient. In TRITON-TIMI 38, patients with a prior history of stroke or transient ischemic attack (TIA) experienced net harm from prasugrel (because of a lack of ischemic benefit and a strong trend toward excessive major bleeding, including intracranial hemorrhage), and patients ≥75 years of age and who weighed <60 kg experienced no net clinical benefit (because of modest ischemic benefit balanced by an increased risk of bleeding). Therefore, prasugrel is contraindicated in patients with a history of stroke or TIA; it can be considered in patients ≥75 years of age who have an increased ischemic risk (e.g., diabetes or prior MI) in whom the potential ischemic benefit may outweigh any increased risk of major bleeding; and a maintenance dose adjustment to 5 mg may be considered in patients weighing <60 kg, as pharmacokinetic modeling suggests that active metabolite exposure with this dose is similar to the 10 mg dose in heavier patients.

NON-THIENOPYRIDINES

Ticagrelor

Ticagrelor, a cyclopentyltriazolopyrimidine, is a reversibly binding oral P2Y12 receptor antagonist (Fig. 8-4). It interacts with the P2Y12

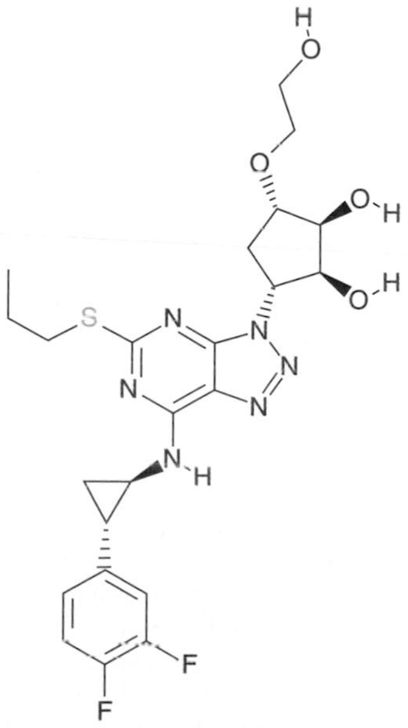

Figure 8-4 Chemical structure of ticagrelor.

receptor at a ligand binding site separate from that for ADP or the thienopyridines and therefore antagonizes ADP-mediated P2Y12 receptor activation noncompetitively.[62] In addition to P2Y12 receptor antagonism, ticagrelor may have off-target effects via inhibition of erythrocyte adenosine reuptake.

Pharmacology and Metabolism. Unlike the thienopyridines, ticagrelor does not require metabolic conversion to an active form to antagonize the P2Y12 receptor. Peak plasma concentration is attained at a median of 90 minutes after administration. The parent compound is metabolized primarily by CYP3A isoenzymes into a metabolite that has a similar potency in inhibiting the P2Y12 receptor; this metabolite is present at approximately 40% of the parent concentration. Elimination of ticagrelor is mainly through hepatic metabolism, and the primary route of elimination of the active metabolite is likely through biliary excretion. CYP3A inhibitors such as ketoconazole or diltiazem increase plasma concentrations of ticagrelor, and ticagrelor increases the exposure to drugs that are CYP3A substrates, such as simvastatin. CYP2C19 genotype has no effect on ticagrelor pharmacodynamics.[63] The mean half-life of ticagrelor and its active metabolite is 7.2 hours and 8.5 hours, respectively.

Pharmacodynamics. Compared with clopidogrel, ticagrelor has a rapid onset of action, achieves more intensive P2Y12 inhibition, and has a relatively faster offset of anti-platelet effect.[64] A ticagrelor 180-mg loading dose provides an IPA with ADP 20 mmol/L of 41% at 30 minutes and 88% at 2 hours after administration compared with 8% and 41% after a clopidogrel 600-mg loading dose, respectively. Maintenance-dose ticagrelor 90 mg twice daily provides an IPA with ADP 20 mmol/L of approximately 75% compared with 50% with clopidogrel 75 mg daily. The extent of inhibition is similar 24 hours after discontinuation of either clopidogrel or ticagrelor because of faster offset with ticagrelor, and the IPA for ticagrelor on day 3 after the last dose is comparable with that for clopidogrel at day 5.

Clinical Studies. The Study of Platelet Inhibition and Patient Outcomes (PLATO) trial randomized 18,624 patients with ACS with or without ST elevation to either ticagrelor or clopidogrel.[65] The primary efficacy endpoint was a composite of death from cardiovascular causes, MI, or stroke; the major safety endpoint was major bleeding as defined by the trial, which was more inclusive than TIMI-defined major bleeding. Initial patient management could be conservative or invasive, and patient randomization was stratified by the intent for early invasive management as indicated by the investigator. Unlike TRITON-TIMI 38, PLATO included both thienopyridine-naïve patients and thienopyridine-treated patients. At 12 months, ticagrelor led to a significant reduction in the primary composite endpoint compared with clopidogrel (9.8% vs. 11.7%; HR 0.84 [95% CI 0.77–0.92], $P < 0.001$). A similar relative reduction in the primary endpoint was observed in the 13,408 patients treated with a planned invasive strategy, 44% of whom had received clopidogrel before randomization and allocation to the study drug.[66] Ticagrelor significantly reduced cardiovascular mortality by an absolute risk reduction of 1.1% and all-cause mortality by 1.4%; however, the statistical validity of this latter finding may be questioned because this endpoint was analyzed in a hierarchical fashion after the rate of stroke, which was not statistically significant between study arms. There was no increase in all-cause major bleeding with ticagrelor. The rate of fatal intracerebral hemorrhage was significantly greater with ticagrelor therapy, but this was balanced by a higher rate of non-intracranial fatal bleeding with clopidogrel, resulting in an overall similar rate of fatal bleeding with the two therapies. Non–CABG-related TIMI major bleeding was significantly more frequent with ticagrelor (HR 1.25 [95% CI, 1.03–1.53], $P = 0.03$). In subgroup analyses according to region, ticagrelor did not provide an ischemic benefit in the North American cohort (HR 1.25 [95% CI, 0.93–1.67], interaction $P = 0.045$). A definitive explanation for this observation has not been identified.

Adverse Effects. Ticagrelor has been associated with dyspnea, hyperuricemia, and ventricular pauses, possibly attributable to interference with adenosine degradation and inhibition of erythrocyte adenosine reuptake. Holter monitoring in a subgroup of patients in the PLATO trial demonstrated that ticagrelor led to an infrequent but greater rate of ventricular pauses ≥3 seconds in the first week of therapy but did not result in significantly increased syncope or pacemaker implantation compared with clopidogrel. An increased rate of the complaint of dyspnea has been consistently observed in phase II and phase III studies. In The Dose Confirmation Study Assessing Anti-Platelet Effects of AZD6140 versus Clopidogrel in Non-ST-segment Elevation Myocardial Infarction (DISPERSE-2), 10.5% of patients receiving ticagrelor 90 mg BID reported dyspnea, compared with 6.4% of patients receiving clopidogrel ($P = 0.07$).[67] In PLATO, dyspnea was reported in 13.5% of ticagrelor-treated patients compared with 7.8% of clopidogrel-treated patients ($P < 0.001$). In a randomized, double-blind phase II study that actively monitored the complaint of dyspnea in 123 patients with stable coronary artery disease, 38.6%, 9.3%, and 8.3% of patients in the ticagrelor, clopidogrel, and placebo groups reported dyspnea, respectively ($P < 0.001$). Most cases of dyspnea occurred within 1 week of starting ticagrelor and were not associated with adverse changes in cardiac or pulmonary function.[68]

Cangrelor. Cangrelor is an intravenous, rapid, and direct-acting, reversible inhibitor of the P2Y12 receptor that has a half-life of approximately 3 minutes (Fig. 8-5). In a phase II study of patients undergoing elective PCI, a dose of 4 mcg/kg/min achieved >95% inhibition of platelet aggregation within 15 minutes of administration. After a bolus dose and infusion, normalization of platelet function occurs within 60 minutes after discontinuation. The Cangrelor versus Standard Therapy to Achieve Optimal Management of Platelet Inhibition (CHAMPION)-PCI and CHAMPION-PLATFORM trials were phase III, randomized, clinical trials comparing cangrelor with clopidogrel administered before or after PCI, respectively.[69,70] Cangrelor was not superior to clopidogrel in either trial with respect to the composite endpoint of death from any cause, MI, or ischemia-driven revascularization at 48 hours. The safety and efficacy of cangrelor is being examined further in the CHAMPION PHOENIX trial (clinicaltrials.gov identifier, NCT01156571).

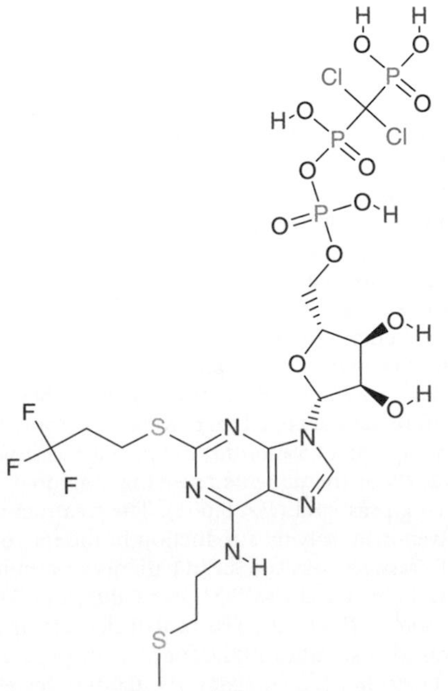

Figure 8-5 Chemical structure of cangrelor.

THROMBIN RECEPTOR ANTAGONISTS

Basic Principles

Thrombin exerts a panoply of effects on thrombosis, hemostasis, and inflammation. Generated at sites of vascular injury, it is the effector protease of the coagulation cascade, converting circulating fibrinogen to fibrin monomer, which polymerizes to form fibrin, the fibrous matrix of thrombus. Thrombin promotes edema by increasing the permeability of the vascular endothelium, induces vasoconstriction in the absence of the endothelium through its action on smooth muscle cells, and stimulates prostaglandin and cytokine production by endothelial cells. Thrombin is also the most potent agonist for platelet activation and provokes shape change, granule secretion, synthesis and release of TXA2, mobilization of p-selectin and CD40 to the platelet surface, and activation of the GP IIb/IIIa receptor.[4] The cellular effects of thrombin are mediated primarily by the activation of protease-activated receptors (PARs). There are two platelet thrombin receptors in humans: PAR1 and PAR4. PAR1 is more important, mediating platelet activation at low thrombin concentrations, whereas PAR4 mediates platelet activation only at high thrombin concentrations. PARs are unique in that each receptor carries its own ligand that is active only after cleavage. Thrombin binds the N-terminus of the PAR1 receptor with high affinity at an extracellular, hirudin-like site and then cleaves the receptor between residues Arg 41 and Ser 42; this unmasks a new N-terminus beginning with the sequence SFLLRN (serine–phenylalanine–leucine–leucine–arginine asparagine). This N-terminus functions as a tethered ligand, docking intramolecularly with the body of the receptor and activating it. The inability of PAR4 to activate platelets at low thrombin concentrations is likely caused by the absence of an extracellular hirudin-like domain. The PAR1 receptor is an attractive candidate for targeted inhibition in patients with cardiovascular disease. PAR mediated signaling appears to be a more important contributor to thrombosis compared with hemostasis. In addition, platelet PAR antagonism maintains the fibrin-generating and protein C functions of thrombin and does not appear to interfere with other platelet-signaling pathways such as those mediated by collagen and ADP (Fig. 8-6). Therefore, unlike other platelet receptor inhibitors, PAR1 antagonists may have a wide therapeutic window between ischemia reduction and bleeding risk. Two PAR1 antagonists, vorapaxar and atopaxar, are currently being examined in clinical trials.

Vorapaxar

Vorapaxar is a synthetic tricyclic 3-phenylpyridine analogue of himbacine. It is a high-affinity, orally active, low-molecular-weight, nonpeptide, competitive PAR1 antagonist that is slowly eliminated, with a half-life of approximately 5 to 11 days. Recovery of platelet function to ≥50% of baseline occurred at 4 weeks after treatment discontinuation in healthy volunteers (Fig. 8-7). The Thrombin Receptor Antagonist (TRA)-PCI trial was a phase II, placebo-controlled, dose-ranging study of the safety and tolerability of vorapaxar in 1030 patients undergoing nonurgent coronary angiography or planned PCI. Patients received a vorapaxar loading dose or placebo at least 1 hour before angiography, and those who subsequently underwent PCI were randomized to maintenance-dose vorapaxar or placebo for 60 days. PCI patients were administered clopidogrel in addition to the study drug. Vorapaxar was not associated with an increase in TIMI major or minor bleeding compared with placebo, although there was an increase in bleeding that did not meet the TIMI criteria. Death and MI occurred less frequently in patients randomized to vorapaxar (7.3% vs. 4.5%), with a signal of a dose-related effect. Within the cohort of 76 patients who underwent CABG rather than PCI, there were no differences between vorapaxar or placebo in chest-tube drainage, the need for re-exploration because of bleeding, or in the number of patients requiring transfusions >2 units. Pharmacodynamic analyses using light transmission aggregometry showed that loading doses of vorapaxar inhibited thrombin-receptor activating peptide (TRAP)–mediated platelet aggregation in a dose-dependent manner. After a 40-mg dose, approximately 90% of patients had ≥80% inhibition by 2 hours. A

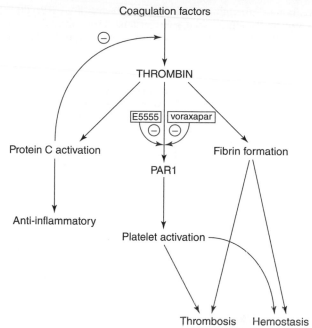

Figure 8-6 **Rationale for platelet protease-activated receptor inhibition in the treatment of cardiovascular disease.** Thrombin acts as a platelet agonist through its activation of the platelet PAR1 and PAR4 receptors; it is the main effector protease of the coagulation cascade and triggers fibrin formation; and, within the environment of the normal endothelium, it activates protein C to terminate its own production. Fibrin(ogen) appears more important than thrombin-induced platelet activation for hemostasis. PAR1 is the primary mediator of thrombin-induced platelet activation, and PAR1 antagonists may have a wide therapeutic window for platelet-dependent processes such as acute coronary syndrome and stent thrombosis by leaving the fibrin generation and protein C functions of thrombin intact. Vorapaxar and atopaxar are PAR1 inhibitors currently under clinical investigation. *PAR,* protease-activated receptor. (*Adapted with permission from Angiolillo DJ Capodanno D, Goto S: Platelet thrombin receptor antagonism and atherothrombosis,* Eur Heart J *31:17 28, 2010.*)

maintenance dose of vorapaxar 2.5 mg daily provided greater than 80% inhibition in all patients at 30 and 60 days. Two phase III studies of vorapaxar are ongoing. The Thrombin Receptor Antagonist for Clinical Event Reduction in Acute Coronary Syndrome trial (TRACER) will evaluate the efficacy and safety of a vorapaxar in addition to standard-of-care in approximately 13,000 patients with non–ST elevation ACS.[71] The Thrombin-Receptor Antagonist in Secondary

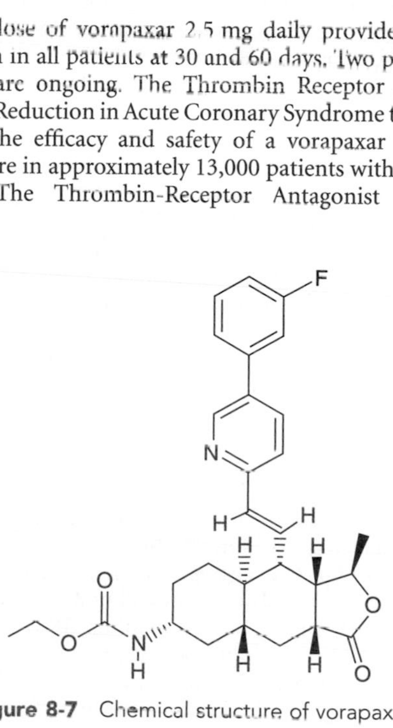

Figure 8-7 Chemical structure of vorapaxar.

Prevention of Atherothrombotic Ischemic Events (TRA 2°P)-TIMI 50 will evaluate the efficacy and safety of long-term vorapaxar in up to 27,000 patients with a history of MI, ischemic stroke, or PAD receiving standard therapy.[72]

Atopaxar

Atopaxar is a low-molecular-weight, orally active, PAR1 antagonist that provides potent inhibition of TRAP-induced aggregation. The safety and efficacy of atopaxar was explored in the phase II, dose-ranging Japanese–Lesson from Antagonizing the Cellular Effect of Thrombin (J-LANCELOT) trial.[73] J-LANCELOT randomized 241 patients with ACS and 263 patients with CAD to either atopaxar or placebo for 12 weeks and 24 weeks, respectively. The incidence of TIMI-criteria major or minor bleeding was similar in the placebo and the combined atopaxar groups, although there was a numerical increase in any TIMI bleeding with the highest dose of atopaxar studied. The rates of major adverse cardiovascular events were similar among groups. Statistically significant dose-related increases in liver function test abnormalities and corrected Q–T interval were observed with atopaxar. Similar findings were observed in LANCELOT-ACS, an international, phase II dose-ranging study of 603 patients with unstable angina or non-STEMI treated with atopaxar or placebo in addition to standard therapy for 12 weeks. In this study, the incidence of CURE-defined bleeding was numerically, but not significantly, higher in the combined atopaxar group, and the incidence of cardiovascular death, MI, or stroke was numerically lower. The incidence of Holter-detected ischemia at 48 hours was significantly lower in the combined atopaxar group (RR, 0.67; 95% CI: 0.48–0.94, $P = 0.02$). Dose-dependent liver function test abnormalities and relative Q–T interval prolongation were observed. Further studies are required to fully establish the safety and efficacy of atopaxar.

PHOSPHODIESTERASE INHIBITORS

Cilostazol

Cilostazol, a selective phosphodiesterase type III (PDE III) inhibitor, increases cAMP levels in platelets, endothelial cells, and smooth muscle cells, thereby resulting in vasodilatory and anti-platelet effects. It was approved by the FDA in 1998 for the treatment of symptoms of intermittent claudication. Pharmacodynamic studies have shown that the addition of cilostazol to aspirin and clopidogrel (triple anti-platelet therapy) results in greater ADP-induced platelet inhibition compared with aspirin and clopidogrel alone.[74] Adjunctive cilostazol therapy in addition to aspirin and clopidogrel has been associated with a reduced risk of stent thrombosis, re-stenosis, and major adverse cardiac events without increased bleeding complications in patients undergoing PCI, including those treated with DESs.[75,76] These benefits have been more marked in complex settings such as in patients with diabetes mellitus and long lesions. The clinical studies of cilostazol in the PCI setting have been conducted primarily in Asia. The most common side effects of cilostazol include headache, tachycardia, palpitations, soft stools, and diarrhea, which may lead to drug discontinuation in up to 15% of cases. Cilostazol should be avoided in patients with congestive heart failure of any severity with or without preserved left ventricular systolic function because of an increased mortality risk with phosphodiesterase inhibitors.

GLYCOPROTEIN IIB/IIIA INHIBITORS

The GP IIb/IIIa receptor is an integrin, a heterodimer consisting of noncovalently associated α- and β-subunits, which mediate the final common pathway of platelet aggregation. In particular, the GP IIb/IIIa receptor consists of the αIIb and β₃ subunits. By competing with fibrinogen and vWF for GP IIb/IIIa binding, GP IIb/IIIa antagonists interfere with platelet cross-linking and platelet-derived thrombus formation (Fig. 8-8). Since the GP IIb/IIIa receptor represents the final common pathway leading to platelet aggregation, these agents are very

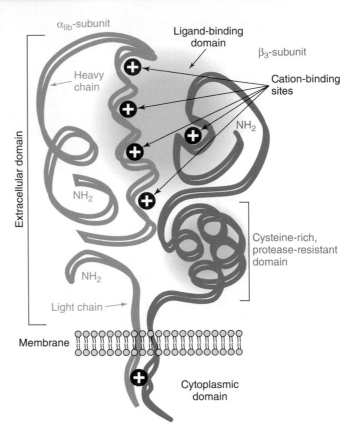

Figure 8-8 **Structure of the glycoprotein (GP) IIb/IIIa receptor.** The GP IIb/IIIa receptor is an integrin, a heterodimer consisting of noncovalently associated α- and β-subunits, which mediate the final common pathway of platelet aggregation. The GP IIb/IIIa receptor consists of the αIIb and β₃ subunits. The α-subunit is a 136-kD molecule with light and heavy chains; the light chain contains a short cytoplasmic tail, a transmembrane region, and a short extracellular domain, and the heavy chain is entirely extracellular. The β-subunit is a 84.5-kD molecule with a short intracellular tail, transmembrane region, and a large extracellular domain. Platelet activation leads to a conformational change in the GP IIb/IIIa receptor, markedly increasing its affinity for its ligands through its binding sites. There are two main binding sites on the GP IIb/IIIa receptor. One recognizes the amino acid sequence arginine-glycine-aspartic acid (Arg-Gly-Asp or RGD) that is found on multiple ligands (fibronectin, von Willebrand factor [vWF], and vitronectin) but, most importantly, on fibrinogen, the major GP IIb/IIIa ligand, in which the RGD sequence occurs twice. The other peptide sequence is the Lys-Gln-Ala-Gly-Asp-Val, which is only located at the carboxyl terminus of the gamma chain of fibrinogen. (*Reproduced with permission from Topol EJ, Byzova TV, Plow EF: Platelet GP IIB/IIIa blockers, Lancet 353:227–231, 1999.*)

effective in inhibiting platelets. Investigations of oral GP IIb/IIIa inhibitors have been stopped because of their lack of benefit and increased mortality in patients with ACS or in those undergoing PCI. The reasons for these negative outcomes remain elusive. Currently, only parenteral GP IIb/IIIa inhibitors are approved for clinical use and recommended only in the setting of patients with ACS who are undergoing PCI. Although GP IIb/IIIa inhibitors have been shown to reduce major adverse cardiac events (death, MI, and urgent revascularization) by 35% to 50% in patients undergoing PCI, their broad use has been limited as they are associated with an increased risk of bleeding.[77]

Pharmacology

There are three parenteral GP IIb/IIIa antagonists approved for clinical use: abciximab, eptifibatide, and tirofiban. Abciximab is a large chimeric monoclonal antibody with a high binding affinity that results in a prolonged pharmacologic effect. In particular, it is a monoclonal antibody that is a Fab (fragment antigen binding) fragment of a chimeric human–mouse genetic reconstruction of 7E3. The Fc portion of the antibody was removed to decrease immunogenicity, and the Fab portion was attached to the constant regions of a human immunoglobulin. Abciximab binding is specific for the β_3-subunit and explains its ability to bind other β_3-receptors such as vitronectin ($\alpha V \beta_3$). Unlike the small-molecule GP IIb/III inhibitors eptifibatide and tirofiban, abciximab interacts with the GP IIb/IIIa receptor at sites distinct from the ligand-binding RGD sequence site and exerts its inhibitory effect noncompetitively. Its plasma half-life is biphasic, with an initial half-life of less than 10 minutes and a second-phase half-life of approximately 30 minutes. However, because of its high affinity for the GP IIb/IIIa receptor, it has a biologic half-life of 12 to 24 hours; and because of its slow clearance from the body, it has a functional half-life up to 7 days. Platelet-associated abciximab can be detected for more than 14 days after the infusion has been stopped. The recommended dose for abciximab is 0.25 mg/kg bolus followed by an intravenous infusion with 0.125 mcg/kg/min for 12 hours. No renal adjustments are required. The small-molecule agents eptifibatide and tirofiban, unlike abciximab, do not induce an immune response and have a lower affinity for the GP IIb/IIIa receptor. Eptifibatide is a reversible, and highly selective heptapeptide with a rapid onset and a short plasma half-life of 2 to 2.5 hours. Its molecular design is based on barbourin, a member of the disintegrin family, which contains a novel Lys-Gly-Asp (KGD) sequence making it highly specific for the GP IIb/IIIa receptor. In the setting of PCI, a double bolus and infusion regimen is recommended (180 mcg/kg, followed by a second 180 mcg/kg bolus, followed by 2 mcg/kg/min for a minimum of 12 hours); peak plasma levels are established shortly after the bolus dose, and a slightly lower concentration is subsequently maintained throughout the infusion period. Since eptifibatide is mostly eliminated through renal mechanisms, a lower infusion dose (1 mcg/kg/min) is recommended in patients with creatinine clearance less than 50 mL/min. Recovery of platelet aggregation occurs within 4 hours of completion of the infusion. Tirofiban is a tyrosine-derived nonpeptide inhibitor that mimics the RGD sequence and is highly specific for the GP IIb/IIIa receptor. Tirofiban is associated with a rapid onset and a short duration of action, with a plasma half-life of approximately 2 hours. Like eptifibatide, substantial recovery of platelet aggregation is present within 4 hours of completion of infusion. It is currently not FDA approved for PCI, although it is both approved and widely used throughout Europe for this indication (bolus 10 mcg/kg followed by infusion 0.15 mcg/kg/min for 18–24 hours). Several studies have documented that this approved bolus and infusion regimen for tirofiban achieves suboptimal levels of platelet inhibition for up to 4 to 6 hours that likely accounted for inferior clinical results in the PCI setting. For this reason, a high-dose bolus regimen (25 mcg/kg) achieving more optimal platelet inhibition has been suggested. Since tirofiban is mostly eliminated through renal mechanisms, dosage adjustment is required for patients with renal insufficiency. Patients treated with GP IIb/IIIa inhibitors have a higher incidence of thrombocytopenia. Severe thrombocytopenia is more commonly associated with abciximab and requires immediate cessation of therapy. The mechanism of thrombocytopenia is unknown. Regardless of its etiology, thrombocytopenia in patients undergoing PCI is associated with more ischemic events, bleeding complications, and transfusions. The platelet count typically falls within hours of GP IIb/IIIa administration. Re-administration of abciximab, but not eptifibatide and tirofiban, is associated with a slightly increased risk of thrombocytopenia.

Clinical Trials with Glycoprotein IIb/IIIa Inhibitors

Before the era of pretreatment with high loading doses of clopidogrel, the safety and efficacy of GP IIb/IIIa inhibition was tested in several clinical studies that included patients with ACS as well as stable CAD. The landmark trial demonstrating the efficacy of GP IIb/IIIa inhibition in the PCI setting was the Evaluation of IIb/IIIa platelet receptor antagonist 7E3 in Preventing Ischemic Complications (EPIC) trial.[78]

In this study, high-risk patients undergoing balloon angioplasty were randomized to abciximab bolus and infusion, or abciximab bolus alone, or placebo. The group treated with abciximab bolus and infusion had a 35% lower rate of death, MI, or unplanned urgent revascularization at 30 days compared with the placebo group. No significant benefit with abciximab bolus alone was observed, suggesting that shorter duration of platelet inhibition was insufficient to favorably affect clinical outcomes. Major bleeding complications occurred in a very high proportion of patients treated with abciximab. A series of procedural modifications, including front-wall arterial puncture, reducing arterial sheath size (from 8F to 6F), reducing heparin dosing (target activating clotting time [ACT] of 200 to 250 seconds rather than >300 seconds), early sheath removal, and abandoning the use of routine venous sheaths, markedly reduced major bleeding complications (~1%–1.5% in future trials). After the EPIC trial, the Evaluation in PTCA to Improve Long-term Outcome with abciximab GP IIb/IIIa blockade (EPILOG) trial was conducted in patients undergoing balloon angioplasty but who were at a lower risk than patients in EPIC.[79] In EPILOG, abciximab was given with lower doses of weight-adjusted heparin and weight-adjusted infusion of abciximab. This study was stopped prematurely because of a significant reduction in the incidence of death or MI in patients treated with abciximab and also because of acceptable bleeding rates. Similar results were reported in the Evaluation of Platelet GP IIb/IIIa Inhibition in Stenting (EPISTENT) trial which was the first randomized trial examining the use of GP IIb/IIIa inhibitors—in this case, abciximab—among patients undergoing stent placement.[80] The Enhanced Suppression of the Platelet IIb/IIIa Receptor with Integrilin (ESPRIT) trial conducted in patients undergoing coronary stenting using eptifibatide was also terminated early because of the superior efficacy of eptifibatide.[81] Major bleeding was rare but occurred more frequently in eptifibatide-treated patients compared with placebo-treated patients. On the basis of these trials, GP IIb/IIIa inhibitors became a cornerstone in the treatment of patients undergoing PCI because of their ability to improve short-term and long-term outcomes, mostly by reducing the occurrence of peri-procedural MI. Subsequently, however, it was shown that a GP IIb/IIIa inhibitor may no longer benefit patients if they had been pretreated with high-dose clopidogrel, particularly those with stable CAD or in the absence of elevated cardiac enzymes. The first Intracoronary Stenting and Antithrombotic Regimen–Rapid Early Action for Coronary Treatment (ISAR-REACT) trial showed that in 2159 low- to intermediate-risk patients undergoing elective PCI, all of whom had been pretreated for at least 2 hours with a 600-mg loading dose of clopidogrel, there was no benefit to abciximab therapy compared with placebo with respect to the incidence of death, MI, and urgent target vessel revascularization at 30 days ($P = 0.8$).[82] The findings were similar in the Intracoronary Stenting and Antithrombotic Regimen–Is Abciximab a Superior Way to Eliminate Elevated Thrombotic Risk in Diabetics (ISAR-SWEET) trial, the first dedicated randomized trial evaluating GP IIb/IIIa blockade in patients with diabetes scheduled for elective PCI.[83] Overall, these studies suggest that GP IIb/IIIa inhibitors offer no clinical benefit in low- to intermediate-risk patients scheduled for PCI, including those with diabetes, if they have been pretreated with clopidogrel. The incremental benefit of GP IIb/IIIa inhibitors for patients with ACS in the current era of treatment with a high loading dose of clopidogrel before PCI was assessed in the ISAR-REACT 2 trial. This trial randomized 2022 patients with ACS pretreated with clopidogrel 600 mg for at least 2 hours to either abciximab or placebo in the catheterization laboratory at the time of PCI.[84] Abciximab significantly reduced the incidence of the primary endpoint of death, MI, or target vessel revascularization at 30 days, but the benefit of abciximab treatment was limited only to those patients who presented with an elevated troponin. Overall, these findings and those from retrospective analyses of other studies suggest that in the modern era of interventional cardiology using high clopidogrel dosing regimens, GP IIb/IIIa inhibition should be reserved only for high-risk patients with ACS and elevated cardiac biomarkers.

Timing of Glycoprotein IIb/IIIa Administration

Two different timing strategies for the administration of GP IIb/IIIa inhibitors have been used in the large randomized GP IIb/IIIa trials: (1) before angiography ("upstream" treatment) or (2) in the cardiac catheterization laboratory in patients about to undergo PCI ("provisional" treatment). These two strategies were compared in the Early Glycoprotein IIb/IIIa Inhibition in Non–ST Segment Elevation Acute Coronary Syndrome (EARLY ACS) trial, which randomized 9492 invasively managed patients with non–ST elevation ACS to either routine upstream eptifibatide or placebo infusion and provisional eptifibatide after angiography.[85] There were no differences between the groups in the primary endpoint, and patients in the early eptifibatide group had significantly higher rates of bleeding and transfusion. These findings do not support the routine use of upstream GP IIb/IIIa inhibition compared with ad hoc GP IIb/IIIa inhibition in patients with ACS undergoing PCI.

Glycoprotein IIb/IIIa Inhibitors in Primary Percutaneous Coronary Intervention

The use of GP IIb/IIIa inhibitors, in particular abciximab, in STEMI patients undergoing primary PCI is supported by a meta-analysis of 11 randomized trials involving a total 27,115 patients; this study found that the administration of abciximab was associated with a significant reduction in the rate of re-infarction as well as mortality rates at 30 days.[86] However, most studies were conducted in patients who had not been pretreated with clopidogrel. In the Third Bavarian Reperfusion Alternatives Evaluation (BRAVE 3) trial, 800 patients with acute STEMI within 24 hours from symptom onset, all of whom were treated with clopidogrel 600 mg, were randomly assigned to receive either upstream abciximab or placebo.[87] Abciximab was not associated with a reduction in the primary endpoint, infarct size, or ischemic endpoints at 30 days, which argued against the routine use of upstream abciximab in clopidogrel pretreated patients undergoing primary PCI. Strategies of facilitated PCI have been developed on the basis of the premise that time-to-reperfusion is a critical determinant of outcome. A series of pilot, small-sized investigations with GP IIb/IIIa inhibitors measuring surrogate markers of ischemic benefit, such as angiographic flow or ST segment resolution, showed promising results. This series set the basis for larger studies to clarify the safety and efficacy of different regimens of facilitated PCI using GP IIb/IIIa inhibitors alone or in combination with a reduced-dose fibrinolytic. In the Facilitated Intervention with Enhanced Reperfusion Speed to Stop Events (FINESSE) trial, 2452 patients with STEMI presenting ≤6 hours after symptom onset were randomized to receive PCI facilitated with early

TABLE 8-3	Terminology Commonly Used to Describe the Antiplatelet Effect of P2Y12 Inhibitors	
Term	**Sampling Requirements**	**Definition**
High on-treatment reactivity High residual platelet reactivity High post-treatment reactivity	Single blood sample after P2Y12 inhibitor exposure or on maintenance therapy	Platelet reactivity while on P2Y12 inhibitor therapy (e.g., % aggregation, PRU, PRI %, AU·min) that is above a particular threshold
Nonresponsiveness	Blood sample before and after P2Y12 inhibitor exposure	Change in platelet reactivity before and after P2Y12 inhibitor exposure below a particular threshold

ADP, adenosine 5'-diphosphate; *PRU*, P2Y12 reaction units; *PRI*, platelet reactivity index; *AU*, aggregation unit.

abciximab and half-dose reteplase (combination-facilitated), PCI with early abciximab alone (abciximab-facilitated), or primary PCI with abciximab at the time of the procedure.[88] The primary endpoint (composite of death from all causes, ventricular fibrillation occurring >48 hours after randomization, cardiogenic shock, and congestive heart failure during the first 90 days after randomization) occurred in 9.8%, 10.5%, and 10.7% of the patients in the combination-facilitated PCI group, abciximab-facilitated PCI group, and primary PCI group, respectively ($P = 0.55$), without significant differences in mortality. These results do not support the use of a facilitated pharmacologic strategy for reperfusion, with either abciximab alone or abciximab plus reduced-dose reteplase, in anticipation of urgent PCI for patients presenting early with STEMI.[88]

PLATELET FUNCTION TESTING

The pharmacodynamic effect of an anti-platelet agent can be defined by the *response* before and after exposure (i.e., the inhibition of platelet aggregation, or IPA) or by the absolute level of platelet reactivity on therapy, termed *on-treatment reactivity* (Table 8-3). On-treatment reactivity has been proposed as a better measure of thrombotic risk because of the variability in platelet reactivity before treatment.[24] The results of several ex vivo platelet function tests have been associated with clinical outcomes after PCI in clopidogrel-treated patients (Table 8-4). Diagnostic cut-offs to identify at-risk patients using the various tests have been proposed using receiver–operator characteristic curve

TABLE 8-4	Methods to Measure the Effect of P2Y12 Antagonists on Platelet Function	
Assay	**Methodology**	**Units of Measurement/Expression of Results**
LTA	Transmission of light through platelet-rich sample compared with platelet-poor sample after exposure to ADP	• *Maximal aggregation* (%)—measurement of on-treatment reactivity • *Final (late) aggregation* (%)—aggregation 5–6 min after induction of ADP; measurement of on-treatment reactivity • *IPA* (%)—relative change in aggregation before and after exposure • Δ *platelet aggregation* (%)—absolute change in aggregation before and after exposure)
VASP	Phosphorylation status of VASP measured by flow cytometry after incubation with ADP, PGE₁, or both	• *Platelet reactivity index* (%)—ratio of PGE1-stimulated VASP phosphorylation to ADP + PGE1 stimulated VASP phosphorylation (i.e., a measure of the reduction of phosphorylated VASP induced by ADP)
VerifyNow P2Y12	Agglutination of fibrinogen-coated beads by platelets in the presence of ADP (20 mmol) and PGE1	• *P2Y12 reaction units (PRU)*—measurement of on-treatment reactivity • %—One minus the ratio of ADP-induced aggregation with iso-TRAP-induced aggregation; surrogate measure of IPA
Multi-plate Analyzer (MEA)	Change in electrical conductance between a pair of electrodes as platelets adhere after exposure to ADP	• *AU·min*—measurement of on-treatment reactivity
PlateletWorks	Ratio of single platelet counts by cell counter after stimulation with ADP versus baseline (no ADP)	• %—measurement of on-treatment reactivity

Each test listed has been associated with clinical outcomes in clopidogrel-treated patients in at least one study.

LTA, light transmittance aggregometry; *IPA*, inhibition of platelet aggregation; *VASP*, vasodilator-stimulated phosphoprotein phosphorylation analysis; *PRI*, platelet reactivity index; *PRU*, P2Y12 reaction units; *MEA*, multiple electrode aggregometry; *AU*, aggregation units; *TEG*, thromboelastography.

TABLE 8-5	Ongoing or Planned Randomized Clinical Trials of Platelet Function Testing in Patients Undergoing Percutaneous Coronary Intervention							
Trial Name	**Clinical Presentation**	**Device**	**Diagnostic Cut-off**	**Control Group**	**Comparator**	**Primary Endpoint**	**Duration**	**Estimated Enrollment (patients)**
TARGET-PCI (NCT01177592)	Elective PCI	VN P2Y12 Verigene CYP2C19	PRU ≥230	Standard of care (no PFT or genotyping)	Prasugrel 60 mg/10 mg	CV death, MI, ischemic stroke, and urgent TVR	6 mo	1500
TRIGGER-PCI (NCT00910299)	Elective PCI	VN P2Y12	PRU ≥208	Clop 75 mg/day	Prasugrel 60 mg/10-mg	CV death, MI	6 mo	2150
DANTE (NCT00774475)	PCI for ACS	VN P2Y12	PRU ≥240	Clop 75 mg/day	Clop 150 mg/day	CV death, MI, TVR	12 mo	442
ARCTIC (NCT00827411)	PCI for stable CAD or ACS	VN PY12	PRU >235 or % ≤15%	Standard of care (no PFT)	PFT-guided (GP IIb/IIIa inhibitor, oral P2Y12 either clop 150 mg/day or prasugrel 10 mg/day)	Death, MI, stroke, urgent TVR, ST	12 mo	2500

PCI, percutaneous coronary intervention; *NCT*, ClinicalTrials.gov identifier; *ACS*, acute coronary syndrome; *VN*, VerifyNow; *PRU*, P2Y12 reaction units; *Clop*, clopidogrel; *PFT*, platelet function testing; *CV*, cardiovascular; *MI*, myocardial infarction; *ST*, stent thrombosis, *TVR*, target vessel revascularization.

analysis.[24] The results of two small randomized trials suggest that in patients with high on-clopidogrel reactivity, intensified anti-platelet therapy with additional clopidogrel or adjunctive GP IIb/IIIa receptor antagonist therapy may reduce peri-procedural ischemic events.[89,90] The Gauging Responsiveness with A VerifyNow assay–Impact on Thrombosis And Safety (GRAVITAS) trial was a large, multi-center, randomized trial that tested whether prolonged high-dose clopidogrel was superior to standard dose clopidogrel in 2214 patients with high on-treatment reactivity to standard treatment 12 to 24 hours after PCI. Patients were randomly assigned to either an additional clopidogrel loading dose followed by 150 mg daily for 6 months or a placebo loading dose followed by 75 mg daily. The VerifyNow P2Y12 test was used to assess clopidogrel effect; 41% of screened patients met the protocol criteria for high on-treatment reactivity (P2Y12 Reaction Units ≥230). At 6 months, the rate of cardiovascular death, MI, or stent thrombosis did not differ between groups (2.3% vs. 2.3%, HR 1.01 [95% CI: 0.58–1.76]; $P = 0.97$), and high-dose therapy was not associated with increased GUSTO severe or moderate bleeding compared with standard-dose therapy (1.4% vs. 2.3%, HR 0.59 [95% CI 0.31–1.11]; $P = 0.10$). The pharmacodynamic effect of high-dose clopidogrel was statistically significant but relatively modest. A potential benefit of high-dose clopidogrel could not be excluded, given the lower-than-expected event rate and the wide confidence intervals, but a clinically meaningful benefit appeared unlikely.[91] Several other large randomized trials of individualized anti-platelet therapy based on platelet function testing are planned or ongoing (Table 8-5). The results of these trials will help determine whether on-treatment reactivity is a risk marker or a modifiable risk factor in patients undergoing PCI.

Conclusion

Dual anti-platelet therapy with aspirin and a P2Y12 receptor antagonist improves outcomes in patients undergoing coronary stent implantation. There is now an ever-increasing array of options for platelet inhibitor therapy during and after PCI, including newer thienopyridines, oral and intravenous non-thienopyridines, and triple therapy with oral PAR1 antagonists, cilostazol, or intravenous GP IIb/IIIa inhibitors. Genotyping and platelet function testing may provide further insight into the optimal treatment strategy for PCI patients. A comprehensive understanding of the mechanistic underpinnings and trial data for each of these agents and approaches is essential for best clinical practice.

REFERENCES

1. Davi G, Patrono C: Platelet activation and atherothrombosis. N Engl J Med 357:2482–2494, 2007.
2. Varga-Szabo D, Pleines I, Nieswandt B: Cell adhesion mechanisms in platelets. Arterioscler Thromb Vasc Biol 28:403–412, 2008.
3. Dorsam RT, Kunapuli SP: Central role of the P2Y12 receptor in platelet activation. J Clin Invest 113:340–345, 2004.
4. Angiolillo DJ, Capodanno D, Goto S: Platelet thrombin receptor antagonism and atherothrombosis. Eur Heart J 31(1):17–28, 2010.
5. Angiolillo DJ, Ueno M, Goto S: Basic principles of platelet biology and clinical implications. Circ J 74:597–607, 2010.
6. King SB, 3rd, Smith SC, Jr, Hirshfeld JW, Jr, et al: 2007 focused update of the ACC/AHA/SCAI 2005 guideline update for percutaneous coronary intervention: A report of the American College of Cardiology/American Heart Association task force on practice guidelines: 2007 writing group to review new evidence and update the ACC/AHA/SCAI 2005 guideline update for percutaneous coronary intervention, writing on behalf of the 2005 writing committee. Circulation 117:261–295, 2008.
7. Jolly SS, Pogue J, Haladyn K, et al: Effects of aspirin dose on ischaemic events and bleeding after percutaneous coronary intervention: Insights from the PCI-cure study. Eur Heart J 30:900–907, 2009.
8. Anderson JL, Adams CD, Antman EM, et al: ACC/AHA 2007 guidelines for the management of patients with unstable angina/non st-elevation myocardial infarction: A report of the American College of Cardiology/American Heart Association task force on practice guidelines (writing committee to revise the 2002 guidelines for the management of patients with unstable angina/non st-elevation myocardial infarction): Developed in collaboration with the American College of Emergency Physicians, the Society for Cardiovascular Angiography and Iinterventions, and the Society of Thoracic Surgeons: Endorsed by the American Association of Cardiovascular and Pulmonary Rehabilitation and the Society for Academic Emergency Medicine. Circulation 116:e148–304, 2007.
9. Price MJ, Teirstein PS: Dynamics of platelet functional recovery following a clopidogrel loading dose in healthy volunteers. Am J Cardiol 102:790–795, 2008.
10. Leon MB, Baim DS, Popma JJ, et al: A clinical trial comparing three antithrombotic-drug regimens after coronary-artery stenting. Stent anticoagulation restenosis study investigators. N Engl J Med 339:1665–1671, 1998.
11. Bouman HJ, Schomig E, van Werkum JW, et al: Paraoxonase-1 is a major determinant of clopidogrel efficacy. Nat Med 17(1):110–116, 2010.
12. Steinhubl SR, Berger PB, Mann JT, 3rd, et al: Early and sustained dual oral antiplatelet therapy following percutaneous coronary intervention: A randomized controlled trial. JAMA 288:2411–2420, 2002.
13. Steinhubl SR, Berger PB, Brennan DM, et al: Optimal timing for the initiation of pre-treatment with 300 mg clopidogrel before percutaneous coronary intervention. J Am Coll Cardiol 47:939–943, 2006.
14. Montalescot G, Sideris G, Meuleman C, et al: A randomized comparison of high clopidogrel loading doses in patients with non-st-elevation acute coronary syndromes: The ALBION (Assessment of the best Loading dose of clopidogrel to Blunt platelet activation, Inflammation, and Ongoing Necrosis) trial. J Am Coll Cardiol 48:931–938, 2006.
15. von Beckerath N, Taubert D, Pogatsa-Murray G, et al: Absorption, metabolization, and antiplatelet effects of 300-, 600-, and 900-mg loading doses of clopidogrel: Results of the ISAR-choice (Intracoronary Stenting and Antithrombotic Regimen: Choose between 3 high oral doses for immediate clopidogrel effect) trial. Circulation 112:2946–2950, 2005.
16. Price MJ, Coleman JL, Steinhubl SR, et al: Onset and offset of platelet inhibition after high-dose clopidogrel loading and standard daily therapy measured by a point-of-care assay in healthy volunteers. Am J Cardiol 98:681–684, 2006.
17. Aleil B, Jacquemin L, De Poli F, et al: Clopidogrel 150 mg/day to overcome low responsiveness in patients undergoing elective percutaneous coronary intervention. J Am Coll Cardiol Intv 1(6):631–638, 2008.
18. Angiolillo DJ, Bernardo E, Palazuelos J, et al: Functional impact of high clopidogrel maintenance dosing in patients undergoing elective percutaneous coronary interventions. Results of a randomized study. Thromb Haemost 99:161–168, 2008.
19. Gurbel PA, Bliden KP, Hiatt BL, et al: Clopidogrel for coronary stenting: Response variability, drug resistance, and the effect of pretreatment platelet reactivity. Circulation 107:2908–2913, 2003.
20. Hochholzer W, Trenk D, Fromm MF, et al: Impact of cytochrome P450 2C19 loss-of-function polymorphism and of major demographic characteristics on residual platelet function after loading and maintenance treatment with clopidogrel in patients undergoing elective coronary stent placement. J Am Coll Cardiol 55:2427–2434, 2010.
21. Siller-Matula JM, Lang I, Christ G, et al: Calcium-channel blockers reduce the antiplatelet effect of clopidogrel. J Am Coll Cardiol 52:1557–1563, 2008.
22. Price MJ, Nayak KR, Barker CM, et al: Predictors of heightened platelet reactivity despite dual-antiplatelet therapy in patients undergoing percutaneous coronary intervention. Am J Cardiol 103:1339–1343, 2009.
23. Shuldiner AR, O'Connell JR, Bliden KP, et al: Association of cytochrome P450 2C19 genotype with the antiplatelet effect and clinical efficacy of clopidogrel therapy. JAMA 302:849–857, 2009.
24. Bonello L, Tantry US, Marcucci R, et al, Working Group on High On-Treatment Platelet Reactivity: Consensus and future directions on the definition of high on-treatment platelet reactivity to adenosine diphosphate. J Am Coll Cardiol 56:919–933, 2010.

25. Yusuf S, Zhao F, Mehta SR, et al: Effects of clopidogrel in addition to aspirin in patients with acute coronary syndromes without ST-segment elevation. *N Engl J Med* 345:494–502, 2001.
26. Sabatine MS, Cannon CP, Gibson CM, et al: Addition of clopidogrel to aspirin and fibrinolytic therapy for myocardial infarction with st-segment elevation. *N Engl J Med* 352:1179–1189, 2005.
27. Sabatine MS, Cannon CP, Gibson CM, et al: Effect of clopidogrel pretreatment before percutaneous coronary intervention in patients with ST-elevation myocardial infarction treated with fibrinolytics: The PCI-clarity study. *JAMA* 294:1224–1232, 2005.
28. Kandzari DE, Berger PB, Kastrati A, et al: Influence of treatment duration with a 600-mg dose of clopidogrel before percutaneous coronary revascularization. *J Am Coll Cardiol* 44:2133–2136, 2004.
29. Widimsky P, Motovska Z, Simek S, et al, on behalf of the P-tI: Clopidogrel pre-treatment in stable angina: For all patients >6 h before elective coronary angiography or only for angiographically selected patients a few minutes before PCI? A randomized multi-centre trial Prague-8. *Eur Heart J* 29:1495–1503, 2008.
30. Di Sciascio G, Patti G, Pasceri V, et al: Effectiveness of in-laboratory high-dose clopidogrel loading versus routine pre-load in patients undergoing percutaneous coronary intervention: Results of the ARMYDA-5 preload (Antiplatelet therapy for Reduction of MYocardial Damage during Angioplasty) randomized trial. *J Am Coll Cardiol* 56:550–557, 2010.
31. von Beckerath N, Kastrati A, Wieczorek A, et al: A double-blind, randomized study on platelet aggregation in patients treated with a daily dose of 150 or 75 mg of clopidogrel for 30 days. *Eur Heart J* 28:1814–1819, 2007.
32. Mehta SR, Bassand JP, Chrolavicius S, et al: Dose comparisons of clopidogrel and aspirin in acute coronary syndromes. *N Engl J Med* 363:930–942, 2010.
33. Mehta SR, Tanguay JF, Eikelboom JW, et al: Double-dose versus standard-dose clopidogrel and high-dose versus low-dose aspirin in individuals undergoing percutaneous coronary intervention for acute coronary syndromes (current-oasis 7): A randomised factorial trial. *Lancet* 376:1233–1243, 2010.
34. Mehta SR, Yusuf S, Peters RJ, et al: Effects of pretreatment with clopidogrel and aspirin followed by long-term therapy in patients undergoing percutaneous coronary intervention: The PCI-cure study. *Lancet* 358:527–533, 2001.
35. Bhatt DL, Fox KA, Hacke W, et al: Clopidogrel and aspirin versus aspirin alone for the prevention of atherothrombotic events. *N Engl J Med* 354:1706–1717, 2006.
36. Bhatt DL, Flather MD, Hacke W, et al: Patients with prior myocardial infarction, stroke, or symptomatic peripheral arterial disease in the CHARISMA trial. *J Am Coll Cardiol* 49:1982–1988, 2007.
37. Park SJ, Park DW, Kim YH, et al: Duration of dual antiplatelet therapy after implantation of drug-eluting stents. *N Engl J Med* 362:1374–1382, 2010.
38. Kushner FG, Hand M, Smith SC, Jr, et al: 2009 focused updates: ACC/AHA guidelines for the management of patients with ST-elevation myocardial infarction (updating the 2004 guideline and 2007 focused update) and ACC/AHA/SCAI guidelines on percutaneous coronary intervention (updating the 2005 guideline and 2007 focused update): A report of the American College of Cardiology Foundation/American Heart Association task force on practice guidelines. *Circulation* 120:2271–2306, 2009.
39. Mega JL, Close SL, Wiviott SD, et al: Cytochrome P450 polymorphisms and response to clopidogrel. *N Engl J Med* 360:354–362, 2009.
40. Pare G, Mehta SR, Yusuf S, et al: Effects of cyp2c19 genotype on outcomes of clopidogrel treatment. *N Engl J Med* 363:1704–1714, 2010.
41. Holmes DR, Jr, Dehmer GJ, Kaul S, et al: ACCF/AHA clopidogrel clinical alert: Approaches to the FDA "Boxed warning": A report of the American College of Cardiology Foundation task force on clinical expert consensus documents and the American Heart Association endorsed by the Society for Cardiovascular Angiography and Interventions and the Society of Thoracic Surgeons. *J Am Coll Cardiol* 56:321–341, 2010.
42. Mega JL, Close SL, Wiviott SD, et al: Genetic variants in ABCB1 and CYP2C19 and cardiovascular outcomes after treatment with clopidogrel and prasugrel in the triton-timi 38 trial: A pharmacogenetic analysis. *Lancet* 376:1312–1319, 2010.
43. Wallentin L, James S, Storey RF, et al: Effect of CYP2C19 and ABCB1 single nucleotide polymorphisms on outcomes of treatment with ticagrelor versus clopidogrel for acute coronary syndromes: A genetic substudy of the plato trial. *Lancet* 376(9749): 1320–1328, 2010.
44. Gilard M, Arnaud B, Cornily JC, et al: Influence of omeprazole on the antiplatelet action of clopidogrel associated with aspirin: The randomized, double-blind OCLA (Omeprazole CLopidogrel Aspirin) study. *J Am Coll Cardiol* 51:256–260, 2008.
45. Angiolillo DJ, Gibson CM, Cheng S, et al: Differential effects of omeprazole and pantoprazole on the pharmacodynamics and pharmacokinetics of clopidogrel in healthy subjects: Randomized, placebo-controlled, crossover comparison studies. *Clin Pharmacol Ther* 89:65–74, 2011.
46. Cuisset T, Frere C, Quilici J, et al: Comparison of omeprazole and pantoprazole influence on a high 150-mg clopidogrel maintenance dose the PACA (Proton Pump inhibitors and Clopidogrel Aassociation) prospective randomized study. *J Am Coll Cardiol* 54:1149–1153, 2009.
47. Ho PM, Maddox TM, Wang L, et al: Risk of adverse outcomes associated with concomitant use of clopidogrel and proton pump inhibitors following acute coronary syndrome. *JAMA* 301:937–944, 2009.
48. Juurlink DN, Gomes T, Ko DT, et al: A population-based study of the drug interaction between proton pump inhibitors and clopidogrel. *CMAJ* 180(7):713–718, 2009.
49. O'Donoghue ML, Braunwald E, Antman EM, et al: Pharmacodynamic effect and clinical efficacy of clopidogrel and prasugrel with or without a proton-pump inhibitor: An analysis of two randomised trials. *Lancet* 374:989–997, 2009.
50. Bhatt DL, Cryer BL, Contant CF, et al: Clopidogrel with or without omeprazole in coronary artery disease. *N Engl J Med* 363:1909–1917, 2010.
51. Southworth MR, Temple R: Interaction of clopidogrel and omeprazole. *N Engl J Med* 363(20):1901–1917, 1977.
52. Hulot JS, Collet JP, Silvain J, et al: Cardiovascular risk in clopidogrel-treated patients according to cytochrome P450 2C19*2 loss-of-function allele or proton pump inhibitor coadministration: A systematic meta-analysis. *J Am Coll Cardiol* 56:134–143, 2010.
53. American College of Cardiology Foundation Task Force on Expert Consensus Documents, Abraham NS, Hlatky MA, Antman EM, et al: ACCF/ACG/AHA 2010 expert consensus document on the concomitant use of proton pump inhibitors and thienopyridines: A focused update of the accf/acg/aha 2008 expert consensus document on reducing the gastrointestinal risks of antiplatelet therapy and nsaid use. *J Am Coll Cardiol* 56:2051–2066, 2010.
54. Varenhorst C, James S, Erlinge D, et al: Genetic variation of CYP2C19 affects both pharmacokinetic and pharmacodynamic responses to clopidogrel but not prasugrel in aspirin-treated patients with coronary artery disease. *Eur Heart J* 30:1744–1752, 2009.
55. Brandt JT, Payne CD, Wiviott SD, et al: A comparison of prasugrel and clopidogrel loading doses on platelet function: Magnitude of platelet inhibition is related to active metabolite formation. *Am Heart J* 153(66):e9–e16, 2007.
56. Mega JL, Close SL, Wiviott SD, et al: Cytochrome P450 genetic polymorphisms and the response to prasugrel: Relationship to pharmacokinetic, pharmacodynamic, and clinical outcomes. *Circulation* 119:2553–2560, 2009.
57. Jernberg T, Payne CD, Winters KJ, et al: Prasugrel achieves greater inhibition of platelet aggregation and a lower rate of non-responders compared with clopidogrel in aspirin-treated patients with stable coronary artery disease. *Eur Heart J* 27:1166–1173, 2006.
58. Wiviott SD, Trenk D, Frelinger AL, et al: Prasugrel compared with high loading- and maintenance-dose clopidogrel in patients with planned percutaneous coronary intervention: The prasugrel in comparison to clopidogrel for inhibition of platelet activation and aggregation-thrombolysis in myocardial infarction 44 trial. *Circulation* 116:2923–2932, 2007.
59. Wiviott SD, Braunwald E, McCabe CH, et al: Prasugrel versus clopidogrel in patients with acute coronary syndromes. *N Engl J Med* 357:2001–2015, 2007.
60. Antman EM, Wiviott SD, Murphy SA, et al: Early and late benefits of prasugrel in patients with acute coronary syndromes undergoing percutaneous coronary intervention: A TRITON-TIMI 38 (TRial to assess Improvement in Therapeutic Outcomes by optimizing platelet iNhibition with prasugrel-Thrombolysis In Myocardial Infarction) analysis. *J Am Coll Cardiol* 51:2028–2033, 2008.
61. Wiviott SD, Braunwald E, McCabe CH, et al: Intensive oral antiplatelet therapy for reduction of ischaemic events including stent thrombosis in patients with acute coronary syndromes treated with percutaneous coronary intervention and stenting in the TRITON-TIMI 38 trial: A subanalysis of a randomised trial. *Lancet* 371:1353–1363, 2008.
62. Van Giezen J, Nilsson L, Berntsson P, et al: Ticagrelor binds to human P2Y(12) independently from ADP but antagonizes ADP-induced receptor signaling and platelet aggregation. *J Thromb Haemost* 7:1556–1565, 2009.
63. Tantry US, Bliden KP, Wei C, et al: First analysis of the relation between CYP2C19 genotype and pharmacodynamics in patients treated with ticagrelor versus clopidogrel: The onset/offset and respond genotype studies. *Circ Cardiovasc Genet* 3:556–566, 2010.
64. Gurbel PA, Bliden KP, Butler K, et al: Randomized double-blind assessment of the onset and offset of the antiplatelet effects of ticagrelor versus clopidogrel in patients with stable coronary disease: The onset/offset study. *Circulation* 120(25):2577–2585, 2009.
65. Wallentin L, Becker RC, Budaj A, et al: Ticagrelor versus clopidogrel in patients with acute coronary syndromes. *N Engl J Med* 361:1045–1057, 2009.
66. Cannon CP, Harrington RA, James S, et al: Comparison of ticagrelor with clopidogrel in patients with a planned invasive strategy for acute coronary syndromes (PLATO): A randomised double-blind study. *Lancet* 375:283–293, 2010.
67. Cannon CP, Husted S, Harrington RA, et al: Safety, tolerability, and initial efficacy of AZD6140, the first reversible oral adenosine diphosphate receptor antagonist, compared with clopidogrel, in patients with non-ST-segment elevation acute coronary syndrome: Primary results of the DISPERSE-2 trial. *J Am Coll Cardiol* 50:1844–1851, 2007.
68. Storey RF, Bliden KP, Patil SB, et al, on behalf of the ONSET/OFFSET Investigators: Incidence of dyspnea and assessment of cardiac and pulmonary function in patients with stable coronary artery disease receiving ticagrelor, clopidogrel, or placebo in the onset/offset study. *J Am Coll Cardiol* 56:185–193, 2010.
69. Harrington RA, Stone GW, McNulty S, et al: Platelet inhibition with cangrelor in patients undergoing PCI. *N Engl J Med* 361:2318–2329, 2009.
70. Bhatt DL, Lincoff AM, Gibson CM, et al: Intravenous platelet blockade with cangrelor during PCI. *N Engl J Med* 361:2330–2341, 2009.
71. The Thrombin Receptor Antagonist for Clinical Event Reduction in acute coronary syndrome (TRA*CER) trial: Study design and rationale. *Am Heart J* 158:327–334, e324, 2009.
72. Morrow DA, Scirica BM, Fox KA, et al: Evaluation of a novel antiplatelet agent for secondary prevention in patients with a history of atherosclerotic disease: Design and rationale for the thrombin-receptor antagonist in secondary prevention of atherothrombotic ischemic events (TRA 2 degrees P)-TIMI 50 trial. *Am Heart J* 158:335–341, e333, 2009.
73. Goto S, Ogawa H, Takeuchi M, et al: Double-blind, placebo-controlled phase II studies of the protease-activated receptor 1 antagonist E5555 (atopaxar) in Japanese patients with acute coronary syndrome or high-risk coronary artery disease. *Eur Heart J* 31:2601–2613, 2010.
74. Angiolillo DJ, Capranzano P, Goto S, et al: A randomized study assessing the impact of cilostazol on platelet function profiles in patients with diabetes mellitus and coronary artery disease on dual antiplatelet therapy: Results of the OPTIMUS-2 study. *Eur Heart J* 29:2202–2211, 2008.
75. Lee SW, Park SW, Kim YH, et al: Drug-eluting stenting followed by cilostazol treatment reduces late restenosis in patients with diabetes mellitus the DECLARE-diabetes trial (a randomized comparison of triple antiplatelet therapy with dual antiplatelet therapy after drug-eluting stent implantation in diabetic patients). *J Am Coll Cardiol* 51:1181–1187, 2008.
76. Chen KY, Rha SW, Li YJ, et al: Triple versus dual antiplatelet therapy in patients with acute ST-segment elevation myocardial infarction undergoing primary percutaneous coronary intervention. *Circulation* 119:3207–3214, 2009.
77. Boersma E, Harrington RA, Moliterno DJ, et al: Platelet glycoprotein IIb/IIIa inhibitors in acute coronary syndromes: A meta-analysis of all major randomised clinical trials. *Lancet* 359:189–198, 2002.
78. Use of a monoclonal antibody directed against the platelet glycoprotein IIb/IIIa receptor in high-risk coronary angioplasty. The EPIC investigation. *N Engl J Med* 330:956–961, 1994.
79. Platelet glycoprotein IIb/IIIa receptor blockade and low-dose heparin during percutaneous coronary revascularization. The EPILOG investigators. *N Engl J Med* 336:1689–1696, 1997.
80. Randomised placebo-controlled and balloon-angioplasty-controlled trial to assess safety of coronary stenting with use of platelet glycoprotein-IIb/IIIa blockade. *Lancet* 352:87–92, 1998.
81. Novel dosing regimen of eptifibatide in planned coronary stent implantation (ESPRIT): A randomised, placebo-controlled trial. *Lancet* 356:2037–2044, 2000.
82. Kastrati A, Mehilli J, Schuhlen H, et al: A clinical trial of abciximab in elective percutaneous coronary intervention after pretreatment with clopidogrel. *N Engl J Med* 350:232–238, 2004.
83. Mehilli J, Kastrati A, Schuhlen H, et al: Randomized clinical trial of abciximab in diabetic patients undergoing elective percutaneous coronary interventions after treatment with a high loading dose of clopidogrel. *Circulation* 110:3627–3635, 2004.
84. Kastrati A, Mehilli J, Neumann FJ, et al: Abciximab in patients with acute coronary syndromes undergoing percutaneous coronary intervention after clopidogrel pretreatment: The ISAR-REACT 2 randomized trial. *JAMA* 295:1531–1538, 2006.
85. Giugliano RP, White JA, Bode C, et al: Early versus delayed, provisional eptifibatide in acute coronary syndromes. *N Engl J Med* 360:2176–2190, 2009.
86. De Luca G, Suryapranata H, Stone GW, et al: Abciximab as adjunctive therapy to reperfusion in acute ST-segment elevation myocardial infarction: A meta-analysis of randomized trials. *JAMA* 293:1759–1765, 2005.
87. Mehilli J, Kastrati A, Schulz S, et al: Abciximab in patients with acute ST-segment-elevation myocardial infarction undergoing primary percutaneous coronary intervention after clopidogrel loading: A randomized double-blind trial. *Circulation* 119:1933–1940, 2009.
88. Ellis SG, Tendera M, de Belder MA, et al: Facilitated PCI in patients with ST-elevation myocardial infarction. *N Engl J Med* 358:2205–2217, 2008.
89. Bonello L, Camoin-Jau L, Arques S, et al: Adjusted clopidogrel loading doses according to vasodilator-stimulated phosphoprotein phosphorylation index decrease rate of major adverse cardiovascular events in patients with clopidogrel resistance: A multicenter randomized prospective study. *J Am Coll Cardiol* 51:1404–1411, 2008.
90. Valgimigli M, Campo G, de Cesare N, et al: Intensifying platelet inhibition with tirofiban in poor responders to aspirin, clopidogrel, or both agents undergoing elective coronary intervention: Results from the double-blind, prospective, randomized tailoring treatment with tirofiban in patients showing resistance to aspirin and/or resistance to clopidogrel study. *Circulation* 119:3215–3222, 2009.
91. Price MJ, Berger PB, Teirstein PS, et al: Standard- vs. high-dose clopidogrel based on platelet function testing after percutaneous coronary intervention: the GRAVITAS randomized trial. *JAMA* 205(11):1097–1105, 2011.

9

Anticoagulation in Percutaneous Coronary Intervention

DEREK P. CHEW

KEY POINTS

- Despite the innovations in anti-platelet therapies among patients with acute coronary syndrome (ACS) undergoing percutaneous coronary intervention (PCI), careful consideration of anticoagulant therapies during coronary intervention remains important for optimizing clinical outcomes and reducing bleeding risk.

- The relationship between bleeding events and mortality is comparable with those seen with ischemic events. Factors such as age, anemia, low body weight, and renal impairment are well recognized risk factors for bleeding.

- Monitoring levels of anticoagulation with modern agents (enoxaparin or direct thrombin inhibitors) have not been correlated with clinical outcomes.

- Enoxaparin is associated with lower bleeding outcomes, with comparable ischemic events when compared with unfractionated heparin among patients undergoing PCI.

- Bivalirudin has been tested as an alternative to heparin and glycoprotein IIb/IIIa inhibition across the spectrum of patients undergoing PCI and has demonstrated consistent reductions in bleeding with comparable ischemic events.

Introduction

Pharmacologic agents for the prevention of peri-procedural ischemic and bleeding complications during PCI continue to evolve, with robust evidence about the anti-thrombin therapies now available to the interventional cardiologist. Clinical trials support novel direct and indirect inhibitors of thrombin across the diverse array of patients undergoing PCI. Recent data have highlighted the importance of suppressing both ischemic adverse outcomes and bleeding in modern interventional cardiology practice. In addition, some of the newer agents are associated with greater ease of use, less need for monitoring, and less bleeding when used in conjunction with more robust platelet inhibition. This chapter will discuss the modern biology of coagulation and its key effector, thrombin; the monitoring of anticoagulants in the catheterization laboratory (cath-lab), as well as the clinical trial evidence supporting the use of both indirect and direct inhibitors of the thrombin as anticoagulants in PCI.

The Biology of Coagulation: Therapeutic Targets

Conceptualization of the coagulation cascade now recognizes the complex interplay between the coagulative proteins, platelets, and cellular phospholipid membranes. While the subsequent discussion will focus on the coagulative factors that serve as targets in modern antithrombotic regimens, additional effects on platelet-mediated thrombosis and vascular tissue function should not be ignored.

THE CENTRAL ROLE OF THROMBIN

The disruption of endothelial integrity and the expression of prothrombotic molecules such as tissue factor lead to the activation of the soluble coagulative proteins (Fig. 9-1). This amplifying cascade converges on the generation of activated factor X (FXa) and the prothrombinase complex, which leads to the conversion of thrombin from its parent molecule prothrombin. Thrombin generation leads to multiple effects influencing the formation of thrombosis.[1] Specifically, thrombin catalyzes the conversion of fibrin from fibrinogen enabling clot formation while also activating factors V, VIII, and X, thus promoting its own generation. In addition, via direct effects on the protease-activated receptor 1 (PAR1), thrombin promotes platelet activation leading to the expression of CD40 ligand, P-selectin, and the glycoprotein (GP) IIb/IIIa receptor, as well as the secretion of vasoactive agents, including adenosine diphosphate, serotonin, and thromboxane A2 (TXA2). The direct effects of thrombin on endothelial cells and smooth muscle cells result in the expression of adhesion molecules enabling platelet and leukocyte attachment, while its effect on endothelial membrane permeability contributes to the transmigration of the cellular and cytokine-mediated inflammatory response within the vascular wall. While thrombin promotes vasodilation in the intact endothelium, it contributes to vasoconstriction where the endothelium is damaged or denuded. Thrombin also appears to promote fibroblast cytokine production and is mitogenic (Fig. 9-2). However, thrombin has a short circulating half-life, and in the context of a normal endothelial barrier, the effects of thrombin are tightly controlled by a negative feedback mechanism. Anti-thrombin is a single-chain plasma glycoprotein produced by the liver. As an inhibitor of coagulation, this molecule has the ability to bind to thrombin, FXa, and FIXa in equimolar concentrations. Anti-thrombin's action is increased over 1000-fold by the binding of pentasaccharide chain–containing heparins. The pentasaccharide sequence enables the binding of heparins to anti-thrombin and augments the binding affinity of thrombin and the other clotting factors. Anti-thrombin is also activated by the glycosaminoglycan heparin sulfate, which is found on the surface of endothelial cells. Other pathways for the inhibition of thrombin exist. These include the binding of thrombin to thrombomodulin and protein C, together with protein S. This inactivates the upstream coagulation proteins, FVa and FVIIIa, and promotes the release of tissue plasminogen activator (TPA). Hence, thrombin plays a central effector role in the vascular response to balloon-induced and stent-induced vascular injuries and remains an important therapeutic target for the prevention of ischemic complications during PCI. A schematic of the structure of the thrombin molecule is presented in Fig. 9-3. Separate substrate recognition sites are involved in the binding of heparin, fibrinogen, and thrombomodulin, and the catalytic site is responsible for the serine protease activity and is blocked by the direct thrombin inhibitors.

Adverse Events Following Percutaneous Coronary Intervention

Improvements in interventional techniques and refinements in antithrombotic therapies have led to a decline in the incidence of ischemic complications following PCI. Hence, further iterations in antithrombotic strategies can be considered a "two-edged sword," with improved prevention of ischemic complications potentially leading to an increase in bleeding complications (Table 9-1). While the relationship between peri-procedural myocardial infarction (MI) has been widely debated, several studies using data from large-scale clinical

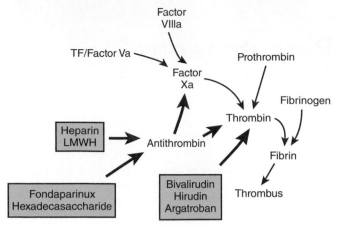

Figure 9-1 Schematic representation of the relationship between coagulation and arterial thrombosis highlighting specific targets for therapy.

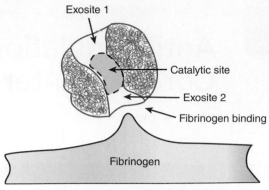

Figure 9-3 Thrombin-binding sites.

trials demonstrate an increased risk of mortality with CK-MB (creatine kinase–muscle brain) elevations of greater than three times the upper limit of normal. In an analysis of patients enrolled in the REPLACE-2 study, CKMB elevation greater than or equal to three times the upper limit of normal was associated with a 3.5-fold increased risk of mortality at 12 months and accounted for 13.2% of all mortality seen by 12 months (Fig. 9-4).[2] Therefore, this underpins the threshold definition for peri-procedural (within 48 hours) MI within many PCI trials of adjunctive pharmacotherapy. Similarly, the clinical significance of postprocedural bleeding events has undergone greater scrutiny over recent years. While these analyses have been hampered by nonstandardized approaches to the recognition and reporting of bleeding events in clinical trials and the lack of routine assessment of blood loss following PCI, a substantial increase in early and late mortality associated with TIMI (thrombolysis in MI) major and minor bleeding following PCI is evident. In an analysis by Kinnard et al., who examined 10,974 patients over a 10-year period, major bleeding events were associated with an approximately 10-fold excess in mortality and approximately three-fold increase in non–Q wave MI.[3] Urgent revascularization and Q-wave MI were also increased. These observations

are supported by analyses of patients enrolled in the ACS trials that report comparable rates of 12-month mortality rates of 12.2% and 11.3% associated with bleeding and ischemic events within 30 days, respectively. In an analysis of the REPLACE-2 study, TIMI minor or major bleeding was associated with a 2.3-fold relative risk of 12 month mortality and accounted for 3.9% of all the mortality observed in this population, while a bleeding event that met the TIMI major criteria was associated with a 6.1-fold increased mortality risk (see Fig. 9-4). In a further analysis of patients with ACS undergoing invasive management in the Acute Catheterization and Urgent Intervention Triage Strategy (ACUITY) study, using a similar methodology, reported that the late mortality hazard was associated with MI, again similar to major bleeding, 2.7-fold and 2.9-fold (both $P < 0.001$), respectively.[4] The clinical characteristics independently associated with bleeding and ischemic events among these ACS patients are displayed in Table 9-2. Within this analysis, more late mortality was attributable to bleeding not associated with coronary artery bypass grafting (CABG) than to MI (11.7% vs. 9.1%), highlighting the greater significance of bleeding events among patients with ACS receiving invasive management. From a clinical perspective, a greater consideration of the relative ischemic and bleeding risks among patients undergoing PCI, especially in the context of ACS, is required when choosing anti-thrombotic agents within modern interventional practice.

Figure 9-2 The central role of thrombin in thrombosis and inflammation. *TF,* tissue factor; *PAR-1,* protease-activating receptor 1.

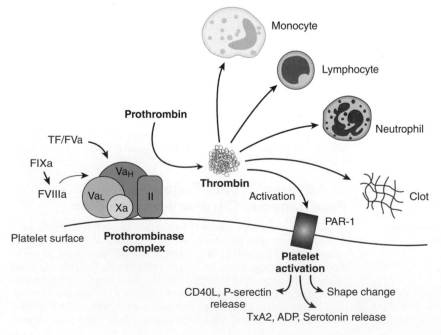

TABLE 9-1	Clinical Endpoint Definitions Bleeding and Ischemia Commonly Used in Clinical Trials of Anti-Thrombotic Agents in Percutaneous Coronary Intervention	
Endpoint	**Definition**
Myocardial infarction (MI) (post-PCI)	Creatine kinase (muscle brain) CK-MB elevation >3 times the upper limit of normal or the development of new Q waves; if CK-MB is unavailable, total CK may be used
Myocardial infarction (post-CABG)	CK-MB elevation >5 times the upper limit of normal and the development of new Q waves, or CK-MB elevation >10 times the upper limit of normal without new Q waves; if CK-MB is unavailable, total CK may be used
Myocardial infarction (non–peri-procedural)	CK-MB elevation >2 times the upper limit of normal or the development of new Q waves; if CK-MB is unavailable, total CK may be used
Thrombolysis in MI (TIMI) major bleeding	Intracerebral hemorrhage, or any bleeding associated with a >5 g/dL fall in hemoglobin or a 15% absolute decrease in hematocrit*
TIMI minor bleeding	Any bleeding event associated with a >3 g/dL fall in hemoglobin or a 10% absolute decline in hematocrit, or a >4 g/dL fall in hemoglobin or a 12% absolute decline in hematocrit in the absence of overt bleeding*
Major bleeding (REPLACE-2 definition)	Intracerebral hemorrhage or any bleeding event associated with a >3 g/dL fall in hemoglobin, or a >4 g/dL fall in hemoglobin in the absence of overt bleeding, or any red cell transfusion of 2 or more units*
GUSTO (Global Use of Strategies to Open Occluded Coronary Arteries) severe or life-threatening bleeding	Intracerebral hemorrhage or bleeding that causes hemodynamic compromise or requires intervention
GUSTO minor bleeding	Bleeding that requires transfusion but does not cause hemodynamic compromise

*All calculations of falls in hemoglobin are adjusted for any transfusion by the Landefeld index

Monitoring of Anticoagulation

Various assays, including the activated clotting time (ACT), ecarin clotting time (ECT), and FXa levels have been used to monitor the therapeutic effect of anticoagulants during PCI. However, the correlation between the levels achieved with these assays with various agents and clinical events have only been studied retrospectively. Furthermore, the relationship between the assay level achieved and clinical events is also influenced by the concomitant anti-platelet therapy. Hence, in the context of unfractionated heparin therapy, increasing levels of ACT are associated with a modest reduction in peri-procedural ischemic events but a moderate increase in bleeding events.[5] In contrast, when heparin is given with abciximab, ischemic events are fewer; there is little further reduction in events at higher ACT levels but a substantial increase in bleeding events occurs (Fig. 9-5). The ACT assay is not as useful for monitoring the efficacy of enoxaparin and the other low-molecular-weight heparins (LMWHs), with lesser degrees of

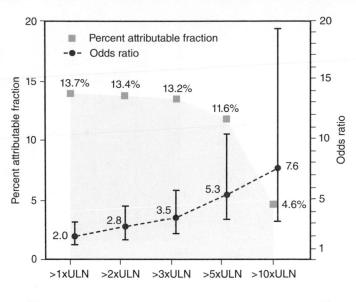

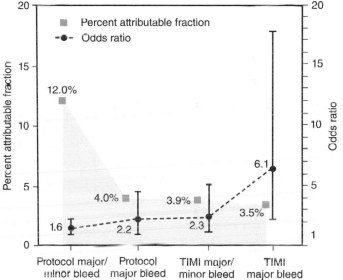

Figure 9-4 The relationship between ischemic events, bleeding events, and late mortality.

prolongation observed in this assay.[6] Traditional laboratory-based FXa assays also remain impractical for cath-lab use. The ENOX assay (Rapidpoint) is a whole-blood, point-of-care assay that correlates with laboratory enoxaparin-induced anti-FXa levels.[7] The Evaluating Enoxaparin Clotting times (ELECT) study explored the relationship

TABLE 9-2	Clinical Factors Associated with Myocardial Infarction and Non–Coronary Artery Bypass Grafting–Related Bleeding Within 30 Days Among Patients with Acute Coronary Syndrome Undergoing Early Invasive Management				
Myocardial Infarction			**Non-CABG Major Bleeding**		
Biomarker elevation	1.66 (1.40–1.97)	$P < 0.001$	Male gender	0.42 (0.36–0.50)	$P < 0.001$
Family history of CAD	1.48 (1.27–1.73)	$P < 0.001$	Anemia (HCT <39% in males and <36% in females)	1.96 (1.63–2.36)	$P < 0.001$
Age per 5 years	1.08 (1.04–1.11)	$P < 0.001$	Age per 5 years	1.14 (1.10–1.19)	$P < 0.001$
ST deviation ≥1.0 mm	1.38 (1.18–1.61)	$P < 0.001$	ST deviation ≥1.0 mm	1.31 (1.10–1.54)	$P < 0.01$
Prior MI	1.28 (1.08–1.50)	$P < 0.001$	Prior PCI	0.70 (0.–0.84)	$P < 0.01$
			Creatinine per 0.1 mg/dL	1.08 (1.05–1.10)	$P < 0.001$
			White cell count per	1.08 (1.05–1.11)	$P < 0.001$
			Prior CVA	1.60 (1.21–2.10)	$P < 0.001$

CABG, coronary artery bypass grafting; *CAD*, coronary artery disease; MI, myocardial infarction; *HCT*, hematocrit; *PCI*, percutaneous coronary intervention; *CVA*, cerebrovascular accident.[4]

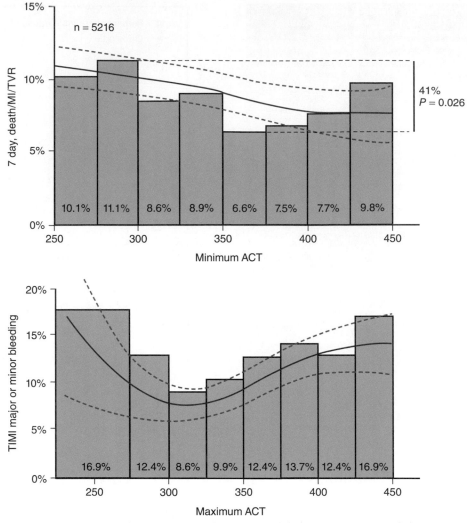

Figure 9-5   Relationship between ACT and outcome with heparin. *ACT,* activated clotting time.

between the ENOX assay results and clinical outcomes among 445 patients receiving subcutaneous enoxaparin, intravenous enoxaparin, or both prior to PCI.[8] There was a nonsignificant and nonlinear association between the ENOX times and ischemic complications, whereas bleeding events increased with greater ENOX times. ENOX times of between 250 and 450 seconds (correlating with anti-FXa levels of between 0.8 and 1.8 international units per milliliters [IU/mL]) for intra-procedural anticoagulation and levels of less than 200 seconds to 250 seconds for sheath removal have been recommended when enoxaparin is used. Similarly, the Hemonox, another point-of-care test of anti-FXa levels, appears to be able to detect suboptimal levels of anti-FXa (<0.5 IU/ml) with modest sensitivity.[9,10] The clinical usefulness of these tests remains to be determined, and they are not in routine clinical use at this time. In contrast to both heparin and LMWH, bivalirudin is generally associated with greater prolongation of ACT. This effect appears to occur in a dose-dependent manner, though no gradient of benefit with respect to ischemic or bleeding events has been observed across the range of ACT values recorded at the doses studied in clinical trials.[11] Furthermore, despite the higher ACT levels, lower rates of bleeding have been consistently observed with bivalirudin, highlighting the limited value of ACT in predicting clinical events with this agent. Hence, ACT provides qualitative but not quantitative information about bivalirudin and is only of value in determining if this agent was effectively administered. As a possible clinical alternative, the monitoring of these agents with the ECT may be more appropriate.

Measurements based on this test appear to better correlate with plasma bivalirudin and hirudin levels.[12] Whether the levels based on this assay relate to clinical events and evolve to recommended targets for therapy remains to be established.

Unfractionated Heparin

HEPARIN PHARMACOLOGY

Unfractionated heparin is a heterogeneous group glycosaminoglycans of various lengths (5000 to 30,000 daltons, mean 15,000 daltons), which exhibit a high affinity for anti-thrombin. This binding augments anti-thrombin's enzymatic inactivation of thrombin, FXa, and FIXa, with the effects on thrombin being the most pronounced. Because of heparin's reliance on anti-thrombin for a therapeutic effect, it is considered an indirect anti-thrombin. The anti-thrombin effect of heparin requires the simultaneous binding of heparin, anti-thrombin, and thrombin. Consequently, molecules with less than18 saccharides lack sufficient length to simultaneously span both anti-thrombin and thrombin and do not exhibit any anti-thrombin activity. These smaller molecules account for up to two thirds of unfractionated heparin preparations. Thrombin inactivation by heparin also occurs via heparin co-factor II, an enzyme with specific activity for thrombin, but requires much higher heparin levels than the heparin–anti-thrombin pathway. However, the anti-FXa effects of heparin are not dependent on simultaneous binding of both anti-thrombin and FXa and therefore anti-thrombin effects are observed across a wider range of saccharide chain lengths. Pharmacokinetic heterogeneity is also observed, as larger heparin molecules are cleared more rapidly, and the attenuation of heparin's anti-thrombin effect is faster relative to its anti-FXa effect. Hence, the activated partial thromboplastin time (APTT) and in vivo anticoagulant effect have an imperfect correlation. The elimination of unfractionated heparin is initially through rapid but saturable metabolism within the endothelial cells and macrophages (zero-order kinetics) followed by slower renal clearance (first-order kinetics). The plasma half-life depends on the dose administered and is approximately 1 hour at doses of 100 IU/kg. In the context of excessive dosing, perforation, or excessive bleeding, unfractionated heparin can be reversed by the administration of protamine. However, the clinical efficacy, safety, and efficacy of this strategy has not been well established. Increasingly, the limitations of heparin have been appreciated. These limitations include the activation of platelets; a dependence on anti-thrombin levels; nonspecific binding to plasma protein; an inability to inhibit clot-bound thrombin; and direct binding to platelet factor 4 contributing to heparin-induced thrombocytopenia (HIT) in 1% to 3% of treated patients. Platelet activation by heparin is evidenced by an increase in the expression of platelet surface adhesion molecules. Nonspecific binding to plasma proteins secreted by platelets and endothelial cells in the setting of inflammation and thrombosis may also contribute to reduced bioavailability. In addition, the heparin–anti-thrombin complex results in a large molecular structure that has limited capacity to access thrombin and FXa bound within a thrombus.

CLINICAL DATA WITH UNFRACTIONATED HEPARIN

Worldwide, unfractionated heparin remains the mainstay anticoagulant for patients undergoing PCI. Despite this fact, there are no prospective randomized data to demonstrate the efficacy of this agent compared with placebo, and current dosing recommendations are empiric. Nevertheless, clinical experience and anecdotal evidence clearly demonstrate the need for some degree of anticoagulation in the setting of balloon-induced and stent-induced vascular injuries. In the absence of prospective randomized data, several studies point toward the benefits and risks associated with greater degrees of anticoagulation with heparin in PCI. Early case control studies in the era of PTCA suggest that patients experiencing acute vessel closure and death or urgent revascularization had lower ACT levels than those not experiencing these complications. Similarly, among 403 patients randomized to either intravenous (IV) heparin 5000 units or 20,000 units IV before balloon angioplasty, those receiving the higher dose experienced a nonsignificant reduction in the rates of death, MI, acute vessel closure, and repeat interventions (8.0% vs. 12.5%, P = ns [not significant]) but an increased rate of bleeding complications (20% vs. 6%, $P < 0.001$).[13] Weight-adjusted dosing has been studied as a strategy to reduce the variability in dose response. In a 400-patient randomized trial assessing weight-adjusted dosing compared with higher fixed dosing, the weight-adjusted dosing strategy was not associated with superior efficacy or safety, though earlier sheath removal was made possible. Nevertheless, a pooled analysis of data from patients treated with heparin only in several randomized clinical trials suggested that there is a gradient of benefit associated with increasing degrees of anticoagulation with commensurate risk of bleeding events. This analysis suggested that ACT levels in excess of 350 seconds are associated with fewer ischemic events, though bleeding rates also increase at these levels.[5] Such levels of anticoagulation are not required when concomitant GP IIb/IIIa inhibition is used, and the relevance of these data in the context of pretreatment with thienopyridines is not known.[14] These observations have also been difficult to demonstrate in smaller studies where the initial heparin doses and, therefore, the ACT levels achieved were lower. In contrast, available data do not support the use of prolonged heparin infusions following PCI for the prevention of subacute ischemic events, where no significant reduction in ischemic events is observed but

there is a clear excess in bleeding events and increased length of hospital stay. This is especially true for patients receiving GP IIb/IIIa inhibition.

Low-Molecular-Weight Heparin

PHARMACOLOGY

The LMWHs are produced by chemical or enzymatic depolymerization of unfractionated heparin resulting in heparin fragments with a mean molecular weight that is approximately 30% of most unfractionated heparin preparations. However, the molecular sizes of heparin molecules still vary, and therefore anticoagulant characteristics remain heterogeneous, though more predictable, when compared with heparin. The principal effect of the LMWHs is the inhibition of anti-FXa via anti-thrombin. In comparison with unfractionated heparin, the LMWHs demonstrate a more consistent dose response as well as less platelet activation; they also demonstrate platelet factor 4 interactions that lead to less HIT. LMWHs have a longer half-life compared with unfractionated heparin. Clearance is by renal excretion, however, and the biologic half-life is increased in patients with renal failure (Table 9-2). Several small studies have explored the various dosing strategies for the use of enoxaparin in PCI. Adequate levels of anti-FXa were observed among patients 2 to 8 hours following subcutaneous dosing of enoxaparin 1 mg/kg twice per day and among those receiving an additional 0.3 mg/kg intravenous dose 8 to 12 hours following subcutaneous dosing at 1.0 mg/kg.[15] Other investigators have suggested that doses as low as 0.5 mg/kg of IV enoxaparin may be safe and efficacious and enable easier sheath management, though a quarter of the patients in this study also received a GP IIb/IIIa inhibitor. Some evidence suggests that enoxaparin may be reversed by the intravenous administration of protamine, but these data are limited.

CLINICAL DATA WITH ENOXAPARIN

Among the available LMWHs, the majority of the data supports the use of enoxaparin in PCI. The initial reported experience with enoxaparin, specifically in PCI, includes a series of studies performed by the National Investigators Collaborating on Enoxaparin (NICE) study group. These studies explored enoxaparin without abciximab (NICE-1) and with abciximab (NICE-4) among patients undergoing PCI and compared these historically with the arms of the EPILOG and EPSI-TENT trials, respectively (Fig. 9-6). In addition, the NICE-3 registry addressed outcomes among patients with ACS receiving the various IV GP IIb/IIIa inhibitors, with use of PCI being left to the discretion of the investigator. The NICE-1 registry assessed enoxaparin 1.0 mg/kg intravenously without a GP IIb/IIIa inhibition before coronary intervention in 828 patients undergoing elective or urgent PCI. The primary study endpoint was in-hospital and 30-day major hemorrhage. Minor bleeding, the need for any transfusion, and the composite ischemic endpoint of death, MI, and urgent revascularization were also examined. Key exclusion criteria were acute MI within 24 hours, recent fibrinolysis (3 days), prior LMWH use within 12 hours, thrombocytopenia less than 100,000 per cubic centimeter (cc), and serum creatinine greater than 2.5 milligram per deciliter (mg/dL). In this patient group, at least one stent was placed in 85% of patients, aspirin was administered to all patients, and clopidogrel pretreatment was left to the discretion of the treating interventionalist. Arteriotomy closure devices were not permitted, and the protocol was prescriptive with respect to the time for sheath removal (4–6 hours). In the study without concomitant GP IIb/IIIa inhibition, major hemorrhage occurred in 1.1% of patients, and minor hemorrhage and transfusions occurred in 6.2% and 2.7% of patients, respectively. The composite ischemic endpoint of death, MI, and urgent revascularization at 30 days was observed in 7.7% of patients, with MI occurring in 5.4% of cases.[16] In the very similar NICE-4 protocol, 818 patients received enoxaparin 0.75 mg/kg and abciximab 0.25 mg/kg bolus and 0.125 microgram per kilogram per

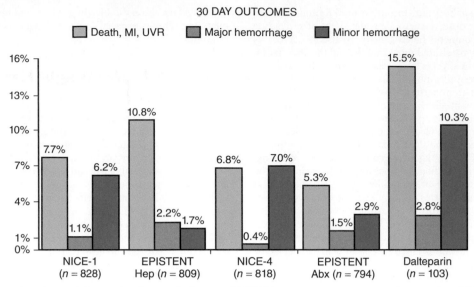

Figure 9-6 Observational studies with low-molecular-weight heparin (LMWH) in percutaneous coronary intervention (PCI) contrasted with events in EPISTENT (Evaluation of Platelet IIb/IIIa Inhibitor for Stenting) trial.

minute (mcg/kg/min) infusion. In this study, 88% of patients received a bare metal stent (BMS). Again, the use of vessel closure devices was not permitted. Inclusion and exclusion criteria and clinical endpoint definitions were similar to those used in the NICE-1 study. In NICE-4, major hemorrhage and minor hemorrhage were reported in 0.4% and 7.0% of patients, respectively, with transfusions required in 1.8% of cases. The composite ischemic endpoint of death, MI, and urgent revascularization at 30 days occurred in 6.8% of patients, suggesting that enoxaparin may confer a similar level of efficacy and safety as observed with unfractionated heparin in the context of abciximab therapy.[16] Again, employing a noncontrolled observational design, the NICE-3 study reported bleeding and ischemic events among 671 patients presenting with ACS and treated with enoxaparin and tirofiban, eptifibatide, or abciximab.[17] Within this population, 43% underwent PCI. By 30 days, the composite endpoint of death, MI, and urgent revascularization was observed in 1.6%, 5.1%, and 6.8% of patients, respectively. The primary endpoint of non-CABG–related major bleeding was reported in 1.9% of patients by 30 days. While numerically higher than the rates observed in other studies, the interpretation of these results is hampered by the noncontrolled nature of the study design. Other observational data in the setting of acute coronary syndromes also suggest that enoxaparin is safe and efficacious among patients with ACS undergoing PCI. A subgroup analysis of 4676 patients undergoing PCI in the ExTRACT-TIMI 25 study suggested that the incidence of death or MI may be reduced more with enoxaparin, compared with heparin, among patients who have received fibrinolysis for ST elevation MI (STEMI) (enoxaparin 10.7% vs. heparin 13.8%, $P = 0.001$), with no significant increase in bleeding complications.[18] Similarly, a larger subgroup analysis of 4687 patients with unstable angina and non–ST elevation ACS undergoing PCI in the Superior Yield of the New Strategy of Enoxaparin, Revascularization and Glycoprotein IIb/IIIa Inhibitors (SYNERGY) study observed a comparable rate of 30-day death or MI with a slight increase in bleeding events.[19]

Two randomized studies have been more optimally designed to examine the relative clinical risks and benefits of enoxaparin among patients undergoing PCI. The CRUISE study randomized 261 patients undergoing elective or urgent PCI to enoxaparin 1 mg/kg IV or heparin, with all patients receiving eptifibatide.[20] This small study reported no difference in the rate of bleeding complications or angiographic complications (6.3% vs. 6.2%, $P = $ ns) during the procedure. Similarly, there were no differences in ischemic endpoints at 48 hours

or 30 days. Several other randomized studies have been too small to demonstrate clear benefits with enoxaparin compared with heparin, with a meta-analysis of these studies demonstrating no difference in the incidence of bleeding or ischemia.[21] The largest study, to date, directly addressing enoxaparin use among patients undergoing PCI was the Safety and Efficacy of Intravenous Enoxaparin in Elective Percutaneous Coronary Intervention: an International Randomized Evaluation (STEEPLE) trial.[22] This study randomized 3528 patients to either IV enoxaparin 0.5 mg/kg ($n = 1070$), IV enoxaparin 0.75 mg/kg ($n = 1228$), or ACT adjusted unfractionated heparin ($n = 1230$). Again, the primary endpoint was non-CABG–related, protocol-defined bleeding by 48 hours (but not using the TIMI or GUSTO [Global Use of Strategies to Open Occluded Coronary Arteries] scales), with the ischemic endpoints at 30 days also reported as secondary endpoints. In this study, GP IIb/IIIa inhibition and thienopyridines were used in approximately 40% and 95% of patients, respectively, with drug-eluting stents (DESs) deployed in 57% of patients; 16% of cases involved multi-vessel intervention. At 48 hours, enoxaparin was associated with a lower rate of protocol-defined major and minor bleeding (enoxaparin 0.5 mg/kg: 6.0% vs. enoxaparin 0.75 mg/kg: 6.6% vs. heparin: 8.7%, $P = 0.0014$), with most of the benefit driven by reductions in major bleeding (enoxaparin 0.5 mg/kg: 1.2% vs. enoxaparin 0.7 5 mg/kg: 1.2% vs. heparin: 2.8%, $P = 0.004$ and $P = 0.007$). However, no difference was seen when the TIMI or GUSTO definition of bleeding was applied. Nor was there a difference in the rate of transfusion. The composite endpoint of death, MI, and urgent revascularization at 30 days favored the unfractionated heparin arm, though these differences did not reach statistical significance and met a broad noninferiority boundary (Fig. 9-7). These results suggest that enoxaparin is a viable alternative to heparin with modest reductions in bleeding risk. To date, no randomized studies have examined the use of enoxaparin versus heparin among patients undergoing primary PCI. In an observational comparison of enoxaparin versus heparin in the FINESSE study of primary PCI versus facilitated PCI, patients receiving enoxaparin experienced a lower rate of death, recurrent MI, and urgent revascularization or refractory ischemia, with a lower overall rate of all-cause mortality at 90 days (3.8% vs. 5.6%, $P = 0.046$).[23] In this study, the choice of anticoagulant was prespecified at each centre, rather than randomized. Similarly, the nonrandomized comparison of outcomes from the MITRA-plus registry of STEMI patients undergoing primary PCI suggested that when compared with heparin, enoxaparin is associated with a hazard ratio of 0.42 (0.2–0.8, $P < 0.001$) for death or recurrent MI,

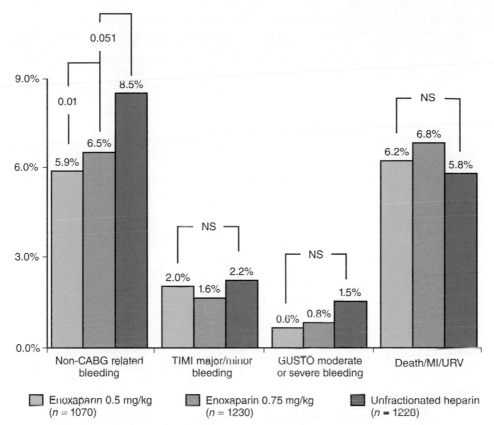

Figure 9-7 Protocol-defined major bleeding and ischemic events in the STEEPLE (Safety and Efficacy of Enoxaparin in Percutaneous Coronary Intervention Patients) trial.

with this benefit being evident with or without the concurrent use of GP IIb/IIIa inhibition.[24]

CLINICAL DATA WITH DALTEPARIN

Data on dalteparin use is limited, with disappointing results suggesting that further clinical development of this agent for use in interventional procedures is unlikely. In a dose ranging study of 107 patients, 4 patients received dalteparin 120 U/kg less than 8 hours before PCI and received either an additional 40 U/kg (1 patient) or no further LMWH (3 patients). The remaining patients were randomized to either 40 U/kg IV (27 patients) or 60 U/kg IV (76 patients) at the beginning of the procedure, with all patients receiving aspirin and abciximab. However, three early thrombotic events led to the decision to unblind the study and terminate the 40-U/kg arm. In this trial, death, MI (Creatine Kinase levels >3 times Upper Limit of Normal), and urgent revascularization was observed in 15.5% of patients overall, and major hemorrhage and transfusion each occurred in 2.8% of patients. Even though the trial was inadequately powered to fully evaluate the clinical usefulness of this agent in PCI, these event rates are higher than commonly seen in modern-day PCI trials; more adequately controlled studies with this agent have not been performed.

PENTASACCHARIDE AND HEXADECASACCHARIDE

Fondaparinux, a pentasaccharide, as well as hexadecasaccharide are both synthetic molecules that mimic the biologically active sequence of heparin in its interaction with anti-thrombin. Given that these molecules are short, their principal effect is the inactivation of FXa. Similarly, these agents have relatively long half-lives and so enable once-daily dosing regimens. These agents are not reversed by protamine and require the administration of FVII concentrates. Given their pharmacokinetic characteristics, the initial interest in these agents has

been for the treatment of patients presenting with ACS. The only large-scale trial evaluating a substantial number of patients undergoing coronary intervention, to date, is the Organization to Assess Strategies in Acute Ischemic Syndromes (OASIS)-5 trial.[25] In this trial of 20,078 patients with ACS randomized to enoxaparin or fondaparinux, 6207 patients underwent coronary intervention. Among these patients, no differences in ischemic complications were observed, though a benefit with fondaparinux was evident with respect to bleeding events, when compared with enoxaparin (enoxaparin: 8.8% vs. fondaparinux: 3.3%, $P < 0.001$). However, a substantial number of patients undergoing PCI received unfractionated heparin in both arms of the study. Furthermore, the protocol was modified during the study to ensure the use of heparin in the fondaparinux arm because of a higher rate of catheter-related thrombosis (enoxaparin: 0.5% vs. fondaparinux: 1.3%, $P = 0.001$). Dedicated randomized trials of these agents, either as stand-alone anti-thrombotic strategies or in combination with other anti-thrombins and anti-platelet agents in PCI, are still awaited.

Direct Thrombin Inhibitors

PHARMACOLOGY

The direct thrombin inhibitor hirudin found in the saliva of the medicinal leech (*Hirudo medicinalis*) is the prototypical molecule of this class. Hirudin is a 65-amino-acid protein that forms a stable noncovalent complex with thrombin. With two domains—the NH_2 terminal core domain and the COOH terminal tail—the hirudin molecule inhibits the catalytic site and the anion-binding exosite in a two-step process. An initial ionic interaction leads to a rearrangement of the thrombin–hirudin complex and the subsequent formation of a tighter irreversible 1:1 bond. This complex and tight binding of hirudin to thrombin helps account for the highly specific effect of hirudin on thrombin. Generally, the direct thrombin inhibitor molecules are smaller than the indirect thrombin inhibitors and demonstrate greater efficacy for the inhibition of clot-bound thrombin, in addition to their effects on fluid-phase thrombin. Two forms of recombinant hirudin (r-hirudin) have been developed, one with a sulfated Tyr63 and the other without this change. The nonsulfated tyrosine molecule appears to have a 10-fold lower affinity for thrombin compared with the naturally occurring compound. The hirudin–thrombin interaction offers a method for categorizing other direct thrombin inhibitors, which have been divided into univalent and bivalent molecules. The univalent molecules dabigatran, agatroban, and melagatran inhibit only the catalytic site and inactivate only fibrin-bound thrombin. The thrombin inhibition provided by these agents is less robust than that observed with hirudin, as dissociation leads to some residual thrombin activity. Of note, argatroban, the only one of these agents approved for use in PCI, binds to the apolar binding site adjacent to the catalytic site and provides competitive inhibition. The bivalent molecules recombinant hirudin and bivalirudin bind to the catalytic site and at least to one of the exosites. While the interaction between hirudin and thrombin is irreversible, the inhibition provided by bivalirudin is more transient. Bivalirudin is a synthetic 20-amino-acid molecule with two domains. These are targeted toward the anion-binding exosite and calaytic sites and are linked by four glycine spacers. Given the shorter amino-acid chain length compared with hirudin, bivalirudin exhibits less avid ionic binding. Furthermore, cleavage of the bivalirudin molecule at the Arg–Pro bond of the amino-terminal extension by thrombin itself enables the release of the thrombin active site for further thrombotic activity. This, in part, accounts for the shorter half-life of bivalirudin compared with hirudin and may also account for some of the reduced bleeding risk seen with this agent. Several other direct thrombin inhibitors have been developed in addition to those discussed, but so far, these have not found a clinical role in the cath-lab. All currently available agents approved for use in PCI require parenteral administration. With the exception of argatroban, these agents are cleared renally, and clearance is attenuated in the setting of reduced renal function. In the setting of excessive dosing or bleeding, these agents can be removed by hemofiltration. Argatroban is primarily eliminated through the hepatic metabolism, and dose reduction is required in the setting of hepatic dysfunction. However, renal function also influences dosing. Bivalirudin also undergoes proteolysis within the plasma, thus contributing to its shorter half-life and relatively constant elimination characteristics even among patients with mild to moderate renal impairment (see Table 9-2). Nevertheless, dose attenuation is required among patients with creatinine clearance that is less than 30 mL/min. These agents are not reversed by protamine. Nonspecific measures such as transfusion of blood products, including fresh frozen plasma, and local measures are recommended in the context of active bleeding.

CLINICAL DATA WITH DIRECT THROMBIN INHIBITORS

Direct thrombin inhibitors, in particular bivalirudin, have emerged as a useful alternative to heparin as anticoagulants for patients undergoing PCI, predominantly as an alternative to GP IIb/IIIa inhibition. Early trials with hirudin focused on the prevention of re-stenosis in the setting of balloon angioplasty. While no anti–re-stenotic effect was evident, reductions in early ischemic events were noted. More recently, these agents have been found to have a role in the management of patients with HIT (argatroban and bivalirudin), and the most recent data suggest that improved thrombin inhibition with bivalirudin enables sparing of GP IIb/IIIa inhibition in the majority of patients undergoing PCI.

Hirudin

The first large-scale randomized trial of direct thrombin inhibition in PCI was the Hirudin in a European Trial Versus Heparin In the Prevention of Restenosis after PTCA (HELVETICA) trial. In this study, 1141 patients with unstable angina undergoing balloon angioplasty received either of two dose regimens of hirudin or unfractionated heparin.

Patients receiving intravenous hirudin experienced a reduction in early cardiac events within 96 hours (hirudin arms combined, relative risk [RR] 0.61; 95% CI, 0.41–0.90; $P = 0.023$). However, in this study, the primary endpoint was event-free survival at 7 months; for this endpoint, there were no differences among the three treatment arms, and similar rates of re-stenosis were observed. Furthermore, in the angioplasty substudy of patients with STEMI in the Global Utilization of Strategies to Open Occluded Coronary Arteries IIb (GUSTO IIb) trial, 503 patients undergoing PTCA were randomized to hirudin or heparin. Hirudin resulted in a 23% ($P = $ ns) reduction in death, MI, or stroke at 30 days. A benefit with hirudin in the setting of PCI is also evident from other observational studies. Among all patients undergoing PCI in the GUSTO IIb (ST elevation [randomized] and non–ST elevation ACS [physician discretion]) a reduction in 30-day MI among the hirudin group ($n = 672$) compared with those receiving heparin ($n = 738$) was seen (4.9% vs. 7.6%, $P = 0.04$), and a nonsignificant increase in bleeding was observed.[26] Similarly, an analysis of the OASIS-2 trial of patients with unstable angina randomized to heparin or hirudin, which assessed outcomes in 172 patients undergoing PCI within 72 hours of randomization came to similar conclusions.[27] Though the study was observational and relatively small, the rate of death or MI at 96 hours was shown to be lower among hirudin-treated patients compared with those receiving heparin (6.4% vs. 21.4%, OR 0.30; 95% CI 0.10–0.88) and 35 days (6.4% vs. 22.9%, OR 0.25; 95% CI 0.07–0.86). However, caution should be exercised when interpreting this nonrandomized comparison. Nevertheless, a meta-analysis of direct thrombin inhibition, which drew data from 2 PCI trials and 9 ACS trials ($N = $ 35,970) and included data on bivalirudin and univalent direct thrombin inhibitors, reported a beneficial effect linked to the timing of PCI.[28] Among patients undergoing PCI with 72 hours of randomization, direct thrombin inhibitors were associated with lower rates of death or MI (OR 0.66; 95% CI 0.48–0.91) compared with heparin. In this analysis, the benefits observed in the PCI trials were driven by a reduction in bleeding (Fig. 9-8). In contrast, a more modest effect was documented when PCI was delayed after 72 hours. No benefit with these agents over heparin was observed in the context of conservative management.

Argatroban

For the widespread application to patients undergoing PCI, agatroban has not currently been studied in large-scale randomized clinical trials. However, as an alternative to heparin among patients with HIT, a small case series totaling 151 patients suggested that this agent is safe.[29,30] Similarly, a small nonblinded, uncontrolled study of argatroban administered to patients treated with abciximab ($n = 150$) and eptifibatide ($n = 2$) suggested that the combinations of these agents is at least feasible.[31]

Bivalirudin

Clinical studies on bivalirudin constitute the majority of modern evidence supporting direct thrombin inhibition in PCI. The first large-scale study with bivalirudin in the context of balloon angioplasty was with the Bivalirudin Angioplasty Study (BAT).[32] The report of the study was first published in 1995, but the trial was conducted before the era of coronary stenting, thienopyridine use, and intravenous GP IIb/IIIa inhibition. In the context of urgent or elective angioplasty, 4312 were patients randomized to bivalirudin 1 mg/kg bolus and 2.5 mg/kg/hr infusion or high-dose unfractionated heparin. A subgroup of 741 patients who had experienced MI underwent stratified randomization to the same treatment arms. Randomization to bivalirudin provided a 22% reduction (6.2% vs. 7.9%, $P = 0.039$) in the composite endpoint of death, MI, or urgent revascularization, and a 62% reduction (3.9% vs. 9.7%, $P < 0.001$) in major bleeding events at 7 days. Among this stratified post-MI subgroup, the triple ischemic endpoint was reduced by 46% by 90 days (OR 0.54; 95% CI 0.36–0.81, $P = 0.009$). However, the advent of GP IIb/IIIa inhibition demanded a reconsideration of bivalirudin's role in patients receiving modern antiplatelet therapies in PCI. The CACHET A/B/C studies explored the role

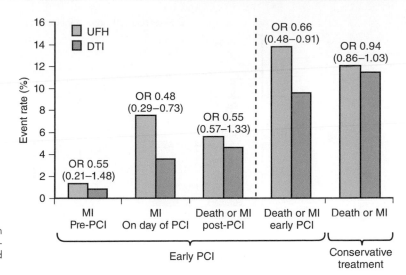

Figure 9-8 The relative impact of direct thrombin inhibition in invasive and conservative management of acute coronary syndromes. *DTI*, direct thrombin inhibitor, *UFH*, unfractionated heparin.

of bivalirudin with either routine or provisional use of abciximab use in 208 patients undergoing coronary angioplasty and stenting, and the studies demonstrated a promising reduction in bleeding events and no increase in ischemic events.[33] The Randomized Evaluation of PCI Linking Angiomax to reduced Clinical Events (REPLACE)-1 study employed a less prescriptive design, randomizing 1056 patients undergoing PCI to either bivalirudin, 0.75 mg/kg and 1.75 mg/kg/hr or heparin 60 to 70 U/kg with GP IIb/IIIa inhibition (abciximab, eptifibatide, or tirofiban) provisionally, routinely, or not at all at the discretion of the interventional cardiologist. Stents and GP IIb/IIIa inhibition was used in approximately 85% and 76% of patients, respectively. A nonsignificant benefit favoring the use of bivalirudin was observed at 48 hours in terms of both ischemic and bleeding complications, despite the liberal use of GP IIb/IIIa inhibition. In the largest trial of antithrombotic therapy in PCI performed to date, the REPLACE-2 study enrolled 6010 elective or urgent patients undergoing modern coronary intervention. Randomization was to bivalirudin (0.75 mg/kg and 1.75 mg/kg/hr IV) and provisional abciximab or eptifibatide versus the planned use of GP IIb/IIIa inhibition and heparin (65 mg/kg IV) conducted in a double-blind, double-dummy manner.[34] The commonly used "triple ischemic endpoint" of death, MI, or urgent revascularization at 30 days was assessed with a noninferiority design. The major exclusions included patients with STEMI undergoing PCI for reperfusion, patients at significant risk of bleeding, or those requiring dialysis. As a result, approximately 50% of patients underwent PCI for ACS, multi-vessel intervention was undertaken in approximately 15% of cases, and saphenous vein graft intervention occurred in 6% of patients. Provisional use of a GP IIb/IIIa inhibitor was encouraged for intraprocedural complications in the bivalirudin arm, and provisional placebo was used in the arm of patients already receiving GP IIb/IIIa inhibition. Among the bivalirudin-treated patients, GP IIb/IIIa inhibition was used in 7.5% of procedures. In contrast, 5.2% of patients treated with heparin or GP IIb/IIIa inhibition received provisional placebo (P = 0.002). Pretreatment with a thienopyridine, mostly clopidogrel, was administered to 86% of patients. Bivalirudin (and provisional GP IIb/IIIa inhibition) was associated with a nonsignificant increase in ischemic events (heparin or GP IIb/IIIa inhibition: 7.6% vs. bivalirudin 7.9%; OR 1.09; 95% CI 0.90–1.32, P = 0.40) but met the boundary for noninferiority. In contrast, bleeding events were significantly reduced when evaluated by the Thrombolysis In Myocardial Infarction criteria or the slightly broader protocol definition that included blood transfusion (heparin or GP IIb/IIIa inhibition: 4.1% vs. bivalirudin 2.4%, P < 0.001). Reduced vascular access site events accounted for a large proportion of this benefit with regard to bleeding. Assessment of 12-month events demonstrated a lower point estimate for mortality with bivalirudin (1.6% vs. 2.5%, P = 0.16).[35] Thus, the

nonsignificant increase in early MI was not associated with an excess in late mortality. These data are further supported by the results of ACUITY, a trial of anti-thrombotic therapy among patients with ACS undergoing PCI. Among this high risk patient population, the strategy of bivalirudin with bailout use of GP IIb/IIIa inhibition was associated with a slight, but nonsignificant increase in ischemic events and a significant reduction in bleeding events (Fig. 9-9).[36] Overall, when considering the combined endpoint of ischemia and bleeding, the use of bivalirudin was "not inferior" to heparin or LMWH and a GP IIb/IIIa inhibitor. These results were maintained for up to 12 months, and no difference in the composite ischemic endpoint (17.8% vs. 19.4% vs. 19.2%, P = ns) or mortality (3.2% vs. 3.3% vs. 3.1%, P = ns) was observed among patients receiving enoxaparin or heparin and GP IIb/IIIa inhibition; bivalirudin and GP IIb/IIIa inhibition; and bivalirudin monotherapy alone, respectively.

The Harmonizing Outcomes With Revascularization and Stents in Acute Myocardial Infarction (HORIZONS-AMI) trial explored the role of bivalirudin monotherapy versus heparin and GP IIb/IIIa inhibition among patients undergoing primary PCI for STEMI.[37] Among the 3602 patients randomized, no difference was observed in adverse cardiac events (death, re-infarction, target vessel revascularization for ischemia or stroke) between the two arms, but a 41% reduction in major bleeding was seen in the bivalirudin arm (bivalirudin 5.0% vs. heparin or GP IIb/IIIa inhibition: 8.4%, P < 0.001). In addition, a reduction in all-cause mortality was evident by 30 days (2.1% vs. 3.1%, P = 0.048). However, a small increase in early stent thrombosis was observed in the bivalirudin arm, though this did not translate to an increase in late cardiac mortality (2.1% vs. 3.8%, P = 0.005) or all-cause mortality (3.5% vs. 4.8%, P = 0.037), with the 12-month analysis favoring bivalirudin. A subsequent subanalysis has suggested that higher loading doses of clopidogrel (600 mg) may mitigate this risk of early stent thrombosis.[38]

Similarly, a large-scale randomized trial compared bivalirudin with unfractionated heparin in 4570 stable or unstable patients without troponin or CK-MB elevation, with 600 mg of clopidogrel administered to all patients at least 2 hours before the procedure.[39,40] This study found no difference in the rates of death, MI, and urgent target vessel revascularization (bivalirudin 5.9% vs. heparin 5.0%, P = 0.23), though a reduction in major bleeding was still evident (3.1% vs. 4.6%, P = 0.008). Hence, with the data considered collectively, the randomized trial experience with bivalirudin demonstrated a clear reduction in bleeding events with rates of ischemic events comparable with clinically relevant alternative strategies across the spectrum of patients undergoing PCI. Furthermore, a reduction in mortality associated with primary PCI is encouraging. These data are supported by observational analyses confirming reductions in bleeding events and suggesting reductions in short-term mortality within routine care.[41]

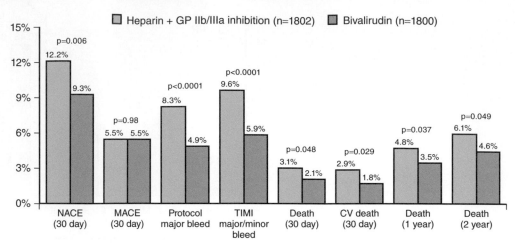

Figure 9-9 Ischemic and bleeding outcomes with bivalirudin versus bivalirudin plus glycoprotein (GP) IIb/IIIa inhibition versus heparin or low-molecular-weight heparin (LMWH) plus GP IIb/IIIa inhibition among patients undergoing percutaneous coronary intervention (PCI) in the ACUITY trial at 30 days.

Special Groups

With the availability of a broad array of therapies, determining the limitations and benefits of each approach is often difficult. In many patients, the use of unfractionated heparin remains a safe and efficacious choice, especially in the context of pretreatment with a thienopyridine and the planned used of GP IIb/IIIa inhibition. Importantly, the effect of unfractionated heparin can be easily reversed with protamine, making it the preferred anti-thrombin for PCI when there is an increased risk of perforation, especially during PCI for chronic total occlusions. However, in specific high-risk populations, the decision to use an alternative anti-thrombotic strategy may be considered.

ST SEGMENT ELEVATION MYOCARDIAL INFARCTION

The efficacy of hirudin has been explored in the context of primary PCI with balloon angioplasty in the GUSTO IIb study (see earlier discussion). Though there are no published randomized studies to optimally evaluate the risks and benefits of using enoxaparin in the context of primary or rescue PCI, several observational studies have suggested a reduction in ischemic events and no increase in bleeding events with or without concurrent GP IIb/IIIa inhibition. The randomized, but yet to be published ATOLL study has also addressed this question and appears to confirm these findings. These studies would suggest that enoxaparin is safe without compromising ischemic outcomes in this context.[23,24] In contrast, the use of bivalirudin is now supported by robust data from the HORIZONS-AMI trial (see earlier discussion).[37,42] Compared with heparin and GP IIb/IIIa inhibition, reductions in bleeding and mortality associated with bivalirudin suggests that this agent has a central role in the anti-thrombotic strategy of catheter-based reperfusion.

TRANSITIONING FROM "UPSTREAM" MANAGEMENT TO THE CATH-LAB

Extrapolation of the clinical experience with unfractionated heparin suggests that the degree of anticoagulation required during PCI is greater than that required during the medical management of patients with ACS. As a result, strategies have evolved to optimize anti-thrombin therapies for these patients who go on to PCI while already receiving one of these agents. Among patients being treated with heparin, an ACT-guided approach is recommended, with an additional 20 to 50 U/kg IV administered to achieve an ACT of approximately 200 to 250 seconds when concomitant GP IIb/IIIa inhibition is planned and around 300 to 350 seconds when heparin is the sole agent. Data on enoxaparin use suggest that PCI can proceed without additional dosing when the procedure is occurring within 8 hours of the subcutaneous dose, but an additional IV bolus of 0.3 mg/kg is recommended when the delay is 8 to 12 hours. Outside this window, a dose of 0.75 mg/kg IV should be administered regardless of GP IIb/IIIa inhibition use, on the basis of the SYNERGY study. Among patients receiving infusions of bivalirudin, an additional bolus of 0.5 mg/kg and an increase in the infusion rate to 1.75 mg/kg was shown to be safe and efficacious in the ACUITY study, again with or without GP IIb/IIIa use (Tables 9-3 and 9-4).[43] Observations from the ACUITY study also suggested that patients receiving bivalirudin after initial heparin or enoxaparin continued to experience a reduced rate of bleeding complications without compromise to ischemic benefits.[43]

DECREASED RENAL FUNCTION

Increased ischemic and bleeding events are observed among patients with renal dysfunction. Analyses of the randomized clinical trial experiences with bivalirudin suggest the relative benefits of this agent in

TABLE 9-3	Pharmacokinetic Characteristics of the Commonly Used Anticoagulants		
Property	**Unfractionated Heparin**	**Enoxaparin**	**Bivalirudin**
Mean molecular weight (daltons)	15,000	5,000	2,180
Dependence on anti-thrombin	Yes	Yes	No
Anti–factor Xa (FXa):anti-FIIa activity	1	2–4	No anti-FXa activity
Half-life (minutes)	~60	~240	25
Bioavailability	+ to +++	++++	++++
Subcutaneous absorption	++	++++	−
Binding to plasma proteins	+++	+	−
Binding to platelets/ Macrophages	++	+	−
Antigenicity/ Heparin-induced thrombocytopenia syndrome (HITS)	++	+	−
Clearance	Renal	Renal	Renal/Proteolysis
Protamine neutralization	++++	++	−

TABLE 9-4	Dosing of the Currently Available Anti-thrombin Agents		
	Unfractionated Heparin	*Enoxaparin*	*Bivalirudin*
No prior treatment	60–100 units/kg intravenous (IV)*	0.5–0.75 mg/kg IV	0.75 mg/kg IV with 1.75 mg/kg/hr infusion
Upstream acute coronary syndrome (ACS) management	60 international units per kilogram (IU/kg) IV and 800–1000 IU/hr infusion	1.0 mg/kg subcutaneously twice daily (SC BID)	0.1 mg/kg IV with 0.25 mg/kg/hr infusion
Additional bolus before percutaneous coronary intervention (PCI)	20–50 IU/kg*	<8 hours since last dose: None 8–12 hours since last SC dose: 0.3 mg/kg IV	0.5 mg/kg IV bolus
Infusion during PCI	None	None	1.75 mg/kg/hr infusion

*Targeting and ACT >200 seconds with concomitant glycoprotein IIb/IIIa inhibition or ACT >300–350 seconds without concomitant glycoprotein IIb/IIIa inhibition.

terms of bleeding complications and ischemic complications are preserved among those patients with reduced renal function.[44,45] Hence, in absolute terms, among patients with at least moderate renal dysfunction (creatinine clearance <60 mL/min), bivalirudin is associated with a greater absolute benefit with respect to bleeding without an increased risk of ischemic events (Fig. 9-10). With enoxaparin and fondaparinux, there are limited data from small studies examining the relative risks and benefits in the context of patients with renal impairment.[46] Reports of relative safety in high-risk patients will need to be confirmed in larger studies.

PATIENTS WITH DIABETES

Subgroup analysis of randomized clinical trials appear to indicate that abciximab provides substantial benefits in terms of reduced repeat revascularization and mortality among patients with diabetes, with comparable effects observed with tirofiban. Clinical trial evidence with bivalirudin supports similar conclusions. In the REPLACE-2 study of bivalirudin plus provisional GP IIb/IIIa inhibition compared with heparin plus GP IIb/IIIa inhibition, bivalirudin-treated patients with diabetes experienced a lower, but nonsignificant, rate of mortality at 12 months (2.3% vs. 3.9%, *P* = ns). No difference in the rate of 30-day bleeding and ischemic outcomes was observed.[47] The long-term effects of enoxaparin-based strategies among patients with diabetes have yet to be reported, and a substantial rate of concomitant GP IIb/IIIa use in these studies will limit the interpretation of these data.

HEPARIN-INDUCED THROMBOCYTOPENIA

Heparin-induced thrombocytopenia syndrome (HITS) precludes the use of unfractionated heparin during PCI. While the rate of HITS is less frequent with the LMWHs, cross-reactivity with these agents is observed and may be associated with increased rates of ischemic and

Figure 9-10 Early and late outcomes in the HORIZONS-AMI trial. *NACE*, Net Adverse Clinical Events = MACE (Major Adverse Cardiovascular Event) and Protocol defined Non-CABG bleeding; *MACE*, Death, re-infarction, ischemia-driven TVR, stroke, or all. Protocol defined bleeding = thrombolysis in myocardial infarction (TIMI) major or minor bleeding, reoperation for bleeding, or blood transfusion.

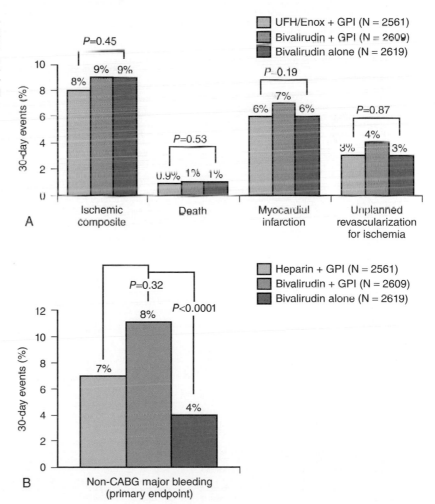

bleeding complications. Whether or not pentasaccharides and hexadecasaccharides are safe and efficacious in this context has yet to be defined. Direct thrombin inhibitors are well suited to the management of patients with HITS requiring PCI. As discussed earlier, observational data with argatroban suggests that this agent can be safely used as an alternative to heparin in these patients. Case reports with recombinant hirudin (lepirudin) suggest that the use of this agent is also feasible.[48] Similarly, a registry of 52 patients with HITS receiving bivalirudin before PCI reported a 96% rate of freedom from death, Q-wave MI, and emergent CABG. Thrombocytopenia (platelet count <50,109/L) was not observed among these patients, which suggests that bivalirudin is also an alternative anticoagulation strategy within this infrequent but high-risk subgroup.[49]

GLYCOPROTEIN IIB/IIIA–SPARING COMBINATION APPROACHES AND ECONOMIC CONSIDERATIONS

When required, combination anti-thrombin strategies, including pretreatment with thienopyridines, IV GP IIb/IIIa inhibition, and direct or indirect thrombin inhibitors appears to be safe. However, given the cost of GP IIb/IIIa inhibition and the increased risk of bleeding events, efforts are ongoing to refine the anti-thrombotic approach and define patient subsets that may not derive incremental benefits from these agents. Optimization of anticoagulation therapies may mitigate the dependence on potent platelet inhibition. To date, with respect to antithrombin therapy and GP IIb/IIIa sparing, the most robust data reside with bivalirudin, given the study designs employed in the REPLACE-2, ACUITY, and HORIZONS-AMI studies. While pretreatment with thienopyridines did not appear to influence this relationship, more potent oral agents such as prasugrel and ticagrelor may provide a further rationale for GP sparing, though this should be formally examined in optimally designed clinical trials.[50] Given the reductions in drug costs and the costs associated with bleeding, the bivalirudin strategy is economically attractive.[51] The increased bleeding risk among older adults and female patients also favors greater absolute benefits with bivalirudin in this context.[52,53] However, therapies associated with reduced bleeding but comparable ischemic outcomes may be of limited value in the context of radial-access PCI, where bleeding risks are substantially lower.[54]

Conclusion

Substantial clinical trial evidence now supports the use of novel coagulants among patients undergoing PCI. These agents demonstrate improved efficacy and safety compared with heparin and enable reduced use of the GP IIb/IIIa inhibition. Questions regarding the optimal anti-thrombotic strategies for treatment of STEMI are likely to be answered in clinical trials that are currently ongoing.

REFERENCES

1. Davie EW, Kulman JD: An overview of the structure and function of thrombin. *Semin Thromb Hemost* 32(Suppl 1):3–15, 2006.
2. Chew DP, Bhatt DL, Lincoff AM, et al: Clinical endpoint definitions following percutaneous coronary intervention and their relationship to late mortality: An assessment by attributable risk. *Heart* 92(7):945–950, 2005.
3. Kinnaird TD, Stabile E, Mintz GS, et al: Incidence, predictors, and prognostic implications of bleeding and blood transfusion following percutaneous coronary interventions. *Am J Cardiol* 92:930–935, 2003.
4. Pocock SJ, Mehran R, Clayton TC, et al: Prognostic modeling of individual patient risk and mortality impact of ischemic and hemorrhagic complications: Assessment from the Acute Catheterization and Urgent Intervention Triage Strategy trial. *Circulation* 121:43–51, 2010.
5. Chew DP, Bhatt DL, Lincoff AM, et al: Defining the optimal activated clotting time during percutaneous coronary intervention: Aggregate results from 6 randomized, controlled trials. *Circulation* 103(7):961–967, 2001.
6. Cavusoglu E, Lakhani M, Marmur JD: The activated clotting time (ACT) can be used to monitor enoxaparin and dalteparin after intravenous administration. *J Invasive Cardiol* 17:416–421, 2005.
7. Saw J, Kereiakes DJ, Mahaffey KW, et al: Evaluation of a novel point-of-care enoxaparin monitor with central laboratory anti-Xa levels. *Thromb Res* 112:301–306, 2003.
8. Moliterno DJ, Hermiller JB, Kereiakes DJ, et al: A novel point-of-care enoxaparin monitor for use during percutaneous coronary intervention. Results of the Evaluating Enoxaparin Clotting Times (ELECT) study. *J Am Coll Cardiol* 42:1132–1139, 2003.
9. El Rouby S, Cohen M, Gonzales A, et al: The use of a HEMOCHRON JR. HEMONOX point of care test in monitoring the anticoagulant effects of enoxaparin during interventional coronary procedures. *J Thromb Thrombolysis* 21:137–145, 2006.
10. Silvain J, Beygui F, Ankri A, et al: Enoxaparin anticoagulation monitoring in the catheterization laboratory using a new bedside test. *J Am Coll Cardiol* 55:617–625, 2010.
11. Cheneau E, Canos D, Kuchulakanti PK, et al: Value of monitoring activated clotting time when bivalirudin is used as the sole anticoagulation agent for percutaneous coronary intervention. *Am J Cardiol* 94:789–792, 2004.
12. Casserly IP, Kereiakes DJ, Gray WA, et al: Point-of-care ecarin clotting time versus activated clotting time in correlation with bivalirudin concentration. *Thromb Res* 113:115–121, 2004.
13. Boccara A, Benamer H, Juliard JM, et al: A randomized trial of a fixed high dose vs a weight-adjusted low dose of intravenous heparin during coronary angioplasty. *Eur Heart J* 18:631–635, 1997.
14. Brener SJ, Moliterno DJ, Lincoff AM, et al: Relationship between activated clotting time and ischemic or hemorrhagic complications: Analysis of 4 recent randomized clinical trials of percutaneous coronary intervention. *Circulation* 110:994–998, 2004.
15. Martin JL, Fry ET, Sanderink GJ, et al: Reliable anticoagulation with enoxaparin in patients undergoing percutaneous coronary intervention: The pharmacokinetics of enoxaparin in PCI (PEPCI) study. *Catheter Cardiovasc Interv* 61:163–170, 2004.
16. Kereiakes DJ, Grines C, Fry E, et al: Enoxaparin and abciximab adjunctive pharmacotherapy during percutaneous coronary intervention. *J Invasive Cardiol* 13:272–278, 2001.
17. Ferguson JJ, Antman EM, Bates ER, et al: Combining enoxaparin and glycoprotein IIb/IIIa antagonists for the treatment of acute coronary syndromes: Final results of the National Investigators Collaborating on Enoxaparin-3 (NICE-3) study. *Am Heart J* 146:628–634, 2003.
18. Gibson CM, Murphy SA, Montalescot G, et al: Percutaneous coronary intervention in patients receiving enoxaparin or unfractionated heparin after fibrinolytic therapy for ST-segment elevation myocardial infarction in the ExTRACT-TIMI 25 trial. *J Am Coll Cardiol* 49:2238–2246, 2007.
19. Ferguson JJ, Califf RM, Antman EM, et al: Enoxaparin vs unfractionated heparin in high-risk patients with non-ST-segment elevation acute coronary syndromes managed with an intended early invasive strategy: Primary results of the SYNERGY randomized trial. *JAMA* 292:45–54, 2004.
20. Bhatt DL, Lee BI, Casterella PJ, et al: Safety of concomitant therapy with eptifibatide and enoxaparin in patients undergoing percutaneous coronary intervention: Results of the Coronary Revascularization Using Integrilin and Single bolus Enoxaparin Study. *J Am Coll Cardiol* 41:20–25, 2003.
21. Borentain M, Montalescot G, Bouzamondo A, et al: Low-molecular-weight heparin vs. unfractionated heparin in percutaneous coronary intervention: A combined analysis. *Catheter Cardiovasc Interv* 65:212–221, 2005.
22. Montalescot G, White HD, Gallo R, et al: Enoxaparin versus unfractionated heparin in elective percutaneous coronary intervention. *N Engl J Med* 355:1006–1017, 2006.
23. Montalescot G, Ellis SG, de Belder MA, et al: Enoxaparin in primary and facilitated percutaneous coronary intervention: A formal prospective nonrandomized substudy of the FINESSE trial (Facilitated INtervention with Enhanced Reperfusion Speed to Stop Events). *JACC Cardiovasc Interv* 3:203–212, 2010.
24. Zeymer U, Gitt A, Zahn R, et al: Efficacy and safety of enoxaparin in combination with and without GP IIb/IIIa inhibitors in unselected patients with ST segment elevation myocardial infarction treated with primary percutaneous coronary intervention. *Eurointervention* 4(4):524–528, 2009.
25. Yusuf S, Mehta SR, Chrolavicius S, et al: Comparison of fondaparinux and enoxaparin in acute coronary syndromes. *N Engl J Med* 354:1464–1476, 2006.
26. Roe MT, Granger CB, Puma JA, et al: Comparison of benefits and complications of hirudin versus heparin for patients with acute coronary syndromes undergoing early percutaneous coronary intervention. *Am J Cardiol* 88:1403–1406, A6, 2001.
27. Mehta SR, Eikelboom JW, Rupprecht HJ, et al: Efficacy of hirudin in reducing cardiovascular events in patients with acute coronary syndrome undergoing early percutaneous coronary intervention. *Eur Heart J* 23:117–123, 2002.
28. Sinnaeve PR, Simes J, Yusuf S, et al: Direct thrombin inhibitors in acute coronary syndromes: Effect in patients undergoing early percutaneous coronary intervention. *Eur Heart J* 26:2396–2403, 2005.
29. Matthai WH, Jr: Use of argatroban during percutaneous coronary interventions in patients with heparin-induced thrombocytopenia. *Semin Thromb Hemost* 25(Suppl 1):57–60, 1999.
30. Lewis BE, Matthai WH, Jr, Cohen M, et al: Argatroban anticoagulation during percutaneous coronary intervention in patients with heparin-induced thrombocytopenia. *Catheter Cardiovasc Interv* 57:177–184, 2002.
31. Jang IK, Lewis BE, Matthai WH, Jr, et al: Argatroban anticoagulation in conjunction with glycoprotein IIb/IIIa inhibition in patients undergoing percutaneous coronary intervention: An open-label, nonrandomized pilot study. *J Thromb Thrombolysis* 18:31–37, 2004.
32. Bittl JA, Chaitman BR, Feit F, et al: Bivalirudin versus heparin during coronary angioplasty for unstable or postinfarction angina: Final report reanalysis of the Bivalirudin Angioplasty Study. *Am Heart J* 142:952–959, 2001.
33. Lincoff AM, Kleiman NS, Kottke-Marchant K, et al: Bivalirudin with planned or provisional abciximab versus low-dose heparin and abciximab during percutaneous coronary revascularization: Results of the Comparison of Abciximab Complications with Hirulog for Ischemic Events Trial (CACHET). *Am Heart J* 143:847–853, 2002.
34. Lincoff AM, Bittl JA, Harrington RA, et al: Bivalirudin and provisional glycoprotein IIb/IIIa blockade compared with heparin and planned glycoprotein IIb/IIIa blockade during percutaneous coronary intervention: REPLACE-2 randomized trial. *JAMA* 289:853–863, 2003.
35. Lincoff AM, Kleiman NS, Kereiakes DJ, et al: Long-term efficacy of bivalirudin and provisional glycoprotein IIb/IIIa blockade vs heparin and planned glycoprotein IIb/IIIa blockade during percutaneous coronary revascularization: REPLACE-2 randomized trial. *JAMA* 292:696–703, 2004.
36. Stone GW, White HD, Ohman EM, et al: Bivalirudin in patients with acute coronary syndromes undergoing percutaneous coronary intervention: A subgroup analysis from the Acute Catheterization and Urgent Intervention Triage strategy (ACUITY) trial. *Lancet* 369:907–919, 2007.
37. Stone GW, Witzenbichler B, Guagliumi G, et al: Bivalirudin during primary PCI in acute myocardial infarction. *N Engl J Med* 358:2218–2230, 2008.
38. Dangas G, Mehran R, Guagliumi G, et al: Role of clopidogrel loading dose in patients with ST-segment elevation myocardial infarction undergoing primary angioplasty: Results from the HORIZONS-AMI (Harmonizing Outcomes with Revascularization and Stents in Acute Myocardial Infarction) trial. *J Am Coll Cardiol* 54:1438–1446, 2009.
39. Kastrati A, Neumann FJ, Mehilli J, et al: Bivalirudin versus unfractionated heparin during percutaneous coronary intervention. *N Engl J Med* 359:688–696, 2008.

40. Kastrati A, Neumann FJ, Mehilli J, et al; ISAR-REACT 3 Trial Investigators: Bivalirudin versus unfractionated heparin during percutaneous coronary intervention. *N Engl J Med* 14;359(7):688–696, 2008.

41. Rassen JA, Mittleman MA, Glynn RJ, et al: Safety and effectiveness of bivalirudin in routine care of patients undergoing percutaneous coronary intervention. *Eur Heart J* 31:561–572, 2010.

42. Mehran R, Lansky AJ, Witzenbichler B, et al: Bivalirudin in patients undergoing primary angioplasty for acute myocardial infarction (HORIZONS-AMI): 1-year results of a randomised controlled trial. *Lancet* 374:1149–1159, 2009.

43. White HD, Chew DP, Hoekstra JW, et al: Safety and efficacy of switching from either unfractionated heparin or enoxaparin to bivalirudin in patients with non-ST-segment elevation acute coronary syndromes managed with an invasive strategy: Results from the ACUITY (Acute Catheterization and Urgent Intervention Triage strategY) trial. *J Am Coll Cardiol* 51:1734–1741, 2008.

44. Chew DP, Bhatt DL, Kimball W, et al: Bivalirudin provides increasing benefit with decreasing renal function: a meta-analysis of randomized trials. *Am J Cardiol* 92:919–923, 2003.

45. Chew DP, Lincoff AM, Gurm H, et al: Bivalirudin versus heparin and glycoprotein IIb/IIIa inhibition among patients with renal impairment undergoing percutaneous coronary intervention (a subanalysis of the REPLACE-2 trial). *Am J Cardiol* 95:581–585, 2005.

46. White HD, Gallo R, Cohen M, et al: The use of intravenous enoxaparin in elective percutaneous coronary intervention in patients with renal impairment: Results from the SafeTy and Efficacy of Enoxaparin in PCI patients, an internationaL randomized Evaluation (STEEPLE) trial. *Am Heart J* 157:125–131, 2009.

47. Gurm HS, Sarembock IJ, Kereiakes DJ, et al: Use of bivalirudin during percutaneous coronary intervention in patients with diabetes mellitus: An analysis from the randomized evaluation in percutaneous coronary intervention linking angiomax to reduced clinical events (REPLACE)-2 trial. *J Am Coll Cardiol* 45:1932–1938, 2005.

48. Manfredi JA, Wall RP, Sane DC, et al: Lepirudin as a safe alternative for effective anticoagulation in patients with known heparin-induced thrombocytopenia undergoing percutaneous coronary intervention: Case reports. *Catheter Cardiovasc Interv* 52:468–472, 2001.

49. Mahaffey KW, Lewis BE, Wildermann NM, et al: The anticoagulant therapy with bivalirudin to assist in the performance of percutaneous coronary intervention in patients with heparin-induced thrombocytopenia (ATBAT) study: Main results. *J Invasive Cardiol* 15:611–616, 2003.

50. Saw J, Lincoff AM, DeSmet W, et al: Lack of clopidogrel pretreatment effect on the relative efficacy of bivalirudin with provisional glycoprotein IIb/IIIa blockade compared to heparin with routine glycoprotein IIb/IIIa blockade: A REPLACE-2 substudy. *J Am Coll Cardiol* 44:1194–1199, 2004.

51. Cohen DJ, Lincoff AM, Lavelle TA, et al: Economic evaluation of bivalirudin with provisional glycoprotein IIB/IIIA inhibition versus heparin with routine glycoprotein IIB/IIIA inhibition for percutaneous coronary intervention: Results from the REPLACE-2 trial. *J Am Coll Cardiol* 44:1792–1800, 2004.

52. Lopes RD, Alexander KP, Manoukian SV, et al: Advanced age, antithrombotic strategy, and bleeding in non-ST-segment elevation acute coronary syndromes: Results from the ACUITY (Acute Catheterization and Urgent Intervention Triage Strategy) trial. *J Am Coll Cardiol* 53:1021–1030, 2009.

53. Lansky AJ, Mehran R, Cristea E, et al: Impact of gender and antithrombin strategy on early and late clinical outcomes in patients with non-ST-elevation acute coronary syndromes (from the ACUITY trial). *Am J Cardiol* 103:1196–1203, 2009.

54. Hamon M, Rasmussen LH, Manoukian SV, et al: Choice of arterial access site and outcomes in patients with acute coronary syndromes managed with an early invasive strategy: The ACUITY trial. *EuroIntervention* 5:115–120, 2009.

Lipid Lowering in Coronary Artery Disease

KAUSIK K. RAY | CHRISTOPHER P. CANNON

KEY POINTS

- Epidemiologic studies suggest a linear relationship between cholesterol and risk for coronary artery disease (CAD).

- There is a linear relationship between the magnitude of low-density lipoprotein cholesterol (LDL-C) reduction and clinical benefit.

- Randomized trials have shown that intensive statin therapy reduces major cardiovascular events by 16% and heart failure by 27% compared with moderate statin therapy.

- In patients with CAD, LDL-C should be less than 70 mg/dL.

- Beyond LDL-C reduction, lowering C-reactive protein (CRP) levels with statins is associated with greater reductions in risk for CAD.

- Raising high-density lipoprotein (HDL) levels appears to be beneficial, and many trials are ongoing.

Epidemiology

CAD is the largest cause of premature death in the Western world (Fig. 10-1). A person is born with an LDL cholesterol (LDL-C) level of 0.8 mmol/L, which increases throughout life (Fig. 10-2, *A*). Several epidemiologic studies have demonstrated a relationship between elevated total cholesterol and LDL-C and an increased risk of death or nonfatal myocardial infarction (MI).[1-4] The relationship between cholesterol and risk of CAD is linear, with no apparent threshold below which risk declines (see Fig. 10-2, *B*), which suggests that interventions that reduce cholesterol the most are also likely to have the greatest impact on CAD risk reduction.[5] The central role of cholesterol in the pathophysiology of CAD has pushed lipid-lowering therapy to the forefront of medical management of this condition. More recently, the largest observational study to date involving over 1 million person-years worth of observation and more that 10,000 cases of fatal or nonfatal MI has shed further light into the relevance of simultaneous assessment of triglycerides (TGs), HDL-cholesterol (HDL-C) and non–HDL-cholesterol (non–HDL-C), which consists of very-low-density lipoprotein (VLDL), intermediate-density lipoprotein (IDL), and LDL-C.[6] Specifically, this shows that after adjustment for non–HDL-C and HDL-C, there is no association between TG and risk of CAD (Fig. 10-3). In contrast, the inverse association between HDL-C and risk persists with some attenuation above 70 mg/dL. One practical implication of this observation is that among individuals with an HDL-C >70 mg/dL use of the TC/HDL-C ratio underestimates cardiovascular (CV) risk in risk calculators. As with LDL-C, a positive relationship is observed between non–HDL-C and risk of CAD with little attenuation. No difference has been observed between fasting and nonfasting levels and risk, suggesting that lipid measurements can be simplified by using non–HDL-C (the difference between TC and HDL-C) and HDL-C levels. Data suggest that TGs are unlikely to be causative factors but markers of risk and that the risk is conferred by concomitant low levels of HDL-C and high levels of non–HDL-C. These latter two factors, rather than TGs, should be the targets of treatment in people with elevated TG levels, providing independent support for the NCEP goals. The LDL-C level incompletely measures atherogenic lipoproteins; measurement of the concentration of apolipoprotein B (apoB), which is a direct measurement of the concentration of proatherogenic particles (e.g., LDL-C, VLDL, IDL), and measurement of apoAI, the major protein in HDL particles, provide alternative approaches to risk prediction. The debate regarding the choice of the best lipid parameter has further intensified with apparently conflicting evidence between prospective studies.[7-9] In approximately 100,000 individuals with about half a million person-years worth of follow-up, it is now clear that overall apoB (the major lipoprotein) in atherogenic particles is equivalent to non–HDL-C and that apoAI, the major protein in HDL particles, is equivalent to HDL-C (Fig. 10-4); this suggests that the choice of assays should be informed by availability and cost. Lipoprotein (a) (Lp[a]) consists of one apoB particle covalently bonded to a protein apolipoprotein via a disulfide bond. It is produced by the liver and is principally under genetic control, which makes it the most reproducible biomarker known. Elevated Lp(a) levels can potentially increase the risk of cardiovascular disease (CVD) (1) via a prothrombotic/anti-fibrinolytic effect as apolipoprotein (a) possesses structural homology with plasminogen and plasmin, and (2) via accelerated atherogenesis as a result of intimal deposition of Lp(a) cholesterol. Observational data from 126,634 individuals suggest a curvilinear association between levels and risk of CAD and stroke even after adjustment for conventional risk factors and other lipid fractions (Fig. 10-5).[10] This association, however, is modest and per 1 SD (standard deviation) difference, that is, about a 60% higher level Lp(a) increases risk by about 13%. It is likely that this factor is causally related and specific for CVD as there is no association with nonvascular deaths (a prior requisite of the Bradford-Hill Criteria for causality); recent mendellian randomization data have provided consistent data for an association of Lp(a) genotype with Lp(a) levels and, in turn, between genotypes and CAD risk.[11]

National Cholesterol Education Program Recommendations

To help reduce the prevalence of elevated blood cholesterol levels in adult Americans, the National Heart, Lung, and Blood Institute (NHLBI) of the National Institutes of Health (NIH) launched the National Cholesterol Education Program (NCEP) in 1985.[12] For the first time, there was a consensus among leading experts in the field on the measurement, detection, and treatment of patients with hypercholesterolemia. The report established criteria that defined candidates with high blood cholesterol levels who should receive medical intervention and provided guidelines on how to detect, set goals, treat, and monitor these patients over time. The NCEP-1 treatment guidelines recommended that all adults older than 20 years have a blood cholesterol measurement at least once every 5 years. Patients with levels greater than 200 mg/dL (5.2 mmol/L), confirmed by a second blood cholesterol measurement, were advised to adopt a Step 1 fat-controlled diet. Patients with cholesterol exceeding 240 mg/dL (6.2 mmol/L) were candidates for intensive treatment with a Step 2 diet and sometimes with drugs, as were those with cholesterol levels in the range of 5.2 to

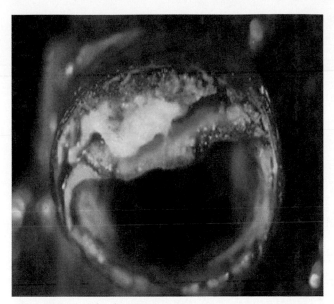

Figure 10-1 Lipid-rich atherosclerotic plaque in a coronary artery.

6.2 mmol/L (200 to 240 mg/dL), who were at especially high risk because they already had CAD or two other risk factors. It was also recommended that drugs for lowering blood cholesterol should be used only when the indication has been confirmed by measuring LDL-C and as a supplement to the dietary treatment. These guidelines were the first steps toward the management of lipids that have become commonplace today.

Early Nonstatin Lipid-Lowering Trials

In the Lipid Research Clinics–Coronary Primary Prevention Trial (LRC CPPT), cholestyramine therapy resulted in a 13% reduction in LDL-C and a significant 19% reduction in fatal and nonfatal MI at 7 years (Table 10-1).[13] During the first 2 years of the trial, higher event rates occurred in the cholestyramine group compared with the placebo group. The Coronary Drug Project evaluated the effects of estrogen, dextrothyroxine, clofibrate, and niacin on recurrent disease in men. Clofibrate resulted in an 8% reduction in total cholesterol and a 25% reduction in triglycerides but no significant reduction on the combined endpoint of cardiac death and nonfatal MI at 5 years.[14] Subjects who were assigned to niacin treatment achieved a 10% reduction in total cholesterol and a 25% reduction in triglyceride levels. At 5 years,

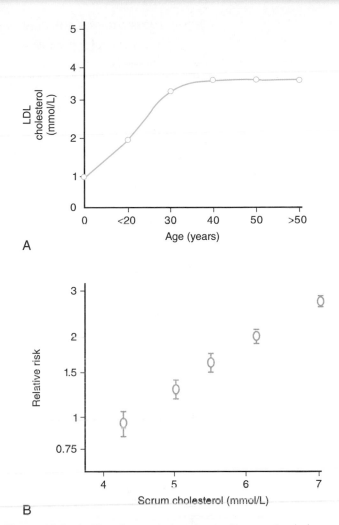

Figure 10-2 A, The change in low-density lipoprotein cholesterol (LDL-C) levels throughout life. **B,** The relationship between cholesterol and long-term risk of coronary heart disease (CHD). (**A,** Data from Freedman DS, Srinivasan SE, Cresanta JL, et al: Cardiovascular risk factors from birth to 7 years of age: The Bogalusa Heart Study. Serum lipids and lipoproteins, Pediatrics 80[Pt 2]:789–796, 1987, and from Webber LS, Srinivasan SF, Wattigney WA, Berenson GD: Tracking of serum lipids and lipoproteins from childhood to adulthood. The Bogalusa Heart Study, Am J Epidemiol 133:884–899, 1991; **B,** Data from Law MR, Wald NJ: Risk factor thresholds: Their existence under scrutiny, BMJ 324:1570–1576, 2002.)

TABLE 10-1	Early Trials of Lipid Lowering with Nonstatin Regimens				
Trial	*Therapy*	*Lipid Differential*	*Outcome Treatment vs. Controls*		*P Value*
Lipid Research Clinics-Coronary Primary Prevention Trial (LRC-CPPT)	Cholestyramine	–9% TC –13% LDL-C	CAD death or MI 7% vs. 8.60%		<0.05
Coronary Drug Project	Clofibrate	–8% TC –25% TG	CAD death 14.1% vs. 16.20%		0.06
Coronary Drug Project	Niacin	–10% TC –25% TG	CAD death 15.9% vs. 16.20%		0.5
Stockholm Ischemic Heart Disease	Niacin + clofibrate	–13% TC –19% TG	CAD death 16.8% vs. 26.40%		<0.01
Helsinki Heart	Gemfibrozil	–10% TC –41% TG	CAD death or MI 7.4% vs. 6.3%		0.14
Veterans Affairs High-Density Lipoprotein Cholesterol Intervention Trial (VA-HIT)	Gemfibrozil	–4% TC –31% TG	CAD death 17.3% vs. 21.70%		0.006
Bezafibrate Infarction Prevention (BIP)	Bezafibrate	–4% TC –21% TG	CAD death or MI 13.6% vs. 15%		0.26

LDL-C, low-density-lipoprotein cholesterol; *TC,* total cholesterol; *TG,* triglycerides.

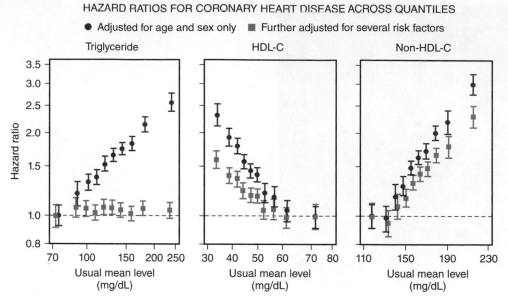

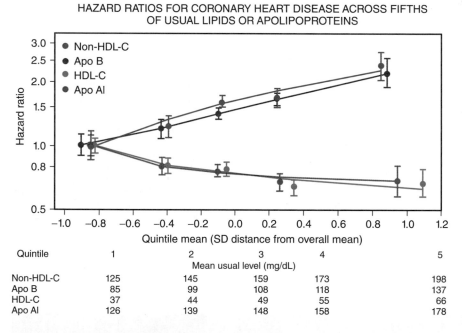

Figure 10-3   Relationship among usual levels of triglyceride (TG), high-density-lipoprotein–cholesterol (HDL-C), and non–HDL-C and incident coronary artery disease (CAD). *(Di Angelantonio E, et al: Major Lipids, apolipoproteins, and risk of vascular disease, JAMA 302(18):1993–2000, 2009.)*

Figure 10-4 Relationship between cholesterol content or lipoprotein level and risk of incident coronary artery disease (CAD). *(Di Angelantonio E, et al: Major Lipids, apolipoproteins, and risk of vascular disease, JAMA 302(18):1993–2000, 2009.)*

Quintile	1	2	3	4	5
			Mean usual level (mg/dL)		
Non-HDL-C	125	145	159	173	198
Apo B	85	99	108	118	137
HDL-C	37	44	49	55	66
Apo AI	126	139	148	158	178

a dose of niacin (3 g/day) was associated with a significant reduction in CAD death or MI (25.6% vs. 30.1%, *P* < 0.005).[15] Benefit was not evident after the second year of therapy. The Stockholm Ischaemic Heart Disease Prevention study evaluated the combination of niacin (3 g/day) and clofibrate (2 g/day).[16] Total mortality and, notably, CAD mortality were significantly reduced in the lipid-lowering therapy group (16.8% and 21.9% vs. the control group rates of 26.4% and 29.7%, *P* < 0.05 and *P* < 0.01, respectively). A significant reduction in nonfatal MI was reported at 44 months (6.8% vs. 13.6%, *P* < 0.01). No significant benefit from gemfibrozil therapy was observed in the secondary prevention arm of the Helsinki Heart Study.[17] However, gemfibrozil therapy did reduce the rates of MI and CAD death in men in the secondary prevention Veterans Affairs High-Density Lipoprotein Cholesterol Intervention Trial (VA-HIT).[18]

▦ Early Secondary Prevention Statin Trials

During a decade of clinical research, successive trials using statins have demonstrated the benefit of lowering serum cholesterol in a wide range of clinical conditions compared with diet alone. The first of these trials was the Scandinavian Simvastatin Survival Study (4S) trial, which randomized 4444 patients with angina pectoris or previous MI and serum cholesterol levels of 215 to 312 mg/dL (5.5 to 8.0 mmol/L) to a lipid-lowering diet or to treatment with simvastatin (average dose of 20 mg/day).[19] Over 5 years, simvastatin produced mean reductions in total cholesterol and LDL-C levels of 25% and 35%, respectively. Statin therapy was associated with an absolute 4% reduction in mortality and a relative risk reduction in all-cause mortality of 30% (*P* = 0.0003).

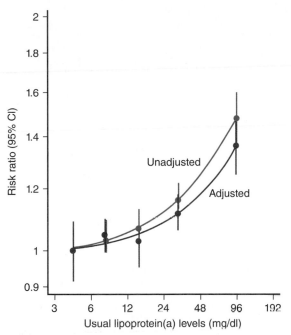

Figure 10-5 Shape of the association between usual lipoprotein (a) [Lp(a)] levels with risk of coronary artery disease (CAD) with and without adjustment for risk factors. *(Erqou S, et al: Lipoprotein(a) concentration and the risk of coronary heart disease, stroke, and nonvascular mortality, JAMA 302(4):412–423, 2009.)*

Significant reductions were also observed for CAD death (42%), major CAD event (34%), and the need for revascularization (37%). This was the first trial in the modern era that provided definitive proof that lipid-lowering therapy was safe and reduced the risk of cardiac death or nonfatal MI. The Cholesterol and Recurrent Events (CARE) trial quickly followed 4S with consistent findings, demonstrating a reduction in major coronary events with pravastatin (40 mg) versus placebo, as well as reductions in the rates of revascularization and stroke in patients with normal cholesterol levels.[20] The Long-Term Intervention with Pravastatin in Ischaemic Disease (LIPID) trial was the largest of the three early secondary prevention trials (N = 9014 patients), and it confirmed the mortality findings of 4S in a population with an overall lower total cholesterol level.[21] LIPID demonstrated that among patients with a history of MI or hospitalization for unstable angina and initial plasma total cholesterol levels of 155 to 271 mg/dL (3.97 to 6.95 mmol/L), pravastatin (40 mg/day) reduced CAD death by 1.9%, resulting in a 24% relative risk reduction (P < 0.001). Similarly, overall mortality was reduced (22%), as were rates for recurrent MI (29%), stroke (19%), and coronary revascularization (20%). These three trials demonstrated the cumulative benefit of statins across a range of baseline cholesterol values.

Heart Protection Study and Cholesterol Treatment Trial Meta-Analysis

The large Heart Protection Study (HPS) demonstrated that the magnitude of benefit from statin therapy (40 mg of simvastatin) was similar at each level of baseline LDL-C, including subjects with an LDL-C level below 100 mg/dL (2.56 mmol/L).[22] HPS studied approximately 20,000 patients who were able to tolerate simvastatin (after a run-in phase) over 5 years and assessed the on-treatment effect (rather than the intention-to-treat effect) of a standard dose of a statin rather than a specific cholesterol or LDL-C target. HPS, however, included a range of patients with CAD; those with prior vascular disease, such

as peripheral vascular disease or stroke; and subjects without prior clinical manifestations of vascular disease who were considered at high risk due to diabetes.[23] The implications of this trial for clinical practice were that physicians did not need to treat to specific targets because subjects with vascular disease all derived similar proportional reductions in risk with simvastatin (40 mg). Preliminary evidence indicated that some overall benefit existed for statin therapy in different circumstances, such as different ages, genders, and different levels of established risk factors, but additional data involving several thousand more patients were needed to provide large-scale evidence of benefit in individual subgroups. The Cholesterol Treatment Trial (CTT) collaborators set out to undertake a prospective meta-analysis of mortality and morbidity from all relevant large-scale, randomized trials of statin therapy.[24] Data on 90,056 individuals were combined. During a mean follow-up of 5 years, there was a significant 12% reduction in all-cause mortality per 38.6-mg/dL (1-mmol/L) reduction in LDL-C, a 19% reduction in coronary mortality, a 24% reduction in the need for revascularization, and a 17% reduction in stroke. Overall, a 38.6-mg/dL (1-mmol/L) reduction in LDL was associated with a 21 to 23% reduction in any major vascular event (Fig. 10-6). Importantly, a similar proportional benefit was observed in different age groups, across genders, at different levels of baseline lipids (including triglycerides and high-density lipoprotein cholesterol [HDL-C]), and equally among those with prior CAD and cardiovascular risk factors and in those without. The CTT meta-analysis collected data on 5103 new cases of cancer, with no evidence that statins increased the overall incidence of any form of cancer (hazard ratio [HR], 1.0; P = 0.9).

These data demonstrate that compared with placebo, statin therapy is safe and reduces the 5-year incidence of major coronary events, coronary revascularization, and stroke among those at high risk for vascular disease or with pre-existing disease. This magnitude of benefit is related to the magnitude of LDL-C reduction and is independent of the initial lipid profile or other presenting characteristics. The absolute benefit correlates chiefly with an individual's absolute risk of cardiovascular events, reinforcing the need to consider long-term statin therapy among all individuals at high risk for any type of major vascular event.

Intensive Statin Therapy for Acute Coronary Syndrome

The early trials looking at treatment of acute coronary syndrome (ACS) (i.e., 4S, CARE, and LIPID) excluded patients within the first 4 6 month period after ACS. The Myocardial Ischemia Reduction with Acute Cholesterol Lowering (MIRACL) trial provided the first evidence that statin therapy initiated early after ACS reduced adverse clinical events by 16 weeks.[25] However, the higher-than-usual dose of statin (80 mg of atorvastatin) and lack of an active comparator coupled with an absence of long-term safety data limited the widespread applicability of its findings.

PROVE IT-TIMI 22 TRIAL

The Pravastatin or Atorvastatin Evaluation and Infection Therapy–Thrombolysis In Myocardial Infarction 22 (PROVE IT-TIMI 22) was the first large-scale study of statin therapy comparing two active comparators. In the PROVE IT-TIMI 22 trial, patients who had been hospitalized for ACS within the preceding 10 days (N = 4162) were randomized to 40 mg of pravastatin (i.e., standard therapy) or 80 mg of atorvastatin daily (i.e., intensive therapy).[26] The primary endpoint was a composite of death from any cause, MI, documented unstable angina requiring rehospitalization, revascularization (performed at least 30 days after randomization), and stroke.

In PROVE IT, the median LDL-C level achieved during treatment was 95 mg/dL (2.46 mmol/L) in the standard-therapy group and 62 mg/dL (1.60 mmol/L) in the high-dose group (P < 0.001). Kaplan-Meier estimates of the rates of the primary endpoint at 2 years were

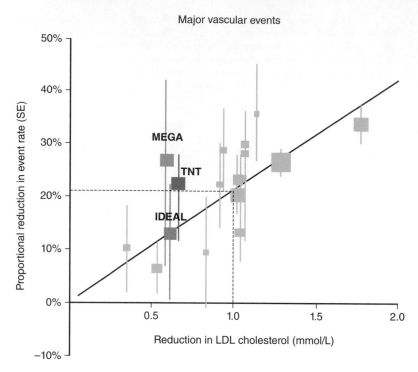

Major vascular events

Figure 10-6 Updated Cholesterol Treatment Trial (CTT) meta-analysis, including the Treating to New Targets (TNT), Individualized Dosing Efficacy versus Flat Dosing to Assess Optimal Pegylated Interferon Therapy (IDEAL), and Management of Elevated Cholesterol in the Primary Prevention Group of Adult Japanese (MEGA) trials, showing the linear relationship between low-density lipoprotein cholesterol (LDL-C) reduction and clinical risk reduction. *(Modified from Baigent C, Keech A, Kearney PM, et al: Efficacy and safety of cholesterol-lowering treatment: Prospective meta-analysis of data from 90,056 participants in 14 randomised trials of statins, Lancet 366:1267–1278, 2005.)*

26.3% for standard therapy and 22.4% for intensive therapy, reflecting a 16% reduction in the hazard ratio (HR) in favor of intensive therapy ($P = 0.005$). Muscle-related side effects were low and not significantly different between groups. There were no cases of rhabdomyolysis.

A TO Z TRIAL

The Aggrastat to Zocor study (A to Z trial) compared an early initiation of an intensive statin regimen with delayed initiation of a less-intensive regimen in patients with ACS.[27] Patients with ACS ($N = 4497$) received 40 mg of simvastatin for 1 month, followed by 80 mg thereafter, which was compared with placebo for 4 months followed by 20 mg of simvastatin. The primary endpoint was a composite of cardiovascular death, nonfatal MI, re-admission for ACS, and stroke. The median LDL-C level on placebo was 122 mg/dL (3.16 mmol/L) at 1 month and 77 mg/dL (1.99 mmol/L) at 8 months with 20 mg of simvastatin. The median LDL-C concentration achieved at 1 month with 40 mg of simvastatin was 68 mg/dL (1.76 mmol/L) and 63 mg/dL (1.63 mmol/L) at 8 months with 80 mg of simvastatin. Overall, 16.7% in the placebo plus simvastatin group experienced the primary endpoint, compared with 14.4% in the simvastatin-only group (40 mg/80 mg), reflecting an HR of 0.89 ($P = 0.14$). Myopathy (i.e., creatine kinase >10 times the upper limits of normal with muscle symptoms) occurred in 9 patients (0.4%) receiving 80 mg of simvastatin, in no patients receiving lower doses of simvastatin, and in 1 patient receiving placebo ($P = 0.02$). The PROVE IT-TIMI 22 and A to Z trials compared similar intensive and moderate statin therapy after ACS, with apparently disparate results. An analysis comparing and contrasting the two trials observed differences between the trials in baseline demographic characteristics, geographic locations, and use of percutaneous coronary intervention (PCI).[28] The LDL-C level difference was greater early in the A to Z trial than in PROVE IT (≤4 months), but the difference was less late in the trials. Significant C-reactive protein (CRP) reduction also occurred earlier in PROVE IT. With common endpoints, an early favorable separation of event curves was seen in PROVE IT but not in the A to Z trial. Clinical endpoint rates and reductions were similar in both trials after 4 months. Factors that may explain this disparity include the statin regimen in the early phase, leading to differences in the magnitude of LDL-C lowering and CRP levels and

differences in the early use of PCI. In summary, the results of these trials support a strategy of early, intensive statin therapy coupled with revascularization when appropriate in patients after ACS.[28]

Intensive Statin Therapy in Stable Coronary Artery Disease

Despite the landmark results from PROVE IT, which led to NCEP recommending an optional LDL-C goal of less than 70 mg/dL in high-risk patients, several questions arose, such as whether intensive statin therapy was safe over a longer period and whether intensive statin therapy was as beneficial in subjects with stable CAD as in ACS patients.[29] The Treating to New Targets (TNT) trial and the Incremental Decrease in Endpoints through Aggressive Lipid Lowering (IDEAL) trial addressed these issues and provided approximately 50,000 patient-years of data on the safety and efficacy of intensive statin therapy.[30,31]

TNT TRIAL

The TNT trial compared a strategy of intensive lipid lowering using 80 mg of atorvastatin with 10 mg of atorvastatin in patients with stable CAD in 10,001 subjects over 5.5 years. The definition of CAD in the study population included patients with previous MI, those with stable angina with objective evidence of atherosclerotic CAD, or patients who had undergone revascularization. After an open-label run-in phase with 10 mg of atorvastatin for 8 weeks, patients were randomized to 10 or 80 mg of atorvastatin (i.e., double-blind period). The primary endpoint of TNT was the time to occurrence of a major cardiovascular event, defined as CAD death, nonfatal MI, resuscitated cardiac arrest, and fatal or nonfatal stroke. During the open-label phase, LDL-C levels fell from 152 mg/dL (3.9 mmol/L) to a mean of 98 mg/dL (2.6 mmol/L). Among those randomized to 80 mg of atorvastatin after the open-label phase, LDL-C fell further by 21.4% to a mean of 77 mg/dL (2 mmol/L). A significant further reduction in triglycerides was observed with the 80-mg dose, but there was no significant difference in HDL-C levels between doses. The primary endpoint occurred in 8.7% of the 80-mg atorvastatin group and in 10.9% of the 10-mg atorvastatin group, reflecting a 22% risk reduction (HR, 0.78; $P < 0.001$). Clinical benefit appeared within 6 months against a background of aggressive medical therapy. This benefit was largely driven by significant reductions in nonfatal MI (HR, 0.78; range, 0.66–0.93; $P = 0.004$) and fatal or nonfatal stroke (HR, 0.75; $P = 0.02$). A trend in favor of cardiovascular death was also observed, which was not significant. Overall, intensive therapy was safe, with no increased risk of adverse effects.

IDEAL TRIAL

The Incremental Decrease in Endpoints through Aggressive Lipid Lowering (IDEAL) trial was a randomized, open-label trial that compared a strategy of achieving an approximately 35% reduction in LDL-C using the 20-mg/40-mg dose of simvastatin versus a strategy of achieving a 55% reduction in LDL-C using 80 mg of atorvastatin in patients with a history of MI. Patients were recruited months to years after the index MI, making IDEAL comparable in design to the 4S and CARE trials.[19,20] Approximately 70% of patients were on statin therapy before study entry, and about 50% of participants had been previously enrolled in the 4S trial. The primary endpoint was coronary death, nonfatal MI, or resuscitated cardiac arrest. IDEAL enrolled 8888 patients and had a mean follow-up period of 4.8 years. During follow-up, the mean LDL-C level was 104 mg/dL (2.69 mmol/L) in the 20-mg/40-mg simvastatin group and 82 mg/dL (2.12 mmol/L) in the 80-mg atorvastatin group. Major coronary events tended to be lower with intensive therapy (HR, 0.89; $P = 0.07$) but did not achieve statistical significance. Major cardiovascular events and any coronary event were significantly reduced by 13% ($P = 0.02$) and 16% ($P < 0.001$), respectively, in the 80-mg atorvastatin group. There was no excess risk of noncardiovascular death with intensive therapy (HR, 0.92; $P = 0.47$). With the exception of transient elevations in liver transaminase levels, there were no significant differences between treatments. The results of the TNT and IDEAL trials further established the important role for intensive statin therapy in the management of patients with stable CAD and extended the observations from PROVE IT-TIMI 22 in ACS patients to patients with stable disease. The IDEAL trial disproved the earlier concerns raised by TNT that intensive statin therapy might be associated with an increased risk of noncardiovascular mortality and provided further safety data on 80 mg of atorvastatin in more than 20,000 patient years of follow-up. Some observers have questioned the importance of TNT and IDEAL, citing that the benefit of intensive therapy in these trials tended to be driven by the so-called soft endpoints, such as recurrent MI or revascularization, compared, for instance, with the landmark 4S trial, in which total mortality was reduced in the statin group compared with placebo. However, in the decade since 4S was completed, the management of CAD has improved dramatically with greater use of additional cardioprotective medication and greater use of revascularization. It is therefore unlikely that a significant benefit in all-cause mortality would be observed with intensive therapy compared with standard therapy unless a much larger trial (perhaps requiring about 50,000 patients) with a longer follow-up is conducted.

SEARCH TRIAL

The Study of the Effectiveness of Additional Reductions in Cholesterol and Homocysteine (SEARCH) trial is the largest and the most recent of the trials in stable coronary disease and randomized 12,064 participants to simvastatin 20 mg versus 80 mg and accrued events over 6.7 years of follow-up.[32] The trial had a lower threshold of total cholesterol (TC) such that individuals had to have a total cholesterol of at least 3.5 mmol/L if they were on statin therapy or 4.5 mmol/L if they were statin naive. At study entry baseline TC was 4.23 mmol/L and LDL-C was 2.50 mmol/L. The average LDL-C difference between more versus less intensive therapy was 0.35mmol/L, which resulted in a nonsignificant 6% reduction in any major vascular event (HR, 0.94; CI 0.88–1.01). Similarly, there were no significant reductions in stroke, coronary death, or coronary revascularizations. The only endpoint to show significant benefit was nonfatal MI, where a 1.1% absolute reduction in risk was observed (7.7% vs. 6.6%).

While consistent with other lower-is-better trials, the data would suggest that simvastatin 80 mg is a far weaker LDL-C lowering regimen than those tested in the TNT and IDEAL trials. Importantly, this trial, by virtue of size and duration, demonstrated the significant increased risk observed from simvastatin 80 mg, not observed with other high-intensity statins. Creatine kinase (CK) elevations >5 upper limit of normal (ULN) and ≤10 × ULN occurred in 1.3% versus 0.5% in the simvastatin 80 mg versus 20 mg doses respectively, and elevations >40 × ULN in 0.4% versus 0%, respectively. Myopathy was also more common occurring at a rate of 90 of 10,000 individuals exposed versus 3 of 10,000 people exposed. These data have resulted in both the U.S. Food and Drug Administration (FDA) and the European Medicines Agency (EMEA) issuing a warning of increased risk of myopathy with simvastatin 80 mg. Atherosclerosis is a chronic disease, and patients who are commenced on statins require this treatment for the remainder of their lives. The benefits of intensive therapy observed over about 5 years are likely to translate into even greater reductions in the number of events over a longer period, providing significant benefits for individuals and health care systems.

Meta-Analysis of Intensive versus Standard Therapy

The four intensive versus standard therapy trials used different endpoints to assess clinical benefit and were each underpowered to assess the historical endpoint of CAD death or nonfatal MI. A literature-based meta-analysis was conducted to obtain consistent large-scale evidence across trials. All eligible trials were required to have at least 1000 participants and a treatment duration of at least 2 years.[33] The four trials discussed previously—PROVE IT-TIMI 22, A to Z, TNT, and IDEAL—were identified, providing information on 27,548 patients and approximately 120,000 patient-years of follow-up data.[26,27,30,31] A separate meta-analysis of the same four trials also assessed the effect of intensive versus standard therapy for reductions in hospitalization with heart failure.[34] The average, pooled baseline LDL-C level in the four trials was 130 mg/dL (3.3 mmol/L), which was reduced on average to 101 mg/dL (2.59 mmol/L). With intensive therapy, the average LDL-C level was lowered further to 75 mg/dL (1.92 mmol/L).[33] This additional reduction in LDL-C was associated with a 16% reduction in the risk of CAD death or MI (OR, 0.84; $P = 0.00003$). Similarly, there was a reduction in the risk of any major cardiovascular event by 16% ($P < 0.0001$). There was a favorable trend toward reduction in CAD death (OR, 0.88; $P = 0.054$) and no excess risk in noncardiovascular mortality was observed (OR, 1.03; $P = 0.73$). Reductions were observed for stroke (OR, 0.82; $P = 0.012$) and for hospitalization for CHF (OR, 0.73; $P < 0.001$).[34] The modest effects overall on all-cause mortality may, in part, reflect contemporary background therapy and also the differential risk between patients with stable CAD and ACS. There is clear evidence of an all-cause mortality benefit within 2 years of ACS from an individual participant meta-analysis of the PROVE IT-TIMI 22 and the A to Z trials.[35] Over approximately 20,000 person-years worth of follow-up intensive statin therapy reduced all-cause mortality by 23% (HR, 0.77; CI 0.63–0.95) and in absolute terms by 1.3% (NNT, 77 over 2 years to prevent one death from any cause) from 4.9% to 3.6%. Statin therapy is now recommended for all patients with established atherosclerotic vascular disease. This meta-analysis extends the earlier findings (i.e., CTT meta-analysis) and demonstrates that beyond standard therapy, additional intensive LDL-C reduction provides a further 16% reduction in risk of CAD or nonfatal MI or any major cardiovascular event, or approximately a 50% reduction compared with placebo.

Given the improvement in standards of medical care and the use of revascularization over the past decade, these additional benefits may seem modest but are achieved over 2 to 5 years. Given the chronic, lifelong nature of these diseases, these benefits throughout an individual's life would be expected to translate into greater absolute benefits by preventing recurrent, multiple events. In addition analytical techniques that take only time to first event into account underestimate the overall benefits of any treatment regimen; as therapies reduce the second and third events among those on more intensive treatments, the real benefit and cost effectiveness of more intensive regimens is even greater. For instance, in the PROVE IT-TIMI 22 trial over 2 years for every 2000 individuals treated, an additional 65 events could be averted by intensive therapy ($P = 0.009$).[36] Similar consistent observations were made in the TNT trial in stable CAD where beyond the first event intensive statin therapy for approximately every 5000 individuals treated for 5 years resulted in 166 fewer second events, 92 fewer third events, 55 fewer fourth events, and 33 fewer fifth events.[37] Taken together, these data support the value of long-term atheroprotection with intensive lipid lowering over time and the need for continuation of therapy.

More recently, the CTT in their second round of analyses provided individual participant data on five trials and 39,612 individuals.[38] Overall, more intensive statin therapy resulted in a 0.53mmol/L lowering of LDL-C and a 15% risk reduction in first major vascular event (RR, 0.85; CI 0.82–0.89), with considerable heterogeneity between studies (χ^2 $P < 0.0001$). However, when studies were standardized per mmol/L lowering in LDL-C, the corresponding risk reduction overall was 28% (RR, 0.72; CI 0.66–0.78) with no significant evidence of heterogeneity across studies (χ^2 $P = 0.05$). Taken together, these data suggest that the differences observed between studies reflect the relative efficacies of the more versus less intensive statin-lowering regimens. On specific endpoints, an incremental 0.53 mmol/L lowering of LDL-C resulted in a 13% reduction in any coronary event (RR, 0.87; CI 0.81–0.93), a 19% reduction in the need for any revascularisation (RR, 0.81; CI 0.76–0.85), and a 14% reduction in any stroke (RR, 0.86; CI 0.77–0.96). Importantly, there was no lower threshold for LDL-C, where a 1 mmol/L additional lowering of LDL-C with intensive therapy over and above standard therapy was not beneficial. For instance, even among those with a baseline LDL-C less than 2.0 mmol/L, a further 1 mmol/L lowering resulted in a 29% risk reduction (RR, 0.71; CI 0.52–0.98) which was similar to the benefit observed among those with an LDL-C greater than 3.5mmol/L (χ^2 $P = 0.2$). Taken together, these results suggest that among high-risk individuals, LDL-C should be lowered as much as possible with no target level.

Observational studies have suggested that among patients with heart failure, a low LDL-C level is associated with an increased risk of adverse events.[39,40] However, it is likely that these observations are confounded, given the results of the meta-analysis, which showed reductions in the risk of the development of heart failure with intensive therapy versus standard therapy. Although the role that lowering LDL-C levels play in reducing the risk of heart failure is not immediately intuitive, results of the latest meta-analysis may reflect the beneficial effects of high-dose statin therapy beyond LDL-C reduction, the so-called *pleiotropic effect*. The data for reduction in heart failure hospitalizations among individuals with coronary disease are in contrast to those from recent trials of statin therapy among individuals with or without ischemic cardiomyopathy in the GISSI HF (HR, 0.97; CI 0.87–1.09) and CORONA trials (HR, 0.92; CI 0.82–1.02).[41,42] This lack of benefit may, in part, be related to the advanced stage of disease. The lack of benefit of statin therapy on major cardiovascular events in this population is likely attributable to the fact that the majority of events are arrhythmic in nature or related to pump failure rather than atherothrombotic events and hence unlikely to be modulated by statins.

Early Benefits of Intensive Statin Therapy for Acute Coronary Syndrome

The risk of adverse clinical events is greatest in the first 6 months after the index ACS event. The early trials of statin therapy in patients with stable CAD suggested that the benefits of statin therapy appeared only after 1 to 2 years.[19,20] Although plaque rupture is a feature of ACS, it has become apparent that ACS is a pancoronary process with multiple vulnerable or ruptured plaques. Although angioplasty and stenting treat a culprit lesion effectively, potent systemic therapy is required to passivate other vulnerable sites.[43] The PROVE IT trial, conducted in patients enrolled within 10 days of experiencing an ACS, demonstrated the superiority of intensive statin therapy versus standard statin therapy in these patients over a period of 2 years, but it was unclear whether this benefit was related principally to a very early benefit, to a late benefit after patients had stabilized, or to a combination of the two. Using a composite endpoint of death, MI, or rehospitalization for recurrent ACS (i.e., the common endpoint in ACS trials), the benefit of intensive statin therapy was assessed in the first 30 days after ACS and in more stable patients from 6 months through end of study.[44] This particular analysis demonstrated that the composite endpoint occurred in 15.7% of patients assigned to 80 mg of atorvastatin and in 20.0% of patients assigned to 40 mg of pravastatin, reflecting a risk reduction of 24% ($P = 0.0002$).

Benefit in favor of 80 mg of atorvastatin was observed as early as 15 days after randomization and was significant by day 30. The composite endpoint occurred in 3.0% of the intensive-therapy group and in 4.2% of the standard-therapy group at 30 days, reflecting a 28% risk reduction at 30 days ($P = 0.046$) with 80 mg of atorvastatin (Fig. 10-7). In

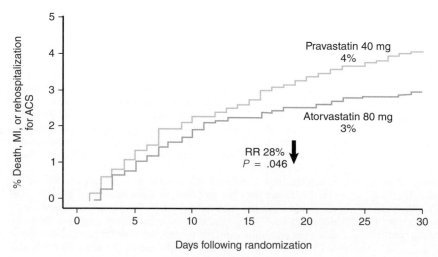

Figure 10-7 Early benefit of intensive standard statin therapy within 30 days after acute coronary syndrome (ACS) in the Pravastatin or Atorvastatin Evaluation and Infection Therapy (PROVE IT) trial. *(Data from Ray KK, Cannon CP, McCabe CH, et al, for the PROVE IT-TIMI 22 Investigators: Early and late benefits of high-dose atorvastatin in patients with acute coronary syndromes: Results from the PROVE IT-TIMI 22 trial, J Am Coll Cardiol 46:1405–1410, 2005.)*

addition to greater reductions in LDL levels, 80 mg of atorvastatin reduced CRP levels to a greater extent than did 40 mg of pravastatin, independent of effects on LDL (1.6 mg/L vs. 2.3 mg/L, $P < 0.0001$). Commencing 6 months after ACS to the end of the study, the composite endpoint occurred in 9.6% of the intensive therapy group and 13.1% of the standard-therapy group, representing a 28% further risk reduction ($P = 0.003$) in favor of high-dose atorvastatin (80 mg). This suggests that among patients who tolerate high-dose statin therapy, continuation of high-dose therapy is beneficial and provides early and late benefits. PROVE IT demonstrated that high-dose statin therapy lowers LDL-C and CRP concentrations at 30 days and is associated with a reduction in clinical events. In contrast, the A to Z trial showed a greater difference in resulting LDL levels between intensive statin regimens versus moderate statin regimens, but no difference in CRP levels at 30 days and, significantly, no early benefit was observed.[27,28] Despite matching for LDL-C at day 30, subjects allocated atorvastatin were less likely to have had an MI or recurrent ACS in the previous 30 days, suggesting that the early benefit is related to effects beyond the concentration of LDL-C and that lowering CRP levels may reduce inflammation and may be more important than lipid lowering with respect to early benefits.[45]

A meta-analysis of 13 randomized trials of early statin therapy for management of ACS assessed the early benefit of statin therapy using cumulative data on 17,963 patients.[46] Only five of the trials enrolled more than 1000 patients, and of these, only three trials had follow-up periods of more than 4 months, and only two trials followed up patients for more than 1 year. This meta-analysis assessed major cardiovascular events, including stroke. In particular, the latter endpoint requires about 2 years to demonstrate a clinical benefit and might have attenuated any observed early composite benefits on CVD. In this analysis, early composite benefit was not observed at 1 month after ACS (HR, 1.02) but appeared by 4 months (HR, 0.84) and was significant by 6 months (HR, 0.76).

Intensive Statin Therapy and Atherosclerosis

Given the clinical impact of statin therapy of cardiovascular event reduction in patients with CAD, it is intuitive to expect that statins would reverse the atherosclerosis disease burden. Several trials used angiography to assess the impact of standard-dose statin therapy on the extent of angiographic disease. Although standard doses of statins reduced LDL-C levels by 20% to 30%, they failed to demonstrate regression of disease burden, and, instead, consistently showed that in the presence of CAD, statins reduce the rate of progression of disease.[47]

REVERSAL TRIAL

The Reversing Atherosclerosis with Aggressive Lipid Lowering (REVERSAL) trial compared the effects of two statin regimens administered for 18 months in 654 patients. Patients were randomized to a moderate-lipid-lowering regimen consisting of 40 mg of pravastatin (licensed in the United States for reducing atherosclerosis progression) or an intensive-lipid-lowering regimen consisting of 80 mg of atorvastatin. The primary efficacy parameter was the percentage of change in atheroma volume (i.e., follow-up value minus baseline). Secondary efficacy parameters included change in total atheroma volume, change in percentage of atheroma volume, and change in atheroma volume in the most severely diseased 10-mm vessel subsegment.

The baseline LDL-C concentration fell from 150.2 mg/dL (3.89 mmol/L) in both treatment groups to 110 mg/dL (2.85 mmol/L) in the pravastatin group and to 79 mg/dL (2.05 mmol/L) in the atorvastatin group ($P < 0.001$). CRP levels decreased 5.2% with pravastatin and 36.4% with atorvastatin ($P < 0.001$). In subjects receiving standard therapy, the percentage of change in atheroma volume from baseline was 2.7% ($P < 0.001$), and in those allocated to intensive therapy, it

was −0.4% ($P = 0.98$; for the difference between groups, $P = 0.02$). Similar differences between groups were observed for secondary efficacy parameters, including change in total atheroma volume ($P = 0.02$), change in percentage of atheroma volume ($P < 0.001$), and change in atheroma volume in the most severely diseased 10-mm vessel subsegment ($P < 0.01$).

ASTEROID STUDY

A Study to Evaluate the Effect of Rosuvastatin on Intravascular Ultrasound-Derived Coronary Atheroma Burden (ASTEROID) assessed whether intensive statin therapy with 40 mg of rosuvastatin could cause regression of atherosclerosis in patients with CAD assessed by intravascular ultrasound (IVUS). A motorized IVUS pullback was used to assess coronary atheroma burden at baseline and after 24 months of treatment in 507 patients. The mean (standard deviation [SD]) baseline LDL-C level of 130.4 mg/dL declined to 60.8 mg/dL; mean HDL-C level at baseline was 43.1 mg/dL, increasing to 49.0 mg/dL; and the median concentration of triglycerides fell from 135 mg/dL to 109 mg/dL. The mean change in percentage of atheroma volume from baseline for the entire vessel was −0.98%. The mean change in atheroma volume in the most diseased 10-mm subsegment was −6.1 mm³ ($P < 0.001$ vs. baseline). Change in total atheroma volume showed a 6.8% median reduction ($P < 0.001$ vs. baseline). These two studies using IVUS confirm that standard statin therapy does not arrest the progression of atherosclerosis and that more intensive therapy is required to stop or even regress pre-existing disease burden (Fig. 10-8). Although the findings in ASTEROID appear more dramatic than the initial findings in REVERSAL, some key differences should be considered. There was no active comparator arm in ASTEROID, so the effect other statin regimens would have had in the same population is not clear. This is particularly important because in REVERSAL, specific subgroups such as those without diabetes and those with lower LDL-C levels appeared to derive greater benefit from 80 mg of atorvastatin. Compared with REVERSAL, there were a greater number of patients in the ASTEROID trial and consequently greater power to demonstrate regression. The ASTEROID population had a lower baseline LDL-C concentration, a lower baseline level of triglycerides, and fewer patients with diabetes, which might have favored demonstration of disease regression resulting from intensive therapy. In ASTEROID, there was higher percentage of patients with no IVUS follow-up for clinical endpoints compared with REVERSAL, highlighting the difficulty of comparing trials. Nevertheless, these trials and similar studies such as the Early Statin Treatment in Patients with Acute Coronary Syndrome: Demonstration of the Beneficial Effect on Atherosclerotic Lesions by Serial Volumetric Intravascular Ultrasound Analysis during Half a Year after Coronary Event (ESTABLISH trial), which studied ACS patients cumulatively, demonstrated the need for intensive lipid reduction to arrest disease progression in subjects with established atherosclerosis.[48,49]

Mechanisms of Benefit

INTENSITY OF LOW-DENSITY LIPOPROTEIN REDUCTION

Given the prior epidemiologic data and clear evidence that a statin is better than placebo and that an intensive statin regimen is better than a standard-dose statin regimen, subjects with CAD who achieved the lowest levels of LDL-C would be expected to be at lowest risk for recurrent events. In the CTT meta-analysis, when all trials were considered and a regression line forced through zero, a linear relationship between lower LDL-C levels and risk reduction was observed. The current intensive statin therapy versus moderate statin therapy trials also fit this regression model, suggesting that the greater the LDL-C difference between two strategies, the greater is the clinical benefit (see Fig. 10-6). However, the long-term efficacy of statin therapy in patients achieving very low LDL-C levels (<100 mg/dL) remained poorly assessed until

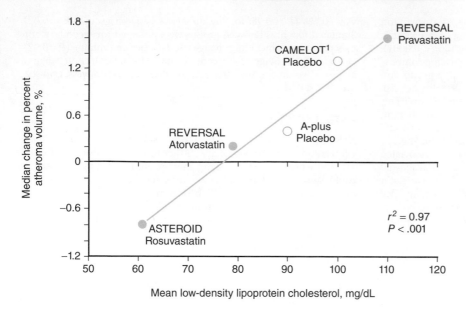

Figure 10-8 Relationship between low-density lipoprotein cholesterol and atherosclerosis progression on intravascular ultrasound in the Reversing Atherosclerosis with Aggressive Lipid Lowering (REVERSAL), Comparison of Amlodipine versus Enalapril to Limit Occurrences of Thrombosis (CAMELOT), Avasimibe and Progression of Coronary Lesions Assessed by Intravascular Ultrasound (A-PLUS), and A Study to Evaluate the Effect of Rosuvastatin on Intravascular Ultrasound-Derived Coronary Atheroma Burden (ASTEROID) trials. *(Data from Nissen SE, Nicholls SJ, Sipayhi I, et al: Effect of very high-intensity statin therapy on regression of coronary atherosclerosis: The ASTEROID trial, JAMA, 295: 1555–1565, 2006.)*

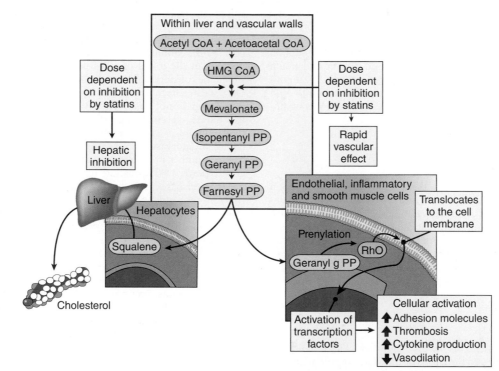

Figure 10-9 Inhibition of hydroxymethyl glutaryl–coenzyme A (HMG-CoA) reductase leads to effects mediated by low-density-lipoprotein–cholesterol (LDL-C) through the liver and nonlipid-related effects in the vessel wall. *(From Ray KK, Cannon CP: The potential relevance of the multiple lipid-independent [pleiotropic] effects of statins in the management of acute coronary syndromes, J Am Coll Cardiol 46:1425–1433, 2005.)*

recently. In an analysis from PROVE IT-TIMI 22, the relationship between achieved LDL-C levels and clinical outcomes with 80 mg of atorvastatin was assessed by dividing these patients into subgroups by achieved LDL-C levels at 4 months (>80–100, >60–80, >40–60, ≤40 mg/dL) and correlating this with risk of subsequent adverse events.[50] Among almost 2000 subjects for whom 4-month LDL-C data were available, about 90% had LDL-C levels less than 100 mg/dL (2.59 mmol/L). Compared with the reference group (LDL-C level of 80 to 100 mg/dL), the hazard of death, MI, stroke, recurrent ischemia, and revascularization was lower among patients with LDL-C levels between greater than 40 and 60 (HR, 0.76) and lowest among those with LDL-C levels less than or equal to 40 mg/dL (HR, 0.61). There

was no increased risk of adverse events at these low levels of LDL-C. It is not necessary to reduce the dose of a statin if the resultant LDL-C levels fall well below guideline recommendations. These results suggest the possibility that further LDL-C lowering beyond the new guideline optimal goal of less than 70 mg/dL (1.8 mmol/L) may translate into additional clinical benefit.

REDUCTION IN CRP LEVELS

Statins possess pleiotropic effects that are mediated by hydroxymethyl glutaryl–coenzyme A (HMG-CoA) reductase but are not dependent on lowering of LDL-C levels (Fig. 10-9). All statins lower CRP levels,

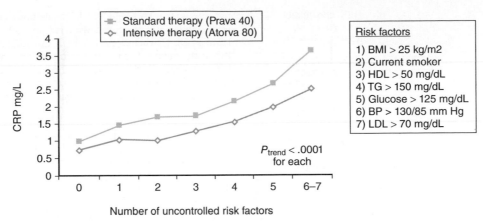

Figure 10-10 Relationships among uncontrolled risk factors, statin therapy, and achieved C-reactive protein (CRP) levels. *(From Ray KK, Cannon CP: The potential relevance of the multiple lipid-independent [pleiotropic] effects of statins in the management of acute coronary syndromes, J Am Coll Cardiol 46:1425–1433, 2005.)*

partly in relation to the statin dose. In PROVE IT, the median levels of CRP were similar in the 80-mg atorvastatin and 40-mg pravastatin groups (12.2 and 11.9 mg/L, respectively; $P = 0.60$) at study entry, but they were significantly lower in the atorvastatin group than in the pravastatin group at 30 days (1.6 vs. 2.3 mg/L, $P < 0.001$), 4 months (1.3 vs. 2.1 mg/L, $P < 0.001$), and the end of the study (1.3 vs. 2.1 mg/L, $P < 0.001$). Although the levels of LDL-C and CRP were reduced by statin therapy at 30 days, the correlation between the achieved values was weak ($R = 0.16$; $P = 0.001$) (i.e., less than 3% of the variance in achieved CRP levels was explained by the variance in achieved LDL). Because there are other known correlates of CRP in statin-naïve subjects, further assessment from PROVE IT performed a cross-sectional analysis of the relationship between on-treatment uncontrolled risk factors and CRP levels.[51] These factors were defined as body mass index (BMI) greater than 25 kg/m² (i.e., World Health Organization's cut-off for overweight), blood pressure higher than 130/85 mm Hg, glucose concentration higher than 110 mg/dL, triglyceride level greater than 150 mg/dL (i.e., Adult Treatment Panel III of the National Cholesterol Education Program's cut-offs), HDL level less than 50 mg/dL, LDL-C level equal to or greater than 70 mg/dL, and smoking. An increase in incremental risk factor burden (i.e., number of uncontrolled risk factors present) was associated with an increase in CRP values (Fig. 10-10). Among patients allocated to standard therapy, the CRP level was 3.8 mg/L (interquartile range [IQR]: 1.9, 7.8) when seven uncontrolled risk factors were present and 1.0 mg/L (IQR: 0.7, 2.1) when none was present ($P < 0.0001$ for trend). However, among patients allocated intensive therapy, the corresponding CRP levels were lower and ranged from 2.4 mg/L (IQR: 1.7, 5.7) to 0.8 mg/L (IQR: 0.4, 1.2) ($P < 0.0001$ for trend). In this population, in which everyone received a statin, prior randomization to 80 mg of atorvastatin was associated with a 27% lower CRP compared with 40 mg of pravastatin ($P < 0.0001$) independently of LDL-C, triglyceride, and HDL levels, and other correlates of CRP such as age, gender, glycemia, blood pressure, smoking, and BMI.[51]

At 30 days, the median LDL concentration was approximately 70 mg/L, and the median CRP level was approximately 2 mg/L. At 30 days, patients in whom statin therapy resulted in LDL-C levels less than 70 mg/dL had lower age-adjusted rates of recurrent MI or CAD death compared with those who did not achieve this goal (2.7 vs. 4.0 events per 100 person-years, $P = 0.008$). Despite the minimal correlation between LDL-C and CRP levels, an identical difference in the age-adjusted rates of events was also observed among patients in whom statin therapy resulted in CRP levels of less than 2 mg/L compared with those in whom statin therapy resulted in higher CRP values (2.8 vs. 3.9 events per 100 person-years, $P = 0.006$). Patients who had achieved LDL-C levels less than 70 mg/dL and CRP levels less than 2 mg/L had the lowest risk of recurrent events, whereas those with LDL-C levels more than 70 mg/dL and CRP levels more than 2 mg/L had the highest risk. Hazard ratios for recurrent events among patients whose values were more than 70 mg/dL for LDL-C and below 2 mg/L for CRP, those whose values were less than 70 mg/dL for LDL and more than 2 mg/L for CRP, and those whose values were more than 70 mg/dL for LDL-C and more than 2 mg/L for CRP, compared with those whose values of achieved LDL-C were less than 70 mg/dL and CRP less than 2 mg/L (i.e., reference group), were 1.3, 1.4, and 1.9, respectively (for trend across groups, $P < 0.001$) (Fig. 10-11, A). Similar data have emerged from the A to Z trial, showing that subjects who achieve a low CRP level with high-dose statin therapy and those who achieve the dual goals of LDL-C levels less than 70 mg/dL and CRP levels less than 2 mg/L are at lower risk for recurrent events (see Fig. 10-11, B).[52] Meta-analysis of achieved CRP levels in the PROVE IT and A to Z trials demonstrated that the adjusted risk of death or recurrent MI of a CRP value greater than 2 mg/L is 1.43 (95% CI: 1.2–1.7). These secondary prevention data demonstrate that using statin therapy to achieve target levels of both LDL-C and CRP decreases the risk of recurrent MI and CAD death among patients with ACS. Whether CRP is causally related to risk or is a marker remains unclear, but several lines of evidence suggest that it is an important player in mediating cardiovascular risk (Fig. 10-12). These data support the hypothesis that therapies designed to reduce inflammation after ACS may improve cardiovascular outcomes.

APOLIPOPROTEINS

Observational data from individuals free from CVD does not support using apolipoproteins over and above traditional lipids. Although the clinical benefits of statins appear to be predominantly related to LDL-C–mediated effects, other lipid markers such as the concentration of apolipoprotein B (apoB), non–HDL-C, total cholesterol to HDL ratio, or apoB/A-I, provide alternative approaches. In statin trials, data about on-treatment lipid values alone explaining the totality of the benefits of statin therapy are conflicting. In the Air Force/Texas Coronary Atherosclerosis Prevention Study (AFCAPS/TexCAPS) trial, on-treatment apoB values appeared to be a superior marker of on-treatment efficacy compared with LDL-C levels, and the on-treatment apoB/A-I ratio appeared to explain the entire benefit of statin therapy in this trial.[53] In contrast, the much larger LIPID trial suggested that the proportion of the treatment effect explained by reductions in LDL-C was 52%,

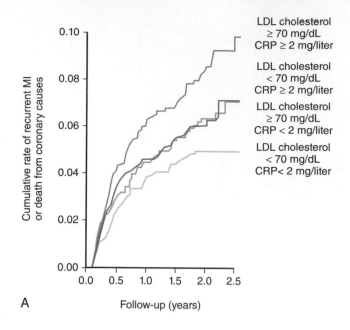

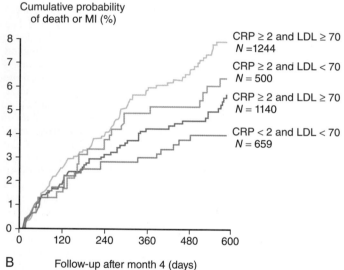

Figure 10-11 Clinical benefit of achieving the dual goals of low-density lipoprotein (LDL) less than 70 mg/dL and C-reactive protein (CRP) levels of less than 2 mg/L with statin therapy in the Pravastatin or Atorvastatin Evaluation and Infection Therapy–Thrombolysis In Myocardial Infarction 22 (PROVE IT-TIMI 22) **(A)** and Aggrastat to Zocor (A to Z) trials **(B)**, showing the benefit of achieving dual goals. (A, *from Ridker PM, Cannon CP, Morrow D, et al, for the Pravastatin or Atorvastatin Evaluation and Infection Therapy–Thrombolysis in Myocardial Infarction 22 (PROVE IT-TIMI 22) Investigators: C-reactive protein levels and outcomes after statin therapy, N Engl J Med 352:20–28, 2005; B, from Morrow DA, de Lemos JA, Sabatine MS, et al: Clinical relevance of C-reactive protein during follow-up of patients with acute coronary syndromes in the Aggrastat-to-Zocor Trial, Circulation 114:281–288, 2006.)*

compared with 67% for apoB, suggesting that nonlipid-related effects may also contribute to the long-term benefit of statins.[54]

In the PROVE IT-TIMI 22 trial, non–HDL-C provided similar information to apoB and neither non–HDL-C nor apoB/AI ratio nor TC/HDL ratio improved risk prediction over and above LDL-C. Risk prediction was improved, however, by the addition of high-sensitivity CRP (hs-CRP) to any lipid component. In contrast to the lipid findings in PROVE IT TIMI 22, in the larger combined dataset of stable

patients in the TNT and IDEAL trials both non–HDL-C and apoB were significantly associated with risk in multi-variable models containing LDL-C, whereas the latter was attenuated and nonsignificant in the same models.[56] Overall, there were no meaningful differences between apoB over non–HDL-C nor in the ratio of TC/HDL over apoB/AI, although these factors were not formally tested in risk prediction models. Reconciling these apparently disparate findings is difficult in the absence of access to primary data. However, one explanation may reside with the high preponderance of individuals with metabolic syndrome, at least in the TNT trial, which indicated that insulin resistance may contribute to higher levels of VLDL and IDL and small dense LDL-C such that LDL-C less closely approximates to non–HDL-C or apoB. However, what is clear is that there is little conclusive evidence to suggest that apoB should be measured as an alternative to non–HDL-C (the optional secondary NCEP III target) in routine clinical practice.

OXIDIZED LOW-DENSITY LIPOPROTEIN

Oxidized phospholipids (OxPLs) exist within atherosclerotic plaques and are bound by lipoprotein(a) in plasma. Circulating levels of oxidized LDL are strongly associated with angiographically documented CAD and therefore may contribute to the pathogenesis of atherosclerosis.[57] In the MIRACL trial, high-dose atorvastatin reduced the total apoB-containing OxPLs by 29.7% as well as reducing apoB levels by 30%. When normalized per apoB-100, compared with placebo, atorvastatin increased the OxPL/apoB level (9.5% versus −3.9%, $P < 0.0001$). These data suggest that atorvastatin treatment results in enrichment of OxPLs on a smaller pool of apoB particles, which may contribute to the reduction in ischemic events after ACS observed in MIRACL.[58]

RAISING HIGH-DENSITY LIPOPROTEIN CHOLESTEROL LEVELS

HDL as a carrier of increased cellular cholesterol in the reverse cholesterol transport pathway is believed to provide protection against atherosclerosis (Fig. 10-13). In reverse cholesterol transport, peripheral tissues (e.g., vessel-wall macrophages) remove their excess cholesterol through the adenosine triphosphate (ATP)–binding cassette transporter A1 (ABCA1) to poorly lipidated apolipoprotein A-I, forming pre-HDL. HDL consists of a heterogeneous class of lipoproteins containing approximately equal amounts of lipid and protein. The various HDL subclasses differ in quantitative and qualitative contents of lipids, apolipoproteins, enzymes, and lipid transfer proteins, resulting in differences in shape, density, size, charge, and antigenicity. Assessment of HDL-C measures the cholesterol content of all these HDL subclasses and is therefore a crude marker of reverse cholesterol transport. The American National Cholesterol Education Program considers HDL-C to be an optional secondary target of lipid treatment, whereas the European Consensus Panel recommend a minimum target for HDL of 40 mg/dL (1.03 mmol/L) in certain patients, such as those with diabetes, but the relevance of the latter recommendation is unclear in light of limited data from clinical trials.[29,59]

CHOLESTEROL ESTER TRANSFER PROTEIN INHIBITION

Humans with CETP deficiency caused by molecular defects in the *CETP* gene have markedly elevated plasma levels of HDL-C and apolipoprotein A-I, suggesting that CETP inhibition may increase HDL-C levels. Preliminary data from phase II trials assessing the relative efficacy of torcetrapib in addition to different doses of atorvastatin at raising HDL showed that the addition of 60 mg of torcetrapib was associated with an increase in HDL of about 55% when added to 80 mg of atorvastatin, compared with about a 40% increase in HDL when used alone. However, in December 2006, Pfizer halted the development of torcetrapib because of a 60% observed increase in deaths in the ILLUMINATE trial.[60] Similar findings of lack of efficacy were

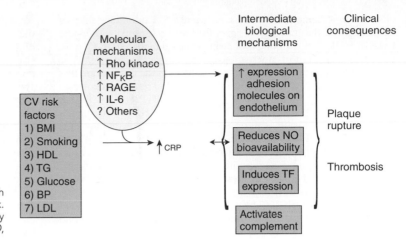

Figure 10-12 Schematic of putative mechanisms by which C-reactive protein (CRP) may mediate cardiovascular (CV) risk. *BMI*, body mass index; *BP*, blood pressure; *HDL*, high-density lipoprotein; *IL-6*, interleukin 6; *LDL*, low-density lipoprotein; *NO*, nitric oxide; *TF*, tissue factor; *TG*, triglycerides.

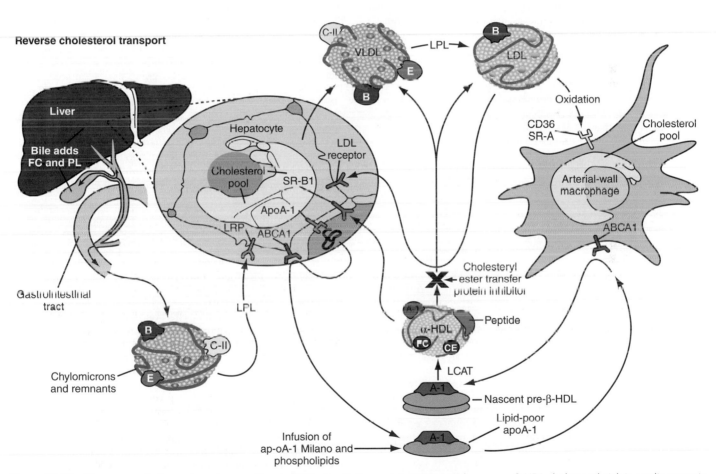

Figure 10-13 The reverse cholesterol transport pathway of high-density lipoprotein (HDL). Lipid-poor pre-β-HDL cholesterol, rich in apolipoprotein A-I (apoA-I), is synthesized by the liver or intestinal mucosa and released into the circulation, where it promotes the transfer of excess cellular-free cholesterol (FC) from macrophages to apoA-I by interacting with the ATP-binding cassette transporter A1 (ABCA1) in arterial wall macrophages. Plasma lecithin-cholesterol acyltransferase (LCAT) converts free cholesterol in pre-β-HDL cholesterol to cholesteryl ester (CE), resulting in the maturation of pre-β-HDL cholesterol to mature α-HDL cholesterol. The α-HDL cholesterol is transported to the liver by a direct or indirect pathway. In the direct pathway, selective uptake of cholesteryl ester by hepatocytes occurs with the scavenger receptor, class B, type 1 (SR-B1). In the indirect pathway, HDL cholesterol cholesteryl ester is exchanged for triglycerides in apolipoprotein B–rich particles (*B*), LDL cholesterol, and very-low-density lipoprotein (VLDL) cholesterol through cholesteryl ester-transfer protein (CETP), with the uptake of cholesteryl ester by the liver through the low-density lipoprotein (LDL) receptor (LDLR). Cholesterol that is returned to the liver is secreted as bile acids and cholesterol. Acquired triglycerides in the modified HDL cholesterol particle are subjected to hydrolysis by hepatic lipase (HL), thereby regenerating small HDL cholesterol particles and pre-β-HDL cholesterol for participation in reverse cholesterol transport. *E*, apolipoprotein-E–rich particles; *PL*, plasma lecithin. *(Modified from Brewer HB, Jr.: Increasing HDL cholesterol levels, N Engl J Med 350:1491–1494, 2004. Copyright 2004 Massachusetts Medical Society. All rights reserved.)*

observed in imaging trials of the same agent.[60–63] Exploratory analyses have suggested that there is no signal for harm associated with higher levels of HDL-C, and among those who achieved higher HDL-C levels, there was regression of atherosclerosis and a lower event rate.[64] The adverse effects now seem to be drug specific with the observation that torcetrapib raises blood pressure and activates the rennin–angiotensin system, including animal species which lack CETP activity, further supporting an off-target effect.[65] The potential for HDL-C raising has received further impetus with observations that anacetrapib not only raises HDL-C by 100% but produces nearly 40% lowering of LDL-C, but does not result in adverse effects on blood pressure.[66,67] This is being tested in a safety study, which may result in a large phase III trial.[68] While the relevance of these biologic changes and the role of CETP inhibition remains unproved, an ongoing phase III trial of dalcetrapib that raises HDL-C by around 30% aims to recruit around 15,000 post-ACS patients with results expected in 2012.[69] To date, no signal for harm has been observed.[70,71] There are important molecular differences between dalcetrapib and anacetrapib. Anacetrapib physically forms a tertiary complex between HDL2 particles and apoB-containing lipoproteins, whereas dalcetrapib is a modulator working in the CETP tunnel and its binding causes conformational change in CETP allowing it to bind to HDL2 particles but not to apoB. Whether these differences contribute to cardiovascular outcomes is a hypothesis that will be answered in the immediate future with the completion of large phase III trials.

NIACIN

A variety of studies have assessed the relative merit of raising HDL-C levels using niacin (discussed previously). A meta-analysis of these data suggests that there is a 1.7% reduction per 1% rise in HDL-C levels with niacin.[72] Niacin raises HDL-C by levels of approximately 28%, but its use has been limited by adverse effects, notably flushing mediated by prostaglandins. Using ultrasound and measurements of carotid intima media thickness, niacin has been shown to attenuate and may reverse atherosclerosis.[73] In a study assessing carotid intima media thickness (ARBITER 6), niacin reduced the progression of atherosclerosis compared with ezetimibe, which was associated with progression ($P = 0.01$).[74] This is particularly interesting, and niacin and ezetimibe both produce about a 20% reduction in LDL-C. This suggests that differences between agents with respect to atherosclerosis may relate more to niacin's 30% rise in HDL-c and 20% lowering of lipoprotein(a). Magnetic resonance imaging (MRI) techniques to image carotid plaques have similarly shown that niacin reduces atheroma burden. An MRI study assessing the effect of 2 g of niacin on carotid atherosclerosis further supported these observations by showing demonstrating regression of atherosclerosis within 12 months.[75] Although niacin did show benefit on all-cause mortality during extended follow-up, the benefit of niacin over contemporary therapy has not been unproven. This concept is being tested in the large-scale 20,000 patient Heart Protection-2 study, in which niacin has been combined with the anti-flushing agent laropripant in a predominantly Chinese population with CAD or a high-risk equivalent. Niacin in a slow-release preparation is being tested versus statin therapy in a post-ACS population in the AIM-HIGH trial (terminated early for futility in 2011).

FIBRATES

Data for fibrates are conflicting. Although some studies such as VAHIT (Veterans Affairs High-Density Lipoprotein Intervention Trial) and the Helsinki Heart study have shown benefit in specific populations, more recent trials have suggested little benefit. Overall, the effects of fibrates on HDL-C levels are modest. This was demonstrated in the Fenofibrate Intervention and Event Lowering in Diabetes (FIELD) trial, in which long-term treatment with fenofibrate to raise HDL-C concentrations and lower triglyceride levels was assessed in subjects with type 2 diabetes and total blood cholesterol

concentrations of less than 251 mg/dL (6.5 mmol/L).[76] At the end of the trial, LDL-C levels fell from 120 mg/dL (3.07 mmol/L) to 95 mg/dL (2.43 mmol/L) in subjects allocated fenofibrate and to 101 mg/dL (2.60 mmol/L) in the placebo group. Triglyceride levels were also lower in the fenofibrate group—131 mg/dL (1.47 mmol/L) versus 166 mg/dL (1.87 mmol/L); however, HDL-C levels were not significantly different—44 mg/dL (1.13 mmol/L) versus 44 mg/dL (1.12 mmol/L)—compared with placebo. The differences in lipid levels between treatment groups decreased during the trial, particularly among patients receiving additional lipid-lowering therapy. Overall, 5.9% of patients on placebo and 5.2% of those on fenofibrate experienced the primary endpoint ($P = 0.16$). There was a significant reduction in nonfatal MI (24%) but a nonsignificant increase in CAD mortality (19%). Total cardiovascular events were significantly reduced by 11%, predominantly reflecting a 21% reduction in coronary revascularization. Overall, the FIELD trial failed to demonstrate a significant benefit of an agent that predominantly reduces triglyceride levels and raises HDL levels modestly in a high-risk population. This finding might have resulted from an unequal, increased use of statin therapy in subjects allocated to placebo.

The Action to Control Cardiovascular Risk in Diabetes (ACCORD) trial assessed whether adding a fibrate to statin therapy reduced cardiovascular risk among diabetics.[77] In this trial, the baseline LDL-C was 2.59 mmol/L, TG was 2.12 mmol/L, HDL-C was 0.98 mmol/L. LDL-C fell in both the placebo group to 2.07 mmol/L and in the fenofibrate group to 2.10 mmol/L with little difference between treatments. TG levels fell in the placebo group to 1.92 mmol/L and to 1.66 mmol/L in the fenofibrate group ($P < 0.001$). HDL-C rose in the placebo group to 1.05 mmol/L and to 1.07 mmol/L in the fenofibrate group ($P = 0.01$). This trial is significant for providing important information on safety, as there were no significant differences in transaminase levels or CK levels >10 × ULN between treatment groups. This reinforces the safety of fenofibrate when combined with a statin. The effect of fenofibrate on the combined endpoint of fatal and nonfatal CAD or stroke was 8% lower but did not reach statistical significance (HR, 0.92; CI 0.79–1.08). A prespecified subgroup analysis showed a significant interaction by gender, with benefit in men and possible harm in women (P interaction 0.01) and a trend toward benefit among subjects with baseline elevated TG and a low HDL-C (P interaction 0.057).

A meta-analysis of 18 fibrate trials, including a mixture of primary and secondary preventions, provided useful new information.[78] This showed a 19% RRR in nonfatal MI (RR, 0.81; CI 0.75–0.89), no effect on stroke (RR, 1.03; CI 0.91–1.16), no effect on cardiovascular death (RR, 0.97; CI 0.88–1.07), and no effect on all-cause mortality (RR, 1.0; CI 0.93–1.08). There was a reduction in the need for revascularization (RR, 0.88; CI 0.78–0.88) and a trend toward increased risk of noncardiovascular deaths (RR, 1.10; CI 1.0–1.21). Taken together, these data suggest modest benefits on nonfatal MI and revascularization only. Among people with an elevated TG greater than 2 mmol/L, there was proportionately greater reduction in coronary events (32% lower vs. 19%; P interaction 0.03); a similar trend was observed in individuals with a baseline HDL less than 1 mmol/L (23% vs. 14%,), although this difference was not statistically significant. These results are derived from access to study-level data only, rather than to individual-level data and require further validation such as that intended in the third cycle of the cholesterol treatment trialists collaboration, which will weight the benefit of fibrates by changes in TG, HDL-C, and non-HDL-C. In a meta-analysis of five trials, there was a greater relative risk reduction in vascular events among those with an atherogenic dyslipidemia profile at baseline (high TG, low HDL; OR 0.65 versus 0.94). Taken together and given the benefits of statin therapy among patients with diabetes in the Collaborative Atorvastatin Diabetes Study (CARDS) trial and in subgroups of other trials, and the CTT meta-analysis of all placebo-controlled trials including subjects with diabetes demonstrates consistent benefits on cardiovascular events among patients with diabetes for major coronary events, for strokes, and for revascularization.[23,79]

EZETIMIBE OR COLESEVELAM

Ezetimibe is a compound that binds to the Niemann Pick receptor in the intestine and reduces the absorption of cholesterol esters. Numerous studies have demonstrated its excellent tolerability and a 20% reduction in LDL-C when administered in addition to statin therapy or as monotherapy. This agent may also be particularly useful in the so-called high-absorber, low-synthesizer groups, where subjects respond poorly to statins with little or no change in LDL-C. However, there is no trial evidence of significant cardiovascular benefit with ezetimibe. The IMPROVE IT trial is assessing the incremental benefit of ezetimibe over statin therapy with respect to clinical outcomes in patients with ACS and compares simvastatin to simvastatin plus ezetimibe. Colesevelam is a bile acid absorption inhibitor, which can be used as monotherapy or combination therapy with statins. As the bile acid pool becomes depleted, the hepatic enzyme, cholesterol 7-α-hydroxylase, is upregulated, which increases the conversion of cholesterol to bile acids. This causes an increased demand for cholesterol in the liver cells, resulting in the dual effect of decreasing transcription and activity of the cholesterol biosynthetic enzyme, HMG-CoA reductase, and increasing the number of hepatic LDL receptors. These compensatory effects result in increased clearance of LDL-C from blood, resulting in decreased serum LDL-C levels. The average LDL-C reduction is in the order of 18% with a rise in HDL-C of 3%.[80] Common adverse effects include flatulence and constipation, and a less common adverse effect is elevation of triglycerides.

GLITAZONES

Glitazones are a novel class of agents that stimulate the PPAR-γ receptor, improve glycemic control, and have favorable effects on dyslipidemia, particularly in reducing triglycerides and raising HDL-C levels. The Prospective Pioglitazone Clinical Trial in Macrovascular Events (PROACTIVE) trial was a placebo-controlled trial that assessed the benefit of a PPAR-γ agonist pioglitazone in subjects with stable type 2 diabetes with evidence of macrovascular disease. Patients with evidence of coronary, cerebral, or peripheral arterial disease and an $HgbA_{1c}$ level greater than 6.5% despite treatment were considered eligible for the study (N = 5238).[81]

Compared with placebo, pioglitazone was associated with a 0.8% versus 0.3% reduction in $HgbA_{1c}$ from baseline (P < 0.0001) and an 11.4% versus 1.8% reduction in triglycerides (P < 0.0001). Significantly, pioglitazone raised HDL-C levels by 19%, compared with 10.1% in the placebo group (P < 0.0001), and reduced the LDL/HDL ratio by 9.5%, compared with 4.2% (P < 0.0001). The primary endpoint of mortality, nonfatal MI, stroke, ACS, coronary or peripheral arterial revascularization, and above-knee amputation tended to be lower in patients allocated pioglitazone (HR, 0.9; P = 0.095). The secondary endpoint of mortality, nonfatal MI, and stroke was reduced by 16% among patients allocated pioglitazone (P = 0.027). The overall findings of PROACTIVE, which included nonacute endpoints such as limb amputation, were neutral. However, a significant reduction in the secondary endpoint of death, nonfatal MI, and stroke was observed, raising the possibility that PPAR-γ agonists may be of value as an adjunctive therapy to statins among patients with diabetes and macrovascular disease. However, these findings require validation in further clinical trials. The differences in glycemic control between treatments were modest, but large differences in HDL-C levels were observed with pioglitazone. It is possible that the beneficial effects of pioglitazone may not be caused just by its effects on glycemia but may also be related to its beneficial effects on atherogenic dyslipidemia or systemic inflammation.[82] A meta-analysis of 16, 390 individuals in pioglitazone trials found an 18% reduction in risk of death, MI, or stroke (CI 0.72–0.94) but a 41% (CI 1.141–1.76) increased risk of heart failure.[83] In the PERISCOPE trial of pioglitazone, there was a lower rate of progression of atherosclerosis in pioglitazone-treated subjects compared with glimepiride on atheroma progression.[84] While the difference in HbA1c in favor of pioglitazone was 0.19% lower, HDL-C was 4.6 mg/dL higher, and TG was 19.6 mg/dL lower. Thus, much of the favorable effects of pioglitazone on atheroma progression are likely related to its beneficial effects on lipids, given the modest differences in HbA_{1c}. The favorable data for pioglitazone are distinctly contradictory to the safety data for rosiglitazone, which was called into consideration by a meta-analysis of randomized trials which suggested an increased risk of MI. In the most recent iteration of 56 trials, which included 35,531 patients, rosiglitazone significantly increased the risk of MI by 28% (CI 1.02–1.63) but had no effect on cardiovascular mortality (OR, 1.03; 95% CI, 0.78–1.36) (*Nissen Archives of Internal Medicine*, epub ahead of print). Rosiglitazone has been removed from the market in Europe, and in the United States it has been put under strict restriction to be used only if all other antidiabetic medications have failed.

Novel Targets for Therapy

PCSK-9

PCSK-9 is a glycoprotein that is expressed at its highest levels in the liver, intestine, and kidney. In humans, this protein degrades the LDL receptor, thus preventing the clearance of LDL-C or apoB-containing lipoproteins from the liver; this leads to higher levels of circulating LDL-C. Nonfunctioning mutations in the *PCSK-9* gene (prevalence of approximately 2% to 3%) lead to lower circulating levels of LDL-C and, in turn, lower risk of CAD in African Americans and in northern European populations.[81,85] These individuals have lifelong lower LDL-C levels that range from 28% in African Americans to 12% in northern Europeans. Interestingly, the observed risk of CAD was much greater than would have been expected for the degree of LDL-C reduction (88% and 28%, in African Americans and northern Europeans, respectively). Statins lead to an increase in the expression of PCSK-9 in a dose-dependent fashion, which perhaps explains why doubling the dose only affords a further 6% reduction in LDL-C. Currently, research is under way to develop inhibitors of PCSK-9, which in combination with statins offers the promise to significantly lower LDL-C levels.

ANTISENSE TO APOLIPOPROTEIN B

Mipomersen is an antisense oligonucleotide designed to reduce apoB100 synthesis by binding to the messenger ribonucleic acid (mRNA) for apoB100, which results in subsequent degradation by ribonuclease H and a reduction in apoB100 and thus in LDL-C. In clinical trials in patients with familial hypercholesterolemia receiving statin injection of mipomersen 200 mg subcutaneously once weekly, LDL-C was reduced by 21% (P < 0.003).[86] The adverse effects relate to a 50% increased risk of injection site reactions and a 12% increase in alanine transaminase (ALT) levels. The risk–benefit ratio needs further evaluation.

THYROID HORMONE ANALOGUES

In individuals with hypothyroidism, thyroxine reduces LDL-C levels by increasing the expression of the LDL receptor. The SRB1 receptor in the liver increases the clearance of cholesterol and its excretion in bile. Eprotirome is a thyroid hormone analogue, which has minimal uptake in extrahepatic tissues and a greater affinity for the T3 β-receptor in the liver, compared with the T3 α-receptor in the heart, which modulates the cardiac effects of T3. In a 12-week dose-ranging study, this compound reduced LDL-C from 3.6 mmol/L to 2.4 mmol/L in statin-treated subjects at the highest dose.[87] Similar proportional reductions were observed in apoB, TG, and lipoprotein(a). The clinical benefits warrant further study.

Conclusion

All patients with CAD benefit from statin therapy, with no apparent threshold below which benefit is absent. Intensive statin therapy reduces cardiovascular events and atherosclerotic disease progression compared with standard therapy and therefore should be considered the standard of care for patients with CAD. In addition to important reductions of LDL-C levels, intensive statin therapy reduces inflammation, which appears to be particularly important with regard to the early benefits observed in patients with ACS and perhaps makes significant contributions thereafter to long-term risk reduction. Beyond statin therapy, the data for other agents that favorably alter lipid profiles are unclear, but potential benefits of agents that raise HDL-C levels or significantly lower triglyceride levels are being investigated.

REFERENCES

1. Kannel WB, Dawber TR, Friedman GD, et al: Risk factors in coronary heart disease. An evaluation of several serum lipids as predictors of coronary heart disease; the Framingham Study. *Ann Intern Med* 61:888–899, 1964.
2. Kannel WB, Castelli WP, Gordon T, et al: Serum cholesterol, lipoproteins, and the risk of coronary heart disease. The Framingham Study. *Ann Intern Med* 74:1–12, 1971.
3. Neaton JD,Wentworth D: Serum cholesterol, blood pressure, cigarette smoking, and death from coronary heart disease. Overall findings and differences by age for 316,099 white men. Multiple Risk Factor Intervention Trial Research Group. *Arch Intern Med* 152:56–64, 1992.
4. Neaton JD, Blackburn H, Jacobs D, et al: Serum cholesterol level and mortality findings for men screened in the Multiple Risk Factor Intervention Trial. Multiple Risk Factor Intervention Trial Research Group. *Arch Intern Med* 152:1490–1500, 1992.
5. Law MR, Wald NJ: Risk factor thresholds: Their existence under scrutiny. *Br Med J* 324:1570–1576, 2002.
6. Emerging Risk Factors Collaboration, Erqou S, Kaptoge S, Perry PL, et al: Lipoprotein(a) concentration and the risk of coronary heart disease, stroke, and nonvascular mortality. *JAMA* 302(4):412–423, 2009.
7. Ridker PM, Rifai N, Cook NR, et al: Non-HDL cholesterol, apolipoproteins A-I and B100, standard lipid measures, lipid ratios, and CRP as risk factors for cardiovascular disease in women. *JAMA* 294:326–333, 2005.
8. Pischon T, Girman CJ, Sacks FM, et al: Non-high-density lipoprotein cholesterol and apolipoprotein B in the prediction of coronary heart disease in men. *Circulation* 112:3375–3383, 2005.
9. Denke MA: Weighing in before the fight: Low-density lipoprotein cholesterol and non-high-density lipoprotein cholesterol versus apolipoprotein B as the best predictor for coronary heart disease and the best measure of therapy. *Circulation* 112:3368–3370, 2005.
10. Emerging Risk Factors Collaboration, Di Angelantonio E, Sarwar N, Perry P, et al: Major lipids, apolipoproteins, and risk of vascular disease. *JAMA* 302(18):1993–2000, 2009.
11. Kamstrup PR, Tybjaerg-Hansen A, Steffensen R, et al: Genetically elevated lipoprotein(a) and increased risk of myocardial infarction. *JAMA* 301(22):2331–2339, 2009.
12. Lowering blood cholesterol to prevent heart disease. National Institutes of Health Consensus Development Conference Statement. *Natl Inst Health Consens Dev Conf Consens Statement* 5:27, 1985.
13. The Lipid Research Clinics Coronary Primary Prevention Trial results. I. Reduction in incidence of coronary heart disease. *JAMA* 251:351–364, 1984.
14. Stamler J: The coronary drug project—findings with regard to estrogen, dextrothyroxine, clofibrate and niacin. *Adv Exp Med Biol* 82:52–75, 1977.
15. Canner P, Berge K, Wenger N, et al: Fifteen year mortality in Coronary Drug Project patients: Long-term benefit with niacin. *J Am Coll Cardiol* 8:1245–1255, 1986.
16. Carlson L, Danielson M, Ekberg I, et al: Reduction of myocardial reinfarction by the combined treatment with clofibrate and nicotinic acid. *Atherosclerosis* 28:81–86, 1977.
17. Frick M, Heinonen O, Huttunen J, et al: Efficacy of gemfibrozil in dyslipidaemic subjects with suspected heart disease. An ancillary study in the Helsinki Heart Study frame population. *Ann Med* 25:41–45, 1993.
18. Rubins HB, Robins SJ, Collins D, et al: Gemfibrozil for the secondary prevention of coronary heart disease in men with low levels of high-density lipoprotein cholesterol. Veterans Affairs High-Density Lipoprotein Cholesterol Intervention Trial Study Group. *N Engl J Med* 341:410–418, 1999.
19. Randomised trial of cholesterol lowering in 4444 patients with coronary heart disease: The Scandinavian Simvastatin Survival Study (4S). *Lancet* 344:1383–1389, 1994.
20. Sacks FM, Pfeffer MA, Moye LA, et al: The effect of pravastatin on coronary events after myocardial infarction in patients with average cholesterol levels. Cholesterol and Recurrent Events Trial Investigators. *N Engl J Med* 335:1001–1009, 1996.
21. Prevention of cardiovascular events and death with pravastatin in patients with coronary heart disease and a broad range of initial cholesterol levels. The Long-Term Intervention with Pravastatin in Ischaemic Disease (LIPID) Study Group. *N Engl J Med* 339:1349–1357, 1998.
22. MRC/BHF Heart Protection Study of cholesterol lowering with simvastatin in 20,536 high-risk individuals: A randomised placebo-controlled trial. *Lancet* 360:7–22, 2002.
23. Collins R, Armitage J, Parish S, et al: MRC/BHF Heart Protection Study of cholesterol-lowering with simvastatin in 5963 people with diabetes: A randomised placebo-controlled trial. *Lancet* 361:2005–2016, 2003.
24. Baigent CA, Keech PM, Kearney L, et al: Efficacy and safety of cholesterol-lowering treatment: Prospective meta-analysis of data from 90,056 participants in 14 randomised trials of statins. *Lancet* 366:1267–1278, 2005.
25. Schwartz GG, Olsson AG, Ezekowitz MD, et al: Effects of atorvastatin on early recurrent ischemic events in acute coronary syndromes: The MIRACL study: A randomized controlled trial. *JAMA* 285:1711–1718, 2001.
26. Cannon CP, Braunwald E, McCabe CH, et al: Intensive versus moderate lipid lowering with statins after acute coronary syndromes. *N Engl J Med* 350:1495–1504, 2004.
27. De Lemos JA, Blazing MA, Wiviott SD, et al: Early intensive vs a delayed conservative simvastatin strategy in patients with acute coronary syndromes: Phase Z of the A to Z Trial. *JAMA* 292:1307–1316, 2004.
28. Wiviott SD, de Lemos JA, Cannon CP, et al: A tale of two trials: A comparison of the post-acute coronary syndrome lipid-lowering trials A to Z and PROVE IT-TIMI 22. *Circulation* 113:1406–1414, 2006.
29. Grundy SM, Cleeman JI, Merz CN, et al: Implications of recent clinical trials for the National Cholesterol Education Program Adult Treatment Panel III guidelines. *Circulation* 110:227–239, 2004.
30. LaRosa JC, Grundy SM, Waters DD, et al: Intensive lipid lowering with atorvastatin in patients with stable coronary disease. *N Engl J Med* 352:1425–1435, 2005.
31. Pedersen TR, Faergeman O, Kastelein JJ, et al: High-dose atorvastatin vs usual-dose simvastatin for secondary prevention after myocardial infarction: The IDEAL study: A randomized controlled trial. *JAMA* 294:2437–2445, 2005.
32. Study of the Effectiveness of Additional Reductions in Cholesterol and Homocysteine (SEARCH) Collaborative Group, Armitage J, Bowman L, Wallendszus K, et al: Intensive lowering of LDL cholesterol with 80 mg versus 20 mg simvastatin daily in 12,064 survivors of myocardial infarction: a double-blind randomised trial. *Lancet* 376(9753):1658–1669, 2010.
33. Cannon CP, Steinberg BA, Murphy SA, et al: Meta-analysis of cardiovascular outcome trials comparing intensive versus moderate statin therapy. *J Am Coll Cardiol* 82:438–445, 2006.
34. Scirica BM, Morrow DA, Cannon CP, et al: Intensive statin therapy and the risk of hospitalization for heart failure after an acute coronary syndrome in the PROVE IT-TIMI 22 study. *J Am Coll Cardiol* 47:2326–2331, 2006.
35. Clarke R, Peden JF, Hopewell JC, et al, PROCARDIS Consortium: Genetic variants associated with Lp(a) lipoprotein level and coronary disease. *N Engl J Med* 361(26):2518–2528, 2009.
36. Murphy SA, Cannon CP, Wiviott SD, et al: Effect of intensive lipid-lowering therapy on mortality after acute coronary syndrome (a patient-level analysis of the Aggrastat to Zocor and Pravastatin or Atorvastatin Evaluation and Infection Therapy-Thrombolysis in Myocardial Infarction 22 trials). *Am J Cardiol* 100(7):1047–1051, 2007.
37. Murphy SA, Cannon CP, Wiviott SD, et al: Reduction in recurrent cardiovascular events with intensive lipid-lowering statin therapy compared with moderate lipid-lowering statin therapy after acute coronary syndromes from the PROVE IT-TIMI 22 (Pravastatin or Atorvastatin Evaluation and Infection Therapy-Thrombolysis In Myocardial Infarction 22) trial. *J Am Coll Cardiol* 54(25):2358–2362, 2009.
38. LaRosa JC, Deedwania PC, Shepherd J, et al, TNT Investigators: Comparison of 80 versus 10 mg of atorvastatin on occurrence of cardiovascular events after the first event (from the Treating to New Targets [TNT] trial). *Am J Cardiol* 105(3):283–287, 2010.
39. Horwich TB, Hamilton MA, Maclellan WR, et al: Low serum total cholesterol is associated with marked increase in mortality in advanced heart failure. *J Card Fail* 8:216–224, 2002.
40. Rauchhaus M, Clark AL, Doehner W, et al: The relationship between cholesterol and survival in patients with chronic heart failure. *J Am Coll Cardiol* 42:1933–1940, 2003.
41. Cholesterol Treatment Trialists' (CTT) Collaboration, Baigent C, Blackwell L, Emberson J, et al: Efficacy and safety of more intensive lowering of LDL cholesterol: A meta-analysis of data from 170,000 participants in 26 randomised trials. *Lancet* 376(9753):1670–1681, 2010.
42. Gissi-HF Investigators, Tavazzi L, Maggioni AP, Marchioli R, et al: Effect of rosuvastatin in patients with chronic heart failure (the GISSI-HF trial): A randomised, double-blind, placebo-controlled trial. *Lancet* 372(9645):1231–1239, 2008.
43. Ray KK, Cannon CP: The potential relevance of the multiple lipid-independent (pleiotropic) effects of statins in the management of acute coronary syndromes. *J Am Coll Cardiol* 46:1425–1433, 2005.
44. Ray KK, Cannon CP, McCabe CH, et al: Early and late benefits of high-dose atorvastatin in patients with acute coronary syndromes: Results from the PROVE IT-TIMI 22 trial. *J Am Coll Cardiol* 46:1405–1410, 2005.
45. Cannon CP, Ray KK, Braunwald E: Reply. *J Am Coll Cardiol* 48:852–853, 2006.
46. Hulten E, Jackson JL, Douglas K, et al: The effect of early, intensive statin therapy on acute coronary syndrome: A meta-analysis of randomized controlled trials. *Arch Intern Med* 166:1814–1821, 2006.
47. Ballantyne CM: Clinical trial endpoints: Angiograms, events, and plaque instability. *Am J Cardiol* 82(6A):5M–11M, 1998.
48. Okazaki S, Yokoyama T, Miyauchi K, et al: Early statin treatment in patients with acute coronary syndrome: Demonstration of the beneficial effect on atherosclerotic lesions by serial volumetric intravascular ultrasound analysis during half a year after coronary event. The ESTABLISH Study. *Circulation* 110:1061–1068, 2004.
49. Hong MK, Lee CW, Kim YK, et al: Usefulness of follow-up low-density lipoprotein cholesterol level as an independent predictor of changes of coronary atherosclerotic plaque size as determined by intravascular ultrasound analysis after statin (atorvastatin or simvastatin) therapy. *Am J Cardiol* 98:866–870, 2006.
50. Wiviott SD, Cannon CP, Morrow DA, et al: Can low-density lipoprotein be too low? The safety and efficacy of achieving very low low-density lipoprotein with intensive statin therapy: A PROVE IT-TIMI 22 substudy. *J Am Coll Cardiol* 46:1411–1416, 2005.
51. Ray KK, Cannon CP, Cairns R, et al: Relationship between uncontrolled risk factors and C-reactive protein levels in patients receiving standard or intensive statin therapy for acute coronary syndromes in the PROVE IT-TIMI 22 trial. *J Am Coll Cardiol* 46:1417–1424, 2005.
52. Morrow DA, de Lemos JA, Sabatine MS, et al: Clinical relevance of C-reactive protein during follow-up of patients with acute coronary syndromes in the Aggrastat-to-Zocor Trial. *Circulation* 114:281–288, 2006.
53. Gotto AM, Jr, Whitney E, Stein EA, et al: Relation between baseline and on-treatment lipid parameters and first acute major coronary events in the Air Force/Texas Coronary Atherosclerosis Prevention Study (AFCAPS/TexCAPS). *Circulation* 101:477–484, 2000.
54. Simes RJ, Marschner IC, Hunt D, et al: Relationship between lipid levels and clinical outcomes in the Long-term Intervention with Pravastatin in Ischemic Disease (LIPID) trial: To what extent is the reduction in coronary events with pravastatin explained by on-study lipid levels? *Circulation* 105:1162–1169, 2002.
55. Ray KK, Cannon CP, Cairns R, et al: Prognostic utility of apoB/AI, total cholesterol/HDL, non-HDL cholesterol, or hs-CRP as predictors of clinical risk in patients receiving statin therapy after acute coronary syndromes: results from PROVE IT-TIMI 22. *Arterioscler Thromb Vasc Biol* 29(3):424–430, 2009.
56. Kastelein JJ, van der Steeg WA, Holme I, et al, IDEAL Study Group: Lipids, apolipoproteins, and their ratios in relation to cardiovascular events with statin treatment. *Circulation*, 117(23):3002–3009, 2008.
57. Tsimikas S, Brilakis ES, Miller ER, et al: Oxidized phospholipids, Lp(a) lipoprotein, and coronary artery disease. *N Engl J Med* 353:46–57, 2005.
58. Tsimikas S, Witztum JL, Miller ER, et al: High-dose atorvastatin reduces total plasma levels of oxidized phospholipids and immune complexes present on apolipoprotein B-100 in patients with acute coronary syndromes in the MIRACL trial. *Circulation* 110:1406–1412, 2004.
59. Chapman MJ, Assmann G, Fruchart JC, et al: Raising high-density lipoprotein cholesterol with reduction of cardiovascular risk: The role of nicotinic acid—A position paper developed by the European Consensus Panel on HDL-C. *Curr Med Res Opin* 20:1253–1268, 2004.
60. Barter PJ, Caulfield M, Eriksson M, et al: Effects of torcetrapib in patients at high risk for coronary events. *N Engl J Med* 357(21):2109–2122, 2007.
61. Nissen SE, Tardif JC, Nicholls SJ, et al, ILLUSTRATE Investigators: Effect of Torcetrapib on the Progression of Coronary Atherosclerosis. *N Engl J Med*, 2007.
62. Kastelein JJ, van Leuven SI, Burgess L, et al, RADIANCE 1 Investigators: Effect of Torcetrapib on Carotid Atherosclerosis in Familial Hypercholesterolemia. *N Engl J Med* 356(16):1620–1630, 2007.

63. Bots ML, Visseren FL, Evans GW, et al, RADIANCE 2 Investigators: Torcetrapib and carotid intima-media thickness in mixed dyslipidaemia (RADIANCE 2 study): A randomised, double-blind trial. *Lancet* 370(9582):153–160, 2007.

64. Nicholls SJ, Tuzcu EM, Brennan DM, et al: Cholesteryl ester transfer protein inhibition, high-density lipoprotein raising, and progression of coronary atherosclerosis: Insights from ILLUS-TRATE (Investigation of Lipid Level Management Using Coronary Ultrasound to Assess Reduction of Atherosclerosis by CETP Inhibition and HDL Elevation). *Circulation* 118(24):2506–2514, 2008.

65. Vergeer M, Bots ML, van Leuven SI, et al: Cholesteryl ester transfer protein inhibitor torcetrapib and off-target toxicity: A pooled analysis of the rating atherosclerotic disease change by imaging with a new CETP inhibitor (RADIANCE) trials. *Circulation* 118(24):2515–2522, 2008.

66. Krishna R, Anderson MS, Bergman AJ, et al: Effect of the cholesteryl ester transfer protein inhibitor, anacetrapib, on lipoproteins in patients with dyslipidaemia and on 24-h ambulatory blood pressure in healthy individuals: Two double-blind, randomised placebo controlled phase I studies. *Lancet* 370(9603):1907–1914, 2007.

67. Bloomfield D, Carlson GL, Sapre A, et al: Efficacy and safety of the cholesteryl ester transfer protein inhibitor anacetrapib as monotherapy and coadministered with atorvastatin in dyslipidemic patients. *Am Heart J* 157(2):352–360, 2009, e2.

68. Cannon CP, Shah S, Dansky HM, et al: Safety of anacetrapib in patients with or at high risk for coronary heart disease. *N Engl J Med* 363(25):2406–2415, 2010.

69. Schwartz GG, Olsson AG, Ballantyne CM, et al, dal-OUTCOMES Committees and Investigators: Rationale and design of the dal-OUTCOMES trial: Efficacy and safety of dalcetrapib in patients with recent acute coronary syndrome. *Am Heart J* 158(6):896–901, 2009, e3.

70. Stroes ES, Kastelein JJ, Bénardeau A, et al: Dalcetrapib: No off-target toxicity on blood pressure or on genes related to the renin-angiotensin-aldosterone system in rats. *Br J Pharmacol* 158(7):1763–1770, 2009.

71. Stein EA, Stroes ES, Steiner G, et al: Safety and tolerability of dalcetrapib. *Am J Cardiol* 104(1):82–91, 2009.

72. Birjmohun RS, Hutten BA, Kastelein JJ, et al: Efficacy and safety of high-density lipoprotein cholesterol-increasing compounds: A meta-analysis of randomized controlled trials. *J Am Coll Cardiol* 45:185–197, 2005.

73. Taylor AJ, Sullenberger LW, Lee HJ, et al: Arterial Biology for the Investigation of the Treatment Effects of Reducing Cholesterol (ARBITER) 2: A double-blind, placebo-controlled study of extended-release niacin on atherosclerosis progression in secondary prevention patients treated with statins. *Circulation* 110:3512–3517, 2004.

74. Villines TC, Stanek EJ, Devine PJ, et al: The ARBITER 6-HALTS Trial (Arterial Biology for the Investigation of the Treatment Effects of Reducing Cholesterol 6-HDL and LDL Treatment Strategies in Atherosclerosis): Final results and the impact of medication adherence, dose, and treatment duration. *J Am Coll Cardiol* 55(24):2721–2726, 2010.

75. Lee JM, Robson MD, Yu LM, et al: Effects of high-dose modified-release nicotinic acid on atherosclerosis and vascular function: A randomized, placebo-controlled, magnetic resonance imaging study. *J Am Coll Cardiol* 54(19):1787–1794, 2009.

76. Keech A, Simes RJ, Barter P, et al: Effects of long-term fenofibrate therapy on cardiovascular events in 9795 people with type 2 diabetes mellitus (the FIELD study): Randomised controlled trial. *Lancet* 366:1849–1861, 2005.

77. ACCORD Study Group, Ginsberg HN, Elam MB, Lovato LC, et al: Effects of combination lipid therapy in type 2 diabetes mellitus. *N Engl J Med* 362(17):1563–1574, 2010.

78. Jun M, Foote C, Lv J, et al: Effects of fibrates on cardiovascular outcomes: a systematic review and meta-analysis. *Lancet* 375(9729):1875–1884, 2010.

79. Colhoun HM, Betteridge DJ, Durrington PN, et al: Primary prevention of cardiovascular disease with atorvastatin in type 2 diabetes in the Collaborative Atorvastatin Diabetes Study (CARDS): Multicentre randomised placebo-controlled trial. *Lancet* 364:685–696, 2004.

80. Davidson MH, Donovan JM, Misir S, et al: A 50-week extension study on the safety and efficacy of colesevelam in adults with primary hypercholesterolemia. *Am J Cardiovasc Drugs* 10(5):305–314, 2010.

81. Cohen JC, Boerwinkle E, Mosley TH Jr, et al: Sequence variations in PCSK9, low LDL, and protection against coronary heart disease. *N Engl J Med* 354(12):1264–1272, 2006.

82. Dormandy JA, Charbonnel B, Eckland DJ, et al: Secondary prevention of macrovascular events in patients with type 2 diabetes in the PROactive Study (PROspective pioglitAzone Clinical Trial In macroVascular Events): a randomised controlled trial. *Lancet* 366(9493):1279–1289, 2005.

83. Lincoff AM, Wolski K, Nicholls SJ, et al: Pioglitazone and risk of cardiovascular events in patients with type 2 diabetes mellitus: A meta-analysis of randomized trials. *JAMA* 298(10):1180–1188, 2007.

84. Nissen SE, Nicholls SJ, Wolski K, et al, PERISCOPE Investigators: Comparison of pioglitazone vs glimepiride on progression of coronary atherosclerosis in patients with type 2 diabetes: The PERISCOPE randomized controlled trial. *JAMA* 299(13):1561–1573, 2008.

85. Benn M, Nordestgaard BG, Grande P, et al: PCSK9 R46L, low-density lipoprotein cholesterol levels, and risk of ischemic heart disease: 3 independent studies and meta-analyses. *J Am Coll Cardiol* 55(25):2833–2842, 2010.

86. Raal FJ, Santos RD, Blom DJ, et al: Mipomersen, an apolipoprotein B synthesis inhibitor, for lowering of LDL cholesterol concentrations in patients with homozygous familial hypercholesterolaemia: A randomised, double-blind, placebo-controlled trial. *Lancet* 375(9719):998–1006, 2010.

87. Ladenson PW, Kristensen JD, Ridgway EC, et al: Use of the thyroid hormone analogue eprotirome in statin-treated dyslipidemia. *N Engl J Med* 362(10):906–916, 2010.

Thrombolytic Intervention

MATTHEWS CHACKO | RANI HASAN

KEY POINTS

- Thrombolytic therapy remains the preferred reperfusion strategy in patients with ST elevation myocardial infarction (STEMI), who present within 3 hours of symptoms onset when timely primary percutaneous coronary intervention (PCI) is not available and no contraindications to thrombolysis are present.

- Adjunctive anti-platelet and anti-thrombotic therapies are critical to the maintenance of epicardial vessel patency and the reduction of downstream microvascular obstruction in patients treated with thrombolytics and have proven survival benefits.

- The routine use of thrombolytics as adjunctive therapy in primary PCI is not supported by clinical evidence and should generally be avoided.

- Early routine coronary angiography and PCI following primary thrombolytic therapy for STEMI should be performed in all high-risk patients.

- Despite the growing availability of primary PCI, thrombolytic therapy will be the most common and important reperfusion strategy for STEMI, given the growing burden of cardiovascular disease worldwide, particularly in developing nations.

Atherosclerotic plaque rupture with subsequent thrombus formation through an intricate series of interactions among the coronary artery endothelium, exposed subendothelium, circulating platelets, and coagulation factors leading to occlusion of an epicardial coronary artery are the pathophysiologic underpinnings of ST-elevation myocardial infarction (STEMI). The "open-artery" hypothesis, which postulates that early reperfusion of the occluded artery translates into myocardial salvage and ultimately improved survival, is the basis of reperfusion therapy. The evidence for the benefit of thrombolytic therapy as a reperfusion strategy in STEMI is indisputable. Pivotal placebo-controlled randomized trials of patients with STEMI from the 1980s, beginning with the GISSI (Gruppo Italiano per lo Studio della Sopravvivenza nell'Infarto Miocardico) and ISIS-2 (Second International Study of Infarct Survival) trials, proved the value of early thrombolysis by reducing mortality by approximately 30% (Table 11-1).[1,2] These studies catalyzed the acceptance of thrombolysis as standard therapy for reperfusion in patients with acute MI and ushered in the *thrombolytic era*, a term that characterized the revolution in attitude among the medical community toward this disease. While primary PCI has superseded thrombolysis as the preferred reperfusion strategy in most instances, the recently updated American College of Cardiology/American Heart Association (ACC/AHA) STEMI guidelines continue to favor thrombolytic therapy over primary PCI as the primary reperfusion strategy in patients who meet the following conditions: (1) present early (<3 hours from symptom onset), (2) have no invasive option (catheterization laboratory [cath-lab] unavailable; vascular access issues), (3) face a significant delay in receiving PCI (prolonged transport time; door-to-balloon minus door-to-needle time of >60 minutes; or door-to-balloon time of >90 minutes), (4) are not in cardiogenic shock, and (5) have no contraindications to thrombolytic therapy (Table 11-2).[1,3] However, because of concerns about bleeding complications, incomplete patency, and early reocclusion rates with thrombolytic therapy, combined with the fact that more primary PCIs are safely and successfully being performed at smaller hospitals without on-site cardiac surgery back-up, thrombolytic therapy has been surpassed by primary PCI as the treatment modality for STEMI associated with better clinical outcomes (Fig. 11-1).[4–7] While PCI has evolved into the preferred reperfusion strategy, particularly at high-volume, experienced centers, approximately 50% of patients with acute MI present to hospitals that are not PCI-capable.[8] Moreover, data from the National Registry of Myocardial Infarction (NRMI-4) suggest that door-to-balloon times remain poor with a median time of 180 minutes for patients transferred from one hospital to another for primary PCI, even within the framework of the current STEMI guidelines, indicating that there are still a substantial number of patients who experience an inordinate delay in mechanical reperfusion therapy in the "real world."[9] This was further evidenced by a cohort study of 68,439 patients presenting to PCI-capable hospitals with STEMI between 1999 and 2002, which suggested that most STEMI patients received reperfusion therapy (68.7% PCI and 54.2% fibrinolysis) during "off hours" (weekdays 5 P.M. to 7 A.M. and weekends) and that these patients experienced significant delays to PCI but not to thrombolytic therapy.[10] Therefore, thrombolytic therapy remains an important tool in the therapeutic armamentarium for treating STEMI, albeit with significant limitations. This chapter reviews the historical basis of thrombolytic intervention, summarizes current thrombolytic agents and adjunctive therapies, and highlights the evidence for its current role in reperfusion therapy for STEMI, laying the groundwork for future progress in this field.

▪ Thrombolytic Agents

Thrombolytic therapy was born in 1933, when Tillett and Garner described the fibrinolytic activity of β-hemolytic streptococci leading to the first therapeutic attempt by Tillett and Sherry in 1948 to dissolve a fibrinous pleural effusion.[11,12] Over 20 years later, in 1971, the results of the first randomized controlled trial demonstrating the benefit of thrombolytic therapy using streptokinase in acute MI were published.[13] In 1981, Rentrop and colleagues showed that intracoronary streptokinase was effective in the lysis of coronary thrombi with the use of coronary angiography, and Markis et al., demonstrated myocardial salvage with the same therapy, thus providing proof of the validity of the concept.[14,15] Shortly thereafter, human tissue plasminogen activator was isolated from a melanoma cell line[16] and was demonstrated to be effective in reducing mortality in acute MI.[17] Current thrombolytic therapy comprises a class of agents known as *plasminogen activators*, which directly or indirectly convert the proenzyme plasminogen into plasmin. Plasmin is a nonspecific serine protease that catalyzes the degradation of fibrin, fibrinogen, prothrombin, and factors V and VII, thus disrupting the coagulation cascade and thrombus generation.[18] Plasminogen activators include the fibrin-specific agents such as *alteplase* (tissue-type plasminogen activator [t-PA]), *single-chain urokinase plasminogen activator* (scu-PA), *tenecteplase* (TNK) and *staphylokinase* (SAK), which enzymatically convert plasminogen into plasmin, as well as the non–fibrin-specific agents such as *streptokinase*, *anistreplase* (anisoylated plasminogen streptokinase activator complex [APSAC]) and *urokinase*. *Reteplase* (recombinant plasminogen activator [r-PA]) and *lanoteplase* (novel plasminogen activator [n-PA]) have intermediate fibrin specificity. Currently, four thrombolytic agents are approved for use by the U.S. Food and Drug Administration (FDA) and are used most commonly worldwide: *streptokinase*, *alteplase*, *reteplase*, and *tenecteplase*. The last three agents were developed via recombinant deoxyribonucleic acid (DNA) technology to improve

TABLE 11-1	Summary of Initial Randomized Clinical Trials for Thrombolytic Therapy in ST Elevation Myocardial Infarction						
Trial	*No. of Sites*	*Agent*	*Dose/Duration*	*Enrollment Dates*	*Placebo/ Blinding*	*Age Criteria (y)*	*Symptom Duration (hr)*
GISSI-1 ($N = 11,806$)	176	SK	1.5 MU/1 hr	2/84–6/85	No	All	<24–<12
ISIS-2 ($N = 17,187$)	417	SK	1.5 MU/1 hr	3/85–12/87	Yes	All	<24
AIMS ($N = 1258$)	39	APSAC	30 U/5 min	9/85–10/87	Yes	<75	<6
ASSET ($N = 5011$)	52	tPA	100 mg/3 hr	11/86–2/88	Yes	<75	<6

APSAC, anisoylated plasminogen streptokinase activator complex; *MU*, million units; *SK*, streptokinase.
Modified from Kiernan TJ, Gersh BJ: Thrombolysis in acute myocardial infarction: Current status, *Med Clin North Am* 91:617–637, 2007.

fibrin-specificity and to increase the duration of activity to enable bolus dosing.[18] The major thrombolytic agents are briefly reviewed with regard to mechanism of action and thrombolytic profile (Table 11-3). Two novel fibrin-specific agents, *monteplase* (MT-PA) and *palmiteplase* (YM866), are modified recombinant tissue plasminogen activators with relatively long half-lives, which have shown potential in preclinical and small-scale clinical studies but have not been tested in larger randomized trials. *Amediplase* [K(2) tu-PA] is a fibrin-specific hybrid plasminogen activator with improved clot penetration in animal models and is undergoing evaluation in Europe for the treatment of STEMI, but no major clinical studies with this agent have been published to date. A novel thrombin-activated plasminogen analogue (BB-10153), which would theoretically be activated only at the site of a developing thrombus, was studied in a small phase II dose-escalation clinical trial in 50 STEMI patients.[19] This trial showed thrombolysis in MI (TIMI) 3 flow in 29% to 43% of patients over a range of bolus doses, with no major cardiovascular adverse events at 30 days of follow-up and relatively few bleeding events (3 TIMI major bleeds, 0 intracranial hemorrhage). The efficacy of this agent will need to be evaluated in larger phase III studies.

Major Historical Comparative Thrombolytic Trials

The GISSI-2/International trial with 20,891 patients with STEMI within 6 hours of symptom onset randomly assigned to either alteplase or streptokinase demonstrated no difference in mortality between streptokinase and alteplase with or without subcutaneous heparin (intravenous heparin was rarely used in this trial) but showed a higher rate of ischemic stroke in the alteplase group.[20] The ISIS-3 trial with

TABLE 11-2	Contraindications to Thrombolytic Therapy in Patients with ST Elevation Myocardial Infarction

Absolute contraindications
- Active internal hemorrhage
- Long-term oral anticoagulant use
- Intracranial neoplasia, aneurysm, or arteriovenous malformation
- Bleeding diathesis
- Recent trauma or intracranial or intraspinal surgery (within 2 mo)
- Major surgery within 2 weeks
- Pregnancy
- Severe hypertension (systolic blood pressure [BP] >180 mm Hg, diastolic BP >110 mm Hg)
- Allergy to streptokinase or previous exposure

Relative contraindications
- Acute pericarditis
- Bacterial endocarditis
- Hemostatic defects caused by severe renal or hepatic disease
- High likelihood of left atrial or ventricular thrombus
- Prolonged cardiopulmonary resuscitation
- Diabetic hemorrhagic retinopathy
- Menstruation

41,299 patients randomized to alteplase, streptokinase, or anistreplase demonstrated equivalence in mortality reduction among the three agents but found that streptokinase was associated with the lowest overall rates of stroke (1.1%) and intracerebral hemorrhage (0.3%).[21] Intravenous heparin was not used in this trial; as it has been borne out collectively through other studies of the fibrin-specific plasminogen activators, adjunctive heparin—while not critical to achieve thrombolysis—is important to sustain infarct vessel patency through the avoidance of rethrombosis. The Global Utilization of Streptokinase and Tissue Plasminogen Activator for Occluded Coronary Arteries I (GUSTO-I) trial with 41,021 patients promulgated the benefit of "accelerated" alteplase plus intravenous heparin in STEMI leading to a 15% relative and 1% absolute reduction in mortality (or 10 lives saved per 1000 patients treated).[22] This study included an angiographic component, which led to the major finding that early and complete infarct vessel patency was tightly linked to a reduction in mortality.[23] The Reteplase (r-PA) Angiographic Phase I International Dose-finding Study (RAPID-I) trial suggested a nonsignificant 30-day mortality benefit with reteplase compared with alteplase (1.9% vs. 3.9%), and the RAPID-II trial showed a significant improvement in coronary artery patency defined as TIMI-2 flow within 90 minutes favoring reteplase over alteplase (85.2% vs. 77.2%, $P = 0.03$).[24,25] The GUSTO III trial with 15,021 patients failed to show true equivalence of reteplase to "accelerated" alteplase but demonstrated a trend toward equivalence, especially for death and disabling stroke. These findings, combined with the more convenient double-bolus administration, rendered reteplase a viable option for thrombolysis.[26] The Assessment of the Safety and Efficacy of a New Thrombolytic 2 (ASSENT-2) trial of 16,949 patients randomized to receive either tenecteplase or alteplase found similar mortality rates, but the highly fibrin-specific tenecteplase was notable for significantly less bleeding compared with alteplase.[27] While this result was tempered by a relatively high rate of intracerebral hemorrhage in both groups, lower rates of overall bleeding (26.1% vs. 28.4%, $P < 0.0003$) and blood transfusions (4.3% vs. 5.5%, $P = 0.0002$) were observed with tenecteplase compared with alteplase.

Timing of Thrombolytic Therapy

EARLY TREATMENT

The degree of myocardial salvage following acute MI is clearly related to timely reperfusion, reinforcing the "time is myocardium" principle with the 2- to 3-hour time point representing the critical window to minimize morbidity and mortality from this disease process (Fig. 11-2).[28] A meta-analysis of six randomized controlled trials of prehospital and in-hospital thrombolysis for acute MI including 6434 patients showed reduced time to thrombolysis (104 vs. 162 minutes, $P = 0.007$) and reduced all-cause hospital mortality (odds ratio [OR], 0.83; 95% confidence interval [CI] 0.70–0.98) with prehospital fibrinolysis.[29] Subsequent randomized trials have reproduced these findings in populations in the United States as well as in Europe and have demonstrated the feasibility of safe and effective prehospital fibrinolysis administered by paramedics.[30–32] Current AHA/ACC guidelines for STEMI management endorse the administration of pre-hospital fibrinolysis by appropriately trained personnel to patients with no contraindications to

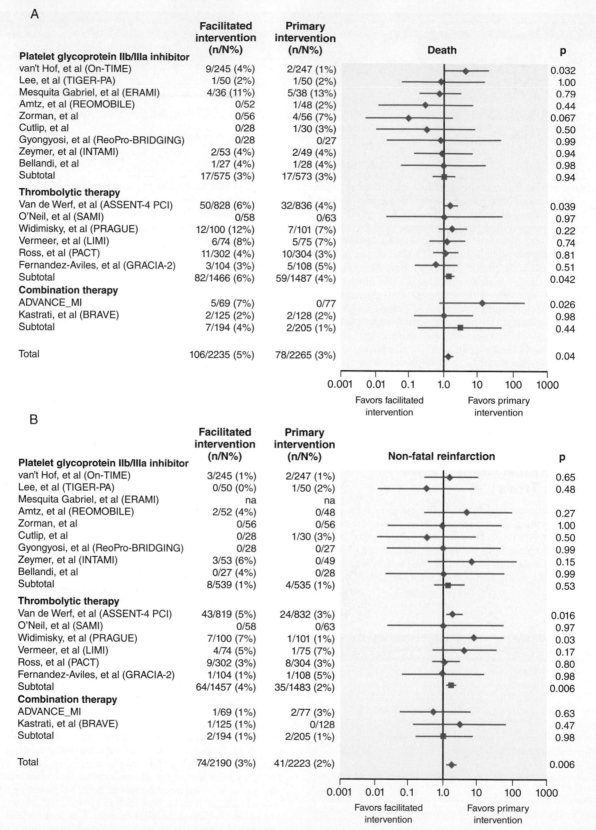

Figure 11-1 A to C, Odds ratios (95% confidence interval) of short term death (A), nonfatal re-infarction (B) and combined death, nonfatal re-infarction and stroke (C) for patients treated with primary percutaneous coronary intervention (PCI) versus thrombolytic therapy for ST elevation myocardial infarction (STEMI). (*Adapted with permission pending from Keeley EC, Boura JA, Grines CL: Primary angioplasty versus intravenous thrombolytic therapy for acute myocardial infarction: A quantitative review of 23 randomized trials, Lancet 361(9351):13–20, 2003.*)

C

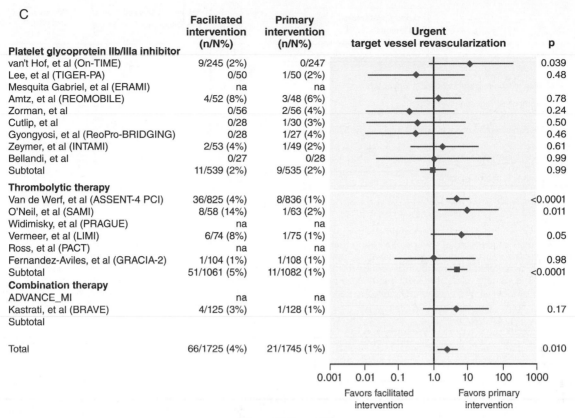

Platelet glycoprotein IIb/IIIa inhibitor	Facilitated intervention (n/N%)	Primary intervention (n/N%)	Urgent target vessel revascularization	p
van't Hof, et al (On-TIME)	9/245 (2%)	0/247		0.039
Lee, et al (TIGER-PA)	0/50	1/50 (2%)		0.48
Mesquita Gabriel, et al (ERAMI)	na	na		
Amtz, et al (REOMOBILE)	4/52 (8%)	3/48 (6%)		0.78
Zorman, et al	0/56	2/56 (4%)		0.24
Cutlip, et al	0/28	1/30 (3%)		0.50
Gyongyosi, et al (ReoPro-BRIDGING)	0/28	1/27 (4%)		0.46
Zeymer, et al (INTAMI)	2/53 (4%)	1/49 (2%)		0.61
Bellandi, et al	0/27	0/28		0.99
Subtotal	11/539 (2%)	9/535 (2%)		0.99
Thrombolytic therapy				
Van de Werf, et al (ASSENT-4 PCI)	36/825 (4%)	8/836 (1%)		<0.0001
O'Neil, et al (SAMI)	8/58 (14%)	1/63 (2%)		0.011
Widimisky, et al (PRAGUE)	na	na		
Vermeer, et al (LIMI)	6/74 (8%)	1/75 (1%)		0.05
Ross, et al (PACT)	na	na		
Fernandez-Aviles, et al (GRACIA-2)	1/104 (1%)	1/108 (1%)		0.98
Subtotal	51/1061 (5%)	11/1082 (1%)		<0.0001
Combination therapy				
ADVANCE_MI	na	na		
Kastrati, et al (BRAVE)	4/125 (3%)	1/128 (1%)		0.17
Subtotal				
Total	66/1725 (4%)	21/1745 (1%)		0.010

0.001 0.01 0.1 1.0 10 100 1000

Favors facilitated intervention   Favors primary intervention

Figure 11-1, cont'd.

thrombolytic therapy (Fig. 11-3).[3] Despite the evidence supporting the potential benefit of prehospital fibrinolysis, logistical challenges, including implementation of systems for rapid prehospital diagnosis and training of personnel in the appropriate administration of thrombolytic agents and adjunctive therapies, have limited the widespread acceptance and adoption of prehospital fibrinolysis.[33,34] On the basis of the current ACC/AHA STEMI guidelines, in-hospital thrombolytic therapy should be administered to those patients who present within 3 hours of symptom onset with a large MI *if* a significant delay in primary PCI (the preferred reperfusion strategy) is anticipated and there is no evidence of cardiogenic shock.[1] In patients who present after 3 hours, primary PCI appears to be superior to both prehospital and in-hospital thrombolysis in terms of myocardial salvage, infarct size, and mortality, possibly because of time-dependent thrombus resistance to thrombolytic agents[35,36] (Fig. 11-4). There appears to be an early and sustained difference in favor of primary PCI versus thrombolysis as a function of time to reperfusion. A large registry study

of 26,205 patients showed that it was not until approximately the 6- to 7-hour mark that age-adjusted 1-year mortality for primary PCI declined to the rates observed with thrombolysis administered within 2 hours (Fig. 11-5).[36] Even if transfer to another facility is required, the benefit of PCI over thrombolysis with regard to the combined reduction in death, re-infarction, and disabling stroke at 30 days (driven primarily by re-infarction) is sustained in those patients with STEMI presenting less than 12 hours from symptom onset.[7,37] However, the net benefit of primary PCI over thrombolysis may be neutralized if the door to balloon time for PCI is 60 minutes longer than door to needle time for thrombolysis, given that every 30-minute delay in the interval from symptom onset to balloon inflation is associated with a 7.5% increased risk of death at 1 year.[38] In patients who present within 3 to 12 hours of symptom onset and when this delay is anticipated, thrombolysis is considered a viable alternative. Ting et al., have developed an evidence-guided approach for selecting the optimal reperfusion strategy based on incurred ischemia time (or transport time) and fixed

TABLE 11-3	Characteristics of Thrombolytic Agents			
	Streptokinase	*Tenecteplase*	*Alteplase*	*Reteplase*
Source	Group C streptococci	Recombinant, human	Recombinant, human	Recombinant, human mutant tissue-type plasminogen activator
Molecular weight (kiloDalton; kDal)	47	57[†]	63–70	39
Fibrin specificity	No	Yes	Yes	Yes
Metabolism	Hepatic	Hepatic	Hepatic	Renal
Half-life (min)	18–23	20–24	3–4	14
Mode of action	Activator complex	Direct	Direct	Direct
Antigenicity	Yes	No	No	No
Estimated hospital cost per dose ($US)*	$300/1.5 MU	$2200	$2200/100 mg	$2200/20 MU

*Costs list U.S. prices of usual dose. Modified from Granger CB, Califf RM, Topol EJ: Thrombolytic therapy for acute myocardial infarction, *Drugs* 44:293–325, 1992 (with permission).

[†]Tucasso NM, Napi JM: Tenecteplase for treatment of acute myocardial infarction, *Ann Pharmacother* 35(10):1233–1240, 2001.

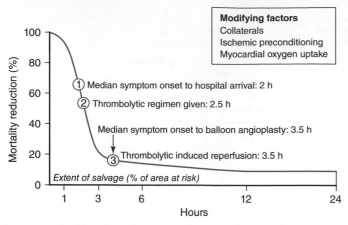

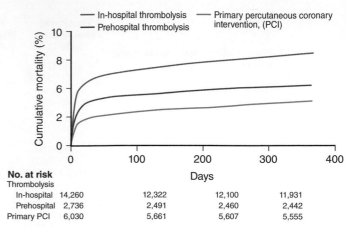

Figure 11-2 Mortality reduction as a function of time with reperfusion therapy and the potential for myocardial salvage illustrating that unless patients present very early into the course of ST elevation myocardial infarction (STEMI), pre–percutaneous coronary intervention (PCI) thrombolysis would have little benefit. (*Adapted with permission pending from Stone GW, Gersh BJ: Facilitated angioplasty: Paradise lost, Lancet 367:543–546, 2006.*)

Figure 11-4 Unadjusted cumulative mortality for 26,205 patients with ST elevation myocardial infarction (STEMI) receiving reperfusion therapy between 1999 and 2004. (*Adapted with permission from Stenestrand U, Lindback J, Wallentin L, for the RIKS-HIA Registry: Long-term outcome of primary percutaneous coronary intervention vs pre-hospital and in-hospital thrombolysis for patients with ST-elevation myocardial infarction, JAMA 296:1749–1756, 2006.*)

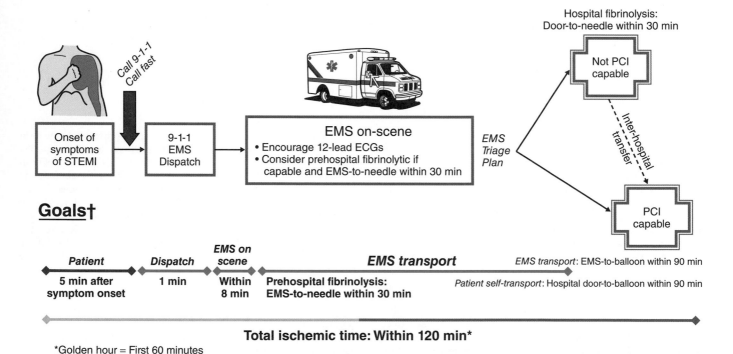

Figure 11-3 Options for transportation of patients with ST elevation myocardial infarction (STEMI) and initial reperfusion treatment goals. (*Adapted from Antman EM, Anbe DT, Armstrong PW, et al: 2007 Focused Update of the ACC/AHA 2004 Guidelines for the Management of Patients With ST-Elevation Myocardial Infarction: A report of the American College of Cardiology/American Heart Association Task Force on Practice Guidelines: developed in collaboration With the Canadian Cardiovascular Society endorsed by the American Academy of Family Physicians: 2007 Writing Group to Review New Evidence and Update the ACC/AHA 2004 Guidelines for the Management of Patients With ST-Elevation Myocardial Infarction, Writing on Behalf of the 2004 Writing Committee, Circulation 117:296–329, 2008.*)

ischemia time (or duration of symptoms) (Table 11-4).[39] In 30% to 40% of patients who fail thrombolysis (<70% ST segment resolution at 90 minutes or ongoing chest pain), rescue PCI should be performed, given the benefit of this strategy (Fig. 11-6).[40–42] There is also accumulating evidence supporting the benefit of performing routine cardiac catheterization and PCI within 24 hours or earlier in select cases regardless of the success of thrombolysis (Fig. 11-7).[43–45] This "pharmaco-invasive" approach is discussed in more detail later in this chapter.

The "facilitated PCI" approach with early administration of a thrombolytic agent in anticipation of mechanical revascularization is also discussed later in this chapter as well as in Chapter 19, Acute MI Intervention.

LATE TREATMENT

Large mega-trials of thrombolytic therapy have suggested that most of the benefit of this strategy is largely confined to the first 12 hours

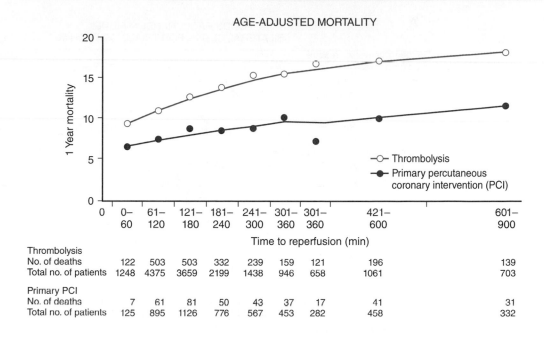

AGE-ADJUSTED MORTALITY

Thrombolysis	0–60	61–120	121–180	181–240	241–300	301–360	301–360	421–600	601–900
No. of deaths	122	503	503	332	239	159	121	196	139
Total no. of patients	1248	4375	3659	2199	1438	946	658	1061	703
Primary PCI									
No. of deaths	7	61	81	50	43	37	17	41	31
Total no. of patients	125	895	1126	776	567	453	282	458	332

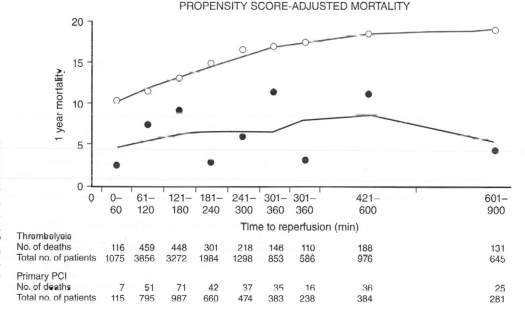

PROPENSITY SCORE-ADJUSTED MORTALITY

Thrombolysis	0–60	61–120	121–180	181–240	241–300	301–360	301–360	421–600	601–900
No. of deaths	116	459	448	301	218	146	110	188	131
Total no. of patients	1075	3856	3272	1984	1298	853	586	976	645
Primary PCI									
No. of deaths	7	51	71	42	37	35	16	36	25
Total no. of patients	115	795	987	660	474	383	238	384	281

Figure 11-5 Age-adjusted mortality according to time to reperfusion and type of therapy in 26,205 patients with ST elevation myocardial infarction (STEMI) receiving reperfusion therapy between 1999 and 2004. *(Adapted with permission from Stenestrand U, Lindback J, Wallentin L, for the RIKS-HIA Registry: Long-term outcome of primary percutaneous coronary intervention vs pre-hospital and in-hospital thrombolysis for patients with ST-elevation myocardial infarction, JAMA 296:1749–1756, 2006.)*

TABLE 11-4	Guide for Selecting a Reperfusion Strategy for Patients with ST Elevation Myocardial Infarction*	
Transport Time (Incurrent Ischemia Time)	**Duration of Onset of Symptoms (Fixed Ischemia Time)**	
	<3 HR	**>3 HR**
<30 min	Primary PCI and GP IIb/IIa	Primary PCI and GP IIb/IIa[†]
30–60 min	Thrombolytic agent and clopidogrel[‡]	Primary PCI and GP IIb/IIa[†]
>60 min	Thrombolytic agent and clopidogrel[‡]	Thrombolytic agent and clopidogrel or Primary PCI and GP IIb/IIa[‡]

*Patients treated with thrombolytic agents should be immediately transferred to a PCI-capable facility in the event of failure to reperfuse. *GP IIb/IIa*, platelet glycoprotein IIb/IIa inhibitor; PCI, percutaneous coronary intervention.
[†]Based on the American Heart Association/American College of Cardiology guidelines.
[‡]Based on clinical trials.
Adapted with permission from Ting HH, Yang EH, Rihal CS: Narrative review: Reperfusion strategies for ST-segment elevation myocardial infarction, *Ann Int Med* 145:610–617, 2006.)

following symptom onset and that many of the complications such as serious bleeding and latent myocardial rupture occur with late thrombolysis. Two specific trials, the Late Assessment of Thrombolytic Efficacy (LATE) trial and the Estudios Multicentrico Estreptoquinasa Republica Americas Sud (EMERAS) trial addressed the issue of late thrombolysis and showed no demonstrable survival benefit beyond the 12-hour mark with alteplase or streptokinase, respectively, with excessive serious bleeding complications in the latter trial.[46,47] The Fibrinolytic Therapy Trialists' Collaboration pooled analysis of 52,892 patients enrolled into eight placebo-controlled trials (excluding LATE) showed significant benefit up to but not beyond 12 hours from symptom onset.[48] The available data provide cogent evidence that there is a "golden" first hour and a "dim" 12th hour after symptom onset, illustrating the narrow therapeutic window for thrombolytic therapy (Fig. 11-8). Health care systems should develop and implement plans to minimize the delays in patient triage and facilitate timely initiation of reperfusion therapy.

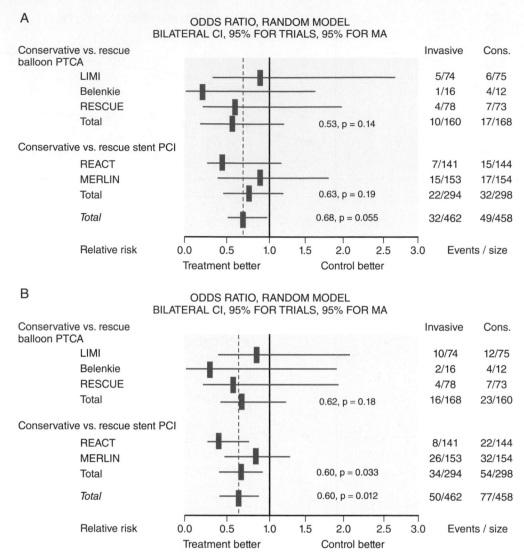

Figure 11-6 **A and B**, Odds ratios for death (*A*) and death or re-infarction (*B*) with rescue PCI versus conservative management of STEMI at 30 days. *PCI*, percutaneous coronary intervention; *LIMI*, LImburg Myocardial Infarction Trial, *MA*, meta-analysis, *MERLIN*, Middlesborough Early Revascularization to Limit Infarction, *PTCA*, percutaneous transluminal coronary angioplasty, *REACT*, REscue Angioplasty versus Conservative Therapy or repeat thrombolysis trial, *RESCUE*, Randomized Evaluation of Salvage Angioplasty with Combined Utilization of Endpoints. (*Adapted with permission pending from Collet JP, Montalescot G, Le May M, Borentain M, Gershlick A: Percutaneous coronary intervention after failed fibrinolysis: A multiple meta-analysis approach according to the type of strategy, J Am Coll Cardiol 48:1326–1335, 2006.*)

Adjunctive Therapies

One of the remaining challenges of contemporary reperfusion therapy is to achieve tissue-level nutrient flow rather than simply restoring the patency of the infarct-related epicardial coronary artery. Microcirculatory reperfusion after thrombolysis is critical, and strategies to reduce platelet aggregation, maintain endothelial integrity, and prevent the downstream effects of an embolized thrombus and atherosclerotic debris through the use of potent anticoagulant, anti-thrombotic, and anti-platelet agents have led to several important clinical trials. To that end, adjunctive therapies aimed at improving epicardial and microcirculatory patency while preserving myocardial function are discussed below.

ASPIRIN

The standard adjuvant pharmacotherapy for all patients with acute MI undergoing thrombolysis should include 162 to 325 mg/day of aspirin in the absence of a documented allergy to aspirin.[1,49] The benefit of aspirin therapy in ISIS-2 resulted in 25 lives saved per 1000 patients

treated as well as preventing 10 nonfatal re-infarctions and 3 strokes per 1000 patients treated.[50] These findings appear to be durable at 10 years of follow-up, making the duration of aspirin therapy in this setting indefinite.[51] Aspirin resistance in patients with stable cardiovascular conditions occurs at a frequency of approximately 5% and confers a significant risk of death, MI, or stroke compared with those with aspirin sensitivity; however, widespread screening remains a controversial issue.[52]

HEPARIN

In the absence of heparin-induced thrombocytopenia or known allergy to heparin, unfractionated heparin should also be part of the standard adjuvant pharmacotherapy for patients with acute MI treated with thrombolysis, given the thrombin-mediated prothrombotic state that is created. The recommended heparin dose by the AHA/ACC Task Force is a 60 units/kg bolus (maximum 4000 units) and a continuous intravenous infusion of 12 units/kg/hr (maximum 1000 units/hr) titrated to keep the activated partial thromboplastin time (aPTT)

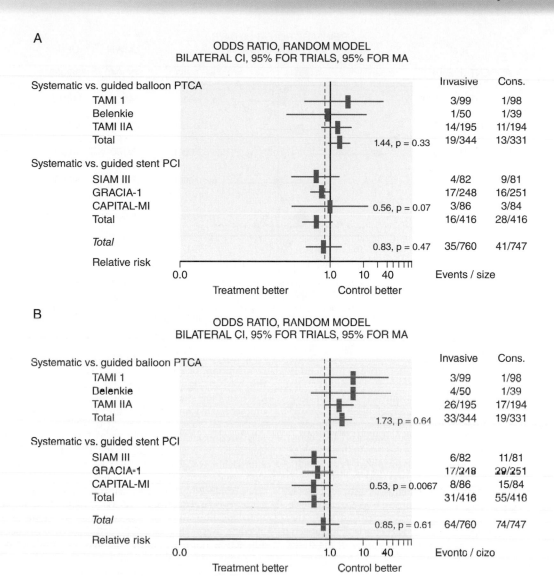

Figure 11-7 **A and B**, Odds ratios for death (A) and death or re-infarction (B) with systematic versus ischemia-guided PCI after STEMI. *PCI*, percutaneous coronary intervention; *STEMI*, ST elevation myocardial infarction; *CAPITAL-MI*, Combined Angioplasty and Pharmacologic Intervention Versus Thrombolytics Alone in Acute Myocardial Infarction, *GRACIA-1*, Randomized trial comparing stenting within 24 hours of thrombolysis versus ischemia-guided approach to thrombolyzed acute myocardial infarction with ST-segment elevation, *MA*, meta-analysis, *PTCA*, percutaneous transluminal coronary angioplasty, *SIAM*, Comparison of Invasive and Conservative Strategies After Treatment with Streptokinase in Acute Myocardial Infarction, *TAMI*, Thrombolysis and Angioplasty in Myocardial Infarction. *(Adapted with permission pending from Collet JP, Montalescot G, Le May M, Borentain M, Gershlick A: Percutaneous coronary intervention after failed fibrinolysis: A multiple meta-analysis approach according to the type of strategy, J Am Coll Cardiol 48:1326–1335, 2006.)*

Figure 11-8 Percent mortality reduction derived from thrombolytic therapy as a function of time from symptom onset to initiation of therapy with clinical trials, from which these data are extrapolated, noted. A greater than 50% reduction in mortality is noted during the first "golden hour" after which the mortality benefit declines to a plateau of approximately 25% reduction until 12 hours, after which there is no apparent survival benefit with thrombolytic therapy. *(With permission from Lincoff AM, Topol EJ: The illusion of reperfusion: Does anyone achieve optimal reperfusion during acute myocardial infarction? Circulation 87:1792–1805, 1993.)*

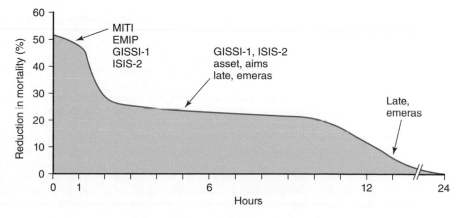

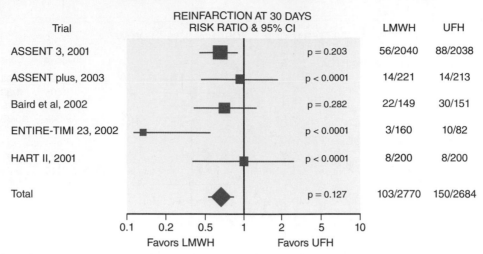

REINFARCTION AT 30 DAYS

Trial	RISK RATIO & 95% CI		LMWH	UFH
ASSENT 3, 2001		p = 0.203	56/2040	88/2038
ASSENT plus, 2003		p < 0.0001	14/221	14/213
Baird et al, 2002		p = 0.282	22/149	30/151
ENTIRE-TIMI 23, 2002		p < 0.0001	3/160	10/82
HART II, 2001		p < 0.0001	8/200	8/200
Total		p = 0.127	103/2770	150/2684

0.1   0.2   0.5   1   2   5   10

Favors LMWH   Favors UFH

Figure 11-9 Rates of re-infarction in patients treated with unfractionated heparin (UFH) versus low-molecular-weight heparin (LMWH) as adjuncts to thrombolysis in ST elevation myocardial infarction (STEMI). *(Adapted with permission from Eikelboom JW, Quinlan DJ, Mehta SR, Turpie AG, Menown IB, Yusef S: Unfractionated and low-molecular-weight heparin as adjuncts to thrombolysis in aspirin-treated patients with ST-elevation acute myocardial infarction: A meta-analysis of the randomized trials,* Circulation *112(25):3855–3867, 2005.)*

between 50 and 70 seconds (class I recommendation).[1] Low-molecular-weight heparin (LMWH) has emerged as an alternative to unfractionated heparin as adjunctive therapy for thrombolysis. The ASSENT III trial assessed two different combination strategies: (1) half-dose tenecteplase plus abciximab and (2) full-dose tenecteplase plus enoxaparin; the investigators compared these strategies with standard tenecteplase with unfractionated heparin in 6095 patients.[53] This demonstrated an impressive reduction in re-infarction in both tenecteplase combination therapy groups, confirming both the potency of the half-dose thrombolytic plus abciximab combination and the efficacy of enoxaparin in this setting. However, this benefit was tempered by an increased rate of bleeding complications requiring blood transfusions in both of the combination therapy groups compared with the tenecteplase plus heparin group. Also disconcerting was the relatively high rate of intracerebral hemorrhage in all three groups of the study (0.8%–0.9%), particularly in older adults. The trial did provide encouraging data for the use of tenecteplase plus enoxaparin rather than heparin to reduce the short-term outcome of re-infarction, even though long-term follow-up at 1 year showed no difference among the treatment groups in terms of mortality.[54] The Enoxaparin as Adjunctive Antithrombin Therapy for ST-elevation Myocardial Infarction (ENTIRE)-TIMI 23 trial evaluated ST-segment resolution at 180 minutes and early angiographic patency using (1) full-dose tenecteplase plus either unfractionated heparin or enoxaparin, or (2) half-dose tenecteplase with abciximab plus either unfractionated heparin or enoxaprarin in 483 patients with acute MI.[55] This study demonstrated a reduction in death or nonfatal MI as well as increased ST-segment resolution in the combined tenecteplase plus abciximab and enoxaparin group compared with tenecteplase and either abciximab or enoxaparin, with no increased bleeding complications. Validating the benefit of enoxaparin in reducing re-infarction, the ExTRACT-TIMI-25 trial compared enoxaparin with unfractionated heparin in 20,506 patients with STEMI undergoing fibrinolysis and demonstrated a 17% relative risk reduction in the primary endpoint of death or nonfatal re-infarction at 30 days (9.9% in the enoxaparin group versus 12.0% in unfractionated heparin group, P < 0.001).[56] This observed benefit was driven primarily by a reduction in nonfatal re-infarction and was sustained at 1-year follow-up with no significant reduction in mortality.[57] However, this benefit occurred at the cost of a significant increase in major bleeding in those treated with enoxaparin (2.1% in the enoxaparin group vs. 1.4% in the unfractionated heparin group, P < 0.001). The CREATE trial of more than 15,000 patients with STEMI treated with thrombolytic therapy randomized to the adjunctive use of the LMWH, reviparin, or placebo demonstrated benefit in favor of

reviparin regarding the primary composite endpoint of death, re-infarction, or stroke at 7 days (9.6% vs. 11%, P = 0.005), though this, too, was offset by a small but significant increase in severe bleeding.[58] In their meta-analysis of randomized trials of LMWH versus unfractionated heparin with thrombolytic therapy in STEMI, Eikelboom et al., suggested a benefit of LMWH in terms of preventing re-infarction at 30 days (Fig. 11-9).[59] However, as highlighted above, this must be weighed against the risk of bleeding with caution in approaching older patients (>75 years old) and patients with significant renal dysfunction. Increasing evidence underscores the importance of bleeding that adversely affects the prognosis of patients with acute coronary syndrome (ACS), as reflected by the directly proportional relationship observed between risk of death and severity of bleeding in these patients.[59] Nonetheless, the evidence of benefit with adjunctive enoxaparin in thrombolytic therapy, with dosing appropriately adjusted for stable renal function, in STEMI in patients under 75 years of age has been recognized with a class I recommendation in the 2007 update to the ACC/AHA STEMI guidelines.[3]

DIRECT THROMBIN INHIBITORS

The deficiencies of heparin and LMWH led to studies of direct thrombin inhibitors such as hirudin and its synthetic peptide congener bivalirudin as adjuncts to thrombolytic therapy. The clot-bound thrombin is quarantined from the inhibition of heparin, where it amplifies its own generation through a positive feedback loop and activates platelets through thromboxane-independent mechanisms, making it an important effector of thrombus formation. Unlike heparin (or LMWH), which potentiates the inhibitory effect of antithrombin III on soluble thrombin and can be highly variable from patient to patient (and even within the same patient), direct thrombin inhibitors directly bind and inactivate both soluble and bound thrombin. A meta-analysis including five trials of thrombolytic therapy in STEMI (N = 9947) showed that bivalent direct thrombin inhibitors, including hirudin (lepirudin) and bivalirudin, reduced the rates of recurrent MI but not mortality, with no such benefit observed with univalent agents such as argatroban.[60] Hirudin was tested against unfractionated heparin in two thrombolytic regimens, including streptokinase and alteplase, in the GUSTO IIb trial with 4000 STEMI patients. Hirudin demonstrated a favorable interaction with streptokinase (but not alteplase) in reducing 30-day death or re-infarction.[61] This study illustrated the crucial role of thrombin generation after streptokinase administration and its relationship to outcomes. The largest dedicated trial using a direct thrombin inhibitor was the Hirulog and Early Reperfusion or Occlusion 2 trial (HERO-2), in which 17,073 patients with STEMI were treated with streptokinase plus either heparin or bivalirudin.[62] This multicenter international trial demonstrated a relatively high overall mortality (10.9% in the streptokinase plus heparin group vs. 10.8% in the streptokinase plus bivalirudin group). The reasons for this remain unclear but may have been related to the use of streptokinase as the thrombolytic agent, the relatively late entry of patients from the time of symptom onset, and underutilization of reperfusion therapies for re-infarction across multiple study sites.[63] While it did show a significant reduction in re-infarction (1.6% in streptokinase plus bivalirudin group vs. 2.3% in the streptokinase plus heparin group, $P = 0.001$), a trend toward increased intracerebral hemorrhage and blood transfusions was noted in the streptokinase plus bivalirudin group. Bivalirudin may be acceptable as an alternative to unfractionated heparin in patients with heparin-induced thrombocytopenia and STEMI treated with streptokinase on the basis of the HERO-2 trial (class IIa recommendation). While recent trials have established the safety and efficacy of bivalirudin as adjunctive therapy to PCI in the management of both non–STEMI and STEMI, no studies have evaluated this agent in combination with newer-generation thrombolytic agents in the treatment of STEMI.[64,65]

GLYCOPROTEIN IIB/IIIA INHIBITOR

The rationale for more potent adjunctive therapies for thrombolysis originated from angiographic studies of thrombolysis monotherapy showing incomplete clot dissolution. This is thought to occur because of platelet activation in the setting of fibrinolysis, which results in residual platelet-rich thrombus that is resistant to pharmacologic thrombolysis. Hence, maximal platelet inhibition remains an important target for adjunctive therapy to thrombolysis in the management of STEMI. The combination of a thrombolytic agent at half-dose with full-dose glycoprotein (GP) IIb/IIIa inhibitor was attractive in light of a number of studies indicating better infarct vessel patency, more complete angiographic clot dissolution, and more ST segment resolution. Most of the available data for the use of the GP IIb/IIIa inhibitors as adjunctive therapy in STEMI involves abciximab and is demonstrated by the GUSTO V trial, which evaluated the combination of half-dose reteplase plus abciximab compared with full-dose reteplase in 16,588 patients.[66] The primary endpoint of 30 day mortality was slightly better with combination therapy (5.6% vs. 5.9%, $P = 0.45$), which fulfilled noninferiority criteria and represented the first combination reperfusion strategy validated as "at least as good as" full-dose thrombolytic therapy. However, there was an increase in bleeding complications that required blood transfusions in 4% of the reteplase-treated patients and 5.7% of the combination-treated patients, most of which occurred in older patients who also had a significantly increased risk of intracerebral hemorrhage (Fig. 11-10). The main findings of the trial suggested that combination therapy may be useful in younger patients (<75 years old), particularly in those with anterior MI. Disappointingly, long-term data highlighted that there was no difference in 1-year mortality between the two strategies.[67] A meta-analysis by De Luca et al., summarized the use of abciximab in this context and showed that abciximab as adjunctive therapy for thrombolysis for STEMI had no mortality benefit at 30 days or long-term, compared with those undergoing primary angioplasty for STEMI. They also showed that though there were similar reductions in re-infarction at 30 days, the bleeding trade-offs with abciximab were significant.[68] Regarding the small molecule GP IIb/IIIa inhibitor tirofiban, in the small randomized dose-finding study FASTER (TIMI 24), the combination of tenecteplase plus tirofiban versus tenecteplase alone demonstrated more rapid and complete ST segment resolution without an increase in major bleeding.[69] The SASTRE (Safety and efficacy of a conjunctive Strategy for Reperfusion Enhancement) investigators demonstrated higher rates of TIMI 3 flow and TIMI grade 3 myocardial perfusion, translating into better clinical outcomes and no increased bleeding risk when tirofiban was used as an adjunct to reperfusion therapy both with thrombolysis (alteplase) and with primary

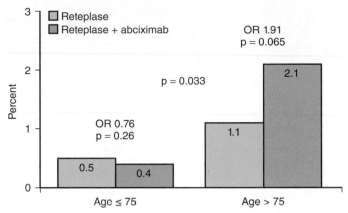

Figure 11-10 GUSTO V trial data. Intra-cranial hemorrhage and treatment by age interaction. *(With permission pending from the GUSTO V Investigators: Reperfusion therapy for acute myocardial infarction with fibrinolytic therapy or combination low dose fibrinolytic therapy and platelet glycoprotein IIb/IIIa inhibition: The GUSTO V Trial, Lancet 357:1905–1914, 2001.)*

PCI in 144 patients.[70] The INTEGRITI (Integrilin and Tenecteplase in Acute Myocardial Infarction) trial evaluating tenecteplase with combinations of eptifibatide in STEMI showed that double-bolus eptifibatide plus half dose tenecteplase improved arterial patency and ST-segment resolution over tenecteplase monotherapy.[71] However, this was at the expense of increased major bleeding and blood transfusions, limiting this as a useful strategy. Hence, large-scale trials showing a survival benefit with the adjunctive use of the small molecule GP IIb/IIIa inhibitors with thrombolysis as primary reperfusion therapy are still lacking. Limited data are available with regard to the role of the GP IIb/IIIa inhibitors in rescue PCI following failed full-dose thrombolytic therapy; the excessive bleeding (despite lower heparin doses), as seen in the subjects in the GUSTO III subgroup who underwent rescue angioplasty with abciximab, is of particular concern.[72] A small series from the stenting era suggests that short-term clinical outcomes may be improved with this strategy with no significant trade-offs in terms of bleeding complications, though caution is certainly warranted.[73]

THIENOPYRIDINES

In COMMIT (Clopidogrel and Metoprolol in Myocardial Infarction Trial) with 45,852 patients, clopidogrel was shown to significantly reduce death (7.5% vs. 8.1%, $P = 0.03$) (Fig. 11-11) and the combined endpoint of death, re-infarction, and stroke (9.2% vs. 10.1%, $P = 0.002$) when given to aspirin-treated patients before thrombolytic therapy for STEMI (Fig. 11-12).[74] The Clopidogrel as Adjunctive Reperfusion Therapy (CLARITY)-TIMI 28 trial also supported the benefit of clopidogrel pretreatment before thrombolysis in patients age 75 or younger with STEMI and demonstrated reduced rates of death and recurrent MI or ischemia at 30 days (Figs. 11-13 and 11-14) as well as significant improvement in coronary blood flow at 48 hours with no excess bleeding with clopidogrel.[75] A substudy of this trial showed significant reductions in the rates of cardiovascular death, MI, and stroke at 30 days from randomization in patients who received clopidogrel pretreatment (300-mg loading dose and thereafter 75 mg daily dose) with thrombolysis followed by coronary angiography and PCI within 1 week compared with patients in whom clopidogrel was initiated at the time of PCI (7.5% vs. 12%, $P = 00.1$), with no difference in bleeding rates.[76] If aspirin allergy or intolerance precludes the use of aspirin with thrombolysis, clopidogrel is considered an acceptable alternative.[1,77] The Harmonizing Outcomes with RevasculariZatiON and Stents in Acute Myocardial Infarction (HORIZONS-AMI) and Clopidogrel Optimal Loading Dose Usage to Reduce Recurrent EveNTs/Optimal Antiplatelet Strategy for InterventionS (CURRENT-OASIS) 7 trials have demonstrated the efficacy and safety of a 600-mg loading dose of

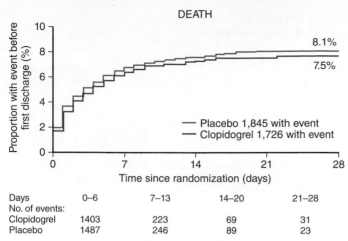

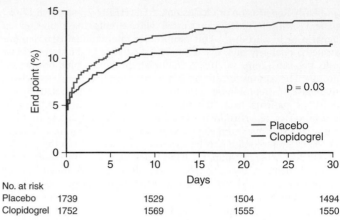

Figure 11-11 Death rates from the COMMIT trial of the addition of clopidogrel to aspirin in 45,852 patients with ST elevation myocardial infarction (STEMI). *(Adapted with permission pending from Chen ZM, Jiang LX, Chen YP, et al: Addition of clopidogrel to aspirin in 45,852 patients with acute myocardial infarction: Randomized placebo-controlled trial, Lancet 366:1607–1621, 2005.)*

Figure 11-13 Cumulative incidence of the combined endpoint of cardiovascular death, recurrent myocardial infarction, or recurrent ischemia leading to the need for urgent revascularization. *(Adapted with permission pending from Sabatine MS, Cannon CP, Gibson CM, et al: Addition of clopidogrel to aspirin and fibrinolytic therapy for myocardial infarction with ST-segment elevation, N Engl J Med 352:1179–1189, 2005.)*

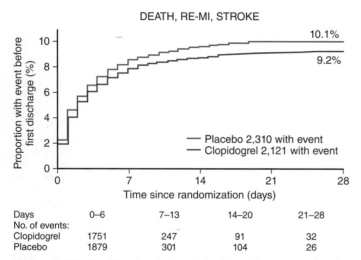

Figure 11-12 Combined endpoint of death, re-infarction, and stroke from the COMMIT trial of the addition of clopidogrel to aspirin in 45,852 patients with ST elevation myocardial infarction (STEMI). *(Adapted with permission pending from Chen ZM, Jiang LX, Chen YP, et al: Addition of clopidogrel to aspirin in 45,852 patients with acute myocardial infarction: Randomized placebo-controlled trial, Lancet 366:1607–1621, 2005.)*

clopidogrel in the treatment of ACS managed with an invasive reperfusion strategy, but no studies to date have evaluated this dosing strategy in combination with thrombolytic therapy.[78,79]

Prasugrel, a novel thienopyridine P2Y12 receptor antagonist with more potent platelet inhibition and possibly less resistance to platelet inhibition was shown to reduce the rate of cardiovascular death, nonfatal MI, and nonfatal stroke at 1 year compared with clopidogrel (9.9% vs. 12.1%, $P < 0.001$) in the Trial to Assess Improvement in Therapeutic Outcomes by Optimizing Platelet Inhibition with Prasugrel-Thrombolysis in Myocardial Infarction (TRITON)-TIMI 38 trial, which included 13,608 patients with moderate- to high-risk ACS managed with PCI.[80] Higher rates of bleeding were also observed with prasugrel compared with clopidogrel (2.4% vs. 1.8%, $P = 0.03$), and no difference in mortality was observed. However, this study suggested a net harm among patients with a history of cerebrovascular disease, age 75 years or over, and weight less than 60 kg. While the FDA has approved prasugrel for use in the management of ACS with PCI, it

remains to be seen whether prasugrel will demonstrate sufficient benefit and safety to be useful as adjunctive therapy with thrombolysis. Ticagrelor is a novel non-thienopyridine P2Y12 receptor antagonist that reversibly inhibits adenosine diphosphate (ADP)–stimulated platelet activation, with more rapid and potent activity than clopidogrel in preclinical studies.[81] The Platelet Inhibition and Patient Outcomes (PLATO) study, a randomized controlled trial that included 18,624 patients, showed a benefit of ticagrelor compared with clopidogrel in the management of ACS with PCI, with a reduction in vascular death, MI, and stroke at 12 months (9.8% vs. 11.7%, $P = 0.001$).[82] There was no difference in overall bleeding, but a higher rate of nonprocedural bleeding was observed with ticagrelor (4.5% vs. 3.8%, $P = 0.03$), including intracerebral hemorrhage. Ticagrelor has yet to be approved by the FDA and has not been studied in conjunction with thrombolytic therapy. However, compared with clopidogrel in the invasive management of ACS, ticagrelor will likely prove to be a useful adjunct in thrombolytic therapy for STEMI.

No meaningful studies have compared ticlopidine, with placebo as adjunctive therapy in STEMI patients undergoing thrombolysis. The Ticlopidine versus aspirin after myocardial infarction (STAMI) trial did address the role of ticlopidine in secondary prevention of cardiovascular events in STEMI patients treated with thrombolysis but found no difference compared with aspirin monotherapy.[83]

FACTOR XA INHIBITORS

The OASIS-6 trial evaluated the adjunctive use of a selective factor Xa inhibitor, fondaparinux, versus unfractionated heparin in 12,092 patients with STEMI and found no benefit in those undergoing primary PCI.[84] This study did demonstrate a significant reduction in death and re-infarction at 30 days and 3 to 6 months in those undergoing thrombolysis treated with fondaparinux, with no increase in severe bleeding, at least after 9 days of therapy. However, an increased frequency of guide catheter thrombosis was observed with fondaparinux. Combined with the OASIS-5 trial in the non-STEMI population, where there was a mortality benefit at 3 and 6 months with less major bleeding with fondaparinux compared with enoxaparin, there appears to be promise for fondaparinux across the spectrum of patients with ACS.[85] The available evidence has garnered a class I recommendation for the use of fondaparinux as adjunctive antithrombotic therapy in thrombolysis-treated patients with STEMI who do not undergo subsequent PCI.[3] However, the prolonged 9-day administration may limit widespread adoption of this therapy.

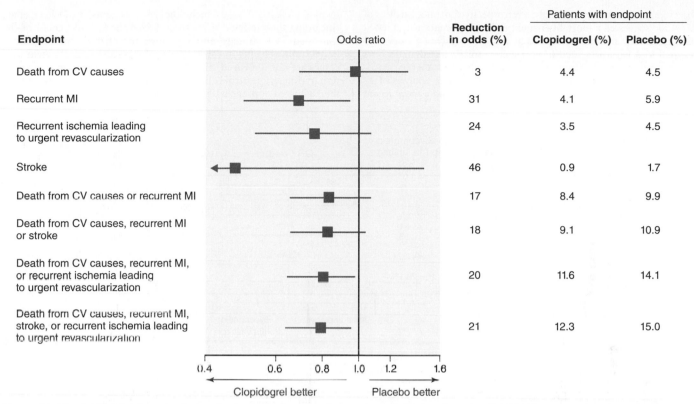

Endpoint	Odds ratio	Reduction in odds (%)	Patients with endpoint	
			Clopidogrel (%)	Placebo (%)
Death from CV causes		3	4.4	4.5
Recurrent MI		31	4.1	5.9
Recurrent ischemia leading to urgent revascularization		24	3.5	4.5
Stroke		46	0.9	1.7
Death from CV causes or recurrent MI		17	8.4	9.9
Death from CV causes, recurrent MI or stroke		18	9.1	10.9
Death from CV causes, recurrent MI, or recurrent ischemia leading to urgent revascularization		20	11.6	14.1
Death from CV causes, recurrent MI, stroke, or recurrent ischemia leading to urgent revascularization		21	12.3	15.0

Figure 11-14 Odds ratios for individual and composite clinical endpoints through 30 days from the CLARITY-TIMI 28 trial. (*Adapted with permission pending from Sabatine MS, Cannon CP, Gibson CM, et al: Addition of clopidogrel to aspirin and fibrinolytic therapy for myocardial infarction with ST-segment elevation, N Engl J Med 352:1179-1189, 2005.*)

Facilitated Percutaneous Coronary Intervention

Considerable attention has been given to the concept of facilitated PCI, which refers to the use of upstream pharmacologic therapy to serve as a "bridge" to primary PCI, given that survival is improved if TIMI 3 flow is present before mechanical reperfusion.[86] The use of full-dose thrombolytic therapy before PCI for STEMI was unhelpful and even harmful in the early major trials that combined thrombolytic therapy with immediate angioplasty.[87] This was thought to be largely because of the prothrombotic effect of plasminogen activators and the showering of platelet-rich micro-thrombi into the microvasculature leading to poorer outcomes. Notably, these early trials were conducted before the routine use of intensive anti-platelet therapy (including the GP IIb/IIIa inhibitor and thienopyridines) and stents, which have improved outcomes with contemporary PCI for STEMI. One of the largest facilitated PCI trials, to date, the ASSENT-4 trial, assessed the role of full-dose tenecteplase with primary PCI.[88] This study was stopped prematurely because of higher in-hospital mortality in the facilitated PCI group compared with the primary PCI group (6% vs. 3%, P = 0.01), with the occurrence of significantly more frequent ischemic complications such as re-infarction and repeat target vessel revascularization in the facilitated group. The strategy of using half-dose thrombolytic therapy plus a full-dose GP IIb/IIIa inhibitor before PCI would seem especially attractive, given the benefit of the GP IIb/IIIa inhibitor in those undergoing primary PCI. The prematurely terminated (because of lack of enrollment) ADdressing the Value of facilitated ANgioplasty after Combination therapy or Eptifibatide monotherapy in acute Myocardial Infarction (ADVANCE MI) trial tested this strategy, comparing eptifibatide plus half-dose tenecteplase to eptifibatide plus placebo before primary PCI for STEMI.[89] This study suggested that eptifibatide plus half-dose

tenecteplase was associated with adverse clinical outcomes and higher bleeding rates despite demonstrating improved pre-PCI coronary flow. The Bavarian Reperfusion AlternatiVes Evaluation (BRAVE) trial addressed the use of upstream abciximab plus half-dose reteplase versus abciximab monotherapy in 253 patients undergoing PCI for STEMI.[90] This trial found no reduction in infarct size by single-photon emission computed tomography (performed between 5 and 10 days after randomization), with nonsignificant trends toward more adverse cardiac events at 6 months and more major bleeding in the abciximab plus reteplase group. The Facilitated Intervention with Enhanced Reperfusion Speed to Stop Events (FINESSE) trial is the largest study to date to evaluate facilitated PCI using thrombolytic therapy.[91] This double-blind international placebo-controlled trial randomized 2452 patients with STEMI undergoing PCI to half-dose reteplase plus abciximab pretreatment (combination-facilitated PCI), abciximab pretreatment (abciximab-facilitated PCI), or abciximab started at the time of PCI (primary PCI). The combination-facilitated PCI group demonstrated more rapid ST segment resolution compared with the abciximab-facilitated PCI and primary PCI groups (43.9% vs. 33.1% and 31.0%, P = 0.01 and P = 0.003, respectively). However, at 90 days of follow-up, no differences were observed between the three groups with regards to the primary composite endpoint of all-cause death, ventricular fibrillation within 48 hours, and new-onset congestive heart failure (9.8%, 10.5%, and 10.7%, respectively, P = 0.55); or mortality (5.2%, 5.5%, and 4.5%, respectively, P = 0.49). Significantly higher rates of all bleeding, intracerebral hemorrhage, and transfusions were observed in the facilitated PCI groups. Specifically, TIMI major or minor bleeding occurred in 14.5% of the combination-facilitated group compared with 10.1% in the abciximab-facilitated group and 6.9% in the primary PCI groups (P < 0.001 for combination-facilitated PCI vs. primary PCI). A 1-year follow-up analysis of the FINESSE trial recapitulated the outcomes observed at 90 days.[92] Interestingly, a retrospective post hoc analysis of this study suggested a mortality benefit of the combination-facilitated PCI in high-risk patients as defined by a TIMI risk score greater than or equal to 3 who presented to non-PCI hospitals less than 4 hours from symptom onset.[93] This suggested a possible role for a pharmaco-invasive strategy in carefully selected patients. A meta-analysis of 17 trials of 4504 patients with STEMI by Keeley et al., and a more recent meta-analysis of 6 trials including 2684 patients by Deluca et al., (including the FINESSE trial) summarized the lack of benefit of the facilitated PCI strategy and demonstrated that despite achieving initial improvements in early metrics of reperfusion, short-term outcomes are not improved and that rates of target vessel revascularization, re-infarction, stroke, bleeding, and death may be increased with the facilitated approach (Figs. 11-15 and 11-16).[94,95] In light of these

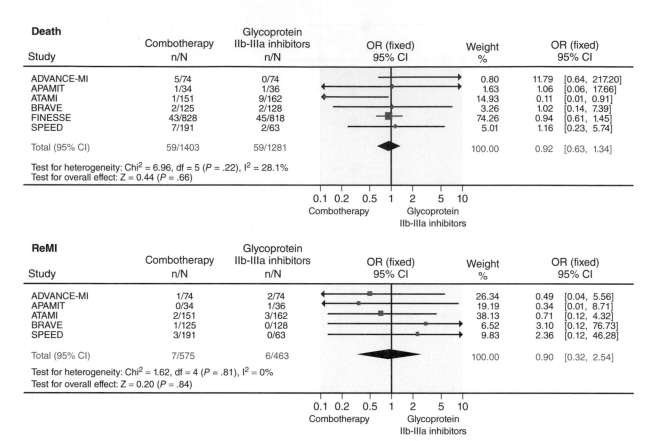

Figure 11-15 Combination facilitated percutaneous coronary intervention (PCI) and benefits in mortality (*upper graph*) and re-infarction (*lower graph*) at 30-day follow-up as compared with early glycoprotein (GP) IIb-IIIa inhibitor administration from a meta-analysis of trials of facilitated PCI, with odds ratios and 95% confidence intervals. The size of the data markers (*squares*) is approximately proportional to the statistical weight of each trial. (*Adapted from De Luca G, Marino P: Facilitated angioplasty with combo therapy among patients with ST-segment elevation myocardial infarction: A meta-analysis of randomized trials, Am J Emerg Med 6:683–690, 2009.*)

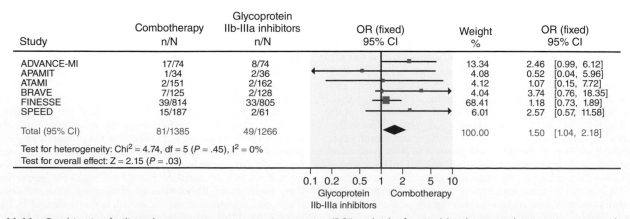

Figure 11-16 Combination facilitated percutaneous coronary intervention (PCI) and risk of major bleeding complications as compared with early glycoprotein (GP) IIb-IIIa inhibitor administration from a meta-analysis of trials of facilitated PCI, with odds ratios and 95% confidence intervals. The size of the data markers (*squares*) is approximately proportional to the statistical weight of each trial. (*Adapted from De Luca G, Marino P: Facilitated angioplasty with combo therapy among patients with ST-segment elevation myocardial infarction: A meta-analysis of randomized trials, Am J Emerg Med 6:683–690, 2009.*)

observations, the updated AHA/ACC STEMI guidelines currently designate facilitated PCI (excluding combination therapy with full-dose thrombolytics) with a class IIb recommendation, suggesting that this strategy may be used in higher-risk patients when PCI is not immediately available and the bleeding risk is low.[1,3]

Facilitated PCI is reviewed in more depth in Chapter 19: Intervention for Acute Myocardial Infarction.

Pharmaco-Invasive Strategy

A growing body of evidence supports the role of routine systematic coronary angiography with PCI following primary thrombolytic therapy for STEMI in selected patients. This pharmaco-invasive strategy is distinct from facilitated PCI in that thrombolytics are not administered as adjunctive or facilitative therapy at reduced doses in combination with other adjunctive pharmacologic agents when primary PCI is planned and available in a timely fashion. Instead, thrombolytics are administered as the primary reperfusion strategy when timely primary PCI is not available, and routine early coronary angiography with provisional PCI is implemented to avoid recurrent ischemia related to incomplete recanalization and propagation of platelet-rich thrombus following fibrinolysis. This strategy is attractive given that many patients with STEMI do not have access to primary PCI within 90 minutes of their first contact with medical care, and it may be important in the management of STEMI patients who may live at some distance from PCI-capable centers. The CARESS-in-AMI trial compared routine coronary angiography and PCI (immediate PCI) with ischemia guided coronary angiography (standard care or rescue PCI) following treatment with half-dose reteplase and adjunctive abciximab, unfractionated heparin, and aspirin in 600 patients with STEMI presenting to non-PCI capable hospitals with at least one high-risk feature, defined as extensive ST-segment elevation, new-onset left bundle branch block, previous MI, Killip class >2, or left ventricular ejection fraction ≤35%.[44] The mean time from symptom onset to thrombolysis was 165 minutes for both groups. PCI was performed in 85.6% of patients in the immediate PCI group compared with 30.3% in the standard care or rescue PCI group, with median times from thrombolysis to angiography of 125 minutes and 200 minutes, respectively ($P < 0.0001$). The primary endpoint of all-cause death, re-infarction, or refractory ischemia at 30 days occurred in 4.4% of the immediate PCI group versus 10.7% of the standard care group, with no difference in bleeding (3.4% vs. 2.3%, $P = 0.47$) or stroke (0.7% vs. 1.3%, $P = 0.50$) between the two groups. This observed benefit was driven primarily by reductions in re-infarction and recurrent ischemia, with a trend toward reduced mortality in the immediate PCI group (Fig. 11-17). The TRANSFER-AMI study randomized 1059 patients with STEMI with at least one high-risk feature, who presented to non-PCI capable hospitals to undergo immediate transfer and PCI within 6 hours of thrombolytic therapy (routine PCI group) or standard treatment with rescue PCI (standard group) following primary reperfusion therapy with full-dose tenecteplase and adjunctive aspirin and UFH or enoxaparin; clopidogrel loading therapy was also encouraged.[45] High-risk features included greater than or equal to 2 mm of ST-segment elevation in two anterior leads, systolic blood pressure less than 100 mm Hg, heart rate higher than 100 beats/min, Killip class II to III, 2-mm or more of ST-segment depression in the anterior leads, or 1 mm or more of ST elevation in right-sided lead V_4 indicative of right ventricular involvement for inferior MIs. The median time from onset of symptoms to thrombolysis was approximately 2 hours in both groups, whereas the median time from tenecteplase administration to angiography was 2.8 hours in the routine PCI group and 32.5 hours in the standard treatment group ($P < 0.001$). PCI was performed in 84.9% of the routine PCI group versus 67.4% of the standard treatment group, and more patients in the routine PCI group received clopidogrel (90.3% vs. 81.4%, respectively, $P < 0.001$) and β-blockers (90.1% vs. 85.4%, respectively, $P = 0.02$). The primary endpoint, a composite of death, re-infarction, recurrent ischemia, new or worsening heart failure, or

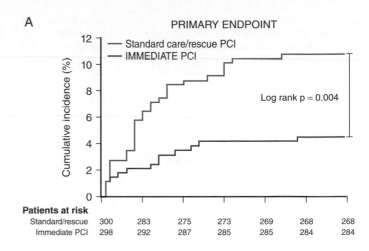

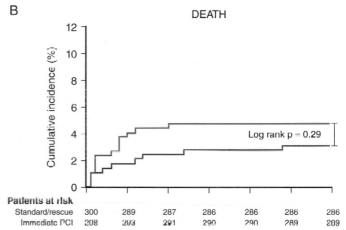

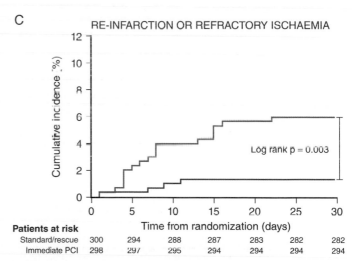

Figure 11-17 A to C, Kaplan-Meier curves for the primary composite endpoint (A), death (B), re-infarction (C), and refractory ischemia in the CARESS-in-AMI trial. (Adapted from Di Mario C, Dudek D, Piscione F, et al: Immediate angioplasty versus standard therapy with rescue angioplasty after thrombolysis in the Combined Abciximab REteplase Stent Study in Acute Myocardial Infarction (CARESS-in-AMI): An open, prospective, randomised, multicentre trial, Lancet 71:559–568, 2008.)

cardiogenic shock at 30 days, occurred in 11.0% of the routine early PCI group and 17.2% of the standard treatment ($P = 0.004$), with no significant difference in significant bleeding between the two groups. Reduction in re-infarction was also observed in the routine PCI group at 6 months of follow-up. In aggregate, these data support the use of pharmaco-invasive strategy with primary thrombolysis followed by routine early angiography and PCI in high-risk STEMI patients who present to non–PCI-capable hospitals. This strategy may also enable more rapid reperfusion with initiation of prehospital therapy in cases that may require prolonged transport times to PCI-capable centers.[96] The pharmaco-invasive strategy was recommended with a class IIa recommendation in the 2009 update to the AHA/ACC STEMI guidelines.[97]

International Perspective

Cardiovascular disease (CVD) remains a major cause of mortality and morbidity globally, and the burden of CVD is only expected to increase in the future. The World Health Organization estimates that by 2030, 23.6 million people will die from CVD, with most of the deaths projected to occur in southeast Asia. Low-income and middle-income countries are disproportionately affected by the global CVD epidemic, with 82% of all CVD deaths around the world occurring among these nations. Many of these individuals will die younger, often in the midst of their productive years, which will result in a significant economic impact, both at the individual family level and at the national level, hampering ongoing economic development. Indeed, from 2006 to 2015, it is estimated that China will sustain a $558 billion loss in income because of costs related to heart disease, stroke, and diabetes.[98] Given that STEMI will continue to comprise a significant proportion of the growing international CVD burden, and most patients in low-income and middle-income countries—as well as significant numbers in the high-income nations—will not have timely access to primary PCI, thrombolysis will serve as the primary reperfusion strategy for the majority of patients with STEMI worldwide. Developing systems for the early recognition and triage of these patients with prompt administration of thrombolytic therapy (unless timely primary PCI is available) and appropriate post-thrombolytic care will be critical in reducing the tremendous global burden of CVD.

Summary

Despite a deeper understanding of the pathophysiology of acute MI as well as the vast improvements in both the pharmacologic and mechanical reperfusion tools available, outcomes with STEMI remain suboptimal. Thrombolytic therapy revolutionized the management of STEMI, ushering in the modern era of reperfusion therapy as the primary treatment modality in acute MI. While thrombolytics were once the mainstay of reperfusion therapy in STEMI, timely primary PCI has evolved to become the favored and recommended strategy at most centers. However, many patients with STEMI do not have access to primary PCI within the critical time interval in which outcomes are maximally preserved with mechanical reperfusion, which underscores the continued importance of thrombolytic therapy in the management of STEMI. Outcomes with thrombolytics will only improve as new fibrinolytic agents are engineered with greater specificity for the actively forming thrombus, potentially reducing the risk of bleeding; more potent adjunctive anti-platelet and anti-thrombotic therapies will possibly reduce thrombolytic-mediated platelet aggregation and distal embolization of thrombus. Furthermore, a pharmaco-invasive approach using thrombolytic therapy as the primary reperfusion strategy with routine subsequent coronary angiography has the potential to improve outcomes in patients with STEMI who do not have access to timely primary PCI. Such a strategy is particularly attractive in light of the fact that the global burden of CVD will continue to grow and disproportionately affect developing nations, where timely primary PCI will not be available to much of the population. Along with innovations in pharmacology and post-thrombolytic management, systems of care will continue to evolve to facilitate rapid and appropriate risk stratification and initiation of reperfusion therapy. Whatever strategy is used, prompt restoration of both epicardial and microvascular flows to limit myonecrosis, preserve left ventricular function, and improve survival is crucial. Thrombolytic agents will continue to play an important role in the management of STEMI, particularly as CVD affects a growing population throughout the world and access to primary PCI remains limited.

REFERENCES

1. Antman EM, Anbe DT, Armstrong PW, et al: ACC/AHA guidelines for the management of ST-elevation myocardial infarction: A report of the American College of Cardiology/American Heart Association Task Force of Practice Guidelines (Committee to Revise the 1999 Guidelines for the Management of Patients with Acute Myocardial Infarction). *Circulation* 110:588–636, 2004.
2. Kiernan TJ, Gersh BJ: Thrombolysis in acute myocardial infarction: Current status. *Med Clin North Am* 91:617–637, 2007.
3. Antman EM, Hand M, Armstrong PW, et al: 2007 Focused Update of the ACC/AHA 2004 guidelines for the management of patients with ST-elevation myocardial infarction: A report of the American College of Cardiology/American Heart Association Task Force on Practice Guidelines: developed in collaboration With the Canadian Cardiovascular Society endorsed by the American Academy of Family Physicians: 2007 Writing Group to Review New Evidence and Update the ACC/AHA 2004 Guidelines for the Management of Patients With ST-Elevation Myocardial Infarction, Writing on Behalf of the 2004 Writing Committee. *Circulation* 117:296–329, 2008.
4. Aversano T, Aversano LT, Passamani E, et al: Thrombolytic therapy vs primary percutaneous coronary intervention for myocardial infarction in patients presenting to hospitals without on-site cardiac surgery. *JAMA* 287(15):1943–1951, 2002.
5. Keeley EC, Boura JA, Grines CL: Primary angioplasty versus intravenous thrombolytic therapy for acute myocardial infarction: A quantitative review of 23 randomized trials. *Lancet* 361:13–20, 2003.
6. Boersma E, for the Primary Coronary Angioplasty Versus Thrombolysis (PCAT)-2 Trialists' Collaborative Group: Does time matter? A pooled analysis of randomized clinical trials comparing primary percutaneous coronary intervention and in-hospital fibrinolysis in acute myocardial infarction patients. *Eur Heart J* 27:779–788, 2006.
7. Andersen HR, Nielsen TT, Rasmussen K, et al, for the DANAMI-2 Investigators: A comparison of coronary angioplasty with fibrinolytic therapy in acute myocardial infarction. *N Engl J Med* 349(8):733–742, 2003.
8. Waters RE, Singh KP, Roe MT, et al: Rationale and strategies for implementing community-based transfer protocols for primary percutaneous coronary intervention for acute ST-segment elevation myocardial infarction. *J Am Coll Cardiol* 43:2153–2159, 2004.
9. Nallamothu BK, Bates ER, Herrin J, et al: Times to treatment in transfer patients undergoing primary percutaneous coronary intervention in the United States: National Registry of Myocardial Infarction (NRMI)-3/4 analysis. *Circulation* 111:761, 2005.
10. Magid DJ, Wang Y, Herrin J, et al: Relationship between time of day, day of week, timeliness of reperfusion, and in-hospital mortality for patients with acute ST-segment elevation myocardial infarction. *JAMA* 294(7):803–812, 2005.
11. Tillett WS, Garner RI: The fibrinolytic activity of hemolytic streptococci. *J Exp Med* 58:485–502, 1933.
12. Tillett WS, Sherry S: The effect in patients of streptococcal fibrinolysin (streptokinase) and streptococcal desoxyribonuclease on fibrinous, purulent, and sanguineous pleural exudations. *J Clin Invest* 28(1):173–190, 1949.
13. European Working Party: Streptokinase in recent myocardial infarction: A controlled multicentre trial. *BMJ* 770:325–331, 1971.
14. Rentrop P, Blanke H, Karsch KR, et al: Selective intracoronary thrombolysis in acute myocardial infarction and unstable angina pectoris. *Circulation* 63:307–317, 1981.
15. Markis JE, Malagold M, Parker JA, et al: Myocardial salvage after intracoronary thrombolysis with streptokinase in acute myocardial infarction. *N Engl J Med* 305:777–782, 1981.
16. Rijken DC, Collen D: Purification and characterization of the plasminogen activator secreted by human melanoma cells in culture. *J Biol Chem* 256:7035–7041, 1981.
17. Van de Werf F, Ludbrook PA, Bergmann SR, et al: Coronary thrombolysis with tissue-type plasminogen activator in patients with evolving myocardial infarction. *N Engl J Med* 310:609–613, 1984.
18. Hilleman DE, Tsikouris JP, Seals AA, et al: Fibrinolytic agents for the management of ST-segment elevation myocardial infarction. *Pharmacotherapy* 27:1558–1570, 2007.
19. Gibson CM, Zorkun C, Molhoek P, et al: Dose escalation trial of the efficacy, safety, and pharmacokinetics of a novel fibrinolytic agent, BB-10153, in patients with ST elevation MI: Results of the TIMI 31 trial. *J Thromb Thrombolysis* 22:13–21, 2006.
20. The International Study Group: In-hospital mortality and clinical course of 20,891 patients with suspected acute myocardial infarction randomized between alteplase and streptokinase with or without heparin. *Lancet* 336:71–75, 1990.
21. ISIS-3 (Third International Study of Infarct Survival) Collaborative Group: ISIS-3: A randomized comparison of streptokinase vs tissue plasminogen activator vs anistreplase and of aspirin plus heparin vs aspirin alone among 41,299 cases of suspected acute myocardial infarction. *Lancet* 339:753–770, 1992.
22. The GUSTO Investigators: An international randomized trial comparing four thrombolytic strategies for acute myocardial infarction. *N Engl J Med* 329:673–682, 1993.
23. The GUSTO Angiographic Investigators: The effects of tissue plasminogen activator, streptokinase, or both on coronary-artery patency, ventricular function, and survival after acute myocardial infarction. *N Engl J Med* 329:1615–1622, 1993.
24. Smalling RW, Bode C, Kalbfleisch J, et al, for the RAPID Investigators: More rapid, complete, and stable coronary thrombolysis with bolus administration of reteplase compared with alteplase infusion in acute myocardial infarction. *Circulation* 91:2725–2732, 1995.
25. Bode C, Smalling RW, Berg G, et al, for the RAPID II Investigators: Randomized comparison of coronary thrombolysis achieved with double-bolus reteplase (recombinant plasminogen activator) and front-loaded, accelerated alteplase (recombinant tissue plasminogen activator) in patients with acute myocardial infarction. *Circulation* 94:891–898, 1996.
26. The GUSTO-III Investigators: An international, multicenter, randomized comparison of reteplase with alteplase for acute myocardial infarction. *N Engl J Med* 337(16):1118–1123, 1997.
27. The Assessment of the Safety and Efficacy of a New Thrombolytic (ASSENT-2) Investigators: Single-bolus tenecteplase compared

with front-loaded alteplase in acute myocardial infarction: The ASSENT-2 double-blind randomized trial. *Lancet* 354(9180):716–722, 1999.
28. Stone GW, Gersh BJ: Facilitated angioplasty: Paradise lost. *Lancet* 367:543–546, 2006.
29. Morrison LJ, Verbeek PR, McDonald AC, et al: Mortality and prehospital thrombolysis for acute myocardial infarction: A meta-analysis. *JAMA* 283:2686–2692, 2000.
30. Morrow DA, Antman EM, Sayah A, et al: Evaluation of the time saved by prehospital initiation of reteplase for ST-elevation myocardial infarction. *J Am Coll Cardiol* 40:71–77, 2002.
31. Wallentin L, Goldstein P, Armstrong PW, et al: Efficacy and safety of tenecteplase in combination with the low-molecular-weight heparin enoxaparin or unfractionated heparin in the prehospital setting: The Assessment of the Safety and Efficacy of a New Thrombolytic Regimen (ASSENT)-3 PLUS randomized trial in acute myocardial infarction. *Circulation* 108:135–142, 2003.
32. Björklund E, Stenestrand U, Lindback J, et al: Pre-hospital thrombolysis delivered by paramedics is associated with reduced time delay and mortality in ambulance-transported real-life patients with ST-elevation myocardial infarction. *Eur Heart J* 27:1146–1152, 2006.
33. Sayah AJ, Roe MT: The role of fibrinolytics in the prehospital treatment of ST-elevation myocardial infarction (STEMI). *J Emerg Med* 34:405–416, 2008.
34. Schull MJ, Vaillancourt S, Donovan L, et al, Canadian Cardiovascular Outcomes Research Team: Underuse of prehospital strategies to reduce time to reperfusion for ST-elevation myocardial infarction patients in 5 Canadian provinces. *CJEM* 5:473–480, 2009.
35. Schömig A, Ndrepepa G, Mehilli J, et al: Therapy-dependent influence of time-to-treatment interval on myocardial salvage in patients with acute myocardial infarction treated with coronary artery stenting or thrombolysis. *Circulation* 108:1084–1088, 2003.
36. Stenestrand U, Lindback J, Wallentin L, for the RIKS-HIA Registry: Long-term outcome of primary percutaneous coronary intervention vs pre-hospital and in-hospital thrombolysis for patients with ST-elevation myocardial infarction. *JAMA* 296:1749–1756, 2006.
37. Widimsky P, Budesinsky T, Vorac D, et al: Long distance transport for primary angioplasty vs immediate thrombolysis in acute myocardial infarction. Final results of the randomized national multicentre trial-PRAGUE-2. *Eur Heart J* 24:94–104, 2003.
38. De Luca G, Suryapranata H, Ottervanger JP, et al: Time delay to treatment and mortality in primary angioplasty for acute myocardial infarction: Every minute of delay counts. *Circulation* 109:1223–1225, 2004.
39. Ting HH, Yang EH, Rihal CS: Narrative review: Reperfusion strategies for ST-segment elevation myocardial infarction. *Ann Int Med* 145:610–617, 2006.
40. Gershlick AH, Stephens-Lloyd A, Hughes S, et al: Rescue angioplasty after failed thrombolytic therapy for acute myocardial infarction. *N Engl J Med* 353:2758–2768, 2005.
41. Patel TN, Bavry AA, Khumbani DJ, et al: A meta-analysis of randomized trials of rescue percutaneous coronary intervention after failed fibrinolysis. *Am J Cardiol* 97(12):1685–1690, 2006.
42. Collet JP, Montalescot G, Le May M, et al: Percutaneous coronary intervention after failed fibrinolysis: A multiple meta-analysis approach according to the type of strategy. *J Am Coll Cardiol* 48:1326–1335, 2006.
43. Fernandez-Aviles F, Alonso JJ, Castro-Beiras A, et al: Routine invasive strategy within 24 hours of thrombolysis versus ischaemia-guided conservative approach for acute myocardial infarction with ST-segment elevation (GRACIA-1): a randomized controlled trial. *Lancet* 364:1045–1053, 2004.
44. Di Mario C, Dudek D, Piscione F, et al: Immediate angioplasty versus standard therapy with rescue angioplasty after thrombolysis in the Combined Abciximab REteplase Stent Study in Acute Myocardial Infarction (CARESS-in-AMI): an open, prospective, randomised, multicentre trial. *Lancet* 71:559–568, 2008.
45. Cantor WJ, Fitchett D, Borgundvaag B, et al: Routine early angioplasty after fibrinolysis for acute myocardial infarction. *N Engl J Med* 360:2705–2718, 2009.
46. Wilcox RG, for the LATE Steering Committee: Late assessment of thrombolytic efficacy with alteplase 6–24 hours after onset of acute myocardial infarction. *Lancet* 342:759–766, 1993.
47. Estudio Multicentrico Estreptoquinasa Republicas de America del Sur (EMERAS) Collaborative Group: Randomized trial of late thrombolysis in patients with suspected acute myocardial infarction. *Lancet* 342:767–772, 1993.
48. Fibrinolytic Therapy Trialists' (FTT) Collaborative Group: Indications for fibrinolytic therapy in suspected acute myocardial infarction: Collaborative overview of mortality and major morbidity results from randomized trials of more than 1000 patients. *Lancet* 343:311–322, 1994.
49. Antithrombotic Trialists' Collaboration. Collaborative meta analysis of randomized trials of antiplatelet therapy for prevention of death, myocardial infarction, and stroke in high-risk patients. *BMJ* 324:71–86, 2002.
50. ISIS-2 (Second International Study of Infarct Survival) Collaborative Group: Randomized trial of intravenous streptokinase, oral aspirin, both or neither among 17,187 cases of suspected acute myocardial infarction: ISIS-2. *Lancet* 2:349–360, 1988.
51. Baigent C, Collins R, Appleby P, et al: ISIS-2:10 year survival among patients with suspected acute myocardial infarction in randomised comparison of intravenous streptokinase, oral aspirin, both, or neither. The ISIS-2 (Second International Study of Infarct Survival) Collaborative Group. *BMJ* 316(7141):1337–1343, 1998.
52. Gum PA, Kottke-Marchant K, Welsh PA, et al: A prospective, blinded determination of the natural history of aspirin resistance among stable patients with cardiovascular disease. *J Am Coll Cardiol* 41(6):961–965, 2003.
53. The Assessment of the Safety and Efficacy of a New Thrombolytic Regimen (ASSENT)-3 Investigators: Efficacy and safety of tenecteplase in combination with enoxaparin, abciximab, or unfractionated heparin: the ASSENT-3 randomized trial in acute myocardial infarction. *Lancet* 358:605–613, 2001.
54. Sinnaeve PR, Alexander JH, Bogaerts K, et al: Efficacy of tenecteplase in combination with enoxaparin, abciximab, or unfractionated heparin: one-year follow-up results of the Assessment of the Safety of a New Thrombolytic-3 (ASSENT-3) randomized trial in acute myocardial infarction. *Am Heart J* 147:993–998, 2004.
55. Antman EM, Louwerenburg HW, Baars HF, et al, for the ENTIRE-TIMI 23 Investigators: Enoxaparin as adjunctive antithrombin therapy for ST elevation myocardial infarction. Results of the ENTIRE-Thrombolysis In Myocardial Infarction (TIMI) 23 Trial. *Circulation* 105(14):1642–1649, 2002.
56. Antman EM, Morrow DA, McCabe CH, et al, the ExTRACT-TIMI 25 investigators: Enoxaparin versus unfractionated heparin with fibrinolysis for ST-segment myocardial infarction. *N Engl J Med* 354(14):1477–1488, 2006.
57. Morrow DA, Antman EM, Fox KA, et al, on behalf of the ExTRACT-TIMI 25 Investigators: One-year outcomes after a strategy using enoxaparin vs. unfractionated heparin in patients undergoing fibrinolysis for ST-segment elevation myocardial infarction: 1-year results of the ExTRACT-TIMI 25 Trial. *Eur Heart J* 31(17):2097–2102, 2010.
58. Yusef S, Mehta SR, Xie C, et al: Effects of reviparin, a low molecular weight heparin, on mortality, re-infarction, and strokes in patients with acute myocardial infarction presenting with ST-segment elevation. *JAMA* 293:427–435, 2005.
59. Eikelboom JW, Mehta SR, Anand SS, et al: Adverse impact of bleeding on prognosis in patients with acute coronary syndromes. *Circulation* 114:774–782, 2006.
60. Direct Thrombin Inhibitor Trialists' Collaborative Group: Direct thrombin inhibitors in acute coronary syndromes: Principal results of a meta-analysis based on individual patients' data. *Lancet* 359:294–302, 2002.
61. The Global Utilization of Strategies to Open Occluded Coronary Arteries (GUSTO) IIb Investigators: A comparison of recombinant hirudin versus heparin for the treatment of acute coronary syndromes. *N Engl J Med* 335:775–782, 1996.
62. HERO-2 Trial Investigators: Thrombin-specific anticoagulation with bivalirudin versus heparin in patients receiving fibrinolytic therapy for acute myocardial infarction: The HERO-2 randomised trial. *Lancet* 358(9296):1855–1863, 2001
63. Edmond JJ, French JK, Aylward PE, et al, for the HERO-2 Investigators: Variations in the use of emergency PCI for the treatment of re-infarction following intravenous fibrinolytic therapy: Impact on outcomes in HERO-2. *Eur Heart J* 28(12):1418–1424, 2007.
64. Stone GW, White HD, Ohman EM, et al, Acute Catheterization and Urgent Intervention Triage strategy (ACUITY) trial investigators: Bivalirudin in patients with acute coronary syndromes undergoing percutaneous coronary intervention: A subgroup analysis from the Acute Catheterization and Urgent Intervention Triage strategy (ACUITY) trial. *Lancet* 369:907–919, 2007.
65. Mehran R, Lansky AJ, Witzenbichler B, et al, HORIZONS-AMI Trial Investigators: Bivalirudin in patients undergoing primary angioplasty for acute myocardial infarction (HORIZONS AMI): 1-year results of a randomised controlled trial. *Lancet* 374:1149–1159, 2009.
66. The GUSTO V Investigators: Reperfusion therapy for acute myocardial infarction with fibrinolytic therapy or combination low dose fibrinolytic therapy and platelet glycoprotein IIb/IIIa inhibition: The GUSTO V Trial. *Lancet* 357:1905–1914, 2001.
67. Lincoff AM, Califf RM, Van de Werf F, et al: Mortality at 1 year with combination platelet glycoprotein IIb/IIIa inhibition and reduced-dose fibrinolytic therapy vs conventional fibrinolytic therapy for acute myocardial infarction: GUSTO V randomized trial. *JAMA* 288:2130–2135, 2002.
68. De Luca G, Suryapranata H, Stone GW, et al: Abciximab as adjunctive therapy to reperfusion in acute ST-segment elevation myocardial infarction: A meta-analysis of randomized trials. *JAMA* 293:1759–1765, 2005.
69. Ohman EM, Van de Werf F, Antman EM, et al, the FASTER (TIMI 24) Investigators. Tenecteplase and tirofiban in ST-segment elevation acute myocardial infarction: results of a randomized trial. *Am Heart J* 150(1):79–88, 2005.
70. Martinez-Rios MA, Rosas M, Gonzalez H, et al, SASTRE Investigators: Comparison of reperfusion regimens with or without tirofiban in ST-elevation acute myocardial infarction. *Am J Cardiol* 93(3):280–287, 2004.
71. Giugliano RP, Roe MT, Harrington RA, et al, the INTEGRITI Investigators: Combination reperfusion therapy with eptifibatide and reduced-dose tenecteplase for ST-elevation myocardial infarction: Results of the integrilin and tenecteplase in acute myocardial infarction (INTEGRITI) Phase II Angiographic Trial. *J Am Coll Cardiol* 41(8):1251–1260, 2003.
72. Miller JM, Smalling R, Ohman EM, et al: Effectiveness of early coronary angioplasty and abciximab for failed thrombolysis (reteplase or alteplase) during acute myocardial infarction (results of the GUSTO-III trial). Global Use of Strategies to Open occluded arteries. *Am J Cardiol* 84(7):779–784, 1999.
73. Gruberg L, Suleiman M, Kapeliovich M, et al: Glycoprotein IIb/IIIa inhibitors during rescue percutaneous coronary intervention in acute myocardial infarction. *J Invasive Cardiol* 18(2):63–64, 2006.
74. Chen ZM, Jiang LX, Chen YP, et al: Addition of clopidogrel to aspirin in 45,852 patients with acute myocardial infarction: Randomized placebo-controlled trial. *Lancet* 366:1607–1621, 2005.
75. Sabatine MS, Cannon CP, Gibson CM, et al: Addition of clopidogrel to aspirin and fibrinolytic therapy for myocardial infarction with ST-segment elevation. *N Engl J Med* 352:1179–1189, 2005.
76. Sabatine MS, Cannon CP, Gibson CM, et al, Clopidogrel as Adjunctive Reperfusion Therapy (CLARITY)-Thrombolysis in Myocardial Infarction (TIMI) 28 Investigators: Effect of clopidogrel pretreatment before percutaneous coronary intervention in patients with ST-elevation myocardial infarction treated with fibrinolytics: The PCI-CLARITY Study. *JAMA* 294:1224–1232, 2005.
77. Patrono C, Bachmann F, Baigent C, et al, the Task Force on the Use of Antiplatelet Agents in Patients Atherosclerotic Cardiovascular Disease: Expert consensus document on the use of antiplatelet agents. *Eur Heart J* 25(2):166–181, 2004.
78. Dangas G, Mehran R, Guagliumi G, et al, HORIZONS-AMI Trial Investigators: Role of clopidogrel loading dose in patients with ST-segment elevation myocardial infarction undergoing primary angioplasty: Results from the HORIZONS-AMI (harmonizing outcomes with revascularization and stents in acute myocardial infarction) trial. *J Am Coll Cardiol* 54:1438–1446, 2009.
79. Mehta SR, Tanguay JF, Eikelboom JW, et al, CURRENT-OASIS 7 trial investigators: Double-dose versus standard-dose clopidogrel and high-dose versus low-dose aspirin in individuals undergoing percutaneous coronary intervention for acute coronary syndromes (CURRENT-OASIS 7): A randomised factorial trial. *Lancet* 376(9748):1233–1243, 2010.
80. Wiviott SD, Braunwald E, McCabe CH, et al, TRITON-TIMI 38 Investigators. Prasugrel versus clopidogrel in patients with acute coronary syndromes. *N Engl J Med* 357:2001–2015, 2007.
81. Storey RF, Husted S, Harrington RA, et al: Inhibition of platelet aggregation by AZD6140, a reversible oral P2Y12 receptor antagonist, compared with clopidogrel in patients with acute coronary syndromes. *J Am Coll Cardiol* 50:1852–1856, 2007.
82. Wallentin L, Becker RC, Budaj A, et al, PLATO Investigators, Freij A, Thorsén M: Ticagrelor versus clopidogrel in patients with acute coronary syndromes. *N Engl J Med* 361(11):1045–1057, 2009.
83. Scrutinio D, Cimminiello C, Marubini E, et al, the STAMI Group: Ticlopidine versus aspirin after myocardial infarction (STAMI) trial. *J Am Coll Cardiol* 37:1259–1265, 2001.
84. Yusuf S, Mehta SR, Chrolavicius S, et al, for the Oasis-6 Trial group: Effects of fondaparinaux on mortality and reinfarction in patients with acute ST-segment elevation myocardial infarction: The OASIS 6 randomized trial. *JAMA* 295:1519–1530, 2006.
85. The Fifth Organization to Assess Strategies in Acute Ischemic Syndromes Investigators (OASIS-5): Comparison of fondaparinaux and enoxaparin in acute coronary syndromes. *N Engl J Med* 354:1464–1476, 2006.
86. Stone GW, Cox D, Garcia E, et al: Normal flow (TIMI-3) before mechanical reperfusion therapy is an independent determinant of survival in acute myocardial infarction. Analysis from the Primary Angioplasty in Myocardial Infarction Trials. *Circulation* 104:636–641, 2001.
87. Topol EJ, Califf RM, George BS, et al, the Thrombolysis and Angioplasty in Myocardial Infarction (TAMI) Study Group: A randomized trial of immediate versus delayed elective angioplasty after intravenous tissue plasminogen activator in acute myocardial infarction. *N Engl J Med* 317(10):581–588, 1987.
88. ASSENT-4 PCI Investigators: Primary versus tenecteplase-facilitated percutaneous coronary intervention in patients with ST-segment elevation acute myocardial infarction (ASSENT-4 PCI): Randomized trial. *Lancet* 367:569–578, 2006.
89. ADVANCE MI Investigators: Facilitated percutaneous coronary intervention for acute ST-segment elevation myocardial infarction: Results from the prematurely terminated ADdressing the Value of facilitated ANgioplasty after Combination therapy or Eptifibatide monotherapy in acute Myocardial Infarction. *Am J Heart* 150(1):116–122, 2005.
90. Kastrati A, Mehilli J, Schlotterbeck K, et al, Bavarian Reperfusion Alternatives Evaluation (BRAVE) Study Investigators: Early administration of reteplase plus abciximab vs abciximab alone in patients with acute myocardial infarction referred for percutaneous coronary intervention: A randomized controlled trial. *JAMA* 291(8):947–954, 2004.
91. Ellis SG, Tendera M, de Belder MA, et al, FINESSE Investigators: Facilitated PCI in patients with ST-elevation myocardial infarction. *N Engl J Med* 358:2205–2217, 2008.
92. Ellis SG, Tendera M, de Belder MA, et al, FINESSE Investigators: 1-year survival in a randomized trial of facilitated reperfusion: results from the FINESSE (Facilitated Intervention with Enhanced Reperfusion Speed to Stop Events) trial. *JACC Cardiovasc Interv* 2:909–916, 2009.
93. Herrmann HC, Lu J, Brodie BR, et al, FINESSE Investigators: Benefit of facilitated percutaneous coronary intervention in high-risk ST-segment elevation myocardial infarction patients presenting to non–percutaneous coronary intervention hospitals. *JACC Cardiovasc Interv* 10:917–924, 2009.

94. Keeley EC, Boura JA, Grines CL: Comparison of primary and facilitated percutaneous coronary interventions for ST-elevation myocardial infarction: Quantitative review of randomized trials. *Lancet* 367(9510):579–588, 2006.

95. De Luca G, Marino P: Facilitated angioplasty with combo therapy among patients with ST-segment elevation myocardial infarction: A meta-analysis of randomized trials. *Am J Emerg Med* 6:683–690, 2009.

96. Thiele H, Scholz M, Engelmann L, et al, Leipzig Prehospital Fibrinolysis Group: ST-segment recovery and prognosis in patients with ST-elevation myocardial infarction reperfused by prehospital combination fibrinolysis, prehospital initiated facilitated percutaneous coronary intervention, or primary percutaneous coronary intervention. *Am J Cardiol* 989:1132–1139, 2006.

97. Kushner FG, Hand M, Smith SC, Jr, et al, American College of Cardiology Foundation/American Heart Association Task Force on Practice Guidelines. 2009 Focused Updates: ACC/AHA Guidelines for the Management of Patients With ST-Elevation Myocardial Infarction (updating the 2004 Guideline and 2007 Focused Update) and ACC/AHA/SCAI Guidelines on Percutaneous Coronary Intervention (updating the 2005 Guideline and 2007 Focused Update): A report of the American College of Cardiology Foundation/American Heart Association Task Force on Practice Guidelines. *Circulation* 120:2271–2306, 2009.

98. World Health Organization Cardiovascular Diseases Factsheet: Available at http://www.who.int/mediacentre/factsheets/fs317/en/index.html: Accessed June 29, 2010.

Other Adjunctive Drugs for Coronary Intervention: β-Blockers, Calcium Channel Blockers, and Angiotensin-Converting Enzyme Inhibitors

VIVEK RAJAGOPAL

KEY POINTS

- β-Blockers reduce myocardial oxygen demand and prevent deleterious myocardial remodeling. These properties explain the protective role of β-blockers in the treatment of acute and chronic ischemic coronary syndromes.

- β-Blockers significantly reduce re-infarction and ventricular fibrillation after myocardial infarction (MI).

- In higher-risk patients with MI, such as those in heart failure or at high risk for developing heart failure, β-blockers increase the risk of cardiogenic shock, counterbalancing the ischemic and arrhythmic benefits.

- As the COMMIT trial demonstrated, intravenous β-blockade provides no overall benefits in patients with acute MI. Nevertheless, patients not at high risk for developing cardiogenic shock do benefit from β-blockade.

- Calcium channel blockers are useful agents in the long-term treatment of hypertension in patients with coronary artery disease (CAD).

- In patients with acute MI, calcium channel blockers should be used only in β-blocker–intolerant patients who are not at high risk for developing heart failure.

- For several decades, β-blockers, calcium channel blockers, and angiotensin-converting enzyme (ACE) inhibitors have been beneficial in a wide spectrum of CAD—stable and unstable angina, non–ST elevation MI (NSTEMI), and ST elevation MI (STEMI). Multiple clinical trials since the 1980s have demonstrated the benefits of these agents, which work either by reducing myocardial oxygen demand or by promoting favorable myocardial remodeling. This chapter will discuss the basic pharmacology of these agents, which will be followed by an in-depth discussion of the randomized trials that used these agents. Finally, we will discuss ongoing research and provide treatment recommendations.

β-Adrenergic Receptors

β-receptors belong to a well-characterized family of receptors known as G protein–coupled receptors.[1] The pathway involves the binding of an agonist (e.g., catecholamines for β-receptors) to an extracellular receptor. Receptor activation causes a coupled G protein to stimulate adenylyl cyclase, which increases intracellular concentrations of cyclic adenosine monophosphate (cAMP). cAMP activates several AMP-dependent protein kinases, which phosphorylate other proteins, resulting in a cellular response. The cellular response for β-receptors differs according to three major subtypes: β_1, β_2, and β_3. Whereas stimulation of β_2 receptors causes bronchodilation and peripheral vasodilation, stimulation of β_1 receptors predominantly affects the heart, increasing contractility and heart rate as well as lipolysis. The β_3 receptor increases heat production in brown adipose tissue, and increases lipolysis in both brown and white adipose tissue.[2,3] Interestingly, the β_3 receptor may play a role in obesity and insulin resistance.[3]

β-ADRENERGIC RECEPTOR BLOCKERS

β-blockers act by directly competing with binding of catecholamines to β-adrenergic receptors. These agents differ in their selectivity, lipid-solubility, metabolism, and partial-agonist ability (intrinsic sympathomimetic ability [ISA]) (Table 12-1).[53] Although some data suggest that these differences might impact efficacy in certain conditions (e.g., chronic congestive heart failure [CHF]), these differences mainly influence side effects, contraindications, and the frequency of dosing. For example, nonselective agents may increase bronchospasm in patients with asthma. Lipophilic agents may have more central nervous system (CNS) effects such as sedation and depression. Type of metabolism will affect plasma half-life in patients with renal or hepatic insufficiency. β-blockers with ISA slow heart rate less than β-blockers without ISA; also, β-blockers with ISA are less likely to decrease high-density lipoprotein (HDL) or increase triglycerides. Despite these pharmacokinetic differences, efficacy in CAD arises primarily from β_1-receptor antagonism. In acute MI, for example, the catecholamine storm decreases the fibrillation threshold, increases myocardial oxygen consumption, and promotes myocardial necrosis. By decreasing heart rate and contractility, blockade of the β_1 receptor lowers myocardial stress, which decreases necrosis. β-blockade also raises the fibrillation threshold. By antagonizing lipolysis, β blockers reduce the concentrations of free fatty acids, causing a greater use of glucose and a lesser use of oxygen. β-blockers, in particular carvedilol, may also inhibit platelet aggregation, but this is still being debated; the mechanism could be membrane interaction instead of β-receptor antagonism.[4] In light of these effects, it is not surprising that numerous clinical trials have demonstrated the benefits of β-blockers in acute coronary syndrome (ACS). Of course, prudence is still required in the use of β-blockers, as they decrease inotropy and slow atrioventricular (AV) conduction, which can be harmful in certain subgroups.

UNSTABLE ANGINA PECTORIS

Because of β-blockers' potent effects in reducing myocardial oxygen demand, treating unstable angina with β-blockers has much intuitive appeal. A few small randomized trials have supported this. Gottlieb and colleagues randomized 81 patients with unstable angina to 4 weeks of propranolol or placebo.[5] All patients received calcium channel blockers, nitrates, or both. Although the incidence of death, MI, or need for urgent coronary artery bypass grafting (CABG) did not differ between groups, propranolol significantly reduced the frequency and severity of recurrent ischemia. In the Holland Interuniversity Nifedipine and Metoprolol Trial (HINT), 338 patients with unstable angina not pretreated with a β-blocker randomly received nifedipine alone, metoprolol alone, or nifedipine and metoprolol.[6] The odds ratios (ORs) for recurrent ischemia or MI by 48 hours were

TABLE 12-1	β-Blockers				
Selective β₁	*Dose (mg)*	*Frequency*	*Excretion*	*Lipid Solubility*	*Intrinsic Sympathomimetic Ability*
Acebutolol	200–600	Q12 Hours	Kidney	Moderate	Low
Atenolol	25–200	Q24 Hours	Kidney	None	None
Betaxolol	20–40	Q24 Hours	Kidney	Moderate	Low
Metoprolol	50–400	Q12 Hours	Liver	Moderate	None
Long-acting		Q24 Hours			
Nonselective β					
Labetolol (α, β₁, β₂)	600–2400	Q6–Q8 Hours	Liver	None	None
Nadolol	80–240	Q24 Hours	Kidney	Low	None
Pindolol	15–45	Q8–Q12 Hours	Kidney	Moderate	Moderate
Propranolol	80–320	Q4–Q6 Hours	Liver	High	None
Long-acting		Q12 Hours			
Timolol	15–45	Q12 Hours	Liver	Moderate	None

Adapted from Griffin B, Topol E, Nair D, Ashley K: *Manual of cardiovascular medicine.* ed 3, Philadelphia, 2008, Lippincott Williams & Wilkins.

1.15 (95% confidence interval [CI] 0.83–1.64) for nifedipine, 0.76 (95% CI 0.49–1.16) for metoprolol, and 0.80 (95% CI 0.53–1.19) for both; not surprisingly, the small numbers limited power of the study, and these differences were not statistically significant. Hohnloser and associates examined the effects of esmolol, a short-acting (half-life 9 minutes) intravenous β-blocker, in a randomized, placebo-controlled trial of 113 patients. The investigators increased esmolol until they reduced the double-product by approximately 25%; thereafter, the esmolol infusion continued for up to 72 hours.[7] Acute MI or urgent revascularization occurred in 9 patients treated with placebo compared with 3 patients treated with esmolol ($P = 0.06$). In a more recent randomized trial, Brunner and colleagues randomized 116 patients with unstable angina to placebo or carvedilol at 25 mg twice a day.[8] Patients received 48-hour Holter monitoring to document ischemia. Carvedilol reduced ischemic time by 75% (204 vs. 49 minutes, $P < 0.05$) with a 66% reduction in number of ischemic episodes (24 vs. 8, $P < 0.05$). Some retrospective data from recent studies also demonstrate the benefit of β-blockers in unstable angina. Ellis and associates pooled data from five randomized trials of abciximab during percutaneous coronary intervention (PCI)—the EPIC, EPILOG, EPISTENT, CAPTURE, and RAPPORT trials.[9] Except for RAPPORT, which had patients with STEMI, the other four trials included patients with unstable angina or NSTEMI. All-cause mortality by 30 days occurred in 0.6% of patients receiving β-blockers compared with 2% in patients not receiving β-blockers. After adjusting for baseline characteristics and propensity score to receive β-blockers, β-blockers remained predictive of lower mortality (hazard ratio [HR] 0.25; 95% CI 0.1–0.57, $P = 0.001$). This mortality difference persisted at 6 months (1.7% vs. 3.7%, adjusted HR 0.53; 95% CI 0.29–0.94, $P = 0.03$). Among patients with unstable angina, β-blockers reduced mortality at 3 months (1.6%–0.6%, $P = 0.029$) and at 6 months (3.1%–1.4%, $P = 0.009$). Similarly, investigators found the mortality benefit of β-blockers in patients enrolled in the American College of Cardiology/American Heart Association Guidelines (CRUSADE) initiative named "Can Rapid Risk Stratification of Unstable Angina Patients Suppress Adverse Outcomes with Early Implementation?".[10] In 72,054 patients with NSTEMI at 509 U.S. hospitals from 2001 to 2004, acute β-blocker use was associated with a lower hospital mortality (adjusted OR 0.66; 95% CI 0.60–0.72, $P < 0.01$). Importantly, nearly all patient subgroups benefited, including patients 80 years or older.

PERCUTANEOUS CORONARY INTERVENTION

Although trials have evaluated adjunctive β-blockade in patients with unstable angina or MI undergoing PCI, less data exist for effect of β-blockade as a specific adjunct to PCI. In fact, most data for adjunctive benefit arise from nonrandomized registries. Sharma and colleagues evaluated 1675 consecutive patients undergoing PCI.[11] None of the patients had had MI before the PCI. The authors did not specify how many patients presented with unstable angina. Creatine kinase–muscle brain (CK-MB) elevation occurred in 13.2% of patients on β-blockers before the procedure compared with 22.1% of patients not on β-blockers ($P < 0.001$). On multivariate analysis, β-blockers remained an independent predictor of lower CK-MB release. Over a mean 15 months follow-up, patients on pre-procedural β-blockers had a mortality of 0.8% compared with 2% for patients not on pre-procedural β-blockers ($P = 0.04$). Chan and colleagues evaluated 4553 consecutive patients without acute or recent MI who underwent PCI, on the basis of whether or not they had been treated with β-blockers at the time of the PCI.[12] Of these patients, 2056 (45%) were on β-blockers at the time of the intervention. Mortality was lower among patients on β-blockers at 30 days (1.3% vs. 0.8%, $P = 0.13$) and at 1 year (6% vs. 3.9%, $P = 0.0014$). After adjusting for differences in the baseline characteristics by propensity analysis, β-blocker therapy remained independently predictive of 1-year survival (HR 0.63; 95% CI 0.46–0.87, $P = 0.0054$). Along with these mortality data, other data suggest the benefit of β-blockers on re-stenosis. Jackson and colleagues followed up 4840 patients undergoing PCI on the basis of whether or not they received β-blockers on discharge.[13] Patients treated with β-blockers had a 5-year clinical re-stenosis rate of 12% versus 14% (adjusted OR 0.83, $P = 0.046$). These data, however, are controversial because a small randomized trial of adjunctive carvedilol failed to show any reduction in re-stenosis in patients undergoing atherectomy.[14] In another small randomized trial, Wang and colleagues examined the effect of intracoronary (IC) propranolol during PCI.[15] In this trial, investigators randomized 150 patients undergoing PCI to placebo or propranolol (15 µg/kg) injected into the distal coronary artery via a balloon catheter positioned across the stenosis. CK-MB elevation occurred in 17% of the propranolol group compared with 36% of the placebo group ($P = 0.01$). The incidence of death, MI, or urgent revascularization by 30 days occurred in 18% of the propranolol group compared with 40% of the placebo group ($P = 0.004$). The relative risk of MI did not differ between the group on prior β-blocker therapy and the group not on prior therapy. Uretsky and colleagues also examined the effect of IC β-blockers during PCI by randomizing 400 patients to IC propranolol or placebo combined with systemic eptifibatide.[16] At 1 year, the composite endpoint of death, postprocedural MI, urgent target lesion revascularization, or MI after hospitalization occurred in 21.5% of the propranolol group and 32.5% of the placebo group ($P < 0.01$); this was driven primarily by lower peri-procedural MI (12.5% propranolol vs. 21.5% placebo; RR reduction 0.43; 95% CI 0.08–0.65, $P = 0.018$).

ACUTE MYOCARDIAL INFARCTION

Early Trials

The data for β-blockade in acute MI come from 26 small trials and two large trials—the Metoprolol in Acute Myocardial Infarction (MIAMI) trial and the First International Study of Infarct Survival (ISIS-1) trial.[17,18]

The MIAMI Trial. Patients with acute MI within 24 hours of symptom onset (N = 5778) were randomized to receive intravenous metoprolol (15 mg) or placebo followed by oral metoprolol (200 mg daily) or placebo for 15 days. β-blockade reduced Q wave infarction significantly from 53.9% to 50.9% (P = 0.024), with a nonsignificant reduction in mortality (4.9%–4.3%, P = 0.29). The MIAMI trial is significantly limited in its applicability to the modern era. Patients enrolled in MIAMI were low risk (e.g., all Killip class I), and the trial occurred in the pre-reperfusion era before routine treatment with ACE inhibition and statins.

The ISIS-1 Trial. Although ISIS-1 was similarly limited by lack of reperfusion, its larger size and power are important. ISIS-1 randomized 16,207 patients with suspected acute MI (mean 5 hours symptom onset) to control or to intravenous atenolol (5–10 mg) followed by 100 mg oral atenolol daily for 7 days. Treatment with atenolol significantly reduced vascular mortality from 4.57% to 3.89% ($P < 0.04$) from days 0 to 7. Atenolol-treated patients also had a significantly lower vascular mortality by 1 year (10.7% vs. 12.0%, $P < 0.01$), although much of this late difference might have arisen because patients randomized to atenolol were more likely to be discharged on β-blockers compared with controls.

Recent Data—The COMMIT Trial

Given that most data for β-blockade in acute MI are several decades old, benefit for β-blockade in the current era—with aggressive use of anti-platelet therapy, thrombolysis or primary angioplasty, statin therapy, and anti–aldosterone therapy—has remained uncertain, and physicians have hoped for trials with modern background therapy to assess the true value of β-blockade. This uncertainty has remained relevant because of persistent fears that β-blockers may exacerbate the condition of some patients with acute MI, particularly those with signs and symptoms of CHF. Fortunately, new data have come recently from the large-scale randomized CLOpidogrel and Metoprolol in Myocardial Infarction Trial (COMMIT).[19] In fact, COMMIT was not only a trial performed in the modern reperfusion era, but it also was the largest trial ever investigating β-blockers in acute MI. As such, it is exceptionally important to have an in-depth understanding of the trial and its implications for patient management. COMMIT (also known as the Second Chinese Cardiac Study—CCS-2) was a placebo-controlled randomized trial with a two-by-two factorial design, randomizing patients with acute MI to metoprolol or placebo as well as to clopidogrel or placebo, with a background therapy of aspirin, anticoagulant therapy (mostly unfractionated heparin), and thrombolysis.

Patient Selection. The scale of the trial was impressive. Between August 1999 and February 2005, COMMIT enrolled 45,852 patients in 1250 Chinese hospitals. Inclusion criteria included left bundle branch block (presumably new), ST elevation, or ST depression within 24-hours of ischemic symptoms. Exclusion criteria included patients scheduled for primary PCI (because of combined aspirin and clopidogrel use that would interfere with the other study arm) or conditions considered high risk for β-blocker therapy—systolic blood pressure <100 mm Hg or heart rate <50 beats per minute (beats/min), heart block, or cardiogenic shock. Interestingly, moderate heart failure (Killip class II or III) was not a contraindication, unlike in trials such as MIAMI.[18]

Study Protocol. Patients randomized to metoprolol received a 5-mg intravenous dose, followed by second and third doses as long as the systolic blood pressure was >90 mm Hg and heart rate was >50 beats/min after each dose. Patients then received 50 mg metoprolol 15 minutes after the last intravenous dose, repeated every 6 hours for 24 hours, followed by 200 mg controlled release metoprolol once daily for up to 4 weeks.

Endpoints. COMMIT had two primary endpoints: (1) all-cause mortality until discharge or day 28, and (2) the composite of death, re-infarction, or cardiac arrest. Secondary endpoints included cardiogenic shock, cardiac arrest, and re-infarction. Prespecified subgroup analyses included effects of metoprolol on primary outcomes according to hospital days and the following subgroups: age, gender, time from symptom onset, fibrinolysis, Killip class, heart rate, systolic blood pressure, and shock risk index (absolute risk of shock calculated from Cox regression model using baseline prognostic characteristics).

Results. Not surprisingly, the large sample size of COMMIT ensured that baseline characteristics between groups were similar (Fig. 12-1). The mean age was 61 years with 26% older than 70 years, and 72% were male. ST elevation occurred in 87%, with left bundle branch block in 6% and ST depression in 7%. Time from symptom onset to treatment was evenly distributed over 24 hours, with approximately one third of patients treated within 6 hours, one third within 6 to 13 hours, and one third within 13 to 24 hours. Although most patients had no signs or symptoms of CHF, a sizable percentage (24%) had Killip class II or III on presentation. Again, this contrasts with the early β-blocker trials that enrolled lower-risk patients with no evidence of CHF. In COMMIT, 54% of patients received thrombolysis, with most of them receiving urokinase. Of those presenting within 12 hours, 68% received thrombolysis; it is unknown how many of the remaining

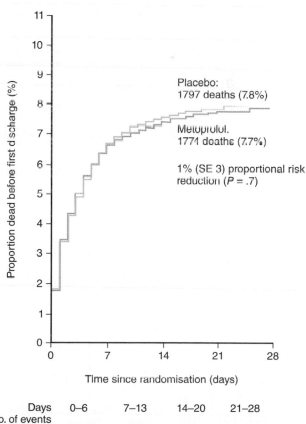

Days	0–6	7–13	14–20	21–28
No. of events				
Metoprolol	1441	220	83	30
Placebo	1449	249	75	24

Figure 12-1 Death in COMMIT.

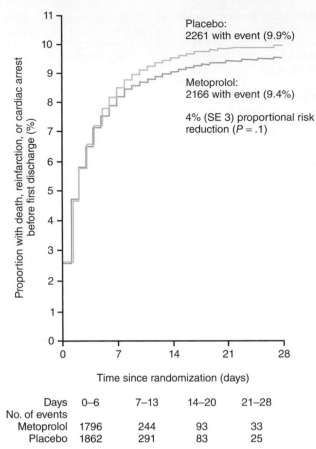

Days	0–6	7–13	14–20	21–28
No. of events			
Metoprolol	1796	244	93	33
Placebo	1862	291	83	25

Figure 12-2   Death, Reinfarction, or Cardiac Arrest in COMMIT.

patients did not receive thrombolytics because of clear contraindications. Notably, slightly fewer metoprolol-treated patients received ACE inhibitors (67.2% vs. 69.3%, $P < 0.0001$). The primary composite outcome of death, re-infarction, or cardiac arrest did not differ between metoprolol-treated patients (9.4%) and placebo-treated patients (9.9%; OR 0.96; 95% CI 0.90–1.01, $P = 0.10$) (Fig. 12-2). Similarly, the co-primary outcome of death did not differ between the metoprolol (7.7%) and placebo (7.8%) groups (see Figure 12-1). Given the prior clinical data supporting early β-blockade in acute MI, reasons for these counterintuitive results require a careful dissection; the questions, in particular, are: Did β-blockade reduce any particular clinical events? Did β-blockade benefit some patients much more than others? β-blockade significantly reduced any re-infarction (2% for metoprolol vs. 2.5% for placebo, $P = 0.001$) and risk of ventricular fibrillation (2.5% vs. 3.0%, $P = 0.001$). The treatment, however, increased the risk of cardiogenic shock by 30% (5.0% vs. 3.9%, $P < 0.0001$). Therefore, although β-blockade significantly reduced arrhythmic death by 22% (1.7% for metoprolol vs. 2.2% for placebo, $P = 0.0002$), β-blockade significantly increased death secondary to cardiogenic shock by 29% (2.2% vs. 1.7%, $P = 0.0002$). Therefore, any benefit in reducing arrhythmic death was counteracted by the harm in increased cardiogenic shock. In absolute terms, metoprolol prevented 5 episodes of ventricular fibrillation and 5 episodes of re-infarction per 1000 treated, but caused 11 episodes of cardiogenic shock per 1000 treated. Interestingly, these effects had differential time courses. In particular, 10 per 1000 increased risk for cardiogenic shock occurred within the first 24 hours. By contrast, reductions in the risk of re-infarction and ventricular fibrillation (VF) began approximately 48 hours after treatment initiation. The propensity of metoprolol to cause cardiogenic shock differed according to baseline characteristics. Metoprolol caused a much higher increase in cardiogenic shock in the

several subgroups: 56.9 per 1000 for patients in Killip class III; 34.6 per 1000 for patients presenting with heart rate >110 beats/min; 23.3 per 1000 per patients presenting with systolic blood pressure <120 mm Hg; 23.1 per 1000 for patients 70 years or older. Not surprisingly, these differences translated into a much higher risk of cardiogenic shock with metoprolol according to baseline risk of shock: 3.7 per 1000 (low risk) versus 16.2 per 1000 (medium risk) versus 56.9 per 1000 (high risk) ($P < 0.0001$). This differential effect on cardiogenic shock translated into a differential effect on mortality according to patients' baseline risk of shock. For patients at high risk of cardiogenic shock, metoprolol caused an absolute increase of 24.8 deaths per 1000 treated. Conversely, treatment caused an absolute *decrease* of 4.2 and 4.3 deaths per 1000 treated in medium-risk and low-risk patients, respectively.

Meta-Analysis Using COMMIT Patients. The COMMIT investigators reported that patients in this trial had a significantly higher risk of shock and mortality compared with patients enrolled in prior trials. Therefore, the investigators examined the effect of β-blockade on patients in COMMIT similar to that in the low-risk patients enrolled in MIAMI (i.e., heart rate >65 beats/min, Killip class I, systolic blood pressure >105 mm Hg). They also pooled these patients with patients from MIAMI, ISIS-1, and 26 small trials (Figure 12-3). The magnitude of benefit in the low-risk COMMIT patients (6.4%–5.7%) was similar to that in the MIAMI patients (4.9%–4.3%). In the analysis of pooled patients (~52,000), β-blockade significantly reduced cardiac arrest (3.1% vs. 3.6%, $P = 0.002$), re-infarction (2.3% vs. 2.8%, $P = 0.0002$), and mortality (4.8% vs. 5.5%, $P = 0.0006$).

Recommendations for β-Blockade during Acute Myocardial Infarction

Given COMMIT's applicability to the modern era and its enormous size (almost twice as many patients as all others combined), the COMMIT data must form the core basis for any recommendations. Accordingly, early intravenous β-blocker therapy for acute MI cannot be recommended for all patients. Nevertheless, the neutrality of the primary endpoints was driven by an increase in cardiogenic shock in patients at higher baseline risk of developing shock. Therefore, it is rational to consider early β-blockade in patients at low risk for shock— age under 70 years, heart rate below 110 beats/min, systolic blood pressure greater than 120 mm Hg, and Killip class I. This is, of course, not supported on a strict scientific basis because such a group was not prespecified. A stronger recommendation can be made for waiting at least 24 hours to determine clinical stability before beginning β-blockade. Because the cardiogenic shock hazard arises within 24 hours, it is possible that waiting could circumvent this hazard, allowing the "fittest for β-blockade" to emerge, giving these patients the benefits of avoiding re-infarction and cardiac arrest, which emerge more slowly over the hospital course.

Chronic Therapy after Myocardial Infarction. ISIS-1 demonstrated a sustained benefit of β-blockade for patients with acute MI; 1-year mortality for atenolol-treated patients was 10.7% versus 12% for patients on placebo ($P < 0.01$). Given that patients randomized to atenolol in this trial were more likely to be discharged on atenolol, the further separation in survival curves at 1 year suggests a beneficial effect of long-term β-blockade after MI. Pooled data from all long-term trials of β-blockade after MI also show a significant protective effect.[20] Long-term β-blockade reduced sudden death from 5.2% to 3.6% ($P < 0.0001$), re-infarction from 7.3% to 5.5% ($P < 0.0001$), and mortality from 9.5% to 7.5% ($P < 0.0001$) over a follow-up of 1 to 3 years. The CAPRICORN trial supported this benefit for patients with recent MI and systolic dysfunction.[21] CAPRICORN randomized 1959 patients with acute MI and left ventricular ejection fraction 40 or less to carvedilol 6.25 mg twice daily (started during hospitalization) or placebo. Carvedilol was titrated up to 25 mg twice daily over 4 to 6 weeks. After a mean follow-up of 15 months, carvedilol treatment reduced all-cause mortality from 15% to 12% (HR 0.77; 95% CI

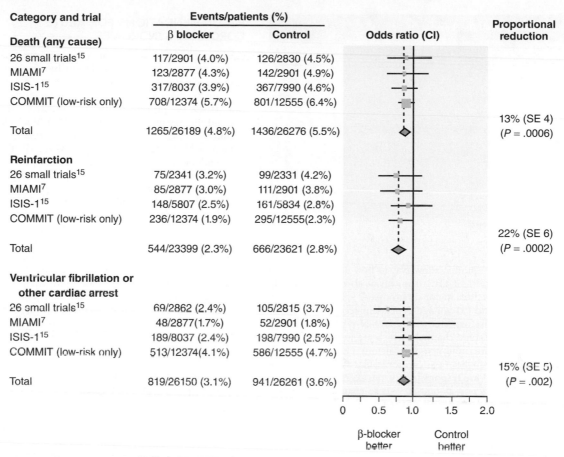

Category and trial	Events/patients (%)		Odds ratio (CI)	Proportional reduction
Death (any cause)	β blocker	Control		
26 small trials[15]	117/2901 (4.0%)	126/2830 (4.5%)		
MIAMI[7]	123/2877 (4.3%)	142/2901 (4.9%)		
ISIS-1[15]	317/8037 (3.9%)	367/7990 (4.6%)		
COMMIT (low-risk only)	708/12374 (5.7%)	801/12555 (6.4%)		
Total	1265/26189 (4.8%)	1436/26276 (5.5%)		13% (SE 4) (*P* = .0006)
Reinfarction				
26 small trials[15]	75/2341 (3.2%)	99/2331 (4.2%)		
MIAMI[7]	85/2877 (3.0%)	111/2901 (3.8%)		
ISIS-1[15]	148/5807 (2.5%)	161/5834 (2.8%)		
COMMIT (low-risk only)	236/12374 (1.9%)	295/12555(2.3%)		
Total	544/23399 (2.3%)	666/23621 (2.8%)		22% (SE 6) (*P* = .0002)
Ventricular fibrillation or other cardiac arrest				
26 small trials[15]	69/2862 (2.4%)	105/2815 (3.7%)		
MIAMI[7]	48/2877 (1.7%)	52/2901 (1.8%)		
ISIS-1[15]	189/8037 (2.4%)	198/7990 (2.5%)		
COMMIT (low-risk only)	513/12374(4.1%)	586/12555 (4.7%)		
Total	819/26150 (3.1%)	941/26261 (3.6%)		15% (SE 5) (*P* = .002)

Figure 12-3 Meta-analysis using COMMIT data.

0.60–0.98, *P* = 0.03). Importantly, the CAPRICORN trial represented modern therapy with aggressive reperfusion, anti-platelet therapy, and anticoagulation; furthermore, all patients received ACE-inhibitors for 48 hours before randomization.

Patient Selection: Role of Genomics. β-blockade does not uniformly benefit all patients after MI, as COMMIT demonstrated, β-blockers may harm certain subgroups while benefiting others. Therefore, clinical trials remain blunt and crude instruments at best. Suppose, for example, that a condition has 100% mortality and that a treatment demonstrates a large absolute reduction in mortality (40%). Thus, 4 of 10 patients given the treatment survived compared with 0 of 10 patients given placebo. This means that 6 treated patients did not receive any benefit. This conundrum presented by clinical trials argues for a finer instrument to determine which of the patients will benefit from the treatment. Given the recent advances in pharmacogenomics, characterization of patients' genetic polymorphisms may be a useful instrument to select the best candidates for β-blocker therapy. Lanfear and colleagues studied polymorphisms in the β_1 and β_2 receptors among patients (*N* = 597) on β-blocker therapy after ACS.[22] No relationship existed between β_1 receptor polymorphisms and mortality in patients treated or not treated with β-blockers. Polymorphisms in β_2 receptors, however, correlated significantly with mortality in patients discharged on β-blockers. In particular, Kaplan-Meier 3-year mortality rates were 6%, 11%, and 16% for three different polymorphisms GG, CG, and CC genotypes, respectively, for polymorphism Gln27Glu (HR 0.24; 95% CI 0.09–0.68 for GG versus CC, *P* = 0.004). Another β_2 receptor polymorphism, Gly16Arg, displayed a relationship between genotypes and mortality: 3-year Kaplan-Meier mortality rates of 10% for the GG and GA genotypes compared with 20% for the AA genotype (HR 0.44; 95% CI 0.22–0.85 for GG vs AA; HR 0.48 95% CI 0.27–0.86

for GA vs. AA, *P* = 0.005 for over all comparison). Importantly, these polymorphisms did not correlate with mortality in patients not treated with β-blockers, indicating a specific interaction of the polymorphisms with β-blocker treatment. Although the mechanism of this interaction is unknown, it is possible that these polymorphisms alter left ventricular remodeling in response to β-blockade, as has been described for β_1 receptor polymorphisms.[23] Similarly, polymorphisms in the peroxisome proliferator-activated receptor α (*PPARα*) gene, which can alter left ventricular remodeling, can interact with β-blocker therapy, affecting rehospitalization rates after ACS.[24] Polymorphisms can also interact differentially with β-blockers in the presence of diabetes. Beitelshees and colleagues followed ACS patients (*N* = 468) and compared those with and without the -866G > A polymorphism in the mitochondrial uncoupling protein 2 (UCP2) gene.[25] Among patients with diabetes with the G/G genotype, β-blocker use reduced cardiac rehospitalization by 80%, whereas β-blocker use *increased* cardiac rehospitalization 11-fold among A-carrier patients with diabetes. These studies, although small, suggest that genomic profiling might help tailor β-blocker therapy in patients with ACS, thereby maximizing benefit and reducing risk. Furthermore, advances in high-throughput genotyping suggest that widespread application is feasible.

Calcium Channels

Intracellular calcium concentrations are tightly regulated by calcium exchangers, ion pumps, and channels. At baseline, cytoplasmic calcium ion concentrations exist at very low levels (<100 nM) compared with extracellular concentrations (>1 mM). When calcium channels open at the plasma membrane or the endoplasmic reticular level, intracellular concentrations of calcium rapidly rise. Adenosine triphosphate (ATP)-dependent pumps restore the Na^+/K^+ gradient across the plasma

TABLE 12-2 Calcium Channel Blockers			
Phenylalkylamine	Vasodilatory Effects	Conduction Effects	Negative Inotropy
Verapamil	+++	++++	+++
Benzothiazepine			
Diltiazem	++	+++	++
Dihydropyridine			
Amlodipine	+++	+	+
Bepridil	+++	+++	++++
Felodipine	++++	+	0
Isradipine	+++	++	0
Nicardipine	++++	+	0
Nifedipine	++++	+	+
Nisoldipine	+++	+	+

0, No activity; ++++, most potent.

membrane, and Na^+/Ca^{2+} pumps allow Na^+ to flow across the membrane for counter-transport of Ca^{2+} from inside to outside the cell. Calcium channels exist as three major subgroups: (1) stretch-operated, (2) receptor-operated, and (3) voltage-dependent receptors. Voltage-dependent receptors exist as three subtypes—N-type, L-type, and T-type; the L-type and T-type channels, which are important to cardiovascular medicine, are inhibited by calcium channel blockers. L-type channels exist throughout the cardiovascular system in cardiac and smooth muscles and are responsible for the slow inward current (plateau phase) of the action potential. T-type channels are found mainly in sinus nodal tissue with very little found in the ventricular myocardium.

CALCIUM CHANNEL BLOCKERS

The three main classes of calcium channel blockers include dihydropyridines, phenylalkylamines, and benzothiazepines (Table 12-2).[53] These classes differ in their vasodilatory and chronotropic effects. In particular, phenylalkylamines (e.g., verapamil) and benzothiazepines (e.g., diltiazem) decrease AV and sinoatrial (SA) conduction, whereas dihydropyridines (e.g., amlodipine) do not. On the other hand, dihydropyridines are more potent vasodilators. Nifedipine, in particular, can cause profound peripheral vasodilation, which results in reflex tachycardia. Despite these differences, all classes of calcium channel blockers have been shown to reduce infarct size in animal models. Some have speculated that calcium channel blockers protect the myocardium via coronary vasodilation and decreased ischemic calcium overload.

ACUTE MYOCARDIAL INFARCTION

Most data for calcium channel blockade after acute MI are over 10 years old. The pivotal trials for early treatment of MI include the Secondary Prevention Reinfarction Israeli Nifedipine Trial (SPRINT-II), the first Danish Study Group on Verapamil in Myocardial Infarction Trial (DAVIT) and three small diltiazem trials.[26] None of these trials showed any significant difference in re-infarction or mortality with calcium channel blockade; in fact, SPRINT-II was stopped prematurely because of increased mortality in the nifedipine group. Recent data are limited and have only served to generate hypotheses. In a recent Japanese trial, investigators randomized 1090 patients after acute MI to β-blocker or calcium channel blocker therapy.[27] At a mean follow-up of 455 days, patients treated with calcium channel blockers did not show any difference in the incidence of cardiovascular death (1.1% vs. 1.7%), re-infarction (1.3% vs. 0.9%), or nonfatal stroke (0.2% vs. 0.7%). Interestingly, the calcium channel blocker group had a significantly lower incidence of CHF (1.1% vs. 4.2%, $P = 0.001$) and coronary spasm (0.2% vs. 1.2%, $P = 0.027$). More data in other populations are required to confirm these differences.

RECOMMENDATIONS FOR ACUTE CORONARY SYNDROMES

Given the lack of large trials demonstrating benefit in acute MI, calcium channel blockers should not be administered routinely, particularly to patients presenting with STEMI. A prominent exception is the patient who presents with ST elevation following cocaine intoxication. Given the prominent role of coronary vasospasm after cocaine use and the possible exacerbation with β-blockade, it is reasonable to administer calcium channel blockers to this group of patients. For patients with unstable angina or non-STEMI, the ACC/AHA guidelines endorse a class I recommendation for some patients with ACS: "In patients with continuing or frequently recurring ischemia when beta-blockers are contraindicated, a non-dihydropyridine calcium antagonist (e.g., verapamil or diltiazem), followed by oral therapy, as initial therapy in the absence of severe left ventricular (LV) dysfunction or other contraindications (Level of Evidence: B)."[28] Furthermore, these guidelines endorse a class IIa recommendation for other patients with ACS with recurrent ischemia, who are already on β-blockers and nitrates: "Oral long-acting calcium antagonists for recurrent ischemia in the absence of contraindications and when β-blockers and nitrates are fully used (Level of Evidence: C)." The guidelines also clearly indicate that short-acting dihydropyridines (e.g., short-acting nifedipine) are contraindicated because of their propensity to decrease blood pressure abruptly and worsen the ischemia or infarction.

CHRONIC THERAPY AFTER MYOCARDIAL INFARCTION

Early Trials

Like the data for acute treatment, many studies investigating chronic treatment are limited by being over 10 years old. These trials started calcium channel blockade weeks to months after MI, continuing these agents over the long term. Data for nifedipine suggest harm, and trials evaluating verapamil and diltiazem showed a nonsignificant reduction in noninfarction, although one large diltiazem trial showed this trend only in patients without CHF.[29] Taken together, the nifedipine trials demonstrate increased mortality with treatment; it is important to note that these trials had small numbers of events and used short-acting, not controlled-release, nifedipine. When the verapamil and diltiazem data are combined, treatment was shown to reduce re-infarction by 22% (95% CI –33%–0.8%, $P < 0.01$).[30]

Recent Trials

Several antihypertensive trials have demonstrated similar outcomes for calcium channel blockers and other agents. Some of these trials have enrolled patients with a history of MI and provide reassuring data.

The CAMELOT Trial. The Comparison of Amlodipine vs Enalapril to Limit Occurrences of Thrombosis (CAMELOT) study randomized 1991 patients with angiographically documented CAD (>20%) to amlodipine 10 mg daily, enalapril 20 mg daily, or placebo.[31] Uniquely, these patients had "normal" blood pressure at baseline (~129/77 mm Hg). The primary outcome was the incidence of adverse cardiovascular events, including cardiovascular death, resuscitated cardiac arrest, nonfatal MI, coronary revascularization, hospitalization for CHF, hospitalization for angina pectoris, stroke or transient ischemic attack (TIA), and any new diagnosis of peripheral vascular disease. The trial had an intravascular ultrasound substudy with the endpoint being percent change in atheroma volume. The mean age of the patients was approximately 57 years, and 38% of the entire study population had a history of MI. The primary endpoint occurred in 23.1% of the placebo group, compared with 20.2% of the enalapril group and 16.6% of the amlodipine group, with significant differences between both the enalapril and amlodipine groups compared with the placebo group (Fig. 12-4). The amlodipine group had a statistical trend for fewer cardiovascular events compared with the enalapril group

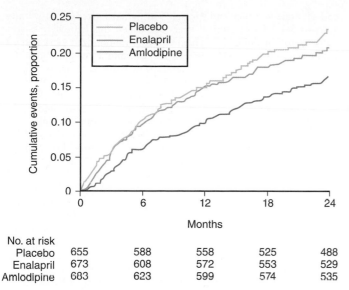

Figure 12-4 Cumulative events in the CAMELOT trial.

No. at risk					
Placebo	655	588	558	525	488
Enalapril	673	608	572	553	529
Amlodipine	683	623	599	574	535

(HR 0.81; 95% CI 0.63–1.04, $P = 0.10$), and amlodipine treatment resulted in significantly fewer hospitalizations for angina (IIR 0.59; 95% 0.42–0.84, $P = 0.003$). Interestingly, amlodipine also displayed a trend for reduced atheroma progression compared with placebo ($P = 0.12$); also, amlodipine-treated patients with baseline blood pressures above mean had significantly reduced atheroma progression compared with the placebo group ($P < 0.001$).

The INVEST Trial. The International Verapamil-Trandolapril Study (INVEST) compared a calcium channel blocker strategy to a non–calcium channel blocker strategy for the treatment of hypertension in patients with CAD.[32] The trial randomized patients to baseline therapy of long-acting verapamil or atenolol. Patients not meeting JNC 7 (the Seventh Report of the Joint National Committee on Prevention, Detection, Evaluation, and Treatment of High Blood Pressure) blood pressure goals received trandolapril, hydrochlorothiazide, or both. The primary endpoint was the incidence of death, MI, or stroke. The 22,576 enrolled patients all had documented CAD, and approximately 32% had history of MI. Because secondary hypertensive therapy was not specified, secondary agents differed between the groups. The verapamil arm received more trandolapril than did the atenolol arm (62.9% vs. 52.4%, $P < 0.001$) but received less hydrochlorothiazide (43.7% vs. 60.3%, $P < 0.001$). At a mean follow-up of 2.7 years, the primary endpoint did not differ between the verapamil and atenolol arms (9.93% for verapamil vs. 10.17% for atenolol; RR 0.98; 95% CI 0.90–1.06). Also, the primary endpoint did not differ according to treatment arm in patients with a history of MI (13.67% for verapamil vs. 14.38% for atenolol; RR 0.95; 95% CI 0.85–1.07). Thus, the INVEST and CAMELOT trials confirmed that long-term calcium channel blockade is safe and efficacious in high-risk patients, even in those with a history of MI. The JNC 7 guidelines recommend that patients receive ACE inhibitors and β-blockers following MI; calcium channel blockers have been given a "compelling indication" for patients with diabetes or a high risk of coronary artery disease. Most patients, of course, require multiple medications for blood pressure control, and all these data suggest that calcium channel blockers are a reasonable part of the treatment plan.[33]

PERCUTANEOUS CORONARY INTERVENTION

As adjunctive therapy to PCI, calcium channel blockers have shown beneficial effects on myocardial perfusion, particularly during a "no-reflow" state, and on re-stenosis.

No-reflow is slow epicardial flow and inadequate myocardial perfusion despite a patent epicardial vessel. Although the mechanisms of no-reflow are incompletely understood, many investigators believe that no-reflow occurs because of widespread microvascular dysfunction from overwhelming thromboembolism and reperfusion injury. Because calcium channel blockers are potent coronary vasodilators, investigators have used these agents in no-reflow states in an attempt to open the plugged microvasculature. Small studies support this idea. In a single-center, nonrandomized study, Hang and colleagues administered intracoronary verapamil to 50 patients with acute MI undergoing primary PCI and compared these patients with 50 historical controls.[34] Myocardial perfusion, as measured by Thrombolysis in Myocardial Infarction Myocardial Perfusion Grade (TMPG), significantly differed with verapamil administration. Specifically, 42% of verapamil-treated patients had TMPG 3 compared with only 14% of control subjects ($P = 0.004$). Moreover, verapamil treatment was an independent predictor of TMPG (OR, 0.26; 95% CI 0.12–0.58; $P = 0.001$). Umemura and colleagues confirmed this benefit of verapamil in patients with acute MI undergoing primary PCI.[35] They performed 99mTc tetrofosmin single photon emission computed tomography (SPECT) before, immediately after, and 1 month after PCI in 101 patients with acute MI. No-reflow occurred in 32 (31%) patients. Verapamil administration independently predicted not only post-PCI thrombolysis in MI (TIMI)-3 flow (OR 22.4, $P = 0.002$) but also lower infarct size by 1 month according to SPECT imaging. In addition to improving no-reflow, calcium channel blockers might also lower the incidence of re-stenosis. Although, thus far, the most effective agents for reducing neointimal hyperplasia have been sirolimus and paclitaxel, some data do exist supporting the beneficial effect of calcium channel blockers in reducing re-stenosis. For example, recent data for benidipine, a dihydropyridine calcium channel blocker, showed that proliferation of vascular smooth muscle cells (VSMC) in culture was significantly reduced by benidipine.[36] The reduction in VSMC proliferation leads to less neointimal hyperplasia. Yamazaki and colleagues showed this by randomizing 63 patients after successful coronary stenting to amlodipine 5 mg/day or quinapril 10 mg/day.[37] Investigators performed quantitative coronary angiography before and immediately after stenting and 3 to 6 months later. Approximately 50% of each group also underwent intravascular ultrasonography at follow-up, and amlodipine-treated patients had a significantly larger minimal lumen diameter (1.52 ± 0.53 mm vs. 1.88 ± 0.64 mm, $P < 0.01$) and a significantly smaller neointimal area (1.9 ± 0.5 mm² vs. 2.7 ± 0.8 mm², $P < 0.01$). This reduction in neointimal proliferation appears to lead to fewer clinical events, as demonstrated by the most recent clinical trial of calcium channel blockade after PCI—the Verapamil Slow-Release for Prevention of Cardiovascular Events After Angioplasty (VESPA) trial.[38] The VESPA investigators randomized 700 patients after PCI to verapamil 240 mg twice daily for 6 months or to placebo. Most patients (83%) received stents, and follow-up was excellent, with 95% having complete clinical follow-up and 94% receiving angiography at 6 months. The primary endpoint, a composite death, MI, or target vessel revascularization by 1 year was 19.3% for placebo patients compared with 29.3% for verapamil patients (RR 0.66; 95% CI 0.48–0.89, $P = 0.002$). The endpoint was driven by a lower risk of target vessel revascularization (26.2% for placebo vs. 17.5% for verapamil, RR 0.67; 95% CI 0.49–0.93, $P = 0.006$). Furthermore, verapamil reduced the incidence of re-stenosis by 75% or more (13.7% vs. 7.8%; RR 0.57; 95% CI 0.35–0.92, $P = 0.014$). Despite being promising, animal and clinical data are limited, and VESPA is a single small trial; furthermore, the advent of drug-eluting stents (DESs) has significantly dampened the enthusiasm toward systemic therapies such as calcium channel blockers.

ANGIOTENSIN-CONVERTING ENZYME

ACE plays an important role in the renin–angiotensin–aldosterone system. When the kidneys sense a decrease in blood volume, the juxtaglomerular apparatus secretes renin, which catalyzes the conversion of angiotensinogen (hepatically produced) to angiotensin I. ACE, secreted by pulmonary and renal endothelial cells, converts angiotensin I to angiotensin II and also degrades bradykinin and other vasoactive peptides. Angiotensin II increases sympathetic activity, promotes aldosterone and antidiuretic hormone release, and increases arteriolar vasoconstriction. Although these actions are helpful counter-regulatory mechanisms (e.g., in acute blood loss), chronic activation of this system promotes atherosclerosis, cardiomyopathy, and nephropathy.[39]

ANGIOTENSIN-CONVERTING ENZYME INHIBITORS

By inhibiting ACE, ACE inhibitors decrease the production of angiotensin II and prevent the degradation of bradykinin. Reduction of angiotensin II lowers arteriolar resistance, which, in turn, lowers blood pressure and increases stroke volume and cardiac output. In addition to their direct hemodynamic effects, ACE inhibitors have pleiotropic actions that promote favorable ventricular remodeling. For example, ACE-I inhibition prevents hypertrophy and apoptosis of cardiac myocytes and decreases myocardial fibrosis through lower collagen type 1 production and altered matrix metalloproteinase activity.[40]

PERCUTANEOUS CORONARY INTERVENTION

Experimental animal models suggest that ACE inhibitors might reduce re-stenosis after coronary intervention, although little clinical data exist to support benefit.[41] For example, Okimoto and colleagues randomized 253 patients after coronary intervention to quinapril or placebo.[42] Binary angiographic re-stenosis occurred in 34.3% of the quinapril group compared with 47.7% of the placebo group ($P < 0.05$). Similarly, Deftereos and colleagues randomized 86 patients to quinapril or placebo after PCI and found a reduction in re-stenosis (9.3% vs. 25.6%, $P = 0.047$).[43] Conversely, in the largest randomized trial of ACE inhibition after PCI, investigators found no reduction in re-stenosis.[44] With the introduction of DESs, high-quality evidence for the true efficacy of ACE inhibitors in reducing re-stenosis will remain elusive.

ACUTE MYOCARDIAL INFARCTION

Numerous trials have demonstrated the benefit of ACE inhibitors after MI. More than two decades ago, several investigators provided evidence that ACE inhibitors greatly attenuate unfavorable remodeling after MI. For instance, Braunwald and colleagues showed decreased end-diastolic volumes and pressures in patients given captopril after anterior MI.[45] Large clinical trials confirmed this benefit in a wide range of patients after MI. The SAVE trial randomized 2231 patients with ejection fraction (EF) 40% or less to captopril or placebo within 3 to 16 days of MI.[46] Captopril significantly reduced recurrent MI (RR 25%; 95% CI 5%–40%, $P = 0.015$), severe heart failure (RR 22%; 95% CI 4%–37%, $P = 0.019$), and all-cause mortality (20% vs. 25%, $P = 0.019$). The Chinese Cardiac Study (CCS-1) also randomized patients ($N = 14,962$) after acute MI to captopril or placebo.[47] Captopril significantly reduced death or heart failure (21.5% vs. 23.1%, $P = 0.02$). Confirming a class effect for ACE inhibitors, the AIRE trial demonstrated that ramipril reduced mortality (RR 27%; 95% CI 11%–40%, $P = 0.002$).[48] Similarly, the GISSI-3, SMILE, and TRACE trials demonstrated comparable benefits of lisinopril, zofenopril, and trandolapril, respectively.[49-51] Complementing these trials was the largest and most definitive ISIS-4 trial. In this extraordinary trial, 58,050 patients within 24 hours of MI (median 8 hours) were randomized in a two-by-two-by-two factorial design to controlled-release mononitrate versus placebo, intravenous magnesium versus placebo, and 1-month oral captopril (6.25 mg titrated up to 50 mg twice daily).[52] At 5 weeks, captopril reduced mortality significantly (7.19% vs. 7.69%, $P = 0.02$). Although the absolute benefit for the entire cohort was modest, higher-risk groups such as those presenting with heart failure or history of previous MI benefited more (up to 10 fewer deaths per 1000 treated).

▣ Conclusion

Although COMMIT suggests caution for acute intravenous β-blockade after MI, the data are strong for the benefit of β-blockers in the subacute and chronic treatment of patients with MI. Indeed, strong recommendations can be made for using β-blockers in all patients after MI, particularly those with left ventricular (LV) dysfunction. Similarly, in stable patients after MI, calcium channel blockers can be a useful adjunct for treating hypertension and angina. Finally, overwhelming evidence supports the routine administration of ACE inhibitors after MI, particularly in those with LV dysfunction. Despite evidence for these therapies, they remain underused. Similarly, other well-established medications, such as anti-platelet agents and statins are under-prescribed for secondary prevention, even to ideal candidates. Therefore, widespread dissemination and re-iteration of evidence-based medicine is critical to maximize benefits for patients in particular, and for public health in general.

REFERENCES

1. Brodde OE, Bruck H, Leineweber K: Cardiac adrenoceptors: Physiological and pathophysiological relevance. *J Pharmacol Sci* 100(5):323–337, 2006.
2. Emorine LJ, Marullo S, Briend-Sutren MM, et al: Molecular characterization of the human beta 3-adrenergic receptor. *Science* 245:1118–1121, 1989.
3. Collins S, Cao W, Robidoux J: Learning new tricks from old dogs: Beta-adrenergic receptors teach new lessons on firing up adipose tissue metabolism. *Mol Endocrinol* 18:2123–2131, 2004.
4. Petrikova M, Jancinova V, Nosal R, et al: Antiplatelet activity of carvedilol in comparison to propranolol. *Platelets* 13:479–485, 2002.
5. Gottlieb SO, Weisfeldt ML, Ouyang P, et al: Effect of the addition of propranolol to therapy with nifedipine for unstable angina pectoris: A randomized, double-blind, placebo-controlled trial. *Circulation* 73:331–337, 1986.
6. The Holland Interuniversity Nifedipine/Metoprolol Trial (HINT) Research Group: Early treatment of unstable angina in the coronary care unit: A randomised, double blind, placebo controlled comparison of recurrent ischaemia in patients treated with nifedipine or metoprolol or both. Report of The Holland Interuniversity Nifedipine/Metoprolol Trial (HINT) Research Group. *Br Heart J* 56:400–413, 1986.
7. Hohnloser SH, Meinertz T, Klingenheben T, et al: Usefulness of esmolol in unstable angina pectoris. European Esmolol Study Group. *Am J Cardiol* 67:1319–1323, 1991.
8. Brunner M, Faber TS, Greve B, et al: Usefulness of carvedilol in unstable angina pectoris. *Am J Cardiol* 85:1173–1178, 2000.
9. Ellis K, Tcheng JE, Sapp S, et al: Mortality benefit of beta blockade in patients with acute coronary syndromes undergoing coronary

intervention: Pooled results from the Epic, Epilog, Epistent, Capture and Rapport Trials. *J Interv Cardiol* 16:299–305, 2003.
10. Miller CD, Roe MT, Mulgund J, et al: Impact of acute beta-blocker therapy for patients with non-ST-segment elevation myocardial infarction. *Am J Med* 120:685–692, 2007.
11. Sharma SK, Kini A, Marmur JD, et al: Cardioprotective effect of prior beta-blocker therapy in reducing creatine kinase-MB elevation after coronary intervention: Benefit is extended to improvement in intermediate-term survival. *Circulation* 102:166–172, 2000.
12. Chan AW, Quinn MJ, Bhatt DL, et al: Mortality benefit of beta-blockade after successful elective percutaneous coronary intervention. *J Am Coll Cardiol* 40:669–675, 2002.
13. Jackson JD, Muhlestein JB, Bunch TJ, et al: Beta-blockers reduce the incidence of clinical restenosis: Prospective study of 4840 patients undergoing percutaneous coronary revascularization. *Am Heart J* 145:875–881, 2003.
14. Serruys PW, Foley DP, Hofling B, et al: Carvedilol for prevention of restenosis after directional coronary atherectomy: Final results of the European carvedilol atherectomy restenosis (EUROCARE) trial. *Circulation* 101:1512–1518, 2000.
15. Wang FW, Osman A, Otero J, et al: Distal myocardial protection during percutaneous coronary intervention with an intracoronary beta-blocker. *Circulation* 107:2914–2919, 2003.
16. Uretsky BF, Birnbaum Y, Osman A, et al: Distal myocardial protection with intracoronary beta blocker when added to a Gp IIb/IIIa platelet receptor blocker during percutaneous coronary intervention improves clinical outcome. *Catheter Cardiovasc Interv* 72:488–497, 2008.
17. Randomised trial of intravenous atenolol among 16027 cases of suspected acute myocardial infarction: ISIS-1. First International

Study of Infarct Survival Collaborative Group. *Lancet* 2:57–66, 1986.
18. Metoprolol in acute myocardial infarction (MIAMI). A randomised placebo-controlled international trial. The MIAMI Trial Research Group. *Eur Heart J* 6:199–226, 1985.
19. Chen ZM, Pan HC, Chen YP, et al: Early intravenous then oral metoprolol in 45,852 patients with acute myocardial infarction: Randomised placebo-controlled trial. *Lancet* 366:1622–1632, 2005.
20. Freemantle N, Cleland J, Young P, et al: beta Blockade after myocardial infarction: Systematic review and meta regression analysis. *BMJ* 318:1730–1737, 1999.
21. Dargie HJ: Effect of carvedilol on outcome after myocardial infarction in patients with left-ventricular dysfunction: The CAPRICORN randomised trial. *Lancet* 357:1385–1390, 2001.
22. Lanfear DE, Jones PG, Marsh S, et al: Beta2-adrenergic receptor genotype and survival among patients receiving beta-blocker therapy after an acute coronary syndrome. *JAMA* 294:1526–1533, 2005.
23. Terra SG, Hamilton KK, Pauly DF, et al: Beta1 adrenergic receptor polymorphisms and left ventricular remodeling changes in response to beta-blocker therapy. *Pharmacogenet Genomics* 15:227–234, 2005.
24. Cresci S, Jones PG, Sucharov CC, et al: Interaction between PPARA genotype and beta-blocker treatment influences clinical outcomes following acute coronary syndromes. *Pharmacogenomics* 9:1403–1417, 2008.
25. Beitelshees AL, Finck BN, Leone TC, et al: Interaction between the UCP2 -866 G>A polymorphism, diabetes, and beta-blocker use among patients with acute coronary syndromes. *Pharmacogenet Genomics* 20:231–238, 2010.

26. Held PH, Yusuf S, Furberg CD: Calcium channel blockers in acute myocardial infarction and unstable angina: An overview. *BMJ* 299:1187–1192, 1989.

27. Comparison of the effects of beta blockers and calcium antagonists on cardiovascular events after acute myocardial infarction in Japanese subjects. *Am J Cardiol* 93:969–973, 2004.

28. Braunwald E, Antman EM, Beasley JW, et al: ACC/AHA 2002 guideline update for the management of patients with unstable angina and non-ST-segment elevation myocardial infarction—summary article: A report of the American College of Cardiology/American Heart Association task force on practice guidelines (Committee on the Management of Patients With Unstable Angina). *J Am Coll Cardiol* 40:1366–1374, 2002.

29. Kaplan NM: The calcium channel blocker controversy. *Hypertens Res* 19:57–64, 1996.

30. Opie LH: Calcium channel blockers in hypertension: reappraisal after new trials and major meta-analyses. *Am J Hypertens* 14:1074–1081, 2001.

31. Nissen SE, Tuzcu EM, Libby P, et al: Effect of antihypertensive agents on cardiovascular events in patients with coronary disease and normal blood pressure: The CAMELOT study. A randomized controlled trial. *JAMA* 292:2217–2225, 2004.

32. Pepine CJ, Handberg EM, Cooper-DeHoff RM, et al: A calcium antagonist vs a non-calcium antagonist hypertension treatment strategy for patients with coronary artery disease. The International Verapamil-Trandolapril Study (INVEST): A randomized controlled trial. *JAMA* 290:2805–2816, 2003.

33. Chobanian AV, Bakris GL, Black HR, et al: The Seventh Report of the Joint National Committee on Prevention, Detection, Evaluation, and Treatment of High Blood Pressure: The JNC 7 report. *JAMA* 289:2560–2572, 2003.

34. Hang CL, Wang CP, Yip HK, et al: Early administration of intracoronary verapamil improves myocardial perfusion during percutaneous coronary interventions for acute myocardial infarction. *Chest* 128:2593–2598, 2005.

35. Umemura S, Nakamura S, Sugiura T, et al: The effect of verapamil on the restoration of myocardial perfusion and functional recovery in patients with angiographic no-reflow after primary percutaneous coronary intervention. *Nucl Med Commun* 27:247–254, 2006.

36. Arakawa E, Hasegawa K: Benidipine, a calcium channel blocker, regulates proliferation and phenotype of vascular smooth muscle cells. *J Pharmacol Sci* 100:149–156, 2006.

37. Yamazaki T, Taniguchi I, Kurusu T, et al: Effect of amlodipine on vascular responses after coronary stenting compared with an angiotensin-converting enzyme inhibitor. *Circ J* 68:328–333, 2004.

38. Bestehorn HP, Neumann FJ, Buttner HJ, et al: Evaluation of the effect of oral verapamil on clinical outcome and angiographic restenosis after percutaneous coronary intervention: The randomized, double-blind, placebo-controlled, multicenter Verapamil Slow-Release for Prevention of Cardiovascular Events After Angioplasty (VESPA) Trial. *J Am Coll Cardiol* 43:2160–2165, 2004.

39. Ferrario CM, Strawn WB: Role of the renin-angiotensin-aldosterone system and proinflammatory mediators in cardiovascular disease. *Am J Cardiol* 98:121–128, 2006.

40. Gajarsa JJ, Kloner RA: Left ventricular remodeling in the post-infarction heart: A review of cellular, molecular mechanisms, and therapeutic modalities. *Heart Fail Rev* 16(1):13–21, 2010.

41. Muller D, Ellis S, Topol E: Experimental models of coronary artery restenosis. *J Am Coll Cardiol* 19:418–432, 1992.

42. Okimoto T, Imazu M, Hayashi Y, et al: Quinapril with high affinity to tissue angiotensin-converting enzyme reduces restenosis after percutaneous transcatheter coronary intervention. *Cardiovasc Drugs Ther* 15:323–329, 2001.

43. Deftereos S, Giannopoulos G, Kossyvakis C, et al: Effect of quinapril on in-stent restenosis and relation to plasma apoptosis signaling molecules. *Am J Cardiol* 105:54–58, 2010.

44. Does the new angiotensin converting enzyme inhibitor cilazapril prevent restenosis after percutaneous transluminal coronary angioplasty? Results of the MERCATOR study: A multicenter, randomized, double-blind placebo-controlled trial. Multicenter European Research Trial with Cilazapril after Angioplasty to Prevent Transluminal Coronary Obstruction and Restenosis (MERCATOR) Study Group. *Circulation* 86:325–327, 1992.

45. Pfeffer M, Lamas G, Vaughan D, et al: Effect of captopril on progressive ventricular dilatation after anterior myocardial infarction. *N Engl J Med* 319:80–86, 1988.

46. Pfeffer M, Braunwald E, Moye L, et al: Effect of captopril on mortality and morbidity in patients with left ventricular dysfunction after myocardial infarction. Results of the survival and ventricular enlargement trial. The SAVE Investigators. *N Engl J Med* 327:669–677, 1992.

47. Oral captopril versus placebo among 14,962 patients with suspected acute myocardial infarction: A multicenter, randomized, double-blind, placebo controlled clinical trial. Chinese Cardiac Study (CCS-1) Collaborative Group. *Chin Med J* 110:834–838, 1997.

48. Effect of ramipril on mortality and morbidity of survivors of acute myocardial infarction with clinical evidence of heart failure. The Acute Infarction Ramipril Efficacy (AIRE) Study Investigators. *Lancet* 342:821–828, 1993.

49. Amborsioni E, Borghi C, Magnani B: The effect of the angiotensin-converting-enzyme-inhibitor zofenopril on mortality and morbidity after anterior myocardial infarction. The Survival of Myocardial Infarction Long-Term Evaluation (SMILE) Study Investigators. *N Engl J Med* 332:80–85, 1995.

50. GISSI-3: Effects of lisinopril and transdermal glyceryl trinitrate singly and together on 6-week mortality and ventricular function after acute myocardial infarction. Gruppo Italiano per lo Studio della Sopravvivenza nell'infarto Miocardico. *Lancet* 343:1115–1122, 1994.

51. Kober L, Torp-Pedersen C, Carlsen J, et al: A clinical trial of the angiotensin-converting-enzyme trandolapril in patients with left ventricular dysfunction after myocardial infarction. Trandolapril Cardiac Evaluation (TRACE) Study Group. *N Engl J Med* 333:1670–1676, 1995.

52. ISIS-4: A randomised factorial trial assessing early oral captopril, oral mononitrate, and intravenous magnesium sulphate in 58,5050 patients with suspected acute myocardial infarction. ISIS-4 (Fourth International Study of Infarct Survival) Collaborative Group. *Lancet* 345:669–685, 1995.

53. Griffin B, Topol E, Nair D, Ashley K: *Manual of cardiovascular medicine*, ed 3, Philadelphia, 2008, Lippincott Williams & Wilkins.

Coronary Intervention

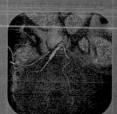

Bare Metal and Drug-Eluting Coronary Stents

GREGG W. STONE | AJAY J. KIRTANE

KEY POINTS

- Bare metal stents overcome many of the drawbacks of balloon angioplasty but are limited by their Achilles' heel, restenosis, which develops in 20% to 40% of cases.

- Drug-eluting stents—which consist of a metallic stent coated with a drug carrier vehicle (usually a polymer) that controls the dose and timing of the elution of an antiproliferative agent—have been shown to significantly reduce in-stent late loss, resulting in reduced rates of angiographic and clinical restenosis.

- First-generation drug-eluting stents, including sirolimus- and paclitaxel-eluting stents, have resulted in similar rates of mortality and myocardial infarction as bare metal stents in a broad spectrum of patients and lesions; however, concern over an increased rate of late stent thrombosis has led to reliance on extended dual antiplatelet therapy.

- Second-generation drug-eluting stents include everolimus-, zotarolimus-, and biolimus A9-eluting stents, which have improved stent platforms and polymers compared with first-generation devices; they provide enhanced deliverability and, in selected cases, improved safety and efficacy.

- The safety and efficacy of drug-eluting stents continue to be explored in specific high-risk and complex situations, including acute myocardial infarction, bifurcation lesions, chronic total occlusions, diabetic patients and saphenous vein grafts; for the most part they have been proven safe and effective compared with their bare metal counterparts. The utility of drug-eluting stents compared with bypass surgery has also become accepted in some but not all cases of left main and multivessel disease.

- The two major limitations of drug-eluting stents continue to be stent thrombosis and restenosis, the etiology of which is multifactorial. New insights into the mechanisms of these events are leading to the development of new, safer, and even more effective DES using bioabsorbable polymers, polymer-free systems, and fully bioabsorbable stents.

Abbreviations

ARC: Academic Research Consortium
BES: biolimus A9-eluting stent
BMS: bare metal stent
CABG: coronary artery bypass grafting
CI: confidence interval
CTO: chronic total occlusion
DES: drug-eluting stent
EES: everolimus-eluting stent
FDA: United States Food and Drug Administration
FFR: fractional flow reserve
FIM: first in man
FKBP-12: FK binding protein-12
HR: hazard ratio
IVUS: intravascular ultrasound
MACE: major adverse cardiac events
MACCE: major adverse cardiac and cerebrovascular events

MI: myocardial infarction
MR: moderate release
mTOR: mammalian target of rapamycin
NS: not significant
PCI: percutaneous coronary intervention
PES: paclitaxel-eluting stent
PES(E): paclitaxel-eluting stent (Express platform)
PES(L): paclitaxel-eluting stent (Liberté platform)
PLLA: poly-L-lactic acid
PTFE: polytetrafluoroethylene
RVD: reference vessel diameter
SES: sirolimus-eluting stent
SR: slow release
STEMI: ST-segment elevation myocardial infarction
SVG: saphenous vein graft
TLF: target lesion failure
TLR: target lesion revascularization
TVF: target vessel failure
TVR: target vessel revascularization
ZES: zotarolimus-eluting stent
ZES(E): zotarolimus-eluting stent (Endeavor platform)
ZES(R): zotarolimus-eluting stent (Resolute platform)

Introduction

The history of percutaneous coronary intervention (PCI) may be described as a series of steps, some transformative (beginning with the introduction of coronary balloon angioplasty), others incremental. Without doubt, however, development of the implantable metallic stent enabled PCI to become a durable approach for the vast majority of patients with coronary artery disease and one that most operators can apply safely. From balloons to atherectomy to lasers to bare metal stents (BMS) and now drug-eluting stents (DES), the evolution of interventional cardiology has progressively and uncompromisingly advanced through the insights and inventions of thousands of physicians and scientists, coupled with the recognition of the importance of optimal adjunctive pharmacotherapy and supported by the performance of worldwide randomized trials and registries that provide an unparalleled evidence base for daily clinical decision making. This chapter traces the evolution and development of the coronary stent from its initial applications to treat balloon angioplasty failures to its widespread global adoption for the treatment of patients with ischemic coronary heart disease.

Overview of Bare Metal Stents

Limitations of Balloon Angioplasty and Development of the Coronary Stent. The performance of the first successful balloon angioplasty by Andreas Grüntzig on September 16, 1977, in Zurich, Switzerland, was a landmark event heralding the inception of percutaneous management of obstructive coronary artery disease. Although this initial procedure set the stage for the millions of PCI procedures that have since taken place, stand-alone balloon angioplasty as performed by Grüntzig and other early pioneers was a highly unpredictable experience. While the majority of vessels tolerate the focal plaque dissections caused by balloon dilatation and heal sufficiently to result in an adequate lumen, the injury to the vessel wall can be excessive and, along with acute recoil and chronic constrictive remodeling, can result in balloon angioplasty's two major limitations: abrupt closure (occurring acutely or within the first several days after angioplasty) and restenosis (occurring later, within months after the procedure). The coronary stent was thus devised as an endoluminal scaffold to create a larger initial lumen, seal dissections, and resist recoil and late vascular remodeling, thereby improving upon the early and late results of balloon angioplasty. The first implantation of stents in human coronary arteries occurred in 1986 when Ulrich Sigwart, Jacques Puel, and their colleagues placed the Wallstent sheathed self-expanding metallic mesh scaffold (Medinvent, Lausanne, Switzerland) in the peripheral and coronary arteries of eight patients.[1] Further experience with this device demonstrated high rates of thrombotic occlusion and late mortality,[2] although patients without thrombosis had a 6-month angiographic restenosis rate of only 14%. This suggested for the first time that stenting could improve late patency in addition to stabilizing the acute results obtained after conventional balloon angioplasty. Contemporaneously, Cesare Gianturco and Gary Roubin developed a balloon-expandable coil stent consisting of a wrapped stainless steel wire resembling a clamshell. Completion of a phase II study using the Gianturco-Roubin stent to reverse postangioplasty acute or threatened vessel closure[3] led to U.S. Food and Drug Administration (FDA) approval for this indication in June 1993. While these stents were being developed and tested, Julio Palmaz designed a balloon-expandable stainless steel stent in 1984 that became the first "slotted tube stent." In this design, rectangular slots were cut into thin-walled stainless steel tubing such that balloon inflation within the stent deformed the rectangular slots into diamond-shaped windows or cells. Although this design allowed for relatively straightforward deployment, the rigidity of the stent made it difficult to deliver it to the coronary vasculature. In 1987 Richard Schatz modified this design by placing a 1-mm central articulating bridge connecting the two rigid 7-mm slotted segments,[4] thus creating the 15-mm Palmaz-Schatz stent (Johnson and Johnson Interventional Systems, Warren, NJ) (Fig. 13-1). The first coronary Palmaz-Schatz stent was placed in a patient by Eduardo Sousa in São Paulo, Brazil, in 1987. The Palmaz-Schatz stent was subsequently investigated in two landmark randomized trials comparing balloon angioplasty to elective stenting. In the

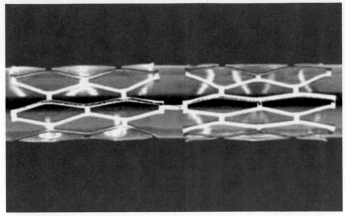

Figure 13-1 The Palmaz-Schatz Stent. Note the articulation between the two slotted tubes.

STRESS and BENESTENT-1 studies, the use of the Palmaz-Schatz stent was associated with a 20% to 30% reduction in clinical and angiographic restenosis compared with conventional balloon angioplasty (Fig. 13-2).[5,6] The Palmaz-Schatz stent also resulted in markedly improved initial angiographic results, with a larger postprocedural minimal luminal diameter and fewer residual dissections, which translated into a lower rate of subacute vessel closure. These results led to approval of the Palmaz-Schatz Stent by the FDA in 1994. Long-term follow-up (through 15 years) has subsequently demonstrated few late clinical or angiographic recurrences from years 1 to 5 after coronary stent implantation,[7,8] with slight and progressive decrements in luminal size thereafter extending beyond 10 years.[9] The mechanisms of this late progression of disease are not entirely known, but as overall stent thrombosis rates remained low in these patients (1.5% at 15 years), the development of new atherosclerosis within the stented segment as a cause of late restenosis has been hypothesized.[9] Despite the success of the Palmaz-Schatz stent in improving the early and late results of conventional balloon angioplasty, widespread adoption of stent technology was initially hindered by high rates of subacute stent thrombosis, necessitating an intense antithrombotic and antiplatelet

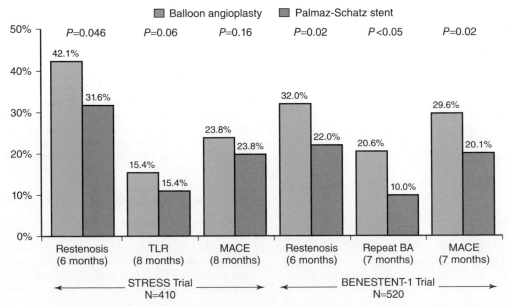

Figure 13-2 The pivotal early stent versus PTCA studies.

regimen (consisting of aspirin, dextran, dipyridamole, heparin, and warfarin). Further refinements in the stent procedure and periprocedural pharmacotherapy regimens were thus required. Antonio Colombo and colleagues demonstrated reduced rates of stent thrombosis with more aggressive intravascular ultrasound (IVUS)-guided deployment techniques, including routine high-pressure adjunctive dilatation (>14 atmospheres),[10] along with the use of aspirin and a second antiplatelet agent (the thienopyridine ticlopidine) rather than prolonged warfarin therapy. These modifications significantly reduced the incidence of stent thrombosis to about 1% to 2%, along with a marked reduction in bleeding and femoral arterial complications.[11] The confirmation of these initial findings in several randomized clinical trials definitively established the superiority of dual antiplatelet therapy (with aspirin and ticlopidine) over anticoagulation with warfarin for the prevention of stent thrombosis and facilitated the widespread adoption of this therapy for coronary stenting by the late 1990s.[12–15]

Stent Design: Impact on Performance and Clinical Outcomes. Coronary stents may be classified based on their composition (e.g., metallic or polymeric), configuration (e.g., slotted tube versus coiled wire), bioabsorption (either inert [biostable] or durable or degradable [bioabsorbable]), coatings (none, or else passive [such as heparin or polytetrafluoroethylene (PTFE) or bioactive [such as those eluting rapamycin or paclitaxel]), and mode of implantation (i.e., self-expanding or balloon-expandable). In theory, the ideal coronary stent would be made of a nonthrombogenic material and have sufficient flexibility in its unexpanded state to allow passage through small guiding catheters and tortuous vessels. It would also have an expanded configuration that provides uniform scaffolding of the vessel wall with low recoil and maximal radial strength while at the same time being conformable on bends. In addition, the stent should be sufficiently radio-opaque to allow fluoroscopic visualization to guide accurate placement and management if restenosis occurs but not so opaque as to obscure important vascular details.

Stent Composition. Until quite recently, the most widely used stent material was 316L stainless steel. Now, however, cobalt chromium and platinum chromium alloys have been employed to provide for lower-profile thin stent struts (75-µm versus 100- to 150 µm in most stainless steel stents) that maintain strength and visibility. Most self-expanding stents utilize nitinol, a nickel-titanium alloy, which, after being baked at a high temperature, maintains shape memory for a preset size and configuration. Other than gold (which has been shown to increase restenosis), there is little evidence that thrombosis or restenosis rates vary with the specific stent metal, although the final stages of surface finishing, smoothing, and purification or passivation may affect early thrombotic and late restenotic processes.[16] There has also been increased interest in polymeric biodegradable stents, which theoretically offer the advantages of increased longitudinal flexibility (though at the expense of radial force), compatibility with noninvasive imaging, and complete bioabsorption over a period of months to a year or longer, thereby restoring underlying vascular reactivity (see Chap. 33, "Biodegradable Stents.")

Stent Configuration and Design. Stents can be assigned to one of three subgroups, based on construction: wire coils, slotted tubes/multicellular, and modular designs. The vast majority of stents in current use are either slotted tube/multicellular or modular in design. Slotted tube/multicellular stents are often classified as having open or closed cells. Open-cell designs tend to have varying cell sizes and shapes, which provide increased flexibility, deliverability, and side branch access, with staggered cross-linking elements to provide radial strength. Closed-cell designs typically incorporate a repeating unicellular element that provides more uniform wall coverage with less tendency for plaque prolapse, but at the expense of flexibility and side branch access. Stent design may significantly impact acute and late vascular responses. Stents that possess better conformability, less

TABLE 13-1	Stent Coatings Designed to Reduce Thrombogenicity
Heparin	
- Multiple formulations incorporating heparin bonding through covalent bonding, ionic bonds, or heparin complexes (Carmeda BioActive Surface (CBAS) covalently heparin-bonded Palmaz-Schatz and BX Velocity stents, Jomed Corline Heparin Surface (CHS) heparin-coated Jostent)	
Carbon	
- Turbostratic (Sorin Carbostent)	
- Silicon carbide (Biotronik Tenax)	
- Diamond-like films (Phytis Diamond and Plasmachem Biodiamond)	
Phosphorylcholine	
- Biocompatibles BiodivYsio stent	
- Medtronic Endeavor drug-eluting stent	
Ionic Oxygen penetration into stent (Iberhospitex Bionert)	
CD34 Antibody to capture endothelial progenitor cells (Orbus-Neich Genous)	
Trifluoroethanol (Polyzene-F coated stent)	
Nanolayer protein coating (SurModics Finale coating on Protex stent)	
Nitric oxide scavengers including titanium-nitric oxide (Hexacath Titan stent)	
Single Knitted PET Fiber Mesh (MGuard)	
Biolinx Polymer (Medtronic Resolute drug-eluting stent)	
Abciximab and other glycoprotein IIb/IIIa inhibitors	
Activated protein C	
Hirudin and bivalirudin	
Prostacyclin	
Gold	

rigidity, and greater circularity experimentally produce less vascular injury, thrombosis, and neointimal hyperplasia.[17,18] Clinical studies have suggested that thin stent struts may be associated with reduced neointimal hyperplasia and lower rates of restenosis.[19]

Stent Coatings. A variety of coatings have been used to attempt to reduce the thrombogenicity or restenosis of metallic stents (Table 13-1). Experimental studies have demonstrated that the coating of stents with inert polymers may reduce surface reactivity and thrombosis,[18] although until recently, most polymers used were found to provoke intense inflammatory reactions.[20] With the advent of the DES came a renewed interest in the study of stent coatings, primarily to act as drug-carrier vehicles. However, concerns regarding the long-term safety of drug-eluting stents and the requirement for extended-duration dual antiplatelet therapy have led to a renewed interest in biocompatible stent coatings. A number of novel stent coatings are currently under investigation. Additionally, covered stents (metallic stents covered by a distensible microporous polytetrafluoroethylene [PTFE] membrane) are of unquestioned clinical utility in treating life-threatening perforations. They are also used for excluding giant aneurysms, pseudoaneurysms, or clinically significant fistulas (see Chap. 27, "Complications of Coronary Intervention.")

Balloon-Expandable versus Self-Expanding Stents. Balloon-expandable stents are mounted onto a delivery balloon and delivered into the coronary artery in their collapsed state. Once the stent is in the desired location, inflation of the delivery balloon expands the stent and embeds it in the arterial wall, following which the stent delivery system is removed. Almost all stents implanted in human coronary arteries are balloon-expandable. Self-expanding stents incorporate either specific geometric designs or nitinol shape-retaining metal to achieve a preset diameter and are released from a restraining sheath once placed in position. Although self-expanding stents are flexible and often easier to deliver compared with their balloon-expandable counterparts, restenosis has remained a concern, thus limiting their use in coronary arteries.[21] Recently, however, a renewed interest in self-expanding stents with reduced outward expansion force for the treatment of patients with acute coronary syndromes or vulnerable plaque has surfaced.[22]

Indications for Coronary Stenting and Comparison with Balloon Angioplasty

Stenting after Failed Balloon Angioplasty. Stents may be used either on a routine (planned) basis or after failed balloon angioplasty for acute or threatened vessel closure ("bail-out" stenting). One of the major benefits of stenting is the ability to reverse abrupt closure due to dissection and recoil, thus eliminating the need for high-risk emergency bypass surgery.[23] These data—coupled with the fact that routine stent implantation compared with balloon angioplasty provides superior acute results and greater event-free survival in almost every patient and lesion subtype studied to date—has for the most part relegated balloon dilation to the rare lesion that is too small (<2.25 mm) for stenting, or to which a stent cannot be delivered because of excessive vessel tortuosity or calcification, or in patients in whom thienopyridines are contraindicated.

Routine Stenting during PCI. The utility of routine stent implantation as a modality to reduce acute vessel closure and late restenosis was first demonstrated in the STRESS and BENESTENT-1 trials, which enrolled patients undergoing PCI of discrete focal lesions.[5,6] As a result, the types of lesions treated in these trials (discrete de novo lesions coverable by one stent, with reference vessel diameter [RVD] 3.0–4.0 mm) became known as "Stress/Benestent" lesions to differentiate them from more complex stenoses. Despite initial concerns regarding the diminished efficacy of coronary stents (which were more costly than balloon angioplasty alone) with more generalized use of these devices,[24] abundant randomized and nonrandomized data now exist comparing stenting to balloon angioplasty across a range of patient and lesion subsets, and they almost universally demonstrate an advantage to coronary stenting over conventional balloon angioplasty.[25-27]

Overview of Drug-Eluting Stents

Limitations of Bare Metal Stents. By the late 1990s, for most patients with coronary artery disease, stent implantation became the prevailing treatment because of their more predictable acute and late angiographic results compared with conventional balloon angioplasty, atherectomy, and laser. Improvements in procedural technique, more effective antiplatelet regimens, and the introduction of increasingly lower-profile, more flexible and deliverable devices additionally contributed to the ascendancy of stenting. With improvements in stent deliverability and reductions in stent thrombosis to <1%, restenosis emerged as the major persistent limitation of coronary stenting. Although coronary stents increase acute luminal diameters to a greater extent than balloon angioplasty (greater acute gain), the vascular injury caused by stent implantation elicits an exaggerated degree of neointimal hyperplasia, resulting in greater late decreases in luminal diameter (late loss) compared with balloon angioplasty alone.[5,6] Importantly, however, in comparing stents with balloon angioplasty, the mean incremental gain in luminal dimensions with stenting is statistically greater than the mean incremental increase in late loss, resulting in a larger net gain in minimal luminal dimensions. This observation led Kuntz and Baim to formulate the "bigger is better" concept: the greater the acute gain, the lower the ultimate rate of restenosis.[28,29] Nonetheless, even with optimal stent implantation, restenosis after BMS implantation still occurred in approximately 20% to 40% of patients within 6 to 12 months, in part because of more complex patient and lesion subsets that were treated with stenting than with balloon angioplasty. Therefore coronary restenosis became known as the Achilles' heel of coronary stenting, with significant resources devoted to its prevention and treatment (see chapter on restenosis).

DES, which maintain the mechanical advantages of BMS while delivering an antirestenotic pharmacological therapy locally to the arterial wall, have been shown to effectively and safely reduce the amount of in-stent tissue that accumulates after stent implantation, resulting in significantly reduced rates of clinical and angiographic restenosis. These devices were designed specifically to prevent the

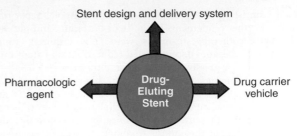

Figure 13-3 Components of a DES.

neointimal hyperplasia resulting after conventional BMS placement and have been highly successful in this regard. In numerous randomized trials, the reduction in neointimal hyperplasia that occurs with DES compared with BMS placement has been shown to result in a marked reduction in binary angiographic restenosis and target lesion revascularization (TLR).[30-32] The initial results of the pivotal randomized trials that led to device approval have been replicated and validated in numerous subsequent trials and real-world registries across the spectrum of disease and lesion subtypes.[33,34]

Components of Drug-Eluting Stents. The three critical components of a DES that must be optimized to ensure its safety and efficacy are as follows: (1) the *stent* itself (including its delivery system), (2) the *pharmacologic agent* being delivered, and (3) the *drug carrier vehicle*, which controls the drug dose and pharmacokinetic release rate (Fig. 13-3).

Designs of Drug-Eluting Stents. The stent component of the DES has typically consisted of a predicate BMS without specific modifications. Indeed, first-generation DES designs often appropriated "off-the-shelf" stent designs in order to expedite device development and regulatory approval. Subsequent DES have incorporated newer, more flexible designs, with resultant improvements in device delivery and performance.[35,36] Additionally, newer dedicated DES designs have included modifications aimed at either optimizing local drug delivery while reducing total drug dose (e.g., abluminal wells engineered into the stent struts) or modifying the stent surface to facilitate direct drug delivery and/or arterial healing following implantation (without a drug carrier vehicle per se).

Basic Pharmacology of Drug-Eluting Stents. Following promising cell culture and in vitro development, the antirestenotic properties of a wide range of pharmacological agents have been tested in humans (Fig. 13-4). Among these, the two most clinically effective classes of agents are the rapamycin-analogue family of drugs and paclitaxel. The principal mechanism of action of rapamycin (also known as sirolimus) and its analogues (including zotarolimus, everolimus, biolimus A9, and novolimus) is inhibition of the mammalian target of rapamycin (mTOR), which prevents cell cycle progression from the G1 to S phase.[37] Two other rapamycin analogues that have been used on DES platforms—tacrolimus and pimecrolimus—have a different mechanism of action, binding directly to FKBP506 and thereby inhibiting the calcineurin receptor with downregulation of cytokines and inhibition of smooth muscle cell activity;[38] unlike the mTOR inhibitors, these agents have not shown significant antirestenotic effects. The other agent that has been used effectively not only in DES, but also on drug-eluting balloons is paclitaxel. By interfering with microtubule function, paclitaxel has multifunctional antiproliferative and anti-inflammatory properties; it prevents smooth muscle migration, blocks cytokine and growth factor release and activity, interferes with secretory processes, is anti-angiogenic, and impacts signal transduction.[39-41] At low doses (similar to those in DES applications), paclitaxel affects the G0-G1 and G1-S phases (G1 arrest), resulting in cytostasis without cell death.[39,42]

Anti-inflammatory, immunomodulators	Anti-proliferative	Smooth muscle cell migration inhibitors, extracellular matrix modulators
Sirolimus (and analogs)	Sirolimus (and analogs)	Batimastat
Paclitaxel, Taxane	Paclitaxel, Taxane	Prolyl hydroxylase inhibitors
Dexamethasone	Actinomycin D	Halofuginone
M-prednisolone	Methothrexate	C-proteinase inhibitors
Interferon γ-1b	Angiopeptin	Probucol
Leflunomide	Vincristine	
Tacrolimus	Mitomycine	
Mycophenolic acid	Statins	
Mizoribine	C MYC antisense	
Cyclosporine	RestenASE	
Tranilast	2-Chloro-deoxyadenosine	
Biorest	PCNA ribozyme	

Figure 13-4 Potential anti-restenotic agents for use with DES. Adapted from Baim and Grossman.

Drug-Eluting Stent Polymers and Drug Carrier Systems. The inability to predictably deliver a specific dose of active drug to the arterial wall over the right time frame led to the failure of early DES programs.[43] To ensure accurate drug dosing, a *drug delivery vehicle* became necessary, which for most first generation stents was a durable (nonerodable) polymer. A wide range of polymer systems have since been developed and are DES-specific (as discussed in subsequent sections of this chapter). While the polymer is instrumental in regulating the pharmacokinetics of drug delivery to the arterial wall (which is necessary for reduced neointimal hyperplasia), the polymer may elicit deleterious vascular responses. Specifically, histopathological studies have demonstrated hypersensitivity and eosinophilic inflammatory reactions as well as delayed endothelialization with DES that were not previously seen with BMS.[44-46] Whether these maladaptive vascular responses are directly related to the polymer or to toxic reactions from the drug itself is speculative, but in animal models these effects can be attenuated by modification of the polymer vehicle.[47] It is believed that in selected patients, excessive inflammation and delayed endothelialization play a role in the development of late stent malapposition, aneurysm formation, and stent thrombosis/restenosis.[44,48] For these reasons, there has been great interest in developing inert and biocompatible polymers, bioabsorbable/biodegradable polymers, and even polymer-free DES.

Generational Classification of Drug-Eluting Stents. Given the rapid evolution of DES technologies, DES are often classified into several generations of development (Table 13-2). First-generation devices include the two DES that were initially approved for clinical use by most regulatory bodies, each of which utilized an early BMS stent platform (suboptimal by today's standards) with a durable polymer (prone to inflammation) to deliver either sirolimus or paclitaxel. Second-generation devices (currently used in the majority of DES procedures) have incorporated more deliverable, thinner-strut stents with polymers designed for biological compatibility. Most second-generation DES utilize rapamycin-analogues, although, as discussed below, there may still be a selective role for paclitaxel-eluting stents (PES). Future-generation DES will continue to undergo iteration, with further modifications of the base stent and use of biodegradable/bioabsorbable or polymer-free drug delivery vehicles.

First-Generation Drug-Eluting Stents

The Cypher Sirolimus-Eluting Stent. The first important DES was the Cypher stent (Cordis, Johnson and Johnson), with initial first-in-human studies as well as subsequent clinical trials leading to its approval in Europe in 2002 and the United States in 2003. Sirolimus is a highly lipophilic, naturally occurring macrocyclic lactone, which was first isolated from *Streptomyces hygroscopicus*, found in a soil sample from Easter Island, and was initially developed as an antifungal agent. Shortly thereafter it was discovered that sirolimus also possessed potent immunosuppressive properties. It was initially approved by the FDA as Rapamune for the prevention of renal transplant rejection in 1999. The primary mechanism of action of sirolimus's inhibition of neointimal hyperplasia is thought to be related to its ability to bind to FK-binding protein-12 (FKBP-12) in cells; the sirolimus-FKBP-12 complex then binds to and inhibits activation of mTOR, preventing progression in the cell cycle from the late G1 to S phase.[37] The sirolimus-eluting stent (SES) was demonstrated to have a marked effect on the suppression of neointimal hyperplasia with low toxicity following implantation in initial small and large animal studies.[49,50] The base stent platform for the Cypher SES is the Bx Velocity stent, a slotted tube with a closed cell design constructed from 316L stainless steel. Prior to mounting, the stent is coated on its luminal as well as its abluminal surface (i.e., conformal coating) with biostable (nonerodible) polymers consisting of poly-n-butyl methacrylate and polyethylene vinyl acetate, which are loaded with 140 mcg/cm² sirolimus. The polymers, which uniformly coat the stent to a thickness of 5 to 10 microns, serve as a drug carrier vehicle, ensuring that the sirolimus is released into the vessel wall in a programmed manner. The slow-release formulation of the Cypher SES employed in clinical practice uses a base coat of blended polymers, which is loaded with sirolimus, as well as a top coat of polymer alone (without sirolimus), which acts as a diffusion barrier and thus reduces the rate of drug release from the base coat into the vessel wall. With this formulation of polymers, most of the sirolimus (approximately 80%) is released within the first month after stent implantation. Human experience with the

TABLE 13-2	Generational Classification of Drug-Eluting Stents		
Generation	**Drug**	**Polymer**	**Stent**
FIRST	**SIROLIMUS OR PACLITAXEL**	**NOT SPECIFICALLY DESIGNED FOR BIOCOMPATIBILITY**	**EARLY BMS PLATFORMS**
Cypher	Sirolimus	Biostable mix of poly-n-butyl methacrylate and polyethylene–vinyl acetate	Bx-Velocity™ (stainless steel)
TAXUS Express	Paclitaxel	Styrene-isobutylene-styrene (SIBS)	Express (stainless steel)
TAXUS Liberté	Paclitaxel	Styrene-isobutylene-styrene (SIBS)	Liberté (stainless steel)
SECOND	**RAPAMYCIN ANALOGUES**	**BIOCOMPATIBLE POLYMERS**	**MORE FLEXIBLE, THINNER-STRUT BMS**
Endeavor	Zotarolimus	Phosphorylcholine	Driver (cobalt chromium)
Resolute	Zotarolimus	Biolinx polymer	Integrity (cobalt alloy)
Xience V (Promus)	Everolimus	Vinylidene fluoride and hexafluoropropylene	Vision (cobalt-chromium)
Biomatrix	Biolimus A9	Abluminal poly-L-lactic acid (bioabsorbable)	S-stent (stainless steel)

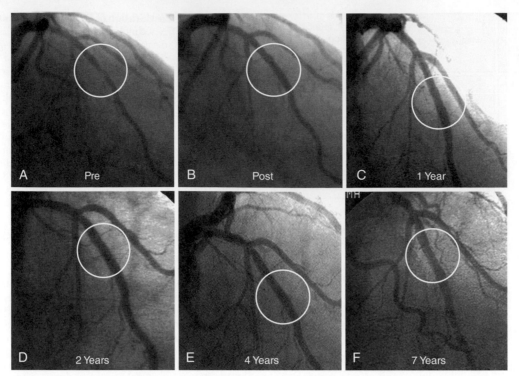

Figure 13-5   Seven-year follow-up of one of the initial SES implantations from Institute Dante Pazzanese of Cardiology in São Paulo, Brazil.

CypherSES was first reported from the first-in-man (FIM) study initiated in 1999 in 45 patients with symptomatic de novo lesions < 18 mm in length with an RVD of 3 to 3.5 mm in native coronary arteries at the Institute Dante Pazzanese of Cardiology in São Paulo, Brazil, and the Thoraxcenter, Rotterdam, The Netherlands. In this study, the SES demonstrated marked suppression of neointimal hyperplasia measured by IVUS and quantitative coronary angiography at 4 months and 1, 2, and 4 years.[51] Serial angiography and IVUS have now been performed at 7 years, showing continued vessel patency without further late loss (Fig. 13-5). Following the success of SES in this initial study, the landmark RAVEL trial was conducted, in which 238 patients outside the United States with relatively simple de novo coronary lesions (lesion length ≤ 18 mm in coronary arteries 2.5–3.5 mm in diameter) were randomized to either the Cypher SES or the uncoated Bx-Velocity stent.[30] In RAVEL, mean late loss at 6 months was markedly lower among SES-treated than BMS-treated patients (-0.01 mm vs. 0.80 mm, $P < 0.001$), with a corresponding reduction in the rate of restenosis (0% vs. 26%, $P < 0.001$). The pivotal U.S. randomized trial that led to FDA approval of SES was the SIRIUS trial, a 1,058-patient randomized trial comparing the Cypher SES with the uncoated Bx-Velocity in patients with vessel diameters of 2.5 to 3.5 mm and lesion lengths of 15 to 30 mm.[52] The primary endpoint, the rate of target vessel failure (TVF: a composite of cardiac death, myocardial infarction [MI], or target vessel revascularization [TVR]) at 9 months, was markedly lower among SES-treated patients (8.6% vs. 21.0%, $P < 0.001$). The rate of major adverse cardiac events (MACE) was similarly lower with SES compared with BMS (7.1% vs. 18.9%, $P < 0.001$). A 60% to 80% relative reduction in composite adverse events with SES versus BMS was observed in all examined subgroups in the trial, including diabetic patients, and did not depend on vessel size or lesion length. Among 703 patients in whom 8-month routine angiographic follow-up was performed, mean in-stent late loss was markedly lower with SES compared with BMS (0.17 mm vs. 1.00 mm, $P < 0.001$), and in-segment angiographic restenosis was greatly reduced with SES (17.6% vs. 50.5%, $P < 0.001$). By IVUS, the in-stent percent volumetric obstruction at 8 months was reduced from 33.4% with the Bx Velocity to 3.1% with the SES ($P < 0.001$). Late stent malapposition was present

in 9.7% of Cypher SES patients versus 0% of Bx Velocity patients ($P = 0.02$). Among patients experiencing restenosis events in SIRIUS, the pattern of restenosis was diffuse in only 13% of patients with SES restenosis versus 58% with BMS restenosis ($P < 0.001$). Thus treatment with repeat PCI for SES restenosis (typically focal) patients was associated with more favorable outcomes than for BMS-restenosis patients (typically diffuse).[53] On the basis of these results, in April 2003 the Cypher SES became the first DES approved by the FDA. To date, this stent has been one of the most studied devices in modern history, with at least 20 randomized trials performed comparing the commercialized Cypher SES to the BMS across a range of patient indications and lesion subsets (Table 13-3). Collectively, these trials demonstrate that the Cypher SES results in a near abolition of in-stent late loss (averaging ~0.15 mm across studies), with an approximate 50% to 75% reduction in angiographic restenosis and clinical recurrence (TLR) compared with bare metal comparators. Longer-term follow-up with this device has extended to 5 years and beyond, particularly for the four major SES trials (RAVEL, SIRIUS, C-SIRIUS, and E-SIRIUS). In these analyses, treatment with SES has resulted in sustained reductions in clinical restenosis endpoints with similar rates of death, MI, and stent thrombosis found in both SES and BMS arms.[54]

The Taxus Paclitaxel-Eluting Stent. Paclitaxel, a highly lipophilic diterpenoid compound, was first isolated in 1963 from the Pacific yew tree (*Taxus brevifolia*) and subsequently developed for its potent antineoplastic properties. Paclitaxel is insoluble in water and has thus been combined with an intravenous oil-based cremophor for intravenous injection as the oncological compound Taxol. The principal action of paclitaxel is to interfere with microtubule dynamics, preventing depolymerization. Because microtubules are ubiquitous, paclitaxel has widespread multicellular and multifunctional activities with dose-dependent effects. Paclitaxel has antiproliferative and anti-inflammatory properties, prevents smooth muscle migration, blocks cytokine and growth factor release and activity, interferes with secretory processes, is antiangiogenic, and impacts signal transduction.[39-41] At low doses (similar to those in DES applications), paclitaxel affects the G0-G1 and G1-S phases (G1 arrest), resulting in cytostasis without cell death

TABLE 13-3	Randomized Controlled Trials Comparing Sirolimus-Eluting Stents with Bare Metal Stents			
Trial Name and Reference	*Study Cohort*	*Number Randomized (planned angiographic follow-up)*	*Latest Follow-up to Date*	*Principal Findings*
RAVEL[276]	Single de novo native coronary lesions	238 (all)	5 years	6-month late loss was significantly lower with SES vs. BMS (−0.01 mm vs. 0.80 mm, $P < 0.001$); no restenosis was seen in the SES group at 6 months.
SIRIUS[31]	Single de novo native coronary lesions	1,058 (approximately 850)	5 years	The 9-month rate of TVF was significantly reduced with SES vs. BMS (8.6% vs. 21.0%, $P < 0.001$), driven by a reduction in TLR. At 5 years, there was a maintained reduction in TLR with SES (9.4% vs. 24.2%, $P < 0.001$), with similar rates of death, MI, and stent thrombosis.
C-SIRIUS[277]	Single de novo native coronary lesions	100 (all)	5 years (in pooled analyses)	SES were associated with greater 8-month in-stent minimum lumen diameter (2.46 mm for SES vs. 1.49 mm with BMS, $P < 0.001$).
E-SIRIUS[278]	Single de novo native coronary lesions	352 (all)	5 years (in pooled analyses)	8-month minimum lumen diameter was greater with SES vs. BMS (2.22 vs. 1.33 mm, $P < 0.001$)
MULTI-STRATEGY[279]	STEMI	745 (none)	8 months	At 8 months, SES were associated with a reduction in TVR compared with BMS (3.2% vs. 10.2%, $P < 0.001$), with no differences observed between stent types in death or MI.
TYPHOON[280]	STEMI	712 (200)	1 year	One-year TVF was lower with SES vs. BMS (7.3% vs. 14.3%, $P = 0.004$). There were no differences between SES and BMS with respect to death, MI, or stent thrombosis.
MISSION![281]	STEMI	310 (all)	3 years	SES were associated with lower in-segment late lumen loss at 9 months than BMS (0.12 mm vs. 0.56 mm, $P < 0.001$). At 3 years, differences in TLR were attenuated (6.3% vs. 12.5%, $P = 0.06$).
SESAMI[282]	STEMI	320 (all)	3 years	SES were associated with lower 1-year binary restenosis rates compared with BMS (9.3% vs. 21.3%, $P = 0.032$). The rate of TLR was lower at 3 years, with no differences in death, MI, or stent thrombosis.
PASEO[283]	STEMI	270 including 90 PES (none)	4 years	SES were associated with lower TLR at 1 year compared to BMS (3.3% vs. 14.4%, $P = 0.016$), which was maintained at 4 years.
STRATEGY[284]	STEMI	175 (all)	5 years	At 8 months, the rate of TLR was lower with SES compared with BMS (6% vs. 20%, $P = 0.006$). This benefit was maintained at 5-year follow up, with no excess in stent thrombosis with SES.
Seville[285]	STEMI	120 (none)	1 year	SES were associated with a non statistically significant different rate of the primary endpoint of cardiac death, MI, or TLR compared with BMS (6.7% vs. 11.%, $P = 0.40$).
SCORPIUS[286]	Diabetic patients	200 (all)	1 year	In-segment late lumen loss was lower with SES compared with BMS (0.18 mm vs. 0.74 mm, $P < 0.001$), with lower rates of MACE.
DIABETES[287]	Diabetic patients	160 (all)	2 years	SES were associated with lower late lumen loss at 9 months (0.06 mm vs. 0.47 mm, $P < 0.001$). At 2 years, SES were associated with a lower rate of TLR compared with BMS (7.7% vs. 35.0%, $P < 0.001$).
DECODE[288]	Diabetic patients	83 (all)	1 year	Mean in-stent late lumen loss at 6 months was lower with SES compared with BMS (0.23 mm vs. 1.10 mm, $P < 0.001$).
SCANDSTENT[289]	Complex CAD	322 (all)	3 years	SES was associated with greater MLD at 6 months than BMS (2.40 mm vs. 1.65 mm, $P < 0.001$). At 3 years the rate of TLR was significantly reduced with SES (4.9% vs. 33.8%, $P < 0.001$).
PRISON II[158]	CTO	200 (all)	4 years	SES had significantly lower 6-month binary in-segment restenosis than BMS (7% vs. 36%, $P < 0.001$). At 4 years, significant reductions in TLR rates were maintained with SES.
SES SMART[290]	Small vessels	257 (all)	2 years	8-month binary in-segment restenosis was lower with SES compared to BMS (9.8% vs. 53.1%, $P < 0.001$). At 2 years, lower rates of TLR and MI were observed with SES compared with BMS.
RRISC[172]	SVG	75 (all)	3 years	6-month in-stent late lumen loss was lower with SES compared with BMS (0.38 mm vs. 0.79 mm, $P = 0.001$). At 3 years, similar rates of TVR were observed with both stent types, with 11 deaths observed with SES vs. 0 deaths with BMS.
Pache et al[291]	Unselected	500 (all)	1 year	SES had lower rates of angiographic restenosis than thin-strut BMS (8.3% vs. 25.5%, $P < 0.001$), with a lower incidence of TVR.
Ortolani et al[292]	Unselected	104 (all)	1 year	SES had less in-stent late loss compared with thin-strut cobalt-chromium BMS (0.18 mm vs. 0.51 mm, $P < 0.001$). At 1 year, rates of TLR were lower with SES, but not to a statistically significant degree.

SES, sirolimus-eluting stent; BMS, bare metal stent; MI, myocardial infarction; MLD, minimal lumen diameter; STEMI, ST-segment elevation myocardial infarction; CTO, chronic total occlusion; SVG, saphenous vein grafts; TLR, target lesion revascularization; TVR, target vessel revascularization; TVF, target vessel failure (cardiac death, MI or TVR).

(probably via the induction of p53/p21 tumor suppression genes).[39,42] Systemic paclitaxel was shown to inhibit restenosis in a rat carotid injury model at levels more than 100-fold lower than those required for tumor cytotoxicity.[40] Neointimal area was greatly reduced in a rabbit balloon injury experiment using local paclitaxel administration,[39] and stent-based paclitaxel elution from polymer-based systems has been shown to profoundly reduce intimal hyperplasia in rabbit iliac arteries for up to 6 months with dose-dependent efficacy and toxicity.[55,56] The TAXUS paclitaxel-eluting stent (PES) (Boston Scientific, Natick, MA) consists of paclitaxel contained within a polyolefin-derivative biostable polymer (styrene-isobutylene-styrene, referred to as SIBS [Translute]), originally coated on the Nir stent and subsequently on the Express open-cell slotted-tube stainless steel stent platform (the device from which most of the randomized clinical trial data for this stent were derived). The base BMS for the current TAXUS stent is the newer Liberté stent, a more flexible, thinner-strutted closed-cell stainless steel slotted-tube stent. Depending on the relative ratio of paclitaxel to polymer, the stent may be formulated with varying release kinetics. The clinically available formulation of the TAXUS PES is the slow-release (SR) formulation, although the moderate-release (MR) formulation has also been tested in moderate-sized clinical trials. The SR stent has relatively more polymer to drug (paclitaxel concentration of 1 mcg/mm^2), with a coat thickness 18 μm and approximately 8% in vivo paclitaxel elution in 30 days. The drug is eluted in a rapid burst phase over the initial 48 hours, followed by a slow, sustained release for the next 10 to 30 days, with the remainder sequestered in the bulk of the polymer matrix below the surface without pathways to the external environment (thus permanently retained on the stent). In a series of porcine experiments at 30, 90, 180, and 360 days involving a total of 350 swine and 800 stents, both SR and MR TAXUS stent formulations were shown to be vasculocompatible, with early development of a thin, mature neointima with low levels of inflammation, microthrombi, and persistent amorphous material deposition (fibrin), no evidence of cytotoxicity, and complete healing and endothelialization within 90 days (data on file, Boston Scientific). The clinical safety and efficacy of the TAXUS PES has been tested in randomized trials in the TAXUS clinical program.[57-61] TAXUS I and II evaluated the TAXUS PES on the Nir stent platform in focal lesions, whereas TAXUS IV, V, and VI investigated the TAXUS Express stent in more complex lesions with longer-term follow-up. All studies have used the SR formulation except for one arm of the TAXUS II trial and TAXUS VI. Collectively, these trials demonstrate a marked decrease of binary restenosis with PES compared with BMS, with a ~60% to 75% reduction in the need for TLR. In the pivotal prospective, randomized, double-blind TAXUS IV study, 1,314 patients with single de novo lesions with visually estimated lengths of 10 to 28 mm in native coronary arteries with an RVD of 2.5 to 3.75 mm were assigned to either a TAXUS SR stent or Express BMS control.[59] At 9 months, the primary endpoint of target vessel revascularization (TVR) was reduced with the TAXUS PES from 12.0% to 4.7% ($P < 0.001$). Follow-up angiography at 9 months demonstrated marked reductions in mean in-stent late loss (0.39 vs. 0.92 mm, $P < 0.001$) and binary in-segment restenosis (7.9% vs. 26.6%, $P < 0.001$). Restenotic lesions were typically focal in nature with PES (mean length 9.8 mm vs. 15.3 mm with BMS, $P < 0.001$). Late coronary aneurysms were infrequent in both groups and not increased with PES. By IVUS, the in-stent percent volumetric obstruction at 8 months was reduced from 29.4% with the BMS to 12.2% with the PES ($P < 0.001$). Late stent malapposition at 9 months was present in 1.1% of PES patients versus 2.2% of BMS patients ($P = 0.62$). Clinical and angiographic efficacy was present across a broad range of patient and lesion subtypes. On the basis of these results, in March 2004 the TAXUS SR stent became the second DES approved by the FDA. Since device approval, the TAXUS PES has been studied in at least 12 randomized trials comparing this device to the BMS across a range of patient indications and lesion subsets (Table 13-4). These studies have demonstrated consistent reductions in measures of neointimal hyperplasia (measured either by angiography or by IVUS), with resultant reductions in clinical restenosis endpoints compared with the BMS. Longer-term follow-up

with this device has extended to 5 years and beyond, particularly for the four major PES trials of the SR stent (TAXUS I, II, IV, and V). In these analyses, treatment with PES results in sustained reductions in clinical restenosis endpoints, with similar rates of death, MI, and stent thrombosis found in both the PES and BMS arms.[59] The currently available PES device is the TAXUS Liberté stent (using the same drug and polymer formulation as the TAXUS Express SR but with an improved stent platform). This device was approved for clinical use based on the TAXUS ATLAS program, in which nonrandomized data from several TAXUS Liberté PES single-arm studies were compared with the treatment arms from prior TAXUS trials with the Express PES.[62] In routine "workhorse" lesions, the Liberté PES was shown to have similar rates of restenosis and safety endpoints compared with the Express PES. However, when used to treat small vessels and long lesions, the Liberté PES was associated with lower rates of TLR compared with a matched sample of Express PES patients. Additionally, in long lesions, there was a lower rate of MI among patients treated with the Liberté PES at 1 year (1.4% vs. 6.5%, $P = 0.02$), a finding that has been maintained up to 3 years.[63]

Comparisons of First-Generation Drug-Eluting Stents and Metanalyses. Following the approval of the TAXUS PES for commercial use, a series of comparisons between the two approved devices (Cypher SES and TAXUS PES) ensued in order to determine whether superiority could be established for a particular DES. A total of 21 randomized comparisons of different sizes have been performed to date in numerous patient and lesion cohorts; they have included a variety of IVUS, angiographic, and clinical endpoints (Table 13-5). In summary, the totality of evidence appears to point to the similar performance of SES and PES stents in routine de novo coronary artery lesions despite a lower amount of neointimal hyperplasia with SES as assessed by IVUS and angiography.[64-67] Among pooled analyses of more complex or "higher restenosis risk" lesion subsets, there may be a clinical benefit to the Cypher SES because of its more potent suppression of neointimal hyperplasia; but validation of these findings would require large-scale, adequately powered clinical trial before any definitive conclusions could be drawn.[68] Concomitant with the large amount of clinical trial data comparing SES, PES, and BMS have come a number of analyses amalgamating trial data across clinical studies to increase overall sample size. In particular, these studies have attempted to address one of the prominent limitations of individual DES studies: the limited power to detect differences in low-frequency safety endpoints, including death, MI, and stent thrombosis. By aggregating data across trials, these DES metanalyses have also served as simple means of summarizing the large number of clinical studies in the published and nonpublished domains. In the largest and most comprehensive metanalysis of DES versus BMS (including 9470 patients from 22 randomized trials and 182,901 patients from 34 observational studies), the use of DES in randomized trials was associated with comparable rates of mortality and MI, with significant reductions in TVR compared with BMS.[33] In another analysis, Stettler and colleagues incorporated comparative data from SES versus BMS trials, PES versus BMS trials, and SES versus PES trials in a statistical "network" of trials to discern treatment effects across all included trials.[69] In this analysis of 38 trials, including data from 18,023 patients, TLR was lower with SES and PES compared with BMS, with similar mortality among patients treated with SES, PES, and BMS. In this analysis, a reduction in the hazard of MI was observed with SES compared with both BMS (hazard ratio [HR] 0.81, 95% credibility interval 0.66–0.97, $P = 0.030$) and PES (HR 0.83, 0.71–1.00, $P = 0.045$). In addition to the Stettler network metanalysis, numerous analyses have focused on the examination of low-frequency safety endpoints in comparing first-generation DES with BMS. More than 50 nonrandomized comparisons between DES and BMS have been published and/or presented. Aside from the initial publication of data from the SCAAR (Swedish Coronary Angiography and Angioplasty Registry) study, the majority of these studies have demonstrated favorable safety for DES compared with BMS. For example, in the largest such analysis of DES safety among 262,700

TABLE 13-4	Randomized Controlled Trials Comparing Paclitaxel-Eluting Stents with Bare Metal Stents			
Trial Name and Reference	**Study Cohort**	**Number Randomized (planned angiographic follow-up)**	**Latest Follow-up to Date**	**Principal Findings**
TAXUS I[57]	Single de novo or restenotic lesions	61 (all)	5 years	6-month percent diameter stenosis was lower with PES compared with BMS (13.6% vs. 27.3%, $P < 0.001$), with improvements in IVUS findings with PES as well.
TAXUS II[58]	Single de novo native coronary lesions	536 (all)	5 years	6-month net volume obstruction was lower with PES slow release vs. BMS (7.9% vs. 23.2%, $P < 0.001$) as well as PES moderate release compared with BMS. Reductions in TLR were maintained at 5 years with both PES formulations with no differences in death, MI, or stent thrombosis.
TAXUS IV[59]	Single de novo native coronary lesions	1,314 (732)	5 years	PES were associated with lower rates of TLR compared with BMS at 9 months (4.7% vs. 12.0%, $P < 0.001$) as well as lower rates of angiographic restenosis. Reductions in TLR were maintained at 5 years with no differences in death, MI, or stent thrombosis.
TAXUS V[60]	Single lesions, including complex lesions	1,156 (all)	5 years	PES reduced 9-month TVR compared with BMS (12.1% vs. 17.3%, $P = 0.02$), with reductions in angiographic restenosis overall and among patients with complex disease. At 5 years, reductions in clinical restenosis have been maintained with similar rates of death, MI, and stent thrombosis.
TAXUS VI[61]	Single long complex lesions	448 (all)	5 years	9-month TVR rate was lower with PES moderate release compared with BMS (9.1% vs. 19.4%, $P = 0.0027$), with lower rates of angiographic restenosis. At 5 years, TVR rates were similar between both stents, although TLR was lower with PES moderate release.
HORIZONS-AMI[293]	STEMI	3006 (1,800)	3 years	PES was associated with lower rates of TLR compared with BMS at 1 year (4.5% vs. 7.5%, $P = 0.002$) and lower binary restenosis at 13 months (10.0% vs. 22.9%, $P < 0.001$). The reduction in TLR was maintained at 3 years, with no significant differences in death, MI, or stent thrombosis observed.
PASSION[294]	STEMI	619 (none)	2 years	PES and BMS were associated with non-statistically significantly different rates of the primary endpoint of TLF (8.8% vs. 12.8%, $P = 0.09$) at 1 year, a finding that was maintained at 2 years.
PASEO[283]	STEMI	270 including 90 SES (none)	4 years	PES were associated with a lower rate of TLR at 1 year compared with BMS (4.4% vs. 14.4%, $P = 0.023$), which was maintained at 4 years.
HAAMU-STENT[295]	STEMI	164 (all)	1 year	Angiographic endpoints were improved with PES compared with BMS, with a trend toward lower TVR at 1 year (3.7% vs. 11%, $P = 0.07$)
SELECTION[296]	STEMI	80 (all)	7 months	Volume of neointimal hyperplasia by IVUS was lower with PES compared with BMS (4.6% vs. 20%, $P < 0.01$), with no differences in late malapposition seen between the stent types.
Erglis et al.[145]	Left main stenosis	103 (all)	6 months	PES were associated with lower rates of binary angiographic restenosis at 6 months compared with BMSs (6% vs. 22%, $P = 0.021$). IVUS measures were also improved with PES.
SOS[171]	SVG	80 (all)	Median 1.5 years	The rate of binary angiographic restenosis was lower with PES compared with BMS (9% vs. 51%, $P < 0.001$). Similar rates of MI and death were observed.

PES, paclitaxel-eluting stent (slow release); BMS, bare metal stent; IVUS, intravascular ultrasound; TVR, target vessel revascularization; MI, myocardial infarction; STEMI, ST-segment elevation myocardial infarction; SVG, saphenous vein grafts; TLR, target lesion revascularization; TVF, target vessel failure (cardiac death, MI, or TVR).

Medicare beneficiaries in the United States, the use of DES was associated with lower rates of death (13.5% vs. 16.5%, $P < 0.001$) and MI (7.5% vs. 8.9%, $P < 0.001$) as well as minimal differences in overall revascularization or bleeding.[70] Similar findings were observed in a metanalysis of observational studies (not including the Medicare analysis), with reductions in death, MI, and TLR seen with DES compared with BMS.[33] Despite the findings from numerous observational registries suggesting that DES may indeed reduce mortality compared with BMS, data from these nonrandomized comparisons of DES versus BMS should be considered exploratory at best and potentially misleading. This observation is based upon several factors: (1) nonrandomized treatment comparisons are subject to significant confounding, which cannot be adequately accounted for using conventional statistical methodology; (2) mortality reductions have never been observed in randomized trials comparing first-generation DES with BMS[31]; and (3) in propensity-matched observational analyses comparing DES to BMS, the majority of benefit of DES compared with BMS was evident within the first 30 days after implantation—a difference that does not have an adequate pathophysiological explanation.[71] These limitations notwithstanding, the abundance of randomized trial and registry study data with first-generation DES has been reassuring, demonstrating the efficacy of both SES and PES in reducing clinical restenosis, and with no major safety concerns compared to BMS.

Second-Generation Drug-Eluting Stents

Pivotal randomized trials have been completed with four second-generation stents: everolimus-eluting stents (EES) (i.e., Xience V/Promus); zotarolimus-eluting stents (ZES) (i.e., Endeavor and Resolute); and biolimus A9-eluting stents (BES) (i.e., Biomatrix). All four polymer-based stents release a rapamycin analogue that binds to cytosolic FKBP12 and subsequently mTOR, thereby blocking the stimulatory effects of the growth factors and cytokines released after vascular injury. However, the underlying stent platform and polymers vary significantly, as do the drug pharmacokinetics and pharmacodynamics, which has resulted in significantly different angiographic and clinical profiles of these devices.

TABLE 13-5	Randomized Controlled Trials Comparing Sirolimus-Eluting Stents and Paclitaxel-Eluting Stents			
Trial Name and Reference	Study Cohort	Number Randomized (planned angiographic follow-up)	Latest Follow-up to Date	Principal Findings
REALITY[64]	1–2 de novo coronary lesions	1,386 (all)	1 year	Despite lower late loss with SES, rates of binary angiographic restenosis were similar with SES and PES (9.1% vs. 11.1%, $P = 0.31$), with similar rates of MACE at 1 year.
Zhang et al.[297]	De novo coronary lesions	673 including 224 Firebird stent (none)	1 year	At 1 year, rates of MACE were similar between SES and PES (8.4% vs. 11.2%).
SORT OUT II[66]	Unselected	2,098 (none)	1.5 years	There were no significant differences between SES and PES in MACE (9.3% vs. 11.2%) or other endpoints, including death, MI, or stent thrombosis.
SIRTAX[298]	Unselected	1,012 (approximately half)	5 years	SES were associated with a lower rate of MACE at 9 months compared with PES (6.2% vs. 10.8%, $P = 0.009$). However, at 5 years, the rates were similar, with an accrual of events in both stent groups.
TAXi[299]	Unselected	202 (none)	3 years	Rates of 6-month MACE were similar with SES and PES (6% vs. 4%, $P = 0.8$), with similar findings at 3 years.
DES-DIABETES[65]	Diabetic patients	400 (all)	2 years	6-month in-segment restenosis was lower with SES compared with PES (3.4% vs. 18.2%, $P < 0.001$). At 2 years, rates of TLR remained lower with SES (3.5% vs. 11.0%, $P = 0.004$).
ISAR-DIABETES[134]	Diabetic patients	250 (all)	5 years (in pooled analyses)	In-segment late lumen loss was lower with SES compared with PES (0.43 mm vs. 0.67 mm, $P = 0.002$), with non-statistically significant rates of TLR at 9 months (6.4% vs. 12.0%, $P = 0.13$).
Kim et al[300]	Diabetic patients	169 (all)	6 months	Late lumen loss was similar with SES and PES (0.26 mm vs. 0.39 mm, $P = 0.36$); rates of TLR were similar at 6 months.
DiabeDES[301]	Diabetic patients	153 (all)	8 months	In-stent late lumen loss was lower with SES compared with PES (0.23 mm vs. 0.52 mm, $P = 0.025$). The rates of TLR and MACE were similar with both types of stents.
CORPAL[302]	Lesions at "high-risk for restenosis"	652 (all)	15 months	Angiographic restenosis rates were similar with SES and PES, with similar rates of TLR.
ISAR LEFT MAIN[146]	Left main stenosis	607 (all)	2 years	Similar rates of angiographic restenosis were observed with SES and PES (19.4% vs. 16.0%, $P = 0.30$), with no differences observed in death, MI, or TLR.
LONG DES II[303]	Long lesions	500 (all)	9 months	In-segment binary restenosis was lower with SES compared with PES (3.3% vs. 14.6%, $P < 0.001$), with a lower rate of 9-month TLR.
Han et al.[304]	Multivessel CAD	416 (all)	19.5 months	Rates of MACE were similar with SES and PES over the follow-up period (6.4% vs. 8.8%), with no differences in minimum lumen diameter.
ISAR-SMART 3[305]	Small vessels	360 (all)	5 years (in pooled analyses)	Late lumen loss at 6–8 months was greater with PES compared with SES (0.56 mm vs. 0.25 mm, $P < 0.001$), with greater TLR (14.7% vs. 6.6%, $P = 0.008$).
Pan et al.[306]	Bifurcation lesions	205 (all)	2 years	SES were associated with lower rates of binary angiographic restenosis, less late lumen loss, and a lower rate of TLR at 2 years compared with PES (4% vs. 13%, $P < 0.021$).
Petronio et al.[67]	Complex lesions	100 (all)	9 months	By IVUS, the area of neointimal hyperplasia was significantly lower with SES than with PES (7.4% vs. 15.4%, $P < 0.001$) at 9 months.
Cervinka et al.[307]	Complex CAD	70 (all)	6 months	IVUS-assessed neointimal hyperplasia volume was lower with SES compared with PES (4.1 mm^3 vs. 17.4 mm^3, $P = 0.001$).
ISAR-DESIRE[263]	BMS restenosis	300 including 100 balloon angioplasty patients (all)	5 years (in pooled analyses)	Angiographic restenosis was lower with both SES (14.3%) and PES (21.7%) compared with balloon angioplasty at 6 months (44.6%). TVR was lower with SES compared with PES (8% vs. 19%, $P = 0.02$).
ISAR-DESIRE 2[265]	SES restenosis	450 (all)	1 year	There were no differences in late lumen loss (0.40 vs. 0.38, $P = 0.85$) or other angiographic or clinical endpoints with SES or PES for the treatment of SES restenosis.
PROSIT[308]	STEMI	308 (all)	1 year	In-segment restenosis was lower with SES compared with PES (5.9% vs. 14.8%, $P = 0.03$), with similar rates of TLR and MACE.
PASEO[283]	STEMI	270 including 90 BMS (none)	4 years	Similar reductions in TLR were seen with SES and PES (relative to BMS); this was maintained throughout the follow-up period.

SES, sirolimus-eluting stent; PES, paclitaxel-eluting stent; MI, myocardial infarction; TLR, target lesion revascularization; TVR, target vessel revascularization; TVF, target vessel failure (cardiac death, MI, or TVR).

Everolimus-Eluting Stents (Xience V/Promus). In the EES (manufactured by Abbott Vascular, Santa Clara, CA and distributed as the Xience V stent—also distributed by Boston Scientific as the Promus stent)—everolimus (100 mcg/cm²) is released from a thin (7.8-μm), nonadhesive, durable, biocompatible fluorocopolymer consisting of vinylidene fluoride and hexafluoropropylene monomers coated onto a low-profile (81 mcg strut thickness) flexible cobalt chromium stent. The release kinetics are similar to those seen with sirolimus from the SES (~80% of the drug released at 30 days, with none detectable after 120 days). The polymer is elastomeric and experiences minimal bonding, webbing, or tearing upon expansion. Fluoropolymers have

been demonstrated to resist platelet and thrombus deposition in blood-contact applications.[72,73] The polymer has also been demonstrated to be noninflammatory in porcine experimental models. The low-profile stent struts facilitate rapid reendothelialization[74] and are fracture-resistant. Preclinical studies have demonstrated more rapid coverage of the stent struts with functional endothelium with EES compared with SES, PES, or ZES.[47] In the small SPIRIT First trial, the EES was shown to markedly reduce the extent of angiographic late loss at 6 and 12 months compared with the otherwise identical cobalt chromium Vision BMS.[75] Subsequently, the safety and efficacy of the EES has been compared with that of the PES, SES, and ZES in 15,426

TABLE 13-6	Randomized Controlled Trials of Everolimus-Eluting Stents				
Trial Acronym and Reference	**Study Cohort**	**EES vs.**	**Number randomized (planned angiographic follow-up)**	**Latest follow-up to Date**	**Principal Findings**
SPIRIT II[75]	Noncomplex CAD; up to 2 lesions	PES(E)	300 (all)	4 years	EES vs. PES(E) resulted in lower 6-month rates of angiographic in-stent late loss (0.11 ± 0.27 mm vs. 0.36 ± 0.39 mm, $P < 0.0001$).
SPIRIT III[84,85]	Noncomplex CAD; up to 2 lesions	PES(E)	1,002 (564)	4 years	EES vs. PES(E) resulted in lower 8-month rates of angiographic in-segment late loss (0.14 ± 0.41 mm vs. 0.28 ± 0.48 mm, $P = 0.004$), noninferior 9-month rates of TVF (7.2% vs. 9.0%, $P = 0.31$), and reduced rates of MACE at 1 year (5.7% vs. 9.9%, $P = 0.01$) and 4 years (12.3% vs. 17.4%, $P = 0.02$).
SPIRIT IV[36,83]	Noncomplex CAD; up to 3 lesions	PES(E)	3,687 (none)	2 years	EES vs. PES(E) resulted in lower 1-year rates of TLF (3.9% vs. 6.6%, $P = 0.0008$) and ischemia-driven TLR (2.3% vs. 4.5%, $P = 0.0008$), with noninferior rates of cardiac death or target-vessel MI (2.2% vs. 3.2%, $P = 0.09$). EES also resulted in lower rates of MI and stent thrombosis (see text). At 2 years TLF occurred in 6.9% of EES patients vs. 9.9% of PES(E) patients ($P = 0.003$).
COMPARE[79,88]	All comers	PES(L)	1,800 (none)	2 years	EES vs. PES(L) resulted in lower 1-year rates of the primary composite endpoint death, MI or TVR (6.2% vs. 9.1%, p = 0.02), and MACE (4.9% vs. 8.2%, p = 0.005). EES also resulted in lower rates of MI, stent thrombosis and TLR (see text). At 2 years the primary composite endpoint occurred in 9.0% of EES patients vs. 13.7% of PES(L) patients (p = 0.002).
SPIRIT V Diabetes[77]	Diabetes	PES(L)	324 (all)	1 year	EES vs. PES(L) resulted in lower 9-month rates of angiographic in-stent late loss (0.19 ± 0.37 mm vs. 0.39 ± 0.49 mm, p = 0.0001).
EXECUTIVE[81]	MVD, otherwise non-complex CAD	PES(L)	200 (all)	9 months	EES vs. PES(L) resulted in lower 9-month rates of angiographic in-stent late loss (0.11 ± 0.27 mm vs. 0.36 ± 0.39 mm, p = 0.008).
ISAR-TEST-4[76]	Simple and complex CAD	SES	1,304 (all)	2 years	EES vs. SES resulted in non-statistically significant rates of in-segment late loss at 24 months (0.29 ± 0.51 mm vs. 0.31 ± 0.58 mm, $P = 0.59$). At 2 years, binary restenosis was lower with EES (12.7% vs. 16.9%, $P = 0.03$). TLF at 2 years was not significantly different between EES and SES (16.0% vs. 18.8%, $P = 0.23$), although TLR tended to be less frequent with EES (9.9% vs. 13.5%, $P = 0.06$).
SORT OUT IV[78]	All comers	SES	2,777 (all)	9 months	EES vs. SES resulted in non-statistically significant different 9-month rates of the composite endpoint of cardiac death, MI, definite stent thrombosis, or TVR (4.9% vs. 5.2%, $P = NS$), and TLR (1.4% vs. 1.7%, $P = 0.64$). The 9-month rates of definite/probable thrombosis were also not different (0.9% in both groups), although definite stent thrombosis was less with EES (0.1% vs. 0.7%, $P = 0.05$).
EXCELLENT[80]	Noncomplex CAD	SES	1,443 (all)	9 months	Noninferiority was present for the primary endpoint of in-segment late loss at 9 months (EES 0.10 ± 0.36 mm vs. SES 0.05 ± 0.34 mm, $P_{NI} = 0.02$). MACE occurred in only ~3.0% of patients in both groups at 9 months.
ESSENCE-Diabetes[86]	Diabetes	SES	300 (all)	1 year	EES vs. SES resulted in lower 8-month angiographic in-segment late loss (mean 0.23 mm vs. 0.37 mm, $P = 0.02$) and lower binary restenosis (0.9% vs. 6.5%, $P = 0.04$).
RESOLUTE-All Comers[87]	All comers	ZES(R)	2,292 (460)	1 year	EES vs. ZES(R) resulted in comparable 1-year rates of TLF (8.3% vs. 8.2%, $P = 0.92$) and TLR (3.4% vs. 3.9%, $P = 0.50$), although less definite stent thrombosis (0.3% vs. 1.2%, $P = 0.01$) and definite/probable stent thrombosis (0.7% vs. 1.6%, $P = 0.05$). EES vs. ZES(R) resulted in non-statistically significant different degrees of in-stent diameter stenosis at 13 months (mean 19.8% vs. 21.7%, $P_{NI} = 0.04$) but less in-segment late loss (mean 0.06 mm vs. 0.15 mm, $P = 0.04$), although comparable rates of binary restenosis (5.2% vs. 6.5%, $P = 0.67$).

EES, everolimus-eluting stents (Xience V/Promus); PES(E), paclitaxel-eluting stents (Taxus Express platform); PES(L), paclitaxel-eluting stents (Taxus Liberté platform); ZES(R), zotarolimus-eluting stents (Resolute platform); CAD, coronary artery disease; MVD, multivessel disease; MI, myocardial infarction; TLR, target lesion revascularization; TVR, target vessel revascularization; TLF, target lesion failure (cardiac death, target-vessel MI, or TLR); TVF, target vessel failure (cardiac death, MI, or TVR); MACE, major adverse cardiac events (cardiac death, MI, or TLR).

patients enrolled in 11 randomized clinical trials[36,76-87] (Table 13-6). Compared with the PES, the EES has been consistently shown to have lower angiographic late loss and restenosis, resulting in less recurrent ischemia, TLR, and TVR. In addition, the EES has been shown to reduce the early and late rates of stent thrombosis and MI compared with the PES. In the large-scale SPIRIT IV trial,[36] 3,687 patients with stable coronary artery disease undergoing PCI of up to three lesions in three vessels were randomized to the EES versus the PES (Express platform). Patients with unstable acute coronary syndromes, MI, thrombus, chronic occlusions, vein graft lesions, and true bifurcation lesions were excluded. The primary endpoint of target lesion failure (TLF)—a composite of cardiac death, target-vessel MI, or ischemia-driven TLR—at 1 year was reduced by 39% (3.9% vs. 6.6%, $P = 0.0008$). EES compared with PES also reduced the 1-year rates of stent thrombosis (0.3% vs. 1.1%, $P = 0.003$), MI (1.9% vs. 3.1%, $P = 0.02$), and TLR (2.3% vs. 4.5%, $P = 0.0008$). These results were sustained at the 2-year follow-up.[83] In the COMPARE trial,[88] 1,800 unrestricted "all comers" patients were randomized to EES versus PES (Liberté platform). The primary endpoint of MACE at 1 year (death, MI, or TVR) was reduced by 31% with the EES (6.2% vs. 9.1%,

$P = 0.02$), driven by reductions in stent thrombosis (0.7% vs. 2.6%, $P = 0.002$), MI (2.8% vs. 5.4%, $P = 0.007$) and TLR (1.7% vs. 4.8%, $P = 0.0002$). Between 1 and 2 years in this high-risk study cohort (in whom only ~15% of patients were maintained on dual antiplatelet therapy), fewer stent thrombosis, MI, and TLR events occurred with EES compared with PES.[79] In contrast to the marked differences between EES and PES, smaller differences have been found between EES and SES in four randomized trials (Table 13-6). In the ISAR-TEST-4 trial,[76] 1,304 patients were randomized to EES versus SES, with routine follow-up angiography planned in all patients at 6 to 8 months and 2 years (an additional 1,229 patients were also randomized to an investigational combination sirolimus/probucol-eluting stent, the results of which are not considered here). EES compared with SES at 2 years resulted in lower rates of binary restenosis (12.7% vs. 16.9%, $P = 0.03$) and ischemia-driven TLR (9.9% vs. 13.5%, $P = 0.06$), with nonsignificant differences in death, MI, and stent thrombosis. In the SORT OUT IV trial,[78] 2,774 unselected patients in Denmark were randomized to EES versus SES and followed through the Danish Civil Registration System and Western Denmark Heart Registry. The primary 9-month endpoint of the composite of cardiac death, MI, definite stent thrombosis, or TVR occurred in a comparable proportion of patients in both groups, although the event rates were lower than expected. Definite stent thrombosis occurred in fewer EES than SES patients (0.1% vs. 0.7%, $P = 0.05$). Similarly, in the EXCELLENT trial,[80] late loss was comparable with EES and SES, and the 9-month MACE rates were extremely low in both groups, although there tended to be fewer stent thromboses with EES (0.4% vs. 0.8%, $P =$ NS). Finally, in the ESSENCE-Diabetes trial,[86] EES compared with SES resulted in lower rates of angiographic late loss and binary restenosis at 8 months in randomized patients with diabetes. In summary, in a broad cross section of patients undergoing PCI, EES have shown marked improvements in safety and efficacy outcomes compared with PES and more modest improvements compared with SES. Long-term follow-up is still ongoing in most of these trials, the results of which are necessary to determine the robustness of these findings. Moreover, larger randomized trials (with careful monitoring) are required to determine with confidence the magnitude of the differences in low-frequency events between different stents eluting rapamycin analogues. The EES has been compared with the Resolute ZES in one large randomized trial,[87] as described below and in Table 13-6.

Zotarolimus-Eluting Stent I (Endeavor). The Endeavor stent (Medtronic, Inc., Santa Rosa, CA) elutes zotarolimus (10 mcg per 1 mm stent length) from a thin layer (5.3 μm) of the biocompatible polymer phosphorylcholine from a flexible, low-profile (91 μm strut thickness) cobalt chromium stent. Phosphorylcholine is a naturally occurring phospholipid found in the membrane of red blood cells that is resistant to platelet adhesion.[89] The potencies of zotarolimus, everolimus, and sirolimus are roughly comparable, and zotarolimus is somewhat more lipophilic. However, the release rate of zotarolimus from Endeavor (~90% within 7 days, 100% within 30 days) is significantly faster than the rate at which everolimus and sirolimus are released from Xience V/Promus and Cypher stents respectively. In the Endeavor I FIM study,[90] the zotarolimus-eluting Endeavor stent (ZES[E]) was implanted in 100 patients with noncomplex coronary lesions. Although TLR was required in only 1% of patients at 1 year, mean in-stent late lumen loss was 0.33 mm at 4 months and 0.61 mm at 12 months. While significantly less than the late mean in-stent loss of 0.8 to 1.0 mm typically experienced with BMS, this degree of late loss would be expected to result in greater rates of binary restenosis and TLR compared with DES such as EES and SES, which achieve more potent suppression of neointimal hyperplasia.[91,92] The ZES(E) was subsequently compared with an otherwise identical BMS in the ENDEAVOR II trial[93,94] in 1,197 randomized patients with noncomplex coronary artery disease. As described in Table 13-7, compared with the BMS, the ZES(E) resulted in significantly reduced rates of TVF and TLR at 9 months, which were sustained for 5 years. Although

the 9-month rate of angiographic in-stent late loss was 0.61 ± 0.46 mm, this was sufficient to reduce in-segment binary restenosis to 13.2% from 35.0% with the BMS ($P < 0.0001$). A series of trials were then performed in which the ZES(E) was compared with other DES. In the ENDEAVOR III trial, the rates of late loss and restenosis were significantly greater with the ZES(E) than the SES.[95] With 436 randomized patients, this study was not powered for clinical endpoints. In contrast, the ENDEAVOR IV trial ($n = 1,548$) demonstrated that despite greater late loss and angiographic restenosis with the ZES(E) compared with the PES, the ZES(E) had noninferior 9-month rates of TVF and comparable 12-month rates of TLR in patients with noncomplex coronary lesions.[35] In addition, with follow-up through 3 years, significant differences have emerged in the rates of cardiac death or MI favoring the ZES(E).[96] Notably, within 1 year, a trend was present for more stent thrombosis (ARC [Academic Research Consortium] definite or probable) with the ZES(E) than the PES. Between 1 and 3 years, however, there was only 1 episode of stent thrombosis with the ZES(E) versus 11 such events with the PES (Fig. 13-6), representing a very favorable late safety profile. Three investigator-sponsored randomized trials have been completed in which the ZES(E) was compared with other DES in unrestricted patient populations. In the SORT OUT III trial,[97] 2,333 unselected patients (nearly 50% of whom presented with acute coronary syndromes) were randomized at five Danish centers to ZES(E) vs. SES. The 9-month primary endpoint of MACE (cardiac death, MI, or TVR) occurred significantly more frequently with the ZES(E)s (6% vs. 3%, $P = 0.0002$). ZES(E) also resulted in higher 9-month rates of MI, stent thrombosis, and TLR, differences that persisted at 18 months (Table 13-7). The ISAR-TEST-2 trial was a three-way 1:1:1 randomized trial in 1,007 patients of an investigational combination sirolimus/probucol-eluting stent versus the ZES(E) and the SES.[98,99] Angiographic follow-up was performed at 6 to 8 months and 2 years. The 674 patients randomized to the ZES(E) had higher rates of late loss, angiographic restenosis (the primary endpoint), and TLR at 6 to 8 months than those assigned to the SES, with similar rates of death, MI, and stent thrombosis (Table 13-7). Greater neointimal hyperplasia and more frequent TLR were evidenced with the SES than the ZES(E) between 6 to 8 months and 2 years, however, such that at the end of 2 years the differences were not as marked. Finally, the ZEST investigators randomized 2,645 patients with simple and complex coronary artery disease to the ZES(E), SES, or PES(L).[100,101] Angiographic follow-up at 9 months demonstrated less late loss and binary restenosis with the SES than the other two stents, with lower rates of TVR and TVF with the SES at 1 and 2 years (Table 13-7). The results with the ZES were intermediate between the SES and the PES(L). There were no significant differences in the 2-year rates of death, MI, or stent thrombosis between the two stents.

Considered collectively, these trials demonstrate that although the ZES(E) has greater late loss than either the SES or PES, it is clearly superior in efficacy to the BMS and likely comparable to other stent platforms in reducing clinical restenosis in simple lesions. In more complex lesions, TLR rates are lower with more potent DES, which have lower rates of late loss. Additional studies are required to determine the relative early and late safety profiles of ZES(E) versus other stents in simple and complex lesions. In this regard the PROTECT trial has completed randomization of 8,800 patients to ZES(E) versus SES and is the first study powered to demonstrate a difference between two stents in the rate of stent thrombosis (the primary endpoint at 3 years' follow-up).

Zotarolimus-Eluting Stent II (Resolute). The Resolute stent (Medtronic, Inc.) is similar to the Endeavor stent in that zotarolimus is eluted from the thin-strut cobalt-chromium Driver (or Integrity) BMS platform. However, instead of the phosphorylcholine coating of the Endeavor stent, the Resolute stent employs the BioLinx tripolymer coating, consisting of a hydrophilic endoluminal component and a hydrophobic component adjacent to the metal stent surface. This polymer serves to slow the elution of zotarolimus, such that 60% of the drug is eluted by 30 days and 100% by 180 days, making this the

TABLE 13-7	Randomized Controlled Trials of Endeavor Zotarolimus-Eluting Stents				
Trial Acronym and Reference	Study Cohort	ZES(E) vs.	Number Randomized (planned angiographic follow-up)	Latest Follow-up to Date	Principal Findings
Endeavor II[93,127]	Noncomplex CAD	BMS	1,197 (600)	5 years	Compared to BMS, ZES(E) reduced the 9-month rates of TVF (the primary endpoint; 15.1% vs. 7.9%, $P < 0.0001$), TLR (11.8% vs. 4.6%, $P < 0.0001$), in-stent late loss (1.03 ± 0.58 to 0.61 ± 0.46 mm, $P < 0.001$), and in-segment binary restenosis (35.0% vs. 13.2%, $P < 0.0001$). The rate of stent thrombosis was 0.5% with ZES(E) vs. 1.2% with BMS ($P = 0.22$). At 5 years TLR was reduced with ZES(E) (16.5% vs. 7.4%, $P < 0.0001$).
Endeavor III[95]	Noncomplex CAD	SES	436 (all)	3 years	Compared to SES, ZES(E) had higher 8-month rates of in-stent late loss (0.60 ± 0.48 vs. 0.15 ± 0.34, $P < 0.001$) and in-segment binary restenosis (11.7% vs. 4.3%, $P = 0.04$).
Endeavor IV[35]	Noncomplex CAD	PES(E)	1,548 (328)	3 years	Compared to PES, ZES(E) were noninferior for the primary endpoint of TVF at 9 months (6.6% vs. 7.1%, respectively ($P_{NI} < 0.0001$, $P_{Sup} = 0.69$). ZES(E) compared to PES resulted in higher rates of angiographic in-stent late loss (0.67 ± 0.49 vs. 0.42 ± 0.50 mm, $P < 0.001$) and a trend toward greater in-segment restenosis (15.3% vs. 10.4%; $P = 0.28$) at 8 months, but comparable rates of TLR at 1 (4.5% vs. 3.2%; $P = 0.23$) and 3 years (6.5% vs. 6.1%, $P = 0.66$). The rates of cardiac death or MI in ZES(E) vs. PES patients was 2.1% vs. 3.1% respectively at 1 year ($P = 0.20$) and 3.6% vs. 7.1% respectively at 3 years ($P = 0.04$). Stent thrombosis after 3 years occurred in 1.1% of ZES(E) patients vs. 1.6% of PES patients ($P = 0.50$).
SORT OUT III[97]	All comers	SES	2,333 (none)	18 months	ZES(E) vs. SES resulted in higher 9-month and 18-month rates of cardiac death, MI or TVR (6% vs. 3%, $P = 0.0002$, and 10% vs. 5%, $P < 0.0001$), MI (2% vs. < 1%, $P = 0.006$, and 2% vs. 1%, $P = 0.03$), stent thrombosis (1% vs. < 1%, $P = 0.048$, and 1% vs. 1%, $P = 0.13$), and TLR (4% vs. 1%, $P < 0.0001$, and 6% vs. 1%, $P < 0.0001$). Mortality was higher at 18 months after ZES(E) (4% vs. 3%, $P = 0.035$).
ISAR TEST 2[98,99]	Simple and complex CAD	SES	674 (all)	2 years	ZES(E) vs. SES resulted in higher 6–8 month rates of late loss (0.58 ± 0.55 vs. 0.24 ± 0.51 mm, $P < 0.001$) and binary restenosis (19.3% vs. 12.0%, $P < 0.01$), and higher 1-year rates of TLR (19.3% vs. 7.2%, $P < 0.01$). With longer-term follow-up to 2 years there was greater late loss with SES compared with ZES, such that the differences in binary restenosis and TLR were not as pronounced (20.9% vs. 18.6%) and TLR (14.3% vs. 10.7%). The rates of death, MI, and stent thrombosis were not significantly different at 9 months or 2 years.
ZEST[100,101]	Simple and complex CAD	SES and PES(L)	2,645 (all)	2 years	For the primary endpoint of TVF at 12 months, ZES(E) was noninferior to SES (10.2% vs. 8.3%, $P_{NI} = 0.01$, $P_{Sup} = 0.17$) and superior to PES(L) (10.2% vs. 14.1%, $P = 0.01$). In-segment binary restenosis at 9 months occurred in 12.1%, 2.4%, and 12.4% of ZES(E), SES, and PES stents ($P < 0.001$). At 24 months the rates of TVF with PES, ZES(E), and SES were 15.3%, 11.2%, and 9.9% ($P = 0.43$ and 0.01 for ZES(E) vs. SES and PES respectively). There were no significant differences in the rates of death, MI, or stent thrombosis at 2 years between the three stents, although there was a difference in TVR (8.6% vs. 6.0% vs. 3.1%, $P = 0.03$ and 0.01 for ZES(E) vs. SES and PES respectively).

ZES(E), zotarolimus-eluting stents (Endeavor platform); PES(E), paclitaxel-eluting stents (Taxus Express platform); PES(L), paclitaxel-eluting stents (Taxus Liberté platform); SES, sirolimus-eluting stents; CAD, coronary artery disease; MI, myocardial infarction; TLR, target lesion revascularization; TVR, target vessel revascularization; TVF, target vessel failure (death, MI, or TVR).

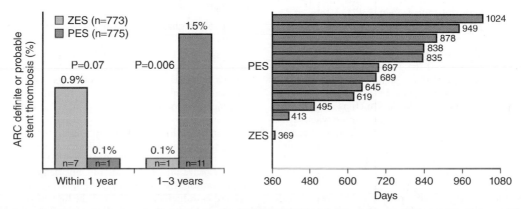

Figure 13-6 Stent thrombosis rates before and after 1 year in the ENDEAVOR IV trial. The right graph shows the timing of the individual occurrences of very late stent thrombosis in the two arms. ZES denotes zotarolimus-eluting stents (Endeavor platform). PES denotes paclitaxel-eluting stents (Taxus Express platform).

slowest rapamycin analogue-eluting DES. In the RESOLUTE trial, the ZES(R) stent was implanted in 139 patients with noncomplex coronary artery disease.[102] The primary endpoint of in-stent late lumen loss at 9 months was 0.22 ± 0.27 mm and the in-segment binary restenosis rate 2.1%, both significantly less than seen with the ZES(E) platform. MACE, TLR, and ARC definite/probable stent thrombosis at 12 months occurred in 8.7%, 0.7%, and 0% of patients respectively. Following these favorable results, 2,292 unselected patients were randomized to ZES(R) versus EES in the RESOLUTE All-Comers trial[87] (Table 13-6). Angiographic follow-up was planned in a subset of 460 patients at 13 months, after the 12-month assessment of the major clinical endpoints. The ZES compared with the EES was noninferior for the primary 1-year endpoint of TLF (8.2% vs. 8.3%, $P_{NI} < 0.001$). Nor were there significant differences between the two devices in the 1-year rates of death, cardiac death, MI, or TLR. Both definite and definite or probable stent thrombosis occurred less frequently with the EES (Table 13-6). At 13 months, restenosis occurred infrequently with both stents, although in-segment late loss was slightly greater with the ZES compared with the EES (0.15 ± 0.43 mm vs. 0.06 ± 0.40 mm, $P = 0.04$). Thus, the ZES (Resolute platform) is the first stent to demonstrate comparable overall safety and efficacy to the EES, although slight differences in angiographic and clinical outcomes between these stent platforms may exist. Larger studies and longer-term follow-up are required to assess the clinical significance of these findings.

Biolimus A9-Eluting Stents (BioMatrix). The BioMatrix stent elutes biolimus A9 (concentration 15.6 mcg/mm), a semisynthetic rapamycin analogue with similar potency but greater lipophilicity than sirolimus, from the stainless steel S-Stent platform (120-µm strut thickness). However, compared with the previously described first- and second-generation DES, the BioMatrix stent is unique in that the drug is eluted from poly-L-lactic acid (PLLA), a biodegradable polymer applied solely to the abluminal stent surface. The biolimus A9 and PLLA are coreleased and the polymer is converted via the Krebs cycle into carbon dioxide and water after a 6- to 9-month period. Conceptually, such a stent might not be prone to the late inflammatory reactions occasionally seen with durable polymers and thus might result in improved outcomes after 1 year. The safety and efficacy of the BioMatrix stent was first tested in the STEALTH trial, in which 120 patients with single de novo coronary lesions received either a BES or a bare metal S-stent.[103] Compared with the BMS, the BES resulted in lower rates of in-stent late loss at 6 months (0.26 ± 0.43 mm vs. 0.74 ± 0.45 mm, $P < 0.001$). The Nobori DES is a similar stent platform that has also been tested against the PES(E) and SES in two modest-sized randomized trials, with favorable angiographic results.[104,105] Following this encouraging early experience, 1,707 "all comer" patients (55% of whom had acute coronary syndromes) were randomized to BES vs. SES in the LEADERS trial.[106] The BMS compared with the SES was noninferior for the primary 9-month composite endpoint of cardiac death, MI, or TVR and demonstrated similar rates of TLR and stent thrombosis (Fig. 13-7). A total of 427 patients were allocated to angiographic follow-up at 9 months, which demonstrated that the BES was noninferior to the SES for the primary angiographic endpoint of in-stent diameter stenosis (mean 20.9% vs. 23.3%, $P_{NI} = 0.001$, $P_{Sup} = 0.26$). Follow-up through 3 years has been reported and demonstrated no significant clinical differences between the BES and the SES[107] (Fig. 13-7), with weak trends favoring the BES over time in safety endpoints such as stent thrombosis. A much larger study will be required to determine whether the BES or other devices with bioabsorbable polymers (or, as discussed below, polymer-free systems or fully bioabsorbable stents) offer clinical advantages to the best-in-class second-generation DES with durable polymers.

Conclusions. In summary, significant progress has been made with second-generation DES compared with their first-generation counterparts in terms of enhanced deliverability (thin-strut cobalt-chromium platforms), safety (in particular lower rates of stent

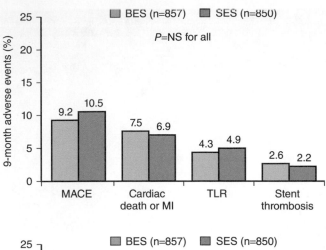

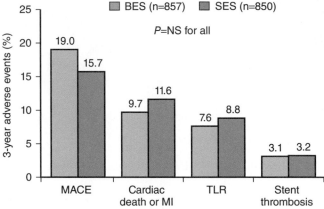

Figure 13-7 Principal clinical endpoints at 9 months (left) and 3 years (right) from the randomized all-comers LEADERS trial. MACE (major adverse cardiac events) denotes cardiac death, myocardial infarction (MI) or clinically indicated target vessel revascularization. Stent thrombosis refers to Academic Research Consortium (ARC) definite or probable events.

thrombosis with EES), and antirestenotic efficacy (EES and ZES[R]). Ongoing studies will demonstrate whether EES, ZES(E), and/or BES have important late safety advantages. As described below, progress is also being made with third-generation stent designs including polymer-free systems and bioabsorbable stents, which promise to further enhance the safety and efficacy of DES.

Drug-Eluting Stents in Specific Situations

Acute ST-Segment-Elevation Myocardial Infarction. Acute ST-segment-elevation myocardial infarction (STEMI) is caused in most cases by rupture of a thin-cap fibroatheroma, a lesion consisting of a lipid-rich necrotic core and an overlying thin (<65 µm), inflamed fibrous cap.[108] Tissue factor and other prothrombotic constituents are released, resulting in thrombotic occlusion of the coronary vessel and subsequent myocardial necrosis. Timely reperfusion with PCI results in improved myocardial salvage and reduced rates of recurrent ischemia, reinfarction, stroke, and death compared with fibrinolytic therapy.[109] As shown in Figure 13-8, compared with balloon angioplasty, the implantation of a BMS in STEMI further reduces subacute vessel closure and restenosis but not death or reinfarction.[110] Stent implantation within or adjacent to a fibroatheroma may result in delayed endothelialization[111] and the highest rates of stent thrombosis have been reported after stent implantation in STEMI, although this risk can be somewhat ameliorated with more potent antiplatelet agents.[112,113]

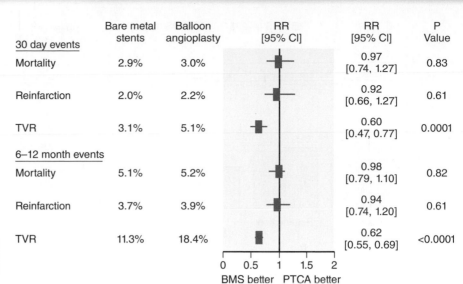

	Bare metal stents	Balloon angioplasty	RR [95% CI]	RR [95% CI]	P Value
30 day events					
Mortality	2.9%	3.0%		0.97 [0.74, 1.27]	0.83
Reinfarction	2.0%	2.2%		0.92 [0.66, 1.27]	0.61
TVR	3.1%	5.1%		0.60 [0.47, 0.77]	0.0001
6–12 month events					
Mortality	5.1%	5.2%		0.98 [0.79, 1.10]	0.82
Reinfarction	3.7%	3.9%		0.94 [0.74, 1.20]	0.61
TVR	11.3%	18.4%		0.62 [0.55, 0.69]	<0.0001

0   0.5   1   1.5   2
BMS better   PTCA better

Figure 13-8 Metanalysis from 13 randomized controlled trials of BMS compared to balloon angioplasty in acute myocardial infarction in 6,922 patients.

The safety and efficacy of SES or PES in STEMI have been reported from at least 13 randomized trials in 7,532 patients and from at least 18 registries in 26,521 patients (Table 13-8). With follow-up ranging between 8 and 24 months, these studies have collectively shown that the use of DES in STEMI is safe, with similar rates of death, reinfarction, and stent thrombosis as with BMS.[114] Moreover, the rates of angiographic restenosis between 6 and 12 months, and clinical restenosis (TLR or TVR) have been consistently reduced with DES compared with BMS in STEMI.[114] However, many of these studies incorporated routine angiographic follow-up, a protocol-specific process that results in revascularization procedures that are not clinically indicated and may artificially overestimate the absolute benefits of DES compared with BMS (the "oculostenotic reflex").[115,116] Moreover, discontinuation of dual antiplatelet therapy within 1 year after DES implantation in STEMI has been strongly associated with subsequent mortality.[117] Future adherence with antiplatelet medications may be difficult to assess in the patient with STEMI. As such, a detailed risk-benefit analysis of DES versus BMS use in STEMI is warranted. In the HORIZONS-AMI trial, 3,002 patients with evolving STEMI were prospectively randomized to PES(E) versus BMS at 123 international centers and followed for 3 years,[118–120] representing the largest DES versus BMS comparative trial to date in any setting. The primary efficacy and safety endpoints were the 12-month rates of ischemia-driven TLR and MACE (a composite of death, reinfarction, stroke, or stent thrombosis) respectively. Routine angiographic follow-up at 13 months (beyond the primary endpoint) was performed in 1,249 patients. At 12 months, PES compared with BMS reduced the rates of ischemia-driven TLR (4.5% vs. 7.5%, HR [95% confidence interval (CI)] = 0.59 [0.43, 0.83], P = 0.002) with similar rates of MACE (8.1% vs. 8.0%, HR [95%CI] = 1.02 [0.76, 1.36], P = 0.92). The 13-month rates of angiographic binary restenosis were reduced from 22.9% with BMS to 10.0% with PES (RR [95%CI] = 0.44 [0.33, 0.57], P < 0.001). In-stent late loss was reduced with PES from 0.82 ± 0.70 mm to 0.41 ± 0.64 mm (P < 0.001), with comparable rates of infarct artery reocclusion, ulceration, ectasia, and aneurysm formation between the two stent types. The greatest reduction in TLR was evident in patients with one or more risk factors for restenosis (RVD < 3.0 mm, lesion length > 30 mm, or insulin-dependent diabetes mellitus), whereas patients without any of these variables had similarly low rates of TLR with BMS as with PES.[120] Clinical follow-up from HORIZONS-AMI at 3 years has been reported[118] and demonstrated statistically nonsignificantly different rates of death, reinfarction, stent thrombosis, and MACE with PES and BMS (Fig. 13-9). At 3 years, TLR was reduced from 15.1% with BMS to 9.4% with PES (HR [95%CI] = 0.60 [0.48, 0.76], P < 0.001), although the absolute benefit of PES was less pronounced in patients in whom routine angiographic follow-up was not performed (12.7% with BMS vs. 8.7% with PES, HR [95%CI] = 0.67 [0.48, 0.93], P = 0.01). Most studies with DES in STEMI have been performed with PES or SES. To date there have been four trials comparing PES, SES, ZES(E), and/or EES (Table 13-9).[121–123] Most have been underpowered to detect differences between these stent platforms, although the COMPARE-AMI trial did report that in 452 randomized patients with STEMI, TLR at 2 years was reduced with EES compared with PES (1.7% vs. 7.6%, P = 0.002), with a trend for less definite stent thrombosis (0.4% vs. 2.6%, P = 0.07).[124] Thus, PES and SES as an alternative to BMS in patients with STEMI undergoing primary PCI have been proven to be safe and effective, with the greatest benefits present in patients at high risk for restenosis after BMS. More experience with second-generation stents in STEMI is required before definitively concluding whether even greater safety and/or efficacy has been achieved.

Diabetes Mellitus. Patients with diabetes have higher rates of angiographic and clinical restenosis after BMS placement than those without

TABLE 13-8	Results of a Metanalysis Drawn from 13 Randomized Trials Comparing Drug-Eluting Stents with Bare Metal Stents In Patients with Acute Myocardial Infarction				
Endpoint	**Drug-Eluting Stent Group [n/N (%)]**	**BMS Group [n/N (%)]**	**Relative Risk [95%CI]**	**P Value**	**Heterogeneity (I²)**
Death	167/4515 (3.7%)	121/2837 (4.3%)	0.89 [0.70, 1.14]	0.36	0%
Reinfarction	153/4515 (3.4%)	108/2837 (3.8%)	0.82 [0.64, 1.05]	0.12	0%
Stent thrombosis	128/4825 (2.6%)	82/3147 (2.6%)	0.97 [0.73, 1.28]	0.81	0%
Target vessel revascularization	241/4515 (5.3%)	326/2837 (11.5%)	0.44 [0.35, 0.55]	<0.001	26%

Adapted from reference 114.

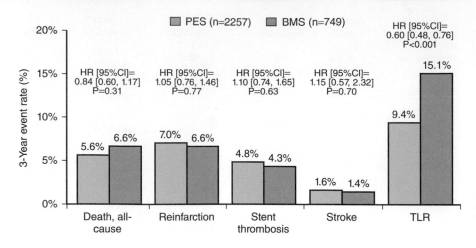

Figure 13-9 Three-year results from the prospective, randomized HORIZONS-AMI trial in which 3,006 patients with STEMI were assigned to TAXUS Expres PES or Express BMS. TLR denotes ischemia-driven target lesion revascularization.

diabetes.[125,126] In general, the pivotal trials in which patients were randomized to DES or BMS revealed comparable relative safety and efficacy with DES in patients either with or without diabetes, although with greater absolute reductions in TLR and TVR in diabetic patients, given their higher baseline risk (Table 13-10).[127–129] Most prior studies have shown comparable rates of in-stent late loss with PES in patients with versus those without diabetes,[130] suggesting that the multiple pathways through which paclitaxel interferes with restenosis (by affecting microtubular function) makes its action relatively independent of the diabetic state.[131] Considerable controversy has existed, however, as to whether the greater suppression of late loss from stents that elute potent rapamycin analogues (such as SES or EES) is preserved in patients with diabetes, given that the effect of rapamycin in interfering with the cell cycle is regulated by glycosylation-dependent enzymes.[132] In this regard, several small to moderate-sized studies have provided conflicting results. For example, among 379 patients with diabetes randomized to SES versus PES(E) in the REALITY trial, the rates of restenosis and clinical events were comparable with both stents.[133] In contrast, in the randomized 250-patient ISAR-Diabetes trial, SES compared with PES resulted in a greater reduction in late loss at 6 months, but statistically nonsignificantly different rates of TLR at 9 months.[134] This issue has more recently been comprehensively addressed by a pooled patient-level analysis from the SPIRIT II, SPIRIT III, SPIRIT IV, and COMPARE trials in which 6,789 patients were randomized to EES versus PES (Express or Liberté platforms). A total of 1,869 of these patients (25%) had diabetes. As shown in Figure 13-10, in patients without diabetes, EES compared with PES produced a marked reduction in the 1-year composite rate of cardiac death, MI, or ischemia-driven TLR.[135] EES compared with PES also markedly reduced the

individual rates of MI, stent thrombosis, and TLR. In contrast, in patients with diabetes, the rates of composite adverse events at 1 year (and their components) were almost identical between the two stent types. A powerful interaction was present between diabetic state and stent platform in the 1-year events. Thus, stents eluting potent rapamycin analogues, especially EES, have been proven to be safer and more effective than PES in patients without diabetes. In patients with diabetes, there is currently no strong evidence to favor one of these stent platforms over the other. Finally, often the most critical revascularization decision in patients with diabetes mellitus is whether to perform PCI or coronary artery bypass grafting (CABG). Four randomized trials have shown comparable 5-year rates of death, MI, or stroke in patients with diabetes treated with BMS or CABG.[136] In the CARDia trial, 510 patients with diabetes mellitus and multivessel disease were randomized to PCI with either SES (69% of patients) or BMS (31% of patents) versus CABG.[13] The primary endpoint of all-cause death, MI, or stroke at 1 year occurred in 10.5% with CABG versus 13.0% with PCI (HR [95%CI] = 1.25 [0.75–2.09], P = 0.39); among the SES subgroup randomization, the 1-year event rates were 12.4% versus 11.6% respectively (HR [95%CI] = 0.93 [0.51–1.71], P = 0.82). Whereas CARDia was insufficiently powered to be definitive, the ongoing FREEDOM trial,[137] which is enrolling more than 2,000 diabetic patients to SES or PES versus CABG, will provide important evidence-based guidance for this high-risk subgroup.

Left Main and Multivessel Disease. Although left main and multivessel disease are distinctly different conditions, revascularization decisions for these patients are often considered together because historically the default strategy has been CABG. Patients with

TABLE 13-9	Comparative Randomized Trials of Drug-Eluting Stents in Acute Myocardial Infarction							
Randomized Trial		**CEZAR** *N* = 400		**ZEST** *N* = 328		**PASEO** *N* = 180		**COMPARE** *N* = 452
DES 1/2/3		SES/PES(E)		SES/PES(L)/ZES(E)		SES/PES(E)		EES/PES(L)
FU Duration		1 year		1 year		4.3 years		2 years
Death	DES 1	3.9%		6.3%	D/MI	7.8%		2.9%
	DES 2	2.7%		4.5%		8.9%		4.2%
	DES 3	—		2.8%				—
Reinfarction	DES 1	2.8%		—		10.0%		4.2%
	DES 2	2.7%		—		8.9%		7.1%
	DES 3	—		—		—		—
Stent thrombosis definite/probable	DES 1	2.7%		3.6%		3.2%		1.7%
	DES 2	2.5%		2.7%		2.2%		3.8%
	DES 3	—		0%				—
Target vessel revascularization	DES 1	6%		5.5%		5.6%	TLR	1.7%	0.002
	DES 2	7%		7.3%		6.7%		7.6%
	DES 3	—		8.3%		—		

FU, Follow-up; TLR, target lesion revascularization; *P* = NS unless otherwise noted.

TABLE 13-10	Comparison from the Three Pivotal Randomized Trials of the Safety and Efficacy of Drug-Eluting Stents Compared with Bare Metal Stents in Patients With versus Without Diabetes Mellitus									
				Patients with Diabetes			**Patients without Diabetes**			
Trial	*DES*	*Duration*	*Endpoint*	DES	BMS	P VALUE	DES	BMS	P VALUE
SIRIUS	SES	9 months	Death, MI, or TVR	12.2%	27.0%	0.003	7.7%	18.6%	<0.001
		9 months	TLR	6.9%	22.3%	<0.001	3.0%	14.1%	<0.001
		9 months	TVR	9.9%	24.3%	0.002	5.2%	16.5%	<0.001
		8 months	In-stent late loss (mm)	0.29 ± 0.54	1.20 ± 0.71	<0.001	0.13 ± 0.40	0.92 ± 0.69	<0.001
TAXUS IV	PES(E)	12 months	Death, MI, or TVR	15.0%	27.2%	<0.001	8.4%	16.9%	<0.001
		12 months	TLR	7.4%	20.9%	<0.001	3.5%	13.2%	<0.001
		12 months	TVR	11.3%	24.0%	0.004	5.9%	14.9%	<0.001
		9 months	In-stent late loss (mm)	0.37 ± 0.52	0.96 ± 0.55	<0.001	0.40 ± 0.49	0.91 ± 0.58	<0.001
ENDEAVOR II	ZES(E)	9 months	TLR	7.5%	15.2%	—	3.9%	10.9%	—

multivessel disease treated with PCI have higher rates of restenosis and stent thrombosis than those with single-vessel disease, especially when diffuse disease, small vessels, and bifurcation lesions requiring treatment are present. In contrast, while restenosis and thrombosis are relatively rare after stenting the relatively short, large-caliber left main segment, PCI failure in the left main jeopardizes a sufficiently large amount of myocardium to entail a high risk of mortality.

Hlatky et al.[138] performed a metanalysis of 10 randomized trials of PCI versus CABG in 7,812 patients with multivessel disease. However, BMS were used in only four of these trials in 3,051 patients[139–142] and no study utilized DES. Follow-up through 5 years[136] demonstrated that compared with CABG, BMS resulted in comparable rates of death, MI, and/or stroke (16.7% vs. 16.9%, HR [95%CI] = 1.04 [0.86–1.27], P = 0.69), with no heterogeneity noted in patients with versus without diabetes or with double- versus triple-vessel disease. The 5-year rates of unplanned revascularization were significantly higher with BMS than with CABG, however (29.0% vs. 7.9%, HR [95%CI] = 0.23 [0.18–0.29] P < 0.001). Prior to the introduction of DES, there had been no randomized trials of PCI versus CABG in patients with unprotected left main disease because observational studies had shown a high rate of procedural failure and late sudden cardiac death with balloon angioplasty[143] as well as unacceptably high restenosis and MACE rates with BMS in this anatomical subgroup.[144] Erglis et al.[145] subsequently randomized 103 patients with left main disease to BMS versus PES and demonstrated that PES resulted in significantly lower 6-month rates of binary restenosis (6% vs. 22%, P = 0.02) and MACE (13% vs. 30%, P = 0.04). The ISAR Left Main investigators then randomized 650 patients with left main disease to PES versus SES[146] and found comparable 1-year rates of composite death, MI, or TLR (13.6%

vs. 15.8%, P = 0.44), definite stent thrombosis (0.3% vs. 0.7%, P = 0.57), and restenosis (16.0% vs. 19.4% P = 0.30) with the two stent types. In a small randomized trial, the LEMANS investigators assigned 105 patients to either PCI with BMS or DES (the latter used in only 35% of patients) versus CABG.[147] The primary endpoint of change in left ventricular ejection fraction (LVEF) 12 months after the procedure was significantly greater with PCI than CABG. PCI also had a significantly better early safety profile.

The most contemporary and relevant examination of the relative safety and efficacy of DES versus CABG in STEMI is the SYNTAX trial, in which 1,800 patients with either triple-vessel disease (n = 1,095) and/or left main disease (n = 705) were randomized to PES(E)s versus CABG.[148] The primary endpoint of SYNTAX—the 1-year composite rate of all-cause mortality, stroke, MI, or unplanned repeat revascularization—occurred significantly less commonly with CABG than with PES (Fig. 13-11, left). However, this was driven by greater rates of revascularization with PCI compared with CABG (although the difference between PCI and CABG was greatly reduced with PES than in the earlier era with BMS). There were no significant differences in the rates of composite death, MI, or stroke nor of death or MI individually between PCI and CABG. However, the 1-year rate of stroke was significantly lower with PCI than CABG. These results were consistent with follow-up through 3 years except that a significant difference emerged for fewer MIs in the CABG group over time[149] (Fig. 13-11, right). Follow-up is ongoing to 5 years.

A borderline interaction (P_{int} = 0.11) was present between the randomization arm and the primary 1-year endpoint for patients with left main versus triple-vessel disease in SYNTAX, such that the primary MACCE endpoint was improved in patients with triple-vessel disease randomized to CABG, whereas there were no significant differences in composite adverse events between PES and CABG for patients with left main disease.[148] Moreover, the selection of the most appropriate revascularization modality in these complex patients may be further discriminated by use of the SYNTAX score (www.syntaxscore.com), an anatomically based risk score that was prospectively defined prior to patient enrollment. Patients undergoing PCI had progressively higher rates of major adverse cardiac and cerebrovascular events (MACCE) with high SYNTAX scores, whereas MACCE outcomes after CABG were independent of SYNTAX score. The 3-year outcomes from the SYNTAX trial, according to the presence of left main disease and SYNTAX score tertile, appear in Table 13-11. These data suggest that CABG might be favored for patients with triple-vessel disease and a high or intermediate SYNTAX score and for patients with left main disease and a high SYNTAX score. Conversely, the 3-year results were equally good or better with PES compared with CABG in patients with triple-vessel disease and a low SYNTAX score and for left main disease and a low or intermediate SYNTAX score. However, given the modest sample sizes of these post hoc subgroups, these impressions should be considered hypothesis-generating only. Moreover, whether other scores incorporating clinical risk factors would have superior discrimination to the SYNTAX score has not been prospectively validated.[150,151] Nonetheless, on the basis of SYNTAX, the most recent U.S. and E.U.

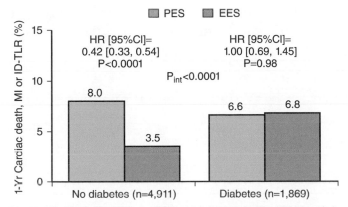

Figure 13-10 Interaction between baseline diabetic status and the composite rate of death, myocardial infarction (MI), or ischemia-driven target lesion revascularization (ID-TLR) at 1 year in patients randomized to everolimus-eluting stents (EES) compared with paclitaxel-eluting stents (PES). From a patient-level pooled metanalysis of the SPIRIT II, III, IV, and COMPARE trials.

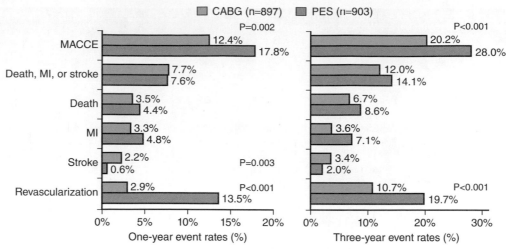

Figure 13-11 One-year (left) and three-year (right) results from the SYNTAX trial in which 1800 patients with triple vessel and/or left main disease were randomized to paclitaxel-eluting stents (PES) versus CABG surgery. MACCE denote, major adverse cardiac or cerebrovascular event; death, myocardial infarction (MI), stroke, or unplanned repeat revascularization. P = NS unless otherwise noted.

guidelines have elevated PCI of the left main to either a class IIb recommendation (U.S. guidelines) or IIa or IIb (E.U. guidelines), depending on the relative risk and complexity for PCI versus CABG.[151,152] The results of PCI in patients with complex coronary artery disease may be further optimized by the use of better stents and pharmacotherapy than were employed in SYNTAX[36,153] and with the regular use of IVUS and fractional flow reserve (FFR) guidance,[154,155] which were rarely utilized in SYNTAX. Many of these issues are being addressed in the ongoing EXCEL trial, in which more than 2500 patients with unprotected left main disease and a low to moderate SYNTAX score are being randomized to PCI with EES versus CABG.

Chronic Total Occlusions. Clinical and angiographic restenosis rates after both balloon angioplasty and stent implantation are increased following PCI of chronic total occlusions (CTO) compared with non-occluded stenoses principally because of an increased incidence of diabetes as well as greater lesion length, plaque mass, and calcification[156,157] (see CTO chapter). It has therefore been hypothesized that the benefits of DES versus BMS in reducing clinical restenosis would be strongly evident in the treatment of CTO lesions. In a 200-patient randomized trial of SES versus BMS, the use of SES resulted in

significant reductions in binary angiographic restenosis (7% vs. 36%, $P < 0.001$) and TLR (4% vs. 19%, $P < 0.001$), with reductions in clinical restenosis maintained through 4 years of clinical follow-up.[158] A large number of retrospective, nonrandomized, and historically controlled comparisons of DES and BMS have similarly demonstrated approximately 60% reductions in clinical restenosis endpoints with DES versus BMS. However, despite similar hazards of mortality and MI with DES versus BMS in a metanalysis aggregating these data, a trend toward increased stent thrombosis was observed with first-generation DES (RR: 2.79, 95%CI: 0.98–7.97, $P = 0.06$), meriting some concern.[159] Additionally, the Cypher SES has been associated with a 16% rate of stent fracture when used in CTO lesions, particularly in when long stents are overlapped in diffusely diseased arterial segments.[160] Studies are ongoing to determine whether these results may be improved upon by second-generation stents that are highly fracture-resistant, such as EES and ZES(R).

Bifurcation Lesions. Bifurcation lesions represent 20% or more of stenoses treated with angioplasty, and PCI of coronary bifurcation lesions is associated with increased procedural complications and worsened long-term outcomes (see bifurcation chapter). Because of the higher rates of clinical restenosis at bifurcation lesions, the use of

TABLE 13-11	Three-Year Outcomes from the SYNTAX Trial, Stratified by Triple-Vessel versus Left Main Disease According to SYNTAX Score Tertile								
	Low SYNTAX Tertile			**Intermediate SYNTAX Tertile**			**High SYNTAX Tertile**		
	PES	CABG	P VALUE	PES	CABG	P VALUE	PES	CABG	P VALUE
Triple-vessel disease	$n = 181$	$n = 171$		$n = 207$	$n = 208$		$n = 155$	$n = 166$	
MACCE	25.8%	22.2%	0.45	29.4%	16.8%	0.003	31.4%	17.9%	0.004
Death, MI, or stroke	11.2%	12.3%	—	16.1%	11.3%	—	17.7%	8.3%	—
Death	7.3%	6.8%	—	10.3%	5.7%	—	11.1%	4.5%	—
MI	5.1%	4.9%	—	8.9%	3.1%	—	7.2%	1.9%	—
Stroke	1.2%	3.2%	—	2.5%	3.6%	—	4.3%	1.9%	—
Revascularization	18.8%	11.6%	—	18.2%	8.4%	—	21.5%	10.5%	—
Left main disease	$n = 118$	$n = 104$		$n = 103$	$n = 92$		$n = 135$	$n = 149$	
MACCE	18.0%	23.0%	0.33	23.4%	23.4%	0.90	37.3%	21.2%	0.003
Death, MI, or stroke	6.9%	11.0%	—	10.8%	15.6%	—	20.1%	15.7%	—
Death	2.6%	6.0%	—	4.9%	12.4%	—	13.4%	7.6%	—
MI	4.3%	2.0%	—	5.0%	3.3%	—	10.9%	6.1%	—
Stroke	0.9%	4.1%	—	1.0%	2.3%	—	1.6%	4.9%	—
Revascularization	15.4%	13.4%	—	15.9%	14.0%	—	27.7%	9.2%	—

MI, myocardial infarction; MACCE, major adverse cardiac or cerebrovascular events (death, MI, stroke, or revascularization); PES, paclitaxel-eluting stent; CABG, coronary artery bypass graft surgery.

a DES for the main vessel of a bifurcation lesion has become the standard of care for bifurcation disease. A strategy of provisional stenting of the side branch is the generally accepted current approach to bifurcation disease unless there is significant high-grade and lengthy disease within the side branch.[161,162] A variety of strategies for the treatment of bifurcation disease with drug-eluting balloons are also currently undergoing evaluation,[163,164] but current data using such balloons in native coronary stenoses are mixed (see drug-eluting balloon chapter). Several dedicated drug-eluting bifurcation stent systems have been designed and are under investigation. Bifurcation stent systems can be classified as those that facilitate access to the side branch to simplify the PCI procedure versus novel stents designed to address the unique geometric challenges of the bifurcated stenosis. Initial experiences with the Devax self-expanding nitinol stent (coated with the bioabsorbable polymer poly-L-lactic acid, which elutes the antiproliferative rapamycin analogue biolimus A9) have demonstrated low rates of restenosis of both the main vessel and side branch in both true bifurcation lesions as well as in the distal bifurcation of the left main coronary artery.[165,166] This "reverse cone" stent is designed to adapt to and cover the main parent vessel and the bifurcation carina; it is used in conjunction with dedicated DES for one or both branches when necessary. Preliminary data have also been published on the use of the Stentys paclitaxel-eluting side branch access stent[167] and the Taxus Petal dedicated bifurcation stent[168]; further clinical data are awaited in order to determine the long-term advantages of these stents for the treatment of bifurcation disease.

Saphenous Vein Grafts. The most common cause of recurrent ischemia following CABG surgery is atheromatous degeneration within the body of a saphenous vein graft (SVG), and BMS have been associated with improved outcomes compared with balloon angioplasty in SVG intervention.[169,170] Although DES have the potential to further lower rates of restenosis of the target lesion within SVG, disease progression at nontarget sites within SVG is frequent (see SVG chapter). Additionally, because of the large caliber of most SVG, the "tolerated late loss" within SVG lesions is typically greater than that within native coronary vessels. Two small randomized trials of DES vs. BMS for critical SVG stenoses have been conducted in patients with SVG lesions and demonstrated lower rates of angiographic restenosis with DES.[171,172] With extended follow-up to a median of 32 months in one of these studies, however, the antirestenotic advantage of SES versus BMS was lost, and the SES was associated with higher mortality.[173] Adequately powered trials examining the potential safety and efficacy of DES for diseased SVG have not been performed. Therefore BMS is recommended for focal disease in large bypass conduits, with DES being reserved for more diffuse graft degeneration (if native coronary artery PCI or repeat surgery is not an option). Finally, a small pilot study of prophylactic "sealing" of moderate, noncritical SVG lesions with PES in order to prevent disease progression within SVG

TABLE 13-12	Academic Research Consortium (ARC) Definitions of Stent Thrombosis
Classification	
Definite	An acute coronary syndrome with angiographic or autopsy evidence of thrombus or occlusion within or adjacent to a stent
Probable	Unexplained death within 30 days after stent implantation or acute myocardial infarction involving the target-vessel territory without angiographic confirmation
Possible	Any unexplained death beyond 30 days after the procedure
Timing	
Acute	Within 24 hours (excluded events within the catheterization laboratory)
Subacute	1–30 days
Early	Within 30 days
Late	30 days–1 year
Very late	After 1 year

demonstrated that DES was superior to medical therapy alone, suggesting a possible preventive role for DES in degenerating SVG lesions prior to their becoming critical.[174] A large randomized trial is required, however, to verify the validity of such an approach.

Stent Failure Mechanisms and Management

Stent Thrombosis. The most feared complication following stent placement is stent thrombosis, which presents as acute MI in more than 80% of patients and results in death within 30 days in 10% to 25% of patients.[175,176] Treatment for stent thrombosis is almost always emergent repeat PCI, although optimal reperfusion is achieved in only two-thirds of patients.[177] Moreover, approximately 20% of patients with a first stent thrombosis experience a recurrent stent thrombosis episode within 2 years.[178] Thus understanding and preventing this complication is of paramount importance. The most widely utilized definition and timing classification of stent thrombosis was developed by the ARC,[179] with definite or probable stent thrombosis considered the best trade-off between sensitivity and specificity (Table 13-12). Stent thrombosis is also classified as primary if it is directly related to an implanted stent or secondary if it occurs at the stent site after an intervening TLR procedure for restenosis. Primary stent thrombosis after BMS placement typically occurs within the first 30 days, although it can rarely occur later.[180] In contrast, primary stent thrombosis after DES placement can occur years afterward, with an annual incidence of 0.2% to 0.3% in patients with noncomplex coronary artery disease,[181,182] and 0.4% to 0.6% after unrestricted use (Fig. 13-12).[183] Thus, rates of primary stent thrombosis are higher with DES than BMS, with the differences emerging predominantly beyond the first year after

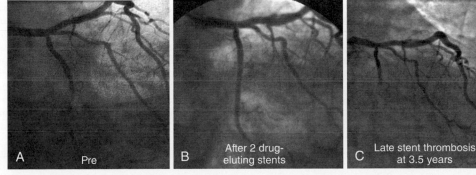

Figure 13-12 A high-grade stenosis is present in the mid portion of the left circumflex artery (left panel). An excellent angiographic result was obtained after placement of two 15 mm long 2.5 mm diameter SES (middle panel). The patient was asymptomatic until 3.5 years later when he presented with acute myocardial infarction to thrombotic occlusion within the prior implanted stents (right panel).

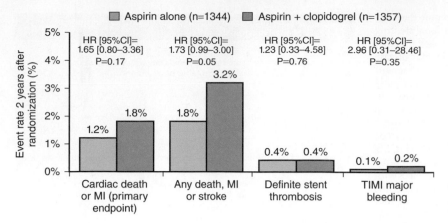

Figure 13-13 Outcomes in the REAL-LATE / ZEST-LATE randomized trial 2 years after 2,701 patients free from adverse cardiovascular events at least 1 year after DES implantation were randomized to aspirin alone versus aspirin plus clopidogrel.

implant.[184] However, after taking into account secondary stent thrombotic events after TLR procedures for restenosis (which occur more commonly after BMS than DES placement), the overall incidence of stent thrombosis (primary plus secondary) does not seem to be increased with DES compared with BMS,[185] and the overall late rates of death and MI are similar with both types of stents.[33] Moreover, the benefits of DES in reducing restenosis and subsequent MACE offset the small excess risk of late primary stent thrombosis with these devices.[186] The mechanisms underlying stent thrombosis are multifactorial and include stent-related factors as well as patient and procedural factors. Stent thrombosis occurs more commonly in complex patients and lesions, especially in patients with acute coronary syndromes and thrombotic lesions (possibly due to stent implantation within or adjacent to necrotic core,[187] diabetes and renal insufficiency, and diffuse disease, small vessels, and bifurcation lesions requiring multiple stents).[175,176,188–191] Hypersensitivity reactions to the DES polymer and vascular inflammation have been associated with stent thrombosis,[46,192] as have stent underexpansion and residual disease at the stent margins.[193–195] Polymers may be inherently thrombogenic and prone to webbing and peeling, thus forming a nidus for thrombosis. Strut fractures (which occur most commonly with stainless steel closed-cell stent designs, such as that of the SES, especially with overlapping stents in the right coronary artery)[160,196] have been pathologically and occasionally clinically linked to stent thrombosis.[197] Whether late acquired stent malapposition is a cause of late stent thrombosis or merely a reflection of underlying vascular toxicity to the drug or polymer, with positive vessel remodeling, is uncertain.[198,199] Finally, the most commonly proposed explanation underlying the increased rate of very late primary stent thrombosis with DES versus BMS is delayed or absent endothelialization of the stent struts. Virmani et al. first observed from autopsy studies that BMS strut endothelialization is 100% complete by 6 months, whereas DES never may achieve > 50% endothelial cell strut coverage even beyond 3 years after implantation.[200] Similar findings have been reported in vivo with angioscopy.[201] Finally, it has been observed that some cases of very late stent thrombosis may be due to the development of neoatherosclerosis within stents, along with new plaque rupture.[202] The rates of stent thrombosis may be decreasing with improvements in stent technology, imaging, and adjunct pharmacology. A large nonrandomized propensity-controlled study has suggested that IVUS guidance may reduce stent thrombosis at both 30 days and 1 year.[203] As discussed above, less reactive, more biocompatible polymers and improvements in stent design have significantly reduced the rates of early (EES) and late (EES and ZES[E]) stent thrombosis. Five randomized trials have demonstrated that stent thrombosis and MACE within 30 days of BMS implantation are markedly reduced by addition of the thienopyridine ticlopidine to aspirin.[12–15,204] In this regard, the efficacy of clopidogrel is similar to that of ticlopidine, with an enhanced safety profile.[205] In patients with acute coronary syndromes, the rates of stent thrombosis have also been reduced with more potent thienopyridines such as prasugrel and ticagrelor.[112,113] Observational studies have uniformly documented that premature thienopyridine discontinuation within 6 months after DES placement is strongly associated with stent thrombosis.[206,207] But whether prolonged dual antiplatelet therapy beyond this time will enhance freedom from stent thrombosis and/or death and MI is unknown, with some studies in support of this hypothesis[207–209] and others against.[206,210] In this regard the potential benefits of prolonged dual antiplatelet therapy, including the prevention of stent-related and non-stent-atherosclerosis-related adverse events must be weighed against the persistent risk of ongoing major bleeding with combination therapy. Only one randomized trial addressing this issue has been completed. In the pooled REAL-LATE / ZEST-LATE trial, 2,701 patients who were MACE-free for at least 1 year after DES (SES, PES, or ZES) placement were randomized to an additional 2 years of clopidogrel along with aspirin or aspirin alone.[211] There were no significant differences between the two groups in the late occurrence of the primary endpoint of cardiac death or MI or of definite stent thrombosis; paradoxically the incidence of the composite endpoint of all-cause death, MI, or stroke tended to be increased with prolonged clopidogrel use (Fig. 13-13). The event rates, however, were lower than expected, and this trial was insufficiently powered to be considered definitive. Several additional randomized trials are ongoing to address the relative safety and efficacy of prolonged dual antiplatelet therapy, the most meaningful of which is the Dual Antiplatelet Therapy (DAPT) Study, in which 20,645 patients free of MACE 1 year after SES, PES, EES, or ZES implantation are being randomized to aspirin alone or aspirin plus a thienopyridine (either clopidogrel or prasugrel), with follow-up for an additional 18 months.

Restenosis. By increasing acute luminal gain[28,29] and eliminating late recoil and negative vessel remodeling,[212] BMS reduce the rates of restenosis compared with balloon angioplasty.[5,6] However, stents induce more arterial injury than balloon angioplasty, which results in a greater absolute amount of neointimal hyperplasia developing over the first 6 to 12 months after the procedure,[213] thereby leading to binary angiographic restenosis in 10% to more than 50% of lesions (depending on patient and lesion complexity). While restenosis most commonly presents with stable angina and exercise-induced ischemia within 1 year of stent implantation, it has become increasingly recognized that restenosis presents as an acute coronary syndrome in as many as 25% of patients, occasionally even with STEMI.[213,214] Numerous studies have demonstrated that the most reproducible determinants of restenosis after BMS implantation are the presence of diabetes mellitus (especially if insulin is required), small RVD, and long lesion length.[125,126,215–218] Other factors associated with restenosis are treatment of ostial and/or calcified lesions, true bifurcation lesions requiring main vessel and sidebranch stents, CTO, and SVG.[219] The same factors are associated with higher rates of DES restenosis. However, angiographic and clinical restenosis (as well as death, MI, and stent thrombosis) after DES placement occurs less frequently in FDA-approved "on label" lesions (generally noncomplex lesions for which safety and efficacy have been established by large-scale randomized trials) than in less well studied and more complex "off label" lesions.[220,221] Nevertheless, in nearly all cases DES have been shown to be more effective than BMS in reducing TLR[33,222,223] (the only possible exceptions being short lesions in large native coronary arteries and possibly SVG with extended follow-up). The timing of angiographic restenosis after BMS placement peaks within approximately 6 months; thereafter, continued organization of the extracellular matrix results in slight luminal enlargement. Serial angiographic and IVUS studies have rarely shown late restenosis,[224,225] although late neoatherosclerosis with plaque rupture has been described as a possible cause of restenosis occurring years after BMS placement.[226] In contrast, a small amount of incremental angiographic late loss has been described for several years after the placement of an SES or EES, although reports on very late loss after PES placement have been conflicting.[76,98,227–230] These observations imply the existence of low-grade chronic vascular inflammation from either the polymer or lack of healing. However, when compared with their BMS counterparts (or with EES vs. PES in the SPIRIT trials), there has been little evidence demonstrating late loss occurring beyond 1 year to be of clinical relevance during extended follow-up of 2 to 5 years.[76,98,181,183,231–233] In the largest randomized trial examining this issue (SIRTAX), 1,012 patients were randomized to PES(E) versus SES and followed for 5 years, with angiographic follow-up performed systematically at 8 months and 5 years.[232] Incremental late loss between these two time periods occurred with both stents, although more so with SES than PES(E). At 1 year, the rate of TLR was less with SES than PES(E); this benefit was somewhat mitigated at 5 years (Table 13-13). The degree to which routine angiographic follow-up triggered late TLR procedures and therefore confounded the clinical results in this study is unknown.[115] Nonetheless, a small degree of angiographic late loss may be expected with polymer-based DES and may contribute to late adverse events in a small proportion of patients. The causes of restenosis after the placement of stents are multifactorial. In addition to excessive late neointimal hyperplasia, restenosis after BMS and DES placement has been associated with stent underexpansion,[234–236] edge dissections and residual untreated disease,[237,238] geographic miss,[239] and strut fractures.[160,196,240] Some[241] but not all[242,243] studies have found an association between nickel allergy and restenosis associated with the placement of BMS or DES. Genetic mutations in the genes encoding mTOR or polymorphisms in the genes encoding proteins involved in paclitaxel metabolism may result in resistance to SES and PES respectively.[244,245] Other genetic polymorphisms have also been associated with restenosis.[246,247] Excessive inflammation from first-generation DES polymers (specifically eosinophilic reactions to PES and granulomatous reactions to SES) may provoke late restenosis.[45,248] And of course the antiproliferative effects of DES depend on both the drug (with rapamycin-analogues being inherently more potent than paclitaxel) and the release kinetics (with extended release of rapamycin-analogues to and possibly beyond 1 month being necessary for maximal efficacy). As discussed above, newer-generation stents—(especially EES and ZES(R)—have been shown to have enhanced efficacy and safety. In addition, by facilitating the operator's ability to achieve larger lumen areas, IVUS may reduce restenosis and improve clinical outcomes after BMS placement.[249] No randomized trial has been adequately powered to demonstrate a reduction in TLR with IVUS after DES implantation, although the recently reported AVIO trial demonstrated that the postprocedural minimal luminal diameter was significantly greater in DES with IVUS guidance.[250] Patients who develop in-stent restenosis are at high risk for recurrence after percutaneous treatment, especially if the pattern of restenosis is diffuse.[251,252] IVUS imaging is highly useful in patients with restenosis to differentiate neointimal hyperplasia from stent underexpansion, geographic miss, strut fracture, and other rare occurrences such as chronic recoil and stent embolization, which require directed approaches to be managed successfully.[253]

Isolated restenosis at the stent edge can often be effectively treated with balloon angioplasty only or an additional short stent. Treatment options for diffuse BMS restenosis due to neointimal hyperplasia have been extensively studied. In the BMS era, neither cutting balloons, directional or rotational atherectomy, or repeat BMS proved better than balloon angioplasty in treating diffuse in-stent restenosis.[254] Vascular brachytherapy with either locally applied beta or gamma radiation was effective in reducing recurrent restenosis within 1 year[255,256] but was logistically complex, and the resultant vascular toxicity with prolonged inflammation and obliteration of normal cell lines resulted in high rates of late stent thrombosis (especially when new BMS were implanted) and restenosis.[257,258] Subsequently, two multicenter randomized trials established that SES and PES(E) significantly reduce angiographic restenosis and improved event-free survival at 9 months compared with either beta or gamma vascular brachytherapy in patients with BMS restenosis[259,260] (Fig. 13-3, left). In these two trials, with follow-up through 2 to 3 years, event-free survival was reduced with PES and noninferior with SES compared with brachytherapy[261,262] (Fig. 13-14, right). In the ISAR-DESIRE trial, 300 patients with BMS restenosis were randomized to balloon angioplasty alone versus SES versus PES(E).[263] Angiographic follow-up at 6 months showed recurrent restenosis after balloon angioplasty in 44.6% of patients versus 14.3% for SES (P < 0.001) and 21.7% for PES (P = 0.001), with TVR rates of 33%, 8%, and 19% respectively (P < 0.001 and P = 0.02 compared with balloon angioplasty, respectively). Based on the results of these trials, treatment with DES (with either PES or rapamycin analogue-eluting stents) has supplanted brachytherapy and other approaches for nearly all cases of BMS restenosis due to intimal hyperplasia except possibly isolated edge stenoses. The optimal treatment for DES restenosis has been less well studied. Compared with BMS restenosis, DES restenosis tends to be focal and is diffuse in less than one-quarter of patients. If the stenosis is isolated to the margin of the stent or is focal within the stent, either balloon angioplasty or implantation of a short DES of the same type is often selected. Management of diffuse DES restenosis has been less well studied. In the CRISTAL trial, 197 patients with diffuse restenosis (mean length ~14 mm) of either SES or PES were randomized to treatment with SES versus balloon angioplasty.[264] Follow-up at 12 months demonstrated a significantly larger minimal lumen diameter (MLD) with SES compared to balloon angioplasty only (2.14 ± 0.62 mm vs. 1.71 ± 0.55 mm, P < 0.0001), with a trend toward less TLR (5.9% vs. 13.1%, P = 0.10). Many operators

TABLE 13-13	Early and Late Results from the SIRTAX Trial			
	Sirolimus-Eluting Stent	*Paclitaxel-Eluting Stent*	*HR [95% CI]*	*P value*
Angiographic in-stent late loss*	(n = 156 lesions)	(n = 195 lesions)		
8 months	0.12 ± 0.36	0.25 + 0.49	—	<0.001
5 years	0.30 ± 0.51	0.37 ± 0.51	—	0.21
Target lesion revascularization	(n = 503 patients)	(n = 509 patients)		
12 months	5.8%	10.4%	0.54 [0.34–0.84]	<0.01
5 years	14.9%	17.9%	0.80 [0.59–1.52]	0.16
1–5 years	—	—	1.15 [0.77–1.73]	0.49

*Paired analysis.

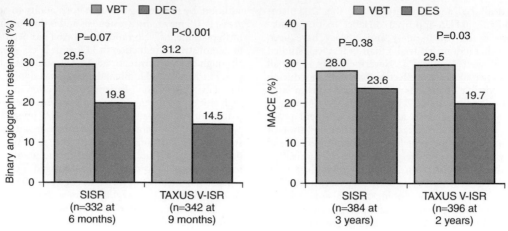

Figure 13-14 Angiographic (left) and clinical (right) results from the SISR trial (sirolimus-eluting stents vs. gamma or beta brachytherapy, $n = 384$) and the TAXUS V-ISR trial (paclitaxel-eluting stents vs. beta brachytherapy, $n = 396$). VBT denotes vascular brachytherapy.

consider diffuse in-stent restenosis after DES (if IVUS demonstrates adequate stent expansion) to represent "drug failure" and will treat with a different class of agent (e.g., PES after SES failure). However, in the ISAR-DESIRE-2 trial, 450 patients with SES restenosis were randomized to SES vs. PES.[265] At 6–8 month follow-up there were no differences between SES and PES in late loss (0.40 ± 0.65 mm vs. 0.38 ± 0.59 mm; $P = 0.85$), binary restenosis (19.6% vs. 20.6%; $P = 0.69$), or TLR (16.6% vs. 14.6%; $P = 0.52$). Finally, recurrent diffuse DES restenosis represents a major clinical challenge. Options that may be considered include cilostazol,[266] brachytherapy,[267] and oral rapamycin.[268] Ultimately, CABG surgery may be required in a small proportion of patients with recurrent DES restenosis.

Conclusions and Future Directions

The development and evolution of the coronary stent has resulted in remarkable progress in the less invasive treatment of coronary artery disease. However, although infrequent, stent thrombosis and restenosis still occur with even the best DES, and the reliance on long-term

dual antiplatelet therapy is a major limitation for many patients, given their cost, complications, and other considerations (e.g., preclusion of surgery or contact sports). Novel DES approaches under active development include stents designed to enhance the rate and completeness of endothelialization,[269] polymer-free stents,[270,271] and fully bioabsorbable stents[272,273] that offer the potential to eliminate late stent thrombosis (see chapter on biodegradable stents). Drug-eluting balloons have been developed and are particularly promising for the treatment of coronary in-stent restenosis[274,275] (see chapter on drug-eluting balloons). Dual-agent DES may also confer improved safety and/or efficacy. In the future, stents will continue to improve in deliverability and ease of use, and adjunctive drugs and devices will enable PCI for the most complex patients and coronary anatomies.

Acknowledgment

The authors gratefully acknowledge Jason Kahn, Kim Dalton, and Scott Wallick for their expert editorial assistance.

REFERENCES

1. Sigwart U, Puel J, Mirkovitch V, et al: Intravascular stents to prevent occlusion and restenosis after transluminal angioplasty. N Engl J Med 316:701–706, 1987.
2. Serruys PW, Strauss BH, Beatt KJ, et al: Angiographic follow-up after placement of a self-expanding coronary-artery stent. N Engl J Med 324:13–17, 1991.
3. George BS, Voorhees WD, III, Roubin GS, et al: Multicenter investigation of coronary stenting to treat acute or threatened closure after percutaneous transluminal coronary angioplasty: clinical and angiographic outcomes. J Am Coll Cardiol 22:135–143, 1993.
4. Schatz RA, Baim DS, Leon M, et al: Clinical experience with the Palmaz-Schatz coronary stent. Initial results of a multicenter study. Circulation 83:148–161, 1991.
5. Fischman DL, Leon MB, Baim DS, et al: A randomized comparison of coronary-stent placement and balloon angioplasty in the treatment of coronary artery disease. Stent Restenosis Study Investigators. N Engl J Med 331:496–501, 1994.
6. Serruys PW, de Jaegere P, Kiemeneij F, et al: A comparison of balloon-expandable-stent implantation with balloon angioplasty in patients with coronary artery disease. Benestent Study Group. N Engl J Med 331:489–495, 1994.
7. Cutlip DE, Chhabra AG, Baim DS, et al: Beyond restenosis: five-year clinical outcomes from second-generation coronary stent trials. Circulation 110:1226–1230, 2004.
8. Kimura T, Abe K, Shizuta S, et al: Long-term clinical and angiographic follow-up after coronary stent placement in native coronary arteries. Circulation 105:2986–2991, 2002.
9. Yamaji K, Kimura T, Morimoto T, et al: Very long-term (15 to 20 years) clinical and angiographic outcome after coronary bare metal stent implantation/clinical perspective. Circulation Cardiovasc Intervent 3:468–475, 2010.
10. Nakamura S, Colombo A, Gaglione A, et al: Intracoronary ultrasound observations during stent implantation. Circulation 89:2026–2034, 1994.

11. Colombo A, Hall P, Nakamura S, et al: Intracoronary stenting without anticoagulation accomplished with intravascular ultrasound guidance. Circulation 91:1676–1688, 1995.
12. Bertrand ME, Legrand V, Boland J, et al: Randomized multicenter comparison of conventional anticoagulation versus antiplatelet therapy in unplanned and elective coronary stenting. The full anticoagulation versus aspirin and ticlopidine (FANTASTIC) study. Circulation 98:1597–1603, 1998.
13. Leon MB, Baim DS, Popma JJ, et al: A clinical trial comparing three antithrombotic-drug regimens after coronary-artery stenting. Stent Anticoagulation Restenosis Study Investigators. N Engl J Med 339:1665–1671, 1998.
14. Schomig A, Neumann FJ, Kastrati A, et al: A randomized comparison of antiplatelet and anticoagulant therapy after the placement of coronary-artery stents. N Engl J Med 334:1084–1089, 1996.
15. Urban P, Macaya C, Rupprecht HJ, et al: Randomized evaluation of anticoagulation versus antiplatelet therapy after coronary stent implantation in high-risk patients: the multicenter aspirin and ticlopidine trial after intracoronary stenting (MATTIS). Circulation 98:2126–2132, 1998.
16. Hehrlein C, Zimmermann M, Metz J, et al: Influence of surface texture and charge on the biocompatibility of endovascular stents. Coronary Artery Dis 6:581–586, 1995.
17. Garasic JM, Edelman ER, Squire JC, et al: Stent and artery geometry determine intimal thickening independent of arterial injury. Circulation 101:812–818, 2000.
18. Rogers C, Edelman ER: Endovascular stent design dictates experimental restenosis and thrombosis. Circulation 91:2995–3001, 1995.
19. Kastrati A, Mehilli J, Dirschinger J, et al: Intracoronary stenting and angiographic results: strut thickness effect on restenosis outcome (ISAR-STEREO) trial. Circulation 103:2816–2821, 2001.
20. van der Giessen WJ, Lincoff AM, Schwartz RS, et al: Marked inflammatory sequelae to implantation of biodegradable and

nonbiodegradable polymers in porcine coronary arteries. Circulation 94:1690–1697, 1996.
21. Han RO, Schwartz RS, Kobayashi Y, et al: Comparison of self-expanding and balloon-expandable stents for the reduction of restenosis. Am J Cardiol 88:253–259, 2001.
22. Shin ES, Garcia-Garcia HM, Okamura T, et al: Comparison of acute vessel wall injury after self-expanding stent and conventional balloon-expandable stent implantation: a study with optical coherence tomography. J Invas Cardiol 22:435–439, 2010.
23. Haude M, Hopp HW, Rupprecht HJ, et al: Immediate stent implantation versus conventional techniques for the treatment of abrupt vessel closure or symptomatic dissections after coronary balloon angioplasty. Am Heart J 140:e26, 2000.
24. Antoniucci D, Valenti R, Santoro GM, et al: Restenosis after coronary stenting in current clinical practice. Am Heart J 135:510–518, 1998.
25. Agostoni P, Biondi-Zoccai GG, Gasparini GL, et al: Is bare-metal stenting superior to balloon angioplasty for small vessel coronary artery disease? Evidence from a meta-analysis of randomized trials. Eur Heart J 26:881–889, 2005.
26. Nordmann AJ, Hengstler P, Leimenstoll BM, et al: Clinical outcomes of stents versus balloon angioplasty in non-acute coronary artery disease. A meta-analysis of randomized controlled trials. Eur Heart J 25:69–80, 2004.
27. Al Suwaidi J, Berger PB, Holmes DR, Jr: Coronary artery stents. JAMA 284:1828–1836, 2000.
28. Kuntz RE, Safian RD, Carrozza JP, et al: The importance of acute luminal diameter in determining restenosis after coronary atherectomy or stenting. Circulation 86:1827–1835, 1992.
29. Kuntz RE, Gibson CM, Nobuyoshi M, Baim DS: Generalized model of restenosis after conventional balloon angioplasty, stenting and directional atherectomy. J Am Coll Cardiol 21:15–25, 1993.

30. Morice MC, Serruys PW, Sousa JE, et al: A randomized comparison of a sirolimus-eluting stent with a standard stent for coronary revascularization. *N Engl J Med* 346:1773–1780, 2002.
31. Moses JW, Leon MB, Popma JJ, et al: Sirolimus-eluting stents versus standard stents in patients with stenosis in a native coronary artery. *N Engl J Med* 349:1315–1323, 2003.
32. Stone GW, Ellis SG, Cox DA, et al: A polymer-based, paclitaxel-eluting stent in patients with coronary artery disease. *N Engl J Med* 350:221–231, 2004.
33. Kirtane AJ, Gupta A, Iyengar S, et al: Safety and efficacy of drug-eluting and bare metal stents: comprehensive meta-analysis of randomized trials and observational studies. *Circulation* 119:3198–3206, 2009.
34. Leon MB, Kandzari DE, Eisenstein EL, et al: Late safety, efficacy, and cost-effectiveness of a zotarolimus-eluting stent compared with a paclitaxel-eluting stent in patients with de novo coronary lesions: 2-year follow-up from the ENDEAVOR IV trial (Randomized, Controlled Trial of the Medtronic Endeavor Drug [ABT-578] Eluting Coronary Stent System Versus the Taxus Paclitaxel-Eluting Coronary Stent System in De Novo Native Coronary Artery Lesions). *JACC Cardiovasc Intervent* 2:1208–1218, 2009.
35. Leon MB, Mauri L, Popma JJ, et al: A randomized comparison of the ENDEAVOR zotarolimus-eluting stent versus the TAXUS paclitaxel-eluting stent in de novo native coronary lesions 12-month outcomes from the ENDEAVOR IV trial. *J Am Coll Cardiol* 55:543–554, 2010.
36. Stone GW, Rizvi A, Newman W, et al: Everolimus-eluting versus paclitaxel-eluting stents in coronary artery disease. *N Engl J Med* 362:1663–1674, 2010.
37. Marx SO, Marks AR: Bench to bedside: the development of rapamycin and its application to stent restenosis. *Circulation* 104:852–855, 2001.
38. Daemen J, Serruys PW: Drug-eluting stent update 2007: part I. A survey of current and future generation drug-eluting stents: meaningful advances or more of the same? *Circulation* 116:316–328, 2007.
39. Axel DI, Kunert W, Goggelmann C, et al: Paclitaxel inhibits arterial smooth muscle cell proliferation and migration in vitro and in vivo using local drug delivery. *Circulation* 96:636–645, 1997.
40. Sollott SJ, Cheng L, Pauly RR, et al: Taxol inhibits neointimal smooth muscle cell accumulation after angioplasty in the rat. *J Clin Invest* 95:1869–1876, 1995.
41. Belotti D, Vergani V, Drudis T, et al: The microtubule-affecting drug paclitaxel has antiangiogenic activity. *Clin Cancer Res* 2:1843–1849, 1996.
42. Hui A, Min WX, Tang J, Cruz TF: Inhibition of activator protein 1 activity by paclitaxel suppresses interleukin-1-induced collagenase and stromelysin expression by bovine chondrocytes. *Arthritis Rheum* 41:869–876, 1998.
43. Lansky AJ, Costa RA, Mintz GS, et al: Non-polymer-based paclitaxel-coated coronary stents for the treatment of patients with de novo coronary lesions: angiographic follow-up of the DELIVER clinical trial. *Circulation* 109:1948–1954, 2004.
44. Finn AV, Joner M, Nakazawa G, et al: Pathological correlates of late drug-eluting stent thrombosis: strut coverage as a marker of endothelialization. *Circulation* 115:2435–2441, 2007.
45. Finn AV, Kolodgie FD, Harnek J, et al: Differential response of delayed healing and persistent inflammation at sites of overlapping sirolimus- or paclitaxel-eluting stents. *Circulation* 112:270–278, 2005.
46. Virmani R, Guagliumi G, Farb A, et al: Localized hypersensitivity and late coronary thrombosis secondary to a sirolimus-eluting stent: should we be cautious? *Circulation* 109:701–705, 2004.
47. Joner M, Nakazawa G, Finn AV, et al: Endothelial cell recovery between comparator polymer-based drug-eluting stents. *J Am Coll Cardiol* 52:333–342, 2008.
48. Cook S, Ladich E, Nakazawa G, et al: Correlation of intravascular ultrasound findings with histopathological analysis of thrombus aspirates in patients with very late drug-eluting stent thrombosis. *Circulation* 120:391–399, 2009.
49. Gallo R, Padurean A, Jayaraman T, et al: Inhibition of intimal thickening after balloon angioplasty in porcine coronary arteries by targeting regulators of the cell cycle. *Circulation* 99:2164–2170, 1999.
50. Suzuki T, Kopia G, Hayashi S-I, et al: Stent-based delivery of sirolimus reduces neointimal formation in a porcine coronary model. *Circulation* 104:1188–1193, 2001.
51. Sousa JE, Costa MA, Abizaid A, et al: Four-year angiographic and intravascular ultrasound follow-up of patients treated with sirolimus-eluting stents. *Circulation* 111:2326–2329, 2005.
52. Moses JW, Leon MB, Popma JJ, et al: Sirolimus-eluting stents versus standard stents in patients with stenosis in a native coronary artery. *N Engl J Med* 349:1315–1323, 2003.
53. Moussa ID, Moses JW, Kuntz RE, et al: The fate of patients with clinical recurrence after sirolimus-eluting stent implantation (a two-year follow-up analysis from the SIRIUS trial). *Am J Cardiol* 97:1582–1584, 2006.
54. Caixeta A, Leon MB, Lansky AJ, et al: 5-year clinical outcomes after sirolimus-eluting stent implantation insights from a patient-level pooled analysis of 4 randomized trials comparing sirolimus-eluting stents with bare-metal stents. *J Am Coll Cardiol* 54:894–902, 2009.
55. Drachman DE, Edelman ER, Seifert P, et al: Neointimal thickening after stent delivery of paclitaxel: change in composition and arrest of growth over six months. *J Am Coll Cardiol* 36:2325–2332, 2000.
56. Farb A, Heller PF, Shroff S, et al: Pathological analysis of local delivery of paclitaxel via a polymer-coated stent. *Circulation* 104:473–479, 2001.
57. Grube E, Silber S, Hauptmann KE, et al: TAXUS I: six- and twelve-month results from a randomized, double-blind trial on a slow-release paclitaxel-eluting stent for de novo coronary lesions. *Circulation* 107:38–42, 2003.
58. Colombo A, Drzewiecki J, Banning A, et al: Randomized study to assess the effectiveness of slow- and moderate-release polymer-based paclitaxel-eluting stents for coronary artery lesions. *Circulation* 108:788–794, 2003.
59. Stone GW, Ellis SG, Cox DA, et al: A polymer-based, paclitaxel-eluting stent in patients with coronary artery disease. *N Engl J Med* 350:221–231, 2004.
60. Stone GW, Ellis SG, Cannon L, et al: Comparison of a polymer-based paclitaxel-eluting stent with a bare metal stent in patients with complex coronary artery disease: a randomized controlled trial. *JAMA* 294:1215–1223, 2005.
61. Dawkins KD, Grube E, Guagliumi G, et al: Clinical efficacy of polymer-based paclitaxel-eluting stents in the treatment of complex, long coronary artery lesions from a multicenter, randomized trial: support for the use of drug-eluting stents in contemporary clinical practice. *Circulation* 112:3306–3313, 2005.
62. Turco MA, Ormiston JA, Popma JJ, et al: Polymer-based, paclitaxel-eluting TAXUS Liberte stent in de novo lesions: the pivotal TAXUS ATLAS trial. *J Am Coll Cardiol* 49:1676–1683, 2007.
63. Turco MA, Ormiston JA, Popma JJ, et al: Reduced risk of restenosis in small vessels and reduced risk of myocardial infarction in long lesions with the new thin-strut TAXUS Liberte stent: 1-year results from the TAXUS ATLAS program. *JACC Cardiovasc Intervent* 1:699–709, 2008.
64. Morice M-C, Colombo A, Meier B, et al: Sirolimus- vs Paclitaxel-Eluting Stents in De Novo Coronary Artery Lesions: The REALITY Trial: A Randomized Controlled Trial. *JAMA* 295:895–904, 2006.
65. Lee SW, Park SW, Kim YH, et al: A randomized comparison of sirolimus- versus Paclitaxel-eluting stent implantation in patients with diabetes mellitus. *J Am Coll Cardiol* 52:727–733, 2008.
66. Galloe AM, Thuesen L, Kelbaek H, et al: Comparison of paclitaxel- and sirolimus-eluting stents in everyday clinical practice: the SORT OUT II randomized trial. *JAMA* 77:494–501, 2011.
67. Petronio AS, De Carlo M, Branchitta G, et al: Randomized comparison of sirolimus and paclitaxel drug-eluting stents for long lesions in the left anterior descending artery: an intravascular ultrasound study. *J Am Coll Cardiol* 49:539–546, 2007.
68. Birkmeier KA, Kastrati A, Byrne RA, et al: Five-year clinical outcomes of sirolimus eluting versus paclitaxel-eluting stents in high-risk patients. *Catheter Cardiovasc Intervent*. 2010.
69. Stettler C, Wandel S, Allemann S, et al: Outcomes associated with drug-eluting and bare-metal stents: a collaborative network meta-analysis. *Lancet* 370:937–948, 2007.
70. Douglas PS, Brennan JM, Anstrom KJ, et al: Clinical effectiveness of coronary stents in elderly persons: results from 262,700 Medicare patients in the American College of Cardiology-National Cardiovascular Data Registry. *J Am Coll Cardiol* 53:1629–1641, 2009.
71. Mauri L, Silbaugh TS, Garg P, et al: Drug-eluting or bare-metal stents for acute myocardial infarction. *N Engl J Med* 359:1330–1342, 2008.
72. Liu T-Y, Lin W-C, Huang L-Y, et al: Surface characteristics and hemocompatibility of PAN/PVDF blend membranes. *Polymers Adv Technol* 16:413–419, 2005.
73. Lin JC, Tiong SL, Chen CY: Surface characterization and platelet adhesion studies on fluorocarbons prepared by plasma-induced graft polymerization. *J Biomater Sci Polym Ed* 11:701–714, 2000.
74. Simon C, Palmaz JC, Sprague EA: Influence of topography on endothelialization of stents: clues for new designs. *J Long Term Eff Med Implants* 10:143–151, 2000.
75. Serruys PW, Ong AT, Piek JJ, et al: A randomized comparison of a durable polymer Everolimus-eluting stent with a bare metal coronary stent: The SPIRIT first trial. *EuroIntervention* 1:58–65, 2005.
76. Byrne RA: ISAR-TEST-4: Two-year clinical and angiographic outcomes from a prospective randomized trial of everolimus-eluting stents and sirolimus-eluting stents in patients with coronary artery disease, Washington, DC, 2010, Transcatheter Cardiovascular Therapeutics.
77. Grube E: SPIRIT V diabetic RCT: 9 month angiographic and 1 year clinical follow-up, Washington, DC, 2010, Transcatheter Cardiovascular Therapeutics.
78. Jensen LO: The SORT OUT IV Trial: A prospective, randomized trial of everolimus-eluting and sirolimus-eluting stents in patients with coronary artery disease, Washington, DC, 2010, Transcatheter Cardiovascular Therapeutics.
79. Smits PC: COMPARE trial: 2-year follow-up, Washington, DC, 2010, Transcatheter Cardiovascular Therapeutics.
80. Kim H-S: EXCELLENT: A prospective randomized trial of everolimus-eluting stents and sirolimus-eluting stents in patients with coronary artery disease, Washington, DC, 2010, Transcatheter Cardiovascular Therapeutics.
81. Ribichini F: EXECUTIVE: A prospective randomized trial of everolimus-eluting stents compared to paclitaxel-eluting stents in patients with multivessel coronary artery disease, Washington, DC, 2010, Transcatheter Cardiovascular Therapeutics.
82. Serruys PW, Ruygrok P, Neuzner J, et al: A randomised comparison of an everolimus-eluting coronary stent with a paclitaxel-eluting coronary stent:the SPIRIT II trial. *EuroIntervention* 2:286–294, 2006.
83. Stone GW: A large-scale randomized comparison of everolimus-eluting and paclitaxel-eluting stents: Two-year clinical outcomes from the SPIRIT IV trial, Washington, DC, 2010, Transcatheter Cardiovascular Therapeutics.
84. Stone GW: Comparison of everolimus-eluting and paclitaxel-eluting stents: First report of the four-year clinical outcomes from the SPIRIT III trial, Washington, DC, 2010, Transcatheter Cardiovascular Therapeutics.
85. Stone GW, Midei M, Newman W, et al: Comparison of an everolimus-eluting stent and a paclitaxel-eluting stent in patients with coronary artery disease: a randomized trial. *JAMA* 299:1903–1913, 2008.
86. Kim Y-H: ESSENCE-DIABETES trial: Randomized comparison of everolimus- eluting stent versus sirolimus-eluting stent implantation for de novo coronary artery disease in patients with diabetes mellitus, Washington, DC, 2010, Transcatheter Cardiovascular Therapeutics.
87. Serruys PW, Silber S, Garg S, et al: Comparison of zotarolimus-eluting and everolimus-eluting coronary stents. *N Engl J Med* 363:136–146, 2010.
88. Kedhi E, Joesoef KS, McFadden E, et al: Second-generation everolimus-eluting and paclitaxel-eluting stents in real-life practice (COMPARE): a randomised trial. *Lancet* 375:201–209, 2010.
89. Whelan DM, van der Giessen WJ, Krabbendam SC, et al: Biocompatibility of phosphorylcholine coated stents in normal porcine coronary arteries. *Heart* 83:338–345, 2000.
90. Meredith IT, Ormiston J, Whitbourn R, et al: First-in-human study of the Endeavor ABT-578-eluting phosphorylcholine-encapsulated stent system in de novo native coronary artery lesions: Endeavor I Trial. *EuroIntervention* 1:157–164, 2005.
91. Mauri L, Orav EJ, Kuntz RE: Late loss in lumen diameter and binary restenosis for drug-eluting stent comparison. *Circulation* 111:3435–3442, 2005.
92. Pocock SJ, Lansky AJ, Mehran R, et al: Angiographic surrogate end points in drug-eluting stent trials: a systematic evaluation based on individual patient data from 11 randomized, controlled trials. *J Am Coll Cardiol* 51:23–32, 2008.
93. Eisenstein EL, Wijns W, Fajadet J, et al: Long-term clinical and economic analysis of the Endeavor drug-eluting stent versus the Driver bare-metal stent: 4-year results from the ENDEAVOR II trial (Randomized Controlled Trial to Evaluate the Safety and Efficacy of the Medtronic AVE ABT-578 Eluting Driver Coronary Stent in De Novo Native Coronary Artery Lesions). *JACC Cardiovasc Intervent* 2:1178–1187, 2009.
94. Fajadet J, Wijns W, Laarman GJ, et al: Randomized, double-blind, multicenter study of the Endeavor zotarolimus-eluting phosphorylcholine-encapsulated stent for treatment of native coronary artery lesions. Clinical and angiographic results of the ENDEAVOR II trial. *Minerva Cardioangiol* 55:1–18, 2007.
95. Kandzari DE, Leon MB, Popma JJ, et al: Comparison of zotarolimus-eluting and sirolimus-eluting stents in patients with native coronary artery disease: a randomized controlled trial. *J Am Coll Cardiol* 48:2440–2447, 2006.
96. Leon MB, Nikolsky E, Cutlip DE, et al: Improved late clinical safety with zotarolimus-eluting stents compared with paclitaxel-eluting stents in patients with de novo coronary lesions: 3-year follow-up from the ENDEAVOR IV (Randomized Comparison of Zotarolimus- and Paclitaxel-Eluting Stents in Patients With Coronary Artery Disease) trial. *JACC Cardiovasc Intervent* 3:1043–1050, 2010.
97. Rasmussen K, Maeng M, Kaltoft A, et al: Efficacy and safety of zotarolimus-eluting and sirolimus-eluting coronary stents in routine clinical care (SORT OUT III): a randomised controlled superiority trial. *Lancet* 375:1090–1099, 2010.
98. Byrne RA, Kastrati A, Tiroch K, et al: 2-year clinical and angiographic outcomes from a randomized trial of polymer-free dual drug-eluting stents versus polymer-based Cypher and Endeavor [corrected] drug-eluting stents. *J Am Coll Cardiol* 55:2536–2543, 2010.
99. Byrne RA, Mehilli J, Iijima R, et al: A polymer-free dual drug-eluting stent in patients with coronary artery disease: a randomized trial vs. polymer-based drug-eluting stents. *Eur Heart J* 30:923–931, 2009.
100. Park DW, Kim YH, Yun SC, et al: Comparison of zotarolimus-eluting stents with sirolimus- and paclitaxel-eluting stents for coronary revascularization: the ZEST (comparison of the efficacy and safety of zotarolimus-eluting stent with sirolimus-eluting and paclitaxel-eluting stent for coronary lesions) randomized trial. *J Am Coll Cardiol* 56:1187–1195, 2010.
101. Park SJ: The ZEST trial: 2-year final outcomes, Washington, DC, 2010, Transcatheter Cardiovascular Therapeutics.
102. Meredith IT, Worthley S, Whitbourn R, et al: Clinical and angiographic results with the next-generation resolute stent system: a prospective, multicenter, first-in-human trial. *JACC Cardiovasc Intervent* 2:977–985, 2009.
103. Grube E, Hauptmann KE, Buellesfeld L, et al: Six-month results of a randomized study to evaluate safety and efficacy of a Biolimus A9 eluting stent with a biodegradable polymer coating. *EuroIntervention* 1:53–57, 2005.
104. Chevalier B, Silber S, Park SJ, et al: Randomized comparison of the Nobori Biolimus A9-eluting coronary stent with the Taxus Liberte paclitaxel eluting coronary stent in patients with stenosis

in native coronary arteries: the NOBORI 1 trial—phase 2. *Circ Cardiovasc Intervent* 2:188–195, 2009.
105. Ostojic M, Sagic D, Beleslin B, et al: First clinical comparison of Nobori -Biolimus A9 eluting stents with Cypher- Sirolimus eluting stents: Nobori Core nine months angiographic and one year clinical outcomes. *EuroIntervention* 3:574–579, 2008.
106. Windecker S, Serruys PW, Wandel S, et al: Biolimus-eluting stent with biodegradable polymer versus sirolimus-eluting stent with durable polymer for coronary revascularisation (LEADERS): a randomised non-inferiority trial. *Lancet* 372:1163–1173, 2008.
107. Serruys PW: LEADERS: Three-year follow-up from a prospective randomized trial of biolimus a9-eluting stents and sirolimus-eluting stents in patients with coronary artery disease, Washington, DC, 2010, Transcatheter Cardiovascular Therapeutics.
108. Virmani R, Burke AP, Farb A, Kolodgie FD: Pathology of the vulnerable plaque. *J Am Coll Cardiol* 47:C13-C18, 2006.
109. Keeley EC, Boura JA, Grines CL: Primary angioplasty versus intravenous thrombolytic therapy for acute myocardial infarction: a quantitative review of 23 randomised trials. *Lancet* 361:13–20, 2003.
110. De Luca G, Suryapranata H, Stone GW, et al: Coronary stenting versus balloon angioplasty for acute myocardial infarction: a meta-regression analysis of randomized trials. *Int J Cardiol* 126:37–44, 2008.
111. Nakazawa G, Finn AV, Joner M, et al: Delayed arterial healing and increased late stent thrombosis at culprit sites after drug-eluting stent placement for acute myocardial infarction patients: an autopsy study. *Circulation* 118:1138–1145, 2008.
112. Cannon CP, Harrington RA, James S, et al: Comparison of ticagrelor with clopidogrel in patients with a planned invasive strategy for acute coronary syndromes (PLATO): a randomised double-blind study. *Lancet* 375:283–293, 2010.
113. Montalescot G, Wiviott SD, Braunwald E, et al: Prasugrel compared with clopidogrel in patients undergoing percutaneous coronary intervention for ST-elevation myocardial infarction (TRITON-TIMI 38): double-blind, randomised controlled trial. *Lancet* 373:723–731, 2009.
114. Brar SS, Leon MB, Stone GW, et al: Use of drug-eluting stents in acute myocardial infarction: a systematic review and meta-analysis. *J Am Coll Cardiol* 53:1677–1689, 2009.
115. Pinto DS, Stone GW, Ellis SG, et al: Impact of routine angiographic follow-up on the clinical benefits of paclitaxel-eluting stents: results from the TAXUS-IV trial. *J Am Coll Cardiol* 48:32–36, 2006.
116. Topol EJ: Coronary angioplasty for acute myocardial infarction. *Ann Intern Med* 109:970–980, 1988.
117. Spertus JA, Kettelkamp R, Vance C, et al: Prevalence, predictors, and outcomes of premature discontinuation of thienopyridine therapy after drug-eluting stent placement: results from the PREMIER registry. *Circulation* 113:2803–2809, 2006.
118. Stone GW: HORIZONS-AMI: three-year follow-up from a prospective randomized trial of antithrombin strategies and drug-eluting stents in patients with acute myocardial infarction undergoing primary angioplasty, Washington, DC, 2010, Transcatheter Cardiovascular Therapeutics.
119. Stone GW, Lansky AJ, Pocock SJ, et al: Paclitaxel-eluting stents versus bare-metal stents in acute myocardial infarction. *N Engl J Med* 360:1946–1959, 2009.
120. Stone GW, Parise H, Witzenbichler B, et al: Selection criteria for drug-eluting versus bare-metal stents and the impact of routine angiographic follow-up: 2-year insights from the HORIZONS-AMI (Harmonizing Outcomes With Revascularization and Stents in Acute Myocardial Infarction) trial. *J Am Coll Cardiol* 56:1597–1604, 2010.
121. Di Lorenzo E, De Luca G, Sauro R, et al: The PASEO (PaclitAxel or Sirolimus-Eluting Stent Versus Bare Metal Stent in Primary Angioplasty) randomized trial. *JACC Cardiovasc Intervent* 2:515–523, 2009.
122. Juwana YB, Suryapranata H, Ottervanger JP, et al: Comparison of rapamycin- and paclitaxel-eluting stents in patients undergoing primary percutaneous coronary intervention for ST-elevation myocardial infarction. *Am J Cardiol* 104:205–209, 2009.
123. Lee CW, Park DW, Lee SH, et al: Comparison of the efficacy and safety of zotarolimus-, sirolimus-, and paclitaxel-eluting stents in patients with ST-elevation myocardial infarction. *Am J Cardiol* 104:1370–1376, 2009.
124. Kedhi E: COMPARE-AMI: Two-year outcomes from a prospective randomized trial of everolimus-eluting stents compared to paclitaxel-eluting stents in patients with STEMI, Washington, DC, 2010, Transcatheter Cardiovascular Therapeutics.
125. Elezi S, Kastrati A, Pache J, et al: Diabetes mellitus and the clinical and angiographic outcome after coronary stent placement. *J Am Coll Cardiol* 32:1866–1873, 1998.
126. Singh M, Gersh BJ, McClelland RL, et al: Clinical and angiographic predictors of restenosis after percutaneous coronary intervention: insights from the Prevention of Restenosis With Tranilast and Its Outcomes (PRESTO) trial. *Circulation* 109:2727–2731, 2004.
127. Fajadet J, Wijns W, Laarman GJ, et al: Randomized, double-blind, multicenter study of the Endeavor zotarolimus-eluting phosphorylcholine-encapsulated stent for treatment of native coronary artery lesions: clinical and angiographic results of the ENDEAVOR II trial. *Circulation* 114:798–806, 2006.
128. Hermiller JB, Raizner A, Cannon L, et al: Outcomes with the polymer-based paclitaxel-eluting TAXUS stent in patients with diabetes mellitus: the TAXUS-IV trial. *J Am Coll Cardiol* 45:1172–1179, 2005.
129. Moussa I, Leon MB, Baim DS, et al: Impact of sirolimus-eluting stents on outcome in diabetic patients: a SIRIUS (SIRolImUS-coated Bx Velocity balloon-expandable stent in the treatment of patients with de novo coronary artery lesions) substudy. *Circulation* 109:2273–2278, 2004.
130. Dawkins KD, Stone GW, Colombo A, et al: Integrated analysis of medically treated diabetic patients in the TAXUS(R) program: benefits across stent platforms, paclitaxel release formulations, and diabetic treatments. *EuroIntervention* 2:61–68, 2006.
131. Mitsuuchi Y, Johnson SW, Selvakumaran M, et al: The phosphatidylinositol 3-kinase/AKT signal transduction pathway plays a critical role in the expression of p21WAF1/CIP1/SDI1 induced by cisplatin and paclitaxel. *Cancer Res* 60:5390–5394, 2000.
132. Rocic P: Differential phosphoinositide 3-kinase signaling: implications for PTCA? *Am J Physiol Heart Circ Physiol* 297:H1970-H1971, 2009.
133. Morice MC, Colombo A, Meier B, et al: Sirolimus- vs paclitaxel-eluting stents in de novo coronary artery lesions: the REALITY trial: a randomized controlled trial. *JAMA* 295:895–904, 2006.
134. Dibra A, Kastrati A, Mehilli J, et al: Paclitaxel-eluting or sirolimus-eluting stents to prevent restenosis in diabetic patients. *N Engl J Med* 353:663–670, 2005.
135. Stone GW, Kedhi E, Serruys PW: Are the Clinical Outcomes with Everolimus-eluting versus Paclitaxel-eluting Coronary Stents Different in Patients With and Without Diabetes? Insights from the SPIRIT II, SPIRIT III, SPIRIT IV and COMPARE Randomized Trials. *Circulation* 122:A17024, 2010.
136. Daemen J, Boersma E, Flather M, et al: Long-term safety and efficacy of percutaneous coronary intervention with stenting and coronary artery bypass surgery for multivessel coronary artery disease: a meta-analysis with 5-year patient-level data from the ARTS, ERACI-II, MASS-II, and SoS trials. *Circulation* 118:1146–1154, 2008.
137. Farkouh ME, Dangas G, Leon MB, et al: Design of the Future REvascularization Evaluation in patients with Diabetes mellitus: Optimal management of Multivessel disease (FREEDOM) Trial. *Am Heart J* 155:215–223, 2008.
138. Hlatky MA, Boothroyd DB, Bravata DM, et al: Coronary artery bypass surgery compared with percutaneous coronary interventions for multivessel disease: a collaborative analysis of individual patient data from ten randomised trials. *Lancet* 373:1190–1197, 2009.
139. Booth J, Clayton T, Pepper J, et al: Randomized, controlled trial of coronary artery bypass surgery versus percutaneous coronary intervention in patients with multivessel coronary artery disease: six-year follow-up from the Stent or Surgery Trial (SoS). *Circulation* 118:381–388, 2008.
140. Hueb W, Lopes NH, Gersh BJ, et al: Five-year follow-up of the Medicine, Angioplasty, or Surgery Study (MASS II): a randomized controlled clinical trial of 3 therapeutic strategies for multivessel coronary artery disease. *Circulation* 115:1082–1089, 2007.
141. Rodriguez AE, Baldi J, Fernandez Pereira C, et al: Five-year follow-up of the Argentine randomized trial of coronary angioplasty with stenting versus coronary bypass surgery in patients with multiple vessel disease (ERACI II). *J Am Coll Cardiol* 46:582–588, 2005.
142. Serruys PW, Ong AT, van Herwerden LA, et al: Five-year outcomes after coronary stenting versus bypass surgery for the treatment of multivessel disease: the final analysis of the Arterial Revascularization Therapies Study (ARTS) randomized trial. *J Am Coll Cardiol* 46:575–581, 2005.
143. O'Keefe JH, Jr, Hartzler GO, Rutherford BD, et al: Left main coronary angioplasty: early and late results of 127 acute and elective procedures. *Am J Cardiol* 64:144–147, 1989.
144. Tan WA, Tamai H, Park SJ, et al: Long-term clinical outcomes after unprotected left main trunk percutaneous revascularization in 279 patients. *Circulation* 104:1609–1614, 2001.
145. Erglis A, Narbute I, Kumsars I, et al: A randomized comparison of paclitaxel-eluting stents versus bare-metal stents for treatment of unprotected left main coronary artery stenosis. *J Am Coll Cardiol* 50:491–497, 2007.
146. Mehilli J, Kastrati A, Byrne RA, et al: Paclitaxel- versus sirolimus-eluting stents for unprotected left main coronary artery disease. *J Am Coll Cardiol* 53:1760–1768, 2009.
147. Buszman PE, Kiesz SR, Bochenek A, et al: Acute and late outcomes of unprotected left main stenting in comparison with surgical revascularization. *J Am Coll Cardiol* 51:538–545, 2008.
148. Serruys PW, Morice MC, Kappetein AP, et al: Percutaneous coronary intervention versus coronary-artery bypass grafting for severe coronary artery disease. *N Engl J Med* 360:961–972, 2009.
149. Wood S: Three-year SYNTAX results extend CABG advantage to intermediate-risk patients. TheHeart.org 2010.
150. Chen SL, Chen JP, Mintz G, et al: Comparison between the NERS (New Risk Stratification) score and the SYNTAX (Synergy between Percutaneous Coronary Intervention with Taxus and Cardiac Surgery) score in outcome prediction for unprotected left main stenting. *JACC Cardiovasc Intervent* 3:632–641, 2010.
151. Garg S, Sarno G, Garcia-Garcia HM, et al: A new tool for the risk stratification of patients with complex coronary artery disease: the clinical SYNTAX score. *Circ Cardiovasc Intervent* 3:317–326, 2010.
152. Wijns W, Kolh P, Danchin N, et al: Guidelines on myocardial revascularization: The Task Force on Myocardial Revascularization of the European Society of Cardiology (ESC) and the European Association for Cardio-Thoracic Surgery (EACTS). *Eur Heart J* 31:2501–2555, 2010.
153. Rassen JA, Mittleman MA, et al: Safety and effectiveness of bivalirudin in routine care of patients undergoing percutaneous coronary intervention. *Eur Heart J* 31:561–572, 2010.
154. Park SJ, Kim YH, Park DW, et al: Impact of intravascular ultrasound guidance on long-term mortality in stenting for unprotected left main coronary artery stenosis. *Circ Cardiovasc Intervent* 2:167–177, 2009.
155. Tonino PA, De Bruyne B, Pijls NH, et al: Fractional flow reserve versus angiography for guiding percutaneous coronary intervention. *N Engl J Med* 360:213–224, 2009.
156. Stone GW, Kandzari DE, Mehran R, et al: Percutaneous recanalization of chronically occluded coronary arteries: a consensus document: part I. *Circulation* 112:2364–2372, 2005.
157. Stone GW, Reifart NJ, Moussa I, et al: Percutaneous recanalization of chronically occluded coronary arteries: a consensus document: part II. *Circulation* 112:2530–2537, 2005.
158. Suttorp MJ, Laarman GJ, Rahel BM, et al: Primary Stenting of Totally Occluded Native Coronary Arteries II (PRISON II): a randomized comparison of bare metal stent implantation with sirolimus-eluting stent implantation for the treatment of total coronary occlusions. *Circulation* 114:921–998, 2006.
159. Colmenarez HJ, Escaned J, Fernandez C, et al: Efficacy and safety of drug-eluting stents in chronic total coronary occlusion recanalization: a systematic review and meta-analysis. *J Am Coll Cardiol* 55:1854–1866, 2010.
160. Kandzari DE, Rao SV, Moses JW, et al: Clinical and angiographic outcomes with sirolimus-eluting stents in total coronary occlusions: the ACROSS/TOSCA-4 (Approaches to Chronic Occlusions With Sirolimus-Eluting Stents/Total Occlusion Study of Coronary Arteries-4) trial. *JACC Cardiovasc Intervent* 2:97–106, 2009.
161. American College of Cardiology/American Heart Association Task Force on Practice Guidelines, Evidence WGtRN, Update the ACC/AHA/SCAI Guideline Update for Percutaneous Coronary Intervention WoBotWC, et al: 2007 Focused Update of the ACC/AHA/SCAI 2005 Guideline Update for Percutaneous Coronary Intervention. *J Am Coll Cardiol* 51:172–209, 2008.
162. Brar SS, Gray WA, Dangas G, et al: Bifurcation stenting with drug-eluting stents: a systematic review and meta-analysis of randomised trials. *EuroIntervention* 5:475–484, 2009.
163. Fanggiday JC, Stella PR, Guyomi SH, et al: Safety and efficacy of drug-eluting balloons in percutaneous treatment of bifurcation lesions the DEBIUT (drug-eluting balloon in bifurcaton utrecht) registry. *Catheter Cardiovasc Intervent* 71:629–635, 2008.
164. Stella PR: Are drug-eluting balloons likely to assist bifurcation stenting? Rationale and the DEBIUT Experience, Washington, D.C., 2010, Transcatheter Cardiovsacular Therapeutics.
165. Hasegawa T, Ako J, Koo BK, et al: Analysis of left main coronary artery bifurcation lesions treated with biolimus-eluting DEVAX AXXESS plus nitinol self-expanding stent: intravascular ultrasound results of the AXXENT trial. *Catheter Cardiovasc Intervent* 73:34–41, 2009.
166. Verheye S, Agostoni P, Dubois CL, et al: 9-month clinical, angiographic, and intravascular ultrasound results of a prospective evaluation of the Axxess self-expanding biolimus A9-eluting stent in coronary bifurcation lesions: the DIVERGE (Drug-Eluting Stent Intervention for Treating Side Branches Effectively) study. *J Am Coll Cardiol* 53:1031–1039, 2009.
167. Verheye S, Grube E, Ramcharitar S, et al: First-in-man (FIM) study of the Stentys bifurcation stent–30 days results. *EuroIntervention* 4:566–571, 2009.
168. Ormiston JA, Lefevre T, Grube E, et al: First human use of the TAXUS Petal paclitaxel-eluting bifurcation stent. *EuroIntervention* 6:46–53, 2010.
169. Hanekamp CE, Koolen JJ, Den Heijer P, et al: Randomized study to compare balloon angioplasty and elective stent implantation in venous bypass grafts: the Venestent study. *Catheter Cardiovasc Intervent* 60:452–457, 2003.
170. Savage MP, Douglas JS, Jr, Fischman DL, et al: Stent placement compared with balloon angioplasty for obstructed coronary bypass grafts. Saphenous Vein De Novo Trial Investigators. *N Engl J Med* 337:740–747, 1997.
171. Brilakis ES, Lichtenwalter C, de Lemos JA, et al: A randomized controlled trial of a paclitaxel-eluting stent versus a similar bare-metal stent in saphenous vein graft lesions the SOS (Stenting of Saphenous Vein Grafts) trial. *J Am Coll Cardiol* 53:919–928, 2009.
172. Vermeersch P, Agostoni P, Verheye S, et al: Randomized double-blind comparison of sirolimus-eluting stent versus bare-metal stent implantation in diseased saphenous vein grafts: six-month angiographic, intravascular ultrasound, and clinical follow-up of the RRISC trial. *J Am Coll Cardiol* 48:2423–2431, 2006.
173. Vermeersch P, Agostoni P, Verheye S, et al: Increased late mortality after sirolimus-eluting stents versus bare-metal stents in diseased saphenous vein grafts: results from the randomized DELAYED RRISC Trial. *J Am Coll Cardiol* 50:261–267, 2007.
174. Rodes-Cabau J, Bertrand OF, Larose E, et al: Comparison of plaque sealing with paclitaxel-eluting stents versus medical therapy for the treatment of moderate nonsignificant saphenous vein graft lesions: the moderate vein graft lesion stenting with the taxus stent and intravascular ultrasound (VELETI) pilot trial. *Circulation* 120:1978–1986, 2009.
175. Holmes DR, Jr, Kereiakes DJ, Garg S, et al: Stent thrombosis. *J Am Coll Cardiol* 56:1357–1365, 2010.

176. Iakovou I, Schmidt T, Bonizzoni E, et al: Incidence, predictors, and outcome of thrombosis after successful implantation of drug-eluting stents. *JAMA* 293:2126–2130, 2005.
177. Burzotta F, Parma A, Pristipino C, et al: Angiographic and clinical outcome of invasively managed patients with thrombosed coronary bare metal or drug-eluting stents: the OPTIMIST study. *Eur Heart J* 29:3011–3021, 2008.
178. van Werkum JW, Heestermans AA, de Korte FI, et al: Long-term clinical outcome after a first angiographically confirmed coronary stent thrombosis: an analysis of 431 cases. *Circulation* 119:828–834, 2009.
179. Cutlip DE, Windecker S, Mehran R, et al: Clinical end points in coronary stent trials: a case for standardized definitions. *Circulation* 115:2344–2351, 2007.
180. Doyle B, Rihal CS, O'Sullivan CJ, et al: Outcomes of stent thrombosis and restenosis during extended follow-up of patients treated with bare-metal coronary stents. *Circulation* 116:2391–2398, 2007.
181. Ellis SG, Stone GW, Cox DA, et al: Long-term safety and efficacy with paclitaxel-eluting stents: 5-year final results of the TAXUS IV clinical trial (TAXUS IV-SR: Treatment of De Novo Coronary Disease Using a Single Paclitaxel-Eluting Stent). *JACC Cardiovasc Intervent* 2:1248–1259, 2009.
182. Weisz G, Leon MB, Holmes DR Jr, et al: Five-year follow-up after sirolimus-eluting stent implantation results of the SIRIUS (Sirolimus-Eluting Stent in De-Novo Native Coronary Lesions) Trial. *J Am Coll Cardiol* 53:1488–1497, 2009.
183. Wenaweser P, Daemen J, Zwahlen M, et al: Incidence and correlates of drug-eluting stent thrombosis in routine clinical practice. 4-year results from a large 2-institutional cohort study. *J Am Coll Cardiol* 52:1134–1140, 2008.
184. Stone GW, Moses JW, Ellis SG, et al: Safety and efficacy of sirolimus- and paclitaxel-eluting coronary stents. *N Engl J Med* 356:998–1008, 2007.
185. Mauri L, Hsieh WH, Massaro JM, et al: Stent thrombosis in randomized clinical trials of drug-eluting stents. *N Engl J Med* 356:1020–1029, 2007.
186. Stone GW, Ellis SG, Colombo A, et al: Offsetting impact of thrombosis and restenosis on the occurrence of death and myocardial infarction after paclitaxel-eluting and bare metal stent implantation. *Circulation* 115:2842–2847, 2007.
187. Finn AV, Nakazawa G, Ladich E, et al: Does underlying plaque morphology play a role in vessel healing after drug-eluting stent implantation? *JACC Cardiovasc Imaging* 1:485–488, 2008.
188. Aoki J, Lansky AJ, Mehran R, et al: Early stent thrombosis in patients with acute coronary syndromes treated with drug-eluting and bare metal stents: the Acute Catheterization and Urgent Intervention Triage Strategy trial. *Circulation* 119:687–698, 2009.
189. Cutlip DE, Baim DS, Ho KK, et al: Stent thrombosis in the modern era: a pooled analysis of multicenter coronary stent clinical trials. *Circulation* 103:1967–1971, 2001.
190. Kuchulakanti PK, Chu WW, Torguson R, et al: Correlates and long-term outcomes of angiographically proven stent thrombosis with sirolimus- and paclitaxel-eluting stents. *Circulation* 113:1108–1113, 2006.
191. Mishkel GJ, Moore AL, Markwell S, et al: Correlates of late and very late thrombosis of drug eluting stents. *Am Heart J* 156:141–147, 2008.
192. Cook S, Ladich E, Nakazawa G, et al: Correlation of intravascular ultrasound findings with histopathological analysis of thrombus aspirates in patients with very late drug-eluting stent thrombosis. *Circulation* 120:391–399, 2009.
193. Fujii K, Carlier SG, Mintz GS, et al: Stent underexpansion and residual reference segment stenosis are related to stent thrombosis after sirolimus-eluting stent implantation: an intravascular ultrasound study. *J Am Coll Cardiol* 45:995–998, 2005.
194. Liu X, Doi H, Maehara A, et al: A volumetric intravascular ultrasound comparison of early drug-eluting stent thrombosis versus restenosis. *JACC Cardiovasc Intervent* 2:428–434, 2009.
195. Okabe T, Mintz GS, Buch AN, et al: Intravascular ultrasound parameters associated with stent thrombosis after drug-eluting stent deployment. *Am J Cardiol* 100:615–620, 2007.
196. Aoki J, Nakazawa G, Tanabe K, et al: Incidence and clinical impact of coronary stent fracture after sirolimus-eluting stent implantation. *Catheter Cardiovasc Intervent* 69:380–386, 2007.
197. Nakazawa G, Finn AV, Vorpahl M, et al: Incidence and predictors of drug-eluting stent fracture in human coronary artery a pathologic analysis. *J Am Coll Cardiol* 54:1924–1931, 2009.
198. Cook S, Wenaweser P, Togni M, et al: Incomplete stent apposition and very late stent thrombosis after drug-eluting stent implantation. *Circulation* 115:2426–2434, 2007.
199. Hassan AK, Bergheanu SC, Stijnen T, et al: Late stent malapposition risk is higher after drug-eluting stent compared with bare-metal stent implantation and associates with late stent thrombosis. *Eur Heart J* 31:1172–1180, 2010.
200. Joner M, Finn AV, Farb A, et al: Pathology of drug-eluting stents in humans: delayed healing and late thrombotic risk. *J Am Coll Cardiol* 48:193–202, 2006.
201. Kotani J, Awata M, Nanto S, et al: Incomplete neointimal coverage of sirolimus-eluting stents: angioscopic findings. *J Am Coll Cardiol* 47:2108–2111, 2006.
202. Higo T, Ueda Y, Oyabu J, et al: Atherosclerotic and thrombogenic neointima formed over sirolimus drug-eluting stent: an angioscopic study. *JACC Cardiovasc Imaging* 2:616–624, 2009.
203. Roy P, Steinberg DH, Sushinsky SJ, et al: The potential clinical utility of intravascular ultrasound guidance in patients undergoing percutaneous coronary intervention with drug-eluting stents. *Eur Heart J* 29:1851–1857, 2008.
204. Hall P, Nakamura S, Maiello L, et al: A randomized comparison of combined ticlopidine and aspirin therapy versus aspirin therapy alone after successful intravascular ultrasound-guided stent implantation. *Circulation* 93:215–222, 1996.
205. Bertrand ME, Rupprecht HJ, Urban P, et al: Double-blind study of the safety of clopidogrel with and without a loading dose in combination with aspirin compared with ticlopidine in combination with aspirin after coronary stenting: the clopidogrel aspirin stent international cooperative study (CLASSICS). *Circulation* 102:624–629, 2000.
206. Airoldi F, Colombo A, Morici N, et al: Incidence and predictors of drug-eluting stent thrombosis during and after discontinuation of thienopyridine treatment. *Circulation* 116:745–754, 2007.
207. van Werkum JW, Heestermans AA, Zomer AC, et al: Predictors of coronary stent thrombosis: the Dutch Stent Thrombosis Registry. *J Am Coll Cardiol* 53:1399–1409, 2009.
208. Brar SS, Kim J, Brar SK, et al: Long-term outcomes by clopidogrel duration and stent type in a diabetic population with de novo coronary artery lesions. *J Am Coll Cardiol* 51:2220–2227, 2008.
209. Eisenstein EL, Anstrom KJ, Kong DF, et al: Clopidogrel use and long-term clinical outcomes after drug-eluting stent implantation. *JAMA* 297:159–168, 2007.
210. Harjai KJ, Shenoy C, Orshaw P, Boura J: Dual antiplatelet therapy for more than 12 months after percutaneous coronary intervention: insights from the Guthrie PCI Registry. *Heart* 95:1579–1586, 2009.
211. Park SJ, Park DW, Kim YH, et al: Duration of dual antiplatelet therapy after implantation of drug-eluting stents. *N Engl J Med* 362:1374–1382, 2010.
212. Mintz GS, Popma JJ, Hong MK, et al: Intravascular ultrasound to discern device-specific effects and mechanisms of restenosis. *Am J Cardiol* 78:18–22, 1996.
213. Chen MS, John JM, Chew DP, et al: Bare metal stent restenosis is not a benign clinical entity. *Am Heart J* 151:1260–1264, 2006.
214. Nayak AK, Kawamura A, Nesto RW, et al: Myocardial infarction as a presentation of clinical in-stent restenosis. *Circ J* 70:1026–1029, 2006.
215. Cutlip DE, Chauhan MS, Baim DS, et al: Clinical restenosis after coronary stenting: perspectives from multicenter clinical trials. *J Am Coll Cardiol* 40:2082–2089, 2002.
216. Kastrati A, Schomig A, Elezi S, et al: Predictive factors of restenosis after coronary stent placement. *J Am Coll Cardiol* 30:1428–1436, 1997.
217. Mercado N, Boersma E, Wijns W, et al: Clinical and quantitative coronary angiographic predictors of coronary restenosis: a comparative analysis from the balloon-to-stent era. *J Am Coll Cardiol* 38:645–652, 2001.
218. West NE, Ruygrok PN, Disco CM, et al: Clinical and angiographic predictors of restenosis after stent deployment in diabetic patients. *Circulation* 109:867–873, 2004.
219. Lemos PA, Hoye A, Goedhart D, et al: Clinical, angiographic, and procedural predictors of angiographic restenosis after sirolimus-eluting stent implantation in complex patients: an evaluation from the Rapamycin-Eluting Stent Evaluated At Rotterdam Cardiology Hospital (RESEARCH) study. *Circulation* 109:1366–1370, 2004.
220. Beohar N, Davidson CJ, Kip KE, et al: Outcomes and complications associated with off-label and untested use of drug-eluting stents. *JAMA* 297:1992–2000, 2007.
221. Win HK, Caldera AE, Maresh K, et al: Clinical outcomes and stent thrombosis following off-label use of drug-eluting stents. *JAMA* 297:2001–2009, 2007.
222. Ko DT, Chiu M, Guo H, et al: Safety and effectiveness of drug-eluting and bare-metal stents for patients with off- and on-label indications. *J Am Coll Cardiol* 53:1773–1782, 2009.
223. Marroquin OC, Selzer F, Mulukutla SR, et al: A comparison of bare-metal and drug-eluting stents for off-label indications. *N Engl J Med* 358:342–352, 2008.
224. Kimura T, Yokoi H, Nakagawa Y, et al: Three-year follow-up after implantation of metallic coronary-artery stents. *N Engl J Med* 334:561–566, 1996.
225. Mintz GS, Weissman NJ: Intravascular ultrasound in the drug-eluting stent era. *J Am Coll Cardiol* 48:421–429, 2006.
226. Hasegawa K, Ito M, Oda M, et al: Intravascular ultrasonic imaging of vulnerable plaque in a bare metal stent 10 years after implantation. *Circulation* 122:1341, 2010.
227. Claessen BE, Beijk MA, Legrand V, et al: Two-year clinical, angiographic, and intravascular ultrasound follow-up of the XIENCE V everolimus-eluting stent in the treatment of patients with de novo native coronary artery lesions: the SPIRIT II trial. *Circ Cardiovasc Intervent* 2:339–347, 2009.
228. Raber L: SIRTAX-LATE: Five-year clinical and angiographic follow-up from a prospective randomized trial of sirolimus-eluting and paclitaxel-eluting stents, Washington, DC, 2010, Transcatheter Cardiovascular Therapeutics.
229. Tsuchida K, Piek JJ, Neumann FJ, et al: One-year results of a durable polymer everolimus-eluting stent in de novo coronary narrowings (The SPIRIT FIRST Trial). *EuroIntervention* 1:266–272, 2005.
230. Tsuchida K, Serruys PW, Bruining N, et al: Two-year serial coronary angiographic and intravascular ultrasound analysis of in-stent angiographic late lumen loss and ultrasonic neointimal volume from the TAXUS II trial. *Am J Cardiol* 99:607–615, 2007.
231. Caixeta A, Lansky AJ, Serruys PW: Clinical follow-up 3 years after everolimus-eluting and paclitaxel-eluting stents. *J Am Coll Cardiol Intervent* 3:1220–1228, 2010.
232. Raber L: SIRTAX-LATE: Five-year clinical and angiographic follow-up from a prospective randomized trial of sirolimus-eluting and paclitaxel-eluting stents, San Francisco, CA, 2009, Transcatheter Cardiovascular Therapeutics.
233. Stone GW: SPIRIT IV: Two-Year Results from a Prospective Randomized Trial of Everolimus-Eluting Stents Compared to Paclitaxel-Eluting Stents in Patients with Coronary Artery Disease, Washington, DC, 2010, Transcatheter Cardiovascular Therapeutics.
234. Doi H, Maehara A, Mintz GS, et al: Impact of post-intervention minimal stent area on 9-month follow-up patency of paclitaxel-eluting stents: an integrated intravascular ultrasound analysis from the TAXUS IV, V, and VI and TAXUS ATLAS Workhorse, Long Lesion, and Direct Stent Trials. *JACC Cardiovasc Intervent* 2:1269–1275, 2009.
235. Morino Y, Honda Y, Okura H, et al: An optimal diagnostic threshold for minimal stent area to predict target lesion revascularization following stent implantation in native coronary lesions. *Am J Cardiol* 88:301–303, 2001.
236. Sonoda S, Morino Y, Ako J, et al: Impact of final stent dimensions on long-term results following sirolimus-eluting stent implantation: serial intravascular ultrasound analysis from the sirius trial. *J Am Coll Cardiol* 43:1959–1963, 2004.
237. Liu J, Maehara A, Mintz GS, et al: An integrated TAXUS IV, V, and VI intravascular ultrasound analysis of the predictors of edge restenosis after bare metal or paclitaxel-eluting stents. *Am J Cardiol* 103:501–506, 2009.
238. Sakurai R, Ako J, Morino Y, et al: Predictors of edge stenosis following sirolimus-eluting stent deployment (a quantitative intravascular ultrasound analysis from the SIRIUS trial). *Am J Cardiol* 96:1251–1253, 2005.
239. Costa MA, Angiolillo DJ, Tannenbaum M, et al: Impact of stent deployment procedural factors on long-term effectiveness and safety of sirolimus-eluting stents (final results of the multicenter prospective STLLR trial). *Am J Cardiol* 101:1704–1711, 2008.
240. Popma JJ, Tiroch K, Almonacid A, et al: A qualitative and quantitative angiographic analysis of stent fracture late following sirolimus-eluting stent implantation. *Am J Cardiol* 103:923–929, 2009.
241. Koster R, Vieluf D, Kiehn M, et al: Nickel and molybdenum contact allergies in patients with coronary in-stent restenosis. *Lancet* 356:1895–1897, 2000.
242. Nakazawa G, Tanabe K, Aoki J, et al: Sirolimus-eluting stents suppress neointimal formation irrespective of metallic allergy. *Circ J* 72:893–896, 2008.
243. Norgaz T, Hobikoglu G, Serdar ZA, et al: Is there a link between nickel allergy and coronary stent restenosis? *Tohoku J Exp Med* 206:243–246, 2005.
244. Hanioka N, Matsumoto K, Saito Y, et al: Functional characterization of CYP2C8.13 and CYP2C8.14: catalytic activities toward paclitaxel. *Basic Clin Pharmacol Toxicol* 107:565–569, 2010.
245. Huang S, Houghton PJ: Mechanisms of resistance to rapamycins. *Drug Resist Update* 4:378–391, 2001.
246. Monraats PS, de Vries F, de Jong LW, et al: Inflammation and apoptosis genes and the risk of restenosis after percutaneous coronary intervention. *Pharmacogenet Genomics* 16:747–754, 2006.
247. Vogiatzi K, Apostolakis S, Voudris V, et al: Interleukin 8 gene polymorphisms and susceptibility to restenosis after percutaneous coronary intervention. *J Thromb Thrombolysis* 29:134–140, 2010.
248. Nakazawa G, Ladich E, Finn AV, et al: Pathophysiology of vascular healing and stent mediated arterial injury. *EuroIntervention* 4(Suppl C):C7–C10, 2008.
249. Sanidas E, Mintz G, Maehara A, et al: Intracoronary Ultrasound for Optimizing Stent Implantation. *Curr Cardiov. Imaging Rep* 3:230–236, 2010.
250. Colombo A: AVIO: A prospective randomized trial of intravascular ultrasound-guided compared to angiography-guided stent implantation in complex coronary lesions, Washington, DC, 2010, Transcatheter Cardiovascular Therapeutics.
251. Elezi S, Kastrati A, Hadamitzky M, et al: Clinical and angiographic follow-up after balloon angioplasty with provisional stenting for coronary in-stent restenosis. *Catheter Cardiovasc Intervent* 48:151–156, 1999.
252. Mehran R, Dangas G, Abizaid AS, et al: Angiographic patterns of in-stent restenosis: classification and implications for long-term outcome. *Circulation* 100:1872–1878, 1999.
253. Mintz GS: Features and parameters of drug-eluting stent deployment discoverable by intravascular ultrasound. *Am J Cardiol* 100:26M-35M, 2007.
254. Mintz GS, Mehran R, Waksman R, et al: Treatment of in-stent restenosis. *Semin Intervent Cardiol* 3:117–121, 1998.
255. Leon MB, Teirstein PS, Moses JW, et al: Localized intracoronary gamma-radiation therapy to inhibit the recurrence of restenosis after stenting. *N Engl J Med* 344:250–256, 2001.
256. Waksman R, Raizner AE, Yeung AC, et al: Use of localised intracoronary beta radiation in treatment of in-stent restenosis: the INHIBIT randomised controlled trial. *Lancet* 359:551–557, 2002.
257. Grise MA, Massullo V, Jani S, et al: Five-year clinical follow-up after intracoronary radiation: results of a randomized clinical trial. *Circulation* 105:2737–2740, 2002.

258. Waksman R, Ajani AE, White RL, et al: Five-year follow-up after intracoronary gamma radiation therapy for in-stent restenosis. *Circulation* 109:340–344, 2004.

259. Holmes DR, Jr, Teirstein P, Satler L, et al: Sirolimus-eluting stents vs vascular brachytherapy for in-stent restenosis within bare-metal stents: the SISR randomized trial. *JAMA* 295:1264–1273, 2006.

260. Stone GW, Ellis SG, O'Shaughnessy CD, et al: Paclitaxel-eluting stents vs vascular brachytherapy for in-stent restenosis within bare-metal stents: the TAXUS V ISR randomized trial. *JAMA* 295:1253–1263, 2006.

261. Ellis SG, O'Shaughnessy CD, Martin SL, et al: Two-year clinical outcomes after paclitaxel-eluting stent or brachytherapy treatment for bare metal stent restenosis: the TAXUS V ISR trial. *Eur Heart J* 29:1625–1634, 2008.

262. Holmes DR, Jr, Teirstein PS, Satler L, et al: 3-year follow-up of the SISR (Sirolimus-Eluting Stents Versus Vascular Brachytherapy for In-Stent Restenosis) trial. *JACC Cardiovasc Intervent* 1:439–448, 2008.

263. Kastrati A, Mehilli J, von Beckerath N, et al: Sirolimus-eluting stent or paclitaxel-eluting stent vs balloon angioplasty for prevention of recurrences in patients with coronary in-stent restenosis: a randomized controlled trial. *JAMA* 293:165–171, 2005.

264. Chevalier B: CRISTAL: A prospective randomized trial of sirolimus-eluting stents compared to balloon angioplasty for restenosis of drug-eluting coronary stents, Washington, DC, 2010, Transcatheter Cardiovascular Therapeutics.

265. Mehilli J, Byrne RA, Tiroch K, et al: Randomized trial of paclitaxel- versus sirolimus-eluting stents for treatment of coronary restenosis in sirolimus-eluting stents: the ISAR-DESIRE 2 (Intracoronary Stenting and Angiographic Results: Drug Eluting Stents for In-Stent Restenosis 2) study. *J Am Coll Cardiol* 55:2710–2716, 2010.

266. Tamhane U, Meier P, Chetcuti S, et al: Efficacy of cilostazol in reducing restenosis in patients undergoing contemporary stent based PCI: a meta-analysis of randomised controlled trials. *EuroIntervention* 5:384–393, 2009.

267. Bonello L, Kaneshige K, De Labriolle A, et al: Vascular brachytherapy for patients with drug-eluting stent restenosis. *J Intervent Cardiol* 21:528–534, 2008.

268. Rodriguez AE, Granada JF, Rodriguez-Alemparte M, et al: Oral rapamycin after coronary bare-metal stent implantation to prevent restenosis: the Prospective, Randomized Oral Rapamycin in Argentina (ORAR II) Study. *J Am Coll Cardiol* 47:1522–1529, 2006.

269. Chong E, Poh KK, Liang S, et al: Two-year clinical registry follow-up of endothelial progenitor cell capture stent versus sirolimus-eluting bioabsorbable polymer-coated stent versus bare metal stents in patients undergoing primary percutaneous coronary intervention for ST elevation myocardial infarction. *J Intervent Cardiol* 23:101–108, 2010.

270. Costa JR Jr, Abizaid A, Costa R, et al: 1-year results of the hydroxyapatite polymer-free sirolimus-eluting stent for the treatment of single de novo coronary lesions: the VESTASYNC I trial. *JACC Cardiovasc Intervent* 2:422–427, 2009.

271. Tada N, Virmani R, Grant G, et al: Polymer-free biolimus a9-coated stent demonstrates more sustained intimal inhibition, improved healing, and reduced inflammation compared with a polymer-coated sirolimus-eluting cypher stent in a porcine model. *Circ Cardiovasc Intervent* 3:174–183, 2010.

272. Ormiston JA, Serruys PW, Regar E, et al: A bioabsorbable everolimus-eluting coronary stent system for patients with single de-novo coronary artery lesions (ABSORB): a prospective open-label trial. *Lancet* 371:899–907, 2008.

273. Serruys PW, Ormiston JA, Onuma Y, et al: A bioabsorbable everolimus-eluting coronary stent system (ABSORB): 2-year outcomes and results from multiple imaging methods. *Lancet* 373:897–910, 2009.

274. Gray WA, Granada JF: Drug-coated balloons for the prevention of vascular restenosis. *Circulation* 121:2672–2680, 2010.

275. Scheller B, Hehrlein C, Bocksch W, et al: Treatment of coronary in-stent restenosis with a paclitaxel-coated balloon catheter. *N Engl J Med* 355:2113–2124, 2006.

276. Morice MC, Serruys PW, Sousa JE, et al: A randomized comparison of a sirolimus-eluting stent with a standard stent for coronary revascularization. *N Engl J Med* 346:1773–1780, 2002.

277. Schampaert E, Cohen EA, Schluter M, et al: The Canadian study of the sirolimus-eluting stent in the treatment of patients with long de novo lesions in small native coronary arteries (C-SIRIUS). *J Am Coll Cardiol* 43:1110–1115, 2004.

278. Schofer J, Schluter M, Gershlick AH, et al: Sirolimus-eluting stents for treatment of patients with long atherosclerotic lesions in small coronary arteries: double-blind, randomised controlled trial (E-SIRIUS). *Lancet* 362:1093–1099, 2003.

279. Valgimigli M, Campo G, Percoco G, et al: Comparison of angioplasty with infusion of tirofiban or abciximab and with implantation of sirolimus-eluting or uncoated stents for acute myocardial infarction: the MULTISTRATEGY randomized trial. *JAMA* 299:1788–1799, 2008.

280. Spaulding C, Henry P, Teiger E, et al: Sirolimus-eluting versus uncoated stents in acute myocardial infarction. *N Engl J Med* 355:1093–1104, 2006.

281. van der Hoeven BL, Liem SS, et al: Sirolimus-eluting stents versus bare-metal stents in patients with ST-segment elevation myocardial infarction: 9-month angiographic and intravascular ultrasound results and 12-month clinical outcome results from the MISSION! Intervention Study. *J Am Coll Cardiol* 51:618–626, 2008.

282. Menichelli M, Parma A, Pucci E, et al: Randomized trial of Sirolimus-Eluting Stent Versus Bare-Metal Stent in Acute Myocardial Infarction (SESAMI). *J Am Coll Cardiol* 49:1924–1930, 2007.

283. Di Lorenzo E, De Luca G, Sauro R, et al: The PASEO (PaclitAxel or Sirolimus-Eluting Stent Versus Bare Metal Stent in Primary Angioplasty) Randomized Trial. *J Am Coll Cardiol Intervent* 2:515–523, 2009.

284. Valgimigli M, Campo G, Arcozzi C, et al: Two-year clinical follow-up after sirolimus-eluting versus bare-metal stent implantation assisted by systematic glycoprotein IIb/IIIa Inhibitor Infusion in patients with myocardial infarction: results from the STRATEGY study. *J Am Coll Cardiol* 50:138–145, 2007.

285. Diaz de la Llera LS, Ballesteros S, Nevado J, et al: Sirolimus-eluting stents compared with standard stents in the treatment of patients with primary angioplasty. *Am Heart J* 154:164 e1–166 e1, 2007.

286. Baumgart D, Klauss V, Baer F, et al: One-year results of the SCORPIUS study: a German multicenter investigation on the effectiveness of sirolimus-eluting stents in diabetic patients. *J Am Coll Cardiol* 50:1627–1634, 2007.

287. Jimenez-Quevedo P, Sabate M, Angiolillo DJ, et al: Long-term clinical benefit of sirolimus-eluting stent implantation in diabetic patients with de novo coronary stenoses: long-term results of the DIABETES trial. *Eur Heart J* 28:1946–1952, 2007.

288. Chan C, Zambahari R, Kaul U, et al: A randomized comparison of sirolimus-eluting versus bare metal stents in the treatment of diabetic patients with native coronary artery lesions: the DECODE study. *Catheter Cardiovasc Intervent* 72:591–600, 2008.

289. Kelbaek H, Thuesen L, Helqvist S, et al: The Stenting Coronary Arteries in Non-stress/benestent Disease (SCANDSTENT) trial. *J Am Coll Cardiol* 47:449–455, 2006.

290. Ardissino D, Cavallini C, Bramucci E, et al: Sirolimus-eluting vs uncoated stents for prevention of restenosis in small coronary arteries: a randomized trial. *JAMA* 292:2727–2734, 2004.

291. Pache J, Dibra A, Mehilli J, et al: Drug-eluting stents compared with thin-strut bare stents for the reduction of restenosis: a prospective, randomized trial. *Eur Heart J* 26:1262–1268, 2005.

292. Ortolani P, Marzocchi A, Marrozzini C, et al: Randomized comparative trial of a thin-strut bare metal cobalt-chromium stent versus a sirolimus-eluting stent for coronary revascularization. *Catheter Cardiovasc Intervent* 69:790–798, 2007.

293. Stone GW, Lansky AJ, Pocock SJ, et al: Paclitaxel-Eluting Stents versus Bare-Metal Stents in Acute Myocardial Infarction. *N Engl J Med* 360:1946–1959, 2009.

294. Laarman GJ, Suttorp MJ, Dirksen MT, et al: Paclitaxel-eluting versus uncoated stents in primary percutaneous coronary intervention. *N Engl J Med* 355:1105–1113, 2006.

295. Tierala I, Syvänne M, Kupari M, for the HAAMU-STENT study group. Comparison of paclitaxel- eluting with bare metal stents in acute myocardial infarction. Accessed online at http://www.tctmd.com/Show.aspx?id=56036.

296. Chechi T, Vittori G, Biondi Zoccai GG, et al: Single-center randomized evaluation of paclitaxel-eluting versus conventional stent in acute myocardial infarction (SELECTION). *J Intervent Cardiol* 20:282–291, 2007.

297. Zhang Q, Zhang RY, Zhang JS, et al: One-year clinical outcomes of Chinese sirolimus-eluting stent in the treatment of unselected patients with coronary artery disease. *Chin Med J (Engl)* 119:165–168, 2006.

298. Windecker S, Remondino A, Eberli FR, et al: Sirolimus-eluting and paclitaxel-eluting stents for coronary revascularization. *N Engl J Med* 353:653–662, 2005.

299. Goy JJ, Stauffer JC, Siegenthaler M, et al: A prospective randomized comparison between paclitaxel and sirolimus stents in the real world of interventional cardiology: the TAXi trial. *J Am Coll Cardiol* 45:308–311, 2005.

300. Kim MH, Hong SJ, Cha KS, et al: Effect of Paclitaxel-eluting versus sirolimus-eluting stents on coronary restenosis in Korean diabetic patients. *J Intervent Cardiol* 21:225–231, 2008.

301. Maeng M, Jensen LO, Galloe AM, et al: Comparison of the sirolimus-eluting versus paclitaxel-eluting coronary stent in patients with diabetes mellitus: the diabetes and drug-eluting stent (DiabeDES) randomized angiography trial. *Am J Cardiol* 103:345–349, 2009.

302. de Lezo JS, Medina A, Pan M: Drug-eluting stent for complex lesions: latest angiographic data from randomized rapamycin versus paclitaxel CORPAL study. *J Am Coll Cardiol* 45(Suppl.):75A, 2005.

303. Kim Y-H, Park S-W, Lee S-W, et al: Sirolimus-eluting stent versus paclitaxel-eluting stent for patients with long coronary artery disease. *Circulation* 114:2148–2153, 2006.

304. Han YL, Wang XZ, Jing QM, et al: [Comparison of rapamycin and paclitaxel eluting stent in patients with multi-vessel coronary disease]. *Zhonghua Xin Xue Guan Bing Za Zhi* 34:123–126, 2006.

305. Mehilli J, Dibra A, Kastrati A, et al: Randomized trial of paclitaxel- and sirolimus-eluting stents in small coronary vessels. *Eur Heart J* 27:260–266, 2006.

306. Pan M, Suarez de Lezo J, Medina A, et al: Drug-eluting stents for the treatment of bifurcation lesions: a randomized comparison between paclitaxel and sirolimus stents. *Am Heart J* 153:15 e1–17 el, 2007.

307. Cervinka P, Costa MA, Angiolillo DJ, et al: Head-to-head comparison between sirolimus-eluting and paclitaxel-eluting stents in patients with complex coronary artery disease: an intravascular ultrasound study. *Catheter Cardiovasc Intervent* 67:846–851, 2006.

308. Lee JH, Kim HS, Lee SW, et al: Prospective randomized comparison of sirolimus- versus paclitaxel-eluting stents for the treatment of acute ST-elevation myocardial infarction: pROSIT trial. *Catheter Cardiovasc Intervent* 72:25–32, 2008.

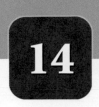

14

Drug-Coated Balloons

BRUNO SCHELLER | WILLIAM A. GRAY

KEY POINTS

- Drug-coated balloon catheters are the most advanced alternative to drug-eluting stents for local intravascular drug delivery.

- Preclinical data indicate effective inhibition of restenosis; however, there is no class effect on drug-coated balloons.

- Randomized clinical trials have shown efficacy and safety in the treatment of coronary in-stent restenosis and treatment of de novo and restenotic lesions in the superficial femoral artery.

- Data from registries identify coronary small vessels; bifurcation lesions; long, diffuse, diseased stenoses; and below-the-knee atherosclerotic disease as potential future indications for drug-coated balloons.

Introduction

Coronary angioplasty was introduced into clinical use by Andreas Grüntzig in 1977.[1] In the field of coronary intervention the most important advance has been the introduction of stents. Stenting overcomes acute recoil and dissection as well as longer-term negative remodeling but not restenosis due to continued neointimal proliferation. Local intravascular drug delivery by drug-eluting stents appears to have addressed this cellular basis of restenosis. However, stents cannot be implanted at all coronary sites where neointimal proliferation may limit the long-term benefit of angioplasty, such as small vessels and bifurcations, and drug-eluting stents have not been found to be effective in the treatment of peripheral vascular disease of the femoropopliteal territory. In the coronary arteries, sometimes delayed or incomplete reendothelialization with the need for long-term dual antiplatelet therapy to reduce the risk of late stent thrombosis can limit the use of this technology in certain patients. Sustained drug release seems to be essential for stent-based local drug delivery owing to the inhomogeneous drug distribution from a drug-eluting stent to the arterial wall,[2] the time course of the inflammation related to the initial trauma of the procedure, as well as the provocation of neointimal hyperplasia due to the implanted prosthesis. About 75% to 85% of the stented vessel wall area is not covered by the stent struts, resulting in low tissue levels of the antiproliferative agent in these areas. Cell culture experiments indicate that low drug concentrations require much longer exposure times to achieve sufficient inhibition of cell proliferation than do higher concentrations.[3] Therefore high drug concentrations on the stent struts, including a controlled and sustained release, are mandatory for stent-based local drug delivery,[4] with the consequence of delayed and incomplete reendothelialization of the stent struts. Autopsy studies show that even beyond 40 months, drug-eluting stents are not always fully covered by endothelium.[5] Furthermore, the polymeric matrices on the stent that are meant to control the release kinetics of the antiproliferative drug can induce inflammation and thrombosis.[6,7] On the other hand, incomplete suppression of neointimal hyperplasia at the stent margins or between the struts may limit the efficacy of drug-eluting stents.[2,8] Alternative approaches to overcome the limitations of drug-eluting stents have included avoiding a sustained drug release from stent struts to allow for earlier reendothelialization, bioerodable polymers or nonpolymeric release mechanisms (such as surface-modified stent struts), and thinner struts

requiring less coverage. Antiproliferative taxanes such as paclitaxel seem to be suitable for the prevention of local intravascular restenosis because of their high lipophilicity and tight binding to various cell constituents, resulting in effective local retention at the site of delivery.[3] The addition of a contrast agent surprisingly resulted in a solubility of taxanes far beyond the concentrations applied in previous investigations.[9] In the porcine coronary model, the intracoronary bolus administration of a taxane-contrast medium formulation led to a significant reduction of neointimal formation after experimental coronary stent implantation despite the short application time.[10,11] Paclitaxel in a contrast agent was better tolerated and led to higher local tissue concentrations than diluted Taxol, indicating the impact of additional compounds for local drug transfer.[12] The surprising discovery was that sustained drug release is not a precondition for long-lasting restenosis inhibition. In 2001, the basic premise of a more lesion- than vessel-specific method of intramural drug delivery became embodied in the concept of a drug-coated balloon. By coating paclitaxel onto the surface of a conventional angioplasty balloon used to dilate the stenotic artery, an exclusively local effect could theoretically be achieved, with the drug transferred to the dilated segment as the balloon was inflated. In this way, an effective local drug concentration is achieved with very low systemic exposure. However, several properties of the balloon coating are crucial for ensuring effective drug delivery to the target site, including (1) its form on the balloon surface; (2) the homogeneity of distribution along the surface of the balloon; (3) its stability during production, handling, and storage; (4) the degree of premature loss while transiting to the target vessel segment; (5) the ability to release during balloon expansion; (6) the transfer efficiency to the vessel wall; and (7) the amount of particulate material released to the distal circulation.

Preclinical Data

Speck and colleagues, using various coating procedures, coated conventional coronary balloon catheters with different doses of paclitaxel. The paclitaxel dose on the coated balloons was 1.3 to 3 µg/mm², corresponding to a total dose of approximately 220 to 650 µg paclitaxel, depending on the balloon size. About 10% of the initial amount of paclitaxel on the balloon was lost while the catheter was being advanced to the lesion through the hemostatic valve and the guiding catheter and about 80% of the dose was released during inflation. Most of the dose released at the target site is distributed as particulate distally in the bloodstream, with less than 20% being directly taken up into the vessel wall. Thus paclitaxel-coated balloons deliver a dose to the target site in a very short time, and this dose is higher than that released by stents over the course of weeks. At 5-week follow-up, the implantation of stents premounted on paclitaxel-coated balloons was found to have caused a marked dose-dependent and statistically significant reduction in late lumen loss and an equally impressive statistically significant increase in minimal lumen diameter compared with controls. Quantitative coronary angiography revealed no edge effects or signs of malapposition or aneurysm. Histomorphometry showed a statistically significant increase in lumen diameter and lumen area and a corresponding decrease in maximal neointimal thickness and neointimal area in the vessels treated with paclitaxel-coated balloons (reduction of neointimal area by 63% in the paclitaxel-coated balloon group vs. the uncoated balloon group).[12,13] Furthermore, the drug is more evenly distributed on the vessel surface compared with that delivered by a

TABLE 14-1	Paclitaxel-Coated Balloons Currently on the Market or in Development			
Company/Origination	*Product*	*Drug Formulation*	*Indication(s)*	*Development/ Launch Status*
University (Charité, Germany)	Paccocath (Prototype)	Paclitaxel with iopromide (Ultravist)	CAD/PAD	Not pursued
B. Braun Melsungen AG (Germany)	SeQuent Please	Modified Paccocath	CAD	CE (since 2009)
MEDRAD Interventional/ Possis (U.S.)	Cotavance	Modified Paccocath	PAD	CE (since 2011)
Eurocor GmbH (Germany)	DIOR I DIOR II	Rough balloon surface Mixture of paclitaxel and shellac	CAD	CE (since 2007)
Lutonix, Inc. (U.S.)	Moxy	Paclitaxel, matrix not disclosed	CAD/PAD	CE submitted
Medtronic Invatec, S.p.A. (Italy)	In.Pact (four different catheters)	Paclitaxel, hydrophilic FreePac	CAD/PAD	CE (since 2009)
Aachen Resonance GmbH (Germany)	Elutax I Elutax II	Structured balloon surface Coating = two layers of paclitaxel (elastic and drug depot)	CAD CAD/PAD	CE (since 2008)
Cook Group, Inc. (U.S.)	Advance 18 PTX	Paclitaxel, matrix not disclosed	PAD	Late stage development
Biotronik AG (Germany)	Pantera Lux	Paclitaxel and butyryl-tri-hexyl citrate matrix	CAD	CE (since 2010)
Angioscore (U.S.)	Coated AngioSculpt	Paclitaxel, matrix not disclosed	CAD/PAD	Early stage development
Cordis (U.S.)	Not disclosed	Sirolimus, matrix not disclosed	?	?
Minvasys (France)	Not disclosed	Not disclosed	?	?

CE, approval in Europe; CAD, coronary artery disease; PAD, peripheral artery disease.

drug-eluting stent.[14] However, studies suggest that the amount of paclitaxel in the arterial tissue varies widely depending on the dose of drug on the balloon and particularly on the coating formulation. An adequate inhibition of neointimal proliferation was observed only when balloons were coated with paclitaxel mixed with the contrast agent iopromide dissolved in acetone. The effect was markedly lower when ethyl acetate was used as a solvent without iopromide. The difference in efficacy of these two coating formulations may be primarily explained by the presence of the hydrophilic iodinated contrast medium in the case of the acetone version, thus suggesting that a proper solubilizing agent is important.[15]

Paclitaxel admixed with a small amount of the hydrophilic contrast medium iopromide (Ultravist) has also been denoted as Paccocath. These balloons are standard angioplasty balloons coated with a paclitaxel dose of 3 µg/mm^2 of balloon surface. The situation in the peripheral arteries is not directly comparable with that in the coronary arteries, and treatment is much more complex in several respects. Compared with the coronary arteries, the incidence of restenosis in the superficial femoral artery is even higher and can reach up to 50% within the first 6 months after intervention. Given the clinical need, it was very encouraging when Albrecht et al. developed early preclinical data demonstrating that local intra-arterial administration of paclitaxel using drug-coated balloons or an admixture of paclitaxel to contrast medium could inhibit in-stent stenosis of peripheral arteries in the porcine overstretch model: in-stent stenosis in the control group was 38% ± 20% (uncoated balloons). In the treatment groups, it was reduced as follows: treatment group I (balloons coated with 330 µg paclitaxel), 18% ± 22%; treatment group II (balloons coated with 480 µg paclitaxel), 12% ± 18%; and treatment group III (6.4 mg paclitaxel dissolved in 50 mL iopromide 370 + 5 mL ethanol), 18% ± 20% ($P < 0.05$).[16] Cremers et al. subsequently evaluated the effects of various inflation times (10, 60, and 2 × 60 seconds) on the efficacy of restenosis inhibition and the safety of different doses (5 µg; 2 × 5 µg paclitaxel/mm^2 balloon surface) in pigs. Treatment with a drug-coated balloon (5 µg paclitaxel/mm^2 balloon surface with iopromide) for 10 seconds reduced the neointimal area to the same extent as contact with the vessel wall for two times 60 seconds (by 57% and 56%, respectively, compared with control). Furthermore, neointimal proliferation and all other parameters characterizing in-stent restenosis were not further decreased by inflating two drug-coated balloons (each containing 5 µg paclitaxel/mm^2 balloon surface) in the same vessel segment for 60 seconds each. These results suggest that balloons coated with the

paclitaxel iopromide formulation release most of the drug rapidly during the first seconds of inflation. Thus, the initial contact of the coated balloon membrane with the vessel wall appears to produce the desired effect of inhibiting neointimal proliferation. The results of this study indicate that it may be sufficient to inflate the balloon for a few seconds only to achieve adequate protection from restenosis. The results also show that doses of up to 10 µg paclitaxel/mm^2 balloon surface applied by the inflation of two drug-coated balloons do not increase the risk of thrombosis or cause aneurysm.[17]

Since this initial research was published, several manufacturers have started commercializing or developing drug-coated balloons. Currently, paclitaxel is the drug of choice, the typical dosage being 3 µg/mm^2 balloon surface. The critical factor enabling successful drug transfer is the formulation used to coat the balloon. Current products range from those with no additive and very tight binding of the drug to the balloon membrane to those applied in conjunction with contrast agents or other beneficial additives. A number of these developers have undertaken extensive research into this issue and believe that the formulation will be critical to successful product performance and adoption (Table 14-1). Still, only scarce data are available on drug-coated balloons other than the Paccocath. The matrix coating of the SeQuent Please balloon catheter (B. Braun Melsungen AG, Germany) for PTCA consists of a mixture of paclitaxel and iopromide, identical in composition to Paccocath. The preclinical data compare very well with the results from the Paccocath program. Granada and colleagues reported histological results showing the Cotavance coating (MEDRAD/Possis, USA, Bayer) an iterative coating formula based on Paccocath, to be superior to an uncoated balloon in treating coronary artery and superficial femoral artery lesions in pigs.[17a] In an additional pilot study, single or overlapping Cotavance balloons were compared with single nonoverlapping balloons coated with a contrast medium (Iopromide) without paclitaxel in a healthy porcine iliofemoral stent model. Balloon angioplasty was followed by self-expandable bare metal stent implantation. After 28 days, Cotavance balloons decreased neointimal proliferation in a dose-dependent manner when assessed by quantitative angiography (late lumen loss with Cotavance single 1.5 ± 0.7 mm vs. Cotavance overlap 0.7 ± 0.6 mm compared with contrast-coated control 1.7 ± 0.4 mm).[18]

FreePac (Medtronic Invatec, Italy) is a proprietary hydrophilic coating formulation with urea serving as the matrix substance. Urea is a nontoxic, ubiquitous endogenous compound commonly used in pharmacy; it is meant to enhance the release of paclitaxel during the short time of contact with the vessel wall. In the porcine coronary model, similar amounts of paclitaxel were transferred to the vessel wall with the Paccocath coating (214 ± 106 µg paclitaxel) and the FreePac coating (175 ± 101 µg paclitaxel) 15 to 25 minutes after stent implantation. Twenty-eight days after balloon dilatation, the original Paccocath coating caused the known strong inhibition of neointimal formation in the porcine coronary model (minimal lumen diameter [MLD]: 2.7 ± 0.3 mm; late lumen loss: 0.3 ± 0.2 mm). The FreePac coating was equally efficacious and equally well tolerated (MLD: 2.7 ± 0.2 mm; late lumen loss: 0.4 ± 0.2 mm). The aim of another study was to determine the minimum effective dose and local toxicity at extremely high doses of the FreePac formulation. The balloons were coated with 1 to 9 µg paclitaxel/mm² balloon surface. In the highest-dose group three balloons each coated with 9 µg paclitaxel/mm² balloon surface were expanded in the same vessel segment. FreePac paclitaxel-coated balloon catheters efficaciously inhibited neointimal proliferation starting with the lowest dose tested (1 µg/mm²) and were well tolerated up to three times the preferred dose of 3 µg/mm². Stent occlusions observed at the highest dose level and repeated treatment (3×9 µg/mm²) indicate that the limit of tolerance was reached.[19]

As early as 2007, a paclitaxel coated balloon catheter called DIOR received approval in Europe (CE mark). A study of first-generation DIOR balloon catheters (Eurocor GmbH, Germany) reported a tissue paclitaxel concentration of the dilated segment in porcine arteries 1.5 hours after dilation of 1.82 ± 1.60 µmol/L, which decreased significantly to 0.73 ± 0.27 ($P = 0.03$), 0.62 ± 0.34, and 0.44 ± 0.31 µmol/L at 12, 24, and 48 hours.[20] In a direct comparison with the Paccocath balloon, the roughened DIOR balloon failed to produce statistically significant effects on angiographic measures of stenosis or morphometric parameters such as maximal neointimal thickness and luminal area. Use of the matrix-coated Paccocath balloon led to a highly significant ($P < 0.01$) reduction in all parameters, indicating neointimal proliferation compared with both uncoated control and DIOR at 28-day follow-up.[21] Only about 50% of the drug coating was released from the roughened balloons during the recommended balloon inflation time of 45 to 60 seconds. In contrast, the iopromide matrix was found to release the full amount of the drug ($4.5\% \pm 0.7$ % of the total paclitaxel dose on balloons after the procedure), which may contribute to its superiority in inhibiting restenosis. The second-generation DIOR II balloon is a coronary dilation balloon for human use with a paclitaxel coating of 3.0 µg/mm² on the balloon surface; this is applied using a completely different coating technique. The drug is mixed with shellac, which is composed of a network of hydroxy fatty acid esters and sesquiterpene acid esters with a molecular weight of about 1,000. The 1 : 1 mixture of paclitaxel and shellac is coated onto regular balloon catheters. A balloon inflation time dependency study in the porcine model of coronary artery overstretch showed almost maximal tissue paclitaxel concentrations after balloon inflation times of 30 seconds and release of 75% of the drug from the balloon surface, which resulted in an up to 20-fold higher tissue concentration compared with the first-generation DIOR. Two weeks after overstretch injury, histomorphometry showed significantly smaller neointimal hyperplasia and neointimal thickness in the DIOR group compared with the conventional uncoated balloon group. Consequently the area of the coronary artery lumen was larger in the DIOR-treated arteries compared with those treated with the conventional balloon (1.20 ± 0.27 mm² vs. 0.5 ± 0.22 mm², $P < 0.001$).[22a]

Elutax (Aachen Resonance, Germany) uses pure paclitaxel without a matrix coated on structured balloon surface. It is difficult to assess it at this point as data from ongoing clinical studies investigating this product in the coronary and peripheral arteries are not yet available. Preclinical data on the Moxy paclitaxel-coated balloon catheter (Lutonix, Inc., USA) were recently presented.[22a] The Lutonix catheters (2 µg/mm² paclitaxel using a proprietary excipient) resulted in inhibition of neointimal proliferation in the porcine coronary overstretch and stent implantation model similar to the effect observed with paclitaxel-coated balloon catheters with an iopromide matrix (Paccocath). Pantera Lux (Biotronik AG, Germany)

uses butyryl-trihexyl citrate (BTHC) as a carrier for paclitaxel. BTHC is used in different medical devices and cosmetics and is approved for blood contact in blood bags. Preclinical data have not yet been published; various clinical studies are ongoing.

A different, alternative mode of local drug delivery into the target artery segment has been developed using the GENIE balloon (Acrostak Corp., Switzerland). Paclitaxel is delivered by a system consisting of a balloon with a distal and proximal occlusive segment and a central segment that allows transfer of paclitaxel to the vessel wall by infusion of paclitaxel solution into the vascular chamber created between the balloons.[23] Preclinical investigations in the coronary arteries of pigs demonstrated that the administration of 10 µM paclitaxel (diluted Taxol, paclitaxel in a mixture of 50% Cremophor EL and 50% ethanol) via GENIE markedly reduced late lumen loss (0.9 ± 0.1 mm) compared with controls (2.2 ± 0.2 mm, $P < 0.001$). The histological examination showed a statistically significant increase in the lumen area (5.2 ± 1.0 mm²) and a corresponding decrease in maximal neointimal thickness (0.1 ± 0.01 mm) and neointimal area (1.0 ± 0.1 mm²) in the stented artery treated with paclitaxel versus the control group (3.0 ± 0.3 mm², 0.3 ± 0.04 mm, 2.4 ± 0.2 mm²).[24] The dose of 2.9 ± 1.6 mL 10 µM paclitaxel in this study equals 24.8 ± 13.7 µg paclitaxel.

The lipophilic nature of the antiproliferative drug zotarolimus makes it a potential candidate for drug-coated balloon applications. A study in pigs aimed at evaluating the safety and efficacy of a novel zotarolimus-coated balloon in comparison with a zotarolimus-eluting stent. In both zotarolimus groups, there was a clear reduction in the neointimal area compared with the control group, which did not receive any drug on the balloon or the stent. The effect of neointimal inhibition was slightly more pronounced with the zotarolimus-coated balloon (control 4.32 ± 1.45 mm², zotarolimus-coated balloon 2.79 ± 1.43 mm², and zotarolimus-eluting stent 3.32 ± 1.11 mm²; $P = 0.001$). The inflammation score was significantly reduced in vessels treated with the zotarolimus-coated balloon.[25]

Clinical Data on Drug-Coated Balloons

At the time of this publication, there were no drug-coated-balloon (DCB) devices approved for human use in the United States or even in clinical trials. In Europe, regulatory approval currently exists for five coronary devices—SeQuent Please (B. Braun, Melsungen, Germany), InPact Falcon (Invatec/Medtronic, Minneapolis, MN), Dior (Eurocor, Bonn, Germany), Elutax (Aachen Resonance, Aachen, Germany), and Pantera Lux (Biotronik, Berlin, Germany)—and also for three peripheral devices—In.Pact Admiral for the superficial femoral artery (SFA) (Invatec/Medtronic), In.Pact Pacific for the SFA (Invatec/Medtronic), and In.Pact Amphirion for infrapopliteal vessels (Invatec/Medtronic). In spite of the multiple device approvals, there is a comparative paucity of data in the literature regarding the clinical safety and utility of DCBs as a stand-alone therapy or in combination with other modalities. The use of DCBs in combination with BMSs or debulking devices has both positive and negative potential: the potential for a better, more secure initial patency but also questions of efficacy, given the potential for edge effect and geographic miss.

Human Pharmacokinetics of Current Drug-Coated-Balloon Technology

Data on the current first generation of DCBs suggest that the amount of drug delivered by the coated balloon to the vessel wall is a minor fraction of the total dose loaded and that the majority of the drug is distributed into the bloodstream either before or during balloon inflation. Therefore defining the possible systemic dose of drug delivered with this technology is important, especially given the requirement to use larger, longer, and possibly multiple coated balloons in certain peripheral vascular applications. In a pharmacokinetic study[25a] 14 patients treated at two sites for femoropopliteal disease with DCB had blood sampling at multiple time intervals before and after treatment with balloons ranging up to 10 cm, with monitoring of vital signs and ECG analysis (which demonstrated no untoward effects). Mean blood levels of paclitaxel in the immediate postintervention phase were roughly an order of magnitude less than the mean chemotherapeutic levels, and blood levels at 2 hours more than half the samples were below the lower limit of quantification. Although the study was small with a considerable heterogeneity of both patients and balloon sizes, nevertheless a reasonable safety margin of systemic paclitaxel was demonstrated. Still to be determined is what, if any, systemic effects the use of longer or multiple balloons in more extensive SFA disease will have.

Data from the Coronary Application of Drug-Coated Balloons

Although DESs are overwhelmingly the choice for most coronary lesions and their efficacy and safety continue to improve to remarkable degrees, specific challenges remain to their delivery and use in specific coronary territories such as bifurcations, small vessels, saphenous vein grafts, long lesions, and diabetic disease, all of which have less robust outcomes with DES than do simpler lesions. In addition, the current need for prolonged dual antiplatelet therapy can be clinically challenging for some patients with medication intolerance or bleeding tendencies. Although improved antiplatelet medication is now available to address the possible consequences of nonresponders to clopidogrel, they trade antiplatelet efficacy for increased bleeding risk. DCB have the potential to improve outcomes regarding difficult vascular stent territories with a more limited duration of dual antiplatelet therapy. While all of the mechanisms of DCB efficacy are yet to be determined, several randomized clinical studies suggest efficacy of the technology in both coronary and peripheral territories. However, it is important to note that not all DCBs have the same formulation, and this can have implications for clinical effectiveness. In the discussion of clinical trial results below, specifics as to the formulations employed are designated for the DCB tested to the extent that they are known. DCB use in humans was first described in a 2006 publication.[26] In this multicenter study, 52 patients with coronary in-stent restenosis (ISR) were randomized to receive angioplasty with either an uncoated balloon or a 3-mcg/mm^2 iopromide-paclitaxel-coated balloon (Paccocath, licensed by Bayer Schering Pharma); aspirin and clopidogrel were given for 1 month, followed by aspirin alone. Baseline demographics, angiography, and short-term procedural outcomes were not different between the two groups. As determined by angiography at 6 months, the Paccocath group demonstrated a clear advantage in the primary endpoint of less in-segment late lumen loss (LLL) (0.74 ± 0.86 vs. 0.03 ± 0.48 mm; $P = 0.002$) as well as in the 6-month secondary endpoints of MLD and binary restenosis. An additional 56 patients with coronary ISR were randomized and the combined cohort of 108 patients was followed for 2 years.[27] The primary endpoint of 6-month angiographic in-segment LLL was similar to that in the original report, with in-segment binary restenosis of only 6% for the DCB group compared with 51% for the standard balloon group; there were no differential effects by gender or diabetes mellitus. Further, a sustained clinical effect of Paccocath was noted at 24 months, as manifest by a significant reduction in target lesion revascularization (TLR) (37% vs. 6%; $P = 0.001$); no subacute thrombosis or other safety issues were seen in the DCB group. Another group of investigators has initiated a series of studies called PEPCAD (Paclitaxel-Eluting PTCA-Catheter in Coronary Disease) to test the same DCB Paccocath formulation (SeQuent Please, licensed by B. Braun) using a variety of coronary therapy comparisons. PEPCAD I was a nonrandomized study investigating the safety and efficacy of the SeQuent Please DCB with provisional BMS implantation in small-vessel (mean reference vessel diameter, 2.36 mm) de novo lesions in 120 patients.[36] At the 6-month follow-up, in-segment LLL was significantly less with DCB alone compared with DCB plus stent (0.18 and 0.73 mm, respectively), with the majority of the restenosis being noted at the stent edges, ostensibly where DCB coverage was inadequate. Although this trial was not adequately powered to assess stent

thrombosis, vessel thrombosis occurred less frequently in the DCB-alone group despite a shorter duration of dual antiplatelet therapy (1 vs. 3 months). PEPCAD II was a multicenter, randomized trial of the SeQuent Please DCB versus the TAXUS Liberté DES in 131 patients with coronary ISR.[28] In the two groups of patients with reference vessels averaging 3.0 mm in diameter, the primary endpoint of 6-month in-segment LLL was significantly less with the DCB compared with the DES (0.17 ± 0.42 vs. 0.38 ± 0.61 mm; $P = 0.03$). At 12 months, TLR trended in favor of the DCB (6% vs. 15%; $P = 0.15$), suggesting that the DCB was at least as effective as the DES for coronary ISR and without the need for repeat stent implantation. Results from the PEPCAD III[28a] multicenter randomized study paired the same SeQuent Please DCB with a BMS and compared it with the Cypher sirolimus-eluting stent (Cordis/Johnson & Johnson, Miami Lakes, FL) in 637 patients with single de novo coronary lesions between 2.5 and 3.5 mm in diameter and <24 mm long. The primary angiographic endpoint of 9-month in-stent LLL was significantly better for the DES compared with the DCB/BMS (0.16 ± 0.39 vs. 0.41 ± 0.51 mm; $P = 0.001$), although there was less difference in in-segment LLL (0.11 ± 0.40 vs. 0.20 ± 0.11 mm; $P = 0.07$). In addition, the 9-month clinical efficacy endpoints of TLR and target vessel revascularization favored the DES approach, however, there was no significant difference in total MACE (15% vs 18%). The investigators concluded that DCB efficacy at the stent margin had been achieved (solving the problem posed by the results of PEPCAD I). But while noninferiority with Cypher DES had not been achieved in the DCB/BMS arm, nevertheless LLL for the combination therapy was comparable to the historical results for paclitaxel-eluting stents. In the PICCOLETO (paclitaxel-eluting balloon versus paclitaxel-eluting stent in small coronary vessel disease) trial[28b] a different paclitaxel-eluting balloon construction that did not involve a carrier molecule was used (first-generation Dior, Eurocor, Bonn, Germany). This single-center trial intended to enroll a total of 80 patients with de novo small-vessel (<2.75 mm) disease, randomizing to either DIOR DCB or TAXUS Liberté DESs. Enrollment was halted after two-thirds of the originally intended number had been enrolled owing to marked outcome differences between the groups. Specifically, among the 57 patients with complete 6-month angiographic and clinical follow-up, the primary endpoint of percent diameter stenosis was significantly worse in the DCB group (43.6 ± 27.4% vs. 24.3 ± 25.1%; $P = 0.029$); additionally, there was significantly less MLD and more binary restenosis in the DCB arm. The investigators concluded that the first-generation DIOR DCB failed to show equivalence to the TAXUS Liberté DES and hypothesized that adjunctive stenting in the DCB may be required to achieve DES-like results. Next in the PEPCAD series of investigations, results are available from the PEPCAD V[28c] single-arm feasibility and safety trial using DCBs (SeQuent Please) for the treatment of coronary bifurcation disease. Specifically, a DCB was used in the main and side branches, then a BMS in the main branch, with a provisional BMS strategy in the side branch. Twenty-eight patients were treated at two sites in Germany with a remarkably low side branch stenting rate (8%) and LLL of 0.38 mm in the main branch and 0.21 mm in the side branch at 9 months. Achievement of the primary endpoint (<30% stenosis in the main branch, <50% stenosis in the side branch) occurred in 97% and 89% of vessels, respectively. Although there were no deaths in the follow-up, two late stent thromboses occurred (1 definite, 1 probable) in the main branch stent. The investigators concluded that there was evidence of efficacy but that the late stent thrombosis noted raised the issue of the safety for DCBs used in combination with BMSs in the setting of bifurcation disease. A corollary pilot effort from a different group of investigators using different balloon formulation was the DEBIUT.[28d] In this study, both first- and second-generation DIOR DCBs (Eurocor, Bonn, Germany) were used. The second-generation device, as contrasted to the first generation employed in the PICCO-LETO trial, is characterized by a 3-mcg/mm^2 concentration of nanoscopic paclitaxel mixed with a proprietary "shellac" excipient. In this multicenter, prospective 3-arm study, 120 patients were randomly assigned to the following main-branch (MB) and side-branch (SB) treatment strategies: BMS in MB/PTCA in SB, DCB and BMS in MB/DCB in SB, and DES in MB/PTCA in SB. Provisional T-stenting was available as needed for all SB therapy, and dual antiplatelet therapy was given for only 3 months in the DCB arms. Although the LLL primary endpoints were not met owing to the unexpectedly strong PTCA results, there were nevertheless strong trends in favor of DCB in comparing efficacy outcomes of DCBs versus BMSs in the MB and DCB versus PTCA in the SB. In addition, the safety profile also favored the DCB. The findings led the investigators to call for a larger, more appropriately powered, study. A nonrandomized single-center trial investigated the treatment of coronary in-stent restenosis with the urea paclitaxel coated In.Pact Falcon DCB (Medtronic Invatec, Italy). A total of 26 restenotic BMSs in 23 patients with a lesion length of 22.8 ± 11.1 mm and a reference vessel diameter of 2.64 ± 0.31 mm were treated. Up to 6 months and including the 6-month angiographic control, only one target lesion revascularization was necessary; in total, the rate of major adverse cardiovascular events up to the 6-month follow-up was 4.3%. In-stent late lumen loss was 0.07 ± 0.37 mm and in-segment late lumen loss 0.02 ± 0.50 mm. Binary restenosis was present in one patient (4.3%).[37]

Clinical Data from the Peripheral Vascular Application of Drug-Coated Balloons

There are a variety of vascular beds for which the DCB technology could be applied, but the focus has largely been on the femoropopliteal and, more recently, the infrapopliteal territories. These vascular territories are the most relevant, with the greatest demonstrated need for reduced restenosis rates. The contiguous SFA and popliteal artery (femoropopliteal) are responsible for most lifestyle-limiting claudication. Taken together, these vessels are the longest nonaortic conduits in the body (at times >300 mm in length) and carry a significant atherosclerotic burden; they are often significantly calcified and chronically occluded throughout their length. As important as their biological descriptors are their physical ones: the vessel is subject not only to the potential for external compression but also other complex forces during hip and knee flexion (bending, torsion, and axial elongation/shortening). Balloon angioplasty has proved to be inferior to stent implantation for moderate-length lesions (<13 cm),[29,30] but 1-year patency rates even with stents is still suboptimal at 63% and is worse for longer lesions. Until recently, DESs have not proved to be effective in reducing restenosis in the femoropopliteal territory; at least two trials with self-expanding nitinol stents coated with either sirolimus[11,12] or everolimus using a durable polymer failed to show efficacy.[32a] Results from a third trial, ZILVER PTX, using paclitaxel without a polymer have demonstrated effectiveness compared to angioplasty alone (PTA) and BMS, but in a relatively constrained ~5- to 6-cm lesion length.[32b] Many involved in this field believe that among the explanations for the failure to date of most of the attempts at DES placement in the femoropopliteal region is the tendency for stents to fracture (because of the forces listed), which appears to be associated with restenosis,[33] the ongoing irritant of a rigid stent interacting with a vessel constantly in motion, and the lack of the correct "formula" of drug dose and duration when accounting for stent provocation of intimal hyperplasia in this unique vessel. Accordingly, many observers anxiously await the 24-month patency data for the ZILVER PTX treatment cohort to establish a durable effect with this device. The development of DCB technology holds the promise of improved outcomes without a permanent stent prosthesis. The first human examination of a DCB in a noncoronary territory, the THUNDER (Local Taxane With Short Exposure for Reduction of Restenosis in Distal Arteries) trial, a multicenter European study involving the three-way randomization of 154 patients with lesions of the femoropopliteal segment to standard balloon angioplasty (control), an iopromide-paclitaxel-coated (3 mcg/mm², Paccocath) balloon, or to paclitaxel mixed with iopromide contrast (0.171 mg/

cm³) and used for a standard balloon procedure up to a maximum dose of 17.1 mg.[34] With a moderate mean lesion length of ~7.5 cm, there was a marked reduction in the iopromide-paclitaxel-balloon group for the primary endpoint of 6-month angiographic LLL compared with both the control balloon and paclitaxel in contrast groups (0.4 ± 1.2 vs. 1.7 ± 1.8 vs. 2.2 ± 1.6 mm; $P < 0.001$ for DCB vs. control). TLR at 6 months was reduced in the DCB group compared with control (4% vs. 29%; $P = 0.001$); again, no effect was seen with the paclitaxel and contrast groups (29%; $P = 0.41$). Importantly, vis-à-vis the prior DES concerns, the comparative benefits of DCBs were sustained at 24-month follow-up. A second study using the same coating technology produced remarkably similar results.[35] In the Fem-Pac (Femoral-Paclitaxel) trial, 87 patients underwent 1:1 randomization between control balloon angioplasty and iopromide-paclitaxel-coated balloon angioplasty in relatively short (~6 cm) lesions in the femoropopliteal arteries. For the primary end point of LLL, the coated balloon arm showed results that were superior to those of the control balloon at 6 months (0.5 ± 1.1 vs. 1.0 ± 1.1 mm; $P = 0.031$), with significantly fewer TLR events (6.7% vs. 33%; $P = 0.002$); this difference in TLR was sustained beyond 18 months. Importantly, no safety issues related to the balloon coating were manifest in either study. Beyond these two Paccocath-based studies, another study, LEVANT I, was recently presented.[35a] Using a different proprietary coating engineered to maximize drug delivery to the tissue while minimizing transit and particulate loss, ~100 patients with femoropopliteal disease were assigned to either a balloon-only strategy or a stent-assisted strategy if it was felt that a bailout stent would be required after initial PTA predilation. Thereafter, each group was randomized to treatment with either a balloon coated with 2 μmcg/mm² paclitaxel or standard PTA. With a reasonable mean lesion length of ~8 cm, at 6 months the DCB groups, both PTA and stent, demonstrated significantly better primary endpoint LLL compared with the PTA group (0.46 ± 1.13 mm vs. 1.09 ± 1.07 mm, $P = 0.016$). Clearly larger trials of DCBs in the peripheral circulation are warranted based on the results in the femoropopliteal territory. The data from the LEVANT I trial in combination with the data using the Paccocath technology now establish that there is a class of DCBs, independent of formulation, that have established early effectiveness in both coronary and peripheral applications.

The Future of Drug-Coated-Balloon Technology

Although there have been data that support the efficacy of DCBs in both the coronary and peripheral circulations, some of the coronary trial outcomes have been less than robust, and it seems to be becoming clearer that not only is the specific coating formulation important in clinical efficacy but also the interaction of the DCB and newly implanted stents, which is still not well understood. Most of the current efforts in DCB development are focused on addressing the potential limitations of the technology. The safety and efficacy of these technologies in certain applications such as overlapping balloons, visceral vessel applications, and in use with adjunctive therapies, including atherectomy and stents, will need to be assessed. Importantly, the risk of particulate embolization of the coating and any unintended effects will need to be better elucidated, especially in visceral applications. In addition, as the mechanism of action of DCBs becomes better understood, the opportunities to modify various aspects of the technology will increase, including improvements in the antiproliferative agents employed, which in combination with different carrier molecules might further extend the tissue residence of the agents and result in more directed deposition of drug into the vessel, with reduced wash-off and distal embolization. Despite the many devices and manufacturers that are involved with DCBs, there remains a paucity of large-scale clinical data sets on the safety and effectiveness of this technology. Fortunately, multiple clinical studies are either under way or are being planned in the near future in Europe involving coronary, femoropopliteal, and infrapopliteal applications. In the

United States, pivotal FDA premarket approval studies of the femoro-popliteal territory using this technology will likely begin in 2011. Most studies in the noncoronary circulation will compare DCBs to PTA, with at least one study examining the effects of adjunctive atherectomy. In addition, the occasional need for stent implantation to maintain short-term vessel patency may limit the application of DCBs in certain territories unless safety and efficacy can be shown in combination with permanent metal prostheses. Finally, there is early developmental work using the application of DCB technology to other areas such as dialysis fistulas, renal arteries, venous circulation, intracranial vessels, and even aortic valvuloplasty.

◼ Summary

Both the preclinical and clinical data to date, albeit with some mixed results in selected coronary applications, support the early effectiveness and safety of DCBs in several vascular territories and validate the concept that the balloon delivery of a short burst of an antiproliferative agent to a targeted vessel segment as feasible. There is still much to learn about the mechanisms of DCBs, with the potential for future improvements after the current early phase of the technology. It is hoped that such advances might enhance delivery efficiency and possibly clinical efficacy of DCBs.

REFERENCES

1. Grüntzig A: Transluminal dilatation of coronary-artery stenosis. *Lancet* 1:263, 1978.
2. Hwang CW, Wu D, Edelman ER: Physiological transport forces govern drug distribution for stent-based delivery. *Circulation* 104:600–605, 2001.
3. Axel DI, Kunert W, Goggelmann C, et al: paclitaxel inhibits arterial smooth muscle cell proliferation and migration in vitro and in vivo using local drug delivery. *Circulation* 96:636–645, 1997.
4. Iofina E, Langenberg R, Blindt R, et al: Polymer-based paclitaxel eluting stents are superior to nonpolymer-based paclitaxel eluting stents in the treatment of de novo coronary lesions. *Am J Cardiol* 98:1022–1027, 2006.
5. Joner M, Finn AV, Farb A, et al: Pathology of drug eluting stents in humans: delayed healing and late thrombotic risk. *J Am Coll Cardiol* 48:193–202, 2006.
6. van der Giessen WJ, Lincoff AM, Schwartz RS, et al: Marked inflammatory sequelae to implantation of biodegradable and nonbiodegradable polymers in porcine coronary arteries. *Circulation* 94:1690–1697, 1996.
7. Virmani R, Guagliumi G, Farb A, et al: Localized hypersensitivity and late coronary thrombosis secondary to a sirolimus eluting stent: should we be cautious? *Circulation* 109:701–705, 2004.
8. Moses JW, Leon MB, Popma JJ, et al: Sirolimus eluting stents versus standard stents in patients with stenosis in a native coronary artery. *N Engl J Med* 349:1315–1323, 2003.
9. Scheller B, Speck U, Schmitt A, et al: Acute cardiac tolerance of current contrast media and the new taxane protaxel using iopromide as carrier during porcine coronary angiography and stenting. *Invest Radiol* 37:29–34, 2002.
10. Scheller B, Speck U, Romeike B, et al: Contrast media as a carrier for local drug delivery: successful inhibition of neointimal proliferation in the porcine coronary stent model. *Eur Heart J* 24:1462–1467, 2003.
11. Scheller B, Speck U, Schmitt A, et al: Addition of paclitaxel to contrast media prevents restenosis after coronary stent implantation. *J Am Coll Cardiol* 42:1415–1420, 2003.
12. Speck U, Scheller B, Abramjuk C, et al: Inhibition of restenosis in stented porcine coronary arteries:uptake of paclitaxel from angiographic contrast media. *Invest Radiol* 39:182–186, 2004.
13. Scheller B, Speck U, Abramjuk C, et al: Paclitaxel balloon coating: a novel method for prevention and therapy of restenosis. *Circulation* 110:810–814, 2004.
14. Speck U, Scheller B, Abramjuk C, et al: Restenosis inhibition by non-stent-based local drug delivery: comparison of efficacy to a drug eluting stent in the porcine coronary overstretch model. *Radiology* 240:411–418, 2006.
15. Scheller B, Speck U, Böhm M: Prevention of restenosis: is angioplasty the answer? *Heart* 93:539–541, 2007.
16. Albrecht T, Speck U, Baier C, et al: Reduction of stenosis due to intimal hyperplasia after stent supported angioplasty of peripheral arteries by local administration of paclitaxel in swine. *Invest Radiol* 42:579–585, 2007.
17. Cremers B, Speck U, Kaufels N, et al: Drug eluting balloon: very short-term exposure and overlapping. *Thromb Haemost* 101:201–206, 2009.
17a. Granada JF: Biological concepts and lessons learned from the Paccocath technology in preclinical animal models. Paper presented at the EuroPCR conference, Paris, France, May 2010.
18. Milewski K, Tellez A, Conditt G, et al: Pilot study of paclitaxel eluting balloon (Cotavance Technology) followed by bare metal stent implantation: effect on neointimal formation in the iliofemoral arterial territory of normal swine. *Am J Cardiol* 104:181-D. Abstract, 2009.
19. Kelsch B, Biedermann M, Scheller B, et al: Dose-response to paclitaxel-coated balloon catheters in the porcine coronary overstretch and stent implantation model. *Invest Radiol* 46:255–263, 2011.
20. Posa A, Hemetsberger R, Petnehazy O, et al: Attainment of local drug delivery with paclitaxel-eluting balloon in porcine coronary arteries. *Coron Artery Dis* 19(4):243–247, 2008.
21. Cremers B, Biedermann M, Mahnkopf D, et al: Comparison of two different paclitaxel-coated balloon catheters in the porcine coronary restenosis model. *Clin Res Cardiol* 98(5):325–330, 2009.
22. Posa A, Nyolczas N, Hemetsberger R, et al: Optimization of drug-eluting balloon use for safety and efficacy: evaluation of the 2nd generation paclitaxel-eluting DIOR-balloon in porcine coronary arteries. *Catheter Cardiovasc Intervent.* DOI 10.1002/ccd. Published online in Wiley InterScience (www.interscience.wiley.com).
22a. Virmani R: Emerging technologies and therapies in endovascular interventions: drug eluting balloon in peripheral vascular interventions—pre-clinical results: insights from a pathologist. Paper presented at the EuroPCR conference, Paris, France, May 2010.
23. Herdeg C, Goehring-Frischholz K, Zuern C, et al: Local catheter-based delivery of antithrombotic or antiproliferative drugs:a new concept for prevention of restenosis. *Thromb Res* 123:236–243, 2008.
24. Dommke C, Haase KK, Süselbeck T, et al: Local paclitaxel delivery after coronary stenting in an experimental animal model. *Thromb Haemost* 98:674–680, 2007.
25. Cremers B, Toner JL, Schwartz LB, et al: Inhibition of coronary neointimal hyperplasia in swine using a novel zotarolimus-eluting balloon catheter. *Eur Heart J* 30(Abstr Suppl):P3206, 2009.
25a. Freyhardt P, Zeller T, Kröncke TJ, et al: Plasma Levels Following Application of Paclitaxel-Coated Balloon Catheters in Patients with Stenotic or Occluded Femoropopliteal Arteries. *Rofo* 183:448–455, 2011.
26. Scheller B, Hehrlein C, Bocksch W, et al: Treatment of coronary in-stent restenosis with a paclitaxel coated balloon catheter. *N Engl J Med* 355:2113–2124, 2006.
27. Unverdorben M, Vallbracht C, Cremers B, et al: Paclitaxel-coated balloon catheter versus paclitaxel-coated stent for the treatment of coronary in-stent restenosis. *Circulation* 119:2986–2994, 2009.
28. Scheller B, Hehrlein C, Bocksch W, et al: Two year follow-up after treatment of coronary in-stent restenosis with a paclitaxel-coated balloon catheter. *Clin Res Cardiol* 97:773–781, 2008.
28a. Pöss J, Jacobshagen C, Ukena C, et al: Hotlines and clinical trial updates presented at the German Cardiac Society Meeting 2010: FAIR-HF, CIPAMI, LIPSIA-NSTEMI, Handheld-BNP, PEPCAD III, remote ischaemic conditioning, CERTIFY, PreSCD-II, German Myocardial Infarction Registry, DiaRegis. *Clin Res Cardiol* 99:411–417, 2010.
28b. Cortese B, Micheli A, Picchi A, et al: Paclitaxel-coated balloon versus drug-eluting stent during PCI of small coronary vessels, a prospective randomised clinical trial. The PICCOLETO study. *Heart* 96:1291–1296, 2010.
28c. Mathey DG, Wendig I, Boxberger M, et al: Treatment of bifurcation lesions with a drug-eluting balloon: the PEPCAD V (Paclitaxel Eluting PTCA Balloon in Coronary Artery Disease) trial. *EuroIntervention* 7:K61–K65, 2011.
28d. Belkacemi A, Agostini P, Voskuil M, et al: Coronary bifurcation lesions treated with the drug-eluting balloon: a preliminary insight from the DEBIUT study. *EuroIntervention* 7:K66–K69, 2010.
29. Schillinger M, Sabeti S, Loewe C, et al: Balloon angioplasty versus implantation of nitinol stents in the superficial femoral artery. *N Engl J Med* 354:1879–1888, 2006.
30. Schillinger M, Sabeti S, Dick P, et al: Sustained benefit at 2 years of primary femoropopliteal stenting compared with balloon angioplasty with optional stenting. *Circulation* 115:2745–2749, 2007.
31. Duda SH, Pusich B, Richter G, et al: Sirolimus eluting stents for the treatment of obstructive superficial femoral artery disease: six-month results. *Circulation* 106:1505–1509, 2002.
32. Duda SH, Bosiers M, Lammer J, et al: Sirolimus eluting versus bare nitinol stent for obstructive superficial femoral artery disease: the SIROCCO II trial. *J Vasc Interv Radiol* 16:331–338, 2005.
32a. Lammer F: First-in-human clinical trial of a nitinol self-expanding everolimus-eluting stent for prevention of restenosis following infrainguinal stenting. Paper presented at the CRISE Meeting, Lisbon, Portugal, September 2009.
32b. Dake M: Paper presented at the Transcatheter Therapeutics meeting, Washington, DC, USA, September 2010.
33. Scheinert D, Scheinert S, Sax J, et al: Prevalence and clinical impact of stent fractures after femoropopliteal stenting. *J Am Coll Cardiol* 45:312–315, 2005.
34. Tepe G, Zeller T, Albrecht T, et al: Local delivery of paclitaxel to inhibit restenosis during angioplasty of the leg. *N Engl J Med* 358:689–699, 2008.
35. Werk M, Langner S, Reinkensmeier B, et al: Inhibition of restenosis in femoropopliteal arteries: paclitaxel-coated versus uncoated balloon: femoral paclitaxel randomized pilot trial. *Circulation* 118:1358–13565, 2008.
35a. Scheinert D: Paper presented at the Transcatheter Therapeutics meeting, Washington, DC, USA, September 2010.
36. Unverdorben M, Kleber FX, Heuer H, et al: Treatment of small coronary arteries with a paclitaxel-coated balloon catheter. *Clin Res Cardiol* 99:165–174, 2010.
37. Cremers B, Clever YP, Schaffner S, et al: Treatment of coronary in-stent restenosis with a novel paclitaxel urea coated balloon. *Minerva Cardioangiol* 58:583–588, 2010.

15

History of Coronary Balloon Angioplasty and Current Indications

JORGE R. ALEGRÍA | DAVID R. HOLMES JR.

KEY POINTS

- Andreas Grüntzig developed the technique of balloon angio plasty of the coronary arteries and revolutionized the treatment of coronary artery disease.
- Complications of balloon angioplasty include coronary artery dissection, abrupt vessel closure, and restenosis.
- Currently balloon angioplasty alone is used only in selected cases, such as small-vessel disease, the treatment of the side branch bifurcation lesions, contraindication to antiplatelet therapy, in-stent restenosis, and in patients with a vein or arterial graft touchdown stenosis.

"There are three stages in the history of every medical discovery. When it is first announced, people say that it is not true. Then, a little later, when its truth has been borne on them, so that it can no longer be denied, they say it is not important. After that, if its importance becomes sufficiently obvious, they say that anyhow it is not new."

Sir James Mackenzie, 1853–1925[1]

Introduction

The treatment of coronary artery disease has multiple facets. It is recognized increasingly that lifestyle changes—a healthier diet, exercise, smoking cessation, and advanced medical therapies including statins, beta blockers, and antiplatelet therapy—are the cornerstones of such treatment. Percutaneous coronary intervention (PCI) has become the preferred approach when revascularization is required. PCI has evolved substantially from the early days of plain balloon angioplasty to bare metal stents, drug-eluting stents, rotational atherectomy, and other interventions for patients with acute coronary syndromes, limiting angina, or significant ischemia and appropriate anatomy. Cardiac surgery for coronary artery disease still has a role when there is severe ischemia, particularly in the setting of abnormal left ventricular function and multivessel disease that is not amenable to PCI. At present, plain balloon angioplasty is utilized only in selected cases; it has been replaced almost completely by stent-based approaches. The objective of this chapter is to offer a historic perspective on the development of balloon angioplasty and its current indications. It is important to state that there are insufficient systematic, randomized data to support evidence-based recommendations on when, in our current era, balloon angioplasty may be used alone. As healthcare costs become increasingly relevant, the use of balloon angioplasty versus stents in selected patients—those at low risk for both acute vessel closure and restenosis—may have to be readdressed.

Historical Overview of Cardiac Catheterization

"History consists of a series of accumulated imaginative inventions."
Voltaire, 1694–1778

Human beings have been affected by the stenosis of luminal conduits across the body throughout history; its treatment has been influenced by the technologies available at specific historical periods (Table 15-1). Interventions that were performed to improve urinary flow by dilating the urethra were recorded by the Egyptians 3000 B.C., using bronze, gold, and silver pipes. Much later, the vascular system was instrumented in cadavers. Around 400 B.C., air and water were pushed through hollow reeds or brass pipes into cadaver aortas to clarify the function of the cardiac valves. In 1651, Harvey catheterized the inferior vena cava in a cadaver, proving that venous blood flows from the periphery to the lungs.[2] In 1844, Claude Bernard, a French physiologist, inserted a mercury thermometer into the carotid artery of a horse and advanced it through the aortic valve into the left ventricle in order to measure blood temperature. Bernard called the procedure cardiac catheterization and continued to perform and improve it over the next four decades, measuring intracardiac pressures in a variety of animals and gaining essential insight on the hemodynamics of the cardiovascular system. Another milestone was passed by Adolph Fick, a German physiologist, in 1870, who estimated cardiac output through oximetric measurements and developed the appropriate calculations. In 1895, Wilhelm Conrad Roentgen discovered x-rays, allowing for the subsequent deeper visualization of the body and blood vessels. Later, in 1901, Roentgen was awarded the first Nobel Prize in physics. In 1929, Werner Forssmann was seeking a "safer approach for intracardiac drug injection", he inserted a catheter into his left basilic vein and advanced it to the right atrium, the first documented catheter placement inside the heart of a living human being. Subsequently, in 1941, Cournand and Richards used the cardiac catheter already described initially by Forssmann and the three of them shared the 1956 Nobel Prize in medicine for development of cardiac catheterization.[3] In the 1950s and '60s, Sones, Ricketts, Abrams, and Judkins developed coronary arteriography, allowing further understanding of the anatomy, physiology, and clinical implications of coronary artery disease.[4] That paved the way for the development of coronary artery bypass grafting in the late 1960s by Kolessov, Green, and Favaloro. It is important to remember that coronary angiography also helped to correlate the clinical symptoms of angina with different degrees of luminal stenosis. In the early 1960s, Charles Dotter and Melvin Judkins, in Portland, Oregon, developed transluminal coronary angioplasty using a wire and coaxial Teflon catheters to "unclog arteries, improving symptoms and peripheral blood flow."[5] Unfortunately Dotter failed to receive support in the United States and was not able to develop the technique further. In the meantime, several investigators and researchers in Europe, especially Zeitler, gained experience in the Dotter technique. In 1974, Andreas Grüntzig, a young German physician, who had trained with Eberhardt Zeitler, modified Dotter's catheter system (Fig. 15-1). Grüntzig developed a double-lumen catheter at the distal end of which was a distensible balloon made of polyvinylchloride (PVC). When inflated, the balloon exerted circumferential pressure on the plaque. Grüntzig achieved 86% patency in the iliac and femoropopliteal arteries and a 3-year patency rate of 73%.[6]

Mechanisms

The basic principles of percutaneous transluminal coronary angioplasty (PTCA) are extensions of Laplace's law. The inflation of the balloon creates a "dilating force" that is a consequence of the diameter

TABLE 15-1	Historical Evolution of Catheterization and Interventions	
3000 BC. The Egyptians performed bladder catheterizations		1946–1947 Dexter studies patients with congenital heart disease.
400 BC. Air and water were pushed through hollow reeds into cadaveric aortas		1947 Zimmerman developed a completely intravascular technique for left heart catheterization
1651 Catheterization of the inferior vena cava by William Harvey		1947 Bing reports the catheterization of the coronary sinus
1665 Wren delivered the first intravenous injection into a dog		1949–1950 Development of cineangiography and imaging intensifier
1667 Major delivered the first intravenous injection into a human		1951 Dotter creates the first balloon-tipped angiographic catheter
1711 Hales performs the first documented cardiac catheterization using a horse		1951 Gorlin and Gorlin develop the formula to calculate stenotic valve areas
1844 Claude Bernard measures blood temperature in the left ventricle of a horse		1952 Facquet and colleagues develop transbronchial left atrial puncture using a rigid bronchoscope
1847 Claude Bernard records intracardiac pressures in a dog.		1953 Bjork performs left atrial puncture using the posterior paravertebral approach
1870 Adolph Fick calculates blood flow by oximetry		
1895 Discovery of x-rays by Roentgen on November 8		1953 Hansen performs left atrial puncture using the suprasternal puncture route
1896 Williams produces fluoroscopic images of the heart		1953 Seldinger develops a percutaneous approach for the introduction of catheters
1896 Haschek and Lindenthal perform the first arteriogram with chalk in the brachial artery in a cadaver		1956 Forssmann, Cournand, and Richards are awarded the Nobel Prize in physiology
1897 Stewart introduces the indicator dilution method to calculate cardiac output using sodium chloride		1956 Brock reports the apical approach to left ventricular puncture
1899 William Baumgarten performs the first coronary angiograms in cadavers		1958 Sones develops coronary angiography at the Cleveland Clinic
1905 Bleichroeder, Unger, and Loeb insert catheters into blood vessels without x-ray		1959 Ross performs the first transseptal left atrial puncture
		1963 Dotter, by serendipity, recanalizes an occluded right iliac artery
1907 Jamin and Merkel publish the first atlas of coronary arteriography from cadavers		1964 Dotter and Judkins perform the first intentional transluminal dilatation in a left popliteal artery
1910 First right-heart angiogram done by Franck and Alwens		1967 Judkins and Amplatz developed catheters for coronary angiography
1919 First angiogram using potassium iodide into the hand veins in a living person performed by Heuser		1968 Schoonmaker and King create the multipurpose catheter
1921 Lipiodol, the first iodinated contrast, is created		1970 The Swan-Ganz catheter is introduced
1929 Werner Forssmann performs the first right heart catheterization		1976 Chazov performs intracoronary lysis with streptokinase
1930 Klein measures cardiac output in humans using the Fick principle		1977 Grüntzig and Myler perform the first human coronary angioplasty during bypass surgery at St. Mary's Hospital in San Francisco
1931 First pulmonary angiogram done by Perez Ara		
1933 Reboul and Racine perform percutaneous ventricular needle puncture		1977 On September 16, Gruentzig performs the first coronary angioplasty in an awake human in Zurich Switzerland
1936 Cournand and Richards begin landmark studies of right-heart physiology		1978 Rentrop performs dislodgement of intracoronary thrombi with guidewires for the treatment of acute myocardial infarction
1942 Catheterization of the right ventricle by Cournand and Richards		
1944 Catheterization of the pulmonary artery by Cournand and Richards		1978 Grüntzig reports the first angioplasty of renal artery stenosis
1945 Lenegre and Maurince perform endocardial electrocardiography		
1945 Richard Bing organizes the first diagnostic cardiac catheterization laboratory		

and length of the balloon; the resulting pressure and dilating force influence the "hoop stress" (Figure 15-2). When properly inflated, the balloon creates contained barotrauma that produces intimal damage, with fissuring or disruption of the plaque, usually more marked at the plaque shoulder; partial dehiscence of the intimal plaque from its underlying media; occasional intramedial dissection; stretching of the media and adventitia; and aneurismal dilatation of the vessel (Table 15-2).[7,8] However, PTCA can induce acute coronary occlusion due to dissection (Fig. 15-3), intraplaque hemorrhage, luminal thrombosis, (Fig. 15-4), and other complications (Table 15-3).

Further insight into the mechanisms of PTCA was gained with the aid of intravascular ultrasound. It was found that plaque fissuring,

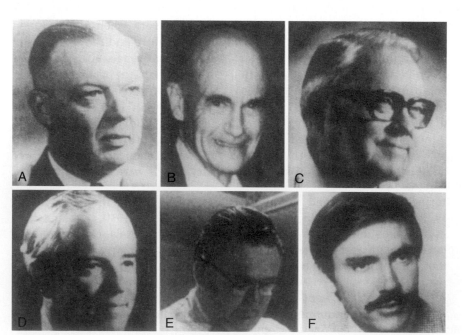

Figure 15-1 Pioneers in interventional cardiology. A. Werner Forssmann (1904–1979). B. Charles T. Dotter (1920–1985). C. Sven I. Seldinger (1921). D. F. Mason Sones (1919–1985). E. Melvin P. Judkins (1922–1985). F. Andreas R. Grüntzig (1939–1985). *From The National Library of Medicine (A); Geddes LA, Geddes LE. The Catheter Introducers. Chicago: Mobium Press, 1993 (B–E); and the Andreas Grüntzig Cardiovascular Center, Emory University, Atlanta, GA (F).*

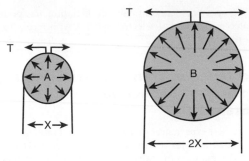

Figure 15-2 Hoop stress (T) is twice as great at an equal pressure in the larger balloon.

medial and adventitial stretching, and separation of the atheroma from the underlying media account for an increase in luminal size as well as the angiographic findings of intraluminal haziness and intimal flap or dissection.[8] In general, multiple mechanisms such as plaque compression and fracture are responsible for the increase in luminal size with PTCA and are relevant to understanding the complications of balloon inflation.[9]

The Development of Coronary Angioplasty

Prior to the development of angioplasty, the armamentarium for treating coronary artery disease with angina and acute coronary syndromes was very limited. There was pain control, attempts at risk factor modification, and prolonged bed rest for patients with myocardial infarction (MI). By the late 1970s, coronary artery bypass grafting (CABG) had become widespread in the United States and its indications were debated. Not uncommonly, surgery was used, but often only as a last resort. The development of interventional cardiology by Andreas Grüntzig revolutionized the treatment of coronary artery disease. Grüntzig did his early work with a peripheral balloon catheter in canine models and later in human cadaver experiments. He visited the United States in 1977 and, in San Francisco with Myler and Hanna, performed coronary angioplasty for the first time on a living human. This was done in the operating room, with patients undergoing multivessel bypass surgery, demonstrating that coronary arteries could be dilated safely in vivo without a significant risk of distal embolization. This previous experience encouraged Grüntzig to perform the first percutaneous transluminal coronary angioplasty in Zurich, Switzerland, on September 16, 1977, a landmark date in the history of medicine (Fig. 15-5). The patient was a 37-year-old insurance salesman with severe exercise-induced angina; angiography established single vessel disease with a proximal stenosis of the left anterior descending artery. The stenosis was located immediately before the takeoff of a large diagonal branch. The patient was informed by Grüntzig about his various options and he was specifically informed that he would be the first patient ever to be treated with this technique. The patient, in the words of Grüntzig, "enthusiastically gave his consent." Grüntzig accessed the right femoral artery and used a Judkins-shaped guiding catheter. There were multiple spectators in the recording booth, including cardiologists, surgeons, anesthesiologists, and cardiology and radiology fellows. The 9-Fr guiding catheter was placed and the procedure, which seemed quite straightforward, was successfully completed. It is important to state that Grüntzig was prepared to perfuse

TABLE 15-2	Mechanisms of Percutaneous Transluminal Coronary Angioplasty
Plaque compression	
Plaque fracture	
Plaque fracture with intimal flaps and localized medial dissection	
Stretching of the disease-free segment	
Stretching with compression	

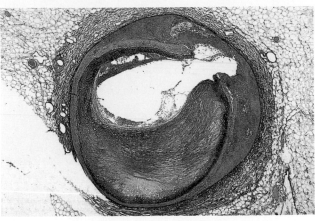

Figure 15-3 Percutaneous transluminal coronary angioplasty with small dissection (Verhoeff-Van Gieson [VVG] stain). *Courtesy W.D. Edwards, MD, Mayo Clinic, Rochester, MN.*

blood into the distal vascular bed in case complete occlusion occurred at the time of dilation. The only abnormality was a transient right bundle branch block, which normalized 4 hours later. It is interesting to read Grüntzig's description of the case, which points out that the patient had lost no time in finding a newspaper reporter who would be ready to spread the news. That certainly could have been a threat to the seriousness of the technique and would have sent the world a message of lack of scientific scrutiny. Grüntzig finally arrived at a "gentleman's agreement" with the reporter to hold the story until more patients had been treated and the first report had been published in a medical journal. His wishes were respected and the first five cases were published in 1978 in the *Lancet*.[10]

On March 1, 1978, Myler in San Francisco and Stertzer in New York introduced coronary angioplasty in the United States. Their research was presented in 1978 and 1979. Grüntzig was very careful about the development of the technique and required a careful analysis of all the cases. This prompted the founding of the National Heart, Lung and Blood Institute (NHLBI) registry for PTCA, which eventually expanded to more than 70 sites worldwide. These early days laid the foundations for what we know today as the "data-driven percutaneous coronary intervention." Also, Grüntzig was an excellent teacher and engaging speaker who captivated his audience in live demonstration courses. The most "educational" time was when Grüntzig dealt with complications. These live courses encouraged the further proliferation of the technique. In the late 1970s and early 1980s, angioplasty was recommended mainly for symptomatic but clinically stable patients who had

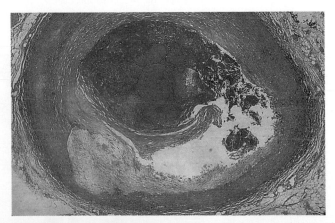

Figure 15-4 Percutaneous transluminal coronary angioplasty with acute thrombosis (hematoxylin and eosin stain). *Courtesy W.D. Edwards, MD, Mayo Clinic, Rochester, MN.*

TABLE 15-3	Potential Complications of Balloon Angioplasty
Complication	
Coronary artery dissection	
Abrupt closure	
Distal embolization, no reflow	
Symptomatic restenosis	
Periprocedural infection	
Coronary perforation	
Need of urgent CABG	
Death	

inducible ischemia with preserved left ventricular function. Such individuals were considered to be good candidates for bypass surgery. The procedure was performed only when stenosis was present (with no occlusions) in proximal, discrete, concentric, and noncalcified lesions in areas that did not involve arterial segments and were not angulated or near the source of a major side branch.[11] In the beginning, around 70% of PTCAs were successful; by 1982 the success rate exceeded 80%. Initially, the catheters were large, 9 or 10 Fr, and were made of solid Teflon. Later, a three-layer catheter was developed that allowed more torque control; the external layer was made of polyurethane for memory. The early experience from Zurich with PTCA was reported in 133 patients who underwent successful PTCA with demonstrated cardiac survival of 96% at 6 years and an enduring improvement in symptoms in 67% of patients. The 10-year follow-up revealed a survival of 90% for patients with single-vessel disease.[12,13] The NHLBI Registry provided relevant information regarding the evolution of patient selection and outcomes. For example, the first registry of PTCA from 1977 to 1981 was compared with the registry from 1985 to 1986, showing that the in-hospital mortality rate (1%) and the rate of nonfatal MI (4.3%) were similar despite a higher-risk population, including older patients with more multivessel disease, decreased ejection fraction, and a more frequent history of MI or previous coronary artery bypass grafting in the registry from 1985 to 1986.[14] The 1980s brought two fundamental changes in technique: first, prolonged balloon inflations came into use because of the availability of perfusion balloon catheters that decreased the rates of coronary dissection and acute closure. Second, "monorail" (i.e., rapid-exchange) catheters with easily expandable guidewires were introduced; these permitted quick withdrawal of the balloon catheters to allow better contrast injection for coronary angiography, thus eliminating the need to perform transstenotic gradients, as had initially been done in the course of documentation. Pretreatment with aspirin during this time was found to decrease the risk of acute coronary artery occlusion during surgery or in the perioperative period.[15] Subsequently angioplasty was attempted in total coronary occlusions, leading to the finding that total occlusion was not an absolute contraindication to coronary angioplasty. Successful balloon dilatation was performed in approximately two-thirds of selected patients with recent total occlusions (<12 months).[16]

Percutaneous Transluminal Coronary Angioplasty of Saphenous Vein Graft Stenosis

One of the earliest experiences in the treatment of saphenous vein graft stenosis included a series of 101 patients between 1981 and 1987. A total of 107 saphenous vein grafts were dilated, with a primary success rate of 91.8%. The risk of MI was 6%, there was a 2% risk of emergency CABG, and a mortality rate of 2%. All of these complications occurred after angioplasty on grafts implanted more than 36 months after surgery.[17]

Clinical Trials of Percutaneous Transluminal Coronary Angioplasty in Coronary Artery Disease

In the multicenter NHLBI Registry of PTCA from 1985 to 1986, the incidence of procedure-related death, nonfatal MI, and CABG were 0.2%, 3.5%, and 2.9% respectively.[18] As previously stated, the initial criteria were very strict for PTCA; using the CASS (Coronary Artery Surgery Study) criteria, only 3.7% of patients would have been eligible for PTCA. The initial success for "simple lesions" was greater than 90%. But the ultimate success of PTCA was determined by patient characteristics, lesion characteristics, technique and devices, and the physician's experience. In the 1985 to 1986 NHLBI Registry, among a total of 1,802 patients without acute MI, single-vessel disease was present in 839, and there was a success rate of 89% for PTCA (the success rate was defined as a reduction of at least 20% in the narrowing of the vessel diameter). Among patients with single-vessel disease, 84% had clinical success and all lesions were dilated without in-hospital death, infarction, or the need of emergency bypass surgery. This was an important study, demonstrating significant progress compared with the PTCA Registry from 1977 to 1981. Other studies included the ACME (angioplasty compared with medical treatment) trial in approximately 212 patients with stable coronary artery disease, single-vessel disease, and positive exercise testing or MI within 3 months and evidence of 70% to 99% stenosis of the proximal vessels. There was a higher rate of complications in the group treated with PTCA (including emergency bypass surgery). The PTCA arm had a higher cost, but with a greater decrease in anginal burden and a decrease of the use of antianginal medications as well as improved exercise tolerance. There was a small group of patients (7) from the PTCA group who required CABG; none of the medically treated patients required this surgery. There was no significant difference in

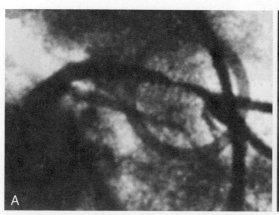
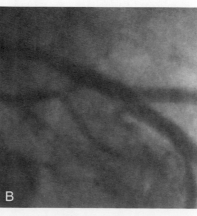

Figure 15-5 A. First percutaneous transluminal coronary angioplasty. B. The 23-year follow-up angiogram. *From Meier B. The first patient to undergo coronary angioplasty—23 year follow-up. N Engl J Med 2001;344: 144–145.*

the rates of death or MI. While there were no differences in rates of death and MI, this study found that patients receiving PTCA had significantly improved exercise duration on treadmill tests and fewer episodes of angina. The EAST (Emory Angioplasty versus Surgery Trial) was a single-center trial with around 400 patients who were randomized to PTCA or CABG. In the PTCA group, 88% of target lesions were treated successfully; in the CABG group, 90% of the patients received an internal mammary artery, and the primary endpoint consisted of a composite of death, Q-wave MI, and large ischemia on thallium imaging at 3 years. There was no difference in the primary endpoint in the two groups (27% for PTCA vs. 26.8% for CABG) or mortality at 3 years (7.1% for PTCA vs. 6.2% for CABG). More than 50% of patients with PTCA required additional revascularization within 3 years, compared with only 13% in the surgical group. Quality-of-life assessment was similar in both groups. At 1 year follow-up, there was no difference in mortality between the two groups, although a trend toward better survival was observed in the CABG-treated patients who had diabetes mellitus with proximal LAD disease. After 3 years, no difference was observed in revascularization rates in the two groups. Subsequently, PTCA was tested in multiple clinical trials, including the GABI trial, the BARI trial, the MASS trial, and the RITA-1 and RITA-2 trials. Overall, all these trials tested different strategies of revascularization, comparing plain balloon angioplasty with medical therapy or CABG. Also, PTCA was tested against thrombolytic therapy in STEMI, demonstrating that PTCA as compared with CABG improved the rates of nonfatal reinfarction. It was also associated with a lower rate of serious bleeding and resulted in at least similar or better ventricular function and a higher patency of the infarct-related artery.[19–21]

Complications of Percutaneous Transluminal Coronary Angioplasty

In the 1977–1983 NHLBI Registry, the mortality rate for PTCA was 0.9%, the rate of emergency CABG was 6.6%, and rate of MI was 5.5%, with a total of 14% of major complications in some 3,000 patients from more than 105 centers. Complications were more frequent in women and in patients with unstable angina. With procedural experience, the rate of MI decreased, but unfortunately the rate of coronary artery dissection or abrupt closure remained unchanged.

CORONARY ARTERY DISSECTION

Coronary artery dissection is the most common complication of PTCA (Fig. 15-3). The majority of dissections do not lead to acute ischemic complications. With smaller dissections, a conservative approach is used. A higher rate of complications is seen with longer dissections, greater degrees of stenosis, and smaller cross-sectional vessel area.[22] Anatomical factors played an important role in the development of coronary artery dissection. For example, PTCA in angulated stenoses resulted in higher initial failure rates and complications. Also, the presence of coronary artery calcification detected by intravascular ultrasound was a predictor of a dissection.

ABRUPT CLOSURE

This is a major complication of PTCA. In clinical studies there were several predictors of this, including proximal vessel tortuosity, eccentricity of the lesion, length, and angulation; but the specific importance of these predictors for the individual patient proved to be unclear. Among the 1,155 patients studied in the first NHLBI Registry, the rate of abrupt closure was 4.5%. Subsequently, in the 1980s and early 1990s, the rates of abrupt closure fluctuated between 4% and 8%, with more than one-fifth of patients requiring emergency bypass surgery despite the use of perfusion devices and longer inflation. This certainly explains the welcoming of stenting in the interventional community, which led to a tremendous decrease in the rate of abrupt closure.

DISTAL EMBOLIZATION

This is a very frequent occurrence in animal models as well as in humans and has been associated with an increase in periprocedural MI, which of course, has an important implication for the no-reflow phenomenon in periprocedural MI.

RESTENOSIS AFTER PERCUTANEOUS TRANSLUMINAL CORONARY ANGIOPLASTY

This usually occurs around 6 months after a procedure. In general, angiographically confirmed restenosis occurred in 30% to 60% of patients after successful PTCA. Among 557 patients who underwent successful PTCA, the NHLBI Registry documented a 34% rate of restenosis,[16] probably due to an acute elastic recoil and chronic negative remodeling of neointimal hyperplasia. This actually represents a response of the vasculature with a component of inflammation, granulation, and excessive matrix remodeling, influencing the degree of restenosis after balloon angioplasty. In a series of 1,758 successful angioplasties at Emory between 1980 and 1984 in patients with single-vessel disease, repeat angiography was done at 6 months and completed in 998 patients (57%). Of the clinical variables only unstable angina predicted stenosis; angiographic variables that predicted restenosis included residual stenosis, total occlusion, and proximal left anterior descending artery location.[23] Throughout the 1980s and 1990s, a greater knowledge of the process of restenosis was obtained. It was with the introduction of antimitotic drug-eluted stents that this problem was significantly evaded.

DEATH

This was studied in a registry of 8,052 PTCA procedures. The incidence of death was 0.4% ($n = 32$), with procedural coronary artery closure, typically from dissection, being the main cause of death. Other predictors were decreased left ventricular function and the jeopardy score or territory at risk.[24] Other complications that occurred with PTCA include vascular-related access problems, particularly hemorrhage, coronary perforation, equipment failure, and embolism.

Influence of Balloon Angioplasty in Interventional Cardiology

Balloon angioplasty allowed the development of interventional cardiology. It first started as an additional technique in the cardiac catheterization laboratory. Subsequently, it evolved into the field of interventional cardiology, which requires board certification by the American Board of Internal Medicine, necessitating a formal training in a fellowship program of the ACGME (Accrediting Council on Graduate Medical Education). The principle of balloon dilation of the coronary arteries has been used and extrapolated to multiple other challenges in the treatment of cardiovascular diseases over the last three decades. These have included balloon dilatation of valves and pulmonary veins as well as balloon occlusion of coronary arteries for alcohol septal ablation and other structural and peripheral interventions.

Current Indications for Balloon Angioplasty

Today percutaneous intervention is performed mostly with stents. The use of balloon angioplasty (Table 15-4) is considered mainly in cases of small-vessel (less than 2 mm in diameter) disease, in the treatment of the side branch in a bifurcation lesion, or when there is allergy to the materials of stents or a contraindication to antiplatelet therapy. Patients who may need to discontinue antiplatelet therapy shortly after intervention, such as imminent surgical procedures with a high

TABLE 15-4	Current Indications for Balloon Angioplasty
Small-vessel disease	
Contraindication to adequate dual antiplatelet therapy	
Inability to cross the lesion with a stent	
Treatment of the side branch bifurcation lesions	
In-stent restenosis	
Vein or arterial graft touchdown stenosis	
Noncardiac surgery within 4 weeks	

bleeding risk, may also be considered candidates for balloon angioplasty. Ostial discrete stenoses that do not allow safe stent placement can be treated with angioplasty. Also when there is a touchdown vein graft stenosis, conventional dilatation may yield excellent, durable results. Patients with an acute coronary syndromes and multivessel disease requiring urgent surgical intervention may also be candidates for treatment with angioplasty of the culprit lesion alone.

Andreas Roland Grüntzig (1939–1985)

Interventional cardiology has a wonderful present and a marvelous, but unpredictable future and was made possible with the development of balloon angioplasty. The technique was developed thanks to the vision and creativity of many, but it was Andreas who invented and developed coronary angioplasty, thus becoming the father of interventional cardiology. It was Grüntzig's genius, creativity, vision, talent, teaching skills, passion, and hard work, among other characteristics, that shaped the development of PTCA, finding worldwide acceptance and helping to reduce the morbidity and mortality related to coronary

artery disease beyond measure. Grüntzig died at the age of only 46, but he left a legacy that lives on today in balloon angioplasty.

Conclusions

Balloon angioplasty of the coronary arteries was developed on the foundations of cardiac catheterization and the tremendous need to treat coronary artery disease. The development of the technique was possible in the late 1970s thanks to the technological advances, creativity, and vision of several pioneers. Among those pioneers, Andreas Grüntzig, who developed balloon angioplasty, helped to create registries and taught the technique in memorable live case demonstrations. Complications of the procedure were seen early on and included acute vessel closure and restenosis. In the 1980s and 1990s the use of multicenter registries allowed the cardiovascular community to gain a better understanding of the indications for PTCA, with significant improvements in technical equipment permitting the treatment of higher-risk patients. Subsequently, stenting revolutionized the history of interventional cardiology in the 1990s. Today balloon angioplasty is rarely performed as the primary PCI method; stent-based approaches have replaced it owing to the risks of abrupt closure and restenosis.

In selected cases plain balloon angioplasty is still performed. Let us not forget that the balloon is a tool to be used and may be continued to be refined for its utility in clinical practice.

Acknowledgments

The authors of this chapter would like to thank Dr. W. Bruce Fye for his comments regarding the historical aspects, to Dr. Debabrata Mukherjee and Dr. John C. Gurley for their suggestions and ideas related to balloon angioplasty, and to the previous authors of the historical chapters of *Topol's Textbook of Interventional Cardiology*.

REFERENCES

1. Wilson R: *The beloved physician: Sir James Mackenzie*, New York, 1926, Macmillan, pp 177.
2. Mueller RL, Sanborn TA: The history of interventional cardiology: cardiac catheterization, angioplasty, and related interventions. *Am Heart J* 129(1):146–172, 1995.
3. Fye WB: Cardiovascular medicine: a historical perspective. In Topol EJ, editor: *Textbook of Cardiovascular Medicine*, Philadelphia, 1998, Lippincott Raven.
4. Fye WB: A historical perspective on atherosclerosis and coronary artery disease. In Fuster V, Ross R, Topol EJ, editors: *Atherosclerosis in Coronary Artery Disease*, Philadelphia, 1996, Lippincott-Raven.
5. Dotter CT, Judkins MP: Transluminal treatment of arteriosclerotic obstruction. description of a new technic and a preliminary report of its application. *Circulation* 30:654–670, 1964.
6. Grüntzig A, Hopff H: [Percutaneous recanalization after chronic arterial occlusion with a new dilator-catheter (modification of the Dotter technique)]. *Dtsch Med Wochenschr* 99(49):2502–2510, 1974.
7. Faxon DP, et al: Acute effects of transluminal angioplasty in three experimental models of atherosclerosis. *Arteriosclerosis* 2(2):125–133, 1982.
8. Soward AL, Essed CE, Serruys PW: Coronary arterial findings after accidental death immediately after successful percutaneous transluminal coronary angioplasty. *Am J Cardiol* 56(12):794–795, 1985.

9. Waller BF: Early and late morphologic changes in human coronary arteries after percutaneous transluminal coronary angioplasty. *Clin Cardiol* 6(8):363–372, 1983.
10. Grüntzig A: Transluminal dilatation of coronary-artery stenosis. *Lancet* 311(8058):263–263, 1978.
11. Myler K, GAR, Stertzer SH: *Coronary Angioplasty*. In Rapaport E (Ed): Cardiology Updated, New York, Elsevier Biomedical 1–66, 1983.
12. Grüntzig A, et al: Long-term follow-up after percutaneous transluminal coronary angioplasty. The early Zurich experience. *N Engl J Med* 316(18):1127–1132, 1987.
13. King SR, Schlumpf M: Ten-year completed follow-up of percutaneous transluminal coronary angioplasty: the early Zurich experience. *J Am Coll Cardiol* 22(2):353–360, 1993.
14. Faxon DP, Ruocco N, Jacobs AK: Long-term outcome of patients after percutaneous transluminal coronary angioplasty. *Circulation* 81(3 Suppl):IV9–IV13, 1990.
15. Schwartz L, et al: Aspirin and dipyridamole in the prevention of restenosis after percutaneous transluminal coronary angioplasty. *N Engl J Med* 318(26):1714–1719, 1988.
16. Holmes DR, Jr. et al: Angioplasty in total coronary artery occlusion. *J Am Coll Cardiol* 3(3):845–849, 1984.
17. Proudfit WL, Shirey EK, Sones FM, Jr: Selective cine coronary arteriography. Correlation with clinical findings in 1,000 patients. *Circulation* 33(6):901–910, 1966.

18. Detre K, et al: Percutaneous transluminal coronary angioplasty in 1985–1986 and 1977–1981. The National Heart, Lung, and Blood Institute Registry. *N Engl J Med* 318(5):265–270, 1988.
19. Zijlstra F, et al. A comparison of immediate coronary angioplasty with intravenous streptokinase in acute myocardial infarction. *N Engl J Med* 328(10):680–684, 1993.
20. Grines CL, et al. A comparison of immediate angioplasty with thrombolytic therapy for acute myocardial infarction. The Primary Angioplasty in Myocardial Infarction Study Group. *N Engl J Med* 328(10):673–679, 1993.
21. Gibbons RJ, et al: Immediate angioplasty compared with the administration of a thrombolytic agent followed by conservative treatment for myocardial infarction. The Mayo Coronary Care Unit and Catheterization Laboratory Groups. *N Engl J Med* 328(10):685–691, 1993.
22. Bell MR, et al: Predictors of major ischemic complications after coronary dissection following angioplasty. *Am J Cardiol* 71(16):1402–1407, 1993.
23. Leimgruber PP, et al: Restenosis after successful coronary angioplasty in patients with single-vessel disease. *Circulation* 73(4):710–717, 1986.
24. Ellis SG, et al: Causes and correlates of death after unsupported coronary angioplasty: implications for use of angioplasty and advanced support techniques in high-risk settings. *Am J Cardiol* 68(15):1447–1451, 1991.

16

Elective Intervention for Stable Angina or Silent Ischemia

GREGORY W. BARSNESS | DAVID E. KANDZARI

KEY POINTS

- Chronic angina is a growing worldwide problem with significant economic and societal costs.

- By reducing the ischemic burden, percutaneous coronary revascularization provides important clinical benefit in patients with established obstructive coronary arterial disease. The foremost effect is prompt symptom control and improved exercise tolerance. Direct evidence for improvement in survival or definitive reduction of major cardiovascular events is lacking in the broad population of patients with chronic, stable symptomatic coronary arterial disease.

- Optimal medical therapy is an essential component of the successful treatment of patients with established coronary disease and those at risk.

- Along with optimal medical therapy, secondary prevention strategies of diet, exercise, and smoking cessation are required elements in the treatment of patients with coronary artery disease and provide important and measurable benefit in this population.

- Patients at elevated risk for adverse events—including those with left ventricular dysfunction, chronic kidney disease, diabetes mellitus, and an extensive ischemic burden—have greater potential for measurable prognostic benefit with revascularization in addition to optimal medical therapy.

Introduction

Angina pectoris affects approximately 9 million of the 16.3 million people with a diagnosis of coronary artery disease in the United States, and the prevalence increases with age for both established and symptomatic coronary disease (Figs. 16-1 and 16-2).[1] In combating this disease, U.S. physicians performed an estimated 6.8 million inpatient cardiovascular procedures in 2007, an increase of 27% over the previous decade, including approximately 622,000 percutaneous coronary revascularization procedures. The mean hospital charge for percutaneous coronary intervention (PCI) was $56,205 in 2008,[1] with average costs near $20,000 for a typical procedure and overnight hospitalization. While costly, appropriate revascularization in patients with chronic angina renders important prognostic benefits, contributing an estimated 5% to the total observed reduction in coronary heart disease mortality between 1980 and 2002.[2] Despite this measurable success in addressing established disease, the incidence and costs associated with symptomatic coronary artery disease continue to grow throughout the world, contributing an ever-increasing proportion to the overall morbidity, mortality, and lost economic productivity in both developed and developing regions. Revascularization is intuitively central to the treatment paradigm for coronary artery disease. A mismatch between myocardial oxygen supply and demand is the predominant mechanism implicated in the development of symptoms associated with obstructive coronary artery disease. Generally, epicardial coronary lesions comprising at least 50% to 79% diameter obstruction (70%-90% by cross-sectional area measurement) are associated with impaired flow and resultant ischemia. When correlated with clinical or objective evidence of ischemia, such lesions are attractive targets for symptom management. However, the realm of patients with symptoms or signs of ischemia may also include those with abnormal coronary endothelial function, coronary vasospasm, microvascular dysfunction, and even silent, asymptomatic myocardial ischemia. In addition, symptoms reminiscent of ischemic angina may be a manifestation of a noncardiovascular process, such as gastrointestinal, musculoskeletal, or neuropsychiatric pathology (generally anything from the navel to the nose), while other patients, especially women and the elderly, may present with symptoms such as fatigue, chronic "soreness," or dyspnea, which may not be immediately recognized as an expression of cardiovascular disease (Tables 16-1 and 16-2).[3] Individuals with significant ischemia may also remain seemingly unaffected by symptoms because of the "self-regulation" of activity, essentially avoiding activities that have previously caused discomfort. Careful attention to individual patient presentation and characteristics, then, is essential for proper diagnostic triage and management. Once recognized, the goals and methods of treatment for this heterogenous syndrome include reduction in both morbidity and mortality, although anticipated benefits depend on patient characteristics and the treatment modality employed. Percutaneous revascularization has, as its principal benefit, the relief of angina. Symptom relief is the direct effect of a reduction in ischemic burden—although, especially in the setting of residual disease or incomplete abrogation of ischemia, additional complex factors no doubt play a role (Fig. 16-3).[4] While improved survival and reduction of major cardiovascular events are important therapeutic objectives, there are limited data to support a major role for percutaneous revascularization in reducing adverse events in the broader population of patients with stable ischemic coronary disease (Fig. 16-4).[5] In fact, a clear survival advantage for revascularization over medical therapy alone has generally been limited to patients at high clinical or anatomical risk, specifically those high-risk patients undergoing surgical revascularization for severe symptomatic triple-vessel disease, left main coronary disease, left ventricular dysfunction, and manifestations of severe ischemia.[6] Numerous advances in the care of patients with established coronary disease have occurred in the interim, however, with the development of advanced medical therapies and surgical and percutaneous revascularization techniques. In the setting of appropriate and optimal medical therapy (OMT), percutaneous revascularization remains an important adjunct for symptom relief and reduction of ischemic burden.

Revascularization in Patients with Chronic Stable Angina

The principles and practice of modern coronary revascularization strategies are rooted in the conduct and results of studies performed in the 1970s and 1980s. These historic investigations set the framework for our current understanding of the role of both surgical and percutaneous coronary revascularization in the treatment armamentarium of chronic symptomatic ischemic coronary artery disease. While these studies provided important insight into the outcome of

TABLE 16-1	Potential Non-Ischemic Diagnoses in Patients with Chest Pain				
Nonischemic Cardiovascular	*Pulmonary*	*Gastrointestinal*	*Chest Wall*	*Psychiatric*	
Aortic dissection	Pulmonary embolus	Esophageal	Costochondritis	Anxiety	
Pericarditis	Pneumothorax	Esophagitis	Fibrositis	Hyperventilation	
	Pneumonia	Spasm	Rib fracture	Panic disorder	
	Pleuritis	Reflux	Sternoclavicular arthritis	Primary anxiety	
		Cholecystitis	Biliary Herpes zoster	Affective disorders	
		Choledocholithiasis		Somatiform disorder	
		Cholangitis			
		Peptic ulcer			
		Pancreatitis			

Reproduced with permission: Gibbons RJ, Abrams J, Chatterjee K, Daley J, Deedwania PC, Douglas JS, et al. ACC/AHA 2002 guideline update for the management of patients with chronic stable angina: a report of the American College of Cardiology/American Heart Association Task Force on Practice Guidelines (Committee to Update the 1999 Guidelines for the Management of Patients with Chronic Stable Angina). Available at: www.accorg/clinical/guidelines/stable/stable.pdf 2002.[3]

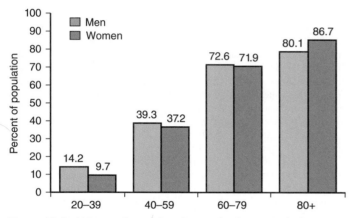

Figure 16-1 U.S. prevalence of cardiovascular disease (including coronary disease, heart failure, stroke, and hypertension) by age and sex. (*Reproduced with permission: Roger VL, Go AS, Lloyd-Jones DM, et al. Heart disease and stroke statistics—2011 update: a report from the American Heart Association. Circulation 2011;1231.*)

TABLE 16-2	Ischemic Provocation or Exacerbating Factors	
Increased Oxygen Demand	*Decreased Oxygen Supply*	
Noncardiac conditions		
Hyperthermia	Anemia	
Hyperthyroidism	Hypoxemia	
Sympathomimetic toxicity (e.g. cocaine)	Sickle cell disease	
Hypertension	Sympathomimetic toxicity	
Anxiety	Hyperviscosity	
Arteriovenous fistulae	Polycythemia	
Cardiac conditions		
Hypertrophic cardiomyopathy	Hypertrophic cardiomyopathy	
Aortic stenosis	Aortic stenosis	
Dilated cardiomyopathy		
Tachycardia		

Reproduced with permission: Gibbons RJ, Abrams J, Chatterjee K, Daley J, Deedwania PC, Douglas JS, et al. ACC/AHA 2002 guideline update for the management of patients with chronic stable angina: a report of the American College of Cardiology/American Heart Association Task Force on Practice Guidelines (Committee to Update the 1999 Guidelines for the Management of Patients with Chronic Stable Angina). Available at: www.accorg/clinical/guidelines/stable/stable.pdf 2002.[3]

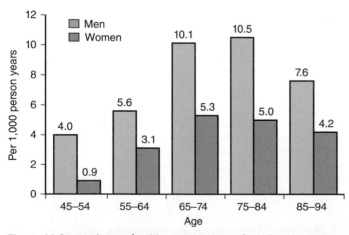

Figure 16-2 Incidence of stable angina pectoris from the Framingham Heart Study (1980–2002/2003) stratified by age and sex. (*Reproduced with permission: Roger VL, Go AS, Lloyd-Jones DM, et al. Heart Disease and Stroke Statistics—2011 update: a report From the American Heart Association. Circulation 2011;1231.*)

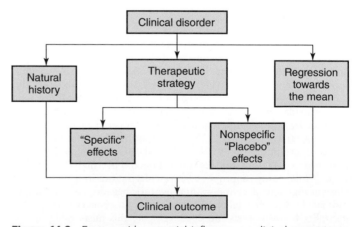

Figure 16-3 Factors with potential influence on clinical response to treatment, including specific, intended effects, such as ischemia reduction after percutaneous coronary intervention, as well as nonspecific effects, often described as "placebo." These effects occur within the context of the natural history of the clinical condition itself, along with the normal "moderation" of effects, or regression toward the mean outcome, that occurs within populations. (*Modified from: Bonetti PO, Holmes DR, Lerman A, Barsness GW. Enhanced external counterpulsation for ischemic heart disease. What's behind the curtain? J Am Coll Cardiol 2003;41(11):1918–1925.*)

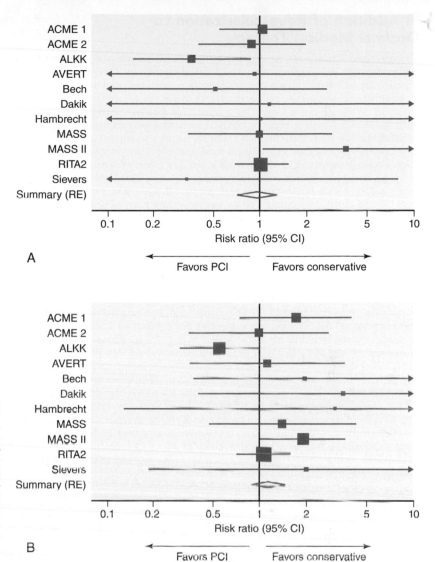

Figure 16-4 A. Point estimates along with 95% confidence intervals and summary statistic for risk of all-cause death after treatment with PCI or medical therapy in 11 studies enrolling patients from 1992 through 2001. *(Reproduced with permission: Katritsis DG, Ioannidis JPA. Percutaneous coronary intervention versus conservative therapy in nonacute coronary artery disease. a meta analysis. Circulation 2005;111(22):2906–2912.)* B. Point estimates along with 95% confidence intervals and summary statistic for risk of cardiac death or myocardial infarction after PCI or medical therapy in 11 studies enrolling patients from 1992 through 2001. From Katritsis DG, Ioannidis JPA. Percutaneous coronary intervention versus conservative therapy in nonacute coronary artery disease. a meta analysis. Circulation 2005;111(22):2906–2912.)*

revascularization and medical therapy using the methodology of the time, great strides have subsequently been made in all areas of treatment, thus decreasing the applicability of these trials to guide therapy in the prevailing healthcare environment. Today, O has been clearly established as the cornerstone of treatment for coronary artery disease. The impact of medical therapy has grown with the introduction of advanced antiplatelet therapy, statins, and angiotensin converting enzyme and receptor inhibition, among other established and evolving therapies that provide important moderation of the inexorable progression of coronary disease. Indeed, appropriate application of evidence-based therapy has had important societal health implications, with a resultant measurable reduction in adverse cardiac events over the past several decades. While appropriate revascularization in patients with chronic angina contributed an estimated 5% to this observed reduction in coronary heart disease mortality between 1980 and 2002, a much larger 50% of the total reduction is attributed to improvement in the risk-factor profiles of those populations in jeopardy, largely thanks to improved agents and the greater application of this medical therapy.[2] While PCI is an important adjunct for symptom control and of established value in reducing both subsequent morbidity and mortality after acute coronary syndromes, both PCI and surgical revascularization are palliative procedures, with lesion progression accounting for significant recurrent morbidity. Recent studies demonstrate the impact of lesion

progression and the need for aggressive concomitant medical therapy in the setting of PCI. Mahn-Won and colleagues[7] retrospectively studied 507 patients undergoing PCI and found that 16% of them underwent clinically driven repeat PCI to treat preexisting nonculprit coronary lesions during the 3-year study period. During the first year after initial PCI, 7.7% of patients in this cohort underwent nonculprit-lesion PCI, with the rate increasing to 16% at 3 years. Greater extent of disease, as manifest by a larger baseline number of significant coronary lesions, independently predicted repeat PCI (odds ratio [OR] 2.29, 95% confidence interval [CI] 1.5–3.5, P < 0.001), as did the baseline risk factors of low levels of high-density lipoprotein (<40 mg/dL; OR 2.01, 95% CI 1.01–3.98, P = 0.046), hypercholesterolemia (total cholesterol >200 mg/dL; OR 1.46, 95% CI 1.22–1.97, P = 0.04), history of PCI (OR 1.24, 95% CI 1.09–1.60, P = 0.003), and increased triglyceride levels (OR 1.003, 95% CI 1.001–1.007, P = 0.038). An additional natural history study[8] of patients who underwent intravascular ultrasound evaluation after PCI for an acute coronary syndrome found that fully one-half of major subsequent adverse events at 3 years occurred at nonculprit sites. Adequate medical therapy and risk modification, then, are essential in the peri- and postinterventional setting to reduce subsequent mortality and morbidity, including symptom recurrence and need for repeat procedures associated with lesion progression and new lesion development.

▦ Addition of Revascularization to Optimal Medical Therapy

The selection of treatment strategies in patients with chronic stable angina depends on symptom status, anatomical complexity, clinical comorbidity, and risk. The main indications for revascularization are to improve symptoms that persist despite O as well as to improve prognosis. While generally suggesting a benefit for revascularization, most randomized trials comparing medical therapy to percutaneous revascularization are limited by their historical nature and entry bias. It is generally agreed that PCI affords rapid and effective symptom relief, a concept borne out in several trials as well as a recent metanalysis[9] of 14 trials, which demonstrated a statistically significant benefit in angina relief with PCI compared with medical therapy (OR 1.69, 95% CI 1.24–2.30). Interestingly, there was important heterogeneity across the trials, with substantially less benefit noted in more contemporary trials of PCI versus OMT, such as COURAGE (Clinical Outcomes Utilizing Revascularization and Aggressive Drug Evaluation),[10] published in 2007 (OR 1.10, 95% CI 0.81–1.49), and OAT (Occluded Artery Trial),[11] published in 2006 (OR 0.83, 95% CI 0.47–1.47). Using meta-regression analysis of the treatment effects of PCI relative to medical therapy, Wijeysundera et al. were able to document an inverse relationship between freedom from angina and the number of "evidence-based" medications utilized during the conduct of a trial (Fig. 16-5).[9] Subgroup analysis of the COURAGE trial[12] confirmed a diminution of angina benefit over time for patients treated with PCI as an initial strategy. While there was a statistically significant difference in rates of freedom from angina between the OMT alone and OMT plus PCI groups at 3 months (42% vs. 53%, P < 0.001), this difference was no longer evident at 3 years (56% vs. 59%, P = 0.30). Although there are numerous potential reasons for this convergence of angina rates during follow-up, including crossover to revascularization from the medical arm, ascertainment bias due to small follow-up populations, and a host of other factors (Fig. 16-3),[4] an important finding is that patients with the most significant anginal burden at baseline obtained the greatest benefit from PCI, whether in OMT alone or OMT-plus-PCI group. In aggregate, these data support a robust, reliable antianginal benefit for PCI in patients with persistent symptoms despite medical therapy. The benefit of percutaneous revascularization on the hard endpoints of death and myocardial infarction is

more controversial and the complexities greater. The relatively low event rates among stable patients with coronary disease, particularly those healthy enough and eligible to be enrolled in randomized prospective trials, limits the discriminatory ability of individual clinical trials to identify treatment effects. Even large metanalytic studies, limited by significant heterogeneity of patient groups and inclusion of antiquated therapies (balloon angioplasty and limited medical options), have provided conflicting results. A metanalysis by Katritsis and colleagues[5] incorporated data from 11 randomized trials of PCI compared with medical therapy in patients with documented coronary artery disease in the absence of a recent acute coronary syndrome. With 2,950 patients included in the analysis, no significant difference could be identified between PCI and medical therapy for overall death (Fig. 16-4A), cardiac death, and myocardial infarction (Figure 16-4B), nonfatal myocardial infarction, or subsequent revascularization. A more recent metanalysis by Schomig and colleagues[13] of 17 trials involving 7,513 patients with chronic stable angina randomized over a 17-year period to PCI or OMT alone again found no significant benefit for PCI over medical therapy with regard to rates of nonfatal myocardial infarction (Fig. 16-6A). However, with selection of cardiac mortality rather than overall mortality as an endpoint, this analysis did suggest a potential advantage for a PCI-based therapeutic strategy for improving long-term outcome (Fig. 16-6B). Further analysis suggested that this benefit was most pronounced in patients who had suffered a recent (<4 weeks) myocardial infarction, as they had about a 35% reduction in the odds of death compared with an estimated risk reduction of 17% for patients with truly stable coronary disease. Both of these metanalyses, however, were limited by several factors, including significant heterogeneity of patient groups and treatments, inclusion of patients with recent acute coronary syndromes, and significant variability in treatments across studies and time periods. Another metanalysis[14] comparing revascularization (surgical or percutaneous) with medical therapy over a 30-year period from 1977 to 2007 confirmed a significant reduction in all-cause mortality associated with revascularization (OR 0.74, 95% CI 0.63-0.88). When this study was stratified by revascularization type, the investigators were also able to show a reduction in mortality with both surgical (OR 0.62, 95% CI 0.50–0.77) and percutaneous (OR 0.82, 95% CI 0.68–0.99) revascularization approaches compared with OMT. This metanalysis, however, like the others, included trials encompassing a broad array of patient populations, including those with recent acute coronary syndromes; it was also limited by the historic nature of treatment algorithms spanning the 30-year study period. Trikalinos and colleagues,[15] in a 20-year network analysis that took into account the evolution of interventional approaches over time, were unable to document a beneficial effect of PCI-based strategies on rates of death or myocardial infarction compared with contemporaneous medical therapy. As previously noted, a major hurdle in the assessment of survival benefits associated with revascularization trials is the relatively low overall event rate. While annualized mortality associated with chronic coronary arterial disease remains approximately 1% to 3% in contemporary series,[14,16,17] the risk of adverse events increases with the degree of left ventricular dysfunction,[18] ischemic burden,[19] and functional limitation (Table 16-3).[20] In addition, risk is increased in the presence of diabetes mellitus, chronic kidney disease, and greater severity of ischemic symptoms[16] and anatomical complexity.[21] It is not surprising, then that a gradient of benefit can be observed for revascularization compared with medical therapy, with greater benefit identified in those patients at greatest risk, whether due to anatomical complexity (Fig. 16-7)[21] or severity of ischemic substrate (Fig. 16-8).[22] Note that in the large cohort of patients identified in the Duke database (n = 18,481) who were treated with an initial strategy of revascularization (either surgical or percutaneous), significant benefit could be demonstrated across the spectrum of disease complexity compared with those patients treated initially with medical therapy alone.[21]

Recent prospective trials have helped to elucidate the potential benefit of percutaneous revascularization across the spectrum of clinical and anatomical risk, along with the continued importance of OMT.

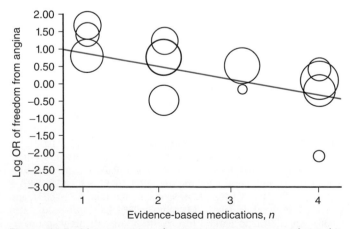

Figure 16-5 Metaregression demonstrating an inverse relationship between freedom from angina and adherence to optimal evidence-based medical regimens within individual trial components of the metanalysis. In more contemporary trials, evidence-based medication was used more frequently and the measurable symptom-relief benefit of PCI was diminished. *(Reproduced with permission: Wijeysundera HC, Nallamothu BK, Krumholz HM, Tu JV, Ko DT. Meta-analysis: effects of percutaneous coronary intervention versus medical therapy on angina relief. Ann Intern Med 2010;152(6):370–379.)*

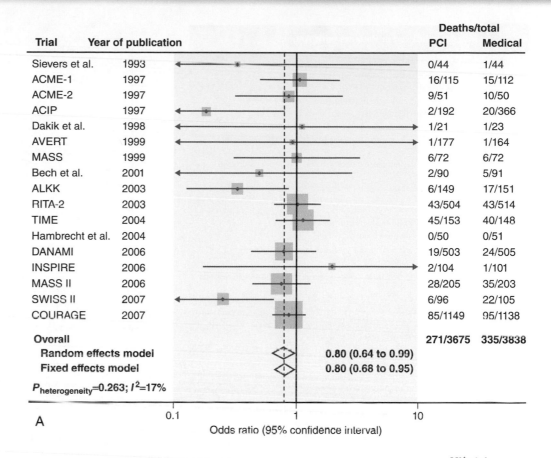

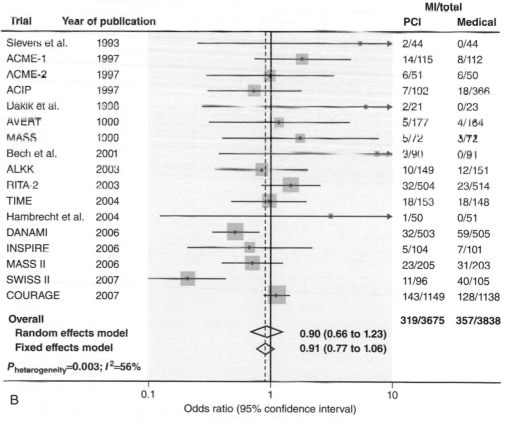

Figure 16-6 A Odds ratios with 95% confidence intervals for risk of cardiac death among 17 randomized trials of PCI or medical therapy with an average follow-up period of 51 months, along with summary statistic. (Reproduced with permission: Schomig A, Mehilli J, de Waha A, et al. A meta-analysis of 17 randomized trials of a percutaneous coronary intervention-based strategy in patients with stable coronary artery disease. J Am Coll Cardiol 2008; 52(11):894–90413. B. Odds ratios with 95% confidence intervals for risk of nonfatal myocardial infarction among 17 randomized trials of PCI or medical therapy with an average follow-up of 51 months, along with summary statistic. Reproduced with permission: Schomig A, Mehilli J, de Waha A, et al. A meta-analysis of 17 randomized trials of a percutaneous coronary intervention-based strategy in patients with stable coronary artery disease. J Am Coll Cardiol 2008;52(11):894–90413.)

TABLE 16-3	Risk Stratification in Patients with Angina

High-risk (>3% annual mortality rate)

1. Severe resting left ventricular dysfunction (LVEF <35%)
2. High-risk treadmill score (score ≤−11)
3. Severe exercise left ventricular dysfunction (exercise LVEF <35%)
4. Stress-induced large perfusion defect (particularly if anterior)
5. Stress-induced multiple perfusion defects of moderate size
6. Large, fixed perfusion defect with LV dilation or increased lung uptake (thallium-201)
7. Stress-induced moderate perfusion defect with LV dilation or increased lung uptake
8. Echocardiographic wall motion abnormality (>2 segments) developing at low dose of dobutamine (less than or equal to 10 mg/kg per minute) or at a low heart rate (<120 beats per minute)
9. Stress echocardiographic evidence of extensive ischemia

Intermediate-risk (1%–3% annual mortality rate)

1. Mild/moderate resting left ventricular dysfunction (LVEF 35%–49%)
2. Intermediate-risk treadmill score (−11–5)
3. Stress-induced moderate perfusion defect without LV dilation or increased lung intake
4. Limited stress echocardiographic ischemia with a wall motion abnormality only at higher doses of dobutamine involving less than or equal to two segments

Low-risk (<1% annual mortality rate)

1. Low-risk treadmill score (score ≥5)
2. Normal or small myocardial perfusion defect at rest or with stress
3. Normal stress echocardiographic wall motion or no change of limited resting wall motion abnormalities during stress

LV, left ventricle; LVEF, left ventricular ejection fraction.

Reproduced with permission: Patel MR, Dehmer GJ, Hirshfeld JW, et al. ACCF/SCAI/STS/AATS/AHA/ASNC 2009 Appropriateness criteria for coronary revascularization: a report of the American College of Cardiology Foundation Appropriateness Criteria Task Force, Society for Cardiovascular Angiography and Interventions, Society of Thoracic Surgeons, American Association for Thoracic Surgery, American Heart Association, and the American Society of Nuclear Cardiology: Endorsed by the American Society of Echocardiography, the Heart Failure Society of America, and the Society of Cardiovascular Computed Tomography. *Circulation* 2009;119(9):1330–1352.

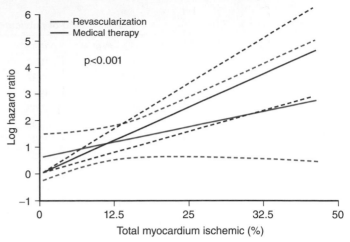

Figure 16-8 Log hazard ratio for 10,627 patients undergoing revascularization or medical therapy for ischemic coronary artery disease as a function of extent of myocardial ischemia. The intersection of curves at an approximate point of inducible ischemia of ≥10% of the myocardium represents the retrospectively identified threshold for survival benefit associated with revascularization. (*Modified with permission: Hachamovitch R, Hayes SW, Friedman JD, et al. Comparison of the short-term survival benefit associated with revascularization compared with medical therapy in patients with no prior coronary artery disease undergoing stress myocardial perfusion single photon emission computed tomography. Circulation 2003;107(23):2900–2907.*)

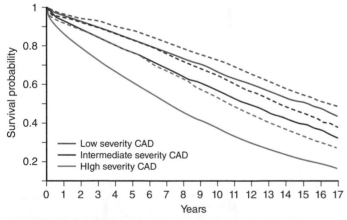

Figure 16-7 Adjusted long-term survival estimates for patients treated with an initial medical (solid lines) or surgical or percutaneous revascularization (dotted lines) approach, stratified by extent of coronary artery disease (CAD) as defined by tertiles of the Duke Index of CAD Severity. High-severity CAD anatomy encompasses those patients with significant (50%-75% stenosis) left main and/or three-vessel coronary artery disease; low-severity CAD includes patients with single-vessel disease or noncritical (<95% stenosis) two-vessel CAD; and intermediate-severity CAD comprises patients with critical proximal LAD disease and the remaining two-vessel disease anatomical subgroups. (*Modified with permission: Smith PK, Califf RM, Tuttle RH, et al. Selection of surgical or percutaneous coronary intervention provides differential longevity benefit. Ann Thorac Surg 2006;82(4):1420–1429.*)

The COURAGE trial[10] is the largest trial yet performed to evaluate whether PCI provides additional clinical benefit over OMT alone. This trial randomized 2,287 patients to OMT or OMT with early percutaneous revascularization (PCI), utilizing predominantly bare metal stents. OMT was intended to include antiplatelet therapy, beta blockade with metoprolol, angiotensin converting enzyme (ACE) inhibition or angiotensin receptor blocker (ARB) therapy, and anti-ischemic measures, including amlodipine and/or nitrate therapy. Diet, exercise, and smoking cessation were also encouraged. All patients underwent entry angiographic evaluation, and those with >70% diameter stenosis in at least one epicardial coronary artery with evidence of ischemia or >80% stenosis and typical anginal symptoms were eligible for inclusion if coronary anatomy was felt to be suitable for PCI. Exclusion criteria included persistent Canadian Cardiovascular Society (CCS) class IV angina, markedly positive stress evaluation, significant heart failure symptoms, left ventricular ejection fraction <30%, or revascularization within the previous 6 months. At a mean follow-up of 4.6 years, there was no significant difference in the primary endpoint of death or myocardial infarction between the PCI and medical treatment groups (OR 1.05, 95% CI 0.87–1.27, P = 0.62), nor was there a difference in overall mortality (7.6% vs. 8.3%, P = 0.38) or freedom from angina (74% vs. 72%, P = 0.35). However, in patients treated with PCI in addition to OMT, freedom from angina was significantly greater up to 3 years, with the medical therapy cohort exhibiting a "catch up" pattern only after the initial 2 years of follow-up (Figure 16-9).[12] Additional early benefits associated with percutaneous intervention included a reduced need for follow-up revascularization during the first year (21% vs. 33%, P < 0.001) with a concomitant reduction in the need for anti-ischemic drug therapy. These results support the widespread use of OMT in patients with established coronary artery disease and suggest that in this setting, early PCI is not associated with reduced long-term event rates. While an initial strategy of OMT alone was not associated with increased rates of death or myocardial infarction, it *was* associated with a significant crossover rate of 30% within the first year of follow-up.[23] In addition, enrolled patients were at relatively low risk, with one-, two-, and three-vessel coronary disease rates of 31%, 39%, and 30%, respectively, and only a 31% incidence of

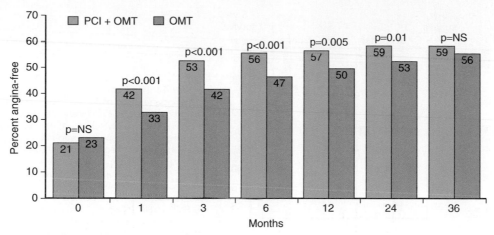

Figure 16-9   Changes in the Angina-Frequency Scale of the Seattle Angina Questionnaire over time within the COURAGE trial cohorts of percutaneous revascularization with optimal medical therapy (PCI plus OMT) and optimal medical therapy alone (OMT). The early anginal benefit demonstrated with PCI plus OMT is reduced over time, as patients within the OMT group experience progressively greater freedom from angina over the initial 3 years of follow-up. *(Modified with permission. Weintraub WS, Spertus JA, Kolm P, et al. Effect of PCI on quality of life in patients with stable coronary disease. N Engl J Med 2008;359(7):677–687.)*

proximal left anterior descending (LAD) disease. Patients also had relatively preserved left ventricular (LV) function, and those with left main coronary disease were not included. Finally, compliance rates with medical therapy at 5 years ranged from 85% for beta blockade to 95% for aspirin or clopidogrel,[10] rates far exceeding the <40% compliance noted in community-based registry studies such as the 40,000-patient "real world" REACH Registry.[24]

The COURAGE Nuclear Substudy[19] evaluated a small but relatively high-risk patient subset of the overall trial. Based on previous work demonstrating the prognostic benefit of coronary revascularization in patients with a significant burden of ischemic myocardium,[22,25] the authors initiated an exploratory evaluation involving 314 consecutive study patients who underwent serial rest/stress myocardial perfusion imaging studies. Based on comparisons of pretreatment ischemic burden and studies performed at 6 to 18 months after randomization, patients in the PCI-plus-OMT group experienced a greater degree of ischemia reduction (≥5% reduction in ischemic myocardium) than those treated with OMT alone (33% vs. 19%, P = 0.0004). The degree of ischemia resolution was also greater in patients with more ischemia at baseline. Importantly, low levels of residual ischemia at follow-up were associated with improved symptom status and better unadjusted survival free of myocardial infarction (P = 0.037), suggesting an important prognostic role for aggressive ischemia reduction in these patients. As with all large randomized trials, the generalizability of these findings is limited by the type of patients enrolled and the already outmoded forms of therapy provided (drug-eluting stents were largely unavailable during recruitment, as were many novel medical therapeutics, including ranolazine). However, the results of this trial provide additional support for the importance of a foundation of OMT while providing confidence in the benefit of percutaneous revascularization as an adjunctive method of symptom and ischemia control. The BARI 2D (Bypass Angioplasty Revascularization Investigation in Type-2 Diabetes) trial[26] addressed a similar question, enrolling 2,368 patients with type 2 diabetes mellitus to early revascularization (coronary bypass surgery or PCI, at the discretion of the treating physician), with OMT and later revascularization as needed for symptom relief. Along with OMT, patients were assigned exercise and risk-factor modification programs with frequent assessment and modification of glycemic control. Patients were included in the trial if they had stable coronary arterial disease (CCS class I or class II in 82%), a positive stress test, and coronary anatomy felt suitable for revascularization. Exclusion criteria included the need for immediate revascularization, left main coronary disease, significant heart failure,

or prior revascularization within a year of study entry. Like the COURAGE trial, the primary endpoint of 5-year all-cause mortality was similar between groups (HR 0.5, 95% CI −2.0–3.1, P = 0.97). Also reminiscent of the COURAGE results, 42% of patients originally assigned to OMT alone crossed over to subsequent revascularization, reinforcing the role of adjunctive revascularization in managing symptoms. Interestingly, because the choice of revascularization was left to the discretion of the treating physician and patient, patients with more extensive disease were generally treated with surgical rather than percutaneous revascularization. In this group of high-risk patients with diabetes mellitus, surgical revascularization offered a significant reduction in nonfatal infarction, with no such advantage noted in those patients selected for PCI over pharmacological therapy.[27] Overall, the results of BARI 2D, like those of the COURAGE trial, support the use of OMT for the treatment of coronary arterial disease, with revascularization providing prompt symptomatic benefit and reduced need for subsequent revascularization, particularly in those patients at greater risk and with symptoms that persist despite aggressive pharmacological therapy. In addition, exploratory subset analysis of both the COURAGE and BARI 2D studies leaves open the possibility that prompt revascularization may provide important prognostic benefit in patients at increased risk because of complex coronary anatomical features or an extensive ischemic substrate. Clearly further study is needed in this area.

■ Selection of Revascularization Strategy

In patients who have persistent anginal symptoms despite aggressive medical therapy or high-risk features of coronary artery disease, revascularization with coronary artery bypass grafting (CABG) or stent-based percutaneous intervention (PCI) is an appropriate consideration. The selection of a specific revascularization strategy depends on numerous factors, including the extent and complexity of the coronary anatomy, presence and severity of comorbidities, and patient and physician preference as well as available scientific evidence. As technology has advanced in the application of both CABG and PCI, this discussion has evolved dramatically. However, while the goals of therapy for both PCI and CABG involve providing symptomatic and prognostic improvement, the methods of achieving these goals continue to be fundamentally different and help to explain the major difference in outcome between the two strategies, that is, the need for more

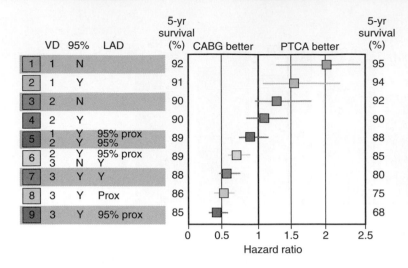

Figure 16-10 Relationship of graded coronary anatomy (GR), including number of vessels with at least 75% stenosis (VD), severity of disease (≥95% stenosis), presence of LAD disease, and differential mortality hazard after either coronary artery bypass grafting (CABG) or percutaneous coronary angioplasty. A gradient of outcome effect is identified, as increased severity of coronary artery disease is associated with improved outcome in CABG-treated patients compared with the outcome associated with PCI in patients with similar high-severity disease. Y indicates yes; N indicates no. *(Modified with permission: Jones RH, Kesler K, Phillips HR III, et al. Long-term survival benefits of coronary artery bypass grafting and percutaneous transluminal angioplasty in patients with coronary artery disease. J Thorac Cardiovasc Surg 1996;111(5):1013–1025.)*

subsequent repeat revascularization in patients undergoing PCI. Because coronary disease is a progressive, incurable condition, both PCI and CABG provide only palliation. Surgical revascularization, however, addresses obstructive coronary disease by providing a perfusion conduit that circumvents a long segment of proximal disease. This allows greater protection from the inexorable development of new and progressive lesions compared with the focal treatment strategy associated with stent placement. In addition, surgical revascularization is associated with more extensive revascularization and a greater likelihood of successful revascularization of all affected territories (full anatomical revascularization),[28] with potential implications for improved survival at follow-up.[28,29] For patients with single-vessel, non-left main coronary artery disease and indications for revascularization, there are few contemporary data to suggest the superiority of CABG over PCI. Revascularization in patients with single-vessel disease generally entails less risk of major morbidity or mortality than that in patients with multivessel disease, and outcomes with PCI have been as good as, or better than those with surgical revascularization. Historically, however, proximal LAD disease has been considered the purview of the surgeon, with randomized and registry data suggesting a survival advantage for surgery in this group (Fig. 16-10).[30] More recent metanalytic studies[31,32] and 10-year follow-up of a randomized trial,[33] however, have failed to confirm a survival benefit for CABG over PCI for the treatment of LAD disease in the modern era. As with other lesion subsets, however, a PCI-based strategy is associated with increased subsequent repeat revascularization, even with the routine application of coronary stents.[33]

Now of largely historical interest, the 1980s and 1990s saw the initiation and completion of several multicenter, randomized trials comparing percutaneous transluminal coronary angioplasty (PTCA) with CABG in patients with multivessel disease. Among nearly 5,000 patients with multivessel coronary disease amenable to either angioplasty or bypass surgery, no difference in death or myocardial infarction, quality of life, or employment status was demonstrated in these trials, suggesting that the primary disadvantage to a primary strategy of angioplasty was the increased need for repeat revascularization. PCI, then, was felt to be a reasonable initial revascularization choice in the setting of preserved ventricular function and technically favorable anatomy.[34] Retrospective database evaluations also confirmed the safety of both modes of revascularization in the majority of patients while documenting a gradient of benefit associated with PTCA or CABG that was dependent upon and correlated directly with the extent and location of coronary stenoses (Fig. 16-10).[30] The evolution of surgical and percutaneous therapies, however, demands recurrent evaluation of comparative outcomes utilizing the best pharmacological and revascularization practices. Contemporary studies of

revascularization in patients with multivessel disease have compared a predominantly stent-based PCI strategy with contemporary surgical techniques, including the judicious use of internal thoracic arterial conduits. The equivalent prognostic impact of bare metal stent (BMS) placement or CABG for the treatment of multivessel disease was confirmed in a pooled patient-level metanalysis of 5-year data from 3,051 patients enrolled in the ARTS (Arterial Revascularization Therapies Study), ERACI-II (Argentine Randomized Trial of Coronary Angioplasty with Stenting versus Coronary Bypass Surgery in Patients with Multivessel Disease), MASS-II (Medicine, Angioplasty or Surgery Study for Multi-Vessel Coronary Artery Disease), and SoS (Stent or Surgery) trials.[35] In this analysis, the 5-year cumulative incidences of death, myocardial infarction, and stroke were similar between patients randomized to PCI with BMS compared with CABG (16.7% vs. 16.9%, HR 1.04, 95% CI 0.86–1.27, P = 0.69). Repeat revascularization, however, occurred significantly more frequently in patients assigned to PCI (29.0% vs. 7.9%, HR 0.23, 95% CI 0.18–0.29) compared with CABG, with a persistent separation of the curves over time (Fig. 16-11). Given the comparable safety of stent-based PCI and CABG in the broad population of patients presenting for multivessel revascularization, the further evolution of drug-eluting stent (DES) technology has provided impetus for further comparative studies. Following the initial positive experience in nonrandomized historical comparisons of outcome after DES, the large SYNTAX (Synergy between Percutaneous Coronary Intervention with TAXUS and Cardiac Surgery) trial was initiated.[36] It randomized 1,800 patients with three-vessel and/or left main coronary artery disease to paclitaxel-eluting stent placement or CABG. The trial was designed as an "all comers" noninferiority trial to evaluate long-term outcomes in patients undergoing revascularization for severe coronary artery disease. Inclusion criteria included patients with previously untreated lesions of ≥50% diameter stenosis with stable or unstable angina or atypical chest pain. If asymptomatic, patients were required to have positive evidence of myocardial ischemia. Exclusion criteria included previous PCI or CABG, acute myocardial infarction (MI), or the need for concomitant cardiac surgery. A separate registry was kept of the 1,275 patients felt to be unsuitable for one of the revascularization options (1,077 CABG patients unsuitable for PCI and 198 PCI patients unsuitable for CABG). At 12 months, the primary endpoint of major cardiac and cerebrovascular events was higher in the group of patients undergoing PCI (17.8% vs. 12.4%, P = 0.002), largely the result of an increased rate of repeat revascularization in the PCI arm (13.5% vs. 5.9%, P < 0.001) despite a mean of 4.6 ± 2.3 stents placed per patient. The trial therefore failed to demonstrate noninferiority for paclitaxel stent-based PCI compared with CABG in this high-risk cohort, although the safety

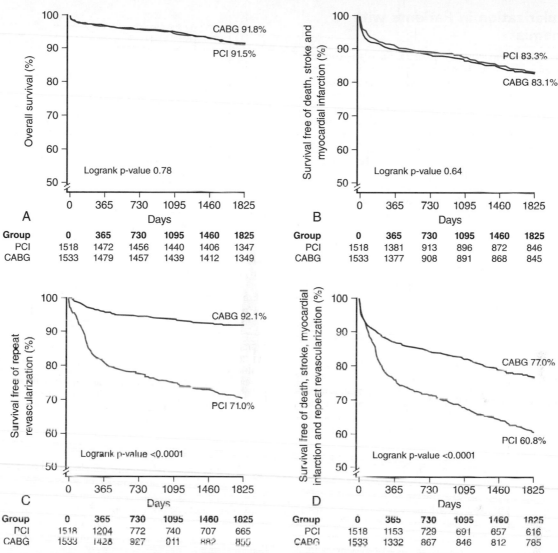

Figure 16-11 **A.** Kaplan-Meier 5-year event-free survival estimates for overall survival. **B.** Survival free of stroke or myocardial infarction. **C.** Survival free of repeat revascularization. **D.** Survival free of major adverse cardiac and cerebrovascular events in a pooled patient level metanalysis of revascularization with coronary artery bypass grafting (CABG) or percutaneous coronary intervention (PCI) with bare metal stents. (With permission: Daemen J, Boersma E, Flather M, et al. Long-term safety and efficacy of percutaneous coronary intervention with stenting and coronary artery bypass surgery for multivessel coronary artery disease: a meta-analysis with 5-year patient-level data from the ARTS, ERACI-II, MASS-II, and SoS trials. Circulation 2008;118(11):1146–1154.)

endpoints were reassuringly similar between groups. In fact, there was no difference between the PCI and CABG groups for the composite of all-cause death, MI, and stroke at 12 months (7.6% vs. 7.7%) and no difference in the individual components of death and MI. There was, however, an excess of stroke after CABG compared with PCI (2.2% vs. 0.6%). Because the SYNTAX trial failed to meet noninferiority for the primary endpoint, additional analysis must be regarded as exploratory and hypothesis-generating. Still, the available information regarding the high-risk subsets of patients with left main coronary artery disease as well as those with diabetes mellitus is of particular interest, as both of these groups have historically done poorly with percutaneous revascularization. Among 705 patients with left main disease in the SYNTAX trial,[37] 1-year major cardiac and cerebrovascular events were similar among the PCI- and CABG-treated groups (15.8% vs. 13.7%, P = 0.44), including similar rates of death (4.2% vs. 4.4%, P = 0.24) or myocardial infarction (4.3% vs. 4.1%), although, as in the overall trial, the rate of stroke was higher in the CABG group than in the PCI group (2.7% vs. 0.3%, P = 0.009).

When scored for anatomical complexity (see below), outcomes for those patients with low or intermediate SYNTAX scores were similar between the PCI and CABG groups. However, in patients in the highest tercile of SYNTAX score, adverse outcomes were significantly higher in patients treated with PCI, driven primarily by increased requirements for repeat revascularization. Another exploratory analysis involving patients with treated diabetes mellitus[38] demonstrated significantly higher event rates in patients undergoing PCI for left main and/or three-vessel disease, related to a marked increase in the need for repeat revascularization in this group (20.3% vs. 6.4%, P < 0.001) at 1 year. While outcomes were similar between treatment groups for both patients with and without diabetes mellitus in the lower tertiles of SYNTAX score, an excess mortality risk was observed in patients with diabetes mellitus in the highest SYNTAX tertile (≥33). The favorable outcomes for both patients with and without diabetes mellitus in the lower SYNTAX tertiles offer an opportunity for further evaluation of the safety and feasibility of PCI in these patient subgroups.

▣ Revascularization in Patients with Silent Ischemia

A primary goal of percutaneous revascularization is the control of medically refractory symptoms. In patients with asymptomatic myocardial ischemia, however, the only reasonable rationale for proceeding to revascularization is to improve prognosis through amelioration of the ischemic burden. Indeed, there is substantial evidence to support the prognostic hazard associated with silent myocardial ischemia. Silent ischemia may be present in 2% to 4% of the general population and travels in the company of numerous risk factors and markers of adverse outcome. Patients with diabetes mellitus, prior myocardial infarction or acute coronary syndrome, chronic renal failure, sudden death episodes, and typical/atypical anginal symptoms may all exhibit evidence of asymptomatic myocardial ischemia on Holter monitor or exercise treadmill testing; prognosis may be impaired in these groups of patients. Unfortunately, it remains unclear in whom or when it is appropriate to screen for silent ischemia. The DIAD (Detection of Ischemia in Asymptomatic Diabetics) trial[39] was a randomized trial to assess the clinical impact of screening for coronary artery disease in asymptomatic adults with diabetes mellitus. The study enrolled 1,123 patients, 522 of whom were randomly assigned to adenosine-stress radionuclide myocardial perfusion imaging and 562 to routine care and follow-up. Of the screening group, 22% had documented silent myocardial ischemia, with 6% exhibiting a significant degree of ischemia. At 5-year follow-up, the overall cardiac event rate was 2.9% (0.6% per year) and was not significantly different between the screened group and the not-screened group (2.7% vs. 3.0%, $P = 0.73$). Among the small group of patients who underwent initial screening and had a significant degree of demonstrable ischemia, event rates were significantly higher than in the overall population (2.4% per year versus 0.4% per year, $P = 0.001$). This trial demonstrated the low yield associated with screening asymptomatic patients, even those with high clinical risk profiles. In addition, although this trial was not intended to evaluate the benefit of revascularization for asymptomatic ischemia and did not regulate additional diagnostic or therapeutic measures beyond protocol-specified nuclear stress imaging, the impact of screening was very minor. Perhaps most remarkable was the dynamic nature of the documented ischemia. At 3-year follow-up, 79% of the patients identified as having asymptomatic myocardial ischemia at baseline no longer exhibited evidence of ischemia, while 10% of patients without previously documented ischemia had developed an abnormal study over that time period. While the potential benefit of diagnostic strategies to evaluate for silent ischemia is unclear, there remain very few data regarding the role of revascularization in patients with documented silent ischemia. The best inferential data for the potential prognostic benefit of revascularization in this clinical setting involve the documentation of an association between degree of myocardial ischemia and poor outcome. Zellweger and colleagues[40] identified just such an association among 3,664 consecutive asymptomatic patients undergoing myocardial perfusion imaging. During an average of 1.9 years of follow-up, 38 patients suffered death or MI. Patients with greater degrees of ischemia at baseline had statistically greater event rates, with patients exhibiting >7.5% ischemic myocardium suffering event rates in excess of 3% per year. Hachamovitch and colleagues[22] similarly followed 10,627 patients without a prior history of coronary disease who had undergone myocardial perfusion imaging. At a mean follow-up of nearly 2 years, cardiac death was observed in 1.4% of patients. These investigators discovered a statistically significant benefit associated with revascularization compared with OMT in patients with an ischemic burden approaching 10% or more of the myocardium, while OMT held the edge at lesser levels of ischemia (Fig. 16-8). The nuclear substudy of the COURAGE trial (see above)[19] also provides fascinating insight into the potential for amelioration of myocardial ischemia to affect outcome. The most direct evidence of a potential role for revascularization in patients with asymptomatic ischemia was documented in the ACIP (Asymptomatic Cardiac Ischemic Pilot) trial.[41] In it, 558 patients with coronary disease suitable for

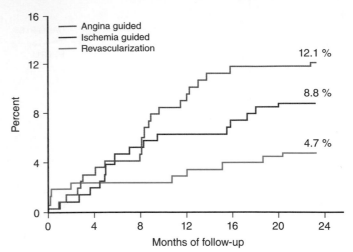

Figure 16-12 Two-year cumulative rates of death or myocardial infarction in 558 patients with ischemia on ambulatory monitoring and stress testing who were treated with revascularization, revascularization in the presence of documented ischemia, or angina-guided revascularization. The outcome of the planned revascularization strategy was significantly different from that of the angina-guided strategy, with a 61% relative risk reduction ($P < 0.01$). The 27% relative risk reduction between the angina-guided and ischemia-guided arms was not significant, nor was the difference between the revascularization and ischemia-guided strategies. *(With permission: Davies RF, Goldberg AD, Forman S, et al. Asymptomatic Cardiac Ischemia Pilot (ACIP) study two-year follow-up: outcomes of patients randomized to initial strategies of medical therapy versus revascularization. Circulation 1997;95(8):2037–2043.)*

revascularization, silent ischemia on Holter monitor, and ischemia on exercise testing were randomized to medical treatment of angina, medical treatment of angina and ambulatory ischemic episodes, or revascularization. At both 1- and 2-year[25] follow-up, survival was best in the routine revascularization arm and worst in the angina-guided arm (61% risk reduction with revascularization, $P = 0.01$), suggesting that amelioration of silent ischemia through prompt revascularization may provide important clinical benefit (Fig. 16-12). Unfortunately there have not been further data in this regard, leaving physicians with as many questions as answers for the appropriate diagnostic and therapeutic strategies in patients suspected to suffer from silent ischemia.

▣ Tools for Selection of Therapy

The growing number and scope of prospective trials of revascularization has provided an important objective structure to guide general discussion of treatment algorithms. However, revascularization decisions for individual patients continue to rely on the subjective "read" by practicing physicians of what is "best" for the patient. Beyond the essential institution of OMT and risk-factor modification programs for all patients, determination of whether or not to offer revascularization, and if so, what type, is often based on the subjective compilation of baseline clinical characteristics and presentation features. Factors such as anginal status, age, gender, and risk-factor profile provide important clues regarding the selection of optimal treatment. In addition, individual patient desires and experience as well as the bias of treating physicians play a significant role in shading discussions and ultimate treatment choice. Several comparative tools are now available to assist physicians and patients in discussing revascularization options. These tools provide guidance through the integration of certain anatomic, functional, and/or baseline clinical components. Some scores, such as the Mayo Clinic risk score[42] and the NCDR risk score,[43] were developed to aid in risk assessment after PCI, while others, such as the Society of Thoracic Surgeons (STS) score[44] (online risk calculator at http://209.220.160.181/STSWebRiskCalc261/de.aspx), euroSCORE[45] (online risk calculator at www.euroscore.org/calc.html), and ACEF[46] score have been validated as independent predictors of adverse events in patients undergoing CABG. While several of these scores have subsequently been evaluated for prognostic ability in patients presenting for either PCI or CABG,[37,46,47] they do not possess proven utility in determining optimal treatment selection. The SYNTAX score,[48] on the other hand, was developed to provide prognostic information regarding outcome after either PCI or CABG in patients with multivessel disease based on the functional impact of angiographically documented coronary disease. The SYNTAX score is a quantitative score that provides a cumulative measure of the extent and complexity of angiographically evident coronary artery disease, taking into account the number, location, and characteristics of lesions identified angiographically as well as the extent of myocardium subserved. Among patients with three-vessel and/or left main disease randomized in the SYNTAX trial,[36] those who were treated with paclitaxel-eluting stent PCI exhibited increasing major adverse cardiovascular and cerebrovascular event (MACCE) rates at 2 years in direct relationship to increased disease complexity as defined by the baseline SYNTAX score. This effect was not identified in patients treated with an initial strategy of CABG. While MACCE rates were not statistically different between patients treated in the PCI or CABG arms when the baseline SYNTAX score was low (0–22) or intermediate (23–32), patients with high SYNTAX scores (>32) experienced lower MACCE rates when treated with CABG compared with those undergoing PCI.[49] Because the SYNTAX score has not shown discriminative ability for risk prognostication among patients undergoing CABG, a mode of revascularization less affected by the complexity of disease, the primary impact of this score is to aid in the identification of patients at undue risk for MACCE after PCI who might therefore benefit from treatment with CABG. Risk scores can provide statistical insight into the population-based risks associated with percutaneous or surgical revascularization but are unable to identify specific risks for an individual patient. To provide additional assistance in risk stratification and treatment selection, national bodies have recently undertaken an initiative to provide guidance through the publication of appropriateness criteria. These documents are essentially an extension of evidence-based guideline documents and serve to fill the gap between known scientific findings and individual patient variability. In the case of the ACCF/SCAI/STS/AATS/AHA/ASNC 2009 Appropriateness Criteria for Coronary Revascularization,[20] nominated technical panelists use a compendium of currently available evidence and current consensus to evaluate the likely benefit and risk associated with revascularization across a broad range of specific patient subtypes. These scenarios are rated on a scale of 1 to 9, first by individual panelists and then collectively. After final review, each scenario is scored as appropriate (scores 7–9: revascularization is generally acceptable and reasonable and is likely to improve the patient's outcome), uncertain (scores 4–6: revascularization may be acceptable or reasonable but further research is necessary for this patient scenario), or inappropriate (scores 1–3: revascularization is not generally accepted or reasonable in this situation and is unlikely to provide prognostic or clinical benefit). In this way, recommendations found in the appropriateness criteria can facilitate discussions with patients, family, and members of the medical team regarding the likely benefits of revascularization strategies (Figs. 16-13 through 16-16).

Summary

Symptomatic coronary artery disease is a growing problem throughout the world, with significant associated economic and societal costs. While there is presently no cure for ischemic coronary artery disease, it is increasingly possible to alter the course of the disease through judicious utilization of the rapidly evolving medical, surgical, and percutaneous therapies currently available. Successful disease management and symptom palliation can be achieved by a robust regimen based on optimal medical management and risk-factor modification through diet and exercise. Percutaneous revascularization also plays an

Low-risk findings on noninvasive study						Asymptomatic					
Symptoms / Med. Rx						**Stress Test / Med. Rx**					
Class III or IV Max Rx	U	A	A	A	A	High Risk Max Rx	U	A	A	A	A
Class I or II Max Rx	U	U	A	A	A	High Risk No.min Rx	U	U	A	A	A
Asymptomatic Max Rx	I	I	U	U	U	Int. Risk Max Rx	U	U	U	U	A
Class III or IV No/min Rx	I	U	A	A	A	Int. Risk No/min Rx	I	I	U	U	A
Class I or II No/min Rx	I	I	U	U	U	Low Risk Max Rx	I	I	U	U	U
Asymptomatic No/min Rx	I	I	U	U	U	Low Risk No/min Rx	I	I	U	U	U
Coronary Anatomy	CTO of 1 vz.; no other disease	1-2 vz. disease; no prox. LAD	1 vz. disease of prox. LAD	2 vz. disease with prox. LAD	3 vz. disease; no left main	**Coronary Anatomy**	CTO of 1 vz.; no other disease	1-2 vz. disease; no prox. LAD	1 vz. disease of prox. LAD	2 vz. disease with prox. LAD	3 vz. disease; no left main

Figure 16-13 Appropriateness ratings for patients without prior coronary bypass with low-risk findings on noninvasive imaging study and asymptomatic. A, appropriate; CTO, chronic total occlusion; I, inappropriate; Int., intervention; Med., medical; Prox. LAD, proximal left anterior descending artery; Rx, treatment; U, uncertain; and vz., vessel. (*Reproduced with permission from: Patel MR, Dehmer GJ, Hirshfeld JW, et al. ACCF/SCAI/STS/AATS/AHA/ASNC 2009 appropriateness criteria for coronary revascularization: a report of the American College of Cardiology Foundation Appropriateness Criteria Task Force, Society for Cardiovascular Angiography and Interventions, Society of Thoracic Surgeons, American Association for Thoracic Surgery, American Heart Association, and the American Society of Nuclear Cardiology: endorsed by the American Society of Echocardiography, the Heart Failure Society of America, and the Society of Cardiovascular Computed Tomography. Circulation 2009;119(9):1330–1352.*)

Intermediate-risk findings on noninvasive study						CCS Class I or II Angina					
Symptoms Med. Rx						**Stress Test** Med. Rx					
Class III or IV Max Rx	A	A	A	A	A		High Risk Max Rx	A	A	A	A	A
Class I or II Max Rx	U	A	A	A	A		High Risk No.min Rx	U	A	A	A	A
Asymptomatic Max Rx	U	U	U	U	A		Int. Risk Max Rx	U	A	A	A	A
Class III or IV No/min Rx	U	U	A	A	A		Int. Risk No/min Rx	U	U	U	A	A
Class I or II No/min Rx	U	U	U	A	A		Low Risk Max Rx	U	U	A	A	A
Asymptomatic No/min Rx	I	I	U	U	A		Low Risk No/min Rx	I	I	U	U	U
Coronary Anatomy	CTO of 1 vz.; no other disease	1-2 vz. disease; no prox. LAD	1 vz. disease of prox. LAD	2 vz. disease with prox. LAD	3 vz. disease; no left main		**Coronary Anatomy**	CTO of 1 vz.; no other disease	1-2 vz. disease; no prox. LAD	1 vz. disease of prox. LAD	2 vz. disease with prox. LAD	3 vz. disease; no left main

Figure 16-14 Appropriateness ratings for patients without prior coronary bypass with intermediate-risk findings on noninvasive imaging study and Canadian Cardiovascular Society (CCS) class I or II angina. A, appropriate; CTO, chronic total occlusion; I, inappropriate; Int., intervention; Med., medical; Prox. LAD, proximal left anterior descending artery; Rx, treatment; U, uncertain; and vz., vessel. *(Reproduced with permission: Patel MR, Dehmer GJ, Hirshfeld JW, et al. ACCF/SCAI/STS/AATS/AHA/ASNC 2009 appropriateness criteria for coronary revascularization: a report of the American College of Cardiology Foundation Appropriateness Criteria Task Force, Society for Cardiovascular Angiography and Interventions, Society of Thoracic Surgeons, American Association for Thoracic Surgery, American Heart Association, and the American Society of Nuclear Cardiology: endorsed by the American Society of Echocardiography, the Heart Failure Society of America, and the Society of Cardiovascular Computed Tomography. Circulation 2009;119(9):1330–1352.)*

High-risk findings on noninvasive study						CCS Class III or IV Angina					
Symptoms Med. Rx						**Stress Test** Med. Rx					
Class III or IV Max Rx	A	A	A	A	A		High Risk Max Rx	A	A	A	A	A
Class I or II Max Rx	A	A	A	A	A		High Risk No.min Rx	A	A	A	A	A
Asymptomatic Max Rx	U	A	A	A	A		Int. Risk Max Rx	A	A	A	A	A
Class III or IV No/min Rx	A	A	A	A	A		Int. Risk No/min Rx	U	U	A	A	A
Class I or II No/min Rx	U	A	A	A	A		Low Risk Max Rx	U	A	A	A	A
Asymptomatic No/min Rx	U	U	A	A	A		Low Risk No/min Rx	I	U	A	A	A
Coronary Anatomy	CTO of 1 vz.; no other disease	1-2 vz. disease; no prox. LAD	1 vz. disease of prox. LAD	2 vz. disease with prox. LAD	3 vz. disease; no left main		**Coronary Anatomy**	CTO of 1 vz.; no other disease	1-2 vz. disease; no prox. LAD	1 vz. disease of prox. LAD	2 vz. disease with prox. LAD	3 vz. disease; no left main

Figure 16-15 Appropriateness ratings for patients without prior coronary bypass with high-risk findings on noninvasive imaging study and Canadian Cardiovascular Society (CCS) class III or IV angina. A, appropriate; CTO, chronic total occlusion; I, inappropriate; Int., intervention; Med., medical; Prox. LAD, proximal left anterior descending artery; Rx, treatment; U, uncertain; vz., vessel. *(Reproduced with permission: Patel MR, Dehmer GJ, Hirshfeld JW, et al. ACCF/SCAI/STS/AATS/AHA/ASNC 2009 appropriateness criteria for coronary revascularization: a report of the American College of Cardiology Foundation Appropriateness Criteria Task Force, Society for Cardiovascular Angiography and Interventions, Society of Thoracic Surgeons, American Association for Thoracic Surgery, American Heart Association, and the American Society of Nuclear Cardiology: Endorsed by the American Society of Echocardiography, the Heart Failure Society of America, and the Society of Cardiovascular Computed Tomography. Circulation 2009;119(9):1330–1352.)*

	CABG			PCI		
	No diabetes and normal LVEF	Diabetes	Depressed LVEF	No diabetes and normal LVEF	Diabetes	Depressed LVEF
Two vessel coronary artery disease with proximal LAD stenosis	A	A	A	A	A	A
Three vessel coronary artery disease	A	A	A	U	U	U
Isolated left main stenosis	A	A	A	I	I	I
Left main stenosis and additional coronary artery disease	A	A	A	I	I	I

Figure 16-16 Appropriateness rating of specific method of revascularization in patients with advanced coronary artery disease deemed to be revascularization candidates. CABG, coronary artery bypass grafting; LAD, left anterior descending artery; LVEF, left ventricular ejection fraction; PCI, percutaneous coronary intervention. (*Reproduced with permission: Patel MR, Dehmer GJ, Hirshfeld JW, et al. ACCF/SCAI/STS/AATS/AHA/ASNC 2009 appropriateness criteria for coronary revascularization: a report of the American College of Cardiology Foundation Appropriateness Criteria Task Force, Society for Cardiovascular Angiography and Interventions, Society of Thoracic Surgeons, American Association for Thoracic Surgery, American Heart Association, and the American Society of Nuclear Cardiology: Endorsed by the American Society of Echocardiography, the Heart Failure Society of America, and the Society of Cardiovascular Computed Tomography. Circulation 2009;119(9).1330-1352.*)

important role in achieving improved quality of life and ultimately prognosis. Indeed, percutaneous revascularization can effectively modulate long-term outcome directly through a reduction of ischemic burden as well as indirectly through symptom control and improved exercise tolerance. As percutaneous technology continues to evolve, which it surely will, promising new indications will be discovered and added to the ever-expanding list of beneficial effects. In the setting of rising healthcare costs and the economic realities of delivering a finite resource, however, efforts to establish and clarify the most appropriate revascularization strategies and candidates will assure the continued availability of these techniques to an ever-growing population of those who may benefit.

REFERENCES

1. Roger VL, Go AS, Lloyd-Jones DM, et al: Heart disease and stroke statistics—2011 update : a report from the American Heart Association. Circulation Feb 123(4):e18–e209, 2011.
2. Ford ES, Ajani UA, Croft JB, et al: Explaining the decrease in U.S. deaths from coronary disease, 1980–2000. N Engl J Med 356(23):2388–2398, 2007.
3. Gibbons RJ, Abrams J, Chatterjee K, et al: ACC/AHA 2002 guideline update for the management of patients with chronic stable angina: a report of the American College of Cardiology/American Heart Association Task Force on Practice Guidelines (Committee to Update the 1999 Guidelines for the Management of Patients with Chronic Stable Angina). Available at: wwwaccorg/clinical/guidelines/stable/stablepdf 2002.
4. Bonetti PO, Holmes DR, Lerman A, et al: Enhanced external counterpulsation for ischemic heart disease. What's behind the curtain? J Am Coll Cardiol 41(11):1918–1925, 2003.
5. Katritsis DG, Ioannidis JPA: Percutaneous coronary intervention versus conservative therapy in nonacute coronary artery disease: a meta-analysis. Circulation 111(22):2906–2912, 2005.
6. Barsness GW, Gersh BJ, Brooks MM, et al: Rationale for the revascularization arm of the Bypass Angioplasty Revascularization Investigation 2 Diabetes (BARI 2D) trial. Am J Cardiol 97(12, Suppl 1):31–40, 2006.
7. Mahn-Won P, Ki-Bae S, Pum-Joon K, et al: Long-term percutaneous coronary intervention rates and associated independent predictors for progression of nonintervened nonculprit coronary lesions. Am J Cardiol 104(5):648–652, 2009.
8. Stone GW, Maehara A, Lansky AJ, et al: A prospective natural-history study of coronary atherosclerosis. N Engl J Med 364(3):226–235, 2011.
9. Wijeysundera HC, Nallamothu BK, Krumholz HM, et al: Meta-analysis: effects of percutaneous coronary intervention versus medical therapy on angina relief. Ann Intern Med 152(6):370–379, 2010.
10. Boden WE, O'Rourke RA, Teo KK, et al: Optimal medical therapy with or without PCI for stable coronary disease. N Engl J Med 356(15):1503–1516, 2007.
11. Hochman JS, Lamas GA, Buller CE, et al: Coronary intervention for persistent occlusion after myocardial infarction. N Engl J Med 355(23):2395–2407, 2006.
12. Weintraub WS, Spertus JA, Kolm P, et al: Effect of PCI on quality of life in patients with stable coronary disease. N Engl J Med 359(7):677–687, 2008.
13. Schomig A, Mehilli J, de Waha A, et al: A meta-analysis of 17 randomized trials of a percutaneous coronary intervention-based strategy in patients with stable coronary artery disease. J Am Coll Cardiol 52(11):894–904, 2008.

14. Jeremias A, Kaul S, Rosengart TK, et al: The impact of revascularization on mortality in patients with nonacute coronary artery disease. Am J Med 122(2):152–161, 2009.
15. Trikalinos TA, Alsheikh-Ali AA, Tatsioni A, et al: Percutaneous coronary interventions for non-acute coronary artery disease: a quantitative 20-year synopsis and a network meta-analysis. Lancet 373(9667):911–918, 2009.
16. Daly CA, De Stavola B, Sendon JLL, et al: Predicting prognosis in stable angina—results from the Euro heart survey of stable angina: prospective observational study. BMJ 332(7536):262–267, 2006.
17. Hjemdahl P, Eriksson SV, Held C, et al: Favourable long term prognosis in stable angina pectoris: an extended follow up of the angina prognosis study in Stockholm (APSIS). Heart 92(2):177–182, 2006.
18. Barsness GW: Managing the patient with severe left ventricular dysfunction. In: Ellis SG, Holmes DR, Jr, editors: Strategic Approaches in Coronary Intervention, ed 3, Philadelphia: Lippincott, 2006, Williams & Wilkins, pp 407–423.
19. Shaw LJ, Berman DS, Maron DJ, et al: Optimal medical therapy with or without percutaneous coronary intervention to reduce ischemic burden: results from the Clinical Outcomes Utilizing Revascularization and Aggressive Drug Evaluation (COURAGE) trial nuclear substudy. Circulation 117(10):1283–1291, 2008.
20. Patel MR, Dehmer GJ, Hirshfeld JW, et al: ACCF/SCAI/STS/AATS/AHA/ASNC 2009 Appropriateness Criteria for Coronary Revascularization: A report of the American College of Cardiology Foundation Appropriateness Criteria Task Force, Society for Cardiovascular Angiography and Interventions, Society of Thoracic Surgeons, American Association for Thoracic Surgery, American Heart Association, and the American Society of Nuclear Cardiology: endorsed by the American Society of Echocardiography, the Heart Failure Society of America, and the Society of Cardiovascular Computed Tomography. Circulation 119(9):1330–1352, 2009.
21. Smith PK, Califf RM, Tuttle RH, et al: Selection of surgical or percutaneous coronary intervention provides differential longevity benefit. Ann Thorac Surg 82(4):1420–1429, 2006.
22. Hachamovitch R, Hayes SW, Friedman JD, et al: Comparison of the short-term survival benefit associated with revascularization compared with medical therapy in patients with no prior coronary artery disease undergoing stress myocardial perfusion single photon emission computed tomography. Circulation 107(23):2900–2907, 2003.
23. Maron DJ, Boden WE, O'Rourke RA, et al: Intensive multifactorial intervention for stable coronary artery disease: optimal medical therapy in the COURAGE (Clinical Outcomes Utilizing

Revascularization and Aggressive Drug Evaluation) trial. J Am Coll Cardiol 55(13):1348–1358, 2010.
24. Steinberg BA, Steg PG, Bhatt DL, et al: Comparisons of guideline-recommended therapies in patients with documented coronary artery disease having percutaneous coronary intervention versus coronary artery bypass grafting versus medical therapy only (from the REACH International Registry). Am J Cardiol 99(9):1212–1215, 2007.
25. Davies RF, Goldberg AD, Forman S, et al: Asymptomatic Cardiac Ischemia Pilot (ACIP) study two-year follow-up: outcomes of patients randomized to initial strategies of medical therapy versus revascularization. Circulation 95(8):2037–2043, 1997.
26. The BARI 2D Study Group: A randomized trial of therapies for type 2 diabetes and coronary artery disease. N Engl J Med 360(24):2503–2515, 2009.
27. Chaitman BR, Hardison RM, Adler D, et al: The Bypass Angioplasty Revascularization Investigation 2 diabetes randomized trial of different treatment strategies in type 2 diabetes mellitus with stable ischemic heart disease: impact of treatment strategy on cardiac mortality and myocardial infarction. Circulation 120(25):2529–2540, 2009.
28. Sarno G, Garg S, Onuma Y, et al: Impact of completeness of revascularization on the five-year outcome in percutaneous coronary intervention and coronary artery bypass graft patients (from the ARTS-II Study). Am J Cardiol 106(10):1369–1375, 2010.
29. Hannan EL, Racz M, Holmes DR, et al: Impact of completeness of percutaneous coronary intervention revascularization on long-term outcomes in the stent era. Circulation 113(20):2406–2412, 2006.
30. Jones RH, Kesler K, Phillips HR, III, et al: Long-term survival benefits of coronary artery bypass grafting and percutaneous transluminal angioplasty in patients with coronary artery disease. J Thorac Cardiovasc Surg 111(5):1013–1025, 1996.
31. Aziz O, Rao C, Panesar SS, et al: Meta-analysis of minimally invasive internal thoracic artery bypass versus percutaneous revascularisation for isolated lesions of the left anterior descending artery. BMJ 334(7594):617, 2007.
32. Kapoor JR, Gienger AL, Ardehali R, et al: Isolated disease of the proximal left anterior descending artery: comparing the effectiveness of percutaneous coronary interventions and coronary artery bypass surgery. J Am Coll Cardiol Cardiovasc Intervent 1(5):483–491, 2008.
33. Goy J-J, Kaufmann U, Hurni M, et al: 10-year follow-up of a prospective randomized trial comparing bare-metal stenting with internal mammary artery grafting for proximal, isolated de novo left anterior coronary artery stenosis: the SIMA (Stenting versus

Internal Mammary Artery grafting) Trial. *J Am Coll Cardiol* 52(10):815–817, 2008.

34. Barsness GW, Holmes DR, Jr, Gersh BJ: Integrated management of patients with diabetes mellitus and ischemic heart disease: PCI, CABG, and medical therapy. *Curr Probl Cardiol* 30(11):583–617, 2005.

35. Daemen J, Boersma E, Flather M, et al: Long-term safety and efficacy of percutaneous coronary intervention with stenting and coronary artery bypass surgery for multivessel coronary artery disease: a meta-analysis with 5-year patient-level data from the ARTS, ERACI-II, MASS-II, and SoS trials. *Circulation* 118(11):1146–1154, 2008.

36. Serruys PW, Morice M-C, Kappetein AP, et al: Percutaneous coronary intervention versus coronary-artery bypass grafting for severe coronary artery disease. *N Engl J Med* 360(10):961–972, 2009.

37. Morice M-C, Serruys PW, Kappetein AP, et al: Outcomes in patients with de novo left main disease treated with either percutaneous coronary intervention using paclitaxel-eluting stents or coronary artery bypass graft treatment in the synergy between percutaneous coronary intervention with TAXUS and cardiac surgery (SYNTAX) trial. *Circulation* 121(24):2645–2653, 2010.

38. Banning AP, Westaby S, Morice M-C, et al: Diabetic and nondiabetic patients with left main and/or 3-vessel coronary artery disease: comparison of outcomes with cardiac surgery and paclitaxel-eluting stents. *J Am Coll Cardiol* 55(11):1067–1075, 2010.

39. Young LH, Wackers FJT, Chyun DA, et al: Cardiac outcomes after screening for asymptomatic coronary artery disease in patients with type 2 diabetes. *JAMA* 301(15):1547–1555, 2009.

40. Zellweger M, Hachamovitch R, Kang X, et al: Threshold, incidence, and predictors of prognostically high-risk silent ischemia in asymptomatic patients without prior diagnosis of coronary artery disease. *J Nucl Cardiol* 16(2):193–200, 2009.

41. Rogers WJ, Bourassa MG, Andrews TC, et al: Asymptomatic Cardiac Ischemia Pilot (ACIP) study: outcome at 1 year for patients with asymptomatic cardiac ischemia randomized to medical therapy or revascularization. *J Am Coll Cardiol* 26(3):594–605, 1995.

42. Singh M, Rihal CS, Lennon RJ, et al: Bedside estimation of risk from percutaneous coronary intervention: the New Mayo Clinic risk scores. *Mayo Clin Proc* 82(6):701–708, 2007.

43. Peterson ED, Dai D, DeLong ER, et al: Contemporary mortality risk prediction for percutaneous coronary intervention: results from 588,398 procedures in the National Cardiovascular Data Registry. *J Am Coll Cardiol* 55(18):1923–1932, 2010.

44. Edwards F, Clark R, Schwartz M: Coronary artery bypass grafting: the Society of Thoracic Surgeons National Database experience. *Ann Thorac Surg* 57(1):12–19, 1994.

45. Nashef SAM, Roques F, Michel P, et al: European system for cardiac operative risk evaluation (EuroSCORE). *Eur J Cardiothorac Surg* 16(1):9–13, 1999.

46. Ranucci M, Castelvecchio S, Menicanti L, et al: Risk of assessing mortality risk in elective cardiac operations: age, creatinine, ejection fraction, and the law of parsimony. *Circulation* 119(24):3053–3061, 2009.

47. Singh M, Gersh BJ, Li S, et al: Mayo Clinic risk score for percutaneous coronary intervention predicts in-hospital mortality in patients undergoing coronary artery bypass graft surgery. *Circulation* 117(3):356–362, 2008.

48. Sianos G, Morel MA, Kappetein AP, et al: The SYNTAX Score: an angiographic tool grading the complexity of coronary artery disease. *EuroIntervention* 1(2):219–227, 2005.

49. Mohr FW, Rastan AJ, Serruys PW, et al: Complex coronary anatomy in coronary artery bypass graft surgery: Impact of complex coronary anatomy in modern bypass surgery? Lessons learned from the SYNTAX trial after two years. *J Thorac Cardiovasc Surg* 141(1):130–140, 2011.

Intervention for Non-ST-Segment Elevation Acute Coronary Syndromes

CURTISS T. STINIS

KEY POINTS

- Risk assessment at admission is vitally important and should be repeated during hospitalization.

- Patients presenting with hemodynamic instability, severe left ventricular dysfunction or overt heart failure, recurrent or persistent rest angina despite intensive medical therapy, mechanical complications, and those with significant electrical instability are deemed to be at extremely high risk for death or a complicated myocardial infarction and should undergo urgent coronary angiography.

- Stable patients are managed by one of two strategies: an initial conservative strategy or an initial invasive strategy.

- Patients with other than low-risk characteristics are generally recommended for an early invasive strategy, which includes intensive medical therapy followed by coronary angiography and revascularization as appropriate.

- Low-risk patients are recommended for an initial conservative strategy and ischemia-guided revascularization.

Introduction

Over the past 31 years percutaneous coronary intervention (PCI) has evolved from a somewhat tenuous and experimental procedure to a durable and mainstream therapy; as a result, the clinical indications for PCI have broadened to include patients with both stable angina pectoris and acute coronary syndrome (ACS).[1-3] ACS comprises the spectrum of clinical signs and symptoms that occur as a result of acute myocardial ischemia and is classified as a non-ST-segment elevation ACS (NSTE-ACS) or as an ST-segment elevation ACS (STE-ACS). NSTE-ACS includes patients with unstable angina (UA) or non-ST-segment elevation myocardial infarction (NSTEMI); STE-ACS includes patients with ST-segment elevation myocardial infarction (STEMI)[4] Various strategies have been proposed for the management of NSTE-ACS, with more recent guidelines and clinical trials increasingly supporting an invasive strategy for high-risk ACS and a less invasive/more conservative strategy for patients deemed to be at lower risk.[5] This chapter discusses PCI for patients with NSTE-ACS, focusing on the pathophysiology, risk stratification, adjunctive treatment during PCI, invasive versus conservative strategy, and the most recent AHA/ACC guidelines for the management of patients with NSTE-ACS.

Background and Rationale for Percutaneous Coronary Intervention in Patients with Non-St-Segment Elevation Acute Coronary Syndrome

Coronary atherosclerosis is a chronic disease in which atheromatous material generally evolves silently over time; it may eventually result in the development of a high-risk (i.e., vulnerable) plaque[6] (Fig. 17-1). Rupture or erosion of this high-risk plaque triggers the formation of intracoronary thrombosis, which can lead to a critical stenosis or occlusion of the coronary artery as well as associated vasospasm. Although the initial stenosis may evolve silently, healing of a ruptured or eroded plaque may lead to more rapid progression of the stenosis; this may remain clinically silent or cause angina pectoris. Thus ACS may have different clinical presentations: UA, NSTEMI, STEMI, and sudden death. All clinical manifestations of ACS share a common pathophysiological pathway (plaque rupture/erosion and some degree of thrombosis and vasoconstriction), but the duration (transient or permanent) and severity (subtotal or total coronary occlusion) are different and associated either with myocardial necrosis (STEMI and NSTEMI) or no evidence of myocardial necrosis (UA) as manifest by negative cardiac biomarkers. It is important to note that within the first few months after an initial episode of coronary instability, there is a strong tendency for repeat instability caused by progression in the severity of the culprit stenosis or that of remote lesions. Although plaque rupture or erosion with associated thrombosis is the most common cause of ACS, it may also be caused by dynamic obstruction (i.e., Prinzmetal's angina or vasospasm secondary to drug abuse), spontaneous coronary artery dissection (most commonly occurring in peripartum women), severe coronary narrowing without thrombus or spasm (i.e., advanced progressive atherosclerosis or severe restenosis from prior PCI), or a precipitating condition extrinsic to the coronary circulation (i.e., fever, sepsis, tachycardia, hypotension, anemia, hypoxemia, etc.).[5] Thus in evaluating individual patients with ACS, it is important to consider the most likely etiology, especially if an invasive strategy is being considered, given that PCI is not necessarily an appropriate therapy for all causes of ACS. Patients with NSTE-ACS have long-term outcomes similar to those of patients with STE-ACS and worse than those of patients with unstable angina.[7] NSTE-ACS patients and STE-ACS patients have similar prognoses, likely due to a high prevalence of multivessel disease as well as a higher incidence of recurrent ischemia (35% vs. 23% at 1 year in the GUSTO IIb trial). The optimal management of unstable angina or NSTEMI, therefore, is twofold: immediate relief of ischemia and the prevention of progression to acute MI or cardiac death. This can be achieved by a combination of anti-ischemic, antiplatelet, and antithrombotic therapy with or without PCI (Fig. 17-1).

RISK STRATIFICATION

Although the risks of individual patients presenting with NSTE-ACS vary widely, several risk scores have been devised to risk-stratify patients and help identify those who may benefit from an early invasive strategy. The TIMI (Thrombolysis in Myocardial Infarction) risk score, which predicts the risk of 14-day all-cause mortality and new or recurrent MI, is a validated risk-prediction model based on data from the TIMI IIB and ESSENCE trials and is the most commonly used. Seven variables at presentation were independently predictive of outcome (Fig. 17-2).[8] The GRACE Registry developed a risk calculator for bedside risk estimation of 6-month mortality for patients after hospitalization for ACS.[9] The overall 6-month mortality rate was 4.8%. Nine predictive variables were identified: older age, previous MI, history of heart failure, increased heart rate, lower systolic blood pressure, serum creatinine level, elevated levels of cardiac biomarkers, ST-segment depression, and no PCI (Figs. 17-3A and 17-3B). The presence of

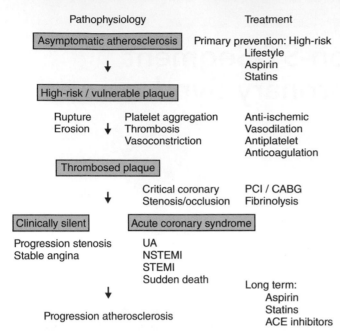

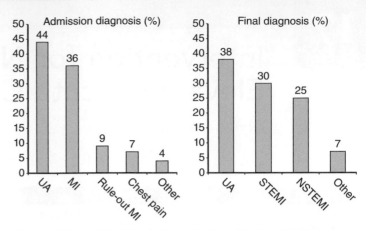

Figure 17-3 A. The risk calculator developed by the GRACE Registry for bedside risk estimation of 6-month mortality in patients after hospitalization for acute coronary syndrome. B. Plot of predicted all-cause mortality.

Figure 17-1 Physiopathological mechanisms underlying acute coronary syndromes. ACE, angiotensin-converting enzyme; CABG, coronary artery bypass grafting; NSTEMI, non-ST-segment elevation myocardial infarction; PCI, percutaneous coronary intervention; STEMI, ST-segment elevation myocardial infarction; UA, unstable angina.

TABLE 17-1	Predictors of Late Troponin Level Rise in Initially Troponin-Negative Patients		
Predictor*	OR	95% CI	P Value
ST-segment deviation	3.52	2.38–5.23	<0.001
Presentation <8 hr from symptom onset	2.91	1.92–4.40	<0.001
No prior percutaneous coronary intervention	2.88	1.54–5.39	0.001
No prior beta blockade	1.74	1.15–2.63	0.008
Unheralded angina	1.65	1.12–2.42	0.01
History of myocardial infarction	1.59	1.06–2.37	0.02

*Late is defined as 12 hours or more.

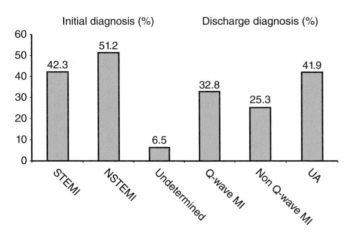

Figure 17-2 The TIMI trial risk score for death or myocardial infarction at 14 days. CAD, coronary artery disease. Score is derived by assigning a value of 0 when a factor is absent and 1 when a factor is present.

elevation in these markers 12 hours later. Of 1,342 patients who were enrolled in the TIMI-IIIB trial, 200 (14.9%) were troponin-negative at baseline but developed an elevated troponin I level (≥0.4 ng/mL) at 12 hours.[10] Six independent predictors were identified (Table 17-1), and a score was derived to identify patients with the highest likelihood to become troponin-positive later during hospital admission (Fig. 17-4). The derived score was tested in 855 patients in the GUSTO IIA (Global Use of Strategies To Open Occluded Arteries in Acute Coronary Syndromes IIA) study and similarly predicted a late rise in troponin T levels. This score, therefore, may be useful to further assist in the risk-stratification of patients who present with NSTE-ACS and initially unremarkable troponin levels.

elevated cardiac biomarkers is a particularly important prognostic indicator, which has been associated with an increased risk for reinfarction and death (discussed further below). It is important to note that although determination of patient risk is vitally important upon initial presentation with NSTE-ACS, individual patient risk often changes during hospitalization and it should be frequently reassessed.

■ Predicting a Late Positive Serum Troponin Level in Initially Troponin-Negative Patients with Non-ST-Segment Elevation Acute Coronary Syndrome

A limitation of the use of the TIMI risk score in identifying patients at higher risk who present with NSTE-ACS is that some patients may initially present with negative cardiac biomarkers, only to demonstrate

■ Adjunctive Treatment during Percutaneous Coronary Intervention for Non-ST-Segment Elevation Acute Coronary Syndrome

ANTIPLATELET TREATMENT

The activation and aggregation of platelets after the rupture of a vulnerable plaque are key components in the pathophysiology of ACS. Aspirin inhibits the cyclooxygenase pathway in platelets and in the endothelium, which prevents the production of thromboxane A2 and therefore inhibits platelet aggregation.[11,12] Multiple studies have shown the benefit of aspirin therapy in coronary artery disease with reduction in angina, death, and MI by 30%.[13,14] Two metanalyses have established that aspirin has efficacy across a wide range of dosages.[13,14] Currently, it is recommended that a dosage of between 162 and 325 mg be given

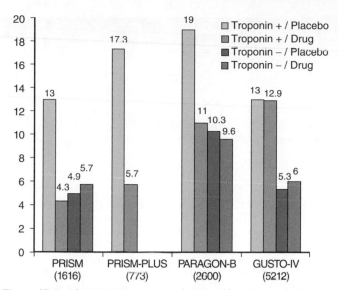

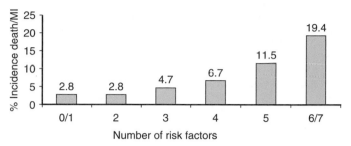

Figure 17-4 The TIMI-IIIB score used to identify patients who become troponin-positive later during hospital admission. MI, myocardial infarction; PCI, percutaneous coronary intervention.

Figure 17-5 Results from the TRITON-TIMI 38 trial.

orally on a daily basis beginning at the acute presentation and continuing for 1 month after PCI when a bare metal stent is used and 3 to 6 months when a drug-eluting stent is used.[5] Thereafter, the dosage may be reduced to between 81 and 150 mg daily on an indefinite basis unless a significant contraindication exists. Although aspirin is certainly an important pharmacological therapy in ACS patients, it does not prevent all thrombotic events.

Thienopyridines—such as ticlopidine, clopidogrel, and prasugrel—exert their antiplatelet effects by blocking the P2Y$_{12}$ receptor and its associated signaling pathway, thereby inhibiting platelet activation. Thienopyridines are administered as an initial loading dose, followed by a maintenance dose because they take longer to exhibit their irreversible antiplatelet effect. It is important to note that their mechanism of action is entirely independent of and complementary to that of aspirin, and the combination of aspirin and a thienopyridine is superior to the use of aspirin alone.[15,16] Ticlopidine in conjunction with aspirin was shown to reduce the rate of vascular death and MI by 46% in NSTE-ACS.[17] Clopidogrel is the most widely studied of the thienopyridine class. The CAPRIE (Clopidogrel versus Aspirin in Patients at Risk of Ischemic Events) trial[18] studied 19,185 patients with atherosclerotic vascular disease and revealed a 9% relative risk reduction in vascular death, MI, or ischemic stroke without a significant increase in bleeding. The CURE (Clopidogrel in Unstable Angina to Prevent Recurrent Events) trial[15] enrolled 12,562 patients and demonstrated a 20% reduction in cardiovascular death, MI, and stroke. A subset of this population who underwent PCI were studied in the PCI-CURE trial,[19] which showed that pretreatment with clopidogrel for a median of 6 days before PCI was associated with a 31% reduction in cardiovascular death or MI. The optimal dosing regimen for clopidogrel is still somewhat a matter of debate. A loading dose of 600 mg achieves maximal platelet inhibition faster than 150 or 300 mg and has lasting benefit of up to 30 days in low- to intermediate-risk patients undergoing elective PCI[20]; however, in higher-risk patients (discussed in detail below), the use of glycoprotein IIb/IIIa inhibitors has an added benefit. An important consideration for the use of clopidogrel in ACS patients is the substantial variability in individual patient response to this drug. Multiple potential hypotheses have been proposed to explain this "clopidogrel resistance," such as differences in clopidogrel dosing, intestinal absorption problems, and varying availability and clearance of the active metabolite.[21] Genetic factors such as polymorphisms of the hepatic CYP pathway (which is responsible for metabolizing

clopidogrel's prodrug into an active metabolite) are becoming increasingly well understood and used in mainstream clinical practice.[22] Testing for CYP mutations, especially of CYP3A, as well as platelet function testing are increasingly being utilized to direct individual patient care.[23] Prasugrel is a newer-generation P2Y$_{12}$ inhibitor that is more potent and more consistent with respect to platelet inhibition. The TRITON-TIMI 38 (Assess Improvement in Therapeutic Outcomes by Optimizing Platelet Inhibition with Prasugrel-Thrombolysis In Myocardial Infarction 38) trial[24] evaluated 13,608 patients with moderate to high risk ACS (NSTE-ACS and STE-ACS) after randomly receiving either prasugrel or clopidogrel during PCI. In this study, prasugrel significantly reduced the composite endpoint of cardiovascular death, nonfatal MI, or nonfatal stroke by 19% as compared with clopidogrel. The TRITON trial showed that prasugrel was associated with a 24% reduction in MI, a 34% reduction in the need for urgent revascularization, and a 52% reduction in stent thrombosis.[25] These benefits, however, were also associated with a 0.5% absolute increase in non-coronary artery bypass graft surgery (non-CABG)-related TIMI major bleeding, a fivefold increase in CABG-related bleeding, and a 0.3% absolute increase in fatal bleeding[24] (Fig. 17-5). A landmark analysis of this trial revealed that patients with a previous transient ischemic attack (TIA) or stroke, those ≥75 years of age, and those who weighed <60 kg were at especially high risk of bleeding.[25-26] Dual antiplatelet therapy with aspirin and a thienopyridine is considered standard pretreatment for patients with NSTE-ACS undergoing PCI with or without stent implantation (ACC/AHA guidelines class 1 recommendation, level of evidence A)[5]; however, the optimal timing for initiation of thienopyridine therapy may still pose a dilemma in actual clinical practice. The frequency of adverse cardiac events is reduced within the first hours of treatment with a thienopyridine; but if the patient is referred for urgent or emergent surgery, this approach may be associated with more perioperative blood loss.[27] However, given the fact that CABG is less likely to be necessary in the contemporary stent era even for high-risk NSTE-ACS patients, early thienopyridine treatment is recommended unless urgent CABG is deemed to be very likely.

ANTICOAGULANT TREATMENT

Since the beginning of PCI, unfractionated heparin (UFH) has been given to prevent thrombosis during intracoronary instrumentation and to minimize thrombosis at the site of the plaque, which is damaged by balloon angioplasty and/or stent implantation. Treatment with UFH in addition to aspirin is usually given based on the data from a metanalysis demonstrating a reduction of the combined death and MI rate of 7.9% for those treated with UFH compared with 10.3% for those treated with aspirin alone.[28] UFH is given as an initial intravenous bolus, usually as 100 IU/kg, and guided by the activating clotting time (ACT) in the range of 250 to 300 seconds. If combined with a GP IIb/IIIa inhibitor, the dose of UFH should be lower: initial intravenous bolus of 50 to 60 IU/kg and ACT in the range of 200 to 250 seconds to prevent excessive bleeding complications. Although the ACC/AHA guidelines recommend that patients with NSTE-ACS receive heparin, the actual duration of heparin therapy is not well established, and most trials that have examined UFH recommend 2 to 5 days of therapy.[5] Low-molecular-weight heparin (LMWH) has also been used in the setting of PCI for NSTE-ACS. In the FRISC (Fast Revascularization during Instability in Coronary Artery Disease) trial,[29] 1,506 patients were randomly assigned to receive dalteparin (120 IU/kg twice daily, with a maximal dose of 10,000 IU) or UFH during the first 5 to 7 days of hospitalization followed by dalteparin (7,500 IU subcutaneously, daily) or placebo for 35 to 45 days. Dalteparin was associated with a 63% relative risk reduction in death or MI during the first 6 days (1.8% in the treatment group versus 4.8% in the placebo group), with persistence of these differences at 40 days. The ESSENCE (Efficacy and Safety of Subcutaneous Enoxaparin in Non-Q-wave Coronary Events) trial[30] evaluated 3,171 UA/NSTE-ACS patients who were randomly assigned to receive enoxaparin (1 mg/kg twice daily) or continuous infusion of UFH (minimum of 48 hours to a maximum of 8 days). The risk of recurrent angina, MI, or death was significantly lower in the enoxaparin patients than in the UFH patients at 14 days (16.6% vs. 19.8%). The benefit persisted at 30 days; however, this came at the cost of increased minor bleeding but no significant difference in major bleeding (6.5% vs. 7%).[30] The TIMI IIB (Thrombolysis In Myocardial Infarction) trial[31] randomized 3,910 patients with UA/NSTE-ACS to receive either enoxaparin or UFH for 3 to 8 days while hospitalized, followed by either enoxaparin or placebo through day 43 on an outpatient basis. At 8 days, a 14.6% risk reduction in the composite endpoint of MI, death, and need for urgent revascularization was noted, and at 43 days a 12.3% risk reduction in the same endpoint was reported. Bleeding was similar in both groups during initial hospitalization, but the risk of major bleeding during the outpatient phase of the study was doubled in the enoxaparin group as compared with placebo. These data suggest that enoxaparin may be more effective than UFH at reducing the risk of ischemic events during the acute management of NSTE-ACS patients without an important increase in major bleeding events. A metanalysis of nearly 22,000 patients with UA/NSTE-ACS enrolled in six randomized trials reported a relative risk reduction of 9% in the composite endpoint of death or MI at 30 days for patients treated with enoxaparin as compared with those treated with UFH and no significant difference in major bleeding at 7 days.[32] These results demonstrate that the use of enoxaparin was beneficial when an early conservative strategy was utilized for patient management. More recent trials have compared UFH with enoxaparin when an early invasive strategy is implemented. The SYNERGY (Superior Yield of the New Strategy of Enoxaparin, Revascularization and Glycoprotein IIb/IIIa Inhibitors) trial[33] studied 10,027 patients with high-risk UA/NSTE-ACS who were treated using an early invasive strategy. In this study, there was no significant difference in the primary endpoint of all-cause mortality or nonfatal MI at 30 days, but patients who received enoxaparin exhibited a 20% increase in TIMI major bleeding in association with invasive procedures, especially CABG.[33] When considered as a whole, the data presented above support the notion that treatment with enoxaparin as compared with UFH appears to be more efficacious at reducing ischemic events in UA/NSTE-ACS patients who are treated with an early conservative strategy. However, it may also result in increased bleeding with invasive procedures. Interpretation of data from the SYNERGY trial and other trials comparing UFH and enoxaparin in UA/NSTE-ACS patients treated with an early invasive strategy must be interpreted carefully, given that many of the patients in these trials had already received one or more other antithrombotic agents before being randomized to a given treatment arm. Thus the high rate of patient crossover is an important confounding factor. The

TABLE 17-2	ACUITY Trial Results			
End Point (30 days)	UFH/Enox + GPI (n = 4603)	Bivalirudin + GPI (n = 4604)	Bivalirduin Alone (n = 4612)	P Value
Net outcome (%)	11.7	11.8	10.1	0.0014
Ischemic composite (%)	7.3	7.7	7.8	NS
Major bleeding (%)	5.7	5.3	3.0	<0.0001

Enox, enoxaprin; GPI, GP IIb/IIIa inhibitor; NS, not significant; UFH, unfractionated heparin.

most recent ACC/AHA guidelines consider enoxaparin to be a reliable alternative to UFH for patients treated both with an early conservative and an early invasive strategy (class 1, level of evidence A).[5] Bivalirudin is a direct thrombin inhibitor and a synthetic analog of hirudin. It reversibly binds thrombin and inhibits clot-bound thrombin. The REPLACE II (Randomized Evaluation in PCI Linking Angiomax to Reduced Clinical Events II) trial[34] demonstrated that bivalirudin could be used as an alternative to UFH plus GP IIb/IIIa blockade in patients at low risk who undergo PCI. The efficacy of bivalirudin was further evaluated in the ACUITY (Acute Catheterization and Urgent Intervention Triage Strategy) trial.[35] It randomized 13,800 patients with moderate- to high-risk unstable angina or NSTEMI undergoing an invasive strategy. There were three treatment groups: group I received UFH or enoxaparin plus GP IIb/IIIa, group II received bivalirudin plus a GP IIb/IIIa inhibitor, and group III received bivalirudin alone. The primary endpoint at 30 days was a net clinical outcome based on an ischemic composite (all-cause mortality, MI, or unplanned revascularization for ischemia) or major bleeding. The net outcome was lower with the bivalirudin-alone strategy, which could be ascribed to a significant reduction in major bleeding in the bivalirudin group (Table 17-2). Fondaparinux is a synthetic polysaccharide that leads to indirect inhibition of factor Xa. Fondaparinux was evaluated in the OASIS-5 (Organization to Assess Strategies for Ischemic Syndromes) trial.[36] In this study, 20,078 patients were randomized to treatment with either fondaparinux (2.5 mg/day) or enoxaparin (1mg/kg twice daily) for a mean of 6 days. Approximately 40% of patients underwent PCI and 15% underwent CABG in both groups. Fondaparinux was equivalent to enoxaparin in terms of the primary efficacy endpoint at 9 days (composite of death, MI, or refractory ischemia), and major bleeding at 9 days was significantly lower with fondaparinux than with enoxaparin (2.2% vs. 4.1%; $P < 0.001$). However, fondaparinux was associated with an increased rate of guide-catheter thromboses; thus it has been recommended that additional anticoagulant with anti-IIa activity also be used.[5]

GLYCOPROTEIN IIB/IIIA INHIBITORS

A critical pathway of platelet activation and aggregation is mediated by a conformational change in the glycoprotein IIb/IIIa (GP IIb/IIIa) receptor from an inactive to an active state. GP IIb/IIIa inhibitors interfere with the ability of the GP IIb/IIIa receptor to bind with target ligands; thus they are potent inhibitors of platelet aggregation.[37] All three currently used GPIIb/IIIa inhibitors (abciximab, eptifibatide, and tirofiban) exhibit different pharmacodynamic and pharmacokinetic properties, different clinical trial outcomes, and as a result have different recommendations for clinical use. Abciximab was the first of the three currently used GPIIb/IIIa inhibitors to be subjected to large-scale clinical trial testing and was first evaluated in the pre-stent era of the early 1990s. The EPIC (Evaluation of c7E3 [later named abciximab] for the Prevention of Ischemic Complications) trial[38] studied high-risk patients with UA, evolving MI, or complex coronary lesion anatomy and showed a 35% reduction in the composite endpoint of death, MI, or recurrent ischemia as compared with placebo. The CAPTURE (c7E3 Fab Antiplatelet Therapy in Unstable Refractory Angina) trial[39] studied

1,265 patients with UA who underwent PCI. In this study, a 30% relative reduction in the primary endpoint of all-cause mortality, MI, or recurrent ischemia requiring urgent revascularization was reported at 30 days. The rate of MI was noted to be lower before, during, and after PCI in patients treated with abciximab, and a subgroup analysis revealed that abciximab facilitated thrombus resolution and prevented recurrent ischemia by continuous ECG monitoring. Abciximab therefore has clearly been shown to be efficacious in the setting of UA/NSTE-ACS patients undergoing PCI. The GUSTO-IV-ACS (Global Use of Strategies to Open Occluded Coronary Arteries IV-Acute Coronary Syndrome) trial,[40] however, studied 7,800 patients with UA/NSTE-ACS who were not scheduled to undergo an early invasive strategy. Patients in this study were randomized to receive an abciximab bolus followed by infusion for either 24 or 48 hours or placebo. In this trial abciximab provided no benefit with respect to the primary composite endpoint of death or MI at 30 days, even in a subgroup of patients with elevated troponin levels. The current ACC/AHA guidelines reflect these results in that abciximab is not recommended for the treatment of patients with UA/NSTE-ACS for whom an initial conservative strategy is planned.[5] Tirofiban was studied in the PRISM (Platelet Receptor Inhibition in Ischemic Syndrome Management) trial,[41] in which 3,232 patients with UA were randomized to receive either UFH or tirofiban for 48 hours. A 32% reduction in the rate of death, MI, or refractory ischemia was noted at 48 hours, but no significant difference was noted at 30 days. The PRISM-PLUS (Platelet Receptor Inhibition in Ischemic Syndrome Management in Patients Limited by Unstable Signs and Symptoms) trial[42] randomized UA and NSTE-ACS patients to receive aspirin plus either heparin, tirofiban, or both. The tirofiban-only arm was stopped early owing to excess death at 7 days (4.6% vs. 1.1% in the heparin-only arm). Patients who received both heparin and tirofiban exhibited the greatest benefit in terms of a reduction in the composite endpoint at 7 days of death, MI, or refractory ischemia. This benefit was sustained at 30 days and at 6 months (27.2% vs. 32% in the heparin-only arm). Eptifibatide was studied in 9,461 patients with NSTE-ACS in the PURSUIT (Platelet Glycoprotein IIb/IIIa in Unstable Angina: Receptor Suppression Using Integrellin Therapy) trial.[43] In this study, treatment with eptifibatide was associated with a 10% reduction in the relative risk of death and MI at 30 days. A meta-analysis[44] confirmed the utility of GPIIb/IIIa inhibitors in the management of patients with moderate- to high risk UA/NSTE-ACS. This analysis pooled 31,402 patients from six different GPIIb/IIIa trials involving ACS patients and showed a 9% reduction in the odds ratio of death or MI for patients treated with a GPIIb/IIIa inhibitor as compared with placebo. Subgroup analysis revealed a 15% reduction in the odds ratio of death or MI for troponin-positive patients and no such reduction in troponin negative patients. Reduction in the odds ratio of death or MI was also noted to be greater in patients who underwent PCI within 5 days.[44] The TARGET (Do Tirofiban and Reopro Give Similar Efficacy Outcomes Trial)[45] study was a direct comparison of the efficacy of abciximab with that of tirofiban. It demonstrated that the primary endpoint (composite of death, nonfatal MI, or urgent revascularization at 30 days) was significantly higher in the tirofiban group compared with those receiving abciximab (7.6% vs. 6.0%), but at 6 months, this difference was no longer statistically significant.[45] Most recently, the EARLY ACS (Early Versus Delayed Provisional Eptifibatide in Acute Coronary Syndromes) trial[46] compared early routine versus delayed provisional administration of eptifibatide in 9,492 patients with NSTE-ACS who were randomly assigned to an invasive strategy. The primary endpoint was the composite of death, MI, recurrent ischemia requiring urgent revascularization, or thrombotic bailout at 96 hours. There was no observed difference in the primary endpoint between the two groups at 96 hours; however, use of early routine eptifibatide was associated with higher rates of non-life-threatening bleeding and transfusions. With the multitude of anti-platelet therapies being administered to ACS patients, there was some concern that the efficacy of GP IIb/IIIa inhibitors might be reduced in patients pretreated with clopidogrel. The ISAR-REACT-2 (Intracoronary Stenting and Antithrombotic Regimen: Rapid Early Action for Coronary Treatment-2) trial[47] addressed this issue. ISAR-REACT-2 was a randomized, double-blind trial that compared treatment with abciximab (*n* = 1012) or placebo (*n* = 1010) in patients with NSTE-ACS[47] who were given a 600-mg loading dose of clopidogrel. The primary endpoint was a composite of death, MI, and urgent target vessel revascularization due to myocardial ischemia at 30 days. There was a significant reduction in the primary endpoint in favor of abciximab in all patients with NSTE-ACS, and this was achieved with no difference in TIMI-defined major bleeding (1.4% vs. 1.4%) (Fig. 17-6). As seen in several other trials, abciximab was highly effective in high-risk NSTE-ACS patients (i.e., troponin-positive) but not effective in troponin-negative patients.

Despite the demonstrated advantages of using GPIIb/IIIa inhibitors in the treatment of patients with NSTE-ACS who undergo PCI, the optimal timing of their initiation is still being clarified. Several trials are currently ongoing that will help to address this question. The most recent ACC/AHA guidelines list therapy with abciximab as a class I indication (level of evidence A) to be used prior to PCI as an "upstream" therapy only if there will be no appreciable delay in proceeding with coronary angiography and PCI is likely to be performed; otherwise therapy with tirofiban or eptifibatide is preferable (level of evidence B).[5]

Early Invasive Strategy versus Conservative Strategy for Patients with Non-ST-Segment Elevation Acute Coronary Syndrome

ACS patients presenting with hemodynamic instability, severe left ventricular dysfunction or overt heart failure, recurrent or persistent rest angina despite intensive medical therapy, mechanical complications (e.g., acute mitral regurgitation and ventricular septal defect), and those with sustained ventricular tachycardia are deemed to be at extremely high risk for death or a complicated MI and thus are recommended to undergo urgent coronary angiography (unless deemed inappropriate for revascularization).[5] For the management of other less overtly ill patients presenting with NSTE-ACS, two strategies have emerged: the initial conservative strategy and the initial invasive strategy. The early conservative strategy entails the use of intensive medical therapy, which includes aspirin, clopidogrel, anticoagulation (UFH, LMWH, or fondaparinux), and beta blockers and/or nitroglycerin (if not contraindicated) (Fig. 17-7). Additional therapy with either eptifibatide or tirofiban (discussed above) is beneficial in patients with elevated biomarkers or with a TIMI risk score ≥4. Patients who become asymptomatic on this regimen are typically observed for 48 to 72 hours and then subjected to cardiac stress testing, which also most typically includes some form of myocardial imaging (nuclear imaging or echocardiography). Patients who manifest signs or symptoms of ongoing ischemia at any time during observation or who demonstrate findings on stress testing that are other than low risk are referred for coronary angiography and subsequent revascularization as appropriate. Patients who demonstrate low-risk stress test findings are not subjected to angiography and are instead treated with aspirin indefinitely (unless contraindicated) and clopidogrel for at least 1 month but ideally for 1 year (in addition to other appropriate pharmacotherapy such as angiotensin converting enzyme [ACE] inhibitors, beta blockers, etc.).[5] Patients managed with an initially invasive strategy are treated with intensive medical therapy including aspirin, anticoagulation (UFH, LMWH, bivalirudin, or fondaparinux), and treated with either clopidogrel or a GPIIb/IIIa inhibitor (or both if high-risk features are present) prior to undergoing coronary angiography and subsequent revascularization as appropriate (Figs. 17-8 and 17-9). The efficacy of these strategies was tested in the earlier days of PCI, before the use of coronary stents and adjunctive treatment with GP IIb/IIIa inhibition. These studies—TIMI IIIB, VANQWISH (Veterans Affairs Non-Q-Wave Myocardial Infarction Strategies In Hospital), and MATE (Medicine versus Angiography in Thrombolytic Exclusion)—showed no

1 Age in years	Points
30 – 39	0
40 – 49	18
50 – 59	36
60 – 69	55
70 – 79	73
80 – 89	91
≥90	100

2 History of congestive
　heart failure 24

3 History of myocardial
　infarction 12

4 Resting heart rate beats / min	Points
50 – 70	3
70 – 90	9
90 – 110	14
110 – 150	23
150 – 200	35
≥200	43

5 Systolic blood pressure mm Hg	Points
≤79.9	24
80 – 99.9	22
100 – 120	18
120 – 140	14
140 – 160	10
160 – 200	4
≥200	0

6 St-segment
　Depression 11

7 Initial serum creatine mg/dL	Points
0 – 0.39	1
0.4 – 0.79	3
0.8 – 1.19	5
1.2 – 1.59	7
1.6 – 1.99	9
2.3 – 3.99	15
≥4	20

8 Elevated cardiac
　enzymes 15

9 No in-hospital percutaneous
　coronary intervention 14

A

Points	
1	..........._
2	..........._
3	..........._
4	..........._
5	..........._
6	..........._
7	..........._
8	..........._
9	..........._

Total risk score _____ (Sum of points)
Mortality risk _____ (from plot)

B

Figure 17-6　Results of the ISAR-REACT 2 trial, comparing abciximab with placebo.

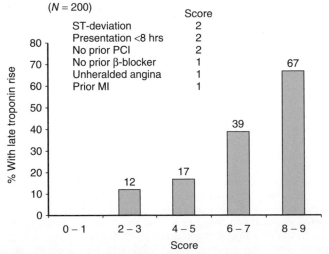

(N = 200)

	Score
ST-deviation	2
Presentation <8 hrs	2
No prior PCI	2
No prior β-blocker	1
Unheralded angina	1
Prior MI	1

Figure 17-7　ACC/AHA guidelines: algorithm for patients with UA/NSTEMI managed by an initial conservative strategy.

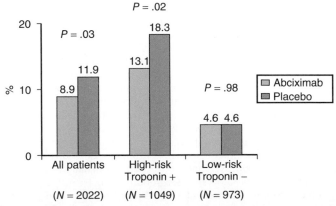

Figure 17-8　ACC/AHA guidelines: algorithm for patients with UA/NSTEMI managed by an initial invasive strategy.

superiority for either strategy.[48–50] After these trials, the outcome of PCI was improved by the use of stents and adjunctive treatment with thienopyridines and GP IIb/IIIa inhibitors. This prompted the initiation of additional randomized trials: the FRISC-II (Fast Revascularization during Instability of Coronary Artery Disease-II) trial, TACTICS-TIMI 18 (Treat Angina with Aggrastat and Determine Cost of Therapy with an Invasive or Conservative Strategy—Thrombolysis in Myocardial

Infarction) trial, VINO (Value of First-Day Angiography/Angioplasty in Evolving Non-ST-Segment Elevation Myocardial Infarction: An Open Multicenter Randomized Trial), RITA-3 (Randomized Intervention Trial of Unstable Angina-3), and ICTUS (Invasive versus Conservative Treatment in Unstable Coronary Syndromes) trial. The characteristics of these trials are presented in Table 17-3.[51–55]

With the invasive strategy approach, early revascularization (in hospital) was achieved in 44% to 76% of the patients, whereas with the conservative strategy, early revascularization was deemed necessary in 9% to 40% of the patients (Fig. 17-6). The contrast in the frequencies

TABLE 17-3	Outcomes of Percutaneous Coronary Intervention in Five Trials				
Characteristic	*FRISC II (N = 2457) (1222/1235)**	*TACTICS (N = 2220) (1114/1106)*	*VINO (N = 131) (64/67)*	*RITA-3 (N = 1810) (895/915)*	*ICTUS(N = 1200) (604/596)*
Mean age (yr)	65	62	66	63	62
Men (%)	70	66	61	62	62
Diabetes (%)	12	28	25	13	14
Previous MI (%)	22	39	26	39	23
Mean follow-up (mo)	24	6	6	24	12
Invasive/selective revascularization					
At end FU	78/43	61/44	73/39	57/28	79/54
PCI at FU	44/21	42/29	52/13	36/16	61/40
CABG at FU	38/23	22/16	35/30	22/12	18/14

*Early invasive versus conservative strategy.

CABG, coronary artery bypass grafting; FRISC-II, Fast Revascularization during Instability of Coronary Artery Disease-II; FU, follow-up; ICTUS, Invasive Conservative Treatment in Unstable Coronary Syndromes; MI, myocardial infarction; PCI, percutaneous coronary intervention; RITA-3, Randomized Intervention Trial of Unstable Angina; TACTICS, Treat Angina with Aggrastat and Determine Cost of Therapy with an Invasive or Conservative Strategy; VINO, Value of First Day Angiography/Angioplasty In Evolving Non-ST-segment Elevation Myocardial Infarction: an Open Multicenter Randomized Trial.

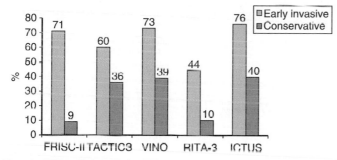

Figure 17-9 Incidence of early (in-hospital) revascularization in several trials.

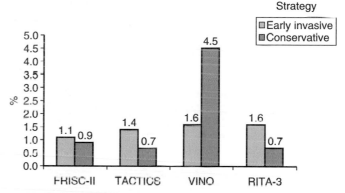

Figure 17-10 Incidence of in-hospital mortality in several trials.

of early revascularization between the early invasive strategy and conservative strategy varied from as low as 24% (TACTICS) to as high as 62% (FRISC-II). Revascularization after hospital discharge was predominantly performed in the patients randomized to an early conservative strategy. The primary endpoint of the various trials, defined as a composite of death and MI with or without rehospitalization, significantly favored the early invasive strategy in all trials except the RITA-3 and ICTUS trials (Table 17-4). The in-hospital mortality and combined in-hospital mortality or nonfatal MI rates are shown in Figures 17-10 and 17-11. The mortality and the combined mortality or nonfatal MI rates at the end of follow-up are presented in Figures 17-12 and 17-13. The RITA-3 trial reported the outcome at a median follow-up of 5 years (Table 17-5).[56] At 1 year, the rates of death and nonfatal MI were not different between the early invasive strategy and the conservative strategy; but at 5 years, there was a significant difference in favor of the early invasive strategy (Fig. 17-14).

OPTIMAL TIMING OF INTERVENTION

The optimal timing of intervention in patients with UA/NSTE-ACS has not been clearly established. The CRUSADE registry (Can Rapid Risk Stratification of Unstable Angina Patients Suppress Adverse Outcomes with Early Implementation of the ACC/AHA Guidelines?) investigated whether the outcomes of early catheterization and later catheterization were different.[57] A total of 56,352 patients were treated at 310 U.S. hospitals and entered into the CRUSADE registry. The patients were retrospectively classified as having very early (23.4 hours) catheterization or later (46.3 hours) catheterization. The difference in delay was introduced because the group of patients with later catheterization was collected at admission during the weekend. The in-hospital

adverse cardiac events occurring in the two groups are presented in Table 17-6. There was no difference between the two groups, but the investigators warned cautiously that they could not exclude an important risk reduction, particularly for early catheterization within 12 hours of presentation. This issue was further addressed in the ISAR-COOL (Intracoronary Stenting with Antithrombotic Regimen COOLing-off) trial.[58] It randomized 410 patients who had symptoms of unstable angina plus ST-segment depression or elevation of cardiac troponin T levels. Patients were randomized to antithrombotic pretreatment for 3 to 5 days (the cooling-off strategy) or very early intervention after pretreatment for less than 6 hours. Antithrombotic pretreatment consisted of heparin, aspirin, clopidogrel, and tirofiban. The outcome is presented in Table 17-7. There was a significant reduction in the combined death and MI rate in favor of the very early intervention strategy. This favorable outcome was predominantly attributable to adverse events occurring before catheterization.

The ELISA (Early or Late Intervention in Unstable Angina) pilot study investigated whether pretreatment with tirofiban was beneficial compared with no pretreatment.[59] A total of 220 patients with NSTE-ACS were randomized to an early strategy (early angiography without tirofiban pretreatment) or to a late strategy (delayed angiography after pretreatment with tirofiban). The primary endpoint was enzymatic infarct size (LDHQ48) as assessed by the area under the lactate dehydrogenase release curve up to 48 hours after symptom onset. The infarct size and clinical outcome at 30 days are presented in Table 17-8. The study showed that delayed angiography with pretreatment with tirofiban was associated with a smaller enzymatic infarct size. There were no differences in clinical outcome at 30 days. The CRUSADE

TABLE 17-4 Early Invasive versus Conservative Strategies in Five Trials					
Trial	*Primary End Point*	*Early Invasive*	*Conservative*	*RR or OR*	*CI 95%, P Value*
FRISC-II	Death/MI at 1 yr	10.4%	14.1%	RR = 0.74	CI: 0.60 to 0.92 P = 0.005
TACTICS	Death/MI/rehosp. for ACS at 6 mo	15.9%	19.4%	OR = 0.78	CI: 0.62 to 0.97 P = 0.025
VINO	Death/MI at 6 mo	6.2%	22.3%		P < 0.001
RITA-3	Death/MI at 1 yr	7.6%	8.3%	RR = 0.91	CI: 0.67 to 1.25 P = 0.58
ICTUS	Death/MI/rehosp. <1 yr	22.7%	21.2%	RR = 1.07	CI: 0.87 to 0.133 P = 0.33

ACS, acute coronary syndrome; FRISC-II, Fast Revascularization during Instability of Coronary Artery Disease-II; ICTUS, Invasive Conservative Treatment in Unstable Coronary Syndromes; MI, myocardial infarction; PCI, percutaneous coronary intervention; RITA-3, Randomized Intervention Trial of Unstable Angina; TACTICS, Treat Angina with Aggrastat and Determine Cost of Therapy with an Invasive or Conservative Strategy; VINO, Value of First Day Angiography/Angioplasty In Evolving Non-ST-segment Elevation Myocardial Infarction: an Open Multicenter Randomized Trial.

TABLE 17-5 RITA-3 Trial Outcomes at a Median Follow-up of 5 Years			
Outcome	*Early Intervention (n = 895)*	*Conservative Strategy (n = 915)*	*RR, 95% CI, and P Value*
Follow-up years			
1 yr death/MI	7.6%	8.3%	0.91 (0.67 to 1.25)
5 yr death/MI	16.6%	20.0%	0.78 (0.61 to 0.99), P = .044
Death	12.1%	15.1%	0.76 (0.58 to 1.0), P = .054
Cardiovasc. death	7.3%	10.6%	0.68 (0.49 to 0.95) P = .026
Cardiovasc. death or MI	12.2%	15.9%	0.74 (0.56 to 0.97) P = .030

MI, myocardial infarction.
From Fox KA, Poole-Wilson P, Clayton TC, et al. 5-Year outcome of an interventional strategy in non-ST-elevation acute coronary syndrome: the British Heart Foundation RITA 3 randomised trial. *Lancet.* 2005;366:914–920.

TABLE 17-6 Timing of Intervention in Patients with NSTEMI Acute Coronary Syndrome in the CRUSADE Registry			
	Timing of Catheterization		
In-Hospital Events	*46.3 HOURS (n = 10,804)*	*23.4 HOURS (n = 45,548)*	*P Value*
Death (%)	4.4	4.1	.23
Recurrent MI (%)	2.9	3.0	.36
Death/MI (%)	6.6	6.6	.86

CRUSADE, Can Rapid Risk Stratification of Unstable Angina Patients Suppress Adverse Outcomes with Early Implementation of the ACC/AHA guidelines [National Quality Improvement Initiative and Registry]; MI, myocardial infarction, NSTEMI, non-ST-segment elevation myocardial infarction.

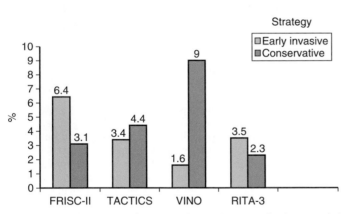

Figure 17-11 Incidence of in-hospital mortality or nonfatal myocardial infarction in several trials.

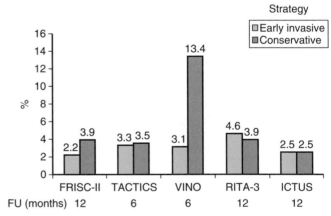

Figure 17-12 Incidence of mortality at the end of follow-up (FU) in several trials.

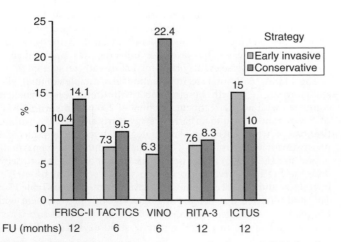

Figure 17-13 Incidence of mortality or nonfatal myocardial infarction at the end follow-up (FU) in several trials.

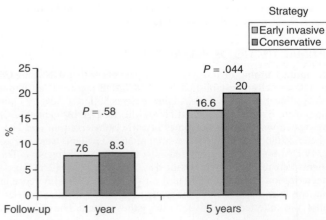

Figure 17-14 Incidence of death or nonfatal myocardial infarction at 5 years' follow-up from the RITA-3 trial.

TABLE 17-7	Outcomes of the ISAR-COOL Trial		
Outcome Characteristic	Prolonged Antithrombotic Pretreatment (%) (n = 207)	Early Intervention (%) (n = 203)	P Value
Definitive treatment			
Conservative	28.0	21.7	
CABG	7.7	7.9	
PCI (stents)	64.3	70.4	
30 Days			
Death/MI	11.6	5.9	.04
Death	1.4	0	.25
Non-fatal MI	10.1	5.9	.12
Q-wave	3.4	2.0	
Non-Q-wave	6.8	3.9	
Major bleeding event	3.9	3.0	.61

CABG, coronary artery bypass grafting; ISAR-COOL, Intracoronary Stenting with Antithrombotic Regimen COOLing-off; MI, myocardial infarction; PCI, percutaneous intervention.

TABLE 17-8	Outcomes of the ELISA Pilot Study	
Outcome Characteristic	Early Strategy* (n = 109)	Delayed Strategy† (n = 111)
Median time to angiography	6 hr	50 hr
Treatment		
PCI (%)	61	58
CABG (%)	14	19
Conservative (%)	25	23
30-Day clinical outcome of death/MI (%)	9.2	9.0
Enzymatic infarct size (LDHQ48)	629 ± 503	432 ± 441 (P = .02)

*Early angiography and no pretreatment.
†Delayed angiography (24–48 hr) and pretreatment with tirofiban
CABG, coronary artery bypass grafting; ELISA, Early or Late Intervention in unStable Angina; LDHQ48, cumulative enzyme release up to 48 hours after symptom onset as assessed by the area under the lactate dehydrogenase release curve; MI, myocardial infarction; PCI, percutaneous intervention.

TABLE 17-9	Outcomes of the CRUSADE Trial: In-Hospital Death or Myocardial Infarction		
Outcome	No Early Invasive Management (n = 9889)	Early Invasive Management (n = 8037)	Adjusted Odds Ratio (95% CI)
Mortality (%)	6.2	2.0	0.63 (0.52 to 0.77)
Post-admission MI (%)	3.7	3.1	0.95 (0.79 to 1.14)
Death or MI (%)	8.9	4.7	0.79 (0.69 to 0.90)

CRUSADE, Can Rapid Risk Stratification of Unstable Angina Patients Suppress Adverse Outcomes with Early Implementation of the ACC/AHA Guidelines; MI, myocardial infarction.

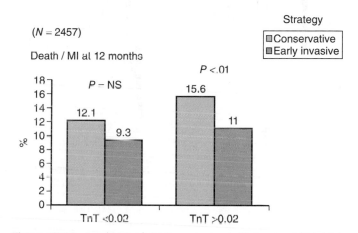

Figure 17-15 Incidence of death or myocardial infarction (MI) in high-risk and low risk groups from the FRISC II trial (N = 2,457). TnT, troponin levels.

quality improvement initiative investigated the use of early invasive management within 48 hours in 17,926 high-risk NSTEMI patients (Table 17-9).[60] A total of 8,037 patients (44.8%) underwent early cardiac catheterization; of these, 75% were revascularized: 4,733 (58.9%) underwent PCI and 1,296 (16.1%) underwent CABG. The unadjusted incidence of in-hospital mortality and postadmission MI was significantly lower for patients who underwent early invasive management than for those not undergoing early invasive management. Patients who underwent early invasive management were younger and had less comorbidity. The adjusted risks for death and MI were lower for patients who underwent early invasive management. In a propensity-matched pair analysis, the mortality rate remained lower for patients who underwent early invasive management (2.5% vs. 3.7%, P < 0.01). More recently, the TIMACS (Timing of Intervention in Acute Coronary Syndromes) trial[61] randomly assigned patients to either an early intervention group (n = 1,593) who underwent coronary angiography within 24 hours of randomization or to a delayed intervention group (n = 1,438) who underwent coronary angiography 36 hours after randomization. The primary endpoint was the first occurrence of a composite of death, new MI, or stroke at 6 months. Results showed that early intervention was associated with a 35% reduction in the primary outcome in high-risk patients (defined as

GRACE risk score >140). The OPTIMA (Immediate Versus Delayed Intervention for Acute Coronary Syndromes; a Randomized Clinical Trial) trial[62] compared patients who were randomly assigned to receive immediate or delayed catheterization. This small study (n = 142) was terminated early due to poor enrolment. However, it demonstrated a significantly lower rate of the composite endpoint of death, nonfatal MI, or unplanned revascularization at 30 days in patients assigned to deferred versus immediate PCI. In a similar fashion, the ABOARD (Immediate vs. Delayed Intervention for Acute Coronary Syndromes: a Randomized Control Trial) trial[63] randomly assigned 352 patients with high-risk NSTE-ACS (TIMI risk ≥3) to receive immediate versus delayed coronary angiography (between 8 to 60 hours postrandomization). In this study there was no significant difference in either the primary outcome of peak hospital troponin I value or the secondary combined outcome of death, MI, or urgent revascularization at 1 month.

PATIENTS WHO DERIVE BENEFIT FROM AN EARLY INVASIVE STRATEGY

Patients with elevated troponin levels (data from FRISC II and TACTICS-TIMI 18, presented in Figs. 17-15 and 17-16), ST-segment depression (data from FRISC II, TACTICS-TIMI 18, and TIMI IIIB), the degree of and number of ECG leads with ST-segment depression (data from FRISC II), and age >65 years (data from TIMI IIIB and TACTICS-TIMI 18) have been clearly shown to benefit from an early invasive strategy. The TIMI risk score applied to TACTICS-TIMI 18 showed that patients at low risk (TIMI risk score 0–2) demonstrated

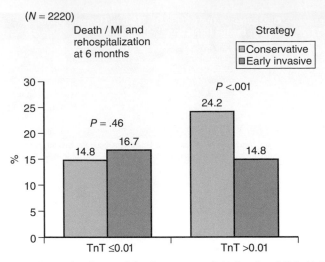

Figure 17-16 Incidence of death or myocardial infarction (MI) in high-risk and low-risk groups from the TACTICS-18 trial.

no difference in outcome (composite of death, MI, or rehospitalization for ACS at 6 months) whether they were treated with an early invasive or an early conservative strategy.[52] Patients at intermediate risk (TIMI risk score 3–4), however, showed better outcomes (as manifest by a significant reduction in the composite of death, MI, or rehospitalization for ACS at 6 months) when treated with an early invasive strategy. Patients at highest risk (TIMI risk score 5–7) showed an even greater improvement in outcomes with an invasive strategy (Table 17-10).[56] Although the presence of elevated cardiac biomarkers and ST-segment depression are each variables in the TIMI risk score, further analysis from the TACTICS-TIMI 18 trial data revealed that the degree of cardiac biomarker elevation and magnitude of ST-segment depression were each independent predictors of poorer outcomes and that these patients benefited from an early invasive strategy.[64]

EARLY INVASIVE STRATEGY IN WOMEN

The benefit of using an early invasive strategy in women is achieved primarily in those with high-risk features such as ST-segment changes or elevated troponin levels. Women who were managed with very early aggressive revascularization had better long-term outcomes than men.[65] The combined endpoint of death and nonfatal MI was significantly reduced at a follow-up of 20 months for women compared with men (OR = 0.65; 95% CI: 0.28–0.92).

TABLE 17-10	Rates of Death, Myocardial Infarction, or Rehospitalization for Acute Coronary Syndrome Stratified by TIMI Risk Score			
	Event Rate (%)			
TIMI Risk Score	INVASIVE	CONSERVATIVE	**OR**	**95% CI**
Low (0–2)	19.8	15.1	1.39	1.02 to 1.88
Intermediate (3–4)	18.2	21.8	0.80	0.64 to 0.99
High (5–7)	22.7	34	0.57	0.38 to 0.87

TIMI, Thrombolysis in Myocardial Infarction trial; MI, myocardial infarction; TACTICS, Treat Angina with Aggrastat and Determine Cost of Therapy with an Invasive or Conservative Strategy trial.
Data from TIMI IIIb and TACTICS-TIMI 18 trials.

Revascularization of Multivessel Disease In Non-ST-Segment Elevation Acute Coronary Syndrome

When patients undergo coronary angiography for NSTE-ACS and are found to have multivessel disease, the interventionalist must decide on an appropriate strategy for revascularization: PCI versus CABG and multivessel PCI versus culprit-vessel PCI. CABG was compared with PCI in patients who were candidates for either procedure based on angiographic findings in AWESOME (the Percutaneous Coronary Intervention versus Coronary Artery Bypass Graft Surgery for Patients with Medically Refractory Myocardial Ischemia and Risk Factors for Adverse Outcomes with Bypass: A Multicenter, Randomized Trial)[66] as well as in the ERACI II (Argentine Randomized Study: Coronary Angioplasty with Stenting versus Coronary Bypass Surgery in Patients with Multivessel Disease) trial.[67] It is important to note that both trials were performed before the advent of drug-eluting stents, which are known to substantially reduce the rate of repeat revascularization, and both trials excluded patients who had clear indications for CABG over PCI (such as left main disease). In the AWESOME trial, 454 patients with medically refractory angina or provocable ischemia after stabilization with medical therapy who were at high risk for increased 30-day postoperative mortality after CABG were randomly assigned to undergo PCI (54% with stenting and 11% with a GPIIb/IIIa inhibitor) or CABG. PCI and CABG were associated with similar mortality rates at 30 days, 3 years, and 5 years; however, survival free of UA or repeat revascularization was lower in the PCI group. A registry of 1,650 patients who were eligible for the AWESOME trial but were not randomized showed similar results (AWESOME registry).[68] In ERACI II, 450 patients with multivessel disease were randomly assigned to CABG or PCI with bare metal stents. Unlike the AWESOME trial, ERACI II showed a significantly lower rate of major adverse events (death, MI, repeat revascularization, and stroke) at 30 days in the PCI group, primarily driven by a reduction in death. At 18 months, mortality remained lower in the PCI group; however, it was noted that the excess deaths seen in the CABG group had all occurred within the first 30 days. PCI was associated with a significant increase in new revascularization procedures at 18 months[67] and 5 years,[69] and a difference in mortality between the PCI and CABG groups was no longer apparent at 5 years.[69] When NSTE-ACS patients are found to have significant multivessel disease by coronary angiography and there are no clear advantages for CABG, the interventionalist is next faced with the decision of whether to perform PCI on the culprit vessel only or to undertake multivessel PCI. In making this decision, it is important to consider from a practical standpoint that it may not always be overtly obvious which lesion is the clear culprit for the ACS event. This is especially the case when a patient has been treated with anticoagulant and antiplatelet therapy for many hours prior to angiography, which may decrease the intracoronary thrombus burden associated with a recently ruptured plaque and make it difficult or impossible to identify. A retrospective analysis of the safety and efficacy of multivessel stenting versus culprit-vessel-only stenting utilizing bare metal stents in 1,240 patients with NSTE-ACS revealed that multivessel stenting was associated with a significant reduction in the composite endpoint of death, MI, or revascularization during a mean follow-up period of 2.3 years.[70] This benefit, however, was entirely attributable to a lower revascularization rate in the patients who had undergone multivessel stenting as compared with those who did not, and there were no differences in safety endpoints between the two groups.[70] The decision to proceed with multivessel PCI versus culprit-vessel-only PCI may be influenced by several factors, including but not limited to angiographic severity/complexity of the lesions present, amount of myocardium supplied by the lesions in question, amount of fluoroscopy time used, and amount of contrast used, which leads to concerns over renal toxicity. In many cases, because of one or more of the previously mentioned factors, an interventionalist may choose to bring a patient back for a staged PCI procedure either during the same hospitalization or at a later time in order to complete the task of total revascularization.

Drug-Eluting Stents for Patients with Non-ST-Segment Elevation Acute Coronary Syndrome

As mentioned above, the primary limitation of multivessel PCI using bare metal stents as compared with CABG has been the higher rate of repeat revascularization. Drug-eluting stents (DESs) are associated with substantially reduced rates of target lesion revascularization (TLR) in those undergoing PCI and are being increasingly used in patients with NSTE-ACS. In various randomized trials comparing the efficacy of DESs with that of bare metal stents to reduce the rates of restenosis and target vessel revascularization, the reported proportions of patients with unstable coronary artery disease were between 30% and 50%.[71-74] Although many variables were studied that predicted early in-hospital complications or target vessel revascularization, the presence of unstable coronary artery disease was not reported as a predictive factor. In a subanalysis of the RESEARCH (Rapamycin-Eluting Stent Evaluated At Rotterdam Cardiology Hospital) registry investigating the safety and efficacy of sirolimus-eluting stents, it was shown that sirolimus stenting in patients with unstable angina and those with stable angina was associated with an almost similar risk reduction in the need for target vessel revascularization compared with bare metal stenting.[75] The hazard ratio at 1 year of clinically driven target vessel revascularization for DES was 0.30 (95% CI: 0.13–0.71; $P < 0.0006$) compared with bare metal stenting. The BASKET (Basel Stent Kosten Effektivitäts Trial) demonstrated that there were fewer adverse cardiac events for patients ($n = 301$) with NSTE-ACS receiving DESs than for those given bare metal stents.[76] A subgroup analysis of the TAXUS IV trial, which examined 450 patients with ACS (80% UA and 20% NSTEMI), revealed a significant reduction in major adverse cardiac events for patients treated with paclitaxel-eluting stents as compared with bare metal stents, with the benefit due entirely to a lower rate of TLR.[77] An analysis of the mandated Massachusetts State PCI Registry showed that in 1,228 matched pairs, the 2-year risk of death or recurrent MI was significantly lower in patients who received DESs, as was the rate of revascularization.[78] It may be concluded, then, that the safety and efficacy of DES implantation is similar in patients presenting with stable or unstable coronary artery disease.

Statins and Percutaneous Coronary Intervention for Non-ST-Segment Elevation Acute Coronary Syndrome

The MIRACL (Myocardial Ischemia Reduction with Aggressive Cholesterol Lowering) trial randomized 3,086 patients with unstable coronary artery disease to early treatment with 80 mg of atorvastatin ($n = 1355$) or placebo ($n = 1384$).[79] At 16 weeks, the primary endpoint (composite of death, nonfatal MI, cardiac arrest, and recurrent ischemia) occurred in 14.8% in the atorvastatin group and 17.4% in the placebo group ($P = 0.048$); however, only 16% of these patients underwent revascularization. In the PROVE IT-TIMI-22 (Pravastatin or Atorvastatin Evaluation and Infection Therapy–Thrombolysis In Myocardial Infarction-22) trial, intensive statin treatment in patients hospitalized for an acute coronary syndrome was compared with standard statin therapy.[80] The combined primary endpoint was death of any cause, MI, documented unstable angina, rehospitalization, revascularization (performed at least 30 days after randomization), and stroke. The trial randomized 4,162 patients to intensive statin treatment

(80 mg of atorvastatin daily, $n = 2,099$) or to pravastatin daily (40 mg, $n = 2,063$). Of these patients, 69% underwent PCI for the treatment of their index acute coronary syndrome before randomization. Three-fourths of these patients underwent an early invasive strategy. The low-density-lipoprotein (LDL) cholesterol levels were 106 mg/dL before treatment in each group. The primary endpoint at the conclusion of follow-up (mean, 24 months) was reached in 22.4% of the intensive atorvastatin group and 26.3% in the standard-dose pravastatin group ($P = 0.005$). The difference in treatment effect started at 30 days, which confirmed the results with statin treatment in the MIRACL trial. In the LIPS (Lescol Intervention Prevention Study), 1,669 patients were randomized to receive 80 mg of fluvastatin or placebo, with treatment starting 2 days after successful PCI.[81] The LIPS study showed that the statin-treated group experienced a significantly lower incidence of adverse clinical events (24.1%) than the placebo group (26.7%, $P = 0.01$).

Early and post-PCI statin therapy is beneficial in reducing the rate of adverse coronary events. According to the ACC/AHA guidelines, LDL cholesterol reduction is recommended when the level is higher than 130 mg/dL or when, after diet, the LDL level is higher than 100 mg/dL for all patients with an ACS, with or without revascularization.[5]

Management Summary of Patients with Non-ST-Segment Elevation Acute Coronary Syndrome

Outlined below is a pragmatic approach consistent with the most recent ACC/AHA and ESC guidelines.[5,82,83] Patients with NSTE-ACS should receive anti-ischemic, antiplatelet, and anticoagulant treatment. An early risk assessment is vitally important in order to identify those who may benefit from an early aggressive approach. This assessment should be based on clinical presentation, age, ECG changes, cardiac enzymes and biomarkers, and clinical course. The risk level is classified as high, intermediate, or low (Tables 17-11, 17-12, and 17-13); further management is guided by risk classification. Patients presenting with NSTE-ACS and evidence of hemodynamic instability or cardiogenic shock, severe left ventricular dysfunction or overt heart failure, recurrent or persistent angina at rest despite intensive medical therapy, acute mitral regurgitation or ventricular septal defect, or sustained ventricular arrhythmias should undergo urgent coronary angiography and appropriate revascularization. Patients who are stable but have a history of prior CABG or PCI within 6 months, new ST segment depression, elevated cardiac biomarkers, angina with minimal activity despite intensive medical therapy, left ventricular ejection fraction <40%, or a TIMI risk score >2 should be managed with an early invasive strategy. Patients with a low TIMI risk score (≤2) and no high-risk features should be managed with an initially conservative strategy. The findings of coronary angiography largely determine whether patients should be referred for PCI or CABG (Fig. 17-17). If PCI is the chosen revascularization modality, it may be performed in the same sitting or in a staged fashion as deemed appropriate by the treating physician. Patients undergoing PCI should receive adjunctive treatment with aspirin, clopidogrel, an anticoagulant (UFH, LMWH, bivalirudin, or fondaparinux), with or without a GP IIb/IIIa antagonist. Lifestyle changes and secondary prevention using aspirin, beta blockers, statins, and ACE inhibitors should be implemented for all survivors of NSTE-ACS as appropriate.

Acknowledgment

The author wishes to thank P. J. de Feyter for his contribution to this chapter in previous editions of this textbook.

TABLE 17-11	ACC/AHA Risk Stratification: Short-Term Risk Stratification of Death or Nonfatal Myocardial Infarction in Patients with NSTEMI Acute Coronary Syndrome		
Feature	High Risk: At Least One of the Following Must Be Present	Intermediate Risk: No High-Risk Feature but Must Have One of the Following	Low Risk: No High- or Intermediate-Risk Feature but May Have Any of the Following
History	Accelerating tempo of ischemic symptoms in preceding 48 hr	Prior MI, peripheral or cerebrovascular disease, or CABG; prior aspirin use	
Character of pain	Prolonged ongoing rest pain (>20 min)	Prolonged (>20 min) rest angina, now resolved, with moderate or high likelihood of CAD. Rest angina (<20 min or relieved with rest or sublingual nitroglycerin)	New-onset or progressive CCS class III or IV angina in the past 2 weeks with moderate or high likelihood of CAD
Clinical findings	Pulmonary edema, most likely related to ischemia. New or worsening MR murmur. S_3 or new or worsening rale. Hypotension, bradycardia, tachycardia. Age >75 yr	Age >70 yr	
ECG findings	Angina at rest with transient ST-segment changes >0.05 mV. Bundle branch block, new or presumed new. Sustained ventricular tachycardia	T-wave inversions >0.2 mV. Pathologic Q waves	Normal or unchanged ECG pattern during an episode of chest discomfort
Cardiac markers	Elevated (e.g., TnT or TnI >0.1 ng/mL)	Slightly elevated (e.g., TnT >0.01 but <0.1 ng/mL)	Normal

ACC/AHA, American College of Cardiology/American Heart Association; CABG, coronary artery bypass grafting; CAD, coronary artery disease; CCS, Canadian Cardiovascular Society; ECG, electrocardiographic; MI, myocardial infarction; MR, mitral regurgitation; NSTEMI, non-ST-segment elevation myocardial infarction; Tn, troponin (I and T forms).

TABLE 17-12	American College of Cardiology and American Heart Association High-Risk Indicators for Non-ST-Segment Elevation Acute Coronary Syndrome

- Recurrent angina or ischemia at rest or with low-level activities despite intensive anti-ischemic treatment
- Elevated troponin levels
- New or presumably new ST-segment depression
- Recurrent angina or ischemia with congestive heart failure symptoms, S_3 gallop, pulmonary edema, worsening rales, or new or worsening mitral regurgitation
- High-risk findings on noninvasive stress testing
- Depressed left ventricular systolic function
- Hemodynamic instability
- Sustained ventricular tachycardia
- Percutaneous coronary intervention within 6 months
- Prior coronary artery bypass grafting

TABLE 17-13	European Society of Cardiology Guidelines for Risk	
	High-Risk Indicators	Low-Risk Indicators
	Elevated troponin levels	Normal troponin levels
	Recurrent ischemia	No recurrent ischemia
	ST-segment depression	No release of creatine kinase MB fraction (CK-MB)
	Early unstable angina after myocardial infarction	Presence of negative or flat T waves
	Diabetes mellitus	Normal electrocardiogram
	Hemodynamic instability	
	Major arrhythmias: ventricular fibrillation, ventricular tachycardia	

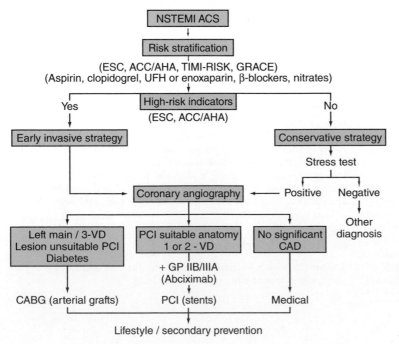

Figure 17-17 ACC/AHA guidelines: management after diagnostic angiography in patients with UA/NSTEMI.

REFERENCES

1. Grüntzig AR, Senning A, Siegenthaler WE: Non-operative dilatation of coronary artery stenosis: Percutaneous transluminal coronary angioplasty. *N Engl J Med* 301:61–68, 1979.
2. de Feyter PJ, Serruys PW, van den Brand M, et al: Emergency coronary angioplasty in refractory unstable angina. *N Engl J Med* 313:342–346, 1985.
3. Sigwart U, Puel J, Mirkovitch V, et al: Intravascular stents to prevent occlusion and restenosis after transluminal angioplasty. *N Engl J Med* 316:701–706, 1987.
4. Alpert JS, Thygesen K, Antman E, Bassand JP: Myocardial infarction redefined—a consensus document of the Joint European Society of Cardiology/American College of Cardiology Committee for the Redefinition of Myocardial Infarction. *J Am Coll Cardiol* 36(3):959–969, 2000.
5. Anderson JL, Adams CD, Antman EM, et al: ACC/AHA 2007 guidelines for the management of patients with unstable angina/non ST-elevation myocardial infarction: a report of the American College of Cardiology/American Heart Association Task Force on Practice Guidelines (Writing Committee to Revise the 2002 Guidelines for the Management of Unstable Angina/non ST-Elevation Myocardial Infarction): developed in collaboration with the American College of Emergency Physicians, the Society for Cardiovascular Angiography and Interventions, and the Society of Thoracic Surgeons: endorsed by the American Association of Cardiovascular and Pulmonary Rehabilitation and the Society for Academic Emergency Medicine. *Circulation* 116(7): e148–e304, 2007.
6. Fuster V, Moreno PR, Fayad ZA, et al: Atherothrombosis and high-risk plaque. Part I. Evolving concepts. *J Am Coll Cardiol* 46:937–954, 2005.
7. Armstrong PW, Fu Y, Chang WC, et al: Acute coronary syndromes in the GUSTO-IIb trial: prognostic insights and impact of recurrent ischemia. The GUSTO-IIb Investigators. *Circulation* 98:1860, 1998.
8. Antman EM, Cohen M, Bernink PJ, et al: The TIMI risk score for unstable angina/non-ST elevation MI: a method for prognostication and therapeutic decision making. *JAMA* 284:835–842, 2000.
9. Eagle KA, Lim MJ, Dabbous OH, et al: A validated prediction model for all forms of acute coronary syndrome: estimating the risk of 6-month postdischarge death in an international registry. *JAMA* 291:2727–2733, 2004.
10. Januzzi JL Jr, Newby LK, Murphy SA, et al: Predicting a late positive serum troponin in initially troponin-negative patients with non-ST-elevation acute coronary syndrome: clinical predictors and validated risk score results from the TIMI IIIB and GUSTO IIA studies. *Am Heart J* 151:360–366, 2006.
11. Patrono C, Coller B, FitzGerald GA, et al: Platelet-active drugs: the relationships among dose, effectiveness, and side effects. the Seventh ACCP conference on Antithrombotic and Thrombolytic Therapy. *Chest* 126(3 Suppl):234S–264S, 2004.
12. Loll PJ, Picot D, Garavito RM: The structural basis of aspirin activity inferred from the crystal structure of inactivated prostaglandin H2 synthase. *Nat Struct Biol* 2(8):637–643, 1995.
13. Collaborative overview of randomized trials of antiplatelet therapy: I. Prevention of death, myocardial infarction, and stroke by prolonged antiplatelet therapy in various categories of patients. Antiplatelet Trialists' Collaboration. *BMJ* 308(6921):81–106, 1994.
14. Antithrombotic Trialists' Collaboration: Collaborative meta-analysis of randomized trials of antiplatelet therapy for prevention of death, myocardial infarction, and stroke in high risk patients. *BMJ* 324(7329):71–86, 2002.
15. Yusuf S, Zhao F, Mehta SR, et al: Clopidogrel in Unstable Angina to Prevent Recurrent Events Trial Investigators. Effects of clopidogrel in addition to aspirin in patients with acute coronary syndromes without ST-segment elevation. *N Eng J Med* 345(7): 494–502, 2001.
16. Bhatt DL, Fox KA, Hacke W, et al: Clopidogrel and aspirin versus aspirin alone for the prevention of atherothrombotic events. *N Engl J Med* 354(16):1706–1717, 2006.
17. Balsano F, Rizzon P, Violi F, et al: Antiplatlet treatment with ticlopidine in unstable angina. A controlled multicenter clinical trial. The Studio della Ticlopidinia nell'Angina Instabile Group. *Circulation* 82(1):17–26, 1990.
18. A randomized, blinded, trial of clopidogrel versus aspirin in patients at risk of ischemic events (CAPRIE). CAPRIE Steering Committee. *Lancet* 348(9038):1329–1339, 1996.
19. Mehta SR, Yusuf S, Peters RJ, et al: Effects of pretreatment with clopidogrel and aspirin followed by long-term therapy in patients undergoing percutaneous coronary intervention: the PCI-CURE study. *Lancet* 358(9281):527–533, 2001.
20. Kandzari DE, Berger PB, Kastrati A, et al: Influence of treatment duration with a 600 mg dose of clopidogrel before percutaneous coronary revascularization. *J Am Coll Cardiol* 44(11):2133–2136, 2004.
21. Oqueli E, Hiscock M, Dick R: Clopidogrel resistance. *Heart Lung Circ* 16(Suppl 3):S17–S28, 2007.
22. Frere C, Cuisset T, Morange PE, et al: Effect of cytochrome p450 polymorphisms on platelet reactivity after treatment with clopidogrel in acute coronary syndrome. *Am J Cardiol* 101(8):1088–1093, 2008.
23. Price MJ. The evidence base for platelet function testing in patients undergoing percutaneous coronary intervention. *Circ Cardiovasc Intervent* 3(3):277–283, 2010.
24. Wiviott SD, Braunwald E, McCabe CH, et al: Prasugrel versus clopidogrel in patients with acute coronary syndromes. *N Eng J Med* 357(20):2001–2015, 2007.
25. Wiviott SD, Braunwald E, McCabe CH, et al: Intensive oral antiplatelet therapy for reduction of ischemic events including stent thrombosis in patients with acute coronary syndromes treated with percutaneous coronary intervention and stenting in the TRITON-TIMI 38 trial: a subanalysis of a randomised trial. *Lancet* 371(9621):1353–1363, 2008.
26. Murphy SA, Antman EM, Wiviott SD, et al: Reduction in recurrent cardiovascular events with prasugrel compared with clopidogrel in patients with acute coronary syndromes from the TRITON-TIMI 38 trial. *Eur Heart J* 29(20):2473–2479, 2008.
27. Yusuf S, Zhao F, Mehta SR, et al: for the Clopidogrel in Unstable Angina to Prevent Recurrent Events Trial Investigators: effects of clopidogrel in addition to aspirin in patients with acute coronary syndromes without ST-segment elevation. *N Engl J Med* 345:494–502, 2001.
28. Oler A, Whooley MA, Oler J, Grady D: Adding heparin to aspirin reduces the incidence of myocardial infarction and death in patients with unstable angina. A meta-analysis. *JAMA* 276:811–815, 1996.
29. Swahn E, Wallentin L: Low molecular-weight heparin (Fragmin) during instability in coronary artery disease (FRISC). FRISC Study Group. *Am J Cardiol* 80(5A):25E–29E, 1997.
30. Cohen M, Demers C, Gurfinkel EP, et al: A comparison of low-molecular-weight heparin with unfractionated heparin for unstable coronary artery disease. Efficacy and Safety of Subcutaneous Enoxaparin in Non-Q-Wave Coronary Events Study Group. *N Eng J Med* 337(7):447–452, 1997.
31. Antman EM, McCabe CH, Gurfinkel EP, et al: Enoxaparin prevents death and cardiac ischemic events in unstable angina/non-Q-wave myocardial infarction. Results of the thrombolysis in myocardial infarction (TIMI) 11B trial. *Circulation* 100(15):1593–1601, 1999.
32. Petersen JL, Mahaffey KW, Hasselblad V, et al: Efficacy and bleeding complications among patients randomized to enoxaparin or unfractionated heparin for antithrombin therapy in non-ST-segment elevation acute coronary syndromes: a systematic overview. *JAMA* 292(1):89–96, 2004.
33. Ferguson JJ, Califf RM, Antman EM, et al: Exoxaparin vs. unfractionated heparin in high-risk patients with non-ST segment elevation acute coronary syndromes managed with an intended early invasive strategy: primary results of the SYNERGY randomized trial. *JAMA* 292(1):45–54, 2004.
34. Lincoff AM, Bittl JA, Harrington RA, et al: Bivalirudin and provisional glycoprotein IIb/IIIa blockade compared with heparin and planned glycoprotein IIb/IIIa blockade during percutaneous coronary intervention: REPLACE-2 randomized trial. *JAMA* 289:853–863, 2003.
35. Stone GW, McLaurin BT, Cox DA, et al: Bivalirudin for patients with acute coronary syndromes. *N Eng J Med* 355:2203–2216, 2006.
36. Yusuf S, Mehta SR, Chrolavicius S, et al: Comparison of fondaparinux and enoxaparin in acute coronary syndromes. *N Eng J Med* 354:1464–1476, 2006.
37. Topol EJ, Byzova TV, Plow EF: Platelet GPIIb-IIIa blockers. *Lancet* 353(9148):227–231, 1999.
38. Use of a monoclonal antibody directed against the platelet glycoprotein IIb/IIIa receptor in high-risk coronary angioplasty. The EPIC Investigation. *N Eng J Med* 330(14):956–961, 1994.
39. Randomised placebo-controlled trial of abciximab before and during coronary intervention in refractory unstable angina: the CAPTURE Study. *Lancet* 349(9063):1429–1435, 1997.
40. Simoons ML and the GUSTO IV-ACS Investigators: Effect of glycoprotein IIb/IIIa receptor blocker abciximab on outcome in patients with acute coronary syndromes without early coronary revascularization: the GUSTO IV-ACS randomized trial. *Lancet* 357(9272):1915–1924, 2001.
41. A comparison of aspirin plus tirofiban with aspirin plus heparin for unstable angina. Platelet Receptor Inhibition in Ischemic Syndrome management (PRISM) study investigators. *N Eng J Med* 338(21):1498–1505, 1998.
42. Inhibition of the platelet glycoprotein IIb/IIIa receptor with tirofiban in unstable angina and non-Q-wave myocardial infarction. Platelet Receptor Inhibition in Ischemic Syndrome Management in Patients Limited by Unstable Signs and Symptoms (PRISM-PLUS) study investigators. *N Eng J Med* 338(21):1488–1497, 1998.
43. Inhibition of platelet glycoprotein IIb/IIIa with eptifibatide in patients with acute coronary syndromes. The PURSUIT trial investigators. Platelet glycoprotein IIb/IIIa in unstable angina: receptor suppression using integrellin therapy. *N Eng J Med* 339(7):436–443, 1998.
44. Boersma E, Harrington RA, Moliterno DJ, et al: Platelet glycoprotein IIb/IIIa inhibitors in acute coronary syndromes: a meta-analysis of all major randomized clinical trials. *Lancet* 359 (9302)189–198, 2002.
45. Moliterno DJ, Yakubov SJ, DiBattiste PM, et al: for the TARGET investigators: Outcomes at 6 months for the direct comparison of tirofiban and abciximab during percutaneous coronary revascularisation with stent placement: the TARGET follow-up study. *Lancet* 360:355–360, 2002.
46. Giugliano RP, White JA, Bode C, et al: Early versus delayed, provisional eptifibatide in acute coronary syndromes. *N Eng J Med* 360:2176–2190, 2009.
47. Kastrati A, Mehilli J, Neumann FJ, et al, for the Intracoronary Stenting and Antithrombotic Regimen Rapid Early Action for Coronary Treatment 2 (ISAR-REACT 2) Trial Investigators: abciximab in patients with acute coronary syndromes undergoing percutaneous coronary intervention after clopidogrel pretreatment: the ISAR-REACT 2 randomized trial. *JAMA* 295:1531–1538, 2006.
48. Effects of tissue plasminogen activator and a comparison of early invasive and conservative strategies in unstable angina and non-Q-wave myocardial infarction. Results of the TIMI IIIB Trial. Thrombolysis in Myocardial Ischemia. *Circulation* 89:1545–1556, 1994.
49. Boden WE, O'Rourke RA, Crawford MH, et al: Outcomes in patients with acute non-Q-wave myocardial infarction randomly assigned to an invasive as compared with a conservative management strategy. Veterans Affairs Non-Q-Wave Infarction Strategies in Hospital (VANQWISH) trial investigators. *N Engl J Med* 338:1785–1792, 1998.
50. McCullough PA, O'Neill WW, Graham M, et al: A prospective randomized trial of triage angiography in acute coronary syndromes ineligible for thrombolytic therapy. Results of the medicine versus angiography in thrombolytic exclusion (MATE) trial. *J Am Coll Cardiol* 32:596–605, 1998.
51. Wallentin L, Lagerqvist B, Husted S, et al: Outcome at 1 year after an invasive compared with a non-invasive strategy in unstable coronary-artery disease: the FRISC II invasive randomised trial. FRISC II Investigators. Fast Revascularisation during Instability in Coronary artery disease. *Lancet* 356:9–16, 2000.
52. Cannon CP, Weintraub WS, Demopoulos LA, et al: Comparison of early invasive and conservative strategies in patients with unstable coronary syndromes treated with the glycoprotein IIb/IIIa inhibitor tirofiban. *N Engl J Med* 344:1879–1887, 2001.
53. Spacek R, Widimsky P, Straka Z, et al: Value of first day angiography/angioplasty in evolving Non-ST segment elevation myocardial infarction: an open multicenter randomized trial. The VINO Study. *Eur Heart J* 23:230–238, 2002.
54. Fox KA, Poole-Wilson PA, Henderson RA, et al: Randomized Intervention Trial of unstable Angina investigators. Interventional versus conservative treatment for patients with unstable angina or non-ST-elevation myocardial infarction: the British Heart Foundation RITA 3 randomised trial. Randomized Intervention Trial of unstable Angina. *Lancet* 360:743–751, 2002.
55. de Winter RJ, Windhausen F, Cornel JH, et al, for the Invasive versus Conservative Treatment in Unstable Coronary Syndromes (ICTUS) Investigators: Early invasive versus selectively invasive management for acute coronary syndromes. *N Engl J Med* 353:1095–1104, 2005.
56. Fox KA, Poole-Wilson P, Clayton TC, et al: 5-Year outcome of an interventional strategy in non-ST-elevation acute coronary syndrome: the British Heart Foundation RITA 3 randomised trial. *Lancet* 366:914–920, 2005.
57. Ryan JW, Peterson ED, Chen AY, et al, for the CRUSADE Investigators: Optimal timing of intervention in non-ST-segment elevation acute coronary syndromes: Insights from the CRUSADE (Can Rapid risk stratification of Unstable angina patients Suppress ADverse outcomes with Early implementation of the ACC/AHA guidelines) Registry. *Circulation* 112:3049–3057, 2005.
58. Neumann FJ, Kastrati A, Pogatsa-Murray G, et al: Evaluation of prolonged antithrombotic pretreatment ("cooling-off" strategy) before intervention in patients with unstable coronary syndromes: a randomized controlled trial. *JAMA* 290:1593–1599, 2003.
59. van't Hof AW, de Vries ST, Dambrink JH, et al: A comparison of two invasive strategies in patients with non-ST elevation acute coronary syndromes: Results of the Early or Late Intervention in unStable Angina (ELISA) pilot study: 2b/3a upstream therapy and acute coronary syndromes. *Eur Heart J* 24:1401–1405, 2003.
60. Bhatt DL, Roe MT, Peterson ED, et al: Utilization of early invasive management strategies for high-risk patients with non-ST-segment elevation acute coronary syndromes: Results from the CRUSADE Quality Improvement Initiative. *JAMA* 292:2096–2104, 2004.
61. Mehta SR, Granger CB, Boden WE, et al: Early versus delayed invasive intervention in acute coronary syndromes. *N Engl J Med* 360(21):2165–2175, 2009.
62. Riezebos RK, Ronner E, Ter Bals E, et al: Immediate versus deferred coronary angioplasty in non-ST-segment elevation acute coronary syndromes. *Heart* 95:807, 2009.
63. Montalescot G, Cayla G, Collet JP, et al: Immediate versus delayed intervention for acute coronary syndromes: a randomized clinical trial. *JAMA* 302:947, 2009.
64. Sabatine MS, Morrow DA, McCabe CH, et al: Combination of quantitative ST deviation and troponin elevation provides independent prognostic and therapeutic information in unstable angina and non-ST-elevation myocardial infarction. *Am Heart J* 151:25, 2006.
65. Mueller C, Neumann FJ, Roskamm H, et al: Women do have an improved long-term outcome after non-ST-elevation acute coronary syndromes treated very early and predominantly with percutaneous coronary intervention: a prospective study in 1,450 consecutive patients. *J Am Coll Cardiol* 40:245–250, 2002.

66. Morrison DA, Sethi G, Sacks J, et al: Percutaneous coronary intervention versus coronary artery bypass surgery for patients with medically refractory myocardial ischemia and risk factors for adverse outcomes with bypass: a multicenter, randomized trial. Investigators of the Department of Veterans Affairs Cooperative Study 385, the Angina With Extremely Serious Operative Mortality Evaluation (AWESOME). *J Am Coll Cardiol* 38:143, 2001.

67. Rodriguez A, Bernardi V, Navia J, et al: Argentine Randomized Study: Coronary Angioplasty with Stenting versus Coronary Bypass Surgery in patients with Multiple-Vessel Disease (ERACI II): 30-day and one year follow-up results. ERACI II investigators. *J Am Coll Cardiol* 37:51, 2001.

68. Morrison DA, Sethi G, Sacks J, et al: Percutaneous coronary intervention versus coronary artery bypass surgery for patients with medically refractory myocardial ischemia and risk factors for adverse outcomes with bypass: the VA AWESOME multicenter registry: comparison with the randomized control trial. *J Am Coll Cardiol* 39:266, 2002.

69. Rodriguez AE, Baldi J, Fernandez Pereira C, et al: Five-year follow-up of the Argentine randomized trial of coronary angioplasty with stenting versus coronary bypass surgery in patients with multiple vessel disease (ERACI II). *J Am Coll Cardiol* 46:582, 2005.

70. Shishehbor MH, Lauer MS, Singh IM, et al: In unstable angina or non-ST-segment acute coronary syndrome, should patients with multivessel coronary disease undergo multivessel or culprit-only stenting? *J Am Coll Cardiol* 49:849, 2007.

71. Morice MC, Serruys PW, Sousa JE, et al: A randomized comparison of a sirolimus-eluting stent with a standard stent for coronary revascularization. *N Engl J Med* 346:1773–1780, 2002.

72. Moses JW, Leon MB, Popma JJ, et al: Sirolimus-eluting stents versus standard stents in patients with stenosis in a native coronary artery. *N Engl J Med* 349:1315–1323, 2003.

73. Colombo A, Drzewiecki J, Banning A, et al: Randomized study to assess the effectiveness of slow- and moderate-release polymer-based paclitaxel-eluting stents for coronary artery lesions. *Circulation* 108:788–794, 2003.

74. Stone GW, Ellis SG, Cox DA, et al, for the TAXUS-IV Investigators: A polymer-based, paclitaxel-eluting stent in patients with coronary artery disease. *N Engl J Med* 350:221–231, 2004.

75. Lemos PA, Serruys PW, van Domburg RT, et al: Unrestricted utilization of sirolimus-eluting stents compared with conventional bare stent implantation in the "real world": The Rapamycin-Eluting Stent Evaluated At Rotterdam Cardiology Hospital (RESEARCH) registry. *Circulation* 109:190–195, 2004.

76. Kaiser C, Brunner-La Rocca HP, Buser PT, et al, for the BASKET investigators: Incremental cost-effectiveness of drug-eluting stents compared with a third-generation bare-metal stent in a real-world setting: Randomised Basel Stent Kosten Effektivitäts Trial (BASKET). *Lancet* 366:921–929, 2005.

77. Moses JW, Mehran R, Nikolsky E, et al: Outcomes with the paclitaxel-eluting stent in patients with acute coronary syndromes: analysis from the TAXUS-IV trial. *J Am Coll Cardiol* 45:1165, 2005.

78. Mauri L, Silbaugh TS, Garg P, et al: Drug-eluting or bare-metal stents for acute myocardial infarction. *N Engl J Med* 359:1330, 2008.

79. Schwartz GG, Olsson AG, Ezekowitz MD, et al, for the Myocardial Ischemia Reduction with Aggressive Cholesterol Lowering (MIRACL) Study Investigators: Effects of atorvastatin on early recurrent ischemic events in acute coronary syndromes: the MIRACL study: aA randomized controlled trial. *JAMA* 285:1711–1718, 2001.

80. Pravastatin or Atorvastatin Evaluation and Infection Therapy-Thrombolysis in Myocardial Infarction 22 investigators. Intensive versus moderate lipid lowering with statins after acute coronary syndromes. *N Engl J Med* 350:1495–1504, 2004.

81. Lescol Intervention Prevention Study (LIPS) Investigators: Fluvastatin for prevention of cardiac events following successful first percutaneous coronary intervention: A randomized controlled trial. *JAMA* 287:3215–3222, 2002.

82. Kushner FG, Hand M, Smith SC, Jr, et al: 2009 focused updates. ACC/AHA guidelines for the management of patients with ST-elevation myocardial infarction (updating the 2004 guideline and 2007 focused update) and ACC/AHA/SCAI guidelines on percutaneous coronary intervention (updating the 2005 guideline and 2007 focused update) a report of the American College of Cardiology Foundation/American Heart Association Task Force on Practice Guidelines. *J Am Coll Cardiol* 54:2205, 2009.

83. Silder S, Albertsson P, Aviles FF, et al: Guidelines for percutaneous coronary interventions. The Task Force for Percutaneous Coronary Interventions of the European Society of Cardiology. *Eur Heart J* 26:804, 2005.

18

Percutaneous Coronary Intervention in Acute ST Segment Elevation Myocardial Infarction

ALBERT SCHÖMIG | **GJIN NDREPEPA** | **ROBERT A. BYRNE** | **ADNAN KASTRATI**

KEY POINTS

- It is estimated that annually 1.25 million Americans experience an acute myocardial infarction (MI) and that ST segment elevation MI (STEMI) accounts for about 30% to 40% of acute MI.

- Catheter-based primary percutaneous coronary intervention (PCI) has become the mainstay of reperfusion therapy, supplanting thrombolytic therapy as reperfusion treatment in patients with STEMI in the United States and in Europe.

- PCI is superior to thrombolytic therapy in reducing death, re-infarction, intracranial bleeding, reocclusion of infarct-related artery and myocardial ischemia in patients with STEMI, irrespective of the patient's risk and whether or not interhospital transfer for PCI is required.

- PCI retains its myocardial salvaging capacity and ability to improve clinical outcome over a wider time window after symptom onset compared with thrombolysis and is the therapy of choice for patients presenting early or late after symptom onset.

- Primary stenting is the preferred primary PCI approach for patients with STEMI; drug-eluting stents (DESs) should be considered the preferred option. Although randomized trials and meta-analyses offer no firm evidence of the effect of DES on mortality (increase or reduction) or recurrent MI, they have demonstrated the clear superiority of DESs in anti–re-stenotic efficacy

- Use of thrombolysis for facilitated PCI as a strategy to promote reperfusion within the time interval from patient presentation to performance of PCI is associated with worse clinical outcome than PCI alone and is not recommended for STEMI patients.

- Available evidence supports the use of clopidogrel, prasugrel, and ticagrelor pre-treatment and glycoprotein (GP) IIb/IIIa receptor inhibitors in patients with STEMI undergoing primary PCI. Bivalirudin, a thrombin receptor blocker, has emerged as an effective and safe anti-thrombotic agent in patients with STEMI undergoing primary PCI and is associated with reduced incidence of bleeding complications and improved survival compared with unfractionated heparin.

- Rescue PCI salvages the ischemic myocardium and improves clinical outcome and thus is recommended in patients with STEMI after failed thrombolysis. In addition, there is evidence in support of routine use of PCI after successful thrombolysis in patients with STEMI.

- Available evidence supports the use of manual aspiration thrombectomy as an adjunctive mechanical strategy in the setting of primary PCI in the majority of patients with STEMI. Mechanical thrombectomy or distal protection devices do not improve the results over conventional PCI in STEMI patients and is not recommended on the basis of current evidence.

- The role of cell-based myocardial repair and regenerative agents in the management of patients with STEMI needs further investigation.

Acute myocardial infarction (MI) can be defined on the basis of a constellation of indices related to clinical, electrocardiographic, biochemical, and pathologic characteristics.[1] According to the most recent American Heart Association (AHA) Heart Disease and Stroke Statistics, it is estimated that annually 1.25 million Americans have an acute MI.[2] Acute MI results mostly from the acute thrombotic occlusion of an epicardial coronary artery, typically occurring as a consequence of atherosclerotic plaque disruption, fissuring, or erosion that leads to exposure of thrombogenic material (plaque lipid content, collagen, and subendothelial extracellular matrix) to circulating blood. Other causative factors of lesser importance include acute plaque expansion (such as that caused by intra-plaque hemorrhage leading to acute closure without or with minimal thrombus formation), embolism, spontaneous dissection, coronary inflammation, and extracoronary factors. In nearly three quarters of all infarct-related arteries, acute thrombosis appears to occur over atherosclerotic plaques causing mild to moderate coronary obstruction; that is, acute thrombotic closure compromises blood supply to an extensive myocardial area.[1] Interruption of coronary blood flow results in myocardial ischemia in the blood deprived myocardial area, which, if severe enough and of sufficient duration, results in myocardial necrosis. Acute ST segment elevation myocardial infarction (STEMI) represents the most malignant presentation of acute coronary syndromes resulting from acute thrombus-mediated closure of an infarct-related coronary artery. Although current evidence suggests that the incidence of STEMI is trending downward (Fig. 18-1) and the STEMI-related mortality has decreased, acute STEMI still represents a severe condition associated with worse short-term prognosis, compared with other less severe presentations of acute coronary syndromes (Fig. 18-2).[3,4] Apart from serving as the pathophysiologic basis for STEMI, acute coronary thrombosis forms the rationale for reperfusion therapy that aims at the prompt restoration of coronary blood flow, which results in myocardial salvage, increased electrical stability, and reduced incidence of fatal ventricular arrhythmias in the acute phase, preserved left ventricular function, and improved short-term and long-term patient survival. Abundant evidence in the past three decades bears witness to the life-saving effect of reperfusion therapy—primary percutaneous coronary intervention (PCI) or thrombolysis—in patients with STEMI. PCI achieves its most impressive life-saving effect in acute STEMI. The objective of this chapter is to summarize recent developments in the field of catheter-based reperfusion therapy for patients with acute STEMI.

Primary Percutaneous Coronary Intervention Versus Thrombolysis

Prompt restoration of coronary blood flow in the occluded coronary artery and the fastest possible myocardial tissue reperfusion form the fundamental principle of early STEMI therapy. Primary PCI refers to a strategy of emergent coronary angiography followed by coronary angioplasty with or without stenting of the infarct-related artery and without prior administration of thrombolytic therapy. In recent years,

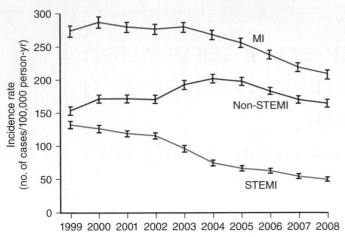

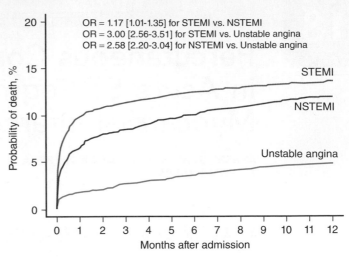

Figure 18-1 Age-adjusted and sex-adjusted incidence rates of acute myocardial infarction from 1999 to 2008. Bars represent 95% confidence intervals. *MI*, myocardial infarction; *STEMI*, ST segment elevation myocardial infarction. *(Yeh RW, Sidney S, Chandra M, Sorel M, Selby JV, Go AS: Population trends in the incidence and outcomes of acute myocardial infarction, N Engl J Med 362:2155–2165, 2010.)*

Figure 18-2 Kaplan-Meier curves of 1-year mortality among patients with acute ST segment elevation myocardial infarction (STEMI), non–ST segment elevation myocardial infarction (NSTEMI), and unstable angina. *(Ndrepepa G, Mehilli J, Schulz S, et al: Patterns of presentation and outcomes of patients with acute coronary syndromes, Cardiology 113:198–206, 2009.)*

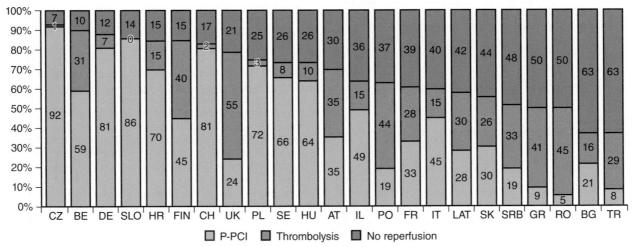

Figure 18-3 In-hospital treatment of acute ST segment elevation myocardial infarction (STEMI) in Europe (data from national registries or surveys). Countries abbreviations: *CZ*, Czech Republic; *SLO*, Slovenia; *DE*, Germany; *CH*, Switzerland; *PL*, Poland; *HR*, Croatia; *SE*, Sweden; *HU*, Hungary; *BE*, Belgium; *IL*, Israel; *IT*, Italy; *FIN*, Finland; *AT*, Austria; *FR*, France; *SK*, Slovakia; *LAT*, Latvia; *UK*, United Kingdom; *BG*, Bulgaria; *PO*, Portugal; *SRB*, Serbia; *GR*, Greece; *TR*, Turkey; *RO*, Romania. *(Widimsky P, Wijns W, Fajadet J, et al: Reperfusion therapy for ST elevation acute myocardial infarction in Europe: Description of the current situation in 30 countries, Eur Heart J 31:943–957, 2010.)*

mechanical reperfusion has become the mainstay reperfusion therapy in patients with STEMI. Current evidence shows that primary PCI has become the dominant reperfusion strategy in patients with STEMI in North America and Europe (Fig. 18-3).[5,6] Multiple lines of evidence from randomized studies reported in recent years firmly suggest that catheter-based mechanical reperfusion in patients with STEMI is superior to pharmacologic thrombolytic therapy in terms of improving of early and late survival as well as in reducing the incidence of re-infarction, intracranial bleeding, reocclusion of the infarct-related artery, and recurrent myocardial ischemia.[7] Primary PCI is expected to become the "dominant default strategy" for prompt early reperfusion in patients with STEMI if growth and diffusion of resource and logistical factors enable its broader application. Several factors may explain the superiority of primary PCI over thrombolysis. Although thrombolytic therapy has been proven to be life saving, it has serious limitations related to high proportions of patients with relative or

absolute contraindications to this therapy; life-threatening bleeding complications disproportionately affecting older patients; a narrow window of therapeutic action after symptom onset because of rapid time-dependent loss of efficacy; limited ability to restore normal blood flow in the infarct-related artery, even if applied in timely fashion; and frequent reocclusions of the infarct-related artery resulting in re-infarction within subsequent months. Apart from being free of these limitations, primary PCI has other advantages over thrombolytic therapy such as restoration of significantly higher rates of thrombolysis in myocardial infarction (TIMI) flow grade 3 in the infarct-related artery (a finding which is both durable because of enhanced stability of the reopened vessel and relatively independent of time from symptom onset) (Fig. 18-4), greater amount of salvaged myocardium, delineation of coronary anatomy and hemodynamic status resulting in risk stratification, and facilitation of patient care and earlier hospital discharge.[8] Lack of availability of care centers equipped to offer timely

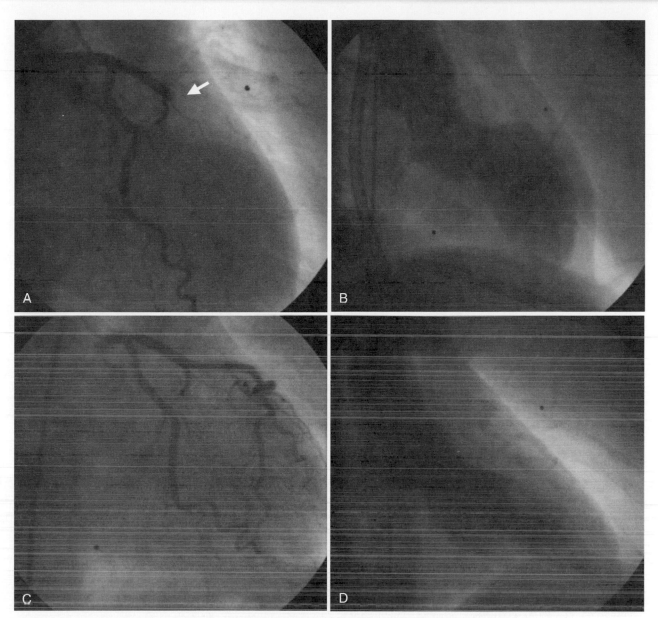

Figure 18-4   Left coronary artery angiography and left ventricular angiogram in the right anterior oblique (RAO) view in a 49-year-old male patient with acute anterior ST segment elevation myocardial infarction (STEMI). **A,** Complete thrombotic occlusion (*white arrow*) of the left anterior descending coronary artery before coronary stenting. **B,** Left ventricular angiogram before coronary stenting. End-systolic frame of the left ventricular angiogram shows an extensive zone of akinesia in the anterior wall. **C,** Left coronary artery angiogram performed 6 months after successful stenting. **D,** End-systolic frame of the left ventricular angiogram performed 6 months after stenting shows a marked regional improvement in the left ventricular function.

catheter-based invasive treatment to patients with STEMI, rather than issues pertaining to clinical effectiveness, is currently perceived as the most important factor that impedes a broader application of this treatment to patients with STEMI. Recent American College of Cardiology/American Heart Association/European Society of Cardiology guidelines define primary PCI as a class I indication (level of evidence: A) in patients with STEMI (including true posterior MI and MI with new or presumably new left bundle branch block [LBBB]) presenting to a hospital with PCI capability if performed within 90 minutes of the first medical contact.[1,9,10] A class I indication (level of evidence: B) is recommended for patients with cardiogenic shock and contraindications to fibrinolytic therapy, irrespective of amount of delay.[1] Numerous additional lines of evidence further establish the superiority of primary PCI over thrombolysis. Primary PCI improves survival even in patients with STEMI who have contraindications to thrombolytic

therapy or in patients presenting outside the therapeutic window of thrombolysis.[11-13] Available evidence suggests that primary PCI is superior to thrombolysis in all studied time intervals. A recent report from the Primary Coronary Angioplasty versus Thrombolysis (PCAT)-2 Trialists' Collaborative Group demonstrated that primary PCI was associated with a 67% reduction in 30-day mortality compared with thrombolysis, which, in absolute terms, translates into 53 lives saved per 1000 patients treated. For PCI-related delays up to 120 minutes, primary PCI was associated with a 26% reduction in mortality compared with thrombolysis or in 19 lives saved per 1000 patients treated (Fig. 18-5).[14] The absolute reduction in mortality with primary PCI widened over time from 1.3% within the first hour to 4.2% after more than 6 hours after symptom onset.[14] The superiority of primary PCI over thrombolysis has been observed particularly in high-risk patients and in centers without on-site cardiac surgery.[15,16] The DANish trial in

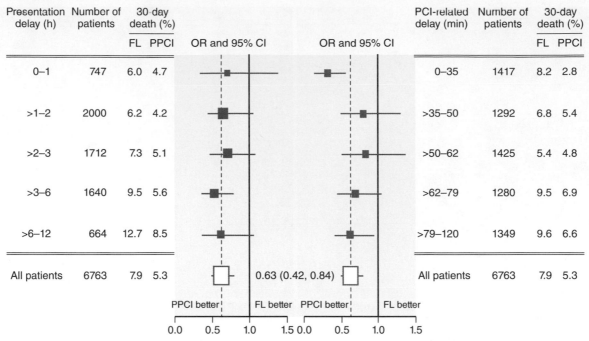

Presentation delay (h)	Number of patients	30-day death (%) FL	30-day death (%) PPCI	OR and 95% CI	OR and 95% CI	PCI-related delay (min)	Number of patients	30-day death (%) FL	30-day death (%) PPCI
0–1	747	6.0	4.7			0–35	1417	8.2	2.8
>1–2	2000	6.2	4.2			>35–50	1292	6.8	5.4
>2–3	1712	7.3	5.1			>50–62	1425	5.4	4.8
>3–6	1640	9.5	5.6			>62–79	1280	9.5	6.9
>6–12	664	12.7	8.5			>79–120	1349	9.6	6.6
All patients	6763	7.9	5.3	0.63 (0.42, 0.84)		All patients	6763	7.9	5.3

Figure 18-5 Thirty-day deaths in patients randomized to primary percutaneous coronary intervention (PPCI) or fibrinolysis (FL). *Left panel:* Thirty-day deaths with odds ratio (OR) and 95% confidence intervals (CI) according to presentation delay. *Right Panel:* Thirty-day deaths with OR and 95% CI according to PCI-related delay. *(Boersma E; Primary Coronary Angioplasty vs. Thrombolysis Group: Does time matter? A pooled analysis of randomized clinical trials comparing primary percutaneous coronary intervention and in-hospital fibrinolysis in acute myocardial infarction patients,* Eur Heart J *27:779–788, 2006.)*

Acute Myocardial Infarction-2 (DANAMI-2) demonstrated that the benefit of PCI is largest in high-risk patients: In patients with TIMI risk scores 5 or greater, there was a significant reduction in the mortality with primary PCI (25.3% vs. 36.2% with thrombolysis; $P = 0.02$), which was not observed in the low-risk group (TIMI risk score 0 to 4).[15] The benefit of primary PCI over thrombolysis was maintained at long-term follow-up. A further report from DANAMI-2 showed that the 8-year composite of death or re-infarction was 34.8% in patients treated with primary PCI versus 41.3% in patients treated with thrombolysis ($P = 0.003$). Of note, primary PCI reduced the risk of re-infarction (13% vs. 18.5%) and mortality (26.7% vs. 33.3%) among patients randomized at referral hospitals.[17] The study reinforced the recommendation that primary PCI should be offered to STEMI patients if transport to invasive care centers can be completed within 120 minutes. A recent meta-analysis of 23 randomized and 32 observational studies reported significant improvement in mortality, stroke, and re-infarction with the use of primary PCI compared with thrombolysis.[18] Current evidence also points out the cost-effectiveness of primary PCI compared with thrombolysis.[19] There is evidence that the use of thrombolytic agents as a reperfusion strategy in patients with STEMI has markedly decreased. Recently, the Global Registry of Acute Coronary Events (GRACE) enrolled, between April 1999 and June 2006,10,954 patients with STEMI or LBBB, who presented within 12 hours of symptom onset; the report from this study documented that the use of primary PCI increased from 15% to 44% and the use of thrombolytic agents decreased from 41% to 16% as reperfusion strategy (Fig. 18-6).[20] At present, it seems that the era of comparative studies between mechanical reperfusion (primary angioplasty or stenting) and pharmacologic thrombolytic therapy is over and the superiority of primary PCI over thrombolysis is almost unanimously accepted. In aggregate, these studies demonstrated that primary PCI is superior to thrombolysis and should be the preferred strategy of reperfusion in patients with STEMI in all clinical situations and patient subsets. However, because the majority of hospitals do not have PCI capability, physicians and hospitals are faced with the challenge of providing

timely primary PCI to patients with STEMI.[21] Recognizing the importance of the problem, several regions in the United States have proposed or established triage and transfer protocols to direct patients with STEMI to hospitals with PCI capability without any delay.[22,23] A series of prehospital timing benchmarks have been proposed, the achievement of which is associated with favorable system performance, that is, achieving an interval from first medical contact to PCI of 90 minutes or less.[24] Available evidence demonstrates significant improvements in the timely provision of reperfusion therapy to patients with STEMI, the safety and efficacy of primary PCI procedures, and the overall management of patients with acute MI.[25]

Time-to-Treatment Interval and Outcome

Time-to-treatment interval is an estimate of overall duration of myocardial ischemia that encompasses the period from the onset of symptoms of coronary occlusion to the initiation of reperfusion therapy—thrombolysis or primary PCI. The time-to-treatment interval has two components: (1) the time from symptom onset to patient arrival at the hospital and (2) the time from patient arrival to the initiation of reperfusion therapy. Apart from disclosing the duration of myocardial ischemia, time-to-treatment interval is an index of the quality and readiness of the health care system to provide reperfusion therapy in timely fashion. Knowledge of the biology of myocardial ischemia and the speed with which it leads to necrosis is important to any understanding of the time-dependent efficacy related to reperfusion regimens and the degree of the benefit of reperfusion therapy in general. Abrupt coronary occlusion results in the drastic reduction of coronary blood flow and in myocardial necrosis that progresses gradually and is typically complete in about 6 hours after the onset of occlusion. A rapid phase of cell death, mostly in the subendocardial region, follows the coronary occlusion; about half the ischemic myocardium that is necrotic at 24 hours has already died at 40 minutes after

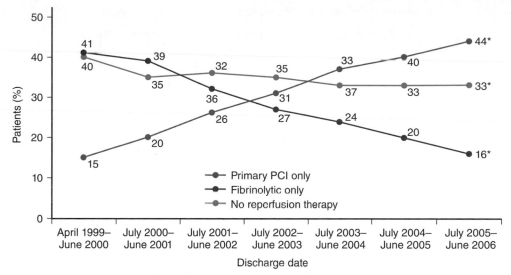

Figure 18-6   Trends in the use of reperfusion therapy in patients with acute myocardial infarction from 1999 to 2006. (*Eagle KA, Nallamothu BK, Mehta RH, et al: Trends in acute reperfusion therapy for ST-segment elevation myocardial infarction from 1999 to 2006: We are getting better but we have got a long way to go, Eur Heart J 29:609–617, 2008.*)

coronary occlusion.[26] A second phase of cell death occurs more slowly in the mid-epicardial myocardium and the subepicardial myocardium. This phase of myocardial necrosis is complete within 6 hours of coronary occlusion and about one third of ischemic myocardium is salvageable at 3 hours.[26]

There are, however, considerable differences between coronary occlusion and acute MI in the experimental setting and spontaneously occurring coronary occlusion and STEMI in the clinical setting. Factors such as the often stuttering course of coronary occlusion, spontaneous recanalization, and persistence of anterograde blood flow in the infarct-related artery, collateral circulation, preconditioning, postconditioning, metabolic need at the time of coronary occlusion, and the effects of initial anti-ischemic (anti-thrombotic) therapy may modify the time-course of the progression of myocardial ischemia to necrosis and may extend the time during which the ischemic myocardium remains viable. Scintigraphic studies have identified viable myocardium in patients with STEMI presenting late (>6 hours) after symptom onset; this viable myocardium appears salvageable if PCI is used as a reperfusion strategy. These studies suggest the existence of two phases of myocardial salvage as well: (1) an early phase of myocardial salvage enabled by early reperfusion (ideally within the first hour) and (2) a late phase of myocardial salvage enabled by later reperfusion. During the early phase, reperfusion is associated with substantial and time-dependent myocardial salvage. However, reperfusion therapy within the first hour following coronary occlusion, which is expected to lead to large amounts of myocardial salvage and the best clinical outcome, is achievable in a very limited number of patients. A prior study has shown that the time-to-treatment interval was less than 2 hours in only 27% of the patients and less than 1 hour in only 3.2%.[27] Reperfusion in the second (later) phase results in a lesser degree of and less time-dependent myocardial salvage. Analysis of the time-to-treatment interval in various studies suggests that most patients are reperfused beyond the golden hour of reperfusion, that is, in the late phase of myocardial salvage, in which a slower progression of the ischemic myocardium to necrosis occurs because of the presence of residual blood flow, collaterals, or other factors that widen the window of myocardial salvage. Nevertheless, these data do not mean that myocardial salvage by primary PCI is not time dependent. They merely indicate that the time window for myocardial salvage is wider with primary PCI than with thrombolysis (Fig. 18-7). Time from onset of symptoms to initiation of reperfusion is an important predictor of myocardial salvage and clinical outcome, whether reperfusion is achieved with thrombolysis

or primary PCI. However, the dependence of myocardial salvage or clinical outcome on the time to-treatment interval in patients with STEMI undergoing PCI still remains controversial. Scintigraphic studies provide valuable information on infarct size and allow assessment of the efficacy of reperfusion in terms of myocardial salvage with a high prognostic value (Fig. 18-8). The BRAVE-2 (Beyond 12 hours Reperfusion AlternatiVe Evaluation) trial demonstrated the potential of primary PCI to salvage the myocardium and reduce the infarct size even in patients with STEMI presenting 12 to 48 hours from symptom onset. The median infarct size was 8% in patients with STEMI who were assigned to primary PCI versus 13% in patients assigned to conservative treatment (*P* < 0.001).[13] A recent update from the BRAVE-2 trial demonstrated a mortality benefit for up to 4 years in patients assigned to invasive treatment (11.1% in patients assigned to invasive treatment vs. 18.9% in patients assigned to conservative therapy; *P* = 0.047; Fig. 18-9).[28] Another recent study involving 396 patients with STEMI demonstrated that late comers (presenting >12 hours from symptom onset) had larger infarct size (14% vs. 7%; *P* = 0.005), lower proportion of initial area at risk salvaged (53% vs. 69%; *P* = 0.05) and lower left ventricular ejection fraction (LVEF; 44% vs. 57%; *P* = 0.04) compared with patients presenting within the first 12 hours from symptom onset. Of note, this study showed that substantial myocardial salvage (more than 50% of initial area at risk) occurred in 41% of late presenters.[29] Together, these studies demonstrated that in patients with STEMI presenting more than 12 hours from symptom onset, a substantial amount of myocardial salvage occurs when primary PCI is used as the reperfusion strategy. A recent meta-analysis of 10 randomized trials (including the Occluded Artery Trial [OAT]) with 3560 patients with acute MI presenting between 12 hours to 60 days after symptom onset demonstrated significant reduction in long-term mortality (6.3% vs. 8.4%, Fig. 18-10). Eight of these 10 studies showed improvements in long-term survival. There was a greater improvement in LVEF over time in patients who received invasive treatment (+4.4% change in LVEF) compared with patients who received medical therapy.[12] With regard to the impact of the time-to-treatment interval on clinical outcome, clinical studies have produced conflicting results. A progressive increase in 1-year mortality with every 15-minute increase in the symptom onset-to-balloon time has been recently reported.[30] Conversely, data from the National Registry for Myocardial Infarction (NRMI) showed no association between symptom onset-to-balloon time and survival in a cohort of 27,080 consecutive patients with acute MI treated with primary angioplasty.[31] Similarly, an analysis

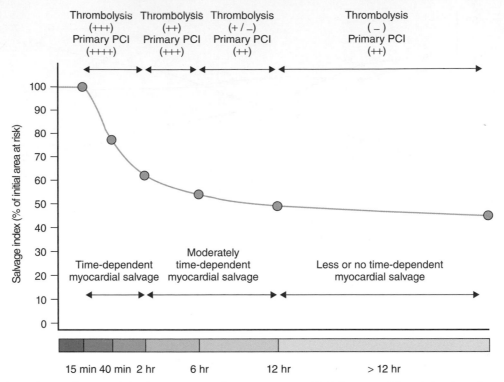

Figure 18-7 Time dependency of myocardial salvage expressed as percentage of initial area at risk and the time dependency of efficacy of thrombolysis or primary percutaneous coronary intervention (PCI). The initial parts of the curve up to 2 hours were reconstructed on the basis of experimental studies. For the first 15 minutes (*15 m*) after coronary occlusion, myocardial necrosis is not observed. At 40 minutes (*40 m*) after coronary occlusion, myocardial cell death develops rapidly, and the myocardial necrosis is confluent. After this point, progression to necrosis is slowed considerably. The other part of the curve showing myocardial salvage from 2 to more than 12 hours from symptom onset is reconstructed on the basis of data from scintigraphic studies in patients with acute myocardial infarction. Efficacy of reperfusion is expressed as follows: (++++) very effective; (+++), effective; (++), moderately effective; (±), uncertainly effective; (−), not effective. *(Reprinted with permission from Schömig A, Ndrepepa G, Kastrati A: Late myocardial salvage: time to recognize its reality in the reperfusion therapy of acute myocardial infarction, Eur Heart J 27:1900–1907, 2006.)*

of 2635 patients enrolled in 10 randomized trials of primary angioplasty versus thrombolytic therapy demonstrated that with increasing time-to-presentation interval, major adverse cardiac event rates increased after thrombolysis but remained relatively stable after angioplasty.[32] A recent publication of the DANAMI-2 trial, involving only the primary PCI substudy showed that 3-year mortality did not differ among patients with symptom onset-to-balloon times greater than 3 hours and 3 to 5 hours.[33] However, the mortality rate was significantly higher in patients presenting 5 hours or later from symptom onset (hazard ratio [HR] 2.36; *P* < 0.001), and the difference in mortality rates remained significant after adjustment for potential confounders. A shorter symptom onset-to-balloon interval was associated with greater rates of TIMI flow grade of 3 after primary PCI and with lower proportions of patients with a LVEF of 40% or less.

Knowledge of the risk distribution alongside the time-to-treatment interval is of importance in understanding the time-dependent efficacy of primary PCI in patients with STEMI. Prior studies have shown that patients presenting early after symptom onset have the highest risk score, which is consistent with the observation that early presenters have the largest cumulated ST-segment elevation, reflecting the largest initial areas at risk and prompting urgent seeking of medical aid.[34,35] This group of patients with STEMI benefit mostly from primary PCI in terms of myocardial salvage, preservation of ventricular function, and survival because of early intervention and the characteristics of the ischemic lesion. Patients who present later after symptom onset may have a smaller initial area at risk producing milder symptoms, and their outcome may be influenced by the survivor–cohort effect; that is, they have already survived the highest risk of death in the early hours after coronary occlusion. Late

presenters may have also a more adverse cardiovascular risk profile. Prior reports show that patients who presented later were older, more often women and diabetic, and had a past history of coronary bypass surgery. Adjusting for these factors considerably attenuates the association between the time-to-treatment interval and mortality (from highly significant in univariable analysis to a borderline significance after adjustment in multivariable model).[30] Patients with a greater delay in admission are also expected to present more frequently with additional adverse characteristics such as impaired renal function, peripheral arterial disease, and greater inflammatory burden—factors not accounted for in the multivariate model. The lack of adjustment for these characteristics further widens the gap between statistical and biologic adjustments with regard to prognosis. Associated comorbidities and the less favorable cardiovascular risk profile may mask the benefits of mechanical reperfusion from myocardial salvage, and the unfavorable outcome after coronary intervention may erroneously be attributed solely to the longer time-to-reperfusion interval. Therefore, it is highly probable that a more adverse baseline risk profile of patients with longer delay to presentation may explain, at least in part, the apparent association between the time-to-treatment interval and mortality. These considerations are important because the apparent reduction of benefit from PCI with increased time to presentation may be interpreted as a poor incentive for prompt intervention in patients with delayed presentation who are badly in need of this treatment.

Although the superiority of primary PCI over thrombolysis for longer time-to-presentation intervals is undeniable, whether primary PCI is superior to thrombolysis when applied early after symptom onset (within 2 hours) is still debated. Most of this controversy was generated after the publication of a subset analysis from the

Before 10 days after
intervention intervention

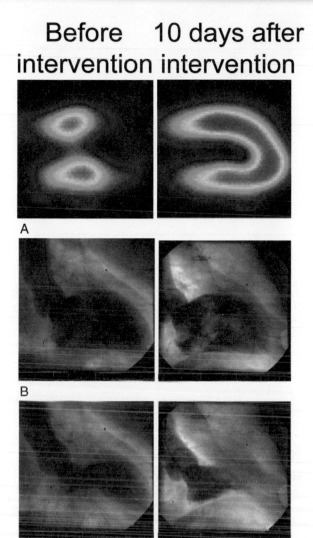

Figure 18-8 Scintigraphic and left ventricular (LV) angiographic images in a 69-year-old patient with acute myocardial infarction treated with coronary artery stenting 16 hours after symptom onset. **A,** Vertical long-axis view of 99m technetium sestamibi scintigraphy **B,** End-diastolic frame of left ventricular angiography in 30-degree right-anterior oblique view. **C,** End systolic frame of left ventricular angiography in 30-degree right-anterior oblique view. *(Kastrati A, Mehilli J, Nekolla S, et al: A randomized trial comparing myocardial salvage achieved by coronary stenting versus balloon angioplasty in patients with acute myocardial infarction considered ineligible for reperfusion therapy, J Am Coll Cardiol 43:734–741, 2004.)*

Comparison of Angioplasty and Prehospital Thrombolysis In acute Myocardial infarction (CAPTIM) trial involving 460 patients; this trial demonstrated that patients with STEMI randomized less than 2 hours after symptom onset had a trend toward lower 30-day mortality with thrombolysis compared with primary PCI (2.2% vs. 5.7%, $P = 0.058$).[36] The reliability of these results is strongly compromised by the fact that they were produced by a subset analysis of a prematurely terminated trial. In fact, a recent meta-analysis by the Primary Coronary Angioplasty versus Thrombolysis (PCAT)-2 Trialists' Collaborative Group based on individual patient data has demonstrated that primary PCI is superior to thrombolysis in terms of reduction of the 30-day mortality even for a presentation delay of less than 2 hours as was the case for 2747 patients (4.3% with PCI vs. 6.2% with thrombolysis, $P = 0.03$).[14] The RISK-HIA (Register of Information and Knowledge about Swedish Heart Intensive Care Admissions) included 26,205 patients

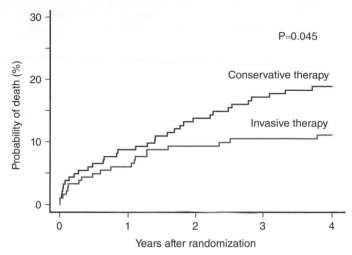

Figure 18-9 Kaplan-Meier curves of 4-year mortality in the invasive and conservative therapy groups of the Beyond 12 hours Reperfusion Alternative Evaluation (BRAVE-2) trial. *(Ndrepepa G, Kastrati A, Mehilli J, Antoniucci D, Schömig A: Mechanical reperfusion and long-term mortality in patients with acute myocardial infarction presenting 12 to 48 hours from onset of symptoms, JAMA 301:487–488, 2009.)*

with STEMI, who received reperfusion therapy within 15 hours of symptom onset. Primary PCI was superior to prehospital thrombolysis or in-hospital thrombolysis with regard to 30-day mortality (mortality rates: 4.9%, 7.6%, and 11.4% respectively) or 1-year mortality (mortality rates: 7.6%, 10.3%, and 15.9%, respectively).[37] Primary PCI was also associated with shorter hospital stay and less re-infarction. Moreover, for treatment delays greater than 2 hours, mortality reductions with prehospital thrombolysis tended to decrease, whereas the benefits with primary PCI persisted, regardless of the amount of delay.[37] On the basis of these data, as well as the negative findings of the studies on early thrombolysis in the settings of the facilitated PCI strategy despite earlier restoration of flow in a considerable number of patients (see section on Facilitated PCI), it is unlikely that the occasionally propagated therapy of prehospital (in-ambulance) thrombolysis will be able to compete with a primary PCI strategy. In addition, prehospital thrombolysis carries the risk of exposing a sizeable proportion of misdiagnosed patients to the hazards of thrombolysis. Therefore, as long as no specifically designed studies have provided evidence in support of prehospital thrombolysis over routine PCI in patients calling for medical assistance within 2 to 3 hours from symptom onset, the application of prehospital thrombolysis strategy should be discouraged.

Recent studies have demonstrated the existence of an association between door-to-balloon interval and survival in patients with STEMI. A report from the National Registry of Myocardial Infarction (NRMI) data, which included a cohort of 29,222 patients with STEMI treated with PCI within 6 hours of presentation, longer door-to-balloon intervals were associated with increased in-hospital mortality.[38] In-hospital mortality was 3%, 4.2%, 5.7%, and 7.4% for door-to-balloon intervals of 90 minutes or less, 91 to 120 minutes, 121 to 150 minutes, and more than 150 minutes, respectively ($P < 0.001$).[38] In a report based on the Danish medical registries of patients with STEMI ($N = 6209$ patients undergoing primary PCI within 12 hours from symptom onset) showed an association and dependence of long-term (median 3.4 years) mortality on the time-to-treatment interval. Thus, for delays 0 to 60 minutes, 61 to 120 minutes, 121 to 180 minutes, and 181 to 360 minutes, long-term mortality was 15.4%, 23.3%, 28.1%, and 30.8%, respectively.[39] In a recent report from the National Cardiovascular Data Registry, which included 43,801 patients with STEMI, median door-to-balloon time was 93 minutes with 57.9% of patients treated within 90 minutes. Longer door-to-balloon times were associated with a higher adjusted risk of in-hospital mortality, which increased in a

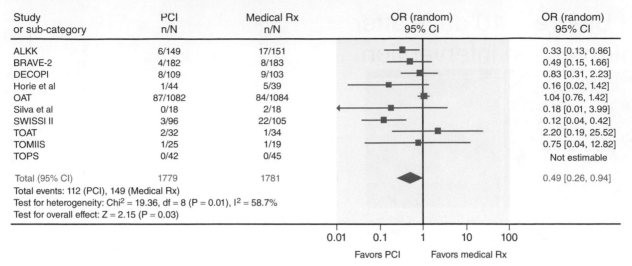

Study or sub-category	PCI n/N	Medical Rx n/N	OR (random) 95% CI	OR (random) 95% CI
ALKK	6/149	17/151		0.33 [0.13, 0.86]
BRAVE-2	4/182	8/183		0.49 [0.15, 1.66]
DECOPI	8/109	9/103		0.83 [0.31, 2.23]
Horie et al	1/44	5/39		0.16 [0.02, 1.42]
OAT	87/1082	84/1084		1.04 [0.76, 1.42]
Silva et al	0/18	2/18		0.18 [0.01, 3.99]
SWISSI II	3/96	22/105		0.12 [0.04, 0.42]
TOAT	2/32	1/34		2.20 [0.19, 25.52]
TOMIIS	1/25	1/19		0.75 [0.04, 12.82]
TOPS	0/42	0/45		Not estimable
Total (95% CI)	**1779**	**1781**		**0.49 [0.26, 0.94]**

Total events: 112 (PCI), 149 (Medical Rx)
Test for heterogeneity: Chi² = 19.36, df = 8 (P = 0.01), I² = 58.7%
Test for overall effect: Z = 2.15 (P = 0.03)

```
0.01    0.1     1     10    100
   Favors PCI    Favors medical Rx
```

Figure 18-10 Individual and pooled risk of death (odds ratios [OR]) with confidence intervals [CI]) comparing late percutaneous coronary intervention (PCI) versus best medical therapy (Rx) only for infarct-related artery occlusion late (>12 h) in the course of acute myocardial infarction. *ALKK, Arbeitsgemeinschaft Leitende Kardiologische Krankenhausärzte; BRAVE-2, Beyond 12 Hours Reperfusion Alternative Evaluation Trial; DEPOCI, Randomized Trial of Occluded Artery Angioplasty After Acute Myocardial Infarction; OAT, Occluded Artery Trial; SWISSI II, Swiss Interventional Study on Silent Ischemia Type II; TOAT, The Occluded Artery Trial; TOMIIS, Total Occlusion Post-Myocardial Infarction Intervention Study; TOPS, Treatment of Post-thrombolytic Stenoses. (Abbate A, Biondi-Zoccai GG, Appleton DL, et al: Survival and cardiac remodeling benefits in patients undergoing late percutaneous coronary intervention of the infarct-related artery: Evidence from a meta-analysis of randomized controlled trials, J Am Coll Cardiol 51:956–964, 2008.)*

continuous nonlinear fashion (door-to-balloon 30 minutes, mortality 3%; 60 minutes, 3.5%; 90 minutes, 4.3%; 120 minutes, 5.6%; 150 minutes 7%; 180 minutes 8.4%; P < 0.001).[40] It appears that both a high-risk profile and a shorter presentation delay may accentuate this association.[41] Despite these data, door-to-treatment times have not decreased significantly in recent years, so greater efforts should be made to improve this parameter.[38] Door-to-balloon time is an important indicator of patient characteristics and of the experience of the institution providing the primary PCI.[35,42] Comorbid conditions, absence of chest pain, delayed presentation after symptom onset, less specific ECG findings, and hospital presentation during off-hours were associated with longer total door-to-balloon times.[35] Longer door-to-balloon times were also encountered in patients with older age, female gender, nonwhite race, and complex medical histories.[43] Door-to-balloon delay also depended heavily on hospital-related characteristics. Thus, presentation at night and treatment at lower-volume facilities were strong independent predictors of longer door-to-balloon interval.[43,44] Greater experience with primary PCI is associated with shorter door-to-balloon times and lower in-hospital mortality in patients with STEMI treated with primary PCI.[42] Notably, primary PCI was found to be superior to thrombolysis irrespective of the door-to-balloon time that the treating institution was able to achieve.[14] A further study demonstrated that a combination of shorter door-to-balloon time (<90 min) with a shorter symptom onset-to-door time (<4 hr) was associated with lowest longer term mortality.[45] Other studies have also demonstrated that short door-to-balloon times (≤90 min) are associated with lower mortality in early presenters but not in late presenters.[46]

In summary, PCI is an efficacious reperfusion treatment option for patients presenting early or late after onset of symptoms. In a clinical scenario in which both reperfusion therapies—thrombolysis and primary PCI—are readily available and can be rapidly applied, current evidence from randomized trials, registries, and meta-analyses strongly support the use of primary PCI as the reperfusion strategy of choice. Even in patients presenting within 1 hour from symptom onset, there is no convincing reason to consider fibrinolysis in preference to primary PCI. Even though the efficacy of primary PCI is reduced over longer time-to-treatment intervals, late comers still benefit from primary PCI in terms of myocardial salvage and clinical outcome. Despite the undeniable importance of prehospital care for the successful management of patients with STEMI, available evidence does not support the routine use of prehospital thrombolysis.

Interhospital Transfer for Primary Percutaneous Coronary Intervention

Two factors—the lack of PCI facilities in the majority of hospitals that receive patients with STEMI and the proven superiority of primary PCI over thrombolysis—have led to the concept of emergency interhospital transfer for primary PCI instead of initial thrombolysis in the presenting hospital in patients with STEMI. Earlier randomized trials of on-site thrombolysis versus interhospital transfer plus PCI performed in the last 10 years or so have confirmed that transfer of patients for primary PCI is a better strategy than thrombolysis at the initial hospital. The results of these trials have been summarized in 2 meta-analyses. The first meta-analysis of six randomized trials performed before 2003, which included 3750 patients, showed that a strategy of patient transfer plus primary PCI was associated with a 42% reduction in the 30-day incidence of the combined endpoint of death, re-infarction, and stroke compared with a strategy of on-site thrombolysis.[47] When the components of primary endpoints were considered separately, the strategy of transfer plus primary PCI was associated with a 68% reduction in re-infarction (P < 0.001), 56% reduction in stroke (P = 0.015), and 19% reduction in mortality (P = 0.08). Other quantitative reviews of studies that have involved patient transfer for PCI have suggested that for every 100 patients treated, primary PCI after interhospital transfer instead of on-site thrombolysis prevented 7 major adverse cardiac events defined as death, nonfatal re-infarction, or nonfatal stroke.[48] Evidence suggests that patient transfer for PCI is also beneficial in patients with acute MI who receive full-dose thrombolytic therapy in a community hospital. In the Streptokinase In Acute Myocardial Infarction (SIAM-III) trial, patients presenting within 12 hours of acute MI were randomized to receive immediate stenting within 6 hours (n = 82) or delayed stenting at 2 weeks (n = 81) after full-dose reteplase. Immediate stenting was associated with a significant reduction of the combined endpoint (death, re-infarction, ischemic events, and target vessel revascularization) at 6 months (25.6% vs. 50.6%, P = 0.001).[49] In keeping with this, recent studies provided further evidence of the benefits of transfer of patients for primary PCI

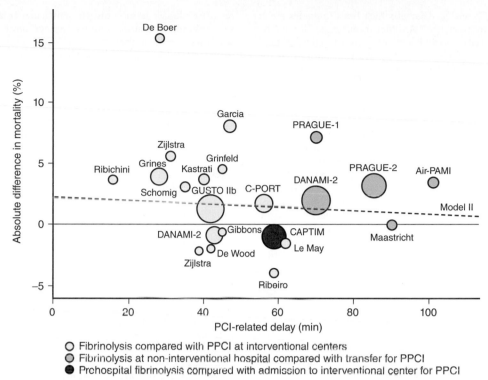

Figure 18-11 Absolute risk reduction in short-term mortality rate achieved by primary percutaneous coronary intervention (PPCI) according to PCI-related delay (extra delay used to perform PPCI instead of initiating fibrinolysis) in various studies. *(Terkelsen CJ, Christiansen EH, Sørensen JT, et al: Primary PCI as the preferred reperfusion therapy in STEMI: it is a matter of time, Heart 95:362–369, 2009.)*

compared with on-site thrombolysis. A recent study randomized 401 patients presenting to community hospitals to a strategy of on-site thrombolysis or to intravenous tirofiban and transport for primary PCI. The delay to reperfusion, defined as the interval from admission to start of thrombolysis or primary PCI, was 35 and 145 minutes, respectively, for the on-site thrombolysis and transport for PCI. The composite endpoint of death, re-infarction, or stroke was lower among patients assigned to the transport for primary PCI strategy at 30 days (0% vs. 15.5%, P = 0.019) and 1 year (11.4% vs. 21.5%, P = 0.006).[50] A recent report of 850 patients with STEMI enrolled in the PRimary Angioplasty in patients transferred from General community hospitals to specialized PTCA Units with or without Emergency thrombolysis (PRAGUE)-2 trial showed that the 5-year composite endpoint of death, re-infarction, stroke, or revascularization was 40% in patients assigned to a strategy of transfer for primary PCI versus 53% in patients assigned to on-site thrombolysis in the presenting hospital (P < 0.001).[51] A large registry that included 16,043 patients with STEMI who were treated with in-hospital thrombolysis, 3078 treated with pre-hospital thrombolysis, and 7084 patients treated with primary PCI, indicated that transfer for PCI is better than prehospital thrombolysis even in early presenters for whom the treatment is initiated within 2 hours.[37] In aggregate, the results of the randomized trials and registries provide clear evidence in favor of the transfer of patients for primary PCI.

A strategy of patient transfer for primary PCI instead of on-site thrombolysis inevitably incurs additional delays imposed by transportation, logistics, and the organizational and technical aspects of PCI procedures. However, primary PCI has been found to be superior to thrombolysis despite these delays.[7] PCI-related delay has become an integral part of treatment algorithms for patients with STEMI, although the evidence in support of this choice is poor and the assessment of this parameter is very difficult. No specific study has addressed this issue, and, in fact, the definition of the time point in PCI-related delay at which thrombolysis and primary PCI are at equipoise (and beyond which primary PCI might become inferior to thrombolysis) was based

almost solely on a post hoc analysis of randomized clinical trials. A prior study that performed a regression analysis of mortality benefit from primary PCI or thrombolysis versus difference in time between application of these therapeutic options defined a PCI-related delay of 60 minutes as the time point beyond which primary PCI was inferior to thrombolysis.[52] Although this analysis was later found to be flawed in several aspects, to a large extent, the 60-minute window for acceptable PCI-related delay is still endorsed in the recent ACC/AHA guidelines for the management of patients with STEMI.[9,53] More recent studies have corrected and expanded the PCI-related delay at which the mortality rates of the two strategies are equal to 110 minutes, and 119 minutes (Fig. 18-11).[53,54] In all these studies, the PCI-related delay was calculated on the basis of published summarized data and not on individual patient data. The most thorough time-based analysis that used individual patient data showed that primary PCI is superior to thrombolysis up to a PCI-related delay of 120 minutes.[14] In this study, even in the group of patients presenting within 1 hour, mortality was lower with primary PCI (4.7% vs. 6%), indicating that even in early presenters with PCI-related delays of 60 minutes or less, there is no reason to prefer thrombolysis over primary PCI as the reperfusion strategy. The Vienna registry reported a comparable in-hospital mortality (8.1% vs. 8.2%) in patients treated with primary PCI versus thrombolysis at a mean PCI-related delay of 138 minutes.[55] In 192,509 patients entered into the NRMI 2–4 registries, the mean PCI-related delay at which mortality benefits of primary PCI and thrombolysis were at equipoise was 114 minutes (95% confidence interval [CI] 96–132 minutes).[56] Of note, the study showed that PCI-related delay was not static and varied considerably, depending on the risk characteristics of patients such as age, symptom duration, and infarct location. Thus, PCI-related delay varied from less than 1 hour for patients under 65 years of age with anterior infarction who presented within 2 hours to almost 3 hours for patients over 65 years of age with nonanterior infarction who presented later than 2 hours from symptom onset. Indeed, a recent regression analysis of 16 randomized trials of primary PCI versus thrombolysis further emphasized the impact of baseline risk on the PCI-related delay at which both therapies are at equipoise with regard to mortality.[57] Another recent regression analysis, which included 27 trials with 4399 patients randomized to primary PCI and 4474 patients randomized to thrombolysis, found that the higher the risk of patients, the larger was the reduction in mortality achieved by primary PCI. It was calculated that for each 10-minute increase of PCI-related delay, there was a 0.75%, 0.45%, and 0% mortality benefit in high, medium, and low risk patients, respectively.[58] Although these studies showed that longer delays reduce the survival benefits of primary PCI, such delays could be acceptable and even beneficial in high-risk STEMI patients. In essence, these studies advocate the use of flexible PCI-related delay according to the risk profile of STEMI patients. However, a longer PCI-related delay is often associated with less experience and inadequate infrastructure at the primary PCI center, which introduces an inevitable bias that is difficult to adjust for in this kind of analysis.[42] Thus, assessment of the relationship between PCI-related time delay and outcome provides helpful information for the optimization of the primary PCI network but contributes little to the discussion about choosing the right reperfusion option for various settings. In an attempt to shorten PCI-related time delays, direct transportation of patients to hospitals that are capable of performing primary PCI rather than to the nearest hospital without PCI facility has also been suggested.[59]

In summary, prompt referral of patients with acute MI to centers with PCI facilities should be the primary objective of the first-contact emergency medical system. This is currently feasible for the large majority of patients with STEMI in the United States and should be attempted in the future for all patients with STEMI seeking medical aid. Nearly 80% of the adult population in the United States lives within 60 minutes of a hospital with PCI facility; even among those living closer to hospitals without PCI facility, almost three fourths would experience less than 30 minutes of additional delay in direct referral to a hospital with PCI facility.[60] The development of regional systems of STEMI care is a matter of utmost importance for improving the treatment of patients with STEMI.[22,23] Although not derived from specifically designed studies, a maximal 90- to 120-minute PCI-related delay seems to be reasonable. A flexible consideration of PCI-related delay, implying acceptance of longer delays for high-risk STEMI patients, seems also justified.

■ Facilitated Percutaneous Coronary Intervention

Facilitated PCI refers to a deliberate strategy of administration of pharmacologic therapy aimed at restoring anterograde flow in the infarct-related artery before proceeding to definitive revascularization with PCI in patients with STEMI. It is conceived as an option for filling the time gap between patient presentation and performance of PCI. The pharmacologic regimen consists of drugs known for their ability to restore blood flow such as full-dose or half-dose thrombolysis or a combination of half-dose thrombolysis with GP IIb/IIIa receptor antagonists. As data about the ability of GP IIb/IIIa receptor antagonists to reopen the infarct-related artery are controversial, the isolated use of these drugs may or may not be part of the strategy of facilitated PCI. Two factors underpin the rationale behind the concept of facilitated PCI: (1) Ventricular function and prognosis have been found to be better in patients with STEMI who present at the time of primary PCI with spontaneous TIMI flow grade 2 and 3 compared with those who have a TIMI flow grade of 0 and 1 in the infarct-related artery; (2) a large proportion of patients with STEMI are unable to receive mechanical reperfusion without a certain amount of delay because of a variety of reasons. Facilitated PCI was hypothesized to offer a reduction in ischemia time, earlier reperfusion, higher TIMI flow rates in the infarct-related artery and facilitated guidewire or balloon passage, decreased clot burden, and lower incidence of distal embolization. The Bavarian Reperfusion Alternatives Evaluation (BRAVE) trial was the first randomized trial to evaluate the impact of facilitated PCI with

reteplase plus abciximab on left ventricular infarct size estimated by single photon emission computed tomography (SPECT). Although the study reported a higher rate of pre-PCI TIMI flow grade 3 in the infarct-related artery in the facilitated PCI group, no reduction in infarct size was observed.[61] These results were confirmed by several subsequent clinical trials on this issue. The Assessment of the Safety and Efficacy of a New Treatment Strategy for Acute Myocardial Infarction (ASSENT)-4 PCI study was a randomized trial of patients with STEMI presenting within 6 hours from symptom onset, who were scheduled to undergo PCI after an anticipated delay of 1 to 3 hours and were assigned to standard PCI ($n = 838$) or to PCI preceded by administration of full-dose tenecteplase ($n = 829$).[62] All patients received aspirin and a bolus without an infusion of unfractionated heparin. The investigators of ASSENT-4 PCI planned to enroll 4000 patients, but the Data and Safety Monitoring Board recommended early cessation because of higher in-hospital mortality in the facilitated PCI group than in the group with standard PCI. The primary endpoint of ASSENT-4 PCI was death, congestive heart failure (CHF), or shock within 90 days from randomization. This occurred in 19% of patients in the facilitated PCI group and 13% in the standard PCI group (relative risk [RR] 1.39; 95% CI 1.11–1.74, $P = 0.005$). There were more in-hospital strokes (1.8% vs. 0%, $P < 0.001$) and higher incidence of ischemic complications such as re-infarction (6% vs. 4%; $P = 0.03$) and repeat target vessel revascularization (7% vs. 3%; $P = 0.004$) among patients treated with facilitated PCI than among those treated with standard PCI. The ASSENT-4 PCI trial concluded that a strategy of facilitated PCI consisting of full-dose thrombolysis (tenecteplase) plus concurrent anti-thrombotic therapy that preceded PCI by 1 to 3 hours was associated with a worse clinical outcome than a strategy of primary PCI alone; therefore, this strategy is not recommended.[62] The meta-analysis of Keeley et al, which included 17 trials of patients with STEMI assigned to facilitated PCI ($n = 2237$) or primary PCI ($n = 2267$), showed that facilitated PCI was associated with significantly worse short-term outcomes (up to 42 days) than primary PCI alone: death (5% vs. 3%), nonfatal re-infarction (3% vs. 2%), urgent target vessel revascularization (4% vs. 1%), major bleeding (7% vs. 5%), hemorrhagic stroke (0.7% vs. 0.1%), and total stroke (1.1% vs. 0.3%).[63] The increased rates of adverse events were observed mainly when thrombolytic therapy was used to facilitate PCI.[63] The recently published FINESSE (Facilitated Intervention with Enhanced Reperfusion Speed to Stop Events) study was another confirmation of the inefficacy and even detrimental effects of facilitated PCI in patients with STEMI.[64] The study enrolled 2452 patients with STEMI presenting within the first 6 hours from symptom onset, who were randomly assigned to facilitated PCI with half-dose reteplase, abciximab versus abciximab alone, or conventional PCI with abciximab given in the catheterization laboratory (cath-lab). All patients received unfractionated heparin or enoxaparin before PCI and a 12-hour infusion of abciximab after PCI. The primary endpoint was the composite of death from all causes, ventricular fibrillation occurring more than 48 hours after randomization, cardiogenic shock, and CHF during the first 90 days after randomization. In the combination therapy–facilitated group, the abciximab-facilitated group, and the primary PCI group, the primary endpoint occurred in 9.8%, 10.5%, and 10.7% of the patients, respectively ($P = 0.55$, Fig. 18-12); 90-day mortality rates were 5.2%, 5.5%, and 4.5%, respectively ($P = 0.49$); early ST segment resolution occurred in 43.9%, 33.1%, and 31% ($P = 0.003$ for combination-facilitated PCI versus primary PCI, and $P = 0.01$ for combination-facilitated PCI versus abciximab-facilitated PCI). Overall, there was a graded increase in the rates of bleeding, intracranial hemorrhage, and transfusions in the PCI-facilitated groups.[64] The evidence offered by the ASSENT-4 PCI trial, the meta-analysis by Keeley et al., and the FINESSE trial discourages the use of thrombolytics either at full dose or at half dose combined with GP IIb/IIIa inhibitors as pharmacologic facilitation of PCI.[62–65] Although the reasons for the failure of facilitated PCI are not entirely clear, pre-PCI thrombolysis may be associated with increased risk of bleeding and enhanced platelet activation. In summary, the failure of thrombolysis to improve the results of subsequent PCI

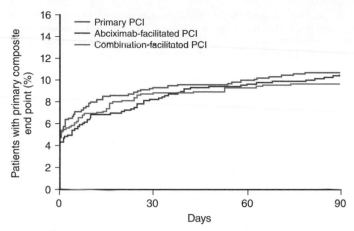

Figure 18-12 Kaplan–Meier estimates of the proportion of patients meeting the composite endpoint in the FINESSE trial. Data are shown for all patients randomly assigned to a treatment group. $P = 0.55$ for the comparison of primary percutaneous coronary intervention (PCI) with reteplase-plus-abciximab–facilitated (combination-facilitated) PCI. $P = 0.86$ for the comparison of primary PCI with abciximab-facilitated PCI. $P = 0.68$ for the comparison of abciximab-facilitated PCI with combination-facilitated PCI. *(Ellis SG, Tendera M, de Belder MA, et al: Facilitated PCI in patients with ST-elevation myocardial infarction, N Engl J Med 358:2205–2217, 2008.)*

represents a further significant reduction in the role that this treatment deserves in the current reperfusion therapy of patients with STEMI. Although facilitation of PCI, in the sense of promoting reperfusion as the patient is directed to the cath-lab, should remain a goal to strive for, available evidence demonstrates that it cannot be achieved with present-day thrombolysis.

Routine Use of Percutaneous Coronary Intervention after Thrombolysis

Thrombolysis followed immediately by PCI was thought to combine the benefits of early reperfusion achieved by thrombolysis (enhanced myocardial salvage) with the benefits of PCI (more complete or fuller reperfusion in case of failed thrombolysis, stability of established blood flow, and prevention of reclosure or thrombosis in case of initially successful thrombolysis). However, earlier studies were not encouraging, and a meta-analysis of studies of PCI immediately after thrombolysis initiated in the late 1980s showed that this therapeutic strategy

was not beneficial, probably because of the use of outdated fibrinolytic agents, anti-thrombotic regimens, and PCI equipment and the increased risk of bleeding that characterized the post-thrombolysis period.[63] Two new trials have supported the use of PCI immediately after thrombolysis. The CARESS-in-AMI (Combined Abciximab REteplase Stent Study in Acute Myocardial Infarction) trial included 600 patients 75 years of age or older with at least one high-risk feature (extensive ST segment elevation, LBBB of new onset, previous MI, Killip class >2, or LVEF ≤35%), who presented within 12 hours from symptom onset and were treated initially in non-PCI hospitals with half-dose reteplase, abciximab, heparin, and aspirin.[65] Patients were randomized to immediate transfer for PCI (299 patients) or standard care with transfer for rescue PCI (301 patients). The primary outcome was a composite of 30-day death, re-infarction, or refractory ischemia. In the group assigned to immediate PCI, 289 patients (97%) underwent angiography, and 255 patients (85.6%) underwent PCI. In the group assigned to standard care, 91 patients (30.3%) underwent rescue PCI. The primary endpoint occurred in 4.4% of patients assigned to immediate PCI and in 10.7% of the patients assigned to standard care with eventual rescue PCI ($P = 0.004$), with no differences in major bleeding (3.4% vs. 2.3%, $P = 0.47$) or stroke (0.7% vs. 1.3%, $P = 0.50$). In the immediate PCI group, the interval from reteplase to angiography or PCI was 2.25 hours. The Trial of Routine Angioplasty and Stenting after Fibrinolysis to Enhance Reperfusion in Acute Myocardial Infarction (TRANSFER-AMI) included 1059 high-risk patients with STEMI, who presented to non-PCI hospitals within 12 hours from symptom onset.[66] Patients were randomized to standard treatment, including rescue PCI (522 patients), or to a strategy of immediate transfer for PCI within 6 hours after thrombolysis (537 patients). All patients received aspirin, tenecteplase, and heparin or enoxaparin; concomitant clopidogrel was strongly encouraged. The primary endpoint was the composite of death, re-infarction, recurrent ischemia, new or worsening CHF, or cardiogenic shock within 30 days. In the group assigned to transfer for PCI, 98.5% underwent coronary angiography, and 84.9% received PCI (2.8 hours after randomization); in the group assigned to standard care, 88.7% underwent coronary angiography, and 67.4% received PCI (32.5 hours after randomization). At 30 days, the primary endpoint occurred in 11% of the patients assigned to immediate PCI and in 17.2% of the patients assigned to standard treatment ($P = 0.004$), with no significant differences in major bleeding. A recent meta-analysis that included seven trials, which included 2961 patients comparing early routine PCI after thrombolysis with standard therapy in patients with STEMI, found that early routine use of PCI after thrombolysis reduced the 30-day rate of re-infarction (2.6% vs. 4.7%, $P = 0.003$), the combined endpoint of death or re-infarction (5.6% vs. 8.3%, $P = 0.004$; Fig. 18-13), and recurrent ischemia (1.9% vs. 7.1%, $P < 0.001$) without affecting the rates of major bleeding (4.9% vs. 5.0%, $P = 0.70$) or stroke (0.7% vs. 1.3%, $P = 0.21$).[67] The benefits

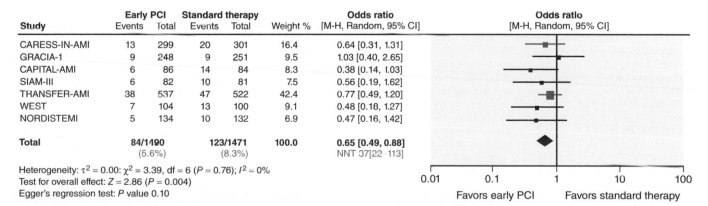

Study	Early PCI Events	Total	Standard therapy Events	Total	Weight %	Odds ratio [M-H, Random, 95% CI]
CARESS-IN-AMI	13	299	20	301	16.4	0.64 [0.31, 1.31]
GRACIA-1	9	248	9	251	9.5	1.03 [0.40, 2.65]
CAPITAL-AMI	6	86	14	84	8.3	0.38 [0.14, 1.03]
SIAM-III	6	82	10	81	7.5	0.56 [0.19, 1.62]
TRANSFER-AMI	38	537	47	522	42.4	0.77 [0.49, 1.20]
WEST	7	104	13	100	9.1	0.48 [0.18, 1.27]
NORDISTEMI	5	134	10	132	6.9	0.47 [0.16, 1.42]
Total	**84/1490** (5.6%)		**123/1471** (8.3%)		**100.0**	**0.65 [0.49, 0.88]** NNT 37[22–113]

Heterogeneity: $\tau^2 = 0.00$; $\chi^2 = 3.39$, df = 6 ($P = 0.76$); $I^2 = 0\%$
Test for overall effect: $Z = 2.86$ ($P = 0.004$)
Egger's regression test: P value 0.10

Figure 18-13 Combined death, re-infarction, or recurrent ischemia in trials comparing early percutaneous coronary intervention versus standard therapy after fibrinolysis for ST segment elevation myocardial infarction. *(Borgia F, Goodman SG, Halvorsen S, et al: Early routine percutaneous coronary intervention after fibrinolysis vs. standard therapy in ST-segment elevation myocardial infarction: A meta-analysis, Eur Heart J 31:2156–2169, 2010.)*

of routine use of PCI after thrombolysis were maintained at 6 to 12 months of follow-up. Another meta-analysis of nine trials with a total of 3325 patients showed a 24% reduction in total mortality ($P = 0.06$), a 45% reduction ($P < 0.001$) in recurrent MI, and a 65% reduction in recurrent ischemia ($P < 0.001$), with no significant difference in the incidence of major bleeding or stroke in patients managed with early or immediate PCI after thrombolysis as opposed to standard care.[68] These studies demonstrated that the approach of routine use of PCI after thrombolysis is beneficial in patients with STEMI. Among factors that seem to have had a positive impact on the outcome of routine use of PCI after thrombolysis are the recent advances in PCI technology and adjunctive pharmacologic therapy.

Rescue Percutaneous Coronary Intervention

Rescue PCI is defined as PCI performed within 12 hours after failure of thrombolysis in patients with continuing or recurrent myocardial ischemia. In the absence of coronary angiography, partial (<50%) resolution of ST segment resolution on the surface electrocardiogram (ECG), continuation of chest discomfort, or both are used as putative markers of failed thrombolysis, even though they are known to be imprecise. Even with the use of the most advanced fibrin-specific thrombolytic agents available, thrombolysis restores optimal epicardial blood flow TIMI grade 3 in just over half the STEMI patients. Furthermore, 5% to 10% of patients will suffer coronary reocclusions after an initial successful thrombolysis. The less-than-optimal results with thrombolysis can be explained by the fact that the plaque–thrombosis ratio at the site of coronary occlusion is, on average, 80% (plaque) to 20% (thrombotic material) and that, not infrequently, plaque expansion contributes more to acute coronary occlusion compared with acute thrombosis.[69,70] These factors and others make the establishment of TIMI flow grade 3 by thrombolysis less likely. The mortality rate is higher in patients with an occluded infarct-related artery (TIMI flow grade 0–1) and those with suboptimal blood flow restoration (TIMI flow 2) compared with that in patients with restoration of TIMI flow grade 3 in the infarct-related artery. It has recently been estimated that annually in the United States nearly 125,000 patients with STEMI will have suboptimal reperfusion with thrombolytic therapy.[71] In the past, patients with failed thrombolysis have been treated with conservative therapy and watchful waiting, repeat thrombolysis, or rescue PCI. Over the years, the concept of rescue PCI as a treatment for failed thrombolysis has evolved from a "conscience tranquillizer" to a valuable therapeutic option with the capacity to improve the health of patients.[72] In the last 5 years, two trials of rescue PCI for failed thrombolysis have been published: (1) the Middlesbrough Early Revascularization to Limit Infarction (MERLIN) trial and (2) the Rescue Angioplasty or Repeat Thrombolysis (REACT) trial.[73,74] The MERLIN trial randomized 307 patients with STEMI and failed thrombolysis (failure of ST segment elevation in the lead with maximal elevation to resolve by 50%) to emergency coronary angiography with or without rescue PCI or conservative therapy. The primary endpoint was all-cause mortality at 30 days. Thirty-day all-cause mortality was similar in the rescue and conservative groups (9.8% vs. 11%, $P = 0.7$). The combined incidence of major adverse cardiac events was reduced in the rescue PCI group (37.3% vs. 50.0%, $P = 0.02$) driven by less subsequent revascularization (6.5% vs. 20.1%; $P = 0.01$). Re-infarction (7.2% vs. 10.4%, $P = 0.03$) and CHF (24.2% vs. 29.2%, $P = 0.3$) were less common among patients undergoing rescue PCI. There was an increased incidence of strokes (4.6% vs. 0.6%, $P = 0.03$) and blood transfusions (11.1% vs. 1.3%, $P = 0.001$) among patients treated by rescue PCI versus those treated by conservative therapy.[73] The REACT trial included 427 patients with STEMI within 6 hours of symptom onset and 90-minute EGM criteria for failed thrombolysis (<50% ST segment resolution in the leads with previous maximal ST segment elevation). Patients were randomly assigned to one of three options: (1) rescue PCI ($n = 144$), (2) repeat thrombolysis ($n = 142$), or (3) conservative therapy ($n = 141$).

Coronary stents were used in 68.5% of patients, and 43.4% of patients received GP IIb/IIIa receptor blockers. The 6-month probability of event-free survival was significantly higher in patients assigned to rescue PCI (84.6%) compared with patients assigned to conservative therapy (70.1%) or repeat thrombolysis (68.7%, $P = 0.004$). Recently, the authors of the REACT trial published their report on the primary composite endpoints of death, recurrent MI, cerebrovascular events, and severe heart failure at 1 year and mortality at a median of 4.4 years.[75] The 6-month advantage in the event-free-survival was maintained at 1 year of follow-up (81.5%, 67.5%, and 64.1% in rescue PCI, conservative therapy, and repeat thrombolysis arms, respectively, $P = 0.004$). The 1-year rate of clinically driven revascularizations was significantly reduced by rescue PCI compared with the other two therapies. Of note, the most important finding of this study was a significant reduction of mortality at a median of 4.4 years: mortality rates were 11.2% in the rescue PCI arm, 22.4% in the conservative therapy arm, and 22.3% in the repeat thrombolysis arm (for rescue PCI vs. conservative therapy: HR 0.43; 95% CI 0.23–0.97; and for rescue PCI vs. repeat thrombolysis: HR 0.41; 95% CI 0.22–0.75). Of importance was the finding that repeat thrombolysis did not offer any benefit compared with conservative therapy.[75] In summary, rescue PCI improves clinical outcome and should be recommended for patients with STEMI after failed thrombolysis.

Technical Aspects of Primary Percutaneous Coronary Intervention

From a technical point of view, primary PCI is not substantially different from elective PCI, although it is characterized by more frequent use of thrombus aspiration devices and direct stenting. However, PCI in the early phase of STEMI can be more difficult and requires more experience than does routine PCI in a stable patient. The goal of primary PCI is to open occluded coronary arteries and restore normal blood flow to the ischemic region. Primary PCI is performed in conditions of increased risk caused by hemodynamic and electrical instability, increased thrombogenicity associated with STEMI, and thrombotic occlusion of stenotic coronary arteries. The latter finding impedes visualization of the coronary artery, makes guidewire and balloon passage through the occluded lesion more difficult, and predisposes to distal embolization of thrombotic material with a potential for further worsening of microcirculation function. Operators performing primary PCI in STEMI must act quickly and as early as possible to restore coronary blood flow in the infarct-related artery to stop evolving ischemia and progression to necrosis and to increase the chances of myocardial salvage and infarct size reduction. Vascular access is achieved via the femoral artery, though radial artery access is increasingly being preferred. Adjunct antithrombotic therapy is used peri-procedurally (see the section on Peri-procedural Anti-thrombotics in Patients with STEMI Undergoing PCI). After the procedure, the patient is monitored continuously; in the absence of complications, the patient is discharged from the hospital within a few days.

Primary Stenting in Patients with ST Elevation Myocardial Infarction

In the early days of mechanical reperfusion for STEMI, balloon angioplasty was the mainstay of therapy. However, although superior to thrombolysis, balloon angioplasty often produces suboptimal results, mostly related to recurring ischemia and reocclusion within the first days and weeks after the procedure, as well as a high incidence of late vessel narrowing (re-stenosis). Despite these limitations of balloon angioplasty, in general, coronary stenting in the setting of STEMI was avoided because of the fear that implantation of a metallic structure within the highly thrombogenic milieu of the infarct-related artery (including thrombotic material and balloon-induced plaque disruption) would predispose to acute stent thrombosis and coronary reocclusion. Furthermore, in the early days of PCI, the profound anticoagulation that was needed to prevent stent thrombosis markedly increased the risk of bleeding, posing additional risk for patients. Refinement in stent technology and advances in peri-procedural and long-term anti-thrombotic therapy transformed primary stenting from an infrequently used therapeutic option, usually in bail-out situations, to the dominant form of primary PCI in patients with STEMI. Primary stenting has been directly compared with primary angioplasty alone. A recent meta-analysis summarized the results of 13 trials, which randomized 6922 patients with acute MI to coronary stenting (3460 patients) or balloon angioplasty alone (3462 patients).[76] In a meta-analysis of five trials that included patients with cardiogenic shock, primary stenting significantly reduced the need for revascularization at 1 year (11.3% vs. 18.3%) but had no effect on mortality (5.1% vs. 5.2%) or re-infarction (3.7% vs. 3.9%). The meta-regression analysis demonstrated a significant association between patient risk profile and mortality benefits from primary stenting at 1 year. No such association was observed for re-infarction.[76] These conclusions, however, are subject to limitations related to significant variations in the cross-over rates and the possible confounding effects of thienopyridine treatment in patients treated with primary stenting. Against this, an analysis of the Primary Angioplasty in Myocardial Infarction (PAMI) trial showed not only better angiographic results with primary stenting but also a sustained benefit in mortality for up to 5 years after MI.[77] Mechanistically, compared with balloon angioplasty, stents achieve a better immediate angiographic result because of a larger postprocedural arterial lumen, fewer early ischemic events, and enhanced longer-term patency durability caused by attenuation of elastic recoil and constrictive remodeling. Currently, primary stenting is the preferred strategy for primary PCI in patients with STEMI, as it may reduce costs, radiation exposure, and potentially the incidence of no-reflow and distal embolization of thrombotic material.[78]

■ Drug-Eluting Stents in Patients with ST Elevation Myocardial Infarction

The development of DESs represented an important milestone in the evolution of PCI. Compared with bare metal stents (BMS), DES have reduced the need for target vessel revascularization by 60% to 70% in the setting of randomized clinical trials. However, DES implantation in patients with STEMI is considered an "off-label" indication (i.e., an indication outside those studied in the trials on which the FDA [U.S. Food and Drug Administration] based its approval). In general, there are still concerns about a possible increase in the incidence of stent thrombosis (especially late events beyond 1 year) after DES implantation because of inhibition or delayed re-endothelization of the stented segment.[79] Specifically, it has been postulated that the risk of stent thrombosis might be higher if DES are implanted in patients with STEMI. Putative mechanisms offered to explain higher rates of stent thrombosis after DES implantation in patients with STEMI include an increased risk of stent malapposition (thrombus jailing and subsequent dissolution, as well as coronary spasm at culprit lesions during the acute event may increase the risk of stent undersizing), a modulation of drug release kinetics by superimposed thrombotic material, and uptake of lipophilic drugs by necrotic core material, which because of very slow turnover, may lead to further prolongation of tissue exposure and exacerbate delayed healing.[79] Despite these still unresolved issues, recent evidence about the use of DES in STEMI has been mostly reassuring, and DES implantation is increasingly being used in the setting of primary PCI. Recent information on the use of DES in patients with STEMI has emerged from registries, randomized trials, and meta-analyses. A recent report comes from the GRACE registry, in which data of 5093 patients with STEMI treated with stenting were analyzed.[80] Unadjusted 2-year mortality was lower in patients who received DES compared with patients who received BMSs (3.9% vs. 5.3%, $P = 0.04$). A time-dependent analysis after propensity and risk adjustment

showed a similar mortality up to 6 months after stent implantation (1.5% in patients with DES vs. 2.2% in patients with BMS, $P = 0.21$) and a close to five-times increase in mortality from 6 months to 2 years (6.3% vs. 1.6%; HR = 4.90, $P = 0.001$) in patients who received DES compared with those who received BMSs. Thus, data from the GRACE registry gave a clear signal of increased risk of late mortality with DES in patients with STEMI.[80] In contrast, Massachusetts state data, which included 7217 patients with acute MI treated with stenting (4016 patients with DES and 3201 patients with BMSs) came to different conclusions.[81] In a matched-pairs analysis, the 2-year risk-adjusted mortality was lower for patients who received DES compared with patients who received BMS in the overall group (10.7% vs. 12.8%, $P = 0.02$) and in patients with STEMI (8.5% vs. 11.6%, $P = 0.008$). Patients with STEMI who received DES had similar 2-year rates of recurrent MI (7% vs. 8%, $P = 0.34$) but significantly lower rates of target vessel revascularization (10.2% vs. 13.9%, $P = 0.003$) compared with patients who received BMS.[81] Despite the fact that registries may include large numbers of patients and their analysis incorporate propensity score adjustment, great caution is warranted when interpreting comparative efficacy on the basis of these studies, mainly because observed outcome differences may simply represent the impact of unmeasured residual confounding.

A number of recent randomized trials have increased markedly the current knowledge on the efficacy and safety of the use of DES in patients with acute MI. The most recent and largest one is the Harmonizing Outcomes with Revascularization and Stents in Acute Myocardial Infarction (HORIZONS-AMI) trial, which randomized in a 3:1 ratio 3006 patients with STEMI to receive paclitaxel-eluting stents (2257 patients) or BMS (749 patients).[82] In addition, a factorial design that allowed initial allocation to heparin and routine GP IIb/IIIa inhibitor versus bivalirudin plus bail-out GP IIb/IIIa inhibitor was used. Patients who received paclitaxel-eluting stents, compared with those who received BMS, had significantly lower 12-month rates of ischemia-driven target lesion revascularization (4.5% vs. 7.5%, $P = 0.002$) and target-vessel revascularization (5.8% vs. 8.7%, $P = 0.006$). The composite of death, re-infarction, stroke, and stent thrombosis (safety endpoint) was similar between paclitaxel-eluting stents and BMS (8.1% vs. 8.0%) with no significant differences with regard to 12-month rates of death (3.5% and 3.5%) or stent thrombosis (3.2% and 3.4%). The 13-month rate of binary re-stenosis was significantly lower with paclitaxel-eluting stents than with BMS (10.0% vs. 22.9%, $P < 0.001$).[82] The extension of follow-up showed that DES maintained their superiority by showing a 40% reduction in target lesion revascularization at 3 years compared with BMS.[83] The results of HORIZONS-AMI clearly demonstrated the advantages of the use of paclitaxel-eluting stents in patients with STEMI. Finally, recent meta-analyses summarizing the results of individual studies—both registries and randomized trials—have been reassuring about the efficacy and safety of DES in patients with acute MI.[84,85] A recent meta-analysis involving 14 randomized trials and 7781 patients showed that treatment with DES resulted in a significant reduction in the hazard of re-intervention (0.41; 95% CI 0.32–0.52), whereas the hazards of death (0.90; 95% CI 0.71–1.15), myocardial infarction (0.81; 95% CI 0.63–1.04), and stent thrombosis (0.84; 95% CI 0.61–1.17) did not differ significantly up to 2 years (Figure 18-14, A and B).[85] Another recent meta-analysis that included 13 randomized trials (7352 patients; HORIZONS-AMI included) and 18 registries (26,521 patients) provided further support for the use of DES in patients with STEMI.[84] New reports on 3-year data from the randomized trials on DES versus BMS in STEMI, including the HORIZONS-AMI trial, showed a durable benefit with DES without compromised long-term safety.[83] In summary, stents with or without drug coating should be considered the preferred approach for patients with STEMI undergoing primary PCI. Ample evidence from multiple sources proves a clear anti–restenotic advantage of DES over BMS in patients with STEMI. Randomized trials and meta-analyses offer no evidence of an effect of DES on mortality (increase or reduction) or recurrent MI.

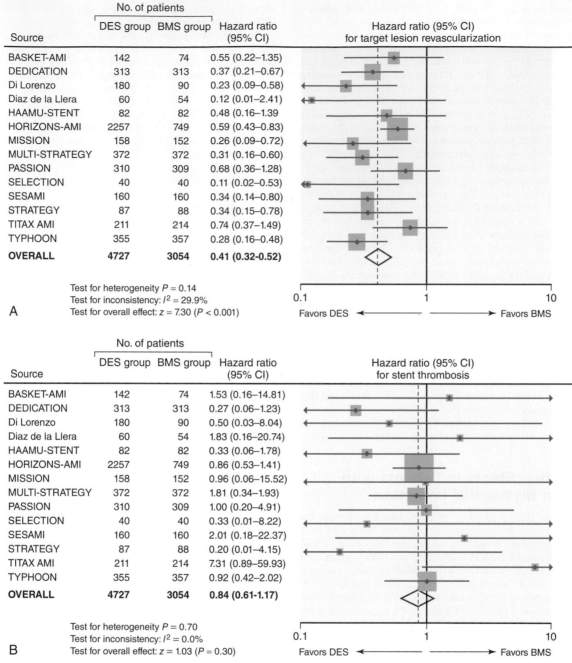

	No. of patients			
Source	DES group	BMS group	Hazard ratio (95% CI)	Hazard ratio (95% CI) for target lesion revascularization
BASKET-AMI	142	74	0.55 (0.22–1.35)	
DEDICATION	313	313	0.37 (0.21–0.67)	
Di Lorenzo	180	90	0.23 (0.09–0.58)	
Diaz de la Llera	60	54	0.12 (0.01–2.41)	
HAAMU-STENT	82	82	0.48 (0.16–1.39)	
HORIZONS-AMI	2257	749	0.59 (0.43–0.83)	
MISSION	158	152	0.26 (0.09–0.72)	
MULTI-STRATEGY	372	372	0.31 (0.16–0.60)	
PASSION	310	309	0.68 (0.36–1.28)	
SELECTION	40	40	0.11 (0.02–0.53)	
SESAMI	160	160	0.34 (0.14–0.80)	
STRATEGY	87	88	0.34 (0.15–0.78)	
TITAX AMI	211	214	0.74 (0.37–1.49)	
TYPHOON	355	357	0.28 (0.16–0.48)	
OVERALL	**4727**	**3054**	**0.41 (0.32–0.52)**	

Test for heterogeneity $P = 0.14$
Test for inconsistency: $I^2 = 29.9\%$
Test for overall effect: $z = 7.30$ ($P < 0.001$)

A

0.1   1   10
Favors DES ⟵   ⟶ Favors BMS

	No. of patients			
Source	DES group	BMS group	Hazard ratio (95% CI)	Hazard ratio (95% CI) for stent thrombosis
BASKET-AMI	142	74	1.53 (0.16–14.81)	
DEDICATION	313	313	0.27 (0.06–1.23)	
Di Lorenzo	180	90	0.50 (0.03–8.04)	
Diaz de la Llera	60	54	1.83 (0.16–20.74)	
HAAMU-STENT	82	82	0.33 (0.06–1.78)	
HORIZONS-AMI	2257	749	0.86 (0.53–1.41)	
MISSION	158	152	0.96 (0.06–15.52)	
MULTI-STRATEGY	372	372	1.81 (0.34–1.93)	
PASSION	310	309	1.00 (0.20–4.91)	
SELECTION	40	40	0.33 (0.01–8.22)	
SESAMI	160	160	2.01 (0.18–22.37)	
STRATEGY	87	88	0.20 (0.01–4.15)	
TITAX AMI	211	214	7.31 (0.89–59.93)	
TYPHOON	355	357	0.92 (0.42–2.02)	
OVERALL	**4727**	**3054**	**0.84 (0.61–1.17)**	

Test for heterogeneity $P = 0.70$
Test for inconsistency: $I^2 = 0.0\%$
Test for overall effect: $z = 1.03$ ($P = 0.30$)

B

0.1   1   10
Favors DES ⟵   ⟶ Favors BMS

Figure 18-14   Hazard ratios of re-intervention associated with drug-eluting stent versus bare metal stent (*A*) and hazard ratios of stent thrombosis associated with drug-eluting stent versus bare metal stent (*B*). *DES*, drug-eluting stent; *BMS*, bare-metal stent; *CI*, confidence interval. The size of the data marker is proportional to the weight of the individual studies. *BASKET-AMI*, Basel Stent Kosten Effektivitäts in Acute Myocardial Infarction trial; *DEDICATION*, The Drug Elution and Distal Protection in Acute Myocardial Infarction Trial; *HAAMUSTENT*, The Helsinki area acute myocardial infarction-treatment re-evaluation—Should the patient get a drug-eluting or a normal stent trial; *HORIZONS-AMI*, Harmonizing Outcomes with Revascularization and Stents in Acute Myocardial Infarction; MISSION A Prospective Randomized Controlled Trial to Evaluate the Efficacy of Drug-Eluting Stents versus Bare-Metal Stents for the Treatment of Acute Myocardial Infarction; MULTI-STRATEGY the Multicentre Evaluation of Single High-Dose Bolus Tirofiban versus Abciximab With Sirolimus-Eluting Stent or Bare-Metal Stent in Acute Myocardial Infarction Study; PASSION the Paclitaxel-Eluting Stent versus Conventional Stent in Myocardial Infarction with ST-Segment Elevation trial; SELECTION Single-Center Randomized Evaluation of Paclitaxel-Eluting Versus Conventional Stent in Acute Myocardial Infarction; SESAMI the Randomized Trial of Sirolimus Stent versus Bare Stent in Acute Myocardial Infarction trial; STRATEGY the Single High Dose Bolus Tirofiban and Sirolimus Eluting Stent versus Abciximab and Bare-Metal Stent in Myocardial Infarction trial; TITAX AMI titanium-nitride-oxide coated stents versus paclitaxel-eluting stents in acute myocardial infarction; TYPHOON the Trial to Assess the Use of the Cypher Stent in Acute Myocardial Infarction Treated with Balloon Angioplasty CABG aorto-coronary bypass surgery, CK creatine kinase, PCI percutaneous coronary intervention. (*Dibra A, Tiroch K, Schulz S, et al: Drug-eluting stents in acute myocardial infarction: updated meta-analysis of randomized trials, Clin Res Cardiol 99:345–357, 2010.*)

Adjunctive Thrombectomy and Distal Protection Devices in Primary Percutaneous Coronary Intervention

Although primary PCI is a highly effective therapy in patients with STEMI, there has been concern that conventional PCI using balloons and stents may dislodge thrombotic material, atherosclerotic plaque debris, or both into the distal microcirculation, resulting in distal embolization and impaired myocardial perfusion. Distal embolization during mechanical reperfusion is considered an important contributor to microvascular dysfunction and no-reflow. Distal embolization does occur during PCI for STEMI, and visible debris has been aspirated in 73% of patients.[86] In recent years, there has been an increased interest in developing thrombectomy and protection systems to reduce the thrombotic burden, limit distal embolization, and improve myocardial perfusion and the clinical outcome. Apart from pharmacologic agents such as GP IIb/IIIa inhibitors, several mechanical devices have been developed and used to prevent distal embolization. In principle, there are two categories of devices that might be employed in an attempt to reduce distal embolization: (1) thrombectomy devices (aspiration thrombectomy, mechanical thrombectomy) and (2) embolic protection devices (distal occlusive devices, proximal occlusive devices and distal embolic filters). Earlier small-scale randomized studies, which included limited numbers of patients, tested the safety, feasibility, and efficacy of various devices and showed that, in general, embolic protection can be safely performed during PCI for STEMI and that some of these devices have positive effects on myocardial reperfusion and outcome. Recent studies using thrombectomy with simple manual aspiration devices have reported encouraging results in terms of clinical outcomes and have led to an increased use of manual aspiration as an adjunctive therapy to primary PCI.[87–89] TAPAS (Thrombus Aspiration during Percutaneous coronary intervention in Acute myocardial infarction Study) is the largest randomized study, to date, in which 1071 patients with STEMI were randomized to aspiration thrombectomy with the 6F-compatible Export catheter plus conventional PCI versus PCI alone. The primary endpoint was a myocardial blush grade of 0 or 1. A myocardial blush grade of 0 to 1 occurred in 17.1% of the patients in the thrombus-aspiration group and in 26.3% of those in the conventional-PCI group (P < 0.001); complete resolution of ST segment elevation occurred in 56.6% and 44.2% of patients, respectively (P < 0.001). There was a trend toward lower 30-day mortality in the group with aspiration thrombectomy (2.1% vs. 4.1%, P = 0.07). There were no significant differences in re-infarction (0.8% vs. 1.9%), target vessel revascularization (4.5% vs. 5.8%), major bleeding (3.8% vs 3.4%) and major adverse cardiac events (6.8% vs 9.4%) at 30 days.[88] At 1 year, all-cause mortality was 4.7% in the thrombus aspiration group and 7.6% in the conventional PCI group (P = 0.04, Fig. 18-15). The 1-year combined incidence of death or nonfatal re-infarction was 5.6% in the thrombus-aspiration group and 9.9% in the conventional-PCI group (P = 0.009).[89] The most important implication of TAPAS is that protection of microvascular function with aspiration thrombectomy is clinically relevant and results in considerable clinical benefit in patients with STEMI, including reduction in cardiac mortality. It has to be remembered, however, that TAPAS was performed in a single, high-volume center and that the very short door-to-aspiration and door-to-balloon times (medians: 28 minutes and 26 minutes, respectively) make the results difficult to generalize. Finally, the fact that the aspiration thrombectomy group received mostly direct stenting and the conventional PCI group received mostly balloon dilation followed by stenting may have led to increased distal embolization in the conventional PCI group. The EXPIRA (Thrombectomy With Export Catheter in Infarct-Related Artery During Primary Percutaneous Coronary Intervention) trial used contrast-enhanced magnetic resonance imaging (MRI) to assess myocardial reperfusion in 175 patients with STEMI, who were randomly assigned to standard PCI (87 patients) or manual thrombectomy plus PCI (88 patients). The primary endpoints were the occurrence of myocardial blush grade 2 or more and the rate of 90-minute ST segment

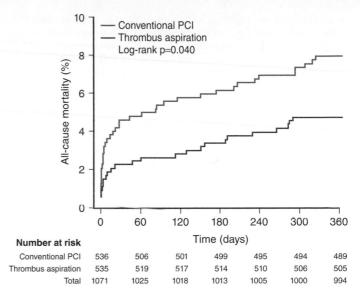

Figure 18-15 Kaplan-Meier curves for all-cause mortality at 1-year follow-up in the TAPAS trial. *(Vlaar PJ, Svilaas T, van der Horst IC, et al: Cardiac death and reinfarction after 1 year in the Thrombus Aspiration during Percutaneous coronary intervention in Acute myocardial infarction Study (TAPAS): A 1-year follow-up study, Lancet 371:1915–1920, 2008.)*

resolution greater than 70%. Myocardial blush grade 2 or more and ST segment resolution occurred more frequently in the manual thrombectomy-plus-PCI group (88% vs. 60%, P = 0.001 and 64% vs. 39%, P = 0.001). In the acute phase, microvascular obstruction was significantly lower in the thrombectomy-PCI group; and at 3 months, the infarct size was significantly reduced only in the manual thrombectomy-plus-PCI group. At 9 months, cardiac death occurred significantly less often in the manual thrombectomy-plus PCI arm (0% vs. 4.6%, P = 0.02).[87] Another recent study showed that thrombus aspiration was associated with higher LVEF and less remodeling at 6 months.[90] In JETSTENT (AngioJET thrombectomy and STENTing for treatment of acute myocardial infarction), 501 patients were randomly allocated to thrombus extraction with a somewhat more complex mechanical (rheolytic) thrombectomy catheter before direct stenting versus direct stenting alone. In terms of the co-primary endpoints, the trial was negative with nonsignificant differences between rheolytic thrombectomy and conventional therapy in ST segment resolution (85.8% vs. 78.8%) and scintigraphic infarct size (11.8% vs. 12.75%). Furthermore, both TIMI flow and TIMI myocardial blush grade tended to be poorer in patients treated with thrombectomy. In contrast, the 6-month incidence of major adverse cardiac events (11.2% vs. 19.4%) and 1-year event-free survival (85.2% vs. 75.0%) were significantly better among patients assigned to rheolytic thrombectomy before direct stenting, which is somewhat difficult to reconcile with the discordant findings related to microcirculatory function.[91] Thus, the apparent benefit associated with thrombus extraction in primary intervention needs to be qualified by the observation that benefit is unlikely to be a class effect. Indeed, in two recent large-scale meta-analyses demonstrating a mortality benefit for patients randomized to thrombus extraction as opposed to those managed with conventional primary intervention, this effect appeared to be confined to patients treated with manual thrombectomy devices.[92,93] This evidence of differential efficacy is reflected in the guidelines, which restrict their endorsement of thrombus extraction to manual aspiration devices only.[10]

Peri-Procedural Anti-Thrombotic Therapy

Pretreatment with aspirin and clopidogrel and peri-procedural heparinization represent the most common forms of adjunct antithrombotic management in patients with STEMI undergoing PCI. Platelet inhibition by various anti-thrombotic agents used before, during, and after PCI is an integral part of PCI in patients with STEMI. The use of anti-thrombotic agents, especially GP IIb/IIIa inhibitors in the setting of facilitated PCI, has been described earlier in this chapter (see the section on Facilitated PCI). Among GP IIb/IIIa inhibitors, abciximab was the agent most commonly used during primary PCI procedures. A retrospective analysis of APEX-AMI showed that GP IIb/IIIa use was associated with a significantly lower 90-day mortality and combined incidence of death, CHF, and shock.[94] A recent meta-analysis of abciximab use in primary stenting, which included high-risk patients with STEMI, showed a significant reduction in the composite endpoint of death or re-infarction with abciximab for up to 3 years of follow-up (12.9% vs. 19.0%, $P = 0.008$); mortality alone was reduced (10.9% vs. 14.3%, $P = 0.052$).[95] Another more recent meta-analysis, which included 16 trials with 10,085 patients, showed that GP IIb/IIIa inhibitors—mostly abciximab—did not reduce 30-day mortality (2.8 vs. 2.9%, $P = 0.75$) or re-infarction (1.5 vs. 1.9%, $P = 0.22$) but were associated with higher risk of major bleeding (4.1 vs. 2.7%, $P < 0.001$). An interaction between patient risk and benefits from GP IIb/IIIa inhibitors in terms of mortality was observed ($P = 0.008$).[96] The recently published BRAVE-3 (the Bavarian Reperfusion Alternatives Evaluation-3) trial included 800 patients, all pretreated with a 600-mg loading dose of clopidogrel, who were randomized to abciximab or placebo. Infarct size measured with sestamibi SPECT imaging at discharge (15.7% vs. 16.6%, $P = 0.47$) or 30-day incidence of death, re-infarction, stroke, or urgent revascularization (5% vs. 3.8%, $P = 0.40$) did not differ significantly between patients assigned to abciximab and those assigned to placebo (Fig. 18-16, *A* and *B*).[97] The trial raises doubts concerning the routine use of abciximab in the setting of primary PCI after pretreatment with clopidogrel.[97] The efficacy of intracoronary abciximab has been recently assessed in the CICERO (Comparison of Intracoronary Versus Intravenous Abciximab Administration During Emergency Reperfusion of ST-Segment Elevation Myocardial Infarction) study, which randomized 534 patients with STEMI to intravenous or intracoronary abciximab infusion.[98] In this trial, intracoronary administration of abciximab did not improve myocardial reperfusion, as assessed by ST segment resolution (the primary endpoint); however, it improved myocardial reperfusion, as assessed by myocardial blush, and reduced the enzymatic infarct size compared with intravenous administration. In summary, the place of GP IIb/IIIa inhibitors in the era of contemporary primary PCI is not fully clear. Apparently, patients who receive immediate high-dose clopidogrel pretreatment on presentation appear to derive little benefit from this therapy. The role of GP IIb/IIIa inhibitors is expected to be further reduced with the introduction of more potent anti-platelet drugs as alternatives to clopidogrel.

In keeping with this, the use of a loading dose of clopidogrel before primary PCI has become a standard approach. A recent report from the HORIZONS-AMI trial showed that the 600-mg clopidogrel loading dose compared with the 300-mg dose reduced significantly the 30-day mortality (1.9% vs. 3.1%, $P = 0.03$), re-infarction (1.3% vs. 2.3%, $P = 0.02$), and definite or probable stent thrombosis (1.7% vs. 2.8%, $P = 0.04$), without incurring higher bleeding rates.[99] In a subgroup analysis of the Trial to Assess Improvement in Therapeutic Outcomes by Optimizing Platelet Inhibition with Prasugrel–Thrombolysis in myocardial Infarction 38 (TRITON-TIMI 38), which included patients with STEMI who underwent primary PCI, prasugrel (60-mg loading dose and 10-mg daily maintenance dose) was associated with a significant 21% risk reduction (10.0% vs. 12.4%, $P = 0.022$) of the composite endpoint of death from cardiovascular causes, nonfatal MI, or nonfatal stroke compared with clopidogrel (300-mg loading dose and 75-mg daily maintenance dose) (Fig. 18-17).[100] Life-threatening bleeding and TIMI major or minor bleeding were also similar with the two treatments; TIMI major bleeding after coronary artery bypass grafting (CABG) was significantly higher with prasugrel (18.8% vs. 2.7%, $P = 0.0033$).[100] In the subset of 7544 patients with STEMI from the Platelet Inhibition and Patient Outcomes (PLATO) trial treated with PCI,

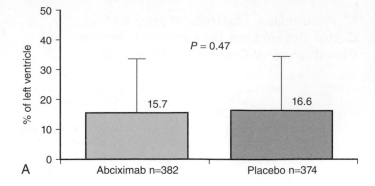

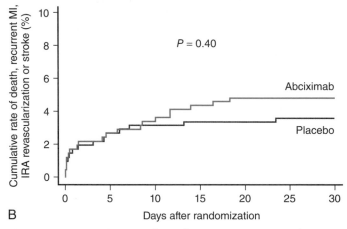

Figure 18-16 A, Scintigraphic infarct size (primary endpoint) in patients randomized to abciximab or placebo in the BRAVE-3 trial. **B,** The 30-day cumulative rate of death, recurrent myocardial infarction, infarct-related artery revascularization, or stroke in patients randomized to abciximab or placebo in the BRAVE-3 trial. *(Mehilli J, Kastrati A, Schulz S, et al: Abciximab in patients with acute ST-segment-elevation myocardial infarction undergoing primary percutaneous coronary intervention after clopidogrel loading: A randomized double-blind trial,* Circulation *119:1933–1940, 2009.)*

ticagrelor (initial 180-mg loading followed by 90 mg twice daily) was compared with clopidogrel (300–600 mg loading followed by 75 mg daily) (Fig. 18-18). The primary endpoint of death from vascular causes, MI, or stroke occurred in 9.4% of the ticagrelor group and 10.8% of the clopidogrel group ($P = 0.07$). There were significant differences between ticagrelor and clopidogrel in all-cause mortality (5.0% vs. 6.1%, $P = 0.05$) with a trend for reduction in cardiovascular mortality (4.5% vs. 5.5%, $P = 0.07$), definite stent thrombosis (1.6% vs. 2.4%, $P = 0.03$), and MI (4.7% vs. 5.8%, $P = 0.03$) without a detectable difference in major bleeding (9.0% vs. 9.2%, $P = 0.76$).[101] Although data concerning the role of prasugrel and ticagrelor in primary PCI are derived from subgroup analyses, both drugs seem promising as anti-thrombotic agents for primary PCI procedures.

Bivalirudin—a direct thrombin inhibitor—has recently been tested in the HORIZONS-AMI trial, which included 3602 patients with STEMI who presented within 12 hours after the onset of symptoms and who were randomized to primary PCI with heparin plus a GP IIb/IIIa inhibitor or bivalirudin alone.[102] Co-primary endpoints—major bleeding and net adverse clinical events (the combined endpoint of major bleeding, death, re-infarction, target-vessel revascularization or stroke) at 30-days—were used to judge the efficacy of treatment. Anticoagulation with bivalirudin alone, compared with heparin plus GP IIb/IIIa inhibitors, was associated with a reduced 30-day rate of net adverse clinical events (9.2% vs. 12.1%, $P = 0.005$) and a lower rate of major bleeding (4.9% vs. 8.3%, $P < 0.001$). Of importance was the

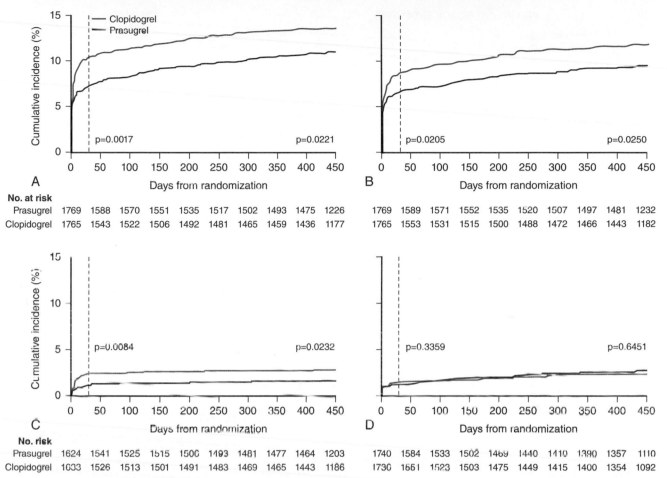

Figure 18-17 Kaplan–Meier estimates for patients randomized to prasugrel or clopidogrel in patients undergoing percutaneous coronary intervention for ST segment elevation myocardial infarction in the TRITON-TIMI 38 trial. **A,** Primary study endpoint (cardiovascular death, nonfatal myocardial infarction, or nonfatal stroke). **B,** Key secondary endpoint (cardiovascular death, nonfatal myocardial infarction, or urgent target vessel revascularization. **C,** Stent thrombosis. **D,** TIMI major bleeding unrelated to CABG surgery. Dotted line represents 30 days. *(Montalescot G, Wiviott SD, Braunwald E, et al: Prasugrel compared with clopidogrel in patients undergoing percutaneous coronary intervention for ST-elevation myocardial infarction (TRITON-TIMI 38). Double-blind, randomised controlled trial, Lancet 373:723–731, 2009.)*

finding that treatment with bivalirudin alone reduced the 30-day incidence of cardiac (1.8% vs. 2.9%, $P = 0.03$) and all-cause mortality (2.1% vs. 3.1%, $P = 0.047$) (Fig. 18-19). The rate of stent thrombosis within the first 24 hours was higher following treatment with bivalirudin (1.3% vs. 0.3%, $P < 0.001$), though this did not persist at 30 days. The benefits of bivalirudin treatment were maintained for up to 3 years of follow-up.[83] These results strongly support the use of bivalirudin as an anticoagulant or anti-thrombotic regimen in the setting of primary PCI. The reduced rate of bleeding complications with bivalirudin is considered to be the driving force behind the reduced rate of adverse clinical events, including mortality. There are no properly designed studies on the value of low-molecular-weight heparins (LMWH) and factor Xa inhibitors in patients with STEMI treated with PCI. A PCI subset analysis from the Organization for the Assessment of Strategies for Ischemic Syndromes (OASIS-6) trial could not show any benefit with the use of fondaparinux.[103]

Adjunct Pharmacologic Therapies to Improve Myocardial Tissue Reperfusion

No-reflow is a frequent finding in patients with STEMI treated with primary PCI, and its presence is associated with reduced myocardial salvage, increased infarct size, impaired left ventricular function and increased risk of short-term and long-term mortality (Figure 18-20, A and B).[104,105] In recent years, various pharmacologic (see the section on Facilitated PCI) and nonpharmacologic approaches (see the section on Adjunctive Thrombectomy and Distal Protection Devices in Primary PCI) have been used as adjunct therapy to PCI to enhance myocardial reperfusion and salvage and to improve outcome in patients with STEMI.

Adenosine—a potent vasodilator of arterioles—and adenosine agonists have been recently tested as adjunctive therapy to PCI in patients with STEMI. It is hypothesized that adenosine, through its effects on microcirculatory function and its consistent protective effects on myocardial ischemic injury, would promote myocardial salvage and improve clinical outcome. In experimental studies, adenosine reduces ischemia-reperfusion injury, limits infarct size, and improves left ventricular function. In the AMISTAD-II (Acute Myocardial Infarction Study of Adenosine) trial, 2118 patients with anterior STEMI receiving thrombolysis or primary angioplasty were randomized to a 3-hour infusion of adenosine 50 or 70 mcg/kg/min or of placebo.[106] Adenosine did not reduce the combined endpoint of death, new heart failure, or first hospitalization for heart failure within 6 months (16.3% with adenosine vs. 17.9% with placebo). Infarct size, measured with sestamibi scintigraphy was reduced with high-dose adenosine (70 mcg/kg/min) but not with low-dose adenosine (50 mcg/kg/min). In a recent trial of 448 patients with STEMI, randomized to double intracoronary

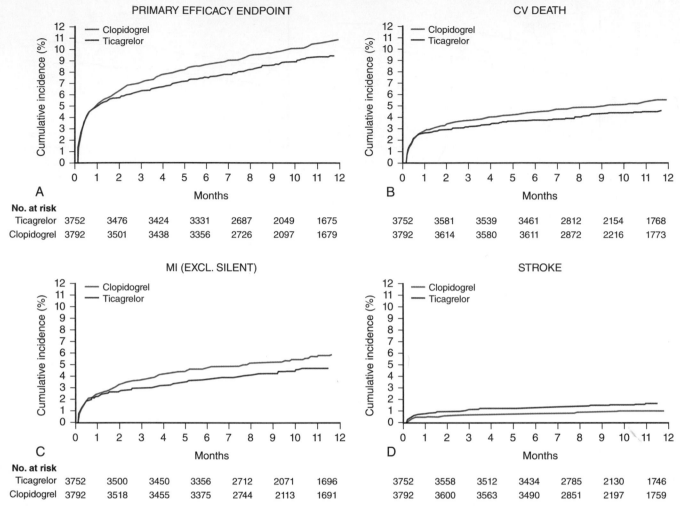

Figure 18-18 **A,** Kaplan–Meier estimates of the time to first occurrence of the primary endpoint (incidence of myocardial infarction [MI], stroke, or vascular death) and each of its components for patients with ST-segment elevation acute coronary syndromes undergoing primary PCI who received ticagrelor or clopidogrel in the Platelet Inhibition and Patient Outcomes (PLATO) trial. **B,** Cardiovascular death. **C,** Myocardial infarction. **D,** Stroke. *(Steg PG, James S, Harrington RA, et al: Ticagrelor versus clopidogrel in patients with ST-elevation acute coronary syndromes intended for reperfusion with primary percutaneous coronary intervention: A Platelet Inhibition and Patient Outcomes (PLATO) trial subgroup analysis,* Circulation *122:2131–2141, 2010.)*

boluses of adenosine (2 × 120 mcg) or placebo, there were no significant differences in ST segment resolution, myocardial blush grade, TIMI flow grade, enzymatic infarct size, or clinical outcome at 20 days.[107] The first bolus was given after thrombus aspiration, whereas the second one was given after stent deployment.

Sodium nitroprusside—a direct nitric oxide donor—has multiple vascular functions, including arteriolar vasodilatation, platelet inhibition, and anti-inflammatory actions. When given as intracoronary repeated doses of 120 mcg before each balloon inflation, sodium nitroprusside reduced no-reflow and improved reperfusion in the infarcted region, as assessed by myocardial blush and corrected TIMI flow count.[108] Another study of 40 patients undergoing primary PCI assigned patients to 4 anti–no-reflow strategies: intracoronary injection of sodium nitroprusside (100–150 mcg), adenosine (60–120 mcg), verapamil (100–500 mcg), or nitroglycerin (200–400 mcg; control group).[109] Sodium nitroprusside was the most beneficial agent in improving the myocardial blush grade and LVEF. A recent randomized trial assigned 98 patients with STEMI to sodium nitroprusside (single dose of 60 mcg injected in the infarct-related artery) or placebo.[110] Although sodium nitroprusside failed to improve coronary flow or tissue reperfusion, the drug reduced the 6-month composite endpoint of death, re-infarction, or target lesion revascularization (6.3% vs. 20%, *P* = 0.05). It has to be mentioned that all studies that assessed the

efficacy of sodium nitroprusside included limited numbers of patients with STEMI, used different doses and routes of drug administration, and had multiple methodologic inconsistencies, so the role of this drug in the management of patients with STEMI is still largely unknown. Based on the experimental evidence that complement system activation may be involved in reperfusion-associated ischemic injury, the effect of pexelizumab—a humanized monoclonal antibody that binds the C5 component of complement—on clinical outcome in patients with STEMI undergoing primary PCI has been evaluated in the APEX-AMI trial.[111] The trial randomized 5745 patients with STEMI (within 6 hours from symptom onset) to receive pexelizumab (2-mg/kg intravenous bolus before PCI followed by 0.05 mg/kg/hr infusion over the subsequent 24 hours) or placebo. No difference in 30-day rate of all-cause mortality (4.06% vs. 3.92%, *P* = 0.78) or in the composite endpoint of death, cardiogenic shock, or CHF at 30 days (8.99% vs. 9.19%, *P* = 0.81) or 90 days (10.24% vs. 10.16%, *P* = 0.91) between pexelizumab and placebo groups was observed.[111] This trial showed that mortality was not affected by pexelizumab. Overall, there is no evidence supporting the use of complement system inhibitors in patients with STEMI undergoing primary PCI. A recent meta-analysis has summarized the effects of the use of nicorandil—a hybrid compound of adenosine triphosphate (ATP)–sensitive potassium channel opener and nitric oxide donor—as adjunctive therapy in patients with STEMI

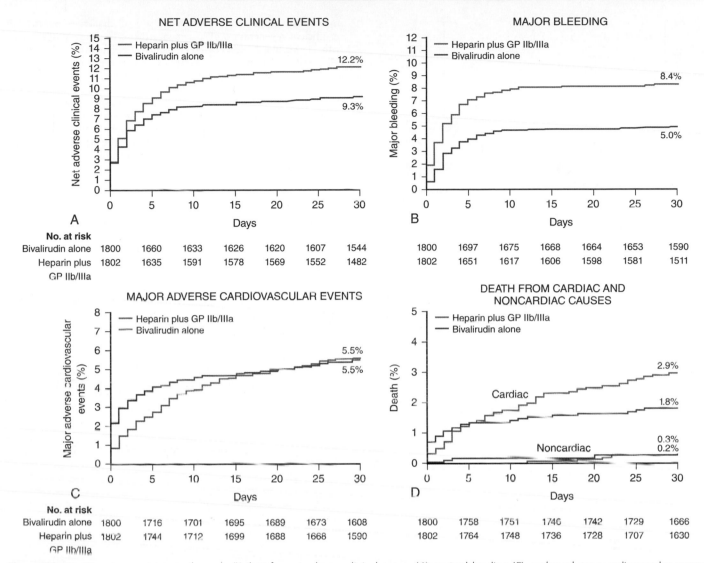

Figure 10-19 Time-to-event curves through 30 days for net adverse clinical events (A), major bleeding (B), major adverse cardiovascular events (C), and death from cardiac and noncardiac causes (D) in the HORIZONS AMI trial comparing bivalirudin with heparin plus glycoprotein IIb/IIIa. (Stone GW, Witzenbichler B, Guagliumi G, et al: Bivalirudin during primary PCI in acute myocardial infarction, N Engl J Med 358:2210–2230, 2008.)

undergoing PCI. The data show that nicorandil treatment reduced the incidence of TIMI flow grade 2 or less, had no effect on peak creatine kinase value, and improved LVEF.[112] However, the studies included are small, and the data are still not sufficient to allow a firm recommendation for the use of ATP-sensitive potassium channel openers in primary PCI. In the CAldaret in patients undergoing primary percutaneous coronary intervention for ST-Elevation Myocardial Infarction (CASTEMI) trial, 387 patients with STEMI were randomized within 6 hours to caldaret (an agent purported to reduce intracellular calcium by inhibiting the sodium–calcium exchanger and enhancing calcium reuptake by the sarcoplasmic reticulum) or placebo. Caldaret was not associated with reduction in infarct size or improvement in left ventricular function, as assessed by gated SPECT imaging.[113] A subsequent publication from the same trial reported that at post-infarct day 30, there was a significant decrease in the incidence of LV dysfunction in patients receiving low and high doses of caldaret versus placebo (8.0%, 6.9% vs. 17.5%, P < 0.05 for both comparisons).[114]

Limited information exists on other agents or approaches used as adjunctive to primary PCI in patients with STEMI. The Acute Myocardial Infarction with Hyperoxemic Therapy (AMIHOT) trial randomized patients with acute MI within 24 hours after primary stenting to intracoronary hyperoxemic reperfusion with aqueous oxygen or controls.[114a] Although the hyperoxemic reperfusion was safe and well tolerated, it did not cause any improvement in ST segment resolution, regional wall motion by serial echocardiography, or reduction in SPECT infarct size. In post hoc analysis, however, patients with anterior MI reperfused within 6 hours showed a greater improvement in regional wall motion and smaller infarct size (9.0% vs. 23% of the left ventricle, P = 0.03) with hyperoxemic reperfusion. These findings were further corroborated in the AMIHOT-II trial, which included 301 patients with STEMI of anterior wall.[116] The trial showed that intracoronary delivery of supersaturated oxygen reduced scintigraphic infarct size (20% vs. 26.5%, adjusted P = 0.03) with noninferior rates of major adverse cardiac events at 30 days, compared with placebo. Active cooling as a means of cardioprotection has also recently been evaluated. The COOL-MI (COOling as an adjunctive therapy to percutaneous intervention in patients with acute Myocardial Infarction) evaluated the effect of systemic hypothermia by randomizing 395 patients with STEMI presenting within 6 hours to primary PCI with mild hypothermia or primary PCI alone.[115] While the procedure was well tolerated, no effect of cooling on final infarct size at 30 days could be demonstrated. A recent small trial randomized 58 patients with STEMI to either an intravenous bolus of 2.5 mg of cyclosporine (a potent inhibitor of the mitochondrial permeability–transition pore)

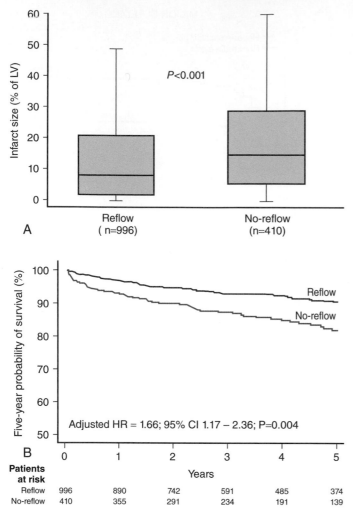

Figure 18-20   Infarct size (medians [25th-75th percentiles]) in the 7–14 days scintigraphy (A) and Kaplan–Meier curves of five-year mortality (B) in patients with reflow and no-reflow after primary percutaneous coronary intervention (PCI) for ST elevation myocardial infarction (STEMI). LV, left ventricle; HR, hazard ratio. (Ndrepepa G, Tiroch K, Fusaro M, et al: 5-year prognostic value of no-reflow phenomenon after percutaneous coronary intervention in patients with acute myocardial infarction, J Am Coll Cardiol 55:2383–2389, 2010.)

per kilogram of body weight or to normal saline immediately before PCI. Infarct size was assessed by measuring the release of creatine kinase and troponin I. In 27 patients, infarct size was measured with MRI on day 5 after infarction. All three estimates showed a reduction in infarct size with cyclosporin; the median infarct size (estimated with MRI) was 37 g in the cyclosporine group and 46 g in the control group (P = 0.04). No adverse effects were reported in patients who received cyclosporine.[117] In summary, although there is still interest in a variety of adjunctive interventions directed at limiting no-reflow, reducing infarct size, and enhancing myocardial perfusion, available evidence is not strong enough to recommend that any of these interventions be routinely used as an adjunct to primary PCI in patients with STEMI.

Cell-Based Therapy and Regenerative Agents after ST Elevation Myocardial Infarction

Reperfusion therapy has proven to be life saving in patients with STEMI; however, progression of the disease toward chronic myocardial dysfunction still remains a real challenge. Because of insufficient regeneration of lost myocardial cells, intuitively, patients with STEMI may be considered as prime candidates for application of cell-based cardiac repair techniques to enhance myocardial recovery after myocardial necrosis by replacing lost myocytes. Animal studies of MI have reported that stem cell transplantation and progenitor cell transplantation have resulted in neoangiogenesis, myogenesis, and improved contractile function. At present, however, it is still unclear whether the beneficial effect from stem cells results from differentiation into myocytes or blood vessels or through the cytokine–paracrine mechanisms that modulate metabolism, inotropism, apoptosis, and inflammation.[118] A number of recent studies, mostly involving limited numbers of patients, have evaluated the use of various stem cell–based techniques for myocardial regeneration in patients with STEMI after PCI. A number of recent meta-analyses have summarized the results of these trials. One meta-analysis included 13 randomized controlled trials with 811 patients.[119] The pooled analysis of trials showed that stem cell therapy demonstrated modest efficacy, with improvement in LVEF by 2.99% (P < 0.001, Fig. 18-21), reduction in left ventricular end-systolic volume by 4.74 mL (P = 0.003), and reduction in myocardial infarct area by 3.51% (P = 0.004) compared with controls. Subgroup analysis revealed that the best results in improving left ventricular function were achieved when bone marrow–derived stem cells were infused within 7 days following acute MI and the cell dose was higher than 108 cells. Moreover, there were trends in favor of benefit for most clinical outcomes, but statistical significance was not achieved. Another recent meta-analysis of intracoronary autologous bone marrow stem cell transfer, which included a total of six trials with 525 patients with STEMI undergoing PCI, showed an absolute increase in LVEF (4.77%, P = 0.005) compared with controls, with no significant difference in end-diastolic left ventricular dimensions or major adverse cardiac events.[120] These summarized data of existing randomized trials show a slight but significant improvement in LVEF but no significant effect of stem cell therapy on clinical outcome.

The ability of granulocyte colony-stimulating factor (G-CSF) to mobilize stem cells from bone marrow (CD34+ mononuclear blood stem cells) and to increase their circulating levels has led to its use for stem cell mobilization (G-CSF injection) in patients with STEMI and for harvesting stem cells for intracoronary delivery. Recent data on this agent have shown conflicting results. A meta-analysis of 10 randomized trials with 445 patients demonstrated a significant improvement of LVEF in the groups treated with G-CSF injection versus placebo with a mean difference of 1.32% (P = 0.36, Fig. 18-22), with no significant difference in infarct size (P = 0.17), target vessel revascularization rates, or mortality at follow-up.[121] On the basis of source studies and the results of this meta-analysis, G-CSF does not represent a useful therapy in patients with STEMI undergoing PCI.

In experimental and small-scale clinical studies, erythropoietin has shown promise as a cardioprotective agent with the capacity to improve the left ventricular function. Randomized studies, so far, have not been promising.[122,123] In a recent randomized study of 138 patients with STEMI treated with primary PCI, erythropoietin (3.33 × 104 units) given 24 to 48 hours after primary PCI failed to reduce scintigraphic infarct size measured at 5 days and 6 months after randomization or to improve LVEF at 6 months. The cumulative 6-month incidence of death, recurrent MI, stroke, or target vessel revascularization was 13.2% in the erythropoietin group and 5.7% in the placebo group (P = 0.15).[122] In another randomized study of 529 patients with STEMI treated with primary PCI, a single dose of erythropoietin (60,000 international units) given within 3 hours of PCI did not improve left ventricular function at 6 weeks. However, less major adverse cardiovascular events occurred in the erythropoietin group (8%) than in the control group (19%, P = 0.032) patients.[123]

In summary, cell-based therapy for cardiac regeneration is still under investigation on multiple fronts, including types of cells used,

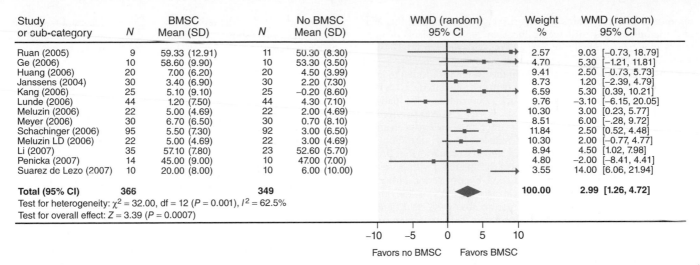

Study or sub-category	N	BMSC Mean (SD)	N	No BMSC Mean (SD)	WMD (random) 95% CI	Weight %	WMD (random) 95% CI
Ruan (2005)	9	59.33 (12.91)	11	50.30 (8.30)		2.57	9.03 [−0.73, 18.79]
Ge (2006)	10	58.60 (9.90)	10	53.30 (3.50)		4.70	5.30 [−1.21, 11.81]
Huang (2006)	20	7.00 (6.20)	20	4.50 (3.99)		9.41	2.50 [−0.73, 5.73]
Janssens (2004)	30	3.40 (6.90)	30	2.20 (7.30)		8.73	1.20 [−2.39, 4.79]
Kang (2006)	25	5.10 (9.10)	25	−0.20 (8.60)		6.59	5.30 [0.39, 10.21]
Lunde (2006)	44	1.20 (7.50)	44	4.30 (7.10)		9.76	−3.10 [−6.15, 20.05]
Meluzin (2006)	22	5.00 (4.69)	22	2.00 (4.69)		10.30	3.00 [0.23, 5.77]
Meyer (2006)	30	6.70 (6.50)	30	0.70 (8.10)		8.51	6.00 [−.28, 9.72]
Schachinger (2006)	95	5.50 (7.30)	92	3.00 (6.50)		11.84	2.50 [0.52, 4.48]
Meluzin LD (2006)	22	5.00 (4.69)	22	3.00 (4.69)		10.30	2.00 [−0.77, 4.77]
Li (2007)	35	57.10 (7.80)	23	52.60 (5.70)		8.94	4.50 [1.02, 7.98]
Penicka (2007)	14	45.00 (9.00)	10	47.00 (7.00)		4.80	−2.00 [−8.41, 4.41]
Suarez de Lezo (2007)	10	20.00 (8.00)	10	6.00 (10.00)		3.55	14.00 [6.06, 21.94]
Total (95% CI)	**366**		**349**			**100.00**	**2.99 [1.26, 4.72]**

Test for heterogeneity: $\chi^2 = 32.00$, df = 12 ($P = 0.001$), $I^2 = 62.5\%$
Test for overall effect: $Z = 3.39$ ($P = 0.0007$)

−10   −5   0   5   10

Favors no BMSC   Favors BMSC

Figure 18-21 Weighted mean difference (WMD; with 95% confidence interval [CI]) in left ventricular ejection fraction (LVEF) in patients treated with autologous bone marrow–derived stem cell (BMSC) compared with controls. Infusion of BMSC significantly improved LVEF by 2.99% ($P = 0.0007$). (*Martin-Rendon E, Brunskill SJ, Hyde CJ, Stanworth SJ, Mathur A, Watt SM: Autologous bone marrow stem cells to treat acute myocardial infarction: a systematic review, Eur Heart J 29:1807–1818, 2008.*)

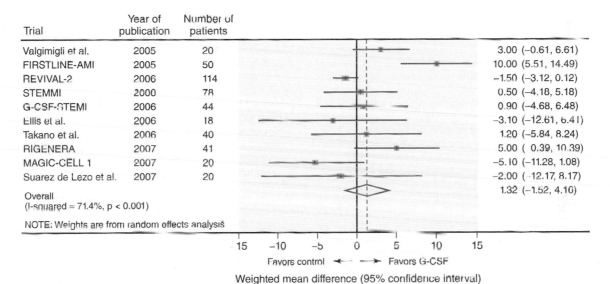

Trial	Year of publication	Number of patients		
Valgimigli et al.	2005	20		3.00 (−0.61, 6.61)
FIRSTLINE-AMI	2005	50		10.00 (5.51, 14.49)
REVIVAL-2	2006	114		−1.50 (−3.12, 0.12)
STEMMI	2006	78		0.50 (−4.18, 5.18)
G-CSF-STEMI	2006	44		0.90 (−4.68, 6.48)
Ellis et al.	2006	18		−3.10 (−12.61, 6.41)
Takano et al.	2006	40		1.20 (−5.84, 8.24)
RIGENERA	2007	41		5.00 (0.39, 10.39)
MAGIC-CELL 1	2007	20		−5.10 (−11.28, 1.08)
Suarez de Lezo et al.	2007	20		−2.00 (−12.17, 8.17)
Overall (I-squared = 71.4%, p < 0.001)				1.32 (−1.52, 4.16)

NOTE: Weights are from random effects analysis

15   −10   −5   0   5   10   15

Favors control   ←   →   Favors G-CSF

Weighted mean difference (95% confidence interval)

Figure 18-22 The effect of stem cell mobilization by granulocyte colony-stimulating factor (G-CSF) on change in left ventricular ejection fraction. Compared with conventional treatment, stem cell mobilization by G-CSF had no additional beneficial effect on change in left ventricular function at follow-up as shown by the weighted mean difference for change in left ventricular ejection fraction between treatment and control groups in individual trials. *FIRSTLINE-AMI,* Front-Integrated Revascularization and Stem Cell Liberation in Evolving Acute Myocardial Infarction trial; *G-CSF-STEMI,* Granulocyte Colony-Stimulating Factor ST-Segment Elevation Myocardial Infarction trial; *MAGIC Cell 1,* Myocardial Regeneration and Angiogenesis in Myocardial Infarction with G-CSF and Intra-Coronary Stem Cell Infusion 1 trial; *REVIVAL-2,* Regenerate Vital Myocardium by Vigorous Activation of Bone Marrow Stem Cells trial; *STEMMI* = Stem Cells in Myocardial Infarction trial. (*Zohlnhöfer D, Dibra A, Koppara T, et al: Stem cell mobilization by granulocyte colony-stimulating factor for myocardial recovery after acute myocardial infarction: a meta-analysis, J Am Coll Cardiol 51:1429–1437, 2008.*)

magnitude of benefit, routes and time of administration, mechanism(s) of action, and possible adverse effects such as arrhythmogenesis, oncogenic transformation, multi-organ seeding, aberrant cell differentiation, and accelerated atherosclerosis. Available evidence does not support the use of G-CSF to mobilize stem cells from bone marrow to enhance cardiac regeneration in patients with STEMI after primary PCI. Further studies are needed to clarify the role of intracoronary injection of bone marrow–derived stem cells in patients with STEMI. Information available on the use of erythropoietin as a regenerative agent in patients with STEMI is not supportive and is limited.

Special Issues of Primary Percutaneous Coronary Intervention

CARDIOGENIC SHOCK

Cardiogenic shock is a serious complication and remains the major cause of death in patients with STEMI. Primary PCI is a class 1 recommendation in patients with STEMI less than 75 years old who develop cardiogenic shock.[1,9] Despite advances in primary PCI technique and adjunctive care, the prognosis of patients with cardiogenic shock that complicates STEMI remains grave. A survey from the NRMI that analyzed the outcome of cardiogenic shock in 293,633 patients demonstrated an increase in PCI rates for patients with shock from 27.4% to 54.4% from 1995 to 2004.[124] The study showed that the increase in PCI rates was associated with a reduction in the overall in-hospital mortality from 60.3% to 47.9%. Of 22,883 patients enrolled in the GUSTO-I Trial (U.S. patients), cardiogenic shock occurred in 1891 patients (8.3%). Of patients with cardiogenic shock, 953 (50.4%) survived 30 days, and 527 (2.8%) survived 11 years after an acute event. Primary PCI was an independent correlate of reduced 30-day mortality. The Should We Emergently Revascularize Occluded Coronaries for Cardiogenic Shock (SHOCK) trial randomized 302 patients with acute MI complicated by cardiogenic shock to receive early revascularization (mostly PCI, $n = 152$) or initial medical stabilization ($n = 150$) treatment.[125] At 1 year of follow-up, there was an absolute 13% difference in survival rates favoring patients assigned to an early revascularization approach. This benefit in survival remained almost unchanged (13.1% and 13.2%, respectively) at 3 years and 6 years of follow-up. The 6-year survival rates for hospital survivors were 62.4% in those assigned to early revascularization and 44.4% in those assigned to initial medical stabilization with annual rates of death of 8.3% and 14.3%, respectively. For 1-year survivors, the annual rates of death were 8% and 10.7%, again favoring patients assigned to early revascularization. The SHOCK trial demonstrated that almost two thirds of hospital survivors with cardiogenic shock complicating acute MI who were treated with early revascularization survived at 6-year follow-up.[125] The trial strongly recommended early revascularization in patients with acute MI complicated by cardiogenic shock. Although evidence from specifically designed studies is still lacking, intra-aortic balloon pumping represents almost a standard treatment in patients with STEMI complicated by cardiogenic shock. Alternative percutaneous left ventricular assist devices are also under investigation in this setting.[126] The recently published TRIUMPH (Tilarginine Acetate Injection in a Randomized International Study in Unstable MI Patients With Cardiogenic Shock) tested the impact of nitric oxide inhibition with tilarginine—a nitric oxide synthase inhibitor—in patients with STEMI who developed cardiogenic shock; 96% of them were treated with PCI. The study randomized 398 patients to tilarginine (1 mg/kg bolus and 1 mg/kg per hour 5-hour infusion) or to placebo. The 30-day (48% vs. 42%, $P = 0.24$) and 6-month (58% vs. 59%, $P = 0.80$) all-cause mortality did not differ between patients assigned to tilarginine or placebo.[127] The study was terminated before completion for reasons of futility. Apart from the failure of nitric oxide inhibition to improve outcome, the study showed that early mortality in patients with cardiogenic shock remains high despite recent advances in mechanical and pharmacologic therapies.

PRIMARY PERCUTANEOUS CORONARY INTERVENTION DURING OFF-HOURS

The relationship between time of day when patients with STEMI present to the hospital and outcomes from primary PCI and in-hospital mortality has been recently addressed. In the CADILLAC trial, which included 2082 patients undergoing primary PCI, 49% of patients presented during off-hours or weekends.[128] Although there was a 21-minute delay in time-to-treatment in those presenting during off-hours, this delay did not impact procedural success, myocardial recovery, or survival after primary PCI. A recent analysis of 102,086 patients with STEMI who underwent reperfusion (68,439 patients underwent thrombolysis, and 33,647 patients underwent PCI) showed that in 67.9% of patients treated with thrombolysis and in 54.2% of patients treated with PCI, reperfusion was performed during off-hours.[44] For patients treated with PCI, door-to-balloon time was 21.3 minutes longer for patients presenting during off-hours than for those presenting during regular hours (116.1 minutes vs. 94.8 minutes). Patients presenting during off-hours and undergoing PCI had a trend to higher in-hospital mortality than did patients presenting during regular hours (odds ratio 1.05; 95% CI 0.95–1.16, $P = 0.30$).[44] A recent study of 747

patients admitted to the Massachusetts General Hospital who underwent primary PCI showed that patients admitted during off-hours had higher in-hospital mortality (8% vs. 3.7%, $P = 0.01$), higher rates of cardiogenic shock (37% vs. 24%, $P < 0.001$), and longer door-to-balloon times (134 vs. 109 minutes, $P < 0.001$) than patients admitted on hours.[129] Along the same lines, a recent report of 685 patients undergoing primary PCI in the NHLBI Dynamic Registry between 1997 and 2006 showed that the composite of in-hospital death, infarction, or target vessel revascularization was significantly higher in off-hours patients (16.2% vs. 6.8%, adjusted $P = 0.002$).[130]

PRIMARY PERCUTANEOUS CORONARY INTERVENTION IN OLDER ADULTS

Older adult patients represent an increasing proportion of those admitted to hospital with STEMI, and advanced age is an important correlate of poor outcome after both PCI and thrombolysis. It is widely accepted that primary PCI in older adults is more challenging for a variety of reasons such as more complex coronary anatomy (multivessel disease, calcified and tortuous coronary arteries with lower rates of TIMI flow grade 3 after the procedure), increased rate of bleeding complications, increased rate of vascular complications because of a higher prevalence of peripheral vascular disease, increased prevalence of comorbidities such as impaired renal function predisposing to contrast nephropathy, delayed presentation, and atypical symptoms. The optimal management of patients with STEMI is still unclear, at least in part because of under-representation of older adults and the very old in trials that have established therapeutic value of primary PCI. The PCAT-2 meta-analysis reported that the absolute reduction of mortality with primary PCI increased with advancing age, from, 1% at ages under 65 years to 6.9% at ages 85 years or over.[14] So far, three randomized trials have assessed the efficacy of primary PCI in older adults. A small study that included 87 patients 75 years of age or older showed that primary PCI was superior to thrombolysis with streptokinase in reducing the composite endpoint of death, re-infarction, or stroke at 1 year (13% vs. 44%, $P = 0.001$).[131] In the Senior Primary Angioplasty in Myocardial Infarction (SENIOR PAMI) trial, 481 patients over 70 years of age were randomized to PCI or thrombolysis. In patients age 70 to 80 years, there was a trend toward reduced 30-day mortality with primary PCI (7.1% vs. 11.3%, $P = 0.17$) and a significant reduction in the composite endpoint of death, re-infarction, or stroke (7.7% vs. 17.0%, $P < 0.01$) with primary PCI compared with thrombolysis. However, none of these endpoints differed between the two treatment options in patients over 80 years of age.[132] The TRIANA (TRatamiento del Infarto Agudo de miocardio eN Ancianos, or Treatment of Acute Myocardial Infarction in the Elderly) study included 266 patients 75 years of age or older who were randomized to primary PCI (134 patients) or thrombolysis (132 patients). The trial reported a trend toward reduction in the 30-day composite endpoint of death, re-infarction, or disabling stroke with primary PCI (18.9% vs. 25.4%, $P = 0.21$).[133] Non-significant reductions were found in the incidence of death (13.6% vs. 17.2%, $P = 0.43$), re-infarction (5.3% vs. 8.2%, $P = 0.35$), or disabling stroke (0.8% vs. 3.0%, $P = 0.18$). Recurrent ischemia was encountered less commonly in primary PCI-treated patients (0.8% vs. 9.7%, $P = 0.001$). It is notable that both Senior-PAMI and TRIANA trials were terminated before completion because of slow recruitment. These results were reinforced by a recent meta-analysis of all three studies (Fig. 18-23).[133]

PRIMARY PERCUTANEOUS CORONARY INTERVENTION AND MULTI-VESSEL INTERVENTION

Multi-vessel coronary artery disease occurs in approximately 50% of patients undergoing primary PCI for STEMI, and its presence is associated with reduced reperfusion success and an adverse prognosis following primary PCI.[134,135] The increased cardiovascular risk in patients with multi-vessel coronary artery disease is explained by a series of factors, including impaired function of the noninfarct zone, impact of

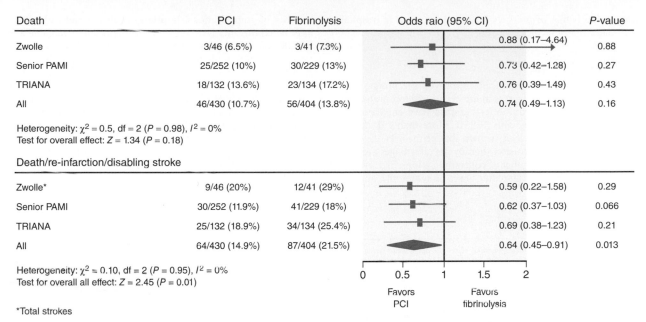

Death	PCI	Fibrinolysis	Odds ratio (95% CI)	P-value
Zwolle	3/46 (6.5%)	3/41 (7.3%)	0.88 (0.17–4.64)	0.88
Senior PAMI	25/252 (10%)	30/229 (13%)	0.73 (0.42–1.28)	0.27
TRIANA	18/132 (13.6%)	23/134 (17.2%)	0.76 (0.39–1.49)	0.43
All	46/430 (10.7%)	56/404 (13.8%)	0.74 (0.49–1.13)	0.16

Heterogeneity: $\chi^2 = 0.5$, df = 2 ($P = 0.98$), $I^2 = 0\%$
Test for overall effect: $Z = 1.34$ ($P = 0.18$)

Death/re-infarction/disabling stroke				
Zwolle*	9/46 (20%)	12/41 (29%)	0.59 (0.22–1.58)	0.29
Senior PAMI	30/252 (11.9%)	41/229 (18%)	0.62 (0.37–1.03)	0.066
TRIANA	25/132 (18.9%)	34/134 (25.4%)	0.69 (0.38–1.23)	0.21
All	64/430 (14.9%)	87/404 (21.5%)	0.64 (0.45–0.91)	0.013

Heterogeneity: $\chi^2 = 0.10$, df = 2 ($P = 0.95$), $I^2 = 0\%$
Test for overall all effect: $Z = 2.45$ ($P = 0.01$)

Favors PCI — Favors fibrinolysis

*Total strokes

Figure 18-23 Odds ratios for mortality and incidence of the combined endpoint in the three randomized trials comparing primary percutaneous coronary intervention and fibrinolysis performed in very old patients with ST segment elevation myocardial infarction. *PCI*, percutaneous coronary intervention.[133]

extensive atherosclerotic disease, presence of stunned and hibernating myocardium, and slow flow in the critically narrowed non–infarct-related arteries. All these factors have contributed to adverse events in prior studies. Most of the recent studies, but not all of them, reported worse clinical outcomes with intervention in nonculprit coronary arteries at the time of primary PCI.[136–139] A report from the APEX-AMI trial showed that multi-vessel disease was present in 2201 of the 5373 patients who underwent primary PCI (41%). Of those with multi-vessel disease, 9.9% underwent multi-vessel intervention, whereas 90.1% underwent PCI of the infarct-related artery alone. At 90 days, death occurred in 12.5% of patients who had multi-vessel intervention and in 5.6% of patients who had PCI of the infarct related artery alone ($P = 0.001$); a composite of death, CHF, or shock occurred in 17.4% of patients who had multi-vessel intervention and in 12% of patients who had PCI of the infarct-related artery alone ($P = 0.02$). In multivariate analysis, multi-vessel intervention was an independent predictor of 90-day mortality (adjusted HR 2.44, $P = 0.001$).[138] In another recent study, 3521 patients with STEMI underwent primary PCI of the culprit vessel during the index procedure; of these, 259 underwent nonculprit vessel intervention at the time of the index procedure, whereas 538 patients underwent staged PCI within 60 days of the index procedure. In patients without hemodynamic compromise, culprit-vessel PCI during the index procedure was associated with lower in-hospital mortality compared with multi-vessel PCI during the index procedure (0.9% vs. 2.4%, $P = 0.04$). Patients undergoing staged multivessel PCI within 60 days after the index procedure had a significantly lower 12-month mortality rate than did patients undergoing culprit-vessel PCI only (1.3% vs. 3.3%, $P = 0.04$).[137] The study discouraged intervention in the nonculprit coronary arteries at the time of primary PCI and suggested that a staged intervention within 60 days after the primary PCI for the infarct-related artery may be a preferable approach. Along the same lines, a recent report from the EUROTRANSFER registry, which included 1598 patients with STEMI and complete angiographic data, showed that non–infarct-related artery PCI during the primary PCI was performed in 9% of patients with multi-vessel disease and was associated with increased 1-year mortality.[134] Finally, the large National Cardiovascular Data Registry showed that patients with STEMI who underwent multi-vessel intervention had higher in-hospital mortality in all patients (7.9% vs. 5.1%, $P < 0.01$) and in

those with cardiogenic shock (36.5% vs. 27.8%, $P = 0.01$).[136] The largest randomized trial, to date, which enrolled 214 patients with STEMI, assigned 84 patients to a strategy of revascularization of the infarct-related artery only; 65 patients to a strategy of in-hospital complete revascularization, including infarct-related and non–infarct-related arteries; and 65 patients to a strategy of post-discharge complete revascularization.[139] During a mean follow-up of 2.5 years, the incidence of major adverse cardiac events was 50% in the group assigned to infarct-related artery revascularization only, 23.1% in the group with in-hospital complete revascularization, and 20% in the group with post-discharge complete revascularization.[139] Current Guidelines from both the European Society of Cardiology and the American College of Cardiology/American Heart Association discourage PCI of non–infarct-related arteries at the time of primary or rescue PCI in stable STEMI patients;[1,10] however, there is a strong need for well-designed studies on this topic.

PRIMARY PERCUTANEOUS CORONARY INTERVENTION IN HOSPITALS WITH AND WITHOUT ONSITE CORONARY ARTERY BYPASS GRAFT SURGERY

Whether PCI should be performed only in hospitals capable of CABG surgery or whether PCI should be expanded also to hospitals without cardiac surgery capability still remains controversial. The problem is of importance because of the expanding number of hospitals performing primary PCI and the potential for worse outcomes because of lower volumes and lack of cardiac surgery backup. In a recent study using 2004–2006 National Cardiovascular Data Registry information, it was reported that off-site PCI centers had similar risk-adjusted in-hospital mortality, procedure success, morbidity, and emergency cardiac surgery rates as did hospitals with cardiac surgery facilities on site.[140] A recent report from the hospitals of New York showed that there was no significant difference in the outcomes of patients with STEMI undergoing primary PCI in centers without or with surgical backup in terms of in-hospital or 30-day mortality (2.3% vs. 1.9%, $P = 0.40$), emergency CABG surgery immediately after primary PCI (0.06% vs. 0.35%, $P = 0.06$), or subsequent revascularization (23.8% vs. 21.5%, $P = 0.52$) or mortality (7.1% vs. 5.9%, $P = 0.07$) at 3 years.[141] The message from these studies is that primary PCI can be performed in hospitals without cardiac surgery facilities on site.

Conclusion

Reperfusion therapies have dramatically improved the prognosis of patients with acute STEMI. Advances in interventional techniques and devices as well as in anti-thrombotic therapies have enhanced the effectiveness of PCI in patients with STEMI. More than a decade of randomized clinical trials has clearly shown that primary PCI is superior to thrombolysis as a reperfusion therapy. Its advantages are conferred by the extremely low number of contraindications, high efficacy in patients presenting early or late after onset of symptoms, and low number of complications. In addition, PCI is not only very helpful after failed thrombolysis but may also represent a valuable adjunct to initially successful pharmacologic reperfusion. Although the proportion of patients with STEMI treated with PCI has been increasing steadily in recent years, major efforts are required to make this therapy available to all patients within a short time from symptom onset. Patients with STEMI who undergo PCI benefit from pretreatment with effective anti-platelet therapies. Additional work is needed to develop new effective adjunct therapies that can promote further myocardial salvage after PCI. Intensive experimental and clinical research aiming at myocardial cell regeneration is ongoing and offers new prospects for the improvement of prognosis and quality of life in patients with STEMI.

REFERENCES

1. Van de Werf F, Bax J, Betriu A, et al: Management of acute myocardial infarction in patients presenting with persistent ST-segment elevation: The Task Force on the Management of ST-Segment Elevation Acute Myocardial Infarction of the European Society of Cardiology. *Eur Heart J* 29:2909–2945, 2008.
2. Lloyd-Jones D, Adams RJ, Brown TM, et al: Heart disease and stroke statistics—2010 update: A report from the American Heart Association. *Circulation* 121:e46–e215, 2010.
3. Yeh RW, Sidney S, Chandra M, et al: Population trends in the incidence and outcomes of acute myocardial infarction. *N Engl J Med* 362:2155–2165, 2010.
4. Ndrepepa G, Mehilli J, Schulz S, et al: Patterns of presentation and outcomes of patients with acute coronary syndromes. *Cardiology* 113:198–206, 2009.
5. Lambert L, Brown K, Segal E, et al: Association between timeliness of reperfusion therapy and clinical outcomes in ST-elevation myocardial infarction. *JAMA* 303:2148–2155, 2010.
6. Widimsky P, Wijns W, Fajadet J, et al: Reperfusion therapy for ST elevation acute myocardial infarction in Europe: description of the current situation in 30 countries. *Eur Heart J* 31:943–957, 2010.
7. Keeley EC, Boura JA, Grines CL: Primary angioplasty versus intravenous thrombolytic therapy for acute myocardial infarction: A quantitative review of 23 randomised trials. *Lancet* 361:13–20, 2003.
8. Keeley EC, Grines CL: Primary coronary intervention for acute myocardial infarction. *JAMA* 291:736–739, 2004.
9. Antman EM, Hand M, Armstrong PW, et al: 2007 focused update of the ACC/AHA 2004 guidelines for the management of patients with ST-elevation myocardial infarction: A report of the American College of Cardiology/American Heart Association Task Force on Practice Guidelines. *J Am Coll Cardiol* 51:210–247, 2008.
10. Kushner FG, Hand M, Smith SC, Jr, et al: 2009 focused updates: ACC/AHA guidelines for the management of patients with ST-elevation myocardial infarction (updating the 2004 guideline and 2007 focused update) and ACC/AHA/SCAI guidelines on percutaneous coronary intervention (updating the 2005 guideline and 2007 focused update): A report of the American College of Cardiology Foundation/American Heart Association Task Force on Practice Guidelines. *J Am Coll Cardiol* 54:2205–2241, 2009.
11. Grzybowski M, Clements EA, Parsons L, et al: Mortality benefit of immediate revascularization of acute ST-segment elevation myocardial infarction in patients with contraindications to thrombolytic therapy: A propensity analysis. *JAMA* 290:1891–1898, 2003.
12. Abbate A, Biondi-Zoccai GG, Appleton DL, et al: Survival and cardiac remodeling benefits in patients undergoing late percutaneous coronary intervention of the infarct-related artery: Evidence from a meta-analysis of randomized controlled trials. *J Am Coll Cardiol* 51:956–964, 2008.
13. Schömig A, Mehilli J, Antoniucci D, et al: Mechanical reperfusion in patients with acute myocardial infarction presenting more than 12 hours from symptom onset: A randomized controlled trial. *JAMA* 293:2865–2872, 2005.
14. Boersma E: Does time matter? A pooled analysis of randomized clinical trials comparing primary percutaneous coronary intervention and in-hospital fibrinolysis in acute myocardial infarction patients. *Eur Heart J* 27:779–788, 2006.
15. Thune JJ, Hoefsten DE, Lindholm MG, et al: Simple risk stratification at admission to identify patients with reduced mortality from primary angioplasty. *Circulation* 112:2017–2021, 2005.
16. Aversano T, Aversano LT, Passamani E, et al: Thrombolytic therapy vs primary percutaneous coronary intervention for myocardial infarction in patients presenting to hospitals without on-site cardiac surgery: A randomized controlled trial. *JAMA* 287:1943–1951, 2002.
17. Nielsen PH, Maeng M, Busk M, et al: Primary angioplasty versus fibrinolysis in acute myocardial infarction: Long-term follow-up in the Danish acute myocardial infarction 2 trial. *Circulation* 121:1484–1491, 2010.
18. Huynh T, Perron S, O'Loughlin J, et al: Comparison of primary percutaneous coronary intervention and fibrinolytic therapy in ST-segment-elevation myocardial infarction: Bayesian hierarchical meta-analyses of randomized controlled trials and observational studies. *Circulation* 119:3101–3109, 2009.
19. Wailoo A, Goodacre S, Sampson F, et al: Primary angioplasty versus thrombolysis for acute ST-elevation myocardial infarction: An economic analysis of the National Infarct Angioplasty project. *Heart* 96:668–672, 2010.
20. Eagle KA, Nallamothu BK, Mehta RH, et al: Trends in acute reperfusion therapy for ST-segment elevation myocardial infarction from 1999 to 2006: We are getting better but we have got a long way to go. *Eur Heart J* 29:609–617, 2008.
21. Jacobs AK, Antman EM, Faxon DP, et al: Development of systems of care for ST-elevation myocardial infarction patients: Executive summary. *Circulation* 116:217–230, 2007.
22. Bonow RO, Masoudi FA, Rumsfeld JS, et al: ACC/AHA classification of care metrics: performance measures and quality metrics: A report of the American College of Cardiology/American Heart Association Task Force on Performance Measures. *Circulation* 118:2662–2666, 2008.
23. Jacobs AK: Regional systems of care for patients with ST-elevation myocardial infarction: Being at the right place at the right time. *Circulation* 116:689–692, 2007.
24. Studnek JR, Garvey L, Blackwell T, et al: Association between prehospital time intervals and ST-elevation myocardial infarction system performance. *Circulation* 122:1464–1469, 2010.
25. Roe MT, Messenger JC, Weintraub WS, et al: Treatments, trends, and outcomes of acute myocardial infarction and percutaneous coronary intervention. *J Am Coll Cardiol* 56:254–263, 2010.
26. Reimer KA, Lowe JE, Rasmussen MM, et al: The wavefront phenomenon of ischemic cell death. 1. Myocardial infarct size vs duration of coronary occlusion in dogs. *Circulation* 56:786–794, 1977.
27. Taher T, Fu Y, Wagner GS, et al: Aborted myocardial infarction in patients with ST-segment elevation: Insights from the Assessment of the Safety and Efficacy of a New Thrombolytic Regimen-3 Trial Electrocardiographic Substudy. *J Am Coll Cardiol* 44:38–43, 2004.
28. Ndrepepa G, Kastrati A, Mehilli J, et al: Mechanical reperfusion and long-term mortality in patients with acute myocardial infarction presenting 12 to 48 hours from onset of symptoms. *JAMA* 301:487–488, 2009.
29. Busk M, Kaltoft A, Nielsen SS, et al: Infarct size and myocardial salvage after primary angioplasty in patients presenting with symptoms for <12 h vs. 12–72 h. *Eur Heart J* 30:1322–1330, 2009.
30. De Luca G, Suryapranata H, Ottervanger JP, et al: Time delay to treatment and mortality in primary angioplasty for acute myocardial infarction: Every minute of delay counts. *Circulation* 109:1223–1225, 2004.
31. Cannon CP, Gibson CM, Lambrew CT, et al: Relationship of symptom-onset-to-balloon time and door-to-balloon time with mortality in patients undergoing angioplasty for acute myocardial infarction. *JAMA* 283:2941–2947, 2000.
32. Zijlstra F, Patel A, Jones M, et al: Clinical characteristics and outcome of patients with early (<2 h), intermediate (2–4 h) and late (>4 h) presentation treated by primary coronary angioplasty or thrombolytic therapy for acute myocardial infarction. *Eur Heart J* 23:550–557, 2002.
33. Maeng M, Nielsen PH, Busk M, et al: Time to treatment and three-year mortality after primary percutaneous coronary intervention for ST-segment elevation myocardial infarction: A DANish Trial in Acute Myocardial Infarction-2 (DANAMI-2) substudy. *Am J Cardiol* 105:1528–1534, 2010.
34. Aquaro GD, Pingitore A, Strata E, et al: Relation of pain-to-balloon time and myocardial infarct size in patients transferred for primary percutaneous coronary intervention. *Am J Cardiol* 100:28–34, 2007.
35. Nallamothu BK, Bates ER, Herrin J, et al: Times to treatment in transfer patients undergoing primary percutaneous coronary intervention in the United States: National Registry of Myocardial Infarction (NRMI)-3/4 analysis. *Circulation* 111:761–767, 2005.
36. Steg PG, Bonnefoy E, Chabaud S, et al: Impact of time to treatment on mortality after prehospital fibrinolysis or primary angioplasty: Data from the CAPTIM randomized clinical trial. *Circulation* 108:2851–2856, 2003.
37. Stenestrand U, Lindback J, Wallentin L: Long-term outcome of primary percutaneous coronary intervention vs prehospital and in-hospital thrombolysis for patients with ST-elevation myocardial infarction. *JAMA* 296:1749–1756, 2006.
38. McNamara RL, Wang Y, Herrin J, et al: Effect of door-to-balloon time on mortality in patients with ST-segment elevation myocardial infarction. *J Am Coll Cardiol* 47:2180–2186, 2006.
39. Terkelsen CJ, Sorensen JT, Maeng M, et al: System delay and mortality among patients with STEMI treated with primary percutaneous coronary intervention. *JAMA* 304:763–771, 2010.
40. Rathore SS, Curtis JP, Chen J, et al: Association of door-to-balloon time and mortality in patients admitted to hospital with ST elevation myocardial infarction: National cohort study. *BMJ* 338:b1807, 2009.
41. Brodie BR, Hansen C, Stuckey TD, et al: Door-to-balloon time with primary percutaneous coronary intervention for acute myocardial infarction impacts late cardiac mortality in high-risk patients and patients presenting early after the onset of symptoms. *J Am Coll Cardiol* 47:289–295, 2006.
42. Nallamothu BK, Wang Y, Magid DJ, et al: Relation between hospital specialization with primary percutaneous coronary intervention and clinical outcomes in ST-segment elevation myocardial infarction: National Registry of Myocardial Infarction-4 analysis. *Circulation* 113:222–229, 2006.
43. Angeja BG, Gibson CM, Chin R, et al: Predictors of door-to-balloon delay in primary angioplasty. *Am J Cardiol* 89:1156–1161, 2002.
44. Magid DJ, Wang Y, Herrin J, et al: Relationship between time of day, day of week, timeliness of reperfusion, and in-hospital mortality for patients with acute ST-segment elevation myocardial infarction. *JAMA* 294:803–812, 2005.
45. Hannan EL, Zhong Y, Jacobs AK, et al: Effect of onset-to-door time and door-to-balloon time on mortality in patients undergoing percutaneous coronary interventions for ST-segment elevation myocardial infarction. *Am J Cardiol* 106:143–147, 2010.
46. Brodie BR, Gersh BJ, Stuckey T, et al: When is door-to-balloon time critical? Analysis from the HORIZONS-AMI (Harmonizing Outcomes with Revascularization and Stents in Acute Myocardial Infarction) and CADILLAC (Controlled Abciximab and Device Investigation to Lower Late Angioplasty Complications) trials. *J Am Coll Cardiol* 56:407–413, 2010.
47. Dalby M, Bouzamondo A, Lechat P, et al: Transfer for primary angioplasty versus immediate thrombolysis in acute myocardial infarction: a meta-analysis. *Circulation* 108:1809–1814, 2003.
48. Zijlstra F: Angioplasty vs thrombolysis for acute myocardial infarction: a quantitative overview of the effects of interhospital transportation. *Eur Heart J* 24:21–23, 2003.
49. Scheller B, Hennen B, Hammer B, et al: Beneficial effects of immediate stenting after thrombolysis in acute myocardial infarction. *J Am Coll Cardiol* 42:634–641, 2003.
50. Dobrzycki S, Kralisz P, Nowak K, et al: Transfer with GP IIb/IIIa inhibitor tirofiban for primary percutaneous coronary intervention vs. on-site thrombolysis in patients with ST-elevation myocardial infarction (STEMI): a randomized open-label study for patients admitted to community hospitals. *Eur Heart J* 28:2438–2448, 2007.
51. Widimsky P, Bilkova D, Penicka M, et al: Long-term outcomes of patients with acute myocardial infarction presenting to hospitals without catheterization laboratory and randomized to immediate thrombolysis or interhospital transport for primary percutaneous coronary intervention. Five years' follow-up of the PRAGUE-2 Trial. *Eur Heart J* 28:679–684, 2007.
52. Nallamothu BK, Bates ER: Percutaneous coronary intervention versus fibrinolytic therapy in acute myocardial infarction: Is timing (almost) everything? *Am J Cardiol* 92:824–826, 2003.

53. Terkelsen CJ, Christiansen EH, Sorensen JT, et al: Primary PCI as the preferred reperfusion therapy in STEMI: It is a matter of time. *Heart* 95:362–369, 2009.
54. Betriu A, Masotti M: Comparison of mortality rates in acute myocardial infarction treated by percutaneous coronary intervention versus fibrinolysis. *Am J Cardiol* 95:100–101, 2005.
55. Kalla K, Christ G, Karnik R, et al: Implementation of guidelines improves the standard of care: the Viennese registry on reperfusion strategies in ST-elevation myocardial infarction (Vienna STEMI registry). *Circulation* 113:2398–2405, 2006.
56. Pinto DS, Kirtane AJ, Nallamothu BK, et al: Hospital delays in reperfusion for ST-elevation myocardial infarction: Implications when selecting a reperfusion strategy. *Circulation* 114:2019–2025, 2006.
57. Tarantini G, Razzolini R, Napodano M, et al: Acceptable reperfusion delay to prefer primary angioplasty over fibrin-specific thrombolytic therapy is affected (mainly) by the patient's mortality risk: 1 h does not fit all. *Eur Heart J* 31:676–683, 2010.
58. De Luca G, Cassetti E, Marino P: Percutaneous coronary intervention-related time delay, patient's risk profile, and survival benefits of primary angioplasty vs lytic therapy in ST-segment elevation myocardial infarction. *Am J Emerg Med* 27:712–719, 2009.
59. Henry TD, Atkins JM, Cunningham MS, et al: ST-segment elevation myocardial infarction: recommendations on triage of patients to heart attack centers: Is it time for a national policy for the treatment of ST-segment elevation myocardial infarction? *J Am Coll Cardiol* 47:1339–1345, 2006.
60. Nallamothu BK, Bates ER, Wang Y, et al: Driving times and distances to hospitals with percutaneous coronary intervention in the United States: Implications for prehospital triage of patients with ST elevation myocardial infarction. *Circulation* 113:1189–1195, 2006.
61. Kastrati A, Mehilli J, Schlotterbeck K, et al: Early administration of reteplase plus abciximab vs abciximab alone in patients with acute myocardial infarction referred for percutaneous coronary intervention: A randomized controlled trial. *JAMA* 291:947–954, 2004.
62. Primary versus tenecteplase-facilitated percutaneous coronary intervention in patients with ST-segment elevation acute myocardial infarction (ASSENT-4 PCI): Randomised trial. *Lancet* 367:569–578, 2006.
63. Keeley EC, Boura JA, Grines CL: Comparison of primary and facilitated percutaneous coronary interventions for ST-elevation myocardial infarction: Quantitative review of randomised trials. *Lancet* 367:579–588, 2006.
64. Ellis SG, Tendera M, de Belder MA, et al: Facilitated PCI in patients with ST-elevation myocardial infarction. *N Engl J Med* 358:2205–2217, 2008.
65. Di Mario C, Dudek D, Piscione F, et al: Immediate angioplasty versus standard therapy with rescue angioplasty after thrombolysis in the Combined Abciximab REteplase Stent Study in Acute Myocardial Infarction (CARESS-in AMI): An open, prospective, randomised, multicentre trial. *Lancet* 371:559–568, 2008.
66. Cantor WJ, Fitchett D, Borgundvaag B, et al: Routine early angioplasty after fibrinolysis for acute myocardial infarction. *N Engl J Med* 360:2705–2718, 2009.
67. Borgia F, Goodman SG, Halvorsen S, et al: Early routine percutaneous coronary intervention after fibrinolysis vs standard therapy in ST-segment elevation myocardial infarction: A meta-analysis. *Eur Heart J* 31:2156–2169, 2010.
68. Desch S, Eitel I, Rahimi K, et al. Timing of invasive treatment after fibrinolysis in ST elevation myocardial infarction—a meta-analysis of immediate or early routine versus deferred or ischemia-guided randomised controlled trials. *Heart* 96:1695–1702, 2010.
69. Brosius FC, 3rd, Roberts WC: Significance of coronary arterial thrombus in transmural acute myocardial infarction. A study of 54 necropsy patients. *Circulation* 63:810–816, 1981.
70. Richardson SG, Allen DC, Morton P, et al: Pathological changes after intravenous streptokinase treatment in eight patients with acute myocardial infarction. *Br Heart J* 61:390–395, 1989.
71. Wijeysundera HC, Vijayaraghavan R, Nallamothu BK, et al: Rescue angioplasty or repeat fibrinolysis after failed fibrinolytic therapy for ST-segment myocardial infarction: A meta-analysis of randomized trials. *J Am Coll Cardiol* 49:422–430, 2007.
72. Eeckhout E: Rescue percutaneous coronary intervention: Does the concept make sense? *Heart* 93:632–638, 2007.
73. Sutton AG, Campbell PG, Graham R, et al: A randomized trial of rescue angioplasty versus a conservative approach for failed fibrinolysis in ST-segment elevation myocardial infarction: The Middlesbrough Early Revascularization to Limit INfarction (MERLIN) trial. *J Am Coll Cardiol* 44:287–296, 2004.
74. Gershlick AH, Stephens-Lloyd A, Hughes S, et al: Rescue angioplasty after failed thrombolytic therapy for acute myocardial infarction. *N Engl J Med* 353:2758–2768, 2005.
75. Carver A, Rafelt S, Gershlick AH, et al: Longer-term follow-up of patients recruited to the REACT (Rescue Angioplasty Versus Conservative Treatment or Repeat Thrombolysis) trial. *J Am Coll Cardiol* 54:118–126, 2009.
76. De Luca G, Suryapranata H, Stone GW, et al: Coronary stenting versus balloon angioplasty for acute myocardial infarction: A meta-regression analysis of randomized trials. *Int J Cardiol* 126:37–44, 2008.
77. Mehta RH, Harjai KJ, Cox DA, et al: Comparison of coronary stenting versus conventional balloon angioplasty on five-year mortality in patients with acute myocardial infarction undergoing primary percutaneous coronary intervention. *Am J Cardiol* 96:901–906, 2005.
78. Loubeyre C, Morice MC, Lefevre T, et al: A randomized comparison of direct stenting with conventional stent implantation in selected patients with acute myocardial infarction. *J Am Coll Cardiol* 39:15–21, 2002.
79. Joner M, Finn AV, Farb A, et al: Pathology of drug-eluting stents in humans: delayed healing and late thrombotic risk. *J Am Coll Cardiol* 48:193–202, 2006.
80. Steg PG, Fox KA, Eagle KA, et al: Mortality following placement of drug-eluting and bare-metal stents for ST-segment elevation acute myocardial infarction in the Global Registry of Acute Coronary Events. *Eur Heart J* 30:321–329, 2009.
81. Mauri L, Silbaugh TS, Garg P, et al: Drug-eluting or bare-metal stents for acute myocardial infarction. *N Engl J Med* 359:1330–1342, 2008.
82. Stone GW, Lansky AJ, Pocock SJ, et al: Paclitaxel-eluting stents versus bare-metal stents in acute myocardial infarction. *N Engl J Med* 360:1946–1959, 2009.
83. Stone GW: HORIZONS-AMI: Three-year follow-up from a prospective randomized trial of antithrombin strategies and drug-eluting stents in patients with acute myocardial infarction undergoing primary angioplasty. *Transcatheter Cardiovascular Therapeutics* Washington, D.C.; 2010.
84. Brar SS, Leon MB, Stone GW, et al: Use of drug-eluting stents in acute myocardial infarction: A systematic review and meta-analysis. *J Am Coll Cardiol* 53:1677–1689, 2009.
85. Dibra A, Tiroch K, Schulz S, et al: Drug-eluting stents in acute myocardial infarction: Updated meta-analysis of randomized trials. *Clin Res Cardiol* 99:345–357, 2010.
86. Stone GW, Webb J, Cox DA, et al: Distal microcirculatory protection during percutaneous coronary intervention in acute ST-segment elevation myocardial infarction: A randomized controlled trial. *JAMA* 293:1063–1072, 2005.
87. Sardella G, Mancone M, Bucciarelli-Ducci C, et al: Thrombus aspiration during primary percutaneous coronary intervention improves myocardial reperfusion and reduces infarct size: The EXPIRA (thrombectomy with export catheter in infarct-related artery during primary percutaneous coronary intervention) prospective, randomized trial. *J Am Coll Cardiol* 53:309–315, 2009.
88. Svilaas T, Vlaar PJ, van der Horst IC, et al: Thrombus aspiration during primary percutaneous coronary intervention. *N Engl J Med* 358:557–567, 2008.
89. Vlaar PJ, Svilaas T, van der Horst IC, et al: Cardiac death and reinfarction after 1 year in the Thrombus Aspiration during Percutaneous coronary intervention in Acute myocardial infarction Study (TAPAS): A 1-year follow-up study. *Lancet* 371:1915–1920, 2008.
90. Liistro F, Grotti S, Angioli P, et al: Impact of thrombus aspiration on myocardial tissue reperfusion and left ventricular functional recovery and remodeling after primary angioplasty. *Circ Cardiovasc Interv* 2:376–383, 2009.
91. Migliorini A, Stabile A, Rodriguez AE, et al: Comparison of AngioJet rheolytic thrombectomy before direct infarct artery stenting with direct stenting alone in patients with acute myocardial infarction. The JETSTENT trial. *J Am Coll Cardiol* 56:1298–1306, 2010.
92. Burzotta F, De Vita M, Gu YL, et al. Clinical impact of thrombectomy in acute ST-elevation myocardial infarction. An individual patient-data pooled analysis of 11 trials. *Eur Heart J* 30:2193–2203, 2009.
93. Tamhane UU, Chetcuti S, Hameed I, et al: Safety and efficacy of thrombectomy in patients undergoing primary percutaneous coronary intervention for Acute ST elevation MI: A meta-analysis of randomized controlled trials. *BMC Cardiovasc Disord* 10:10, 2010.
94. Huber K, Holmes DR, Jr, van't Hof AW, et al: Use of glycoprotein IIb/IIIa inhibitors in primary percutaneous coronary intervention: Insights from the APEX-AMI trial. *Eur Heart J* 31(14):1708–1716, 2010
95. Montalescot G, Antoniucci D, Kastrati A, et al: Abciximab in primary coronary stenting of ST-elevation myocardial infarction: A European meta-analysis on individual patients' data with long-term follow-up. *Eur Heart J* 28:443–449, 2007.
96. De Luca G, Gibson CM, Bellandi F, et al: Early glycoprotein IIb-IIIa inhibitors in primary angioplasty (EGYPT) cooperation: An individual patient data meta-analysis. *Heart* 94:1548–1558, 2008.
97. Mehilli J, Kastrati A, Schulz S, et al: Abciximab in patients with acute ST-segment-elevation myocardial infarction undergoing primary percutaneous coronary intervention after clopidogrel loading: a randomized double-blind trial. *Circulation* 119:1933–1940, 2009.
98. Gu YL, Kampinga MA, Wieringa WG, et al: Intracoronary versus intravenous administration of abciximab in patients with ST-segment elevation myocardial infarction undergoing primary percutaneous coronary intervention with thrombus aspiration the comparison of intracoronary versus intravenous abciximab administration during emergency reperfusion of ST-segment elevation myocardial infarction (CICERO) trial. *Circulation* 122(25):2709–2717, 2010.
99. Dangas G, Mehran R, Guagliumi G, et al: Role of clopidogrel loading dose in patients with ST-segment elevation myocardial infarction undergoing primary angioplasty: Results from the HORIZONS-AMI (harmonizing outcomes with revascularization and stents in acute myocardial infarction) trial. *J Am Coll Cardiol* 54:1438–1446, 2009.
100. Montalescot G, Wiviott SD, Braunwald E, et al: Prasugrel compared with clopidogrel in patients undergoing percutaneous coronary intervention for ST-elevation myocardial infarction (TRITON-TIMI 38): Double-blind, randomised controlled trial. *Lancet* 373:723–731, 2009.
101. Steg PG, James S, Harrington RA, et al: Acute coronary syndromes intended for reperfusion with primary percutaneous coronary intervention. A Platelet Inhibition and Patient Outcomes (PLATO) trial subgroup analysis. *Circulation* 122:2131–2141, 2010.
102. Stone GW, Witzenbichler B, Guagliumi G, et al: Bivalirudin during primary PCI in acute myocardial infarction. *N Engl J Med* 358:2218–2230, 2008.
103. Yusuf S, Mehta SR, Chrolavicius S, et al: Effects of fondaparinaux on mortality and reinfarction in patients with acute ST-segment elevation myocardial infarction: The OASIS-6 randomized trial. *JAMA* 295:1519–1530, 2006.
104. Ndrepepa G, Tiroch K, Fusaro M, et al: 5-year prognostic value of no-reflow phenomenon after percutaneous coronary intervention in patients with acute myocardial infarction. *J Am Coll Cardiol* 55:2383–2389, 2010.
105. Ndrepepa G, Tiroch K, Keta D, et al: Predictive factors and impact of no reflow after primary percutaneous coronary intervention in patients with acute myocardial infarction. *Circ Cardiovasc Interv* 3:27–33, 2010.
106. Ross AM, Gibbons RJ, Stone GW, et al: A randomized, double-blinded, placebo-controlled multicenter trial of adenosine as an adjunct to reperfusion in the treatment of acute myocardial infarction (AMISTAD-II). *J Am Coll Cardiol* 45:1775–1780, 2005.
107. Fokkema ML, Vlaar PJ, Vogelzang M, et al: Effect of high dose intracoronary adenosine administration during primary percutaneous coronary intervention in acute myocardial infarction: A randomized controlled trial. *Circ Cardiovasc Interv* 2:323–329, 2009.
108. Shinozaki N, Ichinose H, Yahikozawa K, et al: Selective intracoronary administration of nitroprusside before balloon dilatation prevents slow reflow during percutaneous coronary intervention in patients with acute myocardial infarction. *Int Heart J* 48:423–433, 2007.
109. Hendler A, Aronovich A, Kaluski E, et al: Optimization of myocardial perfusion after primary coronary angioplasty following an acute myocardial infarction. Beyond TIMI 3 flow. *J Invasive Cardiol* 10:32–36, 2006.
110. Amit G, Cafri C, Yaroslavtsev S, et al: Intracoronary nitroprusside for the prevention of the no-reflow phenomenon after primary percutaneous coronary intervention in acute myocardial infarction. A randomized, double-blind, placebo-controlled clinical trial. *Am Heart J* 152:887, 2006, e889–e814.
111. Armstrong PW, Granger CB, Adams PX, et al: Pexelizumab for acute ST-elevation myocardial infarction in patients undergoing primary percutaneous coronary intervention: A randomized controlled trial. *JAMA* 297:43–51, 2007.
112. Iwakura K, Ito H, Okamura A, et al: Nicorandil treatment in patients with acute myocardial infarction: A meta-analysis. *Circ J* 73:925–931, 2009.
113. Bar FW, Tzivoni D, Dirksen MT, et al: Results of the first clinical study of adjunctive CAldaret (MCC-135) in patients undergoing primary percutaneous coronary intervention for ST-Elevation Myocardial Infarction. The randomized multicentre CASTEMI study. *Eur Heart J* 27:2516–2523, 2006.
114. Tzivoni D, Balkin J, Bar FW, et al: Effect of caldaret on the incidence of severe left ventricular dysfunction in patients with ST-elevation myocardial infarction undergoing primary coronary intervention. *Am J Cardiol* 103:1–4, 2009.
144a. O'Neill WW, Martin JL, Dixon SR, et al: Acute myocardial infarction with hyperoxemic therapy (AMIHOT): a prospective, randomized trial of intracoronary hyperoxemic reperfusion after percutaneous coronary intervention. *J Am Coll Cardiol* Jul 31;50(5):397–405, Epub 2007.
115. O'Neill WW: A prospective, randomized trial of mild systemic hypothermia during PCI treatment of ST elevation MI. Paper presented at Transcatheter Cardiovascular Therapeutics,, Washington, D.C., 2003.
116. Stone GW, Martin JL, de Boer MJ, et al: Effect of supersaturated oxygen delivery on infarct size after percutaneous coronary intervention in acute myocardial infarction. *Circ Cardiovasc Interv* 2:366–375, 2009.
117. Piot C, Croisille P, Staat P, et al: Effect of cyclosporine on reperfusion injury in acute myocardial infarction. *N Engl J Med* 359:473–481, 2008.
118. Gersh BJ, Simari RD, Behfar A, et al: Cardiac cell repair therapy: A clinical perspective. *Mayo Clin Proc* 84:876–892, 2009.
119. Martin-Rendon E, Brunskill SJ, Hyde CJ, et al: Autologous bone marrow stem cells to treat acute myocardial infarction: A systematic review. *Eur Heart J* 29:1807–1818, 2008.
120. Zhang SN, Sun AJ, Ge JB, et al: Intracoronary autologous bone marrow stem cells transfer for patients with acute myocardial infarction: A meta-analysis of randomised controlled trials. *Int J Cardiol* 136:178–185, 2009.
121. Zohlnhofer D, Dibra A, Koppara T, et al: Stem cell mobilization by granulocyte colony-stimulating factor for myocardial

recovery after acute myocardial infarction: A meta-analysis. *J Am Coll Cardiol* 51:1429–1437, 2008.

122. Ott I, Schulz S, Mehilli J, et al: Erythropoietin in patients with acute ST-segment elevation myocardial infarction undergoing primary percutaneous coronary intervention: A randomized, double-blind trial. *Circ Cardiovasc Interv* 3:408–413, 2010.

123. Voors AA, Belonje AM, Zijlstra F, et al: A single dose of erythropoietin in ST-elevation myocardial infarction. *Eur Heart J* 31:2593–2600, 2010.

124. Babaev A, Frederick PD, Pasta DJ, et al: Trends in management and outcomes of patients with acute myocardial infarction complicated by cardiogenic shock. *JAMA* 294:448–454, 2005.

125. Hochman JS, Sleeper LA, Webb JG, et al: Early revascularization and long-term survival in cardiogenic shock complicating acute myocardial infarction. *JAMA* 295:2511–2515, 2006.

126. Seyfarth M, Sibbing D, Bauer I, et al: A randomized clinical trial to evaluate the safety and efficacy of a percutaneous left ventricular assist device versus intra-aortic balloon pumping for treatment of cardiogenic shock caused by myocardial infarction. *J Am Coll Cardiol* 52:1584–1588, 2008.

127. Alexander JH, Reynolds HR, Stebbins AL, et al: Effect of tilarginine acetate in patients with acute myocardial infarction and cardiogenic shock: The TRIUMPH randomized controlled trial. *JAMA* 297:1657–1666, 2007.

128. Sadeghi HM, Grines CL, Chandra HR, et al: Magnitude and impact of treatment delays on weeknights and weekends in patients undergoing primary angioplasty for acute myocardial infarction (the CADILLAC trial). *Am J Cardiol* 94:637–640, A639, 2004.

129. Cubeddu RJ, Cruz-Gonzalez I, Kiernan TJ, et al: ST-elevation myocardial infarction mortality in a major academic center "on-" versus "off-" hours. *J Invasive Cardiol* 21:518–523, 2009.

130. Glaser R, Naidu SS, Selzer F, et al: Factors associated with poorer prognosis for patients undergoing primary percutaneous coronary intervention during off-hours: Biology or systems failure? *JACC Cardiovasc Interv* 1:681–688, 2008.

131. de Boer MJ, Ottervanger JP, van't Hof AW, et al: Reperfusion therapy in elderly patients with acute myocardial infarction: A randomized comparison of primary angioplasty and thrombolytic therapy. *J Am Coll Cardiol* 2002;39:1723–1728, 2008.

132. Grines CL: A prospective randomized trial of primary angioplasty and thrombolytic therapy in elderly patients with acute myocardial infarction (SENIOR-PAMI), Presented at Transcatheter Cardiovascular Therapeutics, Washington, D.C., 2005.

133. Bueno H, Betriu A, Heras M, et al: Primary angioplasty vs. fibrinolysis in very old patients with acute myocardial infarction: TRIANA (TRatamiento del Infarto Agudo de miocardio eN Ancianos) randomized trial and pooled analysis with previous studies. *Eur Heart J* 32(1):51–60, 2010.

134. Dziewierz A, Siudak Z, Rakowski T, et al: Impact of Multivessel Coronary Artery Disease and Noninfarct-Related Artery Revascularization on Outcome of Patients With ST-Elevation Myocardial Infarction Transferred for Primary Percutaneous Coronary Intervention (from the EUROTRANSFER Registry). *Am J Cardiol* 106:342–347, 2010.

135. Sorajja P, Gersh BJ, Cox DA, et al: Impact of multivessel disease on reperfusion success and clinical outcomes in patients undergoing primary percutaneous coronary intervention for acute myocardial infarction. *Eur Heart J* 28:1709–1716, 2007.

136. Cavender MA, Milford-Beland S, Roe MT, et al: Prevalence, predictors, and in-hospital outcomes of non-infarct artery intervention during primary percutaneous coronary intervention for ST-segment elevation myocardial infarction (from the National Cardiovascular Data Registry). *Am J Cardiol* 104:507–513, 2009.

137. Hannan EL, Samadashvili Z, Walford G, et al: Culprit vessel percutaneous coronary intervention versus multivessel and staged percutaneous coronary intervention for ST-segment elevation myocardial infarction patients with multivessel disease. *JACC Cardiovasc Interv* 3:22–31, 2010.

138. Toma M, Buller CE, Westerhout CM, et al: Non-culprit coronary artery percutaneous coronary intervention during acute ST-segment elevation myocardial infarction: Insights from the APEX-AMI trial. *Eur Heart J* 31:1701–1707, 2010.

139. Politi L, Sgura F, Rossi R, et al: A randomised trial of target-vessel versus multi-vessel revascularisation in ST-elevation myocardial infarction: major adverse cardiac events during long-term follow-up. *Heart* 96:662–667, 2010.

140. Kutcher MA, Klein LW, Ou FS, et al: Percutaneous coronary interventions in facilities without cardiac surgery on site: a report from the National Cardiovascular Data Registry (NCDR). *J Am Coll Cardiol* 54:16–24, 2009.

141. Hannan EL, Zhong Y, Racz M, et al: Outcomes for patients with ST-elevation myocardial infarction in hospitals with and without onsite coronary artery bypass graft surgery: The New York State experience. *Circ Cardiovasc Interv* 2:519–527, 2009.

19

Interventions in Cardiogenic Shock

AMR BANNAN | HOWARD C. HERRMANN

KEY POINTS

- Cardiogenic shock (CS) remains the leading cause of death among patients hospitalized with an acute myocardial infarction (AMI).

- Left ventricular dysfunction accounts for the majority of CS in AMI patients. Early restoration of perfusion to the territory supplied by the infarct-related artery is of paramount importance in preventing CS or changing outcomes once it has developed.

- The SHOCK trial and registry demonstrated the mortality benefit of early, immediate revascularization compared with medical stabilization.

- All subgroups demonstrate benefit from the early invasive approach. Revascularization is associated with some benefit at every level of risk.

- Although the subgroup of patients above 75 years of age did not have a survival advantage with early revascularization therapy in SHOCK, other trials and registries have shown benefit in this age group. Therapy has to be individualized in this population, and the functional status of the patient before the AMI is of particular importance.

- Major predictors of improved outcomes with percutaneous coronary intervention (PCI) in CS are time to reperfusion, achievement of vessel patency, and increase in thrombolysis in MI (TIMI) flow grade.

- The majority of patients who present with CS have multi-vessel disease. Despite the absence of supporting data, interventions on non–infarct-related artery (IRA) lesions may be beneficial. Patients with coronary anatomy not deemed suitable for PCI should be surgically revascularized.

- CS is a treatable illness with a reasonable chance of recovery in the primary PCI era. An early invasive approach can increase both short-term and long-term survival, and survivors often regain an excellent quality of life.

Background

CS is the leading cause of mortality among patients hospitalized for AMI.[1] The incidence and mortality of patients with CS in the setting of AMI have remained unchanged for nearly two decades, despite a progressive decline in the overall mortality of AMI, with the development of the coronary care unit and early defibrillation in the 1970s, the routine use of aspirin and β-blockers in the 1980s, and the introduction of reperfusion therapy with thrombolytics in the early 1990s.[2–6] More recently, however, registries collecting data from the mid-1990s have shown a decrease in the incidence and mortality of CS complicating AMI (Figs. 19-1 and 19-2).[7,8] These trends are associated with the increasing use of primary PCI and rescue PCI for STEMI (Fig. 19-3). To understand which of the patients with shock complicating AMI benefit from PCI, it is necessary to define CS, review its pathophysiology, and examine in detail the trials of PCI in shock.

Definition and Pathophysiology

CS is a state of end-organ hypoperfusion caused by cardiac failure. Manifestations may include cold extremities, decreased urine output (less than 30 mL/hr), alteration in mental status, or both in the setting of low systemic arterial blood pressure. Hemodynamically, CS is characterized by low cardiac output and systemic arterial hypotension in the setting of normal or elevated left ventricular filling pressure. Typical hemodynamic parameters of CS are shown in Table 19-1.

CS results from temporary or permanent derangements in the entire circulatory system. Many of these abnormalities are partially or completely reversible, which may explain the positive functional outcome in most survivors. Left ventricular pump failure is the primary insult in most forms of CS. Left ventricular dysfunction may reflect new irreversible injury, reversible ischemia, damage from prior infarction, or a combination of these. The decrease in coronary perfusion as a consequence of the low cardiac output may compromise flow in vessels other than the infarct artery, which leads to ischemia in the territory of the non–infarct-related artery and further decline in left ventricular function. The degree of myocardial dysfunction that initiates CS is variable. It is often, but not always, severe. Thus, other components of the cardiovascular system contribute to the pathophysiology of CS in the setting of AMI. The decrease in cardiac output triggers the release of catecholamines, which constrict the peripheral arterioles to maintain the perfusion of vital organs. This reflex mechanism of increased systemic vascular resistance is not fully effective, as demonstrated by variations in the systemic vascular resistance in trials of CS, in which hemodynamic data were assessed, with median values during CS in the normal range despite vasopressor therapy.[9] These findings are consistent with the observation that MI can cause systemic inflammatory response syndrome (SIRS). Right ventricular dysfunction may also cause or contribute to CS. Predominant right ventricular failure is rare and represents only 5% of cases of shock complicating AMI. Right ventricular failure may limit left ventricular filling via a decrease in cardiac output, ventricular interdependence, or both. Shock caused by isolated right ventricular dysfunction carries nearly as high a mortality risk as shock caused by left ventricular failure. Additionally, the benefit of revascularization was similar in the SHOCK trial and registry in patients with primarily right ventricular dysfunction versus primarily left ventricular dysfunction.[10] Mechanical complications such as ventricular septal rupture and papillary muscle rupture may lead to CS without severe reduction in left ventricular function.[11,12] Finally, most patients with CS complicating AMI develop shock after presenting at the hospital. In some, medication use contributes to the development of shock. Classes of medications used to treat AMI that have been associated with shock include β-blockers, angiotensin-converting enzyme (ACE) inhibitors, nitrates, diuretics, and morphine. In light of the complex pathophysiology of CS, severe impairment of left ventricular contractility does not always lead to shock, and conversely, left ventricular ejection fraction (LVEF) may be only moderately depressed in patients with CS. In fact, the mean LVEF in the SHOCK trial was 30%.[13] However, LVEF remains an important prognostic indicator (Fig. 19-4).[14]

Clinical Presentation

SHOCK TRIAL AND REGISTRY

The SHOCK trial is the largest randomized trial comparing immediate revascularization (accomplished by either PCI or coronary artery bypass grafting [CABG]) and initial medical stabilization (including

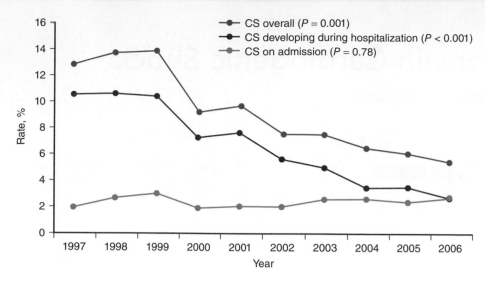

Figure 19-1 Temporal trends of cardiogenic shock (CS) from 1997 to 2006, demonstrating a reduction in the overall incidence of CS and the development of CS during hospitalization in patients presenting with an acute coronary syndrome. (*Redrawn with permission from Jeger RV, Radovanovic D, Hunziker PR, et al, AMIS Plus Registry investigators: Ten-year trends in the incidence and treatment of cardiogenic shock,* Ann Intern Med *149(9):618–626, 2008.*)

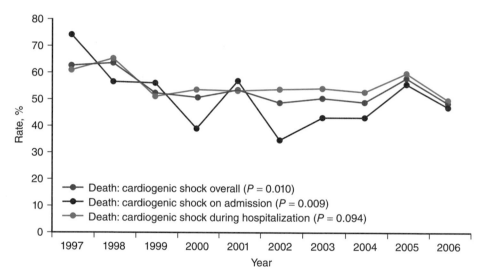

Figure 19-2 Temporal trends in mortality in patients with an acute coronary syndrome and cardiogenic shock (CS) from 1997 to 2006. The data demonstrate a reduction in the rate of death in CS overall, in patients with CS on admission, and in those developing CS during hospitalization. (*Redrawn with permission from Jeger RV, Radovanovic D, Hunziker PR, et al, AMIS Plus Registry investigators: Ten-year trends in the incidence and treatment of cardiogenic shock,* Ann Intern Med *149(9):618–626, 2008.*)

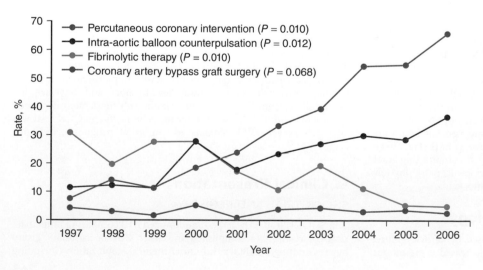

Figure 19-3 Temporal trends of cardiogenic shock (CS) from 1997 to 2006, demonstrating an increase in use of percutaneous coronary intervention (PCI) for revascularization, with a corresponding decrease in the use of fibrinolysis. The use of coronary artery bypass grafting (CABG) remained unchanged during this time period. (*Redrawn with permission from Jeger RV, Radovanovic D, Hunziker PR, et al, AMIS Plus Registry investigators: Ten-year trends in the incidence and treatment of cardiogenic shock,* Ann Intern Med *149(9):618–626, 2008.*)

TABLE 19-1	Typical Hemodynamic Parameters of Cardiogenic Shock	
Cardiac Index	*Less Than 2.2 L/M²*	
Systolic blood pressure	<90 mm Hg with supportive measures, or mean arterial pressure 30 mm Hg less than baseline	
Left ventricular filling pressure	LVEDP > 15 mm Hg	

L/m², liters per meters squared; *LVEDP*, left ventricular end-diastolic pressure.

reperfusion therapy with thrombolytics) in the setting of CS complicating AMI.[13,15] This trial and its registry provide insight into the etiology, risk factors, hemodynamic profile, clinical features, timing, and prognosis of CS complicating AMI. Eligible patients had to have an ST segment elevation myocardial infarction (STEMI) complicated by shock caused by left ventricular failure (mechanical and iatrogenic causes excluded), clinical and hemodynamic confirmation of CS, and shock developing within 36 hours of infarction. Intra-aortic balloon counterpulsation was permitted in both arms. Randomization had to occur within 12 hours of the diagnosis of shock. Patients with severe systemic illness, mechanical complications of MI, dilated cardiomyopathy (DCM), and severe valvular heart disease were excluded. A total of 302 patients were randomized in the SHOCK trial. A simultaneous registry prospectively enrolled patients who did not fulfill the eligibility criteria for entry into the trial. The SHOCK trial and registry included patients with mechanical complications of AMI, patients with shock secondary to medications, patients who presented more than 36 hours after infarction or were not randomized within 12 hours of shock, and patients with shock diagnosed on clinical grounds alone (no hemodynamic confirmation). A total of 1190 patients were enrolled in this prospective, nonrandomized registry.

ETIOLOGY

Among all of the patients enrolled in the SHOCK trial and registry, 78.5% had predominant left ventricular failure, most often with electrocardiogram (ECG) findings consistent with recent anterior MI (58%). Shock complicating inferior MI was less common (34.4%) and was associated with a prior MI in one third of patients or a mechanical cause of shock in the remainder. Mechanical complications accounted

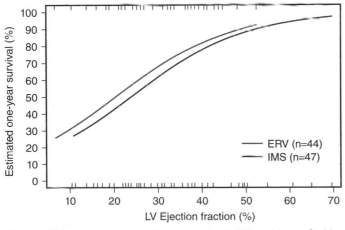

Figure 19-4 One-year survival rates in the SHOCK trial stratified by left ventricular ejection fraction (LVEF). Survival rates increase with increasing ejection fraction (*P* = 0.001), and this relationship is independent of treatment assignment (interaction *P* = 0.778). *ERV*, early revascularization; *IMS*, initial medical stabilization. (*Redrawn with permission from Picard MH, Davidoff R, Sleeper LA, et al: Echocardiographic predictors of survival and response to early revascularization in cardiogenic shock, Circulation 107:279–284, 2003.*)

for a minority of causes of CS. Severe mitral regurgitation was found in 6.9% of cases, ventricular septal rupture in 3.4%, right ventricular infarction in 2.8%, and tamponade and rupture in 1.4%. Additionally, a minority of cases may be iatrogenic, induced by medications such as β-blockers, calcium channel blockers, ACE inhibitors, diuretics, nitrates, and morphine. Risk factors for the development of CS in the context of AMI included older age, anterior MI, hypertension, diabetes mellitus, multi-vessel coronary artery disease (CAD), prior MI or angina, prior diagnosis of heart failure, STEMI, and left bundle branch block (LBBB).

CLINICAL MANIFESTATIONS

Variability exists in the clinical manifestations of CS caused by left ventricular failure in the setting of AMI.[16] Although the majority of patients with predominant left ventricular failure causing CS has classic findings of peripheral hypoperfusion and pulmonary congestion in the setting of arterial hypotension, approximately one quarter of patients manifest hypotension and hypoperfusion in the absence of clinical pulmonary congestion. Consequently, the absence of pulmonary congestion on physical evaluation should not be considered a surrogate for low risk. Clearly, left ventricular compromise can coexist with a normal initial pulmonary evaluation. CS is diagnosed at presentation in only a minority of patients, but the majority of patients who ultimately develop shock following AMI do so within the first 24 hours. In a report from the SHOCK trial and registry that included CS patients with predominant left ventricular failure, only 9% of the patients were diagnosed at the time of presentation (median delay from MI symptom onset to hospital admission was 1.25 hours).[17] About half of the patients (46.6%) who developed CS did so within 6 hours of infarct onset. By 24 hours, 74.1% of the patients who developed CS were diagnosed, and late shock (onset > 24 hours) occurred in 25.9% of the study patients. By implication, then, there is often a therapeutic window that could allow for intervention either before CS develops or early in its course. The median time from hospital admission to shock onset, however, was only 4.6 hours, indicating that the window is relatively narrow for many patients. Other studies have shown a higher incidence of late shock. These studies included CS caused by the mechanical complications of MI, which usually manifests later than CS caused by left ventricular failure.[18] Angiographic data from patients enrolled in the SHOCK trial revealed extensive, severe CAD in the majority. Almost two thirds had three vessel coronary disease, and 21% had left main disease. The left anterior descending coronary artery was the culprit vessel in 49% of the cases, and the right coronary artery (RCA) in 29%.[19] The mortality rates from CS in the modern era (50%–60%) are lower than many clinicians believe and are far lower than the historic figures of 80% to 90%. However, mortality rates can range from 10% to 80%, depending on demographic, clinical, and hemodynamic factors. Specific factors include age, clinical signs of peripheral hypoperfusion, anoxic brain damage, LVEF, and stroke work. Female gender does not appear to be an independent predictor of poor outcome. Hemodynamic data are predictive of short-term mortality but not long-term mortality. However, early revascularization remains the strongest predictor of outcome.

TREATMENT

General Measures

Anti-thrombotic therapy with aspirin and heparin should be given as routinely recommended for STEMI. Clopidogrel may be deferred until after emergency coronary angiography because, on the basis of angiographic findings, CABG may be necessary immediately. Clopidogrel is indicated in all patients who undergo PCI; on the basis of extrapolation of data on patients with MI who were not in shock, clopidogrel should be useful in patients with shock as well. Negative inotropes and vasodilators (including nitroglycerin) should be avoided. Arterial oxygenation and near-normal pH should be maintained to minimize ischemia, with a low threshold to institute mechanical ventilation via mask or endotracheal tube.

Management of Complications and Special Conditions

Recognition of less common causes of CS in the setting of AMI (ventricular septal rupture, papillary muscle rupture causing acute mitral regurgitation, right ventricular infarction, and left ventricular outflow tract [LVOT] obstruction) is of paramount importance. Ventricular septal rupture should be strongly suspected in patients with a small infarction and shock. Papillary muscle rupture leading to mitral regurgitation and right ventricular infarction should be suspected in patients with inferior MI, especially in the absence of prior MI. These diagnoses may affect the revascularization strategy, and if CS is suspected, echocardiography, right heart catheterization, or ventriculography should be performed before making a decision on surgical or percutaneous revascularization.

Mechanical Support

Intra-aortic balloon counterpulsation (IABP) has long been the mainstay of mechanical therapy for CS. Use of IABP improves coronary and peripheral perfusion and augments left ventricular performance. In the large National Registry of Myocardial Infarction (NRMI), IABP use was independently associated with survival at centers with higher rates of IABP use, whether PCI, fibrinolytic therapy, or no-reperfusion had been used; however, no randomized trials have demonstrated benefit.[20] The role of ventricular assist devices in the setting of AMI is discussed elsewhere in this textbook.

Reperfusion

The only way to prevent CS in the setting of AMI appears to be very early reperfusion therapy. In a randomized trial of early, in-ambulance thrombolysis versus primary PCI, the incidence of CS was 0% among patients assigned to prehospital thrombolysis and only 0.5% in the group randomized within 2 hours from symptom onset.[21] However, reperfusion with thrombolytics is inferior to revascularization with PCI in achieving sustained TIMI-3 flow in the infarct-related artery. The survival benefit of early revascularization in CS, reported in several observational studies, was demonstrated convincingly in the randomized SHOCK trial, which demonstrated lower 6-month and 12-month mortality rates with a strategy of early emergency revascularization compared with initial medical stabilization, including IABP placement and thrombolytic therapy.[22–24] There was a 13% absolute increase in 1-year survival in patients assigned to early revascularization (Fig. 19-5).[25] This corresponds to a number-needed-to-treat (NNT) of less than 8 patients to save one life. Numerous registry studies have confirmed the survival advantage of early revascularization in CS, whether percutaneous or surgical, both in the young and in older adults. Although thrombolytic therapy is less effective, thrombolytics should be administered (in the absence of contraindications) when immediate revascularization is not possible. Ideally, such patients should have an IABP and be transferred immediately to a facility that offers revascularization.

Percutaneous Coronary Intervention in Cardiogenic Shock

Multiple trials have demonstrated the superiority of emergency revascularization with PCI compared with fibrinolytics in achieving sustained TIMI-3 flow in STEMI, with improvement in mortality rates and preservation of left ventricular function. In the SHOCK trial, PCI constituted the most frequent mode of revascularization, with 84 of 132 patients randomized to immediate revascularization undergoing immediate PCI.[26] Success with PCI was achieved in 76% (defined as the combination of a residual stenosis <50%, a >20% reduction in stenosis, and TIMI-2 or TIMI-3 flow). Overall survival in the patients selected for PCI was 54% at 30 days and 50% at 1 year. Thirty-day survival was 65% after successful PCI but only 20% if unsuccessful ($P > 0.001$). At 1 year, these values were 61% and 15%, respectively ($P > 0.001$). Post-PCI patency and TIMI-3 flow of the infarct-related

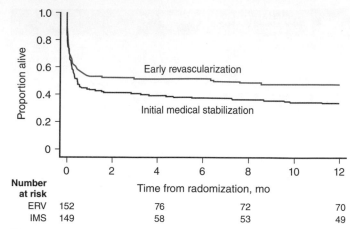

Figure 19-5 Survival rates among patients undergoing early revascularization or initial medical stabilization in the SHOCK Trial. Both 6-month and 12-month survival rates were significantly higher in those randomized to early revascularization. *(Redrawn with permission from Hochman JS, Sleeper LA, White HD, et al, SHOCK investigators: One-year survival following early revascularization for cardiogenic shock, JAMA 285:190–192, 2001.)*

artery was strongly associated with survival, even after adjustment for important clinical and hemodynamic characteristics. No patient who had an occluded infarct-related artery (TIMI flow grade 0 or 1) after PCI survived. Among CS patients undergoing PCI, age, time from symptom onset to PCI, and post-PCI flow grade are independent predictors of mortality. Importantly, revascularization provided benefit at every level of risk.

In the SHOCK trial, the success rate of PCI was relatively low (76%) and not unexpected, given that most patients had diffuse disease and occluded arteries and were hemodynamically unstable. This study predates the era of widespread stenting and adjunctive anti-platelet therapies in the setting of AMI. The majority of these patients underwent balloon angioplasty. Stents were used in 34% of patients, mainly to salvage a failed balloon PCI; the stents were largely first-generation devices implanted without the benefit of current adjunctive therapies. The culprit artery stenting rate increased during the study from 0% in 1993 to 10% in 1996 and to 74% by 1998 ($P > 0.001$). PCI was more often successful in stented patients than in unstented patients (93% vs. 67%, $P < 0.013$), although 1-year survival was similar (54% vs. 48%, $P < 0.82$). This discrepancy between the success rate and the mortality rate for PCI is probably a result of bias, since most stenting was performed following unsuccessful balloon angioplasty. The use of glycoprotein (GP) IIb/IIIa inhibitors (abciximab) also increased during the study period from 0% in 1993 to over 80% by 1998. Although the use of stents and GP IIb/IIIa inhibitors did not improve the mortality rate in the SHOCK trial, more recent data from multiple registries demonstrated that increased use of routine stenting and GP IIb/IIIa inhibitors were independent predictors of procedural success rates, TIMI-3 flow and mortality in patients undergoing PCI for CS.[27] Although 81% of patients in the SHOCK trial had multi-vessel disease, most patients with PCI underwent single-vessel procedures (87%). During the study period, there was an increase in the frequency of multi-vessel procedures from 0% to 23% ($P = 0.018$). One-year survival was 55% after single-vessel PCI but only 20% after a single-stage multi-vessel procedure. More recent data demonstrated no mortality difference between those undergoing only culprit-vessel PCI and those undergoing multivessel PCI in CS despite a high percentage of use of stenting and GP IIb/IIIa inhibitors.[28] Although PCI of the culprit lesion alone has been advocated in the management of AMI, the prevalence of multi-vessel disease and the possibility of ischemia far from the infarct zone and of progressive deterioration in left ventricular function may argue for a strategy of more complete revascularization with multi-vessel PCI or

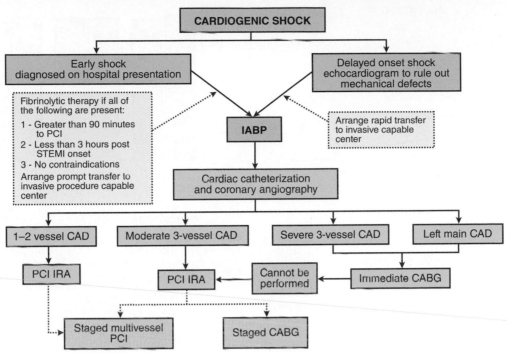

Figure 19-6 Algorithm proposed by the American College of Cardiology to guide the choice of revascularization strategy for patients with cardiogenic shock complicating an acute myocardial infarction. (Redrawn with permission from Ryan IJ, Antman EM, Brooks NH, et al: 1999 update: ACC/AHA guidelines for the management of patients with acute myocardial infarction: A report of the American College of Cardiology/American Heart Association Task Force on Practice Guidelines (Committee on Management of Acute Myocardial Infarction), J Am Coll Cardiol 34:890–911, 1999.)

surgery. As in STEMI without shock, earlier revascularization is better in CS. Presentation 0 to 6 hours after symptom onset was associated with lower mortality rates among CS patients undergoing primary PCI in the Arbeitsgemeinschaft Leitende Kardiologische Krankenhausarzte (ALKK) registry, in which door-to-angiography times were less than 90 minutes in approximately three fourths of patients.[27] In the SHOCK trial, long-term mortality rates appeared to increase as time to revascularization increased from 0 to 8 hours. However, there was a survival benefit as long as revascularization was performed within 48 hours after MI and 18 hours after shock onset. The initial misperception that older patients do not benefit from PCI arose from the interaction between treatment effect and age in the SHOCK trial. The apparent lack of benefit for older adults in the SHOCK trial was likely caused by imbalances between groups in the baseline ejection fraction. Several studies, including the SHOCK trial and registry, have shown the consistent benefit of revascularization in older patients, which suggests that clinicians are capable of identifying older patients who are most appropriate for revascularization.[29] The American College of Cardiology/American Heart Association ACC/AHA guidelines recommend early revascularization in CS for those under 75 years of age (class I) and for suitable candidates over 75 years of age (class IIa).[30] In a certain group of patients, however, additional treatment is futile, particularly when irreversible multiple end-organ failure or anoxic brain damage has occurred. Clearly, the revascularization approach must be individualized. An important consideration, especially for older adults, is functional status before the index event.

Multi-Vessel Disease

The optimal revascularization strategy (i.e., percutaneous or surgical revascularization, single or multi-vessel PCI) for patients with multi-vessel CAD and CS is not clear. This is of particular importance because multi-vessel disease is common; 87% of patients in the SHOCK trial had multi-vessel disease. Both percutaneous and surgical methods of revascularization were permitted in the SHOCK trial.

Thirty-seven percent of patients assigned to the early revascularization strategy underwent CABG at a median of 2.7 hours after randomization.[31] Despite a higher prevalence of triple-vessel or left main disease and diabetes mellitus in patients who underwent CABG compared with PCI, survival and quality of life were similar. The coronary anatomy may be most amenable to CABG in some patients. Immediate CABG is the preferred method of revascularization when severe triple-vessel or left main disease is present and should be performed, as needed, when ventricular septal rupture or severe mitral regurgitation exists. In the SHOCK trial, the rate of multi-vessel PCI increased over the study period, which perhaps suggests that operators had gained experience with PCI in patients with CS. However, this small subset had a worse adjusted outcome than those who had single-vessel PCI. PCI of the infarct-related artery is recommended in the case of single-vessel or double-vessel disease or moderate triple-vessel disease and when CABG is not possible for patients with more extensive disease. Staged multi-vessel PCI may be performed if surgery is not an option, and a single-stage procedure may be considered if the patient remains in shock after PCI of the infarct-related artery and if the other vessels have a flow-limiting lesion and supply a large region at risk. A proposed management algorithm by the American College of Cardiology is shown in Fig. 19-6.

Long-Term Survival and Quality of Life

Long-term survival data from the SHOCK trial were reported recently. Remarkably, the 3-year and 6-year survival rates in the early revascularization group were 41.4% and 32.8%, with persistence of treatment benefit (Fig. 19-7).[32] These findings are consistent with the 11-year survival rate of 55% observed in the Global Utilization of Streptokinase and t-PA for Occluded Coronary Arteries (GUSTO-I) trial with 30-day CS survivors.[33] Furthermore, in GUSTO-I, annual mortality rates after 1 year (2% to 4%) were similar for those with shock and

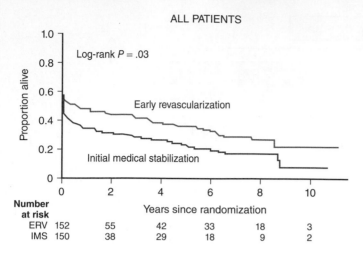

ALL PATIENTS

Log-rank *P* = .03

Early revascularization

Initial medical stabilization

Number at risk					
ERV	152	55	42	33	18	3
IMS	150	38	29	18	9	2

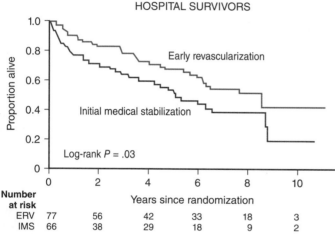

HOSPITAL SURVIVORS

Early revascularization

Initial medical stabilization

Log-rank *P* = .03

Number at risk					
ERV	77	56	42	33	18	3
IMS	66	38	29	18	9	2

Figure 19-7   Long-term survival rates of patients in the SHOCK trial by Kaplan–Meier analysis. The mortality benefit of immediate revascularization persisted during the 6 years of mean follow-up. *(Redrawn with permission from Hochman JS, Sleeper LA, Webb JG, et al, for the SHOCK investigators: Early revascularization and long-term survival in cardiogenic shock complicating acute myocardial infarction, JAMA 295:2511–2515, 2006.)*

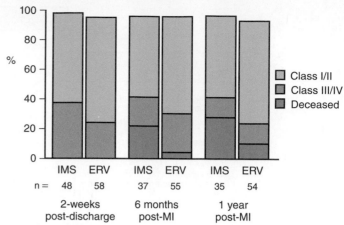

n =	IMS 48	ERV 58	IMS 37	ERV 55	IMS 35	ERV 54

2-weeks post-discharge   6 months post-MI   1 year post-MI

□ Class I/II
▨ Class III/IV
▨ Deceased

Figure 19-8   Graphic representation of the functional status of survivors of cardiogenic shock (CS) in the SHOCK trial at 2 weeks after discharge, 6 months after myocardial infarction (MI), and 1 year after MI. The graphs show that the majority of survivors were New York Heart Association (NYHA) class I or 2 at 2 weeks after discharge. Most of these patients continued to remain in the same functional class at year 1. The percentage of patients who were in class III/IV at 2 weeks after discharge decreased at year 1. *ERV*, early revascularization; *IMS*, initial medical stabilization. *(Redrawn with permission from Sleeper LA, Ramanathan K, Picard MH, et al, for the SHOCK investigators: Functional status and quality of life after emergency revascularization for cardiogenic shock complicating acute myocardial infarction, J Am Coll Cardiol 46:266–273, 2005.)*

those without shock. In survivors, quality of life is at least as important as long-term survival. At 2 weeks after discharge, 75.9% of patients assigned to revascularization and 62.5% of patients assigned to medical stabilization in the SHOCK trial were in New York Heart Association (NYHA) functional class I to II.[34] Among patients who were in NYHA functional class III to IV at 2 weeks, 55% of survivors improved to class I to II by 1 year (Fig. 19-8). Similarly, in a series of patients with CS treated with early revascularization, 80% of survivors were completely asymptomatic at a median of 18 months, and all were in NYHA functional class I to II.[35] Bicycle exercise testing in a subgroup showed age-appropriate exercise capacity in all. Finally, in a series of patients treated with circulatory support, nearly all performed activities of daily living (ADLs) 1 year after the event, and some had even returned to full-time employment.[36]

Conclusion

CS is a treatable illness with a reasonable chance for recovery. The literature has traditionally focused on the very high mortality associated with this diagnosis. It is important to recognize that although patients with CS are at very high risk for early death, great potential exists for salvage. Revascularization is associated with some benefit at every level of risk. An early invasive approach can increase short-term and long-term survival and results in patients regaining an excellent quality of life.

REFERENCES

1. Becker RC, Gore JM, Lambrew C, et al: A composite view of cardiac rupture in the United States National Registry of Myocardial Infarction. *J Am Coll Cardiol* 27(6):1321–1326, 1996.
2. Goldberg RJ, Gore JM, Alpert J, et al: Cardiogenic shock complicating acute myocardial infarction. Incidence and mortality from a community-wide perspective, 1975 to 1988. *N Engl J Med* 325:1117–1122, 1991.
3. Goldberg RJ, Samad NA, Yarzebski J, et al: Temporal trends in cardiogenic shock complicating acute myocardial infarction. *N Engl J Med* 340:1162–1168, 1999.
4. Gruppo Italiano Per Lo Studio Della Streptochinasi Ne'll Infarto Miocardico (GISSI): Effectiveness of intravenous thrombolytic treatment in acute myocardial infarction. *Lancet* 397–401, 1986.
5. ISIS-2 (Second International Study of Infarct Survival) Collaborative Group: Randomized trial of intravenous streptokinase, oral aspirin, both, or neither among 17,187 cases of suspected acute myocardial infarction. ISIS-2. *Lancet* 2:349–360, 1988.
6. Fibrinolytic Therapy Trialists' (FTT) Collaborative Group: Indications for Fibrinolytic therapy in suspected acute myocardial infarction: Collaborative overview of early mortality and major morbidity results from all randomized trials of more than 1000 patients. *Lancet* 343:311–322, 1994.
7. Jeger RV, Radovanovic D, Hunziker PR, et al, AMIS Plus Registry investigators: Ten-year trends in the incidence and treatment of cardiogenic shock. *Ann Intern Med* 149(9):618–626, 2008.
8. Babaev A, Frederick PD, Pasta DJ, et al: Trends in the management and outcomes of patients with acute myocardial infarction complicated by cardiogenic shock. *JAMA* 294:448–454, 2005.
9. Fincke R, Hochman JS, et al, SHOCK investigators: Cardiac power is the strongest hemodynamic correlate of mortality in cardiogenic shock: A report from the SHOCK trial registry. *J Am Coll Cardiol* 44:340–348, 2004.
10. Jacobs AK, Leopold JA, Bates E, et al: Cardiogenic shock caused by right ventricular infarction: A report from the SHOCK registry. *J Am Coll Cardiol* 41:1273–1279, 2003.
11. Menon V, Webb JG, Hillis LD, et al, for the SHOCK investigators: Outcome and profile of ventricular septal rupture with cardiogenic shock after myocardial infarction: A report from the SHOCK trial registry. *J Am Coll Cardiol* 36:1110–1116, 2000.
12. Thompson CR, Buller CE, Sleeper LA, et al, for the SHOCK investigators: Cardiogenic shock due to acute severe mitral regurgitation complicating acute myocardial infarction: A report from the SHOCK trial registry. *J Am Coll Cardiol* 36:1104–1109, 2000.
13. Hochman JS, Sleeper LA, Webb JG, et al: Early revascularization in acute myocardial infarction complicated by cardiogenic shock: SHOCK Investigators: Should We Emergently Revascularize Occluded Coronaries for Cardiogenic Shock. *N Engl J Med* 341:625–634, 1999.
14. Picard MH, Davidoff R, Sleeper LA, et al: Echocardiographic predictors of survival and response to early revascularization in cardiogenic shock. *Circulation* 107:279–284, 2003.
15. Hochman JS, Buller CE, Sleeper LA, et al, for the SHOCK investigators: Cardiogenic shock complicating acute myocardial infarction—etiologies, management and outcome: A report from the SHOCK trial registry. *J Am Coll Cardiol* 36:1063–1070, 2000.

16. Menon V, White H, LeJemtel T, et al: The clinical profile of patients with suspected cardiogenic shock due to predominant left ventricular failure: A report from the SHOCK trial registry. SHould we emergently revascularize Occluded Coronaries in cardiogenic shocK? *J Am Coll Cardiol* 36(3 Suppl A):1071–1076, 2000.

17. Webb JG, Sleeper LA, Buller CE, et al, for the SHOCK investigators: Implications of the timing of onset of cardiogenic shock after acute myocardial infarction: A report from the SHOCK trial registry. *J Am Coll Cardiol* 36:1084–1090, 2000.

18. Lindholm MG, Køber L, Boesgaard S, et al: Cardiogenic shock complicating acute myocardial infarction: Prognostic impact of early and late shock development. *Eur Heart J* 24(3):258–265, 2003.

19. Sanborn TA, Sleeper LA, Webb JG, et al: Correlates of one-year survival in patients with cardiogenic shock complicating acute myocardial infarction: Angiographic findings from the SHOCK trial. *J Am Coll Cardiol* 42:1373–1379, 2003.

20. Chen EW, Canto JG, Parsons LS, et al: Relation between hospital intra-aortic balloon counterpulsation volume and mortality in acute myocardial infarction complicated by cardiogenic shock. *Circulation* 108:951–957, 2003.

21. Steg PG, Bonnefoy E, Chabaud S, et al: Impact of time to treatment on mortality after prehospital fibrinolysis or primary angioplasty: Data from the CAPTIM randomized clinical trial. *Circulation* 108:2851–2856, 2003.

22. Lee L, Bates ER, Pitt B, et al: Percutaneous transluminal coronary angioplasty improves survival in acute myocardial infarction complicated by cardiogenic shock. *Circulation* 78:1345–1351, 1988.

23. Verna E, Repetto S, Boscarini M, et al: Emergency coronary angioplasty in patients with severe left ventricular dysfunction or cardiogenic shock after acute myocardial infarction. *Eur Heart J* 10:958–966, 1989.

24. Moosvi AR, Khaja F, Villanueva L, et al: Early revascularization improves survival in cardiogenic shock complicating acute myocardial infarction. *J Am Coll Cardiol* 19:907–914, 1992.

25. Hochman JS, Sleeper LA, White HD, et al, SHOCK investigators: One-year survival following early revascularization for cardiogenic shock. *JAMA* 285:190–192, 2001.

26. Webb JG, Lowe AM, Sanborn TA, et al, for the SHOCK investigators: Percutaneous coronary intervention for cardiogenic shock in the SHOCK trial. *J Am Coll Cardiol* 42:1380–1386, 2003.

27. Zeymer U, Vogt A, Zahn R, et al: Predictors of in-hospital mortality in 1333 patients with acute myocardial infarction complicated by cardiogenic shock treated with primary percutaneous coronary intervention (PCI): Results of the primary PCI registry of the Arbeitsgemeinschaft Leitende Kardiologische Krankenhausarzte (ALKK). *Eur Heart J* 25:322–328, 2004.

28. Claessen B, Vis MM, Koch KT, et al: Multivessel versus culprit only intervention in patients with multivessel disease complicated with cardiogenic shock. *J Am Coll Cardiol* 5(Suppl 1):A 185.E1734, 2010 (abstract).

29. Dzavik V, Sleeper LA, Cocke TP, et al: Early revascularization is associated with improved survival in elderly patients with acute myocardial infarction complicated by cardiogenic shock: A report from the SHOCK trial registry. *Eur Heart J* 24:828–837, 2003.

30. Ryan TJ, Antman EM, Brooks NH, et al: 1999 update: ACC/AHA guidelines for the management of patients with acute myocardial infarction: A report of the American College of Cardiology/American Heart Association Task Force on Practice Guidelines (Committee on Management of Acute Myocardial Infarction). *J Am Coll Cardiol* 34:890–911, 1999.

31. White HD, Assmann SF, Sanborn TA, et al: Comparison of percutaneous coronary intervention and coronary artery bypass grafting after acute myocardial infarction complicated by cardiogenic shock: Results from the Should We Emergently Revascularize Occluded Coronaries for Cardiogenic Shock (SHOCK) trial. *Circulation* 112:1992–2001, 2005.

32. Hochman JS, Sleeper LA, Webb JG, et al, for the SHOCK investigators: Early revascularization and long-term survival in cardiogenic shock complicating acute myocardial infarction. *JAMA* 295:2511–2515, 2006.

33. Singh M, White J, Hasdai D, et al: Long-term outcome and its predictors among patients with ST-elevation myocardial infarction complicated by shock: Insights from the GUSTO-I trial. *J Am Coll Cardiol* 50:1752–1758, 2007.

34. Sleeper LA, Ramanathan K, Picard MH, et al, for the SHOCK investigators: Functional status and quality of life after emergency revascularization for cardiogenic shock complicating acute myocardial infarction. *J Am Coll Cardiol* 46:266–273, 2005.

35. Ammann P, Straumann E, Naegeli B, et al: Long-term results after acute percutaneous transluminal coronary angioplasty in acute myocardial infarction and cardiogenic shock. *Int J Cardiol* 82:127–131, 2002.

36. Smith C, Bellomo R, Raman JS, et al: An extracorporeal membrane oxygenation-based approach to cardiogenic shock in an older population. *Ann Thorac Surg* 71:1421–1427, 2001.

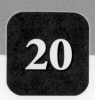

20 Bifurcations and Branch Vessel Stenting

ANTONIO COLOMBO | GORAN STANKOVIC

KEY POINTS

- An ostial lesion should always be considered a possible bifurcation lesion except at an aorto-ostial location.

- A 6 French (6F) guiding catheter is appropriate for most bifurcation procedures; a 7F or 8F guiding catheter should be used, if in doubt.

- Side branch loss should not be risked; the side branch should always be protected with a wire.

- If there are difficulties wiring the side branch, dilating the main branch first should be considered.

- Provisional stenting does not mean accepting a poor final result for an important side branch.

- Treatment of a bifurcation lesion with two stents (main and side branches) as intention to treat is an acceptable approach.

- When implanting two stents, final kissing inflation should always be preceded by high-pressure inflation of the side branch.

- When dedicated drug-eluting stents (DESs) for bifurcation lesions become available, many concepts may change, including a more liberal use of a two-stent strategy,

- Optimal anti-platelet therapy is a key factor for short-term and long-term success of stenting.

Bifurcation Lesions

A bifurcation coronary lesion occurs at or adjacent to a significant division of a major epicardial coronary artery. Coronary bifurcation lesions have been the subject of several classifications with the underlying assumption that each type could be associated with a specific treatment. However, attempts to classify bifurcation lesions have all of the limitations of coronary angiography (different plaque distribution and extent of disease when evaluated by intravascular ultrasound).[1-6] At the present time, there are six different classifications of bifurcation lesions (Fig. 20-1). The most important distinction is to divide bifurcation lesions into "true" bifurcations, where the main branch (MB) and the side branch (SB) are both significantly narrowed (>50% diameter stenosis), and "nontrue" bifurcations, which include all the other lesions involving a bifurcation. In routine practice, the Medina classification is still the simplest and most widely used approach to classify the distribution of atherosclerotic plaque at the bifurcation site.[5] The designation "1" means the presence of stenosis and "0" the absence of stenosis, in each of the three bifurcation segments, starting with proximal MB, distal MB, and proximal SB: the designation "1.1.1" indicates a critical stenosis in all three segments and "1.1.0" when only the proximal and distal MBs are affected; however, many other combinations are possible. A limitation of the Medina classification is that the length of the stenosis involving the SB is not specified; this distinction is, however, a key element to properly plan the treatment. Despite an array of devices available, the use of DESs remains the default approach to treat bifurcation lesions, and the implantation of a single stent on the MB is the most widely used approach.

CONTEMPORARY STUDIES

Several major randomized trials comparing the use of one or two stents in the treatment of coronary bifurcations demonstrated that the implantation of a stent only in the MB remains the preferred strategy. The sirolimus-eluting stent (SES) bifurcation study has been the first attempt to provide specific information in this subset of lesions.[7] Eighty-five patients were randomly assigned to either stenting both branches or stenting the MB only with provisional stenting of the SB. Data were analyzed by actual treatment received, not by intention to treat. The cross-over rate was very high, 51.2% in the provisional group and 4.7% in the two-stent group. Re-stenosis at 6 months did not differ significantly between the two-stent (28.0%) and the stent-plus-percutaneous transluminal coronary angioplasty (PTCA) (18.7%) groups (P = 0.53). During the 6-month follow-up, there was one death in the two-stent group and none in the stent-plus-PTCA group. There was no significant difference between the groups in Q wave myocardial infarction (MI) (1.6% vs. 4.5%), non–Q wave MI (9.5% vs. 4.5%), tricuspid valve regurgitation (TVR) (11.1% vs. 9%), or target vessel failure (19% vs. 13.6%). There were three cases of stent thrombosis, all of which occurred in the stent–stent group. Therefore, this study demonstrated that, compared with historical studies using bare metal stents (BMSs), a clear improvement has been achieved in the treatment of bifurcation lesions when one or two DESs were implanted.[1,8,9] In a second study, Pan and coworkers compared two strategies for the SES treatment of bifurcation lesions in 91 patients with "true" coronary bifurcation lesions.[10] Major adverse cardiac events (MACE) at six months were similar between two groups and occurred in 3 patients in the provisional group (2 non–Q wave MIs and 1 TLR) and in 3 patients in the two-stent group (1 subacute stent thrombosis with subsequent death and 2 TLR). Six-month angiographic re-evaluation was obtained in 80 patients (88%) and the re-stenosis rates of the MB and the SB were also similar in two study groups. A third randomized study was the Nordic Bifurcation Study (Nordic), in which 413 patients were randomized to two stents (n = 206) using crush, culotte, Y, or other techniques or provisional stenting (n = 207) with SES implantation.[11] The cross-over from provisional stenting to two stents was allowed only with thrombolysis in MI (TIMI) flow grade 0 following SB dilation. Procedural success was achieved in 97% of cases in provisional stenting versus 95% in the two-stents group. The cross-over rate was also low, and SB was stented only in 4.3% of the patients in the provisional stenting group. Final kissing balloon inflation was performed in 32% and 74% of the patients, respectively (P < 0.001). At 6 months, there was no difference between the two groups with regard to cardiac death, MI, index lesion MI, TVR, TLR, and stent thrombosis. Fourteen-month follow-up confirmed these results, and 2 months after recommended cessation of dual anti-platelet therapy, the rates of stent thrombosis and MACE were low and similar in the two arms.[12] In a fourth trial, Bifurcations Bad Krozingen (BBK) study, Ferenc et al compared 202 patients randomly allocated to either provisional T stenting or routine T stenting, using SES.[13] Final kissing balloon dilatation was performed in both groups irrespective of whether they were assigned to routine or provisional T stenting; in the provisional T stent arm, cross-over to SB stenting was mandated in case of a flow-limiting dissection or residual stenosis of greater than 75%. The primary endpoint was percent diameter stenosis of the SB at 9-month angiographic follow-up and was similar between the two groups (P = 0.15). The overall 1-year incidence of target lesion re-intervention was 10.9% after provisional T stenting and 8.9% after routine T stenting (P = 0.64), and the primary clinical outcome (death, MI, target lesion revascularization) was

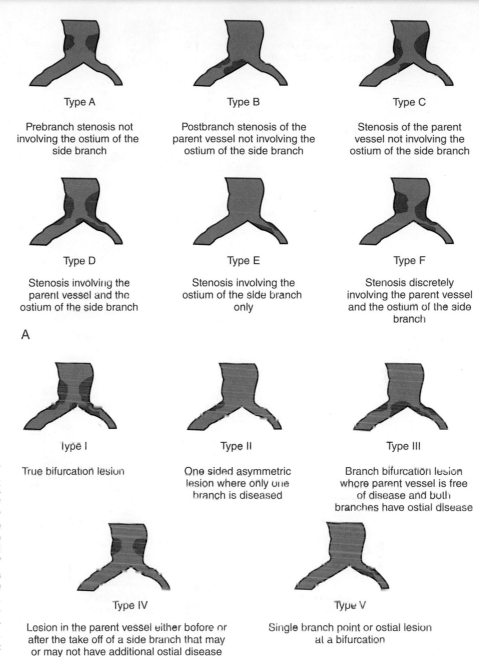

Type A
Prebranch stenosis not involving the ostium of the side branch

Type B
Postbranch stenosis of the parent vessel not involving the ostium of the side branch

Type C
Stenosis of the parent vessel not involving the ostium of the side branch

Type D
Stenosis involving the parent vessel and the ostium of the side branch

Type E
Stenosis involving the ostium of the side branch only

Type F
Stenosis discretely involving the parent vessel and the ostium of the side branch

A

Type I
True bifurcation lesion

Type II
One sided asymmetric lesion where only one branch is diseased

Type III
Branch bifurcation lesion where parent vessel is free of disease and both branches have ostial disease

Type IV
Lesion in the parent vessel either before or after the take off of a side branch that may or may not have additional ostial disease

Type V
Single branch point or ostial lesion at a bifurcation

B

Figure 20-1 Various classifications of bifurcations according to plaque distribution: Duke (A), Sanborn (B), Safian (C), Lefevre (D)1, SYNTAX (SYNergy between percutaneous coronary intervention with TAXus and cardiac surgery study) (E), and Medina (F). *(With permission from Safian RD: Bifurcation Lesions. In Safian RD, Freed M, editors: Manual of interventional cardiology, Royal Oak, CA, 2001, Physicians' Press; Medina A, Suarez de Lezo J, Pan M: A new classification of coronary bifurcation lesions, Rev Esp Cardiol 59:183, 2006; Popma J, Leon M, Topol EJ: Atlas of interventional cardiology, Philadelphia, PA, 1994, Saunders; Spokojny AM, Sanborn TM: The bifurcation lesion. In Ellis SG, Holmes DR, editors: Strategic approaches in coronary intervention, Baltimore, MD, 1996, Williams and Wilkins.)*

equivalent in both groups (12.9% provisional T stenting vs. 11.9% routine T stenting ($P = 0.83$). The fifth trial of interest was the CACTUS trial (Coronary Bifurcations: Application of the Crushing Technique Using Sirolimus-Eluting Stents).[14] In this study, 350 patients were randomly allocated to either provisional T or crush SES implantation, with mandatory final kissing balloon inflation in both groups. Stent implantation in the SB was allowed by the T stenting technique only when at least one of the following conditions was met: (1) residual stenosis 50% or greater, (2) dissection of type B or worse, or (3) thrombolysis in MI (TIMI) flow grade 2 or less. A high proportion of patients (92%) had true bifurcations, and the cross-over rate in the provisional T group was 31%. The primary angiographic endpoint was the in-segment re-stenosis rate, and the primary clinical endpoint was a 6-month rate of major adverse cardiac events (cardiac death, MI, or target vessel revascularization). At 6 months, angiographic

re-stenosis rates were not different between the crush group (4.6% and 13.2% in the MB and SB, respectively) and the provisional stenting group (6.7% and 14.7% in the MB and SB, respectively; P = not significant [NS]). The primary clinical outcome (death, MI, revascularization) was also similar in both groups (15% provisional vs. 15.8% crush, P = NS). Finally, in the BBC ONE study (British Bifurcation Coronary Study: Old, New, and Evolving Strategies), 500 patients were randomly allocated to either a simple strategy (minimalist provisional T) or a complex strategy (either crush or culotte) using paclitaxel-eluting stents (PES).[15] In the simple strategy, the MB was stented, followed by optional kissing balloon dilatation or T stent, using the following criteria: TIMI flow grade less than 3 in the SB, severe ostial pinching of the SB (>90%), threatened SB closure, or SB dissection greater than type A. If one of these criteria existed, the operator could progress to the next stage, but if the SB was stented, final kissing

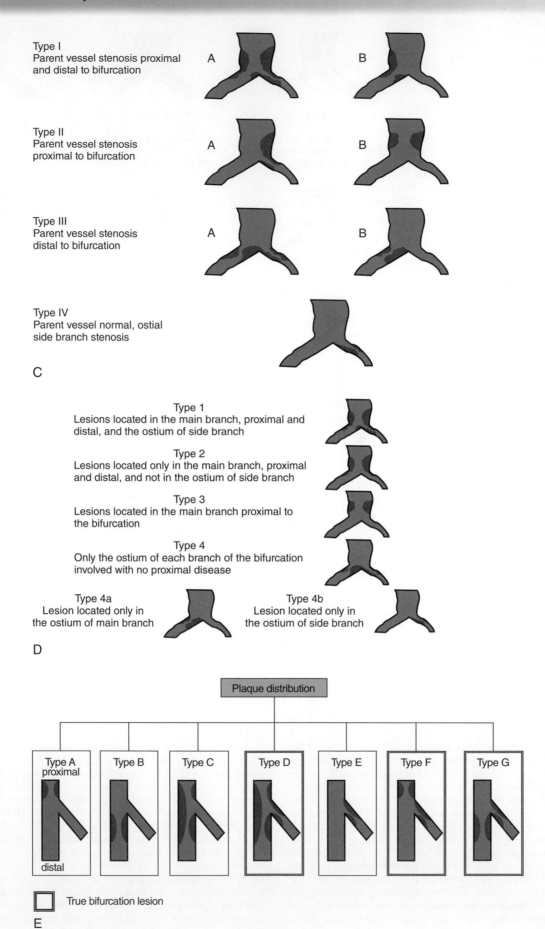

Type I
Parent vessel stenosis proximal
and distal to bifurcation

A   B

Type II
Parent vessel stenosis
proximal to bifurcation

A   B

Type III
Parent vessel stenosis
distal to bifurcation

A   B

Type IV
Parent vessel normal, ostial
side branch stenosis

C

Type 1
Lesions located in the main branch, proximal and
distal, and the ostium of side branch

Type 2
Lesions located only in the main branch, proximal
and distal, and not in the ostium of side branch

Type 3
Lesions located in the main branch proximal to
the bifurcation

Type 4
Only the ostium of each branch of the bifurcation
involved with no proximal disease

Type 4a
Lesion located only in
the ostium of main branch

Type 4b
Lesion located only in
the ostium of side branch

D

Plaque distribution

Type A
proximal

Type B

Type C

Type D

Type E

Type F

Type G

distal

☐ True bifurcation lesion

E

Figure 20-1, cont'd.

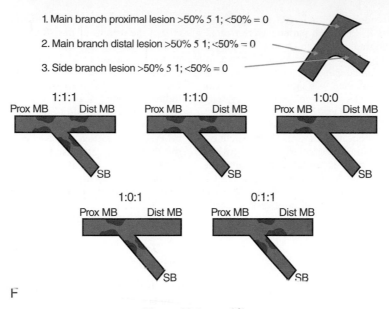

1. Main branch proximal lesion >50% 5 1; <50% = 0

2. Main branch distal lesion >50% 5 1; <50% = 0

3. Side branch lesion >50% 5 1; <50% = 0

1:1:1

Prox MB   Dist MB

SB

1:1:0

Prox MB   Dist MB

SB

1:0:0

Prox MB   Dist MB

SB

1:0:1

Prox MB   Dist MB

SB

0:1:1

Prox MB   Dist MB

SB

F

Figure 20-1, cont'd.

balloon was mandatory. Only 30% of the SB underwent further treatment after MB stenting (27% balloon dilatation and 3% stenting). In the complex strategy, both branches were systematically stented (culotte or crush techniques) with mandatory kissing balloon dilation. At 9 months clinical follow-up, there was a significant difference between the two groups in terms of death, MI, or revascularization (simple 8% vs. complex 15.5%). This difference was largely driven by the higher incidence of MI in the complex group (11.2% vs. 3.6%, $P = 0.001$). It is quite surprising to note the very high number of complications that occurred in patients randomized to the complex strategy. The clinical implication of those trials is that in most cases, provisional stenting rather than elective stenting of the SB should be performed. Provisional stenting seems to be less expensive and simpler and can be performed with less contrast and in a shorter procedural time. At the same time, the evidence of equivalent results in the two arms does not contradict the choice of crush or culotte stenting in selected cases with complex anatomy or with diffuse disease in the SB. The consensus from randomized trial data was that routine two-vessel stenting did not improve either angiographic or clinical outcomes for

most patients with coronary bifurcation lesions, although routine two-vessel stenting did not involve a significant penalty either.

One shortcoming of those trials was that the treatment groups that included two stents were heterogeneous, and the techniques used may have resulted in different clinical outcomes.

Clinical outcomes in randomized trials comparing one-stent versus two-stent strategy that included DESs are presented in Fig. 20-2. To evaluate the impact of a specific two-stent technique, the Nordic complex bifurcation stenting study was performed. In this investigation, 424 patients were randomized to either crush or culotte stenting using SES (77% of which were "true" coronary bifurcation lesions).[16] At 6 months clinical follow-up, there was no difference between the two groups in terms of death, post-procedure MI, or revascularization (the primary endpoint: crush 4.3% vs. culotte 3.7%, $P = 0.87$). However, there was a trend toward higher incidence of peri procedural MI (crush 15.5% vs. culotte 8.8%, $P = 0.08$) and significantly higher occurrence of in stent re-stenosis in the crush group (crush 10.5% vs. culotte 4.5%, $P = 0.046$). To evaluate the impact of a specific DES type on clinical outcome in patients with bifurcation lesions, Pan et al enrolled

Figure 20-2 Clinical outcomes in randomized trials comparing one-stent versus two-stent strategy, using drug-eluting stents. *1S*, single stent; *2S*, two stents.

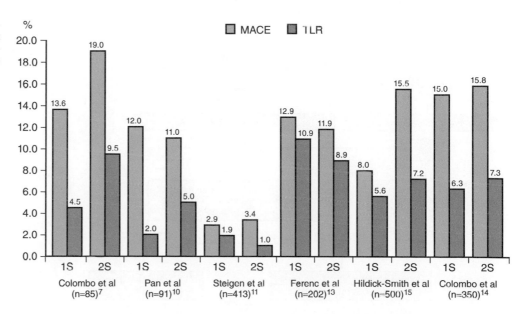

205 patients in a prospective randomized trial; 103 patients were assigned to SES and 102 patients to PES.[17] All patients were treated with provisional T stenting. Angiographic data and immediate procedural results were similar in both groups. There was no difference in the rates of death or MI in hospital and during follow-up. The primary endpoint, the angiographic re-stenosis rate, was significantly lower in the SES group (9% vs. 29%, $P = 0.011$), as was target lesion revascularization at 24 months after stenting (4% vs. 13%, $P = 0.021$). Similar results were obtained in the COBIS (Coronary Bifurcation Stenting) registry, which compared major adverse cardiac events (MACE defined as cardiac death, MI, or target lesion revascularization) between SES and PES.[18] At a mean follow-up of 22 months, treatment with SES resulted in a lower incidence of MACE (HR 0.53; 95% CI 0.32–0.89, $P < 0.01$) and target lesion revascularization (HR 0.55; 95% CI 0.31–0.97, $P = 0.02$) but not of cardiac death and cardiac death or MI.

APPROACH TO TREATMENT OF BIFURCATION LESIONS

Bifurcations vary not only in anatomy (plaque burden, location of plaque, angle between branches, diameter of branches, bifurcation site) but also in the dynamic changes in anatomy during treatment (plaque or carina shift, dissection). Previous pathologic studies demonstrated that atherosclerosis occurs predominantly in low shear–stress regions of bifurcation but that carina (flow divider) involvement by atherosclerosis is extremely unusual. Nakazawa et al recently demonstrated that in nonstented coronary bifurcations, the lateral wall showed significantly greater intima as well as necrotic core thickness compared with the flow divider.[19] After stenting, plaque formation and neointimal growth were also significantly less at the flow divider compared with the lateral wall. Those observations were also confirmed in vivo with the IVUS (intravenous ultrasound) preintervention evaluation of the distal left main coronary artery (LMCA) bifurcations.[20] Oviedo et al showed that bifurcation disease is usually diffuse and, contrary to angiographic classifications, that the carina (flow divider) was spared in all lesions, whereas plaque was present predominantly on the opposite side of the flow divider. However, data presented by van der Giessen et al threw new light on the subject through computed tomographic (CT) angiography, which suggested that the carina does have some atheroma present in 30% of bifurcations, though the volume of that plaque remains small and atheroma was present only if there is significant volume of plaque located at the lateral walls opposite to flow divider (low wall shear–stress areas), indicating that atherosclerotic plaque grows circumferentially.[21] Koo et al evaluated with IVUS and

fractional flow reserve (FFR) the mechanisms of changes in the geometry of the ostium of the SB after MB stenting to test the hypothesis that MB stenting may create worsening of an SB ostial lesion as a result of a combination of MB plaque and carina shift.[22] The investigators concluded that the decrease in plaque volume in the proximal MB, with no associated increase in plaque volume in the distal MB, was indirect evidence of plaque shift from the MB to the SB ostium after stent implantation. Additionally, the increased luminal volume in the distal MB, with no significant decrease in the plaque volume, was believed to be caused by vessel enlargement and provided support to the theory that carina shift is likely to contribute to the degree of luminal narrowing of the SB. As a result of those investigations, it can be concluded that no two bifurcations are identical and that no single strategy can be applied to every bifurcation. Thus, the more important issue in bifurcation PCI is selecting the most appropriate strategy for an individual bifurcation and optimizing the performance of this technique.

GUIDING CATHETER SELECTION

Most bifurcation lesions can be approached with a 6F guiding catheter, since a provisional strategy will be used most of the time. The exception is when, because of lesions characteristics, the operator decides from the very beginning to implant two stents (need of 8F guiding catheter, even if technically a 7F guiding catheter can be used with some new DESs). When there are doubts regarding the optimal treatment and the operator needs to make a decision following predilatation, use of a 7F or 8F guiding catheter is recommended. With the currently available very-low profile balloons, it is possible to insert two balloons inside a large lumen 6F guiding catheter. If two stents are needed and a 6F guiding catheter is employed, it is important to be aware of certain limitations. The two stents can only be inserted and deployed sequentially. The standard crush technique and the V or kissing-stents technique cannot be performed unless a guiding catheter of 8F is used. New second-generation DESs may allow the use of a 7F guiding catheter. When the operator knows a priori that two stents will be implanted, an 8F guiding catheter is the best choice in the view of the authors of this chapter.

GENERAL OUTLINE FOR TREATING A BIFURCATION LESION

Fig. 20-3 summarizes a proposed approach to bifurcation lesions with an attempt to give directions for SB stenting as intention to treat only in cases where disease on the SB extends beyond the ostium and the SB has a significant area of distribution.

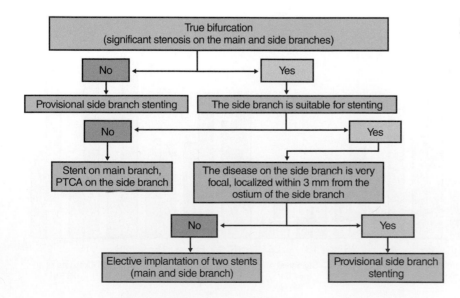

Figure 20-3 Proposed algorithm for stenting bifurcation lesions.

The most frequently used approach is provisional SB stenting, and it is outlined as follows:

1. Placement of two wires (MB and SB)
2. Predilatation, when needed
3. Stenting of the MB
4. Recrossing with a wire into the SB
5. Crossing with a balloon into the SB
6. Performance of kissing balloon inflation with moderate pressure (8 atmosphere [atm]) in the SB, until the balloon is fully expanded
7. Placement of a second stent in the SB only if the result is inadequate

An important aspect when stenting bifurcations is the protection of the SB by inserting a wire to be left in until the stenting procedure on the MB has been completed, including high-pressure stent deployment or postdilatation. These temporary jailed wires can be retrieved, provided care is taken to avoid any trauma to the ostium of the proximal coronary with the guiding catheter, which tends to get pulled in.

In the provisional technique, wire crossing through the distal strut (the "carina strut") following MB stenting is strongly recommended because it creates better SB scaffolding compared with proximal crossing.

To optimize SB access through the carina strut, the POT (proximal optimization) technique is proposed. Optimization of the stent deployment proximal to the carina by using a short, half-size bigger balloon or a spherical balloon may help access the most distal strut during wire exchange. If the result remains unsatisfactory after MB stenting (>75%

residual stenosis, dissection, TIMI flow grade <3 in an SB ≥2.5 mm or FFR <0.75), SB stenting should be performed. SB stenting can be performed with T stenting or TAP (T and Protrusion; see below for description of TAP) stenting, reverse or internal crush and culotte, followed by kissing balloon inflation.

DIFFICULT ACCESS TO THE SIDE BRANCH

After having attempted different types of wires with all sorts of curves and exhausted all personal tactics, the operator may still be unable to advance a wire in the SB. At this point, few options are available: (1) aborting the procedure because the risk of losing the SB will be too high, depending on the size and distribution of the branch (typically an angulated circumflex artery), (2) performing rotational atherectomy on the MB with the intent to remove the plaque that prevents entry toward the SB, (3) dilating the MB with a balloon on the basis of the rationale that plaque modification and, hopefully, a favorable plaque shift will facilitate access toward the SB, (4) using the Venture wire control catheter (VWC-St. Jude Medical, Maple Grove, MN), a low-profile catheter with a tip that can be deflected up to 90 degrees, which facilitates wire orientation and provides excellent backup support (Fig. 20-4).[23] Each of these four options has its rationale, and the specific anatomic condition, the operator's experience, and the clinical scenario may direct the selection of the best strategy. Usually, the third option is the one more frequently employed and is effective most of the time.

Figure 20-4 Baseline angiogram presenting large, eccentric, atherosclerotic plaque which involves the distal part of the left main coronary artery (LMCA) and extends into the ostial segment of the left anterior descending (LAD) artery. Because of a tight LMCA lesion and unfavorable access to ostial LAD (A), a Venture wire control catheter (St. Jude Medical, Maple Grove, MN) (arrow) was used to insert coronary guidewire (thick arrow) (B). After that two guidewires were inserted in the intermediate branch and left circumflex (LCx) artery. Following predilatation of LMCA or ostial LAD lesion a drug-eluting stent was implanted from the ostium of LMCA toward the LAD artery (C), and final kissing balloon inflation was performed with three balloons, positioned from the LMCA to the LAD, intermediate branch, and LCx arteries (D). Panel D presents final angiographic result. NC, non compliant balloon.

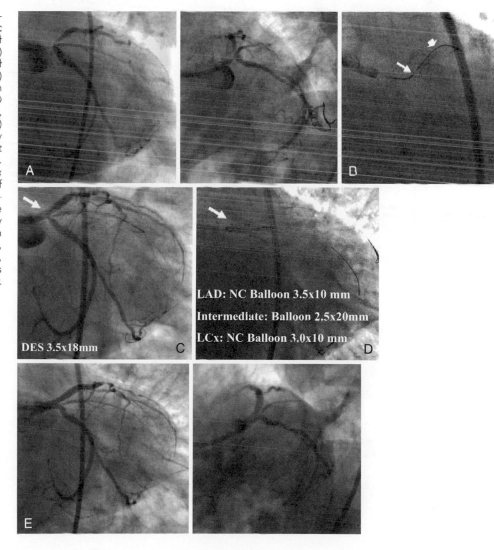

ROLE OF FINAL KISSING BALLOON INFLATION

Final kissing balloon inflation is proposed if the SB is dilated through the MB stent struts to correct MB stent distortion and proximal expansion and to provide better scaffolding of the SB ostium and facilitate future access to the SB. The CACTUS trial subanalysis showed that final kissing balloon inflation was associated with better angiographic results and lower MACE rates when complex stenting was performed and similar results were observed when using a simpler provisional SB stenting technique.[14] Several criteria have been proposed to define lesions in which final kissing balloon inflation is required (>75% residual stenosis at the SB, TIMI flow grade <3, or FFR <0.75). However, there is significant debate on the use of routine kissing inflations following the Nordic III study presentation during the TCT 2009 meeting, which has established that there is no systematic clinical advantage to a routine kissing strategy when a single stent treatment is used (http://www.tctmd.com/show.aspx?id=84126; accessed on June 12, 2010). Therefore, two appropriate strategies are (1) to use a pressure wire to interrogate the significance of the side branch lesion and to treat or not treat, accordingly, or (2) simply to do kissing balloon inflations on all angiographically significant ostial SB lesions, which reduces the proportion of physiologically significant SB ostial lesions; this is supported by information from the Nordic III trial which demonstrated that there appears to be no penalty for doing so.[24] A study by Koo et al has shown that kissing balloon inflation restores normal

FFR.[25] As a general approach, the authors of this chapter favor final kissing balloon inflation.

A SECOND STENT IN THE SIDE BRANCH FOLLOWING THE PROVISIONAL APPROACH

When the results obtained with balloon dilatation of the SB is not satisfactory and there is a need to implant a second stent, the following strategies can be used: T, TAP, culotte, or reverse or internal crush configuration. FFR or new imaging techniques such as optical coherence tomography (OCT) could be of value in the evaluation of the SB result after balloon dilation.

1. *T technique* (Fig. 20-5): Most probably, this technique is the one most frequently used to shift from provisional stenting to stenting the SB.[26,27] The T technique consists of advancing a second stent into the SB (following adequate dilation of the MB stent struts). The stent is positioned at the ostium of the SB in an attempt to minimize any possible gap. A second kissing balloon inflation is also performed. In the authors' view, the T technique is associated with the risk of leaving a small gap between the stent implanted in the MB and the one implanted in the SB. This gap may be a factor contributing to an uneven distribution of the drug, which leads to ostial re-stenosis at the SB. The authors believe that this was a possible concurrent cause for the re-stenosis they noticed at the ostium of the SB when two stents were implanted in the Sirolimus

Figure 20-5 A schematic representation of the T stenting technique.

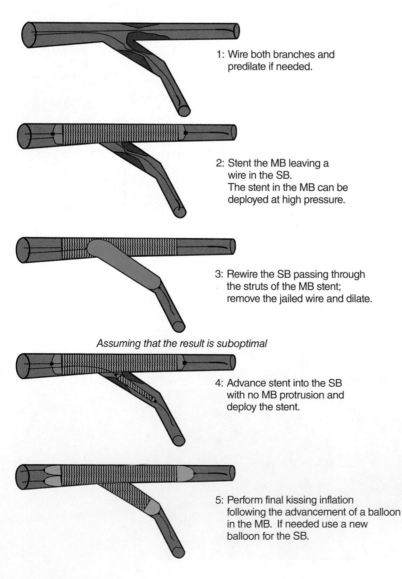

1: Wire both branches and predilate if needed.

2: Stent the MB leaving a wire in the SB.
The stent in the MB can be deployed at high pressure.

3: Rewire the SB passing through the struts of the MB stent; remove the jailed wire and dilate.

Assuming that the result is suboptimal

4: Advance stent into the SB with no MB protrusion and deploy the stent.

5: Perform final kissing inflation following the advancement of a balloon in the MB. If needed use a new balloon for the SB.

bifurcation study. The T technique was, indeed, used when two stents were implanted.[7]

2. *T stenting and small protrusion (TAP)*: The TAP technique is a modification of the T stenting technique and is based on an intentional minimal protrusion of the SB stent within the MB (Fig. 20-6).[28,29] This technique can be described as follows:

   a. A second stent is advanced in the SB in such a way as to protrude minimally (1 or 2 mm) into the MB.
   b. A balloon is advanced in the MB.
   c. The SB stent is deployed as usual (12 atm or more), and the MB balloon is simultaneously inflated at 12 atm or more.
   d. Both balloons are deflated and removed.

   The technique is quite similar to the V stenting technique, but the only difference is that one of the components of the system is a balloon inflated inside a stent previously deployed in the MB.

   Despite some concerns about the stent protrusion in the MB, in the authors' experience, IVUS can be performed in the MB and the

SB, and when needed, additional stents can be advanced distally in the MB and in the SB.

3. *Reverse or internal crush*: The crush is performed after main branch stenting (Fig. 20-7).[30,31] The main purpose in performing the reverse crush is to allow an opportunity for provisional SB stenting. This technique was developed with the intent to minimize any possible stent gap between the MB and SB stents. The reverse crush can be performed using a 6F guiding catheter in the following steps:

   a. A second stent is advanced into the SB and left in position without being deployed.
   b. A balloon, sized according to the diameter of the MB and shorter than the stent already deployed, is advanced in the MB and positioned at the level of the bifurcation, taking care to make it stay inside the stent previously deployed in the MB.
   c. The stent in the SB is retracted about 3 mm or less into the MB and deployed. The deploying balloon is removed, and an angiogram is obtained to verify the absence of any distal dissection and

Figure 20-6 Example of T stenting and small protrusion (TAP) technique. The baseline angiogram presents diffuse disease of the LAD and ostial or proximal segment of diagonal branch (A). Following stent implantation in the proximal and mid-segments of the LAD artery and balloon angioplasty at the diagonal branch the result appears unsatisfactory (B). A second stent is advanced in the diagonal branch to minimally protrude (1 or 2 mm) into the LAD artery, and the balloon is positioned in the LAD artery. The stent in the diagonal branch is deployed, and the balloon in the LAD artery is simultaneously inflated (C). Angiographic view of the final result (D). Transverse and longitudinal views of final intravascular ultrasound in the LAD artery (E) and the diagonal branch (F) confirm optimal stent position in the diagonal branch, with minimal protrusion in the LAD artery. *LAD*, left anterior descending; *NC*, noncompliant balloon; *DES*, drug-eluting stent.

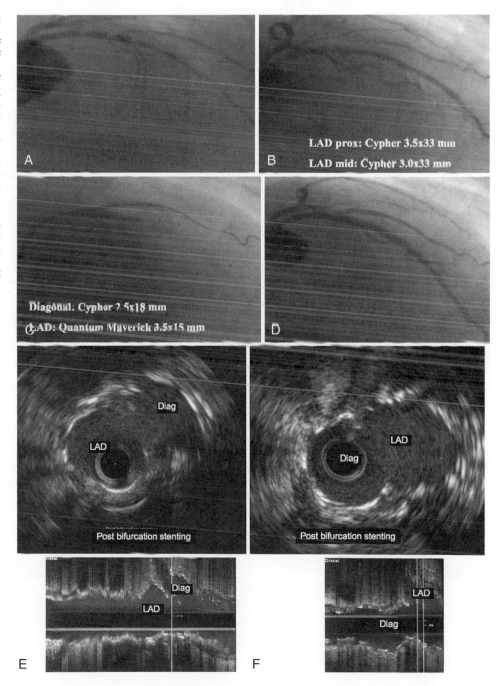

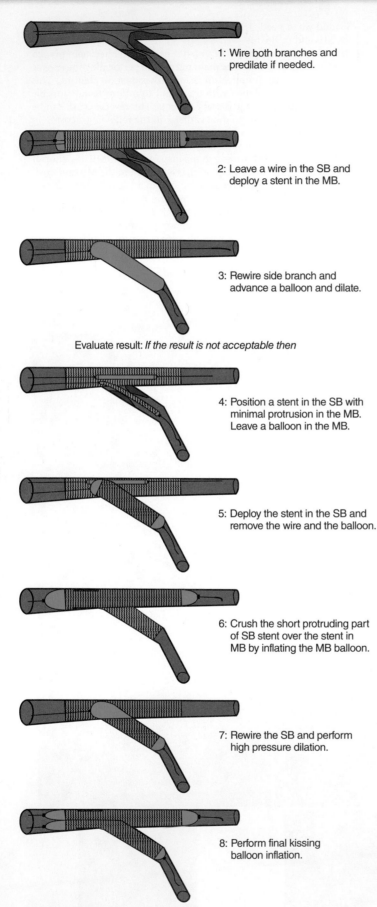

1: Wire both branches and predilate if needed.

2: Leave a wire in the SB and deploy a stent in the MB.

3: Rewire side branch and advance a balloon and dilate.

Evaluate result: *If the result is not acceptable then*

4: Position a stent in the SB with minimal protrusion in the MB. Leave a balloon in the MB.

5: Deploy the stent in the SB and remove the wire and the balloon.

6: Crush the short protruding part of SB stent over the stent in MB by inflating the MB balloon.

7: Rewire the SB and perform high pressure dilation.

8: Perform final kissing balloon inflation.

Figure 20-7 A schematic representation of the reverse or internal crush technique.

the need for an additional stent. If such is the case, the wire from the SB is removed, and the balloon in the MB is inflated at high pressure (12 atm or more).

d. The SB struts are recrossed with a wire and a balloon (a 1.5-mm balloon is sometimes needed). The balloon is sized to the SB reference diameter and inflated at high pressure (12–20 atm).

e. Final kissing balloon is performed.

In the authors, practice, this technique has been completely superseded by the TAP technique.

4. *The provisional culotte technique:* The culotte technique can be proposed as a provisional SB stenting strategy in Y-shaped, angulated bifurcation lesions, as in the original description, although the first stent can be deployed across the most angulated branch, usually the SB (inverted culotte).[32,33]

This technique can be described as follows:

a. After MB stenting, a second stent is advanced in the SB, with the stent protruding into the MB to overlap with the proximal part of the MB stent and expanded following the removal of the MB wire.

b. The MB is rewired through the stent struts and dilated.

c. Finally, kissing balloon inflation is performed.

EUROPEAN BIFURCATION CLUB APPROACH TO BIFURCATION STENTING

The European Bifurcation Club (EBC) was founded in 2004 to devise a common terminology for the description and treatment of bifurcation lesions and to exchange ideas on the clinical, technical, and fundamental aspects of the specific treatment strategies implemented in this setting. A synopsis of these discussions is presented below:[24,34–36]

1. The Medina classification should be used for bifurcation lesions (1,0) and the MADS (Main, Across, Distal, Side, based on the manner in which the first stent has been implanted) classification for bifurcation stenting techniques.

2. Provisional T stenting remains the gold standard technique for most bifurcations.

3. Large SBs with ostial disease extending over 5 mm from the carina are likely to require a two-stent strategy.

4. In the provisional technique, after wiring both branches, the MB should be predilated when required, whereas SBs without severe calcification or long significant lesion (>5 mm) do not require predilatation.

5. The SB wire should be jailed behind the MB stent in true bifurcation lesions.

6. The MB stent is selected according to distal main branch diameter and postdilatation; or kissing balloon inflations are required to optimize the proximal main branch stent diameter.

7. Wire cross through the distal strut following MB stenting is recommended.

8. The POT (proximal optimization) technique—optimization of the stent deployment proximal to the carina by using a short half-size bigger balloon—should be used in any case of difficulty recrossing into an SB with either a wire or a balloon.

9. Kissing balloon inflation for carina reconstruction is mandatory in two-stent techniques.

10. Kissing balloon inflations, or pressure wire interrogation, should be used in provisional stenting when an angiographically significant (>75%) SB lesion persists after main branch stenting.

11. High-pressure proximal stent inflation using a short noncompliant balloon should be considered for the correction of possible proximal stent distortion after kissing balloon inflation.

■ Two Stents as Intention to Treat

If the operator evaluates that a particular bifurcation will need implantation of two stents—one in the MB and the other in the SB—the techniques that are considered suitable in the era of DESs are described below. The two-stent approach will be reserved only for selected "true" bifurcations following evaluation of additional parameters:

SIZE AND TERRITORY OF DISTRIBUTION OF THE SIDE BRANCH

The term *side branch* is sometimes misinterpreted as a vessel of less importance compared with the MB. This statement may be true in most cases, but there are various anatomic conditions in which the SB is as important as the MB with regard to both size and territory of distribution. The LMCA which bifurcates into the left anterior descending (LAD) artery and the left circumflex (LCx) artery, the RCA (right coronary artery) which bifurcates in a posterior descending artery and a number of posterolateral branches, a dominant LCx artery which bifurcates into a distal LCx artery and a large obtuse marginal branch are all examples in which the SBs are important vessels, which may generate a large ischemia if left with a critical narrowing. As shown in Fig. 20-3, the size of the territory supplied by the SB becomes a valuable element to guide the decision to accept a mediocre result at the SB ostium (following balloon angioplasty) versus the need to have almost 0% residual stenosis as following additional SB stenting.

LENGTH OF LESIONS AT THE OSTIUM OF THE SIDE BRANCH

Most of the studies demonstrated that a focal lesion present at the ostium of the SB does not prevent a provisional approach, but the situation may be different when the stenosis extends for several millimeters into the SB.

ANGLE BETWEEN THE MAIN BRANCH AND THE SIDE BRANCH AND THE NARROWING AT THE OSTIUM OF THE SIDE BRANCH

The angle of origin of the SB from the MB can be acute, close to 90 degrees, or obtuse. The narrower the angle between the two branches, the higher will be the risk of plaque prolapse and compromise of the ostium of the SB.[37] Another element to consider when looking at the angle between the two branches is the difficulty to recross into the SB following stenting of the MB. The severity of the narrowing at the ostium of the SB is another factor influencing the placement of two stents. An additional variable to be considered is the result obtained following balloon dilatation of the SB. All these elements mean that the decision to implant a second stent may also be made at an intermediate time, following predilatation of the MB and the SB.

These considerations should not downplay the fact that the decision for one stent, two stents, or sometimes even three (in case of a trifurcation) should be taken as early as possible. An action taken in a timely manner will influence the result positively and help save time and cost and also lower the risks of complications.

It is important to be aware that if the decision is to use one stent (in the MB), there is almost always the possibility of having to place a second stent in the SB in case the result is not optimal or adequate.

◼ Two-Stent Techniques

CULOTTE TECHNIQUE

The culotte technique (Fig. 20-8) uses two stents and results in full coverage of the bifurcation at the expense of an excess of metal covering of the proximal end.[32,33]

The culotte technique probably gives the best coverage of the carina. An important caveat about this approach is that with some closed cells, some stents, for example, the Cypher stent, the opening of the struts toward the branches may only reach a maximum diameter of 3 mm. For this reason, the culotte technique should be used only with stents which have a design (open cells stents) that allows full opening of the

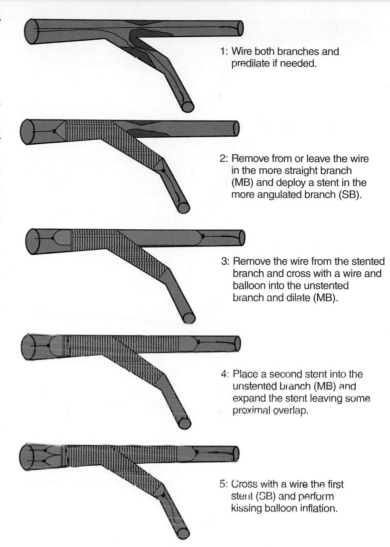

1: Wire both branches and predilate if needed.

2: Remove from or leave the wire in the more straight branch (MB) and deploy a stent in the more angulated branch (SB).

3: Remove the wire from the stented branch and cross with a wire and balloon into the unstented branch and dilate (MB).

4: Place a second stent into the unstented branch (MB) and expand the stent leaving some proximal overlap.

5: Cross with a wire the first stent (SB) and perform kissing balloon inflation.

Figure 20-8 A schematic representation of the culotte technique.

struts toward both branches. The Nordic complex bifurcation stenting study compared crush or culotte stenting using SESs and at 6-month follow up demonstrated no difference between the two groups in terms of death, MI, or repeat revascularization and a significantly higher incidence of peri-procedural MI and in-stent re-stenosis in the crush group.[16]

TECHNIQUE DESCRIPTION

Step one: Both branches are predilated.

Step two: A stent is deployed across the most angulated branch, usually the SB.

Step three: The nonstented branch is rewired through the stent struts and dilated.

Step four: A second stent is advanced and expanded into the nonstented branch, usually the MB.

Step five: Finally, kissing balloon inflation is performed.

This technique is suitable for all angles of bifurcations and provides near-perfect coverage of the SB ostium. Disadvantages are that, similar to the crush technique, the culotte technique leads to a high concentration of metal with a double-stent layer at the carina and in the proximal part of the bifurcation. Other disadvantages of the technique are that rewiring both branches through the stent struts can be difficult and time consuming and there is a limitation in the maximum opening

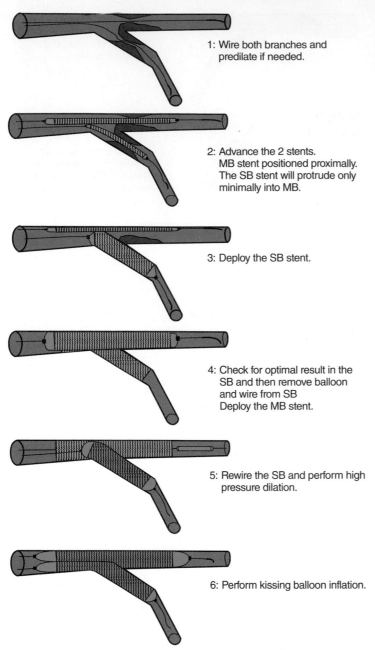

1: Wire both branches and predilate if needed.

2: Advance the 2 stents. MB stent positioned proximally. The SB stent will protrude only minimally into MB.

3: Deploy the SB stent.

4: Check for optimal result in the SB and then remove balloon and wire from SB Deploy the MB stent.

5: Rewire the SB and perform high pressure dilation.

6: Perform kissing balloon inflation.

Figure 20-9 A schematic representation of the mini-crush technique.

achievable when a stent with a closed-cell design such as the Cypher stent is implanted.

MINI-CRUSH TECHNIQUE (SIDE BRANCH STENT CRUSHED BY THE MAIN BRANCH STENT)

The crush technique (Fig. 20-9) was established together with DESs.[38] The recent addition of "mini" highlights the need to decrease, as much as possible, the amount of stent overlap between the SB and the MB, as described by Galassi et al compared with modified T stenting as described by Kobayashi et al.[39,40] The Sirolimus bifurcation study brought to the attention the emerging problem of SB focal re-stenosis despite the use of two Cypher stents (one in the MB and the other in the SB).[7] At that time, the T technique was the default approach when two stents were implanted. The need to obtain full coverage of the ostium of the SB prompted the idea of allowing some protrusion of

the SB stent into the MB. The next step was to flatten the SB stent against the MB stent. The angiographic results following the initial application of this technique, which was solely used with the Cypher stent, were quite optimal, and there was no need for recrossing into the SB to perform a final kissing inflation. Despite a favorable short-term clinical outcome without any event of stent thrombosis, however, there was a 25% incidence of focal re-stenosis at the ostium of the SB. Subsequently, routine recrossing into the SB, inflation of a balloon in the SB, and kissing balloon inflation were performed.[41] The implementation of final kissing balloon inflation was done to allow better strut contact against the ostium of the SB and, therefore, better drug delivery. The crush technique became a sort of a simplified culotte technique.[32] Routine performance of final kissing inflation decreases re-stenosis at the ostium of the SB.[41] Additionally, when re-stenosis occurs, it is usually focal (<5 mm in length) and frequently not associated with symptoms or ischemia.

The main advantage of the crush technique is that immediate patency of both branches is ensured. This objective is notably important when the SB is functionally relevant or difficult to be wired. The main disadvantage is that the performance of final kissing balloon inflation makes the procedure more laborious because of the need to recross multiple struts with a wire and a balloon. Webster et al reported bench testing with three different stent platforms (BX Velocity, from Cordis, a Johnson & Johnson company, Miami Lakes, FL; Express II, from Boston Scientific, Natick, MA; and Driver, from Medtronic, Minneapolis, MN) using the crush technique.[42] These authors stressed the importance of final kissing balloon inflation and concluded that appropriate SB and MB postdilatation is needed to fully expand the stent at the SB ostium, to widen gaps between stent struts overlying the SB (facilitating subsequent access), and to prevent stent distortion. The performance of the crush technique requires a 7F or 8F guiding catheter and the technique commits the operator to implant two stents. A modification of the crush technique, which allows provisional SB stenting and permits performing the same or similar approach using a 6F guiding catheter, is described below. An angiographic example of the crush technique is presented in Fig. 20-10.

When the angle between the MB and the SB is near 90 degrees, it is possible to minimize the gap even without crushing the SB stent and using the modified T technique.

Technique Description

Step one: Both branches are wired and fully dilated. Particular attention is paid to dilate the SB, and a 6-mm long cutting balloon is used if there is evidence that the predilating balloon does not fully expand at the ostium of the SB.

Step two: The stent for the SB is positioned in the SB, and then the MB stent is advanced.

Step three: The SB stent is pulled back into the MB for about 2 to 3 mm. This step is verified in at least two projections.

Step four: The stent in the SB is deployed at a minimum 12 atm. The balloon is deflated and removed from the guiding catheter. An angiogram is taken to verify that the SB has an appropriate lumen and normal flow and that no distal dissection or residual lesions are present. If an additional stent is needed in the SB, this is the time to perform the implantation. Following this check, the wire is removed from the SB, and the stent in the MB is fully deployed at high pressure, usually above 12 atm. An angiogram is taken following the removal of the balloon from the MB.

Step five: A wire is advanced in the SB. This maneuver may be time consuming in the initial experience with this technique. Lately, an average of 2 minutes of fluoroscopy has been used to complete the wire advancement in the SB. Besides trying with the initial floppy wire such as Balance Universal (Abbott Vascular Devices, Redwood City, CA) further attempts should consider using Rinato/Prowater (Asahi Intec, Japan or Abbott Vascular Devices, Redwood City, CA; Crossit 100, Pilot 50 or Pilot 150, Abbott Vascular Devices, Redwood City, CA). Frequently, the initial step is to try to cross through the stent struts into the SB with the smallest balloon

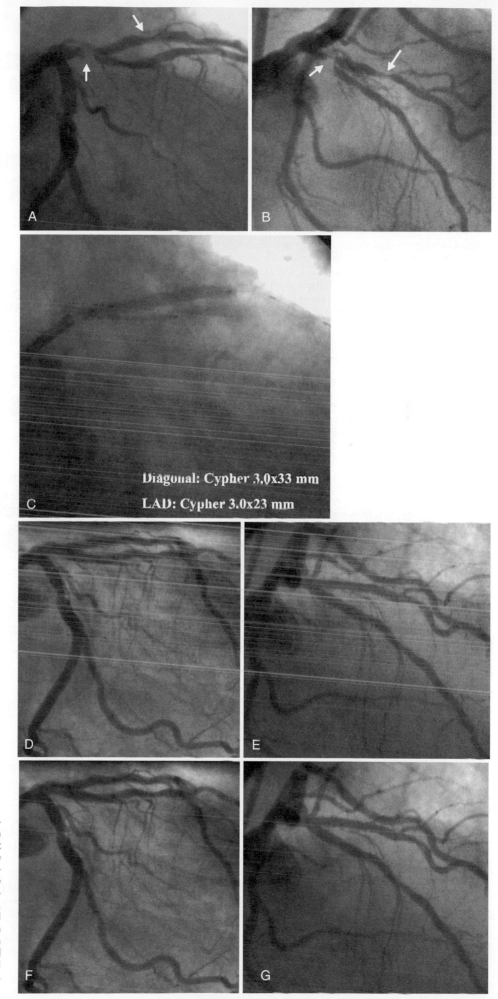

Figure 20-10 Example of the crush stenting technique. **A and B,** Baseline angiogram of a bifurcation lesion, involving the left anterior descending (LAD) artery and a large diagonal branch. **C,** Following lesion predilatation, two stents are positioned with the stent in the LAD artery placed more proximally than the stent in the diagonal branch. A side branch stent is inflated first (diagonal branch). Note that a long stent was chosen for the diagonal branch to also cover a lesion distal to bifurcation site (*arrow*) **D and E,** Optimal final result. **F and G,** The final outcome was maintained at 10-month angiographic follow-up. DES: drug-eluting stent.

Diagonal: Cypher 3.0x33 mm

LAD: Cypher 3.0x23 mm

on the catheterization table; if this balloon fails, a balloon with a 1.5 to 1.25-mm diameter balloon is used. If this very small balloon cannot be crossed, repositioning the wire traversing the stent struts in another spot is considered. If the problem is still present, a fixed wire balloon such as an ACE (Boston Scientific-Scimed, Minneapolis, MN) is tried. It is important to perform a final dilatation on the stent toward the SB with a balloon appropriately sized to the diameter of this branch and inflated at high pressure (12 atm or more).

Step six: A second balloon is advanced over the wire which was left in place in the MB, and kissing balloon inflation is performed at 8 atm or more.

STEP CRUSH

When a two-stent technique is necessary as intention to treat and a 6F guiding catheter is the only available approach (radial approach), the *step crush* or the *modified balloon crush* technique can be used.[43] The final result is basically similar to that obtained with the standard crush technique, except that each stent is advanced and deployed separately. The need for a 6F guiding catheter is the main reason to use this technique. *Double kissing crush technique* and *sleeve technique* are other variants of the crush technique, which may optimize stent deployment and apposition.[44,45]

Technique Description

Step one: This step is the same as step one of the standard crush technique.

Step two: A stent is advanced in the SB, protruding a few millimeters into the MB. A balloon (Maverick balloon, or any other balloon of similar size and features) is advanced in the MB over the bifurcation.

Step three: The stent in the SB is deployed, the balloon is removed, an angiogram is performed, and, if the result is adequate, the wire is also removed. The MB balloon is then inflated (to crush the protruding SB stent) and removed. Optionally, kissing balloon inflation can be performed at that time ("double kissing crush" technique proposed by Chen et al).[44]

Step four: A second stent is advanced in the MB and deployed (usually at 12 atm or more).

The next steps are similar to those of the crush technique and involve recrossing into the SB, SB stent dilatation, and final kissing balloon inflation.

V STENTING AND SIMULTANEOUS KISSING STENT TECHNIQUES

The V and the SKS techniques (Fig. 20-11) are performed by delivering and implanting two stents together.[46,47] One stent is advanced in the SB and the other one in the MB. Both stents are pulled back to create a new carina as close as possible to the original one. The main advantage of the V technique is that the operator will never lose access to any of the two branches. In addition, when final kissing inflation is performed, there is no need to recross any stent. Fig. 20-12 shows an example of V technique performed on the LMCA. When the two stents protrude into the MB with the creation of a double barrel and a very proximal carina, the technique is called the SKS technique.[47] The V technique is preferable for selected bifurcation lesions where the lesions are distal to the bifurcation (Medina 0.0.1); if there is a proximal stenosis in the MB, a different approach is preferred, rather that creating an overlap with the SKS.

Technique Description

Step one: Both branches are wired and fully predilated. It is important to perform adequate predilatation to allow full stent expansion.

Step two: The two stents are positioned into the branches, with a slight protrusion of both stents in the main proximal branch. With different operators, a variable amount of protrusion is possible, which sometimes helps create a rather long (≥5 mm) double barrel in the

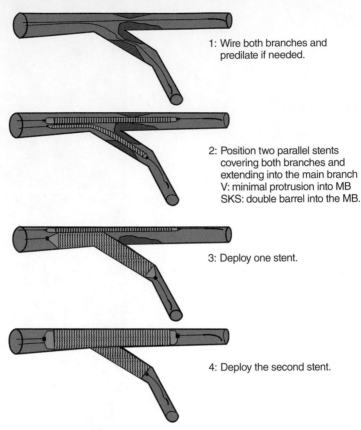

1: Wire both branches and predilate if needed.

2: Position two parallel stents covering both branches and extending into the main branch
V: minimal protrusion into MB
SKS: double barrel into the MB.

3: Deploy one stent.

4: Deploy the second stent.

Some operators deploy the two stents simultaneously

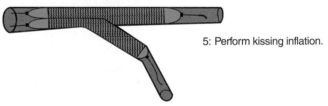

5: Perform kissing inflation.

Figure 20-11 A schematic representation of the V stenting technique.

proximal MB (SKS). It is impossible to be accurate in positioning the stent exactly at the ostium of each branch, but generally limiting the length of the new carina to less than 5 mm is attempted. Sometimes, it is necessary to advance the first stent more distally into the vessel to facilitate the advancement of the second stent. This maneuver is essential when the kissing stent technique is used to stent a trifurcation using three kissing stents (a 9F guiding catheter is necessary for this). Following accurate stent positioning, it is important to verify correct placement in two projections before deploying the stents. Each balloon is first inflated individually at high pressure of 12 atm or more, as operators inflate the balloons simultaneously.

Step three: The next step is to inflate both balloons simultaneously at approximately 8 atm. The sizes of the balloon and the stents are chosen according to the diameter of the vessels to be stented. If the reference vessel size proximal to the bifurcation is relatively small and the operator fears the risk that the two balloons inflated simultaneously may become oversized, kissing inflation is performed at low pressure (4 atm).

Using the V technique, a metallic neocarina is created within the vessel proximal to the bifurcation. Theoretical concerns about the risk of thrombosis related to this new carina have not been confirmed, to date, in the experiences of various operators. The technique has been successfully applied with BMSs and with DESs. The types of lesions

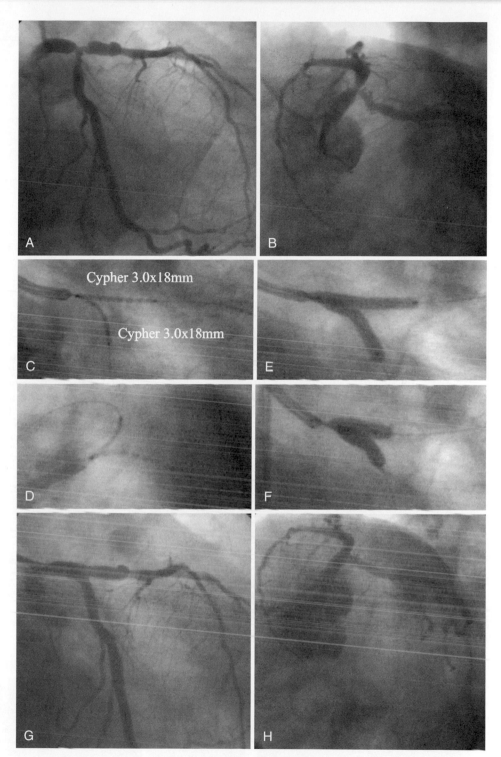

Figure 20-12 Example of the V stenting technique. Baseline angiogram of an LMCA bifurcation lesion, with two large branches, **A and B,** LAD and LCx. V stenting was used because the disease was mainly at the level of the very distal LMCA, and the angle of the two branches was very favorable for the V technique. **C and D,** Stent positioning in two projections. **E and F,** Stent deployment and postdilatation with the 4-mm balloons. **G and H,** Final result. *LMCA,* left main coronary artery; *LAD,* left anterior descending; *LCx,* left circumflex; *DES,* drug-eluting stent.

that are considered most suitable for this technique are very proximal lesions such as bifurcation of a short LMCA free of disease. Ideally, the angle between the two branches should be less than 90 degrees. The V technique is also suitable for other bifurcations, provided the portion of the vessel proximal to the bifurcation is free of disease and there is no need to deploy a stent more proximally. How problematic positioning a stent proximally to the double barrel may be quite intuitive, with an inevitable bias toward one of the two branches and a high likelihood to leave a gap.

"Y" AND "SKIRT" TECHNIQUES

The "Y" technique has a particular historical value because it was the first bifurcation stenting technique demonstrated in a live case course.[48] This technique involves an initial predilatation followed by stent deployment in each branch. If the results are not adequate, a third stent may also be deployed in the MB.[49] To approximate the proximal stent to the previously deployed stents, it is necessary to modify the stent delivery system by placing one stent over two balloons ("skirt" stenting).[50] This technique is the last resort for treating very demanding bifurcations in which there is a need to maintain uninterrupted wire access to both branches.

FLOWER PETAL STENTING

The technique of "flower petal" stenting involves implanting a stent in the SB with single strut protruding into the MB; the protruding strut closest to the carina is wired and dilated to create a larger strut or a "flower petal"; this protruding petal is then flattened and plastered down over the carina with a series of MB inflations, including an MB stent and kissing balloon inflations, thus ensuring complete ostial coverage and scaffolding.[51] The most challenging part of this technique is wiring a single strut close to the carina; in the original description, this required intravascular ultrasound guidance and was not always successful. The technique was modified to allow ex vivo wiring of the proximal strut and subsequent balloon insertion into this strut. This approach needs partial inflation of the proximal segment of the stent performed before stent insertion in the guiding catheter. Although this creates a bulkier two-wire and balloon system, the technique is suitable for a 6F guided catheter and is mainly applied in bifurcation lesions located in the distal left main. The main characteristics of the most frequently used two-stent techniques are summarized in Table 20-1. No definitive statement can be made about the best strategy to be used when there is a need to implant two stents in a bifurcation. Nevertheless, a schematic approach according to the anatomy of the lesion is presented in Fig. 20-13.

CONTROVERSIES IN THE TECHNICAL APPROACH TO ISOLATED OSTIAL LEFT ANTERIOR DESCENDING OR CIRCUMFLEX LESIONS

Approach to Ostial Left Anterior Descending Artery Lesion

The left main 0,1,0 lesion (ostial LAD) is traditionally considered to be unfavorable for percutaneous intervention because of the technical

TABLE 20-1	Main Characteristics of Two-Stent Techniques			
	T/TAP	*Mini-Crush*	*Culotte*	*SKS*
Guiding catheter (Fr)	6	7*	6	7
Provisional side branch (SB) stenting	Yes	No	Possible	No
Preserved GW access main branch (MB)	Yes	Yes	No	Yes
Preserved GW access SB	No	No	No	Yes
Bifurcation angle:				
- <70 degrees	Not ideal	Ideal	Suitable	Suitable
- >70 degrees	Ideal	Not ideal	Not ideal	Not ideal
MB and SB diameters:				
- Similar diameters	Suitable	Suitable	Ideal	Ideal
- Discrepancy in diameters	Suitable	Ideal	Not ideal	Not ideal

GW, guidewire; *TAP*, T and protrusion; *SKS*, simultaneous kissing stent.
*6 French (6F) could be used for balloon "step-crush."

difficulty and potential risk of serious complications. Two interventional strategies are traditionally used in this lesion subset: (1) precise stent implantation at the LAD ostium level or (2) stenting the LMCA towards the LAD artery. IVUS guidance is recommended to assess plaque distribution before deciding which technique should be applied in a specific lesion. Precise stenting of the LAD ostium is feasible in cases with a large bifurcation angle and IVUS documentation of absence of disease in the distal LMCA. Precise LAD ostial stenting consists of scaffolding the counter-carina with a mild protrusion of the stent covering the ostium of the circumflex. In this technique, the proximal stent marker should be positioned just proximal to the angiographic carina (the transducer of the IVUS catheter could be filmed when it is positioned at the carina level to have a reference for subsequent stent placement). Disadvantages of precise ostial LAD stenting are as follows: (1) If the device is positioned too proximally, it

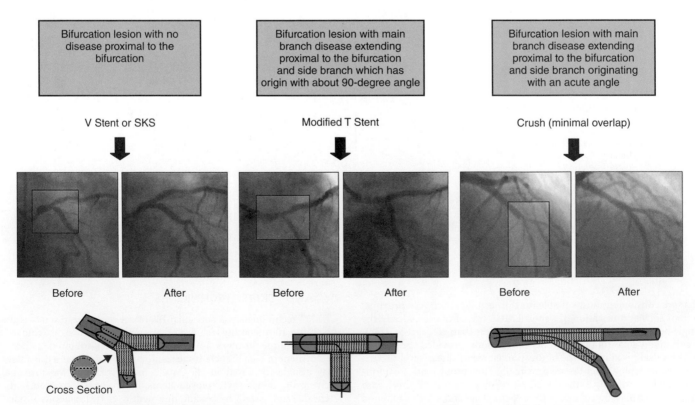

Figure 20-13 Proposed approach when implanting two stents on a bifurcation as intention to treat.

protrudes into the LMCA that may compromise a LCx artery and make repeating of the intervention difficult; (2) if the ostial LAD lesion is not totally covered by the stent, acute recoil and late re-stenosis are likely.[34] Therefore, optimal positioning of the stents is critical for the treatment of this lesion. Furthermore, with branch ostial disease, there is frequent involvement of the distal LMCA, and thus the impending danger of incomplete lesion coverage if stenting is not extended to the involved LMCA. From this perspective, left main branch ostial lesion is necessarily a bifurcation disease and should be treated in a similar manner. Therefore, ostial disease of the LAD and LCx arteries would ideally be treated percutaneously by stenting from the LMCA into the diseased main branch with provisional SB stenting.

Approach to Isolated Non-Left-main Side Branch Ostial (0,0,1) Bifurcation Lesions: Lesions at the Ostium of a Diagonal or Obtuse Marginal or Posterolateral Branch

It is important to focus on these particular lesions which may, in some unlucky conditions, become the origin of a new lesion in the MB. Isolated SB ostial lesions (0,0,1), although not frequent, are very challenging lesions (especially in Y-shaped angulations). Operators should always remember the "sad story of the ostial diagonal lesion" and be aware that a too-aggressive treatment of these lesions may not always be the best approach, as it may lead to trauma to the LAD artery causing a new stenosis on this vessel. Unfortunately, an easy solution to this conundrum cannot be recommended; rather, the operator can only be alerted about this possible risk. Occasionally, a simple cutting balloon dilatation at the ostium of a diagonal branch is a minimalistic approach that could be considered. Brunel et al have developed an "inverted" technique for the treatment of Medina 0,0,1 lesions, derived from the usual provisional T stenting.[52] A stent is implanted from the proximal MB through the SB, with reopening of the strut through the distal MB and systematic final kissing balloon dilatation. Alternative approaches include use of single short stent (precise ostial positioning is very difficult, and complete ostial coverage is difficult or impossible except for 90 degrees bifurcation), shunt technique, or dedicated stents.[34] One strategy to be considered is to evaluate with FFR the functional significance of the lesion located at the SB. Finally, the fact that optimal medical therapy is a reasonable approach should not be dismissed.

DEDICATED BIFURCATION STENTS

The conventional approach to bifurcation PCI still has a number of limitations such as maintaining access to the SB throughout the procedure; MB stent struts jailing the SB ostium, resulting in difficulty in rewiring the SB or passing the balloon or stent into the SB through the stent struts; distortion of the MB stent by SB dilatation; inability to fully cover and scaffold the ostium of the SB; inability of the stent structure to withstand SB balloon dilatation and deformation, and, finally, operator skills and technical experience.[53] Thus far, the main advantage of most of the dedicated bifurcation stents is to allow the operator to perform the procedure on a bifurcation lesion without the need to rewire the SB. Dedicated bifurcation stents can be broadly divided into the following:

1. Stents for provisional side branch stenting that facilitate or maintain access to the SB after MB stenting and which do not require recrossing of MB stent struts (e.g., Petal, former AST stent, from Boston Scientific, Natick, MA; Multi-link Frontier/ Pathfinder from Abbott Vascular Devices, Redwood City, CA; Invatec Twin-Rail from Medtronic/Invatec, Brescia, Italy; Nile Croco/Pax from Minvasys, Genevilliers, France; Antares from Trireme Medical, CA; Y-Med SideKick from Y-Med, San Diego, CA; and Stentys from Stentys SAS, Clichy, France). These stents allow placement of a second stent on the SB, if needed.
2. Stents that usually require another stent implanted in the bifurcation (e.g., Axxess Plus from Devax, Irvine, CA; Sideguard from Cappella, MA; and Tryton from Tryton Medical, MA). The Tryton and Sideguard stents are designed to treat the SB first and require

recrossing into the SB after MB stenting for final kissing inflation. The Axxess Plus stent is the exception, as it is implanted in the proximal MB at the level of the carina and does not require recrossing into the SB but may require the implantation of two more stents in the distal MB and SB to completely treat some types of bifurcation lesions.

The Taxus Petal bifurcation paclitaxel-eluting coronary stent system is made of platinum-enhanced alloy and is designed to pave a uniform layer of metal in the MB as well as extending 2 mm into the SB. It is the short segment stent or "nipple" extending into the SB, from which this device derives the name "Petal." The Taxus Petal bifurcation stent is crimped over two balloons, with the SB balloon positioned underneath the Petal elements. On inflation, the MB balloon deploys the stent into the main artery, and the SB balloon deploys the Petal into the ostium of the SB. The first generation of this stent, called AST Petal, developed by Advanced Stent Technologies, was a 316L stainless steel slotted tube design. Formerly the Frontier System, the Pathfinder everolimus-eluting ABS (Abbott Bifurcation Stent), is a chromium cobalt stent with the Xience V DES platform. ABS stent is crimped onto two balloons. The MB balloon, which is mounted on a rapid-exchange lumen, extends the length of the stent. The SB balloon, which is mounted on an over-the-wire (OTW) lumen, exits the stent at the mid-point. The Twin-Rail is similar to the Multi-link Frontier double-balloon system, except that in the latter, the SB balloon is a short, tapered balloon, and in the Twin-Rail, there is a full dilatation balloon.

The Nile Pax (BMS version Nile Croco) paclitaxel-eluting polymer-free dedicated bifurcation stent is a 6F compatible chromium cobalt stent mounted on two independent Rx PTCA catheters (with specific SB balloon shape). The stent delivery system (SDS) is similar to those of the Multi link Frontier and Twin-Rail stents, but unlike these systems, which are a single catheter with single inflation port, the Nile Croco/Pax has two independent yet joined catheters that require independent manipulation and pressure monitoring. The Antares stent, with automatic SB support deployment, consists of a single-balloon expandable 316L stainless steel stent. It has an SB support structure in the center the stent provided with two radiopaque tantalum markers for positioning and orienting at the bifurcation site. Stent deployment is achieved using a single rapid-exchange balloon catheter and an SB stabilizing wire encased in a peel-away lumen to minimize wire crossing. As the stent approaches the targeted bifurcation, the catheter is torqued to align the stent's central opening with the SB ostium. On expansion of the main stent body, the ostial crown is automatically deployed, with elements protruding approximately 2 mm into the SB to scaffold the ostium. The Antares stent is similar to the Petal stent but has the advantage of tracking over a single wire and unlike the Petal stent, which uses a balloon to expand the SB elements, the SB elements expand automatically with this stent.

The SideKick stent integrates an MB fixed-wire platform with a rapid-exchange steerable SB guidewire designed to preserve SB access during bifurcation stenting. There are three models with different exit ports (proximal, mid, distal) that are selected on the basis of the location of disease in the bifurcation. When the device is close to the carina, a guidewire is passed through the SB exit port and MB stent struts into the SB, thus avoiding recrossing into the SB. Stentys is a self-expanding nitinol stent made of Z-shaped mesh linked by small interconnections. The stent is coated on the abluminal side with paclitaxel on a durable polymer matrix (PESU), a polysulfone that permits controlled drug elution. The unique feature of this stent is the facility to disconnect the stent struts with an angioplasty balloon. Thus, an opening for the SB can be created anywhere in the stent after it is implanted in the vessel, and at the same time, the disconnected struts scaffold the SB ostium.

The Axxess Plus stent (Devax, Irvine, CA) is a self-expanding, nickel–titanium, conically shaped stent that is placed at the level of the carina by means of the skirt technique and was the first of these dedicated bifurcation stents designed to elute an anti–re-stenotic drug (biolimus A9). The Axxess Plus stent has a rapid-exchange delivery system with hydrophilic coating, with controlled deployment on withdrawal of a cover sheath using the actuator. However, the Axxess stent may be limited by the fact that it needs to be precisely nested at the carina to be effective; as well, in most cases, another stent will be needed to treat the bifurcation fully. The sideguard ostium protection device is a self-expanding, trumpet-shaped nitinol stent that is deployed using a special balloon release sheath system. It is currently a BMS, but the next generation will be a DES with a biodegradable polymer. Radiopaque markers located at the distal and proximal ends of the Sideguard delivery system facilitate positioning of the stent at the SB ostium. The stent is deployed using a nominal pressure balloon, which helps tear a protective sheath that keeps the Sideguard in place until deployment. Once released, the Sideguard self-expands into place. The delivery system and the guidewire are then removed from the SB. A conventional stent is then placed in the MB, the SB is reaccessed with a guidewire, and the procedure is completed with a standard final kissing inflation. Tryton SB stent is a slotted tube, cobalt–chromium balloon-expandable stent designed to be implanted in the SB of a bifurcation. The stent consists of three zones: (1) a distal SB zone (that treats the disease in the SB); (2) a transition zone (positioned at the SB ostium); and (3) an MB zone. Treatment of a bifurcation with the Tryton stent generally commits the operator to implanting two stents in the bifurcation, and the technique is identical in approach to that used when performing the culotte technique. The Tryton stent is deployed across the SB ostium first. A standard MB stent is then tracked through the proximal MB zone of the Tryton into the distal MB and deployed. The MB stent struts then have to be recrossed in order to perform final kissing inflation.

Dedicated bifurcation stents may potentially overcome the limitations of conventional stents in bifurcations (SB protection, multiple layers, distortion, SB access, crossing through side of the stent, gaps in scaffolding). However, although efforts to produce dedicated bifurcation stent delivery systems are strongly encouraged and research is fostered, none of the currently available systems can at the moment challenge the results offered by the provisional T stent strategy in the majority of bifurcation lesions.

▣ Role of Adjunctive Procedures

ROTATIONAL ATHERECTOMY

As discussed for ostial lesion, the role of rotablation is important to allow optimal stent expansion in lesions with severe superficial calcifications. Even if no data on the role of this technology with DES are available, it is intuitive to aim for optimal stent expansion and symmetry. In a setting of a highly calcific lesion, this goal can only be obtained with adequate lesion preparation. The main area of discussion is on how frequently a calcific lesion should be pretreated with rotational atherectomy and when, conversely, a high pressure balloon is sufficient. Except for information obtained with IVUS or in circumstances where no balloon would cross the lesion, additional objective guidelines cannot be recommended to make a scientific decision. The operator's judgment often remains the most used tool dictating the choice of rotational atherectomy. Burr size is typically small (1.25 or 1.5 mm) with the intent to modify the plaque and minimize the risk of embolization. SB stent underdeployment because of inadequate

preparation remains the most important cause of re-stenosis at the ostium of the SB.[54]

CUTTING BALLOON

Bifurcation lesions with fibrotic plaque at the SB ostium are an ideal setting for this device. The REDUCE III (REstenosis reDUction by Cutting balloon Evaluation) randomized trial evaluated the role of cutting balloon dilatation before stenting versus standard balloon dilatation in a variety of lesions.[55] This trial reported a lower re-stenosis rate (11.8% vs. 18.8%, $P = 0.04$) when lesions were predilated with the cutting balloon. The fact that the final postprocedure lumen diameter was larger in the cutting balloon arm and that the late loss was 0.74 mm for both strategies seems to indicate that the main advantage was better stent expansion. As just discussed in the context of rotational atherectomy, it is difficult to demonstrate that a niche device has an advantage in every lesion. For this reason, the use of cutting balloon is recommended in selected moderately calcific and fibrotic lesions, especially ones that involve the origin of the SB.

ASSOCIATED PHARMACOLOGIC TREATMENT

When performing bifurcation stenting with one or two stents, the authors of this chapter do not usually change the protocol of peri-procedural heparin administration (100 Units/kg without elective glycoprotein [GP] IIb/IIIa inhibitors and 70 Units/kg with elective GP IIb/IIIa inhibitors). Usage of GP IIb/IIIa inhibitors is reserved for thrombus-containing lesions and for patients with acute coronary syndrome (ACS). GP IIb/IIIa inhibitors are sometimes administered when the final result at the SB appears suboptimal and the operator decides not to implant another stent. Another approach as an alternative to GP IIb/IIIa inhibitors and heparin is bivalirudin. The chapter authors pay a lot of attention to pre-procedural preparation with thienopyridines; when in doubt, a 600-mg loading dose of clopidogrel is administered in the catheterization laboratory.[56] The evaluation of individual responses to clopidogrel, the possibility of doubling the dose, or using other agents such as ticagrelor or prasugrel are being evaluated, and new guidelines will soon be available. In the authors' current practice, the duration of combined thienopyridine and aspirin treatment following stent implantation is usually for a minimum or 6 months and usually extended to 1 year.

▣ Conclusion

With the introduction of DESs, a remarkable improvement has occurred in the treatment of bifurcation lesions. However, several randomized DES trial data showed that routine two-vessel stenting does not improve either angiographic or clinical outcomes for most patients with coronary bifurcation lesions. Therefore, provisional T stenting remains the gold standard technique for most bifurcations. Nevertheless, there are several bifurcation lesions for which two stents need to be implanted as intention to treat, and the operators should be confident in such settings. Finally, specific DESs for different types of bifurcations may further facilitate the conquest of one of the most challenging areas in interventional cardiology.

REFERENCES

1. Lefevre T, Louvard Y, Morice MC, et al: Stenting of bifurcation lesions: Classification, treatments, and results. *Catheter Cardiovasc Interv* 49:274–283, 2000.
2. Safian RD: Bifurcation Lesions. In Safian RD, Freed M, editors: *Manual of interventional cardiology*, Royal Oak, CA, 2001, Physicians' Press.
3. Aliabadi D, Tilli FV, Bowers TR, et al: Incidence and angiographic predictors of side branch occlusion following high-pressure intracoronary stenting. *Am J Cardiol* 80:994–997, 1997.

4. Louvard Y, Lefevre T, Morice MC: Percutaneous coronary intervention for bifurcation coronary disease. *Heart* 90:713–722, 2004.
5. Medina A, Suarez de Lezo J, Pan M: A new classification of coronary bifurcation lesions. *Rev Esp Cardiol* 59:183, 2006.
6. Fujii K, Kobayashi Y, Mintz GS, et al: Dominant contribution of negative remodeling to development of significant coronary bifurcation narrowing. *Am J Cardiol* 92:59–61, 2003.

7. Colombo A, Moses JW, Morice MC, et al: Randomized study to evaluate sirolimus-eluting stents implanted at coronary bifurcation lesions. *Circulation* 109:1244–1249, 2004.
8. Al Suwaidi J, Berger PB, Rihal CS, et al: Immediate and long-term outcome of intracoronary stent implantation for true bifurcation lesions. *J Am Coll Cardiol* 35:929–936, 2000.
9. Yamashita T, Nishida T, Adamian MG, et al: Bifurcation lesions: Two stents versus one stent—immediate and follow-up results. *J Am Coll Cardiol* 35:1145–1151, 2000.

10. Pan M, de Lezo JS, Medina A, et al: Rapamycin-eluting stents for the treatment of bifurcated coronary lesions: A randomized comparison of a simple versus complex strategy. *Am Heart J* 148.857-864, 2004.

11. Steigen TK, Maeng M, Wiseth R, et al: Randomized study on simple versus complex stenting of coronary artery bifurcation lesions: The Nordic bifurcation study. *Circulation* 114:1955–1961, 2006.

12. Jensen JS, Galloe A, Lassen JF, et al: Safety in simple versus complex stenting of coronary artery bifurcation lesions. The Nordic bifurcation study 14-month follow-up results. *EuroIntervention* 4:229–233, 2008.

13. Ferenc M, Gick M, Kienzle RP, et al: Randomized trial on routine vs. provisional T-stenting in the treatment of de novo coronary bifurcation lesions. *Eur Heart J* 29:2859–2867, 2008.

14. Colombo A, Bramucci E, Sacca S, et al: Randomized study of the crush technique versus provisional side-branch stenting in true coronary bifurcations: The CACTUS (Coronary Bifurcations: Application of the Crushing Technique Using Sirolimus-Eluting Stents) Study. *Circulation* 119:71–78, 2009.

15. Hildick-Smith D, de Belder AJ, Cooter N, et al: Randomized trial of simple versus complex drug-eluting stenting for bifurcation lesions: The British Bifurcation Coronary Study: Old, new, and evolving strategies. *Circulation* 121:1235–1243, 2010.

16. Erglis A, Kumsars I, Niemela HJ, et al: Randomized comparison of coronary bifurcation stenting with the crush versus the culotte technique using sirolimus eluting stents: The Nordic stent technique study. *Circ Cardiovasc Interv* 2:27–34, 2009.

17. Pan M, Suarez de Lezo J, Medina A, et al: Drug-eluting stents for the treatment of bifurcation lesions: A randomized comparison between paclitaxel and sirolimus stents. *Am Heart J* 153:15 e1–e7, 2007.

18. Song YB, Hahn JY, Choi SH, et al: Sirolimus- versus paclitaxel-eluting stents for the treatment of coronary bifurcations results: From the COBIS (Coronary Bifurcation Stenting) Registry. *J Am Coll Cardiol* 55:1743–1750, 2010.

19. Nakazawa G, Yazdani SK, Finn AV, et al: Pathological findings at bifurcation lesions: The impact of flow distribution on atherosclerosis and arterial healing after stent implantation. *J Am Coll Cardiol* 55:1679–1687, 2010.

20. Oviedo C, Maehara A, Mintz GS, et al: Intravascular ultrasound classification of plaque distribution in left main coronary artery bifurcations: Where is the plaque really located? *Circ Cardiovasc Interv* 3:105–112, 2010.

21. van der Giessen AG, Wentzel JJ, Meijboom WB, et al: Plaque and shear stress distribution in human coronary bifurcations: A multislice computed tomography study. *EuroIntervention* 4:654–661, 2009.

22. Koo BK, Waseda K, Kang HJ: Anatomic and functional evaluation of bifurcation lesions undergoing percutaneous coronary intervention. *Circ Cardiovasc Interv* 3:113–119, 2010.

23. Aranzulla TC, Sangiorgi GM, Bartorelli A, et al: Use of the Venture wire control catheter to access complex coronary lesions: How to turn procedural failure into success. *EuroIntervention* 4:277–284, 2008.

24. Hildick-Smith D, Lassen JF, Albiero R, et al: Consensus from the 5th European Bifurcation Club meeting. *EuroIntervention* 6:34–38, 2010.

25. Koo BK, Park KW, Kang HJ, et al: Physiological evaluation of the provisional side-branch intervention strategy for bifurcation lesions using fractional flow reserve. *Eur Heart J* 29:726–732, 2008.

26. Carrie D, Karouny E, Chouairi S, Puel J: "T"-shaped stent placement: A technique for the treatment of dissected bifurcation lesions. *Cathet Cardiovasc Diagn* 37:311–313, 1996.

27. Nakamura S, Hall P, Maiello L, Colombo A: Techniques for Palmaz-Schatz stent deployment in lesions with a large side branch. *Cathet Cardiovasc Diagn* 34:353–361, 1995.

28. Burzotta F, Gwon HC, Hahn JY, et al: Modified T-stenting with intentional protrusion of the side-branch stent within the main vessel stent to ensure ostial coverage and facilitate final kissing balloon: The T-stenting and small protrusion technique (TAP-stenting). Report of bench testing and first clinical Italian-Korean two-centre experience. *Catheter Cardiovasc Interv* 70:75–82, 2007.

29. Burzotta F, Sgueglia GA, Trani C, et al: Provisional TAP-stenting strategy to treat bifurcated lesions with drug-eluting stents: One-year clinical results of a prospective registry. *J Invasive Cardiol* 21:532–537, 2009.

30. Hussain F: Provisional reverse "mini-crush" technique for bifurcation angioplasty. *J Invasive Cardiol* 20:E154–E157, 2008.

31. Ormiston JA, Currie E, Webster MW, et al: Drug-eluting stents for coronary bifurcations: Insights into the crush technique. *Catheter Cardiovasc Interv* 63:332–336, 2004.

32. Chevalier B, Glatt B, Royer T, Guyon P: Placement of coronary stents in bifurcation lesions by the "culotte" technique. *Am J Cardiol* 82:943–949, 1998.

33. Kaplan S, Barlis P, Dimopoulos K, et al: Culotte versus T-stenting in bifurcation lesions: Immediate clinical and angiographic results and midterm clinical follow-up. *Am Heart J* 154:336–343, 2007.

34. Stankovic G, Darremont O, Ferenc M, et al: Percutaneous coronary intervention for bifurcation lesions: 2008 consensus document from the fourth meeting of the European Bifurcation Club. *EuroIntervention* 5:39–49, 2009.

35. Legrand V, Thomas M, Zelisko M, et al: Percutaneous coronary intervention of bifurcation lesions: State-of-the-art. Insights from the second meeting of the European Bifurcation Club. *EuroIntervention* 3:44–49, 2007.

36. Thomas M, Hildick-Smith D, Louvard Y, et al: Percutaneous coronary intervention for bifurcation disease. A consensus view from the first meeting of the European Bifurcation Club. *EuroIntervention* 2:149–153, 2006.

37. Brunel P, Lefevre T, Darremont O, Louvard Y: Provisional T-stenting and kissing balloon in the treatment of coronary bifurcation lesions: Results of the French multicenter "TULIPE" study. *Catheter Cardiovasc Interv* 68:67–73, 2006.

38. Colombo A, Stankovic G, Orlic D, et al: Modified T-stenting technique with crushing for bifurcation lesions: Immediate results and 30-day outcome. *Catheter Cardiovasc Interv* 60:145–151, 2003.

39. Galassi AR, Colombo A, Buchbinder M, et al: Long-term outcomes of bifurcation lesions after implantation of drug-eluting stents with the "mini-crush technique." *Catheter Cardiovasc Interv* 69:976–983, 2007.

40. Kobayashi Y, Colombo A, Akiyama T, et al: Modified "T" stenting: A technique for kissing stents in bifurcational coronary lesion. *Cathet Cardiovasc Diagn* 43:323–326, 1998.

41. Ge L, Airoldi F, Iakovou I, et al: Clinical and angiographic outcome after implantation of drug-eluting stents in bifurcation lesions with the crush stent technique: Importance of final kissing balloon post-dilation. *J Am Coll Cardiol* 46:613–620, 2005.

42. Webster MWI, Ormiston JA, Currie E, et al: Drug-eluting stents for coronary bifurcations: Bench-top insights into the "crush" technique [abstract]. *J Am Coll Cardiol* 43(Suppl A):1024–1053, 2004.

43. Collins N, Dzavik V: A modified balloon crush approach improves side branch access and side branch stent apposition during crush stenting of coronary bifurcation lesions. *Catheter Cardiovasc Interv* 68:365–371, 2006.

44. Chen S, Zhang J, Ye F, et al: DK crush (double-kissing and double-crush) technique for treatment of true coronary bifurcation lesions: Illustration and comparison with classic crush. *J Invasive Cardiol* 19:189–193, 2007.

45. Jim MH, Ho HH, Chan AO, et al: Stenting of coronary bifurcation lesions by using modified crush technique with double kissing balloon inflation (sleeve technique): Immediate procedure result and short-term clinical outcomes. *Catheter Cardiovasc Interv* 69:969–975, 2007.

46. Schampaert E, Fort S, Adelman AG, et al: The V-stent: A novel technique for coronary bifurcation stenting. *Cathet Cardiovasc Diagn* 39:320–326, 1996.

47. Sharma SK: Simultaneous kissing drug-eluting stent technique for percutaneous treatment of bifurcation lesions in large-size vessels. *Catheter Cardiovasc Interv* 65:10–16, 2005.

48. Baim DS: Is bifurcation stenting the answer? *Cathet Cardiovasc Diagn* 37:314–316, 1996.

49. Helqvist S, Jorgensen E, Kelbaek H, et al: Percutaneous treatment of coronary bifurcation lesions: A novel "extended Y" technique with complete lesion stent coverage. *Heart* 92:981–982, 2006.

50. Kobayashi Y, Colombo A, Adamian M, et al: The skirt technique: A stenting technique to treat a lesion immediately proximal to the bifurcation (pseudobifurcation). *Catheter Cardiovasc Interv* 51:347–351, 2000.

51. Kinoshita Y, Katoh O, Matsubara T, et al: First clinical experience of "flower petal stenting": A novel technique for the treatment of coronary bifurcation lesions. *JACC Cardiovasc Interv* 3:58–65, 2010.

52. Brunel P, Martin G, Bressollette E, et al: "Inverted" provisional T stenting, a new technique for Medina 0,0,1 coronary bifurcation lesions: Feasibility and follow-up. *EuroIntervention* 5:814–820, 2010.

53. Latib A, Colombo A, Sangiorgi GM: Bifurcation stenting: Current strategies and new devices. *Heart* 95:495–504, 2009.

54. Costa RA, Mintz GS, Carlier SG, et al: Bifurcation coronary lesions treated with the "crush" technique: An intravascular ultrasound analysis. *J Am Coll Cardiol* 46:599–605, 2005.

55. Ozaki Y, Suzuki T, Yamaguchi T, et al: Can intravascular ultrasound guided cutting balloon angioplasty be a substitute for drug eluting stent? Final results of the prospective randomized multicenter trial comparing cutting balloon with balloon angioplasty before stenting (Reduce III) [abstract]. *J Am Coll Cardiol* 43(Suppl A):1138–1166, 2004.

56. Patti G, Colonna G, Pasceri V, et al: Randomized trial of high loading dose of clopidogrel for reduction of periprocedural myocardial infarction in patients undergoing coronary intervention: Results from the ARMYDA-2 (Antiplatelet therapy for Reduction of MYocardial Damage during Angioplasty) study. *Circulation* 111:2099–2106, 2005.

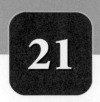

21

Small Vessel and Diffuse Disease

MASAKIYO NOBUYOSHI | HIROYOSHI YOKOI | SHINICHI SHIRAI

KEY POINTS

- In light of the paucity of randomized trial data demonstrating the superiority of any particular device in the treatment of small vessel and diffuse disease, treatment needs to be individualized.

- Rotational atherectomy may provide a rational approach to long-calcified stenoses by rendering them responsive to balloon dilation.

- Given the substantial incidence of re-stenosis despite stent placement in the setting of long lesions, until the problem of in-stent re-stenosis (ISR) can be alleviated, the routine use of stents should be undertaken with extreme caution.

- Although drug-eluting stents (DESs) are associated with a lower rate of ISR compared with bare metal stents (BMSs), until the problem of very late stent thrombosis can be alleviated, the decision to implant a DES or use an alternative revascularization strategy (including a BMS or surgical revascularization) must be made for each patient after consideration of the relative risks and benefits of each therapy.

Small vessels and diffuse coronary disease present considerable challenges to the interventional cardiologist. Compared with discrete stenoses, percutaneous revascularization of small vessel and diffuse disease is associated with decreased rates of procedural success, greater incidence of acute complications, and re-stenosis. Patients with diffuse coronary disease often have other conditions (e.g., diabetes, multivessel disease) that are associated with adverse procedural outcomes. Furthermore, patients with diffuse disease may not be suitable candidates for conventional coronary artery bypass grafting (CABG) because the disease involves the distal vascular territories.

In general, despite enthusiastic and favorable observational reports during the preliminary experience with a variety of new-generation devices, the superiority of ablative and debulking techniques over balloon angioplasty in the treatment of small vessel and diffuse disease has not been confirmed in more recent randomized trials. Likewise, in spite of the significant improvements in both short-term and long-term outcomes of coronary stenting of discrete stenoses, recent data suggest that re-stenosis rates remain substantially high when either long or multiple overlapping stents are used to treat small vessel and diffuse disease. This chapter examines the various potential approaches to the long lesion and emerging concepts regarding the treatment of small vessel and diffuse coronary disease by providing insights through examination of the first-hand experience of treating long lesions at the Kokura Memorial Hospital and by reviewing the worldwide literature.

▨ Pathophysiologic Considerations

The length of a coronary stenosis is an important determinant of its hemodynamic significance that may affect the decision as to whether a particular lesion merits revascularization. Whereas a discrete stenosis of moderate severity may not be flow limiting, a longer stenosis of similar severity may impair distal blood flow. The relationships among stenosis severity, lesion length, and trans-lesional flow in an idealized system are governed by Poiseuille's law, which dictates that flow varies directly as a function of luminal diameter and inversely as a function of lesion length:

$$Flow = \P(\Delta P)(r4)8/(\eta)(l)$$

in which ΔP is the pressure difference across the stenosis, r is the minimal lumen radius of the stenotic segment, η is blood viscosity, and l is the length of the lesion.[1] Because flow across the lesion varies in proportion to the fourth power of radius but only as a first power of length, lesion length would be expected to exert relatively little impact on trans-lesional flow for discrete (e.g., <5 mm long) stenoses. However, as the length of a stenosis increases, for example, from 5 to 25 mm, a fivefold drop in blood flow across the stenosis would occur. It is essential that physicians performing coronary angiography or angioplasty understand this basic concept.[2] Poiseuille's law relates to flow of fluids through cylindrical tubes in well-controlled experimental settings. It does not take into consideration complexities of human coronary artery disease (CAD) such as plaque irregularity and eccentricity, nonlaminar and pulsatile flow, vasoactive properties of the arterial wall, and the potential for compensatory dilation. There is experimental evidence that lesion length has an important physiologic significance. Short, 40% to 60% coronary narrowings in a canine model, with no major resting hemodynamic effects, significantly reduced flows when stenosis length was increased to 10 and 15 mm. The hemodynamic effects of a 15-mm long, 40% to 60% stenosis were similar to those of a discrete 90% narrowing.[3]

COMPARISON OF VARIOUS STENT DESIGNS FOR TREATMENT OF LONG LESIONS

Data on the relative short-term and long-term efficacies of multiple overlapping stents versus placement of a single long stent are currently lacking, although the latter approach certainly provides potential advantages from the standpoint of procedure duration. The relationship between stent design and re-stenosis rates also remains incompletely defined. In an attempt to address these issues, the acute and chronic outcomes of various stents (Palmaz-Schatz, Gianturco-Roubin, and Wallstent) implanted in 148 lesions longer than 20 mm at Kokura Memorial Hospital between June 1990 and December 1995 were analyzed. Cases involving bypass grafts and acute myocardial infarction (MI) were excluded; only lesions that could be fully covered by the stent(s) were considered. Because the conventional Palmaz-Schatz stent was available only in short lengths, all Palmaz-Schatz stents included in this analysis involved the use of multiple stents. Palmaz-Schatz stents were used to treat 70 lesions, the Gianturco-Roubin stent was used for 38 lesions, and the Wallstent was used for 40 lesions. Although the average lesion length was greater than 30 mm for all stents, the Wallstent was typically used for lesions greater than 40 mm. In this nonrandomized comparison, the reference diameter was significantly greater in the Wallstent group, and Gianturco-Roubin stents were used most frequently for failed percutaneous transluminal coronary angioplasty (PTCA). The use of multiple stents was undertaken in 100% of the Palmaz-Schatz group, 44% of the Gianturco-Roubin group, and 40% of the Wallstent group. Procedural success (>50% improvement in vessel narrowing) and freedom from in-hospital complications were independent of stent design. Stent thrombosis occurred in 4.3% of the Palmaz-Schatz group but was not observed in either the

TABLE 21-1	Kokura Hospital Series of Long Lesions: Immediate and Follow-Up Outcome			
Outcomes	Palmaz-Schatz	Gianturco-Roubin	Wallstent	P Value
Procedural success (%)	100	92	93	NS
Clinical success (%)	91	92	85	NS
MLD before treatment (mm)	0.80 ± 0.45	0.72 ± 0.47	0.89 ± 0.44	NS
MLD after treatment (mm)	2.56 ± 0.40	2.30 ± 0.37	2.82 ± 0.63	0001
MLD at follow-up (mm)	1.43 ± 0.85	1.61 ± 0.53	1.32 ± 0.60	NS
Re-stenosis rate (%)	48	37	59	NS

MLD, minimal lumen diameter; *NS*, not significant.

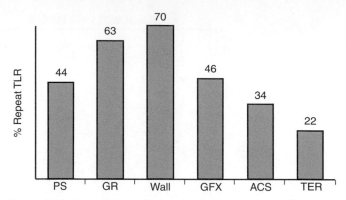

Figure 21-1 Comparison of stent designs to repeat TLR for in-stent re-stenosis. *GR*, Gianturco-Rubin; *PS*, Palmaz-Schatz; *TER*, Terumo; *TLR*, target lesion revascularization.

Gianturco-Roubin or the Wallstent group. Quantitative angiography demonstrated a significantly larger immediate postprocedural minimum luminal diameter (MLD) in the Wallstent group, consistent with the larger reference vessel diameter in these patients. Six-month angiography, conducted in 97% of patients, demonstrated no significant differences in MLD among the groups. Binary re-stenosis rates were high in all groups: 48% for the Palmaz-Schatz stent, 37% for the Gianturco-Roubin stent, and 59% for the Wallstent groups. Repeat target lesion revascularization (TLR) was required in 31%, 20%, and 40%, respectively. Analysis of MLD demonstrated that late loss indices for the Palmaz-Schatz stent and the Wallstent were uniformly high, even though the initial acute gain was large. In contrast, the smaller acute gain in the Gianturco-Roubin group was compensated for by a more moderate degree of late loss (Table 21-1). In summary, although acute results with all stents in the treatment of lesions greater than 20 mm in length were acceptable, the incidence of late renarrowing was substantial regardless of the type of stent examined. A wide variety of newer stent designs are currently undergoing clinical testing. Follow-up studies are needed to determine if these new designs afford re-stenosis benefits over those of the first-generation stents.

NEW GENERATION LONG STENTS

The late outcomes of various new long stents (GFX, ACS multi-link, Terumo) implanted in 211 lesions greater than 20 mm at the Kokura Memorial Hospital between January 1997 and December 2000 were analyzed. GFX long stents (30 mm) were used to treat 76 lesions, the acute coronary syndrome (ACS) multi-link long stent (35 mm) was used for 42 lesions, and the Terumo long stent was used for 93 lesions (30 mm: 65 lesions, 40 mm: 28 lesions). Binary re-stenosis rates remained high when compared with short lesions in all groups: 40.6% for the GFX long stent, 37.5% for the ACS multi-link long stent, and 33.3% for the Terumo long stent. Full-cover stenting of long lesions is likely to give rise to diffuse ISR. Treatment of diffuse ISR remains exceedingly problematic. Recurrent rates of 42% to 80% frequently necessitate multiple additional PTCA procedures and often bypass surgery.[4,5] The diffuse ISR was an independent predictor of long-term outcome after coronary stenting. Angiographically discernible diffuse ISR was observed in 44% of the multiple Palmaz-Schatz stent group, 50% of the Gianturco-Roubin stent group, 59% of the Wallstent group, 64% of the GFX long stent group, 39% of the ACS long stent group, and 38% of the Terumo long stent group. Thus, repeat TLR was required in 44%, 63%, 70%, 46%, 34% and 22%, respectively (Fig. 21-1).

FULL-COVER STENTING VERSUS SPOT STENTING FOR TREATMENT OF LONG LESIONS

Colombo and colleagues have described a strategy to treat discrete high-grade disease within moderately diseased vessels; this strategy, called *spot stenting*, consists of implantation of a short stent only in discrete segments of a long lesion, where intracoronary ultrasound criteria were not satisfied (cross-sectional area >5.5 mm²). With this technique, 96% procedural success and a re-stenosis rate of 17% were obtained.[6] The long-term outcomes of patients with lesions greater than 20 mm undergoing single (spot stenting) or multiple stent (full-cover stenting) therapy at the Kokura Memorial Hospital were analyzed. Of 95 consecutive patients treated with the Palmaz-Schatz stent, multiple stents were used in 62 and single stents in 33. Although there were no significant differences among the two groups with regard to patient and lesion characteristics, the single-stent group contained significantly more emergency cases, and the final dilation pressures were also significantly lower. Postprocedure MLD for the multiple-stent and single-stent groups did not differ significantly, and late angiography also showed no significant differences. Neither re-stenosis rates (44% and 36%) nor the rates of the need for repeat TLR (17% and 17%) were significantly different (Table 21-2). Many reports found that long stent length was associated with an increased frequency of late ISR.[7] If stent length was the only determinant of re-stenosis, spot stenting might be advantageous and would be an appropriate treatment. Conversely, if lesion length is also a factor, using long stents to completely cover the diseased segment might be preferable. NACI investigators have suggested that stenting of long coronary lesions (>20 mm) involves significantly higher rates of the need for repeat TLR than more discrete lesions.[8] In the series by Kastrati and colleagues, multivariate analysis of both binary re-stenosis and late lumen loss demonstrated that lesion length was an independent risk factor for re-stenosis. The risk was further increased by the multiplicity of implanted stents.[9] To evaluate the impact of stent length on late angiographic outcome with coronary stent implantation, 6-month follow-up quantitative coronary angiograms (QCAs) of all consecutive 926 lesions, disregarding length treated with a single coronary stent in native arteries, between September 1999 and March 2000 at the Kokura Memorial Hospital was analyzed. There was no significant relation between the stent length–lesion length ratio and late angiographic outcome; the late angiographic outcome did correlate significantly to lesion length rather than to stent length (Fig. 21-2). Thus, covering the lesion with the least number of nonoverlapping stents might reduce the risks of re-stenosis.

TABLE 21-2	Kokura Hospital Series of Long Lesions: Quantitative Coronary Angiographic Data		
Outcomes	Full-cover Stenting	Spot	P-value
MLD before treatment (mm)	0.57 ± 0.43	0.63 ± 0.30	NS
MLD after treatment (mm)	2.78 ± 0.63	2.62 ± 0.378	NS
MLD at follow-up (mm)	1.72 ± 1.01	1.76 ± 0.95	NS
Re-stenosis rate (%)	44	36	NS

MLD, minimal lumen diameter; *NS*, not significant.

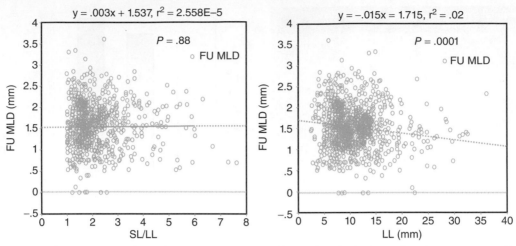

Figure 21-2 Late angiographic outcome—relationship to stent length and lesion length. *LL,* lesion length; *MLD,* minimal lumen diameter; *SL,* stent length.

SUMMARY

From currently available observational data, stent implantation in long stenoses is associated with re-stenosis rates twice as high as those seen when single stents are used to treat discrete lesions. This fact might be the cause of the lower rate of event-free survival of patients receiving multiple stents.[10,11] Long lesions are also significantly more prone to re-stenosis compared with short lesions following balloon angioplasty, but when re-stenosis occurs within stents, the prospects for successful long-term control are poorer. Although still incompletely defined, recurrent re-stenosis rates as high as 80% have been reported following balloon angioplasty for diffuse ISR. Despite these concerns, the use of multiple stents to treat long lesions is a commonplace occurrence in current interventional practice, and several long (>15 mm) stents of various designs have recently been approved for use in the United States. Randomized clinical trials are clearly needed to document the superiority of this yet-untested approach to traditional long balloon angioplasty.

Adjunctive Pharmacologic Treatment for Long Lesions

Despite the various mechanical approaches discussed earlier, percutaneous revascularization of long lesions continues to be associated with increased risks of peri-procedural complications and late recurrence. It stands to reason that the potential benefits afforded by a variety of novel and emerging strategies aimed at increasing the safety of angioplasty, its long-term efficacy, or both may be especially evident in the setting of more complex lesion morphologies such as long lesions. A series of prospective clinical trials has recently demonstrated the efficacy of potent antagonists of the glycoprotein (GP) IIb/IIIa receptor for patients undergoing percutaneous revascularization. Administration of abciximab has significantly reduced the occurrence of acute ischemic events in the setting of both high-risk and low-risk PTCA; and the benefits persist at 3-year follow-up.[12-15] Results of the IIb/IIIa Platelet Receptor Antagonist 7E3 in Preventing Ischemic Complications (EPIC) Trial have been analyzed partially. The benefits of abciximab during angioplasty are not diminished by the presence of adverse lesion characteristics, including lesion length. Because of their propensity to increased late luminal loss, long lesions may be especially responsive to locally delivered ionizing radiation therapy. According to preliminary clinical data, it appears to be especially effective in reducing neointimal hyperplasia following arterial wall injury.[16] Gene-based therapy, currently in the preclinical phase of testing, may also ultimately be of benefit in treating lesion types that are at the highest risk

of restenosis.[17] Deploying drug-eluting stents (DESs) is feasible; the SES elicits minimal neointimal proliferation. Additional placebo-controlled trials are necessary to confirm the promising outcomes.[18]

DRUG-ELUTING STENT

Drug-Eluting Stent for Small Vessel Disease

Previous reports elucidated that percutaneous coronary intervention (PCI) for small coronary artery by balloon angioplasty had a lower primary success rate and high re-stenosis rates (as high as 50%) compared with that for large vessel.[19-21] For small vessel treatment, stent implantation was not demonstrated to be superior to balloon angioplasty, therefore, small vessel stent implantation was a controversial issue in the bare metal stent (BMS) era.[21-23] C-SIRUIS and E-SIRIUS evaluated the efficacy of sirolimus-eluting stent (SES) implantation for diffuse long and small vessel disease.[24,25] Both studies included patients with high re-stenosis risk with long (15–32 mm) lesions and small (2.5–3 mm) vessels. These patients were randomly assigned to SES or bare metal stents (BMS). The binary re-stenosis rates were significantly reduced in SES groups (in C-SIRIUS, 2.3% in SES and 52.3% in BMS [$P = 0.001$]; in E-SIRIUS, 5.9% in SES and 42.3% in BMS [$P = 0.0001$]). Furthermore, the rates of TLR were also remarkably decreased in patients who received DESs compared with patients who received BMS (in C-SIRIUS, 4.0% in SES and 18.5% in BMS [$P = 0.05$]; and in E-SIRIUS, 4.0% in SES and 20.9% in BMS [$P < 0.0001$]). The SES-SMART study was a randomized control study of 257 patients receiving SESs or BMSs in the small coronary artery (diameter ≤2.75 mm). Eight months and 24 months clinical follow-up results were obtained.[26,27] The reference diameter was 2.2 mm, and the lesion length was 11.84 mm. Follow-up angiography revealed that the rates of binary re-stenosis were 53.1% in the BMS group, and 9.8% in the SES group ($P < 0.001$). MACCE (composite of cardiac death, MI, cerebrovascular accident, emergency or elective CABG, or TLR) rates were decreased in DES (9.3%) compared with BMS (31.3%, $P < 0.001$), mainly because of a reduction in TLR (DES 7%, BMS 21.1%) and MI (DES 1.6%, BMS 7.8%, $P = 0.04$). Paclitaxel-eluting stents (PES) were studied in the nonrandomized TAXUS ATLAS trial, which evaluated the efficacy of small stents (TAXUS Liberte of 2.25 mm) compared with the historical control of TAXUS EXPRESS (collecting from TAXUS IV and V).[28] In this study, the TAXUS Liberte 2.25 mm stent significantly reduced the rate of 9-month angiographic re-stenosis (18.5% vs. 32.7%, $P = 0.0219$) and TLR at 12 months (6.1% vs. 16.9%, $P = 0.0039$). The SPIRIT IV (Clinical Evaluation of the XIence V Everolimus Eluting Coronary Stent System in the Treatment of Patients with de novo Native Coronary Artery Lesions) study evaluated the efficacy of Xience V everolimus-eluting stents (EESs) compared with PESs.[29] The primary endpoint of this study was ischemia-driven target lesion failure (composite of cardiac death, target vessel MI, or TLR by either PCI or CABG) at 1 year. In the subgroup analysis, target lesion failure was reduced with the EES group compared with the PES group in vessel diameter greater than 2.75 mm, therefore, the EES for small vessel treatment was effective. In summary, from the randomized and large registry studies, the DES for small vessels is effective in reducing major adverse cardiac events (MACE), mainly because of the reduction in re-stenosis and TLR rates compared with BMSs. Second-generation stents also seems to be effective in improving the outcomes of the treatment for small vessel disease.

Drug-Eluting Stent for Long and Diffuse Lesions

In the BMS era, multiple and long stent implantation for long, diffuse lesions was also associated with a high incidence of re-stenosis, because of diffuse ISR.[30–32] Diffuse ISR is, in turn, the major risk factor for malignant recurrent ISR, and therefore long-segment BMS implantation is associated with a poor clinical outcome.[33,34] Randomized clinical trials and registries which included complex coronary lesions found that DESs reduce the need for revascularization therapy and provide clinical efficacy in routine practice compared with BMSs.[24,25,35–40] Furthermore, in the DES era, interventionalists implant stents to cover the entire atherosclerotic lesion, that is, the stented segment length tends to be longer than the lesion length.[35]

Tsagalou E et al reported the results of multiple DES implantations for 66 patients with diffuse LAD stenosis. In this study, 39 patients were treated with SESs, average length 84 ± 22 mm, and 27 patients with PESs, average length 74 ± 14 mm. The number of stents implanted per patient was 2.8 ± 0.7. Procedural success was achieved in 95% of cases. Eleven (16.6%) patients had in-hospital non–Q wave MI (5 SESs and 6 PESs), and 1 patient developed intra-procedural stent thrombosis. All patients had clinical follow-up, and 52 patients (79%) had angiographic follow-up at 6 months. The MACE rate was 15% (7.5% for SESs and 7.5% for PESs). No patient died, 1 patient had non–Q wave MI, and 10 patients (15%) underwent TVR.[41] J Aoki et al reported the results of multiple DES implantations in 122 consecutive patients with de novo coronary lesions. In this study, 81 patients were treated with SESs (average length 77 mm) and 42 patients with PESs (average length 84 mm). The number of stents implanted per patient was 3.3 ± 1.1, and the mean total stent length was 79 mm. Procedural success was achieved in 96% of cases. At 30 days, 7 patients (5.8%) had an MI, and 1 patient developed subacute stent thrombosis. All patients had 1 year clinical follow-up. The MACE rate was 18% (18.5% for SESs and 17.1% for PESs). Five patients (4.1%) died, 12 patients (10%) had MI, and 9 patients (7.5%) underwent TVR.[42] In the Multicenter Prospective Nonrandomized Registry Study for Drug-Eluting Stents in Very Long Coronary Lesions (Cypher versus Taxus)(Long-DES) trial, a nonrandomized registry compared angiographic and clinical outcomes in 637 patients undergoing stent placement with either BMSs ($n = 177$), SESs ($n = 294$), or PESs ($n = 166$) in long coronary lesions. Baseline characteristics were similar in the three arms, including a number of high-risk patients as well as patients with diabetes. The stent length was similar (42.8 mm in SES vs. 43.1 mm in PES, $P = NS$). The DES group received more stents with longer length compared with the BMS group. Patients with SES had smaller reference vessel diameter (2.80 mm in SES vs. 2.9 mm PES). At 6-month angiographic follow-up, completed in approximately 80% of all patients, there was 65% less in-stent late loss in the SES group compared with the PES group (0.27 mm vs. 0.78 mm, $P < 0.0001$), and 65% less in-segment re-stenosis in the SES group compared with the PES group (7.4% vs. 21.3%, $P < 0.001$). The rate of TLR was significantly lower with DESs compared with BMSs (2.7% SES, 5.4% PES, and 18.6% BMS, $P < 0.001$), but the difference between the SES and PES groups was not statistically significant ($P = 0.14$).[43] The TAXUS ATLAS long lesion trial compared the TAXUS Liberte 38-mm stent for long lesion treatment with historical controls (TAXUS EXPRESS).[28] The rate of MI was reduced with the

long TAXUS Liberte stent compared with TAXUS Express stent (1.4% vs. 6.5%, $P = 0.0246$).

Long-Term Efficacy and Safety Issues

DES implantation for small vessel disease or long lesions with multiple stent is efficacious for reduction of re-stenosis rates and TLR rates compared with BM implantation. However, even with DESs, these lesions are still associated with an increased risk of re-stenosis, need for revascularization, and MACE[38,44–47] from the insight of the large registries of DESs compared with normal or large vessels or short lesions. In the e-Cypher registry, small vessel treatment was one of the predictors of MACE at 12 months.[38] Kastrati also found that the small vessel diameter was one of the strongest predictors of re-stenosis, and a 0.5-mm decrease in vessel size was associated with adjusted odds ratios (ORs) of 1.74 (95% CI, 1.31–2.32) for angiographic re-stenosis and 1.65 (95% CI, 1.22–2.23) for TLR. In patients with full metal jackets (stent length >60 mm), stent length itself and reference diameter were the predictors of re-stenosis.[45] Elezi et al found that patients with small diameter stents were at high risk of re-stenosis compared with normal or large vessel cohorts.[46] Shirai et al reported that according to the stent length, the incidences of target lesion revascularization rates increased in patient and lesion level analyses.[47] In the Synergy between PCI with Taxus and Cardiac Surgery (SYNTAX) trial, it was demonstrated that MACE rates increased as the SYNTAX score increased.[48] Complex procedures with extensive coverage of the coronary artery with DESs are associated with a substantial risk of repeated procedures. The recently reported Fractional flow reserve versus Angiography in Multi-vessel Evaluation (FAME) trial results suggested that PCI guided by physiologic lesion assessment in patients with multivessel disease resulted in fewer lesions treated and improved the clinical outcome.[49] A major long-term concern regarding DESs for long lesions is the potential for late and very late stent thrombosis.[50–53] In the Bern and Rotterdam study, stent thrombosis was reported to occur at a continuous rate of 0.4% to 0.6% per year for up to 4 years without diminution.[54] Previous data, including a meta-analysis of 10 randomized studies, demonstrated that stent length is a risk factor for acute and late stent thrombosis and MACE.[55,56] Orlic et al reported that stent length per lesion and per patient is a powerful indicator for MACE in the treatment of multi-vessel disease with SES implantation at 6 months.[57] Data from the Spanish registry ESTROFA and the Israeli arm of the eCypher registry also showed that stent length is an independent predictor of subacute and late stent thrombosis for up to 3 years.[58,59] The long stent group had an increase in long-term clinical events, including death and MI through 3 years.[47] Suh et al also reported that stent length was one of the predictors of stent thrombosis and that the threshold of stent length for predicting stent thrombosis was 31.5 mm.[60] The SYNTAX trial showed a stent thrombosis rate of 3.3% after 1 year.[48] In this trial, the mean total stent length was 86.1 mm, with 4.6 stents used to cover 3.6 lesions or patients. The 3.3% stent thrombosis rate at 1 year suggests that complex procedures with implantation of longer and multiple stents to treat multi-vessel disease and full-coverage of atherosclerotic lesions may be associated with an increased risk for stent thrombosis. Räber et al reported that angiographic follow-up revealed an increased late loss in DES overlap patients compared with that without stent overlap, and re-stenosis occurred at the zone of stent overlap in 68% of re-stenosis patients.[61] In one study, there was a high incidence of incomplete neointimal coverage and stent malapposition in overlapping DES sites by intravascular ultrasound, angioscopy, and optical coherence tomography.[62–64] In particular, late malapposition seemed to be associated with very late stent thrombosis.[65] Re-stenosis and stent malapposition might have been the result of increased inflammation induced by excessive drug and polymer at the overlap site.[66]

THERAPEUTIC ANGIOGENESIS

Promoting neovascularization by the administration of specific growth factors or genetic material encoding specific endothelial cell mitogen of soluble basic fibroblast growth factor (VEGF) represents another intriguing potential therapeutic approach for patients with diffuse coronary disease.[67] Animal studies have demonstrated, angiographically and histologically, the feasibility of forming collateral channels in ischemic vascular territories and improved blood flow to ischemic limbs by either local or systemic application of such deoxyribonucleic acid (DNA) encoding material.[68-70] Isner and colleagues administered naked plasmid DNA to the diseased territory of patients suffering from severe distal lower extremity peripheral vascular disease and rest pain via hydrogel-coated balloons inflated upstream to the disease. Rapid development of collateral vessels was associated with augmented blood flow to the limb, as assessed by intra-arterial Doppler imaging.[71] Similar results have been achieved in animal models via systemic (intramuscular or intra-arterial) administration of DNA encoding VEGF, which possesses tropism for ischemic tissue.[70] Although therapeutic angiogenesis holds great promise in the treatment of severe, diffuse coronary disease, a number of issues need to be addressed as these techniques enter phase I clinical testing:

Determination of the optimal growth factor or combination thereof to promote neovascularization

Development (if necessary) of effective transfecting DNA vectors

Determination of the relative efficacy of systemic delivery compared with the more invasive and technically cumbersome local delivery techniques

Determination of optimal dosing and the need for and timing of repeat applications

Development of methods to ensure delivery of these potent agents only to appropriate target areas

Determination of the potential for short-term and long-term adverse sequelae related to the administration of these mitogenic, pro-proliferative agents.

SUMMARY

In light of the paucity of randomized trial data demonstrating the superiority of any particular device in the treatment of small vessel and diffuse disease, treatment needs to be individualized. The treatment algorithm used in approaching long lesions at the Kokura Memorial Hospital, based on the presence or absence of various ancillary morphologic features, is presented in Figure 21-3. It should be re-emphasized that, to date, no technique has proven superiority to prevent re-stenosis over that of standard angioplasty using long balloon catheters. In the ERBAC trial, rotational atherectomy was associated with a modest but statistically significant improvement in acute procedural success relative to balloon angioplasty; it might be a rational approach to treating long calcified stenoses by rendering them responsive to balloon dilation. The role of coronary stent placement in the treatment of nondiscrete stenoses remains to be defined. Given the substantial incidence of re-stenosis despite stent placement in the setting of long lesions, until the problem of ISR can be resolved, the routine use of stents

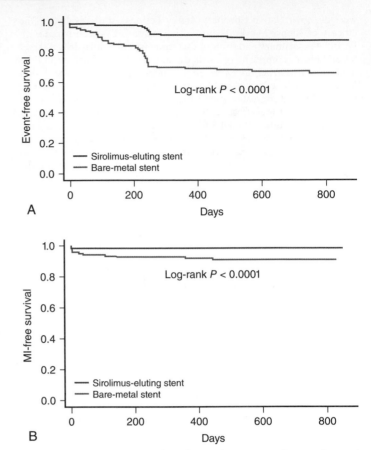

Figure 21-3 A, The use of sirolimus-eluting stent for small vessel disease was associated with a significantly lower incidence of the clinical endpoint (24 months composite of major adverse cardiac and cerebrovascular events (MACCE; death, nonfatal myocardial infarction [MI], target lesion revascularization [TLR] cerebrovascular accident). **B,** The reduction of MACCE was not only caused by a reduction in TLR but also by a reduction in MI.

should be undertaken with extreme caution. Perhaps spot stenting those areas failing to respond adequately within a long diseased segment or failing to develop large dissection flaps following balloon dilation might reduce the problem of ISRs. Despite the advent of new devices during the past decade, long lesions continue to present a difficult challenge. The ultimate solution might depend on the development of novel adjunct strategies such as radiation, gene-based therapy, and DESs, which may substantially reduce the potential for neointimal proliferation and thereby stenosis recurrence.

REFERENCES

1. Berne R, Levy M: *Cardiovascular physiology*, St Louis, 1986, Mosby.
2. Marcus M, Harrison D, White C, et al: Assessing the physiologic significance of coronary obstructions in patients: Importance of diffuse undetected atherosclerosis. *Prog Cardiovasc Dis* 31:39–56, 1988.
3. Feldman R, Nichols W, Pepine C, et al: Hemodynamic significance of the length of a coronary arterial narrowing. *Am J Cardiol* 41:865–871, 1978.
4. Kimura T, Tamura T, Yokoi H, et al: Long-term clinical and angiographic follow-up after placement of Palmaz-Schatz coronary stent: a single-center experience. *J Interv Cardiol* 7:129–139, 1994.
5. Bauters C, Banos JL, Van Belle E, et al: Six-month angiographic outcome after successful repeat percutaneous interventional for in-stent restenosis. *Circulation* 97:318–321, 1998.
6. De Gregorio J, Colombo A, et al: Treatment strategies for long and calcified lesions. *J Interv Cardiol* 11:557–564, 1998.
7. Kobayashi Y, De Gregorio J, Kobayashi N, et al: Stented segment length as an independent predictor of restenosis. *J Am Coll Cardiol* 34:651–659, 1999.

8. Saucedo JF, Kennard ED, Popma JJ, et al: Importance of lesion length on new device angioplasty of native coronary arteries. *Cath Cardiovasc Interv* 50:19–25, 2000.
9. Kastrati A, Elezi S, Dirschinger J, et al: Influence of lesion length on restenosis after coronary stent placement. *J Am Coll Cardiol* 83:1617–1622, 1999.
10. Eccleston D, Belli G, Penn I, et al: Are multiple stents associated with multiplicative risk in the optimal stent era? *Circulation* 94(Suppl I):I-454, 1996.
11. Gaxiola E, Vlietstra R, Browne K, et al: Six-month follow-up of patients with multiple stents in a single coronary artery. *J Am Coll Cardiol* 29(Suppl A):276A, 1997.
12. The EPIC Investigators: Use of a monoclonal antibody directed against the platelet glycoprotein IIb/IIIa receptor in high-risk coronary angioplasty. *N Engl J Med* 330:956–961, 1994.
13. The EPILOG Investigators: Platelet glycoprotein IIb/IIIa receptor inhibition with abciximab with lower heparin dosages during percutaneous coronary revascularization. *N Engl J Med* 336:1689–1696, 1997.

14. Brener S, Barr L, Burchenal J, et al: A randomized, placebo-controlled trial of abciximab with primary angioplasty for acute MI. The RAPPORT trial. *Circulation* 96(Suppl I):I-473, 1997.
15. Topol EJ, Ferguson JJ, Weisman HF, et al: Long-term protection from myocardial ischemic events in a randomized trial of brief integrin beta3 blockade with percutaneous coronary intervention. EPIC Investigator Group. Evaluation of Platelet IIb/IIIa Inhibition for Prevention of Ischemic Complications. *JAMA* 278:479–484, 1997.
16. Teirstein P, Massullo V, Jani S, et al: Catheter-based radiotherapy to inhibit restenosis after coronary stenting. *N Engl J Med* 336:1697–1703, 1997.
17. Bennett M, Schwartz S: Antisense therapy for angioplasty restenosis: Some critical considerations. *Circulation* 92:1981–1993, 1995.
18. Sousa JE, Costa MA, Abizaid A, et al: Lack of neointimal proliferation after implantation of sirolimus-coated stents in human coronary arteries. *Circulation* 103:192–195, 2001.
19. Foley DP, Melkert R, Serruys PW, the CARPORT, MERCATOR, MARCATOR, and PARK Investigators: Influence of vessel size on

renarrowing process and late angiographic outcome after successful balloon angioplasty. *Circulation* 90:1239–1251, 1994.

20. Schunkert H, Harrel L, Palacios IF: Implications of small reference vessel diameter in patients undergoing percutaneous coronary revascularization. *J Am Coll Cardiol* 34:40–48, 1999.

21. Hirshfeld JW, Schwartz JS, Jugo R, et al, the M-HEART Investigators: Restenosis after coronary angioplasty: A multivariate statistical model to relate lesion and procedure variables to restenosis. *J Am Coll Cardiol* 18:647–656, 1991.

22. Elezi S, Kastrati A, Neumann FJ, et al: Vessel size and long-term outcome after coronary stent placement. *Circulation* 98:1875–1880, 1998.

23. Akiyama T, Moussa I, Reimers B, et al: Angiographic and clinical outcome following coronary stenting of small vessels: A comparison with coronary stenting in large vessels. *J Am Coll Cardiol* 32:1610–1618, 1998.

24. Schofer J, Schluter M, Gershlick AH, et al: Sirolimus-eluting stents for treatment of patients with long atherosclerotic lesions in small coronary arteries: Double-blind, randomised controlled trial (E-SIRIUS). *Lancet* 362:1093–1099, 2003.

25. Schampaert E, Cohen EA, Schlüer M, et al: The Canadian Study of the Sirolimus-Eluting Stent in the Treatment of Patients with Long De Novo Lesions in Small Native Coronary Arteries (C-SIRIUS). *JACC* 43:1110–1115, 2004.

26. Ardissino D, Cavallini C, Bramucci E, et al: Sirolimus-Eluting vs Uncoated Stents for Prevention of Restenosis in Small Coronary Arteries.(SES SMART), *JAMA* 29:2727–2734, 2004.

27. Menozzi A, Solinas E, Ortolani P, et al: Twenty-four months clinical outcomes of sirolimus-eluting stents for the treatment of small coronary arteries: The long-term SES-SMART clinical study. *Eur Heart J* 30:2095–2101, 2009.

28. Turco MA, Ormiston JA, Popma JJ, et al: Reduced risk of restenosis in small vessels and reduced risk of myocardial infarction in long lesions with the new thin strut TAXUS Liberté stent 1-year results from the TAXUS ATLAS program. *JACC Interv* 1:699–709, 2008.

29. Stone GW, Rizvi A, Newman W, et al: Everolimus-eluting versus paclitaxel-eluting stents in coronary artery disease. *N Engl J Med* 362:1663, 2010.

30. Kobayashi Y, De Gregorio J, Kobayashi N, et al: Stented segment length as an independent predictor of restenosis *J Am Coll Cardiol* 34:651–659, 1999.

31. Kastrati A, Elezi S, Dirschinger J, et al: Influence of lesion length on restenosis after coronary stent placement. *Am J Cardiol* 83:1617–1622, 1999.

32. Colombo A, Goldberg SL, Almagor Y, et al: A novel strategy for stent deployment in the treatment of acute or threatened closure complicating balloon coronary angioplasty: Use of short or standard (or both) single or multiple Palmaz-Schatz stents. *J Am Coll Cardiol* 22:1887–1891, 1993.

33. Mehran R, Dangas G, Abizaid AS, et al: Angiographic patterns of in-stent restenosis: Classification and implications for long-term outcome. *Circulation* 10:1872–1878, 1999.

34. Shiran A, Mintz GS, Waksman R, et al: Early lumen loss after treatment of in-stent restenosis: An intravascular ultrasound study. *Circulation* 98:200–203, 1998.

35. Moses JW, Leon MB, Popma JJ, et al. Sirolimus-eluting stents versus standard stents in patients with coronary artery disease. *N Engl J Med* 349:1315–1323, 2003.

36. Degertekin M, Arampatzis CA, Lemos PA, et al: Very long sirolimus-eluting stent implantation for de novo coronary lesions. *Am J Cardiol* 93:826–829,2005.

37. Morice M-C, Serruys PW, Sousa JE, et al: A randomized comparison of a sirolimus-eluting stent with a standard stent for coronary revascularization. *N Engl J Med* 346:1773–1780, 2002.

38. Urban P, Gershlick AH, Guagliumi G, et al: Safety of coronary sirolimus-eluting stents in daily clinical practice: One-year follow-up of the e-Cypher registry. *Circulation* 113:1434–1441, 2006.

39. Abbott JD, Voss MR, Nakamura M, et al: Unrestricted use of drug-eluting stents compared with bare-metal stents in routine clinical practice. *J Am Coll Cardiol* 50:2029–2036, 2007.

40. Williams DO, Abbott JD, Kip KE, DEScover Investigators: Outcomes of 6906 patients undergoing percutaneous coronary intervention in the era of drug-eluting stents: Report of the DEScover registry circulation. *Circulation* 114:2154–2162, 2006.

41. Tsagalou E, Chieffo A, Iakovou I, et al: Multiple overlapping drug-eluting stents to treat diffuse disease of the left anterior descending coronary artery. *J Am Coll Cardiol* 45:570–1573, 2005.

42. Aoki J, Ong AT, Rodriguez-Granillo GA, et al: Full metal jacket (stented length >64 mm) using drug-eluting stent for de novo coronary artery lesions. *Am Heart J* 150:994–999, 2005.

43. Kim YH, Park SW, Lee SW, et al: Comparison of sirolimus-eluting stent, paclitaxel-eluting stent, and bare metal stent in the treatment of long coronary lesions. *Catheter Cardiovasc Interv* 67:181–187,2006.

44. Kastrati A, Dibra A, Mehilli J, et al: Predictive factors of restenosis after coronary implantation of sirolimus- or paclitaxel-eluting stents. *Circulation* 113:2293–2300, 2006.

45. Lee CW, Park DW, Lee BK, et al: Clinical and angiographic outcomes after placement of multiple overlapping drug-eluting stents in diffuse coronary lesions. *Am J Cardiol* 97:506–511, 2006.

46. Elezi S, Dibra A, Mehilli J, et al: Vessel size and outcome after coronary drug-eluting stent placement. Results from a large cohort of patients treated with sirolimus- or paclitaxel eluting stents. *J Am Coll Cardiol* 48:1304 –1309, 2006.

47. Shirai S, Kimura T, Nobuyoshi M, et al: Impact of multiple and long sirolimus-eluting stent implantation on three-year clinical outcomes in the j-Cypher registry. *JACC Interv* 3:180–188, 2010

48. Serruys PW, Morice MC, Kappetein AP, et al: Percutaneous coronary intervention versus coronary-artery bypass grafting for severe coronary artery disease. *N Engl J Med* 360:961–972, 2009.

49. Tonino PA, De Bruyne B, Pijls NH, et al, FAME study investigators: Fractional flow reserve versus angiography for guiding percutaneous coronary intervention. *N Engl J Med* 360(3):213–224, 2009.

50. McFadden EP, Stabile E, Regar E, et al: Late thrombosis in drug-eluting coronary stents after discontinuation of antiplatelet therapy. *Lancet* 364:1519–1521, 2004.

51. Lagerqvist B, James SK, Stenestrand U, et al: Long-term outcomes with drug-eluting stents versus bare-metal stents in Sweden. *N Engl J Med* 356:1009–1019, 2007.

52. Daemen J, Wenaweser P, Tsuchida K, et al: Early and late coronary stent thrombosis of sirolimus-eluting and paclitaxel-eluting stents in routine clinical practice: Data from a large two-institutional cohort study. *Lancet* 369:667–678, 2007.

53. Iakovou I, Schmidt T, Bonizzoni E, et al: Incidence, predictors, and outcome of thrombosis after successful implantation of drug-eluting stents. *JAMA* 293.2126 2130, 2005.

54. Wenaweser P, Daemen J, Zwahlen M, et al: Incidence and correlates of drug-eluting stent thrombosis in routine clinical practice 4-year results from a large 2-institutional cohort study. *J Am Coll Cardiol* 52:1134–1140, 2008.

55. Moreno R, Fernandez C, Hernandez R, et al: Drug-eluting stent thrombosis: Results from a pooled analysis including 10 randomized studies. *J Am Coll Cardiol* 45:954–959, 2005.

56. Cutlip DE, Baim DS, Ho KKL, et al: Stent thrombosis in the modern era. A pooled analysis of multicenter coronary stent clinical trials. *Circulation* 103:1967–1971, 2001.

57. Orlic D, Bonizzoni E, Stankovic G, et al: Treatment of multivessel coronary artery disease with sirolimus-eluting stent implantation: immediate and mid-term results. *J Am Coll Cardiol* 43:1154–1160, 2004.

58. de la Torre-Hernandez JM, Alfonso F, Hernandez F, et al: Drug-eluting stent thrombosis. Results from the multicenter Spanish Registry ESTROFA (Estudio ESpañol sobre TROmbosis de stents FArmacoactivo). *J Am Coll Cardiol* 51:986–990, 2008.

59. Planer D, Beyar R, Almagor Y, et al: Long-term (>3 years) outcome and predictors of clinical events after insertion of sirolimus-eluting stent in one or more native coronary arteries (from the Israeli arm of the e-Cypher registry). *Am J Cardiol* 101:953–959, 2008.

60. Suh J, Park DW, Lee JY, et al: The relationship and threshold of stent length with regard to risk of stent thrombosis after a drug-eluting stent implantation. *JACC Interv* 3:383–389, 2010.

61. Räber L, Jüni P, Löffel L, et al: Impact of stent overlap on angiographic and long-term clinical outcome in patients undergoing drug-eluting stent implantation. *J Am Coll Cardiol* 55:1178–1188, 2010.

62. Alfonso F, Pérez-Vizcayno MJ, Ruiz M, et al: Coronary aneurysm after drug-eluting stent implantation. *J Am Coll Cardiol* 53: 2053–2060, 2009.

63. Awata M, Kotani J, Uematsu M, et al: Serial angioscopic evidence of incomplete neointimal coverage after sirolimus-eluting stent implantation. *Circulation* 116:910–916, 2007.

64. Matsumoto D, Shite J, Shinke T, et al: Neointimal coverage of sirolimus-eluting stents at 6-month follow-up: Evaluated by optical coherence tomography. *Eur Heart J* 28:961–967, 2007.

65. Ayman KM, Bergheanu SC, Stijnen T, et al: Late stent malapposition risk is higher after drug-eluting stent compared with bare-metal stent implantation and associates with late stent thrombosis. *Eur Heart J* 31:1172, 2010.

66. Lim SY, Jeong MH, Hong SJ, et al: Inflammation and delayed endothelization with overlapping drug-eluting stents in a porcine model of in-stent restenosis. *Circ J* 72:463– 468, 2008.

67. Isner J: Angiogenesis for revascularization of ischemic tissues. *Eur Heart J* 18:1–2, 1997.

68. Takeshita S, Zheng L, Brogi E, et al: Therapeutic angiogenesis. A single intra-arterial bolus of vascular endothelial growth factor augments revascularization in a rabbit ischemic hind limb model. *J Clin Invest* 93:662–670, 1994.

69. Shou M, Thirumurti V, Rajanayagam S, et al: Effect of basic fibroblast growth factor on myocardial angiogenesis in dogs with mature collateral vessels. *J Am Coll Cardiol* 29:1102 1106, 1997.

70. Tsurumi Y, Takeshita S, Chen D, et al: Direct intramuscular gene transfer of naked DNA encoding vascular endothelial growth factor augments collateral development and tissue perfusion. *Circulation* 94:3281–3290, 1996.

71. Isner J, Pieczek A, Schainfeld R, et al: Clinical evidence of angiogenesis after arterial gene transfer of phVEGF165 in patient with ischemic limb. *Lancet* 248:370–374, 1996.

22

Percutaneous Coronary Intervention for Unprotected Left Main Coronary Artery Stenosis

SEUNG-JUNG PARK | YOUNG-HAK KIM

KEY POINTS

- A significant left main coronary artery (LMCA) stenosis is defined as angiographic diameter stenosis >50%, minimal luminal area <6 mm2, or fractional flow reserve (FFR) <0.80 caused by target stenosis at the LMCA.

- Stenting for unprotected LMCA stenosis is an alternative to bypass surgery, especially for patients at a high surgical risk or emergent clinical situations such as bailout procedure or acute myocardial infarction (AMI).

- Use of intravascular ultrasound is strongly recommended for lesion assessment, treatment selection, optimal stenting, and good prognosis in LMCA stenting.

- Drug-eluting stents (DESs) reduce the incidence of re-stenosis and subsequent need for repeat revascularization with similar risk of death or MI compared with bare metal stents (BMSs).

- A single-stent strategy is recommended for bifurcation LMCA stenosis.

- Standard dual anti-platelet therapy with aspirin and clopidogrel should be administered at least for 1 year after DES implantation for LMCA stenosis.

Introduction

Because of the long-term benefit of coronary artery bypass grafting (CABG) compared with medical therapy, CABG has been the standard treatment for unprotected LMCA stenosis.[1-3] However, with the advancement of technique and equipment, percutaneous coronary intervention (PCI) has been found to be feasible for patients with unprotected LMCA stenosis.[3] In particular, the recent introduction of DESs, together with advances in peri-procedural and postprocedural adjunctive pharmacotherapies, has improved the outcomes of PCI for these complex coronary lesions.[4-29] Therefore, in the recent updated guidelines, PCI for unprotected LMCA stenosis has still been indicated as class IIb for patients at a high surgical risk or emergent clinical situations such as bailout procedure or AMI as an alternative therapy to CABG.[30] Patients with LMCA stenosis have been traditionally classified into two subgroups: (1) protected (a previous patent graft from CABG to one or more major branches of the left coronary artery) and (2) unprotected LMCA disease (without such bypasses). In this review, current outcomes of PCI with DES in a series of research studies conducted across several countries are evaluated.

Definition of Significant Left Main Coronary Artery Stenosis

Coronary angiography has been the standard tool to determine the severity of coronary artery disease. Although a traditional cut-off for significant coronary stenosis has been stenosis diameter of 70% in non-LMCA lesions, its cut-off in LMCA has been stenosis diameter

of 50%. However, because the conventional coronary angiogram is only a lumenogram providing information about lumen diameter but yielding little insight into lesion and plaque characteristics themselves, it has several limitations caused by peculiar anatomic and hemodynamic factors. In addition, the LMCA segment is the least reproducible of all coronary segments with the largest reported intraobserver and interobserver variabilities.[31-33] Therefore, intravascular ultrasound (IVUS) is often used to assess the severity of LMCA stenosis.

The significance of the stenosis at the LMCA necessitating revascularization should be determined by the absolute luminal area, not by the degree of plaque burden or area stenosis. Because of remodeling, a larger plaque burden can exist in the absence of lumen compromise.[34] Abizaid et al reported the results of 1-year follow-up in 122 patients with LMCA stenosis. The minimal lumen diameter by IVUS was the most important predictor of cardiac events, with a 1-year event rate of 14% in patients with a minimal luminal diameter less than 3 mm.[35] Fassa et al reported that the long-term outcomes of patients with LMCA stenosis with a minimal lumen area less than 7.5 mm^2 who did not have revascularization were considerably worse than the outcomes of patients who were revascularized.[36] Practically, it is important to keep the IVUS catheter coaxial with the LMCA and to disengage the guiding catheter from the ostium so that the guiding catheter is not mistaken for a calcific lesion with a lumen dimension equal to the inner lumen of the guiding catheter. When assessing distal LMCA disease, it is important to begin imaging in the most coaxial branch vessel from both branches. Nevertheless, distribution of plaque in the distal LMCA is not always uniform; and it may be necessary to image from more than one branch back into the LMCA.[37,38] FFR may play an adjunctive role in determining significant stenosis at the LMCA. *Fractional flow reserve* is the ratio of the maximal blood flow achievable in a stenotic vessel to the normal maximal flow in the same vessel.[39] A value of fractional flow reserve less than 0.8 is considered a reliable indicator of significant stenosis producing inducible ischemia. In patients with an angiographically equivocal LMCA stenosis, a strategy of revascularization versus medical therapy based on FFR cut-off point of 0.75 was associated with an excellent survival and freedom from events for up to 3 years of follow-up.[40] On the basis of the results of IVUS and FFR, LMCA with IVUS area less than 6 mm^2 or FFR less than 0.80 is generally considered a significant stenosis necessitating revascularization with CABG or PCI.

Outcomes of Drug-Eluting Stents Compared with Bare Metal Stents

SAFETY IN TERMS OF THE RISK OF DEATH, MYOCARDIAL INFARCTION, OR STENT THROMBOSIS

Although there are disputes about the long-term safety of DESs, the possibility of late or very late thrombosis has still been the major factor limiting global use of DESs, especially for unprotected LMCA stenosis. Table 22-1 depicts the results of recent studies demonstrating the outcomes of DES implantation for unprotected LMCA stenosis. It is clear

TABLE 22-1	Outcomes Drug-Eluting Stent for Unprotected Left Main Coronary Artery Stenosis												
	Chieffo et al[4]		Valgimigli et al[6]		Park et al[5]		De Lezo et al[28]	Price et al[11]	Kim et al[20]	Meliga et al[29]	Mehilli et al[42]	
Stent type	SES, PES	BMS	SES, PES	BMS	SES	BMS	SES	SES	SES, PES	SES, PES	PES	SES
Design	Single-center registry		Single-center registry		Single-center registry		Single-center registry	Single-center registry	Single-center registry	Multi-center DELFT registry	Multi-center randomized study	
No. of patients	85	64	95	86	102	121	52	50	63	358	302	305
Age (yr)	63	66	64	66	60	58	63	69	67	66	69	69
Ejection fraction (%)	51*	57	41	42	60	62	57	NA	50	49	53	54
Acute myocardial infarction (%)	NA	NA	17	20*	9.8	6.6	NA	NA	5	8.4	NA	NA
Bifurcation involvement (%)	81*	58	65	66	71*	43	42	94	54	74	63	63
Two-stent technique (%)	74	NA	40*	15	41*	18	18	89	17	43	51	49
Initial clinical outcomes	In-hospital		30 days		In-hospital		In-hospital	In-hospital	In-hospital	In-hospital	30 days	
Death (%)	0	0	11	7	0	0	0	0	0	3	1	2
Myocardial infarction (%)	6	8	4	9	7	8	4	8	10	7	4	4
Stent thrombosis (%)	0	0	0	0	0	0	0	4	0	NA	0.3	0.7
TVR (%)	0	2	0	2	0	0	0	6	0	0.8	0.3 (TLR)	0.7 (TLR)
Any events (%)	NA	NA	15	19	7	8	4	10	10	11	5.0	4.6
Long-term outcomes (%)	Cumulative		Cumulative		Cumulative		Cumulative	After discharge	Cumulative	3 years	2 years	
Mean follow-up, months	6	6	17	12	12	12	12	9	11	NA	NA	NA
Death (%)	4	11	14	16	0	0	0	10	5	9	10	9
Myocardial infarction (%)	NA	NA	4*	12	7	8	1	2	11	9	5	5
Stent thrombosis (%)	0.1	0	NA	NA	0	0	0	0	0.2	0.6	0.3	0.7
TVR (%)	19	31	6*	12	2*	17	2	38	19	14	9 (TLR)	11 (TLR)

BMS, bare metal stent; NA, not available; MACE, major adverse cardiac events including death, myocardial infarction, and TVR; PES, paclitaxel-eluting stent; SES, sirolimus-eluting stent; TVR, target vessel revascularization; TLR, target lesion revascularization.
*P < 0.05 between drug-eluting stent (SES, PES, or both) versus BMS.

that none of the clinical studies showed a significant increase in the cumulative rates of death or MI in DES implantation for unprotected LMCA, compared with BMS implantation. In the three early pilot studies comparing the outcomes of DESs with those of BMSs, the incidences of death, MI, or stent thrombosis were comparable in the two stent types during the procedure and at follow-up.[4-6] Of interest, in the study by Valgimigli et al, DESs were associated with significant reduction in both the rate of MI (hazard ratio [HR] 0.22, $P = 0.006$) and composite of death or MI (HR 0.26, $P = 0.004$) compared with BMSs.[6] Considering that re-stenosis can lead to AMI in 3.5% to 19.4% of patients, a significant reduction of re-stenosis achieved by DESs might contribute to the better outcome of DESs. In fact, a previous study warned that the episode of re-stenosis with the use of BMSs in LMCA stenosis could present as late mortality.[41] In addition, more frequent repeat revascularization to treat BMS re-stenosis, in which CABG is the standard of care for unprotected LMCA, may also be related to the increase in hazardous accidents compared with DESs. A recent meta-analysis supported the safety of DESs by postulating that DESs did not increase the risk of death, MI, or stent thrombosis compared with BMSs.[18] In this meta-analysis including 1278 patients with unprotected LMCA stenosis, for a median of 10 months, mortality rate in DES-based PCI was only 5.5% (range 3.4%-7.7%) and was not higher than BMS-based PCI. Recently, three registry studies assessed the risk of safety outcomes with the use of DESs compared with BMSs over 2 years.[25-27] After rigorous adjustment using the propensity score or the inverse-probability-of-treatment weighting method to avoid selection bias, which was an inherent limitation of registry study, DES was at least not associated with long-term increase of death or MI. Of interest, the report of Palmerini et al showed the survival benefit of DESs over 2 years. These studies supported previous pilot studies that elective PCI with DES for unprotected LMCA stenosis seems to be a safe alternative to CABG. With regard to the risk of stent thrombosis, in the series of DES studies for LMCA stenosis, the incidence of stent thrombosis at 1 year ranged from 0% to 4% and was not statistically different from that with BMS.[4-6] Recently, a multi-center study confirmed this finding that the incidence of definite stent thrombosis at 2 years was only 0.5% in 731 patients treated with DESs.[19] In addition, the DELFT (Drug Eluting stent for LeFT main) multi-center registry, which included 358 patients undergoing LMCA stenting with DES, reported that the incidence of definite, probable, and possible stent thrombosis was 0.6%, 1.1%, and 4.4%, respectively, at 3 years.[29] In recent multi-center large studies for the ISAR-LEFT-MAIN (Intracoronary Stenting and Angiographic Results: Drug-Eluting Stents for Unprotected Coronary Left Main Lesions) study or the MAIN-COMPARE (COMparison of Percutaneous Coronary Angioplasty Versus Surgical Revascularization) study, the incidence of definite or probable stent thrombosis was less than 1%.[21,42] However, because these studies are still underpowered to completely exclude the possibility of increased risk of stent thrombosis in the very long term, further research needs to be performed with such a specific focus. Previous studies assessing the long-term outcomes of DESs for complex lesions showed slightly inhomogeneous outcomes. For example, recent large registries evaluating the safety of DESs for complex lesions showed comparable risks of death or MI for the two stent types.[43,44] The recent large NHLBI (National Heart, Lung, and Blood Institute) registry in the United States reported that the off-label use of DESs, compared with BMSs, for similar indications was associated with a comparable 1-year risk of death and a lower 1-year risk of MI after adjustment.[43] Of interest, a large registry that included 13,353 patients in Ontario (Canada) found that the 3-year mortality rate in a propensity-matched population was significantly higher with BMSs than with DESs.[44] The comparable or lower incidence of death or MI with the use of DESs compared with BMSs, may be attributed, at least in part, to the off-setting risks of re-stenosis versus stent thrombosis.

PROGNOSTIC FACTORS

Several attempts have been made to predict the long-term outcomes of complex LMCA intervention. Predictably, peri-procedural and long-term mortality rates depend strongly on clinical presentation. In the ULTIMA (Unprotected Left Main Trunk Investigation Multicenter Assessment) multi-center registry, which included 279 patients treated with BMSs, 46% of whom were inoperable or high surgical risk, the in-hospital mortality was 13.7%, and the 1-year incidence of all-cause mortality was 24.2%.[45] However, in the 32% of patients with low surgical risk (age <65 years and ejection fraction [EF] >30%), there were no peri-procedural deaths, and the 1-year mortality was 3.4%. Similarly, in DES implantation, high surgical risk represented by high Euro-SCORE or Parsonnet score, was the independent predictor of death or MI.[13,46] Therefore, it is recommended that a lot of attention should continue to be paid in the procedure of patients at high surgical risk. More recently, the SYNTAX (Synergy between PCI with Taxus and Cardiac Surgery) score, which is an angiographic risk stratification model, has been created to predict long-term outcomes after coronary revascularization with either PCI or CABG.[47] In the recent SYNTAX study comparing PCI with paclitaxel-eluting stents (PESs) versus CABG for multi-vessel or LMCA disease, the long-term mortality was significantly associated with the SYNTAX score.[47] Therefore, for patients with high clinical risk profiles or complex lesion morphologies, who are defined using these risk stratification models, the PCI procedures need to be performed by experienced interventionalists with the aid of IVUS, mechanical hemodynamic support, and optimal adjunctive pharmacotherapies, after a judicious selection of patients.

RECURRENT REVASCULARIZATION

Compared with BMSs, DESs reduce the incidence of angiographic re-stenosis and subsequently the need of repeat revascularization in unprotected LMCA stenosis. In early pilot studies, the 1-year incidence of repeat revascularization in DES implantation was 2% to 19% compared with 12% to 31% in BMS implantation (see Table 22-1).[4-6] Fortunately, in a 3-year long-term study, the incidence of repeat revascularization remained steady, and, significantly, the "late catch-up" phenomenon of late re-stenosis was not noted after coronary brachytherapy.[21] Two recent larger registries confirmed the efficacy of DESs.[25,27] The risk of target lesion revascularization over 3 years was

reduced by 60% with use of DES.[27] The risk of re-stenosis was significantly influenced by lesion location. DES treatment for ostial and shaft LMCA lesions had a very low incidence of angiographic or clinical re-stenosis.[14] In a study that included 144 patients with ostial or shaft stenosis in three cardiac centers, angiographic re-stenosis and target vessel revascularization (TVR) at 1 year occurred in only 1 (1%) and 2 (1%) patients, respectively. In contrast, PCI for LMCA bifurcation has been more challenging, although the prevalence had been more than 60% across previous studies.[4-6,10,21] However, repeat revascularization was exclusively performed in patients with PCI for bifurcation stenosis.[4-6] A recent study assessing the outcomes of DESs for LMCA stenosis showed that the risk of target vessel revascularization was six fold in bifurcation stenosis compared with nonbifurcation stenosis (13% vs. 3%).[13] The risk of bifurcation stenosis was mostly highlighted in a recent study by Price et al who reported that the target lesion revascularization (TLR) rate after sirolimus-eluting stent (SES) implantation was 44%.[11] In this study, 94% of patients (47 of 50) had lesions at the bifurcation and 98% underwent serial angiographic follow-up at 3 months, 9 months, or at both time points. This discouraging result cautioned against the efficacy of DESs and emphasized the need for meticulous surveillance with angiographic follow-up after PCI for LMCA bifurcation stenosis. However, this study was limited by the exclusive use of a complex stenting strategy (two stents in both branches) in 84% of patients, which might have increased the need of repeat revascularization. Although there was a debate about this, a current report proposed that the complex stenting technique might be associated with high occurrence of re-stenosis compared with the simple stenting technique.[8,48] A subgroup analysis of the large Italian registry supported this with the hypothesis that a single-stenting strategy for bifurcation LMCA lesions had long-term outcomes comparable with that for nonbifurcation lesions.[24] Taken together, before the novel treatment strategy is established, the simple stenting approach (LMCA to left anterior descending [LAD] artery with optional treatment in the left circumflex [LCx] artery) is primarily recommended in patients with relatively patent or diminutive LCx. Furthermore, future stent platforms specifically designed for LMCA bifurcation lesions may provide better scaffolding and more uniform drug delivery to the bifurcation LMCA stenosis. With regard to the differential benefit of DES type for the prevention of re-stenosis, the two most widely applicable DESs—SESs and PESs—had been evaluated in earlier studies. In an early study comparing the two DESs from a RESEARCH registry showed a comparable incidence of major adverse cardiac events (MACEs) with 25% in SESs (55 patients) and 29% in PESs (55 patients).[12] The recent ISAR-LEFT-MAIN study with a prospective randomized design compared 305 patients receiving SESs and 302 patients receiving PESs.[42] At 1 year, MACEs occurred in 13.6% of the SES group and 15.8% of the SES group with 16% and 19.4% of re-stenosis, respectively (*P* = NS). The subgroup analysis of MAIN-COMPARE registry supported the comparable safety and effectiveness of the two DESs.[49] Use of a second-generation DES is being evaluated in many research studies.

TECHNICAL ISSUES OF LEFT MAIN STENTING

Stenting Techniques

Stenting for ostial or body LMCA lesions seems very simple as the other stenting technique for non-LMCA coronary lesions. For instance, a brief and enough stent expansion is required to get optimal stent expansion and to avoid ischemic complications. In an ostial LMCA lesion, the coronary stent is generally positioned outside of the LMCA for complete lesion coverage of the ostium. Stenting for bifurcation LMCA lesions, however, is technically demanding and should be performed by experienced operators. In general, selection of the appropriate stenting strategy is dependent on the plaque configuration surrounding the LMCA. However, in spite of recent randomized studies comparing single-stent treatment versus two-stent treatment for bifurcation coronary lesions, the optimal stenting strategy for

LMCA bifurcation lesions has not been determined yet.[50,51] The current consensus is that the two-stent strategy does not have long-term advantages in terms of the incidence of any MACE compared with the single-stent strategy. Therefore, a systemic treatment of two-stent strategy for all LMCA bifurcation lesions—such as T stenting, kissing stenting, crush technique, or culotte technique—is not generally recommended. Instead, provisional stenting should be considered as the first-line treatment for LMCA bifurcations without significant side branch (SB) stenosis. Table 22-2 summarizes favorable and unfavorable angiographic morphologies toward single-stent and two-stent techniques for LMCA bifurcation stenosis. Fig. 22-1 is an example of a patient treated with provisional stenting, in which a single stent was placed in the LMCA crossing the LCx artery. However, as shown in Fig. 22-2, a patient with bifurcation LMCA disease involving the ostia of the LCx artery and the LAD arteries was treated with an elective two-stent technique.

Intravascular Ultrasound

The IVUS is considered a useful invasive diagnostic modality in determining anatomic configuration, selecting treatment strategy, and defining optimal stenting outcomes in the BMS or the DES era.[52] Although a retrospective study reported that the clinical impact of IVUS-guided stenting for LMCA with DES did not show a significant clinical long-term benefit compared with angiography-guided procedure, the usefulness of IVUS-guided stenting may not be hampered by this underpowered retrospective study.[53] The information gathered by

TABLE 22-2	Favorable or Unfavorable Anatomic Features for Provisional Stenting in the Treatment of Unprotected Left Main Coronary Artery Stenosis
	Anatomic Features
Favorable	Significant stenosis at the ostial LCx artery with Medina classification 1.1.0. or 1.0.0.
	Large size of LCx artery with ≥2.5 mm in diameter
	Right dominant coronary system
	Narrow angle with LAD artery
	No concomitant disease in LCx artery
	Focal disease in LCx artery
Unfavorable	Insignificant stenosis at the ostial LCx artery with Medina classification 1.1.1., 1.0.1., or 0.1.1
	Diminutive LCx artery with <2.5 mm in diameter
	Left dominant coronary system
	Wide angle with LAD artery
	Concomitant disease in LCx artery
	Diffuse disease in LCx artery

LAD, left anterior descending; *LCx*, left circumflex.

IVUS may be crucial for an optimal stenting procedure in unprotected LMCA stenosis. In fact, angiography has a limitation in assessing the true luminal size of LMCA because the LMCA is often short and lacks a normal segment for comparison. Therefore, the severity of LMCA stenosis is often underestimated by the misinterpretation of the normal

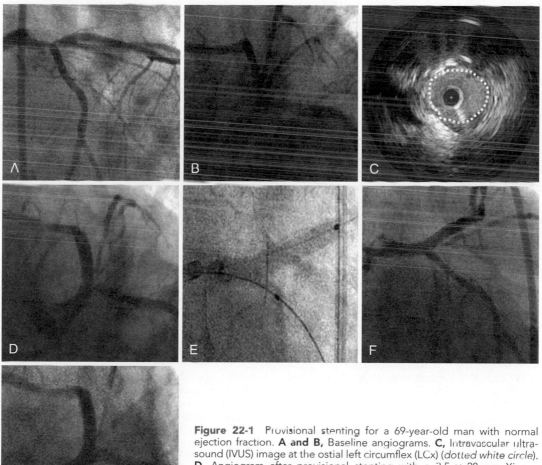

Figure 22-1 Provisional stenting for a 69-year-old man with normal ejection fraction. **A and B,** Baseline angiograms. **C,** Intravascular ultrasound (IVUS) image at the ostial left circumflex (LCx) (*dotted white circle*). **D,** Angiogram after provisional stenting with a 3.5 × 28 mm Xience everolimus-eluting stent (Abbott Vascular, Santa Clara, CA) in the left main coronary artery–left anterior descending artery (LMCA-LAD artery) overlapped with a stent in the middle LAD artery. **E,** Kissing balloon inflation after high-pressure balloon dilation with a 4.5 × 8 mm noncompliant balloon. **F and G,** Final angiograms after kissing balloon inflation with two 3.5 × 15 mm noncompliant balloons.

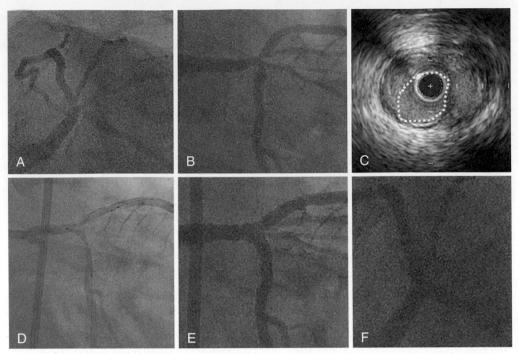

Figure 22-2 Crush stenting for a 66-year-old man with normal ejection fraction. **A and B,** Baseline angiograms. **C,** Intravascular ultrasound (IVUS) image at the ostial left circumflex (LCx) artery (*dotted white circle*). **D,** Positioning of two stents for crush stenting with two 3.5 × 23 mm left anterior descending (LAD) artery and 3.0 × 18 mm (LCx) Cypher sirolimus-eluting stents (Cordis Corp, Johnson & Johnson, Warren, NJ). **E and F,** Final angiograms after sequential high-pressure balloon dilation with a noncompliant balloon of 4 × 18 mm in the LAD artery and a noncompliant balloon of 3.0 × 18 mm in the LCx artery followed by kissing balloon inflation.

segment adjacent to a focal stenosis. In addition to the actual assessment of the LMCA lesion before the procedure, use of IVUS is very helpful to get an adequate expansion of the DES, to prevent stent inapposition, and to achieve full lesion coverage with the DES. A recent subgroup analysis from the MAIN-COMPARE registry reported a very interesting finding that IVUS guidance was associated with improved long-term mortality compared with the conventional angiography-guided procedure.[23] With an adjustment using propensity-score matching, for 201 matched pairs, there was a strong tendency toward lower risk of 3-year mortality with IVUS guidance compared with angiography guidance (6.3% vs. 13.6%, log-rank $P = 0.063$, HR 0.54; 95% CI 0.28–1.03). In particular, for 145 pairs of patients receiving DESs, the 3-year incidence of mortality was lower with IVUS guidance compared with that with angiography guidance (4.7% vs. 16.0%, log-rank $P = 0.048$; HR 0.39; 95% CI 0.15–1.02). Of interest, the mortality rate started to diverge beyond 1 year after the procedure. Therefore, in spite of the inherent limitations of its nonrandomized registry design, this study indicated that IVUS guidance may play a role in reducing very late stent thrombosis and subsequent long-term mortality. In fact, IVUS evaluations of stent underexpansion, incomplete lesion coverage, small stent area, large residual plaque and inapposition have been found to predict stent thrombosis after DES placement.[54–58] Therefore, mandatory use of IVUS in PCI for unprotected LMCA is strongly recommended.

DEBULKING ATHERECTOMY

In the BMS era, debulking coronary atherectomy had been widely used before stenting in an attempt to reduce re-stenosis by removal of the plaque burden. However, after the introduction of the DES, the role of debulking has become limited because of the dramatic benefit for re-stenosis reduction. A study suggested a viable role of debulking atherectomy even in the DES era for 99 coronary bifurcations.[59] Of interest, debulking in the main branch and the SB for LMCA stenoses allowed single stenting in 60 of the 63 LMCA bifurcation stenoses.

Surprisingly, at 1-year follow-up, no serious adverse event had occurred. This study indicated that debulking may be preferred in LMCA bifurcations to aid the provisional single-stenting strategy. In addition, debulking still plays a limited role in facilitating stent delivery. Debulking was used to remove plaque in the LMCA that inhibits advancement of the wire into the LAD artery. Similarly, rotablation has been used before stenting when calcification in the proximal segment prevents stent delivery or a calcified target lesion is not sufficiently dilated. Therefore, although data are limited, debulking atherectomy or rotablation still has a limited role even in DES treatment to improve lesion compliance.

Hemodynamic Support

Patients in an unstable hemodynamic condition need pharmacologic or device-based hemodynamic support during the procedure for LMCA stenosis. Old age, MI, cardiogenic shock, and decreased left ventricular ejection fraction (LVEF) are common clinical conditions requiring elective or provisional hemodynamic support. Among hemodynamic support devices, including the intra-aortic balloon pump, percutaneous hemodynamic support devices, or left ventricular assist devices, the intra-aortic balloon pump has been the most frequently used. Although there is no doubt that the provisional use of the intra-aortic balloon pump in patients with hemodynamic compromise is necessary for a successful procedure, the prevalence of planned use of the balloon pump is widely ranged, as the literature indicates. A study recently suggested the role of support by the intra-aortic balloon pump from 219 elective LMCA interventions.[60] In this study, a prophylactic balloon pump was used for a broad range of patients having distal LMCA bifurcation lesions, low EF (<40%), use of debulking devices, unstable angina, and critical right CAD. In that study, interestingly, although the patients receiving elective intra-aortic balloon pump support had a more complex clinical risk profile, the rate of procedural complications was lower than in those not receiving its support (1.4% vs. 9.3%, $P = 0.032$). Therefore, at least, its elective use needs to be considered for patients in a high-risk condition having multi-vessel disease, complex LMCA anatomy, low EF, or unstable presentations. Hopefully, the new support devices such as Tandem-Heart (CardiacAssist, Pittsburgh, Pennsylvania) or the Impella Recover LP 2.5 System (Impella CardioSystems, Aachen, Germany) may improve the feasibility of implementation and reduce the complication rate related to these devices.

Anti-thrombotics

Although the reported incidence of stent thrombosis in DES treatment for LMCA lesions has been very low, fear of stent thrombosis remains a major concern and therefore prevents more generalized use of DESs.[61] Careful administration of anti-platelet agents is very important to prevent the occurrence of stent thrombosis. In fact, premature discontinuation of clopidogrel was strongly associated with stent thrombosis in several studies.[62,63] Therefore, as generally recommended, dual anti-platelet therapy, which includes aspirin and clopidogrel (or ticlopidine), should be maintained for up to 1 year. If the patients seem to be at high risk, a high loading dose (600 mg) or lifelong administration of clopidogrel needs to be considered. Fortunately, a recent randomized study suggested that 1-year administration of standard dual anti-platelet therapy may be comparably safer in terms of the risk of death, MI, or stroke compared with prolonged therapy beyond 1 year.[64] However, because of the lack of power in LMCA stenting, further research is required to determine the optimal combination and duration of anti-platelet therapy. Aggressive use of anti-thrombotics should also be considered for complex lesion anatomy or an unstable coronary condition. For example, as demonstrated in earlier studies, use of the glycoprotein (GP) IIb/III inhibitor may play a role in reducing procedure-related thrombotic complications, including death or MI.[65] However, the additive role of the GP IIb/IIIa inhibitor cilostazol, low-molecular weight heparin, direct thrombin inhibitor, and other new drugs in DES treatment for LMCA lesions need to be investigated in future studies. Until the collection of evidence has been completed, aggressive combination of anti-thrombotic drugs before, during, and after the procedure to avoid thrombotic complications in high-risk patients has to be considered. Although the features of high risk are not well delineated, off-label use of DESs—such as in diabetes mellitus, multiple stenting, long DES, chronic renal failure, or MI—is a good index of a high-risk procedure.[66]

Comparison with Coronary Artery Bypass Surgery

It is surprising to note that guidelines for unprotected LMCA treatment, in which elective PCI for patients who are treatable with bypass surgery is a contraindication, are based mostly on 20-year old clinical trials.[1-3] These studies demonstrated a definite benefit of survival of CABG in LMCA stenosis compared with medical treatment. However, application of these results to current practice seems inappropriate because the surgical techniques as well as the medical treatments used in these studies are no longer relevant by today's standards and because no randomization studies between PCI and CABG with enough power have been conducted. The lack of data on the current CABG procedure used in unprotected LMCA stenosis further precludes any theoretical comparison of the two revascularization strategies. Table 22-3 lists patient and lesion characteristics favoring PCI or CABG based on current expert opinions and evidence. Several nonrandomized studies describing the better safety and efficacy of DES treatment for unprotected LMCA stenosis compared with CABG have been published (Table 22-4). Chieffo et al compared retrospectively the outcomes of 107 patients undergoing DES placement with 142 patients undergoing CABG.[7] They showed that the DES was associated with a nonsignificant benefit of mortality (odds ratio [OR] 0.331, $P = 0.167$) and a significantly low incidence of the composite of death or MI (0.260, $P = 0.0005$) and death, MI, or cerebrovascular accident (OR 0.385, $P = 0.01$) at 1-year follow-up. Conversely, CABG was correlated with a lower occurrence of target vessel revascularization (3.6% vs. 19.6%, $P = 0.0001$). These findings were supported by the study by Lee et al, which consisted of 50 patients who received DES placement and 123 patients who received CABG.[9] In this study, although the DES group

TABLE 22-3	Features Favoring Percutaneous Coronary Intervention or Coronary Artery Bypass Grafting
Indications in Favor of PCI	
Absolute	Suitable coronary anatomy for stenting with preserved left ventricular function (≥40%)
	Patient who refuses surgery
Relative	Lesion restricted to the LMCA ostium or shaft
	Isolated LMCA lesion
	Bail-out procedure (e.g., dissection at the LMCA complicated during angiography or PCI)
	Acute myocardial infarction at the LMCA, in which emergent revascularization is necessary
	Cardiogenic shock caused by LMCA stenosis, in which emergent revascularization is necessary
	Old age ≥80 years
	Serious comorbid disease (e.g., chronic lung disease, poor general performance, etc.)
	Limited life expectancy of <1 year
	Prior CABG
	Coronary anatomy, unsuitable for CABG (e.g., poor distal run-off)
Indications in Favor of CABG	
Absolute	Patient who refuses PCI
	Contraindication to anti-platelet therapy, including aspirin, heparin, and thienopyridine (ticlopidine or clopidogrel)
	History of serious allergic reaction to stainless steel, drugs coved on drug-eluting stents, and contrast agent
	History of known coagulopathy or bleeding diathesis
	Pregnant women
Relative	Complex coronary anatomies at LMCA, unsuitable for stenting (e.g., severe calcification, severe tortuosity, etc.)
	Total occlusions at other major epicardial coronary arteries (≥2)
	Multi-vessel stenosis, except in the LMCA
	Decreased left ventricular dysfunction (<40%)
	Extensive peripheral vascular disease, in which placement of guiding catheter or intra-aortic balloon pump is not likely to be performed
	In-stent re-stenosis at the LMCA, in which repeat PCI is not likely to be performed

CABG, coronary artery bypass graft surgery; *LMCA*, left main coronary artery; *PCI*, percutaneous coronary intervention.

had a slightly higher surgical risk, the rate of mortality or MI at 30 days was comparable between the two treatments. At 1-year follow-up, the DES group had non-significantly better clinical outcomes compared with CABG, reflected by overall survival (96% vs. 85%) and survival freedom from death, MI, target vessel revascularization, or adverse cerebrovascular events (83% vs. 75%). However, the survival freedom from repeat revascularization at 1 year remained nonsignificantly higher for the CABG group compared with the DES group (95% vs. 87%). The results of a recent multi-center registry were in agreement with the previous two reports with regard to the safety outcomes.[10] The PCI group treated with BMSs or DESs (60%) had similar incidences of death, MI, or both but a higher incidence of target lesion revascularization compared with the CABG group. Safety with the use of PCI was similar to the use of CABG, and this was confirmed also in the case of older patients (age ≥75 years) by Palmerini et al.[15] Recently, a randomized study comparing PCI and CABG was undertaken in 105 patients with unprotected LMCA stenosis.[17] PCI was performed using either BMSs (65%) or DESs (35%). The primary endpoint was the change in LVEF 12 months after the intervention, and a significant increase was noted only in the PCI group (3.3 ± 6.7% after PCI vs. 0.5 ± 0.8% after CABG, $P = 0.047$). In contrast, at 1-year after the procedure, repeat revascularization was significantly lower in the CABG group ($n = 5$) than in the PCI group ($n = 15$), although the incidence of death or MI was comparable between the two groups. However, this study was still underpowered to assess

TABLE 22-4	Comparison of Drug-Eluting Stent to Coronary Artery Bypass Surgery for Unprotected Left Main Coronary Artery Stenosis									
	Chieffo et al[7]		*Lee et al*[9]		*Palmerini et al*[15]		*Buszman et al*[17]		*Seung et al*[21]	
Study design	Registry		Registry		Registry		Randomized study		Registry	
Treatment type	PCI with SES, PES	CABG	PCI with SES	CABG	PCI with SES	CABG	PCI with BMS, DES	CABG	PCI with BMS, DES	CABG
No. of patient	107	142	50	123	157	154	52	53	1102	1138
Age (yr)	64	68	72	70	73*	69	61	61	62	64
Ejection fraction (%)	52	52	51	52	52	55	54	54	62	60
EuroSCORE or Parsonnet score (Lee)	4.4	4.3	18*	13	6*	5	3.3	3.5	NA	NA
Initial clinical outcomes	In-hospital		30 days		30 days		30 days		NA	
Death (%)	0	2	2	5	3.2	4.5	0	0	NA	NA
Myocardial infarction (%)	9	26	0	2	4.5	1.9	1.9	3.8	NA	NA
TVR (%)	0	2	0	1	0.6	0.6	1.9	0	NA	NA
Any MACE (%)	NA	NA	0	8	NA	NA	NA	NA	NA	NA
Cerebrovascular accident	0	1.4	2*	17	NA	NA	0	2	NA	NA
Long-term clinical outcomes	Cumulative after discharge		Kaplan-Meier		Cumulative		At 1 year		Kaplan–Meier at 3 years for propensity-matched cohort	
Mean follow-up, months	12	12	6	6	14	14	NA	NA	33.9	38.4
Death (%)	2.8	6.4	4	13	13.4	12.3	1.9	7.5	7.9	7.8
Myocardial infarction (%)	0.9	1.4	NA	NA	8.3	4.5	1.9	5.7	NA	NA
TVR (%)	19.6*	3.6	7	1	25.5*	2.6	28.8*	9.4	12.6	2.6
Cerebrovascular accident (%)	0.9	0.7	NA	NA	NA	NA	0	3.8	NA	NA
Any events (%)	NA	NA	11	17	NA	NA	NA	NA	NA	NA

BMS, bare metal stent; *DES*, drug-eluting stent; *NA*, not available; *MACE*, major adverse cardiac events including death, myocardial infarction, and TVR; *PCI*, percutaneous coronary intervention; *PES*, paclitaxel-eluting stent; *SES*, sirolimus-eluting stent; *TVR*, target vessel revascularization.

*$P < 0.05$ between percutaneous coronary intervention (PCI) versus coronary artery bypass grafting (CABG).

the long-term clinical effectiveness of PCI compared with CABG. Stronger evidence for the feasibility of PCI as an alternative to CABG comes from the recent, large MAIN-COMPARE study.[21] This registry analyzed data from 2240 patients with unprotected LMCA disease treated at 12 medical centers in Korea. Of these, 318 were treated with BMSs, 784 were treated with DESs, and 1138 underwent CABG. To avoid bias caused by the nonrandomized study design, a novel adjustment was performed by using propensity-score matching in the overall population and in separate periods. In the first and second waves, BMSs and DESs, respectively, were used exclusively. The outcomes of stenting in the overall study population and in each wave were compared with those of concurrent CABG, in which propensity-score matching was performed to reduce potential bias in nonrandomized study, as shown in Fig. 22-3. During 3 years of follow-up, patients treated with stenting were nearly four times as likely to need repeat revascularization compared with those who underwent CABG (HR 4.76; 95% CI 2.80–8.11). However, the rates of death (HR 1.18; 95% CI 0.77–1.80) and the combined rates of death, MI, and stroke (HR 1.10; 95% CI 0.75–1.62) were not significantly higher with the use of stenting compared with CABG. A similar pattern was also observed in patients treated with DESs or BMSs. Given the fact that the recommendation for CABG for unprotected LMCA disease has been based mostly on survival benefit compared with medical treatment, the lack of a statistically significant difference in mortality may support PCI as an alternative option to bypass surgery.[30] In addition, a current recommendation of routine angiographic surveillance at 6 to 9 months after PCI for unprotected LMCA stenosis might increase the unnecessary need of repeat revascularization because of the "oculo-stenotic" reflex. The ultimate proof of the relative values of PCI and CABG for unprotected LMCA stenosis clearly will come from the results of randomized clinical trials comparing the two treatment strategies. The trials will involve a number of technical considerations that could significantly alter the outcomes of angioplasty. The SYNTAX trial compared the outcomes of PCI with those of PESs and CABG for unprotected LMCA stenosis in a subgroup analysis from the randomized study cohort.[67] As shown in the subset of patients with LMCA disease, of which 348 patients received CABG and 357 received PCI, the PCI

group (15.8%) demonstrated equivalent 1-year clinical outcomes of major adverse cardiac and cerebrovascular events (MACCEs), including death, MI, stroke, and repeat revascularization compared with the CABG group (13.7%, P = 0.44). When the patients were stratified according to the vascular involvement, the event rate in the PCI group was numerically higher in patients with two-vessel disease (19.8% vs. 14.4%, P = 0.29) and those with three-vessel disease (19.3% vs. 15.4%, P = 0.42). However, the incidences were numerically lower in the PCI group in patients with isolated LMCA (7.1% vs. 8.5%, P = 1.0) or single-vessel disease (7.5% vs. 13.2%, P = 0.27). Interestingly, the higher rate of repeat revascularization with the use of PCI (11.8% vs. 6.5%, P = 0.02) was offset by a higher incidence of stroke with the use of CABG (2.7% vs. 0.3%, P = 0.01). When the follow-up was extended

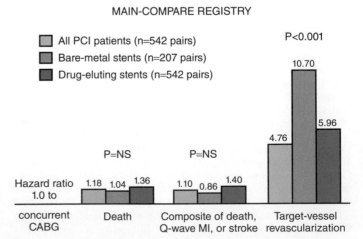

Figure 22-3 The hazard ratios for 3-year death, myocardial infarction (MI), stroke, or target vessel revascularization among patients treated with stenting, compared with those treated with coronary artery bypass grafting (CABG).

to 3 years, the incidence of death, MI, or stroke after PCI or CABG (13.0% vs. 14.3%, $P = 0.60$) did not differ; this result was presented in the Transcatheter Cardiovascular Therapeutics (TCT) 2010 in Washington, D.C., by Serruys. However, the incidence of repeat revascularization was higher in the PCI group than in the CABG group (11.7% vs. 20.0%, $P = 0.004$). When patients were stratified according to the SYNTAX score terciles, the incidence of MACCE did not differ between the PCI and CABG groups in patients with low (0–22) and intermediate (23–32) scores. In spite of the information from the SYNTAX trial, it should be noted that the analysis for LMCA disease was not the primary objective analysis but post hoc hypothesis-generating analysis. A more global randomized trial, the EXCEL (Evaluation of XIENCE PRIME versus Coronary Artery Bypass Surgery for Effectiveness of Left Main Revascularization), is also being performed to compare PCI and CABG in approximately 2500 patients with unprotected LMCA stenosis.

Conclusion

Current studies, although limited by a nonrandomized study design, small sample size, and short-term follow-up, have demonstrated the procedural and mid-term safety and effectiveness of DESs compared with BMSs or CABG. With these attempts, PCI with DES will be increasing and can be recommended as the reliable alternative to bypass surgery for patients with unprotected LMCA stenosis, especially as the first-line therapy for ostial or shaft stenosis. Although bifurcation stenosis remains challenging for the percutaneous approach, further research on the novel procedural technique, new dedicated stent platform, and optimal pharmacotherapies may improve outcomes. Furthermore, as more randomized clinical trials comparing PCI with CABG for unprotected LMCA stenosis are undertaken, confidence in the long-term safety, durability, and efficacy of PCI will grow in the near future.

REFERENCES

1. Takaro T, Hultgren HN, Lipton MJ, et al: The VA cooperative randomized study of surgery for coronary arterial occlusive disease II. Subgroup with significant left main lesions. *Circulation* 54:III107–III117, 1976.
2. Chaitman BR, Fisher LD, Bourassa MG, et al: Effect of coronary bypass surgery on survival patterns in subsets of patients with left main coronary artery disease. Report of the Collaborative Study in Coronary Artery Surgery (CASS). *Am J Cardiol* 48:765–777, 1981.
3. Park SJ, Mintz GS: *Left main stem disease*, Seoul, 2006, Informa Healthcare.
4. Chieffo A, Stankovic G, Bonizzoni E, et al: Early and mid term results of drug-eluting stent implantation in unprotected left main. *Circulation* 111:791–795, 2005.
5. Park SJ, Kim YH, Lee BK, et al: Sirolimus-eluting stent implantation for unprotected left main coronary artery stenosis: Comparison with bare metal stent implantation. *J Am Coll Cardiol* 45:351–356, 2005.
6. Valgimigli M, van Mieghem CA, Ong AT, et al: Short- and long-term clinical outcome after drug eluting stent implantation for the percutaneous treatment of left main coronary artery disease: Insights from the Rapamycin-Eluting and Taxus Stent Evaluated At Rotterdam Cardiology Hospital registries (RESEARCH and T-SEARCH). *Circulation* 111:1383–1389, 2005.
7. Chieffo A, Morici N, Maisano F, et al: Percutaneous treatment with drug eluting stent implantation versus bypass surgery for unprotected left main stenosis: A single-center experience. *Circulation* 113:2542–2547, 2006.
8. Kim YH, Park SW, Hong MK, et al: Comparison of simple and complex stenting techniques in the treatment of unprotected left main coronary artery bifurcation stenosis. *Am J Cardiol* 97:1597–1601, 2006.
9. Lee MS, Kapoor N, Jamal F, et al: Comparison of coronary artery bypass surgery with percutaneous coronary intervention with drug-eluting stents for unprotected left main coronary artery disease. *J Am Coll Cardiol* 47:864–870, 2006.
10. Palmerini T, Marzocchi A, Marrozzini C, et al: Comparison between coronary angioplasty and coronary artery bypass surgery for the treatment of unprotected left main coronary artery stenosis (the Bologna Registry). *Am J Cardiol* 98:54–59, 2006.
11. Price MJ, Cristea E, Sawhney N, et al: Serial angiographic follow-up of sirolimus-eluting stents for unprotected left main coronary artery revascularization. *J Am Coll Cardiol* 47:871–877, 2006.
12. Valgimigli M, Malagutti P, Aoki J, et al: Sirolimus-eluting versus paclitaxel-eluting stent implantation for the percutaneous treatment of left main coronary artery disease: A combined RESEARCH and T-SEARCH long-term analysis. *J Am Coll Cardiol* 47:507–514, 2006.
13. Valgimigli M, Malagutti P, Rodriguez-Granillo GA, et al: Distal left main coronary disease is a major predictor of outcome in patients undergoing percutaneous intervention in the drug-eluting stent era: An integrated clinical and angiographic analysis based on the rapamycin-eluting stent evaluated at Rotterdam Cardiology Hospital (RESEARCH) and TAXUS-Stent Evaluated At Rotterdam Cardiology Hospital (T-SEARCH) registries. *J Am Coll Cardiol* 47:1530–1537, 2006.
14. Chieffo A, Park SJ, Valgimigli M, et al: Favorable long-term outcome after drug-eluting stent implantation in nonbifurcation lesions that involve unprotected left main coronary artery. A multicenter registry. *Circulation* 116:158–162, 2007.
15. Palmerini T, Barlocco F, Santarelli A, et al: A comparison between coronary artery bypass grafting surgery and drug eluting stent for the treatment of unprotected left main coronary artery disease in elderly patients (aged ≥75 years). *Eur Heart J* 28:2714–2719, 2007.
16. Sheiban I, Meliga E, Moretti C, et al: Long-term clinical and angiographic outcomes of treatment of unprotected left main coronary artery stenosis with sirolimus-eluting stents. *Am J Cardiol* 100:431–435, 2007.
17. Buszman PE, Kiesz SR, Bochenek A, et al: Acute and late outcomes of unprotected left main stenting in comparison with surgical revascularization. *J Am Coll Cardiol* 51:538–545, 2008.
18. Biondi-Zoccai GGL, Lotrionte M, Moretti C, et al: A collaborative systematic review and meta-analysis on 1278 patients undergoing percutaneous drug eluting stenting for unprotected left main coronary artery disease. *Am Heart J* 155:274–283, 2008.
19. Chieffo A, Park S-J, Meliga E, et al: Late and very late stent thrombosis following drug-eluting stent implantation in unprotected left main coronary artery: A multicentre registry. *Eur Heart J* 29:2108–2115, 2008.
20. Kim YH, Dangas GD, Solinas E, et al: Effectiveness of drug-eluting stent implantation for patients with unprotected left main coronary artery stenosis. *Am J Cardiol* 101:801–806, 2008.
21. Seung KB, Park DW, Kim YH, et al: Stents versus coronary-artery bypass grafting for left main coronary artery disease. *N Engl J Med* 358:1781–1792, 2008.
22. Tamburino C, Di Salvo ME, Capodanno D, et al: Are drug-eluting stents superior to bare-metal stents in patients with unprotected non bifurcational left main disease? Insights from a multicentre registry. *Eur Heart J* 30(10):1171–1179, 2009.
23. Park SJ, Kim YH, Park DW, et al: Impact of intravascular ultrasound guidance on long-term mortality in stenting for unprotected left main coronary artery stenosis. *Circ Cardiovasc Interv* 2:167–177, 2009.
24. Palmerini T, Sangiorgi D, Marzocchi A, et al: Ostial and midshaft lesions vs. bifurcation lesions in 1111 patients with unprotected left main coronary artery stenosis treated with drug eluting stents: Results of the survey from the Italian Society of Invasive Cardiology. *Eur Heart J* 30:2087–2094, 2009.
25. Tamburino C, Di Salvo ME, Capodanno D, et al: Comparison of drug-eluting stents and bare-metal stents for the treatment of unprotected left main coronary artery disease in acute coronary syndromes. *Am J Cardiol* 103:187–193, 2009.
26. Palmerini T, Marzocchi A, Tamburino C, et al: Two-year clinical outcome with drug-eluting stents versus bare-metal stents in a real-world registry of unprotected left main coronary artery stenosis from the Italian Society of Invasive Cardiology. *Am J Cardiol* 102:1463–1468, 2008.
27. Kim YH, Park DW, Lee SW, et al: Long-term safety and effectiveness of unprotected left main coronary stenting with drug-eluting stent compared with bare-metal stent. *Circulation* 120:4007, 2009.
28. de Lezo JS, Medina A, Pan M, et al: Rapamycin-eluting stents for the treatment of unprotected left main coronary disease. *Am Heart J* 148:481–485, 2004.
29. Meliga E, Garcia-Garcia HM, Valgimigli M, et al: Longest available clinical outcomes after drug-eluting stent implantation for unprotected left main coronary artery disease: The DELFT (Drug Eluting stent for LeFT main) registry. *J Am Coll Cardiol* 51:2212–2219, 2008.
30. Kushner FG, Hand M, Smith SC, et al: 2009 focused updates: ACC/AHA guidelines for the management of patients with ST-elevation myocardial infarction (updating the 2004 guideline and 2007 focused update) and ACC/AHA/SCAI guidelines on percutaneous coronary intervention (updating the 2005 guideline and 2007 focused update) a report of the American College of Cardiology Foundation/American Heart Association Task Force on Practice Guidelines. *J Am Coll Cardiol* 54:2205–2241, 2009.
31. Arnett EN, Isner JM, Redwood DR, et al: Coronary artery narrowing in coronary heart disease: comparison of cineangiographic and necropsy findings. *Ann Intern Med* 91:350–356, 1979.
32. Fisher LD, Judkins MP, Lesperance J, et al: Reproducibility of coronary arteriographic reading in the coronary artery surgery study (CASS). *Cathet Cardiovasc Diagn* 8:565–575, 1982.
33. Isner JM, Kishel J, Kent KM, et al: Accuracy of angiographic determination of left main coronary arterial narrowing. Angiographic–histologic correlative analysis in 28 patients. *Circulation* 63:1056–1064, 1981.
34. Gerber TC, Erbel R, Gorge G, et al: Extent of atherosclerosis and remodeling of the left main coronary artery determined by intravascular ultrasound. *Am J Cardiol* 73:666–671, 1994.
35. Abizaid AS, Mintz GS, Abizaid A, et al: One-year follow-up after intravascular ultrasound assessment of moderate left main coronary artery disease in patients with ambiguous angiograms. *J Am Coll Cardiol* 34:707–715, 1999.
36. Fassa AA, Wagatsuma K, Higano ST, et al: Intravascular ultrasound-guided treatment for angiographically indeterminate left main coronary artery disease. A long term follow-up study. *J Am Coll Cardiol* 45:204–211, 2005.
37. Oviedo C, Maehara A, Mintz GS, et al: Is accurate intravascular ultrasound evaluation of the left circumflex ostium from a left anterior descending to left main pullback possible? *Am J Cardiol* 105(7):948–954, 2010.
38. Oviedo C, Maehara A, Mintz GS, et al: Intravascular ultrasound classification of plaque distribution in left main coronary artery bifurcations: Where is the plaque really located? *Circ Cardiovasc Interv* 3(2):105–112, 2010.
39. Tonino PAL, De Bruyne B, Pijls NHJ, et al: Fractional flow reserve versus angiography for guiding percutaneous coronary intervention. *N Engl J Med* 360:213–224, 2009.
40. Jasti V, Ivan E, Yalamanchili V, et al: Correlations between fractional flow reserve and intravascular ultrasound in patients with an ambiguous left main coronary artery stenosis. *Circulation* 110:2831–2836, 2004.
41. Takagi T, Stankovic G, Finci L, et al: Results and long-term predictors of adverse clinical events after elective percutaneous interventions on unprotected left main coronary artery. *Circulation* 106:698–702, 2002.
42. Mehilli J, Kastrati A, Byrne RA, et al: Paclitaxel- versus sirolimus-eluting stents for unprotected left main coronary artery disease. *J Am Coll Cardiol* 53:1760–1768, 2009.
43. Marroquin OC, Selzer F, Mulukutla SR, et al: A comparison of bare-metal and drug-eluting stents for off-label indications. *N Engl J Med* 358:342–352, 2008.
44. Tu JV, Bowen J, Chiu M, et al: Effectiveness and safety of drug-eluting stents in Ontario. *N Engl J Med* 357:1393–1402, 2007.
45. Tan WA, Tamai H, Park SJ, et al: Long-term clinical outcomes after unprotected left main trunk percutaneous revascularization in 279 patients. *Circulation* 104:1609–1614, 2001.
46. Kim YH, Ahn JM, Park DW, et al: EuroSCORE as a predictor of death and myocardial infarction after unprotected left main coronary stenting. *Am J Cardiol* 98:1567–1570, 2006.
47. Serruys PW, Morice M-C, Kappetein AP, et al: Percutaneous coronary intervention versus coronary-artery bypass grafting for severe coronary artery disease. *N Engl J Med* 360:961–972, 2009.
48. Valgimigli M, Malagutti P, Rodriguez Granillo GA, et al: Single-vessel versus bifurcation stenting for the treatment of distal left main coronary artery disease in the drug-eluting stenting era.

Clinical and angiographic insights into the Rapamycin-Eluting Stent Evaluated at Rotterdam Cardiology Hospital (RESEARCH) and Taxus-Stent Evaluated at Rotterdam Cardiology Hospital (T-SEARCH) registries. *Am Heart J* 152:896–902, 2006.

49. Lee J-Y, Park D-W, Yun S-C, et al: Long-term clinical outcomes of sirolimus- versus paclitaxel-eluting stents for patients with unprotected left main coronary artery disease: Analysis of the MAIN-COMPARE (Revascularization for Unprotected Left Main Coronary Artery Stenosis: Comparison of Percutaneous Coronary Angioplasty Versus Surgical Revascularization) registry. *J Am Coll Cardiol* 54:853–859, 2009.

50. Colombo A, Moses JW, Morice MC, et al: Randomized study to evaluate sirolimus-eluting stents implanted at coronary bifurcation lesions. *Circulation* 109:1244–1249, 2004.

51. Steigen TK, Maeng M, Wiseth R, et al: Randomized study on simple versus complex stenting of coronary artery bifurcation lesions: The Nordic bifurcation study. *Circulation* 114:1955–1961, 2006.

52. Mintz GS, Nissen SE, Anderson WD, et al: American College of Cardiology Clinical Expert Consensus document on standards for acquisition, measurement and reporting of intravascular ultrasound studies (IVUS). A report of the American College of Cardiology Task Force on Clinical Expert Consensus Documents. *J Am Coll Cardiol* 37:1478–1492, 2001.

53. Agostoni P, Valgimigli M, Van Mieghem CAG, et al: Comparison of early outcome of percutaneous coronary intervention for unprotected left main coronary artery disease in the drug-eluting stent era with versus without intravascular ultrasonic guidance. *Am J Cardiol* 95:644–647, 2005.

54. Sonoda S, Morino Y, Ako J, et al: Impact of final stent dimensions on long-term results following sirolimus-eluting stent implantation: Serial intravascular ultrasound analysis from the SIRIUS trial. *J Am Coll Cardiol* 43:1959–1963, 2004.

55. Costa MA, Gigliotti OS, Zenni MM, et al: Synergistic use of sirolimus-eluting stents and intravascular ultrasound for the treatment of unprotected left main and vein graft disease. *Cathet Cardiovasc Interv* 61:368–375, 2004.

56. Fujii K, Carlier SG, Mintz GS, et al: Stent underexpansion and residual reference segment stenosis are related to stent thrombosis after sirolimus-eluting stent implantation: An intravascular ultrasound study. *J Am Coll Cardiol* 45:995–998, 2005.

57. Cook S, Wenaweser P, Togni M, et al: Incomplete stent apposition and very late stent thrombosis after drug-eluting stent implantation. *Circulation* 115:2426–2434, 2007.

58. Okabe T, Mintz GS, Buch AN, et al: Intravascular ultrasound parameters associated with stent thrombosis after drug-eluting stent deployment. *Am J Cardiol* 100:615–620, 2007.

59. Tsuchikane E, Aizawa T, Tamai H, et al: Pre-drug-eluting stent debulking of bifurcated coronary lesions. *J Am Coll Cardiol* 50:1941–1945, 2007.

60. Briguori C, Airoldi F, Chieffo A, et al: Elective versus provisional intraaortic balloon pumping in unprotected left main stenting. *Am Heart J* 152:565–572, 2006.

61. Chieffo A, Park S-J, Meliga E, et al: Late and very late stent thrombosis following drug-eluting stent implantation in unprotected left main coronary artery: A multicentre registry. *Eur Heart J* 29:2108–2115, 2008.

62. Iakovou I, Schmidt T, Bonizzoni E, et al: Incidence, predictors, and outcome of thrombosis after successful implantation of drug-eluting stents. *JAMA* 293:2126–2130, 2005.

63. Park DW, Park SW, Park KH, et al: Frequency of and risk factors for stent thrombosis after drug-eluting stent implantation during long-term follow-up. *Am J Cardiol* 98:352–356, 2006.

64. Park S-J, Park D-W, Kim Y-H, et al: Duration of dual antiplatelet therapy after implantation of drug-eluting stents. *N Engl J Med* 362(15):1374–1382, 2010.

65. Cura FA, Bhatt DL, Lincoff AM, et al: Pronounced benefit of coronary stenting and adjunctive platelet glycoprotein IIb/IIIa inhibition in complex atherosclerotic lesions. *Circulation* 102:28–34, 2000.

66. Tina L, Pinto Slottow RW: Overview of the 2006 Food and Drug Administration Circulatory System Devices Panel meeting on drug-eluting stent thrombosis. *Cathet Cardiovasc Interv* 69:1064–1074, 2007.

67. Morice MC, Serruys PW, Kappetein AP, et al: Outcomes in patients with de novo left main disease treated with either percutaneous coronary intervention using paclitaxel-eluting stents or coronary artery bypass graft treatment in the Synergy Between Percutaneous Coronary Intervention with TAXUS and Cardiac Surgery (SYNTAX) trial. *Circulation* 121:2645–2653, 2010.

23

Complex and Multi-vessel Percutaneous Coronary Intervention

ARASHK MOTIEI | DAVID R. HOLMES, JR.

KEY POINTS

- In patients with less complex angiographic, multi-vessel disease, percutaneous coronary intervention (PCI) is associated with the same frequency of death and myocardial infarction (MI) as coronary artery bypass grafting (CABG).

- Stents significantly reduce the risk of early CABG in patients undergoing multi-vessel PCI.

- The frequency of repeat procedures is reduced with bare metal stents (BMSs) by more than 50% compared with balloon angioplasty.

- There are concerns about late outcomes with drug-eluting stents (DESs) in patients with complex lesions and multi-vessel disease.

Patients with multi-vessel coronary disease represent an important group of patients with coronary artery disease (CAD). Although various definitions of multi-vessel disease have been used in different studies, in clinical terms, this generally refers to the presence of two-vessel or three-vessel disease as delineated by coronary angiography. Patients with three-vessel coronary disease or two-vessel disease with proximal left anterior descending (LAD) artery involvement represent a subgroup of patients with CAD, in whom survival benefit with bypass surgery has been clearly established.[1] Over the years, considerable advances have been made in revascularization techniques by means of CABG and with PCI. With the constant evolution of techniques, there has been a tremendous interest in comparing the outcomes of these modalities with a view to determining appropriate clinical practice. In broad terms, the clinical studies that have compared CABG with PCI can be viewed in terms of three major groups when evaluated from the standpoint of important developments in the history of PCI. With the advent of percutaneous coronary balloon angioplasty (PTCA), multiple studies were conducted to compare PTCA with CABG. These represent the first group of studies comparing PCI with CABG. The development of coronary stents leads to a second series of comparisons of PCI with stenting to CABG. Important lessons have been learned from both these groups of studies, and the findings of the important literature from this period will be presented below. With the arrival of the DES, more recent studies have continued to focus on comparisons of PCI with the DES to CABG. This last group of studies is the most relevant to contemporary clinical practice and will be discussed in detail.

◼ Percutaneous Coronary Balloon Angioplasty Versus Coronary Artery Bypass Grafting

Multiple trials have compared the outcomes of patients with multi-vessel disease revascularized by balloon angioplasty or CABG. Important landmark studies on this subject are summarized below.

BARI

In the BARI (Bypass Angioplasty Revascularization Investigation) trial, symptomatic patients with multi-vessel CAD ($n = 1829$) were randomly assigned to initial treatment with PTCA or CABG. The 10-year survival was 71% for PTCA and 73.5% for CABG ($P = 0.18$). At 10 years, the PTCA group had substantially higher subsequent revascularization rates compared with the CABG group (76.8% vs. 20.3%, $P < 0.001$), but the angina rates for the two groups were similar. In the subgroup of patients who had not been treated for diabetes, survival rates were nearly identical by randomization (PTCA 77% vs. CABG 77.3%, $P = 0.59$). In the subgroup who had been treated for diabetes, the CABG group had higher survival compared with the PTCA group (PTCA 45.5% vs. CABG 57.8%, $P = 0.025$) (Figs. 23-1, 23-2 and 23-3).[2]

RITA

In the RITA (Randomised Intervention Treatment of Angina) trial, 1011 patients with coronary heart disease (45% single-vessel, 55% multi-vessel) were randomly assigned to initial treatment with PTCA or CABG. The median follow-up was 6.5 years. The primary endpoint of death or nonfatal MI occurred in 17% of the PTCA group and 16% of the CABG group ($P = 0.64$). Subsequent nonrandomized CABG was undertaken in 134 (26%) of the PTCA group, and a second CABG was undertaken in 14 (3%) of the CABG group. In the PTCA group, 138 (27%) patients required an additional nonrandomized PTCA at some point; 45 of these also required a nonrandomized CABG. In the CABG group, 47 (9%) required nonrandomized PTCA subsequently; 7 of these also required a second CABG. The prevalence of angina was consistently higher in the PTCA group, with an absolute average 10% increase compared with the CABG group ($P < 0.001$).[3]

GABI

The GABI (German Angioplasty versus Bypass surgery Investigation) trial compared the outcomes in patients 1 year after complete revascularization with CABG or PTCA. A total of 8981 patients with multi-vessel CAD were randomly assigned to undergo CABG (177 patients) or PTCA (182 patients). During the first year of follow-up, further interventions were necessary in 44% of the patients in the PTCA group (repeated PTCA in 23%, CABG in 18%, and both in 3%) but in only 6% of the patients in the CABG group (repeated CABG in 1% and PTCA in 5%, $P < 0.001$). Seventy-four percent of the patients in the CABG group and 71% of those in the PTCA group were free of angina 1 year after treatment.[4]

EAST

The Emory Angioplasty versus Surgery Trial (EAST) was a single-center, randomized comparison of a strategy of initial coronary angioplasty ($n = 198$) or CABG ($n = 194$) for patients with multi-vessel CAD. The primary endpoint (death, MI, or a large ischemic defect at 3 years) was not different, and repeat revascularization was significantly greater in the angioplasty group. Survival at 8 years was 79.3% in the angioplasty group and 82.7% in the surgical group ($P = 0.40$). Patients with proximal LAD artery stenosis and those with diabetes tended to have better rates of late survival with surgical intervention, although not reaching statistical significance. After the first 3 years, repeat interventions remained relatively equal for both treatment groups.[5]

CABRI

The Coronary Angioplasty versus Bypass Revascularization Investigation (CABRI) was a multi-national, multi-centre, randomized trial comparing the strategies of revascularization with CABG and PTCA in patients with symptomatic multi-vessel CAD. Of the 1054 patients recruited, 513 were randomized to CABG and 541 to PTCA. After 1 year of follow-up, 2.7% of those randomized to CABG and 3.9% of those randomized to PTCA had died; this difference was not significant. However, patients randomized to PTCA required significantly more re-interventions; at 1 year, only 66.4% required a single-vessel revascularization procedure compared with 93.5% of patients randomized to CABG (relative risk [RR] = 5.23; 95% confidence interval [CI] 3.90–7.03, $P < 0.001$). The patients in the PTCA group took significantly more medication at 1 year (RR = 1.30; CI 1.18–1.43, $P < 0.001$). They were also more likely to have clinically significant angina (RR = 1.54; CI 1.09–2.16, $P = 0.012$); this association was present in both genders but was significant only in females.[6]

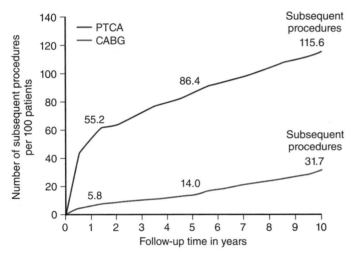

Figure 23-1   Revascularization in BARI. *Blue solid line*, coronary artery bypass grafting (CABG); *Red dashed line*, percutaneous transluminal coronary angiography (PTCA). (*Modified with permission from BARI investigators: The final 10-year follow-up results from the BARI randomized trial*, J Am Coll Cardiol *49(15):1600–1606, 2007.*)

ERACI

In ERACI (Argentine Randomized trial of Percutaneous Transluminal Coronary Angioplasty vs. coronary artery bypass surgery), 127 patients who had multi-vessel CAD and clinical indication of myocardial revascularization were randomized to undergo coronary angioplasty ($n = 63$) or bypass surgery ($n = 64$). At 3 years, freedom from combined cardiac events (death, Q wave MI, angina, and repeat revascularization procedures) was significantly greater for the bypass surgery group compared with the coronary angioplasty group (77% vs. 47%, $P < 0.001$). There were no differences in overall (4.7% vs. 9.5%, $P = 0.5$) and cardiac mortality (4.7% vs. 4.7%) or in the frequency of MI (7.8% vs. 7.8%, $P = 0.8$) between the two groups. However, patients who had bypass surgery were more frequently free of angina (79% vs. 57%, $P < 0.001$) and required fewer additional re-interventions (6.3% vs. 37%, $P < 0.001$) compared with patients who had coronary angioplasty.[7] These early trials, although perhaps no longer directly relevant to current clinical practice, yielded a series of important findings. Firstly, survival in patients with multi-vessel disease was found to be similar for PTCA and CABG except in patients with diabetes, for whom CABG was advantageous. The key difference between the procedures was found to lie in the substantially greater need for revascularization procedures in patients treated with PTCA. With the development of coronary stents, it was clearly established that coronary stenting was associated with a lower risk of repeat revascularization procedures compared with balloon angioplasty alone. This led to a second series of comparisons of CABG with PCI, this time with the use of coronary artery stents. These trials are summarized below.

Percutaneous Coronary Intervention with Bare Metal Stenting Versus Coronary Artery Bypass Grafting

ARTS

In the ARTS (Arterial Revascularization Therapies Study) trial, a total of 1205 patients were randomly assigned to CABG ($n = 605$) or stent implantation ($n = 600$). At 5 years, there was no significant difference in survival between the stent and CABG groups (8% for stents vs. 7.6% for CABG, $P = 0.83$). In a subgroup of 208 patients with diabetes, mortality trended higher in the stent group (13.4%) compared with 8.3% in the CABG group ($P = 0.27$). The overall freedom from death, stroke, or MI was not significantly different between the groups (18.2%

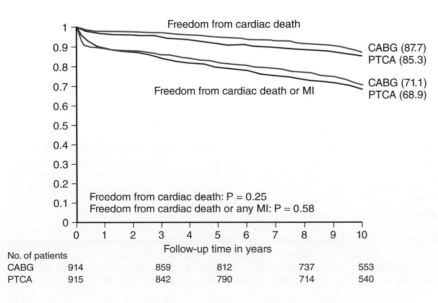

Figure 23-2   Cardiac death; Cardiac death or myocardial infarction (MI) in BARI. *Bold solid line*, coronary artery bypass grafting (CABG), *Red dashed line*, percutaneous transluminal coronary angiography (PTCA). (*Modified with permission from BARI investigators: The final 10-year follow-up results from the BARI randomized trial*, J Am Coll Cardiol *49(15):1600–1606, 2007.*)

No. of patients					
CABG	914	859	812	737	553
PTCA	915	842	790	714	540

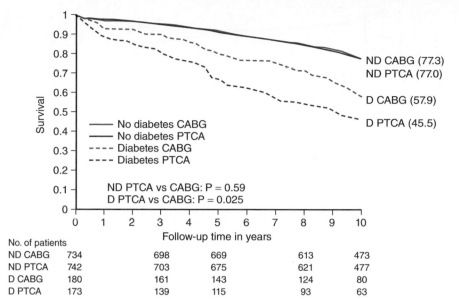

Figure 23-3 Overall survival by diabetes status in BARI. *(Modified with permission from BARI investigators: The final 10-year follow-up results from the BARI randomized trial, J Am Coll Cardiol 49(15):1600–1606, 2007.)*

No. of patients					
ND CABG	734	698	669	613	473
ND PTCA	742	703	675	621	477
D CABG	180	161	143	124	80
D PTCA	173	139	115	93	63

in the stent group vs. 14.9% in the surgical group, $P = 0.14$). However, the incidence of repeat revascularization was significantly higher in the stent group (30.3%) than in the CABG group (8.8%, $P < 0.001$). The composite event-free survival rate was 58.3% in the stent group and 78.2% in the CABG group ($P < 0.0001$). This difference was largely driven by the differences in revascularization rates.[8]

AWESOME

In the AWESOME (Angina With Extremely Serious Operative Mortality Evaluation) study, patients from 16 Veterans Affairs Medical Centers were screened to identify those with myocardial ischemia refractory to medical management and the presence of one or more risk factors for adverse outcome with CABG. A total of 232 patients were randomized to CABG and 222 to PCI. The 30-day survivals for CABG and PCI were 95% and 97%, respectively. At 36 months, there was no significant difference in survival—79% and 80% for CABG and PCI, respectively. However, there was a difference in survival free of revascularization: 66% and 44% for CABG and PCI, respectively ($P = 0.001$).[9]

MASS-II

MASS-II (Medicine, Angioplasty, or Surgery Study II) included 611 patients, who were randomly assigned to undergo CABG ($n = 203$), PCI ($n = 205$), or medical therapy ($n = 203$). The inclusion of the medical therapy arm made this trial different from many of the other studies. The rates of event-free survival, namely, the combined incidence of overall mortality, MI, or refractory angina that required revascularization, were significantly different among patients in the 3 therapeutic groups at 5-year ($P = 0.0026$) and 10-year ($P < 0.0001$) follow-up. Pairwise treatment comparisons of the primary end points at 5-year follow-up demonstrated no significant difference between PCI and medical therapy (hazard ratio [HR] 0.93, 95% CI 0.67 to 1.30). At 10-year follow-up, this comparison continued to demonstrate a nonsignificant difference between the PCI and medical therapy groups (HR 0.79, 95% CI 0.62 to 1.01). After multivariate Cox analysis at 10-year follow-up, a protective effect of CABG compared with medical therapy (HR 0.43, 95% CI 0.32 to 0.58, $P < 0.001$) and PCI (HR 0.53, 95% CI 0.39 to 0.72, $P < 0.001$) was observed.[10,10a]

The cumulative survival rates at 10 years for patients assigned to each group were 74.9% for PCI, 75.1% for CABG, and 69.0% for medical therapy ($p = 0.089$). In terms of non fatal MI, CABG was significantly superior to PCI and medical therapy at 10-year ($P = 0.016$) but not 5-year ($P = 0.785$) follow-up the incidence of uncomplicated MI was 8.3% and 10.3% at 5- and 10-year follow-up, respectively, in the CABG group. In the PCI arm, 11.2% and 13.2% had an uncomplicated MI at 5 and 10 years, respectively. In the medical therapy group 15.3% and 20.7% had an uncomplicated or nonfatal MI during the 5- and 10-year follow-up, respectively.

At 5-year follow-up, 3.4% in the CABG group required PCI compared with 24.1% required for patients in the medical therapy group and 32.2% in the PCI group respectively ($P = 0.021$). At 10-year follow-up, additional interventions were needed in 7.4% in the CABG group compared with 41.5% required for patients in the PCI group and 39.4% in the medical therapy group due to uncontrolled angina ($P < 0.001$). Patients treated with surgery were most likely to be free of angina symptoms after 10 years of follow-up. In the medical therapy group 43% were free of angina symptoms after the 10-year follow-up compared with 64% in the CABG group and 59% in the PCI group.

In terms of cardiac death, 20.7%, 10.8% and 14.1% had died of MI in the medical therapy, CABG, and PCI groups by 10-year follow-up, respectively ($P = 0.019$). The incidence of stroke was similar at 6.9% in the medical therapy arm, 8.4% in the CABG, and 5.4% in the PCI group ($P = 0.550$) at ten years.

SOS

The aim of the Stent or Surgery (SoS) trial was to assess the effect of stent-assisted PCI versus CABG in the management of patients with multi-vessel disease. In 53 centers in Europe and Canada, symptomatic patients with multi-vessel CAD were randomized to CABG ($n = 500$) or stent-assisted PCI ($n = 488$) and then followed up for a median of 2 years. Twenty-one percent ($n = 101$) of patients in the PCI group required additional revascularization procedures compared with 6% ($n = 30$) in the CABG group ($P < 0.001$). At a median follow-up of 6 years, 53 patients (10.9%) died in the PCI group compared with 34 (6.8%) in the CABG group (HR 1.66; CI 1.08–2.55, $P = 0.022$). The incidence of death or Q wave MI was similar in both groups (PCI 9%; [$n = 46$], CABG 10% [$n = 49$], $P = 0.80$). There were fewer deaths in the CABG group than in the PCI group (PCI 5% [$n = 22$], CABG 2% [$n = 8$], $P = 0.01$). This seemed to result, at least in part, from a higher proportion of noncardiovascular deaths in the PCI arm (from cancer) compared with the CABG arm. Additionally, the mortality rate in the CABG group was lower than the rates that had been reported in previous studies. Subsequently, it was seen that at a median follow-up of 6 years, 53 patients (10.9%) had died in the PCI group compared with 34 (6.8%) in the CABG group (HR 1.66; CI 1.08–2.55, $P = 0.022$).[11]

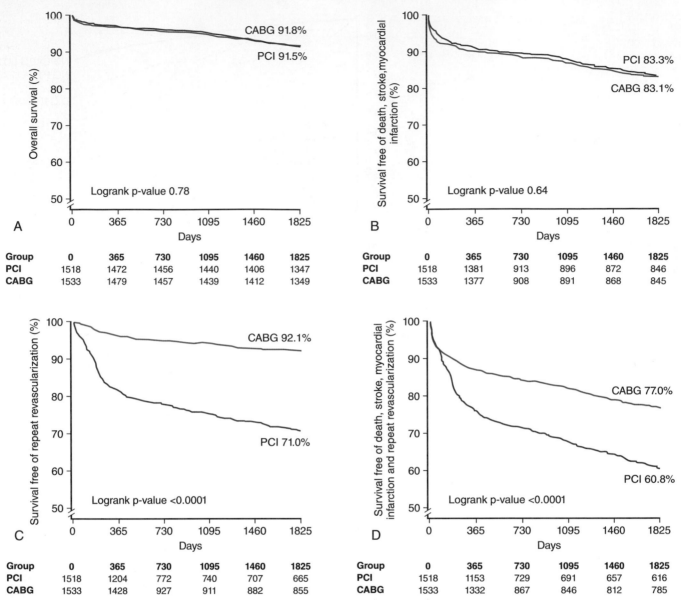

Figure 23-4 Outcomes of percutaneous coronary intervention (PCI) with bare metal stenting versus coronary artery bypass grafting (CABG) in a meta-analysis of four trials. *(Modified with permission from Daemen J, Boersma E, Flather M, et al: Long-term safety and efficacy of percutaneous coronary intervention with stenting and coronary artery bypass surgery for multivessel coronary artery disease: A meta-analysis with 5-year patient-level data from the ARTS, ERACI-II, MASS-II, and SoS trials, Circulation 118(11):1146–1154, 2008.)*

ERACI II

The ERACI II trial randomized a total of 450 patients with multi-vessel disease to undergo either PCI ($n = 225$) or CABG ($n = 225$). At the 5-year follow-up, patients initially treated with PCI had similar survival and freedom from nonfatal acute MI than those initially treated with CABG (92.8% vs. 88.4% and 97.3% vs. 94%, respectively, $P = 0.16$). Freedom from repeat revascularization procedures (PCI or CABG) was significantly lower with PCI compared with CABG (71.5% vs. 92.4%, $P = 0.0002$). Accordingly, driven by a greater need for revascularization, freedom from major adverse cardiac events (MACEs) was also significantly lower with PCI compared with CABG (65.3% vs. 76.4%, $P = 0.013$). However, at 5 years, similar numbers of patients randomized to each revascularization procedure were asymptomatic or with class I angina.[12]

A pooled analysis of the four randomized trials described above (ARTS, ERACI II, SoS and MASS II), with a total of 3051 patients from

all four trials, evaluated the relative safety and efficacy of PCI with stenting and CABG for the treatment of multi-vessel CAD (Fig. 23-4). At 5 years, the cumulative incidence of death, MI, and stroke was similar in the PCI with stenting group and the CABG group (16.7% vs. 16.9%, respectively; HR 1.04; CI 0.86–1.27, $P = 0.69$). Repeat revascularization, however, occurred significantly more often after PCI compared with CABG (29.0% vs. 7.9%, respectively; HR 0.23; CI 0.18–0.29, $P < 0.001$). Major adverse cardiac and cerebrovascular events (MACCEs) were significantly higher in the PCI group than in the CABG group (39.2% vs. 23.0%, respectively; HR 0.53; CI 0.45–0.61, $P < 0.001$).[13] Two additional meta-analyses showed similar findings. Hlatky et al used pooled individual patient data from 10 randomized trials to compare the effectiveness of CABG with that of PCI according to patients' baseline clinical characteristics. Data were available on 7812 patients. PCI was performed with balloon angioplasty in six trials and with BMSs in four trials. Over a median follow-up of 5.9 years, 15% of patients assigned to CABG died compared with 16% of patients assigned to PCI (HR 0.91; CI 0.82–1.02, $P = 0.12$). In patients with diabetes, mortality was substantially lower in the CABG group than in the PCI group (HR 0.70; CI 0.56–0.87); however, mortality was similar between the groups in patients without diabetes (HR 0.98; CI 0.86–1.12, $P = 0.014$ for interaction). In another study, the authors identified 23 randomized controlled trials, in which 5019 patients were randomly assigned to PCI and 4944 to CABG. Again, this study included data from patients treated with PTCA alone and PTCA with stenting. The difference in survival after PCI or CABG was less than 1% at the 10-year follow-up. Survival did not differ between PCI and CABG for patients with diabetes in the six trials that reported on this subgroup. Procedure-related strokes were more common after CABG than after PCI (1.2% vs. 0.6%; risk difference 0.6%, $P = 0.002$). Angina relief was greater after CABG than after PCI, with risk differences ranging from 5% to 8% at 1 to 5 years ($P < 0.001$). The absolute rates of angina relief at 5 years were 79% after PCI and 84% after CABG. Repeated revascularization was more common after PCI than after CABG (risk difference, 24% at 1 year and 33% at 5 years, $P < 0.001$); the absolute rates at 5 years were 46.1% after balloon angioplasty, 40.1% after PCI with stents, and 9.8% after CABG. In comparisons based on observational studies, the CABG–PCI hazard ratio for death favored PCI among patients with the least severe disease and CABG among those with the most severe disease.[14] Overall, in a manner similar to what was observed with the trials of PTCA versus CABG, the use of stenting continued to be associated with a higher frequency of the need for revascularization procedures. However, there was no significant difference in mortality.

The development of DESs represented an important milestone in the history of interventional cardiology. With the reduced risk of re-stenosis associated with the use of these stents, there is ongoing interest in comparisons of PCI using DES with CABG. Some of the important studies that have looked at this are reviewed below.

Percutaneous Coronary Intervention with Drug-Eluting Stents Versus Coronary Artery Bypass Grafting

SYNTAX

In the SYNTAX (SYNergy between percutaneous coronary intervention with TAXus and cardiac surgery) trial, a total of 1800 patients were randomized to undergo CABG or PCI using paclitaxel-eluting stents (PESs).[15,15a] Patients for whom only one of the two treatment options was beneficial because of anatomic features or clinical conditions were entered into a parallel, nested CABG or PCI registry. A noninferiority comparison of the two groups was performed for the primary endpoint—MACCE (i.e., death from any cause, stroke, MI, or repeat revascularization) in the 12-month period after randomization. The 12-month rates of MACCEs were also analyzed on the basis of the SYNTAX score. (The SYNTAX score reflects a comprehensive anatomic assessment, with higher scores indicating more complex CAD; a low score was defined as 22 or less, an intermediate score as 23 to 32, and a high score as 33 or greater). A higher proportion of patients had complete revascularization after CABG than after PCI (63.2% vs. 56.7%, $P = 0.005$). Overall, the rate of complete revascularization was lower in both treatment groups in this study compared with previous studies. This was likely to have resulted from a different definition of completeness of revascularization used in the earlier trials and the more complex anatomic characteristics of the patients in this trial. In the CABG group, off-pump surgery was performed in 15% of patients, one or more arterial grafts were used in 97.3% of patients, and an average of 2.8 conduits and 3.2 distal anastomoses per patient were performed. In the PCI group, 14.1% of patients underwent staged procedures, 63.1% had at least one bifurcation or trifurcation treated, more than four stents on average were implanted per patient, and a third of patients had placement of stents with a total length of more than 100 mm. These characteristics reflect a population of patients with fairly complex anatomy. At 12 months, the incidence of MACCEs

was lower in the CABG group (12.4%) than in the PCI group (17.8%, $P = 0.002$) (Fig. 23-5). This was largely driven by the rate of repeat revascularization at 12 months, which was significantly higher among patients in the PCI group than among those in the CABG group (13.5% vs. 5.9%, $P < 0.001$). Death occurred in 4.4% of the PCI group compared with 3.5% of the CABG group ($P = 0.37$). The rate of death from cardiac causes was greater with PCI than with CABG (3.7% vs. 2.1%, $P = 0.05$); the rate of death from noncardiac causes, although not significant, was higher with CABG (1.4% vs. 0.7%, $P = 0.13$). MI occurred in 3.3% of the CABG group versus 4.8% of the PCI group ($P = 0.11$). Stroke was significantly more likely to occur with CABG (2.2%, vs. 0.6% with PCI, $P = 0.003$). The 12-month rates of symptomatic graft occlusion (in the CABG group) and stent thrombosis (in the PCI group) were similar ($P = 0.89$). In the CABG group, the binary 12-month rates of MACCEs were similar among patients with low SYNTAX scores (0–22; 14.7%), those with intermediate scores (23–32; 12%), and those with high scores ($\geq$33; 10.9%). However, in the PCI group, the rate of MACCEs had increased significantly among patients with high SYNTAX scores (23.4%) compared with those with low scores (13.6%) or intermediate scores (16.7%) ($P = 0.002$ for high vs. low scores; $P = 0.04$ for high vs. intermediate scores) (Fig. 23-6). There was a significant interaction between the SYNTAX score and the treatment group ($P = 0.01$); patients with low or intermediate scores in the CABG group and in the PCI group had similar rates of MACCEs, whereas among patients with high scores, the event rate had increased significantly in the PCI group. The three year results of this trial have recently been published. Total MACCE through 3 years was significantly higher in the PCI arm compared with the CABG arm (CABG 20.2% vs. PCI 28.0%; $P < 0.001$; (Fig. 23-5). This was driven in part by increased repeat revascularization in the PCI arm (CABG 10.7% vs. PCI 19.7%; $P < 0.001$. The composite safety endpoint of death/stroke/MI was not significantly different between treatment groups 3-year post-randomization (CABG 12.0% vs. PCI 14.1%; $P = 0.21$). Death from all causes was not different between the treatment groups at 3 years (CABG 6.7% vs. PCI 8.6%; $P = 0.13$). The cumulative rate of cardiac death was significantly higher in the PCI arm (CABG 3.6% vs. PCI 6.0%; $P = 0.02$). The incidence of stroke was not significantly different between CABG- (3.4%) and PCI-treated patients (2.0%, $P = 0.07$). The MI rate was 3.6% in the CABG and 7.1% in the PCI arm ($P = 0.002$). There were no significant interactions between left main (LM) or three vessel disease (3VD) status and treatment group for 3-year MACCE or any of the components. The treatment effect of PCI compared with CABG was not significantly different between patients in either of these groups.

The rates of MACCE and the individual MACCE components were not significantly different in patients with low SYNTAX scores ($\leq$22) treated with either PCI or CABG (Fig. 23-6). In patients with intermediate SYNTAX scores (23-32), repeat revascularization rates were significantly higher in PCI-treated patients (CABG 10.1% vs. PCI 17.4%, $P = 0.01$), as were MI and MACCE rates (MI: CABG 3.2% vs. PCI 7.6%, $P = 0.02$; MACCE: 18.9 vs. 27.4%, $P = 0.02$). In patients with the most complex anatomical disease (those with SYNTAX scores $\geq$33), MACCE and its components, apart from stroke, were significantly higher in patients treated with PCI (MACCE: CABG 19.5% vs. PCI 34.1%, $P < 0.001$).

Patients with 3VD with SYNTAX scores in the lowest tercile had similar MACCE rates between treatment arms (CABG 22.2% vs. PCI 25.8%, $P = 0.45$). In those 3VD patients with intermediate or high SYNTAX scores, the rate of MACCE was significantly increased in favor of CABG (23-32: CABG 16.8% vs. PCI 29.4%, $P = 0.003$; $\geq$33: CABG 17.9% vs. PCI 31.4%, $P = 0.004$). Myocardial infarction was significantly higher in the PCI arm of the 3VD intermediate SYNTAX score tercile (3.1 vs. 8.9%, $P = 0.01$). In 3VD patients with SYNTAX score $\geq$33, mortality (CABG 4.5% vs. PCI 11.1%, $P = 0.03$) and MI (1.9 vs. 7.2%, $P = 0.02$) were significantly higher in the PCI arm.

Major adverse cardiac and cerebrovascular event rates were not significantly different in patients with LM disease who had low or intermediate SYNTAX scores (0-22: CABG 23.0% vs. PCI 18.0%, $P = 0.33$;

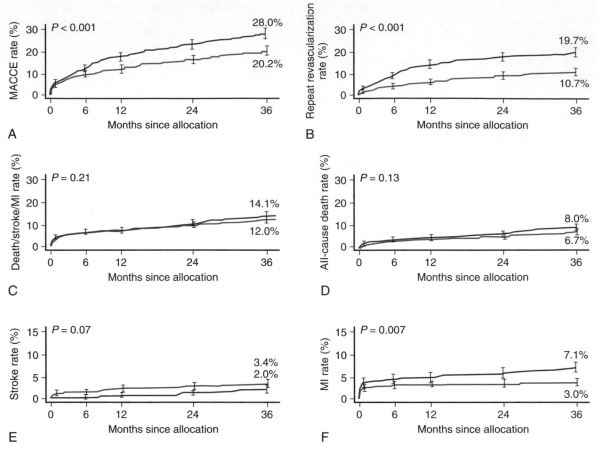

Figure 23-5 Outcomes in the SYNTAX trial. *(Modified with permission from Serruys PW, Morice MC, Kappetein AP, et al: Percutaneous coronary intervention versus coronary-artery bypass grafting for severe coronary artery disease, N Eng J Med 360(10):961–972, 2009.)*

23-32: CABG 23.4% vs. PCI 23.4%, $P = 0.90$). In LM patients with the most complex anatomy (SYNTAX score ≥ 33), MACCE was significantly increased in PCI-treated patients (CABG 21.2% vs. PCI 37.3%, $P = 0.003$) as was repeat revascularization (9.2 vs. 27.7%, $P < 0.001$).

Compared with the first year results some interesting observations can be made about the three year results of this trial. Overall, the trends in MACCE, death/stroke/MI, all-cause death, and repeat revascularization rates seen in the first year of follow-up were sustained through the second and third year. Compared with outcomes after 1 year of follow-up, at three years, cardiac death was found to be significantly increased in the overall PCI-treated patient population, largely in those patients with higher SYNTAX scores. Although stroke was significantly increased at 1 year of follow-up for CABG, no difference in stroke was seen during the interval of 1- and 3-year follow-up. A difference in the MI rate between the two treatment groups was also noted after the first year of follow-up. Two-thirds and one-half of all MIs were periprocedural (occurring within 7 days of the index procedure) in the surgical and PCI cohorts, respectively. The likely cause of the increased MIs in the PCI arm was felt to be due to restenosis and additional revascularization in these patients with advanced diffuse disease or stent thrombosis. When compared with CABG patients, MI rates were higher in the 3VD PCI group and not significantly different in the LM PCI cohort.

Based on these observations, the authors felt that CABG remains the standard for more complex anatomy. Percutaneous intervention in this trial demonstrated similar outcomes to CABG in patients with less complex disease, measured by lower SYNTAX score for 3 vessel disease

and lower and intermediate scores for LM disease. This highlights the emerging importance of the SYNTAX score as an effective risk assessment tool for making decisions about revascularization options.[15a]

ARTS II

As mentioned previously, ARTS I was a randomized trial that included 1205 patients with multi-vessel disease to compare CABG and BMSs. ARTS II was a multi-center, nonrandomized, open-label trial designed to compare the safety and efficacy of sirolimus-eluting stents (SESs) in patients with de novo multi-vessel CAD, compared with the surgical and BMS groups of ARTS I acting as historical controls. The ARTS II trial enrolled 607 patients, with an attempt to enroll at least one third of patients with three-vessel disease. At 5 years, the death–stroke–myocardial infarction event-free survival rate was 87.1% in the ARTS II cohort treated with SESs versus 86% ($P = 0.1$) and 81.9% ($P = 0.007$) in the ARTS I cohorts treated with CABG and BMSs, respectively. The 5-year MACCE rate in ARTS II (27.5%) was significantly higher than in the CABG group in ARTS I (21.1%, $P = 0.02$), and lower than in the BMS group in ARTS I (41.5%, $P < 0.001$). This was largely driven by differences in revascularization rates. During the follow-up period, freedom from revascularization was observed in 91% of the ARTS I–CABG group, 79.2% of ARTS II–SES group, and 69.1% of ARTS I–BMS group ($P < 0.001$ for comparisons of DES vs. CABG and DES vs. BMS). Similar to what was observed in the SYNTAX trial, a significant difference in MACCE-free survival was observed when patients were stratified according to SYNTAX score tertiles. When compared with the lowest SYNTAX score (SYNTAX score <16; 5-year MACE-free

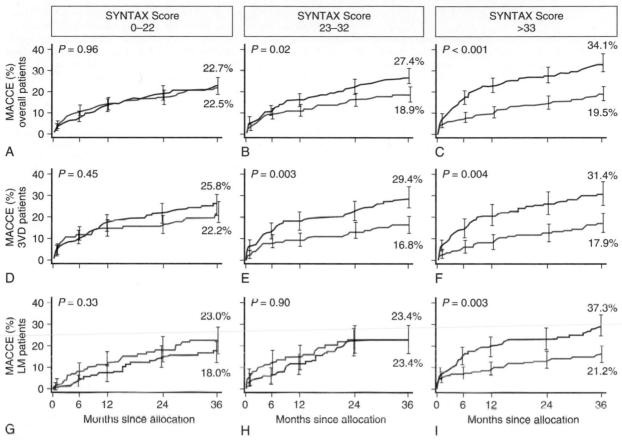

Figure 23-6 Outcomes in SYNTAX according to the SYNTAX score. *(Modified with permission from Serruys PW, Morice MC, Kappetein AP, et al: Percutaneous coronary intervention versus coronary-artery bypass grafting for severe coronary artery disease, N Eng J Med 360(10):961–972, 2009.)*

rate 80.1%), both the intermediate (SYNTAX score 16–24) and high (SYNTAX score >24) syntax score groups demonstrated a lower MACE-free survival rate (intermediate 70.1%, log-rank P = 0.02; high 67.1%, P = 0.001).[16]

ERACI III

In the ERACI III trial, 225 patients with multi-vessel disease who received DESs met clinical and angiographic inclusion criteria for the ERACI II trial and were compared with both ERACI II treatment arms (ERACII–PCI and ERACI II–CABG). At 1 year, freedom from MACCEs was significantly greater in the ERACI III–DES cohort (88%) than in the ERACI II–CABG cohort (80.5%, P = 0.038) and in the ERACI II–PCI cohort (78%, P = 0.006). The ERACI III–DES cohort had freedom from death and acute MI similar to the ERACI II–PCI arm but greater than the ERACI II–CABG arm. Freedom from repeat revascularization was similar between the ERACI III–DES and the ERACI II–CABG (95.1%, P = not significant [NS]) groups, but both were significantly better than those in the ERACI II–PCI arm (91.2% and 83%, P = 0.002 and 0.02, respectively). It was concluded that patients with multi-vessel disease treated with DESs in ERACI III had better 1-year outcomes than those treated with PCI or CABG in ERACI II.[17] The 3-year MACCE rate was lower in ERACI III–DES (22.7%) than in ERACI II–BMS (29.8%, P = 0.015), mainly reflecting less target vessel revascularization (14.2 vs. 24.4%, P = 0.009). MACCE rates at 3 years were similar in DES-treated and CABG-treated patients (22.7%, P = 1.0), in contrast to results at 1 year (12 vs. 19.6%, P = 0.038). MACCE rates in ERACI III–DES were higher in patients with diabetes (RR 0.81; CI 0.66–0.99, P = 0.018). Death or nonfatal MI at 3 years trended

higher in the DES cohort (10.2%) than in the BMS cohort (6.2%, P = 0.08) and lower than in the CABG cohort (15.1%, P = 0.07) Subacute or late-stent thrombosis (>30 days) occurred in nine of the DES group and in none of the BMS group (P = 0.008). It therefore appeared that the initial advantage for PCI with DES over CABG observed at 1 year was not apparent by 3 years. Furthermore, despite the continued lower incidence of MACCEs, the initial advantage over BMS appeared to decrease with time.[18]

CARDIA

The purpose of the CARDia (Coronary Artery Revascularization in Diabetes) study was to compare the safety and efficacy of PCI with stenting against CABG in patients with diabetes and symptomatic multi-vessel CAD. The primary outcome was a composite of all-cause mortality, MI, and stroke, and the main secondary outcome included the addition of repeat revascularization to the primary outcome events. A total of 510 patients with diabetes and multi-vessel or complex single-vessel coronary disease from 24 centers were randomized to PCI plus stenting or to CABG. BMSs were used initially, but a switch to SES (Cypher) was instituted later in the trial. After 12 months of follow-up, the composite rate of death, MI, and stroke was 10.5% in the CABG group and 13% in the PCI group (HR 1.25; CI 0.75–2.09, P = 0.39), all-cause mortality rates were 3.2% and 3.2%, and the rates of death, MI, stroke, or repeat revascularization were 11.3% and 19.3% (HR 1.77; CI 1.11–2.82, P = 0.02), respectively. When the patients who underwent CABG were compared with the subset of patients who received DESs (69%), the primary outcome rates were 12.4% and 11.6% (HR 0.93; CI 0.51–1.71, P = 0.82), respectively.[19]

FREEDOM

The FREEDOM (Future REvascularization Evaluation in patients with Diabetes mellitus: Optimal management of Multivessel disease) trial was a multi-center, open-label, prospective randomized superiority trial of PCI versus CABG in at least 2000 patients with diabetes in whom revascularization was indicated. Consenting patients with multi-vessel disease were randomized on a 1:1 basis to either CABG or multi-vessel stenting using DESs and observed at 30 days, 1 year, and annually for up to 5 years. At the discretion of primary physicians or interventionalists, patients randomized to the PCI–DES arm received any approved DESs. The primary outcome measure was the composite of all-cause mortality, nonfatal MI, or stroke. Patients were observed for a mean of 4 years.[20]

Meta-Analysis

A recent meta-analysis based on ARTS II, CARDIa, ERACI III, and SYNTAX looked at a total of 3895 patients: 1914 in the DES arm and 1981 in the CABG arm. Pooled analysis of data from these four studies showed that in patients treated with DESs, compared with those treated with CABG, there was a similar risk of the combined endpoints of death, MI, and stroke (10.2% vs. 10.8%, respectively; RR 0.94; CI 0.77–1.116, $P = 0.56$), but a significantly higher risk of target vessel revascularization (TVR) (14.6% vs. 6.8%, respectively; RR 2.09; CI 1.72–2.55, $P < 0.001$) and, therefore, a significantly higher risk of MACCEs (21.2% vs. 16.3%, respectively; RR 1.27; CI 1.09–1.48, $P = 0.002$). Interestingly, when MACCE rates at 1 year are used, the risk is equivalent between DES and CABG (14.4% vs. 12.5%, respectively; RR 1.05; CI 0.70–1.57, $P = 0.83$).[21]

Registry Studies

The New York registry study compared 9963 patients receiving DESs and 7437 patients undergoing CABG in terms of death in the hospital; death within 30 days after treatment; and death, MI, and revascularization up to 18 months after treatment.[22] There were no significant differences between the two groups in the risk-adjusted rates of in-hospital or 30-day mortality (adjusted odds ratio [OR] 1.29; CI 0.92–1.81, $P = 0.15$). Of patients who received DESs, 28.4% underwent repeat PCI and 2.2% underwent CABG within 18 months. The respective rates for patients undergoing CABG were 5.1% and 0.1%; both differences were statistically significant ($P < 0.001$). Of patients who received DESs, 12.5% underwent repeat PCI within 30 days and 18.3% underwent repeat PCI within 60 days. The rate of repeat PCI in this registry may be inflated because many patients underwent planned PCI associated with incomplete revascularization during the index admission. Of the 28.4% of patients who underwent repeat PCI during the study period, only a little more than one quarter (7%) underwent TVR. After adjustment for baseline differences the survival in patients with three-vessel disease was 94% in the CABG group and 92.7% in the PCI group ($P = 0.03$). In patients with two-vessel disease, overall survival was 96% in the CABG group compared with 94.6% in the PCI group ($P = 0.003$). There was also a significant difference in freedom from MI—92.1% in the CABG group compared with 89.7% in the PCI group ($P = 0.001$). Among patients with two-vessel disease, 94.5% in the CABG group were free of MI compared with 92.5% in the PCI group ($P = 0.001$). This study has two key limitations. First, it is subject to the selection bias that is inherent to the design of registry studies. Second, patients were studied at a time that predated the recognition of the importance and implementation of prolonged dual anti-platelet therapy. This may account, in part, for the relatively higher frequency of MI and death in the DES group. Furthermore, the limited follow-up is unlikely to capture events related to graft failure in the CABG group.

In another registry, 3720 consecutive patients with multi-vessel disease who underwent isolated CABG surgery or received DESs were identified and comparisons were made in terms of safety (total mortality, MI, and stroke) and efficacy (target-vessel revascularization) during a 3-year follow-up. Patients receiving DESs had considerably higher 3-year rates of TVR. DESs were also associated with higher rates of death (adjusted HR 1.62; CI 1.07–2.47) and MI (adjusted HR 1.65; CI 1.15–2.44). The risk adjusted rate of stroke was similar in the two groups (HR 0.92; CI 0.69–1.51).[23] In a study by Javaid et al, 1080 patients were treated for two-vessel disease (196 with CABG and 884 with PCI) and 600 for three-vessel disease (505 with CABG and 95 with PCI). One-year mortality, cerebrovascular events, Q wave MI, target vessel failure, and composite MACCEs were compared between the CABG and PCI cohorts. Adjusted outcomes showed increased MACCEs with PCI in patients with two-vessel disease (HR 2.29; CI 1.39–3.76, $P = 0.01$) and three-vessel disease (HR 2.90; CI 1.76–4.78, $P < 0.001$). Adjusted outcomes for the subpopulation without diabetes demonstrated equivalent MACCE rates with PCI for two-vessel (HR 1.77; CI 0.96–3.25, $P = 0.07$) and three-vessel disease (HR 1.70; CI 0.77–3.61, P 0.19).[24] Park et al studied 3042 patients with multi-vessel disease who underwent coronary implantation of DES ($n = 1547$) or CABG ($n = 1495$). The primary endpoint was all-cause mortality. After adjustment for baseline differences, the overall risks of death were similar among all patients (HR 0.85; CI 0.56–1.30, $P = 0.45$), patients with diabetes (HR 1.76; CI 0.82–3.78, $P = 0.15$), and patients with compromised ventricular function (HR 1.39; CI 0.41–4.65, $P = 0.60$). In the anatomic subgroups, mortality benefit with DES implantation was noted in patients with two-vessel disease with involvement of the nonproximal LAD artery (HR 0.23; CI 0.01–0.78, $P = 0.016$). The rate of revascularization was significantly higher in the DES group than in the CABG group (HR 2.81; CI, 2.11–3.75, $P < 0.001$).[25] Overall, these registry studies continue to demonstrate a revascularization advantage to CABG. In some studies, there seems to be a higher incidence of death and MI in the PCI arms, and it is not clear if these differences resulted from issues related to stent thrombosis in the setting of abbreviated anti-platelet therapy. In a recent publication, a total of nine observational nonrandomized studies were identified and analyzed, including a total of 24,268 patients with multi-vessel coronary disease who underwent DES–PCI ($n = 13,540$) and CABG ($n = 10,728$). Mean follow-up time was 20 months. Pooled analysis showed that DES–PCI and CABG were comparable in terms of composite occurrence of death, acute MI, and cerebrovascular accidents (HR 0.94; CI 0.72–1.22, $P = 0.66$). However, there was a significantly higher risk of repeat revascularization in the DES–PCI group (HR 4.06; CI 2.64–6.24, $P < 0.001$). The overall MACCE rate in DES–PCI was higher compared with the CABG group (HR 1.86; CI 1.36–2.54, $P < 0.001$).[26]

Recommendations for Clinical Practice

Once multi-vessel disease is diagnosed with coronary angiography, the clinical data should be reviewed in detail with an interventional cardiologist and the referring cardiologist.

- If the coronary anatomy is clearly of the type that would be best treated with bypass surgery, this approach should be adopted.
- If there are patient factors such as advanced comorbidities that would make CABG high risk, PCI should be considered.
- For patients with multi-vessel disease but with very discrete lesions that would require short segments of stenting, PCI should be preferred, since in this situation, the likelihood of requiring a repeat revascularization procedure is lower than with more complex anatomy requiring larger numbers of stents and longer stents.
- The choice of PCI with DES versus CABG in patients with diabetes is being studied, and presently enough data are not available to make a clear recommendation. However, on the basis of the experience of previous trials before the availability of DES, CABG is believed to be the favored revascularization option for these patients.
- If there are clinical circumstances in which the patient cannot take dual anti-platelet therapy for at least 1 year (typically because of a

foreseeable need or an established plan for elective noncardiac surgery or a known history of poor medical compliance), the option of CABG should be encouraged. However, it is important to note that for many of these patients, PCI with a BMS is a good option, and, where appropriate, this needs to be presented to the patient along with the option of CABG.

- Another factor to consider is the age of the patient. When evaluating revascularization strategies for young patients, when CABG and PCI are both technically feasible options, PCI rather than CABG should be preferred. Given that the vast majority of vein grafts are expected to occlude over time, clinical problems resulting from vein graft disease are very likely to be encountered over a young patient's lifetime. With the use of PCI as the first approach in most cases, the CABG option remains reserved for future use, if necessary; the problems with vein graft disease can be avoided or delayed.
- In the subset of patients in which the coronary anatomy and other patient factors allow a consideration of both revascularization

options, a detailed discussion needs to be held with the patient. This discussion should include consultation with an interventional cardiologist and a cardiac surgeon. Every effort should be made to ensure that the patient understands the pros and cons of both revascularization approaches. Patient preference is the cornerstone of determining the appropriate management strategy, particularly since the outcomes of both modalities are similar in terms of the "hard" endpoints of death and MI. Many patients prefer to undergo PCI in view of the lower short-term morbidity while being aware of the higher risk of the need for a repeat procedure. Such patients are willing to undergo more than one PCI, should the need arise, rather than undergo CABG with its substantial short-term morbidity. However, there are many patients who prefer to undergo CABG with a view to having a more "durable" outcome, at least in terms of avoiding repeat procedures. Thorough patient education and counseling are instrumental in helping patients and their health care providers in selecting a treatment strategy.

REFERENCES

1. Yusuf S, Zucker D, Peduzzi P, et al: Effect of coronary artery bypass graft surgery on survival: Overview of 10-year results from randomised trials by the Coronary Artery Bypass Graft Surgery Trialists Collaboration. *Lancet* 344(8922):563–570, 1994.
2. The final 10-year follow-up results from the BARI randomized trial. *J Am Coll Cardiol* 49(15):1600–1606, 2007.
3. Henderson RA, Pocock SJ, Clayton TC, et al: Seven year outcome in the RITA-2 trial: Coronary angioplasty versus medical therapy. *J Am Coll Cardiol* 42(7):1161–1170, 2003.
4. Hamm CW, Reimers J, Ischinger T, et al: A randomized study of coronary angioplasty compared with bypass surgery in patients with symptomatic multivessel coronary disease. German Angioplasty Bypass Surgery Investigation (GABI). *N Eng J Med* 331(16):1037–1043, 1994.
5. King SB, 3rd, Kosinski AS, Guyton RA, et al: Eight-year mortality in the Emory Angioplasty versus Surgery Trial (EAST). *J Am Coll Cardiol* 35(5):1116–1121, 2000.
6. First-year results of CABRI (Coronary Angioplasty versus Bypass Revascularisation Investigation). CABRI Trial Participants. *Lancet* 346(8984):1179–1184, 1995.
7. Rodriguez A, Mele E, Peyregne E, et al: Three-year follow-up of the Argentine Randomized Trial of Percutaneous Transluminal Coronary Angioplasty Versus Coronary Artery Bypass Surgery in Multivessel Disease (ERACI). *J Am Coll Cardiol* 27(5):1178–1184, 1996.
8. Serruys PW, Ong AT, van Herwerden LA, et al: Five-year outcomes after coronary stenting versus bypass surgery for the treatment of multivessel disease: The final analysis of the Arterial Revascularization Therapies Study (ARTS) randomized trial. *J Am Coll Cardiol* 46(4):575–581, 2005.
9. Morrison DA, Sethi G, Sacks J, et al: Percutaneous coronary intervention versus coronary artery bypass graft surgery for patients with medically refractory myocardial ischemia and risk factors for adverse outcomes with bypass: A multicenter, randomized trial. Investigators of the Department of Veterans Affairs Cooperative Study #385, the Angina With Extremely Serious Operative Mortality Evaluation (AWESOME). *J Am Coll Cardiol* 38(1):143–149, 2001.
10. Hueb W, Lopes NH, Gersh BJ, et al: Five-year follow-up of the Medicine, Angioplasty, or Surgery Study (MASS II): A randomized controlled clinical trial of 3 therapeutic strategies for multi-

vessel coronary artery disease. *Circulation* 115(9):1082–1089, 2007.
10a. Hueb W, Lopes N, Gersh BJ, et al: Ten year follow-up survival of the medicine, angioplasty, or surgery study (MASS II): a randomized controlled clinical trial of 3 therapeutic strategies for multivessel coronary artery disease. *JA Circulation* 122(10):949–957, 2010.
11. Booth J, Clayton T, Pepper J, et al: Randomized, controlled trial of coronary artery bypass surgery versus percutaneous coronary intervention in patients with multivessel coronary artery disease: Six-year follow-up from the Stent or Surgery Trial (SoS). *Circulation* 118(4):381–388, 2008.
12. Rodriguez AE, Baldi J, Fernandez Pereira C, et al: Five-year follow-up of the Argentine randomized trial of coronary angioplasty with stenting versus coronary bypass surgery in patients with multiple vessel disease (ERACI II). *J Am Coll Cardiol* 46(4):582–588, 2005.
13. Daemen J, Boersma E, Flather M, et al: Long-term safety and efficacy of percutaneous coronary intervention with stenting and coronary artery bypass surgery for multivessel coronary artery disease: A meta-analysis with 5 year patient-level data from the ARTS, ERACI-II, MASS-II, and SoS trials. *Circulation* 118(11):1146–1154, 2008.
14. Bravata DM, Gienger AL, McDonald KM, et al: Systematic review: The comparative effectiveness of percutaneous coronary interventions and coronary artery bypass graft surgery. *Ann Int Med* 147(10):703–716, 2007.
15. Serruys PW, Morice MC, Kappetein AP, et al: Percutaneous coronary intervention versus coronary-artery bypass grafting for severe coronary artery disease. *N Eng J Med* 360(10):961–972, 2009.
15a. Kappetein AP, Feldman TE, Mack MJ, et al: Comparison of coronary bypass surgery with drug-eluting stenting for the treatment of left main and/or three-vessel disease: 2-year follow up of the SYNTAX trial. *A Eur Heart J* 2011.
16. Serruys PW, Onuma Y, Garg S, et al: 5-year clinical outcomes of the ARTS II (Arterial Revascularization Therapies Study II) of the sirolimus-eluting stent in the treatment of patients with multivessel de novo coronary artery lesions. *J Am Coll Cardiol* 55(11):1093–1101, 2010.
17. Rodriguez AE, Grinfeld L, Fernandez-Pereira C, et al: Revascularization strategies of coronary multiple vessel disease in the drug

eluting stent era: One year follow-up results of the ERACI III Trial. *EuroIntervention* 2(1):53–60, 2006.
18. Rodriguez AE, Maree AO, Mieres J, et al: Late loss of early benefit from drug-eluting stents when compared with bare-metal stents and coronary artery bypass surgery: 3 years follow-up of the ERACI III registry. *Eur Heart J* 28(17):2118–2125, 2007.
19. Kapur A, Hall RJ, Malik IS, et al: Randomized comparison of percutaneous coronary intervention with coronary artery bypass grafting in diabetic patients. 1-year results of the CARDia (Coronary Artery Revascularization in Diabetes) trial. *J Am Coll Cardiol* 55(5):432–440, 2010.
20. Farkouh ME, Dangas G, Leon MB, et al: Design of the Future REvascularization Evaluation in patients with Diabetes mellitus: Optimal management of Multivessel disease (FREEDOM) Trial. *Am Heart J* 155(2):215–223, 2008.
21. From AM, Al Badarin FJ, Cha SS, et al: Percutaneous coronary intervention with drug-eluting stents versus coronary artery bypass surgery for multivessel coronary artery disease: A meta-analysis of data from the ARTS II, CARDia, ERACI III, and SYNTAX studies and systematic review of observational data. *EuroIntervention* 6(2):269–276, 2010.
22. Hannan EL, Wu C, Walford G, et al: Drug-eluting stents vs. coronary-artery bypass grafting in multivessel coronary disease. *N Eng J Med* 358(4):331–341, 2008.
23. Li Y, Zheng Z, Xu B, et al: Comparison of drug-eluting stents and coronary artery bypass surgery for the treatment of multivessel coronary disease: Three-year follow-up results from a single institution. *Circulation* 119(15):2040–2050, 2009.
24. Javaid A, Steinberg DH, Buch AN, et al: Outcomes of coronary artery bypass grafting versus percutaneous intervention with drug-eluting stents for patients with multivessel coronary artery disease. *Circulation* 116(11 Suppl):I200–I206, 2007.
25. Park DW, Yun SC, Lee SW, et al: Long-term mortality after percutaneous coronary intervention with drug-eluting stent implantation versus coronary artery bypass surgery for the treatment of multivessel coronary artery disease. *Circulation* 117(16):2079–2086, 2008.
26. Benedetto U, Melina G, Angeloni E, et al: Coronary artery bypass grafting versus drug-eluting stents in multivessel coronary disease. A meta-analysis on 24,268 patients. *Eur J Cardiothorac Surg* 36(4):611–615, 2009.

24

Chronic Total Occlusion

AHMED A. KHATTAB | BERNHARD MEIER

KEY POINTS

- Chronic total coronary occlusion is a common feature in patients with coronary artery disease and is the most common reason for discarding percutaneous coronary intervention (PCI).

- Clinically, a chronic total coronary occlusion imitates a 90% stenosis without its risk of causing infarction.

- The success rate of percutaneous recanalization is heavily dependent on the patient's age as well as the length and anatomical variables of the occlusion; it also depends on the operator's experience and perseverance.

- Complications are comparable with those of PCI in the case of a nontotal lesion but they are usually not related to the occlusion itself.

- Stiff, polymer-coated coronary guidewires have the highest chance of crossing a chronic total occlusion successfully.

- The technical success rate after successful wire passage is over 90%.

- The standard approach to chronic total occlusions once the wire has passed is balloon predilation and complete coverage with a drug-eluting stent.

- Sophisticated gadgets and techniques may enhance the success rate in selected cases. However, they are not free of complications and should be reserved for use by superspecialists.

- The effect of additional diagnostic tools (intracoronary ultrasound, computed tomography) on the success rate has not been accurately determined but is probably small.

The Role of Percutaneous Coronary Intervention in Chronic Total Occlusions

The initial "chronic" total occlusions tackled by Andreas Grüntzig, the pioneer of percutaneous coronary intervention (PCI), were those that had silently progressed from stenoses while the respective patients had been on the rather long waiting list for PCI typical for the late 1970s. The primary success rate was 62%.[1] A "true" chronic total occlusion is usually defined as a 100% luminal diameter obstruction without flow in that segment of 3 months or more duration. In contrast to interventional cardiologists, cardiac surgeons may even prefer chronic occlusions to stenoses. Both require the same surgical technique, but the occluded coronary artery provides no competitive flow for the graft that might enhance its propensity for attrition. Moreover, an occluded native artery will usually not cause a major clinical problem should the graft occlude. The aspect of reduced risk in dealing with chronic occlusions pertains also to PCI. However, the heightened intricacy of recanalizing a chronic occlusion rather than dilating a stenosis impacts indications for PCI. Hence chronically occluded lesions account for 20% to 40% of patients with angiographically documented coronary artery disease, but they represent only 10% of targets for PCI. Chronic occlusions remain the single most important reason not to attempt PCI, thus favoring, instead, bypass surgery or medical treatment. It appears that the better the surgical program is developed, the less time is invested in recanalization attempts of chronic occlusions by PCI.

Histology and Pathophysiology of Chronic Total Occlusion

HISTOLOGY

A chronic total coronary occlusion has several anatomical components.[2,3] An atherosclerotic plaque is invariably present as a major or a minor part of the luminal obstruction. Thrombus is the complementary element. There may be a single clot of uniform structure and age or layers of clots of disparate structures and ages associated with fibrointimal proliferation. The latter situation signifies the occurrence of prior thrombi secondary to previous plaque fissures that may or may not have been totally occlusive. In cases in which they had been totally occlusive, these fissures were partially recanalized before subsequently reoccluding (Fig. 24-1). The most recent thrombus is assumed to obstruct the last lumen that had been patent up to the final complete occlusion of the particular coronary segment. The recanalization equipment should be passed through this thrombus. The texture of the thrombus is crucial for success or failure of PCI. The older and the more fibrosed and/or calcified a clot, the smaller the chance of crossing it safely. The point of entry to a total occlusion often comprises a thick, hard layer, called the proximal fibrous cap, making guidewire penetration potentially difficult. Similar but usually thinner is the distal fibrous cap, which can make the guidewire exit challenging after having progressed through the entire length of the occlusion. Spontaneous recanalization of a totally occluded segment may occur by lysis of a clot, development of several new channels through the thrombus (intraluminal microchannels), dilation of the adventitial vasa vasorum (bridging collaterals), or a combination of these mechanisms. Microchannels holding a mean diameter of only 0.007 inch are invisible on angiography. Angiographically, such a recanalization (functional occlusion) can be readily distinguished from a true total occlusion by the presence of antegrade flow, which may coexist with retrograde filling of the distal part of the vessel, as is easily demonstrable by angiography in case of ipsilateral collaterals. However, it is not possible to discern which of the aforementioned mechanisms is active for antegrade flow, and functional occlusion is difficult to differentiate from a subtotal stenosis. Tackling a subtotal stenosis that had never been completely occluded before and that shows no collateralization creates the risk of an acute infarction resulting from abrupt vessel closure; tackling a recanalized segment does not. Conversely, it is generally easy to pass a subtotal stenosis with a coronary guidewire, but it may be tedious or impossible, even with sophisticated equipment, to pass a recanalized segment, because the recanalization may consist of several tortuous microchannels in densely fibrosed tissue or be simulated by copious vasa vasorum.

PATHOPHYSIOLOGY

Collaterals and Preservation of Myocardial Function

Well-developed collaterals at the time of an acute occlusion of a coronary artery avoid cell death of the subtended myocardium. Poor collaterals may still limit necrosis to the least perfused layers, usually the subendocardium. The performance of collaterals correlates well with the significance and age of a lesion. In other words, collaterals are quite common in patients with long-standing coronary disease and subtotal stenoses of the vessel in question, but are rare in young patients with mild coronary artery disease suffering an acute thrombotic coronary

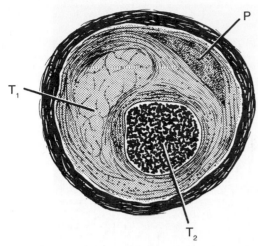

Figure 24-1 Schematic diagram of a cross section of a totally occluded coronary artery segment. There are thrombotic foci (T_1 and T_2) of different ages, indicating a first plaque (P) fissure with an organized and heavily fibrosed thrombus (T_1) and a more recent one causing complete occlusion (I_2). The extent of fibrosis of the most recent thrombus is the decisive factor in determining the chance of successful recanalization.

occlusion from a ruptured insignificant plaque. On the other hand, there is a greater propensity for spontaneous recanalization in the young patient with an occlusion based on an insignificant stenosis. These lesions often present with a recanalized vessel but complete loss of function. The typical chronic occlusion to be tackled is therefore one most often in an elderly patient with established coronary artery disease, a complex anatomy in and around the occlusion, and a fairly well preserved distal myocardium.

COLLATERALS AND ISCHEMIC SYMPTOMS

A total occlusion that is well collateralized is functionally equivalent to a 90% stenosis.[4] It sustains myocardial viability but produces clinically apparent ischemia during periods of increased oxygen demand. Hence the patient with a chronic total coronary occlusion that was collateralized well enough at the time of the acute event to preserve part or all of the dependent myocardium is liable to have exertional angina. Such a patient may also have chest pain at rest because of increased oxygen demand secondary to spells of hypertension or tachycardia but will not face the major risk of unstable angina—i.e., acute occlusion with ensuing myocardial infarction.

Percutaneous Coronary Intervention for Chronic Total Occlusion

Improvement of clinical symptoms and normalization of a positive exercise test or restoration of vitality in the territory of the occluded vessel—together with a reasonable chance of technical success—provide the rationale and ethical basis for PCI in chronic total occlusion.[5,6] Reduced left ventricular remodeling[7] and improved survival[8-13] have been observed after successful catheter-based recanalization. The most conspicuous benefit, however, consists in a significantly lower need for later coronary artery bypass grafting (CABG). Overall, the average left ventricular functional improvement after recanalization of chronic total coronary occlusions is not overwhelming and may escape detection by crude assessment. Moreover it is more likely to be found after recanalizing fairly recent occlusions. Finally, patients with untreated chronic total occlusions face a threefold risk of cardiac mortality or complications in case of future cardiac events.[14]

The case depicted in Figure 24-2 may be anecdotal, but it provides compelling evidence that in an individual case a recanalized artery may provide reverse collaterals to its former donor artery years later, thereby saving the patient's life. These awaited benefits are predicated on persistent patency of the recanalized segment.

OPEN-ARTERY HYPOTHESIS

The debate is ongoing whether an open artery per se provides clinical benefit. This debate is partially ignited by mixing up study results examining different clinical scenarios. In this context, three distinct but heterogeneous clinical settings exist: first, opening an infarct-related artery within a few hours after symptom onset to salvage the jeopardized myocardium and prevent necrosis; second, opening an infarct-related artery several days to a few weeks after the appearance of symptoms to revert residual ischemia in the peri-infarct zone (the original open-artery hypothesis); and third, opening a chronically occluded artery ($\geq$ 3 months occlusion age) that is collateralized and usually occluded without causing a myocardial infarction, in order to restore normal coronary blood flow to the supplied myocardium. Although the evidence supporting recanalization of an infarct-related artery in the acute setting is robust and ascertained, the optimal management strategy for the time beyond the first couple of days is mostly unclear. While previous studies denied a benefit from tackling these occlusions compared with medical treatment alone,[15] common sense and more recent data suggest the contrary. The SWISSI II trial[16] randomized patients within 3 months after myocardial infarction (provided that they had silent ischemia as verified by stress-test imaging and one- or two-vessel disease on angiography amenable for PCI) to either complete revascularization (96 patients) or intensive anti-ischemic drug treatment (105 patients). During a mean follow-up of 10.2 ± 2.6 years, 27 major adverse cardiac events (cardiac death, nonfatal myocardial infarction, or symptom-driven revascularization) occurred in the intervention group and 67 events occurred in the medical therapy group (adjusted hazard ratio [HR], 0.33; 95% confidence interval [CI], 0.20-0.55; $P < 0.001$), which corresponds with an absolute event reduction of 6.3% per year (95% CI, 3.7%-8.9%; $P < 0.001$). Left ventricular ejection fraction remained preserved in revascularized patients (mean of 54% ± 9.9% at baseline and 56% ± 8% at final follow-up) and decreased significantly ($P < 0.001$) in medically managed patients (mean of 60% ± 12% at baseline to 49% ± 8% at final follow-up). Abbate et al[17] performed a systematic review and metanalysis of randomized trials comparing PCI of the infarct-related artery with medical therapy in patients randomized >12 hours to 60 days after acute myocardial infarction. The survival and cardiac remodeling benefits in patients undergoing late PCI of the infarct-related artery are plotted in Figure 24-3. Data supporting a favorable impact of complete revascularization with PCI on survival in patients with at least one chronic total occlusion are accumulating.[8-13] Figure 24-4 shows the influence of success in a recanalization attempt in three large registries with various follow-up periods. Procedure success has shown instrumental for longevity of patients with attempted revascularization of a chronic total occlusion (Table 24-1). Aziz et al.[11] performed a retrospective study comparing the survival of patients with a successful percutaneous revascularization of a chronic total occlusion versus those with a failed procedure between the years 2000 and 2004. Technical success was 69%. During a mean follow-up of 1.7 ± 0.5 years, the mortality rate was 2.5% in the successfully recanalized patients and 7.3% in the failure group. The crude hazard ratio for death with recanalization failure was 3.92 (95% CI 1.56–10.07; $P = 0.004$). The rates of CABG were 3.2% versus 21.7% ($P < 0.001$) for success and failure patients, respectively. Multivariate analysis showed that recanalization failure was an independent predictor of death.

Prasad et al.[12] examined the trends in procedural success and long-term outcomes after PCI for chronic total occlusions over 25 years from the Mayo Clinic registry. The patients were divided into four groups according to the time of their intervention: group 1 (balloon

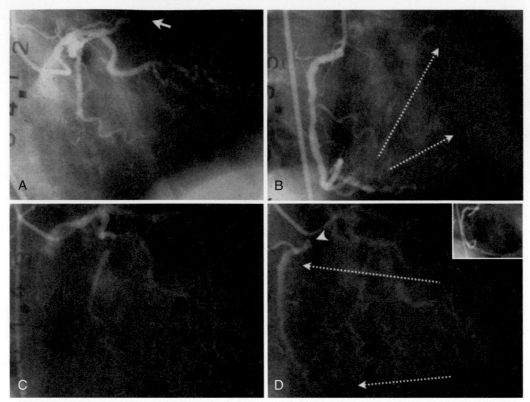

Figure 24-2 Lifesaving recruitment of reverse collaterals after 6 years of dormancy. **A.** Chronic total occlusion of the left anterior descending coronary artery (arrow) in a 58-year-old woman with preserved left ventricular function and stable angina pectoris. **B.** Copious collaterals (dashed arrows) form the mildly diseased right coronary artery. **C.** Successfully recanalized left anterior descending coronary artery. **D.** Complete occlusion of the orifice of the right coronary artery (arrowhead) 6 years later, with resurgence of stable angina after several years without symptoms. The collaterals (dashed arrows) had apparently been immediately recruitable because the left ventricular function was still normal. This time, they functioned in a reverse direction from the left anterior descending coronary artery that had stayed patent to the now occluded right coronary artery. Had the left anterior descending coronary artery not been recanalized 6 years earlier, the occlusion of the right coronary artery would have caused an infarction in the inferior and the anterior wall; the left anterior descending coronary artery would still have depended on the collaterals from the right coronary artery. This would not have been compatible with life. **Insert,** The recanalized right coronary artery.

angioplasty era), group 2 (early bailout stent era), group 3 (elective bare-metal stent era), and group 4 (drug-eluting stent era). Procedural success rates were 51%, 72%, 73%, and 70% ($P < 0.001$ for balloon angioplasty versus stent), respectively, in the four groups. During follow-up, the combined endpoint of death, myocardial infarction, or target lesion revascularization was significantly lower in the two most recent cohorts compared with those patients treated before ($P = 0.001$ for trend). Patients with a technical success did appear to have slightly

greater survival starting at 6 years of follow-up, although technical failure was not an independent predictor of mortality in the multivariate analysis (HR 1.16 [95% CI 0.90–1.5], $P = 0.25$). Patients who underwent a failed recanalization were much more likely to be referred for surgical revascularization (11% vs. 1%). Valenti et al.[13] sought to determine the impact on survival of successful drug-eluting stent-supported PCI for chronic total occlusion among 486 patients with 527 chronic total occlusions between 2003 and 2006. Recanalization of the targeted occlusion was successful in 71% of patients (68% of lesions). Multivessel intervention was performed in 62% of patients in whom recanalization of the chronic total occlusion was unsuccessful and in 71% of patients with successful recanalization of the chronic total occlusion ($P = 0.062$). At a median follow-up of 2 years (1.1–2.8 years), the cardiac survival rate was higher in the successfully recanalized group compared with the failure group (92 ± 2 vs. 87 ± 3%; $P = 0.025$). The survival benefit was also evident among patients with multivessel disease (91 ± 2% for patients with successful recanalization of the chronic total occlusion vs. 87 ± 3% for those with failed recanalization of the chronic total occlusion; $P = 0.021$) and particularly evident when complete revascularization was achieved versus incomplete revascularization (94 ± 2 vs. 84 ± 4%; $P < 0.001$).

INDICATIONS

The indications for a recanalization attempt are based on a projection of difficulties (in particular duration and length of occlusion) balanced against the potential benefit for the patient (current symptoms and limitation of activity) and the amount of viable myocardium at stake.

TABLE 24-1	Predictors of Long-Term Mortality after Attempted Revascularization of a Chronic Total Occlusion*	
Mid-american heart institute (2,013 patients)[10]		
Success	0.7 (0.5–0.8)	
Age >70 years	1.9 (1.5–2.4)	
Ejection fraction <40%	2.1 (1.7–2.7)	
Double vessel disease	1.5 (1.1–2.2)	
Triple vessel disease	1.9 (1.4–2.7)	
Diabetes mellitus	1.4 (1.1–1.8)	
Creatinine >2.0 mg/dL	2.2 (1.3–3.9)	
Unstable angina	1.3 (1.0–1.6)	
Rotterdam thoraxcenter (874 patients)[9]		
Success	0.6 (0.3–1.0)	
Age	1.0 (1.0–1.1)	
Multivessel disease	4.3 (1.9–9.6)	
Diabetes mellitus	2.5 (1.3–4.7)	

*Hazard Ratio (95% confidence interval).

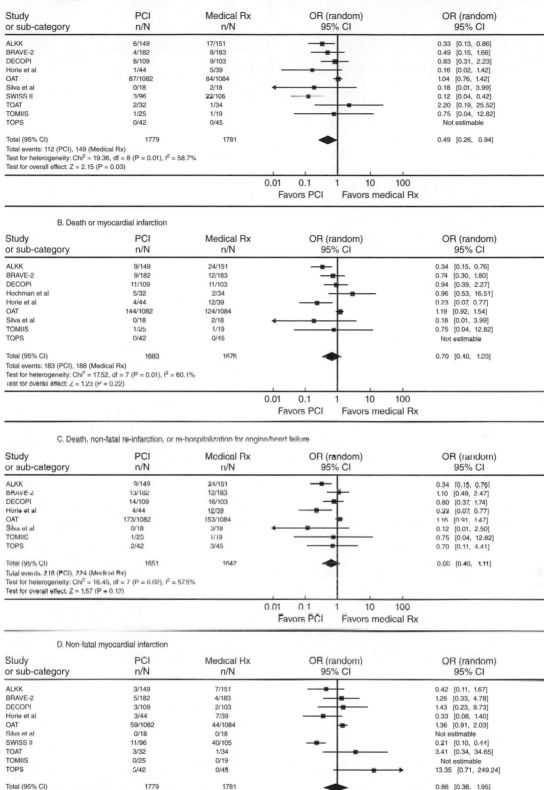

Figure 24-3 Individual and pooled risks of adverse outcomes forest plots showing individual and pooled risks of death **(A)**, death, and nonfatal recurrent myocardial infarction **(B)**, death, nonfatal recurrent myocardial infarction, or rehospitalization for angina/heart failure **(C)**, and nonfatal recurrent myocardial infarction **(D)** comparing late percutaneous coronary intervention (PCI) versus best medical therapy (Rx) only for infarct-related artery occlusion late (>12 hours) in the course of acute myocardial infarction. ALKK = Arbeitsgemeinschaft Leitende Kardiologische Krankenhausärzte; BRAVE-2 = Beyond 12 Hours Reperfusion Alternative Evaluation Trial; CI = confidence interval; DEPOCI = Randomized Trial of Occluded Artery Angioplasty After Acute Myocardial Infarction; OAT = Occluded Artery Trial; OR = odds ratio; SWISSI II = Swiss Interventional Study on Silent Ischemia Type II; TOAT = The Occluded Artery Trial; TOMIIS = Total Occlusion Post-Myocardial Infarction Intervention Study; TOPS = Treatment of Post-thrombolytic Stenoses. *(From Abbate A, Biondi-Zoccai GG, Appleton DL, et al. Survival and cardiac remodeling benefits in patients undergoing late percutaneous coronary intervention of the infarct-related artery: evidence from a meta-analysis of randomized controlled trials. Reproduced with permission. J Am Coll Cardiol 2008;51:956-964.)*

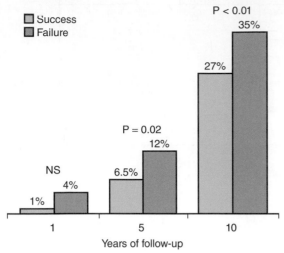

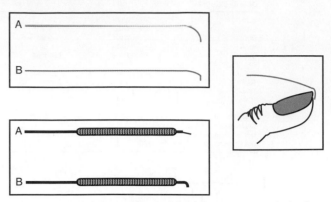

Figure 24-4 Mortality from three different registries with average follow-ups of 1 year (Total Occlusion Angioplasty Study of the Italian Society of Cardiology, TOAST-GISE with 286 successful and 83 failed recanalization attempts),[8] 5 years (Rotterdam Thoraxcenter experience with 576 successful and 309 failed recanalization attempts),[9] and 10 years (Mid-American Heart Institute, Kansas City, Kansas, USA, with 1491 successful and 514 failed recanalization attempts).[10] NS, not significant.

Figure 24-5 Top left panel: For difficult lesions, particularly chronic total occlusions, it is beneficial to add an additional sharp J-bend 1 to 2 mm from the tip of the guidewire **(B)** to the custom end **(A)**. Right panel: This can be achieved by using the dumped nail. Bottom left panel: The wire tip modification from A to B affords steerability even when entering tight lesions, an occluding segment, or when supporting the wire with a catheter advanced far to its tip.

The fact that a patient with a coronary occlusion is suffering enough to opt for CABG if angioplasty is not offered is a strong argument in favor of a PCI recanalization attempt. Indications may be broad if the recanalization attempt is part of the diagnostic coronary angiogram because a failure is less costly and imposes on the patient only a somewhat longer procedure. In multivessel disease, the presence of a chronic total occlusion should in itself not be sufficient reason to switch to CABG; however, the intricacy of recanalizing a chronic occlusion should be taken into consideration. With exceptions, two or more chronic occlusions can be too time-consuming to be attempted. One or two additional nontotal lesions appear to be reasonable for a single session. If the vessel with the additional lesion provides collaterals to the occluded vessel, recanalization of the occluded vessel should be done first. The second vessel PCI should be subject to a good result of the recanalization of the first. However, occasionally patients with a chronic occlusion of the right coronary artery are accepted for angioplasty of the left anterior descending or the left circumflex coronary arteries (or vice versa), disregarding the occluded vessel. Although published results of pertinent series have improved with the judicious use of drug-eluting stents, the increased risk of interventions on the left anterior descending coronary artery when the dominant right coronary artery is occluded (or vice versa) must be underscored. Indications for PCI attempts at chronic total occlusions correlate reciprocally with the local development of CABG. The most aggressive respective centers are in Japan, where overall PCI/CABG ratios are very high (>10/1). But even in that country, these ratios vary from >20/1 to <1/1 in individual centers. This points to the worldwide variations in indications for attempting to deal with chronic total occlusions.

ROUTINE TECHNIQUES

Knowledge about the length of the occlusion and the course of the vessel at and distal to the occlusion is of paramount importance for a transluminal recanalization. A preocclusion angiographic film, if available, should be scrutinized before and, in case of problems, during the recanalization attempt. If the distal segment of the artery is filled by ipsilateral or contralateral collaterals, a late freeze-frame of a contrast medium injection into the donor artery showing the distal part of the occluded vessel can be helpful for guidance, in conjunction with a freeze-frame of the proximal part of the occluded vessel showing the stump. Injections of contrast medium into the donor vessel to visualize the distal vessel segment during the recanalization attempt can be useful and may be achieved by using the same groin for placing the second arterial catheter in the case of contralateral collaterals.

The use of computed tomography has been advocated to predefine an occluded segment before an attempt at dealing with a chronic total occlusion by PCI.[18] A three-dimensional reconstruction of the occluded segments may certainly be helpful. However, the advantage of attempting PCI ad hoc during the diagnostic coronary angiogram and the quest to contain irradiation (already a problem with chronic occlusion PCI) will confine this technique to patients undergoing coronary computed tomography for reasons other than a previously detected chronic total occlusion planned for a PCI procedure. Attempts to recanalize chronic total coronary occlusions call for adapted techniques and materials. Special recanalization wires are commonly recommended and have succeeded in cases where floppy wires failed. Advancement of a balloon catheter (or support catheter) close to the tip of the guidewire to enhance wire manipulation is common practice. Inflation of a balloon in the occlusion stump or a proximal side branch for additional support (beyond that achieved after the optimal guiding catheter has been selected) of the penetrating guidewire is a valid option in selected situations. A simple but often crucial technique consists in custom-shaping an additional bend 1 to 2 mm from the guidewire tip (Fig. 24-5). Once inside the occlusion or with the support catheter far advanced, the conventional J at the tip is straightened out and useless. Steerability is maintained exclusively by this additional bend. The technique of using a polymer-coated, hydrophilic guidewire with a soft tapered tip to enter and cross microchannels is a reasonable initial approach only if there is a hint of forward flow. The penetration and drilling techniques using stiff wires, in a step-up manner, and a microcatheter or an over-the-wire balloon catheter for wire support or exchange are alternatives for true chronic total occlusions. During a retrograde approach, flexible polymer-coated wires should be used for septal collateral navigation and delivery of an exchange catheter to the distal end of the occlusion. Generally, if a false lumen is entered, it may help to introduce a second wire and keep it away from the false lumen marked by the first wire (parallel wire technique).

DEDICATED DEVICES AND TECHNIQUES

Table 24-2 lists devices specifically developed for chronic total occlusion PCI. Some of them have been used since the 1980s and most were used in peripheral arteries before being adapted to the coronary vasculature.

TABLE 24-2	Techniques Designed for Chronic Total Occlusion Angioplasty (in chronological order with principal innovator in parentheses)
High-speed rotational smooth burr*	
Magnum ball-tip wire	
Low-speed rotational smooth burr*	
High-frequency vibrating wire	
Laser wire*	
Ultrasound recanalization	
SafeCross small wire with optical coherence reflectometry/radiofrequency energy	
Frontrunner spreading forceps	
Parallel wire technique	
CART† retrograde technique	
Crosser wire with relatively low frequency vibration	
Tornus crossing catheter	
CiTop tip expanding catheter	
Stingray reentry catheter	

*No longer in use.
†Controlled antegrade and retrograde subintimal tracking.

The Frontrunner, a catheter similar to a myocardial biotome, is advanced into the stump where the front-end forceps is opened to spread the occluded segment apart. The idea behind this technique is that the walls will separate where they are softest—that is, at the occluded thrombus, not unlike a butter sandwich being pulled apart. The bulkiness of this equipment and the possibility of not finding the true lumen with this type of blunt dissection are major limitations that relegate this device to the niche gadgets. The sparse clinical data available reveal a high incidence of coronary perforation.[19] The device was subsequently withheld from coronary application and its use restricted to chronic total occlusions of the lower extremity. The "intelligent" recanalization system called SafeCross is based on optical coherence reflectometry; it is designed to distinguish the impenetrable vessel wall from soft occlusion material, thereby guiding progress. After years of poor acceptance, it has been upgraded with a radiofrequency penetration facilitator, hence the name changed from SafeSteer to SafeCross. A prospective multicenter registry featured 54% device success and could not accomplish a breakthrough in clinical adoption.[20] The Crosser system features a 20-MHz vibration generated at the outside end and transmitted to the tip of a coronary guidewire. This fairly simple concept has been successfully used in small clinical series.[21,22] Technical success was achieved in 63% of procedures in cases where conventional means had previously failed. These figures must be seen in the light of similar success with other short-lived new devices for chronic total occlusion angioplasty when first published and compared in a serial rather than randomized fashion with more conventional approaches. A fairly straightforward idea is that of the Tornus exchange catheter.[23] Albeit rarely, particularly with the introduction of sleek balloons less than 1.5 mm diameter, successful wire passage may be rendered useless by the impossibility of crossing the occlusion with a balloon. For this, a flexible metallic catheter has been developed; it is available in two sizes, with a spiral outer surface structure. It permits advancement through the occlusion with a screwing motion guided by the correctly placed coronary guidewire. Once across, the channel should have been sufficiently enlarged for passage with a balloon catheter in addition to the option of exchanging the coronary guidewire for a stiffer version before withdrawing the Tornus exchange catheter. Alternatively, the rotablator or a laser wire may be used to deal with such nondilatable occlusions.

More recent devices still with limited clinical data include the CiTop crossing system[24] and the Stingray reentry system.[25] CiTop is a 0.014-inch recanalization guidewire with a dilatable tip that permits step-by-step advancement across the occlusion (Fig. 24-6). After its safety and feasibility were demonstrated, further data regarding its efficacy are currently being collected in a multicenter study. The Stingray may facilitate reaching the true distal lumen when the guidewire lands subintimally. This device has two components: first, a self-orienting, winged, flat balloon catheter, giving the device its name, which is advanced over any 0.014-inch guidewire and inflated in the subintimal

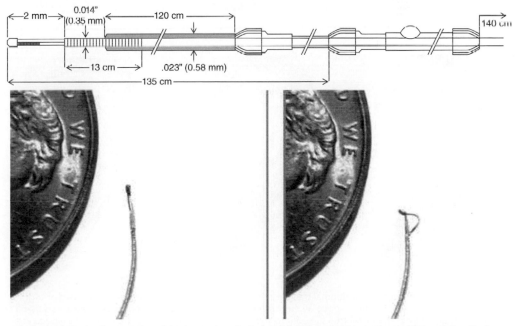

Figure 24-6 A new dedicated device for treating chronic total occlusions. The CiTop guidewire has additional tip dilating capability to create an intraocclusion furrow that allows it to advance forward. Top: schematic description of the device; bottom: distal tip in its operating position. *(From Scheinowitz M, Amrami I, Oppenhaim U, et al. Crossing chronic total occlusions with a new 0.014" CiTop guidewire: proof of concept. Published with permission. Catheter Cardiovasc Intervent 2009;74:278-285).*

space, and, second, a special reentry guidewire used to exit the inflated balloon via one of two lateral ports situated 180 degrees apart in the true distal vessel lumen. No clinical data have as yet been published. The main arena for technical progress in the realm of chronic total occlusion is guidewire technology. Polymer-coated, hydrophilic guidewires and spring-coil guidewires are the two main groups of guidewires for treating chronic total occlusions. While polymer guidewires, also termed plastic jacket wires, always have a hydrophilic coating, spring-coil wires, also known as stiff wires, may have a hydrophilic coating, either throughout or sparing the tip. Stiffness of the tip is often graded by the minimally required deflection force in grams. Polymer-coated guidewires glide through microchannels and tortuous collaterals but may easily deviate in front of hard obstacles into the softer subintimal space and cause dissections or perforations. Perforations may similarly occur after successfully crossing the occlusion if the guidewire tip is left unnoticed as it migrates outside the distal epicardial vessel. On the contrary, the tactile feeling obtained from uncoated stiff wires makes them more controllable. Both guidewire classes may have regular or tapered tips. With a clinically compelling indication, highly accomplished operators may employ the retrograde technique after a failed antegrade recanalization attempt.[26,27] This device implies a retrograde passage to the distal vessel segment with a

polymer-coated guidewire advanced through a particularly well-developed (preferably septal) collateral vessel from the collateral donor artery. The wire is usually shielded by a flexible microcatheter, allowing exchange for stiffer guidewires if needed. Once facing the distal cap, the retrograde wire serves either as an optical guide for the penetrating antegrade wire to reach the distal true lumen or it may be progressed throughout the occlusion length supported by an inflated balloon (after gently predilating the collateral channels to allow retrieval of the balloon) or support catheter. The Corsair microcatheter was developed as a collateral channel dilator to facilitate retrograde approaches. This over-the-wire micro- and support catheter with a spiral structure allows the bidirectional rotation to be transmitted to the distal shaft for crossing small tortuous collateral channels. Landing by the retrograde wire in a false lumen gives the option of switching to the CART technique[28,29] (Controlled Antegrade and Retrograde Subintimal Tracking), in which the antegrade wire is directed into that false lumen after it has been dilated from a retrograde direction, so that the distal true lumen is finally reached (Fig. 24-7). More recently, a reverse CART technique[30] has been applied with success. The kissing wire and knuckle wire techniques[31,32] without balloon dilation are defined as bilateral wiring techniques. Although the retrograde wire can often be passed back into the aorta, grabbing it with a snare to

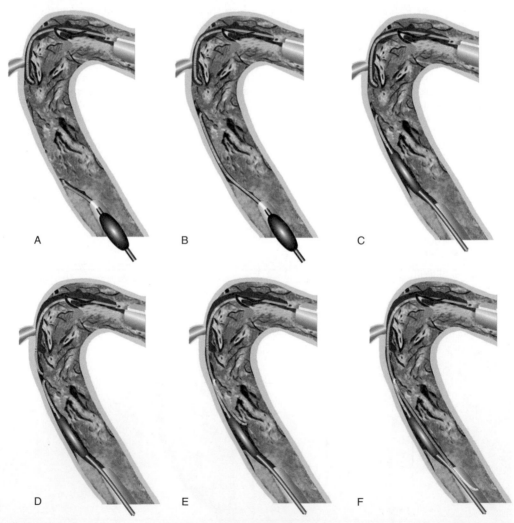

Figure 24-7 Controlled antegrade and retrograde subintimal tracking: the CART technique. First a wire is advanced antegradely from the proximal true lumen into the occlusion then into the subintimal space at the occlusion site. Next a wire is advanced retrogradely till the distal end of the occlusion, then penetrates retrogradely from the distal true lumen into the occlusion and finally into the subintimal space at the occlusion site. The subintimal space is dilated from retrograde to allow easier passage of the antegrade wire along the retrograde wire course to ultimately reach the distal true lumen. The subintimal track is limited to the occlusion site. *(From Surmely JF, Tsuchikane E, Katoh O, et al. New concept for CTO recanalization using controlled antegrade and retrograde subintimal tracking: the CART technique. Reproduced with permission. J Invasive Cardiol 2006;18:334-338.)*

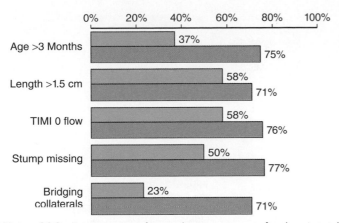

Figure 24-8 Success rates of recanalization attempts for chronic total coronary occlusions with (green bars) or without (purple bars) the most important risk factors. Depending on indications and revascularization techniques, the absolute figures may be higher or lower. However, the relative differences persist. (*Data from Puma JA, Sketch MH Jr, Tcheng JE, et al: Percutaneous revascularization of chronic coronary occlusions: An overview. J Am Coll Cardiol 1995;26:1-11.*)

TABLE 24-3	In-Hospital Adverse Outcomes and Complications for Chronic Total Occlusion PCI	
In-hospital adverse outcomes		**Patients (%)**
All-cause death		2 (0.4)
Cardiac death		1 (0.2)
Q-wave myocardial infarction		1 (0.2)
Non-Q-wave myocardial infarction		10 (2.1)
Stroke		0 (0)
Stent thrombosis		0 (0)
Procedural complications		**Patients (%)**
Cardiac tamponade		2 (0.4)
Emergent PCI		2 (0.4)
Emergent CABG		0 (0)
Blood transfusion		8 (1.6)
Access site surgery		2 (0.4)
Gastrointestinal bleeding		1 (0.2)
Contrast-induced nephropathy		6 (1.2)
Radiation dermatitis		0 (0)

PCI, percutaneous coronary intervention, CABG, coronary artery bypass graft surgery.

Data from the J-CTO Registry (Multicenter chronic total occlusion registry in Japan) including 498 patients with 528 chronic total occlusions (89% success in the first attempt cases and 69% in the retry cases).[34]

produce a wire loop is not recommended. There is a risk of damaging the collaterals or even producing bleeding into the pericardium by such wire manipulations in spite of the protection sheath. Hence the technique is recommended for septal but not epicardial collaterals even by its proponents. The retrograde wire may also create an entry hole for the antegrade wire at the site where it emerges from the occluded segment into the proximal stump. Intracoronary ultrasound has been advocated to help in regaining the true lumen in case a subintimal passage should wind up in a dead end.[33] Again, this technique must be reserved to the few operators who are highly experienced in chronic total occlusion angioplasty and the use of intracoronary ultrasound and have dealt with a high volume of such procedures.

FACTORS PREDICTIVE OF SUCCESS OR FAILURE

Figure 24-8 depicts some of the major factors affecting the technical success of chronic total occlusion recanalization. The absolute figures are likely to vary considerably from operator to operator, depending on his or her determination and utilization of aggressive devices. Yet the significance of the variables persists till today. Duration of occlusion is the key factor. The most rapid decline in the chance of success occurs during the first weeks after the occlusion. For nonspecialized operators, it is wise to accept only angiographically ideal occlusions (a short straight segment in a large vessel with a tapered stump) with a sound clinical indication in the case of an occlusion that is known to be not more than a few months old. Copious local bridging collaterals are an infallible sign of chronicity. The same holds true for the length of the occluded segment or the absence of a proximal stump. Attempts to recanalize venous bypass grafts with old occlusions are unrewarding and should be avoided.[33a]

COMPLICATIONS

The overall risk of angioplasty of occluded vessels lies somewhere between that of diagnostic coronary angiography and PCI of nonoccluded vessels. Statistically it has been shown equal to general PCI.[5] However, the chronic occlusion is most often not directly responsible for a dismal outcome but rather reflects the more advanced disease of the average patient with a chronic occlusion. Many of these patients undergo additional treatment for nonoccluded vessels, or the occlusion has to be approached through significantly diseased coronary arteries. The longer duration of the procedure (implying considerably higher radiation and doses of contrast) and the accidental closure of side branches, collateral channels, or peripheral coronary arteries by stent implantation, distal embolization, or irremediable dissections are at the base of most such complications. The J-CTO registry (multicenter chronic total occlusion registry in Japan), enrolling consecutive patients undergoing PCI for chronic total occlusion from 12 Japanese centers, recently revealed in-hospital clinical outcome data for 498 patients with 528 chronic total occlusions.[34] Complex strategies were utilized (parallel wiring in 31% and a retrograde approach in 25% of cases) and high procedural success rates (89% in the first-attempt cases and 69% in the retry cases) achieved. In-hospital adverse event rates were low, as reflected in Table 24-3. Large amounts of contrast dye (median 293 mL) and long fluoroscopic times (median 45 min) were not associated with serious clinical sequelae (contrast-induced nephropathy 1.2% and radiation dermatitis 0%). It is noteworthy that coronary perforations were frequently documented by angiography (antegrade 7.2% and retrograde 13.6%); all of these occurred during guidewire manipulation. Cardiac tamponade was rare (0.4%).

MORTALITY

Death is a rare complication of chronic total occlusion PCI. Fatal outcomes due to left main coronary artery dissections by the guiding catheter, embolization into a patent vessel of retracted occlusion material by the balloon, inadvertent air injection during device exchanges, or coronary perforation or rupture have been reported.

NEED FOR EMERGENCY CABG

In addition to cardiac tamponade due to perforation during attempted recanalization, an indication for emergency CABG is the occlusion of a non-previously occluded coronary artery either by an inadvertent trauma, an embolus, or an additional PCI attempt. The failure to pass a chronic total occlusion per se or its abrupt reclosure cannot possibly create significant ischemia unless an only collateral has been destroyed in the process. In contrast to some anecdotal reports, this is also a prerequisite for significant ischemia in case of a reclosure of the recanalized segment during follow-up. Collaterals (unless secluded from the recanalized artery by a stent) remain reliably on standby even for years, capable of working in both directions (Fig. 24-2).

INFARCTION

The most likely explanations for an infarction in the wake of a recanalization of a chronically occluded coronary artery are the occlusion of a hitherto patent side branch, distal embolization of occlusion

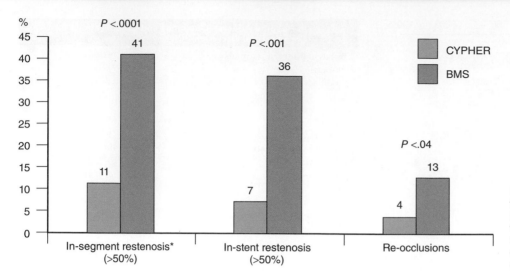

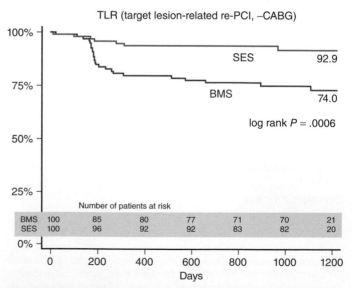

Figure 24-9 Randomized trial comparing the CYPHER sirolimus-eluting stent (SES) to its bare metal platform (BMS) in 200 patients with chronic total occlusion. There is a marked advantage for the CYPHER stent at one year (*stented segment plus proximal and distal 5mm).[35]

material, or irremediable dissection of the distal vessel segment. In retrograde approaches, dissection or thrombus formation in the donor artery may also be of concern.

PERFORATION OR RUPTURE

Guidewire perforation in the occluded segment is usually harmless because the diseased thick vessel walls seal spontaneously. Peripheral perforation in thin-walled normal coronary artery segments, on the other hand, may lead to tamponade, particularly if they are multiple (typical for hydrophilic guidewires). Rupture of the occluded segment due to balloon inflation or stent placement in a subintimal position or oversizing of the balloon secondary to overestimation of the nonvisible size of the vessel or inadvertent entry into a small side branch are fortunately rare but often difficult to treat. The use of bulky atherectomy devices increases the risk of rupture. However, these devices are rarely used in chronic total occlusions because they further complicate the technique of an already intricate procedure. Some of the ruptures drain into a ventricle and are thus clinically innocuous. Some close spontaneously, particularly after antagonizing heparin, or are contained in the muscle. Some can be remedied percutaneously by prolonged balloon inflation, flap patching with a stent, or implantation of a covered stent either to close the hole or disconnect the leaking artery from the inflow. While a noncovered stent may tack back a flap over the hole, it may also increase the leak. Distal perforations may be sealed by coils or microspheres. Some leaks need emergency surgery. If a perforated vessel is also filled via collaterals, it is useful, after sealing the perforation, to inject the collaterals to exclude the presence of retrograde contrast extravasation.

EXTENSIVE DISSECTION

Extensive dissection is almost invariably seen after recanalization of a chronic total occlusion, particularly if the occluded segment was rather long. Therefore the entire segment is usually fitted with one or several stents to the end of a perfect aspect. Randomized studies condone this, as reocclusion and restenosis are significantly reduced by elective stenting of a recanalized chronic total occlusion. Based on the results of several trials, it seems reasonable to use drug-eluting stent implantation after successfully reopening a chronic total occlusion. The first randomized trial, PRISON II (PRimary Intracoronary Stent placement after successfully crossing chronic total OcclusioNs) (Fig. 24-9), comparing the Cypher (sirolimus-eluting) stent to bare metal stenting in total chronic occlusions of 200 patients, found a significant reduction of the restenosis rate from 40% to 10% and of major adverse cardiac events from 20% to 4% with the Cypher stent.[35] This advantage

persisted at >3 years of follow-up[36] (Fig. 24-10). There were no statistically significant differences in death, myocardial infarction, and stent thrombosis according to the Academic Research Consortium criteria between the two groups, although stent thrombosis was numerically higher for the Cypher stent (5% versus 2%). Data from the RESEARCH registry[37] failed, however, to demonstrate an advantage for the Cypher stent at 3 years, in spite of an initially reported clinical benefit at 1 year compared to a historical group of patients treated with bare metal stents.

Significant event prevention in favor of another active stent (the paclitaxel-eluting Taxus stent) was seen in 48 patients compared with matched controls, with a reduction of restenoses from 50% to 10% and of reocclusion from 20% to 2%.[38] Recent data from a prospective multicenter registry including over 8,000 patients, of whom 687 were successfully treated for chronic total occlusions using Cypher stents, demonstrated that procedural factors and stent implantation

Figure 24-10 Target lesion revascularization up to 1,200 days in the PRISON II study of Figure 24-9 comparing the use of the sirolimus-eluting Cypher stent (SES) to its bare metal platform (BMS) in 400 randomized patients with chronic coronary occlusions. There is a sustained marked advantage for the Cypher stent. *(Reproduced with permission. Am Heart J 2009;157:149-155.)*[36]

techniques affect outcome (death and myocardial infarction at 6 months).[39] Overall, the use of drug-eluting stents in chronic total occlusion recanalization is associated with significantly fewer major adverse cardiac events and target vessel revascularization, restenosis, and stent reocclusion as compared with the use of bare metal stents. This was shown in a metanalysis including over 4,000 patients.[40] Dedicated head-to-head randomized trials between different drug-eluting stents in the realm of chronic total occlusion are on the way: PRISON III is currently enrolling 300 patients treated by either sirolimus- or zotarolimus-eluting stents. The primary endpoint is in-segment late loss at 8 months. The ongoing CIBELES (nonacute coronary occlusion treated with everolimus eluting stents) trial is investigating an everolimus-eluting against a sirolimus-eluting stent on angiographic late loss.

In light of the relative innocuousness of a stent thrombosis in a previously chronically occluded lesion and the high relative restenosis rate of bare metal stents in this situation, it is likely that only drug-eluting stents will be used for this indication before long.

Future Perspectives for Percutaneous Coronary Intervention

IN CHRONIC TOTAL OCCLUSIONS

Chronically occluded coronary arteries are a frequent finding in patients needing revascularization. However, with conservative treatment, the risk emanating from the occluded artery itself is low. Future cardiac events may well be more common than in a population without significant coronary artery disease, but they are due to progression of other lesions on the clinical background of an already present occlusion rather than the chronic occlusion itself. Yearly mortality is about 4% in the natural course of patients with a chronic total occlusion of the left circumflex or the right coronary artery. It is about 10% if the occlusion is in the left anterior descending coronary artery. Successful

recanalization reduces this risk by half. The modest primary success rate and moderate clinical improvement to be expected with recanalization of chronic total coronary occlusions warrant moderation on the part of interventional cardiologists in accepting and treating these patients. Even if primary success has been improved by new technologies and skills, the clinical yield will never match that of PCI of stenoses. As a comparatively low-yield intervention, percutaneous recanalization of chronic total coronary occlusions should remain a low-risk, low-cost option. This sets limits as to how sophisticated, complicated, risky, and expensive tools and techniques for percutaneous coronary recanalizations can get. Simple mechanical means have a fairly high potential for revascularization, are user-friendly, and involve relatively little risk. Additionally, they are affordable. Stiff and/ and polymer-coated hydrophilic wires have excelled as the most successful tools for the routine recanalization of totally occluded coronary arteries. They are the first choice at most centers. However, neither stiff nor polymer-coated wires (let alone both) should be used by inexperienced operators who are unaware of their potential for proximal or peripheral dissection (stiff wires) and peripheral perforation (polymer-coated wires), with subsequent severe ischemia or acute or delayed cardiac tamponade. Niche devices like the SafeCross, Crosser, Tornus catheter, and potentially CiTop will continue to be used at highly specialized institutions. The same holds true for techniques employing multiple guidewires, retrograde approaches, or intravascular ultrasound guidance. It is not necessary to uncritically stent all recanalized occlusions and to extend the stents from healthy margin to healthy margin. Many dissected, recanalized segments will heal nicely during follow-up, as in the pre-stent era.[41] The clinical benefit of recanalizing a chronic total occlusion may not always be immediately apparent. However, there is always a possibility that a recanalized vessel will save a patient's life when the prior collateral donor occludes and the myocardium is salvaged thanks to reversed collaterals (Fig. 24-2). This may sanction (albeit late) a recanalization attempt that was frowned upon at the time because of a questionable indication.

REFERENCES

1. Meier B: Chronic total coronary occlusion angioplasty. *Catheter Cardiovasc Diagn* 17:212–217, 1989.
2. Aziz S, Ramsdale DR: Chronic total occlusions—a stiff challenge requiring a major breakthrough: is there light at the end of the tunnel? *Heart* 91:iii42–iii48, 2005.
3. Stone GW, Kandzari DE, Mehran R, et al: Percutaneous recanalization of chronically occluded coronary arteries: a consensus document: part I. *Circulation* 112:2364–2372, 2005.
4. Flameng W, Schwartz F, Hehrlein FW: Intraoperative evaluation of the functional significance of coronary collateral vessels in patients with coronary artery disease. *Am J Cardiol* 42:187–192, 1978.
5. Stone GW, Reifart NJ, Moussa I, et al: Percutaneous recanalization of chronically occluded coronary arteries: a consensus document: part II. *Circulation* 112:2530–2537, 2005.
6. Di Mario C, Werner GS, Sianos G, et al: European perspective in the recanalisation of Chronic Total Occlusions (CTO): consensus document from the EuroCTO Club. *EuroIntervention* 3:30–43, 2007.
7. Kirschbaum SW, Baks T, Gronenschild EH, et al: Addition of the long-axis information to short-axis contours reduces interstudy variability of left-ventricular analysis in cardiac magnetic resonance studies. *Invest Radiol* 43:1–6, 2008.
8. Olivari Z, Rubartelli P, Piscione F, et al: Immediate results and one-year clinical outcome after percutaneous coronary interventions in chronic total occlusions: data from a multicenter, prospective, observational study (TOAST-GISE). *J Am Coll Cardiol* 41:1672–1678, 2003.
9. Hoye A, van Domburg RT, Sonnenschein K, et al: Percutaneous coronary intervention for chronic total occlusions: the Thoraxcenter experience 1992–2002. *Eur Heart J* 26:2630–2636, 2005.
10. Suero JA, Marso SP, Jones PG, et al: Procedural outcomes and long-term survival among patients undergoing percutaneous coronary intervention of a chronic total occlusion in native coronary arteries: a 20-year experience. *J Am Coll Cardiol* 38:409–414, 2001.
11. Aziz S, Stables RH, Grayson AD, et al: Percutaneous coronary intervention for chronic total occlusions: improved survival for patients with successful revascularization compared to a failed procedure. *Catheter Cardiovasc Intervent* 70:15–20, 2007.

12. Prasad A, Rihal CS, Lennon RJ, et al: Trends in outcomes after percutaneous coronary intervention for chronic total occlusions: a 25-year experience from the Mayo Clinic. *J Am Coll Cardiol* 49:1611–1618, 2007.
13. Valenti R, Migliorini A, Signorini U, et al: Impact of complete revascularization with percutaneous coronary intervention on survival in patients with at least one chronic total occlusion. *Eur Heart J* 29:2336–2342, 2008.
14. Moreno R, Conde C, Perez-Vizcayno MJ, et al: Prognostic impact of a chronic occlusion in a noninfarct vessel in patients with acute myocardial infarction and multivessel disease undergoing primary percutaneous coronary intervention. *J Invas Cardiol* 18:16–19, 2006.
15. Hochman JS, Lamas GA, Buller CE, et al: Coronary intervention for persistent occlusion after myocardial infarction. *N Engl J Med* 355:2395–2407, 2006.
16. Erne P, Schoenenberger AW, Burckhardt D, et al: Effects of percutaneous coronary interventions in silent ischemia after myocardial infarction: the SWISSI II randomized controlled trial. *JAMA* 297:1985–1991, 2007.
17. Abbate A, Biondi-Zoccai GG, Appleton DL, et al: Survival and cardiac remodeling benefits in patients undergoing late percutaneous coronary intervention of the infarct-related artery: evidence from a meta-analysis of randomized controlled trials. *J Am Coll Cardiol* 51:956–964, 2008.
18. Mollet NR, Hoye A, Lemos PA, et al: Value of preprocedure multislice computed tomographic coronary angiography to predict the outcome of percutaneous recanalization of chronic total occlusions. *Am J Cardiol* 95:240–243, 2005.
19. Orlic D, Stankovic G, Sangiorgi G, et al: Preliminary experience with the Frontrunner coronary catheter: novel device dedicated to mechanical revascularization of chronic total occlusions. *Catheter Cardiovasc Intervent* 64:146–152, 2005.
20. Baim DS, Braden G, Heuser R, et al: Utility of the Safe-Cross-guided radiofrequency total occlusion crossing system in chronic coronary total occlusions (results from the Guided Radio Frequency Energy Ablation of Total Occlusions Registry Study). *Am J Cardiol* 94:853–858, 2004.
21. Melzi G, Cosgrave J, Biondi-Zoccai GL, et al: A novel approach to chronic total occlusions: the crosser system. *Catheter Cardiovasc Intervent* 68:29–35, 2006.

22. Grube E, Sutsch G, Lim VY, et al: High-frequency mechanical vibration to recanalize chronic total occlusions after failure to cross with conventional guidewires. *J Invas Cardiol* 18:85–91, 2006.
23. Tsuchikane E, Katoh O, Shimogami M, et al: First clinical experience of a novel penetration catheter for patients with severe coronary artery stenosis. *Catheter Cardiovasc Intervent* 65:368–373, 2005.
24. Scheinowitz M, Amrami I, Oppenhaim U, et al: Crossing chronic total occlusions with a new 0.014" CiTop guidewire: proof of concept. *Catheter Cardiovasc Intervent* 74:278–283, 2009.
25. Beyar R, Lotan C: Innovations in cardiovascular interventions 2008—technology parade. *EuroIntervention* 4:676–684, 2009.
26. Surmely JF, Katoh O, Tsuchikane E, et al: Coronary septal collaterals as an access for the retrograde approach in the percutaneous treatment of coronary chronic total occlusions. *Catheter Cardiovasc Intervent* 69:826–832, 2007.
27. Ochiai M: Retrograde approach for chronic total occlusion: present status and prospects. *EuroInterv* 3:169–173, 2007.
28. Surmely JF, Tsuchikane E, Katoh O, et al: New concept for CTO recanalization using controlled antegrade and retrograde subintimal tracking: the CART technique. *J Invas Cardiol* 18:334–338, 2006.
29. Matsumi J, Saito S: Progress in the retrograde approach for chronic total coronary artery occlusion: a case with successful angioplasty using CART and reverse-anchoring techniques 3 years after failed PCI via a retrograde approach. *Catheter Cardiovasc Intervent* 71:810–814, 2008.
30. Rathore S, Katoh O, Tuschikane E, et al: A novel modification of the retrograde approach for the recanalization of chronic total occlusion of the coronary arteries: intravascular ultrasound-guided reverse controlled antegrade and retrograde tracking. *J Am Coll Cardiol Intervent* 3:155–164, 2010.
31. Surmely JF, Katoh O: Bilateral approach. In Waksman R, Saito S, editors: *Chronic Total Occlusions*, West Sussex, UK, 2009, Wiley-Blackwell, pp 107–112.
32. Saito S: Different strategies of retrograde approach in coronary angioplasty for chronic total occlusion. *Catheter Cardiovasc Intervent* 71:8–19, 2008.
33. Kimura BJ, Tsimikas S, Bhargava V, et al: Subintimal wire position during angioplasty of a chronic total coronary occlusion: detec

tion and subsequent procedural guidance by intravascular ultrasound. *Catheter Cardiovasc Diagn* 35:262–265, 1995.

33a. Puma JA, Sketch MH Jr, Tcheng JE, et al: Percutaneous revascularization of chronic coronary occlusions: An overview. *J Am Coll Cardiol* 26:1–11, 1995.

34. Morino Y, Kimura T, Hayashi Y, et al: In–hospital outcomes of contemporary percutaneous coronary intervention in patients with chronic total occlusion: insights from the J–CTO Registry (Multicenter CTO Registry in Japan). *J Am Coll Cardiol Intervent* 3:143–151, 2010.

35. Suttorp MJ, Laarman GJ, Rahel BM, et al: Primary stenting of totally occluded native coronary arteries II (PRISON II study): a randomized comparison of bare metal stent implantation with sirolimus–eluting stent implantation for the treatment of chronic total coronary occlusions. *Circulation* 114:921–928, 2006.

36. Rahel BM, Laarman GJ, Kelder JC, et al: Three–year clinical outcome after primary stenting of totally occluded native coronary arteries: a randomized comparison of bare–metal stent implantation with sirolimus–eluting stent implantation for the treatment of total coronary occlusions (Primary Stenting of Totally Occluded Native Coronary Arteries [PRISON] II study). *Am Heart J* 157:149–155, 2009.

37. García–García HM, Daemen J, Kukreja N, et al: Three–year clinical outcomes after coronary stenting of chronic total occlusion using sirolimus–eluting stents: insights from the rapamycin–eluting stent evaluated at Rotterdam cardiology hospital–(RESEARCH) registry. *Catheter Cardiovasc Interv* 70:635–639, 2007.

38. Werner GS, Krack A, Schwarz G, et al: Prevention of lesion recurrence in chronic total coronary occlusions by paclitaxel–eluting stents. *J Am Coll Cardiol* 44:2301–2306, 2004.

39. Khattab AA, Hamm CW, Senges J, et al: Sirolimus–eluting stent treatment at high–volume centers confers lower mortality at 6–month follow–up: results from the prospective multicenter German Cypher Registry. *Circulation* 120:600–606, 2009.

40. Colmenarez HJ, Escaned J, Fernández C, et al: Efficacy and safety of drug–eluting stents in chronic total coronary occlusion recanalization: a systematic review and meta–analysis. *J Am Coll Cardiol* 55;1854–1866, 2010.

41. Werner GS, Schwarz G, Prochnau D, et al: Paclitaxel–eluting stents for the treatment of chronic total coronary occlusions: a strategy of extensive lesion coverage with drug–eluting stents. *Catheter Cardiovasc Intervent* 67:1–9, 2006.

25

Bypass Graft Intervention

JOHN S. DOUGLAS, JR.

KEY POINTS

- Early postoperative ischemia (<30 days) is often due to graft occlusion or stenosis and percutaneous coronary intervention is frequently feasible.

- Unstable angina or ST-segment elevation myocardial infarction years after coronary artery bypass grafting is most often due to a saphenous vein graft lesion; in such cases native vessel percutaneous coronary intervention is preferred when possible.

- Intravenous thrombolytic therapy is ineffective in saphenous vein graft occlusion/ST-segment elevation myocardial infarction; angiographic evaluation and primary percutaneous coronary intervention is preferred for ST-segment elevation myocardial infarction after coronary artery bypass grafting.

- Embolic protection halves the risk of atheroembolic myocardial infarction during saphenous vein graft percutaneous coronary intervention and should be used routinely in the treatment of de novo saphenous vein graft lesions.

- Multiple diseased or occluded saphenous vein grafts, reduced left ventricular function, and available arterial conduits favor repeat coronary artery bypass grafting; a patent left internal mammary artery to the left anterior descending favors percutaneous coronary intervention.

- Drug-eluting stents reduce restenosis in saphenous vein grafts and native coronary arteries and have become the default strategy for many operators in spite of reduced efficacy in saphenous vein grafts compared with native vessels.

Scope of the Problem

Coronary artery bypass grafting (CABG) is one of the most common surgical procedures. The efficacy of CABG has been enhanced by the use of arterial grafts, off bypass procedures, and minimally invasive surgical techniques; in addition, attempts have been made to improve graft longevity with antiplatelet agents and lipid-lowering therapy. However, the temporary nature of the palliative effect remains a significant healthcare problem. Severe myocardial ischemic syndromes occur in 3% to 5% of patients immediately after surgery; thereafter, recurrent ischemic symptoms appear in 4% to 8% of the millions of surviving post-CABG patients annually. Saphenous vein graft (SVG) attrition, the most common cause, is up to 30% during the first year and is about 4% per year thereafter. At 10 years, only 40% of patent grafts are free of significant stenosis. At Emory University and the Cleveland Clinic, reoperation was required in about 3% of patients by 5 years, 15% by 10 years, and 30% by 15 years. Even in the most experienced centers, the risk of in-hospital death and nonfatal Q-wave myocardial infarction (MI) is triple that of the initial operation. In New York State, in-hospital mortality was 4.1% for initial operations but 11%, 25%, and 39% for first, second, and third reoperations, respectively.[1] In addition to being more risky, reoperative surgery was associated with less complete anginal relief and reduced graft patency. These factors have promoted a conservative approach to reoperation and favored the use of percutaneous coronary intervention (PCI).[2–6] In addition, many symptomatic patients who are candidates for percutaneous methods would not be considered for reoperation because of jeopardy to limited myocardium, risk to patent grafts, lack of

suitable conduits, poor left ventricular (LV) function, advanced age, or coexisting medical problems. In the past decade at Emory University Hospital, approximately 15% of the patients who underwent PCI had had prior CABG, and bypass graft intervention was the most common indication. It is in this difficult group of patients—those requiring bypass graft intervention—that decision making is particularly critical owing to the increased risk and reduced long-term benefit of bypass graft intervention.

Indications for Intervention

Patients who experience recurrent ischemia after coronary bypass surgery have diverse anatomical problems; therefore selection for PCI must be based on careful analysis of the probabilities of outcomes compared with competing strategies. The status of the left anterior descending (LAD) coronary artery and its graft significantly influences revascularization choices because of its impact on long-term outcome and the lack of survival benefit of reoperative surgery to treat non-LAD coronary artery–related ischemia.[7,8] Factors favoring surgical revascularization include multiple vessel involvement, severe vein graft disease, poor LV function, more total occlusions of native coronary arteries, and the availability of arterial conduits (Table 25-1).[8] Because both the choice of percutaneous methods and the relative effectiveness of each are often influenced by the time elapsed since surgery, indications are considered in relation to this factor.

EARLY POSTOPERATIVE PERIOD

The performance of routine intraoperative angiography at the conclusion of CABG at one center and three recent trials in which routine angiography was performed at 6 to 12 months to assess graft patency have provided sobering insights regarding contemporary CABG.[9–12] Among 366 consecutive patients who underwent intraoperative completion angiography, Zhao and colleague found that 12% of bypass grafts had defects important enough to require intervention (open surgical revision 3.4%, open-chest PCI 6%, and minor adjustment 2.8%).[9] In a randomized trial of over 3,000 patients, graft failure at 1 year occurred in 30% of saphenous vein grafts (SVGs),[10] while SVG failure occurred in 23% performed off pump and 16% on pump in another report,[11] and 38% of gastroepiploic artery grafts failed in a third.[12] Graft failure was associated with death, new MI, or repeat revascularization in 26% of patients.[10] Recurrent ischemia within days of surgery is usually related to acute vein graft thrombosis. However, stenosis may exist at proximal or distal anastomoses (Fig. 25-1); a bypass graft may be kinked; the wrong vessel may have been bypassed; or the revascularization may have been rendered incomplete as a result of diffuse disease, stenoses distal to graft insertion, or inaccessible intramyocardial position of a recipient artery. To determine the cause of severe early postoperative myocardial ischemia and define therapeutic options, coronary arteriography has been carried out within a few hours of surgery in 3% to 4% of patients in some centers,[13–15] and this strategy is recommended. PCI in patients with early ischemia after CABG is a class I indication in the American College of Cardiology/American Heart Association/Society for Cardiovascular Angiography and Interventions (ACC/AHA/SCAI) PCI guidelines.[16] Although 44 (29%) of 145 patients catheterized because of ischemia early after surgery had no apparent cause for ischemia, most patients had correctable problems; 30 patients had emergency reoperation, and 44

TABLE 25-1	Significant Predictors of Method of Revascularization in Decreasing Order of Importance Variable Chi-Square Odds Ratio* Confidence Interval (95%)
Number of diseased grafts (2 vs. 0)[†] 133 0.01 0.01–0.03	
Number of occluded grafts (2 vs. 0)[†] 103 0.05 0.03–0.09	
Prior infarct 98 37 18–75	
Chronic obstructive pulmonary disease 82 0.02 0.01–0.04	
Hyperlipidemia 70 0.11 0.06–0.18	
Patent LIMA to LAD 57 6.6 4–11	
EF (50 vs. 40%)[†] 46 1.3 1.1–1.7	
Years from 1995 (4.4 vs. 1.5)[†] 40 3.0 1.9–4.6	
Native artery occlusion (2 vs. 1)[†] 24 0.41 0.229–0.58	
Years from CABG (15 vs. 6)[†] 23 0.44 0.33–0.63	
Maximum LAD stenosis (100 vs. 80%)[†] 13 0.73 0.61–0.86	
Maximum LMT stenosis (60 vs. 0%)[†] 12 0.47 0.31–0.72	
Age (73 vs. 60 years)[†] 12 1.8 1.3–2.6	
Unstable angina 8 2.0 1.2–3.1	
Number of diseased vessels (3 vs. 2)[†] 5 2.1 1.1–4.1	

*Odds ratio > 1 denotes a higher likelihood of PCI.
[†]Odds ratio calculated for 75th vs. 25th percentile for the respective variable in the cohort.
CABG, coronary artery bypass grafting; EF, ejection fraction; LAD, left anterior descending; LIMA, left internal mammary artery; LMT, left main trunk.
From Brener SJ, Lytle BW, Casserly IP, et al. Predictors of revascularization method and long-term outcome of percutaneous coronary intervention or repeat coronary bypass surgery in patients with multivessel coronary disease and previous coronary bypass surgery. Eur Heart J. 2006;27:413–418.

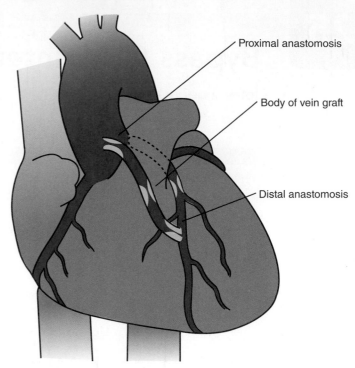

Proximal anastomosis

Body of vein graft

Distal anastomosis

Figure 25-1 Sites of saphenous vein graft stenoses. All lesions between the proximal and distal anastomoses are considered midgraft lesions.

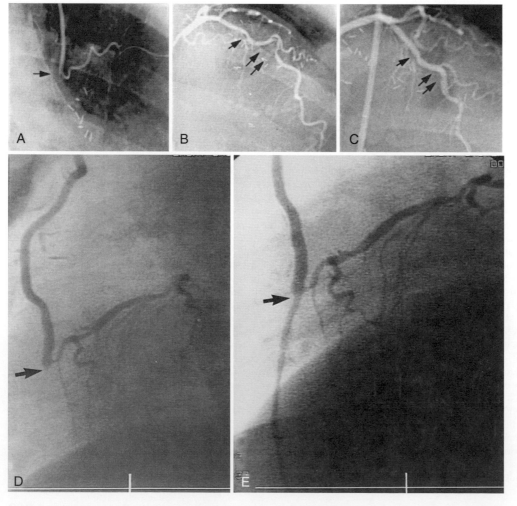

Figure 25-2 Two cases of failure of minimally invasive CABG treated with percutaneous catheter-based intervention. Patient 1: A 78-year-old woman underwent left internal mammary artery (LIMA) to left anterior descending coronary artery (LAD) through a left fourth intercostal incision without cardiopulmonary bypass because of refractory angina and a long stenosis of a tortuous LAD. Angina at rest recurred within a few hours after surgery, and angiography on the second postoperative day revealed occlusion of the LIMA graft about 4 cm from its insertion into the LAD (**A**, arrow). The LAD was tortuous, with multiple, severe stenoses (**B**, arrows), and left ventricular function was normal. Angioplasty and stent implantation in the native vessel yielded an excellent angiographic result (**C**, arrows) and favorable short-term follow-up. Patient 2: Because of disabling angina and a long proximal LAD stenosis, a 60-year-old man underwent minimally invasive LIMA to LAD. About 2 hours after surgery, an ECG showed anterior ST-segment elevation, and emergency coronary arteriography revealed occlusion of the distal LAD at the graft insertion (**D**, left lateral view, arrow). Balloon angioplasty through the LIMA graft was successful (**E**, arrow), and the patient remained asymptomatic at 6-month follow-up.

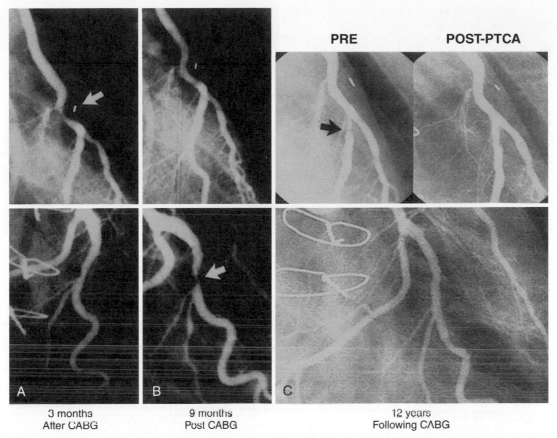

| | PRE | POST-PTCA |

A
3 months
After CABG

B
9 months
Post CABG

C
12 years
Following CABG

Figure 25-3 A 37-year-old woman had placement of saphenous vein grafts to the left anterior descending (LAD) and posterior descending coronary arteries. Unstable angina recurred 3 months later, and high-grade stenosis was present at the junction of the saphenous vein graft to the LAD (**A**, top, arrow). The circumflex coronary artery had minimal disease (**A**, bottom). The saphenous vein graft to the posterior descending coronary artery was patent. Balloon angioplasty of the distal anastomosis was successful. Disabling angina recurred 9 months following CABG. Coronary arteriography (**B**, top) showed a widely patent distal anastomosis but high-grade stenosis of the circumflex coronary artery (**B**, bottom, arrow) unresponsive to nitroglycerin. Balloon angioplasty of the circumflex stenosis was successful (residual stenosis 5%). Twelve years following CABG, angina recurred and recatheterization showed high-grade stenosis of the mid-LAD just beyond the takeoff of a large diagonal (**C**, top left, arrow); the vein graft to the posterior descending coronary artery was occluded. Previous PTCA sites at the distal anastomosis of the vein graft to the LAD and the circumflex artery (**C**, bottom) were widely patent. Balloon angioplasty of the mid-LAD was successful. The patient remained asymptomatic for 4.5 years, when a new thrombotic stenosis in the midportion of the SVG to the LAD led to replacement of this graft with a LIMA. All prior PTCA sites were patent. Surgical benefit was extended over 16 years with three percutaneous procedures.

underwent PCI.[13-15] Graft occlusion or stenosis was present in about 60% of catheterized patients. In 7 patients, focal stenosis was present in a venous or arterial graft distal anastomosis, and balloon dilation across suture lines was safe in these patients. However, in our experience (Fig. 25-2) and in that of others, extreme care is warranted even a few hours after surgery to ensure an intracoronary position of the steerable guidewire. In addition, balloon sizing should be conservative, because we are aware of unreported cases of suture-line disruption and severe hemorrhagic complications. Immediate access to a covered stent is essential should suture line perforation occur. Patients at increased risk for early postoperative ischemia include those undergoing minimally invasive and "off-bypass" techniques and those receiving non-internal mammary artery (IMA) arterial grafts. When ischemia recurs 1 to 12 months after surgery, perianastomotic stenoses are among the most common problems (Fig. 25-3). Stenotic lesions of the distal anastomosis of saphenous vein or arterial grafts can be successfully dilated with balloon angioplasty at this time with little morbidity and good long-term patency in 80% to 90% of patients.[3,17] Stenoses, or in some cases total occlusions, of the middle or distal portions of the IMA or radial artery grafts may be dilated successfully (Fig. 25-4), especially when the presence of a short occlusion can be documented. Stenotic

lesions of mid-SVGs occurring within a year of surgery are usually due to intimal hyperplasia; these lesions can be dilated with balloon angioplasty and/or stented with little risk of distal embolization, but recurrence in about 50% of cases in our experience and periprocedural graft perforation has been observed. Stents, directional atherectomy, and excimer laser angioplasty have all been tried for the treatment of proximal anastomotic lesions with excellent initial results but significant rates of restenosis. There are few data regarding use of drug-eluting stents at this site.

1 TO 3 YEARS AFTER SURGERY

Patients with recurrent ischemia 1 to 3 years after surgery frequently have new stenoses in graft conduits and native coronary arteries that are amenable to percutaneous intervention. Whenever possible, native coronary lesions are targeted. ACC/AHA/SCAI PCI guidelines consider focal ischemia-producing graft lesions in patients 1 to 3 years after CABG with preserved left ventricular function to be a class IIa indication ("conflicting evidence, weight of evidence/opinion in favor of usefulness").

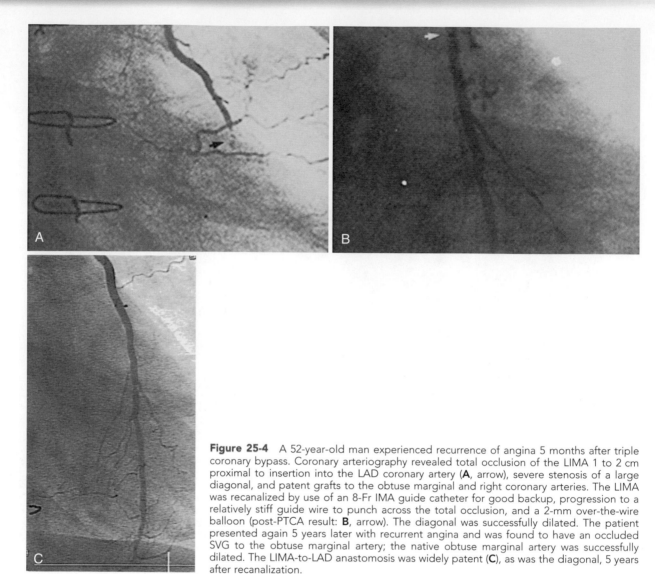

Figure 25-4   A 52-year-old man experienced recurrence of angina 5 months after triple coronary bypass. Coronary arteriography revealed total occlusion of the LIMA 1 to 2 cm proximal to insertion into the LAD coronary artery (**A**, arrow), severe stenosis of a large diagonal, and patent grafts to the obtuse marginal and right coronary arteries. The LIMA was recanalized by use of an 8-Fr IMA guide catheter for good backup, progression to a relatively stiff guide wire to punch across the total occlusion, and a 2-mm over-the-wire balloon (post-PTCA result: **B**, arrow). The diagonal was successfully dilated. The patient presented again 5 years later with recurrent angina and was found to have an occluded SVG to the obtuse marginal artery; the native obtuse marginal artery was successfully dilated. The LIMA-to-LAD anastomosis was widely patent (**C**), as was the diagonal, 5 years after recanalization.

MORE THAN 3 YEARS AFTER SURGERY

Beginning about 3 years after implantation, atherosclerotic lesions appear in vein grafts with increasing frequency. Unstable ischemic syndromes are common, and aggressive invasive evaluation and therapy are indicated. In about 70% of post-CABG patients presenting with acute coronary syndrome, the culprit lesion is located in a SVG. Atherosclerotic plaques in vein grafts contain foam cells, cholesterol crystals, blood elements, and necrotic debris, with less fibrocollagenous tissue and calcification than is present in native coronary arteries (Fig. 25-5). Consequently the plaques in older vein grafts may be softer and more friable as well as being larger than those observed in native coronary arteries, and they frequently have associated thrombus formation (Fig. 25-6). Atheroembolism related to graft intervention may have catastrophic consequences. Consequently bulky vein graft lesions (those with a large potential atheroma mass) should be avoided if possible and embolic protection utilized if not. Improved initial outcome has been reported with stent placement compared with balloon dilation in SVGs. However, long-term results in SVGs, even with stents, have been disappointing. Data on long-term outcomes with drug-eluting stents in SVGs are limited (see below). The role of percutaneous techniques in totally occluded SVGs is controversial. Balloon angioplasty alone has resulted in high complication rates and low patency in most reports. Unfortunately,

prolonged intracoronary thrombolytic therapy has been associated with thromboembolic MI, hemorrhagic complications, and relatively low long-term patency. ACC/AHA/SCAI guidelines consider chronically occluded SVG intervention to be a class III indication ("procedure not useful, may be harmful").

ACUTE MI

After coronary bypass surgery, approximately 3% of patients experience acute MI annually. Because these patients were excluded from early reperfusion trials, therapy has been based on clinical experience and remains controversial. Reports from the National Registry of Myocardial Infarction-2 indicate that patients with prior bypass surgery have a high in-hospital mortality with reperfusion strategies, probably attributable to the presence of multivessel disease, prior MI, advanced age, and comorbidity. In 50% to 70% of patients, the culprit vessel has been found to be a vein graft, and considerable lesion-associated thrombus was a common accompaniment. Intravenous thrombolytic therapy is less effective in SVGs.[18] Most investigators currently favor emergency coronary arteriography if it is feasible, and the option of more specific intervention, including thrombectomy and mechanical recanalization. Kahn and associates[19] reported experience with 72 postbypass patients who underwent direct PCI without

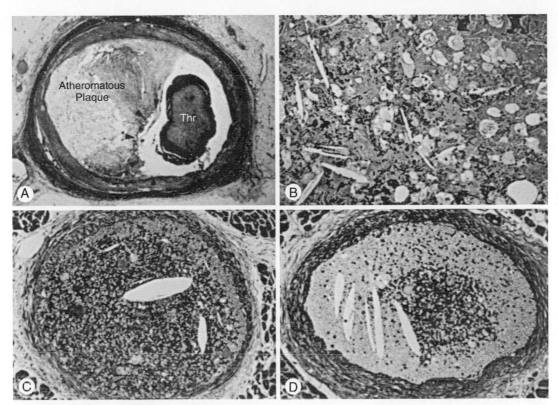

Figure 25-5 **A** and **B**. Vein graft. A. Low-power photomicrograph shows rupture (arrowheads) of atheromatous plaque caused by balloon angioplasty and secondary thrombosis (Thr). Sections taken at adjacent sites were involved by such extensive disruption that luminal boundaries were obliterated. **B**. High power photomicrograph demonstrates nature of plaque, with foam cells, cholesterol clefts, blood elements, and necrotic debris. **C** and **D**. Intramural coronary artery branches. Atheromatous emboli obstruct vessels in anterolateral (**C**) and inferoseptal (**D**) walls of left ventricle (compare with B). *(From Saber RS, Edwards WD, Holmes DR Jr, et al. Balloon angioplasty of aortocoronary saphenous vein bypass grafts: A histopathologic study of six grafts from five patients, with emphasis on restenosis and embolic complications. J Am Coll Cardiol 1988;12:1501–1509.)*

antecedent thrombolytic therapy. There were no urgent bypass operations, strokes, or transfusions. In-hospital survival was 90%. However, in a more recent report of 58 post-CABG patients treated with primary PCI for acute MI in PAMI II, the infarct vessel was a bypass graft in 55% and outcomes were less favorable than in 1,042 patients without prior CABG. At the Mayo Clinic, worse outcomes were also reported in 128 post-CABG patients, about one-third of whom were treated with stents.[20] The ACC/AHA Task Force Report on Early Management of Acute Myocardial Infarction classified primary percutaneous transluminal coronary angioplasty (PTCA) for vein graft recanalization to be a class IIa intervention that is "acceptable, of uncertain efficacy and may be controversial; weight of evidence in favor of usefulness/efficacy."[21]

Technical Strategy

The postoperative patient offers unique challenges to the PCI operator. The selection of a guide catheter to achieve coaxial alignment and provide adequate backup support is often the key to success. Figure 25-7 illustrates the shapes of guide catheters that are commonly used for vein graft interventions; 7-Fr catheters are favored for many vein graft procedures (for optimal visualization, to facilitate stenting, and to accommodate large balloons; embolic protection devices and covered stents are needed to treat bypass graft perforations). Although some have recommended routine use of slightly oversized balloons and stents for vein graft procedures, it is prudent to "size" balloons and stents no larger than the normal reference segment. This is especially true in older vein grafts, in which vein graft rupture has been reported with modest oversizing. In addition, Iakovau et al. reported no benefit of oversizing with respect to target vessel revascularization (TVR)

(31% vs. 26%, $P = 0.3$), and MI was increased (29% vs. 17%, $P < 0.05$).[22] Pichard and colleagues have interestingly reported favorable outcomes using undersized stents in SVGs.[23] In general, most experienced operators stent from "normal to normal." When vein grafts encircling the heart are encountered or in the case of IMA grafts to far distal locations, balloon catheters with extra-long (145-cm) shafts (or shorter guide catheters) may be needed, or the guide catheter can be shortened and a flared, short sheath one size smaller used to close the cut end of the catheter. Embolic protection strategies, a class I indication in PCI guidelines for de novo SVG lesions, have been shown to reduce atheroembolic myocardial infarction by approximately 50% (see "Results," below) and should be used routinely in PCI of de novo SVG lesions.

Results of Intervention

PCI VERSUS REOPERATION

At Emory University between 1980 and 1994, a total of 2,613 postbypass patients underwent catheter-based myocardial revascularization. Compared with 1,561 patients treated with reoperative surgery, in-hospital outcomes were more favorable for mortality (1.1% vs. 6.9%; $P < 0.001$), Q-wave infarction (1.4% vs. 5.4%; $P < 0.001$), stroke (0% vs. 2.8%; $P = 0.27$), length of stay (3.0 vs. 10.5 days; $P < 0.001$), and costs ($8,500 vs. $24,200; $P < 0.01$); in-hospital CABG was required in 2.9% of angioplasty patients. Ten-year survival was better in the angioplasty group. By 5 years, approximately 50% of the angioplasty patients required either repeated PCI or CABG, and survival was better in patients who underwent native vessel compared with graft interventions—an observation not confirmed in the Mayo Clinic

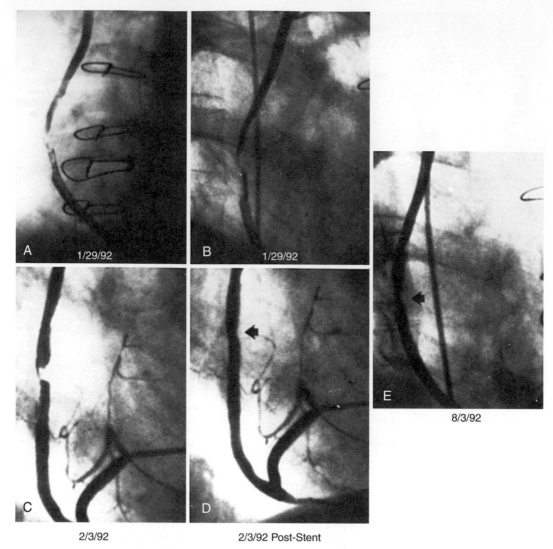

Figure 25-6 A 59-year-old man developed unstable angina 10 years after coronary bypass surgery. **A.** Coronary arteriography revealed high-grade stenosis with thrombus and poor flow in a sequential SVG to the posterior descending and circumflex coronary arteries. No narrowing was present in the left anterior descending coronary artery, diagonal, and large anterior marginal systems. The inferior left ventricular wall was moderately hypokinetic. **B.** After infusion of thrombolytic agent into the graft for approximately 1 hour, flow improved and thrombus was diminished. The patient was maintained on intravenous heparin for 5 days. **C.** Coronary arteriography then showed that an eccentric, high-grade focal stenosis was present in the proximal SVG to the right coronary artery without thrombus. **D.** After placement of a 4.0-mm stent (arrow), the patient became asymptomatic. **E.** Protocol-mandated recatheterization 6 months later revealed excellent patency of the SVG with mild narrowing of approximately 40% at the stent site (arrow). At last follow-up 10 months after intervention, the patient remained asymptomatic. Although the outcome of this patient was favorable, the current availability of thrombectomy and methods of embolic protection make a more direct approach appealing in some patients with extensive SVG thrombus.

experience after correction for baseline differences.[6] In 2,191 post-CABG patients who underwent multivessel revascularization at the Cleveland Clinic between 1995 and 2000, a total of 1,487 had reoperation and 704 PCI.[8] Initial outcomes were more favorable with PCI for completeness of revascularization, 30-day mortality, periprocedural Q-wave infarction, and stroke. At 5 years, unadjusted survival was 79% for CABG and 75% for PCI, $P = 0.008$. The only randomized comparison of PCI and CABG in postbypass patients was reported by Morrison et al., who randomized 143 patients (67 to PCI and 75 to CABG).[24] At 3 years, survival was approximately 75%, comparable to the 5-year survival in the Cleveland Clinic study; there was no significant advantage of one procedure over the other. An Emory University experience with 1,712 diabetic patients who required repeat revascularization between 1985 and 1999 (1,123 with PCI, 589 with reoperation) indicated relatively poor-long term outcomes. Survival at 5 years with PCA and reoperation was about 60%.[25]

VEIN GRAFT BALLOON ANGIOPLASTY

Although PCI for native vessel stenoses has been firmly established and enhanced with drug-eluting stents, conduit lesion interventions have been more controversial. In reports of more than 2,000 patients who underwent balloon angioplasty of SVGs, emergency coronary bypass surgery was needed in 0.3% to 5%; Q-wave MI occurred in 0% to 2.5%; and overall mortality was 0.8%. The most common complication encountered was non-Q-wave MI, which occurred in 13% of 599 patients undergoing 672 vein graft dilations at Emory University. Many of the patients in early series had relatively ideal lesions that were discrete and free of thrombus. Subsequent cardiac events, however, were common. Even when balloon angioplasty of mid-SVG sites was deemed optimal, about half required reintervention within a year in some studies. In 599 consecutive patients who underwent balloon dilation of SVGs at Emory University, 5-year survival was 81%; MI-free survival, 62%; and MI-free, repeated

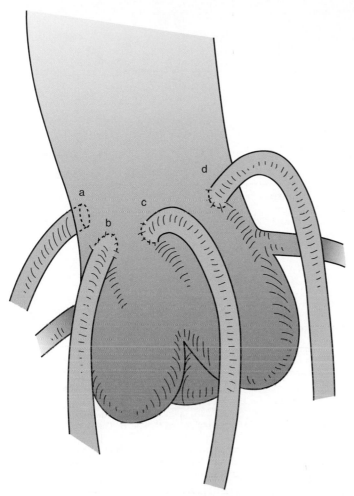

Figure 25-7 Selection of guide catheters in vein graft angioplasty. Obtaining adequate backup becomes more difficult in positions c and d. **A.** Multipurpose shape. **B.** multipurpose, right Judkins. **C.** Hockey stick, left Amplatz, right Judkins. **D.** Hockey stick, left Amplatz.

revascularization-free survival, 31%. Restenosis occurred in 68% of proximal lesions, 61% of midvein graft lesions, and 45% of distal anastomotic lesions. The best long-term results with vein graft interventions occurred with stenoses at the distal implantation site within 1 year of surgery, wherein restenosis was noted in only 22% of patients and late events were rare.

VEIN GRAFT ATHEROABLATION

In an attempt to improve outcome of interventions in SVGs, directional atherectomy was performed initially in observational trials, with encouraging results. However, in a randomized multicenter trial of coronary angioplasty versus directional atherectomy for SVG lesions involving approximately 300 patients, atherectomy was associated with more complications, higher cost, and similar restenosis at 6 months. These factors resulted in a decreased use of directional atherectomy for saphenous vein lesions. Excimer laser angioplasty of SVGs has been reported in several large multicenter trials. In more than 500 lesions, clinical success was achieved in 92% with in-hospital death in 1%, CABG in 1.6%, Q-wave infarction in 2.4%, and non-Q-wave infarction in 2.2%. In 106 consecutive patients subjected to quantitative analysis of procedural and follow-up angiograms, restenosis was noted in 52%, with approximately half having total occlusion, and 1-year mortality was 9%. These observational results have not supported widespread applications of excimer laser angioplasty in SVG lesions.

BARE METAL STENTS

Many different stent designs have been used in SVGs. The self-expanding Wallstent, in our experience, resulted in successful deployment in more than 95% of patients, but stent thrombosis was reported in up to 10% and restenosis in up to 50%. Use of the Palmaz-Schatz coronary stent in SVGs was reported in observational registries, in nonrandomized comparative studies, and in a randomized trial comparing balloon angioplasty with stents.[26] The multicenter registry of the use of the Palmaz-Schatz stent in the United States enrolled 589 patients and reported procedural success in 97%, stent thrombosis in 1.4%, in-hospital mortality in 1.7%, Q-wave infarction in 0.3%, and urgent bypass surgery in 0.9%. Restenosis at 6 months was 18% for de novo lesions and 46% for those with prior procedures, and 12-month event-free survival was 76%. These results were more favorable than in the subsequent randomized trial. In 320 consecutive patients who underwent stenting of SVG aorto-ostial lesions, 43% of whom had debulking (laser or atherectomy) before stent implantation, it was noted that debulking before stenting afforded no benefit regarding complications, 1-year target lesion revascularization, or cardiac event-free survival. A total of 220 patients with new SVG lesions and angina pectoris or objective evidence of myocardial ischemia were randomly assigned to implantation of Palmaz-Schatz stents or standard balloon angioplasty in the SAVED (Saphenous Vein De novo) trial.[26] Patients with lesion length greater than two stents, MI within 7 days, or evidence of intragraft thrombus were excluded. Stented patients received warfarin anticoagulation. Patients assigned to stenting had a higher rate of procedural efficacy, defined as a reduction of stenosis to less than 50% of the vessel diameter with the assigned therapy, than did those assigned to angioplasty (Fig. 25-8), but they experienced more hemorrhagic complications resulting from warfarin anticoagulation. In-hospital complications were otherwise similar in the two groups, although there was a trend toward fewer non-Q-wave infarctions in the stent group. Whether stents have a significant effect in reducing particulate matter embolization is not certain, but it is a possible explanation for this trend. Restenosis occurred in 37% of the stented patients and in 46% of the angioplasty group ($P = 0.24$). Late lumen loss was significantly greater in patients who received high-pressure (≥ 16 atm) stent expansion, suggesting that routine high pressure may be undesirable in SVG stenting. The outcome in the SAVED trial with respect to freedom from death, MI, repeated bypass surgery, or revascularization was significantly better in the stent group (73% vs. 58%; $P = 0.03$). The lack of a significant difference in restenosis rates in the treatment groups was due to the greater late lumen loss in the stent group and the small sample size. Several centers have reported outcomes of more contemporary SVG interventions, but these studies were performed prior to embolic protection and drug-eluting stents. Comparing outcomes of 1990–1994 patients with 1995–1998 patients, Hong and colleagues reported similar initial success rates but improved 1-year event-free survival in the more recent experience (71% vs. 59%; $P < 0.0001$), lower late mortality (6.1% vs. 11.3%; $P < 0.0001$), and a protective effect of stent implantation in both time periods.[27] Five-year outcome data from Emory University in 2,556 patients who underwent PCI of SVGs emphasized the poorer outcome of diabetic compared to nondiabetic patients with respect to survival and event-free survival (Fig. 25-9A and B).[28] When only the patients receiving bare metal stents were considered, in-hospital outcomes among diabetic and nondiabetic patients were not significantly different, but survival was worse in diabetics. Kaplan-Meier survival curves are shown in Figure 25-9C.

DRUG-ELUTING STENTS

Although bare metal stents improve the initial and intermediate-term outcomes of SVG PCI, the impact is modest owing to restenosis and disease progression. A number of published reports of the use of drug-eluting stents (DESs) in SVGs have shown conflicting results, leading some to question their use for this indication.[29] In the first of two

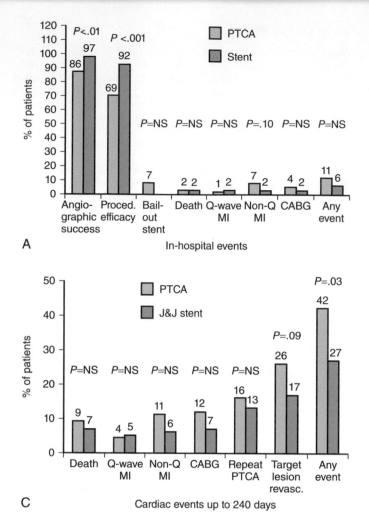

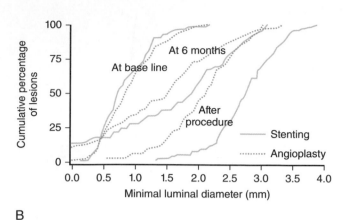

Figure 25-8 Results from the SAVED trial, a randomized comparison of Palmaz-Schatz stenting and standard balloon angioplasty.[26] **A.** Stents were associated with a higher procedural success rate, whereas other in-hospital events were similar. **B.** The minimal luminal diameter at 6 months was larger in the stent group (1.73 vs. 1.49 mm; *P* = 0.01). **C.** Late cardiac events were significantly more common in patients in the PTCA group. (*From Savage MP, Douglas JS Jr, Fischman DL, et al. Stent placement compared with balloon angioplasty for obstructed coronary bypass grafts. Saphenous Vein De novo Trial Investigators. N Engl J Med 1997;337:740–747.*)

randomized comparisons of DESs with bare metal stents (BMSs) in SVGs, Vermeersch et al. implanted sirolimus-eluting stents (SESs) in 38 patients and BMSs in 37. At 6 months, patients receiving SESs had less restenosis (14% versus 33%, *P* = 0.03) and TLR (5% vs. 22%, *P* = 0.047) but similar rates of death and MI.[30] At a median follow-up of 32 months, "late catch up" had occurred and TVR rates were comparable.[31] A second randomized trial compared the outcomes of 41 patients treated with paclitaxel-eluting stents (PESs) with 39 treated with BMSs.[32] Angiographic restenosis at 1 year occurred in 57% of BMS-treated SVGs and 11% of PES-treated with SVGs (*P* < 0.0001), and target lesion revascularization was significantly less common with PES at 1.5 years (5% vs. 28%, *P* = 0.003).[32,33] Several observational registries have been reported describing outcomes of SVG stenting in larger groups of patients followed for up to 3 years.[34–36] These reports, which suffer the limitations of observation data, suggest that DESs in SVG are safe but that benefit in terms of reduced restenosis and need for repeat revascularization during the first year may be lost at 2 to 3 years. In the largest of these studies, even the benefit of lower TVR at 9 months was confined to patients with an SVG diameter <3.5 mm.[34] Roughly 15% of stented SVGs occlude during the first year, thus confounding the assessment of whether the loss of early benefit is due to progression at the stent or at nontarget sites. It has been recognized for almost 3 decades that SVGs may deteriorate rapidly once stenoses begin to occur.[3] Ellis and colleagues reported that patients with moderate untreated SVG lesions had a 45% cardiac event rate compared with 2% in patients without them; these investigators proposed a strategy of "sealing" moderate SVG lesions with stents.[37] Rodes-Cabau et al. extended these ideas in a randomized angiographic and intravascular

ultrasound (IVUS) pilot trial, finding that sealing moderate SVG lesions with PESs safely reduced SVG disease progression and resulted in a trend toward fewer cardiac events at 1 year (3% vs. 19%, *P* = 0.09).[38] This small pilot trial sets the stage for a larger randomized clinical trial, which will be needed to determine the place of this strategy. The data at present indicate that DESs in SVGs are safe; the occurrence of death or MI is equal or less than with BMSs, and there is no difference in stent thrombosis. Choosing DESs over BMSs for the treatment of severe focal SVG stenoses must depend on the assurance of reliable dual antiplatelet therapy and be favored in SVGs < 3.5 mm in diameter and in patients at high risk for restenosis (long lesions, diabetics). The significant occurrence of adverse cardiac events after SVG stenting (annual mortality of 5%-10%, SVG occlusion in 15%) indicates a need for native vessel PCI when possible.

EMBOLIC PROTECTION

Recently, attention has refocused on the importance of periprocedural elevations of CK-MB and troponin, which indicate myocardial necrosis most often due to atheroembolism. Even when mostly straightforward single-lesion, single-stent SVG PCI procedures were carried out prior to the availability of embolic protection, significant creatine kinase elevations were noted in 20% of patients (Fig. 25-5). The rate of myocardial infarction and procedural risk were shown to increase with lesion complexity, length, and estimated plaque volume.[39] In over 1,000 patients who underwent SVG stenting, CK-MB elevation was the most powerful predictor of late mortality. The key role played by atheroembolization and confirmation of effective protective strategies

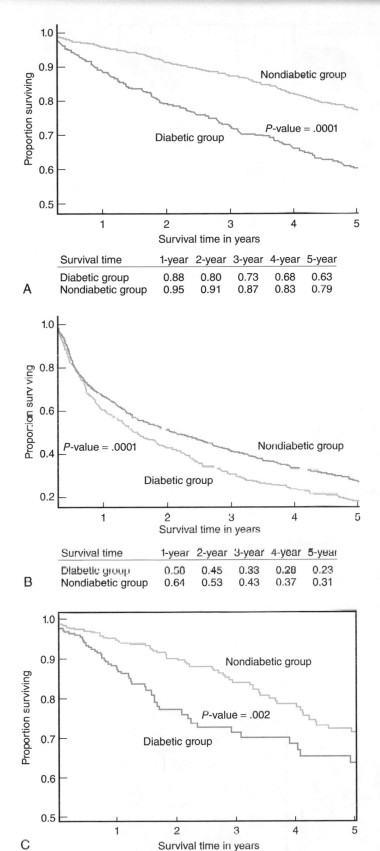

Figure 25-9 **A.** Kaplan-Meier curves showing survival free of death in 2,556 patients who underwent PCI at Emory University Hospital comparing 5 year outcomes of non-diabetics with those with treated diabetes.[28] **B.** Kaplan-Meier curves showing survival free of death, MI, or repeat revascularization. **C.** Kaplan-Meier curves showing survival free of death in 1,045 patients who underwent bare metal stent implantation in SVGs. *(From Ashfaq S, Ghazzal Z, Douglas JS, et al. Impact of diabetes on five-year outcomes after vein graft intervention performed prior to the drug-eluting stent era. J Invas Cardiol 2006;18:100–105.)*

were the products of several observational and randomized studies.[40] The Guardwire system (Medtronic Vascular, Santa Rosa, CA) utilized a hollow 0.014-inch wire incorporating a compliant, inflatable distal occlusion balloon (Fig. 25-10). During inflation of the distally placed balloon, flow in the graft was interrupted; the stent was then implanted, followed by aspiration of the graft using a special monorail catheter and deflation of the balloon, restoring flow. The effectiveness of this strategy in a broad range of patients was confirmed in the SAFER (Saphenous Vein Graft Angioplasty Free of Emboli Randomized) trial, where 801 patients were randomly assigned to stent implantation with or without use of the Guardwire distal protection.[41] Thirty-day major adverse cardiovascular events (MACE) were reduced by 42% with use of the Guardwire (16.5% to 9.6%, $P = 0.004$) primarily because of the lower rates of MI. The Guardwire system, frequently applicable even in the presence of severe stenosis owing to its relatively low profile, captures small particles and soluble vasoactive agents such as endothelin and serotonin and a variety of coagulation components that have been shown to be liberated during SVG PCI. Removal of these vasoactive substances may contribute to improved immediate post-PCI coronary flow and myocardial perfusion. Analysis of the benefit of the Guardwire in relation to lesion length in SAFER showed that even with lesions <10 mm in length, a 77% reduction in 30-day MACE was experienced (2.2% vs 8.1%). The use of the Guardwire increased costs at 30 days by less than $650 per patient, with a cost-effectiveness ratio of $3,700 per year of life, making it highly cost-effective. Disadvantages of the Guardwire include the need to completely occlude the target SVG during stent deployment and aspiration (not always well tolerated), a requirement for a relatively long "parking" segment distal to the lesion, inability to protect side branches, and the complexity of the system. A variety of filters have been applied to SVG interventions (Fig. 25-11). In a 651-patient randomized multicenter trial, the Filter Wire (Boston Scientific, Natick, MA) was compared with the Guardwire. Thirty-day MACE, the primary endpoint, was similar; 9.9% with Filter compared to 11.6% with the Guardwire, and there was no difference in rates of death or MI. Some of the advantages of filters include ease of use, avoidance of ischemia because of preserved coronary flow, and good visualization. Disadvantages include the need to cross the lesion with a somewhat bulky filter, which may cause embolization or require predilation; these sequelae have been shown to increase the occurrence of Q-wave MI. In addition, particles smaller than the 100-micron pore size and soluble agents may not be captured. The former may not be relevant based on studies reporting that filtering was just as efficient as balloon occlusion in particle capture despite pore sizes larger than the majority of embolic particles. Other problems with filters include the long distal parking segment required and the potential for overwhelming the filter, resulting in diminished antegrade flow mimicking no reflow. The optimal strategy should this occur is to aspirate the stagnant dye column, which may contain suspended debris, followed by filter removal and replacement if more interventional work is needed. When the TriActiv distal occlusion balloon device, which incorporates active flush and aspiration (Kensey Nash, Exton, PA), was compared with either the Guardwire or Filter wire, MACE was similar, indicating noninferiority. Proximal protection with the Proxis system (St. Jude, St. Paul, MN) is applicable when there is insufficient room beyond the lesion for distal protection. Proxis involves placement of a hydrophilic coated sheath into the proximal SVG (Fig. 25-12). Inflation of a compliant balloon

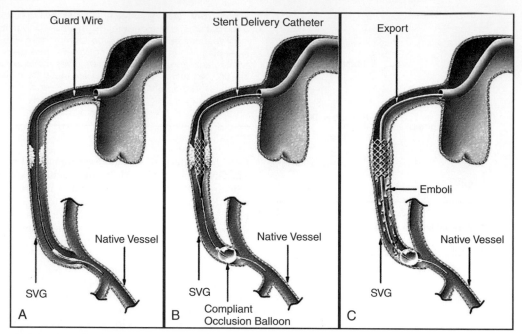

Figure 25-10 The Guardwire device for distal embolic protection. **A.** The lesion is crossed and balloon positioned distally. **B.** Following balloon occlusion the stent is deployed. **C.** The occluded SVG is aspirated, followed by deflation of the distal occlusion balloon, which restores flow.

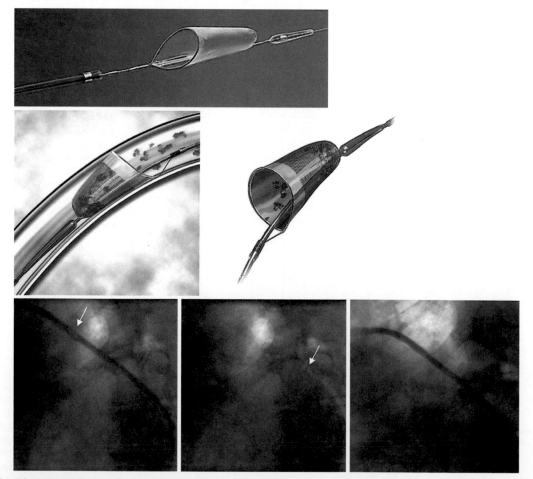

Figure 25-11 The Filter wire. Top panel. The polyurethane nonocclusive filter with 110 micron pore size mounted on a nitinol loop fixed to a guidewire. Middle, left panel. The filter is deployed distal to the lesion and the nitinol expanded to the size of the vessel (3.0 to 5.5 mm). Middle, right panel. Filter removed with large embolic load. Bottom, left panel. Thrombus containing SVG lesion. Bottom, middle panel. Deployed filter. Bottom, right panel. Excellent result post-stenting. *(From Gorog DA, Foale RA, Malik I, et al. Distal myocardial protection during percutaneous coronary intervention. When and where? J Am Coll Cardiol 2005;46:1434–1445.)*

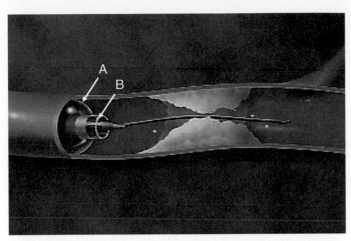

Figure 25-12 The Proxis device consists of a hydrophilic sheath. It is placed into the proximal SVG, followed by inflation of the sealing balloon (A), which occludes the SVG. The lesion is crossed with a guidewire; the lesion is then stented and debris is aspirated by reversing flow in the SVG (B).

surrounding this sheath occludes the vein graft; stent implantation can then be carried out, followed by flow-reversal aspiration of the SVG and subsequent balloon deflation, restoring flow. When Proxis was compared with either Filter wire or Guardwire in a randomized trial, MACE was comparable (9.2% vs. 10%, P = NS). Advantages of the Proxis device include the ability to institute embolic protection before the lesion is crossed with a guidewire, to protect side branches, and to handle large embolic loads; also, the operator can use the guidewire of choice, but the most proximal SVG segment must be disease-free and, of course, the graft must be occluded during the procedure for several minutes. Other filters that have undergone evaluation include the SPIDER (eV3, Plymouth, MN) which was tested in a 732-patient randomized trial, with 30-day MACE, the primary endpoint, occurring in 9.2% of the SPIDER arm and 8.7% of the approved control device arm, indicating noninferiority.

In an analysis of SVG stenting in 3,958 patients from six studies, angiographic variables were potent predictors of 30-day MACE.[40] SVG degeneration score and large estimated plaque volume were the most potent predictors; thrombus, advanced patient age, and active tobacco use also contributed. When the occurrence of MACE was analyzed relative to degeneration score or plaque volume, the use of embolic protection had similar relative treatment benefit across all categories of risk. The almost halving of MACE associated with embolic protection across all risk strata strongly supports its routine use in all PCIs of old SVGs. This contrasts sharply with current practice, where embolic protection is used in only half of SVG PCI procedures (see Chapter 29 for more information regarding embolic protection).

ADJUNCTIVE PHARMACOTHERAPY

Accepted adjunctive therapy during PCI of native and SVG PCI includes antithrombotic measures (aspirin, antithrombin, other antiplatelet agents) and vascular dilators as needed for the prevention and treatment of slow or no reflow. Unfractionated heparin was used in the vast majority of SVG studies reported. Among the 403 SVG patients in REPLACE 1 and 2 randomized to heparin or bivalirudin, logistic regression analysis revealed no difference in the combined endpoint (death, MI, urgent revascularization, or major bleeding), but there was less minor bleeding with bivalirudin.[42] However, a somewhat increased risk of perforation with SVGs makes the use of bivalirudin less appealing in this group of patients. Optimal clopidogrel dosing and duration of therapy following SVG PCI have not been studied. The relatively large embolic burden encountered in SVG procedures provides some explanation of the failure of glycoprotein IIb/IIIa platelet receptor

inhibitors to prevent periprocedural MI in these patients.[40] When data from five large trials (EPIC, EPILOG, EPISTENT, IMPACT II, and PURSUIT) with a total of over 600 SVG PCI patients and data from the Cleveland Clinic registry were analyzed, there was no apparent benefit from IIb/IIIa inhibitors.[40] The use of microvascular dilators to treat no or slow reflow following PCI or prophylactically before the procedure has not been well studied but is an important strategy in SVG PCI (see discussion of no-reflow below).

RESTENOSIS LESIONS IN SVGS

The management of patients with restenosis of SVG stent sites is a topic of considerable interest and a significant clinical problem. As is true in native coronary intervention, treatment of in-stent restenotic lesions in SVGs is safer than treatment of de novo SVG lesions primarily because of reductions in "slow, no reflow" and periprocedural MI. In a double-blind randomized trial including 120 patients with in-stent restenosis receiving gamma radiation with ^{192}Ir or placebo, Waksman reported significantly lower restenosis in the irradiated group at 6 months compared with the control group and a 79% reduction in the need for repeat intervention.[43] However, intracoronary brachytherapy is not currently available in most centers and DESs have become the default strategy in spite of a paucity of data to support this application.

INTERNAL MAMMARY ARTERY GRAFTS

In contrast to SVGs, favorable results have been reported with balloon dilation of IMA graft stenoses. Lesions at the anastomosis of arterial grafts with the native coronary artery behave much like distal anastomotic lesions of SVGs. They usually occur within a few months of surgery and often respond to low-pressure balloon inflations. Successful dilation and stenting of ostial or extremely proximal IMA graft lesions is infrequently required. In a report of PCI of 32 IMA graft lesions, 12 were in the midportion of the artery and 20 were at the anastomosis.[17] Success was obtained in over 90% of approximately 1,000 patients in over 20 reports in the literature. Complications were infrequent, the most common being IMA dissection and spasm. Among 68 patients, 78% had follow-up angiography at a mean of 8 months; restenosis occurred in 15% at the anastomosis of the graft with the coronary artery and in 43% at midgraft. There are no very large series or long-term data regarding stenting in IMA grafts or PCI in gastroepiploic or radial artery grafts.

▓ Complications

Given the known increased risk of coronary bypass reoperation, there has been concern that emergency reoperation for failed PCI would be associated with markedly increased risk. At Emory University from 1980 to 1989, a total of 1,263 patients with prior coronary bypass surgery underwent elective percutaneous intervention; of these patients, 46 (3.6%) underwent reoperation for failed PCI.[44] Three patients (6.5%) died and 11 (24%) had nonfatal Q-wave MI. Actuarial 3-year survival for the 46 patients was 91%. Considering these factors and the high recurrence rate following PCI, some authors have concluded that percutaneous intervention in patients with prior CABG should be restricted to focal lesions in four angiographic situations: (1) unbypassed native coronary artery, (2) distal anastomoses that are less than 3 years old, (3) SVGs less than 3 years old, and (4) distal native coronary artery lesions reached through fully patent grafts.[5] The ACC/AHA/SCAI PCI guidelines are more permissive, however; they extend indications for intervention to include older SVGs, especially when reoperation is not an excellent option.[16]

PERFORATION

Coronary artery perforation is a potential complication of all coronary interventions. It has been attributed to vessel wall penetration with guidewires, inflation of a balloon in a subintimal location or overexpansion of a coronary artery or graft, atheroablative techniques, and stent implantation. SVG perforation is a rare complication of balloon angioplasty. Prolonged balloon inflation and reversal of anticoagulation are effective in stabilizing most patients. However, in spite of the absence of pericardium and the scarring that is present after bypass surgery, vessel perforation may result in extensive hemorrhage, vessel occlusion, and cardiac tamponade, necessitating emergency surgery. Covered stents have had an increasing role in the treatment of perforation. In one report of 35 perforations, a polytetrafluoroethylene (PTFE)-covered stent was successful in sealing 100%.[45] Because of their large diameter, SVGs are favorable conduits for use of this strategy for sealing perforations. Although the use of oversized balloons has been advocated for vein graft dilations, older vein grafts may rupture with only modest oversizing; rupture was documented to occur in one patient with a balloon-to-SVG ratio of 1.1 : 1. Because of this potential risk, it seems wise to size balloons and stents to the normal adjacent vessel or slightly smaller.[23]

NO REFLOW

The cause of slow or no reflow following SVG PCI is multifactoral and probably includes vasospasm and embolization of atheromatous debris and thrombus. The importance of microvascular spasm is suggested by the observation that vasoconstrictors are released during SVG stent procedures, by the reduction in no-reflow when a calcium channel blocker is administrered before SVG PCI, by the apparent treatment effect of small vessel dilators (calcium channel blockers, adenosine, nitroprusside), and by the lack of benefit of nitroglycerin.[46,47] The dominant role of atheroembolism is apparent from the studies of embolic protection and pathology (Fig. 25-5).[40]

The Future of Bypass Graft Intervention

Thorny issues related to bypass graft intervention occupy both ends of the temporal spectrum. Intraoperative angiography has identified significant bypass graft imperfections, the treatment of which may enhance graft patency, improve clinical outcomes, and reduce the need for subsequent ischemia-driven repeat revascularization. Is the information gained worth the added cost? Or is a low threshold for ischemia-driven early angiography sufficient? SVG PCI is encumbered by atheroembolic myocardial infarction and high subsequent cardiac events due to restenosis and progressive vein graft disease. However, embolic protection strategies documented to be beneficial across the entire range of risk strata are markedly underutilized. Will physician education be sufficient to change this practice? Or are technical improvements necessary before wide-scale use occurs? Are DESs sufficiently effective in SVGs to warrant the increased cost associated with their use? Is one DES more effective than others? The data are not compelling. And finally, can disease progression in nontarget sites be retarded? Will the use of "plaque sealing" of moderate SVG lesions by DES implantation, which appeared promising in a pilot trial, be tested in the multicenter study required to corroborate these findings? In the future of bypass graft intervention, there are more questions than answers.

REFERENCES

1. Hannan EL, Kilburn H, O'Donnell JF, et al: Adult open heart surgery in New York State. JAMA 264:2768–2774, 1990.
2. Gruentzig AR, Senning A, Siegenthaler WE: Nonoperative dilatation of coronary-artery stenosis: percutaneous transluminal coronary angioplasty. N Engl J Med 301:61–68, 1979.
3. Douglas JS, Jr, Gruentzig AR, King SB, III, et al: Percutaneous transluminal coronary angioplasty in patients with prior coronary bypass surgery. J Am Coll Cardiol 2:745–754, 1983.
4. Douglas JS, Jr, King SB, III, Roubin GS: Percutaneous transluminal coronary angioplasty in patients with prior coronary artery bypass grafting. J Thorac Cardiovasc Surg 93:272–275.7, 1987.
5. Loop FD, Whitlow PL: Coronary angioplasty in patients with previous bypass surgery. J Am Coll Cardiol 16:1348–1350.9, 1990.
6. Mathew V, Clavell AL, Lennon RJ, et al: Percutaneous coronary interventions in patients with prior coronary bypass surgery: changes in patient characteristics and outcome during two decades. Am J Med 108:127–135, 2000.
7. Subramanian S, Sabik JF III, Houghtaling PL, et al: Decision-making for patients with patent left internal thoracic artery grafts to left anterior descending. Ann Thorac Surg 87:1392–1400, 2009.
8. Brener SJ, Lytle BW, Casserly IP, et al: Predictors of revascularization method and long-term outcome of percutaneous coronary intervention or repeat coronary bypass surgery in patients with multivessel coronary disease and previous coronary bypass surgery. Eur Heart J 27:413–418, 2006.
9. Zhoa DX, Leacche M, Balaguer JM, et al: Routine intraoperative completion angiography after coronary artery bypass grafting and 1-stop hybrid revascularization: results from a fully integrated hybrid catheterization laboratory/operating room. J Am Coll Cardiol 53:232–241, 2009.
10. Alexander JH, Hafley G, Harrington RA, et al: Efficacy and safety of edifoligide, an E2F transcription factor decoy, for prevention of vein graft failure following coronary artery bypass graft surgery: PREVENT IV: a randomized controlled trial. JAMA 294:2446–2454, 2005.
11. Shroyer AL, Grover FL, Hattler B, et al: On-pump versus off-pump coronary-artery bypass surgery. N Engl J Med 361:1827–1837, 2009.
12. Glineur D, D'hoore W, El Khoury G, et al: Angiographic predictors of 6-month patency of bypass grafts implanted to the right coronary artery. J Am Coll Cardiol 51:120–125, 2008.
13. Reifart N, Haase J, Storger H, et al: Interventional standby for cardiac surgery. Circulation 94(Suppl I):I–86, 1996.
14. Rasmussen C, Thiis JJ, Clemmensen P, et al: Management of suspected graft failure in coronary artery bypass grafting. Circulation 94(Suppl I):I–413, 1996.
15. Cutlip DE, Dauerman HL, Carrozza JP: Recurrent ischemia within thirty days of coronary artery bypass surgery: angiographic findings and outcome of percutaneous revascularization. Circulation 94(Suppl I):I-249, 1996.

16. Smith SC, Jr, Feldman TE, Hirschfeld JW, et al: ACC/AHA/SCAI 2005 guideline update for percutaneous intervention: a report of the American College of Cardiology/American Heart Association Task Force on the Guidelines (ACC/AHA/SCAI Writing Committee to Update the 2001 Guidelines for Percutaneous Coronary Intervention). J Am Coll Cardiol 47:1–121, 2006.
17. Shimshak TM, Giorgi LV, Johnson WL, et al: Application of percutaneous transluminal coronary angioplasty to the internal mammary artery graft. J Am Coll Cardiol 12:1205–1214, 1988.
18. Grines CL, Booth DC, Nissen SE, et al: Mechanism of acute myocardial infarction in patients with prior coronary artery bypass grafting and therapeutic implications. Am J Cardiol 65:1292–1296, 1990.
19. Kahn JK, Rutherford BD, McConahay DR, et al: Usefulness of angioplasty during acute myocardial infarction in patients with prior coronary artery bypass grafting. Am J Cardiol 65:698–702, 1990.
20. Suwaidi JA, Velianou JL, Berger PB, et al: Primary percutaneous coronary interventions in patients with acute myocardial infarction and prior coronary artery bypass grafting. Am Heart J 142:452–459, 2001.
21. Ryan TJ, Anderson JL, Antman EM, et al: ACC/AHA guidelines for the management of patients with acute myocardial infarction: A report of the American College of Cardiology/American Heart Association Task Force on Practice Guidelines (Committee on Management of Acute Myocardial Infarction). J Am Coll Cardiol 28:1328–1428, 1996.
22. Iakovau I, Dangas G, Mintz GS, et al: Relation of final lumen dimensions in saphenous vein grafts after stent implantation to outcome. Am J Cardiol 93:963, 2004.
23. Hong TJ, Pichard AD, Mintz GS, et al: Outcome of undersized drug-eluting stents for percutaneous coronary intervention of saphenous vein graft lesions. Am J Cardiol 105:179–185, 2010.
24. Morrison DA, Sethi G, Sacks J, et al: Percutaneous coronary intervention versus repeat bypass surgery for patients with medically refractory myocardial ischemia: AWESOME randomized trial and registry experience with post-CABG patients. J Am Coll Cardiol 40:1951–1954, 2002.
25. Cole JH, Jones EL, Craver JM, et al: Outcomes of repeat revascularization in diabetic patients with prior coronary surgery. J Am Coll Cardiol 40:1968–1975, 2002.
26. Savage MP, Douglas JS, Jr, Fischman DL, et al: Stent placement compared with balloon angioplasty for obstructed bypass grafts. Saphenous Vein De novo Trial Investigators. N Engl J Med 337:740–747, 1997.
27. Hong MK, Mehran R, Dangas G, et al: Are we making progress with percutaneous saphenous vein graft treatment? J Am Coll Cardiol 38:150–154, 2001.

28. Ashfaq S, Ghazzal Z, Douglas JS, et al: Impact of diabetes on five-year outcomes after vein graft intervention performed prior to the drug-eluting stent era. J Invas Cardiol 18:100–105, 2006.
29. Douglas JS, Jr: Are our patients better off with drug-eluting stents in saphenous vein grafts? JACC Cardiovasc Intervent 2:1113–1114, 2009.
30. Vermeersh P, Pierfrancesco A, Verheye S, et al: Randomized double-blind comparison of sirolimus-eluting versus bare-metal stent implantation in diseased saphenous vein grafts: six-month angiographic, intravascular ultrasound, and clinical follow-up of the RRISC trial. J Am Coll Cardiol 48:2423–2431, 2006.
31. Vermeesch P, Agostoni P, Verheye S, et al: Increased late mortality after sirolimus-eluting stetns versus bare-metal stents in diseased saphenous vein grafts. J Am Coll Cardiol 50:261–267, 2007.
32. Brilakis ES, Lichtenwalter C, de Lemos JA, et al: A randomized-controlled trial of a paclitaxel-eluting stent versus a similar bare-metal stent in saphenous vein graft lesions: the SOS (Stenting of Saphenous Vein Grafts). J Am Coll Cardiol 53:919–928, 2009.
33. Lichtenwalter C, De Lemos JA, Roesle M, et al: Clinical presentation and angiographic characteristics of saphenous vein graft failure after stenting. J Am Coll Cardiol Intervent. 2:855–860, 2009.
34. Brodie BR, Wilson H, Stuckey T, et al: for the STENT Group. Outcomes with drug-eluting versus bare-metal stents in saphenous vein graft intervention: results from the STENT (Strategic Transcatheter Evaluation of New Therapies) Group. J Am Coll Cardiol Intervent 2:1105–1112, 2009.
35. Latib A, Ferri L, Ielasi A, et al: Comparison of the long-term safety and efficacy of drug-eluting and bare-metal stent implantation in saphenous vein grafts. Circ Cardiovasc Intervent 3:249–256, 2010.
36. Goswami NJ, Gaffigan M, Berrio G, et al: Long-term outcomes of drug-eluting stents versus bare-metal stents in saphenous vein graft disease: results from the Prairie "Real World" Stent Registry. Catheter Cardiovasc Intervent 75:93–100, 2010.
37. Ellis SG, Brener SJ, DeLuca S, et al: Late myocardial ischemic events after saphenous vein graft intervention: importance of initially "non-significant" vein graft lesions. Am J Cardiol 79:1460–1464, 1997.
38. Rodès-Cabau J, Bertrand OF, Larose E, et al: Comparison of plaque sealing with paclitaxel-eluting stents versus medical therapy for the treatment of moderate nonsignificant saphenous vein graft lesions: the Moderate Vein Graft Lesion Stenting With the Taxus Stent and Intravascular Ultrasound (VELETI) Pilot Trial. Circulation 120:1978–1986, 2009.
39. Liu MW, Douglas JS, Jr, Lembo NJ, et al: Angiographic predictors of a rise in serum creatine kinase (distal embolization) after balloon angioplasty of saphenous vein coronary artery bypass grafts. Am J Cardiol 72:514–517, 1993.

40. Coolong A, Baim DS, Kuntz RE, et al: Saphenous vein graft stenting and major adverse cardiac events. A predictive model derived from a pooled analysis of 3,958 patients. *Circulation* 117:790–797, 2008.

41. Baim DS, Wahr D, George B, et al: Randomized trial of a distal embolic protection device during percutaneous intervention of saphenous vein aorto-coronary bypass grafts. *Circulation* 105:512–590, 2002.

42. Kao J, Lincoff AM, Topol EJ, et al: Direct thrombin inhibition appears to be a safe and effective anticoagulant for percutaneous bypass graft interventions. *Catheter Cardiovasc Intervent* 68:352–356, 2006.

43. Waksman R: Intracoronary gamma radiation for in-stent restenosis in saphenous vein grafts: A multicenter randomized clinical trial (SVG WRIST). *Am Coll Cardiol* 38:597, 2001.

44. Weintraub WS, Cohen CL, Curling PE, et al: Results of coronary surgery after failed elective coronary angioplasty in patients with prior coronary surgery. *J Am Coll Cardiol* 16:1341–1347, 1990.

45. Lansky AJ, Stone GW, Grube E, et al: A multicenter registry of the JoStent PTFE stent graft for the treatment of arterial perforations complicating percutaneous coronary interventions. *J Am Coll Cardiol* 35:26A, 2000.

46. Leineweber K, Bose D, Vogelsang M, et al: Intense vasoconstriction in response to aspirate from stented saphenous vein aortocoronary bypass grafts. *J Am Coll Cardiol* 47:981–986, 2006.

47. Hillegass WB, Dean NA, Liao L, et al: Treatment of no-reflow and impaired flow with the nitric oxide donor nitroprusside following percutaneous coronary interventions: initial human clinical experience. *J Am Coll Cardiol* 37:1335–1343, 2001.

The Thrombus-Containing Lesion

ON TOPAZ

Introduction

Thrombus is a hallmark constituent of active, unstable atherosclerotic plaques commonly found in patients with acute coronary syndromes. Over the past three decades, percutaneous coronary intervention (PCI) has achieved high success rates with the ever-increasing inclusion of complex target lesions.[1] However, despite this impressive progress, one critical component, the thrombus, remains a formidable obstacle to revascularization. It continues to constitute a hazardous element whose presence threatens PCI-related major adverse coronary events (MACE), stent thrombosis, increased rate of in-hospital complications, 6-month recurrent MI, and death.[2-6] Consequently thrombus exerts a major impact on the performance and outcome of primary and rescue interventions[7] (Table 26-1), although the optimal treatment of thrombotic lesions is still enigmatic and controversial. The aim of this chapter

is to present the role of thrombus in the pathophysiology of acute coronary syndromes, describe its unique morphology, outline its impact on interventions and outcomes, present available modalities for its identification, delineate pharmacological therapy, and consider the tools and techniques that may be used for thrombus removal. A specific set of challenging thrombus-containing lesions and their management options is highlighted.

Pathophysiology of Thrombus

An understanding of the structure of thrombus and its multifaceted characteristics is essential for making proper management choices in the revascularization of atherosclerotic lesions and vessels. A thrombus-containing lesion is formed when the fibrous cap of an atherosclerotic plaque develops structural defects.[8] Significant adverse morphological changes in the plaque become manifest by erosion, fissure, or rupture. Such weakening of the plaque's integrity exposes the inner necrotic core, which enables the transfer of plaque material into the arterial lumen. Cholesterol crystals inside the plaque also perforate the tunica intima, triggering further disruption, with the crystal content identified as an independent predictor of thrombus and clinical events.[9] The ensuing contact of exposed, disrupted, and highly thrombogenic subendothelial matrix and plaque with circulating platelets and white blood cells activates the coagulation cascade. The resultant platelet adhesion and aggregation lead to thrombus formation (Fig. 26-1). Furthermore, released tissue factor from the arterial injury directly activates the extrinsic coagulation cascade and promotes fibrin formation. Activated platelets release powerful promoters of vasoconstriction and aggregation, including serotonin, adenosine diphosphate, thromboxane A2, oxygen-derived free radicals, endothelin, and platelet activating factor.[10] As the thrombus accumulates to form a critical obstacle (Fig. 26-2), impaired flow dynamics alongside and distal to the thrombotic lesion develop, frequently accompanied by dynamic vasoconstriction and resultant clinical ischemic events.[11] During PCI, the notorious instability of thrombus is frequently encountered, as thrombi adhere loosely or at times quite firmly to the underlying plaque and the vessel wall while exhibiting marked friability or rigidity in response to the application of balloons and stents. These seemingly contradictory physical properties stem from the cumulative effect of an assortment of components within the thrombus. Structurally, the thrombus is held by a scaffolding platform of fibrin fibers.[12] Two distinct types of branching fibrin fibers are organized in a three-dimensional network. Dense, thin fibers resist deforming mechanical forces and are poorly dissolved by thrombolytic agents. Thick fibrin fibers, on the other hand, are susceptible to the effects of external mechanical forces and readily dissolved by thrombolytic therapy.[13] Platelets, red blood cells, vasoconstrictors and procoagulant compounds are anchored to the matrix of the crisscrossing fibers (Fig. 26-3). Abnormalities in platelet function can persist and predict clinical events following PCI.[14] In patients presenting with acute coronary syndrome, the clot-adhering platelets typically exert a significantly increased contractile force leading to increased platelet aggregation, so that the entire thrombus exhibits increased elastic modulus.[15] The platelets sustain and amplify the coagulant response at the plaque site and release procoagulant platelet-derived microparticles. Various biochemical processes and interactions between activated platelets, red blood cells, fibrinogen, vasoconstrictors, atherosclerotic material, and the vessel wall all have a substantial impact on the fibrin network.

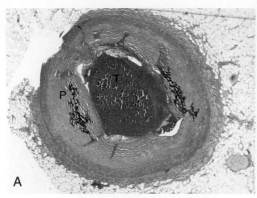
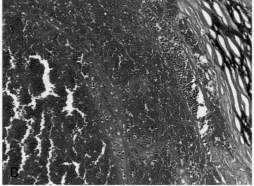

Figure 26-1 High-power view of right coronary artery showing: **A**, layering of acute thrombus (T), **B**, Red blood cells alternate between layers of fibrin (H&E, 20x). *(Courtesy of Shannon Mackey-Bojack MD, Jesse E. Edwards Registry of Cardiovascular Disease Collection, Nasseff Heart Center, United hospitals, University of Minnesota School of Medicine, St. Paul, MN.)*

These constituents account for the thrombus's level of activity, stability, or instability and for the overall "aggressiveness" of the thrombus as encountered during intervention. The presence and ratio of the above-mentioned components lead to the formation of distinct thrombus types, each with unique rheolytic and mechanical properties. The two most prominent are the red and white thrombi. They can be detected by angioscopy[16] (Fig. 26-4), and their angiographic characteristics correlate with the histology of extracted thrombi.[17] The red thrombus has a dense surface with a loose inner core. Transmission or scanning electron microscopy demonstrates loosely packed fibrin and many interspersed red blood cells. The white thrombus consists of a dense structure lacking loose inner spaces, yet it contains a high concentration of platelets with fibrin and only few red blood cells.[18] Based on the histopathological analysis of aspirated thrombotic content, erythrocyte-rich (red) thrombus is found in about 35% of patients, predominately in those presenting with low TIMI flow. The platelet-rich (white) thrombus is identified in 65% of cases, especially in the early hours of acute myocardial infarction.[19] Noteworthy, however, is the fact that in many patients the occlusive thrombus is a mixture of red and white clot, and the frequent resistance upon extraction attempts suggests that certain clots contain layers upon layers of one thrombus type interspersed with the other.[20,21] From a clinical management viewpoint, coronary risk factors such as hypercholesterolemia, smoking, and male gender adversely influence plaque morphology in patients with acute coronary syndromes and are associated with a higher frequency of thrombus.

Detection of Thrombus-Containing Lesions

Various imaging modalities are available for the diagnosis of intracoronary thrombus. Numerous studies have demonstrated the poor sensitivity of angiography, although specificity approaches 100% when

multiple angiographic views are obtained for verification and strict definitions are used. Nevertheless, angiography remains the practical "gold standard" for the recognition of thrombus, demonstrating the classic findings of reduced contrast density, staining, haziness, irregular lesion contour, "filling defect," or a smooth convex meniscus at the site of a total thrombotic occlusion. When a thrombus is suspected but not apparent angiographically, the more sensitive techniques for its detection may be utilized, including angioscopy,[22] intravascular ultrasound[23] (Fig. 26-5), and the recently introduced optical coherence tomography.[24]

Thrombus Grading

Grading systems are essential for adequate assessment of the thrombus burden and management decisions prior to and during interventions. The established, most commonly used thrombus grading classification was introduced by the Thrombolysis In Myocardial Infarction (TIMI) Study Group.[25] This method is based on the visual angiographic assessment of thrombus size, utilizing a score ranging from grades 0 through 5 (Table 26-2, Fig. 26-6). An important modification to this

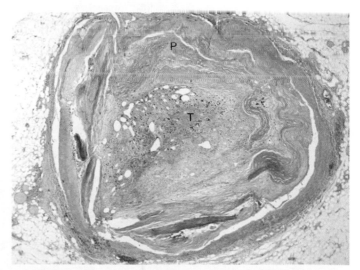

Figure 26-2 Cross section of right coronary artery occluded by calcified, complicated atherosclerotic plaque (P) and organized thrombus (T). (H&E 2x). *(Courtesy of Shannon Mackey-Bojack, MD, Jesse E. Edwards Registry of Cardiovascular Disease Collection, Nasseff Heart Center, United Hospitals, University of Minnesota School of Medicine, St. Paul, MN.)*

TABLE 26-1	The Impact of Thrombus on Percutaneous Coronary Intervention
Requires targeted treatment, which increases costs and may prolong procedures.
Adverse effect on lesion, vessel, and clinical outcome during and after interventions.
Increased procedure-related risk of distal embolization, "no reflow," acute thrombotic occlusion, periprocedural myocardial infarction, need for emergency bypass surgery, myocardial infarction, and death.
Predictor of major adverse coronary events, early and late stent thrombosis, and in-hospital complications, as well as risk of 6-month recurrent myocardial infarction and death.
Predictor of success in selected cases of chronic total occlusion.

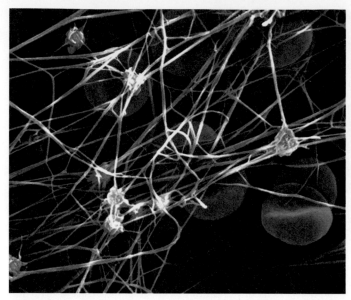

Figure 26-3   Scanning electron microscopy of a thrombus. Note the criss-crossing thick and thin fibrin fibers, which provide a scaffolding system for the thrombus structure. Platelets (violet color) and red blood cells are attached to the fibrin net. *(Courtesy of Marc Carr Jr, MD, PhD, and Hemodyne Inc., Richmond, VA.)*

TABLE 26-2	Thrombus Grading Scores

Definition*

Grade 0: No angiographic characteristics of thrombus.

Grade 1: Possible thrombus: angiographic features include decreased density of contrast, haziness, irregular lesion contour, or a smooth, convex meniscus at the site of total occlusion suggestive but not diagnostic of thrombus.

Grade 2: Definite thrombus present in multiple angiographic views: marked irregular lesion contour with a significant filling defect. The thrombus's greatest dimension is <1/2 vessel diameter.

Grade 3: Definite thrombus in multiple views with greatest dimension >1/2 but <2 vessel diameters.

Grade 4: Definite large thrombus with greatest dimension >2 vessel diameters.

Grade 5: Complete thrombotic occlusion of the vessel: a convex margin that stains with contrast and persists for several cardiac cycles.

Grade 5 reclassification†

Intervention-based: the occlusion is crossed with a guidewire or small balloon. Once antegrade flow is restored, the culprit thrombus undergoes restratification:

Small thrombus, grade 1–3

Large thrombus, grade 4

Thrombus grading by a two-category scale‡

Low thrombus grade corresponds to TIMI thrombus grades 1–3

High thrombus grade corresponds to TIMI thrombus grades 4–5

*Gibson CM et al. *Circulation.* 2001;103:2550–2554.
†Sianos G. et al. *J Am Coll Cardiol.* 2007;50:572–583.
‡Niccoli G et al. *Am J Cardiol.* 2010;105:587–591.

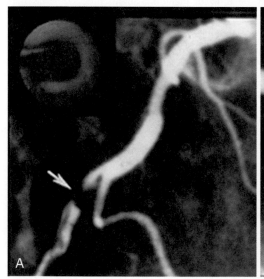
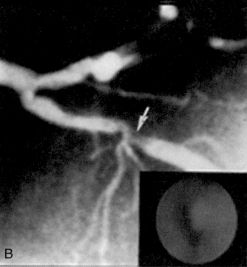

Figure 26-4   A. Angiogram of RCA demonstrating a 1-cm filling defect with a trace amount of contrast crossing the tight atherosclerotic obstruction (arrow). Corresponding angioscopy demonstrates a bulging red thrombus. B. Angiogram demonstrating a hazy eccentric lesion in the obtuse marginal branch (arrow). Angioscopy revealing a white thrombus emerging from a yellow plaque. *(Courtesy of George Abela MD, Division of Cardiology, Michigan State University, East Lansing, MI. From Abela GS et al. Am J Cardiol 1999; 83:96–98. With permission of the authors and Elsevier.)*

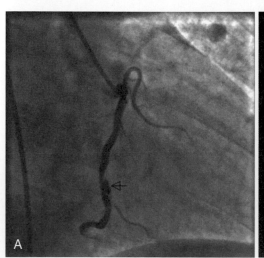
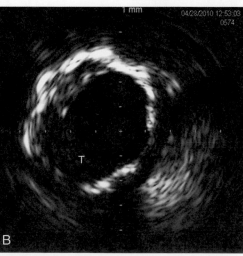

Figure 26-5   A. Ultrasound of thrombus. B. Corresponding RCA angiogram. *(Courtesy of Michael Foster, MD, South Carolina Heart Center, Columbia, South Carolina.)*

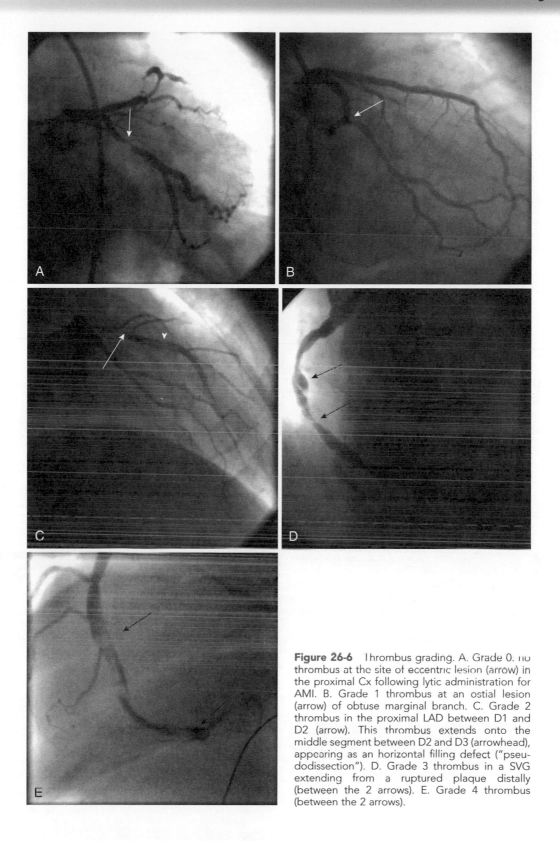

Figure 26-6 Thrombus grading. A. Grade 0. no thrombus at the site of eccentric lesion (arrow) in the proximal Cx following lytic administration for AMI. B. Grade 1 thrombus at an ostial lesion (arrow) of obtuse marginal branch. C. Grade 2 thrombus in the proximal LAD between D1 and D2 (arrow). This thrombus extends onto the middle segment between D2 and D3 (arrowhead), appearing as an horizontal filling defect ("pseudodissection"). D. Grade 3 thrombus in a SVG extending from a ruptured plaque distally (between the 2 arrows). E. Grade 4 thrombus (between the 2 arrows).

scoring system[5] was recently introduced by the Thoraxcenter investigators, who reclassified the highest grade (i.e., grade 5, which consists of TIMI 0 flow and a strong angiographic suspicion of a large thrombus). When this grade is encountered, either a guidewire or a 1.5-mm balloon (inflated or uninflated) is applied to recanalize the suspected thrombus (Fig. 26-7). As soon as antegrade flow is restored, the exposed, apparently thrombotic content undergoes restratification into a small thrombus burden (grade 1-3) or a large thrombus burden (grade 4) and treatment ensues accordingly. Niccoli and colleagues have introduced a minimalistic thrombus categorization whereby a low grade is assigned to the above-mentioned TIMI grades of 1 to 3 and a high grade corresponding to grades 4 and 5.[26] For a

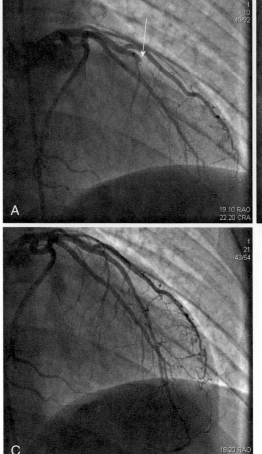

Figure 26-7 Grade 5 thrombus. A. Intervention based reclassification of grade 5 with a guidewire traversing the occlusive LAD thrombus (arrow). B. Guidewire restratification of the thrombus to a small residual burden at the site of the underlying plaque. C. The restratification enabled a revascularization strategy based on treatment with standard balloon intervention and stenting.

more accurate quantitative measurement, Aleong and colleagues have innovatively developed a technique combining edge detection and video densitometry-based quantitative coronary angiography. In early experience with patients exhibiting large intracoronary clots, this modality appeared to quantify the thrombotic volume accurately.[27] The advantages and limitations of these thrombus grading classifications are described in Table 26-3. Factors that account for the formation of a specifically high-grade thrombus are depicted in Table 26-4. Among these, the relationship among hyperglycemia, increased

TABLE 26-4	Factors Favoring Formation of a High-Grade Thrombus in Atherosclerotic Lesions
Lesion-related	
Acute plaque rupture and complex morphology	
Vessel-related	
Slow or stagnant antegrade coronary or SVG flow	
Large anatomical size increases thrombus formation and accumulation in native coronary vessels and SVG	
Morphology: ectasia, aneurysm, old SVG	
Myocardial infarction-related	
Late presentation (>12 hours) after onset of chest pain	
Established Q-wave MI with continuous chest pain and ischemia	
Cardiogenic shock	
Failed thrombolytics	
PCI-related	
Triggering of the plaque and thrombus with guidewire, balloon, or stent—the "angry clot" phenomenon	
Inadequate anticoagulation during intervention	
Inadequate stent apposition to the vessel wall	
Lack of or premature cessation or abrupt termination of thienopyridines therapy	
Underlying factors	
Hypercoagulability	
Heparin-induced thrombocytopenia and thrombosis (HITT)	
Vasculitis	
Increased WBCs	
Hyperglycemia	
Prothrombotic states	
Cocaine and methamphetamine	

TABLE 26-3	Advantages and Limitations of Contemporary Thrombus Grading Classifications
Advantages	
1. Convenient assessment during diagnostic angiography and interventions	
2. Constitute logical grading scales that are readily available and globally applied	
3. High inter- and intraobserver agreement	
4. Correlate well with clinical outcomes	
5. Reliable tools for comparison with previous angiograms	
Limitations	
1. Based solely on visual assessment of the thrombus	
2. Underestimation of thrombus presence and size in comparison with angioscopy and intracoronary ultrasound	
3. Do not differentiate between types of thrombi	
4. Inability to assess the thrombotic content of chronic total occlusions	
5. Do not incorporate quantitation or qualification of the underlying plaque	

white blood cell count, and findings of a high thrombus grade merits special clinical attention.[26] These factors also adversely impact the achievement of proper ST-segment resolution during interventions and are associated with a worse PCI outcome.[28] A plausible direct relationship between high thrombus content and large vessel size has been known for a long time; however, it has not been uniformly confirmed.[26] Intriguingly, despite the convenience of the above-mentioned classifications, most studies of PCI in ischemic coronary syndromes rarely measure, grade, or report the presence of any thrombotic burden.[29] This unfortunate omission occurs despite the growing recognition of the structural complexity of thrombi[30] and its significant impact on PCI outcome.[31,32]

Limitations of Standard PCI in Thrombus-Containing Lesions

In the absence of an apparent thrombus or when only a small thrombus (corresponding to grades 1–2) is detected, the recommended PCI strategy includes standard pharmacotherapy, balloon angioplasty, and stenting.[33] Aspiration catheters can be useful as well in this situation. The management of a significant (grade 3) or heavy thrombotic burden (grades 4–5) is considerably more challenging.[34] In this scenario, dislodgment of friable thrombotic material by balloon and stent deployment is an issue of significant concern. Embolization of fragmented thrombotic particles obstructs flow within distal arterial segments, side branches, and myocardial microvessels. Overall, distal embolization occurs in the range of 6% to 15% of standard PCI for all lesion types in acute coronary syndromes and is associated with up to a sevenfold increase in the rate of periprocedural MI. In most instances, resultant severe ischemia, microinfarctions, inflammatory response, and contractile dysfunction reduce coronary reserve and cause deleterious effects on recovery and salvage.[35] These complications are especially encountered among patients who undergo primary PCI for acute myocardial infarction (AMI).[4,5] This was convincingly shown by the TAPAS investigators, who studied the sequelae of angiographically visible distal embolization after PCI in 883 ST-segment elevation MI (STEMI) patients receiving triple antiplatelet therapy.[4] Those who sustained angiographically evident embolization had significantly worse outcomes than patients without, as expressed by lower myocardial blush grade, impaired ST-segment resolution, and higher level of myocardial enzyme leakage.[4] At 1 year follow-up of these patients, reinfarction occurred in 8.9%, versus 3.0% in those without embolization ($P = 0.018$). Importantly, the size of the aspirated thrombus was larger in patients with evidence of angiographic embolization versus those without ($P = 0.002$), and it more often contained erythrocytes (50% vs. 15.7%, $P < 0.001$, respectively). When compared with the revascularization of thrombus-free lesions, embolization also significantly increases the need for emergency bypass surgery as well as the procedure-related death rate.[36] The considerably limited yield of standard PCI in thrombus-containing lesions is further elucidated by the phenomenon of "illusion of reperfusion."[37] Essentially, this term describes a marked discrepancy between primary PCI-gained TIMI 3 flow versus the disappointing, suboptimal degree of myocardial salvage. Notably, the desired grade 3 myocardial blush score is gained in only 28% to 35% of patients in whom the standard PCI induces a TIMI 3 epicardial flow.[38] The main cause of this marked discrepancy is the prevalent intracoronary thrombus and related distal embolization, microvessel obstruction, no reflow, and myocardial necrosis. Clearly, patients who develop procedure-related "no reflow" sustain larger-sized infarcts, significantly worse left ventricular (LV) function, and a greater risk of adverse cardiac events and death.[39] Thus the thrombus's deleterious impact as a hazardous material that promotes adverse coronary events and suboptimal outcome should be anticipated and dealt with promptly before, during, and after PCI.[32,40] Accordingly, Table 26-5 delineates the indications for a dedicated thrombus removal strategy.

TABLE 26-5	Indications for a Targeted Thrombus Strategy
Pathology	
Atherosclerosis with associated thrombus	
Thrombotic embolus in a coronary artery or SVG	
Intracoronary thrombus accumulation secondary to hypercoagulability	
Clinical	
Unstable and stable angina, STEMI, non-STEMI associated with:	
Need to reduce thrombus burden in clot laden lesions.	
Need to reduce thrombus impairment to forward flow.	
Need to reduce threat of thrombotic embolization.	
Need to reduce risk of "no reflow."	
Targets	
Native coronary arteries, old saphenous vein grafts, chronic total occlusions, stents	

Pharmacotherapy for Thrombus-Containing Lesions

The mainstay pharmacological treatments for the management of thrombus-containing lesions include aspirin, heparin, glycoprotein IIb/IIIa platelet receptor antagonists, thienopyridines (clopidogrel, prasugrel, ticlopidine), and direct thrombin inhibitors. As for the potential benefit of selective administration of intracoronary thrombolytic agents, further exploration and evidence are warranted. Interestingly, a beneficial decrease of the thrombotic burden can be gained with the mainstay agents even before the initiation of an intervention, with resultant improved PCI results and reduced risk of distal thrombotic embolization. Specifically, chronic aspirin therapy has been shown to decrease the thrombotic burden before stent deployment,[26] heparin to reduce fibrin formation and abolish platelet contractile forces,[41] and the glycoprotein IIb/IIIa receptor antagonists to dramatically reduce platelet aggregate size as well as to improve thrombolytic access to the platelet-rich clot's fibrin.[42] However, these agents are less effective in an already formed, active, unstable thrombus,[43] especially when it is a high-grade thrombus. For example, significant limitations of these useful pharmacological therapies are quite apparent during the revascularization of old saphenous vein grafts with a large thrombotic content.[44] Suboptimal PCI results in these thrombotic vessels are manifested by inadequate ST-segment resolution at 60 minutes, limited prevention of distal embolization, and insufficient revascularization. Thus, revascularization of lesions containing a significant clot burden should incorporate a mechanical thrombus removal strategy[45] in order to improve PCI outcome.

Approach to Mechanical Thrombus Removal

ROLE OF ADJUNCTIVE THROMBECTOMY

The recent publication of several landmark studies[5,46] has rekindled interest in mechanical thrombus extraction, especially for the management of STEMI. Contemporary mechanical thrombus removal or dissolution devices can be categorized into four main types, according to their activation mode: (1) manual aspiration catheters, (2) power-sourced thrombectomy, (3) ultrasound-induced sonication, and (4) embolic protection. The potential benefits and limitations of mechanical thrombectomy devices are described in Table 26-6. Technically, thrombus removal devices are user-friendly owing to a relatively small size and convenient rapid delivery. Their efficiency contributes to the reduction of procedure-related radiation exposure. A different classification of these devices defines thrombus extraction modalities as either "simple" (i.e., aspiration-based) or "complex" (i.e., mechanically based).[47] This categorization is supported by a recent metanalysis

TABLE 26-6	Utility of Thrombectomy Devices

Benefits
- Shortening of door-to-thrombus clearance time
- Direct contact for targeted maximal thrombus extraction
- Allow selective infusion of thrombolytics, platelet aggregation inhibitors and vasodilators through the device
- Removal of thrombus-related prothrombotic coagulants and promoters of vasoconstriction and platelet aggregation
- Reduction of distal embolization and "no reflow"
- Restoration or antegrade flow, improved myocardial blush score, and lowering of cTFC (Corrected TIMI Frame Count)
- Enable accurate assessment of the underlying plaque morphology and stenosis
- Facilitate stenting
- Improved post-MI 6-month and 1-year MACE and survival rates

Limitations
- May prolong PCI duration
- Higher dependency on operator's technique
- May not achieve complete thrombus removal
- Can cause distal embolization due to device manipulation
- Do not completely eliminate "no reflow"
- Do not reduce the need for adjunctive stenting
- Increased cost

of 17 randomized trials on thrombus removal versus standard PCI in 3,909 patients,[48] which found that thrombus removal was associated with a significantly greater likelihood of TIMI 3 flow, myocardial blush grade 3, and ST-segment resolution. The investigators concluded that thrombus removal devices appear to improve markers of myocardial perfusion in patients undergoing primary PCI, with no difference in overall 30-day mortality but an increased likelihood of stroke. The clinical benefits of thrombectomy appeared to be influenced by the device type, with a trend toward survival benefit with manual aspiration catheters and worse outcomes with mechanical devices. Facing the large variability of thrombus content and size among patients with acute coronary syndromes, well-trained operators can choose the device according to the angiographic morphological features of the targeted thrombus burden, often achieving excellent results with any of these tools. The last point was recently reemphasized by a large Dutch study of 812 consecutive patients treated with drug-eluting stents for STEMI. The investigators examined the impact of an underlying thrombus size on procedural outcome, demonstrating the direct, proportional effect of the initial and final thrombotic burden on mortality and its role as an independent predictor of postprocedure MACE and stent thrombosis[5] (Fig. 26-8). The TAPAS study investigators[44] found that thrombus aspiration is applicable in a large majority of patients with STEMI, affording better reperfusion and clinical outcomes than PCI without a mechanical thrombus removal strategy. These findings confirm previous observations from smaller trials and provide credence to the notion that manual aspiration protects the microcirculation during primary PCI. However, it is unclear whether these findings are attributed to an immediate reduction in thrombotic burden, facilitation of direct stenting, or a combination of the two.[49]

THROMBUS ASPIRATION CATHETERS

Manual thrombus aspiration of the infarct-related vessel has attracted intense interest as a useful method for the rapid reduction of thrombotic burden, prevention of thrombus embolization, preservation of microvascular integrity, and reduction of infarct size.[50] Most aspiration-based catheters are available in 4- to 6-Fr sizes; they contain an extraction lumen and aspiration syringe. They are user-friendly because of their low crossing profile, hydrophilic coating, flexibility, and tapered distal tip. Among commercially available aspiration catheters are the Export (Medtronic, Minneapolis, MN), Pronto Extraction Catheter (Vascular Solutions, Minneapolis, MN), Diver CE (Invatec, Roncadelle, Italy), Xtract (Volcano, Rancho Cordova, CA), QuickCat (Kensey Nash, Exton, PA), and Fetch (Possis, Minneapolis, MN). Several prospective trials involving these catheters, including the DEAR-MI[51] and REMEDIA,[52] have demonstrated an increased myocardial blush of grade 2 to 3 and adequate ST-segment resolution of >70% in a substantial number of patients who received this treatment versus those who underwent standard PCI. In addition, the manual thrombus aspiration modality improved myocardial tissue-level perfusion as well as LV functional recovery and modeling.[53] It is unclear whether one aspiration catheter provides a significant advantage over the others. In the prospective single-center STEMI study, RETAMI, the investigators found that the use of a certain aspiration catheter before stenting removed more thrombotic burden and provided a greater postintervention epicardial flow and microvascular perfusion as compared with a catheter made by another manufacturer.[54] However, such conclusions strongly depend on operator preference and other factors such as cost. In a study similar to the REMEDIA trial, investigators observed a significant decrease in procedure-related elevation of cardiac enzymes in comparison with patients who did not receive aspiration, as well as only 3% no-reflow versus 15%, respectively. Importantly, aspiration catheters do not increase procedure time and offer a safe, straightforward approach for thrombus removal. Follow-up over 6 months demonstrates a significantly decreased occurrence of LV dilation versus standard PCI.[55] Metanalysis of randomized studies on catheter thrombus aspiration shows a significant benefit of reducing mortality compared with PCI alone, 2.7% versus 4.4% ($P = 0.05$), respectively.[56] However, some investigators failed to find any advantage to the routine use of aspiration catheters in STEMI patients, observing that this approach does not increase myocardial salvage and, in fact, may increase final infarct size.[57] Among the limitations of aspiration catheters are the difficult delivery along tortuous vessels and reduced ability to aspirate at the distal coronary segments; there is also the risk of dissection/perforation in cases where the guidewire is not located within the true lumen. The low, negative aspiration pressure and the small evacuation holes also limit the yield of these catheters in the presence of a large thrombotic volume. Commonly, the application of aspiration catheters results in inadequate clot extraction, leaving at least 30% to 50% residual thrombus volume.[57] The considerable risk of catheter-induced distal embolization, especially during a hurried maneuver, and the need to repeatedly pass across a large thrombus, should be taken into account in planning clot extraction. It is noteworthy that even the sequential use of thrombus aspiration catheters and distal protection filters is associated with insufficient thrombus removal.[56,58,59]

POWER-SOURCED THROMBECTOMY DEVICES

The mainstay representatives of this group of mechanical tools are the rheolytic thrombectomy, the excimer laser, and the X-Sizer. The question of whether power-based mechanical thrombectomy offers any advantage over aspiration catheters is relevant to practical management, although there are no prospective studies with direct comparisons between these two modalities. Some authorities opine that a comparison between power-based mechanical thrombectomy devices and aspiration catheters is not required and, in fact, should be considered unethical in patients with lesions containing large thrombotic burdens.[60] Overall, there is a strong clinical impression that the larger the target thrombus, the higher the extracting yield of a power-based mechanical thrombectomy device.[61,62] The X-Sizer thrombectomy system (eV3, Plymouth, MN) is used mainly in Europe.[63] It consists of a helical cutter enclosed in a protective housing attached to a dual-bore catheter shaft containing a guidewire and vacuum/extraction

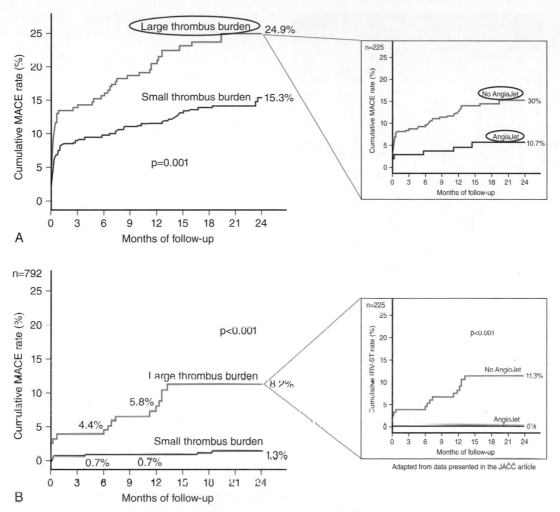

Figure 26-8 A. Large unresolved thrombus increases MACE. B. Large unresolved thrombus increases stent thrombosis. *(From Sianos G, et al: J Am Coll Card 50:572–583, 2007. With permission of the authors and Elsevier.)*

lumens. Activation of the handheld controller simultaneously rotates the helical cutter at 2,100 rpm, which entraps and macerates soft atherosclerotic plaque and thrombus and channels to a vacuum collection bottle. The device operates cutters 1.5, 2.0, and 2.3 mm in diameter and is compatible with 0.014-inch guidewires. Napodano and colleagues studied 92 AMI patients,[64] demonstrating that direct PCI for AMI with X-Sizer thrombectomy followed by stenting significantly improves myocardial reperfusion as assessed by myocardial blush score and ST-segment resolution. The large, prospective X-AMINE multicenter study that followed demonstrated a success rate for the device of 87% and adequate thrombus removal in 95% of the lesions.[65] The AngioJet rheolytic thrombectomy system (AngioJet, Possis/Medrad, Minneapolis, MN), is an FDA-approved device for thrombus-containing lesions encountered in coronary and peripheral interventions. The principle of activation is based on the creation of saline jets inside the catheter that travel backward at high speed to create a negative pressure zone (Venturi effect). Side windows along the catheter's tip optimize fluid flow, drawing thrombus into the catheter for fragmentation and removal (Fig. 26-9). A new AngioJet console, the ULTRA, features automated, rapid setup and support for a wide range of catheters. Multiple rapid-exchange 4- or 5-Fr flexible catheters are available for various target vessels including native coronary arteries, old saphenous vein grafts, and peripheral arteries. Proper thrombectomy technique incorporating slow advancement of the catheter essentially eliminates the need for a temporary pacemaker;

however, some operators recommend it in patients requiring revascularization of a major vessel or in cases with limited myocardial reserve. The AngioJet's ability to treat a large thrombotic burden in STEMI patients and provide more effective myocardial perfusion than that obtained with standard balloon and stenting has been well documented[66,67] (Fig. 26-10). The Thoraxcenter group elegantly demonstrated that AngioJet thrombectomy is a significant independent predictor of reduced risk for stent thrombosis and MACE, specifically when it is applied for the removal of a large thrombotic burden in STEMI patients.[5] In the FAST study, AngioJet was used in 116 AMI patients with extensive thrombus loads, leading to significant improvements in perfusion, as compared with a control group with similar thrombus loads who received standard PCI.[68] The in-hospital rate of MACE for the AngioJet was relatively low at 8%. Further evidence of the excellent safety profile of the AngioJet has been reported repeatedly.[69,70]

Nevertheless, this tool, together with the entire concept of thrombus extraction, sustained a major setback a few years ago when negative results from the AngioJet AIMI multicenter study were published.[71] In retrospect, this study was poorly designed, as the presence of thrombus in the target lesion was not required for enrollment, and operators were required to utilize a technique mandating passive advancement to the distal end of the target vessel, allowing only retrograde thrombectomy. In order to address questions raised by and about the AIMI study, a new prospective, multicenter JetStent study was launched,

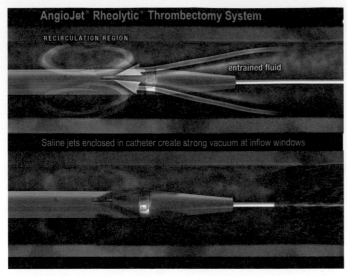

Figure 26-9 AngioJet: scheme of a rheolytic thrombectomy device.

comparing the effect of the AngioJet versus direct stenting on myocardial reperfusion, infarct size, and clinical outcomes in STEMI patients.[72] The JETSTENT trial exclusively focused on AMI patients with angiographically visible thrombus, using only slow, single-pass, antegrade thrombectomy and a narrower temporal definition of early ST-segment resolution (more than 50% within 30 minutes). It enrolled 501 STEMI patients with visible thrombus (grades 1–4) or with a totally occluded infarct-related vessel (thrombus grade 5 with subsequent restratification). At baseline, both groups had a thrombus grade of 3 to 5 in 99% and TIMI 0 flow in 83% of the patients. A platelet receptor antagonist was used in 97% and 98%, respectively. A 93% procedural success rate was achieved in both groups. The results demonstrated improved myocardial reperfusion and short-term clinical endpoints with the AngioJet as determined by higher rates of early ST-segment resolution (86% vs. 79%, respectively, $P = 0.04$). A significant difference in MACE rate was observed between the groups at 1 and 6 months: 3.1% AngioJet versus 6.9% direct stenting ($P = 0.05$), and 12% versus 21% ($P = 0.01$), respectively. No difference was found between the two approaches regarding myocardial blush score and corrected TIMI frame count. Multivariable regression analysis showed that randomization to rheolytic thrombectomy was a predictor of ST-segment resolution (OR 1.7, 95% CI 1.03–2.8, $P < 0.039$) and 6 months MACE rate (HR 0.5, 95% CI 0.31–0.82, $P = 0.06$). Notably, despite the encouraging outcomes of the JetStent study, skepticism regarding the interpretation of results and the chance for wider use of this modality remains.[73] Lasers are mainly used for debulking lesions deemed unsuitable for standard PCI and can be applied for the revascularization of thrombus-containing lesions.[74] The pulsed-wave ultraviolet-wavelength excimer laser (Spectranetics, Colorado Springs, CO) has been successfully applied in patients with acute coronary syndromes, including AMI[75] (Fig. 26-11). The excimer laser light interacts favorably with several components of the occluding thrombus. Laser-generated acoustic shock waves dissolve fibrin fibers[76] and suppress platelet aggregation[77] (Fig. 26-12). The thrombus-dissolution capability of this laser was further examined by the CARMEL multicenter study.[61] The trial enrolled 151 "real world" AMI patients with continuous chest pain and ischemia in the presence of either STEMI or non-STEMI, including those with late presentation, cardiogenic shock (13%), failed thrombolytic therapy (11%), and contraindications for

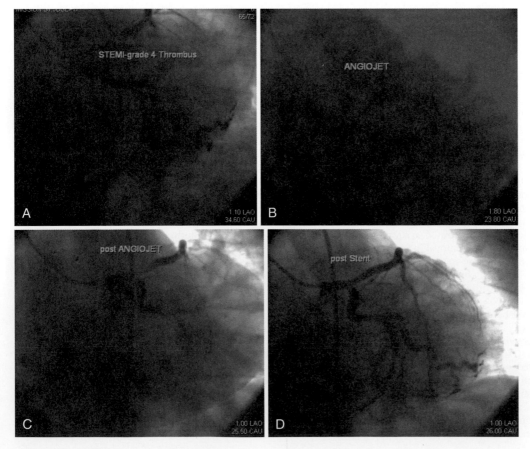

Figure 26-10 Rheolytic thrombectomy in a patient 3 hours after onset of anterior wall STEMI. A. Pre PCI: Grade 4 thrombus at ostial-proximal LAD. TIMI 1 flow observed. At that time the LVEDP was 28 mm Hg. B. Rheolytic thrombectomy performed with a slow antegrade and retrograde technique across the thrombus. C. Post-AngioJet clearance of the thrombus was accompanied by restoration of TIMI 3 flow. D. Final results after stenting with a 4.0/16-mm BMS. *(Courtesy of William B. Abernethy III, MD, Memorial Mission Hospital Heart Center, Asheville, NC.)*

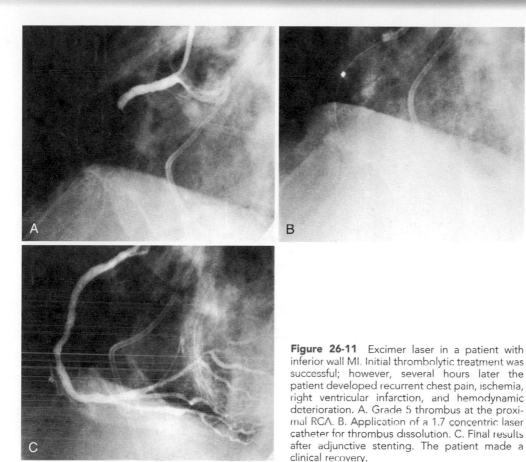

Figure 26-11 Excimer laser in a patient with inferior wall MI. Initial thrombolytic treatment was successful; however, several hours later the patient developed recurrent chest pain, ischemia, right ventricular infarction, and hemodynamic deterioration. A. Grade 5 thrombus at the proximal RCA. B. Application of a 1.7 concentric laser catheter for thrombus dissolution. C. Final results after adjunctive stenting. The patient made a clinical recovery.

this therapy (17%). The target vessel was a coronary artery in 79% and an old bypass graft in 21%. As opposed to many studies, the entire cohort underwent quantitative and statistical analyses by independent core laboratories. The results proved that despite the presence of compromised hemodynamics and a heavy thrombotic burden in as many as 65% of the patients, laser success was achieved in 95%, angiographic success in 97%, and procedural success in 91%. It is noteworthy that thrombus was not identified as a predictor of PCI failure. A baseline TIMI 0 flow of 1.2 ± 1.1 increased to 2.8 ± 0.5 with the laser energy and was followed by final TIMI flow of 3.0 ± 0.2 ($P < 0.001$ vs. baseline) with adjunctive stenting. Distal embolization occurred in only 2%, no reflow in 3%, device-induced small dissection was observed in 4%, and a small perforation in 0.6%. Total MACE was relatively low at 13%. The most important finding attested that maximal removal effect was directly proportional to the baseline thrombus burden (i.e., the larger the initial thrombus burden at the target lesion, the more effective and the greater gain for the laser-induced dissolution (Fig. 26-13). Further subgroup analysis of this trial recognized a specific laser gain among late-presentation patients who exhibited a heavy thrombotic burden and unstable hemodynamic parameters.[78] Thus this study provided the first scientific, quantitative evidence of the considerable benefit of a dedicated mechanical thrombectomy device in thrombus-removal strategy and particularly in AMI.

Ultrasound-induced thrombus dissolution can be offered as adjunctive therapy aimed at increasing the efficacy of common thrombolytic therapies.[79] Ultrasound-producing devices are defined by their different acoustic intensity and frequency, ranging from low (20–400 KHz) to high (0.5–3 KHz). The two main approaches to sonication therapy rely on an external device delivering transcutaneous therapeutic ultrasound energy[80] and on the invasive, intravessel catheter, which delivers sonication directly to the targeted thrombus. Further randomized studies will be required to investigate the promise and safety issues relating to the external mode of delivery and to examine whether it provides improved enhancement of pharmacological thrombolytic agents and superior thrombus dissolution in comparison with the more invasive, direct intracoronary delivery method.

Embolic Protection Devices

These tools are used to prevent the propagation of thrombus or atheromatous debris downstream. They can be classified into three categories: filter-based, proximal occlusion, and distal occlusion devices. The use of embolic protection devices does not require any special preparation of the patient other than the standard anticoagulation therapy for percutaneous intervention. These devices are user-friendly: however, a clear limitation relates to the need to cross the very same clot that requires protection and the need for an adequate length of distal landing zone. Overall, the embolic protection devices are useful adjuncts in primary PCI for acute coronary syndromes and have been shown to efficaciously reduce the rate of periprocedural infarction.[81] These devices have a class I indication for saphenous vein graft (SVG) interventions owing to the prevalence of thrombus-containing lesions.[82] However, in studying the value of distal protection during rescue PCI, the EMERALD investigators found that patients with AMI undergoing rescue PCI compared with primary PCI have similar myocardial perfusion, infarct size, and clinical outcomes, concluding that distal protection apparently does not offer any

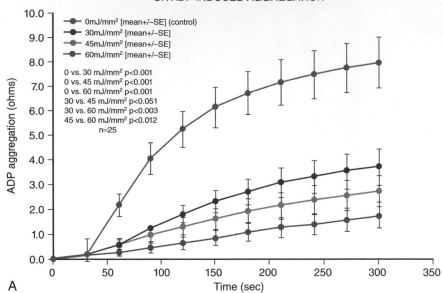

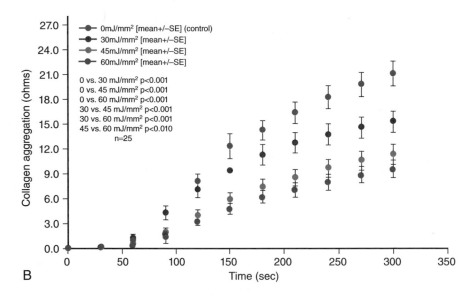

Figure 26-12 A and B. The in vitro effect of ultraviolet wavelength excimer laser on platelet aggregation. (Based on Topaz O, et al: Thromb Haemost 86:1087–1093, 2001. With permission of the authors and Schattauer Publishers, Stuttgart, Germany.)

detectable benefit in this patient population.[83] In fact, there is a concern that the routine use of filter protection for PCI of STEMI may increase the incidence of stent thrombosis, and the clinically driven target lesion and vessel revascularization.[84] All together, a selective rather than routine strategy of protection device utilization should be applied, limited to those patients at the highest risk of clinically relevant embolization.[85]

STENTS WITH THROMBUS CAPTURING MECHANISMS

During PCI, direct stenting of thrombus-containing lesions with either bare metal or drug-eluting stents is a common strategy.[86] Nonetheless, despite the popularity and perceived success of direct stenting, distal embolization and "no flow" do occur, mainly owing to the

mobilization of fragmented clot.[67,87] Conceptually, a dedicated thrombus-trapping stent could offer a targeted approach to the management of thrombus and reduction of embolization. The MGuard stent (Inspire-MD, Tel-Aviv, Israel) was developed for this purpose: it provides a unique stainless steel bare metal stent covered with an ultrathin, micrometer-level (150 × 180 micrometer), flexible mesh net fabricated by circular knitting (Fig. 26-14). During stent deployment, the net stretches and slides over the expanding stent struts, creating custom-designed pores parallel to the vessel wall. Once deployed, the MGuard stent seals the thrombus and accompanying plaque and captures potential embolic debris between the fiber net and the arterial wall[88] (Figs. 26-15 and 26-16). According to a prospective multicenter study with 100 STEMI patients, all with angiographic evidence of thrombus in the infarct-related artery, this unique stent achieved an impressive 90% myocardial blush grade 3 and 90% of complete

QCA PER TIMI THROMBUS

GRADE	0	1	2	3	4
	No thrombus	Small thrombus	Medium thrombus	Large thrombus	Extensive thrombus
# of patients	11	14	28	45	63
MLD: Baseline (mm)	.87±.69	.72±.43	.65±.45	.59±.49	.37±.49
Post laser	1.74±.46	1.48±.49	1.51±.51	1.50±.41	1.62±.62
Laser acute gain	.90±.63	.76±.52*	.84±.60	.94±.48	1.21±.72*
Final	2.97±.60	2.54±.55	2.47±.62	2.62±.55	2.76±.62
.%DS: Baseline	74%±21%	76%±16%	77%±16%	82%±16%	89%±15%
Post laser	47%±13%	51%±11%	52%±15%	51%±13%	53%+17%
Laser acute reduction	27%±18%	25%±15%	25%±19%	31%±16%	36%±20%
Final	16%±17%	15%±13%	22%±14%	16%±17%	22%±16%

* p=0.03

Figure 26-13 Maximal device gain and thrombus dissolution are obtained in the extensive thrombus group. (*Adapted from Topaz O et al. Am J Cardiol. 2004;93:694–701. With permission of the authors and Elsevier.*)

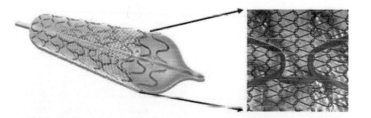

Figure 26-14 MGuard stent, InspireMD, Tel-Aviv, Israel; technical scheme of a thrombus-capturing stent system.

Figure 26-15 81 year old with inferior STEMI. A. Grade 5 thrombus occluding the RCA. B. Post aspiration and balloon dilation, antegrade flow restrored but Grade 2 thrombus is present. C. Deployment of a 3.0/24 mm MGuard thrombus capturing stent D. Final results demonstrating complete patency of the RCA with TIMI 3 blush. ST segment resolved. Courtesy of Ran Kornowski MD, Rabin Medical Center, Israel.

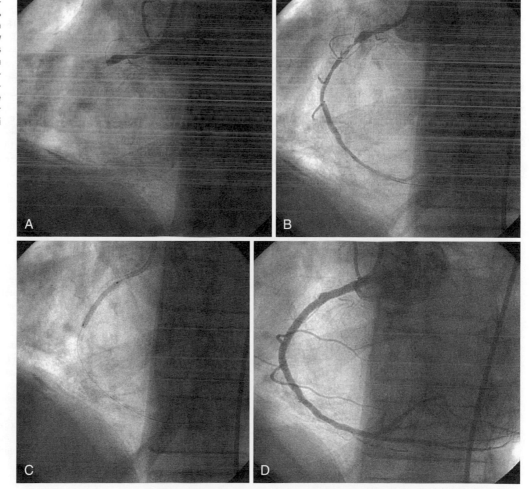

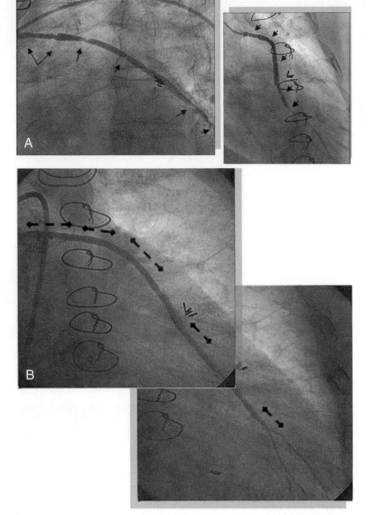

TABLE 26-7	SVG Sculpting—a PCI Technique for Revascularization of Totally Occluded Saphenous Vein Grafts

Steps:

1. Engage the total SVG occlusion with a maximal support guiding catheter and carefully advance a penetrating guidewire.
2. Enhance guidewire advancement along the occluded graft with a dedicated support catheter.
3. Once the guidewire reaches the distal graft or enters the native vessel beyond the anastomosis, exchange with a heavy support guidewire.
4. Apply a mechanical thrombectomy device along the occluded graft in a slow antegrade and retrograde fashion.
5. When restored antegrade flow is angiographically apparent, assesses residual thrombus burden and the exposed underlying lesions.
6. In the presence of significant residual thrombus, inject selectively into the graft 10–20 mg t-PA, allowing 10–15 minutes dwell time for interaction with the thrombus.
7. Repeat thrombectomy for further reduction of residual clot burden.
8. Dilate/stent the cleared underlying graft stenoses as indicated.
9. Protection device can be added at the discretion of the operator.
10. Selection of adjunct pharmacotherapy for SVG sculpting at the discretion of the operator: can include combination of multiple agents such as aspirin, heparin, 2b/3a platelet receptor blocker, direct thrombin inhibitor, thienopyridines, nitroglycerin, adenosine, thrombolytic drugs.

Unique Thrombus-Containing Targets and Related Revascularization Techniques

BYPASS GRAFTS

Myocardial ischemia occurring early after CABG is typically caused by graft thrombosis resulting from surgery-related mechanical issues, while late ischemic events are caused by progression of soft, friable atheromatous plaques in the grafts.[92,93] Collagen-rich (firm) or collagen–poor (soft) thrombus superimposition, an integral component of this process (Fig. 26-18), is found in as many as 80% of old bypass grafts.[94] The thrombotic content is often much greater in vein grafts than in native arteries because of the greater caliber of vein grafts and the lack of side branches, conditions promoting blood stagnation and coagulation. The TARGET investigators clearly demonstrated that, in the current strategy of routine stenting and glycoprotein IIb/IIIa inhibitors, thrombus is still the angiographic characteristic most closely associated with adverse outcome of PCI in SVGs.[43] Thus the revascularization of degenerated, friable old saphenous vein grafts is fraught with technical difficulties and risks.[95] Among those vessels, a unique group can be encountered: it consists of totally occluded grafts that continue to account for ongoing ischemia at their distal perfusion territory. Commonly, the corresponding grafted native coronary artery is occluded by severe atherosclerosis and thrombus that originally migrated from the diseased vein graft.[96] In most cases, percutaneous revascularization of these grafts, whether occluded for a short or long period, provides the only viable treatment option, albeit technically highly demanding.[97] Indeed, traditionally, operators were advised to resist the challenge of opening such occluded old grafts because of the remarkable technical difficulties and concerns for procedure-induced complications.[98] In our experience, a technique termed "SVG sculpting" (Table 26-7) has been utilized, facilitating the revascularization of totally occluded grafts through maximal removal of their thrombotic content and subsequent stenting, as described in Table 26-5. The initial step of this strategy involves careful guidewire entry and recanalization of the occluded graft, followed by targeted removal of the voluminous occlusive thrombus with mechanical thrombectomy. A critical component of this approach incorporates selective intragraft administration of a thrombolytic agent. This is usually followed by final passage with the thrombectomy device for extraction of the postlytic residual thrombotic material. After maximal mechanical removal of the thrombus, final vessel patency is ensured with stenting of the underlying stenosis (Fig. 26-19). Nevertheless, the SVG sculpting technique is not

Figure 26-16 Thrombus capturing in an ischemic patient with degenerated SVG to the obtuse marginal branch. A. 5 consecutive lesions (arrows) along the graft. B. Treatment with 4 consecutive MGuard Stents (3.5 × 24 mm, 3.5 × 15 mm, 3.25 × 12 mm, 2.75 × 12 mm) and a bare metal stent distally. Protection device was not used. Courtesy of Ran Kornowski MD, Rabin Medical Center, Israel.

(>70%) ST-segment resolution.[89] The investigators concluded that the MGuard stent offers a safe and feasible option for PCI in STEMI patients providing a very high perfusion grade and accompanying significant ECG improvement.

POWER THROMBECTOMY

This unique reperfusion strategy is aimed at the treatment of ischemic lesions and vessels laden with very heavy thrombotic burdens and accompanying slow antegrade flow. It combines power-sourced mechanical thrombectomy with selective injection of thrombolytic agents into the target vessels. The thrombolytic agents can be selectively administered during the intervention through a dedicated perfusion balloon such as the ClearPath device (Fig. 26-17). The premise of the power-thrombectomy approach rests on offering combined targeted maceration of the thrombus load by the mechanical device with the benefits stemming from direct interaction of the pharmacotherapy with the underlying clot and a decreased risk of systemic lytic effects.[90,91]

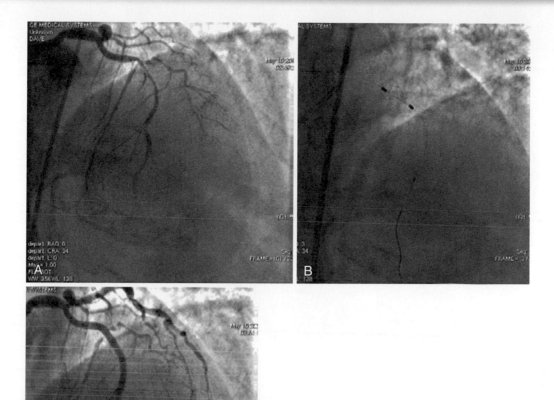

Figure 26-17 A patient with unstable angina and anterolateral ischemia. A. The LAD exhibits a long eccentric thrombotic lesion in the middle segment and TIMI 2 flow. B. A Clearway 2.0/20-mm perfusion balloon was used to selectively deliver intracoronary abciximab and adenosine into the LAD. C. Final angiographic results following stenting. TIMI 3 flow was restored.

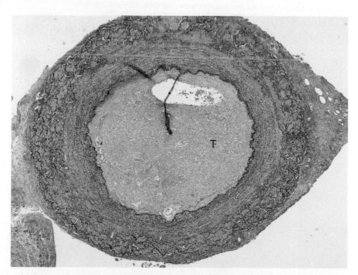

Figure 26-18 Cross-sectional histopathology of a 95% to 99% stenosis of a saphenous vein graft. The lumen is narrowed mainly by organized thrombus (T). The thrombus consists of loose fibrous tissue with small recanalized vascular channels (ELVG 4X). During PCI, such channels enable guidewire crossing, which should be followed by thrombus removal before plaque modification by balloon intervention and stenting. *(Courtesy of Shannon Mackey-Bojack MD, Jesse E. Edwards Registry of Cardiovascular Disease Collection, Nasseff Heart Center, United Hospitals, University of Minnesota School of Medicine, St.Paul, MN.)*

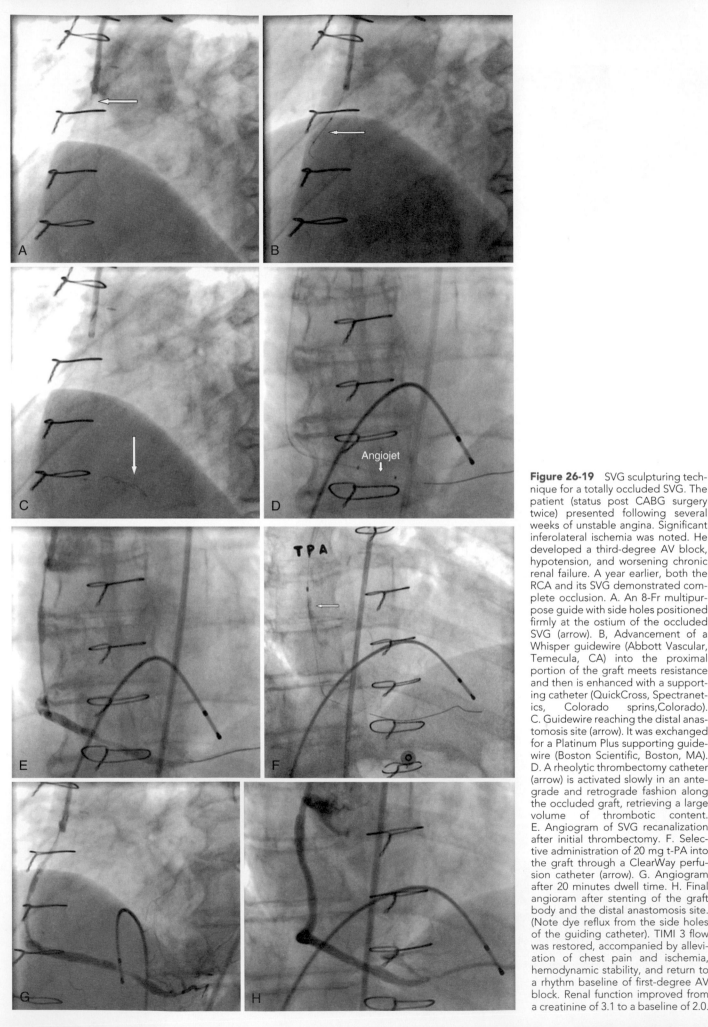

Figure 26-19 SVG sculpturing technique for a totally occluded SVG. The patient (status post CABG surgery twice) presented following several weeks of unstable angina. Significant inferolateral ischemia was noted. He developed a third-degree AV block, hypotension, and worsening chronic renal failure. A year earlier, both the RCA and its SVG demonstrated complete occlusion. A. An 8-Fr multipurpose guide with side holes positioned firmly at the ostium of the occluded SVG (arrow). B, Advancement of a Whisper guidewire (Abbott Vascular, Temecula, CA) into the proximal portion of the graft meets resistance and then is enhanced with a supporting catheter (QuickCross, Spectranetics, Colorado sprins,Colorado). C. Guidewire reaching the distal anastomosis site (arrow). It was exchanged for a Platinum Plus supporting guidewire (Boston Scientific, Boston, MA). D. A rheolytic thrombectomy catheter (arrow) is activated slowly in an antegrade and retrograde fashion along the occluded graft, retrieving a large volume of thrombotic content. E. Angiogram of SVG recanalization after initial thrombectomy. F. Selective administration of 20 mg t-PA into the graft through a ClearWay perfusion catheter (arrow). G. Angiogram after 20 minutes dwell time. H. Final angioram after stenting of the graft body and the distal anastomosis site. (Note dye reflux from the side holes of the guiding catheter). TIMI 3 flow was restored, accompanied by alleviation of chest pain and ischemia, hemodynamic stability, and return to a rhythm baseline of first-degree AV block. Renal function improved from a creatinine of 3.1 to a baseline of 2.0.

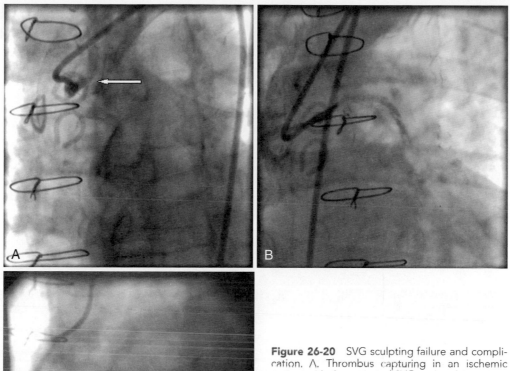

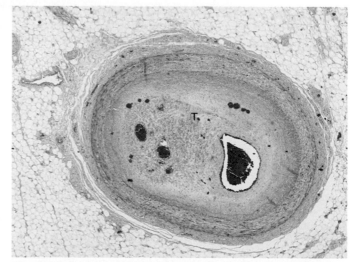

Figure 26-20 SVG sculpting failure and complication. A. Thrombus capturing in an ischemic patient with degenerated SVG to the obtuse marginal branch. A. 5 consecutive lesions (arrows) along the graft. B. Treatment with 4 consecutive MGuard Stents (3.5 × 24 mm, 3.5 × 15 mm, 3.25 × 12 mm, 2.75 × 12 mm) and a bare metal stent distally. Protection device was not used. Courtesy of Ran Kornowski MD, Rabin Medical Center, Israel. B. Post SVG sculpting there is resultant heavy thrombus burden without restoration of antegrade flow. C. Complication of SVG sculpting occurring immediately after stent deployment at the graft's anastomosis with the PDA. The rupture was contained without a need for intervention or further sequelae.

a panacea, device-related failure is a reality, and complications can occur (Fig. 26-20) because of the complex pathology of the target vessels. Other operators recommend a synergistic use of balloon-based distal embolization protection with rheolytic thrombectomy in this challenging context.[99]

CHRONIC TOTAL OCCLUSIONS

Called one of the last frontiers of revascularization, chronic total occlusions (CTOs) remain the most powerful predictors of referral for CABG.[100] The benefits of PCI for this complex lesion include symptom relief, improved LV function, and potentially a survival benefit when compared with failed CTO intervention. Technically, a CTO is considered a highly demanding revascularization target.[101] CTOs frequently contain organized thrombi of various ages in addition to fibrotic tissue, calcifications, and atherosclerotic material. Histopathology demonstrates that the original arterial lumen has been critically narrowed by atherosclerosis and contains an organized thrombus consisting of a vascular plexus through which either no flow or very restricted flow is possible (Fig. 26-21). Commonly, a process of recanalization of the organized thrombus by microchannels occurs, resulting in antegrade flow beyond the plaque, albeit limited.[102] Indeed, despite the recognition of the angiographic hallmark of CTO as 100% stenosis without any dye propagation distally, approximately 50% of these lesions are, in fact, less than 99%

Figure 26-21 Histopathology of a cross section of the RCA which is occluded by an organizing thrombus (T), consisting of loose fibrous tissue with realized vascular channels (H&E x10). *(Courtesy of Shannon Mackey-Bojack MD, Jesse E. Edwards Registry of Cardiovascular Disease Collection, Nasseff Heart Center, United Hospitals, University of Minnesota School of Medicine, St. Paul, MN.)*

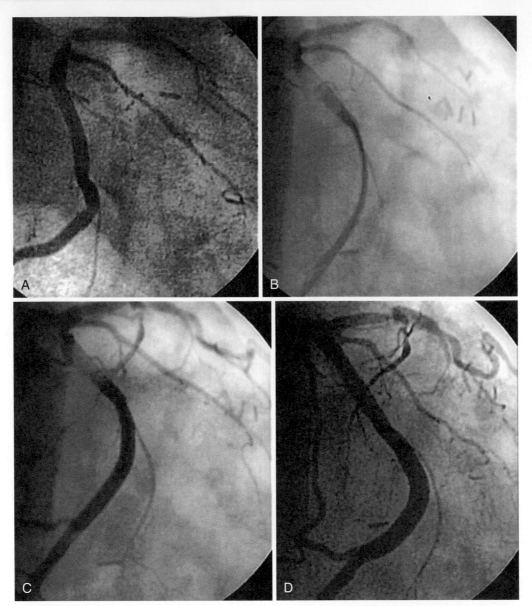

Figure 26-22 The "angry clot" phenomenon: a patient status post CABG surgery presenting with unstable angina, severe ischemia, and hemodynamic compromise. A LIMA graft to a diffusely diseased LAD was patent. A. The left main exhibits critical stenosis with grade 2 thrombus. B. PCI of the left main lesion: the patient received a 2b/3a platelet receptor antagonist, heparin, aspirin, and clopidogrel. However, as soon as the guidewire crossed the left main stenosis and was positioned at the distal Cx artery, rapid and aggressive thrombus accumulation occurred along the entire vessel, resulting in marked narrowing and slow flow. Increased chest pain, ischemia, and hypotension ensued, requiring immediate thrombus dissolution. This was obtained with a 0.9-mm rapid exchange X-80 excimer laser catheter (Spectranetics, Colorado Springs, CO), which was activated at maximal flow (80 mJ/mm2/80 Hz). Angiography after laser debulking and thrombolysis demonstrates restoration of flow, with reversal of the clot accumulation and mild residual clot remaining at the proximal vessel. D. Final results after stenting of the left main were accompanied by a clinical recovery.

stenosed.[103] While all of the above-mentioned morphological constituents account for the marked technical difficulty of crossing CTOs, it is the thrombus that should be considered the main element potentially providing a chance at penetration and revascularization through the total occlusion. Operators should attempt to traverse the thrombus through the above-mentioned vascular microchannels and remove the bulk of it before attempting to dilate or stent the lesion.[104] Thus careful guidewire maneuvering either antegrade or through a retrograde approach into and across these microchannels can lead to successful crossing and the creation of a morphological platform for futher plaque treatment. Unfortunately, efforts to cross a CTO can be hampered by prompting an underlying dormant thrombus to become active and unstable, thus culminating in the rapid formation and accumulation of a large volume—the notorious "angry clot" phenomenon (Fig. 26-22). This adverse process may then threaten the entire outcome of the PCI procedure. Therefore, following guidewire recanalization and distal positioning, a further reduction in the burden of the occlusive thrombus with a mechanical removal device is warranted. Then, with extraction of most of the obstructive thrombotic component, contrast injections can precisely demonstrate the residual underlying plaque, and subsequent balloon dilatation and stenting may be facilitated. Corroborating the benefit of focusing the

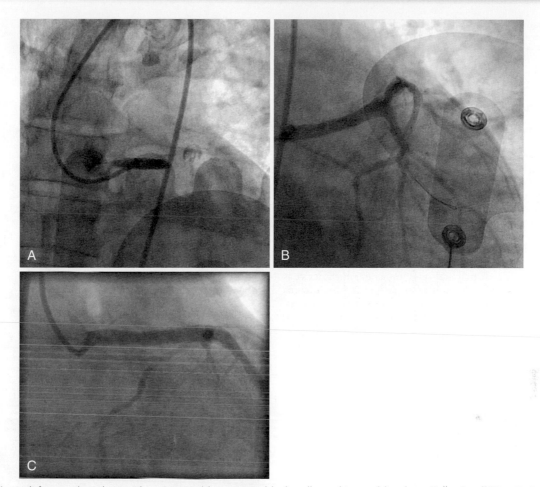

Figure 26-23 Acute left main thrombosis. This 48-year-old patient suddenly collapsed in a public place. Following CPR, anterior wall STEMI was diagnosed. A stormy course during transfer to the medical center included repeated episodes of intense chest pain, hypotension, increased ischemia, and ventricular tachycardia, culminating in full arrest upon entry to the cardiac catheterization suite. At 45 minutes, full code was required, including intubation, defibrillation x17, amiodarone, and epinephrine prior to relative stabilization and catheterization. A. Total occlusion of the left main artery. B. An 0.014-in. ATW guidewire recanalized the occlusion, followed by Export aspiration catheterization, which extracted clot. C. The target left main lesion was dilated and successfully stented with a 5.0/16-mm Liberte stent, yielding a diameter of 5.7 mm. TIMI 3 flow was restored; however, refractory arrhythmias ensued, requiring additional CPR, antiarrhythmics, defibrillation x24, and intra-aortic balloon pump insertion. Following stabilization, the patient received therapeutic hypothermia for 2 days. Repeat cardiac catheterization and IVUS on day 7 demonstrated patency of the stent and adequate coronary flow. The patient was discharged without angina or CHF, with a LVEF of 30%, anterolateral hypokinesis, and no neurological deficit. (Courtesy of William R. Hathaway, MD, and William D. Kuehl, MD, Mission Memorial Heart Center, Asheville, NC.)

revascularization technique on the thrombotic component of CTOs is recent evidence from the National Heart, Lung and Blood Institute registry. Multivariate regression analysis demonstrated that the presence of thrombus is a strong predictor of success in CTO revascularization (adjusted OR 0.31, 95% CI 0.15–0.61, $P = 0.0008$). This finding is of paramount importance, as it attests to the fact that thrombus removal clears the way for subsequent successful dilatation and the ability to deliver adequate stenting.[105]

LEFT MAIN DISEASE

Percutaneous revascularization of left main disease is a topic of great current interest.[106] Thrombus frequently accompanies severe obstructive left main lesions, thus having an additional major impact on clinical and procedure-related risks and complications. Acute thrombosis of an underlying left main plaque predicts grave consequences; in cases of acute total occlusion, an emergency PCI constitutes the

only realistic revascularization option (Fig. 26-23). Prasad and colleagues reported a 28-patient series with unprotected thrombotic left main lesions; these patients underwent standard PCI.[107] It is noteworthy that only a modest angiographic success rate of 83% (24 patients) was achieved, accompanied by a cumulative in-hospital mortality of 36%. These outcomes raise a valid concern that the thrombus-containing stenoses were not treated by a dedicated thrombus-removal approach. For such high-risk interventional scenarios and specifically those aiming to reduce the dreaded risk of distal embolization, our experience indicates a need to first focus on a thrombus-removal strategy, preferably with a mechanical thrombectomy device. Once the thrombus has been treated, the following dilation and stent implantation can be safely and efficiently performed. The merits of this approach include adequate clot clearance, proper exposure and assessment of the associated underlying atherosclerotic plaque, and facilitated stent delivery and deployment. The results of such an approach show a high success rate.[108] For selected symptomatic patients who present with CTO of the left main artery,[109] a PCI can become a viable management option with either antegrade or retrograde recanalization through one of the distinct angiographic collateral channels connecting the RCA with the left coronary system.[110]

STENT THROMBOSIS

Early, late, and very late stent thrombosis is an ominous clinical development that has a significant impact on clinical outcome[111] (Fig. 26-24). Stent thrombosis is often multifactorial.[112] One of the major causes is post-PCI residual thrombus, which then either gradually accumulates over time or rapidly aggregates to form a fully occlusive thrombus. Stent thrombosis can become manifest by serious complications such as nonfatal and fatal AMI[113,114] and marked hemodynamic instability. Expedient thrombus management is key to a favorable outcome, especially for patients who present with STEMI.[112] Primary PCI, including additional stenting with or without thrombectomy, is effective in restoring vessel patency, but reocclusion and restenosis are frequent.[115] The often raised practical question as to which device is best for the management of stent thrombosis can be addressed according to the amount of occlusive thrombus and associated clinical findings.[116,117] While a small to medium thrombus load in a stable patient can be managed with combination therapy of pharmacological agents and an aspiration catheter, a large burden, especially in the presence of hemodynamic instability and ongoing ischemia, calls for enhanced removal by a power-based mechanical thrombectomy device. Nevertheless, even successful PCI for stent thrombosis is associated with a larger infarct and poorer outcome than in patients with de novo STEMI.[116]

MULTIVESSEL CORONARY THROMBOSIS

This is an uncommon occurrence that poses a considerable management challenge. Patients with simultaneous multivessel thrombosis frequently present with ACS, mostly with either STEMI or NSTEMI, accompanied by severe hemodynamic compromise (Fig. 26-25). The pathophysiological process that accounts for this situation begins when plaque ruptures and resultant acute thrombosis of a single artery leads to the development of cardiogenic shock. This, in turn, further decreases coronary perfusion pressure; consequently, multivessel thrombus is formed on other preexisting lesions as well.[118] Another mechanism of multivessel coronary thrombosis involves thrombotic embolization and the occlusion of multiple coronary vessels from a left chamber cardiac tumor.[119] The optimal treatment approach to multivessel coronary thrombosis is unknown, varying considerably from PCI to urgent CABG. In instances where the most critical culprit lesion can be identified with certainty, selective treatment with aspiration catheter, aggressive pharmacotherapy, and subsequent stenting can be beneficial. However, in a case of PCI failure or in patients with continuous global ischemia due to thrombus-laden lesions in the other coronary arteries (especially with accompanying hemodynamic deterioration) urgent CABG is the preferred management option.

◼ Summary

Thrombus-containing plaques play a major role in the pathophysiology and management of acute coronary syndromes. Understanding the structural elements comprising the thrombus and proper assessment of its burden are prerequisites for tailoring successful strategies for revascularization. The useful ACC/AHA guidelines for the management of patients with acute coronary syndromes are readily available, yet developing precise algorithms for PCI management of these multifaceted thrombus-containing lesions remains a difficult task because of the complex characteristics of the coronary thrombus and the

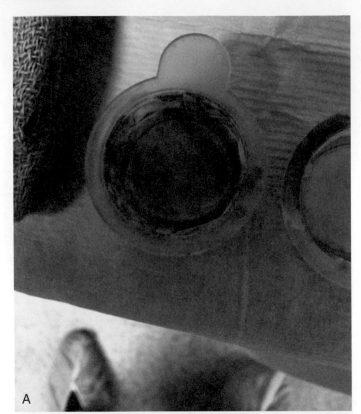

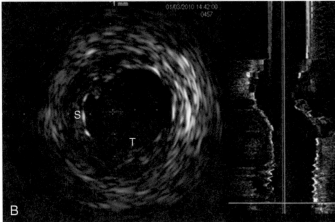

Figure 26-24   Ultrasound of stent (S) thrombosis (T) and corresponding extracted thrombus. (*Courtesy of James Margolis, MD, Miami Beach Florida.*)

morphological features of the associated atherosclerotic plaque and host vessels. While consensus commonly can be found regarding the angiographic classification of a thrombus and its burden, technical experience with removal technologies differs widely among interventionists. Therefore the current management of these challenging lesions diverges considerably. Enhanced capabilities of thrombus-defining diagnostic tools, increased accuracy of thrombus classifications, the discovery of new pharmacotherapeutic agents targeting these lesions, and the further development of specific technologies are warranted. This prospect will undoubtedly lead to a significant improvement in the outcomes of interventions for acute coronary syndromes.

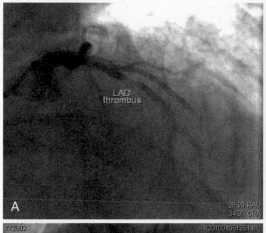

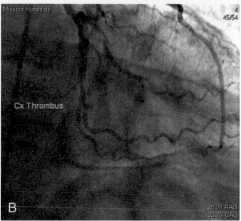

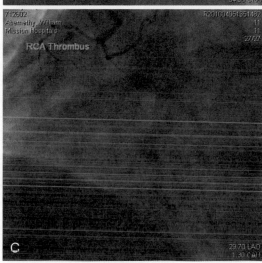

Figure 26-25 Simultaneous multivessel coronary thrombosis in a patient with inferior wall STEMI. A. LAD thrombus. B. Cx thrombus. C. RCA thrombus. PCI of the distal Cx artery was attempted in order to limit the infarct size and serve as a bridge prior to CABG but was not successful. The patient underwent successful emergency CABG. (*Courtesy of Courtesy of William B. Abernethy III,MD, Asheville Cardiology Associates, Memorial Mission Hospital Heart Center, Asheville, NC.*)

REFERENCES

1. Vankitachalam L, Kip KE, Selzer F, et al: Twenty-year evolution of percutaneous coronary intervention and its impact on clinical outcomes. a report from the National Heart Lung and Blood Institute-sponsored,multicenter 1985–1986 PTCA and 1997–2006 dynamic registries. *Circ Cardiovasc Interv* 2:6 12, 2000.
2. Singh M, Berger PB, Ting HH, et al: Influence of coronary thrombus on outcome of percutaneous coronary angioplasty in the current era. *Am J Cardiol* 88;1091–1096, 2001.
3. White CJ, Ramee SR, Collins TJ, et al: Coronary thrombi increase PTCA risk Angioscopy as a clinical tool. *Circulation* 93:253–258, 1996.
4. Fokkema ML, Vlaar PJ, Svilaas T, et al: Incidence and clinical consequences of distal embolization on the coronary angiogram after percutaneous coronary intervention for ST-elevation myocardial infarction. *Eur Heart J* 30(8):908–915, 2009.
5. Sianos G, Papafaklis MI, Daemen J, et al: Angiographic stent thrombosis after routine use of drug eluting stents in ST-segment elevation myocardial infarction. The importance of thrombus burden. *J Am Coll Cardiol* 50:572–583, 2007.
6. Freeman M, Williams AE, Chisholm RJ, et al: Intracoronary thrombus and complex morphology in unstable angina. Relation to timing of angiography and in-hospital cardiac events. *Circulation* 80:17–23, 1989.
7. Topaz O: Revascularization of thrombus laden lesions in AMI: the burden on the interventionalist. *J Invas Cardiol* 19:324–325, 2007.
8. Virmani R, Burke AP, Farb A, et al: Pathology of the unstable plaque. *Prog Cardiovasc Dis* 44:349–356, 2002.
9. Abela GS, Aziz K, Vedre A, et al: Effect of cholesterol crystals on plaques and intima in arteries of patients with acute coronary and cerebrovascular syndromes. *Am J Cardiol* 103:959–968, 2009.
10. Sami S, Willerson JT: Contemporary treatment of unstable angina and non-ST-segment elevation myocardial infarction. *Texas Heart Inst J* 37(2):141–148, 2010.
11. Schwartz SM, Galis SG, Rosenfeld ME, et al: Plaque rupture in humans and mice. *Arterioscler Thromb Vasc Biol* 27:705–713, 2007.
12. Whittaker P, Przyklenk K: Fibrin architecture in clots: a quantitative polarized light microscopy analysis. *Blood Cells Mol Dis* 42:51–56, 2009.

13. Carr ME, Carr SL: Fibrin structure and concentration alter clot elastic modulus but do not alter platelet medicated force development. *Blood Coag Fibrinolysis* 6:79–86, 1995.
14. Kereiakes DJ, Michelson AD: Platelet activation and progression to complications, *Rev Cardiovasc Med* 7:75–81, 2006.
15. Krishnaswami A, Carr ME, Jesse RL, et al: Patients with coronary artery disease who present with chest pain have significantly elevated platelet contractile force and clot elastic modulus. *Thromb Haemost* 88:739–744, 2002.
16. Abela GS, Eisenberg JD, Mittleman MA, et al: Detecting and differentiating white from red coronary thrombus by angiography in angina pectoris and in acute myocardial infarction. *Am J Cardiol* 83:94–97, 1999.
17. Beygui F, Collet JP, Nagaswami C, et al: Architecture of intracoronary thrombi in ST-elevation acute myocardial infarction: time makes the difference. *Circulation* 113:e21–e23, 2006.
18. Johnstone E, Friedl SE, Maheshwari A, et al: Distinguishing characteristics of erythrocyte-rich and platelet-rich thrombus by intravascular ultrasound catheter system. *J Thromb Thrombolysis* 24:233–239, 2007.
19. Vlaar PJ, Svilaas T, Vogelzang M, et al: A Comparison of 2 thrombus aspiration devices with histopathological analysis of retrieved material in patients presenting with ST-segment elevation myocardial infarction. *JACC Cardiovasc Intervent* 1:265–267, 2008.
20. Topaz O: On the hostile massive thrombus and the means to eradicate it. *Catheter Cardiovasc Intervent* 65:280–281, 2005.
21. Zhao Hy, Han HB, Li D, et al: Pathological analysis of aspirated materials from the culprit lesion in patients with acute myocardial infarction. *Zhonghua Xin Xue Guan Bing Za Zhi* 37(9):785–789, 2009.
22. Teirstein PS, Schatz RA, Wong SC, et al: Coronary stenting with angioscopic guidance. *Am J Cardiol* 75:344–347, 1995.
23. Bonello L, De Labriolle A, Lemesle G, et al: Intravascular ultrasound-guided percutaneous coronary interventions in contemporary practice. *Arch Cardiovasc Dis* 102:143–151, 2009.
24. Kubo T, Imanishi T, Kashiwagi M: Multiple coronary lesion instability in patients with acute myocardial infarction as determined by optical coherence tomography. *Am J Cardiol* 105(3):318–322, 2010.

25. Gibson CM, de Lemos JA, Murphy SA, et al: Combination therapy with abciximab reduces angiographically evident thrombus in acute myocardial infarction-a TIMI 14 substudy. *Circulation* 103:2550–2554, 2001.
26. Niccoli G, Spaziani C, Marino M, et al: Effect of chronic aspirin therapy on angiographic thrombotic burden in patients admitted for a first ST-elevation myocardial infarction. *Am J Cardiol* 105(5):587–591, 2010.
27. Aleong G, Vaqueriza D, Del Valle R, et al: Dual quantitative coronary angiography:a novel approach to quantify intracoronary thrombotic burden. *EuroIntervention* 4:475–480, 2008.
28. Pinto DS, Kirtane AJ, Pride YB, et al: CLARITY-TIMI-28 Investigators. Association of blood glucose with angiographic and clinical outcomes among patients with ST-segment elevation myocardial infarction. *Am J Cardiol* 101:303–307, 2008.
29. Topaz O, Topaz A, Polkampally PR: Thrombectomy in acute myocardial infarction. *Intervent Cardiol* 4:86–91, 2009.
30. Furie B, Furie BC: Mechanisms of thrombus formation. *N Engl J Med* 359:038–949, 2008.
31. Listro F, Grotti S, Angioli P, et al: Impact of thrombus aspiration on myocardial tissue reperfusion and left ventricular functional recovery and remodeling after primary angioplasty. *Circ Cardiovasc Intervent* 2:376–383, 2009.
32. Vlaar PJ, Svilaas T, van der Hors IC, et al: Cardiac death and reinfarction after 1 year in the Thrombus Aspiration during Percutaneous coronary intervention in Acute myocardial infarction Study(TAPAS): a 1-year follow-up study. *Lancet* 371:1915–1920, 2008.
33. Kunadian V, Zorkun C, Williams SP, et al: Intracoronary pharmacotherapy in the management of coronary microvascular dysfunction. *J Thromb Thrombolysis* 26:234–242, 2008.
34. Eeckhout E, Kern MJ. The coronary no reflow: a review of mechanisms and therapies. *Eur Heart J* 22:729–739, 2001.
35. Heusch G, Kleinbongard P, Bose D, et al: Coronary microembolization: from bedside to bench and back to bedside. *Circulation* 120(18):1822–1836, 2009.
36. Ohtani T, Ueda Y, Shimizu M, et al: Association between cardiac troponin T elevation and angioscopic morphology of culprit lesion in patients with non-ST segment elevation acute coronary syndrome. *Am Heart J* 150.227–233, 2005.

37. Lincoff AM, Topol EJ: Illusion of reperfusion. Does anyone achieve optimal reperfusion during acute myocardial infarction? *Circulation* 88:1361–1374, 1993.
38. Kaya MG, Arsian F, Abaci A, et al: Myocardial blush grade: a predictor for major adverse cardiac events after primary PTCA with stent implantation for acute myocardial infarction. *Acta Cardiol* 62:445–451, 2007.
39. Brosh D, Assali AR, Mager A, et al: Effect of no-reflow during primary percutaneous coronary intervention for acute myocardial infarction on six-month mortality. *Am J Cardiol* 99:442–445, 2007.
40. Topaz O: Focus on the infarct-related artery: a thrombus runs through it. *Catheter Cardiovasc Intervent* 57:340–341, 2002.
41. Carr ME, Carr SL, Greilich PE: Heparin ablates force development during platelet medicated clot retraction. *Thromb Haemost* 75:674–678, 1996.
42. Collet JP, Montalescot G, Lesty C, et al: Effects of abciximab on the architecture of platelet-rich clots in patients with acute myocardial infarction undergoing primary coronary intervention. *Circulation* 103:2328–2331, 2001.
43. Silva JA: Percutaneous coronary intervention of thrombotic lesions: still challenging! *Catheter Cardiovasc Intervent* 56:8–9, 2002.
44. Kalyanasundaram A, Blankenship JC, Berger P, et al: Thrombus predicts ischemic complications during percutaneous coronary intervention in saphenous vein grafts: results from TARGET trial. *Catheter Cardiovasc Intervent* 69:623–629, 2007.
45. Topaz O: Ischemic coronary syndromes and SVG interventions: do 2b/3a inhibitors miss the target? *Catheter Cardiovasc Intervent* 69:630–631, 2007.
46. Svilaas T, Vlaar PJ, van der Horst IC, et al: Thrombus aspiration during primary percutaneous intervention. *N Eng J Med* 358:557–567, 2008.
47. Mamas MA, Fraser D, Fath-Ordoubadi F: The role of thrombectomy and distal protection devices during percutaneous coronary interventions. *EuroIntervention* 4:115–123, 2008.
48. Tamahane UU, Chetcuti SJ, Hameed I, et al: Safety and efficacy of thrombectomy in patients undergoing primary percutaneous coronary intervention for acute ST elevation MI: a meta-analysis of randomized controlled trials. *BMC Cardiovasc Disord* 10:10, 2010.
49. Srinivasan M, Rihal C, Holmes DR, et al: Adjunctive thrombectomy and distal protection in primary percutaneous coronary intervention. *Circulation* 119:1311–1319, 2009.
50. Sardella G, Mancone M, et al: Thrombus aspiration during primary percutaneous coronary intervention improves myocardial reperfusion and reduces infarct size. The Expira (Thrombectomy with Export Catheter in Infarct-Related artery during primary percutaneous coronary intervention), prospective, randomized trial. *J Am Coll Cardiol* 53:309–315, 2009.
51. Silva-Orrego P, Colombo P, Bigi R, et al: Thrombus aspiration before primary angioplasty improves myocardial perfusion in acute myocardial infarction: the DEAR-MI study. *J Am Coll Cardiol* 48:1552–1559, 2006.
52. Burzotta F, Trani C, Romangnoli E, et al: Manual thrombus-aspiration improves myocardial reperfusion: the randomized evaluation of the effect of mechanical reduction of distal embolization by thrombus aspiration in primary and rescue angioplasty(REMEDIA) trial. *J Am Coll Cardiol* 46:371–376, 2005.
53. Liistro F, Grotti S, Angioloi P, et al: Impact of thrombus aspiration on myocardial tissue reperfusion and left ventricular functional recovery and remodeling after primary angioplasty. *Circ Cardiovasc Intervent* 2:376–383, 2009.
54. Sardella G, Mancone M, Nguyen BL, et al: The effect of thrombectomy on myocardial blush in primary angioplasty: the randomized evaluation of thrombus aspiration by two thrombectomy devices in acute myocardial infarction RETAMI trial. *Catheter Cardiovasc Intervent* 71:84–91, 2008.
55. De Luca L, Sardella G, Davidson CJ, et al: Impact of intracoronary aspiration thrombectomy during primary angioplasty on left ventricular remodeling in patients with anterior ST elevation myocardial infarction. *Heart* 92:951–957, 2006.
56. Bavry AA, Kumbhani,DJ, Bhatt DL: Role of adjunctive thrombectomy and embolic protection devices in acute myocardial infarction: a comprehensive meta-analysis of randomized trials. *Euro Heart J* 29:2989–3001, 2008.
57. Kaltof A, Bottcher M, Nielsen SS, et al: Routine thrombectomy in percutaneous coronary intervention for acute ST segment elevation myocardial infarction. *Circulation* 114:40–47, 2006.
58. Brilakis ES, Banerjee S, Lombardi WL: Retrograde recanalization of native coronary artery chronic occlusions via acutely occluded vein grafts. *Catheter Cardiovasc Intervent* 75:109–113, 2010.
59. Burzotta F, Trani C, Romagnoli E, et al: Feasibility of sequential thrombus aspiration and filter distal protection in the management of very high thrombus burden lesions. *J Invas Cardiol* 19:317–323, 2007.
60. Antoniucci D, Valenti R, Migliorini A: Thrombectomy during PCI for acute myocardial infarction: are the randomized controlled trials data relevant to the patients who need this technique? *Catheter Cardiovasc Intervent* 71:863–869, 2008.
61. Matar F, Anderson D, Rossi P, et al: Benefits of rheolytic thrombectomy in patients with ST-elevation myocardial infarction and high thrombus burden: findings from the cardioquest interventional database. *Cardiovasc Revasc Med* 9:113–114, 2008.
62. Topaz O, Ebersole D, Das T, et al: Excimer laser angioplasty in acute myocardial infarction (the CARMEL multicenter study). *Am J Cardiol* 93:694–701, 2004.
63. Beran G, Lang I, Schreiber W, et al: Intracoronary thrombectomy with the X-Sizer catheter system improves epicardial flow and accelerates ST-segment resolution in patients with acute coronary syndrome: a prospective, randomized controlled study. *Circulation* 105:2355–2360, 2002.
64. Napodano M, Pasquetto G, Sacca S, et al: Intracoronary thrombectomy improves myocardial reperfusion in patients undergoing direct angioplasty for acute myocardial infarction. *J Am Coll Cardiol* 42:1395–1402, 2003.
65. Lefevre T, Garcia E, Reimers B, et al: X-Sizer for thrombectomy in acute myocardial infarction improves ST-segment resolution. *J Am Coll Cardiol* 46:246–252, 2005.
66. Sianos G,Papafaklis MI, Vaina S, et al: Rheolytic thrombectomy in patients with ST-elevation myocardial infarction and largethrombus burden: the Thoraxcenter experience. *J Invas Cardiol* 18:3C–7C, 2006.
67. Antoniucci D, Valenti R, Migliorini A, et al: Comparison of rheolytic thrombectomy before direct infarct artery stenting versus direct stenting alone in patients undergoing percutaneous coronary intervention for acute myocardial infarction. *Am J Cardiol* 93:1033–1035, 2004.
68. Margheri M, Falai M, Vittore G, et al: Safety and efficacy of the AngioJet in patients with acute myocardial infarction: results from the Florence Appraisal Study of Rheolytic Thrombectomy (FAST). *J Invas Cardiol* 18:481–486, 2006.
69. Chinnaiyan K, Grines CL, O`Neill WW, et al: Safety of AngioJet thrombectomy in acute ST segment elevation myocardial infarction: a large, single center experience. *J Invas Cardiol* 18:17C–21C, 2006.
70. Sherev DA, Shavelle DM, Abdelkarim M, et al: Angiojet rheolytic thrombectomy during rescue PCI for failed thrombolysis: a single center experience. *J Invas Cardiol* 18:12C–16C, 2006.
71. Ali A, Cox D, Dieb N, et al: Rheolytic thrombectomy with percutaneous coronary intervention for infarct size reduction in acute myocardial infarction: 30 day results from a multicenter randomization study. *J Am Coll Cardiol* 48:244–250, 2006.
72. Migliorini A, Stabile A, Rodriguez AE, et al: Comparison of AngioJet rheolytic atherectomy before direct infarct artery stenting with direct stenting alone in patients with acute myocardial infarction. *The JETSTENT trial J Am Coll Cardiol* 56:1298–1306, 2010.
73. Kastrati A, Byrne RA, Schomig A: Is it time to jettison complex mechanical thrombectomy in favor of simple manual aspiration devices? *J Am Coll Cardiol* 56:1307–1309, 2010.
74. Topaz O: Laser. In Topol EJ, editor: *Textbook of Interventional Cardiology*, ed 4, Philadelphia, 2003, Saunders, pp 675–703.
75. Topaz O, Bernardo NL, Shah R, et al: Effectiveness of excimer laser coronary angioplasty in acute myocardial infarction or in unstable angina pectoris. *Am J Cardiol* 87:849–855, 2001.
76. Topaz O, Minisi AJ, Morris C, et al: Photoacoustic fibrinolysis: pulsed wave mid infrared laser-clot interaction. *J Thromb Thrombolysis* 3:209–214, 1996.
77. Topaz O, Minisi AJ, Bernardo NL, et al: Alterations of platelet aggregation kinetics with ultraviolet laser emission: the "stunned platelet phenomenon." *Thromb Haemost* 86:1087–1093, 2001.
78. Topaz O, Ebersole D, Dahm JB, et al: Excimer laser in myocardial infarction: a comparison between STEMI paitents with established Q-wave versus patients with non-STEMI (non-Q). *Lasers Med Sci* 23:1–10, 2008.
79. Shen X, Chandra N, Holmberg M, et al: Therapeutic ultrasound-enhanced thrombolysis in patients with acute myocardial infarction. *Angiology* 6(3):253–258, 2010.
80. Cohen MG, Tuero E, Blugermann J, et al: Transcutaneous ultrasound facilitated coronary thrombolysis during acute myocardial infarction. *Am J Cardiol* 92(4):454–457, 2003.
81. Bates ER: Aspirating and filtering atherothrombotic debris during percutaneous coronary intervention. *JACC Cardiovasc Intervent* 1:265–267, 2008.
82. Baim DS, Wahr D, George B, et al: Randomized trial of a distal embolic protection device during percutaneous intervention of saphenous vein aorto-coronary bypass grafts. *Circulation* 105:1285–1290, 2002.
83. Dangas G, Stone GW, Weinberg MD, et al: Contemporary outcomes of rescue PCI for AMI: comparison with primary angioplasty and the role of distal protection devices (EMERALD trial). *Am Heart J* 156(6):1090–1096, 2008.
84. Kaltoft A, Kelbaek H, Klovgaard L, et al: Increased rate of stent thrombosis and target lesion revascularization after filter protection in primary percutaneous coronary intervention for ST-segment elevation myocardial infarction: 15 months follow-up of the DEDICATION (Drug Eluting and Distal Protection in ST Elevation Myocardial Infarction) trial. *J Am Coll Cardiol* 55(9):867–871, 2010.
85. Limbruno U, De Caterina R: EMERALD, AIMI, and PROMISE: is there still a potential for embolic protection in primary PCI? *Eur Heart J* 27:1139–1145, 2006.
86. Timurkaynak T, Ozdemir M, Cengel A, et al: Direct stenting in angiographically apparent thrombus-containing lesions. *J Invas Cardiol* 13:742–747, 2001.
87. Alfonso F, Rodriguez P, Phillips P, et al: Clinical and angiographic implications of coronary stenting in thrombus-containing lesions *J Am Coll Cardiol* 29:725–733, 1997.
88. Assa-Vaknin H, Assali A, Kornowski R: Preliminary experiences using the MGuard stent platform in saphenous vein graft lesions. *Catheter Cardiovasc Intervent* 74:1055–1057, 2009.
89. Piscione F, Danzi GB, Cassese S, et al: Multicenter experience with MGuard net protection stent in ST-elevation myocardial infarction: safety, feasibility and impact on myocardial reperfusion. *Catheter Cardiovasc Intervent* 75:715–721, 2010.
90. Topaz O, Perin EC, Jesse RL, et al: Power thrombectomy in acute coronary syndromes. *Angiology* 54:457–468, 2003.
91. Atar S, Rosenschein U: Perspectives on the role of ultrasonic devices in thrombolysis. *J Thromb Thrombolysis* 17(2):107–114, 2004.
92. Parang P, Arora A: Coronary vein graft disease: pathogenesis and prevention. *Can J Cardiol* 25:e57–e62, 2009.
93. Yong A, Groenestein P, Brieger D, et al: Late thrombotic occlusion of a left internal mammary artery graft causing ST-elevation myocardial infarction. *Int J Cardiol* 23:142–143, 2010.
94. Hata M, Takayama T, Sezai A, et al: Efficacy of aggressive lipid controlling therapy for preventing saphenous vein graft disease. *Ann Thorac Surg* 88:1440–1444, 2009.
95. Veldkamp RF, Valk SDA, van Domburg RT, et al: Mortality and repeat interventions up until 20 years after aorto-coronary bypass surgery with saphenous vein grafts. A follow up of 1041 patients. *Eur Heart J* 21:747–753, 2000.
96. Holmes DR, Jr, Berger PB: Percutaneous revascularization of occluded vein grafts: is it still a temptation to be resisted? *Circulation* 99(1):26–29, 1999.
97. Perin EC, Leite-Sarmento R, Silva GV, et al: Wireless laser recanalization of chronic total coronary occlusions. *J Invas Cardiol* 13:401–405, 2001.
98. Londero HF: Editorial. Totally occluded saphenous vein graft recanalization: a dangerous option. *Catheter Cardiovasc Intervent* 60:218–220, 2003.
99. Gaitonde RS, Sharma N, von der Lohe E, et al: Combined distal embolization protection and rheolytic thrombectomy to facilitate percutaneous revascularization of totally occluded saphenous vein grafts. *Catheter Cardiovasc Intervent* 60:212–217, 2003.
100. Grantham JA, Marso SP, Spertus J, et al: Chronic total occlusion angioplasty in the United States. *JACC Cardiovasc Intervent* 2(6):479–486, 2009.
101. Christofferson RD, Lehmann KG, Martin GV, et al: Effect of chronic total coronary occlusion on treatment strategy *Am J Cardiol* 95(9):1088–1091, 2005.
102. Edwards JE: Atherosclerotic lesions: their distribution and histopathology. In Budinger TF, editor: *Noninvasive Techniques for Assessment of Atherosclerosis in Peripheral, Carotid and Coronary Arteries*, New York, 1982, Raven Press, pp 1–13.
103. Srivatsa SS, Edwards WD, Boos CM, et al: Histologic correlates of angiographic chronic total coronary artery occlusions: influence of occlusion duration on neovascular channel patterns and intimal plaque composition. *J Am Coll Cardiol* 29:955–963, 1997.
104. Topaz O: Revascularization of the impenetrable CTO-in support of the enhanced antegrade approach. *Catheter Cardiovasc Intervent* 73:276–277, 2009.
105. Abbott JD, Vlachos HA, Sawhney N, et al: Recent trends in the percutaneous treatment of chronic total coronary occlusions. *Am J Cardiol* 97:1691–1696, 2006.
106. Kandzari DE, Colombo A, Park SJ, et al: Revascularization for unprotected left main disease: evolution of the evidence basis to redefine treatment standards. *J Am Coll Cardiol* 20:1576–1578, 2009.
107. Prasad SB, Whitbourn R, Maliapan Y, et al: Primary percutaneous coronary intervention for acute myocardial infarction caused by unprotected left main stem thrombosis. *Catheter Cardiovasc Intervent* 73:301–307, 2009.
108. Topaz O, Polkampally PR, Mohanty PK, et al: Excimer laser debulking for percutaneous coronary intervention in left main coronary artery disease. *Lasers Med Sci* 24:955–960, 2009.
109. Topaz O: Total left main coronary artery occlusion: the acute, the chronic and the iatrogenic. *Chest* 101:843–846, 1992.
110. Topaz O, DiSciascio G, Cowley MJ, et al: Complete left main coronary artery occlusion: angiographic evaluation of collateral vessel patterns and assessment of hemodynamic correlates. *Am Heart J* 121:450–456, 1991.
111. Serruys PW, Onuma Y, Garg S, et al: 5-year clinical outcomes of the ARTS 2 of the sirolimus-eluting stent in the treatment of patients with multivessel de novo coronary artery lesions. *J Am Coll Cardiol* 55(11):1093–1101, 2010.
112. Costa JR, Sousa A, Moreira AC, et al: Incidence and predictors of very late major cardiac adverse events in the DESIRE (Drug Eluting Stents in the Real World) late registry. *JACC Cardiovasc Intervent* 3(1):12–18, 2010.
113. Alexopoulos D, Xanthopoulos I, Davlouros P, et al: Mechanisms of nonfatal acute myocardial infarction late after stent implantations: the relative impact of disease progression, stent restenosis and stent thrombosis. *Am Heart J* 159(3):439–445, 2010.
114. Garg S, Serruys P: Benefits and safety concerns associated with drug-eluting coronary stents. *Exp Rev Cardiovasc Ther* 8(3):449–470, 2010.
115. Ergelen M, Gorgulu S, Uyarel H, et al: The outcome of primary percutaneous coronary intervention for stent thrombosis causing ST-elevation myocardial infarction. *Am Heart J* 159(4): 672–676, 2010.
116. Parodi G, Memisha G, Bellandi B: et al. Effectiveness of primary percutaneous coronary interventions for stent thrombosis. *Am J Cardiol* 103(7):913–916, 2009.
117. Topaz O: Late stent thrombosis: is AngioJet rheolytic thrombectomy the preferred revascularization technique? *Catheter Cardiovasc Intervent* 58:18–19, 2003.
118. Turgeman Y, Suleiman K, Atar S: Multivessel acute coronary thrombosis and occlusion: an unusual cause of cardiogenic shock. *J Invas Cardiol* 19(9):E278–E280, 2007.
119. Konagai N, Cho M, Nakamura K, et al: Left atrial myxoma as a cause of acute myocardial infarction. *Texas Heart Inst J* 37(1):125–126, 2010.

27

Complications of Percutaneous Coronary Intervention

MARVIN H. ENG | JEFFERY W. MOSES | PAUL S. TEIRSTEIN

KEY POINTS

- The introduction of stents and superior anticoagulation as with glycoprotein IIb/IIIa inhibitors, thienopyridines, and direct thrombin inhibitors has successfully improved the safety of percutaneous coronary intervention. While less frequent than in the past, major complications such as death (~0.7%) and myocardial infarction (~2%) still occur in these procedures.[1]

- Primary causes for abrupt closure include dissection, thrombus formation, and acute stent thrombosis. Initial treatment for abrupt closure includes balloon redilation, optimization of activated clotting time, and a thorough investigation for the cause of abrupt closure, often using intravascular ultrasound. Ultimately, the patency of the artery must be maintained, most frequently with stent deployment to stabilize a dissection.

- Device embolization (most commonly stent embolization) is associated with periprocedural myocardial infarction and possible emergent referral to surgery, particularly if the device is not retrieved. Techniques to retrieve dislodged coronary stents include inflating small balloons to retrieve the stent into the guide, snaring the stent, entangling the stent with two coronary wires, and deploying or crushing the stent in its embolized location. Referral to coronary bypass surgery remains an option should the stent be dislodged in an unacceptable location for implantation.

- Coronary perforations are most frequently due to distal wire perforations or balloon/stent oversizing and should be treated with balloon occlusion and reversal of anticoagulation. Covered stent implantation may be considered for large perforations in major vessels. Perforations in small vessels that do not resolve with balloon occlusion may be treated with coil or Golfoam embolization. High suspicion for cardiac tamponade with a low threshold for echocardiography should be maintained. Referral to emergent surgery is an option should the perforation not seal

- Emergent referral to bypass surgery is rarely necessary during percutaneous coronary intervention. The morbidity and mortality of such surgery is exceedingly high; therefore there should be an exhaustive search for catheter-based solutions to avoid emergent bypass surgery.

- The incidence of periprocedural myocardial infarction varies depending on the assay and definition used. Large periprocedural myocardial infarctions (> 5 times the upper limit of normal CK-MB elevation) are associated with increased late mortality. Strategies to attenuate periprocedural myocardial infarction include the optimization of platelet inhibition (thienopyridines, glycoprotein IIb/IIIa inhibition), statin therapy, and the use of embolic protection devices during saphenous vein graft interventions.

- When the distal microcirculation is overwhelmed by embolized material, the no-reflow phenomenon can ensue. First-line treatment is with vasodilators such as intracoronary adenosine, nitroprusside, and verapamil. No-reflow can be attenuated with the use of thrombectomy in cases of acute thrombus formation or with embolic protection devices during saphenous vein graft interventions.

- Compulsive flushing of catheters during equipment exchanges prevents the great majority of air embolism. Should air embolism occur, the resolution of any air lock and restoration of antegrade flow in the vessel followed by stabilizing hemodynamics are the top priorities.

- If the presence of contrast allergy is known, reactions can usually be effectively pretreated with antecedent steroids. Anaphylactic reactions are frequently overlooked as a cause of hypotension. Unexplained hypotension should prompt a systematic search for its cause, which should include anaphylaxis (in addition to cardiogenic shock, abrupt closure, perforation with tamponade, air embolism, guide dissection, oversedation with respiratory acidosis, and access site bleeding). Contrast reactions during cardiac catheterization require immediate recognition and should be treated aggressively with intravenous fluids, steroids, and epinephrine if necessary.

Introduction

"Good judgment comes from experience and experience comes from bad judgment."

—**Unknown**

While the best approach to complications of percutaneous coronary intervention (PCI) is avoiding them, unfortunately complications are an important part of the interventional cardiologist's career. The prompt recognition of complications along with a calm and effective response are essential components of successful management. This chapter explores the most common procedural complications.

Abrupt Closure

INCIDENCE

The incidence of abrupt closure (often called acute closure) during percutaneous coronary PCI has steadily decreased from 3% in the balloon angioplasty era to 0.3% in the current era (Fig. 27-1). The trend in decreasing acute closure rates corresponds to the increased utilization of stents and effective antithrombotics, including glycoprotein IIb/IIIa inhibitors, dual antiplatelet therapy, and direct thrombin inhibitors. The decrease in abrupt closure has resulted in emergent coronary artery bypass grafting (CABG) and reduced periprocedural PCI mortality from 1.4% in 1985–1986 to 0.7% in 2006, most recently observed from the National Heart, Lung and Blood Institute (NHLBI) dynamic registry (Fig. 27-2).[1]

MECHANISMS

The most common mechanism of acute closure is dissection and injury to the media (Table 27-1, Fig. 27-3).[2] Intramural hematomas can develop, along with intimal flaps, causing mechanical obstruction. With mechanical obstruction and the exposure of subintimal tissue, thrombus formation is often initiated. Vasoconstriction further complicates this milieu but is rarely a major mechanism of closure.[3] While the predominate causes of acute closure in the pre-stent era were dissection (28%), thrombus (20%), or both (7%),[4] the cause is

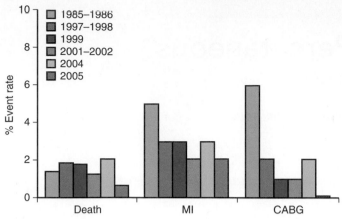

Figure 27-1 Improvements in PCI outcomes through its evolution from balloon angioplasty to the drug-eluting stent era are reflected in the NHLBI dynamic registry. *(Reproduced with permission from Venkitachalam L et al. Circ Cardiovasc Intervent. 2009;2:6–13.)*

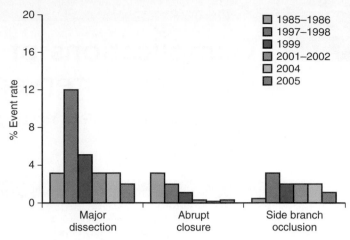

Figure 27-2 Progressive decrease in abrupt closure and major dissection with evolution of PCI to the current era of the drug-eluting stent. *(Reproduced with permission from Venkitachalam L et al. Circ Cardiovasc Intervent. 2009;2:6–13.)*

TABLE 27-1	Classification of Coronary Dissection	
Type	**Description**	**Acute Closure (%)**
A	Minor radiolucencies within lumen during angiography without dye persistence	0–2
B	Parallel tracks or double lumen separated by radiolucent area during angiography without dye persistence	2–4
C	Extraluminal cap with dye persistence	10
D	Spiral luminal filling defects	30
E	New persistent filling defects	9
F	Non-E types leading to impaired flow or total occlusion	69

Reproduced with permission from Klein LW. *Catheter Cardiovasc Intervent.* 2005;64: 395–401.

TABLE 27-2	ACC/AHA Lesion Classification System
Type A	
Discrete (<10 mm length)	
Concentric	
Readily accessible	
Nonangulated segment, <45 angle	
Smooth contour	
Little or no calcification	
Less than totally occlusive	
Not ostial in location	
No major side-branch involvement	
Absence of thrombus	
Type B	
Tubular (10–20 mm length)	
Eccentric	
Moderate tortuosity of proximal segment	
Moderately angulated segment, >45 degrees, <90 degrees	
Irregular contour	
Moderate to heavy calcification	
Total occlusions <3 months old	
Ostial in location	
Bifurcation lesions requiring double guide wires	
Some thrombus present	
Type C	
Diffuse (>2 cm length)	
Excessive tortuosity of proximal segment	
Extremely angulated segments >90 angle	
Total occlusion >3 months old	
Inability to protect major side branches	
Degenerated vein grafts with friable lesions	

B1, one adverse characteristic; B2, ≥2 adverse characteristics.

indeterminate in almost 50% of patients.[4,5] Patient factors predictive of abrupt closure include unstable angina, multivessel disease, and female gender.[6,7] In examining the angiographic risk factors of dissection-mediated acute closure, proximal tortuosity was the strongest predictor, followed by American College of Cardiology (ACC) lesion grade C (Table 27-2), longer lesion length, and de novo stenosis. Similarly, risks of thrombotic closure include the presence of preexisting thrombus, degenerated vein grafts, and recent myocardial infarction.[7] In the drug-eluting stent (DES) era, common causes of acute closure are stent-edge dissection and acute stent thrombosis. Stent-edge dissection occurs with oversizing of stents or aggressive balloon dilation at the edges, while acute stent thrombosis occurs either because of inadequate platelet inhibition or underexpansion of the stent.[8] Recent analysis of the ACUITY trial found that independent predictors of early stent thrombosis included minimal luminal diameter, diabetes mellitus, and preprocedural administration of thienopyridines.[9] Air embolism and the no-reflow phenomenon are also part of the differential diagnosis of abrupt closure (see sections for No Reflow and Air Embolism).

PROGNOSTIC SIGNIFICANCE

Most data regarding outcomes of patients experiencing abrupt closure are derived from the pre-stent era. In studies from the balloon angioplasty era, 6% of patients died, 36% suffered nonfatal myocardial infarction, and 30% were referred for emergency CABG.[4]

TREATMENT

Abrupt closure results in acute ischemia, which may become manifest by dramatic ECG changes, hypotension, hypertension, chest pain, ventricular arrhythmias, and/or bradycardia.

The first priorities are to stabilize hemodynamics and relieve ischemia. Vasopressors, ionotropes and possibly intra-aortic balloon pump (IABP) insertion should be considered for hemodynamic instability. Extreme vagal reactions may also cause bradycardia or hypotension and should be treated with atropine, intravenous fluid boluses, and vasopressors if necessary. Immediate recognition and treatment of

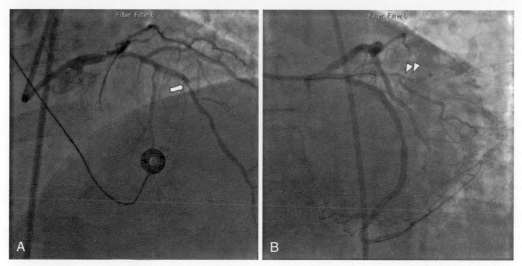

Figure 27-3 Coronary dissection. **A.** Flow-limiting dissection in the left anterior descending artery (arrow). **B.** Flow-limiting spiral dissection of the obtuse marginal branch with incomplete distal filling (arrowheads).

electrical instability with antiarrhythmic medications and cardioversion is imperative.[3] Expeditious balloon inflation to reestablish antegrade flow must be quickly attempted. Urgent stenting is usually required to stabilize the dissection. Glycoprotein IIb/IIIa antagonists can be helpful if thrombus is responsible for the acute closure. Prospective use of abciximab in elective or urgent PCI was compared in both balloon angioplasty and stenting cohorts in the EPISTENT trial, showing that abciximab decreases rates of abrupt closure and side-branch loss in both cohorts.[10] The utility of glycoprotein IIb/IIIa inhibitors as a bailout is controversial, as the data support its use upstream to PCI.[10,11] In the case of persistent acute closure, one should consider the use of intravascular ultrasound (IVUS) to more clearly define the pathology. IVUS can document the presence and extent of dissection. Multiple stents may be required to restore patency and achieve an adequate result. If the IVUS findings are suspicious for thrombus, aspiration thrombectomy may be valuable and the addition of a glycoprotein IIb/IIIa inhibitor should be considered. Intracoronary thrombolytic delivery has been used as a bailout for abrupt closure, but it is associated with significant morbidity and is not recommended.[6]

Factors affecting the inflow and outflow should be investigated. The use of multiple angiographic views, IVUS, and selective distal injections may better delineate the anatomy. IVUS is particularly helpful in confirming suspected stent-edge dissections or stent underexpansion. Guide-catheter dissections may cause poor inflow and can easily be overlooked. Pressure dampening, ventricularization, ECG changes, or severe ischemic pain may point to ostial guide catheter dissection. Distal wire dissections that occlude outflow may require stenting even if the distal vessel is of small caliber. In the pre-stent, balloon angioplasty era, approximately 40% of cases with acute closure ultimately achieved procedural success.[6] The predominate treatment was repeat balloon dilation with prolonged inflation facilitated by autoperfusion balloon catheters. Historically, the use of stents as bailout devices for abrupt or impending closure dramatically decreased the need for emergent CABG.[12] Although no randomized trial has been performed, the dramatic decrease in urgent and emergent CABG, from 3% to 0.7% in the NHLBI dynamic registry, was clearly associated with the use of stents and more effective anticoagulation, primarily glycoprotein IIb/IIIa inhibitors.[1] Clearly in the case of edge dissections, additional stents are required to cover the dissection and maintain vessel patency. Acutely thrombosed stents due to underexpansion require immediate dilation to achieve stent apposition and repeat IVUS to verify optimal stent deployment. Patients with a successful outcome following treatment of abrupt closure require close monitoring in an intensive care setting. If needed, intra-aortic balloon counterpulsation should be

initiated until the patient is stable. Serial cardiac enzyme assessments, ECGs, and echocardiography to assess the extent of myocardial damage are also recommended (see Fig. 27-4 for an algorithm outlining the management of acute vessel closure).

UNSUCCESSFUL OUTCOME

If recanalization is unsuccessful, the interventionist is faced with the choice of referral for emergent coronary bypass surgery or medical management. Medical management is essentially acceptance that the patient will sustain a myocardial infarction. The quantity of myocardium subtended by the closed vessel and the likelihood of a successful surgical result are the most important factors in deciding between surgical or medical management of abrupt closure. Care must be taken to distinguish "refractory closure" from "no reflow," since CABG is ineffective in the latter.

Coronary Perforation

INCIDENCE

Coronary perforation is a serious complication with an incidence ranging from 0.19% to 3% of cases (Table 27-3). Lesions associated with perforation are more complex in nature. ACC type B or C, calcified lesions, or chronic total occlusions are more likely to sustain perforation.[13,14] Women and the elderly are at greater risk of perforation.[4]

MECHANISM

There are two basic mechanisms of perforation: guide wire penetration and vessel rupture. Vessel rupture is usually caused by balloon or stent mismatch with oversizing of the dilatation catheter. Occasionally, an appropriate sized catheter will result in perforation, due to extensive dissection, lack of vessel wall integrity, or calcification. Early balloon angioplasty studies found that when the balloon:artery ratio became greater than 1.2:1, the risk of perforation increased.[4] Use of atherectomy devices such as eximer laser or rotational atherectomy also increases the risk of perforation.[15] Recanalization of chronic total occlusions has become a common setting for perforation, usually owing to small guidewire perforations, particularly with the increasing use of stiffer and hydrophilic guidewires.[13] Ellis-graded perforations (Table 27-4) fall into three classes of severity ranging from small endovascular leaks into the adventia (grade I) to frank extravasation into the pericardial space (grade III). Grade I perforations are frequently

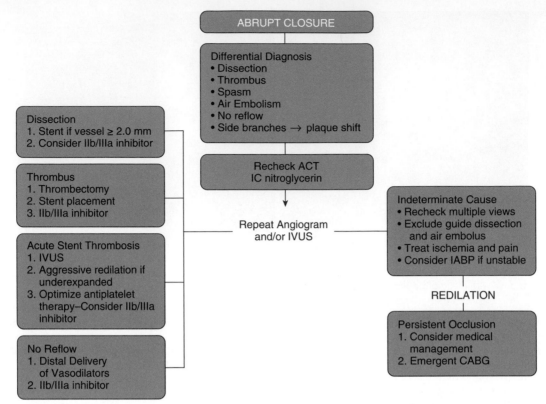

Figure 27-4 Suggested algorithm for the management of abrupt closure. *(Adapted with permission from Klein LW. Catheter Cardiovasc Intervent. 2005;64:395–401.)*

TABLE 27-3	Incidence and Outcome of Coronary Perforation Across Reported Studies					
Author	*Number of Procedures*	*Perforation Incidence*	*Tamponade (%)*	*CABG (%)*	*MI (%)*	*Death (%)*
Aljuni SC et al. (1988–1992)[18]	8,932	0.4%	17	37	26	9
Dippel EJ et al. (1995–1999)[15]	6,214	0.58%	22	22	NA	11
Ellis SG et al. (1990–1991)[94]	12,900	0.4%	24	24	16	5
Fasseas P et al. (1990–1991)[14]	16,298	0.58%	11.6	10.5	12.6	7.5
Gruberg L et al. (1990–1999)[16]	30,746	0.27%	31	39	34	10
Gunning MG et al. (1995–2001)[17]	6,245	0.8%	46	15	NA	12
Javaid A et al. (1996–2005)[95]	38,559	0.19%	19	35	NA	17
Kiernan JT et al. (2000–2008)[13]	14,281	0.48%	18	3	7.4	5.9
Shimony A et al. (2001–2008)[19]	9,568	0.59%	15.8	7	NA	7
Stankovic G et al. (1993–2001)[96]	5,728	1.5%	12	13	18	8
Ramana RK et al. (2001–2004)[97]	4,886	0.5%	4	20	32	8
Witzke CF et al. (1995–2003)[98]	12,658	0.3%	18	5	5	2.6

NA = not available.

caused by guidewires, but atheroablative devices as well as stents can cause small endovascular leaks. Occasionally guidewires can cause very large distal perforations; therefore extreme vigilance should be maintained, particularly in using stiff and hydrophilic guidewires in distal tortuous vessels. Grade II and III perforations are usually caused by high-pressure balloon inflations, oversized balloon catheters or stents, or the use of atheroablative devices (Fig. 27-5).

PROGNOSIS

Perforation severity correlates with worsening prognosis. Grade III perforations can quickly result in cardiac tamponade, rapid

hemodynamic collapse, myocardial infarction (MI), and/or death[4,13–19] (Table 27-3). Referral for emergency CABG is often indicated.

DIAGNOSIS

Given the dire consequences of coronary perforation, the interventionist must be especially attuned to recognizing this complication early. Patients may experience severe chest pain, dizziness, or nausea disproportional to symptoms typically associated with balloon inflation. There may be persistent ST-segment changes after balloon inflation. Vasovagal reactions may also accompany perforations, along with severe bradycardia and hypotension.[20] Awareness and vigilance post-PCI is vital, since cardiac tamponade as late as 24 hours post-PCI has been reported.[4,21] Late tamponade risk can be minimized with careful "final" angiograms visualizing all instrumented vessels and their branches.

MANAGEMENT

Grade I perforations can generally be treated with reversal of anticoagulation and/or prolonged balloon inflation at or proximal to the perforated vessel segment. Guidewire perforations are often best treated by balloon occlusion but can also be treated with the delivery of occlusive coils, fat, or beads. Occasionally, grade I perforations can resolve without an intervention, but small endovascular leaks may persist and require the use of a covered stent or referral to emergent CABG. Grade III perforations are catastrophic and more likely require urgent pericardiocentesis, deployment of a polytetraflouroethylene (PTFE)-covered stent, and/or referral for emergent surgery.[20]

Once a perforation occurs, the first step is to remain calm and advance a balloon from the guide catheter across the perforation without losing guidewire position. If the perforation has resulted from a guidewire, balloon inflation proximal to the perforation is indicated. This highlights an essential fundamental rule of interventional cardiology: a balloon should remain in the guide or within the lesion following any inflation until angiography confirms that there is no perforation. When perforation is recognized, balloon expansion to a pressure sufficient to occlude flow (usually 2–4 atm) is the first and most urgent step. Once the vessel is occluded, the patient's hemodynamics may normalize; however, aggressive treatment with intravenous fluids, atropine, vasopressors, and perhaps an intra-aortic balloon pump may be required. In treating perforations, anticoagulation is immediately discontinued. If heparin was used as the anticoagulant, reversal with protamine is usually indicated. Glycoprotein IIb/IIIa inhibitors must also be stopped and abciximab should be reversed with an infusion of platelets. The effects of tirofiban and eptifibatide cannot be reversed with platelet infusions, but these agents have a shorter half-life. Although IIb/IIIa inhibitors can increase bleeding complications, they do not increase the incidence or severity of perforations.[15] Direct thrombin inhibitors such as bivalirudin are increasingly utilized for peri-PCI anticoagulation, and the short half-life of this anticoagulant is advantageous in sealing wire perforations. Infusion of fresh frozen plasma is the only means of reversing anticoagulation with bivalirudin; this, however, requires a time delay to thaw the blood products.[22]

The presence of coronary perforation should also trigger urgent echocardiography. If a large pericardial effusion is present associated with cardiac tamponade physiology, emergent pericardiocentesis is indicated. Should echocardiography not be available, the diagnosis of tamponade on clinical grounds, use of right heart catheterization, or fluoroscopy of the heart's borders may be helpful. A major advance in the treatment of coronary perforation is the availability of PTFE membrane-covered stents. Prior to the advent of PTFE stents, the presence of a grade III perforation often required emergency CABG, which carried significant mortality.[21] The currently available PTFE stent is a distensible microporous PTFE membrane layered between two bare metal stents. Deployment of the stent graft excludes the perforation, possibly at the cost of occluding side branches. The initial experience using PTFE grafts was reported in a small case series demonstrating a decrease in cardiac tamponade and emergency CABG.[23] PTFE-covered stents are bulky and delivery into tortuous vessels can be challenging. A separate guide catheter for delivery of the PTFE-covered stent may be needed, as most guide catheters cannot accommodate both an angioplasty balloon and PTFE-stent graft (Fig. 27-6). Therefore a two-guide technique has been developed wherein contralateral access is established and a separate guide catheter is used to deliver the stent. A wire from the second guide catheter is advanced down the coronary vessel and the angioplasty balloon is momentarily deflated to allow guidewire passage. The PTFE stent is then quickly advanced across the

	Ellis Classification of Coronary Perforations	
Classification	**Description**	**Possible Clinical Sequelae**
I	Focal extraluminal crater without extravasation; limited to media or adventitia	Usually benign, may rarely cause delayed cardiac tamponade
II	Pericardial or myocardial blush without contrast in pericardium; limited extravasation producing patch of blushing or staining within the myocardium or pericardium	
III	Persistent extravasation with streaming or jet of contrast	High risk, increased morbidity and mortality
IIIA	Directed toward pericardium	High risk of acute cardiac tamponade
IIIB	Directed toward myocardium (e.g., ventricular cavity)	More benign course: possible fistula formation

Reproduced with permission from Klein LW. *Catheter Cardiovasc Intervent.* 2006;68: 713-717.

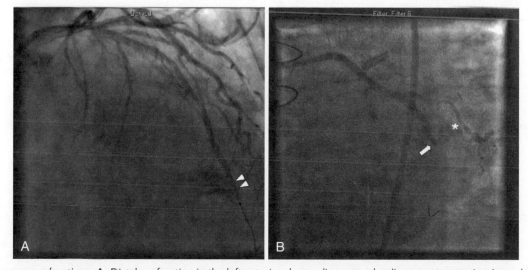

Figure 27-5 Coronary perforations. **A.** Distal perforation in the left anterior descending artery leading to extravasation (arrowheads) during treatment of a severe plaque. **B.** Perforation in a mid-obtuse marginal branch due to rotational atherectomy with extravasation into the pericardium (*).

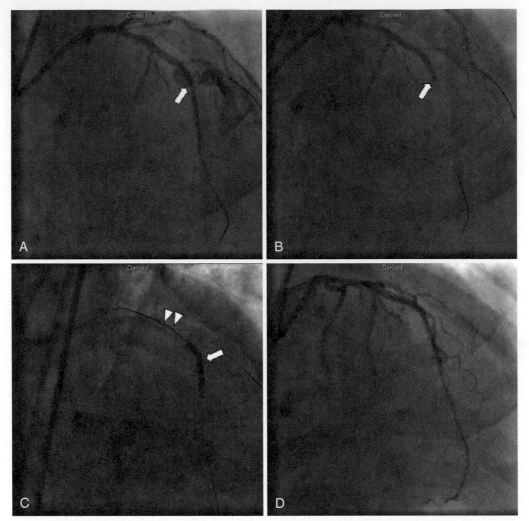

Figure 27-6 Successful exclusion of a coronary perforation with a PTFE-covered stent graft. **A.** An Ellis class III perforation at the mid-left anterior descending artery (LAD) with streaming into the pericardial space (arrow). **B.** Balloon tamponade of the perforation. **C.** The dual-guide technique is shown as the original coronary wire is withdrawn (arrowheads) while a JoStent (arrow) (Abbott Vascular, Santa Rosa CA) covered stent graft is deployed in the mid-LAD to exclude the perforation. **D.** Final angiogram demonstrating no extravasation after stent graft deployment.

perforation and deployed after the removal of the angioplasty balloon. This technique employing two guide catheters has been documented to decrease the rate of adverse events.[24] Side-branch vessels near the perforation site may be excluded by the PTFE-covered stent, which may result in a periprocedural MI.[23] IVUS should be used routinely to verify adequate expansion of the covered stent, since deploying this dual stent layer may require aggressive (≥18 atm) but judicious post-dilation. Occasionally, collateral filling may cause persistent extravasation despite exclusion of the perforation with a stent graft and surgical management, or occlusion of the supplying collateral may be required. Perforations in small vessels can be addressed with either additional prolonged balloon inflations or the injection of thrombin, polyvinyl alcohol, Gelfoam, collagen, or the embolization of microcoils or beads.[25,26] (See Fig. 27-7 for a suggested strategy for the management of coronary perforation.)

Device Embolization

INCIDENCE

Embolization of equipment such as coronary stents and guidewire fragments is a potentially catastrophic complication of PCI. Stents are the most common devices embolized, with an incidence ranging from 3% for first-generation hand-crimped devices to a much lower 0.32% for current stent delivery systems.[27,28]

MECHANISM

Extreme tortuosity and calcification increase the risk of stent embolization due to dislodgement from delivery balloons. For this reason, stents are more frequently lost in the right coronary and circumflex arteries and less commonly in the left anterior descending artery.[27,29] In the initial experience using Palmaz-Shatz stents, manually crimped stents were found to have a relatively high embolization rate of 3%.[28]

TREATMENT

There are numerous approaches to the removal of embolized stents. If possible, maintain guidewire position through the center of the stent. This will facilitate retrieval using one of many commercially available snares (Fig. 27-8). Another option is to advance a small-diameter balloon through the unexpanded stent and attempt to drag it back into the guide catheter. A third approach is to pass a second wire alongside the embolized stent, attempting to enter one of the struts, and then to attach a single torquing device to both

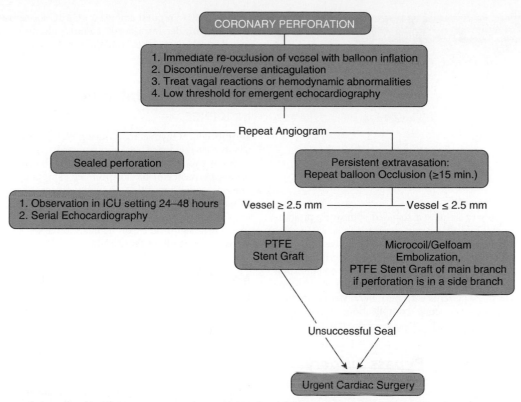

Figure 27-7 Suggested algorithm for the management of coronary perforation. *(Reproduced with permission from Klein LW. Catheter Cardiovasc Intervent. 2006;68:713–717.)*

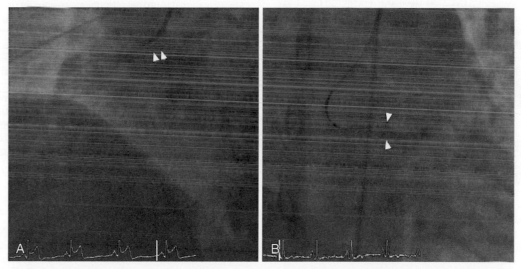

Figure 27-8 Snaring of an embolized coronary stent at the right coronary ostium. **A.** A coronary stent (arrowheads) was stripped from the balloon and is located at the right coronary ostium. **B.** Using a gooseneck snare, the stent is retrieved and retracted into the guide.

wires used in order to twist the wires together. Then the wire-wrapped stent is withdrawn from the artery. A fourth approach is to deploy the embolized stent in its unintended location. Retrieval devices such as biliary forceps or bioptomes can easily damage the arterial wall and should be avoided or handled with great care. Deploying a new stent alongside the embolized stent such that the dislodged stent is embedded into the arterial wall is a reasonable option should retrieval be difficult, but this technique may be associated with an elevated risk of periprocedural MI, death, and referral to CABG.[30]

RETAINED COMPONENTS OF PERCUTANEOUS CORONARY ANGIOPLASTY EQUIPMENT

The incidence of retained components of percutaneous coronary angioplasty equipment is reported to be 0.2% in a single-center series.[31] Things such as angioplasty balloons and guidewire fragments have embolized down coronary vessels. The successful recovery of such fragments utilizes techniques similar to those for retrieving embolized stents.[32,33] In one report, four patients with retained guidewire fragments and a gold band from a balloon catheter did not suffer ischemic complications.

TABLE 27-5	Coronary Stent Embolization is Associated with Significant Major Adverse Cardiac Events				
	Incidence	N	Death (%)	MI (%)	CABG (%)
Brilakis ES et al.[27]	0.32%	38	3%	11%	5%
Bolte J et al.[30]	1.7%	387	6.2%	3.9%	17%
Cantor WJ et al.[99]	8.3%	108	2.8%	5%	16%
Eggebrecht H et al.[100]	0.9%	20	15%	NA	15%

NA, not available.

PROGNOSIS

The embolization of coronary stents is associated with worse prognoses and an increased risk of adverse cardiac events (Table 27-5).[27,29,30] Successful retrieval is associated with good prognoses; however, unsuccessful management or retrieval results in high rates of periprocedural MI, emergent referral to CABG, and death.[30] Peripheral embolization of stents is rarely associated with significant clinical sequelae. In one noninvasive assessment of 20 patients with peripheral stent embolization there were no peripheral vascular complications over a mean duration of 5 years.[29]

◼ Emergency Coronary Bypass Surgery

INCIDENCE

The incidence of emergency CABG has steadily decreased; it was 1.5% to 2.9% in the balloon angioplasty era and is 0.14% to 0.41% in the stent era[34-36] (Table 27-6). Data from the NHLBI dynamic registry describe an incidence of 0.7% for early CABG ≤ 30 days from PCI.[1] Patient characteristics associated with emergent CABG included cardiogenic shock, acute MI, multivessel disease, and a prior history of MI. Procedural variables distinguishing patients referred for emergent CABG include ACC type C lesions, placement of an intra-aortic balloon pump (IABP), dissection, perforation, and abrupt closure. Analysis from one single-center study found that most patients referred for CABG had at least one or two high-risk characteristics and those with four high-risk factors had a 9.3% incidence of emergent CABG.[36]

PROGNOSIS

Emergent CABG following PCI is associated with significant morbidity and mortality. The death rate ranged between 7.8% and 14% in three single-center studies. Q-wave MIs, stroke, and/or renal insufficiency commonly complicate postemergent CABG procedures.[34] Q-wave MI accounts for most of the patient deaths, followed by cardiac arrhythmias, suggesting that delay in perfusion while transitioning to surgery is the most common mechanism of demise.[34] Therefore it is advisable to attempt all possible solutions expeditiously and, if success does not

TABLE 27-6	Unadjusted Rates of MACE following Emergent CABG for Failed PCI in Contemporary Retrospective Single-Center Registries					
	Time Period	Incidence	N	Death	MI	Stroke
Seshadri N et al.[35]	1992–2000	0.6%	113	15%	12%	53%
Roy P et al.[36]	1994–2008	0.4%	90	7.8%	5.7%	10%
Yang EH et al.[34]	1995–2003	0.5%	77	13%	NA	NA

MACE, major adverse cardiovascular events; NA, not available.

appear likely, to request emergency CABG sooner rather than later and strongly consider intra-aortic counterpulsation and aggressive pharmacological support to maintain perfusion pressure en route to surgery.

◼ Myocardial Infarction

INCIDENCE

Periprocedural myonecrosis during PCI is common, occurring with a 0% to 47% incidence based on reported series.[37] The definition of MI varies between studies with respect to biomarker assay, threshold values, frequency of blood specimen sampling, and use of ECG data among studies, resulting in wide ranges of reported incidence.[38] Whether myonecrosis is directly responsible for late adverse outcomes or is simply a symptom of disease severity is debated. However, the prognostic significance of higher biomarker values is reproducible across many studies (Table 27-7).

MECHANISM

Obvious causes of periprocedural MI include side-branch occlusion, distal macroembolization, no reflow, abrupt occlusion, prolonged balloon inflations, and hypotension (Table 27-8). Distal microembolization occurs frequently, and the extent of myonecrosis has been shown to be proportional to the plaque burden and degree of calcification.[39] Microvascular embolization is reflected by worsening myocardial perfusion grade, and impaired perfusion grade is directly proportional to a larger infarct size by magnetic resonance imaging (MRI).[40] Doppler coronary flow studies give further credence to the importance of distal embolization and microvascular obstruction as the cause of most post-PCI biomarker elevation, supported by delayed-enhancement MRI studies.[41,42] Of note, in optimizing stent expansion, greater cross-sectional areas were linked to greater CK-MB elevation postprocedure, suggesting that aggressive stent expansion increases the risk of distal embolization.[43] The process of advancing and implanting bulkier devices such as stents has been associated with more numerous periprocedural MIs.[10] The use of glycoprotein IIb/IIIa inhibitors significantly decreased the rate of MIs following stenting.[44,45] The use of mechanical atherectomy devices is more likely to result in periprocedural MI. As coronary lesions are debulked, plaque is "pulverized" and sent downstream into the intracoronary vascular bed. While most embolized particles are small and pass harmlessly through the coronary microcirculation, atherectomy is associated with a somewhat increased periprocedural MI as measured by CK-MB elevations and the no-reflow phenomenon as compared with balloon angioplasty.[46]

PROGNOSIS

Periprocedural enzyme elevation measured as CK-MB and troponin elevation is directly related to adverse events including death, and Q-wave MI (QWMI)[47,48] (Table 27-7, Fig. 27-9). This has been observed in multicenter trials, as well as in meta-analysis of multiple acute coronary syndrome (ACS) and stable coronary disease trials.[49]

PREVENTIVE PHARMACOTHERAPY

Periprocedural myocardial necrosis appears to be part of the "collateral damage" that occurs when PCI is undertaken, but numerous pharmacological and device developments have emerged to lower the incidence of this complication. Agents such as glycoprotein IIb/IIIa inhibitors, PY12 receptor inhibitors, and statins decrease periprocedural MI. The use of distal embolic protection during vein graft interventions has been shown to reduce periprocedural MI significantly.

Glycoprotein IIb/IIIa inhibitors target the common final receptor for platelet cross-linking and thrombus formation. Abciximab, a murine monoclonal antibody specific for platelet IIb/IIIa receptors,

TABLE 27-7	Incidence and Implication of Periprocedural Myocardial Infarction from Major Studies				
Authors	**N**	**Cardiac Marker Cutoff Level**		**Incidence (%)**	**Follow-up Implication**
Abdelmeguid et al.[101]	4,484	CK 1-2x ULN		5.8	Death (RR 1.27)
Abdelmeguid et al.[102]	4,664	CK 2-5x ULN		2.6	Death (RR 2.19)
Kong et al.[103]	2,812	CK 5x ULN		1.3	Death (RR 1.05)
		CK 1-1.5x ULN		2.3	
		CK 1.5-3x ULN		3.8	
		CK > 3x ULN		2.9	
Ghazzal et al.[104]	15,637	CK 1-2x ULN		4.6	Death (OR 1.84)
		CK 2-3x ULN		1.1	
		CK > 3x ULN		1.6	
Tardiff et al.[105]	1,616	CK-MB > 1x ULN		18.0	Death/MI/Revasc. 6 month endpoint 1-3x ULN 32.4% 3-5x ULN 37.9% 5-10x ULN 35.3% >10x ULN 43.6%
Waksman et al.[106]	3,265	CK-MB > 2x ULN, ST/T changes or CP		4.7	Death 7.8%
Simoons et al.[107]	5,025	CK-MB 1-3x ULN		13.2	Death (log enzyme ratio OR 1.82)
Roe et al.[108]	2,384	CK-MB > 3x ULN		6.6	Death (OR 1.06)
		CK-MB 1-3x ULN		21.3	
		CK-MB 3-5x ULN		6.0	
		CK-MB 5-10x ULN		7.1	
		CK-MB > 10x ULN		9.5	
Mehran et al.[39]	2,256	CK-MB >4 ng/mL		25.8	NR
Stone et al.[109]	7,147	CK-MB >4 ng/mL		14	Death (adjusted OR 8.00)
Dangas et al.[110]	4,085	CK-MB >4 ng/mL		36.9	Death (OR 1.5)
Ajani et al.[111]	1,326	CK-MB >4 ng/mL		45	Death/MI/TVR (OR 1.57)
Brener et al.[112]	3,478	CKMB >8.8 ng/mL		24	Death (OR 1.89)
Ellis et al.[113]	8,409	CK-MB >8.8 ng/mL		17.2	Death
Brener et al.[114]	3,573	CK-MB >8.8 ng/mL		38	Death (HR 1.1)
Hong et al.[115]	1,693	CK-MB 4-20 ng/mL		32.1	Death (OR 5.5)
		CK-MB >20 ng/mL		15.2	
Natarajan et al.[116]	1,128	cTNI 1-4x ULN		7.6	NR
		cTNI > 5x ULN		9.1	
Nallamothu et al.[117]	1,157				Death
		cTnI 1- < 3x ULN		16	cTnI 5- < 8x ULN OR
		cTnI 3- < 5x ULN		4.6	3.4
		cTnI 5- < 8x ULN		2	cTnI ≥ 8x ULN OR 2.7
		cTnI ≥ 8x ULN		6.5	
Fuchs et al.[118]	1,129	TnI 1-3x ULN		15	
		TnI > 3x ULN		15.5	Death/MI/TVR TnI > 3x ULN 6.4%
Cavallini et al.[119]	3,494	cTnI >0.15 ng/dL		44.2	Death (OR 1.9)
		CK-MB >5 ng/mL		16.0	

CP, chest pain; HR, hazard ratio; OR, odds ratio; NR, not recorded; RR, relative risk; TVR, target vessel revascularization; ULN, Upper limit of normal; cTnI, cardiac tronponin I; TnI, troponin I.

Reproduced with permission from Herrman J. *Eur Heart J.* 2005;26: 2493–2519.

TABLE 27-8	Mechanisms of Periprocedural Myonecrosis
Procedure-related complications	
Side-branch occlusion	
Flow-limiting dissection	
Abrupt closure	
Macroscopic embolization	
No reflow	
Microscopic embolization	
Lesion-specific characteristics	
Large thrombus burden	
Plaque volume	
Plaque vulnerability	
Patient-specific characteristics	
Arterial inflammation	
Aspirin resistance	
Genetic predisposition	

Reproduced with permission from Bhatt DL, Topol EJ. *Circulation.* 2005;112:906–922.

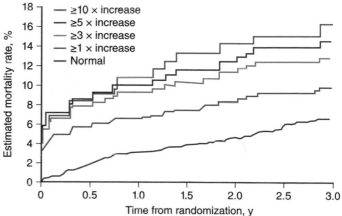

Figure 27-9 Mortality for patients with 1- to 10-fold increases in periprocedural creatinine kinase elevation. The *P* values for comparisons are ≥1x *P* = 0.02, ≥3x *P* < 0.001, ≥5x *P* < 0.001, and ≥10x *P* < 0.001. (*Reproduced with permission from Topol EJ et al. JAMA. 1997;278: 479–484.*)

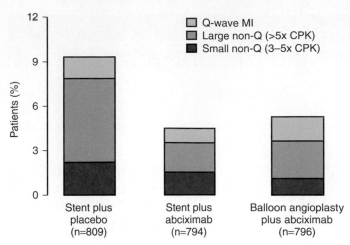

Figure 27-10 Incidence and type of myocardial infarction for each treatment group. *(Reproduced with permission from the EPISTENT investigators. Lancet. 1998; 352:87–92.)*

TABLE 27-9	TIMI Grading System for Describing Coronary Flow
TIMI Grade	
0	No antegrade flow beyond the point of occlusion.
I	Contrast material is able to pass through the area of obstruction but fails to opacify the distal coronary bed.
II	Contrast is able to penetrate the area of obstruction and fills the distal coronary bed; however, it is perceptibly slower than other coronary vessels unaffected by the coronary obstruction.
III	Antegrade flow into distal coronary bed of the obstructed artery is as prompt as the flow in an uninvolved coronary vessel.

causes an 80% blockade of platelet function[50] and, during PCI in the EPIC trial, first demonstrated a reduction in periprocedural MI (8.6% vs. 5.2%; $P = 0.013$) in association with balloon angioplasty or atherectomy.[51] These results were consistently reproduced during the implantation of stents, as demonstrated in the EPISTENT, EPILOG, and the CAPTURE trials, each showing greater than 50% reductions in periprocedural MI as opposed to PCI with heparin and aspirin alone[10,45,52] (Fig. 27-10). Similar reductions in periprocedural MI were observed with synthetic small-molecule glycoprotein IIb/IIIa inhibitors such as eptifibatide and tirofiban. A 40% reduction in MI was seen at 48 hours (5.4% vs. 9.0%; $P = 0.0015$) in the ESPRIT trial, and most of the clinical benefit of eptifibatide in the PURSUIT trial was attributed to reductions in periprocedural MI.[53,54] Tirofiban was observed to reduce periprocedural MI when administered in a high-dose fashion in the ADVANCE trial.[55] Adequate platelet inhibition appears to be the key to success with respect to preventing periprocedural MI and inhibiting PY12 receptors. This was first observed with pretreatment using ticlodipine and then with clopidogrel in the PCI subset of the CURE trial, where a 44% reduction in MI was seen at 30 days.[56,57] Preprocedural loading with 300 mg of clopidogrel was found to reduce the primary endpoint of MI, death, and target vessel revascularization (TVR) by 38% if this agent was given at least 6 hours prior to PCI.[58,59] A high loading dose (600 mg) of clopidogrel caused a 50% reduction in periprocedural MI, likely because therapeutic inhibition of platelets was achieved more rapidly.[60] As expected, resistance to either aspirin or clopidogrel confers an increased risk of periprocedural MI.[61] Tailoring anticoagulation strategies by adding eptifibatide in the treatment of patients without an optimal response to clopidogrel may reduce periprocedural MI.[62] In addition to optimizing antiplatelet therapy prior to PCI, pretreatment with statins appears to prevent myocardial injury in patients undergoing either elective or emergent PCI.[63,64] Loading patients with atorvastatin 40 mg for 1 week prior to PCI caused a 72% reduction in periprocedural MI (3% vs. 18%; $P = 0.025$) during elective PCI in the ARMYDA study.[63] The mechanism of myonecrosis attenuation may be related to the decreased expression of VCAM-1 and ICAM-1 post-PCI.[65] Even if patients were receiving chronic statin therapy, reloading with high doses of statins led to a further reduction of periprocedural MI.[66]

Since many periprocedural MIs are caused by distal embolization, the use of embolic protection devices has been extensively studied, mainly in such interventions. In the SAFER trial, a total of 801 patients undergoing elective saphenous vein graft PCI were randomized to distal protection using the Guardwire (Medtronic Vascular, Santa Rosa, CA), causing a 41% reduction in periprocedural MI.[67] Proximal protection and aspiration using the PROXIS (St. Jude Medical, MN) produced comparable rates of periprocedural MI, and its use was found to be noninferior to distal embolic protection devices when used in saphenous vein graft interventions.[68] The benefits of distal embolic protection have not been reproduced in native coronary vessels. The EMERALD trial randomized 501 patients to receiving either distal embolic protection using the Guardwire Plus distal protection device (Medtronic Vascular, Santa Rosa, CA) combined with aspiration thrombectomy or usual care for ST-segment elevation MI (STEMI).[69] Despite the use of the Guardwire Plus and aspiration thrombectomy, no differences were observed with respect to death, MI, or infarct size. Lack of efficacy of distal embolic protection devices in the setting of STEMI is likely attributable to the increased door-to-balloon time seen in the treatment group. Similarly in the PROMISE study, use of Filterwire EX (Boston Scientific, Natick, MA) distal protection during ACSs did not lead to any decrease of infarct size or reduction in MACE.[70] Periprocedural MI remains a common complication that predicts future adverse outcomes. Judicious revascularization, optimization of pharmacological therapy, and the use of embolic protection devices when appropriate may reduce its incidence.

Coronary No-Reflow

INCIDENCE AND DIAGNOSIS

Coronary no-reflow is the inability to perfuse myocardium after opening a previously occluded or stenosed epicardial coronary artery.[71] No-reflow is suspected to result from a combination of endothelial damage, platelet and fibrin embolization, vasospasm, and tissue edema that overwhelms the coronary microcirculation. Reperfusion-related injury is hypothesized to contribute to no-reflow via infiltration of the microcirculation with neutrophils and platelets. The incidence of no-reflow ranges from 0.6% to 2% and is more frequently observed with the use of stents, atherectomy, and PCI in saphenous vein grafts.[72,73] Risk factors for no-reflow include the angiographic presence of thrombus, cardiogenic shock, increased reperfusion time, hyperglycemia, and leukocytosis.[74–76] Diagnosis of no reflow is made angiographically by assessing flow, usually using the TIMI grading system (Table 27-9); however, there are other ways of measuring microcirculatory myocardial perfusion, as with myocardial blush score, TIMI frame count, and contrast echocardiography.

PREVENTION

To some degree, the no-reflow phenomenon can be minimized or prevented during coronary intervention with diligent pharmacological and mechanical pre- and post treatment (Table 27-10). Pretreatment with intracoronary calcium channel blockers is a helpful adjunct to the treatment of saphenous vein grafts.[77] Use of distal protection devices in the context of saphenous vein graft PCI in the SAFER trial decreased the rate of no-reflow to 4.8%, compared with 9.7% in performing PCI without distal protection.[67] Rates of no-reflow increase with the use of rotational atherectomy arc likely due to the embolization of pulverized plaque into the microcirculation. In one study, the use of preemptive intracoronary adenosine and nitroglycerin during rotational atherectomy decreased the rate of no-reflow from 11.4% to 1.4%.[77,78] Administration of abciximab prior to PCI for STEMI increased the proportion of patients with TIMI III flow both before and after PCI in the ADMIRAL trial.[79] This increase in TIMI III flow translated into higher patient LVEF and decreased the composite endpoint of death, target vessel revascularization, and reinfarction among patients receiving abciximab. The most recent development in preventing no-reflow and optimizing perfusion in the setting of STEMI is aspiration thrombectomy. The TAPAS trial was a prospective trial randomizing 1,071 patients to either routine aspiration thrombectomy prior to coronary stenting versus usual care.[80] Aspiration thrombectomy improved markers of reperfusion such as myocardial blush score and ST-segment resolution, but outcomes with respect to death, reinfarction, target vessel revascularization, and composite major adverse cardiovascular events (MACE) were not found to be different at 30 days. Rates of MACE correlated with the degree of perfusion as measured by myocardial blush score and ST-segment resolution (Fig. 27-11). At 1 year, routine aspiration thrombectomy reduced the rate of cardiac death to 3.4% compared with 6.7% in association with routine PCI (Fig. 27-12).[81] Benefits of adjunctive thrombectomy during STEMI were reproduced in both meta-analysis and in a pooled patient analysis of 11 randomized clinical trials for both 30 day and 1 year major adverse cardiovascular and cerebrovascular events (MACCE) respectively.[82,83]

TREATMENT

First-line treatment for no-reflow primarily consists of delivery of vasodilators, especially adenosine, calcium channel blockers, and nitroprusside into the coronary microcirculation (Table 27-11). Should the dye column stop at midvessel, distal injections through balloons or microcatheters should be performed to exclude dissection. Injection of vasodilators through an infusion catheter close to the distal bed may improve microcirculatory drug delivery. There is no role for emergent coronary bypass surgery or thrombolytic therapy. If the stenosis is widely patent by angiography or IVUS, additional coronary stenting is not helpful. Cases involving cardiogenic shock may require intra-aortic

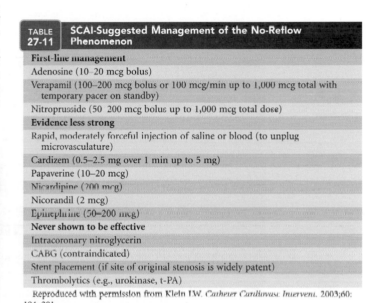

TABLE 27-11	SCAI-Suggested Management of the No-Reflow Phenomenon
First-line management	
Adenosine (10–20 mcg bolus)	
Verapamil (100–200 mcg bolus or 100 mcg/min up to 1,000 mcg total with temporary pacer on standby)	
Nitroprusside (50–200 mcg bolus up to 1,000 mcg total dose)	
Evidence less strong	
Rapid, moderately forceful injection of saline or blood (to unplug microvasculature)	
Cardizem (0.5–2.5 mg over 1 min up to 5 mg)	
Papaverine (10–20 mcg)	
Nicardipine (200 mcg)	
Nicorandil (2 mcg)	
Epinephrine (50–200 mcg)	
Never shown to be effective	
Intracoronary nitroglycerin	
CABG (contraindicated)	
Stent placement (if site of original stenosis is widely patent)	
Thrombolytics (e.g., urokinase, t-PA)	

Reproduced with permission from Klein LW. *Catheter Cardiovasc Intervent.* 2003;60:194–201.

TABLE 27-10	Prevention of No-Reflow
Use of distal protection devices in treating saphenous vein graft lesions	
In performing rotational atherectomy, routine use of nitroglycerin, verapamil and heparin in combination with the flush solution	
Consider pretreatment with a glycoprotein IIb/IIIa inhibitor during PCI in patients with acute coronary syndromes	
Minimize balloon inflation and consider direct stenting in patients with bulky atheromas or saphenous vein grafts	
Pretreatment with verapamil or adenosine	
Aspiration thrombectomy for thrombus-laden lesions	

Figure 27-11 Cardiac death, all-cause mortality, and the combined endpoint are inversely proportional to myocardial blush score and degree of ST-segment resolution, proving that outcomes are directly related to the quality of perfusion. *(Reproduced with permission from Vlaar PJ et al. Lancet. 2008;371:1915–1920.)*

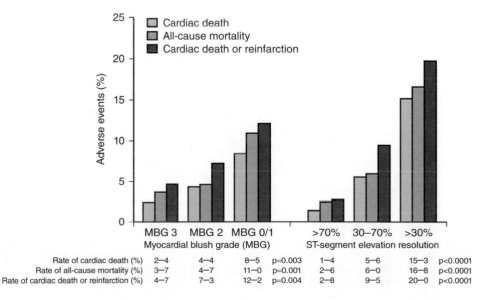

	MBG 3	MBG 2	MBG 0/1		>70%	30–70%	>30%	
Rate of cardiac death (%)	2–4	4–4	8–5	p=0.003	1–4	5–6	15–3	p<0.0001
Rate of all-cause mortality (%)	3–7	4–7	11–0	p=0.001	2–6	6–0	16–8	p<0.0001
Rate of cardiac death or reinfarction (%)	4–7	7–3	12–2	p=0.004	2–8	9–5	20–0	p<0.0001

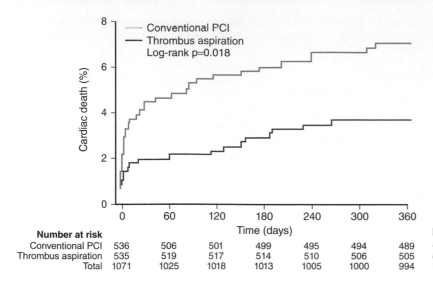

Figure 27-12 Significant reduction of cardiac death by aspiration thrombectomy to 3.6% compared with 6.7% with delivering usual care. *(Reproduced with permission from Vlaar PJ et al. Lancet. 2008;371:1915–1920.)*

Number at risk

Conventional PCI	536	506	501	499	495	494	489
Thrombus aspiration	535	519	517	514	510	506	505
Total	1071	1025	1018	1013	1005	1000	994

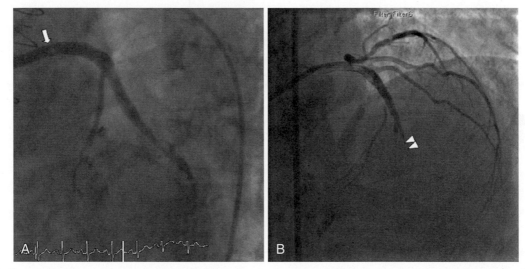

Figure 27-13 **A.** Air embolism (arrow) from inadequate flushing of a distal protection filter. **B.** "Air lock" created by a large air embolus, causing cessation of flow in the left anterior descending artery (arrowheads).

balloon counterpulsation to maintain adequate systemic perfusion pressure.

PROGNOSIS

No-reflow is associated with larger infarct size, reduced left ventricular ejection fraction (LVEF), and death.[84–86] Retrospective analysis has shown that patients with no-reflow undergoing primary PCI have an in-hospital and 6-month mortality increase of 6-fold and 10-fold respectively. The adjusted odds for death at 6 months was 5.4 times higher in patients with no-reflow.[86]

Air Embolism

INCIDENCE

Injection of air into the coronary artery is potentially fatal, resulting in "air lock," causing abrupt occlusion of the vessel, possible cardiac

arrest, and MI. Almost always iatrogenic, the incidence of this complication is approximately 0.1% to 0.3%.[87] Air embolism usually results from the inadequate aspiration of catheters or the entrainment of air during equipment exchanges. Occasionally, rupture of an inadequately prepared coronary balloon or introduction of air through an intracardiac defect can lead to paradoxical embolism into the coronary circulation.

DIAGNOSIS

The degree of danger associated with air embolism is directly related to the amount of air that enters the coronary circulation. Once air is injected, air lock can develop. preventing perfusion of the distal coronary bed (Fig. 27-13). Air embolism may manifest as chest pain, hypotension, transient ECG changes consistent with myocardial ischemia, arrhythmias (bradycardia, heart block, ventricular tachycardia and ventricular fibrillation), and even cardiac arrest. The diagnosis of air

TABLE 27-12	Treatment of Air Embolism
Ventilate with 100% oxygen	
Aggressive treatment with IV fluids, atropine, or vasopressors for hemodynamic support	
Consider intra-aortic balloon pump counterpulsation for hemodynamic support	
Dissipate the "air lock" with wires or balloon catheters	
Consider catheter aspiration or air embolus	
Treat no-reflow phenomenon with standard vasodilators (adenosine, verapamil, nitroprusside)	

TABLE 27-13	Commonly Used Pretreatment Regimen for Contrast Allergy
Prednisone 50 mg orally 13, 7, and 1 hours(s) prior to procedure or hydrocortisone 100 mg IV 1 hour prior to procedure	
Cimetidine 300 mg orally 1 hour prior	
Diphenhydramine 50 mg orally 1 hour prior	
Montelukast 10 mg orally 1 hour prior	
Nonionic low or iso-osmolar contrast agent	

embolism is made fluoroscopically and the bolus generally divides into smaller bubbles, causing the slow-flow phenomenon in epicardial vessels.[87]

TREATMENT

Resolution of air embolism can be accomplished fastest by ventilating with 100% oxygen (Table 27-12). Increasing the mean arterial pressure will assist in forcing air bubbles into the coronary microcirculation and overcoming the air lock. Forceful injection of saline or contrast can also assist in dissipating air lock. Balloons can be used to pulverize large bubbles. Thrombectomy catheters can be used to aspirate bubbles from the epicardial vessel. While waiting for an air embolus to resolve, the patient will often become profoundly hypotensive and complain of chest discomfort. Expedient treatment of hypotension with a systemic vasopressor such as norepinephrine or phenylephrine can be lifesaving. Intra-aortic balloon counterpulsation may also be useful. Of course the most efficacious means of dealing with air embolism is prevention and fastidious aspiration and flushing of catheters between equipment exchanges.[88]

⬛ Radiocontrast Hypersensitivity

INCIDENCE AND PROGNOSIS

Allergy to contrast media is a common but rarely serious complication in the cardiac catheterization laboratory. Since the advent of low-osmolar nonionic agents, contrast intolerance has significantly declined. The risk of allergy to contrast agents is estimated to be 4% to 12% and 1% to 3% for ionic and nonionic contrast agents respectively.[89] The reported incidence of severe contrast reactions is 0.23%, with a mortality of one per 55,000 cases.[90] Reactions from contrast media include minor events such as nausea, vomiting, and localized urticaria with pruritus. Moderate reactions include laryngeal or facial edema and mild bronchospasm. Severe reactions are true emergencies and manifest as respiratory or cardiac arrest and shock. Occasionally contrast allergy may manifest solely as persistent hypotension during a cardiac procedure. Approximately 2% to 5% of patients may develop delayed reactions characterized by rash 1 hour to 1 week after contrast exposure.[91] Patients may experience pruritus, maculopapular rash, urticaria, angioedema, and fever. Often, identification of the agent responsible for the allergy may be confounded by the concomitant delivery of antibiotics or treatment with an antithrombotic agent such as clopidogrel. The greatest hazard of anaphylactic reactions is delayed recognition and treatment, since the diagnosis of anaphylaxis is easily overlooked. When hypotension arises during PCI, the search for the cause should be systematic and include anaphylactic reactions in addition to the more common causes of shock such as access-site bleeding, abrupt vessel closure, perforation with tamponade, air embolism, guide dissection, arrhythmias, and oversedation with respiratory acidosis.

TABLE 27-14	Treatment of Anaphylactoid Reactions to Contrast Media
Mild	
Nausea, vomiting, and localized urticaria with pruritus, self-limiting	
Observation	
Moderate	
Laryngeal or facial edema and mild bronchospasm	
Epinephrine	
1:1,000 dilution at 0.1–0.3 mL IM	
1:10,000 dilution at 1–3 mL IV	
Diphenhydramine 25–50 mg IV	
Severe	
Respiratory or cardiac arrest and anaphylactoid shock	
ACLS resuscitation (airway, breathing, circulation)	
Epinephrine drip at 10–20 mcg/min up to 30 minutes after symptom resolution	
Aggressive intravenous fluids	

Reproduced with permission from Nayak K et al. *J Invas Cardiol.* 2009;21:548–551.

PREVENTION AND TREATMENT

Prophylactic measures can decrease the incidence and severity of contrast reactions but do not entirely eliminate the risk of their occurrence. Pretreatment of patients with contrast allergy usually consists of corticosteroids and antihistamines (Table 27-13). Mild reactions may be treated with a similar regimen; however, moderate reactions such as laryngeal edema, bronchospasm and hypotension require the immediate administration of intramuscular (IM) epinephrine 0.1 to 0.3 mL (1:1000 dilution) or intravenous epinephrine 1 mg (1:10,000 dilution) to prevent the progression of symptoms.[92] Severe bronchospasm, laryngeal edema, or cardiac arrest is treated with intravenous (IV) diluted epinephrine diluted 1:10,000 at a dose of 1 to 3 mL (Table 27-14). An overdose of IV epinephrine may manifest as tachycardia, tremor, pallor, and hypertensive emergency. Preexisting beta-blocker therapy may blunt the response of epinephrine and increase the risk of a severe reaction. Supplemental oxygen, endotracheal intubation, aggressive fluid resuscitation, administration of corticosteroids, and the use of an epinephrine drip may be required to stabilize the patient. Such patients should be monitored in the intensive care unit until the reaction subsides.[93]

⬛ Conclusion

Avoidance, recognition, and management of procedural complications are central to maintaining competence as an interventional cardiologist. Although the specific complications described in this chapter represent some of the most important and common mishaps, this is not an exhaustive listing. Complications can never be completely avoided. No matter how experienced the interventionist, complications will teach humility and be a source of continuing education throughout his or her career.

REFERENCES

1. Venkitachalam L, Kip KE, Selzer F, et al: Twenty-year evolution of percutaneous coronary intervention and its impact on clinical outcomes: a report from the National Heart, Lung, and Blood Institute-sponsored, multicenter 1985–1986 PTCA and 1997–2006 dynamic registries. *Circ Cardiovasc Intervent* 2:6–13, 2009.
2. Huber MS, Mooney JF, Madison J, et al: Use of a morphologic classification to predict clinical outcome after dissection from coronary angioplasty. *Am J Cardiol* 68:467–471, 1991.
3. Lloyd WK: Coronary complications of percutaneous coronary intervention: a practical approach to the management of abrupt closure. *Catheter Cardiovasc Intervent* 64:395–401, 2005.
4. Ellis SG, Roubin GS, King SB, et al: Angiographic and clinical predictors of acute closure after native vessel coronary angioplasty. *Circulation* 77:372–379, 1988.
5. Lincoff AM, Popma JJ, Ellis SG, et al: Abrupt vessel closure complicating coronary angioplasty: clinical, angiographic and therapeutic profile. *J Am Coll Cardiol* 19:926–935, 1992.
6. de Feyter PJ, de Jaegere PPT, Murphy ES, et al: Abrupt coronary artery occlusion during percutaneous transluminal coronary angioplasty. *Am Heart J* 123:1633–1642, 1992.
7. Ellis SG: Coronary lesions at increased risk. *Am Heart J* 130:643–646, 1995.
8. Colombo A, Hall P, Nakamura S, et al: Intracoronary stenting without anticoagulation accomplished with intravascular ultrasound guidance. *Circulation* 91:1676–1688, 1995.
9. Aoki J, Lansky AJ, Mehran R, et al: Early stent thrombosis in patients with acute coronary syndromes treated with drug-eluting and bare metal stents: the Acute Catheterization and Urgent Intervention Triage Strategy Trial. *Circulation* 119:687–698, 2009.
10. Topol EJ: Randomised placebo-controlled and balloon-angioplasty-controlled trial to assess safety of coronary stenting with use of platelet glycoprotein-IIb/IIIa blockade. *Lancet* 352:87–92, 1998.
11. Boersma E, Harrington RA, Moliterno DJ, et al: Platelet glycoprotein IIb/IIIa inhibitors in acute coronary syndromes: a meta-analysis of all major randomised clinical trials. *Lancet* 359:189–198, 2002.
12. Schomig A, Kastrati A, Mudra H, et al: Four-year experience with Palmaz-Schatz stenting in coronary angioplasty complicated by dissection with threatened or present vessel closure. *Circulation* 90:2716–2724, 1994.
13. Kiernan TJ, Yan BP, Ruggeiro N, et al: Coronary artery perforations in the contemporary interventional era. *J Intervent Cardiol* 22:350–353, 2009.
14. Fasseas P, Orford JL, Panetta CJ, et al: Incidence, correlates, management, and clinical outcome of coronary perforation: analysis of 16,298 procedures. *Am Heart J* 147:140–145, 2004.
15. Dippel EJ, Kereiakes DJ, Tramuta DA, et al: Coronary perforation during percutaneous coronary intervention in the era of abciximab platelet glycoprotein IIb/IIIa blockade: An algorithm for percutaneous management. *Catheter Cardiovasc Intervent* 52:279–286, 2001.
16. Gruberg L, Pinnow E, Flood R, et al: Incidence, management, and outcome of coronary artery perforation during percutaneous coronary intervention. *Am J Cardiol* 86:680–682, 2000.
17. Gunning MG, Williams IL, Jewitt DE, et al: Coronary artery perforation during percutaneous intervention: incidence and outcome. *Heart* 88:495–498, 2002.
18. Ajluni S, Glazier S, Blankenship L, et al: Perforations after percutaneous coronary interventions: clinical, angiographic, and therapeutic observations. *Catheter Cardiovasc Diagn* 32:206–212, 1994.
19. Shimony A, Zahger D, Van Straten M, et al: Incidence, risk factors, management and outcomes of coronary artery perforation during percutaneous coronary intervention. *Am J Cardiol* 104:1674–1677, 2009.
20. Klein LW: Coronary artery perforation during interventional procedures. *Catheter Cardiovasc Intervent* 68:713–717, 2006.
21. Fejka M, Dixon SR, Safian RD, et al: Diagnosis, management, and clinical outcome of cardiac tamponade complicating percutaneous coronary intervention. *Am J Cardiol* 90:1183–1186, 2002.
22. Annapoorna SK, Oana CR, Kunal S, et al: Changing outcomes and treatment strategies for wire induced coronary perforations in the era of bivalirudin use. *Catheter Cardiovasc Intervent* 74:700–707, 2009.
23. Lansky AJ, Yang Y-m, Khan Y, et al: Treatment of Coronary Artery Perforations Complicating Percutaneous Coronary Intervention With a Polytetrafluoroethylene-Covered Stent Graft. *Am J Cardiol* 98:370–374, 2006.
24. Ben-Gal Y, Weisz G, Collins MB, et al: Dual catheter technique for the treatment of severe coronary artery perforations. *Catheter Cardiovasc Intervent* 75:708–712, 2009.
25. Gaxiola E, Browne K: Coronary artery perforation repair using microcoil embolization. *Catheter Cardiovasc Diagn* 43:474–476, 1998.
26. Pravin KG: Delayed and repeated cardiac tamponade following microleak in RCA successfully treated with intra arterial sterile glue injection. *Catheter Cardiovasc Intervent* 73:797–800, 2009.
27. Brilakis ES, Best PJM, Elesber AA, et al: Incidence, retrieval methods, and outcomes of stent loss during percutaneous coronary intervention. *Catheter Cardiovasc Intervent* 65:333–340, 2005.
28. Schatz R, Baim D, Leon M, et al: Clinical experience with the Palmaz-Schatz coronary stent. Initial results of a multicenter study. *Circulation* 83:148–161, 1991.
29. Kammler J, Leisch F, Kerschner K, et al: Long-term follow-up in patients with lost coronary stents during interventional procedures. *Am J Cardiol* 98:367–369, 2006.
30. Bolte J, Neumann U, Pfafferott C, et al: Incidence, management, and outcome of stent loss during intracoronary stenting. *Am J Cardiol* 88:565–567, 2001.
31. Hartzler GO, Rutherford BD, McConahay DR: Retained percutaneous transluminal coronary angioplasty equipment components and their management. *Am J Cardiol* 60:1260–1264, 1987.
32. Patel T, Shah S, Pandya R, et al: Broken guidewire fragment: a simplified retrieval technique. *Catheter Cardiovasc Intervent* 51:483–486, 2000.
33. Hung C, Tsai C, Hou CJ-Y: Percutaneous transcatheter retrieval of retained balloon catheter in distal tortuous coronary artery. *Catheter Cardiovasc Intervent* 62:471–475, 2004.
34. Yang EH, Gumina RJ, Lennon RJ, et al: Emergency coronary artery bypass surgery for percutaneous coronary interventions: changes in the incidence, clinical characteristics, and indications from 1979 to 2003. *J Am Coll Cardiol* 46:2004–2009, 2005.
35. Seshadri N, Whitlow PL, Acharya N, et al: Emergency coronary artery bypass surgery in the contemporary percutaneous coronary intervention era. *Circulation* 106:2346–2350, 2002.
36. Roy P, de Labriolle A, Hanna N, et al: Requirement for emergent coronary artery bypass surgery following percutaneous coronary intervention in the stent era. *Am J Cardiol* 103:950–953, 2009.
37. Herrmann J: Peri-procedural myocardial injury: 2005 update. *Eur Heart J* 26:2493–2519, 2005.
38. Thygesen K, Alpert JS, White HD, et al: Universal definition of myocardial infarction. *Circulation* 116:2634–2653, 2007.
39. Mehran R, Dangas G, Mintz GS, et al: Atherosclerotic plaque burden and CK-MB enzyme elevation after coronary interventions: intravascular ultrasound study of 2256 patients. *Circulation* 101:604–610, 2000.
40. Choi JW, Gibson CM, Murphy SA, et al: Myonecrosis following stent placement: association between impaired TIMI myocardial perfusion grade and MRI visualization of microinfarction. *Catheter Cardiovasc Intervent* 61:472–476, 2004.
41. Bahrmann P, Werner GS, Heusch G, et al: Detection of coronary microembolization by doppler ultrasound in patients with stable angina pectoris undergoing elective percutaneous coronary interventions. *Circulation* 115:600–608, 2007.
42. Porto I, Selvanayagam JB, Van Gaal WJ, et al: Plaque volume and occurrence and location of periprocedural myocardial necrosis after percutaneous coronary intervention: insights from delayed-enhancement magnetic resonance imaging, thrombolysis in myocardial infarction myocardial perfusion grade analysis, and intravascular ultrasound. *Circulation* 114:662–669, 2006.
43. Iakovou I, Merhan R, Mintz G, et al: Increased CKMB release is a trade-off for optimal stent implantation: an intravascular ultrasound study. *J Am Coll Cardiol* 39:28–29, 2002.
44. Topol EJ, Mark DB, Lincoff AM, et al: Outcomes at 1 year and economic implications of platelet glycoprotein IIb/IIIa blockade in patients undergoing coronary stenting: results from a multicentre randomised trial. *Lancet* 354:2019–2024, 1999.
45. The EPILOG Investigators: Platelet glycoprotein IIb/IIIa receptor blockade and low-dose heparin during percutaneous coronary revascularization. *N Engl J Med* 336:1689–1697, 1997.
46. Topol EJ, Leya F, Pinkerton CA, et al: A comparison of directional atherectomy with coronary angioplasty in patients with coronary artery disease. *N Engl J Med* 329:221–227, 1993.
47. De Labriolle A, Lemesle G, Bonello L, et al: Prognostic significance of small troponin I rise after a successful elective percutaneous coronary intervention of a native artery. *Am J Cardiol* 103:639–645, 2009.
48. Javaid A, Buch AN, Steinberg DH, et al: Does creatine kinase-MB (CK-MB) isoenzyme elevation following percutaneous coronary intervention with drug-eluting stents impact late clinical outcomes? *Catheter Cardiovasc Intervent* 70:826–831, 2007.
49. Nienhuis MB, Ottervanger JP, Bilo HJG, et al: Prognostic value of troponin after elective percutaneous coronary intervention: a meta-analysis. *Catheter Cardiovasc Intervent* 71:318–324, 2008.
50. Gold HK, Gimple LW, Yasuda T, et al: Pharmacodynamic study of F(ab')2 fragments of murine monoclonal antibody 7E3 directed against human platelet glycoprotein IIb/IIIa in patients with unstable angina pectoris. *J Clin Invest* 86:651–659, 1990.
51. The EPIC Investigators: Use of a monoclonal antibody directed against the platelet glycoprotein IIb/IIIa receptor in high-risk coronary angioplasty. *N Engl J Med* 330:956–961, 1994.
52. Randomised placebo-controlled trial of abciximab before and during coronary intervention in refractory unstable angina: the CAPTURE study. *Lancet* 349:1429–1435, 1997.
53. The PURSUIT Trial Investigators: Inhibition of platelet glycoprotein IIb/IIIa with eptifibatide in patients with acute coronary syndromes. *N Engl J Med* 339:436–443, 1998.
54. Novel dosing regimen of eptifibatide in planned coronary stent implantation (ESPRIT): a randomised, placebo-controlled trial. *Lancet* 356:2037–2044, 2000.
55. Valgimigli M, Percoco G, Barbieri D, et al: The additive value of tirofiban administered with the high-dose bolus in the prevention of ischemic complications during high-risk coronary angioplasty: the ADVANCE trial. *J Am Coll Cardiol* 44:14–19, 2004.
56. Steinhubl SR, Lauer MS, Mukherjee DP, et al: The duration of pretreatment with ticlopidine prior to stenting is associated with the risk of procedure-related non-Q-wave myocardial infarctions. *J Am Coll Cardiol* 32:1366–1370, 1998.
57. Mehta SR, Yusuf S, Peters RJG, et al: Effects of pretreatment with clopidogrel and aspirin followed by long-term therapy in patients undergoing percutaneous coronary intervention: the PCI-CURE study. *Lancet* 358:527–533, 2001.
58. Steinhubl SR, Berger PB, Mann JT, III, et al: Early and sustained dual oral antiplatelet therapy following percutaneous coronary intervention: a randomized controlled trial. *JAMA* 288:2411–2420, 2002.
59. Hochholzer W, Trenk D, Bestehorn H-P, et al: Impact of the degree of peri-interventional platelet inhibition after loading with clopidogrel on early clinical outcome of elective coronary stent placement. *J Am Coll Cardiol* 48:1742–1750, 2006.
60. Patti G, Colonna G, Pasceri V, et al: Randomized trial of high loading dose of clopidogrel for reduction of periprocedural myocardial infarction in patients undergoing coronary intervention: results from the ARMYDA-2 (Antiplatelet therapy for Reduction of MYocardial Damage during Angioplasty) study. *Circulation* 111:2099–2106, 2005.
61. Chen W-H, Lee P-Y, Ng W, et al: Aspirin resistance is associated with a high incidence of myonecrosis after non-urgent percutaneous coronary intervention despite clopidogrel pretreatment. *J Am Coll Cardiol* 43:1122–1126, 2004.
62. Cuisset T, Frere C, Quilici J, et al: Glycoprotein IIb/IIIa inhibitors improve outcome after coronary stenting in clopidogrel nonresponders: a prospective, randomized study. *J Am Coll Cardiol Intervent* 1:649–653, 2008.
63. Pasceri V, Patti G, Nusca A, et al: Randomized trial of atorvastatin for reduction of myocardial damage during coronary intervention: results from the ARMYDA (Atorvastatin for Reduction of MYocardial Damage during Angioplasty) study. *Circulation* 110:674–678, 2004.
64. Patti G, Pasceri V, Colonna G, et al: Atorvastatin pretreatment improves outcomes in patients with acute coronary syndromes undergoing early percutaneous coronary intervention: results of the ARMYDA-ACS randomized trial. *J Am Coll Cardiol* 49:1272–1278, 2007.
65. Patti G, Chello M, Pasceri V, et al: Protection from procedural myocardial injury by atorvastatin is associated with lower levels of adhesion molecules after percutaneous coronary intervention: results from the ARMYDA-CAMs (Atorvastatin for Reduction of MYocardial Damage during Angioplasty-Cell Adhesion Molecules) substudy. *J Am Coll Cardiol* 48:1560–1566, 2006.
66. Di Sciascio G, Patti G, Pasceri V, et al: Efficacy of atorvastatin reload in patients on chronic statin therapy undergoing percutaneous coronary intervention: results of the ARMYDA-RECAPTURE (Atorvastatin for Reduction of Myocardial Damage During Angioplasty) randomized trial. *J Am Coll Cardiol* 54:558–565, 2009.
67. Baim DS, Wahr D, George B, et al: Randomized trial of a distal embolic protection device during percutaneous intervention of saphenous vein aorto-coronary bypass grafts. *Circulation* 105:1285–1290, 2002.
68. Mauri L, Cox D, Hermiller J, et al: The PROXIMAL trial: proximal protection during saphenous vein graft intervention using the proxis embolic protection system: a randomized, prospective, multicenter clinical trial. *J Am Coll Cardiol* 50:1442–1449, 2007.
69. Stone GW, Webb J, Cox DA, et al: Distal microcirculatory protection during percutaneous coronary intervention in acute ST-segment elevation myocardial infarction: a randomized controlled trial. *JAMA* 293:1063–1072, 2005.
70. Gick M, Jander N, Bestehorn H-P, et al: Randomized evaluation of the effects of filter-based distal protection on myocardial perfusion and infarct size after primary percutaneous catheter intervention in myocardial infarction with and without ST-segment elevation. *Circulation* 112:1462–1469, 2005.
71. Rezkalla SH, Kloner RA: No-reflow phenomenon. *Circulation* 105:656–662, 2002.
72. Abbo KM, Dooris M, Glazier S, et al: Features and outcome of no-reflow after percutaneous coronary intervention. *Am J Cardiol* 75:778–782, 1995.
73. Piana R, Paik G, Moscucci M, et al: Incidence and treatment of "no-reflow" after percutaneous coronary intervention. *Circulation* 89:2514–2518, 1994.
74. Yip HK, Chen MC, Chang HW, et al: Angiographic morphologic features of infarct-related arteries and timely reperfusion in acute myocardial infarction: predictors of slow-flow and no-reflow. *Chest* 122:1322–1332, 2002.
75. Kojima S, Sakamoto T, Ishihara M, et al: The white blood cell count is an independent predictor of no-reflow and mortality following acute myocardial infarction in the coronary interventional era. *Ann Med* 36:153–160, 2004.
76. Iwakura K, Ito H, Kawano S, et al: Predictive factors for development of the no-reflow phenomenon in patients with reperfused anterior wall acute myocardial infarction. *J Am Coll Cardiol* 38:472–477, 2001.
77. Klein LW, Kern MJ, Berger P, et al: Society of cardiac angiography and interventions: Suggested management of the no-reflow phenomenon in the cardiac catheterization laboratory. *Catheter Cardiovasc Intervent* 60:194–201, 2003.

78. Moses JW, Whitlow PL, Kuntz RE, et al: Myocardial infarction after rotational atherectomy: predictors and influence on late outcome in the STRATAS trial. *J Am Coll Cardiol* 31:455, 1998.

79. Montalescot G, Barragan P, Wittenberg O, et al: Platelet glycoprotein IIb/IIIa inhibition with coronary stenting for acute myocardial infarction. *N Engl J Med* 344:1895–1903, 2001.

80. Svilaas T, Vlaar PJ, van der Horst IC, et al: Thrombus aspiration during primary percutaneous coronary intervention. *N Engl J Med* 358:557–567, 2008.

81. Vlaar PJ, Svilaas T, van der Horst IC, et al: Cardiac death and reinfarction after 1 year in the Thrombus Aspiration during Percutaneous coronary intervention in Acute myocardial infarction Study (TAPAS): a 1-year follow-up study. *Lancet* 371:1915–1920, 2008.

82. De Luca G, Dudek D, Sardella G, et al: Adjunctive manual thrombectomy improves myocardial perfusion and mortality in patients undergoing primary percutaneous coronary intervention for ST-elevation myocardial infarction: a meta-analysis of randomized trials. *Eur Heart J* 29:3002–3010, 2008.

83. Burzotta F, De Vita M, Gu YL, et al: Clinical impact of thrombectomy in acute ST-elevation myocardial infarction: an individual patient-data pooled analysis of 11 trials. *Eur Heart J* 30:2193–2203, 2009.

84. Gibson CM, Murphy SA, Rizzo MJ, et al: Relationship between TIMI frame count and clinical outcomes after thrombolytic administration. *Circulation* 99:1945–1950, 1999.

85. Ross AM, Coyne KS, Moreyra E, et al: Extended mortality benefit of early postinfarction reperfusion. *Circulation* 97:1549–1556, 1998.

86. Mehta RH, Harjai KJ, Boura J, et al: Prognostic significance of transient no-reflow during primary percutaneous coronary intervention for ST-elevation acute myocardial infarction. *Am J Cardiol* 92:1445–1447, 2003.

87. Khan M, Schmidt DH, Bajwa T, et al: Coronary air embolism: incidence, severity, and suggested approaches to treatment. *Catheter Cardiovasc Diagn* 36:313–318, 1995.

88. Dib J, Boyle AJ, Chan M, et al: Coronary air embolism: a case report and review of the literature. *Catheter Cardiovasc Intervent* 68:897–900, 2006.

89. Canter LM: Anaphylactoid reactions to radiocontrast media. *Allergy Asthma Proc* 26:199–203, 2005.

90. Goss J, Chambers C, Heupler F, Jr: Systemic anaphylactoid reactions to iodinated contrast media during cardiac catheterization procedure: guidelines for prevention, diagnosis and treatment. *Catheter Cardiovasc Diagn* 34:99–104, 1995.

91. Yasuda R, Munechika H: Delayed adverse reactions to nonionic monomeric contrast-enhanced media. *Invest Radiol* 33:1–5, 1998.

92. Sampson HA, Munoz-Furlong A, Bock SA, et al: Symposium on the definition and management of anaphylaxis: summary report. *J Allergy Clin Immunol* 115:584–591, 2005.

93. Nayak KR, White AA, Cavendish JJ, et al: Anaphylactoid reactions to radiocontrast agents: prevention and treatment in the cardiac catheterization laboratory. *J Invas Cardiol* 21:548–551, 2009.

94. Ellis SG, Ajluni S, Arnold AZ, et al: Increased coronary perforation in the new device era. Incidence, classification, management, and outcome. *Circulation* 90:2725–2730, 1994.

95. Javaid A, Buch AN, Satler LF, et al: Management and outcomes of coronary artery perforation during percutaneous coronary intervention. *Am J Cardiol* 98:911–914, 2006.

96. Stankovic G, Orlic D, Corvaja N, et al: Incidence, predictors, in-hospital, and late outcomes of coronary artery perforations. *Am J Cardiol* 93:213–216, 2004.

97. Ramana R, Arab D, Joyal D, et al: Coronary artery perforation during percutaneous coronary intervention: incidence and outcomes in the new interventional era. *J Invas Cardiol* 17:606–608, 2005.

98. Witzke C, Martin-Herro F, Clarke SC, et al: The changing pattern of coronary perforation during percutaneous coronary intervention in the new device era. *J Invas Cardiol* 16:297–301, 2004.

99. Cantor WJ, Lazzam C, Cohen EA, et al: Failed coronary stent deployment. *Am Heart J* 136:1088–1095, 1998.

100. Eggebrecht H, Haude M, Birgelen CV, et al: Nonsurgical retrieval of embolized coronary stents. *Catheter Cardiovasc Intervent* 51:432–440, 2000.

101. Abdelmeguid AE, Topol EJ, Whitlow PL, et al: Significance of mild transient release of creatine kinase–MB fraction after percutaneous coronary interventions. *Circulation* 94:1528–1536, 1996.

102. Abdelmeguid AE, Ellis SG, Sapp SK, et al: Defining the appropriate threshold of creatine kinase elevation after percutaneous coronary interventions. *Am Heart J* 131:1097–1105, 1996.

103. Kong TQ, Jr, Davidson CJ, Meyers SN, et al: Prognostic implication of creatine kinase elevation following elective coronary artery interventions. *JAMA* 277:461–466, 1997.

104. Ghazzal Z, Ashfaq S, Morris DC, et al: Prognostic implication of creatine kinase release after elective percutaneous coronary intervention in the pre-IIb/IIIa antagonist era. *Am Heart J* 145:1006–1012, 2003.

105. Tardiff BE, Califf RM, Tcheng JE, et al: Clinical outcomes after detection of elevated cardiac enzymes in patients undergoing percutaneous intervention. *J Am Coll Cardiol* 33:88–96, 1999.

106. Waksman R, Ghazzal Z, Baim DS, et al: Myocardial infarction as a complication of new interventional devices. *Am J Cardiol* 78:751–756, 1996.

107. Simoons ML, van den Brand M, Lincoff M, et al: Minimal myocardial damage during coronary intervention is associated with impaired outcome. *European Heart Journal* 20:1112–1119, 1999.

108. Roe MT, Mahaffey KW, Kilaru R, et al: Creatine kinase-MB elevation after percutaneous coronary intervention predicts adverse outcomes in patients with acute coronary syndromes. *Eur Heart J* 25:313–321, 2004.

109. Stone GW, Mehran R, Dangas G, et al: Differential impact on survival of electrocardiographic Q-wave versus enzymatic myocardial infarction after percutaneous intervention: a device-specific analysis of 7147 patients. *Circulation* 104:642–647, 2001.

110. Dangas G, Mehran R, Feldman D, et al: Postprocedure creatine kinase-MB elevation and baseline left ventricular dysfunction predict one-year mortality after percutaneous coronary intervention. *Am J Cardiol* 89:586–588, 2002.

111. Ajani AE, Waksman R, Sharma AK, et al: Usefulness of periprocedural creatinine phosphokinase-MB release to predict adverse outcomes after intracoronary radiation therapy for in-stent restenosis. *Am J Cardiol* 93:313–317, 2004.

112. Brener SJ, Ellis SG, Schneider J, et al: Frequency and long-term impact of myonecrosis after coronary stenting. *Eur Heart J* 23:869–976, 2002.

113. Ellis SG, Chew D, Chan A, et al: Death following creatine kinase MB elevation after coronary intervention: identification of an early risk period: importance of creatine kinase-MB level, completeness of revascularization, ventricular function, and probable benefit of statin therapy. *Circulation* 106:1205–1210, 2002.

114. Brener SJ, Lytle BW, Schneider JP, et al: Association between CK-MB elevation after percutaneous or surgical revascularization and three-year mortality. *J Am Coll Cardiol* 40:1961–1967, 2002.

115. Hong MK, Mehran R, Dangas G, et al: Creatine kinase-MB enzyme elevation following successful saphenous vein graft intervention is associated with late mortality. *Circulation* 100:2400–2405, 1999.

116. Natarajan MK, Kreatsoulas C, Velianou JL, et al: Incidence, predictors, and clinical significance of troponin-I elevation without creatine kinase elevation following percutaneous coronary interventions. *Am J Cardiol* 93:750–753, 2004.

117. Nallamothu BK, Chetcuti S, Mukherjee D, et al: Prognostic implication of troponin I elevation after percutaneous coronary intervention. *Am J Cardiol* 91:1272–1274, 2003.

118. Fuchs S, Kornowski R, Mehran R, et al: Prognostic value of cardiac troponin-I levels following catheter based coronary interventions. *Am J Cardiol* 85:1077–1082, 2000.

119. Cavallini C, Savonitto S, Violini R, et al: Impact of the elevation of biochemical markers of myocardial damage on long-term mortality after percutaneous coronary intervention: results of the CK-MB and PCI study. *European Heart Journal* 26:1494–1498, 2005.

ABBREVIATIONS

ACC: American College of Cardiology

ADVANCE: Additive Value of Tirofiban Administered With the High-Dose Bolus in the Prevention of Ischemic Complications During High-Risk Coronary Angioplasty

ADMIRAL: Abciximab before Direct Angioplasty and Stenting in Myocardial Infarction Regarding Acute and Long-Term Follow-up

ARMYDA: Atorvastatin for Reduction of Myocardial Damage during Angioplasty

CABG: coronary artery bypass grafting

CADILLAC: Controlled Abciximab and Device Investigation to Lower Late Angioplasty Complications

CAPTURE: c7E3 FAB antiplatelet therapy in unstable refractory angina

CURE: The Clopidogrel in Unstable Angina to Prevent Recurrent Events Trial Investigators

ECG: electrocardiogram

EPISTENT: Evaluation of Platelet IIb/IIIa inhibitor for Stenting

EMERALD: Enhanced Myocardial Efficacy and Recovery by Aspiration of Liberated Debris

EPIC: Evaluation of 7E3 for the Prevention of Ischemic Complications

EPILOG: Evaluation in PTCA to Improve Long-Term Outcome with Abciximab GP IIb/IIIa Blockade

ESPRIT: Enhanced Suppression of the Platelet IIb/IIIa Receptor with Integrilin Therapy

IABP: intra-aortic balloon pump

IM: intramuscular

LVEF: left ventricular ejection fraction

MI: myocardial infarction

MRI: magnetic resonance imaging

NHLB – National Heart, Lung and Blood Institute

PCI: percutaneous coronary interventions

PTFE: polytetraflourethylene

PURSUIT – Platelet Glycoprotein IIb/IIIa in Unstable Angina: Receptor Suppression Using Integrilin Therapy

PROMISE: Protection Devices in PCI Treatment of Myocardial Infarction for Salvage of Endangered Myocardium

QWMI: Q wave myocardial infarction

SAFER: Saphenous Vein Graft Angioplasty Free Of Emboli Randomized trial

STEMI: ST-elevation myocardial infarction

TAPAS: Thrombus Aspiration during Percutaneous Coronary Intervention in Acute Myocardial Infarction Study

TVR: target vessel revascularization

28

Periprocedural Myocardial Infarction and Embolism Protection Devices

KHALED ZIADA | DEBABRATA MUKHERJEE

KEY POINTS

- The contemporary definition of PMI is based on the rise and fall of biomarkers (such as total CK, CK-MB, and/or troponin) after PCI.

- The incidence of PMI is ~25%; this varies according to the biomarker and the preset threshold for diagnosis.

- The primary underlying mechanism of PMI is embolization into the microcirculation distal to the PCI target segment, with platelet aggregation/activation playing a significant role in subsequent myonecrosis.

- Risk factors for the development of PMI include acute presentation, heightened systemic inflammation, and advanced coronary/noncoronary atherosclerotic disease. Atheroablation devices (directional or rotational) are associated with higher rates of PMI, followed by stents and then balloon angioplasty.

- Abrupt vessel closure and/or compromised side branches are associated with PMI, although most PMIs are diagnosed after "apparently" uncomplicated procedures.

- PMI is associated with increased late mortality, the association being more robust when the CK-MB or troponin levels are > 5x ULN.

- Potent antiplatelet therapies (intravenous GP IIb/IIIa inhibitors, direct thrombin inhibitors, and/or oral thienopyridine inhibitors) decrease the incidence of PMI, especially in high-risk procedures.

- Pretreatment with statins reduces the incidence of PMI because of the anti-inflammatory effects of these agents.

- Embolism protection devices have been proven to reduce PMI in saphenous vein graft PCI.

- Bivalirudin appears to provide the best balance of reducing PMI without also increasing bleeding.

Introduction

Over the last decade, major acute ischemic complications of percutaneous coronary intervention (PCI) have been significantly reduced by advances in pharmacological therapies and interventional devices. Q-wave myocardial infarction (MI), need for emergent bypass grafting, and/or in-hospital mortality have been reduced to 1% to 2% of PCI procedures.[1,2] The reduced incidence of these complications can be attributed in large part to the invaluable role of coronary stents in the treatment of abrupt closure and also to the aggressive antiplatelet therapies that have been more commonly utilized over the last decade. This improvement in outcomes is remarkable considering the ever-increasing number and complexity of patients and lesions undergoing PCI today versus 10 or 20 years ago. However, the periprocedural release of cardiac biomarkers is still observed in a considerable proportion of patients undergoing otherwise successful PCI procedures.[2,3] Although the etiology and clinical significance of the periprocedural release of cardiac markers are topics for debate, the rise and fall in serum levels of cardiac biomarkers can be described only as a procedure-related acute MI.[3]

Definition

The definition of periprocedural MI (PMI) has been a subject of debate and evolution over the last decade. Traditionally, PMI was defined along the same lines as an acute MI not related to revascularization—that is, it had to meet at least two of three criteria: prolonged chest pain, electrocardiographic Q waves, and a rise in serum markers. Subsequently, numerous publications demonstrated that CK and CK-MB elevations have prognostic implications, even in the absence of pathological Q waves. The cutoff values of CK and/or CK-MB used to define PMI in these studies varied widely. Numerous investigators used the cutoff value of three times the upper limit of normal (ULN) of CK or CK-MB (3x ULN) as the defining threshold of PMI, although it has been traditional to report > 1x ULN, > 5x ULN, and occasionally > 8x ULN values as well.[4,5] More contemporary studies have used troponin and myoglobin levels, which are considered to be more sensitive markers for myonecrosis, to define PMI. With the consensus redefinition of acute MI,[3] it is now accepted that any elevations of biomarkers above the 99th percentile URL (upper reference limit) after PCI, assuming a normal baseline troponin value, are indicative of a PMI. Pending further data and by arbitrary convention, it is suggested to designate increases more than three times the 99th percentile URL as PCI-related MI (type 4a) in those with elevated troponin levels.[6] The definition of PMI is further complicated by the current practice of earlier referral of patients with ST or non-ST segment elevation to the catheterization laboratory. In those situations, the detection of abnormal levels of cardiac markers after PCI may not necessarily be related to the procedure but simply constitute a reflection of the ongoing myonecrosis caused by thrombosis and/or distal embolization that have led to the procedure. In patients with acute coronary syndrome, biomarker levels may rise after an initially negative sample, which commonly coincides with the time when angiography and PCI are performed.[7] Such a rise and fall in biomarker levels at the time of PCI is not a "mere" laboratory finding; there is solid evidence of irreversible myocardial injury that correlates with the rise in serum level of the biomarker both qualitatively and quantitatively. In a small study utilizing contrast-enhanced magnetic resonance imaging (MRI) to visualize areas of myonecrosis directly, Riccardi et al. reported evidence of hyperenhancement (equivalent to approximately 2 g of myocardium) in 9 of 9 patients in whom there was minor procedure-related CK-MB elevation (approximately 2x ULN). In the 5 control patients who did not have any CK-MB elevation, there was no MRI evidence of hyperenhancement in the target vessel's perfusion territory. Importantly, none of the patients in whom hyperenhancement was detected as evidence of myonecrosis developed electrocardiographic Q waves.[8] In a more contemporary and rigorous study, 48 patients underwent cardiac MRI before and after PCI to detect newly developed hyperenhancement as evidence of procedure-related myonecrosis.[9] Half the patients underwent a third MRI scan at a median of 8 months. Findings were correlated with serum troponin levels recorded 24 hours after the index PCI. All patients were preloaded with clopidogrel and received abciximab at the time of PCI, but the incidence of troponin elevation above ULN was 37% (14 patients). There was evidence of new MRI hyperenhancement in the target vessel's territory in all 14 patients. In patients with no troponin elevation after PCI, there was no evidence of hyperenhancement on MRI. There was

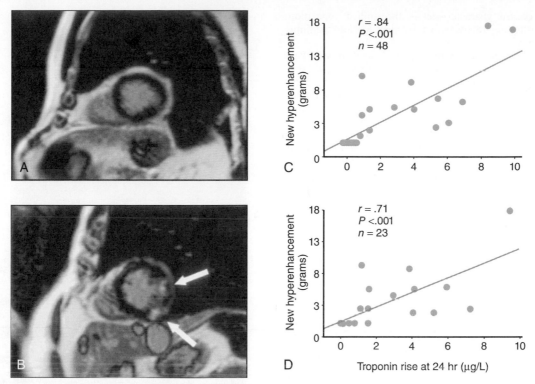

Figure 28-1 Apical ventricular short-axis image (A) in a patient before left circumflex/obtuse marginal bifurcation PCI showing no hyperenhancement. B. This image shows two regions of new hyperenhancement in the distribution of the obtuse marginal branch artery after PCI (arrows). Correlation between 24-hour post-PCI troponin I value versus mass of new myocardial hyperenhancement both early (C) and late (D) after PCI. (From Selvanayagam JB et al. Circulation. 2005;111(8):1027–1032.)

also a linear correlation between the troponin level at 24 hours post-PCI and the mass of newly hyperenhanced myocardium (measured in grams) both on the early post-PCI scan and on the delayed 8-month scan, thus confirming the correlation between periprocedural biomarker release and irreversible myocardial damage (Fig. 28-1).[9]

In addition to confirming the irreversible nature of the myocardial injury, the location of MRI hyperenhancement in relation to the PCI target segment may give insight into the pathophysiological mechanism underlying PMI. In cases where the hyperenhancement is visualized in proximity of the treated segment, side-branch occlusion is the more likely explanation. But when the myocardial injury/damage is downstream from the treated segment, PMI can best be explained by distal microembolization and adverse platelet and inflammatory reactions in the microcirculation.[8,10]

Incidence

As with its definition, the reported incidence of PMI has varied widely from one published report to another (Table 28-1). This variation can be attributed to several factors: the choice of biomarker assayed, the threshold value used to define PMI, and routine versus clinically driven biomarker assays. When the incidence of PMI is reported for a consecutive series of patients undergoing PCI (irrespective of their clinical condition after the procedure), it is invariably higher than in other series in which biomarkers were assayed only in patients who developed certain symptoms or signs of ischemia. This is the result of detection of a fairly larger proportion of clinically silent events with small-magnitude biomarker release.[11] The PCI guidelines update published in 2005 by American College of Cardiology (ACC), American Heart Association (AHA), and European Society of Cardiology (ESC) experts recommend the routine assay of CK-MB and/or troponin in every patient undergoing PCI 8 to 12 hours after the procedure irrespective of presence or absence of symptoms of MI.[2] In nonselected patient series excluding those with initially positive markers, the average incidence of PMI using CK-MB, troponin T, and troponin I >

ULN was 23 ± 12 %, 23 ± 12%, and 27 ± 12%, respectively.[10] Using a lower biomarker cutoff value to define PMI increases the proportion of patients labeled to have PMI.[12,13] Similarly, a higher incidence of PMI (up to 44%) was reported with troponin assays, when compared to studies defining PMI by the traditional CK or CK-MB levels.[14] Other important factors that contribute to the heterogeneity of the conclusions of the various published series include the widely disparate

TABLE 28-1	Incidence of PMI in Selected Large Patient Series			
Reference	N	Type of PCI	Biomarker Definition of PMI	Incidence of PMI (%)
Abdelmeguid et al.[11]	4,664	PTCA, DCA	CK 2-5x ULN	2.6
Ghazzal et al.[15]	15,637	PCI	CK 1-2x ULN	4.6
			CK > 3x ULN	1.6
Harrington et al.[16]	1,012	PTCA DCA	CK-MB x2 ULN	3.8
				10.3
Simoons et al.[17]	5,025	PTCA	CK-MB 1-3x ULN	13.2
Roe et al.[12]	2,384	PCI	CK-MB 1-3x ULN	21.3
			CK-MB 3-5x ULN	6.0
			CK-MB 5-10x ULN	7.1
			CK-MB > 10x ULN	9.5
Stone et al.[18]	7,147	PTCA Stent Ablation Ablation + stent	CK-MB > 4	25.1
				34.4
				37.8
				48.8
Ellis et al.[19]	8,409	PCI	CK-MB > 8.8	17.2
Ntarajan et al.[20]	1,128	PCI	Tn I > 0.5	16.8
Nallamothu et al.[13]	1,157	PCI	Tn I 1-3x ULN	16.0
			Tn I 3-5x ULN	4.6
			Tn I 5-8x ULN	2.0
			Tn I ≥ 8x ULN	6.5
Cavallini et al.[14]	3,494	PCI	Tn I > 0.15	44.2
			CK-MB > 5	16.0

baseline and procedural characteristics in the studied populations, inclusion or exclusion of patients with antecedent MI, and the timing of blood sampling.[7,10]

There may be discrepancies in the reported incidences of PMIs according to the time frame in which various reports were published, the anticoagulation/antiplatelet therapy, and the devices used for PCI. Large Q-wave PMIs were reduced from 2.1% in the BARI trial population to 0.8% in BARI-like patients selected from the more contemporary National Heart, Lung and Blood Institute (BNHLBI) dynamic registry. The reduction was primarily driven by liberal use of stents in the registry, which effectively treated abrupt closure and flow-limiting dissections.[21] Additionally, in the EPISTENT randomized controlled trial, use of abciximab reduced Q-wave PMIs during stenting by more than 40% (1.4% vs. 0.8%).[22]

Underlying Pathophysiological Mechanisms

MRI of the myocardium in patients who develop biomarker release after PCI has revealed two different types of PMI, according to the distribution of hyperenhancement indicative of acute injury. In the more commonly seen "distal" type of PMI, hyperenhancement is in the distal distribution downstream from the treated segment. In the "proximal" type of PMI, the injury is primarily detected adjacent to the treated segment.[8,23] Proximal PMI is usually linked with flow impairment in a side branch arising from the treated segment, whereas the more commonly seen distal PMI results from microvascular obstruction in the distribution of the artery subjected to PCI.

DISTAL EMBOLIZATION AND PERIPROCEDUAL MYOCARDIAL INFARCTION

Although distal embolization associated with endothelial injury has been recognized for years, the importance of this phenomenon in relation to PCI was not fully appreciated until the last decade.[24] Using filter devices, platelet aggregates have been identified in the distal microcirculation and atherosclerotic debris retrieved from arteries downstream from the site of angioplasty (Fig. 28-2). Clinically, intravascular ultrasound (IVUS) studies have provided further insight into the relationship between embolization of plaque material and PMI. Prati and coworkers examined the relationship between change in plaque volume before and after stenting and the degree of CK-MB release in 54 patients. In patients with unstable angina, there was a more significant reduction in plaque volume. More importantly, however, such reduction significantly correlated with CK-MB release even after adjusting for other variables influencing PMI.[25] A more recent and sophisticated analysis by Porto et al. of 62 patients undergoing complex PCI demonstrated a significant association between the change in target lesion plaque area by IVUS and the mass of myonecrosis assessed by hyperenhancement on MRI imaging post-PCI.[23] The authors also correlated impaired microvascular flow (TIMI perfusion grade 0 or 1) with MRI evidence of hyperenhancement downstream from the treated segment, hence suggesting that particulate matter from the atherosclerotic plaque disrupted by angioplasty drifts downstream, leading to microvascular obstruction and myonecrosis. The development and clinical utilization of embolism protection devices provided additional evidence of distal embolization, since particulate matter from the atherosclerotic plaque subjected to angioplasty could be collected, measured, and analyzed. The embolized material primarily consists of debris (atherosclerotic plaque and thrombotic elements), with particles ranging in size from ~50 to >600 μm. Neutrophils and macrophages are also identified. Although these devices are more frequently used in the setting of PCI in saphenous vein grafts, distal embolization in routine native vessel PCI is probably just as frequent, with debris that is very similar in quantity and composition.[26,27]

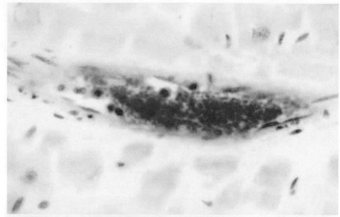

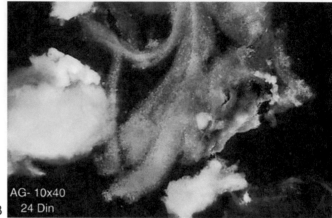

Figure 28-2 A. Histological specimen of intramyocardial microvessel filled with platelets, stained positive for platelet glycoprotein IIb/IIIa, from a patient who experienced sudden cardiac death. B. Atherosclerotic particulate embolic material retrieved from percutaneous coronary revascularization with Angioguard guidewire filter. (*From Topol EJ, Yadav JS. Recognition of the importance of embolization in atherosclerotic vascular disease. Circulation. 2000;01(5):570–580.*)

THE ROLE OF THE PLATELET

Platelet activation plays a critical role in the development and perpetuation of coronary microvascular obstruction following PCI. By definition, the interventional devices used to treat an epicardial stenosis will result in a break in the endothelial surface and release of debris into the coronary bloodstream. The exposed intraplaque contents stimulate platelet activation and aggregation at the site of PCI but probably in the downstream microvasculature as well. Thus the platelet aggregates plugging the microcirculation not only cause mechanical obstruction but also lead to biochemical responses owing to their interaction with the injured endothelium, the neutrophils, and more platelets. The release of vasoactive substances such as serotonin and endothelin-1 from the activated platelets and the injured endothelium lead to intense microvascular vasoconstriction, which accentuates the ischemic injury and resultant myonecrosis.[10,24] One study of aspirin resistance emphasized the role of platelet aggregation in the pathophysiology of PMI. Patients deemed to be resistant to aspirin therapy were found to have a significantly higher incidence of PMI, defined as any increase in CK-MB (51.7% vs. 24.6%, $P = 0.006$).[28] The odds of developing PMI in this cohort of 151 patients presenting for nonurgent PCI increased threefold if they were found to be aspirin-resistant prior to the procedure.[28]

OTHER PATHOPHYSIOLOGICAL MECHANISMS

Distal embolization of plaque debris and platelet activation, with all its local metabolic consequences, probably are the primary mechanisms leading to distal PMI in absence of PCI complications such as side-branch closure or flow-limiting dissections. However, there are other intriguing mechanisms that may interact with embolism and platelet activation. These have been suggested by analysis of coronary sinus blood samples obtained before and after PCI, thus reflecting the local metabolic derangements that result from the intervention. For instance, there is evidence of neutrophil activation in the coronary sinus samples collected post-PCI, as well as an increase in serum levels of C-reactive protein (CRP) and interleukin-6 (IL-6). The increase in the levels of inflammatory markers was associated with post-PCI troponin release.[29] This demonstrates a local inflammatory response at the level of the myocardium in response to PCI and suggests a potential contribution to the process of myocyte damage.[10,29] Concentration of isoprostanes (stable end products of oxygen free radical mediated-lipid peroxidation) also increased in coronary sinus blood following PCI, which demonstrates an increase in the production of free radicals during PCI.[30] The extent to which this inflammatory response and increased oxidative stress contribute to myonecrosis remains unclear.

Risk Factors Predisposing to Periprocedural Myocardial Infarction

Clinical trials examining the role of newer interventional devices and/or glycoprotein (GP) IIb/IIIa inhibitors as well as patient series investigating the incidence and significance of PMI have identified certain subsets of patients who are at higher risk of PMI. These subsets can be identified on the basis of clinical, lesion-related, procedural, or device-related variables.

CLINICAL CHARACTERISTICS

The risk of PMI is significantly increased in patients with evidence of more severe atherosclerotic disease. Multivessel and/or more diffuse coronary artery disease is associated with an approximately 50% increase in the relative risk of developing PMI.[12,15,31] IVUS evidence of increased plaque burden is also a risk factor for development of PMI.[23,25] This may explain why diabetics are at a higher risk of PMI.[32] Interestingly, evidence of advanced noncardiac atherosclerotic disease has been associated with an even higher relative risk of PMI.[31] The clinical presentation at the time of PCI may also play a role in determining the risk of PMI and other adverse events during and after the procedure. Patients with acute coronary syndromes are more likely to develop PMI.[10] However, studies examining the incidence of PMI in this patient population have been limited by certain methodological difficulties. First, it is difficult and more controversial to define PMI when patients present with elevated markers prior to PCI. Therefore most of the studies on this topic excluded these patients from the analysis. Second, even if patients with elevated markers are excluded, it is conceivable that those with negative markers who were referred to PCI within a few hours of presentation may have been having a spontaneous infarction that was appreciated only after the PCI.[10,12] A heightened systemic inflammatory state prior to PCI is also a major predictor of adverse outcomes, including PMI. Most of the evidence supporting this hypothesis is based on correlations between pre-PCI CRP levels and evidence of PMI. A small study of 85 patients with stable angina undergoing PCI demonstrated that PMI (defined by an elevated troponin level) is significantly more frequent in patients with elevated CRP (46% of those with elevated CRP but only 18% of those with a normal CRP developed the complication).[33] Chew and colleagues examined the relationship between preprocedural CRP and the adverse events (death and MI) in the first 30 days following PCI in a larger series of 727 consecutive patients. The highest quartile of CRP was predictive of worse outcome (odds ratio [OR] 3.68, confidence interval [CI] 1.5–9.0), and that association persisted even after adjusting for other variables influencing outcome. The event-free survival curves separated within 24 hours and were primarily driven by a reduction in MI, suggesting that patients with elevated CRP are more susceptible to development of PMI (Fig. 28-3).[34]

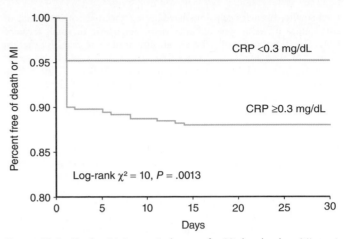

Figure 28-3 Kaplan-Meier survival curves for 30-day death or MI stratified by baseline CRP. The majority of the events and the separation of the curves occurs within the first 1–2 days; i.e., the difference is primarily driven by the incidence of PMI. (*From Chew DP et al. Incremental prognostic value of elevated baseline C-reactive protein among established markers of risk in percutaneous coronary intervention.* Circulation. 2001;104:992–997.)

LESION-RELATED RISK FACTORS

Saphenous vein graft lesions are notorious for the risk of development of PMI, probably because of the increased incidence of both macro- and microembolization with subsequent slow flow and no reflow. In absence of embolism protection devices, the risk of PMI (defined as CK-MB > 3x ULN) in the contemporary era can be as high as 13.7%. This rate almost doubles if the threshold cutoff value to define PMI is any increase in CK-MB.[35] The introduction of embolism protection devices in the last few years has significantly reduced the risk of PMI in those patients.[35–37] Several lesion characteristics are traditionally associated with a higher risk of PMI, primarily those features suggestive of lesion instability (e.g., eccentricity, irregular contour, visible thrombosis). Complex lesions (ACC/AHA type C) usually contain one or more of those features and are thus associated with a significantly increased risk of PMI.[4,11] Lesions involving the ostium of a major side branch are usually among the more complex lesion types and more prone to result in PMI owing to the higher risk of side-branch closure. Other lesion characteristics that confer a higher risk of PMI include those features that suggest a higher plaque burden, such as a multiplicity of lesions, long lesions, and diffusely diseased arteries.

PROCEDURAL COMPLICATIONS AND RISK OF PERIPROCEDURAL MYOCARDIAL INFARCTION

Side-branch occlusion, flow-limiting dissections, and transient abrupt closure have been the most recognizable procedural complications resulting in relatively large PMIs.[4,11,15,38] However, these complications are rare and most detected PMIs follow routine procedures with no obvious angiographic complications.[10,24] With the routine use and universal availability of stents, abrupt closure has become quite rare: <1% cases in contemporary PCI.[24] The effectiveness of stenting and the availability of potent antiplatelet therapies are probably the primary mechanisms by which large (Q-wave) PMIs and the need for emergent coronary surgery have been reduced by almost 50%.[21,39] Abrupt closure or no reflow have not been found to affect outcome when treated promptly, with no subsequent PMI.[38] Side-branch occlusion (SBO) has been and remains the most common angiographically recognizable procedural complication resulting in PMI.[11,15] Unlike abrupt closure, the incidence of SBO has not decreased with the routine use of coronary stenting. In fact, with increasing stent use, SBO has become the most likely cause of acute occlusion during PCI.[40] Major SBOs can be associated with large (possibly Q-wave) infarctions, but even smaller branch occlusions have been associated with evidence of small areas of MRI hyperenhancement, diagnostic of small areas of PMI. The distribution of hyperenhancement in these cases is different from that seen with distal embolization downstream of the target lesion for PCI. With SBO, hyperenhancement is "adjacent" rather than "distal" to the location of the PCI. The likelihood of developing a new hyperenhancement increases 16-fold when an SBO can be recognized angiographically.[23] There have been some intriguing observations regarding SBO and PMI in the era of PCI of complex lesions using drug-eluting stents. In the TAXUS V trial, which randomized 1,172 patients to receive either paclitaxel-eluting or bare metal stents, complex lesion subsets (more than 35% type C) were treated in both groups and >30% of patients received more than one stent. In the subgroup of patients receiving multiple stents, the incidence of 30-day MI was significantly higher with paclitaxel-eluting stents (8.3% vs. 3.3%, $P = 0.047$). Core laboratory angiographic analysis of this patient subset revealed a significantly higher incidence of side-branch compromise or occlusion with paclitaxel-eluting stents than with bare metal stents (42.6% vs. 30.6%, $P = 0.03$), resulting in a higher incidence of < TIMI 3 flow in the paclitaxel-eluting stent group. Why paclitaxel-eluting stents are associated with more side-branch compromise and subsequent PMI remains unclear. Possible explanations include the increasing thickness of the stent struts caused by the drug-eluting polymer, increased platelet deposition, and/or paclitaxel-induced spasm.[41] A comparison of paclitaxel-eluting and everolimus-eluting stents demonstrates the importance of the strut and polymer thickness. A post-hoc analysis of the SPIRIT III randomized trial compared the incidence of PMI in 113 patients receiving the thinner strut/thinner polymer everolimus-eluting stent with that in 63 patients receiving the paclitaxel-eluting stent, in whom a small side branch was "jailed" by the deployed stent. PMI, defined as any increase in CK-MB above ULN, was much lower in the everolimus group (9.0% vs. 29.7%, $P = 0.01$).[42]

RISK OF PERIPROCEDURAL MYOCARDIAL INFARCTION BY INTERVENTIONAL DEVICE

Some of the earliest investigations sparking interest in PMI and its significance were in the context of comparing newer interventional devices with standard balloon angioplasty. Data from the CAVEAT-I trial demonstrated that directional atherectomy (DCA) was associated with more abrupt closure, evidence of PMI, and a subsequently higher rate of clinical adverse events compared with balloon angioplasty.[16,43] These findings were confirmed in the BOAT trial, in which a more refined technique of DCA was supposed to demonstrate its superiority to PTCA. However, the incidence of PMI was still significantly higher with DCA than with balloon angioplasty (16% vs. 6%).[44] DCA is associated with more distal embolization, particularly in saphenous vein graft interventions.[45] There is also evidence of a higher degree of platelet activation with DCA,[46] with its subsequent mechanical obstruction as well as thrombotic and inflammatory responses in the downstream microcirculation. Similarly, rotational atherectomy is associated with more platelet activation and distal embolization of plaque debris than balloon angioplasty owing to its mechanism of action.[47] Although the routine use of coronary stents has dramatically reduced the incidence of most PCI complications (abrupt closure, flow-limiting dissections, need for emergent bypass surgery, and restenosis), stenting increases the incidence of PMI compared with balloon angioplasty, with a relative risk increase of ~20%.[10,24,48] In patients undergoing PCI of the left anterior descending artery randomly assigned to balloon angioplasty or stenting, there was evidence of a higher degree of platelet and neutrophil surface activation after stenting.[49] High-pressure inflations aiming to overexpand stents and reduce restenosis can actually lead to higher CK-MB levels. In a study of approximately 1,000 patients undergoing IVUS-guided stenting, the incidence of PMI (defined as CK-MB 3x ULN) was 16%, 18%, and 25% in three groups of patients in whom the final stent-to-reference lumen area was <70%, 70% to 100%, and >100%, respectively.[50]

■ Prognostic Implications of Periprocedural Myocardial Infarction

Although there is much controversy about the definition and prevalence of PMI with everyday PCI, there is no dispute that significant PMI is associated with an increased mortality risk. There remains controversy about the pathophysiological mechanisms underlying this association as well as the definition and the size of PMI that would confer such increased risk. However, there is convincing evidence that any PMI is associated with some degree of increased risk of death, particularly with longer follow-up. The pioneering work of Abdelmeguid and coworkers had demonstrated that CK and CK-MB elevation post-PCI (primarily balloon angioplasty and DCA in this report) are associated with an approximately 30% relative increase in 3-year mortality.[11] Three-year follow-up of the EPIC trial patients (undergoing angioplasty and DCA as well) revealed an incremental long-term risk of death with increasing degrees of PMI. Among the 2,001 patients enrolled in the trial, the mortality risk increased from 7.3% in those with no CK elevation to 13.1% when CK was > x3 ULN and again to 16.5% with CK > 10x ULN.[51] In the EPISTENT trial, in which stenting was routinely employed in two-thirds of the patients, the 1-year mortality doubled between patients with no or minimal PMI (CK-MB > 1x ULN) to those with CK-MB > 3 to 10x ULN (1.5% vs. 3.4%).[22] Subsequently, similar conclusions were reached by examining outcomes of patients enrolled in PCI clinical trials and large-scale single-center patient registries (Table 28-1).[12,15,16,19,22,52] Although the association between PMI and mortality has not been disputed, the mechanisms that can explain this association are not clear. The magnitude of myonecrosis is limited, but it may provide a nidus for arrhythmogenesis. On the other hand, it has been suggested that the association between PMI and late mortality merely represents a reflection of increased risk in a group of patients with more advanced disease.[7] The latter hypothesis can be criticized by the fact that aggressive preprocedural platelet inhibition (by thienopyridine pretreatment or intravenous GP IIb/IIIa inhibitors) reduces PMI and the subsequent risk of death and adverse events, suggesting that this is a modifiable risk. The threshold above which a PMI is considered prognostically significant has been a subject of some debate. It has been traditional to consider a PMI when the CK-MB is > 3x ULN, although the recent PCI guidelines suggest CK-MB > 5x ULN should be the threshold for defining a PMI.[2] In the large series of Ghazzal and colleagues, minor elevation of total CK (< 3x ULN) did not confer a statistically significant increase in risk of late mortality.[15] Brener and coworkers suggested that only massive CK-MB release (> 10x ULN) predicts an increased risk of death over a 3-year period.[53] However, there has been strong evidence that smaller CK-MB elevations are associated with increasing risk of death. Abdelmeguid and colleagues examined that question specifically and concluded that any increase in CK-MB above normal limits confers some degree of risk.[11] In later meta-analysis, any increase in CK-MB, even < 3x ULN, was associated with a statistically significant increase in the risk of death (OR 1.5). Patients with CK-MB levels between 3x and 5x ULN and those with levels > 5x ULN had an even higher relative risk of dying over the 3-year follow up.[54] Similarly, in the large metanalysis of Roe and colleagues, an increased mortality risk was associated with increasing CK-MB expressed as a continuous variable—that is, with no specific thresholds above or below which the risk changes (Fig. 28-4).[12] Frequently, very large PMIs (i.e., with CK-MB levels > 8x-10x ULN) are associated with significant complications or an unsuccessful procedural result. The association between PMI and mortality has been attributed to the impact of unsuccessful procedures on mortality and not to an independent effect. In a study of approximately 6,000 patients, the incidence of PMI was three times more frequent when the procedure was unsuccessful, and the size of the infarction was also significantly larger. After adjusting for the success of the procedure (defined as residual stenosis <50%; achievement of TIMI 3 flow; and absence of significant residual dissection, need for urgent revascularization, or stent thrombosis within 24 hours), the presence or absence of PMI was not statistically related to

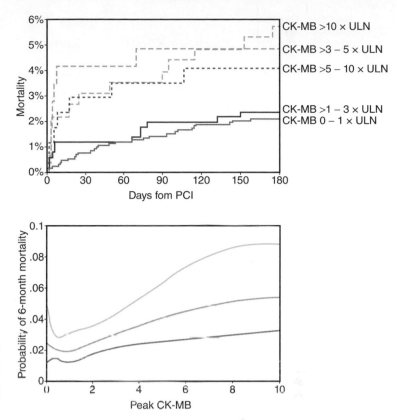

Figure 28-4 Top. Kaplan-Meier curves for 6 months unadjusted mortality after PCI for increments of post-PCI CK-MB. Bottom, continuous unadjusted relationship between peak CK-MB (as xULN) and 6 months mortality. The thin lines represent the 95% confidence intervals. (From Roe M.T. et al. Eur Heart J 2004 25:313 321.)

1-year mortality.[55] However, the study examined only 1-year mortality, and in many investigations examining PMI, the effect on mortality was observed only with longer-term follow-up. In addition, the initial studies by Abdelmeguid et al., which established a relationship between PMI and death, excluded unsuccessful procedural results from the analyses.[4,11] In the recent CK-MB and PCI study examining the significance of post-PCI troponin elevation, unsuccessful procedures doubled the odds of 2-year mortality, yet the effect of post-PCI CK-MB levels remained a strong and significant predictor of mortality.[11] The association between mortality and PMI defined by elevated serum troponin levels is less robust. The updated PCI guidelines propose that a PMI becomes clinically significant if the troponin level is > 5x ULN.[2] In a study of 1,157 patients (>77% receiving stents), 1-year mortality risk increased only in the group of patients with troponin I levels ≥ 8x ULN (≥16 ng/mL).[13] However, in the largest multicenter prospective study (almost 3,500 patients) addressing the significance of post-PCI troponin levels, there was no statistically significant association between troponin I elevation and 2-year mortality. As expected, the incidence of troponin I elevation post-PCI was significantly higher than that of CK-MB, indicating the higher sensitivity of that marker in detecting myonecrosis. Yet, this high sensitivity appears to reduce the ability of troponin elevation to predict prognosis.[14] A contemporary analysis on the prognostic significance of PMI in patients from the ACUITY (Acute Catheterization and Urgent Intervention Triage Strategy) trial suggested that PMI is a marker of baseline risk, atherosclerosis burden, and procedural complexity but in most cases does not appear to have independent prognostic significance.[56]

Prevention and Management of Periprocedural Myocardial Infarction

In the majority of cases of PMI, the event is clinically silent and the diagnosis is made on the basis of routine collection of cardiac biomarkers after PCI. Therefore little can be done to treat the event by any specific measures different from those that should be employed with any patient undergoing PCI—that is, effective beta blockade, antiplatelet therapy, lipid lowering, and aggressive risk-factor control. In the event of a relatively large PMI (e.g., CK-MB ≥ 5x ULN), an additional day of telemetry monitoring and more adequate beta blockade (with a target heart rate of about 60 beats per minute) may be indicated. Given the adverse prognostic implications, it is significantly more important to develop strategies to prevent rather than treat PMI. Successful strategies to prevent PMI include pharmacological and nonpharmacological approaches. The primary pharmacological interventions that achieved significant success include aggressive antiplatelet therapy (primarily intravenous GP IIb/IIIa inhibitors and oral thienopyridine inhibitors) and statin therapy. Nonpharmacological approaches include the use of embolism protection devices in the setting of saphenous vein graft intervention.

INTRAVENOUS GLYCOPROTEIN IIB/IIIA PLATELET INHIBITORS

Periprocedural utilization of these agents provides immediate and near complete inhibition of platelet aggregation. The intravenous administration of the appropriate doses and the targeting of the final common receptor for the aggregation process (the IIb/IIIa receptor) ensure both an extremely high bioavailability and a very predictable and complete response. Abciximab, the prototype of this class of antiplatelet agent, has been shown in multiple clinical trials to reduce the incidence of post-PCI myonecrosis. In the seminal trials (EPIC, EPILOG, and EPISTENT), the cutoff threshold for defining PMI was CKMB 3x ULN. The relative risk reduction in MI at 30 days ranged between 40% and 60%, with the curves separating as early as the first day, thus indicating a significant reduction in PMI (Fig. 28-5).[21,40] In the CAPTURE trial, patients with refractory unstable angina were randomized to receive abciximab or placebo many hours before PCI and during the procedure. In this trial, the incidence of PMI was reduced by >50% in the abciximab arm (2.6% vs. 5.5%, P = 0.009).[57] With rotational

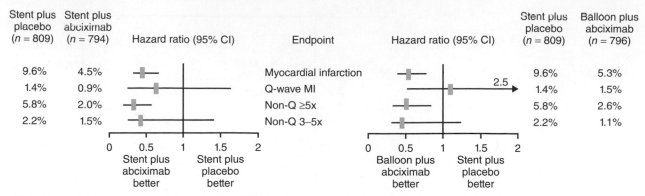

Figure 28-5 Kaplan-Meir estimates and hazard ratios (95% CI) for myocardial infarction in the EPISTENT trial. *(From the EPISTENT investigators. Lancet. 1998;352:87–92.)*

atherectomy, which consistently results in distal microembolization, abciximab bolus and infusion demonstrated a significant advantage over anticoagulation alone in reducing the rise in postprocedural CK and CK-MB.[47] Similar effects have been demonstrated with the synthetic small-molecule IIb/IIIa inhibitors eptifibatide and tirofiban. The impact of eptifibatide on PMI was significantly greater when the dosing regimen was adjusted from one bolus in the PURSUIT-PCI trial to the double-bolus regimen followed in the ESPRIT trial, thus emphasizing the importance of the near complete inhibition that is required if an impact on distal embolization is to be expected. In the PURSUIT trial, the incidence of PMI was reduced by 25%, whereas the reduction with the double-bolus regimen was 40%. In both trials, PMI was defined as CKMB > 3x ULN and the incidence of PMI in the placebo group was very similar in both trials: ~9%.[58,59] Similarly, in the RESTORE trial examining the role of tirofiban in patients with acute coronary syndromes, there was a small but significant reduction in PMI at the 48-hour mark. However, there was no statistically significant difference in the incidence of the primary endpoint (30-day death, MI, or revascularization for recurrent ischemia, use of stents for threatened or abrupt closure) between tirofiban and placebo.[60] With a higher-dose tirofiban bolus, a small study of 202 high-risk patients undergoing PCI demonstrated that PMI defined by troponin rise decreased by ~34% and average CKMB level (expressed in absolute units) was reduced by >50%.[61]

DIRECT THROMBIN INHIBITORS (BIVALIRUDIN)

Although it has been clearly established that intensive platelet inhibition results in reduced PMI, there has been concern about the excess bleeding risk caused by this strategy. The resulting focus on bleeding complications has pointed to the significant adverse prognostic implication of periprocedural bleeding on outcome, with convincing evidence of increased 1-year mortality in patients who suffer an early bleeding complication.[62] This recognition has encouraged the use of the direct thrombin inhibitor bivalirudin as a primary anticoagulant during PCI over the last several years. Large trials comparing bivalirudin to a combination of heparin and GP IIb/IIIa inhibitors has demonstrated the noninferiority of bivalirudin in reducing PMI and its clear superiority in reducing bleeding complications. It thus appears to provide the best balance of reduced PMI with a favorable effect on bleeding complications. In the REPLACE-2 trial examining the role of bivalirudin in low-risk PCI patients, the incidence of MI was slightly higher in the bivalirudin arm: 7.0% compared with 6.2% in the control arm of heparin and GP IIb/IIIa inhibitors. That difference was not statistically significant.[63] In another large randomized trial on over 4,500 low-risk PCI patients (those with stable clinical presentations), bivalirudin therapy was compared with unfractionated heparin, with both groups preloaded with oral aspirin and clopidogrel. Neither anticoagulant strategy was found superior in reducing ischemic complications (PMI 5.6% with bivalirudin vs. 4.8% with heparin), but bleeding complications were reduced in the bivalirudin arm (3.1% vs. 4.6%, P = 0.008).[64] In the ACUITY trial, approximately 14,000 patients with acute coronary syndromes (ACSs) were randomized to one of three antithrombotic regimens: unfractionated or low-molecular-weight heparin plus a GP IIb/IIIa inhibitor; bivalirudin plus a GP IIb/IIIa inhibitor; or bivalirudin alone. All patients were treated using an early invasive strategy, with most subsequently undergoing PCI or coronary artery bypass grafting (CABG), but some were treated medically after angiographic stratification. Comparing those receiving heparin and GP IIb/IIIa inhibitors with those receiving bivalirudin alone, there was no difference in ischemic events, but bleeding complications were reduced by almost 50% at 30 days (5.7% vs. 3.0%, P < 0.001 for noninferiority, P < 0.001 for superiority).[65] In a prespecified analysis, the outcomes of the 7,789 ACUITY patients who underwent PCI were analyzed according to the anticoagulation regimen they received. The results mirrored those of the main trial: no difference in PMI or other ischemic events, with a statistically significant reduction in bleeding complications, leading to improved net clinical benefit in favor of bivalirudin alone. A post-hoc analysis of this subset demonstrated an important interaction between clopidogrel pretreatment and the choice of anticoagulant strategy. Of the 7,789 PCI patients, 129 did not receive clopidogrel, while 3,493 received clopidogrel before angiography, 1,572 at the time of PCI, and 814 after PCI. Patients who received clopidogrel before angiography or within 30 minutes of PCI had similar ischemic complications, whether they were randomized to bivalirudin or heparin-GP IIb/IIIa inhibitors. However, when clopidogrel was not given or given more than 30 minutes after PCI, those randomized to bivalirudin experienced a higher incidence of ischemic events, mostly in the form of PMI (14.1% vs. 8.5%, risk ratio [RR] 1.7, 95% CI 1.05–2.63).[66] This interaction between the timing of clopidogrel therapy and bivalirudin use emphasizes the need for an effective antiplatelet therapy when direct thrombin inhibitors are used during PCI.

P2Y12 PLATELET INHIBITORS

The undisputed effect of GP IIb/IIIa platelet inhibitors in reducing PMI further supports the central role of platelet aggregation/activation in the pathophysiology of PMI. This is also further emphasized by the very high incidence of PMI and other adverse cardiac events in patients with aspirin resistance. Thus dual antiplatelet therapy using thienopyridine platelet inhibitors, namely ticlopidine and clopidogrel, has been advocated. As with other antiplatelet agents, the timing and dosing of these agents seems to have a dramatic impact on their value in reducing PMI and other post-PCI adverse events. Steinhubl et al. reported a significant reduction in the incidence of PMI with the pre-PCI administration of ticlopidine. The longer the duration of therapy, the lower the incidence was; also, among patients pretreated

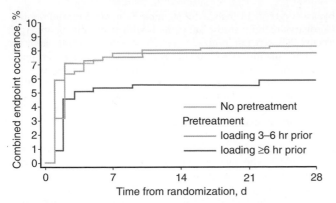

Figure 28-6 The 28-day combined endpoint (death, MI, urgent revascularization) in the CREDO trial, stratified by use and timing of clopidogrel loading dose. The curves separate within 48 hours, primarily owing to differences in incidence of PMI. *(From Steinhubl, SR et al. JAMA. 2002;288:2411–2420.)*

with ticlopidine, the odds ratio for the development of PMI was 0.18 when the duration of pretreatment was ≥3 days.[67] Subsequently, the questions of dosing and duration of pretreatment with clopidogrel, another thienopyridine inhibitor, were addressed in the CREDO trial. The study randomized patients undergoing elective PCI to receive a 300-mg clopidogrel loading dose or placebo 3 to 24 hours prior to PCI. All patients were on aspirin and most of them did undergo PCI. A second randomization to 28 days versus 9 months of dual antiplatelet therapy was performed for those in the clopidogrel arm. The results demonstrated a reduction in 30-day major adverse events (primarily early MIs) only in patients who received the loading dose ≥6 hours prior to PCI (Fig. 28-6).[68] Thus the timing of the loading dose significantly affected the beneficial effect of thienopyridine on PCI outcomes. In the PCI-CURE trial, 30% of patients underwent PCI at the discretion of the treating cardiologists. The subgroup of the larger trial included 2,658 patients with non-ST-segment elevation MI from non-U.S. centers where the time between admission for acute coronary syndrome and PCI averaged 10 days. In this setting, the 30-day incidence of MI was reduced by >50% in patients receiving clopidogrel (2.9% vs 6.2%), suggesting that a longer duration of pretreatment, particularly in high-risk patients, is associated with better protection against procedure-related MI.[69] Several groups have demonstrated that a higher loading dose (600 mg) of clopidogrel can achieve two important goals: it can reach higher levels of platelet inhibition and achieve that target within 2 hours of oral administration.[70] The improved efficacy of the higher loading dose is at least partly attributed to the fact that about one-third of patients do not adequately respond to the inhibitory effect of the 300-mg dose.[70] The ARMYDA-2 trial established the superiority of the 600-mg loading dose of clopidogrel in reducing PMI and improving 30-day outcomes. This study enrolled 255 patients undergoing PCI and randomized them to 300-mg versus 600-mg loading doses of clopidogrel 4 to 8 hours prior to PCI. The primary endpoint of death, MI, or urgent revascularization at 30 days was reduced by 66% in the high-loading-dose arm (4% vs. 12%, $P = 0.04$). This benefit was almost entirely due to the marked reduction in PMI; this was a reduction of approximately 50% in a multivariate model adjusting for all variables influencing the incidence of PMI (OR 0.48, 95% CI 0.15 to 0.97, $P = 0.044$).[71] It remains controversial whether a higher loading dose of clopidogrel (900 mg) can lead to further improvements in PMI and other ischemic complications.[72,73] The main criticism of the routine clopidogrel preloading strategy in patients undergoing coronary angiography is that a fraction of the patients will be referred to bypass surgery; these patients will have an increased risk of bleeding unless their bypass surgery is postponed for at least 5 days. Thus, the ARMYDA-5 PRELOAD trial tested the strategy of high-dose

clopidogrel loading in the catheterization laboratory against high-dose preloading that had previously been established. A total of 409 patients were randomized to receive a 600-mg preloading dose 4 to 8 hours prior to PCI or a 600-mg loading dose in the catheterization laboratory after obtaining diagnostic angiograms. The study revealed no difference in the incidence of PMI between the two strategies (8.8% in laboratory vs. 9.3% preload groups, $P = 0.99$).[74] Point-of-care testing demonstrated that platelet reactivity remained high during the PCI and for the 2 hours that followed in patients treated in the catheterization laboratory, which is not consistent with the previously established association between better platelet inhibition and reduced incidence of PMI. The study was also criticized for the small sample size, which makes it underpowered to detect a difference between the groups.[75] As the evidence for the effectiveness of platelet inhibition with clopidogrel mounted, questions arose regarding the need for the more expensive intravenous GP IIb/IIIa inhibitors in PCI. In sequential investigations (the ISAR-REACT trials), the interaction between clopidogrel loading and abciximab infusion for peri-PCI platelet inhibition was examined in low-risk and then higher-risk patient populations. In ISAR-REACT 1, more than 1,000 stable patients were randomized to receive clopidogrel loading plus placebo versus clopidogrel loading plus abciximab bolus and infusion. At 30 days, there was no statistically significant difference between the two groups in the incidence of MI or death.[76] However, the very low incidence of adverse events in the placebo group diminished the statistical power of the study to detect differences between the groups. In the following study, ISAR-REACT 2, more than 2,000 patients with non-ST-segment elevation ACSs were enrolled. All patients received clopidogrel pretreatment, then half of them were randomized to abciximab bolus plus infusion. Unlike ISAR-REACT 1, there was a significant reduction in the 30-day composite endpoint in favor of abciximab. This included a >20% reduction in infarctions, most of which were PMI (8.1% vs. 10.5%). Based on the results of those two investigations, it seems that a more complete degree of platelet inhibition is needed in patients at higher risk of PMI and other procedural complications. In addition to the more complete platelet inhibition ensured by the use of abciximab, its cross-reactivity with αvβ3 (vitronectin) and αMβ2 (Mac-1) receptors may provide potent anti-inflammatory effects. This appears to be associated with a significant reduction in the degree of rise of inflammatory markers such as CRP, IL-6, and TNF-α in the 1 to 2 days following PCI, an effect that may contribute to the reduction in PMI seen with abciximab use during PCI.[77] The association of more effective platelet inhibition and improved outcomes in patients with ACSs treated invasively has been further supported by results of clinical trials comparing prasugrel and ticagrelor with clopidogrel. Although the incidence of PMI was not directly reported, both agents were associated with statistically significantly lower incidence of ischemic events in the early phase after PCI, which are traditionally driven by periprocedural events.[78,79]

IMPACT OF STATIN THERAPY

The inflammatory response of distal embolization and platelet aggregate interaction with leukocytes contributes to the myonecrosis that is frequently seen after PCI. The observations made in PCI registries have demonstrated a reduction in PMI in patients who received statins at the time of their PCI.[80] Proposed mechanisms to explain this finding include an anti-inflammatory effect and the ability of statins to enhance nitric oxide production.[81] In an analysis of 803 patients undergoing rotational atherectomy, the incidence of myonecrosis was reduced by statin therapy from 52% to 24% and the incidence of PMI (CK-MB ≥ 3x ULN) from 22% to 7.5%.[82] These observations were eventually confirmed in two prospective randomized trials. In both, statin therapy was started several days before scheduled PCI in the active therapy arm. In one report on 451 patients, statin therapy was not restricted to any specific agents. Median post-PCI troponin level was 0.13 ng/mL in the statin group and 0.21 ng/mL in the control group ($P = 0.03$). Similarly, the incidence of troponin I > 5x ULN was significantly reduced with statin therapy (23.5% vs. 32% in the control group, $P = 0.04$).[83] In the similarly designed ARMYDA trial, a smaller number of stable angina patients were randomized to receive atorvastatin versus placebo. There was >50% reduction in incidence of PMI as measured by CK-MB, troponin I, or myoglobin in the atorvastatin group.[84] In ARMYDA-2, there was an incremental benefit of statin and high-dose loading of clopidogrel, leading to a more impressive 80% reduction in PMI.[71] A subgroup analysis of the ARMYDA trial confirmed the anti-inflammatory role of statins in reducing myonecrosis post-PCI. In 138 patients, serum levels of adhesion molecules (ICAM, VCAM, E-selectin) were similar in patients in the atorvastatin group and the placebo group before PCI. Yet, post-PCI, the rises in ICAM and E-selectin were significantly attenuated with atorvastatin therapy. This attenuated rise in adhesion molecules paralleled the protective effect against myonecrosis, providing some evidence that the anti-inflammatory effect of statins contributes to its observed protective effect against myonecrosis and early mortality, which cannot be attributed to its inhibitory effect on 3-hydroxy-3-methyl-glutaryl-CoA reductase (HMG-CoA reductase).[85] The impact of high-dose statin therapy can be demonstrated within days, confirming the existence of mechanisms of action other than lipid lowering. The NAPLES (Novel Approaches for Preventing or Limiting Events) II trial has reported that a single high (80-mg) loading dose (within 24 hours) of atorvastatin reduces the incidence of PMI in elective PCI. The incidence of PMI was 9.5% in the atorvastatin group and 15.8% in the control group (OR 0.56; 95% CI 0.35–0.89; $P = 0.014$).[86]

Since most patients undergoing PCI are already taking statins, the question of pretreatments seemed irrelevant. However, the pleiotropic and anti-inflammatory effects of statins seem to diminish with time. The ARMYDA-RECAPTURE clinical trial randomized more than 380 patients undergoing PCI to an intensive "reloading" of atorvastatin (80 mg 12 hours before and 40 mg immediately before PCI) and a standard therapy group (on a standard daily dose of atorvastatin). All patients were pretreated with clopidogrel and aspirin. At 30 days, there was a significant reduction in the composite endpoint in favor of atorvastatin reloading. The incidence of postprocedure elevation in CK-MB and troponin was significantly lower in the reloading group (13% vs. 24%, $P = 0.017$ and 37% vs. 49%, $P = 0.021$, respectively).[87] Like observations made with abciximab, the benefit of intensive atorvastatin therapy was restricted to patients presenting with ACSs, probably because of the higher underlying risk of PMI.

OTHER PHARMACOLOGICAL INTERVENTIONS

Controversy still exists about the role of preprocedural beta-blocker therapy and PMI. There is evidence that beta blockade has a favorable impact on survival after PCI. Ellis et al. supported this finding in a study of 6,200 patients undergoing PCI, concluding that beta-blocker therapy improved survival in post-PCI patients. However, after adjustment for multiple variables and using propensity analysis, there was no evidence that patients taking beta blockers had a reduced risk for PMI or a reduced size of PMI.[88]

NONPHARMACOLOGICAL APPROACHES

Very few mechanical options to prevent PMI are currently available. Direct stenting (without balloon predilation) has been proposed to reduce plaque trauma and distal embolization. A small study comparing direct stenting with conventional predilation followed by stent deployment demonstrated a significant reduction in PMI.[89] Subsequent larger trials did not confirm any concrete advantages of this approach to reducing myonecrosis or any other adverse events.[90]

The concept of ischemic preconditioning (ICP) and its role in myocyte protection is an intriguing one. Transient and repeated episodes of ischemia followed by reperfusion of the myocardium can provide some protection against myocardial damage when a prolonged episode of ischemia occurs. This pre-conditioning limits reperfusion injury and has been shown to limit infarct size in patients undergoing

bypass surgery.[91] In the CRISP (Remote Ischemic Preconditioning in Coronary Stenting) study, 242 patients with stable angina undergoing elective PCI were randomized to receive remote IPC (induced by three 5-minute inflations of a blood pressure cuff to 200 mm Hg around the upper arm, followed by 5-minute intervals of reperfusion) or control (an uninflated cuff around the arm) before their arrival in the catheterization laboratory. The primary outcome was cTnI at 24 hours after PCI. The median cTnI at 24 hours after PCI was lower in the remote IPC group compared with the control group (0.06 vs. 0.16 ng/mL; $P = 0.040$). After PCI, 42% of patients who underwent remote IPC had a normal TnI level, compared with 24% of the control group ($P = 0.01$).[92] The mechanisms of protection induced by remote ischemic preconditioning are multifactorial; there is evidence of an early opening of mitochondrial potassium channels[93] and a later anti-inflammatory effect mediated by modified gene expression.[94] Embolism protection devices have been the only significant nonpharmacological interventions with a proven advantage in reduction of periprocedural myonecrosis, particularly in saphenous vein graft intervention. These devices are discussed in detail in the following section.

Conclusions

PMI is not uncommon after an apparently uncomplicated PCI. The reported incidence varies according to the biomarker used, the threshold for diagnosis, and the timing of sample collection. Distal embolization of atherosclerotic debris and platelet aggregates is the most plausible mechanism underlying PMI. Overall, the data suggest that PMI is associated with late mortality, and the larger the PMI, the more robust is the association. Potent platelet inhibitor therapy (intravenous or oral), statins (as anti-inflammatory agents), and embolism protection devices (in saphenous vein graft PCI) had the most success in reducing the incidence of PMI. When used as the primary anticoagulant for PCI procedures, the direct thrombin inhibitor bivalirudin may provide the best balance of reduced incidence of PMI without increased bleeding.

Embolism Protection Devices

KEY POINTS

- Embolism protection devices include distal occlusive balloons, filter devices, and proximal flow-reversal systems, all aiming to trap embolized debris from the site of angioplasty before it reaches the distal microvascular bed.

- Clinical trials have demonstrated that the use of these devices during vein graft percutaneous coronary intervention leads to a significant reduction in periprocedural myocardial infarction and is cost-effective; it is now the standard of care during these procedures.

- Several randomized trials have failed to show any benefit of embolism protection in the setting of percutaneous coronary intervention and acute myocardial infarction, thus highlighting the complexity of the mechanisms of myonecrosis and injury in such settings.

- There is good evidence that embolism protection reduces cerebral embolism during carotid stenting, but there has been no conclusive randomized trial based on clinical endpoints to confirm this benefit.

- Comparison of carotid stenting with embolism protection in carotid endarterectomy remains controversial, with some evidence of similar outcomes in patients with asymptomatic disease and in the hands of experienced operators.

- Small clinical trials testing the potential advantages of using embolism protection devices during interventions in other vascular beds (e.g., renal and peripheral) show promising results.

With the wider acceptance of the significance of distal embolization during PCI, efforts to reduce the incidence and impact of this phenomenon have been under way. As discussed earlier, effective antiplatelet therapy with IIb/IIIa inhibitors and thienopyridine inhibitors has resulted in significant progress in reducing procedure-related myonecrosis. Despite routine use of these pharmacological agents, a small PMI is not uncommon even after an uncomplicated procedure. This is of particular concern in the setting of saphenous vein graft interventions, which have a high propensity for distal embolization, the no-reflow phenomenon, and PMI. Lesions with high thrombotic burdens are another subgroup in which interventional procedures of any kind pose a higher risk of distal embolization. The prototype of such procedures is PCI in the setting of acute MI. Over the last few years, several innovative designs for embolism protection devices (EPDs) have been developed to improve outcomes in this subset of patients as well as in other clinical settings. EPDs are of three basic types, those comprising (1) distal occlusion balloons, (2) distal filters, and (3) proximal occlusion devices (Fig. 28-7). Table 28-2 summarizes the differences between the various concepts for EPDs.

DISTAL OCCLUSION DEVICES

The PercuSurge GuardWire system (Medtronic Inc.), the prototype of the balloon occlusion devices, consists of a 0.014-in. hollow guidewire with an occlusion balloon toward the distal end and a 2.5-cm steerable tip beyond the balloon (Fig. 28-7). The GuardWire is used to cross the lesion and the balloon is positioned distal to the lesion in a relatively disease-free segment. Then the balloon is inflated at a low pressure of about 1 atm in order to create a seal; the occlusion diameter ranges from 3 to 6 mm. Angioplasty, stenting, and postdilation are all performed as necessary. The aspiration catheter is then advanced over the wire and any dislodged debris is removed with a slow

TABLE 28-2	Characteristics of Different Concepts in Embolism Protection Devices		
	Distal Filter	**Distal Balloon Occlusion**	**Proximal Occlusion**
Antegrade perfusion	Uninterrupted	Temporarily interrupted*	Temporarily interrupted*
Visualization of the distal vessel	Unhindered	Not possible during inflation	Possible via the inner sheath
Efficacy of emboli protection	May allow passage of emboli < pore size (100 μm)†	Once inflated, traps all emboli	All particles can be aspirated
Vasoactive substances	Pass unimpeded	Can be aspirated completely	Can be aspirated completely
Crossing profile	0.040–0.050 in.	0.026–0.033 in.	No crossing, deployed proximal to the lesion
Embolization during device positioning	Likely to occur	Less likely to occur	None, since device does not cross the lesion
Retrieval profile	Occasionally difficult if filter full of debris	Not a problem after balloon deflation	Not a problem, device is proximal to the lesion
Flexibility of guidewire use	None, since filter is attached to wire	None, since balloon is attached to wire	Excellent, device can be used with any wire
Effect of distal disease on device	May not be feasible if no disease-free segment	May not be feasible if no disease-free segment	Device is proximal, distal disease irrelevant

*Transient ischemia while the embolism protection system is being used unless there are adequate retrograde collaterals.
†In reality, the filter can trap particles smaller than its pore size due to clumping of particles. There have been numerous trials that demonstrated no clinically significant differences between distal balloon occlusion and distal filter concepts.

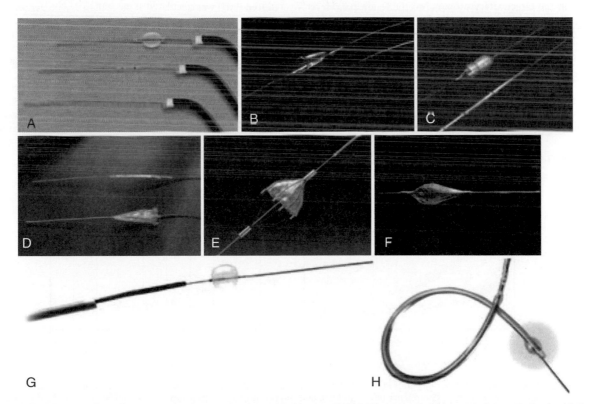

Figure 28-7 Embolism protection devices. A. Medtronic Percusurge Guidewire. B. BSC Filterwire. C. Abbott MedNova Emboshield. D. eV3 Spider. E. Cordis Angioguard. F. Abbott Accunet. G. Mo.ma or Ultra Proximal Cerebral Protection Device by Invatec, Italy. H. St. Jude Proxis catheter. *(Modified and adapted from Mauri L. et al. Circulation. 2006;113:2651-2656.)*

distal-to-proximal pullback. The balloon is deflated and the Guard-Wire is withdrawn. Angiography is performed to confirm distal flow.

DISTAL FILTER DEVICES

All the nonocclusive devices comprise a guidewire and filter. The AngioGuard filter wire (Cordis Inc.), the prototype of the filter devices, consists of a 0.014-in. wire that has a filter basket near its distal end (Fig. 28-7). Beyond the filter a short portion of guidewire protrudes, which can be shaped. The currently used version has pores that are 100 μm in diameter. The smallest nominal filter basket size is currently 4 mm, which would be used for vessels that are >3.0 mm but ≤3.5 mm in diameter, while the largest basket size is 8 mm. As a general principle, the filter should be oversized by about 0.5 to 1.0 mm compared with the vessel reference diameter. Before introducing the wire into the guiding catheter, it is pulled into a sheath under water in order to collapse the filter basket and get rid of the air bubbles. Once the wire crosses the lesion and the filter basket is in a relatively disease-free portion of the artery, the sheath is retracted and the basket is released to deploy in the artery. The sheath is removed over the wire, which then serves as a standard angioplasty wire. During the intervention, blood flow through the pores of the filter is preserved and the injection of contrast for visualization is not affected by the deployed filter. When the interventional procedure is complete, a retrieval sheath is advanced over the wire and used to collapse the filter basket securely. The retrieval sheath and the collapsed filter trapping the embolic debris within it are then removed as one unit.

PROXIMAL OCCLUSION DEVICES

The Proxis system (St. Jude Medical) is the most commonly used device of this type in the United States. The system contains an inner working sheath that is about 6 Fr in diameter; it is advanced through a 7- or 8-Fr guiding catheter. An inflatable balloon is attached to the end of the device and the external surface of the inner sheath. Inflation of this balloon in the target artery proximal to the lesion provides a seal that prevents antegrade flow through the target artery. After the system is in place, the intervention can be performed through the inner working sheath using the wire, balloon, and stent of choice. Small contrast injections for visualization are feasible. At the end of the procedure, the interventional devices are removed and the stagnant blood in the target artery is aspirated via the working sheath. The final step is to deflate the balloon and remove the working sheath, leaving the guiding catheter in the artery after debris and vasoactive substances have been aspirated.

Saphenous Vein Graft Percutaneous Coronary Intervention

Traditionally, vein graft PCI is considered a high-risk procedure owing to the increased risk of distal macro- and microembolization, with subsequent slow flow or no reflow and PMI. More importantly, one of the most potent interventions to reduce risk of PMI in native coronary PCI, namely the use of GP IIb/IIIa inhibitors, appears to be ineffective in the setting of vein graft PCI. A pooled analysis of several GP IIb/IIIa inhibitor trials as well as large registry data have demonstrated that the addition of intravenous IIb/IIIa inhibitors to standard anticoagulation regimens was not associated with any significant reduction in ischemic complications (including PMI) in patients undergoing vein graft PCI.[95,96]

Several small studies testing the efficacy of EPDs (particularly the Percusurge GuardWire) have demonstrated that particulate matter can be aspirated in the majority of cases with an associated reduction in no-reflow and PMI.[97] Based on these findings, 801 patients from 47 centers were randomized to undergo vein graft PCI with the Guard-Wire protection versus no EPD in the SAFER (SVG Angioplasty Free of Emboli Randomized) trial.[35] The primary endpoint was death, Q-wave MI, non-Q-wave MI (CK-MB > 3x ULN), emergent bypass surgery, or target vessel revascularization within 30 days. Almost 40% of patients had angiographic thrombi present. Technical success was achieved with the device in 90.1% of the cases. The primary endpoint was significantly reduced with use of the PercuSurge GuardWire (from 16.5% to 9.6%; $P = 0.004$), primarily driven by the ~50% reduction in non-Q-wave MI from 13.7% to 7.4% (Fig. 28-8). A number of important secondary endpoints were also favorably influenced, most importantly the no-reflow phenomenon, which was reduced dramatically (9.0% vs. 3.0%; $P = 0.02$).[35] Moreover, a cost-effectiveness analysis of the SAFER trial demonstrated that the reduction in ischemic complications leads to shorter hospital stays and a reduction in early costs, thus compensating for most of the added expense of the EPD. The projected improved survival on the basis of reduced early complications (namely, reduced PMI) was calculated at more than $4,000 per year of life saved, which makes the use of EPD in vein graft PCI a very cost-effective strategy.[98] This significant improvement in outcome with the use of the GuardWire occlusion device ushered a new era in which EPD use has become the standard of care with vein graft PCI. Thus the randomized controlled trials leading to FDA approval of other EPDs for use in vein graft PCI were designed as noninferiority trials, with the GuardWire used in the "active" control arm. In a controlled trial, 651 patients undergoing vein graft PCI were randomized to receive the FilterWire EX versus the GuardWire. Use of GP IIb/IIIa inhibitors was

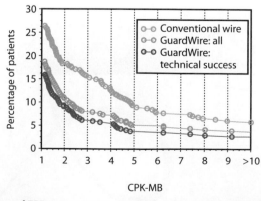
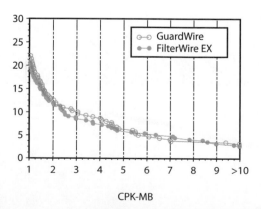

Figure 28-8   Impact of EPD use on PMI in vein graft PCI. Left, the SAFER trial: cumulative distribution function curve of peak cardiac enzyme values after assignment to placebo (395 patients), GuardWire (406 patients), and the per-protocol subgroup with technically successful GuardWire use (366 patients). The CPK-MB is represented as multiples of the upper limit of normal. There is a significantly lower incidence of PMI of any size with Guardwire use. Right, the FIRE trial: a similar plot for patients randomized to distal protection with the FilterWire EX versus the GuardWire, showing noninferiority of the FilterWire. *(From Baim DS et al. Circulation. 2002;105:1285–1290, and Stone GW et al. Circulation. 2003;108:548–553.)*

left to the discretion of the operators. The primary endpoint was a composite similar to that used in the SAFER trial. At 30 days, there was no difference in the incidence of MI, with a trend toward a reduction in the 1-year endpoint in the FilterWire arm (9.9% vs. 11.6%, $P = 0.53$ for superiority, $P = 0.0008$ for noninferiority) (Fig. 28 8).[37] Interestingly, a further examination of these results demonstrated a favorable interaction between the use of both GP IIb/IIIa inhibitors and the FilterWire but not with the GuardWire. This may be related to the improved flow seen with GP IIb/IIIa inhibitors in patients receiving FilterWire protection, probably owing to the reduced degree of platelet aggregation and deposition on the surface of the filter.[99] A more complex study design was used to demonstrate noninferiority of the Proxis system. A total of 639 target vein grafts in 594 patients were prospectively randomized to a test group (using proximal protection when possible, distal protection when not) or a control group (using distal protection when possible). The 30-day composite endpoint was similar to that used for the SAFER trial. The study demonstrated noninferiority of proximal protection when the analysis was performed by intention to treat or by actual device use.[100] Noninferiority trials were similarly designed to test the efficacy of the Triactiv device (Kensey Nash, Exton, PA), MedNova Emboshield (Abbott Vascular Inc, Santa Clara, CA), the AVE Interceptor (Medtronic Cardiovascular, Minneapolis, MN), and the Spider device (eV3 Endovascular, Inc, Plymouth, MN). In those trials, the 30-day primary endpoint was reached in 8% to 11% of patients, achieving the preset standard for noninferiority in comparison with the GuardWire or FilterWire in all studies.[101,102] Despite the convincing evidence of efficacy and cost-effectiveness, adoption of EPD for vein graft interventions in the United States has been sluggish. Data from the National Cardiovascular Data Registry (NCDR) on >19,000 vein graft interventions between 2004 and 2006 demonstrate that EPDs were used in 22% of cases, with 19% of centers not using EPDs and 41% using them in <10% of cases.[103] More recently, analysis of the SoS (Stenting of Saphenous Vein Grafts) trial demonstrated that EPDs were used in 54% of cases. While some of the lack of use was dictated by anatomical considerations, there is evidence that operator preference still contributes to this underutilization of EPDs,[104] These findings suggest a clear need for continuing education and training of interventionists on the value of these devices in reducing morbidity and mortality as well as intensifying efforts to develop more affordable devices that are easier to use.

PERCUTANEOUS CORONARY INTERVENTION FOR ACUTE MYOCARDIAL INFARCTION

The concept of EPD use in primary PCI is both attractive and intuitive. These are the prototypical thrombotic lesions with a very high likelihood of distal embolization. The success of EPDs in vein graft PCI led to clinical trials examining the feasibility of the concept. In a small study, use of the PercuSurge GuardWire during primary stenting of infarct-related arteries resulted in improved flow and subsequently improved ventricular function as compared with procedures performed without EPD use.[105] However, these larger randomized trials did not confirm the initial favorable impression regarding the use of EPDs in primary PCI. The EMERALD (Enhanced Myocardial Efficacy and Removal by Aspiration of Liberated Debris) trial was an international multicenter prospective randomized trial enrolling 501 patients with ST-segment elevation MI undergoing primary or rescue PCI. Patients were randomized to PCI with Percusurge GuardWire distal protection versus PCI without EPD. Two coprimary endpoints were prespecified: ST-segment resolution after PCI by continuous Holter monitoring and infarct size measured by nuclear imaging between days 5 and 14. Secondary endpoints included major adverse cardiac events. Among 252 patients assigned to GuardWire protection, debris was retrieved in 73% of cases. Disappointingly, there was no difference between the two groups in any of the primary or secondary endpoints (ST-segment resolution in 63% vs. 62%, infarct size 12% vs. 9.5%, P = NS for both).[106] The PROMISE (Protection Devices in PCI treatment of Myocardial Infarction for Salvage of Endangered Myocardium) trial

tested the efficacy of the FilterWire in the setting of PCI for acute MI. This study included patients with non-ST-segment elevation MI and used different surrogate endpoints: coronary flow velocity measured by an intravascular Doppler and the size of the infarction measured by hyperenhancement on MRI scans 3 days after the procedure. As in the case of the EMERALD trial, FilterWire protection provided no additional benefit.[107] Other trials examining filter-based EPDs in the setting of primary angioplasty have not demonstrated any clinical benefit to this approach.[108] There are several potential explanations for the disappointing results of EPD use in primary angioplasty. The use of EPDs may delay restoration of epicardial flow and the devices may cause further embolization while crossing the lesion, thus negating any favorable effects of subsequent protection. The incomplete aspiration of liberated debris or leaking of vasoactive substances released from the ruptured plaques may lead to further downstream damage at the time of EPD removal. Embolization into side branches may play a role, particularly in cases of acute thrombotic occlusion, leading to initial TIMI flow grade 0 and absence of visualization of the distal artery at the time of EPD positioning. Importantly, these results also indicate a relative underestimation of the degree of existing damage and the role of reperfusion injury in determining the final infarct size after primary PCI.[109]

CAROTID STENTING

Although the clinical implications of embolization were first elucidated for coronary interventions, the paradigm is applicable and relevant in angioplasty procedures in other arterial beds. Interventional procedures in the carotid and renal arteries are two areas where embolization may be particularly significant. Embolization appears to occur more frequently after carotid stenting than carotid endarterectomy (CEA). Using transcranial Doppler (TCD) monitoring, microscopic embolization was found to occur at least eight times more frequently with carotid angioplasty and stenting than with carotid endarterectomy.[110] Indeed, the vast majority of patients undergoing carotid stenting have TCD evidence of microembolization (Fig. 28-9). As in the case of embolization related to coronary interventions, it appears that evidence of a systemic inflammatory response can lead to more embolization. In a small study of 43 patients undergoing carotid stenting with TCD monitoring of the ipsilateral middle cerebral artery, there was a positive correlation between TCD identified microembolism and preprocedural leukocyte count (a marker of systemic inflammation). This correlation remained significant even after adjusting for age, gender, comorbidities, medical therapy, and use of EPDs.[111] Even small embolic particles may be poorly tolerated by the cerebral microcirculation.[112] In an ex vivo model of carotid angioplasty, particles generated from

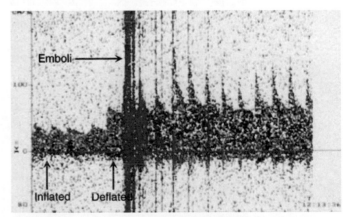

Figure 28-9 Transcranial Doppler monitoring of middle cerebral artery flow during elective carotid artery stenting. The high-intensity transients observed at the time of balloon deflation represent a surge of microemboli from the extracranial site of angioplasty to the intracranial circulation. (*From Topol EJ. et al. Circulation. 2000;101:570–580.*)

human carotid plaques were injected into the cerebral circulation of rats. Interestingly, stenting produced almost twice as much embolization as balloon angioplasty in this model; passage of the guidewire also produced embolization, though only about a quarter as many emboli as balloon angioplasty. Particles <200 μm in size did not cause cerebral ischemia during the first 3 days after the procedure, whereas particles of 200 to 500 μm did cause neuronal death. However, at 7 days, injury due to fragments of both sizes was detected. Thus, if smaller sizes of emboli are relevant in humans, an occlusion device may be better than a filter device. Although filters can be designed with smaller pores, the disadvantage is that this can increase the risk of thrombosis by the filter itself and decrease distal flow. Thus several EPDs were designed for use in conjunction with carotid angioplasty and stenting in the hope of reducing the incidence of procedure-related strokes. Reimers et al. reported their initial experience with three different filter designs (AngioGuard, NeuroSheild, and FilterWire) in 84 patients undergoing carotid stenting.[113] Macroscopic debris was collected in 53% of filters and histological analysis of the debris revealed lipid-rich macrophages, fibrin, and cholesterol clefts. The early experience with the balloon occlusion variety of EPD (PercuSurge GuardWire) was reported in a series of 75 patients. In this series, macroscopic debris was collected from all cases (100%) and histological analysis was very similar to that of particles obtained from filter devices.[114]

In addition to the retrieval of macroscopic and microscopic debris, there is additional evidence that the use of EPD during carotid stenting effectively reduces embolism to the cerebral microcirculation. These data have been gleaned from studies utilizing magnetic resonance diffusion-weighted imaging (DWI), which is the most sensitive imaging modality for the detection of early cerebral ischemia.[115,116] Comparison of DWI scans before and after carotid stenting reveals that the use of EPDs significantly reduces both the incidence and number of new lesions identified on the post-procedure scan. Most new lesions were small (<10 mm) and asymptomatic (Fig. 28-10). In a study of 206 patients, there was no difference in the incidence of stroke between patients who did and did not receive embolism protection, but the number of DWI new lesions was significantly higher in patients who underwent unprotected carotid stenting.[116] Although there has been no randomized trial comparing the outcomes of carotid stenting with and without EPD protection, evidence from large multicenter

registries demonstrates that EPD use has resulted in a significant reduction in neurological adverse events. In a systematic review of published reports, Kastrup et al. compared the outcomes of 2,357 patients undergoing carotid stenting without EPD use to those of 839 patients in whom stenting was performed with an EPD in place. There was a significant reduction in 30-day rate of death and/or stroke with EPD use (1.8% vs. 5.5%, $P < 0.001$). Both minor and major strokes were significantly reduced in patients receiving embolism protection (minor stroke 0.5% vs. 3.7%, $P < 0.001$; major stroke 0.3% vs. 1.1%, $P < 0.05$). The larger carotid stent global registry surveys the major interventional centers worldwide and collects self-reported data on technical details and outcomes. In the most recent update, 6,753 patients were reported to have undergone stenting without EPD use, while 4,221 did receive embolism protection. The 30-day incidence of stroke and procedure-related death was reduced by >50% from 5.3% to 2.2%. Despite EPD protection, symptomatic patients remained at higher risk for developing stroke or procedure-related death compared with the asymptomatic subgroup (2.7% vs. 1.75%).[117]

Few randomized trials have compared contemporary carotid artery stenting with carotic endarterectory (CEA). The SAPPHIRE (Stenting and Angioplasty with Protection in Patients at High Risk for Endarterectomy) trial randomized patients to either endarterectomy or carotid stenting with the AngioGuard filter device. Both symptomatic and asymptomatic patients were included if they had a coexisting condition that placed them at a higher risk of complications during carotid endarterectomy. The primary composite endpoint was death, stroke, or MI at 30 days plus death due to neurologic causes or ipsilateral stroke between day 31 and 1 year. The trial was terminated after 334 patients were randomized because of slowing recruitment. In this high-risk population, the primary composite endpoint was reduced in the stent group compared with the surgical group (12.2% vs. 20.1%, $P = 0.004$ for noninferiority, $P = 0.053$ for superiority). At 30 days, the incidence of stroke was 3.6% and 3.1% in the stent and CEA arms, respectively. This reduction in the primary endpoint was driven primarily by a reduction in MI in the stent arm rather than by differences in cerebral events.[118] To gain FDA approval, several manufacturers of EPD and stent designs initiated a group of large patient registries to demonstrate the safety and efficacy of their novel devices. Most of the enrolled patients were at high risk for complications, as in the

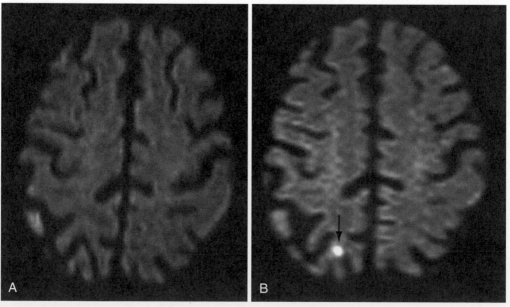

Figure 28-10 Preprocedural (A) and postprocedural (B) axial DWI of the brain. Despite carotid stenting with the use of embolism protection, an ipsilateral hyperintense lesion (arrow) related to silent cerebral embolism is appreciable at the cortical-subcortical junction of right parietal lobe. (*From Cosottini M et al. Stroke. 2005;36:2389–2393.*)

SAPPHIRE design. The low incidence of death or stroke compared with historic adverse event rates in CEA resulted in eventual FDA approval of many of these devices.[119,120] Two European randomized trials attempted to demonstrate noninferiority of carotid stenting compared with endarterectomy: the SPACE (Stent-Supported Percutaneous Angioplasty of the Carotid Artery versus Endarterectomy) and EVA-3S (Endarterectomy vs. Angioplasty in Patients with Symptomatic Severe Carotid Stenosis) trials. Both studies included patients with symptomatic carotid stenosis and attempted to demonstrate the noninferiority of stenting.[121,122] The endpoints were similar: death or stroke at 30 days. Neither study emphasized EPD use; it was employed with only 25% of patients in SPACE. In EVA-3S, EPD use was mandated only after evidence of excess stroke in the first 80 patients.[123] Both studies failed to demonstrate noninferiority, with evidence of excess stroke (mostly minor) in the stenting arm. More recently, reports from two larger randomized trials comparing carotid stenting to endarterectomy were published: the ICSS (International Carotid Stenting Study) and CREST (Carotid Endarterectomy vs. Stenting Trial). The ICSS enrolled 1,713 symptomatic patients, emphasized the use of EPDs (80%), and has a primary endpoint of fatal or disabling stroke at 3 years. At 120 days, the investigators reported an excess of minor strokes in the stenting arm (7.6% vs. 4.1% in endarterectomy group) and an excess of laryngeal nerve palsy in the endarterectomy arm.[124] Alternatively, CREST randomized 2,502 patients with both symptomatic and asymptomatic disease, making it the largest study to date to address this question. The primary composite endpoint was periprocedural stroke, death, or infarction plus ipsilateral stroke within 4 years. All stenting procedures included EPD use. At 30 days, the stroke rate was 4.1% for stenting and 2.3% for endarterectomy, with major strokes <1% in both groups. The study showed no difference between the groups in the composite endpoint and no difference between symptomatic and asymptomatic patients. There was an excess in minor strokes with stenting, balanced by an excess of myocardial infarctions in the endarterectomy group.[125] Based on the totality of evidence, several factors can be seen to have a significant impact on outcomes of carotid stenting: symptomatic status, EPD use, and operator experience. In the two trials that mandated the use of EPDs and restricted enrollment to experienced operators (SAPPHIRE and CREST), there is more evidence of similarity between stenting and endarterectomy. Of note, both studies included asymptomatic patients, who are considered to be lower risk for adverse events. On the other hand, trials that did not mandate EPD use on a large scale and/or included interventional operators with no or minimal experience (SPACE, EVA-3S, and ICSS) had higher event rates with stenting, albeit these trials focused on symptomatic patients. A report on a large single-center experience using a novel proximal protection device (the Mo.Ma Ultra Proximal Cerebral Protection Device by Invatec, Italy) raises hopes of a better future for EPDs in carotid stenting. This device incorporates two occlusion balloons that seal the external and common carotid arteries, thus eliminating antegrade flow (Fig. 28-7). After the procedure is performed, the stagnant blood column is aspirated before the occlusive balloons are deflated. In a series of 1,300 patients, the incidence of death and stroke was a surprisingly low 1.38%.[126] While this may not be reproducible in a larger multicenter trial with less experienced operators, it does give hope that the ceiling of EPD protection in carotid stenting may not have been reached.

RENAL AND PERIPHERAL INTERVENTIONS

Although there are fewer data demonstrating the importance of atheroembolism in the renal vasculature, emboli are also detrimental in this arterial bed. A study by Krishnamurthi and colleagues examined the impact of embolization after surgical revascularization for renal artery stenosis.[127] In this series, evidence of atheroembolism was detected in 16 of 44 patients. In those patients, 5-year survival was significantly worse than that in patients with no evidence of distal embolism (54% vs. 85%, $P = 0.001$), thus suggesting that this phenomenon is clinically relevant to the outcome of renal revascularization.[127] Although difficult to prove, there is little doubt that embolization also occurs in the setting of percutaneous renal revascularization and is likely also associated with worse patient outcomes. It is estimated that 25% of patients have worse renal function after renal intervention. Although the reason for this decrease in renal function is probably multifactorial, embolization is likely part of the problem. The PercuSurge GuardWire and the FilterWire systems have been used successfully during renal intervention. In one series, 65 renal arteries in 56 hypertensive patients were successfully stented with embolism protection (Guardwire, FilterWire, and Angioguard devices). Visible debris was aspirated in 100% of the cases with Guardwire protection and 80% of those in whom filter devices were used. Mean particle number and diameter were 98.1 ± 60.0 per procedure (range, 13–208) and 201.0 +/− 76.0 microm (range, 38.6–206), respectively. At 3 years, only two patients developed worsening renal function.[128] Despite the growing number of renal artery procedures in the last few years, there is no conclusive evidence that the indiscriminate use of this procedure is better than medical therapy in all patients. There is some evidence suggesting an improved renal function with use of abciximab and EPD,[129] although that will require further confirmation. Early experiences with EPD in lower extremity percutaneous revascularization procedures have been reported as well.[130,131] In most cases, filter devices were deployed and retrieved successfully. There was macro- and microscopic debris in all cases, suggesting a potential benefit of these devices in procedures involving the lower extremity, particularly in cases of acute or subacute ischemia with large thrombotic burdens and a high risk of distal showering.

Conclusions

Embolism protection devices have gained widespread acceptance in the interventional cardiology and vascular community over the last decade. There is solid evidence that they are safe to use and effective in reducing distal embolism during interventional procedures. Clinical outcomes have been excellent in vein graft PCI and embolism protection is now considered the standard of care. For various reasons, the results of using embolism protection devices in the setting of primary and rescue PCI have been disappointing, and at this time there does not seem to be a future for those devices in acute MI intervention. Controversy remains regarding the role of carotid stenting and the use of embolism protection devices during such procedures, although there is reasonable evidence that carotid stenting with embolism protection represented an advance in this field. With more innovation in the design of these devices and as ongoing clinical trials are completed, there is potential for future application of embolism protection devices in other settings of coronary and peripheral interventions.

Acknowledgement

The authors wish to acknowledge the work of Julie Hoffman, editorial assistant, for her work on this chapter.

REFERENCES

1. Togni M, Balmer F, Pfiffner D, et al: Percutaneous coronary interventions in Europe 1992–2001. *Eur Heart J* 25(14):1208–1213, 2004.
2. Smith SC, Jr, Feldman TE, Hirshfeld JW, Jr, et al: ACC/AHA/SCAI 2005 guideline update for percutaneous coronary intervention: a report of the American College of Cardiology/ American Heart Association Task Force on Practice Guidelines (ACC/AHA/SCAI Writing Committee to Update 2001 Guidelines for Percutaneous Coronary Intervention). *Circulation* 113(7):e166-e286, 2006.
3. Alpert JS, Thygesen K, Antman E, et al: Myocardial infarction redefined—a consensus document of The Joint European Society of Cardiology/American College of Cardiology Committee for the redefinition of myocardial infarction. *J Am Coll Cardiol* 36(3):959–969, 2000.
4. Abdelmeguid AE, Ellis SG, Sapp SK, et al: Defining the appropriate threshold of creatine kinase elevation after percutaneous coronary interventions. *Am Heart J* 131(6):1097–1105, 1996.

5. Califf RM, Abdelmeguid AE, Kuntz RE, et al: Myonecrosis after revascularization procedures. *J Am Coll Cardiol* 31(2):241–251, 1998.
6. Thygesen K, Alpert JS, White HD: Universal definition of myocardial infarction. *J Am Coll Cardiol* 50(22):2173–2195, 2007.
7. Cutlip DE, Kuntz RE: Does creatinine kinase-MB elevation after percutaneous coronary intervention predict outcomes in 2005? Cardiac enzyme elevation after successful percutaneous coronary intervention is not an independent predictor of adverse outcomes. *Circulation* 112(6):916–922, 2005, discussion 922.
8. Ricciardi MJ, Wu E, Davidson CJ, et al: Visualization of discrete microinfarction after percutaneous coronary intervention associated with mild creatine kinase-MB elevation. *Circulation* 103(23):2780–2783, 2001.
9. Selvanayagam JB, Porto I, Channon K, et al: Troponin elevation after percutaneous coronary intervention directly represents the extent of irreversible myocardial injury: insights from cardiovascular magnetic resonance imaging. *Circulation* 111(8):1027–1032, 2005.
10. Herrmann J: Peri-procedural myocardial injury: 2005 update. *Eur Heart J* 26(23):2493–2519, 2005.
11. Abdelmeguid AE, Topol EJ, Whitlow PL, et al: Significance of mild transient release of creatine kinase-MB fraction after percutaneous coronary interventions. *Circulation* 94(7):1528–1536, 1996.
12. Roe MT, Mahaffey KW, Kilaru R, et al: Creatine kinase-MB elevation after percutaneous coronary intervention predicts adverse outcomes in patients with acute coronary syndromes. *Eur Heart J* 25(4):313–321, 2004.
13. Nallamothu BK, Chetcuti S, Mukherjee D, et al: Prognostic implication of troponin I elevation after percutaneous coronary intervention. *Am J Cardiol* 91(10):1272–1274, 2003.
14. Cavallini C, Savonitto S, Violini R, et al: Impact of the elevation of biochemical markers of myocardial damage on long-term mortality after percutaneous coronary intervention: results of the CK-MB and PCI study. *Eur Heart J* 26(15):1494–1498, 2005.
15. Ghazzal Z, Ashfaq S, Morris DC, et al: Prognostic implication of creatine kinase release after elective percutaneous coronary intervention in the pre-IIb/IIIa antagonist era. *Am Heart J* 145(6):1006–1012, 2003.
16. Harrington RA, Lincoff AM, Califf RM, et al: Characteristics and consequences of myocardial infarction after percutaneous coronary intervention: insights from the Coronary Angioplasty Versus Excisional Atherectomy Trial (CAVEAT). *J Am Coll Cardiol* 25(7):1693–1699, 1995.
17. Simoons ML, van den Brand M, Lincoff M, et al: Minimal myocardial damage during coronary intervention is associated with impaired outcome. *Eur Heart J* 20(15):1112–1119, 1999.
18. Stone GW, Mehran R, Dangas G, et al: Differential impact on survival of electrocardiographic Q-wave versus enzymatic myocardial infarction after percutaneous intervention: a device-specific analysis of 7147 patients. *Circulation* 104(6):642–647, 2001.
19. Ellis SG, Chew D, Chan A, et al: Death following creatine kinase-MB elevation after coronary intervention: identification of an early risk period: importance of creatine kinase-MB level, completeness of revascularization, ventricular function, and probable benefit of statin therapy. *Circulation* 106(10):1205–1210, 2002.
20. Natarajan MK, Kreatsoulas C, Velianou JL, et al: Incidence, predictors, and clinical significance of troponin-I elevation without creatine kinase elevation following percutaneous coronary interventions. *Am J Cardiol* 93(6):750–753, 2004.
21. Srinivas VS, Brooks MM, Detre KM, et al: Contemporary percutaneous coronary intervention versus balloon angioplasty for multivessel coronary artery disease: a comparison of the National Heart, Lung and Blood Institute Dynamic Registry and the Bypass Angioplasty Revascularization Investigation (BARI) study. *Circulation* 106(13):1627–1633, 2002.
22. Randomised placebo-controlled and balloon-angioplasty-controlled trial to assess safety of coronary stenting with use of platelet glycoprotein-IIb/IIIa blockade. The EPISTENT Investigators. Evaluation of Platelet IIb/IIIa Inhibitor for Stenting. *Lancet* 352(9122):87–92, 1998.
23. Porto I, Selvanayagam JB, Van Gaal WJ, et al: Plaque volume and occurrence and location of periprocedural myocardial necrosis after percutaneous coronary intervention: insights from delayed-enhancement magnetic resonance imaging, thrombolysis in myocardial infarction myocardial perfusion grade analysis, and intravascular ultrasound. *Circulation* 114(7):662–669, 2006.
24. Topol EJ, Yadav JS: Recognition of the importance of embolization in atherosclerotic vascular disease. *Circulation* 101(5):570–580, 2000.
25. Prati F, Pawlowski T, Gil R, et al: Stenting of culprit lesions in unstable angina leads to a marked reduction in plaque burden: a major role of plaque embolization? A serial intravascular ultrasound study. *Circulation* 107(18):2320–2325, 2003.
26. Rogers C, Huynh R, Seifert PA, et al: Embolic protection with filtering or occlusion balloons during saphenous vein graft stenting retrieves identical volumes and sizes of particulate debris. *Circulation* 109(14):1735–1740, 2004.
27. Angelini A, Rubartelli P, Mistrorigo F, et al: Distal protection with a filter device during coronary stenting in patients with stable and unstable angina. *Circulation* 110(5):515–521, 2004.
28. Chen WH, Lee PY, Ng W, et al: Aspirin resistance is associated with a high incidence of myonecrosis after non-urgent percutaneous coronary intervention despite clopidogrel pretreatment. *J Am Coll Cardiol* 43(6):1122–1126, 2004.
29. Bonz AW, Lengenfelder B, Jacobs M, et al: Cytokine response after percutaneous coronary intervention in stable angina: effect of selective glycoprotein IIb/IIIa receptor antagonism. *Am Heart J* 145(4):693–699, 2003.
30. Iuliano L, Pratico D, Greco C, et al: Angioplasty increases coronary sinus F2-isoprostane formation: evidence for in vivo oxidative stress during PTCA. *J Am Coll Cardiol* 37(1):76–80, 2001.
31. Kini A, Marmur JD, Kini S, et al: Creatine kinase-MB elevation after coronary intervention correlates with diffuse atherosclerosis, and low-to-medium level elevation has a benign clinical course: implications for early discharge after coronary intervention. *J Am Coll Cardiol* 34(3):663–671, 1999.
32. Zairis MN, Ambrose JA, Ampartzidou O, et al: Preprocedural plasma C-reactive protein levels, postprocedural creatine kinase-MB release, and long-term prognosis after successful coronary stenting (four-year results from the GENERATION study). *Am J Cardiol* 95(3):386–390, 2005.
33. Saadeddin SM, Habbab MA, Sobki SH, et al: Association of systemic inflammatory state with troponin I elevation after elective uncomplicated percutaneous coronary intervention. *Am J Cardiol* 89(8):981–983, 2002.
34. Chew DP, Bhatt DL, Robbins MA, et al: Incremental prognostic value of elevated baseline C-reactive protein among established markers of risk in percutaneous coronary intervention. *Circulation* 104(9):992–997, 2001.
35. Baim DS, Wahr D, George B, et al: Randomized trial of a distal embolic protection device during percutaneous intervention of saphenous vein aorto-coronary bypass grafts. *Circulation* 105(11):1285–1290, 2002.
36. Naidu SS, Turco MA, Mauri L, et al: Contemporary incidence and predictors of major adverse cardiac events after saphenous vein graft intervention with embolic protection (an AMEthyst trial substudy). *Am J Cardiol* 105(8):1060–1064, 2010.
37. Stone GW, Rogers C, Hermiller J, et al: Randomized comparison of distal protection with a filter-based catheter and a balloon occlusion and aspiration system during percutaneous intervention of diseased saphenous vein aorto-coronary bypass grafts. *Circulation* 108(5):548–553, 2003.
38. Abdelmeguid AE, Whitlow PL, Sapp SK, et al: Long-term outcome of transient, uncomplicated in-laboratory coronary artery closure. *Circulation* 91(11):2733–2741, 1995.
39. Yang EH, Gumina RJ, Lennon RJ, et al: Emergency coronary artery bypass surgery for percutaneous coronary interventions: changes in the incidence, clinical characteristics, and indications from 1979 to 2003. *J Am Coll Cardiol* 46(11):2004–2009, 2005.
40. Almeda FQ, Nathan S, Calvin JE, et al: Frequency of abrupt vessel closure and side branch occlusion after percutaneous coronary intervention in a 6.5-year period (1994 to 2000) at a single medical center. *Am J Cardiol* 89(10):1151–1155, 2002.
41. Stone GW, Ellis SG, Cannon L, et al: Comparison of a polymer-based paclitaxel-eluting stent with a bare metal stent in patients with complex coronary artery disease: a randomized controlled trial. *JAMA* 294(10):1215–1223, 2005.
42. Applegate R: Evaluation of the effects of everolimus-eluting and paclitaxel-eluting stents on target lesions with jailed side branches: 2-year results from the SPIRIT III randomized trial. *Catheter Cardiovasc Intervent* 2010.
43. Topol EJ, Leya F, Pinkerton CA, et al: A comparison of directional atherectomy with coronary angioplasty in patients with coronary artery disease. The CAVEAT Study Group. *N Engl J Med* 329(4):221–227, 1993.
44. Baim DS, Cutlip DE, Sharma SK, et al: Final results of the Balloon vs Optimal Atherectomy Trial (BOAT). *Circulation* 97(4):322–331, 1998.
45. Lefkovits J, Holmes DR, Califf RM, et al: Predictors and sequelae of distal embolization during saphenous vein graft intervention from the CAVEAT-II trial. Coronary Angioplasty Versus Excisional Atherectomy Trial. *Circulation* 92(4):734–740, 1995.
46. Dehmer GJ, Nichols TC, Bode AP, et al: Assessment of platelet activation by coronary sinus blood sampling during balloon angioplasty and directional coronary atherectomy. *Am J Cardiol* 80(7):871–877, 1997.
47. Kini A, Reich D, Marmur JD, et al: Reduction in periprocedural enzyme elevation by abciximab after rotational atherectomy of type B2 lesions: Results of the Rota ReoPro randomized trial. *Am Heart J* 142(6):965–969, 2001.
48. Bhatt DL, Topol EJ: Does creatinine kinase-MB elevation after percutaneous coronary intervention predict outcomes in 2005? Periprocedural cardiac enzyme elevation predicts adverse outcomes. *Circulation* 112(6):906–915; discussion 923, 2005.
49. Inoue T, Sohma R, Miyazaki T, et al: Comparison of activation process of platelets and neutrophils after coronary stent implantation versus balloon angioplasty for stable angina pectoris. *Am J Cardiol* 86(10):1057–1062, 2000.
50. Iakovou I, Mintz GS, Dangas G, et al: Increased CK-MB release is a "trade-off" for optimal stent implantation: an intravascular ultrasound study. *J Am Coll Cardiol* 42(11):1900–1905, 2003.
51. Topol EJ, Ferguson JJ, Weisman HF, et al: Long-term protection from myocardial ischemic events in a randomized trial of brief integrin beta3 blockade with percutaneous coronary intervention. EPIC Investigator Group. Evaluation of Platelet IIb/IIIa Inhibition for Prevention of Ischemic Complication. *JAMA* 278(6):479–484, 1997.
52. Tardiff BE, Califf RM, Tcheng JE, et al: Clinical outcomes after detection of elevated cardiac enzymes in patients undergoing percutaneous intervention. IMPACT-II Investigators. Integrilin (eptifibatide) to Minimize Platelet Aggregation and Coronary Thrombosis-II. *J Am Coll Cardiol* 33(1):88–96, 1999.
53. Brener SJ, Lytle BW, Schneider JP, et al: Association between CK-MB elevation after percutaneous or surgical revascularization and three-year mortality. *J Am Coll Cardiol* 40(11):1961–1967, 2002.
54. Ioannidis JP, Karvouni E, Katritsis DG: Mortality risk conferred by small elevations of creatine kinase-MB isoenzyme after percutaneous coronary intervention. *J Am Coll Cardiol* 42(8):1406–1411, 2003.
55. Jeremias A, Baim DS, Ho KK, et al: Differential mortality risk of postprocedural creatine kinase-MB elevation following successful versus unsuccessful stent procedures. *J Am Coll Cardiol* 44(6):1210–1214, 2004.
56. Prasad A, Gersh BJ, Bertrand ME, et al: Prognostic significance of periprocedural versus spontaneously occurring myocardial infarction after percutaneous coronary intervention in patients with acute coronary syndromes: an analysis from the ACUITY (Acute Catheterization and Urgent Intervention Triage Strategy) trial. *J Am Coll Cardiol* 54(5):477–486, 2009.
57. Randomised placebo-controlled trial of abciximab before and during coronary intervention in refractory unstable angina: the CAPTURE Study. *Lancet* 349(9063):1429–1435, 1997.
58. Inhibition of platelet glycoprotein IIb/IIIa with eptifibatide in patients with acute coronary syndromes. The PURSUIT trial investigators. platelet glycoprotein IIb/IIIa in unstable angina: receptor suppression using integrilin therapy. *N Engl J Med* 339(7):436–443, 1998.
59. Novel dosing regimen of eptifibatide in planned coronary stent implantation (ESPRIT): a randomised, placebo-controlled trial. *Lancet* 356(9247):2037–2044, 2000.
60. Effects of platelet glycoprotein IIb/IIIa blockade with tirofiban on adverse cardiac events in patients with unstable angina or acute myocardial infarction undergoing coronary angioplasty. The RESTORE Investigators. Randomized Efficacy Study of Tirofiban for Outcomes and REstenosis. *Circulation* 96(5):1445–1453, 1997.
61. Valgimigli M, Percoco G, Barbieri D, et al: The additive value of tirofiban administered with the high-dose bolus in the prevention of ischemic complications during high-risk coronary angioplasty: the ADVANCE Trial. *J Am Coll Cardiol* 44(1):14–19, 2004.
62. Ndrepepa G, Berger PB, Mehilli J, et al: Periprocedural bleeding and 1-year outcome after percutaneous coronary interventions: appropriateness of including bleeding as a component of a quadruple end point. *J Am Coll Cardiol* 51(7):690–697, 2008.
63. Lincoff AM, Bittl JA, Harrington RA, et al: Bivalirudin and provisional glycoprotein IIb/IIIa blockade compared with heparin and planned glycoprotein IIb/IIIa blockade during percutaneous coronary intervention: REPLACE-2 randomized trial. *JAMA* 289(7):853–863, 2003.
64. Kastrati A, Neumann FJ, Mehilli J, et al: Bivalirudin versus unfractionated heparin during percutaneous coronary intervention. *N Engl J Med* 359(7):688–696, 2008.
65. Stone GW, McLaurin BT, Cox DA, et al: Bivalirudin for patients with acute coronary syndromes. *N Engl J Med* 355(21):2203–2216, 2006.
66. Lincoff AM, Steinhubl SR, Manoukian SV, et al: Influence of timing of clopidogrel treatment on the efficacy and safety of bivalirudin in patients with non-ST-segment elevation acute coronary syndromes undergoing percutaneous coronary intervention: an analysis of the ACUITY (Acute Catheterization and Urgent Intervention Triage strategY) trial. *JACC Cardiovasc Intervent* 1(6):639–648, 2008.
67. Steinhubl SR, Lauer MS, Mukherjee DP, et al: The duration of pretreatment with ticlopidine prior to stenting is associated with the risk of procedure-related non-Q-wave myocardial infarctions. *J Am Coll Cardiol* 32(5):1366–1370, 1998.
68. Steinhubl SR, Berger PB, Mann JT, III, et al: Early and sustained dual oral antiplatelet therapy following percutaneous coronary intervention: a randomized controlled trial. *JAMA* 288(19):2411–2420, 2002.
69. Mehta SR, Yusuf S, Peters RJ, et al: Effects of pretreatment with clopidogrel and aspirin followed by long-term therapy in patients undergoing percutaneous coronary intervention: the PCI-CURE study. *Lancet* 358(9281):527–533, 2001.
70. Muller I, Besta F, Schulz C, et al: Prevalence of clopidogrel non-responders among patients with stable angina pectoris scheduled for elective coronary stent placement. *Thromb Haemost* 89(5):783–787, 2003.
71. Patti G, Colonna G, Pasceri V, et al: Randomized trial of high loading dose of clopidogrel for reduction of periprocedural myocardial infarction in patients undergoing coronary intervention: results from the ARMYDA-2 (Antiplatelet therapy for Reduction of MYocardial Damage during Angioplasty) study. *Circulation* 111(16):2099–2106, 2005.
72. von Beckerath N, Taubert D, Pogatsa-Murray G, et al: Absorption, metabolization, and antiplatelet effects of 300-, 600-, and 900-mg loading doses of clopidogrel: results of the ISAR-CHOICE (Intracoronary Stenting and Antithrombotic Regimen: Choose Between 3 High Oral Doses for Immediate Clopidogrel Effect) trial. *Circulation* 112(19):2946–2950, 2005.
73. Montalescot G, Sideris G, Meuleman C, et al: A randomized comparison of high clopidogrel loading doses in patients with non-ST-segment elevation acute coronary syndromes: the

ALBION (Assessment of the Best Loading Dose of Clopidogrel to Blunt Platelet Activation, Inflammation and Ongoing Necrosis) trial. *J Am Coll Cardiol* 48(5):931–938, 2006.

74. Di Sciascio G, Patti G, Pasceri V, et al: Effectiveness of in-laboratory high-dose clopidogrel loading versus routine preload in patients undergoing percutaneous coronary intervention: results of the ARMYDA-5 PRELOAD (Antiplatelet therapy for Reduction of MYocardial Damage during Angioplasty) randomized trial. *J Am Coll Cardiol* 56(7):550–557, 2010.
75. Stankovic G, Zivkovic M: In-laboratory high-dose clopidogrel loading: do we need a mirror of diamond for "Armida's garden"? *J Am Coll Cardiol* 56(7):558–560, 2010.
76. Kastrati A, Mehilli J, Schuhlen H, et al: A clinical trial of abciximab in elective percutaneous coronary intervention after pretreatment with clopidogrel. *N Engl J Med* 350(3):232–238, 2004.
77. Lincoff AM, Kereiakes DJ, Mascelli MA, et al: Abciximab suppresses the rise in levels of circulating inflammatory markers after percutaneous coronary revascularization. *Circulation* 104(2):163–167, 2001.
78. Wiviott SD, Braunwald E, McCabe CH, et al: Intensive oral antiplatelet therapy for reduction of ischaemic events including stent thrombosis in patients with acute coronary syndromes treated with percutaneous coronary intervention and stenting in the TRITON-TIMI 38 trial: a subanalysis of a randomised trial. *Lancet* 371(9621):1353–1363, 2008.
79. Wallentin L, Becker RC, Budaj A, et al: Ticagrelor versus clopidogrel in patients with acute coronary syndromes. *N Engl J Med* 361(11):1045–1057, 2009.
80. Chang SM, Yazbek N, Lakkis NM: Use of statins prior to percutaneous coronary intervention reduces myonecrosis and improves clinical outcome. *Catheter Cardiovasc Intervent* 62(2):193–197, 2004.
81. Jones SP, Gibson MF, Rimmer DM, III, et al: Direct vascular and cardioprotective effects of rosuvastatin, a new HMG-CoA reductase inhibitor. *J Am Coll Cardiol* 40(6):1172–1178, 2002.
82. Gurm HS, Breitbart Y, Vivekanathan D, et al: Preprocedural statin use is associated with a reduced hazard of postprocedural myonecrosis in patients undergoing rotational atherectomy—a propensity-adjusted analysis. *Am Heart J* 151(5):1031, 2006, e1031–1036.
83. Briguori C, Colombo A, Airoldi F, et al: Statin administration before percutaneous coronary intervention: impact on periprocedural myocardial infarction. *Eur Heart J* 25(20):1822–1828, 2004.
84. Pasceri V, Patti G, Nusca A, et al: Randomized trial of atorvastatin for reduction of myocardial damage during coronary intervention: results from the ARMYDA (Atorvastatin for Reduction of MYocardial Damage during Angioplasty) study. *Circulation* 110(6):674–678, 2004.
85. Patti G, Chello M, Pasceri V, et al: Protection from procedural myocardial injury by atorvastatin is associated with lower levels of adhesion molecules after percutaneous coronary intervetnions: results from the ARMYDA-CAMs (Atorvastatin for Reduction of MYocardial Damage during Angioplasty-Cell Adhesion Molecules) substudy. *J Am Coll Cardiol* 48(8):1560–1566, 2006.
86. Briguori C, Visconti G, Focaccio A, et al: Novel approaches for preventing or limiting events (Naples) II trial: impact of a single high loading dose of atorvastatin on periprocedural myocardial infarction. *J Am Coll Cardiol* 54(23):2157–2163, 2009.
87. Di Sciascio G, Patti G, Pasceri V, et al: Efficacy of atorvastatin reload in patients on chronic statin therapy undergoing percutaneous coronary intervention: results of the ARMYDA-RECAPTURE (Atorvastatin for Reduction of Myocardial Damage During Angioplasty) randomized trial. *J Am Coll Cardiol* 54(6):558–565, 2009.
88. Ellis SG, Brener SJ, Lincoff AM, et al: beta-blockers before percutaneous coronary intervention do not attenuate postprocedural creatine kinase isoenzyme rise. *Circulation* 104(22):2685–2688, 2001.
89. Ballarino MA, Moreyra E, Jr, Damonte A, et al: Multicenter randomized comparison of direct vs conventional stenting: the DIRECTO trial. *Catheter Cardiovasc Interv* 58(4):434–440, 2003.
90. AJ IJ, Serruys PW, Scholte A, et al: Direct coronary stent implantation does not reduce the incidence of in-stent restenosis or major adverse cardiac events: six month results of a randomized trial. *Eur Heart J* 24(5):421–429, 2003.
91. Hausenloy DJ, Mwamure PK, Venugopal V, et al: Effect of remote ischaemic preconditioning on myocardial injury in patients undergoing coronary artery bypass graft surgery: a randomised controlled trial. *Lancet* 370(9587):575–579, 2007.
92. Hoole SP, Heck PM, Sharples L, et al: Cardiac Remote Ischemic Preconditioning in Coronary Stenting (CRISP Stent) study: a prospective, randomized control trial. *Circulation* 119(6):820–827, 2009.
93. Loukogeorgakis SP, Williams R, Panagiotidou AT, et al: Transient limb ischemia induces remote preconditioning and remote postconditioning in humans by a K(ATP)-channel dependent mechanism. *Circulation* 116(12):1386–1395, 2007.
94. Konstantinov IE, Arab S, Kharbanda RK, et al: The remote ischemic preconditioning stimulus modifies inflammatory gene expression in humans. *Physiol Genomics* 19(1):143–150, 2004.
95. Roffi M, Mukherjee D, Chew DP, et al: Lack of benefit from intravenous platelet glycoprotein IIb/IIIa receptor inhibition as adjunctive treatment for percutaneous interventions of aortocoronary bypass grafts: a pooled analysis of five randomized clinical trials. *Circulation* 106(24):3063–3067, 2002.
96. Karha J, Gurm HS, Rajagopal V, et al: Use of platelet glycoprotein IIb/IIIa inhibitors in saphenous vein graft percutaneous coronary intervention and clinical outcomes. *Am J Cardiol* 2006;98(7):906–910, 2006.
97. Webb JG, Carere RG, Virmani R, et al: Retrieval and analysis of particulate debris after saphenous vein graft intervention. *J Am Coll Cardiol* 34(2):468–475, 1999.
98. Cohen DJ, Murphy SA, Baim DS, et al: Cost-effectiveness of distal embolic protection for patients undergoing percutaneous intervention of saphenous vein bypass grafts: results from the SAFER trial. *J Am Coll Cardiol* 44(9):1801–1808, 2004.
99. Jonas M, Stone GW, Mehran R, et al: Platelet glycoprotein IIb/IIIa receptor inhibition as adjunctive treatment during saphenous vein graft stenting: differential effects after randomization to occlusion or filter-based embolic protection. *Eur Heart J* 27(8):920–928, 2006.
100. Mauri L, Cox D, Hermiller J, et al: The PROXIMAL trial: proximal protection during saphenous vein graft intervention using the Proxis Embolic Protection System: a randomized, prospective, multicenter clinical trial. *J Am Coll Cardiol* 50(15):1442–1449, 2007.
101. Mauri L, Rogers C, Baim DS: Devices for distal protection during percutaneous coronary revascularization. *Circulation* 113(22):2651–2656, 2006.
102. Kereiakes DJ, Turco MA, Breall J, et al: A novel filter-based distal embolic protection device for percutaneous intervention of saphenous vein graft lesions: results of the AMEthyst randomized controlled trial. *JACC Cardiovasc Interv* 1(3):248–257, 2008.
103. Mehta SK, Frutkin AD, Milford-Beland S, et al: Utilization of distal embolic protection in saphenous vein graft interventions (an analysis of 19,546 patients in the American College of Cardiology-National Cardiovascular Data Registry). *Am J Cardiol* 100(7):1114–1118, 2007.
104. Badhey N, Lichtenwalter C, de Lemos JA, et al: Contemporary use of embolic protection devices in saphenous vein graft interventions: insights from the stenting of saphenous vein grafts trial. *Catheter Cardiovasc Intervent* 76(2):263–269, 2010.
105. Nakamura T, Kubo N, Seki Y, et al: Effects of a distal protection device during primary stenting in patients with acute anterior myocardial infarction. *Circ J* 68(8):763–768, 2004.
106. Stone GW, Webb J, Cox DA, et al: Distal microcirculatory protection during percutaneous coronary intervention in acute ST-segment elevation myocardial infarction: a randomized controlled trial. *JAMA* 293(9):1063–1072, 2005.
107. Gick M, Jander N, Bestehorn HP, et al: Randomized evaluation of the effects of filter-based distal protection on myocardial perfusion and infarct size after primary percutaneous catheter intervention in myocardial infarction with and without ST-segment elevation. *Circulation* 112(10):1462–1469, 2005.
108. Cura FA, Escudero AG, Berrocal D, et al: Protection of distal embolization in high-risk patients with acute ST-segment elevation myocardial infarction (PREMIAR). *Am J Cardiol* 99(3):357–363, 2007.
109. Ali OA, Bhindi R, McMahon AC, et al: Distal protection in cardiovascular medicine: current status. *Am Heart J* 152(2):207–216, 2006.
110. Jordan WD, Jr, Voellinger DC, Doblar DD, et al: Microemboli detected by transcranial Doppler monitoring in patients during carotid angioplasty versus carotid endarterectomy. *Cardiovasc Surg* 7(1):33–38, 1999.
111. Aronow HD, Shishehbor M, Davis DA, et al: Leukocyte count predicts microembolic Doppler signals during carotid stenting: a link between inflammation and embolization. *Stroke* 36(9):1910–1914, 2005.
112. Rapp JH, Pan XM, Sharp FR, et al: Atheroemboli to the brain: size threshold for causing acute neuronal cell death. *J Vasc Surg* 32(1):68–76, 2000.
113. Reimers B, Corvaja N, Moshiri S, et al: Cerebral protection with filter devices during carotid artery stenting. *Circulation* 104(1):12–15, 2001.
114. Whitlow PL, Lylyk P, Londero H, et al: Carotid artery stenting protected with an emboli containment system. *Stroke* 33(5):1308–1314, 2002.
115. Cosottini M, Michelassi MC, Puglioli M, et al: Silent cerebral ischemia detected with diffusion-weighted imaging in patients treated with protected and unprotected carotid artery stenting. *Stroke* 36(11):2389–2393, 2005.
116. Kastrup A, Nagele T, Groschel K, et al: Incidence of new brain lesions after carotid stenting with and without cerebral protection. *Stroke* 37(9):2312–2316, 2006.
117. Wholey MH, Al-Mubarek N, Wholey MH: Updated review of the global carotid artery stent registry. *Catheter Cardiovasc Intervent* 60(2):259–266, 2003.
118. Yadav JS, Wholey MH, Kuntz RE, et al: Protected carotid-artery stenting versus endarterectomy in high-risk patients. *N Engl J Med* 351(15):1493–1501, 2004.
119. Gray WA, Hopkins LN, Yadav S, et al: Protected carotid stenting in high-surgical-risk patients: the ARCHeR results. *J Vasc Surg* 44(2):258–268, 2006.
120. White CJ, Iyer SS, Hopkins LN, et al: Carotid stenting with distal protection in high surgical risk patients: the BEACH trial 30 day results. *Catheter Cardiovasc Interv* 67(4):503–512, 2006.
121. Ringleb PA, Allenberg J, Bruckmann H, et al: 30 day results from the SPACE trial of stent-protected angioplasty versus carotid endarterectomy in symptomatic patients: a randomised non-inferiority trial. *Lancet* 368(9543):1239–1247, 2006.
122. Mas JL, Chatellier G, Beyssen B, et al: Endarterectomy verus stenting in patients with symptomatic severe carotid stenosis. *N Engl J Med* 355:1660–1671, 2006.
123. Mas JL, Chatellier G, Beyssen B: Carotid angioplasty and stenting with and without cerebral protection: clinical alert from the Endarterectomy Versus Angioplasty in Patients With Symptomatic Severe Carotid Stenosis (EVA-3S) trial. *Stroke* 35(1):e18–e20, 2004.
124. Ederle J, Dobson J, Featherstone RL, et al: Carotid artery stenting compared with endarterectomy in patients with symptomatic carotid stenosis (International Carotid Stenting Study): an interim analysis of a randomised controlled trial. *Lancet* 375(9719):985–997, 2010.
125. Brott TG, Hobson RW, II, Howard G, et al: Stenting versus endarterectomy for treatment of carotid-artery stenosis. *N Engl J Med* 363(1):11–23, 2010.
126. Stabile E, Salemme L, Sorropago G, et al: Proximal endovascular occlusion for carotid artery stenting: results from a prospective registry of 1,300 patients. *J Am Coll Cardiol* 55(16):1661–1667, 2010.
127. Krishnamurthi V, Novick AC, Myles JL: Atheroembolic renal disease: effect on morbidity and survival after revascularization for atherosclerotic renal artery stenosis. *J Urol* 161(4):1093–1096, 1999.
128. Henry M, Henry I, Klonaris C, et al: Renal angioplasty and stenting under protection: the way for the future? *Catheter Cardiovasc Intervent* 60(3):299–312, 2003.
129. Cooper CJ, Haller ST, Colyer W, et al: Embolic protection and platelet inhibition during renal artery stenting. *Circulation* 117(21):2752–2760, 2008.
130. Wholey MH, Toursarkissian B, Postoak D, et al: Early experience in the application of distal protection devices in treatment of peripheral vascular disease of the lower extremities. *Catheter Cardiovasc Intervent* 64(2):227–235, 2005.
131. Siablis D, Karnabatidis D, Katsanos K, et al: Outflow protection filters during percutaneous recanalization of lower extremities' arterial occlusions: a pilot study. *Eur J Radiol* 55(2):243–249, 2005.

29

Access Management and Closure Devices

FERNANDO CURA

KEY POINTS

- The most common catheterization problems are access-site complications, which can also increase hospital stay and medical costs.

- Selection of the appropriate access site is frequently a key issue for the successful completion of coronary or peripheral vascular procedures. Selection depends on the target vessel or structural intervention, the patient's preferences, and the operator's skills.

- The operator should be careful in choosing the site of the femoral artery cannulation. Ideally, the femoral artery is to be entered about 1 to 2 cm below the inguinal ligament.

- The most commonly used femoral closure devices provide two types of mechanisms for percutaneously controlling bleeding: deploying sutures or staples to close the femoral puncture site or using resorbable collagen plugs to temporarily seal the arteriotomy.

- Hemostasis accelerators, which are based on the electrical attractive forces between the patch and the erythrocytes, produce more rapid clot formation.

- Vascular closure devices have improved patient comfort by enabling early ambulation, and their use has decreased the burden on the medical staff, but they have not demonstrated a reduction in groin complication rates.

Introduction

The steady increase in percutaneous interventional procedures for the treatment of cardiovascular diseases in a variety of vascular territories is associated with closer attention to access-site management. The more aggressive level of anticoagulation used during therapeutic procedures requires the achievement of safe and reliable hemostasis of the access site. Coronary interventions are usually performed by the femoral approach; however, to reduce complications and increase patient comfort, radial access is increasingly used and is becoming the preferred access site by many interventionalists.[1] Patients undergoing the femoral approach are usually immobilized overnight, which may result in significant discomfort because of increased back pain and the need for analgesics. Noncompliance of patients regarding strict bed rest after the procedure has been reported to be a substantial factor for femoral complications. During the last decade, there has been a rapid increase in the percutaneous treatment of aortic aneurysms, aortic dissections, and aortic valve replacement using much larger sheaths that require special attention to the access site. The most common catheterization problem involves the access site.[2,3] Additionally, major access-site complications increase the length of hospital stay and medical costs. Moreover, vascular complications are also associated with an increased risk of nonfatal myocardial infarction or death in the year following the procedure, in particular when accompanied by significant bleeding.[4] The use of manual or mechanical compression was until recently the only way to control bleeding by allowing clot formation at the arteriotomy site. The clinical use of vascular closure devices for rapid hemostasis after femoral access was first reported in 1991. Since then, these devices have improved patient comfort by enabling early ambulation, and their use has decreased the burden of the medical staff. However, they have not produced a reduction in groin complication rates. This chapter summarizes the concepts of arterial access puncture, the use of arterial closure devices, and postprocedural management.

Planning Access

The selection of an appropriate access site is frequently a key issue for the successful completion of coronary or peripheral vascular procedures. Proficiency with all available vascular puncture techniques is therefore a basic requirement for the interventionist. It is important to review clinical reports and perform preprocedural vascular assessment of the quality of all peripheral pulses, presence of bruits, blood pressure difference between arms, and other pertinent findings, such as skin color, trophic changes, ulcerations, or the presence of intermittent claudication. Body habitus, such as extreme obesity, may dictate the use of the radial artery instead of the femoral approach. This important decision deserves full analysis of the target vessel for treatment, consideration of the patient's preference, and assessment of the interventionist's skills. Some aspects of the vascular access are crucial to the safety and success of the procedure.

Retrograde femoral access and radial access, with the choice based on the patient's limitations or the operator's preferences, are the two preferred approaches for coronary interventions. There are several techniques for endovascular peripheral therapies according to the target treatment vessel: the crossover femoral approach for contralateral iliofemoral treatment; anterograde femoral puncture for ipsilateral treatment of below-the-knee arteries; femoral retrograde access for aortic, carotid, iliac, and renal vessels; and local puncture for dialysis access treatment. Moreover, the common femoral artery is the preferred access for aortic artery and aortic valve interventions.

RETROGRADE PUNCTURE TECHNIQUE FOR THE FEMORAL ARTERY

The common femoral artery is preferred for percutaneous arterial cannulation because it is large, accessible, and easily compressible. However, strict adherence to meticulous vascular access technique is necessary to avoid vascular complications while using manual compression or femoral closure devices, in particular when larger sheaths are being used. The mean luminal diameter of the common femoral artery is between 6 and 7 mm. This is theoretically large enough to comfortably accommodate the typical range of femoral sheath sizes for most diagnostic and interventional procedures. Diabetics and women have disproportionately smaller common femoral arteries. The vascular access is generally the only painful part of the procedure. Patient sedation and generous local anesthesia are needed, as well as adequate pressure and rhythm monitoring. The operator should be careful in choosing the site of cannulation of the femoral artery. In drawing an imaginary line between the anterosuperior iliac spine and the pubis, arterial pulsation is near or at the midpoint of the line. It is important not to rely on the inguinal crease to select the puncture site because the distance from the inguinal ligament to the inguinal crease varies, particularly in overweight patients. Fluoroscopy should be used to ascertain the relative location of the femoral head and pelvic brim in this subgroup of patients. Puncture at or just above the center of the femoral head is particularly important.

Ideally, the femoral artery is entered about 1 or 2 cm below the inguinal ligament (Fig. 29-1). If cannulation of the artery is too low, the chance of entering the superficial femoral artery rather than the common femoral artery is increased. This entry site may predispose to dissection, arterial occlusion, pseudoaneurysm, bleeding, and arteriovenous fistula formation. Entering the artery above the inguinal ligament may lead to problems in compressing the artery against the inguinal ligament, thus increasing the risk of hematoma formation and favoring retroperitoneal hemorrhage. The use of femoral closure devices is contraindicated in higher or lower femoral punctures. The other important aspect is careful puncture of only the anterior wall of the femoral artery with open-bore needles, which have the advantage of demonstrating blood return immediately. Appropriate vascular hemostasis can be achieved with the use of manual compression or femoral closure devices (Fig. 29-2). A reduction in the sheath size was presumed to result in fewer access complications, but there was no clear association with a decrement in the bleeding rate. Retrograde femoral access can be considered the standard technique for coronary, renal, iliac, and crossover for contralateral femoral interventions (Fig. 29-3). Endovascular repair of abdominal and thoracic aortic aneurysms has become the standard of care for anatomically appropriate patients. All the devices developed to date are deployed through relatively large (12- to 24-Fr) sheaths. Moreover, transcatheter aortic valve implantation is a rapidly emerging treatment option for patients with aortic valve stenosis and high surgical risk. Different access routes have been proposed, including transapical, transsubclavian, and transfemoral, with percutaneous transfemoral being preferred because it is the least invasive and potentially nonsurgical. However, vascular access-site complications due to the large-bore (18- to 24-Fr) delivery catheters remain an important clinical issue, particularly with respect to elderly patients. Traditionally, this access has required arterial exposure with open cut-down; but with the development of suture-mediated arterial closure devices, there is an increasing trend toward percutaneous endovascular repair. This is an effective and safe approach in a select group of patients. The procedure should be performed in a sterile operating room environment with the support of vascular surgeons in the event that the closure device should fail to close the arteriotomy. The need for larger sheaths for these interventions requires a meticulous puncture technique in the anterior wall of the common femoral artery.

PUNCTURE TECHNIQUE FOR THE RADIAL ARTERY

Miniaturization of the procedural equipment has led to a revival of the transradial approach. Despite the considerable training needed, this approach remarkably improves patient comfort and decreases bleeding

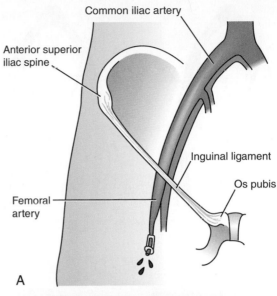

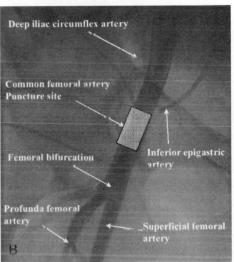

Figure 29-1 Accessing the femoral artery. A. An imaginary line between the superoanterior crest and the pubis is constructed. This imaginary line usually corresponds to the location of the inguinal ligament. The needle should enter approximately 1 cm below the imaginary line while advancing at a 30- to 45-degree angle. B. An excellent method for localizing the puncture site is to use fluoroscopy of the femoral head. The needle point should be over the lower inner quadrant.

Figure 29-2 The femoral artery must be entered using a large-bore needle with backflow of blood. As soon as the needle passes into the vessel through the anterior wall, brisk pulsatile flow occurs. The guidewire is advanced. It prevents occult bleeding through the posterior wall.

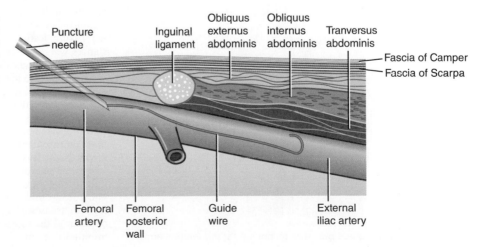

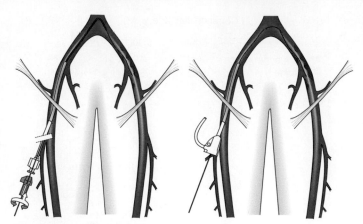

Figure 29-3 Retrograde femoral access for a contralateral approach.

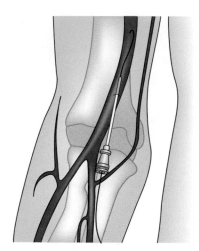

Figure 29-4 Puncture technique for the brachial artery.

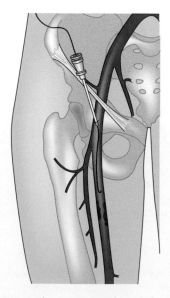

Figure 29-5 Anterograde puncture technique for the femoral artery.

complications, particularly among patients with aggressive anticoagulation regimens. This approach provides an alternative for coronary angiography and angioplasty and for vertebral and internal mammary interventions. It is addressed in Chapter 30.

PUNCTURE TECHNIQUE FOR THE BRACHIAL ARTERY

Brachial access is an alternative technique that can be used for coronary, renal, and lower limb interventions. However, radial access is usually preferred because of a higher rate of complications at the brachial access site, such as artery occlusion or hematoma. Puncture of the brachial artery should be performed in its distal part above the antecubital fossa, where the artery is relatively superficial. At this level, after sheath removal, the artery can be compressed against the humerus to obtain hemostasis (Fig. 29-4). Direct puncture of the axillary artery, which has been performed in the past, has largely been abandoned.

ANTEROGRADE PUNCTURE TECHNIQUE FOR THE FEMORAL ARTERY

The anterograde puncture technique provides more direct access to many lesions in the femoropopliteal segment and the infraglenoidal arteries. It allows for the use of a lower volume of contrast and provides stronger support for chronic occlusions of the superficial femoral artery. However, anterograde puncture is technically far more challenging. Although a high puncture of the common femoral artery is required to allow enough space in which to navigate the guidewire into the superficial femoral artery, suprainguinal puncture should be avoided because of the higher risk of retroperitoneal bleeding (Fig. 29-5). Injection of contrast through the needle usually helps to identify the femoral bifurcation anatomy.

PUNCTURE TECHNIQUE FOR THE POPLITEAL ARTERY

Transpopliteal access becomes useful when the superficial femoral artery cannot be crossed using other techniques. The patient is placed in a prone position. The puncture is performed with the assistance of road-map fluoroscopy after the injection of contrast from an ipsilateral femoral sheath (Fig. 29-6). Particular attention should be paid to achieving complete hemostasis after intervention. The incidence of access-site complications is potentially higher with transpopliteal access than with conventional techniques.[5]

TRANSAPICAL LEFT VENTRICULAR PUNCTURE

Percutaneous interventions are becoming increasingly complex, but in some instances the target lesion may be difficult to reach using conventional transvenous or transarterial access.

Transapical left ventricular puncture gives direct access to the left ventricle; although it was frequently used in the past for diagnostic reasons, it has largely been abandoned in favor of transvenous-transatrial or retrograde access because these routes are associated with fewer complications. Nevertheless, there are multiple clinical circumstances where direct transapical access is required for diagnostic or interventional indications, including access to the left ventricle in the setting of double mechanical valves, inaccessible percutaneous mitral paravalvular leak repair, complex congenital heart disease, percutaneous valve implantation, and many others.[6,7] Percutaneous transthoracic puncture is appealing for an interventional cardiologist but can be complicated by lung puncture, resulting in pneumothorax or hemothorax due to damage to the internal mammary and subcostal arteries or persistant leak after sheath withdrawal. Damage to the coronary artery can be avoided by doing selective coronary angiography before puncture. However, most of these complications can be minimized by puncturing "under direct vision" after a minithoracotomy. Transthoracic or transesophageal cardiac ultrasound is useful in guiding the operator to the access site either for direct puncture or to perform the minithoracotomy.

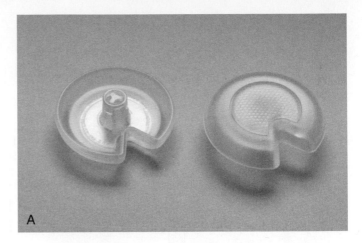

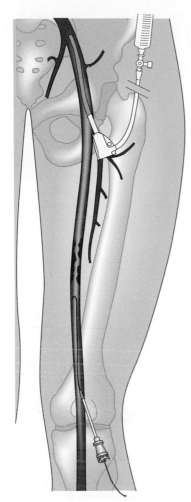

Figure 29-6 Puncture technique for the popliteal artery.

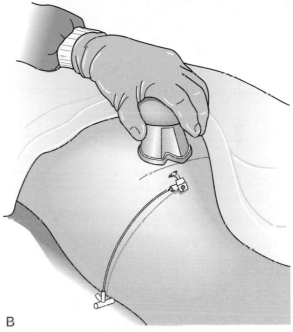

Figure 29-7 A. The Compass compression assist device. B. The Compass is placed over the femoral sheath before pulling it. Then more comfortable manual pressure is applied. *(Photo courtesy of Advanced Vascular Dynamics, Vancouver, WA, 2006.)*

🔲 Hemostatic Methods after Percutaneous Cardiovascular Procedures

Proper technique is essential for achieving successful femoral artery hemostasis without complications. Methods used to achieve hemostasis after a percutaneous procedure include manual compression, mechanical compression, vascular plugs, percutaneous vascular suturing or staples, and topical hemostasis accelerators.

MANUAL COMPRESSION

Digital compression should be considered the "gold standard" of compressive methods. Performed properly, it can prevent bleeding and maintain distal perfusion. This procedure may be performed by a physician, nurse, or technician who has received formal training.

Before sheath removal, the distal pulses and the access site are assessed for signs of a hematoma. The duration of manual compression and the time of immobilization are proportional to the size of the introducer sheath and the level of anticoagulation. Although the manual compression technique is effective with smaller sheath sizes, it becomes more challenging and hazardous with increasing sheath sizes. The recommended compression time should be 10 minutes of firm pressure, 2 to 5 minutes of less firm pressure, and 2 minutes of light pressure while placing the pressure dressing. If bleeding continues, another 15 minutes of pressure should be applied. Risk factors for prolonged bleeding include severe atherosclerosis at the puncture site

and a loss of elasticity without adequate approximation of the vessel edges after the sheath is removed. Other risk factors for bleeding include sheath size, anticoagulation level at the time of sheath removal, aortic regurgitation, elevated blood pressure, obesity, and older age. The use of manual compression has the advantage of continuous observation and modulation of vascular compression. However, it has the disadvantage of requiring a staff member to be available, prolonged immobilization, and bed rest, thus increasing patient discomfort and length of hospital stay. The Compass System (Advanced Vascular Dynamics, Vancouver, WA) is a manual compression-assist device developed to enhance comfort for patients and practitioners. It includes a handle and detachable sterile, disposable disk. Practitioners apply external pressure using the Compass in much the same way that they would apply manual pressure (Fig. 29-7). A vascular C-clamp (Advanced Vascular Dynamics) may be substituted for manual compression (Fig. 29-8). It consists of a flat metal base; a pivoting metal shaft attached to the base; and an adjustable arm lever to impose the desired degree of pressure. Disposable plastic compression disks, which

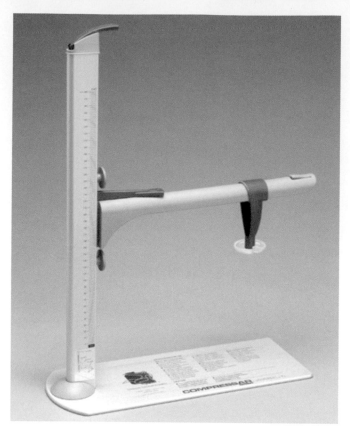

Figure 29-8 The C-clamp is a mechanical compressor system for femoral puncture sites. The disk that applies pressure rests on the vessel entry point. (*Photo courtesy of Advanced Vascular Dynamics, Vancouver, WA, 2006.*)

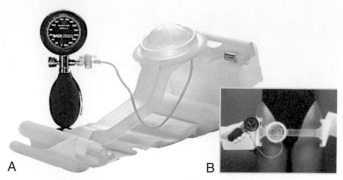

Figure 29-9 A. The Femo-Stop pressure system with the sphygmomanometer. B. The belt should be aligned with the puncture site equally across both hips.

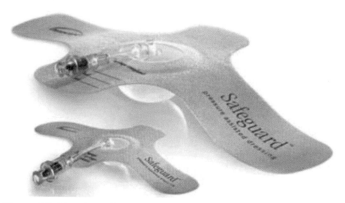

Figure 29-10 The Safeguard dressing is applied with the access site visible under the plastic window. The center bulb is inflated with air to the desired amount of pressure and the syringe is removed.

are attached to the arm, apply pressure over the desired area. This approach has the advantage of freeing up personnel for other functions. It provides pressure over a relatively small area. Its limitations include the inability to modulate pressure easily and some discomfort from the device. The Femo-Stop (RADI Medical Systems, Reading, MA) is a pneumatic pressure device using a clear plastic compression bag that molds itself to skin contours (Fig. 29-9). The Femo-Stop is composed of a plastic arch, inflatable transparent dome, connection tubing, stopcock, elastic or adjustable belt, and handheld manometer. It is held in place by straps that pass around the hips. The amount of applied pressure may be modulated and observed with a sphygmomanometer gauge. It allows visualization of the puncture site. The Femo-Stop is frequently indicated for compression in the repair of pseudoaneurysms. The Safeguard (Datascope Interventional, Mahwah, NJ) is designed for posthemostasis puncture-site management; combining a built-in inflatable bulb and a sterile dressing, it provides adjustable pressure to the site. The device has a clear window that allows staff to assess the site easily without removing the device. Safeguard is ideal for noncompliant patients or those who are overweight (Fig. 29-10).

FEMORAL CLOSURE DEVICES

The most commonly used hemostasis devices provide two types of mechanisms for percutaneously controlling bleeding: deploying sutures or staples to close the femoral puncture site or using resorbable collagen plugs to seal the arteriotomy temporarily. A third group of devices are hemostasis accelerators that are based on the electrical attractive forces between the closure device and the erythrocytes, leading to more rapid clot formation. Arteriotomy closure devices have emerged as an alternative to traditional mechanical compression after percutaneous cardiovascular intervention. These devices have the potential to reduce the time to hemostasis, facilitate patient mobilization, decrease hospital length of stay, and improve patient satisfaction.

Although older, single-center studies and randomized trials have shown mixed results regarding the safety of arterial closure devices compared with manual compression, later data show decreased complications with closure devices. This difference may be due to increased operator experience with arterial closure devices and improved device technology. A metanalysis including 30 selected studies comprising a total of 37,066 patients (12,596 and 24,470 patients in the device and control groups, respectively) found no significant risk with respect to vascular complications between closure devices and mechanical compression in the setting of diagnostic or interventional procedures. The complication rate appears similar for the leading products, Angioseal and Perclose, with a higher complication rate seen with the VasoSeal device for interventional procedures.[8–10] A multivariate analysis performed for 156,853 patients undergoing diagnostic or interventional procedures using suture- or collagen-based closure devices demonstrated a lower risk of serious adverse events relative to manual compression, especially with respect to hemorrhagic complications and pseudoaneurysm (Table 29-1).[11] Serious adverse events were reported in 1.56% of patients in the entire population. Complications were more frequent in women than in men (relative risk [RR] = 2.13;

TABLE 29-1	Risk of Adverse Events after Cardiac Catheterizations by Hemostasis Device in 2001: The American College of Cardiology–National Cardiovascular Disease Registry				
Complications	*Incidence in the Whole Population*	*Collagen Plug*	*Suture Device*	*Manual Compression*	*P Value*
Bleeding (%)	1.13	0.78	1.15	1.20	<0.001
Vessel occlusion (%)	0.07	0.07	0.07	0.07	NS
Dissection (%)	0.02	0.01	0.02	0.03	NS
Pseudoaneurysm (%)	0.37	0.17	0.24	0.45	<0.001
Arteriovenous fistula (%)	0.05	0.04	0.05	0.06	NS
Associated death (%)	0.09	0.03	0.10	0.10	<0.001
Any vascular complication (%)	1.56	1.05	1.48	1.70	<0.001

NS, not significant.

TABLE 29-2	Risk of Adverse Events after Cardiac Catheterizations by Gender in 2001: The American College of Cardiology–National Cardiovascular Disease Registry		
Complications	*Male Gender*	*Female Gender*	*P Value*
Bleeding (%)	0.78	1.70	<0.001
Vessel occlusion (%)	0.05	0.10	<0.001
Dissection (%)	0.02	0.03	0.03
Pseudoaneurysm (%)	0.25	0.56	<0.001
Arteriovenous fistula (%)	0.05	0.06	NS
Associated death (%)	0.05	0.14	<0.001
Any vascular complication (%)	1.09	2.32	<0.001

NS, not significant.

TABLE 29-3	Risk of Adverse Events after Cardiac Catheterizations by Procedure in 2001: The American College of Cardiology–National Cardiovascular Disease Registry		
Complications	*Diagnostic*	*Interventional*	*P Value*
Bleeding (%)	0.59	1.55	<0.001
Vessel occlusion (%)	0.07	0.07	NS
Dissection (%)	0.02	0.03	NS
Pseudoaneurysm (%)	0.21	0.49	<0.001
Arteriovenous fistula (%)	0.07	0.10	0.03
Associated death (%)	0.07	0.10	0.03
Any vascular complication (%)	0.91	2.07	<0.001

NS, not significant.

$P < 0.001$) (Table 29-2). Possible reasons for this may include smaller vessel size in women and hormonal differences. Complications were also more frequent in patients who had interventional cardiac catheterization (RR = 2.26; $P < 0.0001$); they were less frequent in patients in whom the collagen plug devices (RR = 0.62; $P < 0.001$) were used or the suture device (RR = 0.87; $P = 0.02$) compared with manual compression (Table 29-3).[11] Several studies comparing the benefits and cost-effectiveness of closure devices and manual compression found that the use of closure devices was safe and cost-saving.[12,13] All closure devices have been reported to be safe in patients receiving glycoprotein IIb/IIIa inhibitors.[14] However, some reports have raised concerns about an increased risk of bleeding complications with the use of vascular closure devices versus manual compression among patients treated with a combination of anticoagulation drugs such as enoxaparin, clopidogrel, aspirin, and GP IIb/IIIa inhibitors. Despite advances in techniques and the introduction of new products, vessel closure technologies have failed to penetrate most diagnostic and interventional cases.[15]

SUTURE-BASED CLOSURE DEVICES

The percutaneous suture-mediated closure device represents one of several attempts to develop a method to achieve arteriotomy hemostasis in a safe and timely manner. Several studies have shown the efficacy of percutaneous suture-mediated closure devices in decreasing time to hemostasis and time to ambulation without increasing the rate of access-site complications. However, experience suggests that these devices may result in infrequent but challenging vascular complications of the groin, such as retroperitoneal hemorrhage, arterial thromboses, infections, dissections, and large pseudoaneurysms. Proper training and operator skills are necessary for the successful use of these devices. The use of standard aseptic techniques in all cases, along with a single dose of prophylactic intravenous antibiotics during placement of the percutaneous suture-mediated closure device in high-risk patients, appears to prevent infectious complications. The Perclose

(Abbott Vascular Devices, Redwood City, CA) was the first suture-based closure device on the market, and it is based solely on sutures (Fig. 29-11). The main advantage of Perclose compared with other closure devices is that no material is left at the puncture site except for the nonabsorbable sutures. Needles are used to guide the sutures through the vessel wall. The Prostar device uses four needles and two sutures while the Perclose devices use two needles and one suture. These devices can be used with 6- to 10-Fr sheaths. Perclose consists of several components, including a 0.035-in. guidewire, an automatic knot-pushing tool, and the suture-containing device itself. This tool consists of a sheath connected to a handle by a guide that is introduced into the vessel by means of the 0.035-in. guidewire after the angioplasty sheath has been removed. When the intravascular position has been achieved, the device is secured by pulling the lever and releasing the anchor. Using the needle plunger, needles are inserted through the vessel wall and grip the sutures. The needles are then retracted until they are outside of the skin with the sutures. Each of the two suture ends can be retrieved, tied together, and pulled down to the surface of the artery with the help of a knot pusher. This improved device has shortened the time of deployment and improved handling. After it is apparent that hemostasis will be achieved, the guidewire is removed with further sequential tightening of the suture pairs. This device is being used for even larger sheaths by the preclosure technique,[16] which allows for the off-label use of the Prostar device to achieve hemostasis with larger sheaths. After accessing the common femoral artery with an 8- to 10-Fr sheath, the Prostar suture-mediated closure devices is deployed without tying it. After the intervention is finalized, the preloaded sutures are tied over the large sheath while it is removed. The modified preclosure technique is a feasible alternative for hemostasis after using larger sheaths (12- to 18-F) to avoid an open surgical cutdown and diminish the need for general anesthesia. However, there is still an unmet need for dedicated percutaneous femoral closure devices for these large arteriotomies. The Starclose (Abbott Vascular Devices, Redwood City, CA) represents a new concept of extravascular, clip-based femoral closure devices (Fig. 29-12).[17,18] The clips are made of

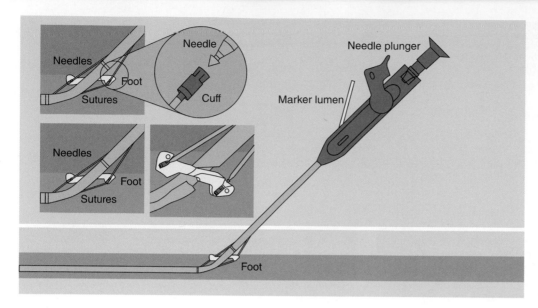

Figure 29-11 Perclose closure device.

nitinol alloy and are deployed through the existing procedural sheath. The extravascular approach closes by apposing the tissue at and above the arteriotomy site, leaving nothing in the arterial lumen. The artery may be accessed again shortly after hemostasis has been achieved.

PLUG-BASED SEALING DEVICES

Collagen is considered one of the most thrombogenic components of vascular wall. It attracts and binds platelets. Collagen also plays an important role in healing wounds by carrying growth factors and providing a matrix for cellular proliferation. Because it is highly compatible and easily manufactured in many different forms, collagen is an ideal component for hemostasis products. It can be used alone to plug the vessel wall or tissue tract or it can be combined with thrombin or Gelfoam. Thrombin converts fibrinogen to fibrin, thus accelerating and strengthening clot formation. The Angioseal (St. Jude Medical, St. Paul, MN)[19] mechanically closes the site by sandwiching the arteriotomy site between a bioabsorbable polymer anchor inside the vessel and an extravascular collagen sponge covering the arterial surface within the skin tract (Fig. 29-13). It consists of four components within a delivery device: anchor, collagen plug, connecting suture, and tamper. All three components deployed into the patient are completely resorbable. The small plug contains only about 15 mg of collagen, and the anchor is made of polyglycolic and polylactic acids. Before Angioseal deployment, the access site should be assessed by injecting contrast through the sheath under fluoroscopy. If the introducer enters the femoral artery above the inguinal ligament, at the bifurcation, at a branch vessel, or at an atherosclerotic vessel, there is an increased risk of device failure or embolization; in such cases an alternative method for hemostasis should be used. Proper technique must be followed to avoid bleeding complications, anchor embolization, thrombosis, and infection. The ExoSeal (Cordis, Johnson & Johnson, USA) consists of a feltlike plug made of polyglycolic acid (PGA) that completely dissolves into carbon dioxide and water over about 3 months. It can be used following diagnostic angiography or interventional procedures and is anchored in place on top of the puncture in the femoral artery, after the catheter is removed. The device uses an indicator nitinol wire to locate the arterial anterior wall to ensure extravascular plug placement. The wire is removed before the plug is delivered. Because no part of the plug is inserted into the artery itself, it does not interfere with blood flow.[20] The Mynx (AccessClosure, Inc. Mountain View, CA) uses an extravascular, bioinert sealant to provide immediate hemostasis of the puncture site. The device has met the challenge of simultaneously sealing the puncture hole in the artery and in the tissue

track by generating a thrombus (Fig. 29-14). It incorporates a unique, low-profile balloon-positioning catheter in combination with a biological procoagulant compound.[21] The Cardiva Catalyst III (Cardiva Medical, Inc., Sunnyvale, CA) is intended to promote hemostasis at an arteriotomy site as an adjunct to manual compression in heparinized patients. It consists of a sterile disposable wire and a sterile disposable clip. After completion of the catheterization procedure, the Catalyst III Wire is inserted into the artery through the existing introducer sheath. The distal tip of the wire is then deployed, which opens the biconvex, low-profile disk within the lumen of the femoral artery distal to the introducer sheath tip.[22] Tension between the disk and the clip creates a site-specific compression of the arteriotomy and establishes temporary hemostasis. Additionally, the Cardiva biocompatible coating includes a minimal amount of protamine sulfate to locally neutralize heparin. The Cardiva Catalyst III is indicated for use in patients undergoing diagnostic and/or interventional femoral artery catheterization procedures using 5-, 6- or 7-Fr introducer sheaths.

ELECTRICITY-BASED SEALING PADS

The patch technologies are a new form of biologically active, superficially applied therapies that accelerate local hemostasis at the puncture site.[23] The use of noninvasive closure devices for interventional procedures has rapidly increased in the past few years.[24] One of the substances used in these pads is chitosan, derived from the deacetylation of chitin. Chitin is obtained from the shells of lobsters, crabs, and shrimp. It has a slightly positive charge and chitosan has a strong positive charge, but erythrocytes and platelets are negatively charged. Because of their positive charges, chitin and chitosan attract negatively charged platelets and red blood cells to the applied area. Other hemostatic pads are impregnated with chemicals such as bovine thrombin or potato starch. These agents, combined with effective manual compression, may result in a shorter time to hemostasis and a stronger blood clot at the puncture site. These devices are effectively used for adjunctive closure devices or as hemostatic accelerators for manual compression of the access site. The simple application and the low cost make this system attractive. The reliability of these devices, however, still needs to be evaluated in larger numbers of patients. The Chito-Seal Topical Hemostasis Pad (Abbott Vascular Devices, Redwood City, CA) is intended for use in the management of bleeding wounds such as vascular access sites. The pad is coated with chitosan gel, which is a powerful hemostatic agent twice as chemically active as chitin. The Clo-sur P.A.D. (Scion Cardio-Vascular, Miami, FL) is a pad consisting of hydrophilic, naturally occurring biopolymer polyprolate acetate.

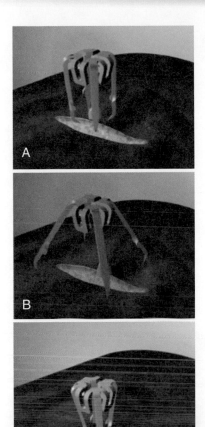

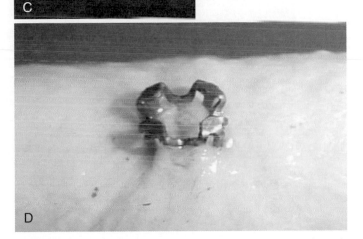

Figure 29-12 Expanding staple-based closure device. A. Staple tracks small through a sterile delivery system, reducing the chance of touch contamination. B. The device expands wide above the arteriotomy to close the arteriotomy. C. It purses the arteriotomy closed to promote healing. It does not remodel the vessel and has no intraluminal components to impede flow. D. The staple gathers the full thickness of the vessel media and adventitia for a secure mechanical closure. *(Photograph courtesy of Medtronic, Minneapolis, MN, 2006.)*

It also activates electrical interference between erythrocytes and the pad, leading to red blood cell agglutination and clot formation. The SyvekPatch (Marine Polymer Technologies, Danvers, MA), an external device used to control bleeding from vascular access sites, consists of a poly-*N*-acetyl glucosamine polymer, which is isolated from a microalgae. The mechanism of action involves clot formation and local vasoconstriction as part of its hemostatic effect.

Access-Site Complications

Local vascular complications at the site of catheter insertion constitute the most common adverse events after cardiovascular interventions. Vascular complications can extend the patient's length of hospitalization and increase the associated procedural costs. Vascular access complications include external bleeding, hematoma, pseudoaneurysm, arteriovenous fistula, vessel dissection, acute vessel closure, retroperitoneal hemorrhage, neural damage, infection, and venous thrombosis. One way to prevent femoral access complications is to carefully select patients and access sites. The American College of Cardiology-National Cardiovascular Data Registry (ACC-NCDR) reported an overall in-hospital serious adverse event rate related to vascular access of 1.56% among 166,680 patients after manual compression or the use of hemostasis devices (Table 29-1). Before placement of a vascular closure device, a femoral artery angiogram through the sheath should be obtained to assess the puncture site, vessel diameter, and presence and severity of atherosclerosis. It can help to identify patients at higher risk for groin complications. Femoral closure devices should be avoided when the artery diameter is less than 5 mm and in cases of higher or lower femoral punctures. Bleeding complications occur more frequently while obtaining access and positioning sheaths or early after removal when local pressure is not properly achieved. Several comorbid conditions have been associated with groin complications. The presence of peripheral vascular disease, renal failure, myocardial infarction, emergency indication for the procedure, and shock as an indication for the procedure demonstrated statistically significant associations with access-site bleeding complications. Hematoma is considered a significant complication when it has a diameter of more than 6 cm. The incidence of local hematoma varies from 1% to 5%, and most hematomas require only observation and no further intervention. Retroperitoneal hemorrhage remains an infrequent but occasionally devastating consequence of percutaneous cardiovascular intervention. The incidence of retroperitoneal hemorrhage is 0.6%; of these patients, 73% require blood transfusions and 10% die during hospitalization.[25] Retroperitoneal hemorrhage was independently associated with "high femoral artery stick" when femoral artery sheaths are placed superior to the inferior epigastric artery, female gender, the use of an Angioseal device, use of a glycoprotein IIb/IIIa inhibitor, a presentation of acute myocardial infarction, and inversely with the patient's weight.[25] Other studies have confirmed three factors to be predictive for retroperitoneal hemorrhage (female gender, low body weight, and high femoral puncture), whereas the use of a glycoprotein IIb/IIIa inhibitor, sheath size, and the use of a closure device did not correlate with bleeding complications.[26] Bleeding complications should be considered when a patient has a new onset of hypotension, flank pain, or decreased hematocrit level. Strict adherence to meticulous vascular access technique, the judicious use of closure devices, and appropriate and rapid management when this complication is suspected should lessen the occasionally serious consequences related to this problem. A major cause of retroperitoneal bleeding is a puncture above the inguinal ligament. When the posterior arterial wall is punctured, blood can spread into the retroperitoneal space. The location of the inferior epigastric artery may be helpful in judging the location of the puncture with regard to the inguinal ligament. The inferior border of this vessel defines the border of the inguinal ligament and represents a marker by which femoral punctures can be assessed for possible risk of retroperitoneal bleeding. The inferior epigastric artery arises from the distal external iliac artery just before it crosses under the inguinal ligament to enter the thigh and become the femoral artery. It typically originates opposite the deep iliac circumflex branch and bears a direct relation to the inferior extent of the peritoneal transversalis fascia (Fig. 29-15). When the entry site of the sheath is superior to the origin of the inferior epigastric artery, the sheath passes through various layers of the anterior abdominal wall, including superficial fascia and muscles, before entering the artery (Fig. 29-16). The collagen plug-based closure devices may not reach the wall of the artery in some cases, and the operator should be careful in choosing the site of cannulation of the

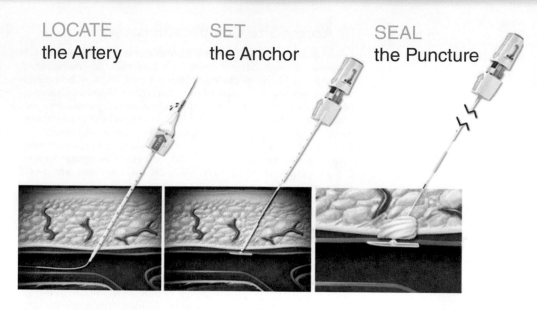

LOCATE the Artery   SET the Anchor   SEAL the Puncture

Figure 29-13 Angioseal hemostasis system. The anchor is deployed, and retraction of the system secures the anchor against the anterior vessel wall. The collagen plug is deployed outside of the artery. The suture is cut at the skin line, leaving the subcutaneous vascular closure components hidden. (*Image courtesy of St. Jude Medical, St. Paul, MN, 2006.*)

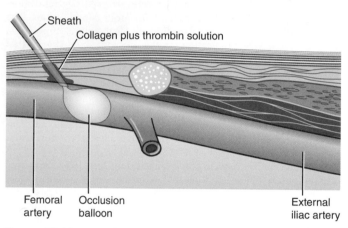

Figure 29-14 Mynx hemostatic device uses a low-profile balloon-positioning catheter in combination with a biological procoagulant-containing bovine collagen and thrombin solution.

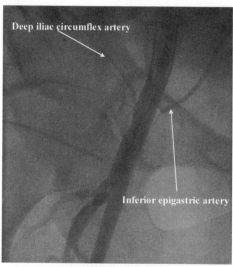

Figure 29-15 Angiogram through the sheath to assess the femoral artery and puncture location. The right anterior oblique, 30-degree projection of a typical femoral artery access site shows the inferior epigastric artery in relation to its surrounding anatomy. The inferior epigastric artery arises from the distal external iliac artery just before it crosses under the inguinal ligament. The inferior border of this vessel defines the border of the inguinal ligament.

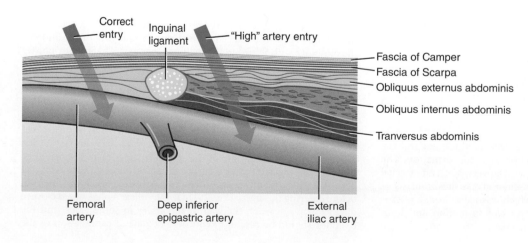

Figure 29-16 The diagram depicts the relation between the high entry and the correct puncture site related to the inguinal ligament and inferior epigastric artery. Placement of the sheath in a high puncture site crosses over the fascia of Camper, fascia of Scarpa, obliquus externus abdominis muscle, obliquus internus abdominis muscle, and the transversus abdominis muscle.

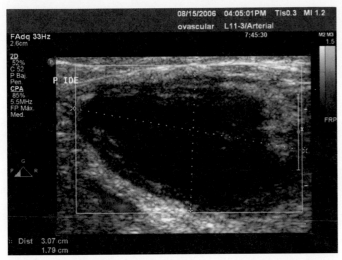

Figure 29-17 A pseudoaneurysm arising from the common femoral artery is assessed by duplex ultrasound.

femoral artery. Fluoroscopy can be used to ascertain the relative location of the femoral head and pelvic brim in that endeavor (Fig. 29-1). The retroperitoneal space appears to be able to sequester large amounts of blood. Volume and blood product support and correction of thrombin and platelet inhibition are central to management when this complication is suspected. Although computed tomography or other forms of imaging are occasionally useful in diagnosing retroperitoneal hemorrhage, this modality is usually not required and may delay treatment. Peripheral vascular surgery or endovascular treatment is appropriate if blood product transfusion does not result in hemodynamic stabilization or if there is clinically significant organ or nerve compression. The incidence of iatrogenic femoral pseudoaneurysms after percutaneous procedures ranges from 0.5% for diagnostic procedures to 1% to 2% for therapeutic interventions. A pseudoaneurysm is a hematoma that remains in continuity with the artery, allowing flow in and out of the hematoma. It can be differentiated from a simple hematoma by the presence of a bruit and a palpable pulsatile mass. Pseudoaneurysms are normally detected by ultrasound (Fig. 29-17). Older age, obesity, female gender, larger sheath size, peripheral vascular disease, a low arterial puncture site below the common femoral bifurcation, and the level of anticoagulation are associated with this complication. A pseudoaneurysm larger than 3 cm in diameter is usually treated by mechanical compression, thrombin injection, or surgery. Smaller pseudoaneurysms can be followed by serial ultrasound. Ultrasound-guided manual or mechanical compression is often used to convert the pseudoaneurysm to a thrombosed hematoma by compressing the neck connecting it to the artery. Ultrasound-guided low-dose thrombin injection appears to be more effective in reducing the need for surgical repair, is better tolerated by the patients, and requires a shorter hospital stay.[27] Arteriovenous fistula is defined as an abnormal connection between an artery and vein. This may be caused by trauma, improper removal of adjacent arterial and venous sheaths, or inadvertent puncture of a vein while accessing an artery. It is an uncommon and low-risk groin complication that is suspected by the detection of a continuous bruit at the access site; it is diagnosed by ultrasound. In cases of arterial insufficiency, the fistula can be treated with ultrasound-guided compression, endovascular stenting, or surgical repair. Occasionally, hematoma-mediated femoral nerve compression accompanying limb weakness may occur. It resolves spontaneously within 2 to 3 weeks. Vessel occlusion associated with manual compression may occur because of excessive occlusive pressure during the compression process. Patients with diabetes, female patients, or those with peripheral vascular disease have arteries with reduced luminal diameters and may be more susceptible to this complication. Vessel occlusion is characterized by a sudden onset of pain and possible paresthesia. The affected limb is cyanotic and cool; it has diminished or absent pulses. Treatment methods for vessel occlusion include administration of heparin or lytic agents or an endovascular or surgical thrombectomy procedure. Although relatively uncommon, vascular closure device-related infection is an emerging and serious phenomenon with a high morbidity rate. It requires aggressive medical and surgical intervention to achieve cure.[28] Access-site infections manifest with high fever, femoral abscess, septic thrombosis, and mycotic aneurysm. The predominant source of pathogens is the endogenous flora of the patient's skin. Attention to skin preparation is part of the infection prevention strategy. Diabetes mellitus and obesity are the most common associated comorbidities. Infectious groin complications are significantly increased with suture-based closure devices. Surgical removal of the percutaneous closure device and debridement to normal arterial wall are recommended for all patients with suspected femoral endarteritis. Before inserting a closure device, it is recommended to again prepare the skin insertion site and remove any pooled blood before beginning the arterial closure, especially in the case of a prolonged procedure. If compromise of sterile technique is suspected, the operator should consider a change of gloves before beginning the arterial closure and a change of towels around the skin insertion site, especially if the drape has become saturated with blood. Some interventionists routinely administer one or more doses of intravenous antibiotics when using a vascular closure device. Although some differences may exist regarding local complications with the use of femoral closure systems, no device has been shown to reduce major local complications.

Conclusions and Future Trends

Several femoral access closure technologies are on the market, and more on the horizon offer at least equivalent patient outcomes compared with manual compression. The ease of use is continuing to improve. Sealing and suturing closure devices have been shown to shorten hemostasis time, reduce the discomfort of manual or mechanical compression, and allow earlier ambulation after cardiovascular procedures without increasing vascular complications compared with conventional compression techniques. Improved devices that assist manual compression are also continuing to evolve. The patch technologies are a new form of biologically active, superficially applied therapies that have found acceptance in many practices. Ultimately, the acceptance of femoral closure devices will depend on which device provides a simple approach with reliable hemostasis at a cost that can justify its incorporation into routine practice. There is still a special need for dedicated femoral closure devices for larger arteriotomies for aortic endovascular repair and aortic valve replacement.

REFERENCES

1. Jolly SS, Amlani S, Hamon M, et al: Radial versus femoral access for coronary angiography or intervention and the impact on major bleeding and ischemic events: a systematic review and meta-analysis of randomized trials. *Am Heart J* 157(1):132–140, 2009.
2. Applegate RJ, Sacrinty MT, Kutcher MA, et al: Propensity score analysis of vascular complications after diagnostic cardiac catheterization and percutaneous coronary intervention 1998–2003. *Catheter Cardiovasc Intervent* 67(4):556–562, 2006.
3. Nikolsky E, Mehran R, Dangas G, et al: Development and validation of a prognostic risk score for major bleeding in patients undergoing percutaneous coronary intervention via the femoral approach. *Eur Heart J* 28(16):1936–1945, 2007.
4. Applegate R, Sacrinty M, Little W, et al: Prognostic implications of vascular complications following PCI. *Catheter Cardiovasc Intervent* 74(1):64–73, 2009.
5. Kluge A, Rauber K, Breithecker A, et al: Puncture of the popliteal artery using a Doppler-equipped (SMART) needle in transpopliteal interventions. *Eur Radiol* 13(8):1972–1978, 2003.
6. Nietlispach F, Johnson M, Moss RR, et al: Transcatheter closure of paravalvular defects using a purpose-specific occluder. *JACC Cardiovasc Intervent* 3(7):759–765, 2010.
7. Brown SC, Boshoff DE, Rega F, et al: Transapical left ventricular access for difficult to reach interventional targets in the left heart. *Catheter Cardiovasc Intervent* 74(1):137–142, 2009.
8. Park Y, Roh HG, Choo SW, et al: Prospective comparison of collagen plug (Angio-Seal) and suture-mediated (the Closer S) closure devices at femoral access sites. *Korean J Radiol* 6(4):248–255, 2005.
9. Nikolsky E, Mehran R, Halkin A, et al: Vascular complications associated with arteriotomy closure devices in patients undergoing percutaneous coronary procedures: a meta-analysis. *J Am Coll Cardiol* 44(6):1200–1209, 2004.

10. Arora N, Matheny ME, Sepke C, et al: A propensity analysis of the risk of vascular complications after cardiac catheterization procedures with the use of vascular closure devices. *Am Heart J* 153(4):606–611, 2007.

11. Tavris DR, Dey S, Albrecht-Gallauresi B, et al: Risk of local adverse events following cardiac catheterization by hemostasis device use: phase II. *J Invas Cardiol* 17(12):644–650, 2005.

12. Resnic FS, Arora N, Matheny M, et al: A cost-minimization analysis of the angio-seal vascular closure device following percutaneous coronary intervention. *Am J Cardiol* 99(6):766–770, 2007.

13. Rickli H, Unterweger M, Sutsch G, et al: Comparison of costs and safety of a suture-mediated closure device with conventional manual compression after coronary artery interventions. *Catheter Cardiovasc Intervent* 57(3):297–302, 2002.

14. Exaire JE, Tcheng JE, Kereiakes DJ, et al: Closure devices and vascular complications among percutaneous coronary intervention patients receiving enoxaparin, glycoprotein IIb/IIIa inhibitors, and clopidogrel. *Catheter Cardiovasc Intervent* 64(3):369–372, 2005.

15. Bangalore S, Arora N, Resnic FS: Vascular closure device failure: frequency and implications: a propensity-matched analysis. *Circ Cardiovasc Intervent* 2(6):549–556, 2009.

16. Kahlert P, Eggebrecht H, Erbel R, et al: A modified "preclosure" technique after percutaneous aortic valve replacement. *Catheter Cardiovasc Intervent* 72(6):877–884, 2008.

17. Tay EL, Co M, Tai BC, et al: Clinical experience of StarClose vascular closure device in patients with first and recurrent femoral punctures. *J Intervent Cardiol* 21(1):67–73, 2008.

18. McTaggart RA, Raghavan D, Haas RA, et al: StarClose vascular closure device: safety and efficacy of deployment and reaccess in a neurointerventional radiology service. *AJNR Am J Neuroradiol* 31(6):1148–1150, 2010.

19. Applegate RJ, Sacrinty M, Kutcher MA, et al: Vascular complications with newer generations of angioseal vascular closure devices. *J Interv Cardiol* 19(1):67–74, 2006.

20. Wong SC, Bachinsky W, Cambier P, et al: A randomized comparison of a novel bioabsorbable vascular closure device versus manual compression in the achievement of hemostasis after percutaneous femoral procedures: the ECLIPSE (Ensure's Vascular Closure Device Speeds Hemostasis Trial). *JACC Cardiovasc Intervent* 2(8):785–793, 2009.

21. Scheinert D, Sievert H, Turco MA, et al: The safety and efficacy of an extravascular, water-soluble sealant for vascular closure: initial clinical results for Mynx. *Catheter Cardiovasc Intervent* 70(5):627–633, 2007.

22. Doyle BJ, Godfrey MJ, Lennon RJ, et al: Initial experience with the Cardiva Boomerang vascular closure device in diagnostic catheterization. *Catheter Cardiovasc Intervent* 69(2):203–208, 2007.

23. Hirsch JA, Reddy SA, Capasso WE, et al: Non-invasive hemostatic closure devices: "patches and pads." *Tech Vasc Intervent Radiol* 6(2):92–95, 2003.

24. Applegate RJ, Sacrinty MT, Kutcher MA, et al: Propensity score analysis of vascular complications after diagnostic cardiac catheterization and percutaneous coronary intervention using thrombin hemostatic patch-facilitated manual compression. *J Invasive Cardiol* 19(4):164–170, 2007.

25. Ellis SG, Bhatt D, Kapadia S, et al: Correlates and outcomes of retroperitoneal hemorrhage complicating percutaneous coronary intervention. *Catheter Cardiovasc Intervent* 67(4):541–545, 2006.

26. Farouque HM, Tremmel JA, Raissi Shabari F, et al: Risk factors for the development of retroperitoneal hematoma after percutaneous coronary intervention in the era of glycoprotein IIb/IIIa inhibitors and vascular closure devices. *J Am Coll Cardiol* 45(3):363–368, 2005.

27. Olsen DM, Rodriguez JA, Vranic M, et al: A prospective study of ultrasound scan-guided thrombin injection of femoral pseudoaneurysm: a trend toward minimal medication. *J Vasc Surg* 36(4):779–782, 2002.

28. Geary K, Landers JT, Fiore W, et al: Management of infected femoral closure devices. *Cardiovasc Surg* 10(2):161–163, 2002.

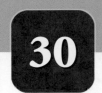

30

Transradial Percutaneous Coronary Intervention for Major Reduction of Bleeding Complications

FARZIN BEYGUI | GILLES MONTALESCOT

KEY POINTS

- Bleeding complications after percutaneous coronary intervention (PCI) are associated with poor outcomes, including mortality.

- The trans-radial approach to PCI is associated with a reduction in the risk of access-site complications, virtually no access-site bleeding, and subsequent reduction of major adverse cardiovascular events (MACEs).

- After an initial learning curve, the procedural success rates of the trans-radial approach become similar to those of the trans-femoral approach.

- The trans-radial approach could be used in any clinical condition for all procedures and devices compatible with 5, 6, or 7 French (5F, 6F, or 7F) guiding catheters.

Both diagnostic coronary angiography and PCI are most commonly performed via the trans-femoral access in a majority of catheterization laboratories. Initial reports in the late 1980s demonstrated the feasibility and security of diagnostic coronary angiography via the trans-radial approach.[1] The development of highly active anti-thrombotic regimens associated with a major reduction of thrombotic complications of PCI, in part resulting in a significant increase in femoral access site–related bleeding complications, led to the development of the trans-radial approach to PCI in the past decade. The use of 6F and more recently 5F guiding catheters, with the generalization of 6F compatible or 5F-compatible balloons, coronary stents, and other approaches such as rotational atherectomy, thrombectomy, or distal protection devices allow treatment of complex lesions, for example, multi-vessel PCI, bifurcation lesions, and so on. These approaches are used in complex situations such as PCI for acute coronary syndrome (ACS), including primary or rescue PCI via the trans-radial approach, following a relatively short and easy learning curve. Although still used rarely in the United States (1.3% of procedures), the use of PCI via the trans-radial approach is growing to an impressive extent in Asia and Europe as was recently reported.[2] In the setting of ACS more than 80% of procedures were performed through the radial access.[3] Similarly primary PCI is more and more frequently performed through a radial access as recently shown in the international randomized ATOLL study, where 66% of procedures used the radial artery.[4]

Rationale for the Trans-Radial Approach

ANATOMIC CONSIDERATION

The radial artery, as well as the ulnar artery, is usually a terminal branch of the brachial artery, originating below the elbow. In some cases, the radial artery originates from the upper brachial artery or even directly from the axillary artery. It follows the external margin of the forearm to reach the wrist, where it divides into two branches and joins the branches of the ulnar artery through the superficial and deep palmar arches. The palmar arches may also be irrigated by the branches of the common inter-osseous artery, a high originated branch of the ulnar artery itself. Quite superficial along its course, the radial artery is covered by the brachioradialis muscle proximally. It becomes extremely superficial and accessible at its 3- to 5-cm distal portion before the wrist, which is the ideal puncture site. Moreover, the satellite radial nerve changes direction at this final portion, making puncture-related nerve injury very rare. The absence of major veins around the radial artery also reduces the risk of arteriovenous fistula. Because of such anatomy, the trans-radial approach to PCI appears to be significantly safe.

FEASIBILITY

The feasibility and security of the trans-radial approach to coronary diagnostic or interventional procedures have been widely demonstrated. Data from such studies are summarized in Table 30-1. Even in the case of experienced operators, the trans-radial approach requires a learning curve to achieve higher rates of procedural success and shorter duration of the procedure and x-ray exposure.[5] Overall, the feasibility of the trans-radial approach for diagnostic or interventional coronary procedures is high (>90%), especially in experienced centers (>95%). In a series of 1119 consecutive patients in South Korea, the mean radial artery diameter measured by ultrasound was 2.6 ± 0.41 mm in men and 2.43 ± 0.38 mm in women.[6] In another series of 250 patients in Japan, the radial artery diameter was larger than 7F and 8F catheters in 71.5% and 44.9% of male patients and 40.3% and 24% of female patients respectively.[7] Although such data may not be totally generalizable to all other populations, they underscore the fact that the trans-radial approach could potentially be used in a majority of patients with 5F, 6F, and even 7F catheters. In some patients with sufficiently large artery diameters, 8F catheters may also be used, if needed. The trans-radial approach has been used for different types of procedures with various devices such as intravascular ultrasound (IVUS)–guided stenting, coronary brachytherapy, distal protection, embolectomy, rotational atherectomy, myocardial biopsy, and bifurcated stents. The approach is incompatible with the intra-aortic balloon pump and all other devices or procedures that need larger than 8F access. Recently, the use of sheathless guiding catheters, with smaller outer diameters—6.5F and 7.5F catheters with introducers of less than 5F and 6F diameters, respectively—has been reported to be feasible and safe. Although their use is infrequent, such catheters may allow complex procedures such as simultaneous kissing stenting.

The Trans-Radial Approach Versus the Trans-Femoral Approach for PCI

The trans-femoral approach represents an easily accessible superficial arterial access point, through which large catheters delivering all types of devices could be introduced.

Compared with the trans-femoral approach, the trans-radial access is associated with fewer vascular complications, more comfort for

TABLE 30-1	Major Trans-radial Percutaneous Coronary Intervention Feasibility Studies					
Author	*Type of Procedure*	*N*	*Catheter Size*	*Success Rate*	*Access Site Complication*
Kiemeneij[47]	Stenting	20	6 French (6F)	100%	0%
Kiemeneij[26]	POBA (plain old balloon angioplasty)	100	6F	94%	2%
Kiemeneij[48]	Stenting	100	6F	96%	3%
Saito[7]	Unselected patient percutaneous coronary intervention (PCI)	1360	6F/7F/8F	92%	0.2%
Kim[23]	Primary PCI	30	6F	90%	0%
Louvard[49]	Primary PCI	277	6F	95%	0%
Mulukutla[50]	Primary PCI (glycoprotein [GP] IIb/IIIa inhibitors in 75%)	41	6F	100%	0%
Valsecchi[24]	Primary PCI	163	6F	97%	0%
Valsecchi[25]	Unselected				
	≥70 years old	323	6F	98.8	0.4%
	<70 years old	80	6F	99	0%

TABLE 30-2	Randomized Trials Comparing Trans-radial and Trans-femoral Approaches for Percutaneous Coronary Intervention						
			Successful Procedure (%)		Access Site Complication (%)		
Author	*Type of Procedure*	*N*	TR	TF	TR	TF	*Other Endpoints*
Mann[51]	POBA	152	91	96	0	5	TR reduced the length of hospital stay and total cost
Kiemeneij[19]	POBA	600	92	91	0	2	Similar procedure, hospital stay, and x-ray exposure durations
Benit[20]	Elective stenting	112	89	98	0	10	Similar procedure, hospital stay, and x-ray exposure durations
Mann[52]	Stenting in ACS	152	96	96	0	4	TR reduced the length of hospital stay and total cost
Mann[53]	Stenting TR versus TF with Perclose®	218			0	3.4	TR reduced the length of procedure, hospital stay, and total cost Perclose: inadequate in 18%; failure of hemostasis in 10% of patients
Louvard[54]	Diagnostic ± ad hoc PCI in about 43%	210	100	100	2	6	TR reduced the length of hospital stay and total cost and was patient preferred, but increased x-ray exposure duration
Saito[55]	Primary stenting	149	96	97	0	3	Comparable in-hospital MACE rates
Louvard[11]	PCI in >80 years	371	89	91	1.6	6.6	Trend to longer TR procedure duration
Cantor[12]	Primary or rescue PCI	50	99.6	100	0.4	0.4	Similar fluoroscopy time and contrast media quantity
Slagboom[56]	Outpatient PCI	644	96	97	0	6	Similar rates of major bleeding, higher rates of same day discharge, and lower rates of minor bleeding with TR
Brasselet[57]	Primary PCI with abciximab	114	91.6	96.5	3.5	19.3	Similar rates of bleeding, transfusion, and MACEs; higher fluoroscopy time, and earlier ambulation with TR
Li[58]	Primary PCI	370	98.4	98.9	2	7	Similar procedure times
Achenbach[59]	PCI in patients age >75 years	307	91	100	1.3	9	Higher examination time with TR, but similar fluoroscopy time, number of catheters, and amount of contrast media
Agostoni meta-analysis[8]	Diagnostic or PCI	2845	93	98	0.3	2.8	Shorter hospital stay, lower hospital costs, longer fluoroscopy times with TR
Rival trial[19]	Diagnostic and/or PCI for ACS	7021	92.4	98	1.4	3.7	Comparable rates of the primary endpoint death, myocardial infarction, stroke and major bleeding at 30 days, significantly higher rates of femoral access sight complications
Jolly meta-analysis[9]	PCI	7020	95	97	0.05	2.3	Significant 73% reduction in major bleeding; trend toward less 30-days mortality and MACEs, significantly shorter hospital stay with TR

TR, TF, trans-radial, trans-femoral; *PCI,* percutaneous coronary intervention; *ACS,* acute coronary syndrome; *POBA,* plain old balloon angioplasty; *MACEs,* major acute coronary events.

patients, the possibility of rapid ambulation, less procedure cost, and shorter hospital stay. Several randomized trials comparing the advantages and disadvantages of each method are summarized in Table 30-2. A meta-analysis of 11 published and unpublished randomized controlled trials, which included 3224 patients, showed that the overall rates of postprocedure major ischemic coronary events are comparable in both methods, the procedural success rate is higher with the trans-femoral approach (98% vs. 93%, $P = 0.0009$), and all of these studies and the pooled analysis demonstrated the significant advantage of the trans-radial approach in terms of bleeding complications, mainly an 89% risk reduction for entry site complications (0.3% vs. 3%, $P < 0.0001$).[8] The previous meta-analysis also showed a clear ongoing

trend toward equalization of procedural success rates between the two approaches through the years. Such finding is probably explained by technologic advancements in materials and improvement in operators' skills and experience following the learning curve. The average duration of exposure to x-ray was, nevertheless, longer for the trans-radial approach (8.9 vs. 7.8 minutes, $P < 0.001$). Another, more recent meta-analysis of 23 published and unpublished randomized trials, which included 7020 patients undergoing coronary angiography or PCI concordantly, showed a significant reduction (73%, $P < 0.001$) in the rate of major bleeding in those undergoing PCI as well as a trend toward lower rates of the combined endpoint of death, myocardial infarction (MI), or stroke (odds ratio [OR] 0.71, $P = 0.058$) and death

TABLE 30-3	Jolly's Meta-analysis (9 of 23 Randomized Trials)						
	Trans-radial			**Trans-femoral**		**OR(95%CI) trans-radial vs. trans-femoral approach**	**P value**
Endpoint	*n*/Total	%		*n*/Total	%		
Death	22/1906	1.2		28/1565	1.8	0.74(0.42–1.30)	0.29
Death/Myocardial infarction/Stroke	56/2209	2.5		71/1784	3.8	0.71(0.49–1.01)	0.058
Major bleeding	13/2390	0.05		48/2068	2.3	0.27(0.16–0.45)	<0.001
Access-site cross-over	150/2542	5.9		34/2460	1.4	3.82(2.83–5.15)	<0.001
Failure to cross lesion	60/1274	4.7		40/1186	3.4	1.31(0.87–1.96)	0.20

(OR 0.74, $P = 0.29$). The major findings of the study are summarized in Table 30-3. Although access site cross-over was higher in the trans-radial approach, the procedure failure rate was not significantly lower and was particularly similar among operators who preferred the trans-radial approach, and there was a trend toward higher failure ($P = 0.07$) among less experienced operators. Such advantages make the trans-radial approach the method of choice for outpatient PCI, which has been reported to be highly feasible and safe. The trans-radial approach is also of particular interest with regard to patients at high risk for bleeding (older adults, women, patients with renal failure, obese persons, or patients on multiple anti-thrombotic agents, especially glycoprotein [GP] IIb/IIIa inhibitors); for example, it has been reported to be associated with fewer vascular complications in obese patients (multivariate OR 0.12; 95% confidence interval [CI] 0.02–0.94, $P = 0.043$) in a retrospective series of 5234 diagnostic or interventional (56.6%) procedures, as well as in older adults (1.6% vs. 6.5%, $P = 0.03$).[10,11] Other patients who benefited from the obvious advantages of the radial approach over the femoral approach are those with severe peripheral arterial disease (PAD), proximal PAD, or both; patients with bilateral aorto-femoral bypass graft; patients with aortic aneurysms; and patients with a prior history of femoral complications after catheterization. The trans-radial approach is also of particular interest in the setting of primary PCI (see Tables 30-1 and 30-2) performed by experienced operators in patients treated with aggressive anti-thrombotic regimens, in whom life-threatening access-site bleeding complications and the subsequent MACEs may be avoided with the trans-radial approach. In such a setting, there is growing evidence that the trans-radial approach is associated with overall similar door-to-balloon times, lower rates of vascular complications and bleeding in the presence of triple anti-platelet therapy, and even reduced 30-day mortality compared with the femoral approach.[12-16] It may also be of interest in patients with chronic kidney disease, as in the British Columbia cohort of 69,214 patients who underwent catheterization. Compared with the radial access, the femoral access was associated with an adjusted odds ratio of 4.36 (2.48–7.66) for the development of the composite endpoint of new dialysis or new chronic kidney disease.[17] Such findings may be related to the reduced risk of atheroembolism in the trans-radial approach. Finally, when considering recent PCI registries such as the RIVIERA (Registry on IntraVenous anticoagulation In the Elective and primary Real world of Angioplasty) registry, which prospectively included 7962 unselected patients, the trans-radial approach appeared as an independent predictor of better in-hospital outcome (OR for death or MI 0.16; CI 0.05–0.50) as well as the only variable correlated to less bleeding.[18] Similar results were also reported by the Canadian MORTAL (Mortality benefit Of Reduced Transfusion after percutaneous coronary intervention via the Arm or Leg) registry; which included 38,872 procedures (20.5% by the trans-radial approach); this registry showed a significant reduction of 30-day mortality (adjusted OR 0.71; CI 0.61–0.82) and 1-year mortality (adjusted OR 0.83; CI 0.71–0.98) by the latter approach. The superiority of the trans-radial approach in the prior study appears to be entirely linked to the reduced rates of transfusion. The major study comparing

the trans-radial and trans-femoral approaches is the very recently published RIVAL trial.[18a] The RIVAL trial included in 7021 ACS patients randomly assigned to each of the approaches for angiography and/or PCI. Indications for angiography were STEMI in 27.2% and 28.5% and NSTEMI in 28.5% and 25.8% in trans-radial and trans-femoral groups respectively. Angiography was performed in 99.8% and PCI in approximately 66% of patients in both groups. PCI success rates were comparable between the 2 groups (95.4% versus 95.2%), with higher access site crossover rates in the transradial group (7.6% versus 2%, $P < 0.0001$). The rates of primary endpoint the composite of death, myocardial infarction, stroke, or non-CABG bleeding at 30 days occurrence were comparable between the trans-radial and trans-femoral groups (3.7% and 4%), as well as each of the individual components. However the secondary endpoint of major vascular complications occurred more often in the trans-femoral group (1.4% versus 3.7%, $P < 0.0001$). Moreover all post-hoc exploratory outcomes including ACUITY-defined major bleeding, the composite of death, myocardial infarction or ACUITY major bleeding, and the composite of major non-CABG bleeding and vascular complications were more frequent in the trans-femoral group.

Although RIVAL failed to show a difference between the 2 groups regarding its primary endpoint, 2 major findings in the subgroup analysis should be underlined: First, in the STEMI subgroup of the study, trans-radial approach was not only associated with a significant reduction of the primary endpoint (HR 0.6 [95%CI 0.38–0.94]) but also of mortality (HR 0.39 [95%CI 0.20–0.76]). Second, the primary endpoint was also significantly reduced by the trans-radial approach in the centers with the highest radial PCI volume (HR 0.49 [95%CI 0.28–0.87] highlighting the importance of the learning curve for the trans-radial approach. The latter finding also points a limit of the study where an experience of only 50 procedures within the previous year was sufficient to validate the expertise for the trans-radial approach.

The Trans-Radial Approach Versus the Trans-Brachial Approach

Two of the randomized trials mentioned above also included a group of patients who underwent PCI through the trans-brachial approach. The ACCESS study reported comparable procedural success rates, equipment consumption, and procedural and fluoroscopy times among the three approaches for PCI.[19] The trans-brachial approach was associated with higher rates of vascular complications compared with the trans-radial approach (2% vs. 0%, $P = 0.035$). The BRAFE (Brachial, RAdial, or Femoral approach for Elective Palmaz-Schatz stent) study compared the trans-radial and trans-femoral approaches to a trans-brachial cut-down approach and reported no local vascular complication with the latter approach.[20] Such brachial approach is not commonly used and appears unacceptably aggressive. The brachial access does not need a cut-down and can be obtained with a classic percutaneous approach; but the brachial access is usually preferred when neither femoral nor radial approaches are possible.

The Trans-Radial Approach Versus the Trans-Ulnar Approach

The PCVI-CUBA (22) study randomized 413 patients with a normal direct or reverse Allen's test to undergo coronary angiography with or without subsequent PCI through the trans-radial approach versus the trans-ulnar approach. The two methods were associated with similar rates of access success (96% vs. 93%), PCI success (96% vs. 95%), and asymptomatic access-site artery occlusion (5% vs. 6%) rates.[21] Vascular complications occurred only in two patients in the trans-ulnar group. If confirmed by further data, the trans-ulnar approach would be an alternative to the trans-radial approach for PCI, although the ulnar artery is usually less superficial and its compression may be little more difficult technically.

Cost-Effectiveness

Although based on small studies, there is systematically concordant evidence that because of shorter hospital stay, reduced nursing workload, reduced rates of complications, and absence of need for closure devices, the trans-radial approach is associated with significant cost reduction in both diagnostic angiography and PCI settings.[22]

Practical Considerations for the Trans-Radial Approach

CONTRAINDICATIONS TO THE TRANS-RADIAL APPROACH

Contraindications to the trans-radial approach include the presence of a forearm arteriovenous fistula or proven absence of collateral ulnar circulation, which could be evaluated as described further below. The trans-radial approach should be considered with precaution and after assessing the balance between other access-site complications and the risk of radial access in patients with end-stage renal disease with potential need for forearm arteriovenous fistula and in patients with small or heavily calcified radial arteries.

ASSESSMENT OF ULNO-PALMAR ARTERIAL ARCHES

Classically, the assessment of collateral ulnar circulation is recommended before undertaking the trans-radial approach to PCI. Early postprocedure occlusion of the radial artery could occur in 0% to 19% of patients, depending on the clinical or ultrasound assessment of the patency of the radial artery, the diagnostic or interventional type of procedure, whether or not anticoagulation is used, and the size of the catheters.[7,23-25] In 40% to 60% of cases, the pulse could be re-detected within hours to weeks after the occlusion, which remains asymptomatic in virtually all patients.[26,27] Nevertheless, incomplete palmar arches and very rare cases of transient or definitive hand or finger ischemia have been reported, which justifies the evaluation of the ulno-palmar arch before the radial puncture. Although assessment of the collateral ulnar circulation is recommended, the low specificity of Allen's test and the absence of symptomatic ischemic complications in the abundant literature have made this recommendation obsolete in many experienced radial centers.

Allen's Test

A simple way of testing the adequacy of the collateral ulnar circulation clinically is the modified Allen's test (Fig. 30-1). The test consists of the simultaneous compression of radial and ulnar arteries, followed by several flexion–extension movements of fingers, which would lead to loss of color in the palm. The ulnar compression is then removed. The re-coloration time of the palm after removal of the ulnar artery compression defines Allen's test: normal less than 5 seconds, intermediate 5 to less than 10 seconds, abnormal 10 seconds or more. The reverse Allen's test comprises all of the above steps except that transient radial compression instead of ulnar compression could be used with the trans-ulnar approach. In clinical practice, the trans-radial approach could be attempted in normal or intermediate patient groups. While the prognostic relevance of Allen's test is still being debated, a recent study demonstrated reduced blood flow and increased capillary lactate levels in the thumb following 30-minute occlusive compression of the radial artery in patients with abnormal result of Allen's test compared with those with a normal result.[28] Although such findings are suggestive of potential ischemic complications in patients with abnormal results, the association with the safety of the procedure has never been shown.

Plethysmo-oxymetric Test (Video 30-1 📹)

The plethysmo-oxymetric test may be a potentially more accurate method for the evaluation of the ulno-palmar arch (see Fig. 30-1, C and D). The radial artery is compressed after the detector is positioned on the thumb. The persistent damping of the plethysmographic curve and a decrease of blood oxygen saturation are signs of inadequate ulnar collateral circulation. Barbeau et al compared this method with Allen's test in 1010 consecutive patients. The study showed that 6.3% of patients were to be excluded on the basis of Allen's test results, whereas only 1.5% had abnormal results from the plethysmo-oxymetric test.[29] Because of the rare occurrence of radial artery occlusion and the exceptionally symptomatic character of such a complication, the prognostic value of neither of these tests has been proven, so many operators use the trans-radial approach without prior evaluation of the ulno-palmar arch. Nevertheless, when Allen's test is performed, an abnormal result should be confirmed with the plethysmo-oxymetric test; the result can then be considered a contraindication to the trans-radial approach and another access point can be chosen.

RIGHT TRANS-RADIAL APPROACH VERSUS LEFT TRANS-RADIAL APPROACH

The left trans-radial access may have some advantages over the right trans-radial approach. Such reported advantages are:
- More patient comfort and less risk in case of hand ischemia for the right-handed majority of patients
- Easier coronary cannulation using standard Judkin's catheters
- Less guidewire use
- Lower rates of unusual artery branching or vessel tortuosity and thus less catheter manipulation
- Shorter procedure and fluoroscopy times
- Selective opacification of left internal thoracic artery bypass grafts

In a randomized trial comparing 232 left and 205 right trans-radial diagnostic procedures, the left-sided approach was associated with shorter duration of catheter manipulation, procedure, and fluoroscopy and lower rates of guidewire use, which suggests increased procedural efficacy.[30] Nevertheless, the right trans-radial approach is clearly more ergonomic for the majority of operators, and the differences between the two approaches may not be of clinical relevance. The choice of the side remains mainly a matter of operator preference.

Bi-Internal thoracic artery–coronary artery bypass graft is a specific situation where a double left-and-right radial approach could be used, allowing direct access to the ostia of internal thoracic arteries for further intervention through the grafts.

PATIENT PREPARATION, ARTERIAL PUNCTURE AND SHEATH INSERTION (Video 30-2 📹)

Explanations and premedication should be given to patients according to local practice. As excessive patient anxiety may cause radial artery spasm, premedication may be used for radial artery puncture. When possible, local anesthesia of the puncture site with an anesthetic cream 30 to 60 minutes before the puncture may improve patient comfort and reduce the risk of radial artery spasm and thus cannulation failure.

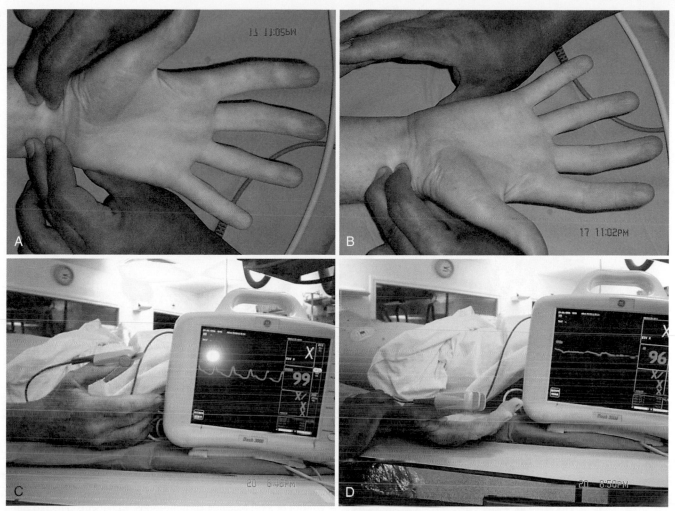

Figure 30-1 Ulno-palmar arch assessment. **A,** Allen's test: compression of both radial and ulnar arteries. **B,** Allen's test: homogenous re-coloration of the palm after cessation of ulnar artery compression in a patient with normal palmar arch. **C,** Plethysmo-oxymetric test: before radial artery compression. **D,** Plethysmo-oxymetric test: dumping of the plethysmographic curve and decrease of oxygen saturation of the thumb after radial compression in a patient with incomplete palmar arch.

Some operators also recommend local vasodilatation by apposition of a nitrate patch or paste on the puncture site. The forearm should be shaved, if necessary, and aseptically prepared. Usually, the groins are also prepared in case of possible failure of the radial access or if larger than 7F catheters are needed. The patient's arm and wrist should rest on an arm-rest. A roll of gauze could be placed under the wrist to make the puncturing easier. Before puncturing, a small dose of subcutaneous lidocaine 1% or 2% solution (0.5–2 mL) is injected at the puncture site. The artery is punctured either with a short 18 G or 19 G entry needle or a 20 G venous type catheter entry needle usually at a 30-degree angle with the horizontal plane. The needle is advanced until blood appears and the bleeding stops. The inner needle is then retrieved if a venous-type needle is used. The needle or the catheter is then retrieved until a pulsatile blood flow appears. A 0.025-inch straight, preferably hydrophilic-coated, guidewire is introduced through the needle or the catheter, which are then removed. Eventually, a very small superficial skin incision is made and a 70-mm long, arterial, hydrophilic-coated sheath is introduced on the wire. Figures 30-2, *A* through *C*, show single right-radial, left-ulnar, and bilateral radial sheaths, respectively, in place. The use of hydrophilic-coated sheaths (Fig. 30-3) as well as the smallest sheath size—4F for diagnostic procedures, and 5F for PCI, with further upsizing, if needed, to 6F, 7F, or even 8F—recommended as they are associated with less radial artery occlusion and spasm and less extraction force at removal.[31]

PREVENTION OF RADIAL ARTERY SPASM

An intra-arterial spasmolytic drug or cocktail is injected through the sheath after its introduction. Different cocktails have been evaluated on the basis of various treatments—nitroglycerin, nitroprusside, molsidomine, phentolamine, diltiazem or verapamil, alone or in combination. In a randomized trial that included 406 patients, the rates of clinical radial artery spasm, angiographic radial artery spasm, or both were significantly reduced by the intra-arterial injection of nitroglycerin 100 mcg with or without combination therapy with verapamil 1.25 mg (3.8% and 4.4%, respectively) compared with placebo (20.4%).[32] However, the effect of nitrates depends on the dose used, and a high dose is recommended when it is used alone. In another randomized trial that included 1219 patients, the combination of verapamil 2.5 mg and molsidomine 1 mg was associated with less radial spasm (4.9%) compared with verapamil 2.5 mg, 5 mg (8.3% and 7.9%), or molsidomine 1 mg (13.3%) alone and placebo (22.2%).[33] In another randomized trial, verapamil 2.5 mg alone was more effective in the prevention of radial artery spasm compared with the α-blocker phentolamine 2.5 mg (spasm rates 13.8% and 23.2%, respectively).[34] The intra-arterial injection of verapamil, nitroglycerin, or a combination of the two seems to be associated with the lowest spasm rates and could be recommended in all patients after the introduction of the sheath in the radial artery.

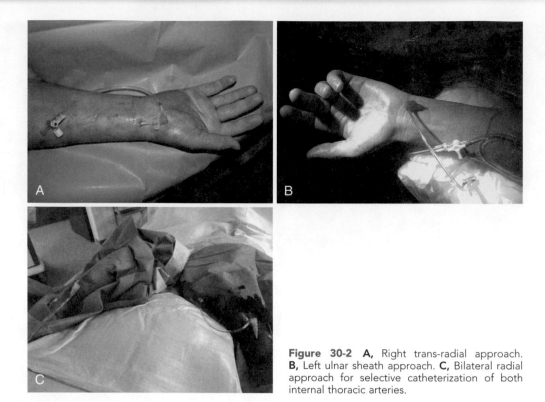

Figure 30-2 A, Right trans-radial approach. **B,** Left ulnar sheath approach. **C,** Bilateral radial approach for selective catheterization of both internal thoracic arteries.

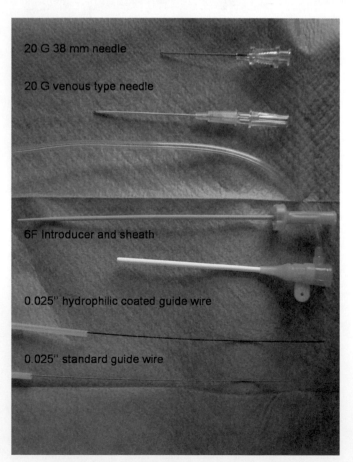

Figure 30-3 Trans-radial approach kit (Terumo®).

ANTICOAGULATION

Because of the potential risk of radial artery occlusion and for full control of local bleeding complications, all patients undergo full-dose anticoagulation therapy after the arterial sheath is placed in the radial artery before both diagnostic and interventional procedures in patients who are not already on anticoagulation therapy. In a series of 415 consecutive patients, Spaulding et al found a high correlation between heparin therapy and postprocedure radial artery occlusion in 71% of untreated patients, 24% of patients receiving 2000 international units (IU) to 3000 IU, and only 4.3% of those receiving 5000 IU of unfractionated heparin.[35] No specific data concerning other regimens of anticoagulation in the specific setting of the trans-radial PCI are available. A small pilot study has reported the feasibility and security of an ad hoc PCI strategy with bivalirudin after initial angiography with low-dose unfractionated heparin (1000 or 2500 IU).[36] Such strategy remains to be validated by further studies. Overall, full anticoagulation is recommended in all patients undergoing trans-radial procedures, and different regimens—fixed dose, weight-adjusted or ACT-adjusted unfractionated heparin, weight-adjusted low-molecular-weight heparin, bivalirudin, and so on—should be considered on the basis of validated guidelines and local practice. Anticoagulants may be injected through the arterial sheath or through a venous access.

GLYCOPROTEIN IIB/IIIA INHIBITORS AND FIBRINOLYTICS

Because of its extremely low vascular-site complication rates, the trans-radial approach to PCI is clearly the method of choice in the setting of PCI with highly active anti-thrombotic regimens and early or rescue PCI after thrombolysis. In a series of mostly patients with ACS undergoing PCI with abciximab through trans-radial access ($n = 83$) or trans-femoral access ($n = 67$), the 1-month major acute coronary events rate was similar in the two approaches, but bleeding complications occurred in 0% of the trans-radial group versus 7.4% of the trans-femoral group ($P = 0.04$).[37]

In another consecutive series of 119 patients undergoing primary PCI with systematic GP IIb/IIIa inhibition with abciximab, compared with the trans-femoral approach ($n = 55$) the trans-radial approach ($n = 67$) was associated with less major access-site complication (5.5% vs. 0%, $P = 0.03$), shorter hospital stay, comparable procedural time but higher x-ray exposure time, and dose-product.[38] In a retrospective analysis of post-thrombolysis rescue PCI with adjuvant GP IIb/IIIa inhibition in 111 patients, of whom 47 had a trans-radial approach, lower rates of access-site bleeding (0% versus 9%, $P = 0.04$) and lower rates of transfusion (4% versus 19%, $P = 0.02$) were reported, as compared with the trans-femoral access. Fluoroscopy time, contrast media volume, and time to first balloon inflation were comparable between the two approaches.[39] Finally, a small randomized pilot trial comparing the trans-radial and trans-femoral approaches for urgent PCI in 50 patients after thrombolysis (66% of patients), GP IIb/IIIa inhibition (94%), or both reported comparable results in procedural success rates (only one failure in the trans-radial group) and vascular complication rates (one pseudo-aneurysm in each group) but slightly longer average local anesthesia to first balloon time in the trans-radial group (32 vs. 26 minutes, $P = 0.04$).[12] In the noninferiority randomized EASY (Trans-radial Coronary Stenting with a Single Abciximab Bolus) trial comparing trans-radial PCI either with same-day discharge and abciximab bolus or hospitalization and abciximab infusion in 1005 patients, of whom 66% had unstable angina, the 30-day composite endpoint of death, MI, urgent revascularization, major bleeding, repeat hospitalization, access-site complications, or severe thrombocytopenia was comparable. The overall rates of access-site complication (4.8% vs. 4.2%), major bleeding (0.8% vs. 0.2%), and transfusion were impressively low.[40] Despite the absence of adequately sized randomized trials in the specific setting of trans-radial PCI with GP IIb/IIIa inhibitors or after thrombolysis, the extremely low rate of access site–related bleeding complications in this approach firmly recommends its use in patients with these highly active anti-thrombotic therapies.

GUIDING CATHETERS

The guidewire used for the trans-radial approach is usually a standard 0.032-inch to 0.035-inch guidewire. In case of anatomic difficulties such as radial or subclavian loops, a hydrophilic-coated guidewire could be used. The progression of the guidewire should be done under fluoroscopic control, especially with hydrophilic-coated guidewires. The catheter exchange could be done using a long 260- to 300-cm exchange guidewire or with a wire placed in the aortic root using a flush syringe in the catheter. The syringe and the catheter are retrieved during the flush injection, under fluoroscopic control (Video 30-3). Such exchange methods are extremely useful when anatomic access is difficult. The cannulation of coronary arteries via the left or right trans-radial approach could be done using standard Judkin's right and left catheters in the majority of patients. The cannulation of both right and left coronary ostia is very similar in the left trans-radial and transfemoral approaches, and all standard catheters could be used through such access. In a series of 412 consecutive left trans-radial diagnostic procedures, only 5.5% of left main and 3% of the right coronary ostia needed to be cannulated by catheters other than the standard left or right Judkin's catheter.[35] For the right trans-radial approach, both left and right Judkin's catheters end up usually in the right coronary or the noncoronary sinuses. Judkin's right catheters should be manipulated as in trans-femoral access, intubating the right coronary ostia after a slight clockwise rotation. For the cannulation of the left main coronary ostium, an initial clockwise rotation is needed, and this is followed by a gentle pull or push first and then a slight anti-clockwise rotation. In most high volume centers, the guiding catheters used are the long-tip Extra-backup 4F or 3.5F for left and right Judkin's catheters and 4F for right coronary PCI. Several other guiding catheters have been used for trans-radial PCI such as the Amplatz left 2F, Champ

TABLE 30-4	Guiding Catheters Used for Trans-radial Percutaneous Coronary Intervention		
Guiding Catheter (curves)	**Left Coronary**	**Right Coronary**	**Bypass Grafts**
Standard catheters			
Judkin's left (3.5F or 4F)	+	– (+ 3.5 curve)	–
Judkin's right (4F)	–	++++	Left/ right IMA
Amplatz left (2F)	++	+	Left SVG
Amplatz right	–	+	–
Extra-backup (3F or 3.5F)	++++	–	–
Multipurpose	+	+	Right SVG
Internal mammary	–	–	Left/right IMA
LCB/RCB	–	–/+	Left/right SVG
Ikari L	+	+	
Specific catheters (manufacturer)			
Kimny (Boston scientific)	+	+	–
MUTA L/R (Boston scientific)	+	+	–
Radial curve (Boston scientific)	+	+	
Fajadet's L/R (Cordis)	+	+	
Mann IM (Boston scientific)	–	–	Left or right IMA
Barbeau L/R (Cordis)	+	+	–
Brachial type K (Terumo)	+	+	
Tiger II (Terumo)	+	+	–

F, French; *IMA*, internal mammary artery; *LCB*, left coronary bypass; *RCB*, right coronary bypass; *SVG*, saphenous vein graft; *–*, unsuitable; *+*, suitable; *++*, very suitable; *++++*, recommended; *–/+*, suitable in some cases.

or the Multi-purpose used for both left and right trans-radial approaches. Finally, specific trans-radial guiding catheters have been developed, although the large majority of operators use standard guiding catheters. A list of guiding catheters used for the trans-radial approach is provided in Table 30-4. The diameter of the guiding catheters is also to be considered as 6F guiding catheters are more often associated with spasm and radial artery occlusion than are 5F catheters. The limitations of 5F catheters compared with 6F catheters are weaker backup because of the higher flexibility of the catheters and incompatibility with some devices (rotational atherectomy, thrombectomy, and distal protection devices, >4 mm coronary stents) or procedures (kissing stent or balloon for bifurcation lesions). Special attention should also be paid to the possibility of bubble formation from the Venturi effect when balloons or devices are rapidly removed from the catheter. Deep, but precautious, arterial intubation can be performed with 5F catheters when needed, that is, for crossing calcified coronary arteries.

DIFFICULT ANATOMY

Frequent variations are encountered in the arterial circulation of the upper limb among patients. During the initial phase of the learning curve, failure of the trans-radial approach usually occurs because of puncture failure, but with experienced operators, failure is more often related to difficult radial artery anatomy.

In a series of 1191 consecutive cases, the following anatomic situations were reported:[6]

- Anomalous upper branching of the radial artery: 3.2%
- High origin of the radial artery: 2.4%
- Radial or brachial artery tortuosity: 4.2% (S and Ω shape in 31% each)

In another series of 2211 consecutive patients, the authors reported a 98.9% success rate; in this series, 22.8% of patients had anatomic variations, including tortuosity (3.8%), stenosis (1.7%), hypoplasia (7.7%), abnormal origin of the radial artery (8.3%), and retro-oesophageal (lusoria) subclavian artery (0.45%).[41] Interestingly, the

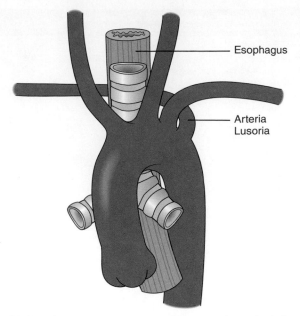

Figure 30-4   Schematic representation of retro-esophageal subclavian artery (arteria lusoria).

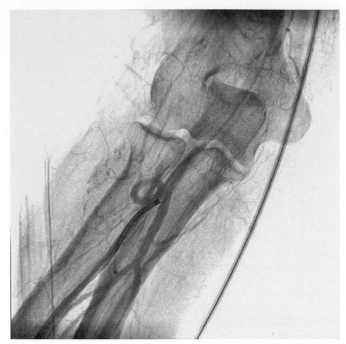

Figure 30-5   Radial artery Ω-shaped complete loop.

TABLE 30-5	**Anatomic Abnormalities**	
Anatomical Difficulties	*Solution*
Forearm	
Lateral position of the radial artery on the wrist	Change puncture site or access site
Hypoplasic radial artery	Change access site
Radial artery remnants	Guidewire progression under angiographic control
Radial artery loops	Hydrophilic-coated guidewires under angiographic control, 0.014 inch angioplasty guidewires
	Change access site in case of calcified "un-loopable" loops
Arm	
Brachial artery remnants	Guidewire progression under angiographic control
High origin of the radial artery	
Brachial artery loops	Hydrophilic-coated guidewires under angiographic control, 0.014 inch angioplasty guidewires
	Change access site in case of calcified "un-loopable" loops
Shoulder–Thorax	
Axillary or subclavian artery loops	Hydrophilic-coated guidewires under angiographic control; deep inspiration
Arteria lusoria (retro-oesophageal right subclavian artery)	Change access site in case of calcified "un-loopable" loops
Brachiocephalic arterial trunk abnormalities	Guidewire progression under angiographic control; deep inspiration
Posterior origin	Guidewire progression under angiographic control; deep inspiration; catheters adapted to aortic angulation
Bicarotidian trunks	
Thoracic aortic rotations	

rates of success in this experienced radial center were high in all anatomic variations (83% to 96.7% success rate) except in the case of the lusoria subclavian artery (60% success rate), which should be considered a contraindication to the trans-radial approach (Fig. 30-4). The most common anatomic variations and difficulties are listed in Table 30-5, and some examples are shown in Figures 30-5 through 30-8 and Videos 30-4 through 30-6 📹.

REPETITION OF TRANS-RADIAL PROCEDURES

Because of the risk of postprocedure radial artery occlusion (Video 30-7 📹), although such complication is rare and usually asymptomatic, the repetition of such procedures may be questioned. In a Japanese series of 812 patients with a first successful trans-radial access, the rates of access failure through the same radial artery in men and women were 3.5% and 7.9%, respectively, for the second attempt, 10% and 20% for the third attempt, and 30% and 50% for the fifth attempt.[42] Such data should be considered with caution as the number of patients with multiple procedures was very low in this series. Furthermore, in another series of 117 repeated ipsilateral trans-radial procedures, the success rate for the second procedure was similar to the first, although the rates of postprocedure radial artery occlusion assessed by ultrasound were higher after the second procedure (2.6% vs. 0%, $P = 0.01$).[43] Furthermore, both pathology examinations of radial arteries used for coronary artery bypass graft and optical coherence tomography have provided evidence of acute and chronic injury—intimal and medial tears and dissection, intimal thickening—especially in those who underwent repeat trans-radial interventions.[44] Such findings have led some to recommend that the trans-femoral approach be considered in patients with a low risk of femoral access–site complications and a high risk of repeated procedures, such as those with complex multi-vessel, high–re-stenosis–risk lesions or heart transplant recipients undergoing systematic annual angiography. However, this is not a concern at centers with high-volume trans-radial procedures.

COMPLICATIONS

The trans-radial access is associated with very low major access site–related complications. The most common complications are (1) radial artery spasm (Figs. 30-9 and 30-10 and Videos 30-7 and 30-8 📹) often related to painful procedures or excessive catheter manipulations and (2) asymptomatic, often reversible radial artery occlusion (Video 30-9 📹), which may occur in 3.8% to 22% and 0% to 19% of patients, respectively.[7,25,26,45] Female gender, diabetes, small body surface area, smoking history, diameter of the radial artery, and 6F versus 5F catheters have been related to radial artery spasm, and the reported

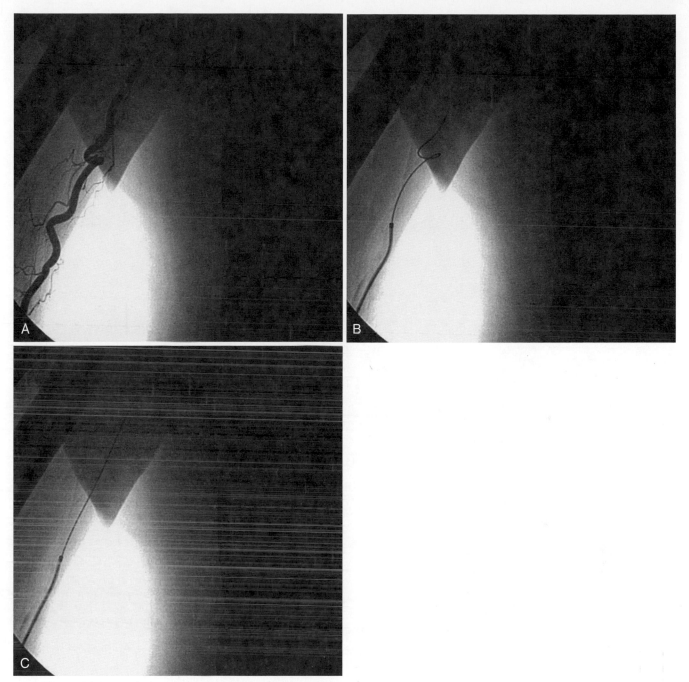

Figure 30-6 Brachial artery loop. **A,** Before wiring. **B,** During wiring. **C,** Artery unlooped by a hydrophilic-coated guidewire.

predictors of radial artery occlusion are small radial artery diameter, small difference between radial artery and sheath diameters, diabetes, no or low-dose anticoagulation, and repeat procedures using the same access site.[43,45,46] A list of reported trans-radial access–related complications is provided in Table 30-6.

Conclusion

Bleeding complications, including death, after PCI have been associated with higher rates of hard clinical events. The trans-radial approach is associated with a dramatic reduction in the risk of entry-site

complications compared with the trans-femoral approach and appears to be the easiest, safest, and most cost-effective way to control bleeding complications and improve clinical outcome after PCI. Growing evidence in large observational studies tends to show significant reduction in MACEs when the trans-radial approach to PCI especially in the setting of ST elevation myocardial infarction as recently demonstrated in the randomized trial RIVAL. Trans-radial access is associated with easy entry-point hemostasis, more comfort for patients, quick postprocedure ambulation, and the possibility of outpatient procedures.

The only "theoretical" contraindication to the trans-radial approach is the inadequate ulnar collateral circulation detected by

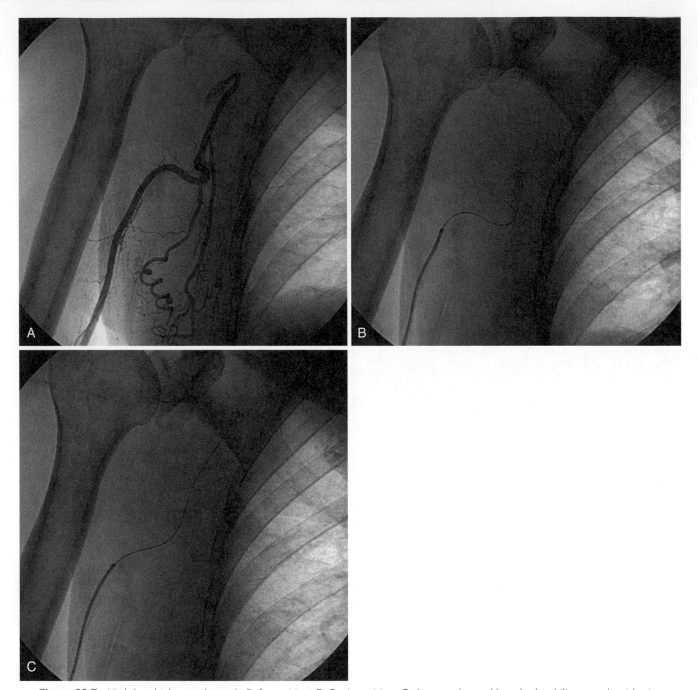

Figure 30-7   High brachial artery loop, **A,** Before wiring. **B,** During wiring. **C,** Artery unlooped by a hydrophilic-coated guidewire.

Allen's test, which continues to be recommended before the procedure, although many operators proceed without such a test because of its unknown value in predicting postprocedure complications. Even though the trans-radial access site seems to be more difficult, compared with the femoral artery initially during an learning curve, once the operator becomes aware of potential anatomic difficulties and ways to overcome such difficulties, the procedural success rates of the trans-radial approach become virtually identical to those of the trans-femoral approach, but without the access-site complications of the latter. There is a need for academic educational programs promoting the trans-radial approach among interventionalists so that this technique can be further developed. The trans-radial approach, once considered an alternative to the trans-femoral approach, is already the preferred method for PCI in many centers, and many believe that its generalization as the first-line method is just a matter of time.

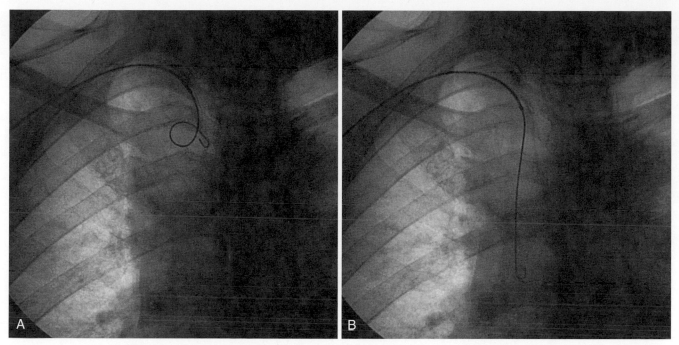

Figure 30-8 Subclavian loop. **A,** Before wiring. **B,** Artery unlooped by a standard preshaped guidewire.

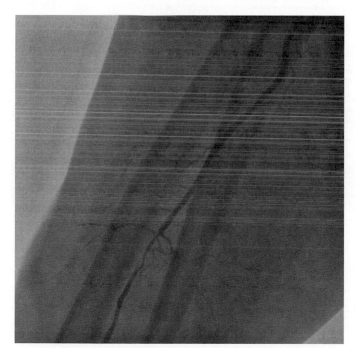

Figure 30-9 Radial artery spasm.

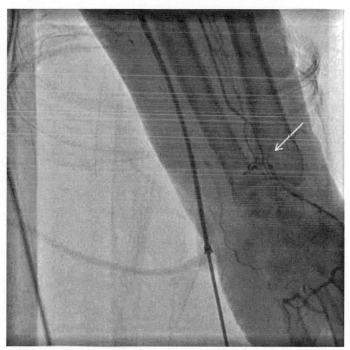

Figure 30-10 Radial artery stenosis (visualized after trans-ulnar opacification).

TABLE 30-6 Trans-radial Approach–Related Reported Complications			
Complications	**Frequency**	**Prevention**	**Solution**
Asymptomatic loss of radial pulse (reversible in approximately 50% of cases)	0%–9%	Spasmolytic cocktail 5 French (5F) catheters	—
Radial artery spasm	4%–23%	Lidocaine cream before puncture Anxiolytic preparation Avoid excessive catheter manipulation and change Preventive spasmolytic cocktail Hydrophilic-coated sheath guidewires and catheters	Spasmolytic cocktail General sedation
Radial artery extraction (refractory spasm)	Exceptional	Avoid excessive force to remove catheter or sheath	Spasmolytic cocktail General sedation
Radial artery false aneurysm	Exceptional	—	Local compression/Surgery
Arterio-venous fistula	Exceptional	Avoid perforation	Local compression/Surgery
Symptomatic finger/hand ischemia	Exceptional	Avoid radial puncture, if inadequate Allen's test 5F catheters Adequate anti-thrombotic cocktails Spasmolytic cocktails	Anticoagulation/Surgery
Bleeding at the puncture site	0%–2%	—	Local compression
Forearm hematoma and compartment syndrome	Exceptional	Control progression of guidewire, long arterial sheath to stop the bleeding in case of perforation; covered stent in case of uncontrollable perforation	Surgery/Leeches
Vascular injury/dissection (radial, brachial, subclavian, carotid arteries)	Exceptional	Control progression of guidewire—especially hydrophilic coated-wires	Anticoagulation/Stent/Surgery

REFERENCES

1. Campeau L: Percutaneous radial artery approach for coronary angiography. *Cathet Cardiovasc Diagn* 16(1):3–7, 1989.
2. Rao SV, Ou FS, Wang TY, et al: Trends in the prevalence and outcomes of radial and femoral approaches to percutaneous coronary intervention: A report from the National Cardiovascular Data Registry. *J Am Coll Cardiol* 1(4):379–386, 2008.
3. Montalescot G, Cayla G, Collet JP, et al: Immediate vs delayed intervention for acute coronary syndromes: A randomized clinical trial. *JAMA* 302(9):947–954, 2009.
4. Montalescot G, Zeymer U, Cohen M, et al: ATOLL: An international randomized study comparing IV enoxaparin to IV UFH in primary PCI. *Eur Heart J* 31:2042, 2010.
5. Hildick-Smith DJ, Lowe MD, Walsh JT, et al: Coronary angiography from the radial artery—experience, complications and limitations. *Int J Cardiol* 64(3):231–239, 1998.
6. Yoo BS, Yoon J, Ko JY, et al: Anatomical consideration of the radial artery for transradial coronary procedures: Arterial diameter, branching anomaly and vessel tortuosity. *Int J Cardiol* 101(3):421–427, 2005.
7. Saito S, Miyake S, Hosokawa G, et al: Transradial coronary intervention in Japanese patients. *Cathet Cardiovasc Interv* 46(1):37–41; discussion 42, 1999.
8. Agostoni P, Biondi-Zoccai GG, de Benedictis ML, et al: Radial versus femoral approach for percutaneous coronary diagnostic and interventional procedures: Systematic overview and meta-analysis of randomized trials. *J Am Coll Cardiol* 44(2):349–356, 2004.
9. Jolly SS, Amlani S, Hamon M, et al: Radial versus femoral access for coronary angiography or intervention and the impact on major bleeding and ischemic events: A systematic review and meta-analysis of randomized trials. *Am Heart J* 157(1):132–140, 2009.
10. Cox N, Resnic FS, Popma JJ, et al: Comparison of the risk of vascular complications associated with femoral and radial access coronary catheterization procedures in obese versus nonobese patients. *Am J Cardiol* 94(9):1174–1177, 2004.
11. Louvard Y, Benamer H, Garot P, et al: Comparison of transradial and transfemoral approaches for coronary angiography and angioplasty in octogenarians (the OCTOPLUS study). *Am J Cardiol* 94(9):1177–1180, 2004.
12. Cantor WJ, Puley G, Natarajan MK, et al: Radial versus femoral access for emergent percutaneous coronary intervention with adjunct glycoprotein IIb/IIIa inhibition in acute myocardial infarction—the RADIAL-AMI pilot randomized trial. *Am Heart J* 150(3):543–549, 2005.
13. Cruden NL, Teh CH, Starkey IR, et al: Reduced vascular complications and length of stay with transradial rescue angioplasty for acute myocardial infarction. *Cathet Cardiovasc Interv* 70(5):670–675, 2007.
14. Hetherington SL, Adam Z, Morley R, et al: Primary percutaneous coronary intervention for acute ST-segment elevation myocardial infarction: Changing patterns of vascular access, radial versus femoral artery. *Heart* 95(19):1612–1618, 2009.
15. Pancholy S, Patel T, Sanghvi K, et al: Comparison of door-to-balloon times for primary PCI using transradial versus transfemoral approach. *Cathet Cardiovasc Interv* 2010;75(7):991–995.

16. Vorobcsuk A, Konyi A, Aradi D, et al: Transradial versus transfemoral percutaneous coronary intervention in acute myocardial infarction: Systematic overview and meta-analysis. *Am Heart J* 158(5):814–821, 2009.
17. Vuurmans T, Byrne J, Fretz E, et al: Chronic kidney injury in patients after cardiac catheterisation or percutaneous coronary intervention: A comparison of radial and femoral approaches (from the British Columbia Cardiac and Renal Registries). *Heart* 96(19):1538–1542, 2010.
18. Montalescot G, Ongen Z, Guindy R, et al: Predictors of outcome in patients undergoing PCI. Results of the RIVIERA study. *Int J Cardiol* 129(3):379–387, 2008.
18a. Jolly SS, Yusuf S, Cairns J, et al: Radial versus femoral access for coronary angiography and intervention in patients with acute coronary syndromes (RIVAL): a randomised, parallel group, multicentre trial. *Lancet* 377(9775):1409–1420, 2011.
19. Kiemeneij F, Laarman GJ, Odekerken D, et al: A randomized comparison of percutaneous transluminal coronary angioplasty by the radial, brachial and femoral approaches: The access study. *J Am Coll Cardiol* 29(6):1269–1275, 1997.
20. Benit E, Missault L, Eeman T, et al: Brachial, radial, or femoral approach for elective Palmaz-Schatz stent implantation: A randomized comparison. *Cathet Cardiovasc Diagn* 41(2):124–130, 1997.
21. Aptecar E, Pernes JM, Chabane-Chaouch M, et al: Transulnar versus transradial artery approach for coronary angioplasty: The PCVI-CUBA study. *Cathet Cardiovasc Interv* 67(5):711–720, 2006.
22. Roussanov O, Wilson SJ, Henley K, et al: Cost-effectiveness of the radial versus femoral artery approach to diagnostic cardiac catheterization. *J Invasive Cardiol* 19(8):349–353, 2007.
23. Kim MH, Cha KS, Kim HJ, et al: Primary stenting for acute myocardial infarction via the transradial approach: A safe and useful alternative to the transfemoral approach. *J Invasive Cardiol* 12(6):292–296, 2000.
24. Valsecchi O, Musumeci G, Vassileva A, et al: Safety, feasibility and efficacy of transradial primary angioplasty in patients with acute myocardial infarction. *Ital Heart J* 4(5):329–334, 2003.
25. Valsecchi O, Musumeci G, Vassileva A, et al: Safety and feasibility of transradial coronary angioplasty in elderly patients. *Ital Heart J* 5(12):926–931, 2004.
26. Kiemeneij F, Laarman GJ, de Melker E: Transradial artery coronary angioplasty. *Am Heart J* 129(1):1–7, 1995.
27. Nagai S, Abe S, Sato T, et al: Ultrasonic assessment of vascular complications in coronary angiography and angioplasty after transradial approach. *Am J Cardiol* 83(2):180–186, 1999.
28. Greenwood MJ, Della-Siega AJ, Fretz EB, et al: Vascular communications of the hand in patients being considered for transradial coronary angiography: Is the Allen's test accurate? *J Am Coll Cardiol* 46(11):2013–2017, 2005.
29. Barbeau GR, Arsenault F, Dugas L, et al: Evaluation of the ulnopalmar arterial arches with pulse oximetry and plethysmography: Comparison with the Allen's test in 1010 patients. *Am Heart J* 147(3):489–493, 2004.
30. Kawashima O, Endoh N, Terashima M, et al: Effectiveness of right or left radial approach for coronary angiography. *Cathet Cardiovasc Interv* 61(3):333–337, 2004.

31. Rathore S, Stables RH, Pauriah M, et al: Impact of length and hydrophilic coating of the introducer sheath on radial artery spasm during transradial coronary intervention: A randomized study. *J Am Coll Cardiol* 3(5):475–483, 2010.
32. Chen CW, Lin CL, Lin TK, et al: A simple and effective regimen for prevention of radial artery spasm during coronary catheterization. *Cardiology* 105(1):43–47, 2006.
33. Varenne O, Jegou A, Cohen R, et al: Prevention of arterial spasm during percutaneous coronary interventions through radial artery: The SPASM study. *Cathet Cardiovasc Interv* 68(2):231–235, 2006.
34. Ruiz-Salmeron RJ, Mora R, Masotti M, et al: Assessment of the efficacy of phentolamine to prevent radial artery spasm during cardiac catheterization procedures: A randomized study comparing phentolamine vs. verapamil. *Cathet Cardiovasc Interv* 66(2):192–198, 2005.
35. Spaulding C, Lefevre T, Funck F, et al: Left radial approach for coronary angiography: Results of a prospective study. *Cathet Cardiovasc Diagn* 39(4):365–370, 1996.
36. Venkatesh K, Mann T: Transitioning from heparin to bivalirudin in patients undergoing ad hoc transradial interventional procedures: A pilot study. *J Invasive Cardiol* 18(3):120–124, 2006.
37. Choussat R, Black A, Bossi I, et al: Vascular complications and clinical outcome after coronary angioplasty with platelet IIb/IIIa receptor blockade. Comparison of transradial vs transfemoral arterial access. *Eur Heart J* 21(8):662–667, 2000.
38. Philippe F, Larrazet F, Meziane T, et al: Comparison of transradial vs. transfemoral approach in the treatment of acute myocardial infarction with primary angioplasty and abciximab. *Cathet Cardiovasc Interv* 61(1):67–73, 2004.
39. Kassam S, Cantor WJ, Patel D, et al: Radial versus femoral access for rescue percutaneous coronary intervention with adjuvant glycoprotein IIb/IIIa inhibitor use. *Can J Cardiol* 20(14):1439–1442, 2004.
40. Bertrand OF, De Larochelliere R, Rodes-Cabau J, et al: A randomized study comparing same-day home discharge and abciximab bolus only to overnight hospitalization and abciximab bolus and infusion after transradial coronary stent implantation. *Circulation* 114(24):2636–2643, 2006.
41. Valsecchi O, Vassileva A, Musumeci G, et al: Failure of transradial approach during coronary interventions: Anatomic considerations. *Cathet Cardiovasc Interv* 67(6):870–878, 2006.
42. Sakai H, Ikeda S, Harada T, et al: Limitations of successive transradial approach in the same arm: The Japanese experience. *Cathet Cardiovasc Interv* 54(2):204–208, 2001.
43. Yoo BS, Lee SH, Ko JY, et al: Procedural outcomes of repeated transradial coronary procedure. *Cathet Cardiovasc Interv* 58(3):301–304, 2003.
44. Yonetsu T, Kakuta T, Lee T, et al: Assessment of acute injuries and chronic intimal thickening of the radial artery after transradial coronary intervention by optical coherence tomography. *Eur Heart J* 31(13):1608–1615, 2010.
45. Coppola J, Patel T, Kwan T, et al: Nitroglycerin, nitroprusside, or both, in preventing radial artery spasm during transradial artery catheterization. *J Invasive Cardiol* 18(4):155–158, 2005.
46. Hildick-Smith DJ, Walsh JT, Lowe MD, et al: Transradial coronary angiography in patients with contraindications to the femoral

approach: An analysis of 500 cases. *Cathet Cardiovasc Interv* 61(1):60–66, 2004.

47. Kiemeneij F, Laarman GJ: Percutaneous transradial artery approach for coronary Palmaz-Schatz stent implantation. *Am Heart J* 128(1):167–174, 1994.

48. Kiemeneij F, Laarman GJ: Transradial artery Palmaz-Schatz coronary stent implantation: Results of a single-center feasibility study. *Am Heart J* 130(1):14–21, 1995.

49. Louvard Y, Ludwig J, Lefevre T, et al: Transradial approach for coronary angioplasty in the setting of acute myocardial infarction: A dual-center registry. *Cathet Cardiovasc Interv* 55(2):206–211, 2002.

50. Mulukutla SR, Cohen HA: Feasibility and efficacy of transradial access for coronary interventions in patients with acute myocardial infarction. *Cathet Cardiovasc Interv* 57(2):167–171, 2002.

51. Mann JT, 3rd, Cubeddu MG, Schneider JE, et al: Right radial access for PTCA: A prospective study demonstrates reduced com-plications and hospital charges. *J Invasive Cardiol* 8(Suppl D): 40D–44D, 1996.

52. Mann T, Cubeddu G, Bowen J, et al: Stenting in acute coronary syndromes: A comparison of radial versus femoral access sites. *J Am Coll Cardiol* 32(3):572–576, 1998.

53. Mann T, Cowper PA, Peterson ED, et al: Transradial coronary stenting: Comparison with femoral access closed with an arterial suture device. *Cathet Cardiovasc Interv* 49(2):150–156, 2000.

54. Louvard Y, Lefevre T, Allain A, et al: Coronary angiography through the radial or the femoral approach: The CARAFE study. *Cathet Cardiovasc Interv* 52(2):181–187, 2001.

55. Saito S, Tanaka S, Hiroe Y, et al: Comparative study on transradial approach vs. transfemoral approach in primary stent implantation for patients with acute myocardial infarction: Results of the test for myocardial infarction by prospective unicenter randomization for access sites (TEMPURA) trial. *Cathet Cardiovasc Interv* 59(1):26–33, 2003.

56. Slagboom T, Kiemeneij F, Laarman GJ, et al: Outpatient coronary angioplasty: Feasible and safe. *Catheter Cardiovasc Interv* 64(4): 421–427, 2005.

57. Brasselet C, Tassan S, Nazeyrollas P, et al: Randomised comparison of femoral versus radial approach for percutaneous coronary intervention using abciximab in acute myocardial infarction: Results of the FARMI trial. *Heart* 93(12):1556–1561, 2007.

58. Li WM, Li Y, Zhao JY, et al: Safety and feasibility of emergent percutaneous coronary intervention with the transradial access in patients with acute myocardial infarction. *Chinese Med J* 120(7): 598–600, 2007.

59. Achenbach S, Ropers D, Kallert L, et al: Transradial versus trans-femoral approach for coronary angiography and intervention in patients above 75 years of age. *Cathet Cardiovasc Interv* 72(5):629–635, 2008.

31 The Role of the Cardiac Surgeon

G. RUSSELL REISS | MATTHEW R. WILLIAMS

KEY POINTS

- The role of the cardiac surgeon in the catheterization laboratory (cath lab) has been traditionally one of providing surgical backup or standby for the interventional cardiologist. The need for such service waxes and wanes parallel to the development and mastery of each new interventional procedure and also correlates with improvement in medical device technology and the total product life cycle.

- Although the incidence has become very low, emergency revascularization surgery for failed percutaneous catheter intervention (PCI) still persists and portends mortality rates approaching 15% in some centers. Performance of elective or high-risk PCI is not recommended without surgical backup or without a defined plan for expeditious surgical intervention at the same institution or, in select cases, at a nearby center of excellence.

- New interventional procedures are often founded on open surgical approaches, converted first to minimally invasive procedures by surgeons, and later translated to percutaneous techniques by interventionalists. These procedures take a defined pathway from conception to clinical acceptance as standard of care. This pathway requires collaboration among surgeons, interventionalists, medical device makers, and the U.S. Food and Drug Administration (FDA), in addition to the execution of well-designed clinical trials.

- With cardiac surgeons opting to be more minimally invasive, integrating percutaneous methods in their daily routine, and interventional cardiologists striving to definitively treat more complex structural heart disease such as aortic stenosis and mitral regurgitation in the cath lab, the clinical paths of the surgeon and the interventional cardiologist have intersected and begun to overlap significantly. This has promoted the cross-pollination of the two disciplines, which is essential for continued innovation in cardiovascular medicine. As a result, the "heart team" model should be considered the standard of care in cardiac centers of excellence.

- The future of interventional cardiology and cardiovascular surgery will require closer collaboration between the surgeon and the cardiologist than has been seen in decades. An overlapping clinical training pathway incorporating certain fundamental principles and skills from both surgical and medical training programs will need to be developed to ensure the appropriate training of the future cardiovascular interventionalist.

- Building a hybrid cardiovascular interventional program in which patients can receive expert treatment from both surgeons and interventionalists in the same setting requires multi-disciplinary input from cardiology, surgery, anesthesia, and radiology, in addition to technical and ancillary staff from both the operating room and the cath lab. Certain pitfalls during the creation of the hybrid infrastructure can be avoided by heeding lessons learned from existing experienced hybrid centers.

The role of the cardiac surgeon in the cath lab can be broadly described in three categories. First, the surgeon has been traditionally viewed as a standby operator backing up the interventional cardiologist in case of any untoward complication or emergency requiring surgical intervention. The need for this role waxes and wanes with the advent and subsequent mastery of each new procedure adopted in the cath lab. Formal surgical standby for routine PCI, where a surgeon is preemptively notified and is waiting in the hospital, no longer exists in most centers, as complications requiring surgical intervention have become quite uncommon in established centers. However, current published guidelines for elective PCI still recommend the availability of an experienced surgical team that can be activated quickly in the event of a cath lab emergency.[1] Some evidence exists that primary PCI performed at certain highly experienced centers without an existing aortocoronary bypass program may be reasonable and have some benefit over the alternative use of fibrinolytic therapy for acute myocardial infarction (MI).[2] This concept is currently not promoted by the consensus of the cardiovascular community.

The second role the cardiac surgeon plays in the cath lab is that of an interventionalist or hybrid cardiac surgeon. The hybrid cardiac surgeon takes a very active role in the cath lab and, in some cases, has formally cross-trained in interventional cardiology. This establishes a new identity for the cardiac surgeon who has traditionally remained outside the cath lab waiting for surgical referrals or the occurrence of a cardiovascular emergency. Still far from the norm, but increasing in numbers, hybrid cardiac surgeons serve an important function in today's more complex interventional procedures such as transcatheter aortic valve replacement (TAVR), combined coronary artery bypass grafting (CABG)/PCI, and hybrid Valve/PCI procedures. As time moves forward and the "heart team" model becomes widely adopted, hybrid surgeons will play a bigger part in shaping the cath lab of the future. As the convergence of cardiology and cardiac surgery continues, the need to have simultaneous skill sets present at the interventional table will become more commonplace and, in many instances, required.

The third role of the cardiac surgeon is that of an innovator. The cardiovascular surgeon's intraoperative experience with structural heart disease and strict adherence to applied surgical principles cannot be underestimated. It provides a unique perspective that can only be gained by years of performing open-heart surgery and mastering a true three-dimensional understanding of the anatomy of the heart and the great vessels. The cardiac surgeon will contribute valuable insight to the conception of new techniques and procedures, their development, and their refinement to art forms, which will ultimately be performed in the interventional suite by the cardiovascular interventionalist of tomorrow.

Historical Perspective

Throughout history, alongside their colleagues in cardiology, radiology, and other disciplines, surgeons have participated in pioneering the majority of invasive procedures and technical innovations in cardiovascular medicine. The input of the surgeon has always been regarded as the gold standard for advice on the anatomic aspects and physiologic practicality of a proposed invasive procedure. With their surgical feasibility proven, new clinical techniques have been adopted by the medical community and have spawned numerous specialties based on the initial curiosity and investigation of the surgeon and his colleagues. Not unique to cardiovascular medicine, this evolution and translation of skill sets has occurred in several areas such as gastroenterology with endoscopy; pulmonary critical care with intensive care, bronchoscopy, and ventilator management; and most recently with interventional radiologists performing vascular intervention, tumor biopsy, thoracostomy, abscess drainage, and more. The field of interventional cardiology has likewise evolved with surgical advancement. Before the advent of modern angiography, surgeons routinely performed their own angiograms in order to define the vascular anatomy prior to embarking on surgical intervention. The concept of having proper imaging or a "roadmap" before open-heart surgery has been a well-accepted practice in cardiovascular surgery for decades. Looking back, in 1929, Werner Forssmann, a surgical trainee at the time, passed a urinary catheter through the vein in his own arm to his heart and subsequently irradiated himself in spite of the reprimand of his department and his lab assistant's discouragement. After successfully demonstrating the catheter to be in the right atrium, Forssmann was credited with performing the first cardiac catheterization.[3] Forssmann received the Nobel Prize in 1956 along with Andre Coumand and Dickinson Richards, for "the role of heart catheterization and angiocardiography in the advancement of medicine."[4] In 1953, Sven-Ivar Seldinger, who was briefly trained as a surgeon before becoming a radiologist, developed a percutaneous approach for the introduction of vascular catheters for both right and left heart catheterization.[5] This technique is now the most common percutaneous approach used for gaining access to the vascular tree. In 1977, Andreas Gruentzig, along with his surgical colleague Richard Myle, inflated the first catheter-guided balloon in a coronary artery intraoperatively during a coronary bypass operation.[3,6] Gruentzig's novel procedure eventually became known as percutaneous transluminal catheter angioplasty (PTCA) and set the stage for modern interventional cardiology and PCI.[7] The list of events and milestones that illustrates how surgeons have remained steadfast beside their nonsurgical colleagues as a fundamental part of developing and advancing nearly every invasive discipline in medicine is quite impressive. Today, the cardiac surgeon is likewise a key team member in any successful and innovative interventional program. The magnitude and activity of the surgeon's role in the day-to day proceedings of the interventional suite is not always a steady one; rather, it usually depends on the risk of each intervention to the patient and the learning curve associated with the introduction of each new procedure, along with the level of the hands-on interest of the individual surgeon. As new procedures that propose to alter the current standard of care, for example, trans-catheter aortic valve implantation (TAVI), are adopted into practice, it is critical for the surgeon's role to be increased while a new comfort zone of safety and efficacy is reached by the entire interventional team.

Surgical Standby

During the early years of PTCA and PCI, surgeons, by necessity, were compelled to remain in house and on "surgical standby" for any urgent consultations and surgical emergencies that resulted from early interventional procedures. Fraught with technical pitfalls and clinical unknowns, more often than not, early complications in the cath lab necessitated an emergent trip to the operating room, often with a patient in extreme cardiogenic shock.[8-10] As a result, indications for emergency CABG after failed PCI became well established over time. The most common indications include abrupt vessel closure, dissection, incomplete revascularization, perforation, and unsuccessful dilation or PCI in addition to other miscellaneous clinical scenarios (Table 31-1).[11] As angiography, PTCA, and surgical techniques improved and medical equipment became more advanced, surgeons were no longer required to remain in such proximity to the cath lab.[12,13] This was particularly true with the introduction of the Gianturco–Roubin stent and its rapid adoption as a "bailout catheter" by the interventional cardiology community.[14,15] Almost uniformly, and for decades, active PCI centers have enjoyed a steady reduction in the percentage of cases requiring emergency CABG after failed PCI (Fig. 31-1).[16] However, it still must be carefully noted that despite universal trends demonstrating decreased morbidity and mortality from PCI, the consequences of complications in the interventional suite remain potentially catastrophic. Thus, it is still common practice today, and also recommended by the ACC/AHA/SCAI Practice Guidelines, that the majority of elective PCI be performed at centers with an active open-heart surgery program, as certain interventional decisions must be discussed with a cardiac surgeon before proceeding with PCI.[1] In the event of

TABLE 31-1	Indications for Emergency Coronary Bypass Surgery after Failed Percutaneous Coronary Intervention		
Periods	1979–1994	1995–1999	2000–2003
Indication	(n = 258 of 8905)	(n = 56 of 7605)	(n = 21 of 6577)
Abrupt vessel closure	55 (21%)	2 (4%)	3 (14%)
Dissection	88 (34%)	12 (22%)	3 (14%)
Incomplete revascularization	26 (10%)	7 (13%)	4 (19%)
Perforation	1 (0.5%)	1 (2%)	2 (9%)
Unsuccessful dilation	67 (26%)	28 (50%)	7 (33%)
Other	21 (8%)	6 (10%)	2 (9%)

Modified from Yang EH, Gumina RJ, et al: Emergency coronary artery bypass for percutaneous interventions: Changes in the incidence, clinical characteristics, and indications from 1979 to 2003, *J Am Coll Cardiol* 46:2004–2009, 2005.

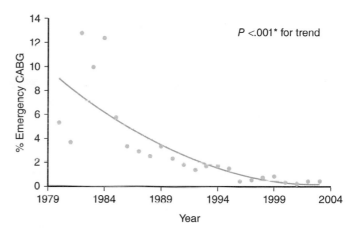

Figure 31-1 Percentage of patients requiring emergency coronary artery bypass grafting (CABG) after percutaneous coronary intervention (PCI) from 1979 to 2003 (n = 23,087). The Armitage test for trend is indicated by an asterisk. (*From Yang EH, Gumina RJ, et al: Emergency coronary artery bypass for percutaneous interventions: Changes in the incidence, clinical characteristics, and indications from 1979 to 2003, J Am Coll Cardiol 46:2004–2009, 2005.*)

emergent need for aortocoronary bypass, outcomes have been shown to be better in centers with an open-heart surgery program (Table 31-2; Fig. 31-2).[11,16] According to current guidelines, on-site surgical backup should provide emergency hemodynamic support and expeditious revascularization to deal with complications that cannot be addressed in the cath lab (Table 31-3). Often, these complications during PCI are life threatening in terms of hemodynamic stability and are associated with prolonged periods of ischemia. Such emergencies require the availability of a cardiac surgery team experienced in emergency aortocoronary operations. Thus, on-site cardiac surgical backup should provide readily available cardiac surgical support in the event of a hemodynamic or ischemic emergency. On-site cardiac surgical backup is also a surrogate for an institution's overall capability to provide a highly experienced and promptly available team to respond to a cath lab emergency.[1] The issues of cardiac surgical backup and the level of committed resources that are needed are frequently revisited; most centers today use the "first-available operating room" model to remain efficient and to maximize resources. Some centers rely on off-site surgical backup, but this is the exception rather than the rule, and such practice exposes the patient to a finite, but potentially fatal, risk and is deemed unnecessary in most areas of the country. Recommendations for primary PCI for ST elevation myocardial infarction (STEMI) without on-site cardiac surgery are given in Table 31-4.[17] The apparent success of centers performing PCI without on-site cardiac

TABLE 31-2 Coronary Artery Bypass Grafting and Mortality Rates Following Percutaneous Coronary Intervention at Hospitals without and with On-site Coronary Artery Bypass Grafting Surgery					
	No. of Patients (%)				
Outcomes	**WITHOUT ON-SITE CABG SURGERY**	**WITH ON-SITE CABG SURGERY**	*Unadjusted P value*	*Adjusted Odds Ratio (95% CI)**	*Adjusted P value*
All PCIs					
No. of patients	8,168	617,686		621,530[†]	
Mortality	492 (6)	20,393 (3.3)	<0.001	1.29 (1.14–1.47)	<0.001
CABG surgery	160 (2)	8,321 (1.4)	<0.001	1.05 (0.87–1.27)	0.59
Primary/rescue PCI					
No. of patients	1,795	34,537		36,235[†]	
Mortality	202 (11.3)	4,209 (12.2)	0.24	0.93 (0.80–1.08)	0.34
CABG surgery	82 (4.6)	1,772 (5.1)	0.29	0.95 (0.73–1.22)	0.67
Non-primary/rescue PCI					
No. of patients	6,373	583,149		585,295[†]	
Mortality	290 (4.6)	16,184 (2.8)	<0.001	1.38 (1.14–1.67)	0.001
CABG surgery	78 (1.2)	6,549 (1.1)	0.45	0.92 (0.73–1.17)	0.52

CABG, coronary artery bypass graft; *CI*, confidence interval; *PCI*, percutaneous coronary intervention.

*Adjusted for age, gender, race, year, Charlson comorbidity score, primary diagnosis of acute myocardial infarction, acuity, multi-vessel PCI, and stent use.

[†]Adjusted models excluded 4324 patients (0.7%) missing on patient covariates; 45 (4 among primary/rescue PCI) among patients without on-site CABG surgery and 4279 (93 among primary/rescue PCI) among patients with on-site CABG surgery.

Wennberg DE, Lucas FL, Siewers AE, Kellett MA, Malenka DJ: Outcomes of percutaneous coronary interventions performed at centers without and with on-site coronary artery bypass graft surgery, *JAMA* 292:1965, 2004.

TABLE 31-3 Role of On-site Cardiac Surgical Back-Up for Percutaneous Coronary Intervention
Class I
Elective PCI should be performed by operators with acceptable annual volume (at least 75 procedures per year) at high-volume centers (more than 400 procedures annually) that provide immediately available on-site emergency cardiac surgical services. (Level of Evidence: B)
Primary PCI for patients with STEMI should be performed in facilities with on-site cardiac surgery. (Level of Evidence: B)
Class III
Elective PCI should not be performed at institutions that do not provide on-site cardiac surgery. (Level of Evidence: C)*

*Several centers have reported satisfactory results on the basis of careful case selection with well-defined arrangements for immediate transfer to a surgical program (333–337; 348–353). Wennberg et al, found higher mortality in the Medicare database for patients undergoing elective PCI in institutions without on-site cardiac surgery (6.0% versus 3.3% respectively. Adjusted P Value <.001). This recommendation may be subject to revision as clinical data and experience increase.

Wennberg DE, Lucas FL, Siewers AE, Kellett MA, Malenka DJ: Outcomes of percutaneous coronary interventions performed at centers without and with onsite coronary artery bypass graft surgery, *JAMA* 292:1965, 2004.

TABLE 31-4 Primary Percutaneous Coronary Intervention for ST Elevation Myocardial Infarction without On-site Cardiac Surgery
Class IIb
Primary percutaneous coronary intervention (PCI) for patients with ST elevation myocardial infarction (STEMI) might be considered in hospitals without on-site cardiac surgery provided that appropriate planning for program development has been accomplished. This should include appropriately experienced physician operators (more than 75 total PCIs and, ideally, at least 11 primary PCIs per year for STEMI); an experienced catheterization team on an all-day, all-week call schedule; and a well-equipped catheterization laboratory with digital imaging equipment, a full array of interventional equipment, and intra-aortic balloon pump capability. A proven plan for rapid transport to a cardiac surgery operating room in a nearby hospital with appropriate hemodynamic support capability for transfer should be in place. The procedure should be limited to patients with STEMI or MI with new or presumably new left bundle branch block on electrocardiogram (ECG) and should be performed in a timely fashion (goal of balloon inflation within 90 minutes of presentation) by persons skilled in the procedure (at least 75 PCIs per year) and at hospitals performing a minimum of 36 primary PCI procedures per year. (Level of Evidence: B)
Class III
Primary PCI should not be performed in hospitals without on-site cardiac surgery and without a proven plan for rapid transport to a cardiac surgery operating room in a nearby hospital or without appropriate hemodynamic support capability for transfer. (Level of Evidence: C)

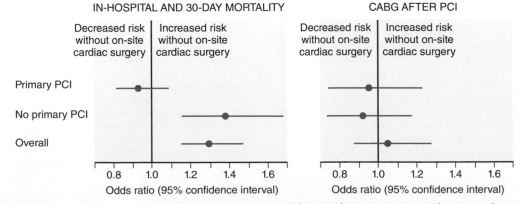

IN-HOSPITAL AND 30-DAY MORTALITY — CABG AFTER PCI

Figure 31-2   The increased risk of post–percutaneous coronary intervention (PCI) mortality in institutions without a cardiac surgery program persisted after adjustment for differences in case mix. Overall, the odds of death for patients having their PCIs in hospitals without on-site cardiac surgery was 29% higher than for patients having PCIs in hospitals with cardiac surgery (odds ratio [OR] 1.29; 95% confidence interval [CI]). (*From Wennberg DE, Lucas FL, Siewers AE, Kellett MA, Malenka DJ: Outcomes of percutaneous coronary interventions performed at centers without and with onsite coronary artery bypass graft surgery, JAMA 292:1965, 2004.*)

TABLE 31-5	Patient Selection for Primary Percutaneous Coronary Intervention and Emergency Aortocoronary Bypass at Hospitals without On-site Cardiac Surgery

Avoid intervention in hemodynamically stable patients with:

- Significant (≥60%) stenosis of an unprotected left main coronary artery upstream from an acute occlusion in the left coronary system that might be disrupted by the angioplasty catheter
- Extremely long or angulated infarct-related lesions with TIMI grade 3 flow
- Infarct-related lesions with TIMI grade 3 flow in stable patients with three-vessel disease
- Infarct-related lesions of small or secondary vessels
- Hemodynamically significant lesions in other than the infarct artery

Transfer for emergency aortocoronary bypass surgery patients with:

- High-grade residual left main or multi-vessel coronary disease and clinical or hemodynamic instability present after primary PCI of occluded vessels, preferably with IABP support.

IABP, intra-aortic balloon pump; *PCI*, percutaneous coronary intervention; *TIMI*, thrombolysis in myocardial infarction.
Wharton TP, Jr., McNamara NS, Fedele FA, Jacobs MI, Gladstone AR, Funk EJ: Primary angioplasty for the treatment of acute myocardial infarction: Experience at two community hospitals without cardiac surgery, *J Am Coll Cardiol* 33:1257–1265, 1999.

TABLE 31-6	Criteria for the Performance of Primary Percutaneous Coronary Intervention at Hospitals without On-site Cardiac Surgery

- The operators must be experienced interventionalists who regularly perform elective PCI at a surgical center (≥75 cases per year). The catheterization laboratory must perform a minimum of 36 primary PCI procedures per year.
- The nursing and technical catheterization laboratory staff must be experienced in handling acutely ill patients and must be comfortable with using interventional equipment. They must have acquired experience in dedicated interventional laboratories at a surgical center. They participate in an all-day, all-year call schedule.
- The catheterization laboratory itself must be well equipped, with optimal imaging systems, resuscitative equipment, and IABP support, and must be well stocked with a broad array of interventional equipment.
- The cardiac care unit nurses must be adept in hemodynamic monitoring and IABP management.
- The hospital administration must fully support the program and enable the fulfillment of the above institutional requirements.
- There must be formalized written protocols in place for immediate and efficient transfer of patients to the nearest cardiac surgical facility that are reviewed or tested on a regular (quarterly) basis.
- Primary PCI must be performed routinely as the treatment of choice round the clock for a large proportion of patients with AMI, to ensure streamlined care paths and increased case volumes.
- Case selection for the performance of primary PCI must be rigorous. Criteria for the types of lesions appropriate for primary PCI and for the selection for transfer for emergency aortocoronary bypass surgery are shown in Table 31-5.
- There must be an ongoing program of outcomes analysis and formalized periodic case review.
- Institutions should participate in a 3- to 6-month period of implementation, during which time a formalized primary PCI program that includes establishment of standards, training of staff, detailed logistic development, and creation of a quality-assessment and error-management system is developed and instituted.

AMI, acute myocardial infarction; *IABP*, intra-aortic balloon pump; *PCI*, percutaneous coronary intervention.
Wharton TP, Jr., McNamara NS, Fedele FA, Jacobs MI, Gladstone AR, Funk EJ: Primary angioplasty for the treatment of acute myocardial infarction: Experience at two community hospitals without cardiac surgery, *J Am Coll Cardiol* 33:1257–1265, 1999.

TABLE 31-7	Surgical Procedures Currently Performed in the Interventional Suite

- Angiography
- Right and left heart volume pressure evaluation
- Temporary and long-term venous access
- Pacemaker implantation
- Atrial fibrillation surgery (maze procedure)
- Vena cava filter implantation
- Valvuloplasty
- Congenital heart defect repairs
- Atrial septal defect (ASD) and patent foramen ovale (PFO) closure
- Arterial and venous stenosis
- Carotid endarterectomy
- Abdominal aortic aneurysm repair
- Thoracic aortic aneurysm repair
- Peripheral arterial disease interventions
- Temporary left ventricular assist device implantation
- Aortic valve replacement
- Mitral valve repair
- Gene and stem cell therapy

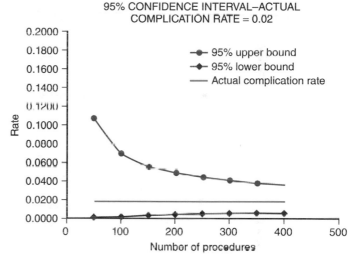

Figure 31-3 Plot of an actual adverse event rate of 2% over a procedure number range from 25 to 400. The horizontal line at 0.02 represents the actual adverse event rate. The curved lines above and below the horizontal line represent the upper and lower bounds of the 95% confidence interval of the estimate of the adverse event rate. Note that as the number of procedures decreases, the range between the upper and lower bounds increases, which indicates lack of stability of any adverse event rate estimate at procedure numbers below 200. *(From Smith SC, Jr., Feldman TE, Hirshfeld JW, Jr., et al: ACC/AHA/SCAI 2005 guideline update for percutaneous coronary intervention: A report of the American College of Cardiology/American Heart Association Task Force on Practice Guidelines (ACC/AHA/SCAI Writing Committee to Update 2001 Guidelines for Percutaneous Coronary Intervention), Circulation 113.e199, 2006.)*

surgery programs, among other things such as operator experience and volume, can be attributed to fairly strict patient selection (Table 31-5) and criteria (Table 31-6).[18] It should be noted that in low-volume centers (<200 PCIs per year), adverse event estimates lose stability and may therefore be unreliable (Fig. 31-3).[1]

The Surgical Interventionalist

Today, many surgical procedures which used to be performed as openheart surgeries exclusively by surgeons are now routinely performed percutaneously (or with cut-down) in the cath lab or in the interventional suite by interventionalists of various disciplines, including surgeons. These procedures are numerous and varied and include pacemaker insertion, mechanical ablation of atrial fibrillation (AF; maze procedure), closure of patent foramen ovale (PFO), and repair of atrial septal defect (ASD), in addition to endovascular alternatives to open carotid endarterectomy, repair and resection of abdominal and thoracic aortic aneurysms, and peripheral artery bypass (Table 31-7). The most recent surgical procedures performed with a closed or percutaneous interventional approach include TAVI and mitral valve repair or clipping. Although not as prevalent as vascular surgeons now performing many of their traditionally open-heart surgeries percutaneously in the interventional suite (i.e., endovascular abdominal aneurysm repair [EVAR]), analogous procedures such as thoracic endovascular aortic repair (TEVAR) are performed more and more in the cath lab by cardiac surgeons. A few hybrid cardiac surgeons have actually gained coronary angiography and PCI skills sufficient for hospital privileging. Now, with TAVI a reality in Europe and with ongoing clinical trials in the United States, cardiac surgeons are required to be part of the percutaneous valve team performing these high-risk procedures.[19] However, because of the rapid development and miniaturization of valve deployment technology, growing worldwide experience, and the usually rapid adoption of new technology by interventional cardiologists, the trans-femoral approach used for TAVI (also known as TF-TAVI) will likely remain exclusively in the domain of the interventional cardiologist if enough cardiac surgeons do not gain the appropriate training and adopt this procedure soon as part of their future practice. In contrast to TF-TAVI and inherent to the design of the procedure, trans-apical trans-catheter aortic valve implantation, also known as TA-TAVI, can be performed in the interventional suite only in the presence of a trained cardiac surgeon, who can gain exposure to and manage surgical control of the left ventricle. A strong case can also be made for the ready availability of the cardiopulmonary bypass machine and an experienced perfusionist.

In this procedure, a small right anterolateral thoracotomy is made over the point of maximal impulse (PMI) on the anterolateral chest wall to gain control of the apex of the left ventricle (Fig. 31-4, *A*). This allows the surgeon to place a circular series of pledgeted sutures in the myocardium before the apical puncture and the placement of a guidewire using the Seldinger technique (see Fig. 31-4, *B*). Once control of the LV apex is attained and guidewire placement across the aortic valve

is confirmed, a long sheath is placed, and a balloon aortic valvuloplasty (BAV) is performed (see Fig. 31-4, *C*). Following the BAV, the balloon-expandable bioprosthesis is deployed in the aortic position (see Fig. 31-4, *D*). The integrity and position of the newly placed bioprosthesis is confirmed intraoperatively by both aortography and transesophageal echocardiography (TEE) before the chest is closed. In this high-risk patient population, minimal amounts of aortic insufficiency and perivalvular leak before the end of the procedure and before awakening the patient from anesthesia are acceptable. It is with procedures such as the TA-TAVI, which will ultimately be combined with PCI in the same setting, that the new cardiac interventionalist will come into his or her own. One will be hard pressed to find a more attractive alternative for the aging and increasingly frail population in the United States than to have well-trained cardiovascular interventionalists who can perform open-heart surgical procedures or minimally invasive and percutaneous or cut-down procedures expeditiously in one setting, thus eliminating the need for multiple costly hospital visits and repeated exposures to anesthesia.

The Cardiac Surgeon's Role in Cardiovascular Innovation

New interventional procedures are largely founded on open-heart surgical approaches, converted first to minimally invasive procedures by surgeons, and later translated to percutaneous techniques by interventionalists. These procedures take a defined pathway from conception to clinical acceptance as the standard of care. This pathway requires collaboration among surgeons, interventionalists, medical device makers, and the FDA, in addition to the execution of well-designed clinical trials.

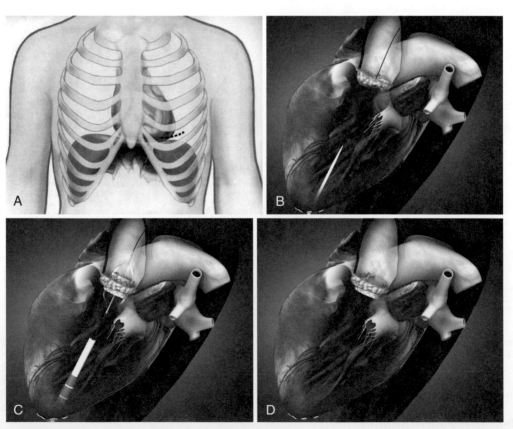

Figure 31-4 Trans-apical transcatheter aortic valve insertion (TA-TAVI). **A,** Keyhole left anterolateral thoracotomy for apical access. **B,** Seldinger technique used for wire insertion and dilation of transmural myocardial track before balloon aortic valvuloplasty. **C,** Balloon expansion of percutaneous aortic valve. **D,** Well-seated percutaneous bioprosthesis in the aortic position.

CREATION AND DEVELOPMENT OF INTERVENTIONAL PROCEDURES

As new ideas come to light in the operating room, a surgical hypothesis is formulated. A prototype is quickly developed; it is often makeshift and primitive at first but is functional to the point of proving a basic concept with a degree of feasibility. As the validation process progresses, more prototyping equipment and instruments needed for the new procedure are developed either in a laboratory or, in some cases, in the clinical theater. The latter, however, can only take place in a setting where the new procedure can be performed with little modification of existing applications or through a combination of existing medical devices used in a similar homologous approach. At this point, a new procedure or medical device is born, and the pathway forward can take a variety of directions. A simple modification based on existing art or a predicate device currently in clinical use can often be placed into practice with an expedited regulatory pathway known in the United States as *510K*. However, for most, the regulatory pathway is much more involved and can require an expensive and lengthy premarket approval (PMA) process or investigational device exemption (IDE) that can take years and tens of millions of dollars before the adoption of the device in the marketplace. This process is often less challenging outside of the United States. Once prototyped and proven feasible, and before receiving regulatory approval, a new technology is usually tested in the laboratory, on rodents or large animals. This allows refinement of the prototype and its materials in terms of size, cost, and efficiency. It also allows exploration of the tolerance extremes a device may be subject to in the clinical setting. After a device application has been thoroughly investigated in a preclinical animal model, it needs to be tested systematically in humans. First-in-human studies are followed by safety and feasibility phase I trials and larger phase II trials, which are usually randomized, all with constant communication and approval from the FDA. In the United States, the regulatory process alone can take years and quickly exhaust vast resources and capital. If and when a device does gain initial FDA regulatory approval and is appropriately financed through the commercialization stage, it still needs to be championed by the end users—in this case, surgeons and interventional cardiologists. Adoption of a procedure as standard of care by this community is ultimately based on clinical efficacy, safety, and cost. If not minimally invasive or percutaneous at first, these approaches will be further developed on the basis of similar sound surgical principles as the open-heart surgical approach. New technology and innovation developed to assist with the conversion of a procedure to a more minimally invasive technique continues as a device progresses through its total clinical product life cycle. This cycle of continual refinement of interventional tools and equipment requires close collaboration among surgeons, interventionalists, and industry partners to constantly provide state-of-the-art care to cardiovascular patients.

THE HYBRID SUITE

For most hospitals, the decision to create a hybrid room is one largely based on return on investment in addition to usefulness for clinicians. With variable economics among medical centers, several models have emerged. The first approach is to perform a retrofit to allow the hybrid team to carry out endovascular interventions and structural heart procedures in existing facilities. This can be done through two separate pathways starting with either an existing cath lab or an existing operating room. An existing cath lab suite can be outfitted with formal anesthesia equipment, appropriate HVAC (heating, ventilating, and air conditioning), scrub sinks, substerile areas and fully stocked with instruments and disposables most often used by hybrid surgeons. Note that multiple disciplines are interested in using hybrid rooms today, so stocking for all these specialties can escalate costs quickly in addition to making space utilization challenging. In the case of preparing a hybrid cath lab room for major cardiac surgical interventions, including aortocoronary bypass and open valve procedures, additional space

and storage are also required for a perfusion team and for equipment, which are essential for ensuring the best outcome during a planned cardiac hybrid case or a "conversion to open" emergency scenario. As an alternative to converting a cath lab to a hybrid room, an operating room can be retrofitted with the appropriate cath lab equipment and imaging technology to become a functional hybrid suite as well. The minimum set of equipment comprises an image intensifier (I-I) for high-quality fluoroscopy and digital cineography, with corresponding flat screens, monitors, interventional table, lead shielding, as well as a full stock of wires, balloons, stents, and other disposables (Fig. 31-5). The additional space needed to accommodate such a retrofit cannot be underestimated, as often the hybrid team finds itself suddenly constricted in an ill-planned, undersized operating theater. This can, at times, be potentially unsafe in the case of challenging cardiovascular procedures, as one has to be constantly prepared to convert to an open-chest approach. The gold standard is to design a hybrid suite from scratch during a major renovation or initial construction of an operating room or cath lab. Few hospitals have this luxury, but more and more, hybrid suites are being recognized as a necessity in larger centers of excellence. In addition, there is a small but growing body of literature discussing the proper methodology and construction of such

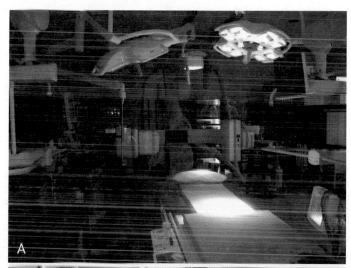

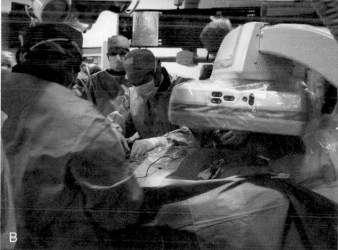

Figure 31-5 Hybrid suite. **A,** Hybrid interventional suite. **B,** Transapical transcatheter aortic valve implantation (intraoperative photo). Note the cardiac surgeon in the foreground in proximity to the left mini-thoracotomy used to access and control the left ventricular apex. Interventional cardiologists prepare the groin for instrumentation on the far side of the operating table.

<table>
<tr><td colspan="2">TABLE 31-8   List of Lessons and Pitfalls in Hybrid Construction</td></tr>
</table>

- Consider input from all those who potentially will be working in the room. This includes staff from anesthesiology, nurses from both the operating room and the catheterization laboratory (cath lab), and technical staff from both as well.
- It is imperative to make the hybrid room large enough and to consider patterns of entry and egress of personnel in light of the additional and cumbersome clinical equipment such as the image intensifier (I-I) and the perfusion machine. Accommodations should be made for space and pathways used for additional clinical equipment and personnel that may not always be present during every case, such as intra-aortic balloon pump apparatus and staff.
- Proper ceiling height that is adequate to allow flat screens and monitors to retract reasonably above head level should be ensured. This can be quite costly and require significant engineering input, as routing of modern HVAC (heating, ventilating, and air conditioning) and air-handling systems need to be considered.
- Plan carefully for anesthesia personnel and equipment (including echo), in particular with regard to the placement of the I-I.
- Develop a plan for preparing and draping the patient in advance to accommodate both the surgeon and the interventional cardiologist. This often requires stocking a combination of standard prep packs from both the cath lab and the operating room in the hybrid suite.
- Use of radiolucent defibrillator pads and careful placement of all lines, tubes, and wires so that they are not within the path of the I-I are important. This requires repeated education of all staff, including frequently rotating residents and fellows who often position and prep the patient.
- Ensure connectivity of all imaging and monitoring equipment, including echocardiography equipment. All imaging should be readily visible in real time to the operating staff and those in the control room.
- Development and continued updating of standard operating procedures (SOPs) and the operations manual.

hybrid suites based on the extensive trial-and-error experiences of some of the earliest and most experienced hybrid centers.[20–22] The authors' own experiences at New York Presbyterian–Columbia University Medical Center led to several lessons, most of which could only have been realized after the construction and extensive use of the four hybrid rooms at this center (Table 31-8). The most important part of creating and running a successful hybrid suite occurs long before actual construction and lies in the extensive multi-disciplinary coordinated planning and includes extensive input from ancillary staff. No one relishes large committee meetings during the purchasing and construction of new clinical equipment and resources; however, because the new hybrid suites will be used for procedures not yet developed, an ounce of prevention is worth a pound of cure. It is important to remember that this burgeoning field is not just providing opportunities for innovation to surgeons and interventional cardiologists but that anesthesia, radiology, nursing, and technical staff will all be faced with new challenges that will arise out of the necessity for resolution, new inventions, processes, and methods. Trivial details that are often taken for granted in the cath lab and operating room can easily be overlooked in the day-to-day operation of the hybrid suite, bringing major high-risk procedures to a screeching halt while staff scramble to make adjustments so that the procedure can continue. Invariably, these delays often occur at the most inconvenient time and while treating a patient who is very ill; therefore, it is wise to perform only routine, low-risk procedures in the beginning while the shortcomings of the hybrid suite can be realized and corrected. Routine parts of any hybrid procedure, for example, prepping and draping the patient, should be well thought out before commencing any hybrid procedure so that both the interventional cardiologist and the surgeon can work without hindering each other. Even the simplest detail, for example, having the operating room staff remember to position defibrillator pads out of the path of the image intensifier or using a radiolucent variety, can avoid costly time and risks in the hybrid room. For the above reasons, the authors recommend that a standard operating procedure (SOP) for each hybrid procedure be created, assembled, and integrated into a formal operations manual containing all SOPs for a particular hybrid

room and made available to all hybrid staff. This type of rigid organization has been shown to improve quality of care, quality assurance (QA), and quality control (QC) and also helps those planning complex clinical interventions that require high-level coordination among a large team in an unfamiliar setting such as the hybrid suite.

Convergence of Surgery and Interventional Cardiology

Unfortunately, the discipline of cardiac surgery will remain too complex for practicing interventional cardiologists to cross-train without completing a lengthy formal residency in surgery. However, focused and well-thought-out surgical rotations integrated throughout medical residency training and cardiology fellowship could prepare one to perform more complex and minimally invasive techniques in conjunction with surgical colleagues. It is important to note, however, that as one violates the integument in an increasingly invasive manner, the risk and magnitude of major complications escalates rapidly, and there is no substitute for the complete mastery of grounded surgical principles and technique. Likewise, presuming that much of the discipline of interventional cardiology can be mastered in short courses that claim to impart interventional "wire" skills is an equal misconception fraught with great hazard. The true mastery of such a specialized discipline requires intense study and unparalleled understanding of coronary artery disease (CAD) and structural heart disease at a level that can be gained only through a formal interventional cardiovascular fellowship, which is currently almost exclusively available through the traditional cardiology pathway. At New York Presbyterian–Columbia University Medical Center, collaboration between cardiology and cardiovascular surgery has been taken forward aggressively. Currently, a formal Hybrid Interventional Cardiology fellowship is available for cardiac surgeons; this is administered jointly by the Departments of Surgery and Medicine and requires the fellow to function clinically in the Division of Cardiac Surgery as well as in the Cardiology Center for Interventional Vascular Therapy (CIVT). The advanced fellowship is 1 year in length and imparts an excellent experience in all aspects of general Interventional Cardiology, including diagnostic angiography, PCI, TAVI, endovascular graft techniques, and hybrid cardiac surgery procedures. Hybrid procedures that have gained the most acceptance today include hybrid coronary revascularization (HCR), hybrid valve surgery with PTCA or PCI, and hybrid procedures for AF. In addition, some centers have also undertaken hybrid therapies for CAD associated with carotid artery disease and aortic arch pathology. In centers with busy hybrid programs, HCR most often refers to minimally invasive direct coronary artery bypass (MIDCAB), in which the anastomosis of the left internal mammary artery (LIMA) to the left anterior descending artery (LADA) is the focus of the surgical portion of the operation and is combined with PCI with drug-eluting stents (DESs) to the non-LADA targets.[22–25] This approach accepts the notion that the surgical LIMA–LADA anastomosis is the most durable form of revascularization available today but also recognizes that the patency rates of traditional saphenous vein grafts (SVG) are less than robust with their ability to remain open in the long term being greatly inferior to the LIMA approach.[26–28] In the era of the modern DES, the SVG as a conduit for CABG must become suspect. Whereas excellent data exist demonstrating 10- to 20-year patency for the LIMA-to-LADA anastomosis, similar data on SVG patency are quite discouraging; thus DES is now an attractive alternative.[29] The LIMA–to–LADA portion of the HCR procedure can be performed in a variety of ways, including totally endoscopic atraumatic CABG, robotically assisted CABG, or CABG performed through a keyhole incision. In these approaches, the LIMA is taken down either endoscopically or robotically, and a LIMA–LADA anastomosis is either performed by hand or with robotic assistance on an arrested heart or a beating heart. The design and techniques for these procedures are still evolving, but several dedicated operators have made great progress toward bringing them to the forefront of mainstream cardiovascular medicine. Table 31-9 summarizes the

TABLE 31-9	Results of Hybrid Coronary Revascularization for Series Using Only Drug-Eluting Stents for Percutaneous Coronary Intervention						
Author, Publication Year	No. Patients	30-Day Mortality	In-Hospital Morbidity, %	LIMA Patency Rate Immediate, %	Mean Follow-Up, Months	Stent Re-stenosis, %	Event-Free Survival, %
MIDCAB and PCI							
Gilard et al, 2007	70	1.4	4.2	N/A	33	2.3	97
Kon et al, 2008	15	0	0	100	12	3	93
TECAB and PCI							
Vassiliades et al, 2006	47	0	0	99	7	6.6	90
Bonatti et al, 2007	5	0	0	100	6	0	100

LIMA, left internal mammary artery; *MIDCAB*, minimally invasive direct coronary artery bypass; ; *N/A*, not available; *PCI*, percutaneous coronary intervention; *TECAB*, totally endoscopic coronary artery bypass.
Leacche M, Umakanthan R, Zhao DX, Byrne JG: Surgical update: Hybrid procedures. Do they have a role? *Circ Cardiovasc Interv* 3:512, 2010.

TABLE 31-10	Results of Hybrid Valve Surgery or Percutaneous Coronary Intervention							
Author, Publication Year	No. Patients	Age, Years*	Acute Coronary Syndrome, %	Congestive Heart Failure, %	Reoperative Procedure, %	Minimally Invasive Procedure, %	Operative Mortality, %
PTCA ± PCI and MVR, AVR, or both							
Byrne et al, 2005	26	72 (53 91)	92	N/A	42	30.8	3.8
PCI and AVR							
Brinster et al, 2006	18	75 (56–89)	N/A	N/A	27.8	100	5.6
PCI and MVR							
Umakanthan et al, 2009	32	69 (44–85)	15	43	38	100	3

AVR, aortic valve replacement; *MVR*, mitral valve replacement; *N/A*, not available; *PCI*, percutaneous coronary intervention; *PTCA*, percutaneous transluminal coronary angioplasty.
*Data presented as median (range).
Leacche M, Umakanthan R, Zhao DX, Byrne JG: Surgical update: Hybrid procedures. Do they have a role? *Circ Cardiovasc Interv* 3:514, 2010.

results of a recently published series on HCR that used only DES.[22–25,30] The reported stent re-stenosis, at an average follow-up of 6 to 33 months, is quite low at 0% to 6.6%, and the incidence of major adverse cardiac events (MACEs) is between 0% and 4.2%.[30] Clearly, larger randomized trials need to be undertaken, but these data are strong evidence to support the continued exploration of this type of hybrid approach. With the aging population, the hybrid alternative to the traditional CABG or valve operation has also become a reality.[31–33] Following the same premise that the LIMA–to–LADA is the most durable method of surgical coronary revascularization, with SVG being a distant contender, valve surgery with PCI with DES to non-LADA targets is now quite a viable option. This is especially true in the case of frail older adults who have already undergone cardiac surgery. This approach allows the surgeon to perform minimally invasive valve surgery using only a mini-thoracotomy or partial sternotomy to replace or repair the valve, thus minimizing overall morbidity. The non-LADA coronary revascularization portion of the procedure can be done with PCI with DES either in the same setting or during a second-stage procedure. The results of published series of hybrid valve surgery or PCI are summarized in Table 31-10.[30–33] Again, more investigation needs to take place, but the benefits derived from the current hybrid approach for treating valvular disease seem quite apparent at this initial stage.

■ The Cardiovascular Interventionalist

With time, certain elective open-heart surgical procedures will become less prevalent. Unfortunately, complications and challenging scenarios such as hostile chest entry and difficult intravascular access to vital structures will remain. Because of this, a need for surgeons who are facile with open-heart surgical techniques and who can proceed expeditiously with prowess will persist, especially in the patient presenting in extremis. With this stated, the future cardiovascular surgeon will likely become more of a cardiovascular interventionalist than currently envisioned. Related fields such as vascular surgery have shown that additional formal endovascular training can and must be seamlessly integrated into fellowship programs to achieve excellence. Despite ongoing clinical domain disputes with interventionalists from other disciplines such as interventional radiology, today's vascular surgical community is comfortable in the interventional suite performing complex vascular interventions that combine percutaneous, endovascular, and cut-down approaches to achieve the desired clinical result. Cardiovascular surgery must follow suit to maintain excellence and safety in treating the growing aging, more complex patient population. Surgeons across the board have continued to perform open-heart surgeries while keeping their eyes on more minimally invasive approaches. In terms of cardiac surgery, femoral cannulation allows major operations to be performed through "mini-sternotomies" or via keyhole thoracotomy incisions. Very fine surgical instruments with fine jaws and extended hand pieces that facilitate even the most delicate maneuvers required for complex open heart surgical procedures such as mitral valve reconstruction are now available. Despite these strides toward less invasive techniques, some patients still remain better served without the trauma of surgery altogether, in particular surgery involving cardiopulmonary bypass. Advancing in parallel to their surgical colleagues, interventional cardiologists, for decades, have been performing all their cath lab procedures through the percutaneous approach. They have been extremely successful in traversing the peripheral vasculature to perform a spectrum of cardiovascular procedures ranging from very delicate coronary interventions for CAD to stenting of larger proximal and distal vessels for peripheral vascular disease and to now replacing the aortic valve via the femoral artery. With both disciplines working from opposite directions—surgeon from open to minimally invasive and the interventional cardiologist from straightforward PTCA to complete aortic valve replacement—it has now become clear that the two disciplines are poised to intersect and converge, overlapping in an unprecedented way. It is only through close collaboration and open recognition of each other's unique, yet complementary, skill set that the field of cardiovascular medicine can advance and new therapies can be born.

REFERENCES

1. Smith SC, Jr, Feldman TE, Hirshfeld JW, Jr, et al: ACC/AHA/SCAI 2005 guideline update for percutaneous coronary intervention: A report of the American College of Cardiology/American Heart Association Task Force on Practice Guidelines (ACC/AHA/SCAI Writing Committee to Update 2001 Guidelines for Percutaneous Coronary Intervention). *Circulation* 113:e166–e286, 2006.
2. Aversano T, Aversano LT, Passamani E, et al: Thrombolytic therapy vs primary percutaneous coronary intervention for myocardial infarction in patients presenting to hospitals without on-site cardiac surgery: A randomized controlled trial. *JAMA* 287:1943–1951, 2002.
3. Bourassa MG: The history of cardiac catheterization. *Can J Cardiol* 21:1011–1014, 2005.
4. Forssmann-Falck R: Werner Forssmann: A pioneer of cardiology. *Am J Cardiol* 79:651–660, 1997.
5. Seldinger SI: Catheter replacement of the needle in percutaneous arteriography: A new technique. *Acta radiol* 39:368–376, 1953.
6. Roubin GS, Gruentzig AR, Casarella WJ: Percutaneous coronary angioplasty: Technique, indications, and results. *Cardiovasc Intervent Radiol* 9:261–272, 1986.
7. Anderson HV, Roubin GS, Leimgruber PP, et al: Primary angiographic success rates of percutaneous transluminal coronary angioplasty. *Am J Cardiol* 56:712–717, 1985.
8. Parsonnet V, Fisch D, Gielchinsky I, et al: Emergency operation after failed angioplasty. *J Thorac Cardiovasc Surg* 96:198–203, 1988.
9. Greene MA, Gray LA, Jr, Slater AD, et al: Emergency aortocoronary bypass after failed angioplasty. *Ann Thorac Surg* 51:194–199, 1991.
10. Lazar HL, Jacobs AK, Aldea GS, et al: Factors influencing mortality after emergency coronary artery bypass grafting for failed percutaneous transluminal coronary angioplasty. *Ann Thorac Surg* 64:1747–1752, 1997.
11. Yang EH, Gumina RJ, Lennon RJ, et al: Emergency coronary artery bypass surgery for percutaneous coronary interventions: Changes in the incidence, clinical characteristics, and indications from 1979 to 2003. *J Am Coll Cardiol* 46:2004–2009, 2005.
12. Barakate MS, Bannon PG, Hughes CF, et al: Emergency surgery after unsuccessful coronary angioplasty: A review of 15 years' experience. *Ann Thorac Surg* 75:1400–1405, 2003.
13. Seshadri N, Whitlow PL, Acharya N, et al: Emergency coronary artery bypass surgery in the contemporary percutaneous coronary intervention era. *Circulation* 106:2346–2350, 2002.
14. Sutton JM, Ellis SG, Roubin GS, et al: Major clinical events after coronary stenting. The multicenter registry of acute and elective Gianturco-Roubin stent placement. The Gianturco-Roubin Intracoronary Stent Investigator Group. *Circulation* 89:1126–1137, 1994.
15. Dean LS, George CJ, Roubin GS, et al: Bailout and corrective use of Gianturco-Roubin flex stents after percutaneous transluminal coronary angioplasty: Operator reports and angiographic core laboratory verification from the National Heart, Lung, and Blood Institute/New Approaches to Coronary Intervention Registry. *J Am Coll Cardiol* 29:934–940, 1997.
16. Wennberg DE, Lucas FL, Siewers AE, et al: Outcomes of percutaneous coronary interventions performed at centers without and with onsite coronary artery bypass graft surgery. *JAMA* 292:1961–1968, 2004.
17. Smith SC, Jr, Feldman TE, Hirshfeld JW, Jr, et al: ACC/AHA/SCAI 2005 Guideline Update for Percutaneous Coronary Intervention–summary article: A report of the American College of Cardiology/American Heart Association Task Force on Practice Guidelines (ACC/AHA/SCAI Writing Committee to Update the 2001 Guidelines for Percutaneous Coronary Intervention). *Circulation* 113:156–175, 2006.
18. Wharton TP, Jr: Nonemergent percutaneous coronary intervention with off-site surgery backup: An emerging new path to access. *Crit Pathw Cardiol* 4:98–106, 2005.
19. Leon MB, Smith CR, Mack M, et al: Transcatheter aortic-valve implantation for aortic stenosis in patients who cannot undergo surgery. *N Engl J Med* 363:1597–1607, 2010.
20. Nollert G, Wich S: Planning a cardiovascular hybrid operating room: The technical point of view. *Heart Surg Forum* 12:E125–E130, 2009.
21. Sikkink CJ, Reijnen MM, Zeebregts CJ: The creation of the optimal dedicated endovascular suite. *Eur J Vasc Endovasc Surg* 35:198–204, 2008.
22. Bonatti J, Vassiliades T, Nifong W, et al: How to build a cath-lab operating room. *Heart Surg Forum* 10:E344–E348, 2007.
23. Gilard M, Bezon E, Cornily JC, et al: Same-day combined percutaneous coronary intervention and coronary artery surgery. *Cardiology* 108:363–367, 2007.
24. Kon ZN, Brown EN, Tran R, et al: Simultaneous hybrid coronary revascularization reduces postoperative morbidity compared with results from conventional off-pump coronary artery bypass. *J Thorac Cardiovasc Surg* 135:367–375, 2008.
25. Vassiliades TA, Jr, Douglas JS, Morris DC, et al: Integrated coronary revascularization with drug-eluting stents: Immediate and seven-month outcome. *J Thorac Cardiovasc Surg* 131:956–962, 2006.
26. Alexander JH, Hafley G, Harrington RA, et al: Efficacy and safety of edifoligide, an E2F transcription factor decoy, for prevention of vein graft failure following coronary artery bypass graft surgery: PREVENT IV: A randomized controlled trial. *JAMA* 294:2446–2454, 2005.
27. Balacumaraswami L, Taggart DP: Intraoperative imaging techniques to assess coronary artery bypass graft patency. *Ann Thorac Surg* 83:2251–2257, 2007.
28. Puskas JD, Williams WH, Mahoney EM, et al: Off-pump vs conventional coronary artery bypass grafting: Early and 1-year graft patency, cost, and quality-of-life outcomes: A randomized trial. *JAMA* 291:1841–1849, 2004.
29. Tatoulis J, Buxton BF, Fuller JA: Patencies of 2127 arterial to coronary conduits over 15 years. *Ann Thorac Surg* 77:93–101, 2004.
30. Leacche M, Umakanthan R, Zhao DX, et al: Surgical update: Hybrid procedures. Do they have a role? *Circ Cardiovasc Interv* 3:511–518, 2010.
31. Brinster DR, Byrne M, Rogers CD, et al: Effectiveness of same day percutaneous coronary intervention followed by minimally invasive aortic valve replacement for aortic stenosis and moderate coronary disease ("hybrid approach"). *Am J Cardiol* 98:1501–1503, 2006.
32. Byrne JG, Leacche M, Unic D, et al: Staged initial percutaneous coronary intervention followed by valve surgery ("hybrid approach") for patients with complex coronary and valve disease. *J Am Coll Cardiol* 45:14–18, 2005.
33. Umakanthan R, Leacche M, Petracek MR, et al: Combined PCI and minimally invasive heart valve surgery for high-risk patients. *Curr Treat Options Cardiovasc Med* 11:492–498, 2009.

32

Restenosis

KEVIN J. CROCE | MARCO A. COSTA | DANIEL I. SIMON

KEY POINTS

- The mechanisms of re-stenosis are different among balloon angioplasty, bare metal stents (BMSs), and drug-eluting stents (DESs).

- Intimal hyperplasia with smooth muscle cell proliferation represents the key mechanism of re-stenosis after BMSs.

- The biology of re-stenosis after drug-eluting stents is variable and may have different cellular composition (T lymphocytes) and fibrin deposition.

- The relative contribution of procedural and mechanical factors in the development of clinical re-stenosis is amplified after DESs.

- The re-stenosis rate and in-stent late lumen loss are lower with DESs compared with BMSs.

- The incidence and patterns of re-stenosis differ among currently available DES platforms.

- The best treatment of DES re-stenosis remains to be determined.

- Emerging anti–re-stenosis strategies include catheter-based drug delivery systems and biodegradable stents with or without combination drug therapy.

"Nature does nothing without purpose or uselessly."

Aristoteles, 384–322 B.C.

Re-stenosis is the arterial wall healing response to mechanical injury, which has plagued cardiologists since the introduction of balloon angioplasty by Gruntzig and collaborators.[1] This chapter will describe the clinical features, mechanisms, and new facets of BMS and DES re-stenosis in contemporary percutaneous coronary intervention (PCI).

Definitions

ANGIOGRAPHIC RE-STENOSIS

Angiographically detected obstruction of 50% diameter stenosis (DS) or more at the site of a previously treated coronary segment has been historically defined as *re-stenosis*.[2] This apparently arbitrary cut-off point was, in fact, founded on good scientific evidence from physiologic experimental studies, which demonstrated that when the arterial lumen diameter is reduced to 50% or less, the coronary flow reserve becomes impeded.[3] For purposes of scientific studies, many definitions of angiographic re-stenosis have been used, although the classic binary definition based on percentage DS is the most widely accepted. Unfortunately, percentage DS does not depict the degree of deterioration in lumen diameter and does not convey a measure of the vessel response to injury.[4,5] The use of the term *percentage DS* itself carries with it the assumption of normal-appearing reference segments, which is known to be an erroneous assumption, given the diffuse aspect of coronary disease and neointimal proliferation.[6] Finally, binary re-stenosis assumes that a patient with 51% DS and another one with 49% DS have different intimal hyperplasia responses and outcomes, which, of course, is not the case.

In view of these considerations, clinical re-stenosis studies have been adopting a more comprehensive approach to reporting findings from both perspectives (categorical and continuous) to determine whether the agent under investigation had restraining or inhibitory effect and whether the ultimate clinical or angiographic outcome has been improved by the use of any new therapy. However, the more subtle facets of potent anti-proliferative devices such as DESs challenge the validity of conventional angiographic parameters. Advanced imaging techniques such as intravascular ultrasound (IVUS) and optical coherence tomography (OCT) have greatly improved the ability to visualize re-stenosis and make quantitative assessments of neointimal thickness, neointimal volume, and minimal luminal diameter (MLD).[7-12] Late loss (LL) is a continuous angiographic measure of lumen deterioration. LL is conventionally calculated by subtracting the MLD value at follow-up (FU) from postprocedural MLD. These computations are made irrespective of the locations of MLD measurements. LL has traditionally served as a major outcome measure in BMS trials and continues to play a similar role in the era of DESs.[13,14] It represents a surrogate marker of neointimal hyperplasia when measurements are performed within stented segments because stents abolish the remodeling component of the re-stenotic process (see below).[4,15] However, conventional LL measurements may be methodologically flawed because of changes in the location of MLD between postprocedure and follow-up measurements.[9,16] As a result, LL frequently derives from measurements performed in different (unmatched) locations in the target segment. Sites with higher degrees of lumen deterioration and neointimal proliferation may be overlooked, which potentially leads to inaccurate conclusions about the anti-proliferative efficacy of a given device. Angiographic re-stenosis parameters have been reported in two ways: in-lesion analysis and in-stent analysis (Fig. 32-1). In-lesion analysis encompasses the stented segment 5 mm distally and proximally in an attempt to depict edge re-stenosis. It is important to note that in-lesion LL will not necessarily be higher than in-stent LL. These somewhat confusing data occur because of the MLD relocation phenomenon. Furthermore, in-lesion LL is affected by vascular remodeling or vessel spasm and cannot be used as a surrogate for intimal hyperplasia or to determine anti-proliferative device efficacy.

Quantitative coronary angiography (QCA) has been largely used to determine re-stenosis parameters in the clinical context, since visual assessment may lead to overestimation of the degree of narrowing in "severe" lesions and underestimation of the severity in "mild or moderate" lesions.[17,18] Clinical and research assessment of re-stenosis has also been markedly improved by IVUS and OCT, which enable high-fidelity measurement of re-stenotic areas, neointimal volume, and MLD, in addition to enabling three-dimensional rendering of the re-stenotic segments. OCT may be a useful technology for the evaluation of stent healing. By using light rather than ultrasound, OCT produces high-resolution in vivo images of coronary arteries and deployed stents with 10 to 15 μm resolution compared with the 150 to 200 μm resolution of IVUS. Although limited in its ability to image deep into the blood vessel wall, OCT increases the diagnostic accuracy of luminal atherosclerosis imaging, thus enabling visualization of small structures such as the thin fibrous caps associated with plaque rupture; it also increases the diagnostic accuracy of stent and re-stenosis imaging, enabling high-resolution assessment of lumen features and neointima (Fig. 32-2).[12] In initial clinical trials, OCT outperformed IVUS in the detection of small degrees of neointimal hyperplasia and was more sensitive

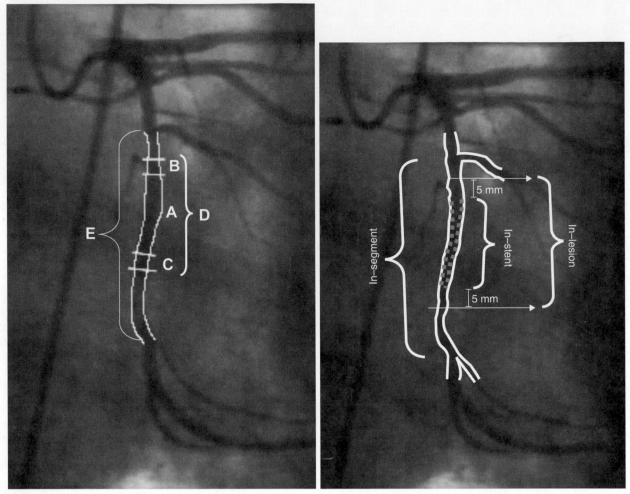

Figure 32-1 Coronary angiography and schematic model illustrating a segmental approach to analyze and report the effects of drug-eluting stents on coronary arteries. *Right panel:* **A,** In-stent, which better describes the anti-proliferative effect of the biologic agent. **B,** Proximal edge (5 mm). **C,** Distal edge (5 mm). **D,** In-lesion, which determines potential paradoxical effects of low drug concentrations at traumatized stent edges ("edge effect"). **E,** In-segment, which is the ultimate determinant of angiographic success from a patient's perspective. *(Reprinted with permission from Sousa JE Serruys PW, Costa MA: New frontiers in cardiology: Drug-eluting stents, Part II, Circulation 107(18):2383–2389, 2003.)*

in detecting stent malapposition.[19,20] In addition, OCT-based single-stent, strut-level analysis provides clear assessment of stent–strut coverage and apposition, which are important clinical parameters that have been linked to DES-induced delayed arterial healing and risk of stent thrombosis.[21–23]

CLINICAL RE-STENOSIS

Although angiography has been widely used as the guiding tool in the management of coronary artery disease (CAD), the clinician should also consider functional, invasive or noninvasive fractional flow reserve, assessment of the re-stenotic lesion before referring the patient to additional coronary revascularization. Gruntzig et al observed that most clinical ischemic events related to vessel renarrowing occurred between 3 and 9 months after balloon angioplasty. This seminal observation illustrates the delay between the biologic process and the symptomatic presentation of re-stenosis, which results in a 70% increase in the incidence of repeat revascularization between 6 and 12 months after the procedure.[24,25] Potent anti-proliferative strategies may delay the biologic response to injury and extend the time frame to develop clinical signs of re-stenosis. Indeed, intimal proliferation following brachytherapy seems to have a different time course.[26] Likewise, re-stenosis after DES may be delayed, although a late catch-up re-stenotic phenomenon has not been observed in clinical studies.[27,28]

Re-stenosis may cause no symptoms in up to 50% of patients, although silent ischemia may be present.[29] Exercise electrocardiographic testing has limited value to detect "silent" re-stenotic lesions, and the detection of re-stenosis by computed tomographic angiography (CTA) can be unreliable because of stent metal radiographic artifacts.[30–32] Other noninvasive tests such as thallium scintigraphy and cardiac and stress echocardiography have been used to improve the sensitivity and specificity of noninvasive assessment of re-stenosis.[33] On the other end of the clinical spectrum, re-stenosis may present itself in the form of acute coronary syndrome (ACS) in up to one third of patients, which challenges the notion that re-stenosis is a benign condition.[34,35] Re-stenosis is of particular concern following left main PCI because of the potential risk of sudden cardiac death (SCD) associated with early "silent" re-stenosis. Despite this theoretical risk, after reviewing clinical data, the writing group for the *2009 Focused Update: ACC/AHA/SCAI Guidelines on Percutaneous Coronary Intervention* decided that the prior class IIa recommendation for angiographic follow-up after left main PCI should be omitted from the 2009 updated guidelines. In making this recommendation, the writing group focused on the inability of angiography to predict a situation that might be prone to acute, sudden stent thrombosis, as well as the risk associated with angiography in a patient who has undergone placement of a left main stent.[36] Target lesion revascularization (TLR), defined as any repeat PCI of the treated coronary segment or bypass surgery of the target vessel, has been

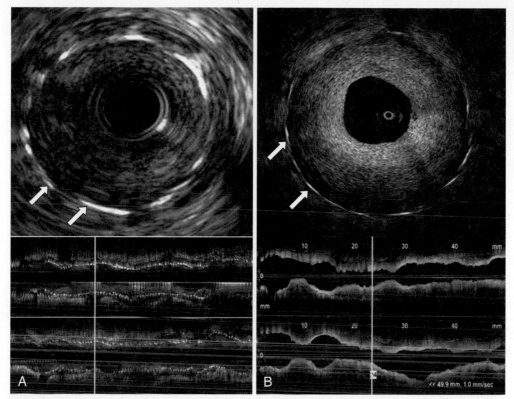

Figure 32-2 Intravascular ultrasound (IVUS) and optical coherence tomography (OCT) imaging of bare metal stent re-stenosis: Six months after implantation in a human coronary artery, a 3.0 × 32 mm Liberté™ stent was evaluated by IVUS with the Boston Scientific Atlantis™ IVUS Catheter (*panel A*) or by OCT with the Light Lab-M3 TD-OCT™ catheter (*panel B*). Stent struts (*white arrows*) are clearly visible in the cross-sectional images (*top panels*). The higher resolution OCT system enables markedly better visualization and quantification of neointimal tissue compared with IVUS in both cross-sectional (A, B, top panels) and longitudinal representations (A, B, bottom panels). In addition, compared with IVUS (0.097"), the smaller profile of the TD OCT imaging catheter (0.016") enables visualization and quantification of neointimal stenosis in areas of critical narrowing where the neointimal tissue completely contacts the IVUS catheter.

proposed as the most specific clinical re-stenosis endpoint among other clinical markers (i.e., death, myocardial infarction [MI], symptoms recurrence, or combined major adverse cardiac events [MACEs]).[4] Target vessel revascularization (TVR) expands the definition of TLR to include repeat PCI of the target vessel, irrespective of the location of the stenosis within the treated segment. In routine clinical practice, noninvasive assessment of recurrence of re-stenosis (symptomatic status and ischemia tests) appears an appropriate approach. This latter recommendation is based on a series of previous observations: (1) Routine angiographic follow-up may have increased morbidity and mortality, albeit to a small extent; (2) asymptomatic patients with nonfunctional angiographic re-stenosis experience a benign course; and (3) the so-called occulo-stenotic reflex leads to a higher rate of repeat revascularization with no clear clinical benefit at 12 months after the initial intervention.[37,38]

Mechanisms of Re-Stenosis

The pathophysiology of re-stenosis is characterized by neointimal proliferation and negative vascular remodeling. The latter contributes only to re-stenosis after PCI without stent implantation, as the scaffolding properties of stents abolish the remodeling process. It is, nevertheless, important to note that the proliferative vascular response is enhanced by the persistent stimuli of rigid metallic struts in the vessel wall. Neointimal hyperplasia has been originally proposed as a general wound healing response.[39] Platelet aggregation, inflammatory cell infiltration, release of growth factors, medial smooth muscle cell (SMC) modulation and proliferation, proteoglycan deposition, and extracellular matrix remodeling were identified as the major milestones in the temporal sequence of this response. It is now recognized that inflammation plays a key role in promoting SMC proliferation, which is central to the pathobiology of re-stenosis.

SMOOTH MUSCLE CELL PROLIFERATION AND RE-STENOSIS

The SMC has long been implicated in the healing process after arterial injury because of its ability to migrate, proliferate, and synthesize extracellular matrix (ECM) on stimulation. After shifting from the contractile to the synthetic phenotype, SMCs may proliferate from 24 hours to 2 to 3 months after vascular injury, returning to the contractile phenotype after this period. Adventitial myofibroblasts (an α-actin staining cell) also proliferate and migrate into the neointima and appear to play an important role in supplying the intimal layer with proliferative cellular elements for new lesion formation.[40] Through fracture of the internal elastic membrane, these adventitial cells migrate into the intima, where they may continue to proliferate and synthesize ECM, which will ultimately constitute the bulk of the re-stenotic lesion. ECM is composed of various collagen subtypes and proteoglycans and actually constitutes the major component of the re-stenotic lesion; neointimal hyperplasia has been shown to be predominately a low-cellular tissue.[41,42] Assessment of cellular proliferation status in atherectomy specimens of re-stenotic lesions has been enabled by use of antibodies to proliferating cell nuclear antigen (PCNA), cyclin E, and cyclin-dependent kinase (CDK), and there is evidence that cells of monocyte or macrophage lineage (HAM-56–positive) proliferate within human in-stent re-stenotic tissue.[2,43,44] The central role of vascular cells in the re-stenotic process provided the basis for anti–re-stenosis pharmacologic strategies targeting cell cycle division early after stent implantation (Fig. 32-3).

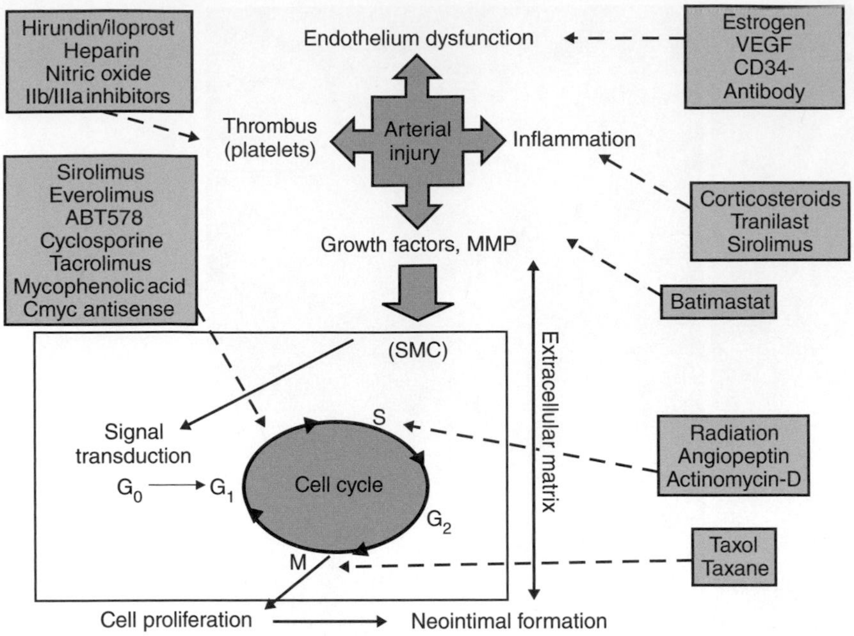

Figure 32-3 The leading processes of re-stenosis (*solid lines*) and corresponding inhibitory (*dashed lines*) effects of different anti–re-stenosis agents. (*Reprinted with permission from Sousa JE, Serruys PW, Costa MA: New frontiers in cardiology: Drug-eluting stents, Part I, Circulation 107(17):2274–2279, 2003.*)

CELL CYCLE AND RE-STENOSIS

The cell cycle is a common hub of the different phases of the re-stenosis process. The unprecedented clinical successes of recent anti–restenosis approaches targeting cellular division pathways illustrate its central role in the formation of neointimal hyperplasia. Currently available DES technologies deliver high concentrations of immunosuppressive or anti-tumor agents locally into the vessel wall. The specific molecular and cellular effects of these agents have been discussed in detail elsewhere.[7] SMCs are quiescent and exhibit very low levels of proliferative activity. However, mechanical injury triggers the progress of SMCs through the G_1 or G_S transition of the cell cycle.[45] The different phases of the cell cycle of eukaryotic cells are regulated by a series of protein complexes composed of cyclins (D, E, A, B), CDKs (CDKs, CDK4, CDK2, p34cdc2), and cyclin-dependent inhibitors (CKIs, p27Kip1, p70, p16 INK4). The function of CKIs is regulated by changes in their concentration as well as in their localization in the cell.[46] p27Kip1 is downregulated after arterial injury when cell proliferation increases. p21Cip1 is not observed in normal arteries but is upregulated along with p27Kip1 in the later phases of the arterial healing response and is associated with a significant decline in cell proliferation and an increase in procollagen and transforming growth factor beta (TGF-β) synthesis.[46] These findings suggest that p27Kip1 and p21Cip1 are endogenous regulators of G_1 transit in vascular SMCs and inhibit cell proliferation after arterial injury. p27Kip1 and p21Cip1 bind and alter the activities of cyclin D–, cyclin E–, and cyclin A–dependent kinases (CDK2) in quiescent cells, leading to failure of G_1 or G_S transition and cell cycle arrest.[47,48] Overexpression of p27Kip1 results in cell cycle arrest in the G_1 phase. Conversely, inhibition of p27Kip1 increases the number of cells in the G_S phase.[49] Consistent with its regulatory role in SMC proliferation and the pathobiology of re-stenosis, polymorphisms in p27Kip1 that enhance the production of this cell cycle inhibitor are associated with reduced SMC proliferation and decreased risk of re-stenosis following PCI.[50]

INFLAMMATION AND RE-STENOSIS

The central role of autocrine and paracrine inflammatory mediators on SMC proliferation is generally well accepted. Leukocyte recruitment and infiltration occur early at sites of vascular injury, where the lining endothelial cells have been denuded and platelets and fibrin have been deposited. The initial tethering and rolling of leukocytes on platelet P-selectin are followed by their firm adhesion and trans-platelet migration, processes that are dependent on leukocyte Mac-1 and platelet glycoprotein (GP) I_b.[51–53] The precise cellular and molecular mechanisms of inflammation following arterial injury are highly dependent on the specific type of injury (i.e., stent versus balloon mechanical versus atherogenesis). Experimental stent deployment in animal arteries causes sustained elevation of monocyte chemoattractant protein-1 (MCP-1) after injury (~14 days) compared with balloon-injured arteries (<24 hours).[54] Antibody-mediated blockade of chemokine receptor 2 (CCR-2), a primary leukocyte receptor for MCP-1, markedly diminished neointimal thickening after stent-induced injury, but not balloon-induced injury, in nonhuman primates.[55] Experimental observations support a causal relationship between inflammation and experimental re-stenosis. Antibody-mediated blockade or selective absence of Mac-1 diminished leukocyte accumulation and limited neointimal thickening after experimental angioplasty or stent implantation. Corticosteroids have long been shown to reduce the influx of mononuclear cells, to inhibit monocyte and macrophage function, and to influence SMC proliferation.[56–59] However, clinical trials with systemic steroid therapy to prevent re-stenosis have shown disappointing results.[60]

REMODELING AND RE-STENOSIS

The term *remodeling* has been applied largely to describe either vascular shrinkage or vascular enlargement. The definition proposed by Schwartz et al, in which remodeling is characterized in a continuous spectrum by any change in vascular dimension, may better describe this compensatory phenomenon.[61] Studies using intravascular ultrasound (IVUS) provided the first evidence of the key role of negative remodeling (vessel shrinkage) on lumen deterioration after nonstented PCI.[62,63] Adventitial myofibroblasts, which are capable of collagen synthesis and tissue contraction, as seen in wound healing, may play an important role in the negative vessel remodeling observed in re-stenosis after balloon angioplasty.[64,65] Nevertheless, remodeling is virtually absent after stenting as observed by volumetric IVUS (Fig. 32-4).[66,67] The superior outcomes of BMSs compared with angioplasty result mainly from the scaffolding property of these metallic prostheses, which prevents vessel shrinkage (elastic recoil and negative remodeling) despite inducing an enhanced neointimal hyperplasia response.

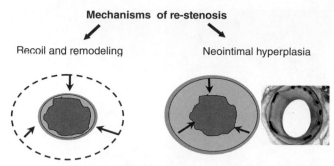

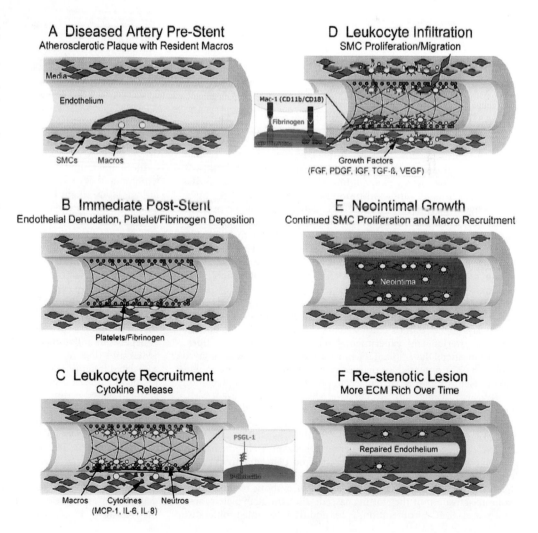

Figure 32-4 Illustration of the two main mechanisms of re-stenosis. Negative vessel remodeling and elastic recoil are mainly observed after balloon angioplasty, whereas in-stent re-stenosis is mainly associated with intimal hyperplasia (in-stent re-stenosis histology, *right panel*).

SPECIFIC MECHANISMS OF BARE METAL STENT RE-STENOSIS

The initial consequences immediately following stent placement are de-endothelialization; crush of the plaque often with dissection into the tunica media and, occasionally, adventitia; and stretch of the entire artery.[68] A layer of platelets and fibrin is then deposited at the injured site. Activated platelets on the surface expressing adhesion molecules such as P-selectin attach to circulating leukocytes via platelet receptors such as P-selectin glycoprotein ligand (PSGL-1) and begin a process of leukocyte rolling along the injured surface. Leukocytes then bind tightly to platelets through the interaction of leukocyte Mac-1 with platelet GP Ibα and through leukocyte integrin cross-linking with fibrinogen, which is bound to the platelet GP IIb/IIIa receptor. Migration of leukocytes across the platelet–fibrin layer and diapedesis into the tissue are driven by the chemical gradients of chemokines released from SMCs and resident macrophages. This is followed by a granulation or cellular proliferation phase. Growth factors are subsequently released from platelets, leukocytes, and SMCs and stimulate the migration of SMCs from the media and adventitia into the intimal layer. The resultant neointima consists of SMCs, ECM, and macrophages recruited over a period of several weeks. Cellular division takes place in this phase, which appears to be essential for the subsequent development of re-stenosis. Over a longer period, the artery enters a phase of remodeling involving ECM protein degradation and resynthesis (Fig. 32-5). Accompanying this phase is a shift to less cellular elements and greater production of ECM. In stented arteries, re-endothelialization of the surface of the stented vessel occurs in parallel with the proliferative processes described above.

SPECIFIC MECHANISMS OF DRUG-ELUTING STENT RE-STENOSIS

Despite almost a decade of clinical experience with DES technologies in human PCI, current understanding of the mechanisms of DES re-stenosis remains somewhat limited. Compared with BMS re-stenosis, the biology of re-stenosis is probably altered by the potent

Figure 32-5 Schematic representation of an integrated cascade of re-stenosis. **A,** Atherosclerotic vessel before intervention. **B,** Immediate result of stent placement with endothelial denudation and platelet or fibrinogen deposition. **C and D,** Leukocyte recruitment, infiltration, and smooth muscle cell (SMC) proliferation and migration in the days after injury. **E,** Neointimal thickening in the weeks after injury, with continued SMC proliferation and monocyte recruitment. **F,** Long-term (weeks to months) change from a predominantly cellular plaque to a less cellular and more extracellular matrix–rich plaque. (*Reprinted with permission from Frederick GP, Welt FGP, Rogers C: Inflammation and restenosis in the stent era, Arterioscler Thromb Vasc Biol 22:1769–1776, 2002.*)

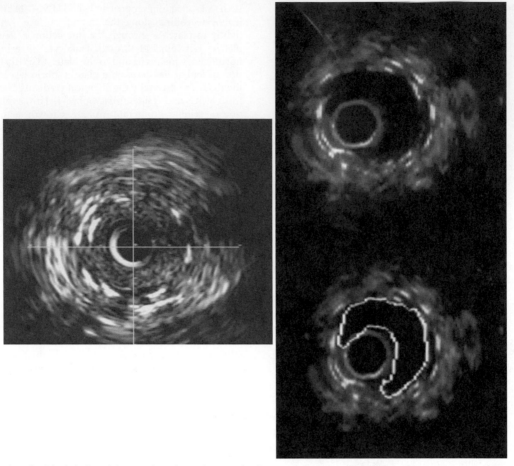

Figure 32-6 Example of a black hole (*delineated in the right panel*) after implantation of sirolimus-eluting stent, as detected by intravascular ultrasound (IVUS). The black hole has a homogeneous black appearance, but its differentiation from the lumen requires careful evaluation of the IVUS image. *Right panel*, A typical IVUS appearance of intimal hyperplasia after bare metal stent implantation.

anti-proliferative agents released from DES devices. The cellular composition of human DES re-stenotic tissue may vary from a T lymphocyte–prominent cellular infiltrate to a predominantly SMC- and ECM-rich tissue similar to BMS re-stenosis. Several lines of evidence suggest that vascular responses, in general, are altered by DESs compared with BMSs. An echolucent intimal hyperplasia, named *black hole*, has been identified by IVUS in patients treated with DESs (Fig. 32-6).[69,70] The molecular mechanisms involved in the development of the black hole are not yet understood but likely represent an altered cellular response to vascular injury. One possible explanation is the preservation of the secretion properties of few resident SMCs and inflammatory cells in spite of the impairment of cell cycle division. Regions of acelullar plasma-like collections have been observed at 30 and 90 days after sirolimus-eluting stent (SES) implantation in porcine coronary arteries; and experimental models show increased fibrin deposition after DES implantation, which is associated with delayed healing.[71,72] The potential for delayed re-endothelialization and inhibition of vascular repair is particularly important following implantation of DES because the anti-proliferative agents used to prevent SMC proliferation also delay re-endothelialization in the stented segment.[72,73] Angioscopic and pathologic evidence, indeed, demonstrates delayed arterial healing with DESs compared with BMSs, as DES-treated arteries have evidence of incomplete re-endothelialization, chronic inflammatory cell infiltration, fibrin deposition, and platelet activation.[72–76] It is important to recognize that inflammatory and thrombotic systems share common signaling pathways and that thrombotic responses that promote activation of the clotting cascade also stimulate platelet activation and SMC proliferation.[77] In addition to anti-proliferative

drug-associated delayed healing with DESs, stent-induced or polymer-induced inflammation has also been identified as a possible contributor to DES re-stenosis and stent thrombosis. Polymer-induced inflammation might be especially operant in cases where there is late DES failure (re-stenosis >6 months after implantation) or late stent thrombosis (>12 months after implantation) occurring long after the DES anti-proliferative dugs have eluted from the polymer.[78–80] Inflammatory responses to the drug, stent, or polymer may result from non-specific innate immune responses that have a predominance of monocyte or macrophage infiltrates or may be related to antigen-specific adaptive immune hypersensitivity responses typified by infiltration of eosinophils, B cells, and T cells.[81] With regard to the inflammatory effects of the stent metal, a recent study demonstrated that ions from the corrosion of stent material activate thrombospondin 1–dependent inflammatory and proliferative signaling pathways in SMCs and thus may promote persistent BMS-associated and DES-associated inflammation and re-stenotic processes.[80] Further evidence for altered arterial healing with DESs comes from studies that demonstrate impaired endothelial function in arterial segments distal to the stented sites in DES-treated arteries compared with BMS-treated arteries.[82,83] DES-associated abnormalities in endothelial function could be related to delayed vascular repair and not to the DES drug itself because the kinetics of the DES are such that the drugs are completely eluted within months after stent implantation.[84–87] It is possible, however, that in certain circumstances, drug accumulation in the arterial wall and in the lipophilic core of the stented atheroma results in prolonged drug retention or release and ongoing vascular dysfunction.[88] The mechanism of DES-associated endothelial dysfunction has not been

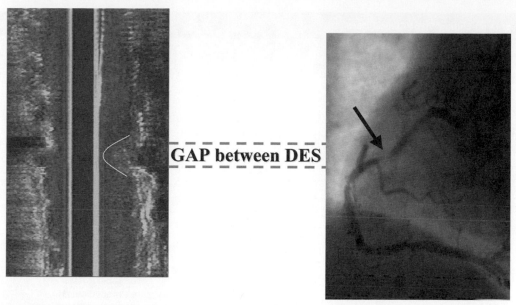

Figure 32-7 Longitudinal intravascular ultrasound (IVUS) image showing a focal intimal hyperplasia formation (delineated) in a gap between two sirolimus-eluting stents. Note the lack of intimal hyperplasia within the stents. Right panel shows the corresponding focal angiographic re-stenosis (*black arrow*). Mechanical and procedure-related factors are key determinants of re-stenosis after implantation of drug-eluting stents.

established, and other than the direct effect of lingering drug, potential etiologies may be related to decreased nitric oxide bioavailability, abnormal release of vasoactive autacoids, or both. Recent studies have demonstrated that there is variability in the severity of DES associated endothelial dysfunction among specific DES agents.[89–91] It is unclear if DES-associated vascular dysfunction influences clinical outcomes following DES implantation. One small study demonstrated impaired endothelial function in patients presenting with in-stent re-stenosis compared with matched controls; however, this association requires validation in larger prospective investigations.[92]

Procedural Factors Associated with Re-Stenosis: the Importance of Interventional Effectiveness

The "bigger is better" philosophy, in which the lumen size obtained after PCI will ultimately determine the occurrence of re-stenosis, has been largely accepted in the BMS era.[93] Somewhat paradoxically, the potent anti-proliferative effects of DESs exposed the mechanical and procedure-related factors as major causes of re-stenosis. Neointimal hyperplasia is mostly abolished within the DES. As a result, the clinical signs of neointimal proliferation or negative remodeling secondary to vessel trauma or untreated disease at the segments adjacent to the DES become amplified (Fig. 32-7). The SLLR (Prospective evaluation of the impact of stent deployment techniques on clinical outcomes of patients treated with the cypheR™ stent) was a large scale (*n* = 1567; 43 participating institutions) study prospectively investigating SES deployment technique and its relationship to clinical outcomes in the modern PCI era. This study reported a high incidence of geographical miss, as defined by the mismatching of lesion and injury vascular targets with subsequent SES treatment deployment sites, and provided the first scientific evidence of the negative impact of procedure-related factors on clinical re-stenosis. Other mechanical failures that may trigger re-stenosis include stent underexpansion and strut fracture, which are both associated with higher rates of TLR.[94,95]

Clinical Factors Linked to Re-Stenosis

Identification of factors associated with higher risk of re-stenosis may be useful in counseling patients on selecting PCI or other therapeutic strategies (clinical treatment or bypass surgery). Unfortunately, there have been inconsistencies in linking re-stenosis to baseline demographic and clinical characteristics. Diabetes mellitus has consistently been demonstrated to be an important clinical risk factor for re-stenosis after angioplasty and BMS implantation.[96] Some anatomic features have also been implicated with the increased likelihood of re-stenosis: saphenous vein graft disease, small vessel diameter, long lesions and chronic total occlusion, which have been associated with higher incidence of angiographic re-stenosis after BMS.[97–101] Although prior knowledge of the subset of patients at higher risk of re-stenosis may be useful for clinical decision making, angiographic and IVUS studies have extensively demonstrated that the principal determinant of re-stenosis is the lumen size achieved at the end of the procedure.[102,103] While the DES has drastically reduced angiographic and clinical re-stenosis across broad patient subsets, certain anatomic and clinical scenarios, such as patients with diabetes mellitus, re-stenotic lesions after brachytherapy or DES implantation, bypass graft disease, and bifurcations continue to be problematic.[104–107]

Incidence and Patterns of Re-Stenosis

The incidence of binary re-stenosis and late loss in key stent clinical trials are described in table 32-1.[14,107–118] One should consider differences in time of follow-up assessment, percentage of patients with angiographic follow-up data, and patient population when interpreting clinical trial re-stenosis data. In-stent re-stenosis has been characterized angiographically as focal (≤10 mm in length), diffuse (>10 mm), proliferative (>10 mm extending outside the stent), or total occlusion in patients treated with Palmaz–Schatz BMSs. This classification correlated with outcomes of re-intervention and was largely adopted in the era of BMSs.[119] Focal re-stenosis occurred in 42% of patients, diffuse in 21%, proliferative in 30%, and total occlusion in 7% after Palmaz–Schatz stent implantation.[119,120] Mid-stent articulation, which provides less scaffolding support, was likely associated with the somewhat high frequency of focal re-stenosis in Palmaz–Schatz stents. The same classification has been used to evaluate re-stenosis after DES implantation, although modern stents do not have articulation and longer stents are used more frequently. Nevertheless, the pattern of in-stent re-stenosis has changed with DESs and appears to be specific for each type of device. For example, re-stenoses after SESs are mostly (>90%) focal and usually located at the stent edges, whereas diffuse

TABLE 32-1	**Summary of Drug-Eluting Stent Clinical Data**				
Study (n)	*Randomized*	*Drug/Agent*	*Device type*	*In-Stent Late Loss** (time of follow-up)	*In-Lesion Re-stenosis* (time of follow-up)
Pivotal Stent trials					
STRESS (n = 410)	Yes	None	Palmaz–Schatz™	0.74-mm (6-month)[†]	31.6% (6-month)
			Balloon angioplasty	0.38-mm (6-month)[†]	42.1% (6-month)
BENESTENT (n = 520)	Yes	None	Palmaz–Schatz™	0.65-mm (6-month)[†]	22% (6-month)
			Balloon angioplasty	0.32-mm (6-month)[†]	42% (6-month)
MUSIC (n = 161)	No	None	IVUS-guided, Palmaz–Schatz™	0.77-mm (6-month)	8.3% (6-month)
Pivotal DES trials					
RAVEL (n = 238)	Yes	Sirolimus	BX Velocity™	−0.01-mm (6-month)	0% (6-month)
			BX Velocity™	0.8-mm (6-month)	26.6% (6-month)
SIRIUS (n = 1058)	Yes	Sirolimus	BX Velocity™	0.17-mm (8-month)	8.9% (9-month)
		None	BX Velocity™		
TAXUS IV (n = 1314)	Yes	Paclitaxel	Express 2™	0.39-mm (SR, 9-month)	7.9% (9-month)
		None	Express 2™	0.92-mm (9-month)	26.6% (9-month)
ENDEAVOR II (n = 1197)	Yes	Zotarolimus	Driver™	0.61-mm (9-month)	13.2% (9-month)
		None	Driver™	1.03-mm (9-month)	35% (9-month)
Head-to-Head Trials					
REALITY (n = 1386)	Yes	Sirolimus	BX Velocity™	0.09-mm (8-month)	9.6% (8-month)
		Paclitaxel	Express 2™	0.31-mm (8-month)	11.1% (8-month)
SIRTAX (n = 1012)	Yes	Sirolimus	BX Velocity™	0.13-mm (9-month)	6.7% (9month)
		Paclitaxel	Express 2™	0.25-mm (9-month)	11.9% (9-month)
Spirit IV (n = 1002)	Yes 2:1	Everolimus	Vision™	0.14-mm (8-month)	8.9% (8-month)
		Paclitaxel	Express 2™	0.28-mm (8-month)	4.7% (8-month)
Diabetes Trials					
DIABETES-I (n = 160)	Yes	Sirolimus	BX Velocity™	0.08 (9-month)	7.7% (9-month)
		None	BX Velocity™	0.66-mm (9-month)	33% (9-month)
DIABETES-II (n = 80)	No	Paclitaxel	Express 2™	0.42-mm (9-month)	7.6% (9-month)
ISAR-DIABETES (n = 250)	Yes	Sirolimus	BX Velocity™	0.19-mm (6-month)	6.9% (6-month)
	Yes	Paclitaxel	Express 2™	0.49-mm (6-month)	16.5% (6-month)

*Pivotal trials data provided for the active treatment groups only.

[†]"In-lesion" late loss is provided for bare metal stent studies because "in-stent" angiography measurements were not applied. Drug-eluting stent figures reflect "in-stent" late loss.

FR, fast release; *SR*, slow release.

intimal proliferation or total occlusion accounts for approximately half of the re-stenosis cases with paclitaxel-eluting stents (PESs).[121–123] Assuming that intimal hyperplasia is almost completely blocked in patients without diabetes, with de novo, short (<20-mm) stenoses located in nonbifurcated native coronary arteries, one should expect that re-stenosis is likely caused by technique-related failures. As a result, re-stenosis would be mostly focal and observed at the stent edges or gaps between stents in these noncomplex cases (see Fig. 32-7). In contrast, biologic and/or mechanical would be more likely to cause diffuse patterns of in-stent. An exception to this rule is re-stenosis after bifurcation PCI, which should be classified separately because it is frequently associated with focal stenosis at the ostium of the side branch.[124]

Treatment of Re-Stenosis

Re-stenosis after balloon angioplasty has a relatively benign outcome after PCI. The low (<20%) rate of repeat re-stenosis in patients with balloon angioplasty re-stenosis treated with BMSs compares favorably with data after treatment of de novo lesions (Table 32-1).[125] Conversely, treatment of in-stent re-stenosis has been associated with high (>35%) rates of repeat target lesion revascularization.[126] At 4 years follow-up, event-free survival was 69% after repeat BMS implantation and 64% after balloon angioplasty.[127] Intracoronary radiation therapy was the sole therapeutic approach that proved its efficacy clinically in the treatment of BMS re-stenosis.[128] However, the treatment paradigm for in-stent re-stenosis has changed and DES implantation is currently the treatment of choice for BMS re-stenosis. Both SESs and PESs have been shown to be superior to brachytherapy in the treatment of BMS re-stenosis.[129–131] Despite its lower frequency compared with BMS

re-stenosis, DES re-stenosis is a particularly vexing problem, and the most appropriate treatment strategy for DES re-stenosis has yet to be defined. A recent randomized investigation study that used 6- to 8-month angiographic follow-up demonstrated that SESs and PESs were equally effective at treating DES re-stenosis; however, late loss (approximately 0.40 mm), binary re-stenosis (approximately 20%), and TLR rates (approximately 15.5%) were relatively high.[132] Re-stenosis outcomes appear to be associated with the pattern of the stenosis, with the highest repeat re-stenosis rates being observed in patients with diffuse patterns.[133,134] Although the strategy of repeat DES has been used widely, the long-term safety of exposing the vessel wall to another potent anti-proliferative therapy such as radiation or implantation of a second DES has yet to be determined, and there is potential for markedly aberrant vascular healing and higher rates of late and very late stent thrombosis. The use of IVUS or OCT may be helpful in defining the mechanism associated with DES re-stenosis and should be considered. If mechanical failures are encountered and the stenosis is discrete, properly sized balloon angioplasty may suffice. If the disease is mostly outside the stent, that is, edge re-stenosis, another DES could be effective. However, a safe and effective strategy for the rare cases of diffuse or proliferative DES re-stenosis has yet to be established.

Future Directions

Future anti–re-stenosis strategies will need to reconcile anti-proliferative strategies with pro-healing effects. Investigators have pursued diverse strategies, including pharmacologic combination, tissue engineering, gene and stem cell therapies, and even procedural modifications (i.e., direct stenting) to limit endothelial injury, accelerate endothelial cell regeneration, or both.[135-137] Further, the use of anti-thrombotic agents in combination with current cell cycle inhibitors may improve the safety of current DESs.[138] The catheter-based drug delivery approach has been resurrected recently. Local drug delivery systems may provide high concentrations of anti-proliferative drugs at the site of vascular injury, without the undesirable persistence of a metallic prosthesis, which may remain prone to thrombosis if re-endothelialization does not occur. However, initial catheter-based local drug delivery therapies were unsuccessful in the treatment of human coronary stenoses because of the rapid washout of the drug downstream into the coronary circulation and the potential flow or pressure-mediated vessel wall injury.[139] Recently, the use of new balloon coating technology and hydrophobic drugs, which may minimize stent-induced injury and increase drug retention, produced satisfactory results in patients with in-stent re-stenosis.[140] However, balloon-based PCI does not provide scaffolding support and may be prone to dissection and abrupt vessel closure. The predictability of the acute results of stent-based PCI is likely the main reason for the widespread acceptance of BMSs in the early days. However, the combination of balloon-based strategies and stents may play an important role in the future. Anti-thrombotic or pro-healing agents may be used in conjunction with BMSs or DESs. Alternatively, the balloon may be coated with potent anti-proliferative agents for early release, and the stents could carry pro-healing drugs to trigger re-endothelialization. The next generations of DESs are attempting to reduce the possibility of polymer-induced inflammation, delayed arterial healing, re-stenosis, and stent thrombosis through use of polymers that have better biocompatibility, are biodegradable, or both. Nonpolymeric delivery systems have been shown to be associated with less peri-stent inflammation in experimental animal studies; early experience with the first biolimus-eluting stent (BES) that has a bioerodable polymer demonstrated good results with noninferiority for a composite endpoint of cardiac death, MI, or clinically induced target vessel revascularization at 9 months compared with standard SES (BES 9% vs. SES 11%; 95% CI 0.64-1.19).[141,142] When the bioerodable polymer BES was studied specifically in long lesions, the MACE rates for the BES and SES were similar (BES 17% vs. SES 14.6%; $P = 0.62$); however, there was a trend toward higher clinically driven TLR (BES 10.5% vs. SES 5.3%; hazard ratio [HR] 1.94; $P = 0.13$).[143] In an OCT substudy of this bioerodable BES long lesion trial, strut coverage at 9 months was more complete in patients allocated to a bioerodable polymer BES versus a durable polymer SES, which suggested improved healing with BESs.[144] The impact of this difference in strut coverage on clinical outcomes and, in particular, on the risk of late stent thrombosis has yet to be determined. It is also difficult to compare the effect or benefit of bioabsorbable polymers versus non-erodable polymers in these aforementioned BES-SES head-to-head trials because the stents have different platforms, drugs, and release kinetics. The benefit of a bioabsorbable polymer will be better assessed in future studies comparing the currently approved durable polymer SES with the Nevo stent (Johnson and Johnson), which has a bioabsorbable drug reservoir that releases sirolimus in a controlled fashion and has kinetics similar to the non-erodable polymer stent. Initial clinical experience with Nevo demonstrated a nonsignificant trend toward improved MACE rates compared with PES (6.1% Nevo vs. 10.8% paclitaxel, $P = 0.14$).[145] Further investigation will be necessary to determine if this bioabsorbable polymer strategy will have better long-term re-stenosis and thrombosis rates and safety profiles compared with currently available stents with non-erodable polymers. Finally, biodegradable DES, which "dissolve" slowly after implantation, represent the ultimate stent technology. Theoretically, biodegradable or erodable stents provide initial scaffolding support to prevent vessel recoil and negative remodeling, without the undesirable continuous vessel injury caused by a permanent rigid foreign body. Although initial iterations of bioabsorbable stents did not fare well compared with the existing stents, probably because the stent biodegraded too quickly, the newest generation of bioabsorbable stents have been made with greater radial strength.[116,147] Initial and 2-year results of studies using newer-generation bioabsorbable EESs are promising, demonstrating reduction in plaque, zero stent thrombosis, and no MACEs at 6 months to 2 years.[148,149] Multimodal imaging also demonstrated the successful absorption of this stent and restoration of coronary artery vasomotor responses 8 to 12 months following implantation.[149]

Summary

The DES certainly represents a major breakthrough in the treatment of CAD and in the prevention of re-stenosis. However, the problem of re-stenosis has not been completely eradicated, and the best treatment strategy for diffuse DES re-stenosis remains controversial. With regard to better deliverability and biodegradable devices, DES platforms can improve considerably in the future, and the current challenge is to further establish the long-term safety of PCI devices while developing new strategies that will both treat obstructive atherosclerosis and promote arterial healing.

REFERENCES

1. Gruntzig AR, Senning A, Siegenthaler WE: Nonoperative dilatation of coronary-artery stenosis: Percutaneous transluminal coronary angioplasty. *N Engl J Med* 301:61–68, 1979.
2. Roubin GS, King SB, 3rd, Douglas JS, Jr: Restenosis after percutaneous transluminal coronary angioplasty: The Emory University Hospital experience. *Am J Cardiol* 60:39B–43B, 1987.
3. Gould KL, Lipscomb K, Hamilton GW: Physiologic basis for assessing critical coronary stenosis. Instantaneous flow response and regional distribution during coronary hyperemia as measures of coronary flow reserve. *Am J Cardiol* 33:87–94, 1974.
4. Kuntz RE, Baim DS: Defining coronary restenosis. Newer clinical and angiographic paradigms. *Circulation* 88:1310–1323, 1993.
5. Rensing BJ, Hermans WR, Deckers JW, et al: Which angiographic variable best describes functional status 6 months after successful single-vessel coronary balloon angioplasty? *J Am Coll Cardiol* 21:317–324, 1993.
6. Guedes A, Tardif JC: Intravascular ultrasound assessment of atherosclerosis. *Curr Atheroscler Rep* 6:219–224, 2004.
7. Costa MA, Simon DI: Molecular basis of restenosis and drug-eluting stents. *Circulation* 111:2257–2273, 2005.
8. Sousa JE, Costa MA, Tuzcu EM, et al: New frontiers in interventional cardiology. *Circulation* 111:671–681, 2005.
9. Costa MA, Sabate M, Angiolillo DJ, et al: Relocation of minimal luminal diameter after bare metal and drug-eluting stent implantation: Incidence and impact on coronary angiographic late loss. *Catheter Cardiovasc Interv* 69(2):181–188, 2006.
10. Garcia-Garcia HM, Shen Z, Piazza N: Study of restenosis in drug eluting stents: New insights from greyscale intravascular ultrasound and virtual histology. *EuroIntervention* 5(Suppl D):D84–D92, 2009.
11. Yamamoto M, Takano M, Murakami D, et al: Optical coherence tomography analysis for restenosis of drug-eluting stents. *Int J Cardiol* 146(1):100–103, 2011.
12. Bezerra HG, Costa MA, Guagliumi G, et al: Intracoronary optical coherence tomography: A comprehensive review clinical and research applications. *JACC Cardiovasc Interv* 2:1035–1046, 2009.
13. Mehilli J, Kastrati A, Wessely R, et al: Randomized trial of a nonpolymer-based rapamycin-eluting stent versus a polymer-based paclitaxel-eluting stent for the reduction of late lumen loss. *Circulation* 113:273–279, 2006.
14. Morice MC, Serruys PW, Sousa JE, et al: A randomized comparison of a sirolimus-eluting stent with a standard stent for coronary revascularization. *N Engl J Med* 346:1773–1780, 2002.
15. Strauss BH, Serruys PW, de Scheerder IK, et al: Relative risk analysis of angiographic predictors of restenosis within the coronary wall stent. *Circulation* 84:1636–1643, 1991.
16. Sabate M, Costa MA, Kozuma K, et al: Methodological and clinical implications of the relocation of the minimal luminal diameter after intracoronary radiation therapy. Dose finding study group. *J Am Coll Cardiol* 36:1536–1541, 2000.
17. Brown BG, Bolson E, Frimer M, et al: Quantitative coronary arteriography: Estimation of dimensions, hemodynamic resistance, and atheroma mass of coronary artery lesions using the arteriogram and digital computation. *Circulation* 55:329–337, 1977.
18. Fleming RM, Kirkeeide RL, Smalling RW, et al: Patterns in visual interpretation of coronary arteriograms as detected by quantitative coronary arteriography. *J Am Coll Cardiol* 18:945–951, 1991.
19. Takano M, Inami S, Jang IK, et al: Evaluation by optical coherence tomography of neointimal coverage of sirolimus-eluting stent three months after implantation. *Am J Cardiol* 99:1033–1038, 2007.
20. Bouma BE, Tearney GJ, Yabushita H, et al: Evaluation of intracoronary stenting by intravascular optical coherence tomography. *Heart* 89:317–320, 2003.
21. Gonzalo N, Garcia-Garcia HM, Serruys PW, et al: Reproducibility of quantitative optical coherence tomography for stent analysis. *EuroIntervention* 5:224–232, 2009.
22. Finn AV, Kolodgie FD, Harnek J, et al: Differential response of delayed healing and persistent inflammation at sites of overlapping sirolimus- or paclitaxel-eluting stents. *Circulation* 112:270–278, 2005.
23. Hassan AK, Bergheanu SC, Stijnen T, et al: Late stent malapposition risk is higher after drug-eluting stent compared with bare-metal stent implantation and associates with late stent thrombosis. *Eur Heart J* 31:1172–1180, 2010.
24. Serruys PW, Luijten HE, Beatt KJ, et al: Incidence of restenosis after successful coronary angioplasty: A time-related phenomenon. A quantitative angiographic study in 342 consecutive patients at 1, 2, 3, and 4 months. *Circulation* 77:361–371, 1988.
25. Cutlip DE, Chauhan MS, Baim DS, et al: Clinical restenosis after coronary stenting: Perspectives from multicenter clinical trials. *J Am Coll Cardiol* 40:2082–2089, 2002.

26. Teirstein PS, Massullo V, Jani S, et al: Three-year clinical and angiographic follow-up after intracoronary radiation: Results of a randomized clinical trial. *Circulation* 101:360–365, 2000.
27. Sousa JE, Costa MA, Abizaid A, et al: Four-year angiographic and intravascular ultrasound follow-up of patients treated with sirolimus-eluting stents. *Circulation* 111:2326–2329, 2005.
28. Fajadet J, Morice MC, Bode C, et al: Maintenance of long-term clinical benefit with sirolimus-eluting coronary stents: Three-year results of the RAVEL trial. *Circulation* 111:1040–1044, 2005.
29. Ruygrok PN, Webster MW, de Valk V, et al: Clinical and angiographic factors associated with asymptomatic restenosis after percutaneous coronary intervention. *Circulation* 104:2289–2294, 2001.
30. Andersen K, Steinthorsdottir SD, Haraldsdottir S, et al: Clinical evaluation and stress test have limited value in the diagnosis of in-stent restenosis. *Scand Cardiovasc J* 43:402–407, 2009.
31. Kumbhani DJ, Ingelmo CP, Schoenhagen P, et al: Meta-analysis of diagnostic efficacy of 64-slice computed tomography in the evaluation of coronary in-stent restenosis. *Am J Cardiol* 103:1675–1681, 2009.
32. de Graaf FR, Schuijf JD, van Velzen JE, et al: Diagnostic accuracy of 320-row multidetector computed tomography coronary angiography to noninvasively assess in-stent restenosis. *Invest Radiol* 45:331–340, 2010.
33. Wijns W, Serruys PW, Simoons ML, et al: Predictive value of early maximal exercise test and thallium scintigraphy after successful percutaneous transluminal coronary angioplasty. *Br Heart J* 53:194–200, 1985.
34. Chen MS, John JM, Chew DP, et al: Bare metal stent restenosis is not a benign clinical entity. *Am Heart J* 151:1260–1264, 2006.
35. Rathore S, Kinoshita Y, Terashima M, et al: A comparison of clinical presentations, angiographic patterns and outcomes of in-stent restenosis between bare metal stents and drug eluting stents. *EuroIntervention* 5:841–846, 2010.
36. Kushner FG, Hand M, Smith SC, Jr, et al: 2009 focused updates: ACC/AHA guidelines for the management of patients with ST-elevation myocardial infarction (updating the 2004 guideline and 2007 focused update) and ACC/AHA/SCAI guidelines on percutaneous coronary intervention (updating the 2005 guideline and 2007 focused update): A report of the American College of Cardiology Foundation/American Heart Association Task Force on Practice Guidelines. *Circulation* 120:2271–2306, 2009.
37. Popma JJ, van den Berg EK, Dehmer GJ: Long-term outcome of patients with asymptomatic restenosis after percutaneous transluminal coronary angioplasty. *Am J Cardiol* 62:1298–1299, 1988.
38. Ruygrok PN, Melkert R, Morel MA, et al: Does angiography six months after coronary intervention influence management and outcome? Benestent II investigators. *J Am Coll Cardiol* 34:1507–1511, 1999.
39. Forrester JS, Fishbein M, Helfant R, et al: A paradigm for restenosis based on cell biology: Clues for the development of new preventive therapies. *J Am Coll Cardiol* 17:758–769, 1991.
40. Scott NA, Cipolla GD, Ross CE, et al: Identification of a potential role for the adventitia in vascular lesion formation after balloon overstretch injury of porcine coronary arteries. *Circulation* 93:2178–2187, 1996.
41. Riessen R, Isner JM, Blessing E, et al: Regional differences in the distribution of the proteoglycans biglycan and decorin in the extracellular matrix of atherosclerotic and restenotic human coronary arteries. *Am J Pathol* 144:962–974, 1994.
42. Schwartz RS, Huber KC, Murphy JG, et al: Restenosis and the proportional neointimal response to coronary artery injury: Results in a porcine model. *J Am Coll Cardiol* 19:267–274, 1992.
43. Kearney M, Pieczek A, Haley L, et al: Histopathology of in-stent restenosis in patients with peripheral artery disease. *Circulation* 95:1998–2002, 1997.
44. Rogers C, Seifert P, Edelman ER: The neointima provoked by human coronary stenting: Contributions of smooth muscle and inflammatory cells and extracellular matrix in autopsy specimens over time. *Circulation* 98:I182, 1998.
45. Nabel EG, Boehm M, Akyurek LM, et al: Cell cycle signaling and cardiovascular disease. *Cold Spring Harb Symp Quant Biol* 67:163–170, 2002.
46. Tanner FC, Yang ZY, Duckers E, et al: Expression of cyclin-dependent kinase inhibitors in vascular disease. *Circ Res* 82:396–403, 1998.
47. Polyak K, Kato JY, Solomon MJ, et al: P27kip1, a cyclin-cdk inhibitor, links transforming growth factor-beta and contact inhibition to cell cycle arrest. *Genes Dev* 8:9–22, 1994.
48. Sherr CJ, Roberts JM: Cdk inhibitors: Positive and negative regulators of g1-phase progression. *Genes Dev* 13:1501–1512, 1999.
49. Coats S, Flanagan WM, Nourse J, et al: Requirement of p27kip1 for restriction point control of the fibroblast cell cycle. *Science* 272:877–880, 1996.
50. van Tiel CM, Bonta PI, Rittersma SZ, et al: P27kip1-838c>a single nucleotide polymorphism is associated with restenosis risk after coronary stenting and modulates p27kip1 promoter activity. *Circulation* 120:669–676, 2009.
51. McEver RP, Cummings RD: Role of psgl-1 binding to selectins in leukocyte recruitment. *J Clin Invest* 100:S97–S103, 1997.
52. Diacovo TG, Roth SJ, Buccola JM, et al: Neutrophil rolling, arrest, and transmigration across activated, surface-adherent platelets via sequential action of p-selectin and the beta 2-integrin cd11b/cd18. *Blood* 88:146–157, 1996.
53. Simon DI, Chen Z, Xu H, et al: Platelet glycoprotein Ib-alpha is a counterreceptor for the leukocyte integrin mac-1 (cd11b/cd18). *J Exp Med* 192:193–204, 2000.
54. Welt FG, Tso C, Edelman ER, et al: Leukocyte recruitment and expression of chemokines following different forms of vascular injury. *Vasc Med* 8:1–7, 2003.
55. Horvath C, Welt FG, Nedelman M, et al: Targeting ccr2 or cd18 inhibits experimental in-stent restenosis in primates: Inhibitory potential depends on type of injury and leukocytes targeted. *Circ Res* 90:488–494, 2002.
56. Rogers C, Edelman ER, Simon DI: A Mab to the beta$_2$-leukocyte integrin Mac-1 (cd11b/cd18) reduces intimal thickening after angioplasty or stent implantation in rabbits. *Proc Natl Acad Sci U S A* 95:10134–10139, 1998.
57. Wang Y, Sakuma M, Chen Z, et al: Leukocyte engagement of platelet glycoprotein Ib-alpha via the integrin Mac-1 is critical for the biological response to vascular injury. *Circulation* 112:2993–3000, 2005.
58. Simon DI, Chen Z, Seifert P, et al: Decreased neointimal formation in mac-1(-/-) mice reveals a role for inflammation in vascular repair after angioplasty. *J Clin Invest* 105:293–300, 2000.
59. Berk BC, Gordon JB, Alexander RW: Pharmacologic roles of heparin and glucocorticoids to prevent restenosis after coronary angioplasty. *J Am Coll Cardiol* 17:111B–117B, 1991.
60. Holmes DR, Jr, Savage M, LaBlanche JM, et al: Results of prevention of restenosis with tranilast and its outcomes (PRESTO) trial. *Circulation* 106:1243–1250, 2002.
61. Schwartz RS, Topol EJ, Serruys PW, et al: Artery size, neointima, and remodeling: Time for some standards. *J Am Coll Cardiol* 32:2087–2094, 1998.
62. Di Mario C, Gil R, Camenzind E, et al: Quantitative assessment with intracoronary ultrasound of the mechanisms of restenosis after percutaneous transluminal coronary angioplasty and directional coronary atherectomy. *Am J Cardiol* 75:772–777, 1995.
63. Mintz G, Popma J, Pichard A, et al: Arterial remodeling after coronary angioplasty: A serial intravascular ultrasound study. *Circulation* 94:35–43, 1996.
64. Staab ME, Srivatsa SS, Lerman A, et al: Arterial remodeling after experimental percutaneous injury is highly dependent on adventitial injury and histopathology. *Int J Cardiol* 58:31–40, 1997.
65. Labinaz M, Pels K, Hoffert C, et al: Time course and importance of neoadventitial formation in arterial remodeling following balloon angioplasty of porcine coronary arteries. *Cardiovasc Res* 41:255–266, 1999.
66. Dussaillant GR, Mintz GS, Pichard AD, et al: Small stent size and intimal hyperplasia contribute to restenosis: A volumetric intravascular ultrasound analysis. *J Am Coll Cardiol* 26:720–724, 1995.
67. Costa MA, Sabaté M, Kay IP, et al: Three-dimensional intravascular ultrasonic volumetric quantification of stent recoil and neointimal formation of two new generation tubular stents. *Am J Cardiol* 85:135–139, 2000.
68. Welt FG, Rogers C: Inflammation and restenosis in the stent era. *Arterioscler Thromb Vasc Biol* 22:1769–1776, 2002.
69. Costa MA, Sabate M, Angiolillo DJ, et al: Intravascular ultrasound characterization of the "black hole" phenomenon after drug-eluting stent implantation. *Am J Cardiol* 97:203–206, 2006.
70. Costa Jde R, Jr, Mintz GS, Carlier SG, et al: Frequency and determinants of black holes in sirolimus-eluting stent restenosis. *J Invasive Cardiol* 18:348–352, 2006.
71. Carter AJ, Aggarwal M, Kopia GA, et al: Long-term effects of polymer-based, slow-release, sirolimus-eluting stents in a porcine coronary model. *Cardiovasc Res* 63:617–624, 2004.
72. Joner M, Finn AV, Farb A, et al: Pathology of drug-eluting stents in humans: Delayed healing and late thrombotic risk. *J Am Coll Cardiol* 48:193–202, 2006.
73. Nakazawa G, Finn AV, Joner M, et al: Delayed arterial healing and increased late stent thrombosis at culprit sites after drug-eluting stent placement for acute myocardial infarction patients: An autopsy study. *Circulation* 118:1138–1145, 2008.
74. Kotani J, Awata M, Nanto S, et al: Incomplete neointimal coverage of sirolimus-eluting stents: Angioscopic findings. *J Am Coll Cardiol* 47:2108–2111, 2006.
75. Finn AV, Joner M, Nakazawa G, et al: Pathological correlates of late drug-eluting stent thrombosis: Strut coverage as a marker of endothelialization. *Circulation* 115:2435–2441, 2007.
76. Finn AV, Nakazawa G, Joner M, et al: Vascular responses to drug eluting stents: Importance of delayed healing. *Arterioscler Thromb Vasc Biol* 27:1500–1510, 2007.
77. Croce K, Libby P: Intertwining of thrombosis and inflammation in atherosclerosis. *Curr Opin Hematol* 14:55–61, 2007.
78. Nebeker JR, Virmani R, Bennett CL, et al: Hypersensitivity cases associated with drug-eluting coronary stents: A review of available cases from the research on adverse drug events and reports (radar) project. *J Am Coll Cardiol* 47:175–181, 2006.
79. Virmani R, Guagliumi G, Farb A, et al: Localized hypersensitivity and late coronary thrombosis secondary to a sirolimus-eluting stent: Should we be cautious? *Circulation* 109:701–705, 2004.
80. Pallero MA, Talbert Roden M, Chen YF, et al: Stainless steel ions stimulate increased thrombospondin-1-dependent TGF-beta activation by vascular smooth muscle cells: Implications for in-stent restenosis. *J Vasc Res* 47:309–322, 2010.
81. Byrne RA, Joner M, Kastrati A: Polymer coatings and delayed arterial healing following drug-eluting stent implantation. *Minerva Cardioangiol* 57:567–584, 2009.
82. Fuke S, Maekawa K, Kawamoto K, et al: Impaired endothelial vasomotor function after sirolimus-eluting stent implantation. *Circ J* 71:220–225, 2007.
83. Shin DI, Kim PJ, Seung KB, et al: Drug-eluting stent implantation could be associated with long-term coronary endothelial dysfunction. *Int Heart J* 48:553–567, 2007.
84. Tesfamariam B: Drug release kinetics from stent device-based delivery systems. *J Cardiovasc Pharmacol* 51:118–125, 2008.
85. Kamath KR, Barry JJ, Miller KM: The taxus drug-eluting stent: A new paradigm in controlled drug delivery. *Adv Drug Deliv Rev* 58:412–436, 2006.
86. Waugh J, Wagstaff AJ: The paclitaxel (taxus)-eluting stent: A review of its use in the management of de novo coronary artery lesions. *Am J Cardiovasc Drugs* 4:257–268, 2004.
87. McKeage K, Murdoch D, Goa KL: The sirolimus-eluting stent: A review of its use in the treatment of coronary artery disease. *Am J Cardiovasc Drugs* 3:211–230, 2003.
88. Raman VK, Edelman ER: Coated stents: Local pharmacology. *Semin Interv Cardiol* 3:133–137, 1998.
89. Shin DI, Seung KB, Kim PJ, et al: Long-term coronary endothelial function after zotarolimus-eluting stent implantation. A 9 month comparison between zotarolimus-eluting and sirolimus-eluting stents. *Int Heart J* 49:639–652, 2008.
90. Kim JW, Suh SY, Choi CU, et al: Six-month comparison of coronary endothelial dysfunction associated with sirolimus-eluting stent versus paclitaxel-eluting stent. *JACC Cardiovasc Interv* 1:65–71, 2008.
91. Hamilos MI, Ostojic M, Beleslin B, et al: Differential effects of drug-eluting stents on local endothelium-dependent coronary vasomotion. *J Am Coll Cardiol* 51:2123–2129, 2008.
92. Thanyasiri P, Kathir K, Celermajer DS, et al: Endothelial dysfunction and restenosis following percutaneous coronary intervention. *Int J Cardiol* 119:362–367, 2007.
93. Kuntz RE, Safian RD, Carrozza JP, et al: The importance of acute luminal diameter in determining restenosis after coronary atherectomy or stenting. *Circulation* 86:1827–1835, 1992.
94. Castagna MT, Mintz GS, Leiboff BO, et al: The contribution of "mechanical" problems to in-stent restenosis: An intravascular ultrasonographic analysis of 1090 consecutive in-stent restenosis lesions. *Am Heart J* 142:970–974, 2001.
95. Popma JJ, Tiroch K, Almonacid A, et al: A qualitative and quantitative angiographic analysis of stent fracture late following sirolimus-eluting stent implantation. *Am J Cardiol* 103:923–929, 2009.
96. Abizaid A, Kornowski R, Mintz GS, et al: The influence of diabetes mellitus on acute and late clinical outcomes following coronary stent implantation. *J Am Coll Cardiol* 32:584–589, 1998.
97. Hirshfeld JW, Jr, Schwartz JS, Jugo R, et al: Restenosis after coronary angioplasty: A multivariate statistical model to relate lesion and procedure variables to restenosis. The m-heart investigators. *J Am Coll Cardiol* 18:647–656, 1991.
98. Foley DP, Melkert R, Serruys PW: Influence of coronary vessel size on renarrowing process and late angiographic outcome after successful balloon angioplasty. *Circulation* 90:1239–1251, 1994.
99. Violaris AG, Melkert R, Serruys PW: Long-term luminal renarrowing after successful elective coronary angioplasty of total occlusions. A quantitative angiographic analysis. *Circulation* 91:2140–2150, 1995.
100. Kastrati A, Schomig A, Elezi S, et al: Predictive factors of restenosis after coronary stent placement. *J Am Coll Cardiol* 30:1428–1436, 1997.
101. Kastrati A, Elezi S, Dirschinger J, et al: Influence of lesion length on restenosis after coronary stent placement. *Am J Cardiol* 83:1617–1622, 1999.
102. de Feyter PJ, Kay P, Disco C, et al: Reference chart derived from post-stent-implantation intravascular ultrasound predictors of 6-month expected restenosis on quantitative coronary angiography. *Circulation* 100:1777–1783, 1999.
103. Serruys PW, Kay IP, Disco C, et al: Periprocedural quantitative coronary angiography after Palmaz-Schatz stent implantation predicts the restenosis rate at six months: Results of a meta-analysis of the Belgian Netherlands Stent Study (BENESTENT) I, BENESTENT II pilot, BENESTENT II and MUSIC trials. Multicenter ultrasound stent in coronaries. *J Am Coll Cardiol* 34:1067–1074, 1999.
104. Lemos PA, Hoye A, Serruys PW: Recurrent angina after revascularization: An emerging problem for the clinician. *Coron Artery Dis* 15(Suppl 1):S11–S15, 2004.
105. Costa M, Angiolillo DJ, Teirstein P, et al: Sirolimus-eluting stents for treatment of complex bypass graft disease: Insights from the secure registry. *J Invasive Cardiol* 17:396–398, 2005.
106. Lemos PA, Hoye A, Goedhart D, et al: Clinical, angiographic, and procedural predictors of angiographic restenosis after sirolimus-eluting stent implantation in complex patients: An evaluation from the rapamycin-eluting stent evaluated at Rotterdam Cardiology Hospital (research) study. *Circulation* 109:1366–1370, 2004.
107. Kastrati A, Dibra A, Eberle S, et al: Sirolimus-eluting stents vs paclitaxel-eluting stents in patients with coronary artery disease: Meta-analysis of randomized trials. *JAMA* 294:819–825, 2005.
108. Serruys PW, de Jaegere P, Kiemeneij F, et al: A comparison of balloon-expandable-stent implantation with balloon angioplasty in patients with coronary artery disease. Benestent study group. *N Engl J Med* 331:489–495, 1994.
109. Fischman DL, Leon MB, Baim DS, et al: A randomized comparison of coronary-stent placement and balloon angioplasty in the treatment of coronary artery disease. Stent restenosis study investigators. *N Engl J Med* 331:496–501, 1994.

110. de Jaegere P, Mudra H, Figulla H, et al: Intravascular ultrasound-guided optimized stent deployment. Immediate and 6 months clinical and angiographic results from the multicenter ultrasound stenting in coronaries study (music study). *Eur Heart J* 19:1214–1223, 1998.

111. Moses JW, Leon MB, Popma JJ, et al: Sirolimus-eluting stents versus standard stents in patients with stenosis in a native coronary artery. *N Engl J Med* 349:1315–1323, 2003.

112. Stone GW, Ellis SG, Cox DA, et al: A polymer-based, paclitaxel-eluting stent in patients with coronary artery disease. *N Engl J Med* 350:221–231, 2004.

113. Fajadet J, Wijns W, Laarman GJ, et al: Randomized, double-blind, multicenter study of the endeavor zotarolimus-eluting phosphorylcholine-encapsulated stent for treatment of native coronary artery lesions: Clinical and angiographic results of the ENDEAVOR II trial. *Circulation* 114:798–806, 2006.

114. Sabate M, Jimenez-Quevedo P, Angiolillo DJ, et al: Randomized comparison of sirolimus-eluting stent versus standard stent for percutaneous coronary revascularization in diabetic patients: The diabetes and sirolimus-eluting stent (diabetes) trial. *Circulation* 112:2175–2183, 2005.

115. Colombo A, Drzewiecki J, Banning A, et al: Randomized study to assess the effectiveness of slow- and moderate-release polymer-based paclitaxel-eluting stents for coronary artery lesions. *Circulation* 108:788–794, 2003.

116. Windecker S, Remondino A, Eberli FR, et al: Sirolimus-eluting and paclitaxel-eluting stents for coronary revascularization. *N Engl J Med* 353:653–662, 2005.

117. Morice MC, Colombo A, Meier B, et al: Sirolimus- vs paclitaxel eluting stents in de novo coronary artery lesions: The REALITY trial. A randomized controlled trial. *JAMA* 295:895–904, 2006.

118. Stone GW, Midei M, Newman W, et al: Comparison of an everolimus-eluting stent and a paclitaxel-eluting stent in patients with coronary artery disease: A randomized trial. *JAMA* 299:1903–1913, 2008.

119. Mehran R, Dangas G, Abizaid AS, et al: Angiographic patterns of in stent restenosis: Classification and implications for long-term outcome. *Circulation* 100:1872–1878, 1999.

120. Alfonso F, Cequier A, Angel J, et al: Value of the American College of Cardiology/American Heart Association angiographic classification of coronary lesion morphology in patients with in-stent restenosis. Insights from the restenosis intra-stent balloon angioplasty versus elective stenting (RIBS) randomized trial. *Am Heart J* 151:681 e681–e689, 2006.

121. Lemos PA, Saia F, Ligthart JM, et al: Coronary restenosis after sirolimus-eluting stent implantation: Morphological description and mechanistic analysis from a consecutive series of cases. *Circulation* 108:257–260, 2003.

122. Colombo A, Orlic D, Stankovic G, et al: Preliminary observations regarding angiographic pattern of restenosis after rapamycin-eluting stent implantation. *Circulation* 107:2178–2180, 2003.

123. Corbett SJ, Cosgrave J, Melzi G, et al: Patterns of restenosis after drug-eluting stent implantation: Insights from a contemporary and comparative analysis of sirolimus- and paclitaxel-eluting stents. *Eur Heart J* 27:2330–2337, 2006.

124. Steigen TK, Maeng M, Wiseth R, et al: Randomized study on simple versus complex stenting of coronary artery bifurcation lesions: The Nordic bifurcation study. *Circulation* 114:1955–1961, 2006.

125. Erbel R, Haude M, Hopp HW, et al: Coronary-artery stenting compared with balloon angioplasty for restenosis after initial balloon angioplasty. Restenosis stent study group. *N Engl J Med* 339:1672–1678, 1998.

126. Alfonso F, Zueco J, Cequier A, et al: A randomized comparison of repeat stenting with balloon angioplasty in patients with in-stent restenosis. *J Am Coll Cardiol* 42:796–805, 2003.

127. Alfonso F, Auge JM, Zueco J, et al: Long-term results (three to five years) of the restenosis intrastent: Balloon angioplasty versus elective stenting (ribs) randomized study. *J Am Coll Cardiol* 46:756–760, 2005.

128. Waksman R, Ajani AE, White RL, et al: Five-year follow-up after intracoronary gamma radiation therapy for in-stent restenosis. *Circulation* 107:24–27, 2003.

129. Sousa JE, Costa MA, Abizaid A, et al: Sirolimus-eluting stent for the treatment of in-stent restenosis: A quantitative coronary angiography and three-dimensional intravascular ultrasound study. *Circulation* 107:24–27, 2003.

130. Holmes DR, Jr, Teirstein P, Satler L, et al: Sirolimus-eluting stents vs vascular brachytherapy for in-stent restenosis within bare-metal stents: The SISR randomized trial. *JAMA* 295:1264–1273, 2006.

131. Stone GW, Ellis SG, O'Shaughnessy CD, et al: Paclitaxel-eluting stents vs vascular brachytherapy for in-stent restenosis within bare-metal stents: The taxus V ISR randomized trial. *JAMA* 295:1253–1263, 2006.

132. Mehilli J, Byrne RA, Tiroch K, et al: Randomized trial of paclitaxel- versus sirolimus eluting stents for treatment of coronary restenosis in sirolimus-eluting stents: The ISAR-DESIRE 2 (intracoronary stenting and angiographic results: Drug eluting stents for in-stent restenosis 2) study. *J Am Coll Cardiol* 55:2710–2716, 2010.

133. Lemos PA, van Mieghem CA, Arampatzis CA, et al: Post-sirolimus-eluting stent restenosis treated with repeat percutaneous intervention: Late angiographic and clinical outcomes. *Circulation* 109:2500–2502, 2004.

134. Cosgrave J, Melzi G, Biondi-Zoccai GG, et al: Drug-eluting stent restenosis the pattern predicts the outcome. *J Am Coll Cardiol* 47:2399–2404, 2006.

135. Rogers C, Parikh S, Seifert P, et al: Endogenous cell seeding: Remnant endothelium after stenting enhances vascular repair. *Circulation* 94:2909–2914, 1996.

136. Kawamoto A, Gwon HC, Iwaguro H, et al: Therapeutic potential of ex vivo expanded endothelial progenitor cells for myocardial ischemia. *Circulation* 103:634–637, 2001.

137. Kutryk MJ, Foley DP, van den Brand M, et al: Local intracoronary administration of antisense oligonucleotide against c-myc for the prevention of in-stent restenosis: Results of the randomized investigation by the Thoraxcenter of antisense DNA using local delivery and IVUS after coronary stenting (ITALICS) trial. *J Am Coll Cardiol* 39:281–287, 2002.

138. Lin CE, Garvey DS, Janero DR, et al: Combination of paclitaxel and nitric oxide as a novel treatment for the reduction of restenosis. *J Med Chem* 47:2276–2282, 2004.

139. Lincoff AM, Topol EJ, Ellis SG: Local drug delivery for the prevention of restenosis. Fact, fancy, and future. *Circulation* 90:2070–2084, 1994.

140. Scheller B, Hehrlein C, Bocksch W, et al: Treatment of coronary in-stent restenosis with a paclitaxel-coated balloon catheter. *N Engl J Med* 355:2113–2124, 2006.

141. Tada N, Virmani R, Grant G, et al: Polymer-free biolimus, a 9-coated stent demonstrates more sustained intimal inhibition, improved healing, and reduced inflammation compared with a polymer-coated sirolimus-eluting Cypher stent in a porcine model. *Circ Cardiovasc Interv* 3:174–183, 2010.

142. Windecker S, Serruys PW, Wandel S, et al: Biolimus-eluting stent with biodegradable polymer versus sirolimus-eluting stent with durable polymer for coronary revascularisation (LEADERS): A randomised non-inferiority trial. *Lancet* 372:1163–1173, 2008.

143. Wykrzykowska JJ, Raber L, de Vries T, et al: Biolimus-eluting biodegradable polymer versus sirolimus-eluting permanent polymer stent performance in long lesions: Results from the leaders multicentre trial substudy. *EuroIntervention* 5:310–317, 2009.

144. Barlis P, Regar E, Serruys PW, et al: An optical coherence tomography study of a biodegradable vs. Durable polymer-coated limus-eluting stent: A LEADERS trial sub-study. *Eur Heart J* 31:165–176, 2010.

145. Abizaid A: *The Nevo RES-I: Twelve-month outcomes*, Paris, France, May 25, 2010, Presented at EuroPCR.

146. Waksman R, Erbel R, Di Mario C, et al: Early- and long-term intravascular ultrasound and angiographic findings after bioabsorbable magnesium stent implantation in human coronary arteries. *JACC Cardiovasc Interv* 2:312–320, 2009.

147. Tanimoto S, Serruys PW, Thuesen L, et al: Comparison of in vivo acute stent recoil between the bioabsorbable everolimus-eluting coronary stent and the everolimus-eluting cobalt chromium coronary stent: Insights from the ABSORB and SPIRIT trials. *Catheter Cardiovasc Interv* 70:515–523, 2007.

148. Ormiston JA, Serruys PW, Regar E, et al: A bioabsorbable everolimus-eluting coronary stent system for patients with single de-novo coronary artery lesions (absorb): A prospective open-label trial. *Lancet* 371:899–907, 2008.

149. Serruys PW, Ormiston JA, Onuma Y, et al: A bioabsorbable everolimus-eluting coronary stent system (ABSORB): 2-year outcomes and results from multiple imaging methods. *Lancet* 373:897–910, 2009.

33

Bioabsorbable Stents

DEBABRATA MUKHERJEE

One of the major advances in the field of interventional cardiology has been the development of coronary stents. By providing mechanical scaffolding to the vessel, a conventional metallic stent prevents abrupt closure of the vessel, which is a major safety concern with balloon angioplasty. Disruption of the endothelium invariably ensues following angioplasty or stenting and in most cases, approximately 12 weeks are needed for complete re-endothelialization and intimal healing.[1] Although stents have significantly reduced acute vessel closure compared with angioplasty, there are several drawbacks. Besides leaving a permanent implant, stenting in the long term may also prevent favorable arterial remodeling.[2] Stenting of long lesions, as commonly performed now, may preclude future surgical or percutaneous revascularization, when needed, and may interfere with image interpretations of MRA and CTA because of metallic artifacts. As conventional metallic stents provide stimuli for smooth muscle cell proliferation, neointimal hyperplasia leading to in-stent re-stenosis occurs in up to 30% of patients at 6 months.[3–5] Drug-eluting stents (DESs), on the platform of metallic stents, markedly reduce the rate of in-stent re-stenosis by eluting anti-proliferative drugs such as rapamycin, everolimus, zotarolimus, and paclitaxel.[6,7] Though DESs have significantly overcome the hurdles of in-stent re-stenosis and have reduced the rate of revascularization, they may cause an increase in stent thrombosis, both early and late, because of either long-term ongoing inflammation or other factors.[8–10] Combination anti-platelet therapy with aspirin and clopidogrel is therefore recommended for at least 12 months after a DES to minimize the risks of stent thrombosis.[11,12] A significant step forward in stent technology is the development of biodegradable or bioabsorbable stents, which may eliminate some of the concerns and drawbacks of traditional metallic stents. Bioabsorbable stents are made up of materials capable of gradual degradation in the body and thus leave no residual implant within the arteries. A bioabsorbable stent should provide adequate scaffolding for a clinically relevant period (ideally about 6 months) and then disappear. This avoids the potential disadvantages of a permanent metallic implant, may reduce or elimante stent thrombosis stent thrombosis, makes future imaging with CTA or MRA possible, facilitates re-intervention, and may restore vasomotion and prevent side branch obstruction by jailing from metallic struts.[13] An effective bioabsorbable stent will perform acutely like a current-generation metallic DES with the same or better long-term safety profile. Only after these criteria have been met will the advantages of bioabsorption encourage the widespread adoption of bioabsorbable stents. A successful design is a combination of numerous factors, including material selection, absorption profile, drug efficacy, deliverability of the stent system, and acute mechanical performance of the stent. Table 33-1 lists the advantages and disadvantages of bioabsorbable stents compared with traditional metallic stents.

Bioabsorbable Materials

Beginning with absorbable sutures in the 1960s, bioabsorbable polymers have been employed in a wide variety of medical devices. Polymers manufactured from lactide and glycolide-based polymers are the most commonly used materials for clinically approved devices. The safety of these polymers, as both vascular and nonvascular device ingredients, has been well demonstrated, with hundreds of devices being approved for human use over the past four decades. The mechanical properties of a polymer are tensile strength, modulus and strain-to-failure affect recoil, expansibility, flexibility, and deliverability of a stent. Thus, a suitable polymer should have high tensile strength, high modulus, and optimal elongation to allow the creation of a low-profile, balloon-expandable stent design. The degradation rate and the degradation products of the polymer affect the duration of vessel support and the degree of tissue reaction. Chemical and thermal properties determine the type of degradation products and the type of processing and sterilization methods that can be used. The characteristics of a suitable polymer for intravascular stenting are listed in Table 33-2; these include optimal mechanical strength, degradation profile, and biocompatibility.[14] The bioabsorbable stents currently under investigation do not meet all of the criteria to be considered optimal. The physical properties of a polymer are determined by its hydrophilicity, crystallinity, molecular-weight distribution, and end groups and the presence of residual monomers or additives.[15–17] Table 33-3 lists the physical properties of commonly used biodegradable polymers. Polyglycolic acid (PGA), the polymer of glycolic acid, is the simplest linear aliphatic polyester. PGA is highly crystalline with a high melting point and a degradation period of 6 to 12 months. Polylactide (PLA) is the polymer of lactic acid. Lactic acid has two optical isomers— L-lactic acid, the naturally occurring isomer, and D-lactic acid. Poly D,L-lactic acid (PDLLA) contains both D-lactide and L-lactic acid.

TABLE 33-1	Advantages and Disadvantages of Bioabsorbable Stents	
Advantages		**Disadvantages**
Long lengths of vessel can be treated without worries of formation of a permanent "full metal jacket," resulting in more physiologic repair		Loss of scaffolding too early may lead to re-stenosis from vessel remodeling
Provide scaffolding only when needed during vessel healing		May cause local tissue reaction with inflammation and neointimal proliferation, leading to re-stenosis
Avoid long-term complications of permanent stent implant, such as late remodeling		Visibility poor on x-ray without markers or contrast embedding
Restore local vascular compliance or vasomotion		Sensitivity to heat and solvents may limit choices of drug or coating
Will not interfere with cardiac magnetic resonance angiography (MRA) or computed tomographic angiography (CTA) imaging		Thick struts needed to improve mechanical strength; may impede deliverability of the stents in smaller vessels
May reduce or eliminate the risk of late stent thrombosis		Malapposition more frequent
Will not preclude future surgical or percutaneous revascularization and will allow re-intervention		Possible embolization of bulky stent particles during degradation may cause watershed infarcts
May afford new treatment options for diffuse disease, and unstable or vulnerable plaque		
May be used repetitively in a single vessel, as there will be no permanent implant or need for re-intervention.		
Suitable for pediatric use and also for use in the younger population		
May be suitable for vessels with complex anatomy and vessels of lower extremities		
Freedom from persistent side branch obstruction by struts		

Poly-L-lactic acid (PLLA) is the homopolymer of L-lactide. The degradation time of PLLA is much slower than that of PDLLA. As PDLLA is amorphous, with low tensile strength, higher elongation time, and rapid degradation rate, it is highly suitable for a drug delivery system. Table 33-4 lists the ideal properties of a polymer suitable for drug elution. In contrast, PLLA is semi-crystalline, with a slower degradation rate and higher tensile strength and thus seems to be ideal for use as a stent. Tissue response to the degradation products depends on the rate of degradation, size and site of the implant, and local tissue microenvironment (pH, acidity, etc.). Lactide-based and glycolide-based polymers undergo degradation by hydrolysis, which leads to the formation of water-soluble, low molecular-weight components, which are metabolized into carbon dioxide and water. Bulk erosion occurs when the rate at which water penetrates the device exceeds that at which the polymer is converted into water-soluble materials, which results in erosion throughout the device. Strongly hydrophobic polymers undergo mostly surface erosion, a process that occurs when the rate at which water penetrates the device is slower than the rate of conversion of polymer into water-soluble material, which leads to device thinning over time but maintains its bulk integrity.[19,20] Figures 33-1 and 33-2 portray the degradation process of bioabsorbable polymers. Limitations of a polymer-based bioabsorbable stent include potential for inflammation and a bulkier profile compared with metallic stents. The search for potential alternatives to bioabsorbable polymers as stent materials has led scientists to investigate the scope of absorbable metals. An ideal absorbable metal stent should have mechanical properties similar to conventional metal stents, have sustained mechanical integrity, have steerable kinetics, induce normal endothelial function with minimal or zero inflammatory or thrombogenic response, and degrade into nontoxic byproducts. Magnesium and iron meet most of these criteria and have been further evaluated. These two metals, even at high doses, were found to have no cytotoxic or genotoxic effects, are devoid of acute systemic toxicity, and are hemocompatible with no chronic toxicity. In general, metallic stents are found to have higher collapse pressure and lesser degree of recoil, thus providing efficient scaffolding.[21]

TABLE 33-2	Characteristics of an Ideal Bioabsorbable Stent Material

- The stent material should have a moderate degradation rate in a predictable fashion over a finite period (within 6 to 12 months) leaving no residual matrices.
- The degradation products should be biocompatible, nontoxic, and not cause significant inflammatory reaction.
- The stent material should have high tensile strength and strain-to-failure before degradation to allow creation of low-profile, balloon-expandable design for easy deliverability and flexibility.
- The stent material should possess adequate radial strength and mechanical properties for vessel support during local healing.
- The stent material should not be thrombogenic and should release no emboli that may cause watershed infarcts.
- The stent material should perform acutely and over the long term like metal stents and should be equal to or better than drug-eluting metal stents with respect to re-stenosis and clinical outcomes.
- The stent material should be easily processed and sterilizable.
- The stent material should have an acceptable shelf life.

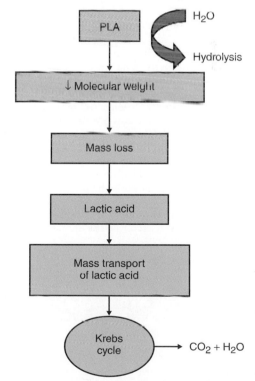

Figure 33-1 Metabolic pathways of bioabsorbable polymers. Bioabsorbable polymers are degraded in the body by hydrolysis into carbon dioxide and water.

TABLE 33-3	Physical Properties of Bioabsorbable Polymers Currently Used for Bioabsorbable Stents						
Polymer	Crystallinity	Tensile Strength (MPa)	Tensile Modulus (GPa)	Melting Point °C	Elongation (%)	Degradation Rate (Months)	Degradation Products
PGA	Semi-crystalline	60–80	7.0	225–230	15–20	6 to 12	Glycolic acid
PLLA	Semi-crystalline	60–70	2.7	173–178	5–10	>24	Lactic acid
PDLLA	Amorphous	40–50	1.9	–	3–10	12–16	Lactic acid

PGA, polyglycolic acid; *PLLA*, poly-L-lactic acid; *PDLLA*, Poly-D,L,-lactic acid.

Adapted from Ormiston JA, Serruys PW, Regar E, et al: A bioabsorbable everolimus-eluting coronary stent system for patients with single de-novo coronary artery lesions (ABSORB): A prospective open-label trial, *Lancet* 371(9616):899–907, 2008.

Polymer-Based Bioabsorbable Stents

The first biodegradable stent, made of a polymer of poly-L-lactide (PLLA) was developed in the early 1980s by Stack et al and implanted in animal models at Duke University in the 1990s.[22] Although this stent could withstand up to 1000 mm Hg of crush pressure, almost twice as much compared with a Palmaz–Schatz stent, could maintain its radial strength for 1 month, and degraded completely by 9 months, further progress in the research of this polymeric stent was somewhat slow. The Duke bioabsorbable stent was the prototype of the PLA stent used in canine femoral arteries and was self-expanding. The long-term degradation of this stent caused little thrombotic response, minimal neointimal hyperplasia, and minimal inflammatory reaction.[22] The Kyoto University biodegradable stent, made of polyglycolic acid, developed a few years after the Duke stent, was more thrombogenic when implanted in a canine model.[23] The Cleveland clinic–Mayo–Thoraxcenter biodegradable stent consisting of five different biodegradable polymers (PDLLA, polyorthoester, poly-hydroxybutyrate/hydroxyvalerate, polycaprolactone, and polyethelene oxide) exhibited marked inflammatory reaction with neointimal proliferation in porcine coronary arteries.[24] This intense local reaction—as demonstrated by a marked inflammatory reaction, neointimal proliferation, medial necrosis, and pseudo-aneurysm formation—was observed in the case of both bioabsorbable and biodurable polymers. Thus, the observed response (at 28 days) was not caused by the formation of degradation products. The inflammatory response was most likely caused by the use of nonsterile implants and a less-than-ideal geometry. When the results obtained in this study are compared with the low-thrombotic and low-inflammatory response obtained with the Duke PLLA stent, it becomes apparent that vessel response is driven by a combination of parameters. An effective bioabsorbable stent must therefore combine an ideal material, adequate sterilization techniques, and an optimal design to achieve desirable results. In a further evaluation of bioabsorbable stents, Lincoff et al demonstrated that the differential degree of local reaction in a porcine coronary injury model was dependent on the size of the polymers, with the lighter PLLA polymers (molecular mass about 80 kiloDaltons [kDa]) being more inflammatory and the heavier polymers (molecular mass about 321 kDa) being less so.[25] Yamawaki et al coated the biodegradable stent with an anti-proliferative drug, a tyrosine kinase inhibitor (tranilast), to suppress this local reaction and found that there was a reduced risk of stenosis with the drug–polymer combination.[26]

TABLE 33-4	Ideal Characteristics of a Drug-Eluting Bioabsorbable Polymer

- Linear degradation profile
- Fast degradation rate (<6 months)
- Compatibility with hydrophilic and hydrophobic drugs
- Stable under different pH conditions
- Good film-forming properties
- Solubility in common solvents
- No toxic metabolic end products

Poly L-Lactic Acid Bioabsorbable Stents

CORONARY STENTS

The collapse pressures of PLLA stents are nearly equal to that of stainless steel metal stents, which makes these polymers suitable for bioabsorbable stents.[20] The Igaki–Tamai stent (Igaki Medical Planning Company, Kyoto, Japan), a mono-filamentous, PLLA-based, 183-kDa biodegradable stent, was the first bioabsorbable stent implanted in humans (Fig. 33-3). It has been improved from its earlier versions with a zigzag, helical coiled design that may minimize tissue injury and thereby reduce local tissue reaction and thrombus formation.[27-29] A combination of the heat-expandable and balloon-expandable properties of the stent allowed its initial self-expansion in response to heat (transmitted by a delivery balloon inflated with 70°C contrast-water mixture and 50°C at the balloon site) and subsequent re-expansion with a moderate degree of balloon inflation (at 6 to 14 atmosphere). Continued expansion of the stent to its normal size over 20 to 30 minutes at 37°C generated a radial strength similar to that of the Palmaz–Schatz stent. As PLLA is radiolucent, gold markers at each end provide radiopacity for stent identification. Following initial success with implantation in animal models, characterized by minimal inflammatory response, Tamai et al extended their experience to humans and implanted 25 of these stents in 19 lesions in 15 patients electively, with angiographic follow-up by intravascular ultrasound (IVUS) at day 1, 3 months, and 6 months.[28,29] Angiographic re-stenosis rates of 5.3% and 10.5% with a loss index of 0.44 mm and 0.48 mm at 3 and 6 months, respectively, were reported. The study reported no deaths, myocardial infarction (MI), or coronary artery bypass grafting (CABG). Although the self-expansion of the stent continued up to the third month after implantation, the stent maintained its scaffolding even at 6 months. Subsequently, Tamai et al reported long-term outcomes of 63 lesions in 50 patients, who underwent elective stenting; this revealed a low complication rate, with 1 in-hospital stent thrombosis causing a Q wave MI, 1 noncardiac death, and 18% repeat percutaneous coronary intervention (PCI), and no surgical revascularization at 4-year follow up.[30] No further human coronary studies have been performed, and the focus is now on a peripheral application. This stent is primarily of historical importance in the evolution of bioabsorbable coronary stents.

DRUG-ELUTING STENTS

Tranilast Stents

In an attempt to reduce inflammatory reaction at the site of stent implantation, Yamawaki et al incorporated ST638 (tranilast, a specific tyrosine kinase inhibitor) or ST494 (an inactive metabolite of ST638) into the Igaki–Tamai PLLA stents and evaluated the stents in a porcine coronary artery model for 21 days.[26] Three weeks after the implantation of the stents, coronary stenosis was assessed by coronary angiography followed by histologic examination. Coronary stenosis was significantly less with the ST638 stent compared with the ST494 stent. Histologic examination of the vessels also showed less neointimal

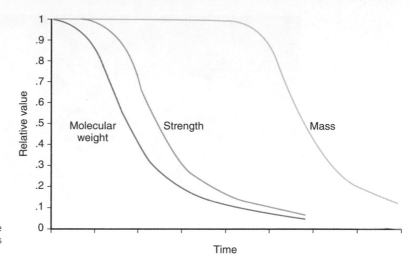

Figure 33-2 During the degradation process, bioabsorbable polymers first undergo reduction in molecular weight, then loss of strength, and finally mass loss.

proliferation and a lesser degree of geometric remodeling at the ST638 sites compared with the ST494 stent sites.[26] Thus, incorporating antiproliferative agents into bioabsorbable stents appears to be an effective way of minimizing tissue inflammatory reactions, thereby reducing the degree of subsequent re-stenosis.

Paclitaxel Stents

Vogt et al developed a novel balloon-expandable, biodegradable double-helical PDLLA stent using controlled expansion of saturated polymers (CESP) for better integration of thermally sensitive polymers and longer drug delivery.[31] Twelve paclitaxel-loaded (170 mcg paclitaxel with release rate of 5–8 mcg initially tapering to 1 mcg at 4 weeks and 0 mcg at 3 months) PDLLA stents, 12 unloaded PDLLA stents, and 12 bare metal stents (316L) were implanted in 36 porcine coronary arteries. Six animals of each group were sacrificed at 3 weeks and 3 months, respectively. During this follow-up, coronary stenosis was significantly reduced with paclitaxel-eluting stents (PES) compared with unloaded and bare metal stents (BMS).[31] Although early endothelialization of the stents was evident and mechanical integrity was maintained at 3 months, a local inflammatory response to the polymer stent was the major concern from this animal study.

Everolimus Stents

The Bioabsorbable Vascular Solutions (BVS) everolimus-eluting stent (EES) is a major advancement in the field of bioabsorbable stents and is the first bioabsorbable DES to undergo clinical studies. The BVS stent is a fully bioabsorbable balloon-expandable DES that performs acutely like a metallic DES. Hence, no special techniques are required to deliver and deploy the stent. With its thin struts, a fairly low profile, and a plastic-like polymeric material, the BVS stent is a highly deliverable and conformable stent. It is a high-molecular-weight PLLA-based stent, with a PDLLA coating serving as a bioabsorbable matrix for an everolimus-eluting layer. Mounted on the ML Vision SDS balloon, the

stent includes two platinum radiopaque markers on the end rings of the stent for enhanced visibility. In addition, the polymeric material of the BVS stent allows it to be visible with MRA and CTA, offering the potential for noninvasive patient follow-up in the future. The BVS everolimus-eluting coronary stent system contains 100 mcg of everolimus per square centimeter of surface area. The vascular response of the BVS everolimus-eluting stent in porcine and rabbit arterial models was characterized by a thin, well-healed neointima comprising compact smooth muscle cells in a proteoglycan–collagen matrix (data obtained from Abbott Vascular, Santa Clara, CA).The ABSORB (A bioabsorbable everolimus-eluting coronary stent system for patients with single de novo coronary artery lesions) trial—the BVS stent system's first in-human clinical trial—was a prospective, open-labeled trial enrolling 30 patients with visually estimated nominal vessel diameter of 3 mm.[32] The design of the BVS stent revision 1.0 used in cohort A of the ABSORB trial included circumferential out-of-phase zigzag hoops, strut thickness of 150 µm, and linkage either directly or by straight bridges (Fig. 33-4). Revision 1.1 (see Figure 33-4) for cohort B of the ABSORB trial was constructed from the same polymer material, but different methods of processing were used to increase the duration of radial support to months and to retain the same total absorption time of about 2 years.[13] In cohort A of the ABSORB first-in-man trial, 3-mm diameter BVS stents, either 12 mm or 18 mm in length, were implanted in 30 patients with simple, de novo, native coronary artery stenoses. The procedure was a success in all 30 patients, and there was successful delivery of the BVS device in 94% (29 of 31 attempts). The device was safe for 2 years with only 1 ischemia-driven major adverse cardiac event (MACE), which was a non-Q myocardial infarction. At 6 months, IVUS revealed no vessel shrinkage (no change in the area within the external elastic lamina), but there was reduction of 11% to 12% in the stent area.[32,33] The in-stent late loss reported on indirect comparison was similar to that reported with polymeric metallic PESs, more than that with metallic EESs, and less than that seen with a polymeric zotarolimus-eluting stent (Fig. 33-5). Another important finding in a small number of patients tested was the return of normal vasoreactivity in the stented segment.[33] Of concern was the fact that 7% of 671 struts in 13 stents showed malapposition at follow-up; the risk of bulky stent particles emblazing and causing watershed infarct was not appropriately investigated with imaging studies.[34] This second phase of the ABSORB clinical trial (cohort B) enrolled 101 patients from 12 centers in Europe, Australia, and New Zealand and incorporated device enhancements designed to improve deliverability and vessel support. Patients treated with the Bioabsorbable Vascular Solutions (BVS) stent, demonstrated no occurrence of stent thrombosis, no need for repeat procedures (ischemia-driven target lesion revascularization), and a very low rate of MACEs of 2% at 30 days.[35] Although this cohort demonstrated the safety of the new revision of BVS, the overall safety

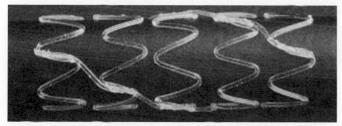

Figure 33-3 The Igaki–Tamai stent is a premounted, balloon-expandable poly L-lactic acid (PLLA) stent with the ability for self-expansion and has a helical zigzag design.

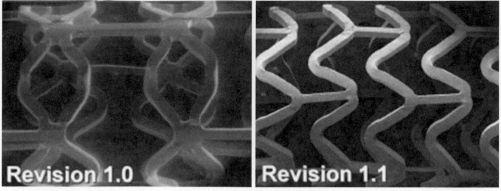

Figure 33-4 Bioabsorbable vascular solution everolimus-eluting stent is a balloon-expandable, drug-eluting (everolimus) bioabsorbable stent composed of polylactide polymers and co-polymers mounted on a standard delivery system.

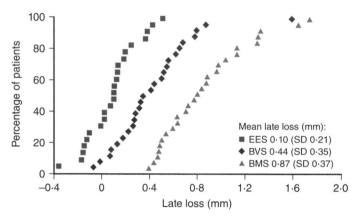

Mean late loss (mm):
■ EES 0·10 (SD 0·21)
◆ BVS 0·44 (SD 0·35)
▲ BMS 0·87 (SD 0·37)

Figure 33-5 Cumulative frequency distribution curve of in-stent late loss in the ABSORB trial (BVS stent) and in the bare-metal stent and metallic drug-eluting stent of the SPIRIT FIRST trial. *BMS*, bare metal stent; *EES*, everolimus-eluting stent. (*Adapted from Ormiston JA, Serruys PW, Regar E, et al: A bioabsorbable everolimus-eluting coronary stent system for patients with single de-novo coronary artery lesions (ABSORB): A prospective open-label trial, Lancet 371(9616):899–907, 2008.*)

of these devices requires further confirmation in large event-driven clinical trials. The ABSORB–EXTEND trial is a single-arm study that is currently enrolling patients at nearly 100 centers in Europe, Asia Pacific, Canada, and Latin America and will enroll approximately 1000 patients, including those with more complex coronary artery disease (CAD).

Non-PLLA Bioabsorbable Coronary Stents

A tyrosine-derived polycarbonate is the bioabsorbable polymer of the stent developed by REVA pharmaceutics (Reva Medical Inc, San Diego, CA). This polymer, developed at Rutgers University, delivers good stent performance and also doubles as a drug-delivery matrix with complete drug release from the polymer. The stent has iodine to allow x-ray visibility, polyethelene glycol to make the material less adhesive to components and less thrombogenic, and an acidic co-monomer to control biodegradation. The non-deforming nature of its "slide and lock" design (Fig. 33-6) results in a stent with good strength, flexibility, expansion without material deformation yet with reduced stent strut thickness and conformability to the vessel wall. It also allows for standard balloon deployment. As the stent is resorbed, the degradation

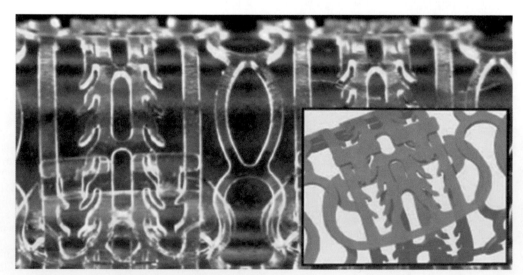

Figure 33-6 Photograph of the REV, a bioabsorbable stent.

products are safely excreted from the body. Radiopacity is provided by impregnation with iodine. Its struts are relatively thick (200 µm); when it is balloon mounted, its crossing profile is 1.7 mm requiring at least a 7F (7 French) guiding catheter. The RESORB first-in-man trial with a non–DES version was a prospective, nonrandomized single-arm safety study that enrolled 27 patients. The primary endpoints were MACEs at 30 days, and secondary endpoints were quantitative coronary angiographic and IVUS parameters at 6 months. At 30 days, 2 patients had experienced a Q wave MI, and 1 had target lesion revascularization. Preliminary results suggested unfavorable outcomes between 4 and 6 months after implantation, with a higher-than-anticipated target lesion revascularization rate driven mainly by reduced stent diameter.[13] Additional studies after design modification are being planned.

Non–Polymer-Based Bioabsorbable Stents

Bioabsorbable polymer stents need to be bulkier and have thicker struts compared with BMSs to generate adequate mechanical properties for their sustenance in the vessels; as an alternative, biodegradable metallic stents may be quite promising. Only two bioabsorbable metal alloys have so far been considered for this application: magnesium and iron. Both metals being essential elements in the human body, the degradation products are likely to be less toxic and more biocompatible compared with the drugs in metallic DES.

MAGNESIUM CORONARY STENTS

Magnesium is one of the most important micronutrients in the human body. The physiologic plasma magnesium concentration is 1.4 to 2.1 mEq/L (0.70–1.05 mmol/L), and the metabolic conversion of magnesium to its chloride, oxide, sulfate, or phosphate salts are well tolerated. The biodegradation products of magnesium in the body are unlikely to cause any serious adverse effects. Magnesium can also act as a systemic and coronary vasodilator. It is a physiologic calcium antagonist and prevents intracellular calcium load during ischemia and platelet aggregation. In addition, magnesium may prevent endothelin-induced vasoconstriction and inhibit endothelin production and has been found to be safe in patients undergoing elective PCI.[36,37] Magnesium alloys contain 3 to 6 mg of magnesium per stent, depending on the stent length and variable amounts of other metals. The magnesium alloy AE21 contains 2% aluminum and 1% rare earth elements (cerium [Ce], praseodymium [Pr], neodymium [Nd]) with an anticipated mass loss of only 50% in 6 months. In the first animal model with this magnesium alloy stent, 20 stents were

implanted in coronaries of 16 pigs via 8F guiding catheters and followed up for up to 56 days with angiograms, IVUS and histopathologic evaluation. The initial procedural success rate was 100%, and there was no evidence of any thromboembolic events during follow-up; however, there was a significant 40% loss of perfused lumen diameter between days 10 and 35 because of neointima formation and a significant 25% luminal re-enlargement between days 35 and 56 because of vascular remodeling from loss of stent integrity. Moreover, uneven and asymmetrical expansion of the stent with protrusion of the stent struts within the adventitia caused inflammation and exaggerated intimal hyperplasia in areas with the greatest concentration of degradation products.[38] Further improvements of the stent by prolonging the rate of metal degradation and enhancing its mechanical integrity were therefore necessary. The Lekton Magic coronary stent (Biotronik, Bulach, Switzerland) was an upgrade from the earlier magnesium alloy stent, comprising WE43 magnesium alloy with zirconium (<5%), yttrium (<5%), and rare earth elements (<5%). The stent has circumferential noose-shaped elements connected by unbowed cross-links along its longitudinal axis (Fig. 33-7). The first-in-man absorbable magnesium stent was evaluated in the PROGRESS-AMS (Clinical performance and angiographic results of coronary stenting with absorbable magnesium stents) trial of 63 patients from seven European centers with stable or unstable angina pectoris without MI.[21] The primary endpoint of the study was a composite of death, nonfatal MI, and ischemia-driven target lesion revascularization. The expected degradation of the stent was 2 to 3 months, and follow-up IVUS had demonstrated complete endothelialization at 2 to 3 months. The designated noninferiority criterion was less than 30% of the primary endpoint, and the study reported 23% of patients meeting the primary endpoint. Although the stent was completely absorbed within 2 months, radial support was lost much earlier so that, perhaps within days, there was an insufficient radial strength to counter the early negative remodeling forces after PCI. At 4 months, there was a high re-stenosis rate of almost 50%, and at 1 year, target vessel revascularization was 45%.[21] Newer designs to assess prolongation of radial support and potential for drug coating are being planned.

MAGNESIUM PERIPHERAL STENTS

Bioabsorbable magnesium stents (AMS) were also studied in the PROGRESS trial for critical limb ischemia from high grade infrapopliteal stenoses (80%–100%) in 20 patients.[39] Angiographic procedural success was achieved in 100% of the patients. Primary clinical patency was maintained in 90% and 78% of patients at 3 and 6 months, respectively. No major or minor amputation was needed in any of the patients at 3 months, and at 6 months, 1 patient had undergone amputation of the index limb. Duplex ultrasound and MRA

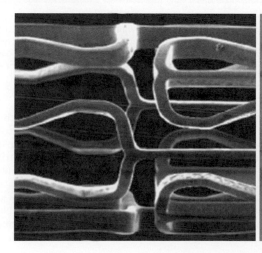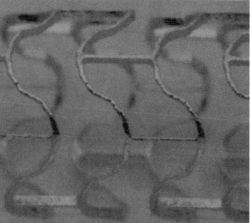

Figure 33-7 A bioabsorbable magnesium stent unexpanded in the left panel and expanded in the right panel at different magnifications. It is a laser cut from tubular magnesium WE-43 and has sinusoidal in-phase hoops linked by straight bridges. Strut thickness is 170 µm but crossing profile for the 3-mm stent is only 1.2 mm. The arterial coverage by expanded stent is similar to conventional metallic stents at 10%. It is balloon expandable, does not have a drug coating, and is radiolucent.

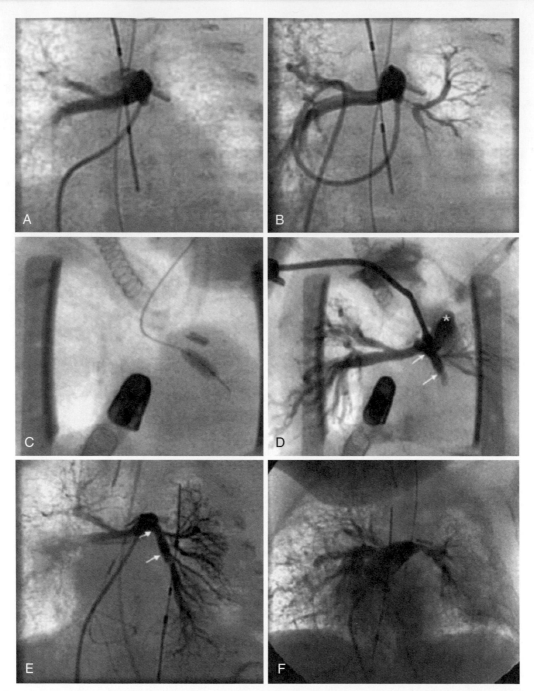

Figure 33-8 **A,** Complete occlusion of the left pulmonary artery after debanding and closure of the arterial duct with a clip (the device with three markers is for calibration purposes). **B,** After crossing the stenosis with a guidewire, angiography revealed reperfusion. **C,** Implantation procedure with a contrast-filled balloon catheter. **D,** Immediately after implantation, only minimal perfusion of the left upper lobe artery was detectable by angiography. The left lower lobe artery was still completely occluded at 4 mm distal to the stent. Both ends of the stent are marked by arrows. The asterisk marks some extravascular contrast agent. **E,** At 1-week follow-up, the left lung was reperfused. **F,** At latest follow-up (33rd day after stent implantation), after the circumferential integrity of the stent had resolved, left lung perfusion persisted with a curved course within the stented area.

demonstrated complete absorption of the stents at 3 months. The average improvement in Rutherford class was 2.3 at 3 months. These pilot results were encouraging, and may open up avenues for the treatment of critical limb ischemia with bioabsorbable metal stents.

DRUG-ELUTING ABSORBABLE METAL STENT SYSTEM

Although absorbable metal stents were found to have adequate mechanical strength, the lack of superior efficacy in reducing re-stenosis has been disappointing. Thus, a strategy of impregnating an anti-proliferative agent into the magnesium stents to prevent the rate of stenosis is warranted. The concept of drug-eluting absorbable metal stents led to the impregnation of bioabsorbable magnesium alloy with a bioabsorbable polymer matrix carrying discrete drug-delivery reservoirs with pimecrolimus. Pimecrolimus, an anti-inflammatory agent (not an MTOR [mammalian target of rapamycin] inhibitor), binds with high affinity to FKBP-12 and inhibits calcineurin, which, in turn, inhibits T cell activation by blocking the transcription of early cytokines.[40] The GENESIS (Randomized, Multicenter Study of the Pimecrolimus-Eluting and Pimecrolimus/ Paclitaxel-Eluting Coronary

TABLE 33-5 A Comparison of the Properties of Five Absorbable Stents and Two Permanent Drug-Eluting Stent Systems

Stent	Strut Material	Coating Material	Design	Absorption Products	Drug Elution	Stent Radio-Opacity	Deployment	Total Strut Thickness (Strut+Coating), μm	Crossing Profile, mm	Stent-to-Artery Coverage, %	Duration Radial Support	Absorption Time
Igaki-Tamai	Polymer–poly-L-lactic acid	Nil	Zigzag helical coils with straight bridges	Lactic acid, carbon dioxide (CO_2), and water (H_2O)	Nil	Gold markers	Self-expanding and heated balloon	170	?	24	6 mo	2 y
Bioabsorbable magnesium alloy	Metal–magnesium alloy	Nil	Sinusoidal in-phase hoops linked by straight bridges	Not applicable	Nil	Nil	Balloon	165	1.2	10	Days or weeks	<4 mo
BVS (Bioabsorbable Vascular Solutions)	Polymer–poly-L-lactic acid	Poly-D,L-lactic acid	Cohort A: out-of-phase sinusoidal hoops with straight and direct links; cohort B: in-phase hoops with straight links	Lactic acid, CO_2, and H_2O	Everolimus	Platinum markers	Balloon	156	1.4	25	Cohort A: weeks; cohort B: 3 mo	2 y
REVA	Polymer–tyrosine-derived polycarbonate polymer	Nil	Side and lock	Amino acids, ethanol, CO_2	Nil	Iodine impregnated	Balloon	200	1.7	55	3 to 6 mo	2 y
BTI (Bioabsorbable Therapeutics Incorporated)	Polymer salicylate + linker	Salicylate + different linker	Tube with laser-cut voids	Salicylate, CO_2, and H_2O	Sirolimus salicylate	Nil	Balloon	200	2.0	65	3 mo	6 mo
Xience V metallic drug-eluting stent	Metal–cobalt chromium	Fluoropolymer	In-phase sinusoidal hoops with curved bridges	Nil	Everolimus	Yes	Balloon	96.2	1.085	10.7	Permanent	Permanent
Cypher metallic drug-eluting stent	Metal–stainless steel	Polyethylene-co-vinyl acetate + poly(n-butyl methacrylate)	Out-of-phase sinusoidal hoops with curved bridges	Nil	Sirolimus	Yes	Balloon	165.2	1.220	12.9	Permanent	Permanent

Adapted from Ormiston JA, Serruys PW: Bioabsorbable coronary stents, *Circ Cardiovasc Interv* 2(3):255-260, 2009.

Stent System in Patients with De Novo Lesions of the Native Coronary Arteries) trial, which was the first large clinical trial of pimecrolimus-eluting stents in a bioerodable polymer, was suspended early because of an increase in target vessel revascularization in the pimecrolimus-eluting stent group (35.5%); these stents are therefore unlikely to be a viable option.[41]

MAGNESIUM STENTS FOR NONCORONARY APPLICATIONS

Conventional stents leave a permanent implant at the vessel site; in the pediatric population, these may be outgrown soon as the vessel size grows appropriately with age. This may lead to a fixed mechanical obstruction of the vessel with the implanted metal stents, which may necessitate surgical intervention. Because they avoid permanent implantation and any casting of the index vessel, bioabsorbable stents may offer an attractive alternative for PCIs for congenital heart diseases, which have been treated mostly by surgical procedures thus far. Recent case reports of successful and uneventful deployment of absorbable magnesium stents in the treatment of a ligated pulmonary artery in a preterm baby and for relief of critical re-coarctation of the aorta in a newborn (Fig. 33-8) reaffirms these promises.[42,43]

ABSORBABLE IRON STENTS

Iron is one of the essential nutrients required by the human body and acts as an essential co-factor for a multitude of enzymes involved in oxygen binding, deoxyribonucleic acid (DNA) synthesis, and redox enzyme activity. The process of iron degradation involves ferrous ion to be oxidized to ferric ion or interaction with nearby cells. Iron ions released from biodegradable iron stents have been shown to reduce the rate of vascular smooth muscle cell proliferation by influencing growth-related gene expression and thus may play a potential role in reducing re-stenosis in vivo.[44] The degradation rate of iron is slow. This slow degradation and small amount of iron in a stent (40 mg) in relation to the iron load of the whole body (400–500 mg/L) make any systemic toxicity unlikely. Corrodible iron thus appears to offer an attractive concept for the formulation of bioabsorbable stents. Peuster and colleagues used corrodible iron (>99.8% iron) to produce iron stents (NOR-I) and implanted these stents in the native descending aorta of 16 New Zealand White Rabbits (mean luminal diameter 3.4 mm; ratio of balloon diameter to vessel diameter 1:13).[45] During the 6–18-month follow-up, no adverse events and no thromboembolic complications were reported, and all the stents were patent in follow-up angiographic evaluations at 6, 12, and 18 months. Moreover, these stents had produced no systemic iron toxicity, no local inflammation, and no neointimal proliferation. In another preclinical study, Waksman et al demonstrated that stents made of biocorrodible iron were safe; measured parameters such as intimal thickness, intimal area, and percentage occlusion showed a trend in favor of the iron stents compared with cobalt chromium stents.[46] Thus, iron stents appear to be promising and feasible on the basis of preliminary animal data but need to be evaluated in clinical studies. Issues with the slow degradation time for iron-based devices and theoretical concerns regarding systemic iron-related toxicity have hampered clinical development so far.

◼ Conclusion and Future Directions

The idea of a coronary prosthesis that does its job and then disappears is intrinsically appealing. Bioabsorbable stents, therefore, have the potential to usher in the next revolution in percutaneous coronary and endovascular interventions. However, adequately powered robust clinical trials are needed to assess the risk–benefit ratio of this platform critically. Significant refinement of drug delivery and stent mechanics is needed; available preliminary data with regard to this appear encouraging. A number of different materials ranging from magnesium, iron, and a variety of polymers have been used to construct bioabsorbable

stents (Table 33-5). The best outcomes, to date, have been with the BVS everolimus-eluting PLLA stent. Impregnation of bioabsorbable stents with anti-proliferative and anti-inflammatory drugs to decrease inflammation and re-stenosis by synergistic effects for the reduction of tissue reaction following bioabsorbable stent implantation appears very promising. The expectation is that a healed, normally functioning vessel free of foreign body and re-stenosis will be free of the risk of late thrombosis and have normal vaso-reactivity. There is tremendous interest in this technology, and the field appears quite crowded with numerous contenders (Table 33-6). However, it remains to be proven whether bioabsorbable stents will stand the test of critical scientific review and time. These stents may offer particular promise in the realm of congenital heart disease and superficial femoral artery interventions.

TABLE 33-6	List of Bioabsorbable Stents Currently in Development
Company	**Product**
Igaki–Tamai	Poly-L-lactic acid (PLLA) material
	Polycaprolactone coating
	Drug-eluting stent (DES) preclinical studies with ST638, ST494
	Balloon-expandable with covered sheath system
Abbott	PLLA stent (BVS)
	Poly-D-L-lactic acid (PDLLA) coating
	Everolimus drug
Reva	Tyrosine-based polycarbonate
	Paclitaxel abluminal delivery
	Slide-and-lock design
Biotronik	Magnesium alloy (93% Mg)
	7 new alloys and 3 new designs considered
	Pimecrolimus-eluting stent failed to show efficacy
	Iron stents in preclinical phase
BTI	Salicylic acid–based surface eroding stent
	Sirolimus eluting
Cordis	Poly-lactic-co-glycolic acid (PLGA)/Poly-caprolactone-co-glycolide (PCL-PGA)
	Balloon-expandable
	Longer drug elution than Cypher stent
	Under development
ART	PLLA stent made from amorphous polymer
	Balloon-expandable
	Claim of positive remodeling
Biosensors	Poly-L-lactic acid (PLLA)/Poly-D-lactide (PLDA) stent
	Self-expanding with retractable sheath
	Elutes everolimus
OrbusNeich	Poly-lactic-co-glycolic acid (PLGA)/Poly-caprolactone-co-glycolide (PCL-PGA) stent
	Elutes a prohealing drug on the abluminal surface
	EPC capturing antibodies on the luminal surface
Bioabsorbable Therapeutics	Incorporates salicylic acid into the backbone of a polyanhydride ester (PAE) polymeric stent
	Surface is coated with sirolimus
	IDEAL™ Stent
Endovasc-TissueGen	PLLA stent
	Spiral helical design
	Claim of growth factors/enzymes delivery
Tepha	Combination of polyester based-"TephaFLEX" and PLLA for additional strength
Sahajanand	PLLA and heparinized PLLA stent with genistein drug
	Balloon expandable
Amaranth	PLLA stent
	Self-expanding stent
	Multiple drug delivery
	Peripheral indication

REFERENCES

1. Grewe PH, Deneke T, Machraoui A, et al: Acute and chronic tissue response to coronary stent implantation: pathologic findings in human specimen. *J Am Coll Cardiol* 35(1):157–163, 2000.
2. Hoffmann R, Mintz GS, Popma JJ, et al: Chronic arterial responses to stent implantation: A serial intravascular ultrasound analysis of Palmaz-Schatz stents in native coronary arteries. *J Am Coll Cardiol* 28(5):1134–1139, 1996.
3. Ellis SG, Savage M, Fischman D, et al: Restenosis after placement of Palmaz-Schatz stents in native coronary arteries. Initial results of a multicenter experience. *Circulation* 86(6):1836–1844, 1992.
4. Fischman DL, Leon MB, Baim DS, et al: A randomized comparison of coronary-stent placement and balloon angioplasty in the treatment of coronary artery disease. Stent Restenosis Study Investigators. *N Eng J Med* 331(8):496–501, 1994.
5. Serruys PW, de Jaegere P, Kiemeneij F, et al: A comparison of balloon-expandable-stent implantation with balloon angioplasty in patients with coronary artery disease. Benestent Study Group. *N Eng J Med* 331(8):489–495, 1994.
6. Moses JW, Leon MB, Popma JJ, et al: Sirolimus-eluting stents versus standard stents in patients with stenosis in a native coronary artery. *N Eng J Med* 349(14):1315–1323, 2003.
7. Stone GW, Ellis SG, Cox DA, et al: A polymer-based, paclitaxel-eluting stent in patients with coronary artery disease. *N Eng J Med* 350(3):221–231, 2004.
8. Farb A, Burke AP, Kolodgie FD, et al: Pathological mechanisms of fatal late coronary stent thrombosis in humans. *Circulation* 108(14):1701–1706, 2003.
9. Ong AT, McFadden EP, Regar E, et al: Late angiographic stent thrombosis (LAST) events with drug-eluting stents. *J Am Coll Cardiol* 45(12):2088–2092, 2005.
10. Pfisterer M, Brunner-La Rocca HP, Buser PT, et al: Late clinical events after clopidogrel discontinuation may limit the benefit of drug-eluting stents: an observational study of drug-eluting versus bare-metal stents. *J Am Coll Cardiol* 2006;48(12):2584–2591.
11. Grines CL, Bonow RO, Casey DE, Jr, et al: Prevention of premature discontinuation of dual antiplatelet therapy in patients with coronary artery stents: a science advisory from the American Heart Association, American College of Cardiology, Society for Cardiovascular Angiography and Interventions, American College of Surgeons, and American Dental Association, with representation from the American College of Physicians. *Circulation* 115(6):813–818, 2007.
12. Zimarino M, Renda G, De Caterina R: Optimal duration of antiplatelet therapy in recipients of coronary drug-eluting stents. *Drugs* 65(6):725–732, 2005.
13. Ormiston JA, Serruys PW: Bioabsorbable coronary stents. *Circ Cardiovasc Interv* 2(3):255–260, 2009.
14. Zidar J, Lincoff A, Stack R: Biodegradable stents. In Topol E, editor: *Textbook of interventional cardiology*, ed 2, Philadelphia, 1994, Saunders.
15. Eberhart RC, Su SH, Nguyen KT, et al: Bioresorbable polymeric stents: Current status and future promise. *J Biomaterials Sci* 14(4):299–312, 2003.
16. Middleton JC, Tipton AJ: Synthetic biodegradable polymers as orthopedic devices. *Biomaterials* 21(23):2335–2346, 2000.
17. Pietrzak WS, Sarver D, Verstynen M: Bioresorbable implants—practical considerations. *Bone* 19(1 Suppl):109S–119S, 1996.
18. Grabow N, Schlun M, Sternberg K, et al: Mechanical properties of laser cut poly(L-lactide) micro-specimens: Implications for stent design, manufacture, and sterilization. *J Biomechanical Engineering* 127(1):25–31, 2005.
19. Grizzi I, Garreau H, Li S, et al: Hydrolytic degradation of devices based on poly(DL-lactic acid) size-dependence. *Biomaterials* 16(4):305–311, 1995.
20. Venkatraman S, Poh TL, Vinalia T, et al: Collapse pressures of biodegradable stents. *Biomaterials* 24(12):2105–2111, 2003.
21. Erbel R, Di Mario C, Bartunek J, et al: Temporary scaffolding of coronary arteries with bioabsorbable magnesium stents: A prospective, non-randomised multicentre trial. *Lancet* 369(9576):1869–1875, 2007.
22. Stack RS, Califf RM, Phillips HR, et al: Interventional cardiac catheterization at Duke Medical Center. *Am J Cardiol* 62(10 Pt 2):3F–24F, 1988.
23. Susawa T, Shiraki K, Shimizu Y: Biodegradable intracoronary stents in adult dogs. *J Am Coll Cardiol* 21(Suppl):483A, 1993.
24. van der Giessen WJ, Lincoff AM, Schwartz RS, et al: Marked inflammatory sequelae to implantation of biodegradable and nonbiodegradable polymers in porcine coronary arteries. *Circulation* 94(7):1690–1697, 1996.
25. Lincoff AM, Furst JG, Ellis SG, et al: Sustained local delivery of dexamethasone by a novel intravascular eluting stent to prevent restenosis in the porcine coronary injury model. *J Am Coll Cardiol* 29(4):808–816, 1997.
26. Yamawaki T, Shimokawa H, Kozai T, et al: Intramural delivery of a specific tyrosine kinase inhibitor with biodegradable stent suppresses the restenotic changes of the coronary artery in pigs in vivo. *J Am Coll Cardiol* 32(3):780–786, 1998.
27. Colombo A, Karvouni E: Biodegradable stents: "Fulfilling the mission and stepping away". *Circulation* 102(4):371–373, 2000.
28. Tamai H, Igaki K, Kyo E, et al: Initial and 6-month results of biodegradable poly-l-lactic acid coronary stents in humans. *Circulation* 102(4):399–404, 2000.
29. Tamai H, Igaki K, Tsuji T: A biodegradable poly-L-lactic acid coronary stent in porcine coronary artery. *J Interv Cardiol* 12:443–449, 1999.
30. Tamai H: Biodegradable stents: Four-year follow up. *Circulation* 68(Suppl):135–138, 2005.
31. Vogt F, Stein A, Rettemeier G, et al: Long-term assessment of a novel biodegradable paclitaxel-eluting coronary polylactide stent. *Eur Heart J* 25(15):1330–1340, 2004.
32. Ormiston JA, Serruys PW, Regar E, et al: A bioabsorbable everolimus-eluting coronary stent system for patients with single de-novo coronary artery lesions (ABSORB): A prospective open-label trial. *Lancet* 371(9616):899–907, 2008.
33. Serruys PW, Ormiston JA, Onuma Y, et al: A bioabsorbable everolimus-eluting coronary stent system (ABSORB): 2-year outcomes and results from multiple imaging methods. *Lancet* 373(9667):897–910, 2009.
34. Di Mario C, Ferrante G: Biodegradable drug-eluting stents: Promises and pitfalls. *Lancet* 371(9616):873–874, 2008.
35. Claessen BE, Henriques JP, George JC, et al: Society for Cardiovascular Angiography and Interventions 2010 and EuroPCR 2010: An update in interventional cardiology. *J Am Coll Cardiol Interv* 3(8):882–884, 2010.
36. Rukshin V, Azarbal B, Shah PK, et al: Intravenous magnesium in experimental stent thrombosis in swine. *Arterioscler Thromb Vasc Biol* 21(9):1544–1549, 2001.
37. Rukshin V, Santos R, Gheorghiu M, et al: A prospective, nonrandomized, open-labeled pilot study investigating the use of magnesium in patients undergoing nonacute percutaneous coronary intervention with stent implantation. *J Cardiovasc Pharmacol Ther* 8(3):193–200, 2003.
38. Heublein B, Rohde R, Kaese V, et al: Biocorrosion of magnesium alloys: A new principle in cardiovascular implant technology? *Heart (British Cardiac Society)* 89(6):651–656, 2003.
39. Peeters P, Bosiers M, Verbist J, et al: Preliminary results after application of absorbable metal stents in patients with critical limb ischemia. *J Endovasc Ther* 12(1):1–5, 2005.
40. Donners MM, Daemen MJ, Cleutjens KB, et al: Inflammation and restenosis: Implications for therapy. *Ann Med* 35(7):523–531, 2003.
41. Verheye S, Agostoni P, Dawkins KD, et al: The GENESIS (Randomized, Multicenter Study of the Pimecrolimus-Eluting and Pimecrolimus/Paclitaxel-Eluting Coronary Stent System in Patients with De Novo Lesions of the Native Coronary Arteries) trial. *J Am Coll Cardiol* 2(3):205–214, 2009.
42. Schranz D, Zartner P, Michel-Behnke I, et al: Bioabsorbable metal stents for percutaneous treatment of critical recoarctation of the aorta in a newborn. *Catheter Cardiovasc Interv* 67(5):671–673, 2006.
43. Zartner P, Cesnjevar R, Singer H, et al: First successful implantation of a biodegradable metal stent into the left pulmonary artery of a preterm baby. *Catheter Cardiovasc Interv* 66(4):590–594, 2005.
44. Mueller PP, May T, Perz A, et al: Control of smooth muscle cell proliferation by ferrous iron. *Biomaterials* 27(10):2193–2200, 2006.
45. Peuster M, Wohlsein P, Brugmann M, et al: A novel approach to temporary stenting: degradable cardiovascular stents produced from corrodible metal-results 6–18 months after implantation into New Zealand white rabbits. *Heart (British Cardiac Society)* 86(5):563–569, 2001.
46. Waksman R, Pakala R, Baffour R, et al: Short-term effects of biocorrodible iron stents in porcine coronary arteries. *J Interv Cardiol* 21(1):15–20, 2008.

Role of Adjunct Devices: Cutting Balloon, Laser, Ultrasound, and Atherectomy

JOHN A. BITTL

The past 25 years have seen several mechanical approaches that ablate or section atheromatous plaque during percutaneous coronary intervention (PCI) to optimize acute results and reduce re-stenosis. Despite promising results from hundreds of small mechanistic studies, dozens of large randomized trials have failed to achieve predefined clinical and angiographic outcomes, and thus the routine use of atheroablative methods during PCI has not found support.[1] In specific circumstances, however, the use of atheroablative devices has been beneficial and in selected cases the only means of achieving procedural and clinical success. This chapter analyzes the results of clinical trials and illustrates the use of adjunctive atheroablative therapies in contemporary practice.

Historical Background

Before the modern era of coronary stenting, the search for treatments to overcome the limitations of PTCA was based on experimental studies, which showed that the healing response of treated coronary arteries was directly proportional to the degree of imposed injury.[2] This was supported by angiographic analyses, which suggested that the degree of late re-stenosis was directly proportional to the gain achieved acutely during treatment and that the proportion between late loss and acute gain was consistent for a broad range of interventional devices.[3] The decades-long search for a mechanical approach to excise or section atheromatous plaque emerged from the concept that

plaque excision would improve clinical outcomes and lower the rate of re-stenosis after coronary intervention. Directional coronary atherectomy (DCA) entered clinical trials in 1987. Excimer laser coronary angioplasty (ELCA), percutaneous transluminal rotational atherectomy (PTRA), and transluminal extraction coronary atherectomy (TEC) were introduced in 1988. Holmium laser angioplasty (HLA) premiered in 1990, and cutting balloon angioplasty (CBA) debuted in 1991. Although each device used a different mechanism for modifying thrombus or atheromatous plaque, the common goal was to obtain larger acute gains and lower re-stenosis rates than could be achieved with PTCA. Evidence from randomized trials (Table 34-1),[1,4–30] however, challenged the hypothesis that routine atheroablation during PCI is beneficial. The introduction of coronary stenting, particularly the use of drug-eluting stents (DESs; Chapter 13), rapidly replaced atheroablative therapies. Although atheroablative therapies may facilitate stent delivery and enhance stent expansion, the development of lower-profile, trackable, high-pressure balloon catheters (Chapter 15) has made PTCA the default method for lesion preparation before and after coronary stenting, and in many cases no lesion preparation is required at all before stent implantation.[31–33]

Cutting Balloon Angioplasty

Cutting balloon angioplasty (CBA), or atherotomy, is a variation of conventional PTCA. In CBA, three or four sharp metal microtomes which are mounted on a noncompliant balloon, incise and score the coronary atheroma during the process of balloon dilation. The purpose of using cutting balloon atherotomy is to reduce the risk of uncontrolled longitudinal tears in the vessel wall caused by conventional balloon dilatation.

MECHANISM OF ACTION

Compared with conventional PTCA, CBA makes controlled microincisions in the atheromatous plaque at lower pressures to reduce barotrauma. In an effort to overcome hoop stress, conventional PTCA stretches and dissects vascular tissue. After the balloon is deflated, the artery undergoes elastic recoil. Small mechanistic studies have suggested that lesions can be dilated at lower pressures with cutting balloon catheters than with conventional PTCA.[21] In one study of 180 lesions, lumen enlargement was achieved at lower balloon pressures after CBA than after PTCA, and the increase in the cross-sectional area of plaque plus media measured by intravascular ultrasound (IVUS) was larger after CBA.[34] In calcified lesions, CBA achieved larger lumen gain than did PTCA.

EQUIPMENT

The Cutting Balloon Ultra-2™ is a monorail device, and the Flextome™ Cutting Balloon (Boston Scientific, Natick, MA) has two catheter designs (Fig. 34-1). The Flextome device contains a flex point every 5 mm along the length of the atherotomes (cutting blades) for greater flexibility and deliverability. It is available in over-the-wire and

TABLE 34-1	Acronyms of Randomized Trials Comparing Atheroablative or Thrombectomy Devices						
Acronym	*Definition*	*Primary Endpoint**	*Patients (n)*	*Year†*	*Indications*	*Comparison*
AMIGO (4)	Atherectomy before Multi-Link® Improves Luminal Gain and Clinical Outcomes	Binary re-stenosis	753	2002	Native vessel	DCA vs. PTCA
AMRO (5)	Amsterdam Rotterdam Randomised Trial	6-month MACE	308	1993	Native vessel	ELCA vs. PTCA
ARTIST (6)	Angioplasty/Rotational Atherectomy for Treatment of Diffuse In-Stent Restenosis Trial	6-month MACE	298	2002	ISR in native vessel	PTRA vs. PTCA
ATLAS (7)	Acolysis During Treatment of Lesions Affecting Saphenous Vein Bypass Grafts)	Successful procedure	189	2000	Infarct artery	UT vs. PTCA
BETACUT (8)	Beta Radiation Assisted by Cutting Balloon Angioplasty for In-Stent Restenosis	Binary re-stenosis	100	2002	ISR in native vessel	CBA vs. PTCA before BT
BOAT (9)	Balloon/Optimal Atherectomy Trial	Binary re-stenosis	989	1995	Native vessel	DCA vs. PTCA
CAPAS (10)	Cutting balloon atherotomy vs. Plain Old Balloon Angioplasty Study	Binary re-stenosis	232	1997	Native vessel	CBA vs. PTCA
CARAT (11)	Coronary Angioplasty and Rotablator Atherectomy Trial	Postprocedure diameter stenosis	222	2000	Native vessel	PTRA vs. PTRA
CAVEAT-I (12)	Coronary Angioplasty Versus Excisional Atherectomy Trial I	Binary re-stenosis	1012	1992	Native vessel	DCA vs. PTCA
CAVEAT-II (13)	Coronary Angioplasty Versus Excisional Atherectomy Trial II	Binary re-stenosis	305	1993	SVG	DCA vs. PTCA
CBASS (16)	Cutting Balloon for Small Size Vessels‡	Binary re-stenosis	99	1999	Native vessels <2.6 mm	CBA vs. PTCA
CCAT (14)	Canadian Coronary Atherectomy Trial	Binary re-stenosis	274	1992	LAD	DCA vs. PTCA
COBRA (15)	Comparison of Balloon Angioplasty/Rotational Atherectomy	Binary re-stenosis	502	1996	Native vessel	PTRA vs. PTCA
CUBA (16)	Cutting Balloon Versus Conventional Balloon Angioplasty Trial‡	Binary re-stenosis	306	1997	Native vessel	CBA vs. PTCA
DART (17)	Dilation/Ablation Revascularization Trial	Binary re-stenosis	446	1998	Small vessel	PTRA vs. PTCA
DESIRE (18)	Debulking and Stenting in Restenosis Elimination‡	Binary re-stenosis				
DOCTORS (19)	Debulking of CTO with Rotational or directional atherectomy before Stenting	Binary re-stenosis	266	2003	Native vessel CTO	PTRA or DCA vs. PTCA
ERBAC (20)	Excimer Rotablator Balloon Angioplasty Comparison	Procedural success	454	1996	Native vessel	ELCA vs. PTCA
ERBAC (20)	Excimer Rotablator Balloon Angioplasty	Procedural success	453	1996	Native vessel	PTRA vs. PTCA
GRT (22)	Global Randomized Trial	Binary re-stenosis	1238	1997	Native vessel	CBA vs. PTCA
LAVA (25)	Laser Angioplasty/ Coronary Angioplasty	6-month MACE	215	1997	Native vessel	HLA vs. PTCA
REDUCE (11)	Restenosis Reduction by Cutting Balloon Evaluation 1†	Binary re-stenosis	802	2001	Native vessel	CBA vs. PTCA
REDUCE (216)	Restenosis Reduction by Cutting Balloon Evaluation 2‡	Binary re-stenosis	492	2002	ISR	CBA vs. PTCA
REDUCE (326)	Restenosis Reduction by Cutting Balloon Evaluation 3	Binary re-stenosis	521	2003	Stenting	CBA vs. PTCA
RESCUT (27)	Restenosis Cutting Balloon Evaluation	Binary re-stenosis	428	2002	ISR	CBA vs. PTCA
ROSTER (28)	Rotational Atherectomy Versus Balloon Angioplasty for Diffuse In-Stent Restenosis	Target lesion revascularization	200	2001	ISR	PTRA vs. PTCA
SPORT (1)	Stenting Post Rotational Atherectomy Trial‡	30-day MACE	735	1999	Stenting in calcified vessels	PTRA vs. PTCA
STRATAS (29)	Study to Determine Rotablator System and Transluminal Angioplasty Strategy	Acute success	497	2000	Native vessel	PTRA vs. PTRA

BT, brachytherapy; *CBA*, cutting balloon atherotomy; *CTO*, chronic total occlusion; *DCA*, directional coronary atherectomy; *ELCA*, excimer laser coronary angioplasty; *HLA*, holmium laser angioplasty; *ISR*, in-stent re-stenosis; *PTCA*, percutaneous transluminal coronary angioplasty; *LAD*, proximal segment of the left anterior descending artery; *MACE*, major adverse cardiac event (death, myocardial infarction, or revascularization); *modified MACE*, death, Q-wave myocardial infarction, revascularization, stroke or stent thrombosis; *PTRA*, percutaneous transluminal rotational atherectomy; *STEMI*, ST-elevation myocardial infarction, *successful procedure (ATLAS)*, final diameter stenosis of 30% or less by quantitative coronary angiography, achievement of Thrombolysis In MI (TIMI) 3 flow (by quantitative coronary angiography), and freedom from MACE (a composite of cardiac death, Q-wave and non–Q-wave MI, emergency bypass, repeat target lesion revascularization, and disabling stroke) within 30 days of treatment, *SVG*, saphenous vein graft; *UT*, ultrasound thrombolysis.

*If the primary endpoint was not stated or if multiple primary endpoints were listed, the endpoint used in power calculations for sample size estimation was used.

†Year patient recruitment was completed. Otherwise, the year study was reported or published.

‡Unpublished, with data approved by investigators where cited.

(Bittl JA, Chew DP, Topol EJ, Kong DF, Califf RM: Meta-analysis of randomized trials of percutaneous transluminal coronary angioplasty versus atherectomy, cutting balloon atherotomy, or laser angioplasty, *J Am Coll Cardiol* 43:936–942, 2004.)

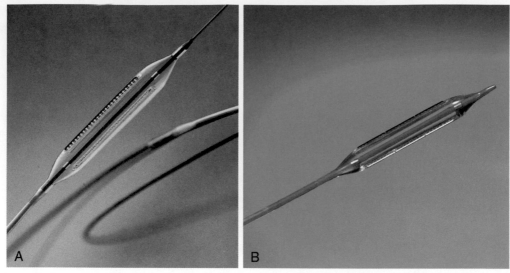

Figure 34-1 The Cutting Balloon Ultra-2™ (*A*) is a monorail device, and the Flextome™ Cutting Balloon (*B*) is available as either a monorail or an over-the-wire catheter. (*Boston Scientific, Natick, MA.*)

monorail configurations. Cutting balloons are available in balloon lengths of 6 mm, 10 mm, and 15 mm. The atherotomes are mounted longitudinally along the balloon surface. They are not directly affixed to the balloon but bonded to a pad mounted on the balloon. The double bond allows flexibility and ensures that the atherotomes remain firmly fixed in place. The number of atherotomes is determined by balloon diameter. Three atherotomes are on 2-mm and 3.25-mm balloons, and four are on 3.5-mm and 4-mm balloons.

TECHNIQUE

The guidewires, catheters, and techniques used for cutting balloon angioplasty are similar to those for conventional PTCA (Chapter 16). However, cutting balloon catheters are less compliant and do not track as well as conventional balloon catheters. CBA may not be feasible when the proximal anatomy is tortuous. The risk of blade fracture or retention may be minimized by slowly inflating and deflating the balloon and by avoiding balloon pressures at or above the rated burst pressures.[35]

CLINICAL RESULTS

Several small but largely positive trials of CBA, all involving less than 200 patients, reported that the use of CBA reduced re-stenosis by 41% to 69% compared with PTCA (Fig. 34-2).[10,16,21,23,24] Other small studies evaluated CBA as pretreatment before brachytherapy for in-stent re-stenosis (ISR) and found no difference in re-stenosis rates between CBA and rotational atherectomy or between CBA and PTCA.[8,30] Several large trials of CBA have been carried out (see Fig. 34-2). The GRT[22] randomized 1238 patients and reported no difference in angiographic re-stenosis between CBA (31.4%) and PTCA (30.4%). The RESCUT study enrolled 428 patients with ISR and reported no difference in re-stenosis between CBA (29.8%) and PTCA (31.2%).[27] The REDUCE 1 study enrolled 802 patients and reported slightly higher re-stenosis rates with CBA than with PTCA (32.7% vs. 25.5%).[1] The REDUCE 2 study enrolled 416 patients and also observed a trend toward higher re-stenosis rates (52.1% vs. 44.2%). The REDUCE 3 study randomized 453 patients undergoing coronary stenting and reported lower re-stenosis rates after the use of CBA than after PTCA (11.8% vs. 19.6%).[16,26]

LESION SELECTION

Several reports have suggested that CBA may be appropriate in small vessels bifurcation lesions or ostial stenoses.[16,21] Bifurcation lesions have been a challenge for PTCA because of plaque shift and high re-stenosis rates, and CBA produced lower re-stenosis rates than PTCA (40% vs. 67%) in a small nonrandomized series of 87 patients with bifurcation lesions.[36] Many interventional cardiologists use CBA for ostial lesions, but evidence of benefit for this indication has been elusive.[37] The technical advantage of CBA is reduced slippage, especially for the treatment of ISR, which constitutes a common use of CBA.[22,26,27,37,38]

COMPLICATIONS

The risk of coronary perforation (Fig. 34-3) is slightly higher after the use of CBA than after conventional PTCA (0.8% vs. 0.0%), as reported in the GRT.[22]

SCORING BALLOON CATHETER

The AngioSculpt® scoring balloon catheter (AngioScore Inc., Fremont, Ca) is an alternative to the cutting balloon. The scoring balloon contains a flexible nitinol scoring ribbon with three rectangular spiral struts to incise the atheromatous plaque at pressures up to 18 atmosphere (atm). The system, which has a low crossing profile (2.7 French [2.7F] maximum), is promoted as a more flexible alternative to the cutting balloon but no multi-center randomized trials of the device have been reported.

▣ Ultrasound

PRINCIPLES

The frequency of therapeutic ultrasound (19 to 50 kHz) is several orders of magnitude lower than the frequency of ultrasound commonly used for diagnostic purposes (20 to 30 MHz). Higher power intensities and lower frequencies result in higher amplitudes of probe motion (20 to 110 μm), producing mechanical effects such as tissue disruption, cavitation, and heating not seen with diagnostic ultrasound.

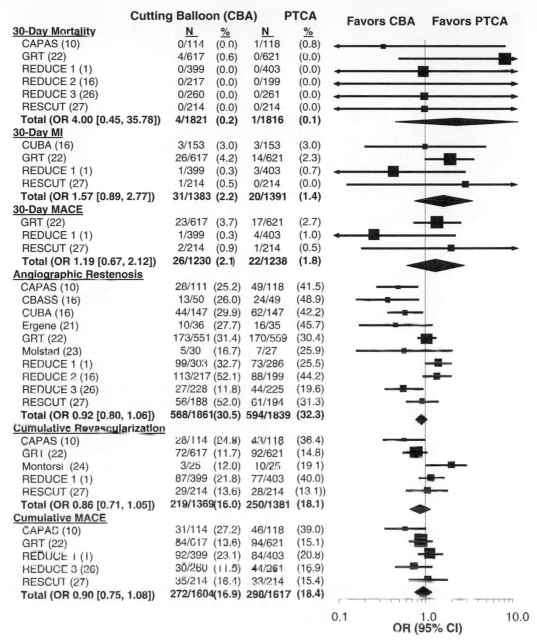

30-Day Mortality	Cutting Balloon (CBA)		PTCA	
	N	%	N	%
CAPAS (10)	0/114	(0.0)	1/118	(0.8)
GRT (22)	4/617	(0.6)	0/621	(0.0)
REDUCE 1 (1)	0/399	(0.0)	0/403	(0.0)
REDUCE 2 (16)	0/217	(0.0)	0/199	(0.0)
REDUCE 3 (26)	0/260	(0.0)	0/261	(0.0)
RESCUT (27)	0/214	(0.0)	0/214	(0.0)
Total (OR 4.00 [0.45, 35.78])	**4/1821**	**(0.2)**	**1/1816**	**(0.1)**
30-Day MI				
CUBA (16)	3/153	(3.0)	3/153	(3.0)
GRT (22)	26/617	(4.2)	14/621	(2.3)
REDUCE 1 (1)	1/399	(0.3)	3/403	(0.7)
RESCUT (27)	1/214	(0.5)	0/214	(0.0)
Total (OR 1.57 [0.89, 2.77])	**31/1383**	**(2.2)**	**20/1391**	**(1.4)**
30-Day MACE				
GRT (22)	23/617	(3.7)	17/621	(2.7)
REDUCE 1 (1)	1/399	(0.3)	4/403	(1.0)
RESCUT (27)	2/214	(0.9)	1/214	(0.5)
Total (OR 1.19 [0.67, 2.12])	**26/1230**	**(2.1)**	**22/1238**	**(1.8)**
Angiographic Restenosis				
CAPAS (10)	28/111	(25.2)	49/118	(41.5)
CBASS (16)	13/50	(26.0)	24/49	(48.9)
CUBA (16)	44/147	(29.9)	62/147	(42.2)
Ergene (21)	10/36	(27.7)	16/35	(45.7)
GRT (22)	173/551	(31.4)	170/559	(30.4)
Molstad (23)	5/30	(16.7)	7/27	(25.9)
REDUCE 1 (1)	99/303	(32.7)	73/286	(25.5)
REDUCE 2 (16)	113/217	(52.1)	88/199	(44.2)
REDUCE 3 (26)	27/228	(11.8)	44/225	(19.6)
RESCUT (27)	56/188	(52.0)	61/194	(31.3)
Total (OR 0.92 [0.80, 1.06])	**568/1861**	**(30.5)**	**594/1839**	**(32.3)**
Cumulative Revascularization				
CAPAS (10)	28/114	(24.8)	43/118	(36.4)
GRT (22)	72/617	(11.7)	92/621	(14.8)
Montorsi (24)	3/25	(12.0)	10/25	(19.1)
REDUCE 1 (1)	87/399	(21.8)	77/403	(40.0)
RESCUT (27)	29/214	(13.6)	28/214	(13.1)
Total (OR 0.86 [0.71, 1.05])	**219/1369**	**(16.0)**	**250/1381**	**(18.1)**
Cumulative MACE				
CAPAS (10)	31/114	(27.2)	46/118	(39.0)
GRT (22)	84/617	(13.6)	94/621	(15.1)
REDUCE 1 (1)	92/399	(23.1)	84/403	(20.8)
REDUCE 3 (26)	30/260	(11.5)	44/261	(16.9)
RESCUT (27)	35/214	(16.4)	33/214	(15.4)
Total (OR 0.90 [0.75, 1.08])	**272/1604**	**(16.9)**	**298/1617**	**(18.4)**

Figure 34-2 Systematic overview of randomized trials of cutting balloon angioplasty (CBA) versus percutaneous transluminal coronary angioplasty (PTCA). Pooled odds ratios (OR) and 95% confidence intervals (CI) were calculated to estimate the overall effect of CBA versus that of PTCA using an empirical Bayes model. Trial abbreviations are given in Table 34-1. (*Updated and reprinted from Bittl JA, Chew DP, Topol EJ, Kong DF, Califf RM: Meta-analysis of randomized trials of percutaneous transluminal coronary angioplasty versus atherectomy, cutting balloon atherotomy, or laser angioplasty, J Am Coll Cardiol 43:936–942, 2004. Copyright (2004), with permission from The American College of Cardiology Foundation.*)

CLINICAL STUDY

The ATLAS (Assessment of Treatment with Lisinopril And Survival) trial compared coronary ultrasound thrombolysis with abciximab treatment in 181 patients undergoing saphenous vein graft (SVG) PCI for acute coronary syndrome (ACS).[7] The primary endpoint of a successful procedure and freedom from major adverse cardiac events (MACEs) was achieved in 63% of patients treated with ultrasound thrombolysis and in 82% of patients treated with abciximab (P = 0.008). The incidence of MACEs at 30 days was 25% with ultrasound thrombolysis and 12% with abciximab (P = 0.036). The use of ultrasound for native-vessel total occlusions is discussed in Chapter 24.

Laser

The use of laser in medicine has broad appeal for the lay population. However, the systematic study of laser–tissue interactions has revealed that all medical laser systems produce unexpected photoacoustic effects and collateral damage (Fig. 34-4).[39]

TECHNIQUE

The size of laser catheters used for angioplasty should be approximately 1.0 mm smaller than the reference diameter of the target vessel. For severe stenoses, the smallest laser catheters are recommended to

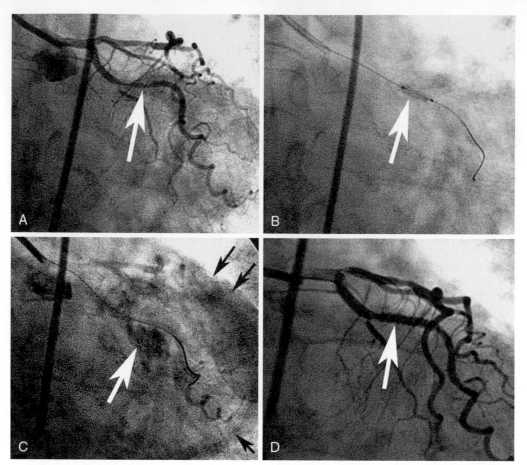

Figure 34-3 Perforation after cutting balloon angioplasty. The first marginal branch had been stented with a 3-mm bare stent showing moderate re-stenosis 7 months later (*A, arrow*) associated with angina. A 3-mm cutting balloon was positioned within the stented segment (*B, arrow*), but inflation was complicated by free perforation (*C, white arrow*), circumferential hemo-pericardium (*C, black arrows*), and cardiac tamponade. The patient was rapidly stabilized with pericardiocentesis and placement of a polytetrafluoroethylene-covered stent to seal the coronary perforation.

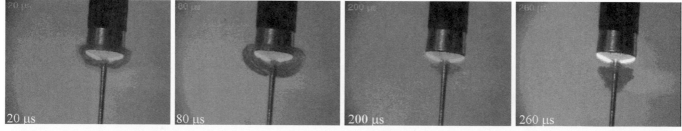

Figure 34-4 Bubble formation during excimer laser angioplasty. Excimer laser light is absorbed by tissue in a disc-shaped layer about 100 microns deep with an area equal to that of the beam, typically the diameter of the catheter. Although some energy is converted into the process of photochemical dissociation, most of it is converted into heat. The steam forms a rapidly expanding vapor bubble that is typically two times the diameter of the catheter tip. After reaching a maximum diameter within approximately 100 microseconds after the laser pulse, the bubble implodes.

increase the likelihood of successful crossing. The elimination of blood and contrast from the coronary artery during excimer laser coronary angioplasty (ELCA) has reduced the extent of collateral damage during angioplasty.[40] This may be achieved by flushing all the lines with saline and, as done in some laboratories, injecting saline through the guiding catheter at a rate of 2 to 3 mL per second during laser activation. A slow catheter advancement rate of 0.2 mm per second yields maximal ablation of plaque (Fig. 34-5). If advancement through the lesion cannot be maintained at a steady pace, increasing the fluence or firing rate should be tried. If no advancement is apparent after several seconds, forceful pushing should be avoided because it may increase the risk of vessel perforation.

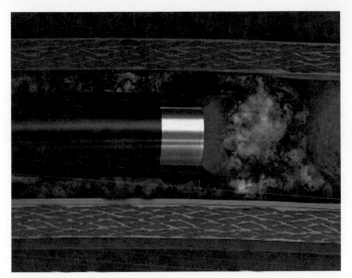

Figure 34-5 Schematic rendition of excimer laser angioplasty procedure. *(Spectranetics, Colorado Springs, CO.)*

CLINICAL RESULTS

Several randomized studies have compared pulsed-wave lasers with other treatment modalities, but none have shown a benefit over conventional PTCA (Fig. 34-6).[5,20,25]

LESION SELECTION

Although ELCA has been approved for seven lesion types (long lesions, moderately calcified lesions, ISR before brachytherapy, SVG lesions, ostial lesions, total occlusions, and undilatable lesions), some interventional cardiologists reserve its use for nondilatable lesions (Fig. 34-7). The photomechanical effects of ELCA can be enhanced by eliminating the saline-flush technique to treat lesions that are difficult to dilate with balloon angioplasty.[41-43]

▣ Directional Coronary Atherectomy

Directional coronary atherectomy (DCA) device was approved by the U.S. Food and Drug Administration (FDA) in 1990 as the first non-balloon PCI device (Fig. 34-8) based on uncontrolled multi-center

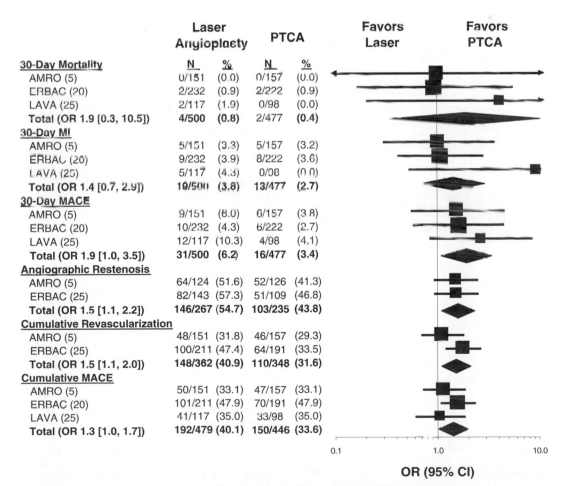

	Laser Angioplasty		PTCA		
	N	**%**	**N**	**%**	
30-Day Mortality					
AMRO (5)	0/151	(0.0)	0/157	(0.0)	
ERBAC (20)	2/232	(0.9)	2/222	(0.9)	
LAVA (25)	2/117	(1.9)	0/98	(0.0)	
Total (OR 1.9 [0.3, 10.5])	**4/500**	**(0.8)**	**2/477**	**(0.4)**	
30-Day MI					
AMRO (5)	5/151	(3.3)	5/157	(3.2)	
ERBAC (20)	9/232	(3.9)	8/222	(3.6)	
LAVA (25)	5/117	(4.3)	0/98	(0.0)	
Total (OR 1.4 [0.7, 2.9])	**19/500**	**(3.8)**	**13/477**	**(2.7)**	
30-Day MACE					
AMRO (5)	9/151	(6.0)	6/157	(3.8)	
ERBAC (20)	10/232	(4.3)	6/222	(2.7)	
LAVA (25)	12/117	(10.3)	4/98	(4.1)	
Total (OR 1.9 [1.0, 3.5])	**31/500**	**(6.2)**	**16/477**	**(3.4)**	
Angiographic Restenosis					
AMRO (5)	64/124	(51.6)	52/126	(41.3)	
ERBAC (25)	82/143	(57.3)	51/109	(46.8)	
Total (OR 1.5 [1.1, 2.2])	**146/267**	**(54.7)**	**103/235**	**(43.8)**	
Cumulative Revascularization					
AMRO (5)	48/151	(31.8)	46/157	(29.3)	
ERBAC (25)	100/211	(47.4)	64/191	(33.5)	
Total (OR 1.5 [1.1, 2.0])	**148/362**	**(40.9)**	**110/348**	**(31.6)**	
Cumulative MACE					
AMRO (5)	50/151	(33.1)	47/157	(33.1)	
ERBAC (20)	101/211	(47.9)	70/191	(47.9)	
LAVA (25)	41/117	(35.0)	33/98	(35.0)	
Total (OR 1.3 [1.0, 1.7])	**192/479**	**(40.1)**	**150/446**	**(33.6)**	

Favors Laser   Favors PTCA

OR (95% CI)   0.1   1.0   10.0

Figure 34-6 Systematic overview of randomized trials of laser angioplasty (LA) versus percutaneous transluminal coronary angioplasty (PTCA). Pooled odds ratios (OR) and 95% confidence intervals (CI) were calculated to estimate the overall effect of laser angioplasty versus that of PTCA. Trial abbreviations are given in Table 34-1, and credits are given in the legend to Figure 34-2.

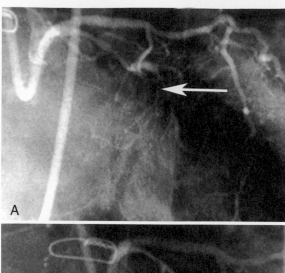

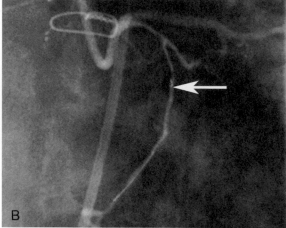

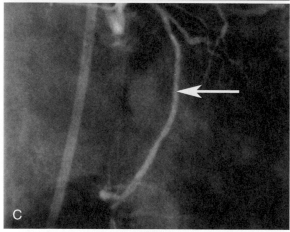

Figure 34-7 Long, undilatable lesion treated with excimer laser angioplasty. The occluded left circumflex coronary artery (*A, arrow*) was crossed with a guidewire and treated with a 1.4-mm excimer laser catheter (*B, arrow*), followed by percutaneous transluminal coronary angioplasty (PTCA) (*C, arrow*).

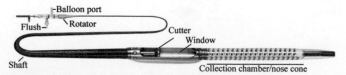

Figure 34-8 Flexi-Cut Directional Debulking System® for atherectomy. (*Abbott Vascular, Chicago.*)

registry data defining the safety and efficacy of the approach. At the current time, catheters for DCA are no longer marketed in the United States.

A novel "plaque excision system," called the SilverHawk (Fox-Hollow Technologies, Redwood City, CA), based on the concept of atherectomy has had extensive uncontrolled experience in the treatment of peripheral artery disease (PAD; Chapter 38) and preliminary experience in human CAD cases.[44] Several randomized trials have evaluated DCA versus PTCA with and without stenting (Fig. 34-9). The failure of optimal atherectomy to achieve better clinical outcomes compared with PTCA in randomized trials was attributed to several factors, including peri-procedural myocardial infarction (MI) or the difficulty in achieving optimal debulking (Fig. 34-10).[4,45]

Percutaneous Transluminal Rotational Atherectomy

MECHANISM

Rotational atherectomy involves the excavation of plaque in a manner similar to that achieved by a dental drill, which can bore into enamel but leaves the pulp unharmed. Based on the theory of differential cutting, rotational atherectomy cuts inelastic atherosclerotic tissue inside coronary arteries and retains the integrity of the elastic artery wall. Rotary ablation attacks hard or calcified atherosclerotic plaque, which is not able to deflect, and produces microfissures at the zone of contact with the burr. The hard plaque is abraded into particles, most of which are smaller than 5 μm in diameter, and taken up by the reticuloendothelial system.

EQUIPMENT

The Rotablator® (Scimed, Boston Scientific, Natick, MA) system includes (1) an advancer that houses the air turbine, drive shaft, and burr; (2) a console to monitor and control the rotation by regulating the air supply to the advancer; and (3) the DynaGlide foot pedal. The abrasive tip is welded to a long flexible drive shaft covered by a plastic sheath and tracks along a central flexible guidewire. The Rotalink® burr catheter is 135 cm in length and contains a 0.058-inch outer sheath. The nickel-coated brass burr is elliptical in shape with 2000 to 3000 microscopic diamond crystals on the leading face (Fig. 34-11). The diamond crystals are 20 μm in size, with only 5 μm protruding from the nickel coating. The trailing edge of the burr is smooth. The burrs are available in various sizes for coronary use in 0.25-mm increments from 1.25 to 2.50 mm in diameter. Rotational energy is transmitted by a compressed air motor that drives the flexible helical shaft at speeds up to 200,000 revolutions per minute (rpm). The number of revolutions per minute is measured by a fibroptic light probe and displayed on a control panel. The speed of rotation and the speed of advancement of the burr are controlled by the operator. During rotation, saline solution irrigates the catheter sheath to lubricate and cool the rotating parts. The burr and the drive shaft move freely over a central coaxial guidewire (0.009 inches diameter, 3 meters length) with a flexible radiopaque platinum spring tip (20 mm long) that does not rotate with the burr during abrasion. The wire and the burr can be advanced independently, which allows the wire to be placed in a safe distal location before the burr is advanced into the diseased artery. With the Rotalink system and a single advancer, multiple burrs can be used. Thus, the exchange of burrs is easier, saves time, and expedites the use of the multiple-burr approach. A console displays the rotational speed in revolutions per minute. The Advancer has preset delimiters for retraction and advancement. The WireClip® torquer and guide wires are critical components of the system. RotaGlide™ lubricant is useful for crossing resistant lesions.

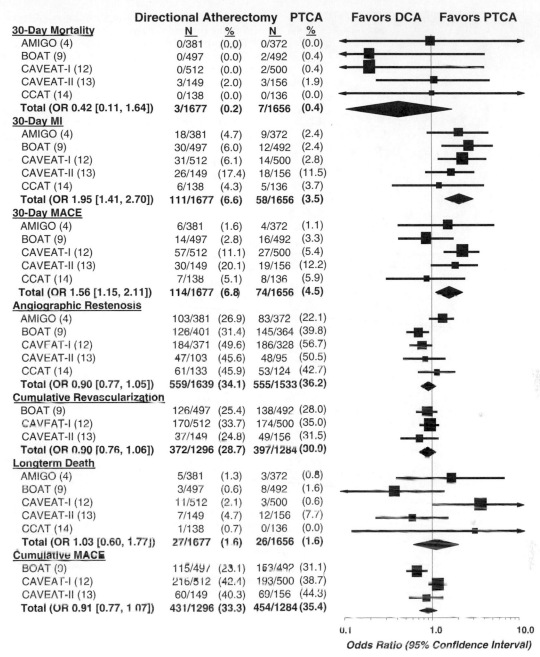

Figure 34-9 Systematic overview of randomized trials of directional coronary atherectomy (DCA) versus percutaneous transluminal coronary angioplasty (PTCA). Pooled odds ratios (OR) and 95% confidence intervals (CI) were calculated to estimate the overall effect of directional coronary atherectomy versus that of PTCA. Trial abbreviations are given in Table 34-1, and credits are given in the legend to Figure 34-2.

PROCEDURE

A sheath is inserted into the femoral artery under local anesthesia, and 6F, 7F, or 8F guiding catheters are used, depending on the size of the burr. The 1.25-mm, 1.50-mm, and 1.75-mm burrs advance through the 0.070-inch inner lumen of the 6F Runway Guide (Boston Scientific, Natick, MA), allowing conversion to salvage rotational atherectomy if undilatable or uncrossable lesions are encountered. The 2-mm and 2.15-mm burrs require a 7F guide, and the 2.25-mm burr requires an 8F guiding catheter. Rotary ablation is preceded by advancing the RotaWire across the target lesion and by parking the unfolded wire tip in a straight segment of the distal vessel. When treating large coronary arteries, particularly the right coronary artery, many cardiologists insert a prophylactic temporary pacemaker because of the high frequency of bradyarrhythmias. Before advancing the burr into the guiding catheter, the rotational speed of the burr should be checked outside the body at the Y-adaptor with flush running. An outside-body

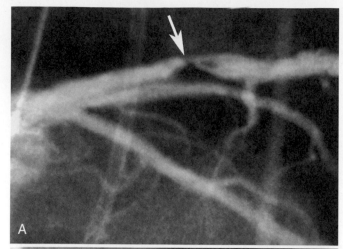

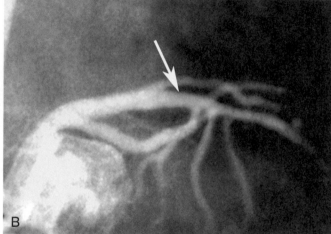

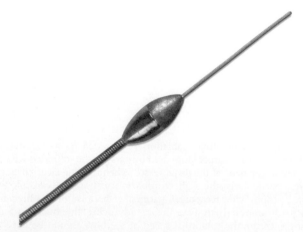

Figure 34-10 Directional coronary atherectomy for complex eccentric lesion (*A, arrow*) followed by balloon angioplasty (*B, arrow*).

Figure 34-11 Rotablator burr. (*Boston Scientific, Natick, MA.*)

speed of 155,000 translates to an unimpeded speed of 140,000 rpm within the coronary artery.

The burr and the drive shaft are manually advanced over the guidewire to the proximal segment of the target vessel. Before rotablation, a three-point checklist should be completed to prevent abrupt burr advancement and vessel dissection. First, the advancer knob is loosened and moved back and forth approximately 5 mm to unload stored tension on the drive cable. Second, the Y-adaptor is loosened to unload stored tension in the Rotablator sheath. And third, the DynaGlide mode is activated at 35,000 for 1 second to unload any residual tension within system. The rotating burr is advanced slowly to the target lesion with a rotational speed of 140,000 rpm. The burr is advanced through the lesion in a back-and-forth pecking motion. The lower rotational speed of 140,000 rpm may be associated with less heat generation and platelet activation than higher speeds. Runs should be limited to 20 seconds. Decelerations of more than 5,000 rpm below the platform speed must be avoided because they increase the risk of vessel trauma, release large particles, and lead to ischemic complications caused by frictional heat. Several slow polishing passes are usually required to achieve maximum plaque removal. If resistance is encountered, the tip is never advanced forcefully. If the lesion cannot be crossed after five attempts, the rotational speed may be increased to 160,000 rpm. If the procedure is unsuccessful and because the lesion cannot be crossed downsizing of the burr may be required.

CLINICAL RESULTS

The STRATAS (Study to determine Rotablator and Transluminal Angioplasty Strategy) trial compared an aggressive PTRA strategy using a burr-to-artery ratio of 0.7 to 0.9 followed by balloon inflation of less than 1 atm (or none at all) versus a moderate debulking strategy using a burr-to-artery ratio of less than 0.7 followed by conventional balloon angioplasty.[29] The clinical success was similar, but the aggressive strategy caused more MIs (11% vs. 7%) and a higher rate of re-stenosis (58% vs. 52%). The CARAT (Coronary Angioplasty and Rotablator Atherectomy Trial) study compared a large-burr strategy with a burr-to-artery ratio of greater than 0.7 with a small-burr strategy using a burr-to-artery ratio of less than 0.7.[11] The large-burr strategy achieved similar immediate lumen enlargement and rate of target vessel revascularization as the small-burr strategy but caused more angiographic complications (12.7% vs. 5.2%, $P < 0.05$). In a series of multi-center randomized trials, the primary endpoint of angiographic re-stenosis was identical in the PTRA and PTCA groups (Fig. 34-12).[1,6,15,17,20] In the single-center ROSTER (Rotational Atherectomy Versus Balloon Angioplasty for Diffuse In-stent Restenosis) trial, the primary endpoint of target lesion revascularization was lower after PTRA than after PTCA (32% vs. 45%, $P = 0.04$).[28] Rotational atherectomy has been recommended as a strategy before stenting of bifurcation lesions, but no evidence exists to support this as a routine approach.[31,32,37]

LESION SELECTION

About 1% to 3% of lesions that can be crossed with guidewires are uncrossable with balloon catheters or undilatable at balloon pressures higher than 20 atm. Rotational atherectomy successfully increases the compliance of most of these resistant lesions, allowing balloon dilatation and stent implantation to be completed successfully (Fig. 34-13). For long calcified lesions, it is recommended that small burrs be used to modify the compliance of the vessel, the procedure be completed with balloon inflations, and spot stenting be performed on the segments with dissection (Fig. 34-14). Thus, in contemporary practice, rotational atherectomy plays an important role to facilitate the dilation or stenting of lesions that might not be crossed or expanded with balloon angioplasty.[46,47] Certain precautions about PTRA require

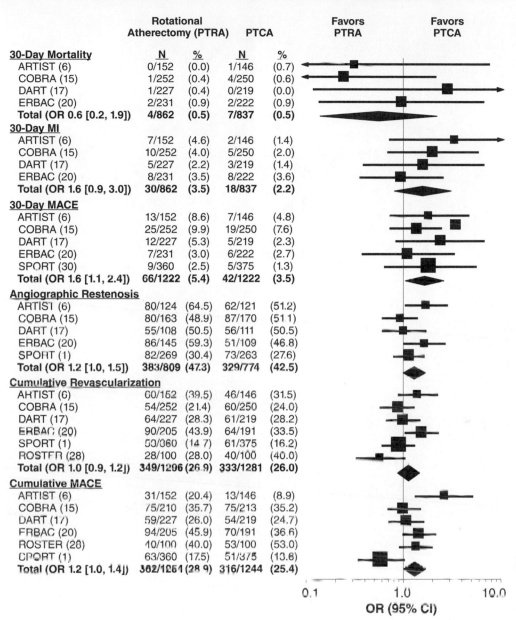

	Rotational Atherectomy (PTRA)		PTCA		Favors PTRA	Favors PTCA
30-Day Mortality	N	%	N	%		
ARTIST (6)	0/152	(0.0)	1/146	(0.7)		
COBRA (15)	1/252	(0.4)	4/250	(0.6)		
DART (17)	1/227	(0.4)	0/219	(0.0)		
ERBAC (20)	2/231	(0.9)	2/222	(0.9)		
Total (OR 0.6 [0.2, 1.9])	**4/862**	**(0.5)**	**7/837**	**(0.5)**		
30-Day MI						
ARTIST (6)	7/152	(4.6)	2/146	(1.4)		
COBRA (15)	10/252	(4.0)	5/250	(2.0)		
DART (17)	5/227	(2.2)	3/219	(1.4)		
ERBAC (20)	8/231	(3.5)	8/222	(3.6)		
Total (OR 1.6 [0.9, 3.0])	**30/862**	**(3.5)**	**18/837**	**(2.2)**		
30-Day MACE						
ARTIST (6)	13/152	(8.6)	7/146	(4.8)		
COBRA (15)	25/252	(9.9)	19/250	(7.6)		
DART (17)	12/227	(5.3)	5/219	(2.3)		
ERBAC (20)	7/231	(3.0)	6/222	(2.7)		
SPORT (30)	9/360	(2.5)	5/375	(1.3)		
Total (OR 1.6 [1.1, 2.4])	**66/1222**	**(5.4)**	**42/1222**	**(3.5)**		
Angiographic Restenosis						
ARTIST (6)	80/124	(64.5)	62/121	(51.2)		
COBRA (15)	80/163	(48.9)	87/170	(51.1)		
DART (17)	55/108	(50.5)	56/111	(50.5)		
ERBAC (20)	86/145	(59.3)	51/109	(46.8)		
SPORT (1)	82/269	(30.4)	73/263	(27.6)		
Total (OR 1.2 [1.0, 1.5])	**383/809**	**(47.3)**	**329/774**	**(42.5)**		
Cumulative Revascularization						
ARTIST (6)	60/152	(39.5)	46/146	(31.5)		
COBRA (15)	54/252	(21.4)	60/250	(24.0)		
DART (17)	64/227	(28.3)	61/219	(28.2)		
ERBAC (20)	90/205	(43.9)	64/191	(33.5)		
SPORT (1)	53/360	(14.7)	61/375	(16.2)		
ROSTER (28)	28/100	(28.0)	40/100	(40.0)		
Total (OR 1.0 [0.9, 1.2])	**349/1296**	**(26.9)**	**333/1281**	**(26.0)**		
Cumulative MACE						
ARTIST (6)	31/152	(20.4)	13/146	(8.9)		
COBRA (15)	75/210	(35.7)	75/213	(35.2)		
DART (17)	59/227	(26.0)	54/219	(24.7)		
ERBAC (20)	94/205	(45.9)	70/191	(36.6)		
ROSTER (28)	40/100	(40.0)	53/100	(53.0)		
SPORT (1)	63/360	(17.5)	51/375	(13.6)		
Total (OR 1.2 [1.0, 1.4])	**362/1254**	**(28.9)**	**316/1244**	**(25.4)**		

0.1   1.0   10.0

OR (95% CI)

Figure 34-12 Systematic overview of randomized trials of percutaneous transluminal rotational atherectomy (PTRA) versus percutaneous transluminal coronary angioplasty (PTCA). Pooled odds ratios (OR) and 95% confidence intervals (CI) were calculated to estimate the overall effect of percutaneous transluminal rotational atherectomy versus that of percutaneous transluminal coronary angioplasty (PTCA). Trial abbreviations are given in Table 34-1, and credits are given in the legend to Figure 34-2.

emphasis. Angulated lesions located in a bend of more than 60 degrees are a relative contraindication to the use of PTRA, and lesions in a bend greater than 90 degrees are a strong contraindication because of the risk of dissection or perforation. When PTRA is performed in nonangulated lesions, the rotating burr should never be advanced to the point of contact with the spring tip of the RotaWire. The rotating burr should not be allowed to remain in one location within the artery; a gentle retraction and re-advancement motion is needed to avoid dissection formation. The rotating burr should not be advanced within the guiding catheter. Rotational atherectomy should be avoided in dissected segments after balloon angioplasty, in lesions with visible thrombus, and in degenerated SVGs.

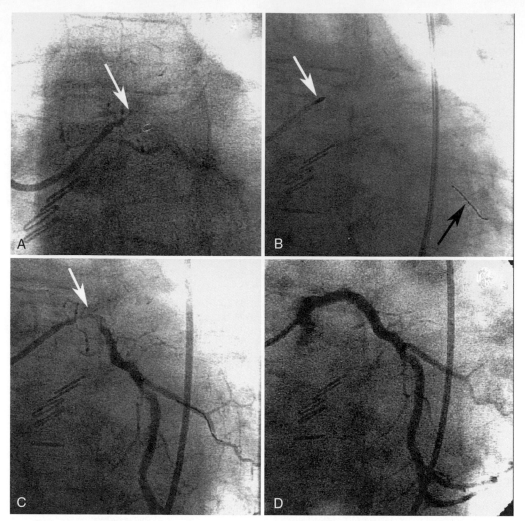

Figure 34-13   Rotational atherectomy for uncrossable left main stenosis. The left main occlusion jeopardized a large un-bypassed left circumflex coronary artery, could be crossed with a guidewire, but could not be crossed with a balloon a catheter (*A, arrow*). After placement of a RotaWire with tip positioned distally (*B, black wire*) a 1.25-mm burr was advanced through the left main occlusion (*B, white arrow*). The residual stenosis (*C, arrow*) was successfully treated with a sirolimus-eluting stent and post-dilated to 4 mm, achieving the final result (*D*).

Conclusion

This chapter reviewed the results of dozens of randomized trials designed to establish the superiority of ablative therapies over PTCA. Systematic analysis suggests that ablative techniques have not been able to achieve prospectively defined endpoints. Although randomized trials are considered to be the gold standard for establishing evidence in interventional cardiology, they produce only general principles about treatment effects and not the fine details of how the treatment should be used. Randomized trials may not be the optimal venue for assessing complex ablative techniques that are dependent on operator expertise and careful patient selection. In a busy interventional practice, familiarity with ablative therapies such as rotational atherectomy and cutting balloon angioplasty is required for successful results to be obtained for commonly encountered challenges such as heavily calcified lesions, ostial disease, bifurcation stenoses, and undilatable lesions.

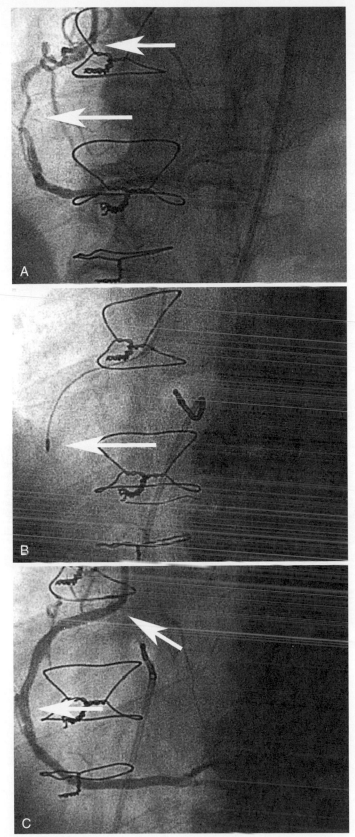

Figure 34-14 Rotational atherectomy for uncrossable lesions in the right coronary artery. Proximal and mid-portion stenoses (*A, arrows*) could not be crossed with low-profile balloon catheters but were successfully treated with a 1.25-mm burr (*B*), leaving dissections that were successfully treated with stents (*C*).

REFERENCES

1. Bittl JA, Chew DP, Topol EJ, et al: Meta-analysis of randomized trials of percutaneous transluminal coronary angioplasty versus atherectomy, cutting balloon atherotomy, or laser angioplasty. *J Am Coll Cardiol* 43:936–942, 2004.

2. Schwartz RS, Huber KC, Murphy JC, et al: Restenosis and the proportional neointimal response to coronary artery injury: Results in a porcine model. *J Am Coll Cardiol* 18:267–274, 1992.

3. Kuntz RE, Gibson CM, Nobuyoshi M, et al: A generalized model of restenosis following conventional balloon angioplasty, stenting, and directional atherectomy. *J Am Coll Cardiol* 21:15–25, 1993.

4. Stankovic G, Colombo A, Bersin R, et al: Comparison of directional coronary atherectomy and stenting versus stenting alone for the treatment of de novo and restenotic coronary artery narrowing. *Am J Cardiol* 93(8):953–958, 2004.

5. Appelman YEA, Piek JJ, Strikwerda S, et al: Randomised trial of excimer laser versus balloon angioplasty for treatment of obstructive coronary artery disease. *Lancet* 347:79–84, 1996.

6. vom Dahl J, Dietz U, Haager PK, et al: Rotational atherectomy does not reduce recurrent in-stent restenosis: Results of the angioplasty versus rotational atherectomy for treatment of diffuse in-stent restenosis trial (ARTIST). *Circulation* 105:583–588, 2002.

7. Singh M, Rosenschein U, Ho KK, et al: Treatment of saphenous vein bypass grafts with ultrasound thrombolysis: A randomized study (ATLAS). *Circulation* 107(18):2331–2336, 2003.

8. Schlüter M, Tübler T, Lansky AJ, et al: Angiographic and clinical outcomes at 8 months of cutting balloon angioplasty and ß-brachytherapy for native vessel in-stent restenosis (BETACUT): Results from a stopped randomized controlled trial. *Catheter Cardiovasc Interv* 66:320–326, 2005.

9. Baim DS, Simonton CA, Feldman RL, et al: A randomized trial comparing balloon angioplasty with optimal atherectomy: The Balloon versus Optimal Atherectomy Trial. *Circulation* 83(12):1611–1616, 1999.

10. Izumi M, Tsuchikane E, Funamoto M, et al: Final results of the CAPAS trial. *Am Heart J* 142:782–789, 2001.

11. Safian RD, Feldman T, Muller DW, et al: Coronary angioplasty and Rotablator atherectomy trial (CARAT): Immediate and late results of a prospective multicenter randomized trial. *Catheter Cardiovasc Interv* 53(2):213–220, 2001.

12. Topol EJ, Leya F, Pinkerton CA, et al: A comparison of balloon angioplasty with directional atherectomy in patients with coronary artery disease. *N Engl J Med* 329:221–227, 1993.

13. Holmes DR, Jr, Topol EJ, Califf RM, et al: A multicenter, randomized trial of coronary angioplasty versus directional atherectomy for patients with saphenous vein bypass graft lesions. CAVEAT-II Investigators. *Circulation* 91(7):1966–1974, 1995.

14. Adelman AG, Cohen EA, Kimball BP, et al: A comparison of coronary atherectomy with coronary angioplasty for lesions of the proximal left anterior descending coronary artery. *N Engl J Med* 329:228–233, 1993.

15. Dill T, Dietz U, Hamm CW, et al: A randomized comparison of balloon angioplasty versus rotational atherectomy in complex coronary lesion (COBRA study). *Eur Heart J* 21:1759–1766, 2000.

16. Chin K: Cutting balloons. In Ellis SG, Holmes DR, Jr, editors: *Strategic approaches in coronary intervention*, ed 3, Philadelphia, 2006, Lippincott Williams & Wilkins.

17. Mauri L, Reisman M, Buchbinder M, et al: Comparison of rotational atherectomy with conventional balloon angioplasty in the prevention of restenosis of small coronary arteries: Results of the Dilatation vs Ablation Revascularization Trial Targeting Restenosis (DART). *Am Heart J* 145:847–854, 2003.

18. Aizawa T: The debulking and stenting in restenosis elimination trial (DESIRE). *Circulation* 104:2954A, 2001.

19. Tsuchikane E, Suzuki T, Asakura Y, et al: Debulking of chronic total occlusions with rotational or directional atherectomy before stenting: final results of DOCTORS study. *Int J Cardiol* 125:397–403, 2008.

20. Reifart N, Vandormael M, Krajcar M, et al: Randomized comparison of angioplasty of complex coronary lesions at a single center. Eximer Laser, Rotational Atherectomy, and Balloon Angioplasty Comparison (ERBAC) Study. *Circulation* 96:91–98, 1997.

21. Ergene O, Seyithanoglu BY, Tastan A, et al: Comparison of angiographic and clinical outcome after cutting balloon and conventional balloon angioplasty in vessels smaller than 3 mm in diameter: A randomized trial. *J Invasive Cardiol* 10(2):70–75, 1998.

22. Mauri L, Bonan R, Weiner BH, et al: Cutting balloon angioplasty for the prevention of restenosis: Results of the Cutting Balloon Global Randomized Trial. *Am J Cardiol* 90:1079–1083, 2002.

23. Molstad P, Myreng Y, Golf S, et al: The Barath Cutting Balloon versus conventional angioplasty. A randomized study comparing acute success rate and frequency of late restenosis. *Scand Cardiovasc J* 32(2):79–85, 1998.

24. Montorsi P, Galli S, Fabbiocchi F, et al: Randomized trial of conventional balloon angioplasty versus cutting balloon for in-stent restenosis. Acute and 24-hour angiographic and intravascular ultrasound changes and long-term follow-up. *Ital Heart J* 5(4):271–279, 2004.

25. Stone GW, de Marchena E, Dageforde D, et al: Prospective, randomized, multicenter comparison of laser-facilitated balloon angioplasty versus stand-alone balloon angioplasty in patients with obstructive coronary artery disease. The Laser Angioplasty Versus Angioplasty (LAVA) Trial Investigators. *J Am Coll Cardiol* 30:1714–1721, 1997.

26. Ozaki Y, Yamaguchi T, Suzuki T, et al: Impact of cutting balloon angioplasty (CBA) prior to bare metal stenting on restenosis: A prospective randomized multicenter trial comparing CBA with balloon angioplasty (BA) before stenting (Reduce III). *Circ J* 71:1–8, 2007.

27. Albiero R, Silber S, Di Mario C, et al: Cutting balloon versus conventional balloon angioplasty for the treatment of in-stent restenosis: results of the restenosis cutting balloon evaluation trial (RESCUT). *J Am Coll Cardiol* 43(6):943–949, 2004.

28. Sharma SK, Kini A, Mehran R, et al: Randomized trial of Rotational Atherectomy Versus Balloon Angioplasty for Diffuse In-stent Restenosis (ROSTER). *Am Heart J* 147(1):16–22, 2004.

29. Whitlow PL, Bass TA, Kipperman RM, et al: Results of the Study to Determine Rotablator and Transluminal Angioplasty Strategy (STRATAS). *Am J Cardiol* 87:699–705, 2001.

30. Lee S-W, Park S-W, Hong M-K, et al: Comparison of angiographic and clinical outcomes between rotational atherectomy and cutting balloon angioplasty followed by radiation therapy with a rhenium 188-mercaptoacetyltriglycine-filled balloon in the treatment of diffuse in-stent restenosis. *Am Heart J* 150:577–582, 2005.

31. Moses JW, Carlier SG, Moussa I: Lesion preparation prior to stenting. *Rev Cardiovasc Med* 5(Suppl 2):S16–S21, 2004.

32. Sharma S, Bagga RS, Kini AS: Debulking approaches prior to stenting in interventional cardiology. In Ellis SG, Holmes DR, Jr, editors: *Strategic approaches in coronary intervention*, ed 3, Philadelphia, 2006, Lippincott Williams & Wilkin.

33. Tsuchikane E, Aizawa T, Tamai H, et al: Pre-drug-eluting stent debulking of bifurcated coronary lesions. *J Am Coll Cardiol* 50:1941–1945, 2007.

34. Okura H, Hayase M, Shimodozono S, et al: Mechanisms of acute lumen gain following cutting balloon angioplasty in calcified and noncalcified lesions: An intravascular ultrasound study. *Catheter Cardiovasc Interv* 57(4):429–436, 2002.

35. Haridas KK, Vijayakumar M, Viveka K, et al: Fracture of cutting balloon microsurgical blade inside coronary artery during angioplasty of tough restenotic lesion: A case report. *Catheter Cardiovasc Interv* 58(2):199–201, 2003.

36. Takebayashi H, Haruta S, Kohno H, et al: Immediate and 3-month follow-up outcome after cutting balloon angioplasty for bifurcation lesions. *J Interv Cardiol* 17(1):1–7, 2004.

37. Smith SC, Jr, Feldman TE, Hirshfeld JW, Jr, et al: ACC/AHA/SCAI 2005 guideline update for percutaneous coronary intervention: A report of the American College of Cardiology/American Heart Association Task Force on Practice Guidelines (ACC/AHA/SCAI Writing Committee to Update the 2001 Guidelines for Percutaneous Coronary Intervention). *J Am Coll Cardiol* 47(1):e1–e121, 2006.

38. Silber S, Albertsson P, Aviles FF, et al: Guidelines for percutaneous coronary interventions: The task force for percutaneous coronary interventions of the European society of cardiology. *Eur Heart J* 26:804–847, 2005.

39. Bittl JA: Physical aspects of excimer laser angioplasty for undilatable lesions. *Catheter Cardiovasc Interv* 71:808–809, 2008.

40. Deckelbaum LI, Natarajan MK, Bittl JA, et al: Effect of intracoronary saline on dissection during excimer laser coronary angioplasty: A randomized trial. *J Am Coll Cardiol* 26:1264–1269, 1995.

41. Ahmed WH, Al-Anazi MM, Bittl JA: Excimer laser facilitated angioplasty for undilatable coronary narrowings. *Am J Cardiol* 78:1045–1047, 1996.

42. Goldberg SL, Colombo A, Akiyama T: Stent under-expansion refractory to balloon dilatation: A novel solution with excimer laser. *J Invasive Cardiol* 10:269–273, 1998.

43. Noble S, Bilodeau L: High energy excimer laser to treat coronary in-stent restenosis in an underexpanded stent. *Catheter Cardiovasc Interv* 71:803–807, 2008.

44. Ikeno F, Hinohara T, Robertson GC, et al: Early experience with a novel plaque excision system for the treatment of complex coronary lesions. *Catheter Cardiovasc Interv* 61(1):35–43, 2004.

45. Baim DS, Cutlip DE, Sharma SK, et al: Final results of the Balloon vs Optimal Atherectomy Trial. *Circulation* 97:322–331, 1998.

46. Brogan WR, Popma JJ, Pichard AD, et al: Rotational coronary atherectomy after unsuccessful coronary balloon angioplasty. *Am J Cardiol* 71(10):794–798, 1993.

47. Kobayashi Y, Teirstein P, Linnemeier T, et al: Rotational atherectomy (stent ablation) in a lesion with stent underexpansion due to heavily calcified plaque. *Cath Cardiovasc Interv* 52:208–211, 2001.

35

Support Devices for High-Risk Percutaneous Coronary Interventions

SRIHARI S. NAIDU | HOWARD C. HERRMANN

KEY POINTS

- The clinical characteristics of the high-risk patient include older age, history of myocardial infarction (MI), low ejection fraction, congestive heart failure (CHF), recent hemodynamic instability, renal insufficiency, and peripheral vascular disease.

- High-risk angiographic characteristics include left main coronary artery (LMCA) disease, last patent conduit, or multi-vessel coronary artery disease, complex lesions (calcified, tortuous, bifurcation), decreased pre-procedure thrombolysis in MI (TIMI) flow and thrombotic lesions.

- The decision to use a circulatory support device should be made within the context of the risk profile of the specific patient for peri-procedural clinical decompensation, after obtaining surgical consultation, when appropriate.

- Intra-aortic balloon pump (IABP) support provides up to 0.5 liter per minute (L/min) of cardiac output; this is supported by a large amount of experiential data in patients with stable cardiac rhythm undergoing high-risk percutaneous coronary intervention (PCI), but recently presented randomized data question a benefit.

- Cardiopulmonary support (CPS) can completely support the circulation, irrespective of cardiac rhythm, and can be instituted quickly by experienced practitioners; but it leads to high rates of vascular and access site complications and does not unload the left ventricle (LV).

- The TandemHeart device indirectly unloads the LV, provides an intermediate level of support reaching flows of up to 3.5 L/min, and can be used for an extended period; however, it is limited by the complex insertion technique and relatively meager clinical data.

- The percutaneous Impella device directly unloads the LV, can provide up to 2.5 l/min of circulatory support, and can also be used for an extended period. It has gained more widespread use because of the easier insertion technique and relatively robust observational data.

Introduction and Rationale

Complications of balloon angioplasty that threaten coronary blood flow, termed *acute and threatened occlusion*, usually require urgent surgical intervention and are the main causes of procedure-related morbidity and mortality. Before the advent of stents as a bail-out treatment for impending vessel closure, this complication occurred in about 6% of balloon angioplasty procedures. Patients who required emergent surgery in this setting had a 50% likelihood of suffering MI, with mortality rates as high as 10%.[1] In these early studies, patient characteristics including compromised ventricular function, LMCA disease and multi-vessel disease, and older age were identified as risk factors for balloon angioplasty related mortality.[2,3] With the development of coronary stents and advanced pharmacotherapy to seal dissections and improve blood flow in thrombotic lesions, respectively, the need for urgent surgery was reduced with a concomitant reduction in PCI-related morbidity and mortality.[4]

In the current era, studies have demonstrated that the need for urgent surgery after PCI has been reduced to less than 1% with a marked reduction in procedure-related mortality.[5] In one comparison of patients treated in 1997–1998 with those treated in 1985–1986, the rate of in-hospital deaths, MI, and coronary artery bypass grafting (CABG) fell from 7.9% to 4.9%, despite the treatment of more complex lesions and stent use in only 71% of patients.[6] Most of the difference between these periods was accounted for by the reduction in the need for emergent CABG from 3.7% to 0.4%.[6] Nonetheless, morbidity and mortality among patients who required emergent CABG remained high.[5] Moreover, the increased confidence afforded by stents and improved operator techniques and experience have prompted interventions on more complex lesions and patients with more severe cardiac and noncardiac diseases. In particular, results of the SYNTAX (SYNergy between percutaneous coronary intervention with TAXus and cardiac surgery) trial now suggest reasonable outcomes in select patients with LMCA disease or multi-vessel coronary disease, while completed and ongoing trials of high-risk PCI with cardiac assist device placement indicate that extremely high-risk patient populations are, indeed, being increasingly considered for PCI.[7,8] Given the large amount of the myocardium in jeopardy in these subsets, as well as the baseline comorbidities (including reduced ventricular reserve), the potential for severe clinical decompensation in such patients is a real concern. It has therefore become essential to precisely identify the predictors of risk and to consider the use of hemodynamic support for patients at high risk for procedural complications and in-hospital mortality. Although a number of investigators have used common sense definitions to classify patients at high risk, two studies systematically developed risk models which will be discussed in more detail.[9-12] In the Mayo Clinic model, clinical and angiographic variables were used to predict in hospital complications after PCI.[9] The variables were age, shock, renal insufficiency, urgent procedures, heart failure, thrombus, and LMCA disease and multi-vessel disease. A score based on these factors predicted the risk of complications and identified a highest risk group with an event rate that exceeded 25%.[12] In a similar study using 46,000 procedures in the New York State Hospital required PCI reporting system, investigators included nine factors in a risk score: (1) ejection fraction, (2) previous MI, (3) gender, (4) age, (5) hemodynamic state, (6) peripheral arterial disease (PAD), (7) CHF, (8) renal failure, and (9) LMCA disease. Using this risk score, a graded risk for in-hospital mortality was derived and validated. About 2% of all patients had a greater than 5% risk for in-hospital death, and about 4% of patients had a greater than 3% risk.[11] Other studies have confirmed these risk factors for PCI-related complications.[3,13,14] However, neither model may accurately represent the higher risk patient populations undergoing intervention in the current era. In addition to these clinical risk factors, angiographic factors of lesion complexity (thrombus, calcification, bifurcations) have been shown to be associated with more dissections, distal embolization, and side-branch occlusions resulting in a threefold increase for in-hospital death.[15]

Several patient characteristics deserve separate discussion. Although female gender was initially associated with complications in early studies of balloon angioplasty, more recent studies have failed to demonstrate a very important effect on outcome.[11,12,16,17] Similarly, patients with diabetes have more complex lesion characteristics and risk factors

TABLE 35-1	Predictors of Risk during Percutaneous Coronary Intervention	
Factor		**Reference**
Clinical and Patient-Related		
Older age		3, 11, 12, 49
Cardiogenic shock		6, 11, 12, 49
Recent myocardial infarction (MI)		6, 11, 12, 49
Congestive heart failure		11–13, 49
Prior coronary artery bypass grafting (CABG)/ revascularization		79
Peripheral vascular disease		11, 49
Chronic renal insufficiency		11–12, 49
Angiographic		
Left main coronary artery/multi-vessel disease		11, 12, 49, 80, 81
Complex lesions (bifurcation, calcification, total occlusion)		15
Decreased thrombolysis in MI (TIMI) flow		82
Left ventricular dysfunction		6, 11, 13, 14, 49
Thrombus		12, 15

but no increase in in-hospital mortality after multivariable adjustment.[18] More recently, baseline left ventricular dysfunction and extent of the myocardium in jeopardy during the procedure have re-emerged as perhaps the strongest clinical risk factors for intra-procedural decompensation and in-hospital mortality. Accordingly, recent studies on high-risk PCI have used the combination of severe ventricular dysfunction (represented by ejection fraction <30% to 35%) and either LMCA disease, last patent conduit, or multi-vessel disease as high-risk PCI inclusion criteria.[19] Thus, it is clear that despite major advances in the technical and procedural performance of modern PCI, clinical and angiographic predictors of significant morbidity and mortality can be identified (Table 35-1). Moreover, it appears likely that increasing numbers of patients will be undergoing high-risk PCI, including the very old and those with LMCA disease, multi-vessel disease, and significant ventricular dysfunction. In many cases, bypass surgery is not a viable option, leaving PCI as the only remaining possible mechanism to improve ventricular function and reduce ischemic symptoms. Together, these data provide the rationale and impetus for the increased use of hemodynamic support during complex or high-risk PCI in the current era. The remainder of this chapter will discuss the approach to such patients, the devices that are currently available to provide support, and the results that may be achieved by using them.

Approach to the Patient

Mechanical circulatory support at the time of PCI has historically been instituted in one of two settings: (1) electively for presumed high-risk intervention and (2) emergently for peri-procedural hemodynamic instability. Specific indications, however, remain unclear because of limitations in performing large-scale, randomized trials and evaluating specific devices in individual patient subsets. Nevertheless, a review of existing literature and ongoing clinical trials provides a framework for patient selection and device selection when evaluating patients for elective or emergent support. Electively placed mechanical support is aimed at improving procedural success by minimizing myocardial ischemia and maintaining hemodynamic stability, thereby reducing clinical decompensation and resultant mortality in high-risk preselected patient subsets, as discussed in the previous section. In this setting, prophylactic insertion of the intra-aortic balloon pump (IABP) or the Impella ventricular assist device appear to have the most robust observational data for improving procedural success with a minimal increase in complications.[19–25] Despite encouraging registry data, however, a recently completed randomized controlled trial failed to show clinical benefit to routine prophylactic IABP insertion in

patients undergoing high-risk PCI.[26] Whether the more powerful Impella device is able to provide benefit within the confines of a randomized controlled trial remains to be seen.[8] The use of mechanical circulatory support in the emergent setting for patients with documented hemodynamic instability or cardiogenic shock is more familiar to interventional cardiologists. Instability may be present before PCI (as in acute MI with compromised ventricular function) or may develop as a consequence of procedural complications such as coronary dissection, poor coronary reflow, or thromboembolism. A common underlying finding in most of these patients is ventricular dysfunction. Although a large randomized clinical trial has not been performed, a pooled meta-analysis of IABP use in patients with acute ST elevation myocardial infarction (STEMI) found no benefit to IABP in conjunction with primary angioplasty, with some benefit seen in those receiving thrombolytic therapy.[27] Available percutaneous ventricular assist devices appear to improve hemodynamic parameters in patients with acute clinical decompensation, but only registry data are available to suggest improved outcome.[28] As a result, determining whether and which device to use in specific settings remains controversial and is primarily guided by experience. Device selection is based on several factors, including ease and rapidity of institution, level of invasiveness and complications, physician familiarity, requisite technical expertise, level of anticipated circulatory support, and available supportive clinical trial data. IABP is the least invasive and most familiar device and may be instituted rapidly, but it provides the least support, averaging 0.5 L/min augmentation in cardiac output.[29] It may be left in place for several days, with a low vascular complication rate.[30] Conversely, full CPS is significantly more invasive, requiring timely surgical and perfusionist collaboration for institution and removal, but can produce greater improvement in cardiac output approximating normal physiology. CPS cannot be maintained indefinitely, however, as hematologic and pulmonary complications increase as bypass time approaches 6 hours.[30] Percutaneous ventricular assist devices (PVADs) such as the TandemHeart or the Impella provide an intermediate level of support approaching 2.5 to 4 L/min and can be placed emergently in the catheterization laboratory (cath lab) without surgical backup, which has prompted their increased use recently. Unlike the Impella, the TandemHeart requires trans-septal puncture to deliver the inflow cannula into the left atrium and requires a somewhat larger arterial cannula. Thus, only patients with larger femoral arterial diameter are able to accommodate device placement, which can be performed only by those skilled in the trans-septal technique. In both devices, the cannulae are larger than an IABP and may result in significant vascular morbidity. However, unlike full CPS, the use of PVAD has been successful for intermediate lengths of time, that is, up to 14 days. Relatively smaller cannulae, as with the Impella, are likely to reduce femoral complications. Historically, elective high-risk PCI has been performed safely with either provisional or prophylactic IABP support. As described above, however, preliminary randomized controlled trial data have suggested that routine prophylactic IABP support may offer little meaningful benefit in these patients.[26] In those select patients who appear to require additional circulatory support, as defined by the inclusion criteria of completed and ongoing randomized trials, PVAD may be considered, with the caveat that the inherent increase in delay and invasiveness (particularly access site complications) may partially offset the benefit and that supportive randomized clinical trials still need to be completed.[8] For patients who develop severe hemodynamic instability, cardiogenic shock, or frank arrest during PCI, bail-out use of the IABP appears beneficial and is certainly the most familiar and rapid strategy. Cath labs experienced in rapid PVAD placement may opt for these larger, more powerful devices. Developing data on hemodynamic parameters that might predict meaningful recovery, such as cardiac power output, would at least theoretically support their use.[31] Although full CPS may be considered in catheterization laboratories equipped and staffed for timely initiation, its clinical use has now been relegated to anecdotal experience. Thus, in emergent settings, PVADs appear more promising but require specialized technical expertise.

Description of Devices

INTRA-AORTIC BALLOON PUMP

The IABP was first used clinically in cardiogenic shock by Kantrowitz in 1968.[32] As its application expanded to include refractory angina, severe hemodynamic compromise, and postcardiotomy pump failure, and with the advent of percutaneous insertion, the IABP was one of the first hemodynamic devices used to support high-risk PCIs.[32-34]

The rapid filling of the balloon in early diastole augments diastolic pressure and thus leads to increased coronary perfusion pressure, whereas deflation of the balloon at end-diastole reduces effective aortic volume and decreases aortic systolic pressure leading to lower left ventricular afterload. The net effect is a decrease in myocardial oxygen requirements from lower systolic wall tension and an increase in coronary perfusion pressure, improving the myocardial supply-and-demand balance. Cardiac output increases because of the improved myocardial contractility as a result of the increased coronary blood flow and the reduced afterload.[35,36]

Insertion Technique

Evaluation of the iliac and femoral arteries is recommended to exclude significant arterial disease. Access in the common femoral artery is obtained via the Seldinger technique. The balloon can be inserted through an 8 or 9 French (F) sheath or directly in a sheath-less fashion. Before insertion, all the air in the balloon should be evacuated with a large syringe attached to the one way valve to maintain the lowest possible profile during insertion. The balloon catheter is advanced under angiographic guidance over a stiff 0.021-inch guidewire until the radiopaque tip marker reaches a level just distal to the left subclavian artery. After removal of the guidewire, the central lumen is flushed and connected to a pressure transducer. The balloon is then connected to the console, the system is purged with helium, and counterpulsation is started. Proper placement and inflation of the balloon should be done fluoroscopically, and the timing of inflation and deflation should be optimized by either the surface electrocardiogram (ECG) or the transduced pressure tracing to achieve optimal hemodynamic support.

Clinical Trials

Much of the data on the use of IABP as well as other circulatory support devices during high-risk PCI comes from the pre-stent era of coronary interventions. Voudris et al showed that support with IABP during elective high-risk angioplasty is both safe and feasible.[22] During a 13-month period (in 1987-1988), 27 patients considered high risk because of decreased left ventricular function or multi-vessel disease underwent angioplasty with IABP support. Primary success, according to contemporary American College of Cardiology (ACC) guidelines, was achieved in all 27 patients. There were no major cardiac events during hospitalization, and there was only one IABP-related vascular complication. After a mean follow-up period of 13 months, there were 2 deaths, 1 cardiac transplantation, and 6 cases of symptom-driven target vessel revascularization (TVR, 22% rate of recurrent angina), which was also successfully performed with IABP support.[22] Similar outcomes were reported by Kahn et al in a group of 28 high-risk patients during the same period.[21] The most common high-risk feature in this cohort of patients was severe left ventricular dysfunction, but some patients had critical stenoses in the left main coronary artery (LMCA) or a single remaining coronary artery. Procedural success was 96% (90 of 94 lesions were successfully dilated). There were 11 cases of intra-procedural hypotension, although the augmented diastolic pressure was maintained over 90 mm Hg in all cases and angioplasty was completed in all patients. Vascular complications associated with the IABP occurred in 11% of the patients. In another series of 21 patients with similar high-risk features, 90% of lesions attempted were successfully dilated without hemodynamic compromise.[23] Device-related complications (hematoma) occurred in 10% of the cases, and procedure-related complications occurred in 14% of the cases.[23] The beneficial effects of IABP support were also shown in high-risk coronary rotational atherectomy.[37] In this retrospective analysis, 28 patients

scheduled to undergo rotational atherectomy were placed on IABP support before the coronary intervention. This group was compared with 131 patients with high-risk coronary lesions who did not have an IABP placed a priori. The group that received a planned IABP comprised patients who were older, had more left ventricular dysfunction, and had a higher incidence of multi-vessel disease. While systolic hypotension occurred in 11% of the patients in the study group, diastolic pressure augmentation provided by the IABP allowed successful completion of the procedure in all patients. Hypotension necessitating IABP placement occurred in 7% of the patients in the comparison group. Slow flow occurred at a similar rate in both groups; however, 27% of the patients in the comparison group who experienced slow flow developed a non–Q wave MI compared with none in the study group. There were no differences in the rate of transfusion requirements or vascular complications.[37] In a more recent study by Brodie et al, IABP was shown to reduce peri-procedural events.[2] The group in this study consisted of 213 patients who presented with acute MI and received an IABP. In contrast to the earlier studies discussed, the majority of patients in this study were treated with stents, and about a third were treated with abciximab, reflecting more contemporary treatments. While the indication for the IABP in most cases was cardiogenic shock, there were 80 patients who were hemodynamically stable but were considered high risk because of left ventricular dysfunction. In this group, the use of IABP support led to a decreased incidence of prolonged hypotension, cardiac arrest, and ventricular fibrillation; however, the difference was not statistically significant because of the low number of patients in this group. IABP use was associated with an increased risk of major bleeding and higher transfusion rates. While IABP use during high-risk coronary interventions has been shown, at least in registry and case series data, to be effective in supporting the circulation, the increased rates of vascular and hemorrhagic complications associated with its use demands careful patient selection.[2,21,22,21,37] For this reason, a strategy of provisional IABP support was compared with prophylactic placement of IABP in high-risk interventions in a retrospective, non-randomized study.[38] Sixty-one patients who received elective IABP were compared with 72 patients in whom support was initiated only when clinically necessary. The patients in the elective IABP group were slightly older, but other high-risk features were similar, including severity of left ventricular dysfunction (ejection fraction [EF] <30%) and rates of multi-vessel disease and unstable angina. Rates of stent and glycoprotein inhibitor use were similar between the two groups. The rates of slow flow were similar in both groups, but hemodynamic deterioration occurred only in patients (15%) in the provisional IABP group, and all received urgent IABP support. Rates of vascular complications were low in this study, with only two patients in the provisional IABP group developing groin hematomas. There were no cases of major bleeding. Although not statistically significant, three deaths occurred in the provisional IABP group in patients who required urgent placement of an IABP compared with one death in the elective group.[38] Most recently, however, routine prophylactic use of IABP in high-risk PCI has come into question, following the preliminary results of a large randomized trial.[26] These findings, if confirmed, highlight the need for randomized controlled trial data to fully elucidate the proper role of any cardiac assist device in high-risk PCI. A summary of the published observational trials using IABP during high-risk PCI is shown in Table 35-2.

PERCUTANEOUS CARDIOPULMONARY SUPPORT

The introduction of the portable Bard CardioPulmonary Bypass Support (CR Bard, Inc., Murray Hill, NJ) system in 1985 expanded the application of percutaneous CPS.[39] While the most common application for temporary circulatory support is for patients who cannot be weaned from cardiopulmonary bypass after cardiac surgery, CPS has also been implemented in the cath lab either emergently as a bridge to cardiac surgery or prophylactically to support high-risk coronary interventions. Full CPS incorporates a heat exchanger, an adjustable blood reservoir, a pump, and an oxygenator and can temporarily

TABLE 35-2	Intra-aortic Balloon Pump Clinical Trials					
Study	*Year*	*Coronary Intervention*	*Number of Patients*	*Revascularization Success Rate (%)*	*Device-Related Complication Rate (%)*	*In-Hospital Mortality Rate*
Anwar A[20]	1990	PTCA	97	85.6	2	1
Kahn JK[21]	1990	PTCA	28	96	11	7.1
Voudris V[22]	1990	PTCA	27	100	3.7	0
Kreidieh I[23]	1992	PTCA	21	90	9.5	0
Kaul U[54]	1995	PTCA	20	95	0	5
O'Murchu B[37]	1995	Atherectomy/PTCA	28	100	7.1	0
Schreiber TL[55]	1998	PTCA	91	87	27	8.7
Brodie BR[2]	1999	PTCA/Stent*	108[†]	89.8	8[‡]	37[§]
Briguori C[38]	2003	PTCA/Stent	61	94	0	8

*Stents used in the last three year of the study.
[†]Includes patients with shock or congestive heart failure (CHF), number of patients undergoing high-risk coronary intervention not defined.
[‡]Includes patients that received intra-aortic balloon pump (IABP) after percutaneous transluminal coronary angioplasty (PTCA).
[§]30-day mortality that includes patients with cardiogenic shock.

substitute for the entire circulation, irrespective of cardiac rhythm. Because blood comes in contact with various biomaterials in the perfusion circuit, activation of blood proteins and cells leads to morbidity that limits the length of time it can be maintained. Other more simplified strategies employ only a blood pump and extracorporeal membrane oxygenator (ECMO).

CPS unloads the right ventricle but does not unload the LV.[39] Pulmonary and systolic aortic pressures have been shown to decrease, whereas diastolic and mean systemic arterial pressures remain unchanged.[39,40] In normal functioning hearts, the reduction in preload and a small increase in afterload produced by the arterial inflow reduces wall stress and produces smaller end-diastolic left ventricular volumes because the LV is able to eject the blood it receives. However, in dilated and poorly contracting hearts, especially after cardiac arrest, the increase in afterload may impair left ventricular emptying and another means of assisting emptying of the LV (e.g., IABP) may be necessary. Another very simple approach is to provide an external cardiac compression approximately every minute while the patient is on CPS. Studies have also shown that CPS does not increase coronary perfusion in the setting of an occlusion, so bypass surgery should be considered if circulation cannot be restored percutaneously. For these reasons, CPS may, at least in theory, be a poor choice for patients undergoing high-risk PCI, in whom unloading the LV and maintaining antegrade coronary blood flow is a primary concern.

Insertion Technique

Before arterial cannulation, angiography of the ilio-femoral arteries is performed to exclude significant arterial disease. Care should be taken to access the artery below the inguinal ligament in the common femoral artery. Invasive monitoring with a pulmonary artery catheter is recommended during support. Once venous access and arterial access are obtained with a flexible 0.038-inch guidewire and an 8F dilator, anticoagulation is started with an anti-thrombin agent. The flexible wire is replaced with a stiff 0.038-inch guidewire, and both the vein and the artery are progressively dilated with a 12F and a 14F dilator. Finally, 18F cannulae are placed, with the inflow at the level of the right atrium and the outflow at the level of the aortic bifurcation. The cannulae are then clamped before being connected to the primed perfusion circuit. Priming of the circuit should be performed by a perfusionist while access is being obtained. After carefully de-airing the system, the cannulae are connected to the perfusion circuit, and support is started at 2 L/min and progressively advanced by 0.5 L/min increments as needed.[40] After successful coronary intervention, CPS is weaned quickly, usually over 15 minutes, by gradually reducing the flow rate. Volume is infused to increase the LV filling pressure to at least 8 to 10 mm Hg or to pre-bypass levels (whichever is less). If necessary, inotropic agents may be used to facilitate the weaning of support. An intra-aortic balloon can also be used if weaning causes

difficulties for the client. The Bard percutaneous CPS system (CR Bard, Murray Hill, NJ) is a portable, battery-operated system that consists of a centrifugal pump (Biomedicus pump), a heat exchanger, and a membrane oxygenator. Venous inflow is achieved by active suction, not by gravity as in the classic cardiopulmonary bypass system, which makes it essential that patients be well hydrated. To prevent air embolism, central venous access should be avoided while the pump is operating. Percutaneous cardiopulmonary support can only be performed for 6 hours. After 6 hours, platelet aggregation, hemolysis, and increased capillary permeability with plasma loss become major complications.

Clinical Trials

Early reports on small numbers of patients showed that using CPS for high-risk angioplasty was feasible, even though it had high rates of femoral access site complications.[41-43] The national registry of elective supported angioplasty reported data on 801 patients who underwent elective angioplasty with CPS in 25 centers from 1988 to 1992. The suggested inclusion clinical criteria were the presence of severe or unstable angina, at least one likely dilatable coronary artery stenosis, and either left ventricular ejection fraction (LVEF) less than 25% or a target vessel supplying more than half of the viable myocardium, or both.[44] Although the initial angioplasty success rate was high in this registry, the rates of device-related complications were also high. The strategy was thus changed to one of standby support for these high-risk interventions. Prophylactic support was implemented in 73% of the patients, and the last 27% of the patients registered had standby support. The overall primary success rate was 93%, and the success rate in the group that had standby support was 91%.[45] The rates of vascular complications (15% vs. 6.1%) and transfusions (31% vs. 14%) decreased with the change in strategy from prophylactic support to standby support. The mortality rate (6.3% vs. 6% in the prophylactic and standby groups, respectively) and the rate of emergent bypass surgery (2.5% vs. 3.2%) did not change, however, reflecting the high-risk profile of the patients in the registry. Only 16 of 217 patients (7.4%) in the standby strategy group required emergency initiation of bypass support. Of these 16 patients, 75% had successful angioplasty without need for bypass surgery, which suggested that standby support reduced the need for emergency bypass surgery. The only group of patients demonstrating a clear benefit to using prophylactic support was the group with an LVEF of 20% or less. In these patients, those treated with prophylactic placement of CPS before coronary intervention had a lower mortality compared with those who had CPS on standby (7% vs. 18%, $P < 0.05$). A separate analysis of the 42 patients in the registry with 60% or more LMCA stenosis who underwent angioplasty was performed, and the results were compared with those for high-risk patients who had another vessel dilated.[46] The hospital mortality was 14.3% in patients who had angioplasty of the LMCA, notably higher than the 4.6% hospital mortality in patients who did not have significant LMCA disease and had angioplasty of another vessel ($P < 0.001$).[46]

In the pre-stent era, additional support with CPS did not improve the outcome of percutaneous intervention in LMCA disease. As the insertion technique evolved from requiring surgical cut-down to a percutaneous approach, as described by Shawl, the experience with CPS continued to grow in the cath lab.[47] His group reported one of the largest series of supported angioplasty from 1988 to 1991.[47-49] Among the first 51 patients, 94% had three-vessel disease, 70% had LVEF 35% or less, and the majority had been turned down for bypass surgery.[47] All the patients tolerated the coronary intervention with the mean coronary stenosis improving from 89% to 21%. The hospital mortality was 6%, which compared well with the 6.9% mortality in patients undergoing CABG with ejection fraction 35% or less at that time.[50] The most frequent complication was bleeding requiring transfusion, which occurred in 40% of the patients. Other complications included pseudo-aneurysm (8%), hematoma (2%), and femoral nerve weakness (8%). With improvement in the cannula removal technique, the requirement for transfusion decreased in later patients to 4% and eliminated the occurrence of femoral nerve injury.[48] In patients with particularly high risk (mean LVEF $\leq$19.5% $\pm$ 3.5%; 54% with dilation of the single remaining patent artery; 17% with dilation of an unprotected LMCA), CPS showed promising short-term and long-term results.[49] Angiographic success was achieved in 98.7% of the arteries attempted in 105 patients. Despite the occurrence of asystole in 5 patients (4.6%) and of electromechanical dissociation in 40 (37%) with balloon inflation, there were no procedural deaths, and all patients were weaned off CPS after the angioplasty. The hospital mortality was 4.7%. After a mean follow-up of 24 $\pm$ 13 months, 97% of patients were in Canadian Cardiovascular Society (CCS) functional class I or II, compared with only 3% before the intervention ($P < 0.001$).[49]

Because of the high rate of complications, attention was turned to using CPS on a standby basis. Two retrospective analyses showed that the incidence of hemodynamic collapse requiring support during angioplasty was less than 1%.[43,51] Subsequently, the National Registry of Elective Cardiopulmonary Support compared the usefulness of prophylactic percutaneous CPS with stand-by percutaneous CPS in patients undergoing high-risk angioplasty.[52] Mortality rates were similar, 6.4% in the prophylactic group and 6.1% in the standby group. The rates of procedural success were also similar in the two groups. However, morbidity was significantly higher in the prophylactic CPS group, with 42% of patients having femoral access site complications that necessitated blood transfusions compared with only 11.7% of patients in the standby group. Of 180 patients in the standby group, only 13 (7.2%) suffered irreversible hemodynamic collapse, and emergency CPS was initiated in less than 5 minutes in 12 of these 13 patients. The patients who did benefit from prophylactic CPS were those with an ejection fraction 20% or less, having a lower mortality with support initiated before angioplasty (4.8% vs. 18.8%, $P < 0.05$).[52] A more recent European study evaluated the usefulness of CPS during the stent era.[53] The report included two groups of patients: (1) group I comprised 68 patients undergoing elective high-risk coronary intervention, and (2) group II consisted of 24 patients presenting with acute MI and cardiogenic shock. In the elective group, primary success was achieved in 66 (97%) patients, with complete revascularization obtained in 44% of the group. Four patients (6%) developed femoral artery complications, and one patient (1.4%) died before discharge. After 28 $\pm$ 19 months of follow-up, major adverse cardiac events (MACEs) occurred in 30% of patients and included 7 deaths (10%). Compared with the previous literature on angioplasty supported by CPS, this study demonstrated that CPS could be used effectively during coronary stenting and also showed an improvement in the rate of complications. Two studies compared CPS and IABP for high-risk coronary interventions. One prospective trial randomized patients to either CPS or IABP support during PCI that was considered high risk because of the presence of unstable angina with poor left ventricular function in a target vessel supplying more than half of the remaining viable myocardium.[54] Between June 1991 and November 1993, 40

patients were randomized. All patients had a history of a prior MI, the majority had three-vessel disease, and the mean ejection fraction in both groups was lower than 25%. All patients were treated with angioplasty using balloon inflations lasting longer than 2 minutes. Patients in both groups tolerated balloon inflations lasting 2 to 3 minutes without hemodynamic decompensation. Primary success was achieved in 19 of 20 patients in both groups with similar angiographic results. There were no vascular or hemorrhagic complications in the IABP group, whereas two patients assigned to CPS developed vascular complications requiring surgical repair, and five other patients required blood transfusions.[54] There was one death in each group thought to be caused by acute vessel closure after discontinuation of support. The study authors concluded that both IABP and CPS were effective in supporting high-risk coronary interventions in the pre-stent era, with IABP having lower rates of complications. Schreiber et al reported retrospective observational data comparing outcomes in a larger group of patients who had undergone high-risk PCI with hemodynamic support.[55] Over a 4-year period, 149 patients who had high-risk PCIs underwent prophylactic placement of either an IABP ($n = 91$) or CPS ($n = 58$). Patients presenting with acute MI, unstable angina, and stable angina were included if they were hemodynamically stable before the procedure. Patients were considered high risk if they had poor ventricular function, had a culprit vessel supplying the majority of the myocardium, or required multi-vessel PCI. Patients who received CPS were more likely to be male (91% vs. 73%, $P < 0.01$), have a history of chronic angina (91% vs. 69%, $P = 0.003$), have CHF (59% vs. 35%, $P = 0.008$), and have a lower mean ejection fraction (26% $\pm$ 13% vs. 32% $\pm$ 14%, $P < 0.01$). Multi-vessel PCI was performed more often in the CPS group (40% vs. 20%, $P < 0.01$). Despite the higher severity of disease in the CPS group, angioplasty was successful more often in the CPS group compared with the IABP group (99% vs. 87% of lesions, $P = 0.005$). MACEs (MI, need for CABG, stroke, death) occurred at similar rates in both groups, although the rate of CABG trended higher in the IABP group without reaching statistical significance (1.7% vs. 6.5%, $P = 0.33$). Of note, the rate of death was high in both groups (12% in the CPS group, 8.7% in the IABP group, $P = 0.71$).[55] As in Kaul's study, access site complications and transfusions occurred more frequently in the CPS group. The higher angioplasty success rate in the CPS group is likely explained by the longer duration of balloon inflation tolerated by this group. This difference would likely not exist with the use of stents. Use of CPS for high-risk PCI has decreased recently with the advent of minimally invasive PVADs. The studies describing CPS in high-risk PCI are summarized in Table 35-3. Complications of prolonged use of CPS and ECMO include bleeding, infection, thrombocytopenia, and compromised perfusion to the lower extremity. The complexity of therapy and the requirements for a surgeon and a bedside perfusionist are the drawbacks to this therapy. Nonetheless, the high level of support may be the only option for some patients experiencing full cardiopulmonary collapse requiring intervention.

PERCUTANEOUS LEFT VENTRICULAR ASSIST DEVICES

Left Atrial Artery–to–Femoral Artery Bypass

A recent innovation in circulatory support available to interventionalists is the percutaneous left ventricular assist device (LVAD). The left atrial artery–to–femoral artery bypass strategy, first described in 1962 by Dennis, was initially used in patients who could not be weaned from cardiopulmonary bypass after surgery.[56-58] More recently, a dedicated system with a compact centrifugal pump (TandemHeart pVAD) was developed to allow relatively rapid percutaneous institution of left atrial artery–to–femoral artery bypass (Fig. 35-1). The pump cycles oxygenated blood from the left atrium to the femoral artery without the need for an external oxygenator or a heat exchanger.

The left atrial artery–to–femoral artery bypass system indirectly unloads the LV and decreases cardiac filling pressures, cardiac workload, and myocardial oxygen demand.[59,60] Previous studies have shown

TABLE 35-3	**Percutaneous Cardiopulmonary Support Clinical Trials**							
Study	*Year*	*Coronary Intervention*	*Number of Patients*	*Revascularization Success Rate (%)*	*Device-Related Complication Rate (%)*	*Transfusion Rate (%)*	*In-Hospital Mortality Rate (%)*	*Bypass Time (min)*
Vogel RA[83]	1988	PTCA	9	100	11	100	11.0	NR
Shawl FA[47]	1989	PTCA	51[1]	100	14	38	5.8	37
Shawl FA[48]	1990	PTCA	121[2]	NR	9.9	29.7	NR	37[3]
Teirstein PS[52]	1993	PTCA	389[4]	88.7	12.6	39	6.4	NR
Sivananthan MN[42]	1994	PTCA	13	83	83	100	7.7	92.8 ± 46
Kaul U[54]	1995	PTCA	20	95	10	25	5	NR
Vogel RA[45]	1995	PTCA	801[5]	93	15[6]	31[6]	6.9	NR
Shawl FA[49]	1996	PTCA	107	98	4.7	1.9	4.7	46 ± 30
Schreiber TL[55]	1998	PTCA	58	99	50	60	12	60 ± 45
de Lezo JS[84]	2002	PTCA	68[7]	97	6	NR	1.5	NR

[1]Includes 20 patients with left ventricular ejection fraction (LVEF) ≤25%, which are included in the 1996 report.
[2]A total of 121 patients reported, 101 of which underwent elective coronary interventions.
[3]Time reported for the elective interventions.
[4]Number of patients with prophylactic percutaneous cardiopulmonary support (CPS) device placement.
[5]27% of patients were treated with a standby strategy.
[6]Complication and transfusion rate reported for the group with percutaneous CPS device placed prophylactically.
[7]A total of 92 patients were reported, 68 of whom had elective procedures.

a decrease in infarct size in the acutely ischemic myocardium with the use of a trans-septal LVAD. Predominant right ventricular failure is a contraindication to the use of a trans-septal LVAD.

Insertion Technique

After angiography of the distal aorta and iliac vessels to exclude significant arterial occlusive disease, access in the femoral vein is obtained. After a trans-septal puncture is performed, the inter-atrial septum is dilated in two stages with 14F and 21F dilators, and the 22F inflow cannula is advanced to the left atrium under angiographic and echocardiographic guidance.[59,61] The outflow 15F to 17F cannula is then inserted by using the Seldinger technique over a stiff guidewire and advanced to the common iliac artery. The cannulae are de-aired and connected to the pump.

The TandemHeart pVAD (Cardiac Assist Inc., Pittsburgh, PA) is a continuous-flow centrifugal pump that operates at 7500 revolutions per minute (rpm) and provides up to 3.5 L/min of blood flow. The pump contains a single moving part (impeller) suspended by

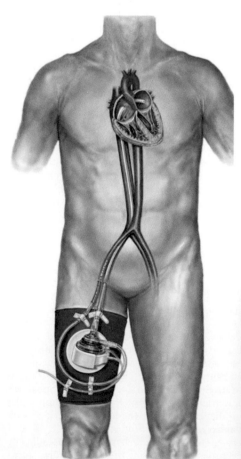
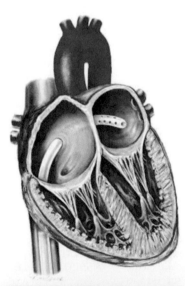
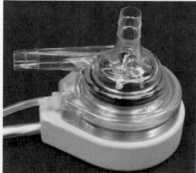

Figure 35-1 TandemHeart percutaneous left ventricular assist device. The inflow cannula to the centrifugal pump is inserted trans-septally to the left atrium, and the outflow is inserted in the femoral artery. See the text for details.

TABLE 35-4	Left Atrial–Femoral Artery Bypass Clinical Trials						
Study	Year	Number of Patients	Insertion Time (min)	Revascularization Success Rate (%)	Mean Support Duration	In-Hospital Mortality (n)	Other Complications
Glassman E[65]*	1993	13	†	100	43 ± 17 min	0	- Transfusion in 1 of 13 patients - Small left-to-right shunts in 2 of 13 patients
Lemos PA[61]	2003	7‡	31 to 69	92.3	55 ± 96 hours	1	- Bleeding in 4 of 7 patients - Hypothermia in 2 of 7 patients
Aragon J[59]	2005	8	†	100	§	1	- Acute renal failure requiring dialysis in 1 of 8 patients
Kar B[64]	2006	5	†	100	107 min¶	1	- Blood transfusions in all patients - Groin hematomas in 2 of 5 patients
Al-Husami W[85]	2008	6	36.5	100	†	1	- No vascular complications (all devices removed in the operating room) - 1 of 6 possible transient ischemic attacks [TIA]/seizure
Vranckx P[66]	2008	23	35	91.3	31 ± 49.8 hours	5	- Bleeding in 27% - Hypothermia in 6/23
Vranckx P[86]	2009	9	27	100	93 minutes	0	- Vascular complications 44.4%
Thomas JL[67]	2010	37	†	100	†	11	- 82% transfusion rate

*The device used in this series was not the Tandemheart pVAD (percutaneous ventricular assist devices).
†Not reported.
‡Five patients were hemodynamically stable prior to insertion of the pVAD.
§Not reported, but all patients had the pVAD removed in the catheterization laboratory at the end of the coronary intervention. The mean procedure time was 169 ± 21 minutes.
¶Excludes duration of support for one patient who required support for an additional 48 hours because of persistent poor left ventricular function.

a magnetic force on a thin lubricating film of fluid.[62] A continuous infusion of heparinized saline solution provides this hydrodynamic bearing for the pump, as well as local anticoagulation and cooling of the motor. Full systemic anticoagulation with heparin is required.

Clinical Trials

A small prospective feasibility study evaluated the hemodynamic effects of the TandemHeart pVAD in short-term stabilization of patients with cardiogenic shock.[60] The device was safely implanted in 18 patients, with a mean duration of support of 4 ± 3 days. Hemodynamic indices, including pulmonary capillary wedge pressure (PCWP), pulmonary arterial pressure (PAP), cardiac output, and systemic blood pressure, showed a significant improvement on TandemHeart pVAD support. During support, there was negligible hemolysis, bleeding requiring transfusion occurred in 5 patients, and two with PAD required surgical placement of an antegrade perfusion cannula to relieve limb ischemia.

To date, there are only a few case reports and small series on the experience with the left atrial artery–to–femoral artery bypass system to support high-risk coronary interventions[59,61-65] (see the case study example below); there is no completed or ongoing large randomized trial. In early series, the device was shown to be easily implanted by interventionalists experienced in trans-septal puncture and to provide circulatory support to allow high-risk coronary interventions to be done successfully in a controlled fashion (Table 35-4). Two case series were recently published.[66-67] In one, between 2000 and 2006, 23 patients with mean age 59 years underwent high-risk PCI using the Tandem Heart device. Implantation was successful in all patients, and PCI was successful in 21 patients (91.3%). Hemodynamic parameters improved, including PCWP and systemic arterial pressure. Five patients died with the device in place, primarily from pre-existing cardiogenic shock. There was mild to moderate access site bleeding in 27% of patients. In the other series, 37 patients received the device for high-risk PCI or cardiogenic shock. The mean age was 73 years, and 97% were in New York Heart Association (NYHA) class III CHF or cardiogenic shock. There was technical PCI success in all patients, but 82% of patients required blood transfusion after the procedure. Overall, however, 71% of patients in this extremely high-risk group survived to discharge.

Subsequently, two small randomized trials have compared the TandemHeart to IABP in patients with cardiogenic shock.[68,69] Although there was benefit in terms of hemodynamic parameters, a small meta-analysis combining both studies did not suggest an effect on survival with use of the device.[70] Because of the trans-septal puncture required, the TandemHeart pVAD may ultimately be best suited for elective initiation of hemodynamic support as insertion times tend to be longer compared with IABP and with other PVAD devices (Impella).

CASE STUDY

An 80-year-old man with severe chronic obstructive pulmonary disease (COPD), chronic renal insufficiency, and carotid artery disease presented with unstable angina. Echocardiography revealed severe left ventricular dysfunction (EF 10%), anterior wall akinesis, and moderate mitral regurgitation. Positron emission tomography (PET) showed lateral wall ischemia and high anterolateral viability. Cardiac catheterization revealed 95% distal LMCA disease involving the ostia of both the left anterior descending (LAD) and left circumflex (LCx) arteries (Fig. 35-2), and a 50% stenosis in the mid-right coronary artery. The patient was thought to be at high risk for surgical revascularization, and thus hemodynamically supported LMCA intervention with the TandemHeart pVAD was undertaken. After trans-septal placement of a 21F inflow cannula in the left atrium, and placement of a 15F outflow cannula in the right common iliac artery, left atrial artery–to–distal aorta bypass was achieved with a nonpulsatile flow rate of 3 L/min. Bifurcation stenting of the LAD and LCx arteries was performed with two sirolimus-eluting stents deployed simultaneously using the "kissing" technique (Figs. 35-3 and 35-4). There was a significant decrease in aortic pulse pressure because of diminished stroke volume, but the mean perfusion pressure was maintained and the patient remained hemodynamically stable without angina or arrhythmia (Fig. 35-5). The patient was discharged 2 days after the procedure and remained angina-free at 1 month follow-up.

The case study is adapted from Naidu SS, Rohatgi S, Herrmann HC, Glaser R: Unprotected left main "kissing" stent implantation with a percutaneous ventricular assist device, J Invasive Cardiol 16(11):683–684.

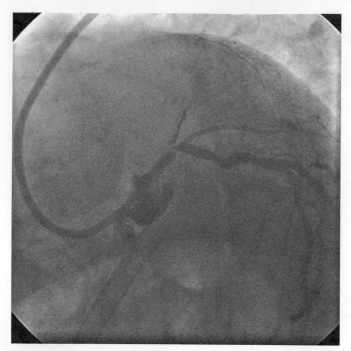

Figure 35-2   Baseline angiography showing distal left main coronary artery (LMCA) stenosis and subtotal occlusion of the proximal left anterior descending (LAD) artery.

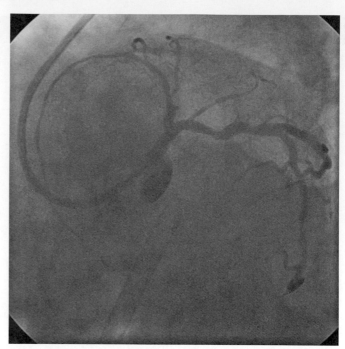

Figure 35-4   Final angiography showing reconstruction of the distal left main coronary artery (LMCA), proximal left anterior descending (LAD) artery, and left circumflex (LCx) coronary artery.

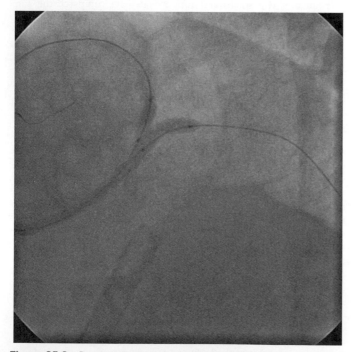

Figure 35-3   Percutaneous coronary intervention using two sirolimus-eluting stents in a "kissing" technique.

TRANS-VALVULAR LEFT VENTRICULAR ASSIST DEVICES

In 1988, Wampler et al described a new catheter-mounted trans-valvular LVAD, which was initially placed surgically via the femoral artery.[71] Development of a smaller (13F/14F) system allowed percutaneous insertion of the device. Two investigational devices, the Impella and Hemopump, have been tested clinically, although only the Impella

is currently available for clinical use. The Impella Recover LP 2.5 (Abiomed, Inc., Danvers, MA) is a microaxial rotary blood pump that unloads the LV by expelling blood from the LV to the aorta (Fig. 35-6). The device can deliver an output of up to 2.5 L/min. The Impella device has been shown to directly unload the LV by decreasing the end-diastolic pressure, decreasing the end-diastolic and end-systolic volumes, and increasing the combined (device plus native heart) cardiac output, simultaneously improving coronary blood flow.[72,73] A larger Impella 5.0 device with greater hemodynamic benefits is also available, but it typically requires surgical cut-down for placement.

Insertion Techniques

Before the procedure, an echocardiogram should be performed to exclude the presence of a left ventricular thrombus or critical aortic stenosis. Angiography of the distal aorta and iliac vessels should also be performed before insertion of the femoral sheath. The Impella 2.5 percutaneous device has a maximal outer diameter of 12F. After inserting an appropriate-sized (usually 13F) sheath in the femoral artery, an exchange length (300 cm) 0.014-inch guidewire is delivered to the LV with an end-hole angiographic catheter (JR4, MPA, etc.). The device is then advanced over the wire and positioned across the aortic valve under fluoroscopic guidance. Recently, a wireless insertion technique has also been described. Proper placement is critical to ensure unimpeded outflow of blood and catheter stability. The proximal part of the catheter connects to a portable mobile console that provides power and allows control of the pump.[73] The Impella Recover LP 2.5 device is mounted on a 9F pigtail catheter (see Fig. 35-1), which sits in the left ventricular cavity. The device provides flows up to 2.5 L/min at its maximal rotational speed of 50,000 rpm and can be safely left in place for up to 5 days.[72] A heparinized 20% dextrose solution continuously lubricates the pump. For prolonged support, heparin infusion to activated clotting time (ACT) of 160 to 180 seconds is required.

Clinical Trials

Initial case studies evaluating the Impella 2.5 device in high-risk PCI suggested safety, feasibility, and minimal complications, with one report suggesting no significant benefit.[74] This was followed by the

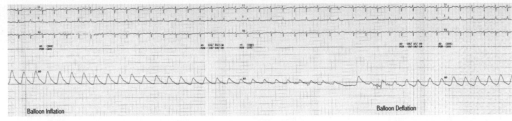

Figure 35-5 Aortic pressure tracing during balloon inflation showing significant decrease in pulse pressure caused by diminished stroke volume with preserved mean perfusion pressure via the TandemHeart bypass circuit.

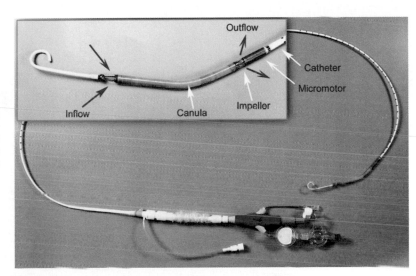

Figure 35-6 Impella Recover LP 2.5 device. *(Adapted from Valgimigli M, Stoendijk P, Sianos G, et al: Left ventricular unloading and concomitant total cardiac output increase by the use of percutaneous Impella Recover LP 2.5 assist device during high-risk coronary intervention, Catheter Cardiovasc Interv 65(2).263-267, 2005.)*

PROTECT 1 (the Prospective Randomized Oral Therapy Evaluation in Crohn's disease Trial) study, the primary safety and feasibility study of 20 patients in the United States.[19] Enrolling patients with LMCA or sole remaining conduit and severe left ventricular dysfunction, the device was technically successful in all cases with a low complication rate. As a result, the multi-center PROTECT 2 superiority trial randomized patients with similar inclusion criteria to prophylactic IABP or Impella 2.5 support. To date, this is the largest randomized controlled trial of high-risk PCI ever performed, and should help clarify the role of this percutaneous cardiac assist device. Several smaller registries have reported on use of the Impella 2.5 device in high-risk PCI, but the largest published series is the multi-center EuroPella Registry.[25,29,75] The baseline characteristics of the 144 patients suggested that these patients were, indeed, at high risk, with 70% having ejection fraction less than 30%, 36% with recent MI, 42% with prior surgical revascularization, 76% with previous MI, 20% with prior stroke, 26% with chronic lung disease, and 62% with diabetics. In addition, 55% had more than three target lesions, with 52.8% having LMCA disease, 17.4% having last remaining patent vessel intervention, and 43.1% having refused CABG. The logistic Euroscore was 15 +/− 12.2, further indicating the high-risk nature of this population. Despite this, overall mortality was 5.5% at 30 days. Another 5.5% required blood transfusion, and 0.7% required surgery for bleeding. No MI or need for emergent CABG was noted. Stroke occurred in 0.7% and vascular complication in 4%.[25] Recently, the results of the multi-center USPella Registry described outcomes in 251 patients using the Impella 2.5 device for a variety of real-world indications, including 178 for high-risk PCI. Of these, 63% were in NYHA class III

or IV heart failure, and 62% had an ejection fraction less than 30% before intervention. In addition, 56% of patients did not qualify for CABG because of excessive comorbidities. Results showed a 96% survival at 30 days, with an MACE rate of 8%. In addition, only 30% of patients remained in NYHA class III or IV heart failure, consistent with an absolute increase in mean ejection fraction from 31% to 37%. This latter improvement resulted in a 29% reduction in the anticipated need for implantable cardioverter defibrillators (ICDs), as the percent of patients with ejection fraction less than 30% was reduced from 62% to 44%.[28] Thus, in real-world practice, Impella use appeared safe, feasible, and efficacious in improving signs and symptoms of heart failure and ventricular dysfunction. Table 35-5 provides a summary of these trials. The other trans-valvular assist device, the Hemopump system (Medtronic Inc., Minneapolis, MN), also expels blood from the LV to the aorta by using a rotating turbine that imparts both rotational and longitudinal velocities to the blood. This device has been shown to increase cardiac output and reduce mean PAP in clinical trials.[76,78] However, the Hemopump was not shown to significantly affect coronary blood flow velocities before or after angioplasty.[77] Small feasibility trials have shown the Hemopump to be safe in supporting high-risk interventions.[76-78] However, to date, the Hemopump is not available clinically.

Conclusion

With the development of stents, and technical improvements in coronary wires, guiding catheters, and balloons, the rates of abrupt closure and hemodynamic collapse during percutaneous interventions have

TABLE 35-5	Transvalvular Left Ventricular Assist Device Clinical Trials					
Study	*Year*	*Number of Patients*	*Revascularization Success Rate*	*Major Adverse Cardiac Events (MACE)*	*Hemolysis*	*Support Duration (hr)*
Dens J*[75]	2006	23	100%	17%	22%	2.1 ± 1.6
Valgimigli M[74]	2006	10	100%	30%[†]	60%	2.4 ± 1.5
Henriques JP[29]	2006	19	100%	5%	§	2.0[‡]
Burzotta F[87]	2008	10	100%	0%	§	§
Dixon SR[19]	2009	20	100%	20%	10%	1.7 ± 0.6
Sjauw KD[25]	2009	144	100%	12.5%	<1%	1.45 ± 0.8
O'Neill W[28]	2010	178	100%	7.9%	0%	1.0

*Revascularization strategy included percutaneous coronary intervention (PCI) and off-pump coronary artery bypass (OPCAB).
[†]4/10 patients also received a transfusion.
[‡]Maximum support time reported.
§Not reported.

TABLE 35-6	Comparison of Circulatory Support Modalities						
	Insertion Technique	*Major Complications*	*Effect on Circulation*	*Length of Support*	*Advantages*	*Limitations*	*Contraindications*
Intra-aortic balloon pump (IABP)	- Percutaneous or surgical	- Limb ischemia - Stroke	- Augment CO by up to 0.5 L/min	- Days to weeks	- More prolonged support duration - Unloads the left ventricle (LV)	- Requires stable rhythm - Lowest level of hemodynamic support	- Moderate to severe aortic insufficiency (AI) - Aortic disease - Uncontrolled sepsis - Coagulopathy - Peripheral arterial disease (PAD)
Cardiopulmonary support (CPS)	- Percutaneous or surgical	- Bleeding, hemolysis - Stroke - Embolus	- Provides complete circulatory support	- Up to 6 hours	- Independent of rhythm - Allows controlled transfer to the OR - Full support	- Limited duration of support - Requires perfusionist - Does not unload the LV	- Moderate to severe AI - PAD - Coagulopathy
Left artery to femoral artery (LA-FA) percutaneous ventricular assist device (pVAD)	- Percutaneous or surgical	- Pericardial tamponade - Aortic puncture - Limb ischemia	- Augment CO by up to 3.5 L/min	- Up to 14 days	- Prolonged support duration - Partial LV support	- Large arterial cannulae - Requires transseptal puncture	- Ventricular septal defect (VSD) - PAD - Right ventricle (RV) failure
Left ventricle-aorta (LV-AO) pVAD	- Percutaneous or surgical	- Limb ischemia	- Augment CO by up to 2.5 L/min	- Up to 14 days	- Prolonged support duration - Partial LV support - Unloads the LV - Ease of use	- Relatively large arterial cannula	- LV thrombus - VSD - Aortic stenosis

decreased. The improved technology has also allowed for higher-risk procedures, which, in the early days of coronary angioplasty, would have been referred for bypass surgery. Moreover, recent clinical trials have suggested that PCI may be a reasonable option in some patients with LCMA or multi-vessel coronary disease, many of whom are very old or have concomitant ventricular dysfunction. As a result, the field of high-risk PCI has evolved to include the use of cardiac assist devices to minimize peri-procedural risk and improve short-term and long-term ventricular function and survival. To date, no formal guidelines for the use of circulatory support devices during high-risk coronary interventions are available. The decision to implement them, therefore,

remains up to the individual interventionalist and is based on the cumulative experience of completed and ongoing clinical trials. A thorough understanding of the high-risk clinical characteristics discussed in this chapter and the procedural and angiographic factors that portend high risk of decompensation and mortality is the first step to use support devices properly. The choice of these devices should be based on the level of support provided by each device, the level of complexity of device insertion and maintenance of support, specific device-related risks, benefits and contraindications, and a working knowledge of the increasing evidence supporting their clinical use (Table 35-6).

REFERENCES

1. Herrmann H, Hirshfeld J: Emergent stenting for failed percutaneous transluminal coronary angioplasty. In Herman HC, editor: *Clinical Use of the Palmaz-Schatz intracoronary stent*, Mount Kisco, NY, 1993, Futura Publishing Co.
2. Brodie BR, Stuckey TD, Hansen D, et al: Intra-aortic balloon counterpulsation before primary percutaneous transluminal coronary angioplasty reduces catheterization laboratory events in high-risk patients with acute myocardial infarction. *Am J Cardiol* 84(1):18–23, 1999.
3. Cohen HA, Williams Do, Holmes DR, Jr, et al: Impact of age on procedural and 1-year outcome in percutaneous transluminal coronary angioplasty: A report from the NHLBI Dynamic Registry. *Am Heart J* 146(3):513–519, 2003.
4. Herrmann HC, Buchbinder M, Clemen MW, et al: Emergent use of balloon-expandable coronary artery stenting for failed percutaneous transluminal coronary angioplasty. *Circulation* 86(3):812–819, 1992.
5. Seshadri N, Whitlow PL, Acharya N, et al: Emergency coronary artery bypass surgery in the contemporary percutaneous coronary intervention era. *Circulation* 106(18):2346–2350, 2002.
6. Williams DO, Holubkov R, Yeh W, et al: Percutaneous coronary intervention in the current era compared with 1985–1986: The National Heart, Lung, and Blood Institute Registries. *Circulation*, 102(24):2945–2951, 2000.
7. Serruys PW, Morice MC, Kappetein AP, et al: Percutaneous coronary intervention versus coronary artery bypass grafting for severe coronary artery disease. *N Engl J Med* 360(10):961–972, 2009.
8. Syed AI, Karkar A, Torguson R, et al: Prophylactic intra-aortic balloon pump for high-risk percutaneous coronary intervention: will the Impella LP 2.5 device show superiority in a clinical randomized study? *Cardiovasc Revasc Med* 11(2):91–97, 2010.
9. Hartzler GO, Rutherford BD, McConahay DR, et al: "High-risk" percutaneous transluminal coronary angioplasty. *Am J Cardiol* 61(14):33G–37G, 1988.
10. Block PC, Peterson ED, Krone R, et al: Identification of variables needed to risk adjust outcomes of coronary interventions: Evidence-based guidelines for efficient data collection. *J Am Coll Cardiol* 32(1):275–282, 1998.
11. Wu C, Hannan EL, Walford G, et al: A risk score to predict in hospital mortality for percutaneous coronary interventions. *J Am Coll Cardiol* 47(3):654–660, 2006.
12. Singh M, Rihal CS, Selzer F, et al: Validation of Mayo Clinic risk adjustment model for in-hospital complications after percutaneous coronary interventions, using the National Heart, Lung, and Blood Institute Dynamic Registry. *J Am Coll Cardiol* 42(10):1722–1728, 2003.
13. Holper EM, Blair J, Selzer F, et al: The impact of ejection fraction on outcomes after percutaneous coronary intervention in patients with congestive heart failure: An analysis of the National Heart, Lung, and Blood Institute Percutaneous Transluminal Coronary Angioplasty Registry and Dynamic Registry. *Am Heart J* 151(1):69–75, 2006.
14. Keelan PC, Johnston JM, Koru-Sengul T, et al. Comparison of in-hospital and one-year outcomes in patients with left ventricular ejection fractions < or = 40%, 41% to 49% and > or = 50% having percutaneous coronary revascularization. *Am J Cardiol* 91(10):1168–1172, 2003.
15. Wilensky RL, Selzer F, Johnston J, et al: Relation of percutaneous coronary intervention of complex lesions to clinical outcomes (from the NHLBI Dynamic Registry). *Am J Cardiol* 90(3):216–221, 2002.
16. Bergelson BA, Jacobs AK, Cupples LA, et al: Prediction of risk for hemodynamic compromise during percutaneous transluminal coronary angioplasty. *Am J Cardiol* 70(20):1540–1545, 1992.
17. Myler RK, Shaw RE, Stertzer SH, et al: Lesion morphology and coronary angioplasty: Current experience and analysis. *J Am Coll Cardiol* 19(7):1641–1652, 1992.
18. Laskey WK, Selzer F, Vlachos HA, et al: Comparison of in-hospital and one-year outcomes in patients with and without diabetes mellitus undergoing percutaneous catheter intervention (from the National Heart, Lung, and Blood Institute Dynamic Registry). *Am J Cardiol* 90(10):1062-1067, 2002.
19. Dixon SR, Henriques JP, Mauri L, et al: A prospective feasibility trial investigating the use of the Impella 2.5 system in patients undergoing high risk percutaneous coronary intervention (The PROTECT I Trial): initial US experience. *JACC Cardiovasc Interv* 2(2):91–96, 2009.
20. Anwar A, Mooney MR, Stertzer SH, et al: Intra-aortic balloon counterpulsation support for elective coronary angioplasty in the setting of poor left ventricular function: A two center experience. *J Invasive Cardiol* 2(4):175–180, 1990.
21. Kahn JK, Rutherford BD, McConahay DR, et al: Supported "high risk" coronary angioplasty using intraaortic balloon pump counterpulsation. *J Am Coll Cardiol* 15(5):1151–1155, 1990.
22. Voudris V, Marco J, Morice MC, et al: "High-risk" percutaneous transluminal coronary angioplasty with preventive intra-aortic balloon counterpulsation. *Cathet Cardiovasc Diagn* 19(3):160–164, 1990.
23. Kreidieh I, Davies DW, Lim R, et al: High-risk coronary angioplasty with elective intra-aortic balloon pump support. *Int J Cardiol* 35(2):147–152, 1992.
24. Osterne EC, Alexim GA, da Motta VP, et al: Intraaortic balloon pump support during coronary angioplasty. Initial experience. *Arq Bras Cardiol* 73(2):191–200, 1999.
25. Sjauw KD, Konorza T, Erbel R, et al: Supported high-risk percutaneous coronary intervention with the Impella 2.5 device: The Europella registry. *J Am Coll Cardiol* 54(25):2430–2434, 2009.
26. Redwood S: *BCIS-1 clinical presentation*, paper presented at the Transcatheter Cardiovascular Therapeutics Conference 2009, San Francisco, CA.
27. Sjauw KD, Engstrom AE, Vis MM, et al: A systematic review and meta-analysis of intra-aortic balloon pump therapy in ST elevation myocardial infarction: Should we change the guidelines? *Eur Heart J* 30(4):389–390, 2009.
28. O'Neill W: *USPella Registry Presentation*, paper presented at the Euro PCR Conference 2010, Paris, France.
29. Henriques JP, Remmelink M, Baan J, Jr, et al: Safety and feasibility of elective high-risk percutaneous coronary intervention procedures with left ventricular support of the Impella Recover LP 2.5. *Am J Cardiol* 97(7):990–992, 2006.
30. Mulukutla SR, Pacella JJ, Cohen A: Percutaneous mechanical assist devices for severe left ventricular dysfunction. In Hasdai E, et al, editors: *Contemporary cardiology: Cardiogenic shock: Diagnosis and treatment*, Totowa, NJ, 2002, Humana Press, Inc.
31. Mendoza DD, Cooper HA, Panza JA: Cardiac power output predicts mortality across a broad spectrum of patients with acute cardiac disease. *Am Heart J* 153(3):366–370, 2007.
32. Kantrowitz A, Tjonneland S, Freed PS, et al: Initial clinical experience with intraaortic balloon pumping in cardiogenic shock. *JAMA* 203(2):113–118, 1968.
33. Bolooki H: Current status of circulatory support with an intraaortic balloon pump. *Cardiol Clin* 3(1):123–133, 1985.
34. Bregman D, Casarella WJ: Percutaneous intraaortic balloon pumping: Initial clinical experience. *Ann Thorac Surg* 29(2):153–155, 1980.
35. Weber KT, Janicki JS: Intraaortic balloon counterpulsation. A review of physiological principles, clinical results, and device safety. *Ann Thorac Surg* 17(6):602–636, 1974.
36. Buckley MJ, Leinbach RC, Kastor JA, et al: Hemodynamic evaluation of intra-aortic balloon pumping in man. *Circulation* 41(5 Suppl):II130–II136, 1970.
37. O'Murchu B, Foreman RD, Shaw RE, et al: Role of intraaortic balloon pump counterpulsation in high risk coronary rotational atherectomy *J Am Coll Cardiol* 26(5):1270–1275, 1995.
38. Briguori C, Sarais C, Pagnotta P, et al: Elective versus provisional intra-aortic balloon pumping in high-risk percutaneous transluminal coronary angioplasty. *Am Heart J* 145(4):700–707, 2003.
39. Litzie A. Extracorporeal Cardiopulmonary bypass support: A historical and current perspective. In Shawl F, editor: *Supported complex and high risk coronary angioplasty*, Boston, MA, 1991, Kluwer Academic Publishers.
40. Shawl F: Percutaneous cardiopulmonary bypass support. Technique, indications and complications. In Shawl F, editor: *Supported complex and high risk coronary angioplasty*, Boston, MA, 1991, Kluwer Academic Publishers.
41. Vogel RA: The Maryland experience: Angioplasty and valvuloplasty using percutaneous cardiopulmonary support. *Am J Cardiol* 62(18):11K–14K, 1988.
42. Sivananthan MU, Rees MR, Browne TF, et al: Coronary angioplasty in high risk patients with percutaneous cardiopulmonary support. *Eur Heart J* 15(8):1057–1062, 1994.
43. Ferrari M, Scholz KH, Figulla HR: PTCA with the use of cardiac assist devices: Risk stratification, short and long-term results. *Cathet Cardiovasc Diagn* 38(3):242–248, 1996.
44. Vogel RA, Shawl F, Tommaso C, et al: Initial report of the National Registry of Elective Cardiopulmonary Bypass Supported Coronary Angioplasty. *J Am Coll Cardiol* 15(1):23–29, 1990
45. Vogel RA: Cardiopulmonary bypass support of high risk coronary angioplasty patients: Registry results. *J Interv Cardiol* 8(2):193–197, 1995.
46. Tommaso CL, Vogel JH, Vogel RA: Coronary angioplasty in high-risk patients with left main coronary stenosis: Results from the National Registry of Elective Supported Angioplasty. *Cathet Cardiovasc Diagn* 25(3):169–173, 1992.
47. Shawl FA, Domanski MJ, Punja S, et al: Percutaneous cardiopulmonary bypass support in high-risk patients undergoing percutaneous transluminal coronary angioplasty. *Am J Cardiol* 64(19):1258–1263, 1989.
48. Shawl FA, Domanski MJ, Wish MH, et al. Percutaneous cardiopulmonary bypass support in the catheterization laboratory: Technique and complications. *Am Heart J* 120(1):195–203, 1990.
49. Shawl FA, Quyyumi AA, Bajaj S, et al: Percutaneous cardiopulmonary bypass-supported coronary angioplasty in patients with unstable angina pectoris or myocardial infarction and a left ventricular ejection fraction < or = 25%. *Am J Cardiol* 77(1):14–19, 1996.
50. Alderman EL, Fisher LD, Litwin P, et al: Results of coronary artery surgery in patients with poor left ventricular function (CASS). *Circulation* 68(4):785–795, 1983.
51. Guarneri EM, Califano JR, Schatz RA, et al: Utility of standby cardiopulmonary support for elective coronary interventions. *Catheter Cardiovasc Interv* 46(1):32–35, 1999.
52. Teirstein PS, Vogel RA, Dorros G, et al: Prophylactic versus standby cardiopulmonary support for high risk percutaneous transluminal coronary angioplasty. *J Am Coll Cardiol* 21(3):590–596, 1993.
53. Suarez de Lezo J, Pan M, Medina A, et al. Percutaneous cardiopulmonary support in critical patients needing coronary interventions with stents. *Catheter Cardiovasc Interv* 57(4):467–475, 2002.
54. Kaul U, Sahay S, Bahl VK, et al: Coronary angioplasty in high risk patients. Comparison of elective intraaortic balloon pump and percutaneous cardiopulmonary bypass support—a randomized study. *J Interv Cardiol* 8(2):199–205, 1995.
55. Schreiber TL, Kodali UR, O'Neill WW, et al: Comparison of acute results of prophylactic intraaortic balloon pumping with cardiopulmonary support for percutaneous transluminal coronary angioplasty (PCTA). *Cathet Cardiovasc Diagn* 45(2):115–119, 1998.
56. Killen DA, Piehler JM, Borkon AM, et al: Bio-medicus ventricular assist device for salvage of cardiac surgical patients. *Ann Thorac Surg* 52(2):230–235, 1991.
57. Pavie A, Leger P, Nzomvuama A, et al: Left centrifugal pump cardiac assist with transseptal percutaneous left atrial cannula. *Artif Organs* 22(6):502–507, 1998.
58. Edmunds LH, Jr, Herrmann HC, DiSesa VJ, et al: Left ventricular assist without thoracotomy: Clinical experience with the Dennis method. *Ann Thorac Surg* 57(4):880–885, 1994.
59. Aragon J, Lee MS, Kar S, et al: Percutaneous left ventricular assist device: "TandemHeart" for high-risk coronary intervention. *Catheter Cardiovasc Interv* 65(3):346–352, 2005.
60. Thiele H, Lauer B, Hambrecht R, et al: Reversal of cardiogenic shock by percutaneous left atrial-to-femoral arterial bypass assistance. *Circulation* 104(24):2917–2922, 2001.
61. Lemos PA, Cummins P, Lee CH, et al: Usefulness of percutaneous left ventricular assistance to support high-risk percutaneous coronary interventions. *Am J Cardiol* 91(4):479–481, 2003.
62. Vranckx P, Foley DP, de Feijter PJ, et al: Clinical introduction of the Tandemheart, a percutaneous left ventricular assist device, for circulatory support during high-risk percutaneous coronary intervention. *Int J Cardiovasc Interv* 5(1):35–39, 2003.
63. Kar B, Butkevich A, Civitello AB, et al: Hemodynamic support with a percutaneous left ventricular assist device during stenting of an unprotected left main coronary artery. *Tex Heart Inst J* 31(1):84–86, 2004.
64. Kar B, Forrester M, Gemmato C, et al: Use of the TandemHeart percutaneous ventricular assist device to support patients undergoing high-risk percutaneous coronary intervention. *J Invasive Cardiol* 18(3):93–96, 2006.
65. Glassman E, Chinitz LA, Levite HA, et al: Percutaneous left atrial to femoral arterial bypass pumping for circulatory support in high-risk coronary angioplasty. *Cathet Cardiovasc Diagn* 29(3):210–216, 1993.
66. Vranckx P, Meliga E, De Jaegere PP, et al: The TandemHeart, percutaneous transseptal left ventricular assist device; a safeguard in high-risk percutaneous coronary interventions. The six-year Rotterdam experience. *EuroIntervention* 4(3);331–337, 2008.
67. Thomas JL, Al-Ameri H, Economides C, et al: Use of a percutaneous left ventricular assist device for high-risk cardiac interventions and cardiogenic shock. *J Invasive Cardiol* 22(8):360–364, 2010.
68. Burkhoff D, Cohen H, Brunckhorst C, et al: A randomized multicenter clinical study to evaluate the safety and efficacy of the TandemHeart percutaneous ventricular assist device versus conventional therapy with intraaortic balloon pumping for treatment of cardiogenic shock. *Am Heart J* 152(3):469–478, 2006.
69. Thiele H, Sick P, Boudriot E, et al: Randomized comparison of intra-aortic balloon support with a percutaneous left ventricular assist device in patients with revascularized acute myocardial infarction complicated by cardiogenic shock. *Eur Heart J* 26(13):1276–1283, 2005.
70. Sjauw KD, Engstrom AE, Henriques JP: Percutaneous mechanical cardiac assist in myocardial infarction. Where are we now, where are we going? *Acute Cardiac Care* 9(4):222–230, 2007.
71. Wampler RK, Moise JC, Frazier OH, et al: In vivo evaluation of a peripheral vascular access axial flow blood pump. *ASAIO Trans* 34(3):450–454, 1988.
72. Valgimigli M, Steendijk P, Sianos G, et al: Left ventricular unloading and concomitant total cardiac output increase by the use of percutaneous Impella Recover LP 2.5 assist device during high-risk coronary intervention. *Catheter Cardiovasc Interv* 65(2):263–267, 2005.
73. Reesink KD, Dekker AL, Van Ommen V, et al: Miniature intracardiac assist device provides more effective cardiac unloading and circulatory support during severe left heart failure than intraaortic balloon pumping. *Chest* 126(3):896–902, 2004.
74. Valgimigli M, Steendijk P, Serruys PW, et al: Use of Impella Recover LP 2.5 left ventricular assist device during high-risk percutaneous coronary interventions: Clinical, haemodynamic and biochemical findings. *EuroIntervention* 2:91–100, 2006.
75. Dens J, Meyns B, Hilgers RD, et al: First experience with the Impella Recover LP 2.5 micro axial pump in patients with cardiogenic shock or undergoing high-risk revascularization. *EuroIntervention* 2:84–90, 2006.
76. Scholz KH, Dubois-Rande JL, Urban P, et al: Clinical experience with the percutaneous hemopump during high-risk coronary angioplasty. *Am J Cardiol* 82(9):1107–1110, A6, 1998.
77. Dubois-Rande JL, Teiger E, Garot J, et al: Effects of the 14F hemopump on coronary hemodynamics in patients undergoing high-risk coronary angioplasty. *Am Heart J* 135(5 Pt 1):844–849, 1998.
78. Smalling RW, Sweeney M, Lachterman B, et al: Transvalvular left ventricular assistance in cardiogenic shock secondary to acute

myocardial infarction. Evidence for recovery from near fatal myocardial stunning. *J Am Coll Cardiol* 23(3):637–644, 1994.

79. Bourassa MG, Detre M, Johnston JM, et al: Effect of prior revascularization on outcome following percutaneous coronary intervention: NHLBI Dynamic Registry. *Eur Heart J* 23(19):1546–1555, 2002.

80. Lee RJ, Lee SH, Shyu KG, et al: Immediate and long-term outcomes of stent implantation for unprotected left main coronary artery disease. *Int J Cardiol* 80(2–3):173–177, 2001.

81. Silvestri M, Barragan P, Sainsous J, et al: Unprotected left main coronary artery stenting: Immediate and medium-term outcomes of 140 elective procedures. *J Am Coll Cardiol* 35(6):1543–1550, 2000.

82. Mehta RH, Harjai KJ, Cox D, et al: Clinical and angiographic correlates and outcomes of suboptimal coronary flow inpatients with acute myocardial infarction undergoing primary percutaneous coronary intervention. *J Am Coll Cardiol* 42(10):1739–1746, 2003.

83. Vogel RA, Tommaso CL, Gundry SR: Initial experience with coronary angioplasty and aortic valvuloplasty using elective semipercutaneous cardiopulmonary support. *Am J Cardiol* 62(10 Pt 1):811–813, 1988.

84. de Lezo JS, Medina A, Romero M, et al: Effectiveness of percutaneous device occlusion for atrial septal defect in adult patients with pulmonary hypertension. *Am Heart J* 144(5):877–880, 2002.

85. Al-Husami W, Yturralde F, Mohanty G, et al: Single-center experience with the TandemHeart percutaneous ventricular assist device to support patients undergoing high-risk percutaneous coronary intervention. *J Invasive Cardiol* 20(6):319–322, 2008.

86. Vranckx P, Schultz CJ, Valgimigli M, et al: Assisted circulation using the TandemHeart during very high-risk PCI of the unprotected left main coronary artery in patients declined for CABG. *Catheter Cardiovasc Interv* 74(2):302–310, 2009.

87. Burzotta F, Paloscia L, Trani C, et al: Feasibility and long-term safety of elective Impella-assisted high-risk percutaneous coronary intervention: a pilot two-centre study. *J Cardiovasc Med* 9(10):1004–1010, 2008.

36

Regional Centers of Excellence for the Care of Patients with Acute Ischemic Heart Disease

DEAN J. KEREIAKES | TIMOTHY D. HENRY

KEY POINTS

- Coronary artery disease (CAD) is the leading cause of death and disability in the United States. Specialized centers of care have been established for the treatment of patients with trauma or stroke. The number of specialized centers of care for patients with acute ischemic heart disease, however, is not commensurate with the magnitude of this public health problem.

- "Regional" care for patients with acute coronary syndrome (ACS) implies meaningful networking associations between community hospitals and rural hospitals that do not provide tertiary cardiovascular services and a tertiary cardiovascular service provider. The definition of networking ranges from being a merged affiliate (same hospital system) to sharing common patient care protocols as well as tracking, reporting, and auditing clinical practice guideline compliance, core measures, and clinical outcomes.

- A direct relationship exists between annual volumes of cardiovascular procedures (coronary bypass surgery, coronary angioplasty, or stenting) for physicians or operators as well as for hospitals or facilities—and optimal clinical outcomes, including survival. Those doctors and hospitals that perform the highest annual volumes of procedures have the best outcomes.

- Medical resources are limited, and a critical shortage of both sub-specialized nurses for intensive cardiovascular care and cardiovascular physician providers is an ongoing issue. The current trend toward proliferation of smaller "heart centers," supposedly for patient convenience, is counter to the well-established link between higher procedural volumes and better clinical outcomes and also further taxes the already limited resource pools of sub-specialty nurses and doctors.

- The prehospital phase of acute ST elevation myocardial infarction (STEMI) is critically important. The performance and transmission of a 12-lead electrocardiogram (ECG) by emergency medical service providers in the field at the point of first medical contact has been demonstrated to significantly reduce delays to the initiation of treatment for STEMI with either fibrinolytic therapy or primary percutaneous coronary intervention (PCI) and, thus, to reduce mortality.

- The current American College of Cardiology/American Heart Association (ACC/AHA) Clinical Practice Guidelines recommend that both "door-to-needle" (<30 minutes) and "door-to-balloon" (<90 minutes) treatment times not represent the "optimal" delays for treatment, but should be considered the "longest acceptable" delays for initiating therapy.

- Most concerns about the strategies to regionalize the care of patients with ACS have focused on the lack of a clear consensus regarding the specific nature of regionalization as well as on the economic and market impacts of such a strategy. The most likely initial focus of a regionalized strategy for ACS care would appear to be STEMI, which has more definitive electrocardiographic and clinical diagnosis criteria and represents a more widely acknowledged "medical emergency" for which efficacy of treatment is time dependent. The process for the credentialing of systems of care for STEMI patients has been developed by the American Heart Association as the *Mission: Lifeline* initiative, with individual states charged with the responsibility for creating regionalized centers and systems for excellence in care.

The past decade has witnessed a remarkable evolution both in our understanding of the pathogenesis of ACS and in therapeutic innovation for catheter-based technologies and adjunctive pharmacotherapies. Spontaneous plaque rupture is followed by platelet adherence, activation, and aggregation, with fibrin incorporation leading to thrombus propagation.[1] The severity of the resultant clinical syndrome is manifest in direct proportion to the degree of restriction in coronary blood flow and ranges from asymptomatic (insignificant restriction) to non–ST elevation ACS (NSTEACS), including unstable angina and non–ST elevation myocardial infarction (NSTEMI), which are associated with severe coronary flow restriction, as well as STEMI, which is usually secondary to complete coronary occlusion.[2] As the pathogenesis of coronary flow restriction is multi-factorial (platelets, thrombus, vasomotion, and mechanical obstruction), it is best addressed by a multi-modal approach to therapy (anti platelet, anticoagulant, and fibrinolytic therapies and catheter-based PCI) implemented in a timely manner. Indeed, the rapid restoration of normal coronary blood flow—via pharmacologic and mechanical recanalization of an occluded coronary artery—limits the extent of myocardial necrosis and reduces mortality. However, a concerted, integrated approach to the therapy for ACS is complicated by the diversity and extent of resources required for the comprehensive treatment of this disease spectrum and by the various settings (urban/suburban and rural) in which care is delivered. The concept of regional centers of excellence for the care of patients with ACS has rapidly evolved and has become the focus of a collaborative initiative involving the American Heart Association and the American College of Cardiology as well as individual states which have been charged with regional organization. It is important to clearly define "regional" so that all of the constituents involved in the care of patients with ACS understand the concept and the implications. The term *regional* implies meaningful networking associations between community hospitals, rural hospitals, or both, which do not provide tertiary cardiovascular services (including PCI), and a tertiary cardiovascular service provider. The definition of "meaningful networking" includes, at one end of the spectrum, being a merged affiliate (same hospital system) and, at the other, merely sharing common protocols for patient care as well as tracking, auditing, and reporting clinical practice guideline compliance, core measures, and clinical outcomes. These "networks" should have well-defined and rehearsed systems for patient transport that will differ, depending on care being delivered in an urban, suburban, or rural setting.

Scope of the Problem

The approach of creating specialized centers of care for treating victims of trauma and, more recently, stroke has been shown to improve clinical outcomes.[3] Trauma victims treated in trauma centers had significantly lower mortality compared with patients treated in a non–trauma center. Specialized centers for the care of patients who had suffered a stroke have been instituted with the standard of care established by the American Heart Association and with a formal process provided through the Joint Commission on Accreditation of Healthcare

Organizations (JCAHO) for the certification of primary stroke centers.[4] Interestingly, the number of deaths from CAD in the United States alone exceeds sevenfold the number for all-cause trauma and fourfold that for stroke in the general population; the number of deaths is twentyfold and fivefold higher for trauma and stroke, respectively, for persons older than 65 years.[5] In addition, of the 865,000 new or recurrent heart attacks which occurred in the United States (U.S.) during 2003, 35% to 40% were attributed to STEMI.[6] In this context, the number of specialized regional centers of care for patients with acute ischemic heart disease is not commensurate with the magnitude of this public health problem.

The Case for Regionalized Care

Both where and how patients with acute ischemic heart disease are treated has been the subject of an ongoing debate. The divergence of opinion ranges from belief that "the real issue is not whether the creation of specialized centers for care of ACS patients would provide an important advance, but how to create them," to the contention that "clear, compelling evidence of the benefits of ACS regionalization within the United States and a better understanding of its potential consequences are needed before implementing a national policy of regionalized ACS care."[7-11]

Proponents assert that the treatment of patients with ACS at regional centers with dedicated facilities will save lives by providing higher-quality care and by improving access to new technologies as well as to specialist physicians.[7-9] These beliefs are, in large part, based on prior experiences with regard to trauma and stroke treatments in the United States as well as on experiences gleaned from multiple European countries, where regionalized systems for ACS care are in place.[12-14] Although efficiency of process and high quality of outcomes have been demonstrated in several European systems, the "generalizability" of these data to current practice in the United States has been questioned.[10,11] As European health systems are characterized by centralized financing as well as control of hospital and emergency transportation organizations, they avoid many of the financial reimbursement "barriers" present in the U.S. health care system. Furthermore, the logistics of providing regionalized care in the United States, where the population is more geographically dispersed, present additional challenges. Nevertheless, several states and municipalities have initiated programs for the regionalized care of patients with ACS.[15] The American Heart Association (AHA), in conjunction with the American College of Cardiology (ACC), has initiated a national program (*Mission: Lifeline*) to provide timely primary PCI to more patients with STEMI and to create both systems and centers of care, with the goal of reducing deaths from CAD and stroke by 25% by the year 2010.[16] These initiatives have been, in part, prompted by recent studies that demonstrated shortfalls in the use of quality-assured, guideline-driven care for patients with ACS as well as wide variability in treatments administered on the basis of age, gender, race, geographic location, and time of presentation.[17-19]

A treatment–risk "paradox" has, indeed, been demonstrated with regard to the use of both proven, guideline-based medical therapies (specifically early administration of thienopyridines, platelet glycoprotein [GP] IIb/IIIa inhibitors, or both) and early angiography and coronary revascularization in patients who present with NSTEACS.[20,21] Although randomized clinical trials have demonstrated that the benefit of an early invasive treatment strategy in NSTEACS is directly proportional to patient risk profile, the propensity to receive such treatment has been greatest in those patients at lower risk. Similarly, treatment with clopidogrel, platelet GP IIb/IIIa inhibitors, or both, in addition to transfer for angiography at a non–PCI capable facility, is inversely proportional to patient risk strata.[22-24] This observation may have arisen from physician misconceptions about benefit–harm trade-offs or concerns about treatment complications. Indeed, one analysis suggests that at least 25% of opportunities to initiate guideline-based care are missed in contemporary community practice.[25] Finally, the process of care for patients with ACS has been further complicated by

the fact that for many U.S. hospitals, the provision of treatment for CAD is the major determinant of their financial well-being. Profitability from a cardiovascular service line is often used to offset deficits incurred by the provision of other important but less profitable services such as mental health, obstetrics, and emergency medicine.[16]

Potential Advantages of Regional Centers

PRACTICE MAKES PERFECT: RELATIONSHIP BETWEEN VOLUME AND OUTCOMES

In general, a patient experiences a better clinical outcome when treated in a center that frequently encounters the particular health problem that the patient has ("Practice makes perfect").[26,27] A direct relationship has been demonstrated between physician–operator as well as facility procedural volumes and optimal clinical outcomes with both elective or primary PCI and coronary bypass surgery.[28-32] A similar relationship has been demonstrated between hospital ACS patient volume and clinical outcomes as well as adherence to ACC/AHA guidelines.[33,34] Doctors and hospitals performing the highest volumes of procedures demonstrate the best clinical outcomes, including survival benefit. Higher-volume PCI centers demonstrate lower risk-adjusted in-hospital mortality as well as less frequent need for emergency coronary artery bypass grafting (CABG), even in the current era of coronary stenting.[31,32,35] Indeed, the relative benefit of primary PCI versus fibrinolysis for the treatment of STEMI may be completely lost when primary PCI is performed in a low-volume institution.[28,36] Data from the New York statewide database demonstrate that physician–operator volume significantly influences the success rate of primary PCI procedures and that hospital volume influences (by 50%) in-hospital mortality following the procedure.[37] These observations have led to the belief that PCI "generally should not be conducted in low-volume hospitals unless there are substantial overriding concerns about geographic or socioeconomic access" and to recommendations for hospitals performing primary PCI for STEMI to satisfy specific minimum requirements for volume of procedures.[30,38]

A pooled analysis of multiple studies involving over one million PCI procedures confirms the relationship between lower procedural volumes (<200 cases) with an increase in both in-hospital mortality and the requirement for emergency CABG following PCI.[32] Other studies have suggested that institutional volumes more than 200 cases yearly may be too low. For example, an analysis of 37,848 PCI procedures, performed at 44 centers in 2001–2002 as part of the Greater Paris area PTCA (percutaneous transluminal coronary angioplasty) registry, demonstrated an increased incidence of major adverse cardiovascular events (MACEs) following elective as well as primary PCI procedures in centers performing less than 400 procedures yearly.[35] In addition, in-hospital mortality increased following primary PCI procedures in lower-volume (<400 PCI/year) programs. These investigators concluded that "tolerance of low-volume thresholds for angioplasty centers with the purpose of providing primary PCI in acute myocardial infarction should not be recommended, even in underserved areas."[11,35] More recently, the relationship between institutional volume and clinical outcomes has been demonstrated in centers providing primary PCI without on-site cardiac surgical facilities. No differences in outcomes were observed in the ACC-NCDR (National Cardiovascular Data Registry) among primary PCI centers stratified on the basis of cardiac surgical capability (with vs. without).[39] However, a significant reduction in risk-adjusted mortality was observed in the highest tertile of primary PCI institutional volume (mean, 83 processes per year) among centers without surgical capability in C-PORT (Community Hospital–Based, Prospective, Randomized Trial).[40] Thus, the established link between procedural volumes and quality outcomes persists despite the advent of coronary stenting and improvements in adjunctive pharmacotherapies. Finally, mortality was reduced among patients with

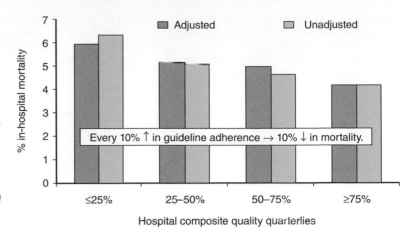

Figure 36-1 Hospital composite quarterly quartiles for adherence to American College of Cardiology/American Heart Association (ACC/AHA) guidelines correlated with in-hospital mortality, both adjusted (for age, gender, body mass index, race, insurance status, family history of coronary disease, hypertension, diabetes, smoking, hypercholesterolemia, prior myocardial infarction/angioplasty/coronary bypass surgery/ congestive heart failure/stroke, renal insufficiency, blood pressure, heart rate, ST segment shift, positive cardiac biomarkers) and unadjusted. Increments in adherence to clinical practice guidelines are associated with a reduction in mortality. (*Reproduced with permission from Peterson FD, Roe MT, Mulgund J, et al: Association between hospital process performance and outcomes among patients with acute coronary syndromes, J Am Med Assn 295:1912–1920, 2006.*)

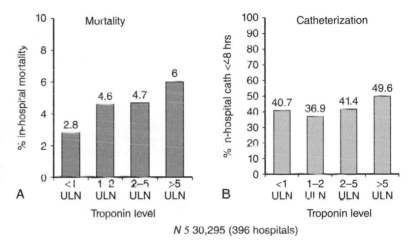

Figure 36-2 Relationship between in-hospital mortality (*A*) and the frequency of in-hospital cardiac catheterization within 48 hours of hospital admission (*B*) stratified by the presence and degree of troponin level elevation. A graded relationship exists between the presence and magnitude of troponin elevation and in-hospital mortality. No significant relationship between the presence or magnitude of troponin elevation and the performance of early (<48 hours) cardiac catheterization is defined. Data are derived from the CRUSADE registry for non ST elevation acute coronary syndrome. (*Adapted from Roe MT, Peterson ED, Li Y, et al. Relationship between risk stratification by cardiac troponin level and adherence to guidelines for non-ST-segment elevation acute coronary syndromes, Arch Intern Med 165:1870–1876, 2005.*)

ADHERENCE TO PRACTICE GUIDELINES

The process of care as measured by ACC/AHA guideline adherence has been linked to both in-hospital and late (6–12 month) survival following presentation of ACS.[42,43] An analysis of hospital composite guideline adherence quartiles demonstrated an inverse relationship between the adherence to guideline-compliant care and the risk adjusted in-hospital mortality rate.[25] For every 10% increase in guideline adherence, a 10% relative reduction in in-hospital mortality was observed (Fig. 36-1).[25] This observation supports the central hypothesis of hospital quality improvement—that better adherence with evidence-based care practices will result in better outcomes for patients.[44] The current system of nonregionalized care has been suboptimal in promoting and achieving guideline adherence, even in the case of those ACS patients who present with "high-risk" indicators.[45] For example, only 33.8% and 44.2% of patients with elevated serum troponin levels in the CRUSADE (Can Rapid Risk Stratification of Unstable angina patients Suppress Adverse outcomes with Early implementation of the ACC/AHA guidelines) registry received early (<24 hours) GP IIb/IIa inhibition or early (<48 hours) cardiac catheterization, respectively.[46] Similarly, although a direct correlation exists between the presence and magnitude of serum troponin elevation and in-hospital mortality, no correlation was observed between troponin

levels and the performance of early (<48 hours) coronary angiography (Fig. 36-2), which has a class I ACC/AHA guideline recommendation for patients with NSTEACS with "high-risk" indicators (including elevated troponin).[46] Both compliance with clinical practice guidelines and the ability to monitor or audit adherence to guidelines appear to be enhanced in higher-volume, regional programs.[43,47] Adherence to guidelines was improved following establishment of an integrated, regional program for ACS care and was highest among the cohort of patients who received revascularization through PCI.[48] Finally, guideline-adherent care of patients without STEMI was significantly greater in centers with cardiac surgical capabilities compared with those without those capabilities.[41] Lower-volume, small community hospitals are unlikely to allocate their capital resources and personnel to adequately track, collate, and report clinical outcomes or process measures (guideline compliance). Certainly, from the perspectives of national and regional payers and the Centers for Medicare and Medicaid Services, monitoring and auditing data derived from multiple small hospitals versus those from fewer, larger networked systems have different levels of complexity. Indeed, in a recent survey commissioned by the AHA, only slightly more than half the hospitals queried were systematically tracking times to STEMI treatment ("door-to-needle" or "door-to-balloon" times), infection rates, re-admission or stroke rates (to 30 days after the procedure), recurrent MI, or mortality following either PCI or coronary bypass surgery.[16] This observation is made more meaningful by the fact that multiple national initiatives such as Get with the Guidelines, the Cardiac Hospitalization Atherosclerosis Management (CHAMPS), the

Guidelines Applied to Practice (GAP) project, the National Registry of Myocardial Infarction (NRMI), and the CRUSADE (ACTION) registry have recently placed emphasis on system quality through systematic measurement of both care processes and clinical outcomes.[9] The positive impact of these programs may be reflected in increased compliance with guidelines for early (≤24 hours) as well as predischarge medical therapies, in addition to the use of diagnostic angiography and revascularization.[41] Similarly, the door-to-balloon (D2B) alliance, initiated in November 2006, has resulted in increased use of recommended strategies for process improvement as well as a greater portion of patients being treated within the recommendations of the guidelines.[49]

PERCUTANEOUS CORONARY INTERVENTION CENTERS WITHOUT ON-SITE CARDIAC SURGICAL FACILITIES

The current trend toward the proliferation of "PCI centers" which lack on-site cardiac surgical facilities for the performance of primary PCI in STEMI may be associated with suboptimal clinical outcomes. In an analysis of 625,854 Medicare patients who underwent PCI, in-hospital and 30-day mortality was significantly increased in those centers without on-site cardiac surgical facilities and was primarily confined to hospitals performing a low number (≤50) of PCI procedures in Medicare patients.[50] Even in the context of a completely integrated community hospital–tertiary hospital system, the performance of primary PCI without on-site cardiac surgical facilities was associated with a trend toward increased hospital mortality compared with primary PCI performed at the tertiary center despite exclusion of the sickest patients (with refractory cardiogenic shock or ventricular arrhythmias) from PCI at the community center.[51] Although single-center studies have reported excellent outcomes in patients undergoing primary PCI at hospitals without on-site cardiac surgical facilities, the one randomized trial that compared fibrinolysis to primary PCI at hospitals without surgery on-site was flawed by an inadequate sample size and by a majority of patients enrolled at a single site.[52,53] More recently, large registry data suggested a similar risk for mortality following both primary PCI and nonprimary PCI performed at hospitals with versus without cardiac surgical facilities.[39] Nonetheless, a significant mortality benefit following primary PCI in nonsurgical centers was achieved only by those institutions in the highest tertile of procedural volumes.[40] Furthermore, the requirement for repeat revascularization appears to be increased at both 30 days and 1 year following primary PCI at hospitals without on-site cardiac surgical facilities.[54] On the basis of these and other data, the current ACC/AHA guidelines for the performance of PCI designate a class III (practice may be harmful and is not recommended) indication for elective PCI and a class IIb (usefulness is less well established by evidence or opinion) for primary PCI in hospitals without on-site cardiac surgical facilities and point out the need for additional evidence base.[38]

LIMITED MEDICAL RESOURCES

The current trend toward the proliferation of small "heart centers" supposedly for patient convenience is counter to the well-established link between higher procedural volumes and better clinical outcomes; in addition, this taxes the already critically limited resource pools, including specialized nurses and subspecialty-trained physician–providers.[55] Patients with more complex cardiovascular diseases (congestive heart failure [CHF], acute myocardial infarction [AMI]) fare better with care from subspecialty physicians (cardiologists) compared with care provided by generalists.[8,9,56] One strategy for dealing with the mismatch between the emerging evidence in favor of an interventional (catheter-based) approach to the treatment of ACS and the current availability of such care is to establish regionalized centers for ACS care.[8,9,23,57] Such centers would provide state-of-the-art radiographic equipment, a broad array of interventional supplies, and an experienced ancillary staff. Both subspecialty nurses and trained cardiologists are in limited supply.[55,58,59] The proliferation of small "heart centers" that focus on PCI, with duplication of services, further taxes the limited resource pools and undermines the ability of established tertiary care centers to provide quality care. Indeed, the development of more PCI programs, particularly those without on-site cardiac surgical facilities, appears unnecessary in the context that the majority (>80%) of the adult U.S. population lives within a 60 minute commute to an existing PCI center.[60] In fact, a recent study indicated that the expansion of PCI-capable hospitals was generally confined to urban and suburban regions and that this had a limited effect on increasing patient access to such care.[61]

Benefit of Catheter-Based Therapy for Acute Coronary Syndrome

ST ELEVATION MYOCARDIAL INFARCTION

The current ACC/AHA guidelines for the treatment of STEMI promotes reperfusion therapy (both fibrinolysis and PCI), with the choice of strategy based on resource availability and the anticipated time course for treatment implementation.[62] The relative advantage of PCI versus fibrinolytic therapy depends on several factors. First, as primary PCI entails an obligate delay for implementation (versus fibrinolysis), the relative advantage of PCI depends on the relative delay to definitive treatment (balloon inflation). Pooled analyses of multiple randomized controlled trials suggest that the survival advantage in favor of PCI is inversely proportional to the relative delay in PCI implementation and that the advantage may be lost if the PCI-related delay (door-to-balloon minus door-to-needle time) exceeds 60 to 110 minutes.[63,64] Differences between these analyses may be explained by differences in patient risk profile. Indeed, a survival advantage in favor of PCI is evident only when the risk of death at 30 days following fibrinolytic therapy exceeds approximately 4%.[65] Longer relative delays may still be associated with a PCI-related survival advantage in those patients at highest risk for death following fibrinolysis.[66] Thus, accurate risk assessment should be part of any STEMI treatment triage algorithm. The relative survival advantage of PCI versus fibrinolysis is also dependent on the case volume experience of both the operator (cardiologist) and the hospital facility.

As noted previously, the best clinical outcomes and the greatest relative advantage of PCI are obtained by the highest-volume operators and institutions.[67] The link between case volume and optimal outcomes has been established both for physician operators and hospitals and is evident with or without the availability of on-site cardiac surgical facilities.[31,40,67] Transport to a center capable of performing PCI yields superior clinical outcomes compared with on-site (community hospital) fibrinolytic therapy when the randomization (treatment decision) to balloon time approximates 90 to 120 minutes.[68] Importantly, no adverse outcomes related to patient transport have been observed in these analyses. Despite the observation that the vast majority (>80%) of individuals in the United States who experienced STEMI in the year 2000 lived within a 60-minute commute to an established PCI center, more recent data regarding patients who first present with STEMI to a community hospital (non-PCI facility) and are subsequently transported to a PCI facility demonstrate excessive delays to definitive treatment.[60,69,70] Indeed, initial presentation to a non-PCI center has been identified as a major determinant of prolonged door-to-balloon times and reflects the lack of a well-defined integrated system with protocol-driven algorithms for care and dedicated transport facilities.[71] Of concern is the fact that door-to-door-to-balloon times (door at non-PCI facility to balloon at PCI facility) for patients requiring transport were a median of 180 minutes and only 15% received PCI within 120 minutes from initial presentation.[69]

Not surprisingly, although the diagnosis of STEMI as well as in-hospital mortality rates associated with STEMI have declined over

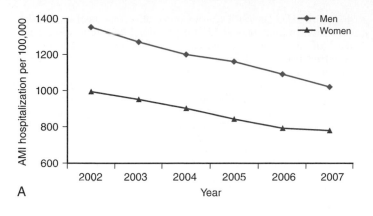

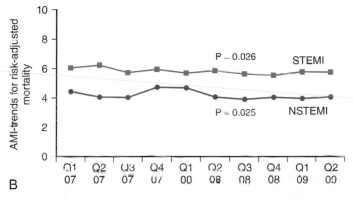

Figure 36-3 **A,** Hospitalization for acute myocardial infarction in Medicare beneficiaries (Medicare fee for service) over time stratified by gender. **B,** Trends in risk-adjusted hospital mortality for acute myocardial infarction over time stratified by infarction type (ST elevation or non–ST elevation) from the ACC/NCDR ACTION Registry. A progressive decline in both the diagnosis as well as hospital mortality associated with myocardial infarction has been observed. (*A, Reproduced with permission from Chen J, Normand SL, Wang Y, et al: Recent declines in hospitalizations for acute myocardial infarction for Medicare fee-for-service beneficiaries: Progress and continuing challenges,* Circulation *121:1322–1328, 2010; B, Reproduced with permission from Roe MT, Messenger JC, Weintraub WS, et al: Treatments, trends, and outcomes of acute myocardial infarction and percutaneous coronary intervention,* J Am Coll Cardiol *56:254–263, 2010.)*

the past 8 to 15 years, mortality rates remain higher for those STEMI patients who require transfer for PCI versus those who do not and likely reflect protracted delays in treatment (Fig. 36-3).[70,72,73] This "gap" exists despite the availability of technology that allows emergency medical systems (EMS) to transmit a pre-hospital 12-lead ECG and makes the diagnosis of STEMI evident at the point of first medical contact. The integration of EMS and the incorporation of the pre-hospital phase for ACS evaluation and diagnosis are integral components of any regionalized system for STEMI care. Earlier STEMI diagnosis via a transmitted pre-hospital 12-lead ECG facilitates in-hospital STEMI treatment with either fibrinolysis or PCI.[74-76] Hospitals which demonstrate the shortest door-to-balloon times incorporate pre-hospital STEMI diagnosis (transmitted ECG) with a multi-disciplinary "team" approach, in which the emergency physician activates the cardiac catheterization laboratory (cath lab) before cardiology consultation.[77] Indeed, the facilitation of in-hospital PCI treatment for STEMI patients with a transmitted pre-hospital ECG has resulted in a significant reduction in door-to-balloon times as well as improvement in survival.[78-80] The consistent, significant relationships among earlier STEMI diagnosis, more rapid treatment, and improved outcomes have prompted a national heart, lung, and blood institute

consensus recommendation for the implementation of pre-hospital 12-lead ECG systems by all EMS providers.[81]

The rapid transport of patients with STEMI to the nearest PCI-capable facility for care may, however, be limited by several factors. First, only a minority (≤5%) of EMS-transported patients with chest pain actually have STEMI.[82] Second, only a minority (~10%) of EMS systems have 12-lead ECG capabilities.[82] Third, a precedent "mandate" exists for the transport of patients with suspected STEMI to the nearest facility, even when fibrinolysis may be contraindicated and the facility does not provide primary PCI. Fourth, evolution toward a more integrated process of pre-hospital care is complicated by the fact that there are 329 different EMS regions in the United States with more than 993 hospital-based EMS systems.[16,82] Remarkably, hospital-based EMS systems represent only 6.5% of all EMS providers, with the remainder comprising private, third-party systems (48.6%) and fire station–based systems (44.9%).[16] Although the transport time to a specialized PCI center may appear long, it can be more than counterbalanced by an integrated EMS system with pre-notification. A doubling of the recommended transport time has been proposed for patients with suspected STEMI who are transported to a "center of excellence" where the target door-to-balloon time is 60 minutes or less.[58] Such efficiency of process can be achieved only through an integrated system for STEMI care that incorporates pre-hospital ECG for earlier diagnosis and expedited triage. Indeed, recent data involving ambulance-based diagnosis of STEMI in the field with pre-hospital activation of the cath lab and direct transport to the interventional center have demonstrated reduced symptom onset-to-balloon times and improved survival.[83] Finally, more uniform evolution toward integration in process of STEMI care has been impeded by diverging incentives, the lack of coordinated objectives, and ostensibly competing strategies. For example, in many regions particularly those without requirements for a state-regulated certificate of need—there has been a proliferation of new cath labs for the provision of primary PCI in centers without on-site cardiac surgical support. Conversely, other regions, including Minneapolis, North Carolina, Los Angeles, and Boston, have developed integrated EMS systems with focus on pre-hospital diagnosis and triage to an established center of excellence proficient in primary as well as elective PCI.

The competing strategies—one focused on building more small PCI centers and the other on more efficient and effective use of existing PCI centers through pre-hospital–EMS integration—have drawn support from divergent financial incentives among different stakeholders in the process of care. Only recently have sophisticated modeling techniques been used to compare the relative efficacy and cost of these "build more" versus "use more effectively" strategies for PCI facilities as they specifically pertain to the care of STEMI patients.[84] Interestingly, and importantly, the strategy focused on EMS integration, pre-hospital diagnosis, and triage and better use of already existing PCI facilities was found to be more effective and less costly than the strategy of proliferating new PCI facilities (Fig. 36-4).[84] The coordination of strategies as well as the integration of essential pre-hospital and hospital resources for ACS care at the state level has been the focus of the national *Mission: Lifeline* initiative of the AHA in conjunction with the ACC.

NON–ST ELEVATION ACUTE CORONARY SYNDROME

Despite therapy with aspirin, unfractionated or low-molecular-weight heparin, nitrates, and β-blockers, patients with NSTEACS remain at appreciable risk for death (~6%), recurrent MI (~11%), or need for coronary revascularization (~50%–60%) for up to 1 year following diagnosis.[85] In the context of therapeutic innovation in catheter-based technology and adjunctive pharmacotherapy, the cumulative weight of data from randomized controlled trials supports the use of an early invasive treatment strategy (angiography followed by revascularization, if feasible) versus conservative treatment strategy (medical therapy with angiography for spontaneous or provoked ischemia). Furthermore, the ACC/AHA guidelines clearly recommend risk assessment before triage for invasive treatment.[62] The relative benefit of invasive (versus conservative) treatment is directly proportional to patient risk profile as reflected by the Thrombolysis in Myocardial Infarction (TIMI) study group; PURSUIT (Platelet GP IIb/IIIa in Unstable Angina: Receptor Suppression using Integrilin); and, GRACE (Global Registry of Acute Coronary Events) risk stratification schemes.[85] In addition, the magnitude of benefit attributable to the invasive (versus conservative) treatment strategy appears to be inversely correlated with the duration of delay from presentation to revascularization and directly correlated with both the relative extent of revascularization in the active treatment (versus the control or conservative) groups as well as the duration of clinical follow-up.[86-91] Recent data suggest that earlier (≤24 hours following presentation) revascularization provides greater benefit as reflected by a reduction in the occurrence of cardiovascular death, MI, or stroke compared with later (≥36 hours) revascularization, particularly in patients with NSTEACS at highest risk.[87] Similarly, pooled patient-level data from the FRISC II (Fast Revascularization during InStability in Coronary disease), ICTUS (Invasive versus Conservative Treatment in Unstable coronary Syndromes), and RITA-3 (Randomized Intervention Treatment of Angina 3) randomized trials show durable long-term (5 years) relative clinical benefit for the invasive (versus conservative) treatment strategy (Fig. 36-5).[91] The major source of controversy is no longer the choice of treatment strategy (invasive versus conservative) but rather the fact that although the benefit of an early invasive strategy is proportional to patient risk, the propensity to receive such treatment is greatest in patients at lower risk.[45,46,92,93] This treatment–risk paradox may be caused by physician misconceptions regarding benefit–harm tradeoffs or concerns about treatment complications and has been observed in relationship to the performance of angiography, PCI, or both as well as the use of platelet inhibitor therapies. Finally, the transport of patients from a non-PCI facility to one capable of performing PCI for NSTEACS was also inversely proportional to patient risk strata.[24] The importance of the treatment–risk paradox is further magnified by the observation that compliance with the current ACC/AHA guidelines (including early angiography) is inversely correlated with in-hospital mortality for ACS.[25] Furthermore, evidence-based therapies (anti-platelet agents, β-blockers, lipid-lowering agents, angiotensin-converting enzyme [ACE] inhibitors) initiated before hospital discharge are associated with an incremental survival advantage in follow-up. The fact that performance measures (compliance with guidelines) relate process of care to mortality presents an opportunity to define strategies that enhance compliance and use of current guidelines.

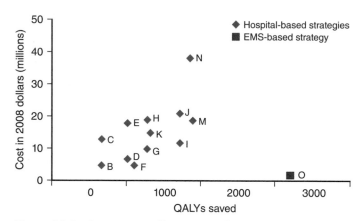

Figure 36-4 Comparative effectiveness of ST elevation myocardial infarction regionalization strategies. Hospital-based (expansion of PCI-capable facilities) versus EMS-based (regionalization with EMS integration for existing PCI facilities) demonstrates that the EMS-based strategy is less costly and more effective. PCI, percutaneous coronary intervention; EMS, emergency medical system; QALYs, quality-adjusted life years. *(Reproduced with permission from Concannon TW, Kent DM, Normand SL, et al: Comparative effectiveness of ST-segment elevation myocardial infarction regionalization strategies, Circ Cardiovasc Qual Outcomes 3:1–8, 2010.)*

Regional Centers of Care for Patients with ST Elevation Myocardial Infarction

The technology available to EMS providers that allows transmission of a pre-hospital 12-lead ECG makes the diagnosis of STEMI evident at the time and place of first medical contact. The integration of EMS and the incorporation of the pre-hospital phase for ACS evaluation and diagnosis are integral components of a regionalized system for STEMI care. In addition, STEMI is the logical initial objective for a regionalized ACS treatment strategy in that five of Medicare's 10 quality indicators focus on STEMI care.[16] Thus, several system process or quality measures are already in place to provide a performance incentive to define "regional networks" for STEMI care. The development of such regional networks for STEMI care should facilitate adherence to guidelines as well as the ability to monitor, audit, and evaluate data. As previously noted, combinations of evidence-based therapies (anti-platelet agents, β-blockers, lipid-lowering agents, ACE inhibitors) provide incremental survival advantage to 1 year following

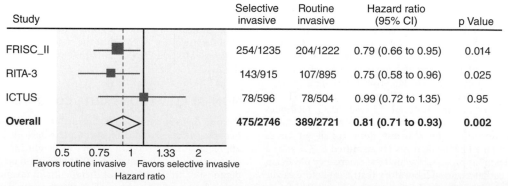

Figure 36-5 Long-term (5-year) impact of routine versus elective invasive approach for non–ST elevation acute coronary syndrome: a meta-analysis of individual patient data from the FIR collaboration. The composite occurrence of cardiovascular death or myocardial infarction to 5-year follow-up was significantly reduced by the routine invasive therapeutic strategy. *FRISC-II*, Fast Revascularization during InStability in Coronary disease; *ICTUS*, Invasive versus Conservative Treatment in Unstable coronary Syndromes; *RITA-3*, Randomized Intervention Treatment of Angina 3. *(Reproduced with permission from Fox KA, Clayton TC, Damman P, et al: Long-term outcome of a routine versus selective invasive strategy in patients with non–ST-segment elevation acute coronary syndrome: a meta-analysis of individual patient data, J Am Coll Cardiol 55:2435–2445, 2010.)*

presentation of ACS, especially STEMI.[42,43] Greater adherence to guidelines has been observed in hospitals with higher volumes of STEMI cases, in centers with on-site cardiovascular surgical facilities, and following the implementation of national process of care and quality initiatives (D2B Alliance).[33,41,49] Smaller centers are unlikely to allocate the resources necessary to optimally track, audit, and report these measures.

MODEL SYSTEMS OF CARE

A regionalized approach to the provision of primary PCI therapy for STEMI has been successfully implemented in major metropolitan areas of the United States, for example, Minneapolis.[26,94] Through partnership with community hospitals in standardized protocol-driven algorithms for care, designated transport systems, and enhanced multidisciplinary communication (among the EMS, the emergency physician, and the interventional cardiologist), the Minneapolis Heart Institute at Abbott Northwestern Hospital has demonstrated the ability to promptly assess and treat STEMI patients coming from a broad area

(90–120 minute transit). By focusing on collaboration and integration of resources, community hospitals initiate adjunctive pharmacotherapies in patients who present with STEMI and emergently transport these patients to the interventional team waiting at Abbott Northwestern Hospital (Fig. 36-6). These data demonstrate regional systems in the United States can achieve results equivalent to those of smaller European centers with organized transfer systems (Table 36-1). Similar results have been duplicated in other regional STEMI systems.[80,95-97] A statewide approach is being used in North Carolina with RACE (Reperfusion of Acute Myocardial Infarction in North Carolina Emergency Department).[98] The Initiative uses standardized protocols and integrated systems for the treatment and timely transfer of patients with STEMI in five regions in North Carolina. The RACE program demonstrated a significant improvement in time to treatment at both PCI and non-PCI hospitals, resulting in increased timely access to PCI on a statewide level.[98] The significance of these regional programs resulted in a new class I recommendation in the recent ACC/AHA guidelines for STEMI that "each community should develop a STEMI system of care."[99,100] This experience stands in stark contrast to the National

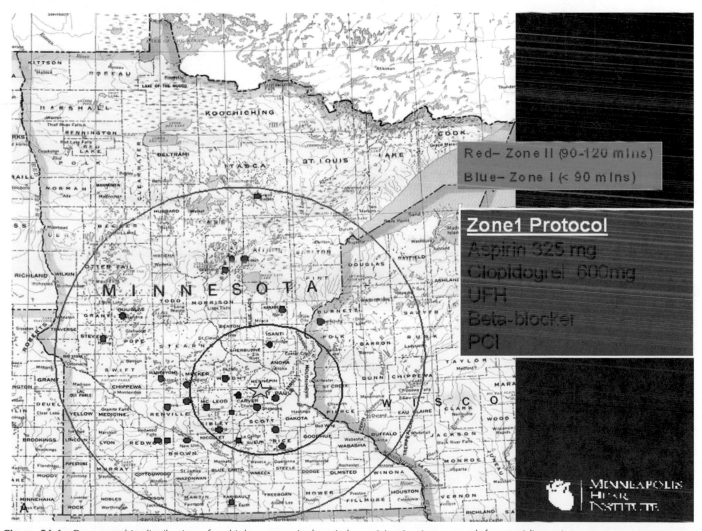

Figure 36-6 Demographic distribution of multiple community hospitals participating in a network for providing primary percutaneous coronary intervention (PCI) for ST elevation myocardial infarction with Minneapolis Heart Institute in Minneapolis, MN. A protocol-driven algorithm for adjunctive pharmacotherapies is illustrated for patients originating within a 90-minute radius for ground transport (Zone 1) (*A*) or for those patients originating within a 90- to 120-minute radius (Zone 2) (*B*). Participating centers have an established, rehearsed mechanism for patient transport. Angiographic and clinical outcomes following transport are comparable with those observed in patients admitted directly to the Abbott Northwestern Hospital in Minneapolis (see Table 36-1).

Continued

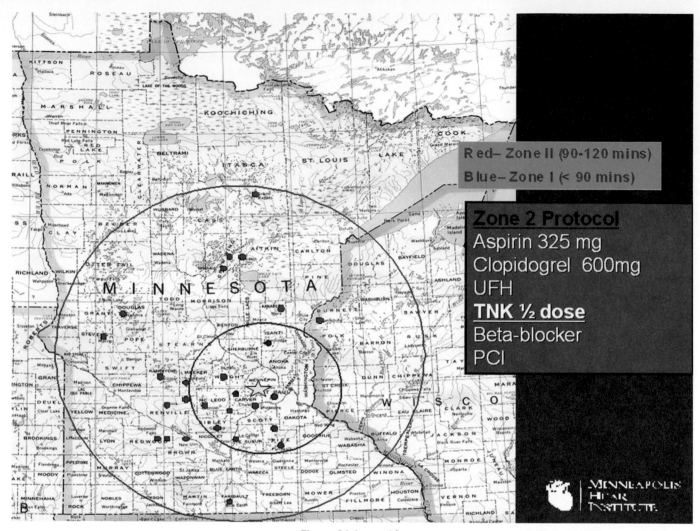

Figure 36-6, cont'd.

TABLE 36-1	Time to Treatment and 30-day Mortality for Minneapolis and Iowa Heart Centers Regional STEMI Programs at Minneapolis and Iowa Heart Centers			
		Minneapolis Heart	*Iowa Heart*	*P Value*
Total time to treatment	PCI	64 (44, 83)	59 (46, 71)	0.02
	Zone 1	95 (81, 117)	102 (90, 121)	0.0008
	Zone 2	123 (101, 152)	136 (122, 167)	0.0001
30-day mortality (%)	PCI	5.4	5.7	0.86
	Zone 1	5.3	3.4	0.21
	Zone 2	6.6	5.8	0.68

PCI, percutaneous coronary intervention.

Results from the Minneapolis Heart Institute and Iowa Heart regional STEMI networks, which include the PCI center at Abbott Northwestern Hospital in Minneapolis and the Mercy Medical Center in Des Moines, Iowa, in Zone 1 hospitals ($N = 21$) up to 60 minutes from the PCI center. These patients have an expected door-to-balloon time of <90 minutes and are treated with aspirin 325 mg, clopidogrel 600 mg, unfractionated heparin, and primary PCI. Zone 2 patients are treated with a pharmaco-invasive approach, which includes the medications above plus half-dose tenecteplase ($N = 32$ hospitals from 60 to 120 miles in Iowa or 60 to 210 miles from the PCI center in Minnesota).

Total time to treatment and 30-day mortality by zone in Minnesota and Iowa are shown. Despite geographic differences, overall time to treatment and 30-day mortality rates are remarkably similar and demonstrate the ability to expand the benefits of primary PCI for up to 210 miles from a PCI center.

Printed with permission from Smith L, Duval S, Tannenbaum MA, et al: Regional ST-elevation myocardial infarction systems expand access to primary percutaneous coronary intervention [abstract], *Circulation* 120:S959, 2009.

Registry of Myocardial Infarction 3 (NRMI 3) and NRMI 4 data regarding patients with STEMI who first present to a community hospital and are subsequently transported to a tertiary facility for PCI.[69] In the absence of a well-defined, integrated system with protocol-driven algorithms for care and dedicated transport facilities, the median door-to-balloon time from NRMI 3 and NRMI 4 is 180 minutes, and only 15% of patients receive PCI therapy within 120 minutes.[69] The discrepancy between current practice and what can be achieved through collaboration and avoidance of duplication of services calls for the development of an optimal process for ACS care.

The striking limitations of the current process for STEMI care is evidenced by the absence of any improvement in times to treatment despite widespread dissemination of "benchmark" goals for therapy (door-to-fibrinolytic infusion time or door-to-balloon time) in the form of guidelines.[101] Indeed, these recommended times to treatment (30 minutes for door-to-fibrinolytic infusion; 90 minutes for door-to-balloon) are not "ideal" times but, rather, the longest times that should be considered acceptable by the medical system.[102,103] Nevertheless, little improvement in overall times to treatment or that portion of patients who received CPG compliant care has been observed with the current process for ACS care in the authors' institution.[95,101] Considering the direct relationship between treatment delays and both short-term and long-term mortality following infarction, the need for improvement in the current process for ACS care is obvious.[104] The realization that "all hospitals are not equal" for the care of patients with STEMI and the demonstration of improved patient outcomes in specialized centers for care of both trauma and stroke have shattered the antiquated concept that patients with suspected MI should be transported to the nearest hospital.[105] Several U.S. cities, including Boston and Los Angeles, have begun directing public EMS to transport such patients only to a limited few "centers of excellence" for heart attack care.[106,107]

In addition to concentrating high-volume expertise and technology, these centers are also integrated with the EMS so that the diagnosis of infarction can be made more rapidly and the "system" for providing PCI is more responsive. The pre-hospital care for ACS, especially STEMI, is critically important. The hospitals with the shortest door-to-balloon times in the United States integrate pre-hospital diagnosis (transmitted ECG) with a multi-disciplinary "team" approach, in which the emergency physician activates the cardiac cath lab before cardiology consultation.[77] Indeed, the facilitation of in-hospital PCI treatment for those patients with a transmitted pre-hospital ECG has resulted in a significant reduction in door-to-balloon times as well as improvement in survival.[78,80,83] Recent multi-center data indicate that the use of centers that receive patients with STEMI along with pre-hospital ECG has resulted in 86% of patients being treated with door-to-balloon times less than 90 minutes in diverse regions across the United States.[107]

FUTURE CARE OF PATIENTS WITH ST ELEVATION MYOCARDIAL INFARCTION

At present, the lack of a coordinated system of care denies many patients the benefit of primary PCI. A coordinated system for the provision of PCI could prevent an estimated 6 to 8 MACEs, major adverse cardiovascular and cerebrovascular events (MACCEs) per 100 patients with STEMI treated, which might affect 35,000 patients yearly.[16,82] However, the current scheme for reimbursement for cardiovascular treatments could penalize community hospitals without cardiac cath labs when patients are transferred or admitted directly to a regional center.[16] Therefore, there is a need to make adjustments to the reimbursement strategy, possibly to include regional "networks" of partnering community and tertiary care centers. Non–PCI-capable hospitals could be motivated to risk-stratify and transfer patients with STEMI on the basis of not only risk but also transport time and distance. Such contractually defined networks could provide similar quality-assured, monitored, and protocol-driven algorithms for care and predefined systems for prompt patient transport.

Issues of case mix index could be defined by a system rather than by an individual hospital. Credentialing and criteria for the development of a "level I heart attack center" should include established ability to provide pre-hospital diagnosis of STEMI with a transmitted 12-lead ECG via integration with local or regional EMS.[16,82] Suggested criteria for both PCI-capable and non–PCI-capable heart attack centers are listed in Tables 36-2 and 36-3. To be successful, a system for the care of patients with STEMI should comprise multiple integral components, including a patient care focus, enhanced operational efficiency, appropriate system incentives ("pay for performance" or "pay for value"), and specific outcome and process measures, as well as mechanisms for quality review and continuous quality improvement. Professional societies and organizations are in the process of developing credentialing criteria for these centers. State and local government agencies may be charged with monitoring the legitimacy of regional

TABLE 36-2	State of Ohio Mission: Lifeline Credentialing Criteria for Non–Percutaneous Coronary Intervention Hospitals and ST Elevation Myocardial Infarction Referral Centers

- Appropriate protocols and standing orders should be in place for the identification of ST elevation myocardial infarction (STEMI). At a minimum, these protocols should be present in the Intensive Care Unit/Coronary Care Unit and Emergency Department (ED).
- Each ED should maintain a standardized reperfusion STEMI care pathway that designates primary percutaneous coronary intervention (PCI) as the preferred reperfusion strategy if transfer of patients to a primary PCI hospital/STEMI–receiving center can be achieved within times consistent with ACC/AHA (American College of Cardiology/American Heart Association) guidelines.
- Each ED should maintain a standardized reperfusion STEMI care pathway that designates fibrinolysis in the ED (for eligible patients) when the system cannot achieve times consistent with ACC/AHA guidelines for primary PCI.
- If reperfusion strategy is for primary PCI transfer, a streamlined, standardized protocol for rapid transfer and transport to a STEMI–receiving center should be operational.
- If reperfusion strategy is for primary PCI transfer, all patients should be transported to the most appropriate STEMI–receiving center, where the expected first door-to-balloon (first device used) time should be within 90 minutes (considering ground versus air transport, weather, traffic).
- When transferring a patient to a primary PCI hospital, the mean or medium door-to-door-to-balloon time should be within 90 minutes.
- The STEMI–referral center should have an ongoing quality improvement process, including data measurement and feedback, for the STEMI population and collect and submit *Mission: Lifeline* required data elements (using the ACTION Registry–GWTG Limited Form*).
- A program should be in place to track and improve treatment (acutely and at discharge) with ACC/AHA guideline–based class I therapies.
- A multi-disciplinary STEMI team, including the EMS, should review hospital-specific STEMI data on a quarterly basis.
- Door-to-first electrocardiogram (ECG) time: The goal should be less than 10 minutes.
- The proportion of STEMI-eligible patients receiving any reperfusion (PCI or fibrinolysis) therapy (goal approximately 100%)
- STEMI–referral center ED door-to-ED discharges (goal within 30 minutes)
- STEMI–referral center ED door-to-balloon (first device used) time should be within 120 minutes (including transport time).
- Each hospital should install synchronized clocks (preferably atomic clocks) in the ED, synchronize the ECG machine times to the atomic clocks, daily and educate team members to use only the atomic clocks when documenting time segments.
- The TIMI (thrombolysis in MI) risk score, a simple risk stratification tool that categorizes a patient's risk of death and ischemic events, should be used to provide a basis for therapeutic decision making.

*This pared down version of the ACTION Registry-GWTG is a 50% reduction in the data collection and was created to allow more hospitals to participate in the registry as well as in the AHA's *Mission: Lifeline* Program. Current registry participants and new participants, who choose the more comprehensive version, will be designated as ACTION Registry-GWTG Premiere participants. ACTION Registry-GWTG Premier, which includes the registry's most robust set of data elements, will remain the most comprehensive choice for monitoring data in ACS, looking at all the acute MI (AMI) performance measures and all test measures, including dosing errors and lipid metrics.

Ohio Mission: Lifeline Coalition: Ohio *Mission: Lifeline* Criteria. (Adapted from National Mission: Lifeline Criteria, American Heart Association, 2010.)

TABLE 36-3	State of Ohio Mission: Lifeline Credentialing Criteria for Primary PCI Hospital / STEMI-Receiving Centers

- Protocols for triage, diagnosis, and cardiac catheterization laboratory activation should be established within the primary PCI hospital/STEMI–receiving center. A single activation phone call should alert the STEMI team. Criteria for EMS activation of the Cardiac Catheterization Laboratory should be established in conjunction with EMS offices.
- The STEMI–receiving center should be available 24 hours/7 days a week to perform primary PCI.
- The cardiac catheterization laboratory staff, including an interventional cardiologist, should arrive within 30 minutes of the activation call.
- There should be universal acceptance of patients with STEMI (no diversion). There should be a plan for triage and treatment for simultaneous presentation of patients with STEMI.
- The interventional cardiologist should meet ACC/AHA criteria for competence. Interventional cardiologists should perform at least 11 primary PCI procedures per year and 75 total PCI procedures per year.
- The STEMI–receiving center should meet ACC/AHA criteria for volume; and a minimum of 36 primary PCI procedures and 200 total PCI procedures should be performed annually.
- For patients presenting at the primary PCI hospital, the mean or medium door-to-balloon time should be within 90 minutes.
- When transferring a patient from a non-PCI hospital, the mean or medium door-to-door-to-balloon time should be within 90 minutes.
- The STEMI–receiving center should participate in the *Mission: Lifeline*–approved data collection tool, ACTION Registry–GWTG.
- A program should be in place to track and improve treatment (acutely and at discharge) with ACC/AHA guideline–based class 1 therapy.
- There should be a recognized STEMI–receiving center liaison or system coordinator in the system and a recognized physician champion.
- There should be regularly scheduled (i.e., monthly) multidisciplinary team meetings to evaluate outcomes and quality improvement data. Operational issues should be reviewed, problems identified, and solutions implemented. The following measurements should be evaluated on an ongoing basis:
  - Door-to-balloon (first device used) time, non-transfer, within 90 minutes
  - STEMI–referral center ED door-to-balloon (first device used) time, transfer within 90 minutes
  - First Medical contact to balloon inflation (first device used), non-transfer, within 90 minutes
  - First medical contact to balloon inflation (first device used) transfer
  - Proportion of eligible patients receiving reperfusion therapy
  - Proportion of eligible patients administered guideline–based class I therapies
  - Proportion of patients with field diagnosis of STEMI and activation of the cardiac catheterization laboratory for intended primary PCI that:
    - Do not undergo acute catheterization because of misdiagnosis
    - Undergo acute catheterization and are found to have no elevation in cardiac biomarkers and no revascularization in the first 24 hours

In-Hospital Mortality

- Each hospital should install synchronized clocks (preferably atomic clocks) in the ED and catheterization laboratory, synchronize the ECG machine and the atomic clocks daily, and educate team members to use only the atomic clocks when documenting time segments.
- The TIMI risk score, a simple risk stratification tool that categorizes a patient's risk of death and ischemic events, should be used to provide a basis for therapeutic decision making.
- All primary PCI hospitals should commit to a level of financial support for the implementation and sustainability of regional coordinators.
- All primary PCI hospitals should be involved in education outreach to non-PCI hospitals and local EMS agencies. Hospitals should also be involved in education of the public about recognition of signs and symptoms and activation of 9-1-1 services.

ACC, American College of Cardiology; *AHA*, American Heart Association; *ECG*, electrocardiogram; *EMS*, emergency medical system; *GWTG*, Get With The Guidelines; *PCI*, percutaneous coronary intervention; *STEMI*, ST elevation myocardial infarction; *TIMI*, thrombolysis in MI.

Ohio Mission: Lifeline Coalition: Ohio *Mission: Lifeline* Criteria. (Adapted from National *Mission: Lifeline* Criteria, American Heart Association, 2010.)

STEMI networks. Monitoring adherence to guidelines may be performed by established "systems" rather than by individual hospitals or centers. Treatment, outcome, and performance data acquisition and analysis will be standardized, with appropriate and timely feedback to participating systems and centers. Individual states have been charged with development of regional coordinators to provide oversight, monitoring, and support for participating systems and centers.

The process for the "development of systems of care for patients with STEMI" has, indeed, been initiated already by the AHA and is the subject of ongoing stakeholder meetings. The AHA has issued a call to action to improve the implementation and timeliness of infarct reperfusion with primary PCI; the ideal system from the perspective of each constituent, including the patient, the physician, the EMS, the non–PCI-capable hospital, the PCI-capable center, and the payer, is carefully considered. Given the importance of time to treatment for STEMI, the ideal system of care will likely be different for various geographic locales (urban/suburban versus rural) and will take into account the risk of MI for each patient. Recommendations for additional research and the requisite changes in policy to support the construction and implementation of systems that will improve quality care and outcomes for patients with STEMI should be forthcoming.

REFERENCES

1. Fuster V, Badimon L, Badimon JJ, et al: The pathogenesis of coronary artery disease and the acute coronary syndromes. *N Engl J Med* 326:242–250, 1992.
2. Braunwald E, Antman EM, Beasley JW, et al: American College of Cardiology/American Heart Association Task Force on Practice Guidelines (Committee on the Management of Patients With Unstable Angina). ACC/AHA guideline update for the management of patients with unstable angina and non-ST-segment elevation myocardial infarction-2002: Summary article: A report of the American College of Cardiology/American Heart Association Task Force on Practice Guidelines (Committee on the Management of Patients With Unstable Angina). *Circulation* 106:1893–1900, 2002.
3. MacKenzie EJ, Rivara FP, Jurkovich GJ, et al: A national evaluation of the effect of trauma-center care on mortality. *New Engl J Med* 354:366–378, 2006.
4. Schwamm LH, Pancioli A, Acker JE, III, et al: American Stroke Association's task force on the development of stroke systems. Recommendations for the establishment of stroke systems of care: Recommendations from the American Stroke Association's task force on the development of stroke systems. *Circulation* 111:1078–1091, 2005.
5. Anderson RN: *Deaths: Leading causes for 1999, National Vital Statistics Report*, Vol 49, No. 11, Hyattsville, MD: National Center for Health Statistics. October 12, 2001.
6. American Heart Association: Heart disease and stroke statistics—2006 update. *Circulation* 113:e85–e151, 2006.
7. Willerson JT: Centers of excellence. *Circulation* 107:1471–1472, 2003.
8. Topol EJ, Kereiakes DJ: Regionalization of care for acute ischemic heart disease–a call for specialized centers. *Circulation* 107:1463–1466, 2003.
9. Califf RM, Faxon DP: Need for centers to care for patients with acute coronary syndromes. *Circulation* 107:1467–1470, 2003.
10. Rathore SS, Epstein RJ, Volpp KGM, et al: Regionalization of care for acute coronary syndromes—more evidence is needed. *J Am Med Assn* 293:1383–1387, 2005.
11. Rathore SS, Epstein AJ, Nallamouthu BK, et al: Regionalization of ST-segment elevation acute coronary syndromes care—putting a national policy in proper perspective. *J Am Coll Cardiol* 47:1346–1349, 2006.
12. Widimsky P, Groch L, Zelizko M, et al: Multicenter randomized trial comparing transport to primary angioplasty vs. immediate thrombolysis vs. combined strategy for patients with acute myocardial infarction presenting to a community hospital without a catheterization laboratory. The PRAGUE study. *Eur Heart J* 21:823–831, 2000.

13. Widimsky P, Budesinsky T, Vorac D, et al: Long distance transport for primary angioplasty vs. immediate thrombolysis in acute myocardial—PRAGUE-2. *Eur Heart J* 24:94–104, 2003.
14. Andersen HR, Nielsen TT, Rasmussen K, et al: A comparison of coronary angioplasty with fibrinolytic therapy in acute myocardial infarction. *N Engl J Med* 349:733–742, 2003.
15. Williams DO: Treatment delayed is treatment denied. *Circulation* 109:1806–1808, 2004.
16. Jacobs AK, Antman EM, Ellrodt G, et al: Recommendation to develop strategies to increase the number of ST-segment elevation myocardial infarction patients with timely access to primary percutaneous coronary intervention—The American Heart Association's acute myocardial infarction (AMI) Advisory Working Group. *Circulation* 113:2152–2163, 2006.
17. Vaccarino V, Rathor SS, Wenger NK, et al: Sex and racial differences in the management of acute myocardial infarction, 1994 through 2002. *New Engl J Med* 353:671–682, 2005.
18. Magid DJ, Wang Y, Herrin J, et al: Relationship between time of day, day of week, timeliness of reperfusion, and in-hospital mortality for patients with acute ST-segment elevation myocardial infarction. *J Am Med Assn* 294:803–812, 2005.
19. Rathore SS, Masoudi FA, Havranek EP, et al: Regional variations in racial differences in the treatment of elderly patients hospitalized with acute myocardial infarction. *Am J Med* 117:811–812, 2004.
20. Yan AT, Yan RT, Tan M, et al: Despite the temporal increases, coronary angiography and revascularization remain paradoxically directed towards low risk non-ST elevation acute coronary syndrome patients[abstract]. *J Am Coll Cardiol* 45:190A, 2005.
21. Roe MT, Peterson ED, Newby LK, et al: The influence of risk status on guideline adherence for patients with non-ST-segment elevation acute coronary syndromes. *Am Heart J* 151:1205–1213, 2006.
22. Banihashemi B, Goodman SG, Yan RT, et al: Global Registry of Acute Coronary Events (GRACE/GRACE(2)) Investigators. Underutilization of clopidogrel and glycoprotein IIb/IIIa inhibitors in non-ST-elevation acute coronary syndrome patients: The Canadian global registry of acute coronary events (GRACE) experience. *Am Heart J* 158:917–924, 2009.
23. Cohen MG, Filby SJ, Roe MT, et al: The paradoxical use of cardiac catheterization in patients with non-ST-elevation acute coronary syndromes: Lessons from the Can Rapid Stratification of Unstable Angina Patients Suppress Adverse Outcomes With Early Implementation of the ACC/AHA Guidelines (CRUSADE) Quality Improvement Initiative. *Am Heart J* 158:263–270, 2009.
24. Roe MT, Chen AY, Delong ER, et al. Patterns of transfer for patients with non-ST-segment elevation acute coronary syndrome from community to tertiary care hospitals. *Am Heart J* 156:185–192, 2008.
25. Peterson ED, Roe MT, Mulgund J, et al: Association between hospital process performance and outcomes among patients with acute coronary syndromes. *J Am Med Assn* 295:1912–1920, 2006.
26. Henry TD, Atkins JM, Cunningham MS, et al: ST-segment elevation myocardial infarction: recommendations on triage of patients to heart attack centers—is it time for a national policy for the treatment of ST-segment elevation myocardial infarction? *J Am Coll Cardiol* 47:1339–1345, 2006.
27. Nallamothu BK, Wang Y, Magid DJ, et al: Relation between hospital specialization with primary percutaneous coronary intervention and clinical outcomes in ST-segment elevation myocardial infarction: National Registry of Myocardial Infarction–4 analysis. *Circulation* 113:222–229, 2006.
28. Magid DJ, Calonge GN, Rumsfeld JS, et al: Relation between hospital primary angioplasty volume and mortality for patients with acute MI treated with primary angioplasty vs. thrombolytic therapy. *J Am Med Assn* 284:3131–3138, 2000.
29. Moscucci M, Share D, Smith D, et al: Relationship between operator volume and adverse outcome in contemporary percutaneous coronary intervention practice: An analysis of a quality-controlled multicenter percutaneous coronary intervention clinical database. *J Am Coll Cardiol* 456:625–632, 2005.
30. Jollis JG, Romano PS. Volume-outcome relationship in acute myocardial infarction: the balloon and the needle. *J Am Med Assn* 284:3169–3171, 2000.
31. Hannan EL, Wu C, Walford G, et al: Volume-outcome relationships for percutaneous coronary interventions in the stent era. *Circulation* 112:1171–1179, 2005.
32. Keeley EC, Grines CL: Should patients with acute myocardial infraction be transferred to a tertiary center for primary angioplasty or receive it at qualified hospitals in the community? The case for emergency transfer for primary percutaneous coronary intervention. *Circulation* 112:3520–3532, 2005.
33. Lewis WR, Sorof SA, Super DM. Practice makes perfect: ACC/AHA guideline adherence is higher in hospitals with high acute myocardial infarction volume [abstract]. *J Am Coll Cardiol* 47:255A, 2006.
34. Kugelmass A, Brown P, Becker E, et al: How do acute percutaneous coronary intervention complication rates vary in hospitals ranked in the top versus the bottom quartiles of hospitals? [abstract]. *J Am Coll Cardiol* 45:339A, 2005.
35. Morice MC, Spalding C, Lancelin B, et al: Does hospital PTCA volume influence mortality and complication rates in the era of PTCA with systematic stenting? Results of the Greater Paris Area PTCA registry [abstract]. *J Am Coll Cardiol* 47:192A, 2006.
36. Cannon CP, Gibson CM, Lambrew CT, et al: Relationship of symptom-onset-to-balloon time and door-to-balloon time with mortality in patients undergoing angioplasty for acute myocardial infarction. *J Am Med Assn* 283:2941–2947, 2000.
37. Vakili BA, Brown DL: 1995 Coronary angioplasty reporting system of the New York State Department of Health. Relation between hospital primary angioplasty volume and mortality for patients with acute MI treated with primary angioplasty vs. thrombolytic therapy. *Am J Cardiol* 91:726–728, 2003.
38. Srinivas VS, Hailpern SM, Koss E, et al: Effect of physician volume on the relationship between hospital volume and mortality during primary angioplasty. *J Am Coll Cardiol* 53:574–579, 2009.
39. Smith S, Feldman TD, Hirshfeld JW, et al: ACC/AHA/SCAI 2005 Guideline update for percutaneous coronary intervention—summary article. A report of the American College of Cardiology/American Heart Association Task Force on Practice Guidelines (ACC/AHA/SCAI Writing Committee to update the 2001 Guidelines for Percutaneous Coronary Intervention). *Circulation* 113:156–175, 2005.
40. Kutcher MA, Klein LW, Ou FS, et al: National Cardiovascular Data Registry. Percutaneous coronary interventions in facilities without cardiac surgery on site: A report from the National Cardiovascular Data Registry (NCDR). *J Am Coll Cardiol* 54:16–24, 2009.
41. Aversano T: Relationship between institutional primary percutaneous coronary intervention volume and mortality in hospitals without on-site cardiac surgery: The C-PORT experience [abstract]. *Circulation* 118:S-1076, 2008.
42. Pride YB, Canto JG, Frederick PD, et al; NRMI Investigators: Outcomes among patients with non-ST-segment elevation myocardial infarction presenting to interventional hospitals with and without on-site cardiac surgery. *JACC Cardiovasc Interv* 2:944–952, 2009.
43. Mukherjee D, Fang J, Chetcuti S, et al: Impact of combination evidence-based medical therapy on mortality in patients with acute coronary syndromes. *Circulation* 109:745–749, 2004.
44. Tay E, Chan MY, Tan WD, et al: Impact of combination evidence-based medical therapy on mortality following myocardial infarction in patients with and without renal dysfunction [abstract]. *J Am Coll Cardiol* 47:161A, 2006.
45. Califf RM, Peterson ED, Gibbons RM, et al: Integrating quality into the cycle of therapeutic development. *J Am Coll Cardiol* 40:1895–1901, 2002.
46. Roe MT, Peterson ED, Newby LK, et al: The influence of risk status on guideline adherence for patients with non-ST-segment elevation acute coronary syndromes. *Am Heart J* 151:1205–1213, 2006.
47. Roe MT, Peterson ED, Yu L, et al: Relationship between risk stratification by cardiac troponin level and adherence to guidelines for non-ST-segment elevation acute coronary syndrome. *Arch Intern Med* 165:1870–1876, 2005.
48. Lewis WR, Sorof SA, Super DM: Practice makes perfect: ACC/AHA guideline adherence is higher in hospitals with high acute myocardial infarction volume [abstract]. *J Am Coll Cardiol* 47:255A, 2006.
49. Corbelli JC, Janicke DM, Cziraky MJ, et al: Acute coronary syndrome emergency treatment strategies: Improved treatment and reduced mortality in patients with acute coronary syndrome using guideline based critical care pathways. *Am Heart J* 157:61–68, 2009.
50. Bradley EH, Nallamothu BK, Herrin J, et al: National efforts to improve door-to-balloon time results from the Door-to-Balloon Alliance. *J Am Coll Cardiol* 54:2423–2429, 2009.
51. Wennberg DE, Lucas FL, Siewers AD, et al: Outcomes of percutaneous coronary interventions performed at centers without and with onsite coronary artery bypass graft surgery. *J Am Med Assn* 292:1961–1968, 2004.
52. Ting HH, Raveendran G, Lennon RJ, et al: A total of 1,007 percutaneous coronary interventions without onsite cardiac surgery: Acute and long-term outcomes. *J Am Coll Cardiol* 47:1713–1721, 2006.
53. Wharton TP, Jr: Should patients with acute myocardial infraction be transferred to a tertiary center for primary angioplasty or receive it at qualified hospitals in community? The case for community hospital angioplasty. *Circulation* 12:3509–3520, 2005.
54. Aversano T, Aversano LT, Passamani E, et al: Thrombolytic therapy vs primary percutaneous coronary intervention for myocardial infarction in patients presenting to hospitals without on-site cardiac surgery: A randomized controlled trial. *JAMA* 287:1943–1951, 2002.
55. Anis A, Normand ST, Wolf RE, et al: Primary percutaneous coronary intervention with or without cardiac surgery on-site: Massachusetts' experience [abstract]. *Circulation* 120:2154, 2009.
56. Kereiakes DJ, Willerson JT: The United States cardiovascular care deficit. *Circulation* 109:821–823, 2004.
57. Greenfield S, Kaplan SH, Kahn R, et al: Profiling care provided by different groups of physicians: Effects of patient case-mix (bias) and physician-level clustering on quality assessment results. *Ann Intern Med* 136:111–121, 2002.
58. Jacobs AK: Primary angioplasty for acute myocardial infarction: Is it worth the wait? *N Engl J Med* 349:798–800, 2003.
59. Bonow RO, Smith SC: Cardiovascular manpower—the looming crisis. *Circulation* 109:817–820, 2004.
60. Fye WB: Cardiology's workforce shortage—implications for patient care and research. *Circulation* 109:813–816, 2004.
61. Nallamothu BK, Bates ER, Wang Y, et al: Driving times and distances to hospitals with percutaneous coronary intervention in the United States—implications for pre-hospital triage of patients with ST-elevation myocardial infarction. *Circulation* 113:1189–1195, 2006.
62. Buckley JW, Bates ER, Nallamothu BK: Primary percutaneous coronary intervention expansion to hospitals without on-site cardiac surgery in Michigan: A geographic information systems analysis. *Am Heart J* 155:668–672, 2008.
63. Antman EM, Anbe DJ, Armstrong PW, et al: ACC/AHA guidelines for the management of patients with ST-elevation myocardial infarction: A report of the American College of Cardiology/American Heart Association Task Force on Practice Guidelines (Committee to Revise the 1999 Guidelines for the Management of Patients with Acute Myocardial Infarction). *Circulation* 110(9):e82–e292, 2004.
64. Nallamothu BK, Bates RK: Percutaneous coronary intervention versus fibrinolytic therapy in acute myocardial infarction: is timing (almost) everything? *Am J Cardiol* 92:824–826, 2003.
65. Betriu A, Masotti M: Comparison of mortality rates in acute myocardial infarction treated by percutaneous coronary intervention versus fibrinolysis. *Am J Cardiol* 95:100–101, 2005.
66. Tarantini G, Razzolini R, Ramondo A, et al: Explanation for the survival benefit of primary angioplasty over thrombolytic therapy in patients with ST-elevation acute myocardial infarction. *Am J Cardiol* 1:1503–1505, 2005.
67. Tarantini G, Razzolini R, Napodano M, et al: Editor's Choice: Acceptable reperfusion delay to prefer primary angioplasty over fibrin-specific thrombolytic therapy is affected (mainly) by the patient's mortality risk: 1 h does not fit all. *Eur Heart J* 31:676–683, 2010.
68. Dalby M, Bouzamondo A, Lechat P, et al: Transfer for primary angioplasty versus immediate thrombolysis in acute myocardial infarction: A meta-analysis. *Circulation* 108:1809–1814, 2003.
69. Nallamothu BK, Bates ER, Herrin J, et al: Times to treatment in transfer patients undergoing primary percutaneous coronary intervention in the United States: National Registry of Myocardial Infarction (NRMI)-3/4 analysis. *Circulation* 111;761–767, 2005.
70. Gibson CM, Pride YB, Frederick PD, et al: Trends in reperfusion strategies, door-to-needle and door-to-balloon times, and in-hospital mortality among patients with ST-segment elevation myocardial infarction enrolled in the National Registry of Myocardial Infarction from 1990 to 2006. *Am Heart J* 156:1035–1044, 2008.
71. Blankenship JC, Scott TD, Skelding KA, et al: Presentation to non-PCI center is major modifiable factor associated with delayed door-to balloon time in HORIZONS-AMI [abstract]. *Circulation* 118:S-903, 2008.
72. Chen J, Normand SL, Wang Y, et al. Recent declines in hospitalizations for acute myocardial infarction for Medicare fee-for-service beneficiaries: Progress and continuing challenges. *Circulation* 121:1322–1328, 2010.
73. Roe MT, Messenger JC, Weintraub WS, et al. Treatments, trends, and outcomes of acute myocardial infarction and percutaneous coronary intervention. *J Am Coll Cardiol* 56:254–263, 2010.
74. Kereiakes DJ, Gibler WB, Martin LH, et al: Relative importance of emergency medical system transport and the pre-hospital electrocardiogram on reducing hospital time delay to therapy for acute myocardial infarction: A preliminary report from the Cincinnati Heart Project. *Am Heart J* 123:835–840, 1992.
75. Diercks DB, Kontos MC, Chen AY, et al: Utilization and impact of pre-hospital electrocardiograms for patients with acute ST-segment elevation myocardial infarction: Data from the NCDR (National Cardiovascular Data Registry) ACTION (Acute Coronary Treatment and Intervention Outcomes Network) Registry. *J Am Coll Cardiol* 53:161–166, 2009.
76. Curtis JP, Portnay EL, Wang Y, et al: National Registry of Myocardial Infarction-4: The pre-hospital electrocardiogram and time to reperfusion in patients with acute myocardial infarction, 2000-2002: Findings from the National Registry of Myocardial Infarction-4. *J Am Coll Cardiol* 47:1544–1552, 2006.
77. Bradley EH, Roumanis SA, Radford, MJ, et al: Achieving door-to-balloon times that meet quality guidelines: How do successful hospitals do it? *J Am Coll Cardiol* 46:1236–1241, 2005.
78. Bjorklund E, Stenestrand U, Landback J, et al: A pre-hospital diagnostic strategy reduced time to treatment and mortality in real life patients with ST-elevation myocardial infarction treated with primary percutaneous coronary intervention [abstract]. *J Am Coll Cardiol* 47:192A, 2006.
79. Pedersen SH, Galatius S, Hansen PR, et al: Field triage reduces treatment delay and improves long-term clinical outcome in patients with acute ST-segment elevation myocardial infarction treated with primary percutaneous coronary intervention. *J Am Coll Cardiol* 54:2296–2302, 2009.
80. Le May MR, So DY, Dionne R, et al: A citywide protocol for primary PCI in ST-segment elevation myocardial infarction. *N Engl J Med* 358:231–240, 2008.
81. Garvey JL, MacLead BA, Dopko G, et al: Pre-hospital 12-lead electrocardiography programs: a call for implementation by emergency medical services systems providing advanced life support—National Heart Attack Alert Program (NHAAP) Coordinating Committee; National Heart, Lung, and Blood Institute (NHLBI); National Institutes of Health. *J Am Coll Cardiol* 47:485–491, 2006.
82. Jacobs AK, Antman EM, Faxon DP, et al: Development of systems of care for ST-elevation myocardial infarction patients: Executive summary. *Circulation* 116:217–230, 2007.

83. Dieker HJ, Liem SSB, Aidi HE, et al: Pre-hospital triage for primary angioplasty. *JACC Card Interv* 3:705–711, 2010.

84. Concannon TW, Kent DM, Normand SL, et al: Comparative effectiveness of ST-segment elevation myocardial infarction regionalization strategies. *Circ Cardiovasc Qual Outcomes* 3:1–8, 2010.

85. Kereiakes, DJ, Antman EM: Clinical guidelines and practice: In search of the truth. *J Am Coll Cardiol* 48:1129–1135, 2006.

86. Tricoci P, Lokhnygina Y, Berdan LG, et al: Time to coronary angiography and outcomes among patients with non ST-segment elevation acute coronary syndromes: Results from the SYNERGY trial. *Circulation* 116:2669–2677, 2007.

87. Mehta SR, Granger CB, Boden WE, et al: Early versus delayed invasive intervention in acute coronary syndromes. *N Engl J Med* 360:2165–2175, 2009.

88. Sorajja P, Gersh BJ, Cox DA, et al: Impact of delay to angioplasty in patients with acute coronary syndromes undergoing invasive management: Analysis from the ACUITY (Acute Catheterization and Urgent Intervention Triage strategY) trial. *J Am Coll Cardiol* 55:1416–1424, 2010.

89. Bavry AA, Kumbhani DJ, Rassi AN, et al: Benefit of early invasive therapy in acute coronary syndromes: A meta-analysis of contemporary randomized clinical trials. *J Am Coll Cardiol* 48:1319–1325, 2006.

90. Lagerqvist B, Husted S, Kontny F, et al: Fast revascularization during InStability in coronary artery disease (FRISC-II) Investigators. *Lancet* 368:998–1004, 2006.

91. Fox KA, Clayton TC, Damman P, et al: Long-term outcome of a routine versus selective invasive strategy in patients with non-ST-segment elevation acute coronary syndrome a meta-analysis of individual patient data. *J Am Coll Cardiol* 55:2435–2445, 2010.

92. Fox KA, Anderson FA, Jr, Dabbous OH, et al: Intervention in acute coronary syndromes: Do patients undergo intervention on the basis of their risk characteristics? The Global Registry of Acute Coronary Events (GRACE). *Heart* 93:177–182, 2007.

93. Tarantini G, Ramondo A, Razzolini R, et al: Patient's risk profile and benefit from invasive approach in initial management of non ST-segment elevation acute coronary syndrome: A meta-regression analysis [abstract]. *Circulation* 114:II-346 (#1757), 2006.

94. Henry TD, Sharkey SE, Burke MN, et al: A regional system to provide timely access to percutaneous coronary intervention for ST-elevation myocardial infarction. *Circulation* 116:721–728, 2007.

95. Aguirre FV, Varghese JJ, Kelley MP, et al: Rural interhospital transfer of ST-elevation myocardial infarction patients for percutaneous coronary revascularization: The Stat Heart Program. *Circulation* 117:1145–1152, 2008.

96. Ting HH, Rihal CS, Gersh BJ, et al: Regional systems of care to optimize timeliness of reperfusion therapy for ST-elevation myocardial infarction: The Mayo Clinic STEMI Protocol. *Circulation* 116:729–736, 2007.

97. Smith L, Duval S, Tannenbaum MA, et al: Regional ST-elevation myocardial infarction systems expand access to primary percutaneous coronary intervention [abstract]. *Circulation* 120:S959, 2009.

98. Jollis JG, Roettig ML, Aluko AO, et al: Implementation of a statewide system for coronary reperfusion for ST-segment elevation myocardial infarction. *JAMA* 298:2371–2380, 2007.

99. Henry TD, Gibson CM, Pinto DS: Moving toward improved care for the STEMI patient: A mandate for systems of care. *Circ Cardiovasc Qual Outcomes* 3(5):441–443, 2010.

100. Kushner FG, Hand M, Smith SC, Jr, et al: American College of Cardiology Foundation/American Heart Association Task Force on Practice Guidelines. 2009 Focused Updates: ACC/AHA guidelines for the management of patients with ST-elevation myocardial infarction (updating the 2004 Guideline and 2007 Focused Update) and ACC/AHA/SCAI guidelines on percutaneous coronary intervention (updating the 2005 Guideline and 2007 Focused Update): A report of the American College of Cardiology Foundation/American Heart Association Task Force on Practice Guidelines. *Circulation* 120:2271–2306, 2009.

101. McNamara RL, Herrin J, Bradley EH, et al; NRML Investigators: Hospital improvement in time to reperfusion in patients with acute myocardial infarction, 1999 to 2002. *J Am Coll Cardiol* 47:45–51, 2006.

102. Rathore SS, Curtis JP, Chen J, et al: Primary percutaneous coronary intervention door-to-balloon time and mortality in patients hospitalized with ST-elevation myocardial infarction: Is 90 minutes fast enough? [abstract]. *Circulation* 118:S-1074 (#6174), 2008.

103. O'Neill WW, Grines CL, Dixon SR, et al: Does a 90-minute door-to-balloon time matter? Observations from four current reperfusion trials [abstract]. *J Am Coll Cardiol* 45:225A, 2005.

104. Brodie BR, Hansen C, Stuckey TD, et al: Door-to-balloon time with primary percutaneous coronary intervention for acute myocardial infarction impacts late cardiac mortality in high-risk patients and patients presenting early after the onset of symptoms. *J Am Coll Cardiol* 47:289–295, 2006.

105. Weaver WD: All hospitals are not equal for treatment of patients with acute myocardial infarction. *Circulation* 108:1768–1771, 2003.

106. Moyer P, Feldman J, Levine J, et al: Implications of the mechanical (PCI) vs. thrombolytic controversy for ST segment elevation myocardial infarction on the organization of emergency medical services. *Crit Pathways in Cardiol* 3:53–61, 2004.

107. Rokos IC, French WJ, Koenig WJ, et al: Integration of pre-hospital electrocardiograms and ST-elevation myocardial infarction receiving center (SRC) networks: Impact on door-to-balloon times across 10 independent regions. *JACC Cardiovasc Interv* 2:339–346, 2009.

Peripheral Vascular Interventions

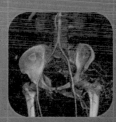

37

Lower Extremity Interventions

DEBABRATA MUKHERJEE

KEY POINTS

- Despite recent advances in the noninvasive evaluation of peripheral arterial disease of the lower extremity, contrast angiography remains the "gold standard" for definitive evaluation.

- Occlusive disease confined to the iliac arteries appears to occur in relatively young patients and may have a significant impact on productivity and lifestyle.

- The excellent intermediate to long-term patency rates following percutaneous intervention in peripheral arterial disease of the lower extremity has led to its emergence as an attractive alternative to surgery in patients with suitable lesions.

- A strategy of primary stenting as opposed to provisional stenting is generally recommended for aorto-ostial lesions.

- The technical and clinical success rates of endovascular intervention for iliac artery stenosis exceed 90%—with a fairly comparable intermediate and long-term patency to that of surgical revascularization—making this the initial therapy of choice for most iliac stenoses.

- While controversial, surgery remains the preferred strategy for patients with obstructive disease of the common femoral and proximal profunda femoris arteries.

- The lower durability of percutaneous intervention may be offset by the less invasive nature of endovascular interventions and resultant decreased morbidity and mortality compared with vascular surgery.

- Interventions can be repeatedly done if they fail, but repeat surgery is technically more challenging and may be limited by the availability of conduit.

- In patients with anatomically appropriate lesions, most practitioners use endovascular interventions preferentially as the initial therapy of choice.

Introduction

Peripheral arterial disease (PAD) of the lower extremity is a common health problem. Epidemiological studies have mostly used intermittent claudication (IC) as a symptomatic marker of the disease and an abnormal ankle-brachial index (ABI) to define the burden of asymptomatic PAD. The prevalence of the disease is dependent on the age of the population studied and the underlying atherosclerotic risk profile of the cohort. It is estimated that the overall disease prevalence is in the range of 3% to 10%, increasing to about 15% to 20% in persons older than 70 years. More than half of all patients with lower extremity PAD may be asymptomatic.[1-7] History (including standardized questionnaires such as the Rose claudication questionnaire used in the Framingham Heart Study) and physical examination may grossly underestimate the true burden of lower extremity PAD.[1] Criqui et al. evaluated the prevalence of lower extremity PAD in a population of 613 men and women in southern California utilizing four different modalities (the Rose questionnaire, pulse examination, ABI, and pulse-wave velocity). The detection rate of PAD with ABI and pulse-wave velocity was 2 to 7 times higher than the detection rate of the Rose questionnaire. Of interest, clinical examination of the pulse overestimated the prevalence of PAD by twofold.[8] To optimally manage patients with lower extremity PAD, whether symptomatic or asymptomatic, it is important to understand the global vascular disease burden, the natural history of the disease process, its impact on the patient's lifestyle, and the risk factors for an individual patient. Such knowledge is key to reducing the mortality and morbidity of the individual patient.

Vascular Anatomy of the Lower Extremity

The abdominal aorta bifurcates at the level of the fourth lumbar vertebra into two branches, the right and the left common iliac arteries. The common iliac arteries divide into the external iliac artery, which normally follows the same axis of the common iliac artery, and the internal iliac arteries, which take a posteromedial track in relation to the common iliac artery. In addition to its terminal branches, the common iliac artery gives off branches to the surrounding tissues, peritoneum, psoas muscle, ureter, and nerves. Occasionally, the common iliac artery provides accessory renal arteries to a normal or ectopic kidney. Figure 37-1 depicts the arterial circulation of the lower extremity. The external iliac arteries are larger than the internal iliac arteries. They descend along the medial border of the psoas major muscle, entering the thigh posterior to the inguinal ligament and becoming the common femoral arteries. The inferior epigastric artery arises medially from the distal external iliac artery and ascends behind the rectus abdominis muscle. This vessel is a useful landmark in predicting higher bleeding risk in arterial punctures proximal to its origin.[9] The external iliac artery gives off other branches; namely the deep circumflex, cremasteric, and several muscular and cutaneous branches, before it continues as the common femoral artery. Together the common iliac and external iliac arteries contribute to the inflow of the lower extremity. The common femoral artery starts as continuation of the external iliac artery, giving off multiple branches to surrounding tissues, such as the pudendal arteries and the superficial circumflex artery. Then, after giving rise to the arteria profunda femoris (roughly 3.5 cm distal to the inguinal ligament), it becomes the superficial femoral artery (SFA). The profunda femoris arises laterally and posteriorly from the common femoral artery while the SFA continues its pathway to end as the popliteal artery, when it passes through the abductor canal. The profunda gives off perforating branches (usually three, with the end of the profunda as the fourth perforating branch), the circumflex (lateral and medial) arteries, and muscular branches. The popliteal artery continues through the abductor's canal and, after giving off muscular, cutaneous, genicular and sural branches, terminates in the anterior tibial artery and the tibioperoneal trunk. The common femoral artery, the SFA, the profunda femoris, and the popliteal artery comprise the outflow of the lower extremity. The anterior tibial artery runs between the two heads of the tibialis posterior muscle; then it passes through the upper part of the interosseous membrane to the front of the leg, medial to the head of the fibula. It descends down to the ankle and then continues to the dorsum of the foot, where it becomes the dorsalis pedis artery. The posterior tibial artery arises from the popliteal artery distal to the origin of the anterior tibial artery as the tibioperoneal trunk. After giving rise to the peroneal artery, the tibioperoneal trunk continues as the posterior tibial artery behind the leg and passes behind the medial malleolus. It ends by giving rise to the arteries of the foot, namely the calcaneal, which anastomoses with

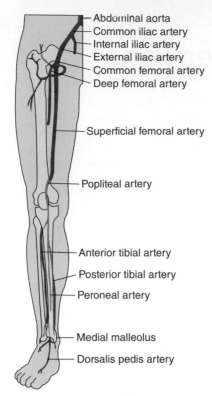

- Abdominal aorta
- Common iliac artery
- Internal iliac artery
- External iliac artery
- Common femoral artery
- Deep femoral artery
- Superficial femoral artery
- Popliteal artery
- Anterior tibial artery
- Posterior tibial artery
- Peroneal artery
- Medial malleolus
- Dorsalis pedis artery

Figure 37-1 Arterial tree of the lower extremity.

TABLE 37-1	Classification of Lower Extremity Peripheral Arterial Disease by Fontaine's Stages and Rutherford's Categories			
		Rutherford		
Stage	**Fontaine Clinical**	**GRADE**	**CATEGORY**	**Clinical**
I	Asymptomatic	0	0	Asymptomatic
IIa	Mild claudication	I	1	Mild claudication
IIb	Moderate-severe claudication	I	2	Moderate claudication
		I	3	Severe claudication
III	Ischemic rest pain	II	4	Ischemic rest pain
IV	Ulceration or gangrene	III	5	Minor tissue loss
		IV	6	Ulceration or gangrene

Reproduced with permission from Dormandy JA, Rutherford RB. Management of peripheral arterial disease (PAD). TASC Working Group. TransAtlantic Inter-Society Concensus (TASC). *J Vasc Surg.* 2000;31:S1–S296.

TABLE 37-2	Grading Lower Extremity PAD by ABI*	
	Supine Resting ABI	**Post-exercise ABI**
Normal	>1.0	>1.0
Mild	0.8–0.9	>0.4
Moderate	0.4–0.8	>0.2
Severe	<0.4	<0.2

*Post exercise ABIs are measured following treadmill exercise at 1 to 2 mph, 10% to 12% grade, for 5 minutes or symptom-limited.

Reprinted with permission Mukherjee D, Yadav JS. Update on peripheral vascular diseases: from smoking cessation to stenting. *Cleve Clin J Med.* 2001;68(8):723–733.

the calcaneal and malleolar branches of the peroneal, and the medial and lateral plantar arteries. The anterior tibial artery, posterior tibial artery, and the peroneal artery are considered the runoff vessels.

Diagnosis of Lower Extremity Peripheral Artery Disease

HISTORY AND PHYSICAL EXAMINATION

Patients with lower extremity PAD may be asymptomatic (detected during physical examination or screening tests) or may present with IC, rest pain, nonhealing ulcers, or intractable foot infections. In light of the limitations of clinical assessment in defining patients with asymptomatic PAD, additional assessment of patients with risk factors for atherosclerosis may be required in identifying those with asymptomatic advanced PAD. Symptomatic patients can be classified according to the severity of ischemia as based on either the Fontaine or Rutherford categories (Table 37-1).

Ankle-Brachial Index

Ankle-brachial index (ABI) is a ratio of the blood pressure in the dorsalis pedis or the posterior tibial artery (whichever is higher) to the blood pressure in the brachial arteries. ABI measurement is one of the most cost-effective methods in assessing PAD of the lower extremity and typically is done with a handheld Doppler ultrasound device. This is a noninvasive, fairly reproducible, inexpensive test. The most widely accepted definition of lower extremity PAD is a resting ABI of <0.9. This ABI is usually associated with a 50% or greater angiographic arterial stenosis with a reported sensitivity of 95% and close to 100% specificity.[7] A resting ABI of 0.4 to 0.9 is suggestive of mild to moderate PAD and an ABI of <0.4 is suggestive of severe PAD (Table 37-2). Resting ABI measurement can be artifactually high in the setting of the calcification of the tibial arteries that is usually seen in diabetic patients. In that setting the use of toe brachial index (TBI) may be used. A TBI of <0.7 is considered abnormal. The use of exercise ABI may be helpful

in equivocal cases. For this the patient walks on the treadmill at a constant speed of 1 to 2 miles per hour at a 10% to 12% incline for 5 minutes, or the exercise can be done with active pedal plantarflexion. A decrease of at least 15 mm Hg in the ankle systolic pressure following the exercise challenge is considered an abnormal test. Patients with no significant PAD are expected to have an increase or no change in their ankle systolic pressure.

Pulse Volume Recording

Plethysmography is used to detect volumetric changes in blood flow to the lower extremity; it is performed at various segments of the lower extremity with pressure cuffs inflated to 60 to 65 mm Hg. Normal tracing will have a rapid systolic upstroke and downstroke with a prominent dicrotic notch. This pattern changes as PAD develops and progresses, with a noted attenuation and widening of the arterial waveform. Ultimately, the waveform becomes flat (nonpulsatile) in patients with advanced PAD (Fig. 37-2).

Segmental Blood Pressure

For this test a series of blood pressure cuffs are placed at the level of the thigh (one or two cuffs), calf, ankle, foot, and big toe. These cuffs are then inflated sequentially to about 20 mm Hg above the systolic pressure in that segment. The cuff pressure is then released slowly and a continuous-wave Doppler probe is used to obtain the pressure at each segment. A decrease between two consecutive levels of 30 mm Hg or more indicates the presence of a stenosis in the segment proximal to the blood pressure cuff. Also the presence of a 20- to 30-mm Hg difference in the pressure at one limb as compared with the contralateral limb at the same level is suggestive of a significant PAD proximal to the cuff in that limb.

Duplex Ultrasonography

Duplex ultrasound uses a 5- to 7.5-MHz transducer to assess and characterize supra- and infrainguinal PAD with high sensitivity and

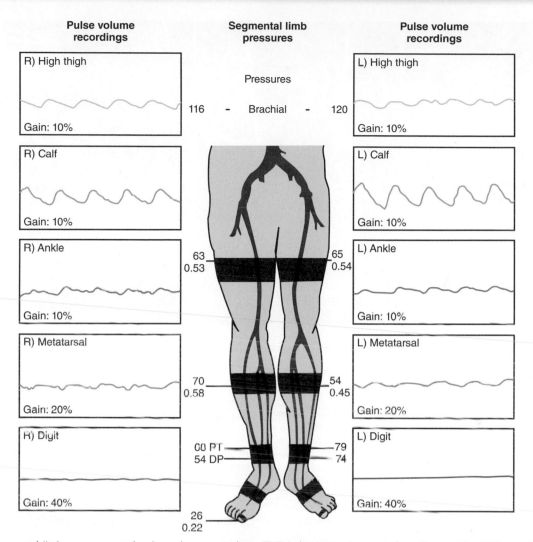

Figure 37-2 Segmental limb pressures and pulse volume recordings (PVRs) demonstrating aortoiliac disease. The PVR waveforms in the thigh segment are dampened and the segmental pressures in the thigh are decreased when compared with the brachial pressures. *(Reproduced with permission from Rajagopalan S, Mukherjee D, Mohler E. Manual of Vascular Diseases. Philadelphia, PA: Lippincott Williams & Wilkins, 2004.)*

specificity (over 90%). Doppler velocities are obtained (60-degree Doppler angle) to complement two-dimensional ultrasonography. Traditionally, arteries are classified on the basis of the degree of stenosis into five categories (normal; 1% to 19%, 20% to 49%, 50% to 99% stenoses; and total occlusions). Duplex ultrasonography may be useful to operators in planning access to a lesion that is amenable to endovascular therapy. It is also very helpful in identifying iatrogenic traumatic lesions and pseudoaneurysms. Direct ultrasound-guided compression or thrombin injection to repair femoral artery pseudoaneurysms is widely used in treating such lesions without the need for surgical procedures. One important limitation of duplex ultrasonography is that it may overestimate residual stenosis following interventions, thus limiting its usefulness as a follow-up tool in this setting.

Computed Tomography Angiography

The use of spiral CT angiography (CTA) in assessing lower extremity PAD has 93% sensitivity and 96% specificity in detecting >50% stenosis with high accuracy when compared with digital subtraction angiography. A recent systematic review and metanalysis suggested that CTA is highly accurate for assessment of PAD in all regions of the lower extremity arteries.[10] CTA correctly identified hemodynamically significant lesions and also accurately distinguished between >50% stenoses and occlusions. Some 94% of occlusions and 87% of nonoccluded segments with more than 50% stenosis detected by contrast angiography were correctly identified by CTA.[10] The accuracy of CTA may actually be even higher than reported in this study because all studies used contrast angiography as the reference standard but did not report whether biplanar views were used routinely. Because CTA reconstructions allow three-dimensional assessment, significant disease may be detected by CTA but not be recognized by angiography, which may lead to underestimation of specificity. CTA has advantages over magnetic resonance angiography (MRA) in the case of patients with pacemakers and defibrillators and in those with metal clips, stents, or prostheses (no significant artifact is seen in CTA as opposed to MRA) and is significantly faster to perform as compared with MRA. However, CTA requires the use of iodinated contrast and entails exposure to ionizing radiation. Dose-saving algorithms are very effective in reducing radiation exposure and should be used whenever possible.[11]

Magnetic Resonance Angiography

The use of gadolinium-enhanced MR angiography (GEMRA) (Fig. 37-3) in the assessment of lower extremity PAD has been compared with standard catheter angiography with a reported sensitivity and specificity of about 90% and 100%, respectively, for detecting stenosis >50%. Most contemporary studies report an agreement of 91% to 97% between MRA and catheter angiography. GEMRA is superior to duplex ultrasound in detecting >50% stenotic lesions (sensitivity of 98% vs. 88% and specificity of 96% vs. 95%).[7] Limitations of this technology

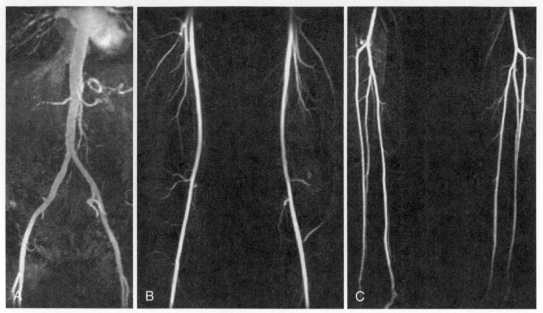

Figure 37-3 Maximal intensity projection images of a normal lower extremities runoff 3D contrast-enhanced MRA. *(Reproduced with permission from Rajagopalan S, Mukherjee D, Mohler E. Manual of Vascular Diseases. Philadelphia, PA: Lippincott Williams & Wilkins, 2004.)*

include the tendency to overestimate the severity of stenosis, metal clips may give the impression of total occlusion, and metal stents can also obscure vascular flow. In addition to these limitations, there are certain subset of patients who cannot be studied with MRA, such as those with pacemakers and defibrillators and those with certain types of cerebral aneurysm clips.[7] The principal role of MRA is in the initial evaluation for PAD, especially in patients with inflow disease, using "bolus chase" three-dimensional imaging, where a single bolus of contrast is followed to the foot.

Contrast Angiography

Despite recent advances in the noninvasive evaluation of lower extremity PAD, contrast angiography remains the gold standard. Traditionally, a pelvic/abdominal aortogram in the anteroposterior projection is done using a straight pigtail catheter (5 or 6 Fr) placed at the level of the L1-L2 vertebrae. Approximately 10 to 15 mL of iso-osmolar contrast is injected at a rate of 15 mL/s with digital subtraction angiography (DSA) technology. This provides an excellent view of the distal aorta and the origin of the common iliac arteries and the external iliac and common femoral arteries. Angulated views (LAO of 30 degrees) can then be used to visualize the iliac and femoral bifurcations without overlap. Then the pigtail catheter is placed above the aortic bifurcation (L3-L4) and digital subtraction with bolus chase, 8 mL/s for 10 seconds, is used to assess the outflow and distal runoff. Selective injections and sheath injections can then be used as needed to further define the territory of interest. "Roadmap" technology can be employed subsequently to help operators in their intervention and the placement of balloons and stents. Contrast angiography remains the most easily used and widely available imaging technique in patients with PAD of the lower extremity when revascularization is contemplated. Noninvasive technologies, such as MRA or CTA, may be used prior to contrast angiography to help identify the potential culprit lesion and plan the best approach to study such lesion (access point, catheter selection, etc.) invasively.[7] Contrast angiography may be associated with vascular access complications (bleeding, infections, pseudoaneurysms, and vascular disruption), atheroembolism, and contrast nephropathy as well as contrast-induced anaphylactoid reactions. These complications, although rare, should be considered in the decision-making process with regard to the assessment of PAD.

Interventions

Percutaneous or surgical interventions are indicated for severe lifestyle-limiting symptoms, to reduce tissue breakdown in the context of critical limb ischemia, or for salvage in the context of acute limb ischemia.

ILIAC ARTERY INTERVENTION (INFLOW DISEASE)

Indications

The indications for iliac artery (or aortoiliac) percutaneous intervention include symptom relief in patients with IC who have failed medical therapy, management of critical limb ischemia (rest pain, ulceration, or gangrene), prior to planned distal lower extremity bypass surgery to restore or to preserve the inflow to the lower extremity, or in preparation for other invasive procedures such as the placement of an intra-aortic balloon pump and the treatment of flow-limiting dissections following invasive catheterization-based procedures.

Revascularization Options

Occlusive disease confined to the iliac arteries appears to occur in relatively young patients and may therefore have a greater impact on productivity and lifestyle. For instance, the mean age of the cohort in the Dutch Iliac Stent Trial was approximately 59 years.[12] These patients (>90% were smokers) were otherwise healthy compared with those with infrainguinal disease or more diffuse PAD. In general, any type of revascularization for this subset of patients can offer satisfactory long-term results. Historically, aortobifemoral bypass surgery has been the gold standard for PAD involving the iliac arteries, as this procedure is associated with excellent long-term patency rates (85%–90% at 5 years, 75%–80% at 10 years, and 60% at 20 years); however, it may be associated with an intraoperative mortality of roughly 1% to 3%, and a major complication rate of 5% to 10%. This, combined with the excellent intermediate to long-term patency rates following percutaneous intervention, has led to the emergence of percutaneous revascularization as an attractive alternative to surgery in patients with suitable lesions for such intervention. In the Swedish randomized controlled trial, where 37% of randomized patients had iliac artery stenosis, there

TABLE 37-3	Recommendations of the TransAtlantic Inter-Society Consensus (TASC) Working Group for the Revascularization Strategy of Aortoiliac Femoropopliteal Lesions*	
Type	**Iliac Disease**	**Femoral Lesions**
TASC A	Single <3 cm of CIA or EIA (unilateral/bilateral)	Single <3 cm in length, not involving SFA or popliteal
TASC B	1. Single 3–10 cm, not extending into the CFA 2. Two stenoses <5 cm long in CIA and/or EIA not extending to CFA 3. Unilateral CIA occlusion	1. Single stenoses or occlusion 3–5 cm long, not involving the distal popliteal artery 2. Heavily calcified ≤3 cm or multiple stenoses or occlusions, each <3 cm 3. Single or multiple lesions in the absence of continuous tibial runoff
TASC C	1. Bilateral 5–10 cm stenosis of CIA and/or EIA, not extending to CFA 2. Unilateral EIA occlusion or stenosis not extending into the CFA 3. Bilateral CIA occlusion	1. Single stenosis/occlusion >5 cm 2. Multiple stenoses or occlusions 3–5 cm, with or without heavy calcification
TASC D	1. >10 cm lesions or diffuse, multiple unilateral stenoses involving the CIA, EIA, and CFA 2. Unilateral occlusion involving both the CIA and EIA 3. Bilateral EIA occlusions 4. Diffuse disease involving the aorta and both iliac arteries or lesions in a patient requiring aortic or iliac surgery (AAA)	Complete CFA or SFA occlusions

CIA, Common iliac artery; EIA, external iliac artery; SFA, superficial femoral artery; CFA, common femoral artery; AAA, abdominal aortic aneurysm.

*Endovascular procedure is the treatment of choice for type A; surgery is the procedure of choice for type D. At present, endovascular treatment is more commonly used in type B lesions, and surgical treatment is more commonly used in type C lesions.

Reproduced with permission from Dormandy JA and Rutherford RB, Management of peripheral arterial disease (PAD), TASC Working Group. TransAtlantic Inter-Society Consensus (TASC). *J Vasc Surg.* 2000;31:S1 S296.

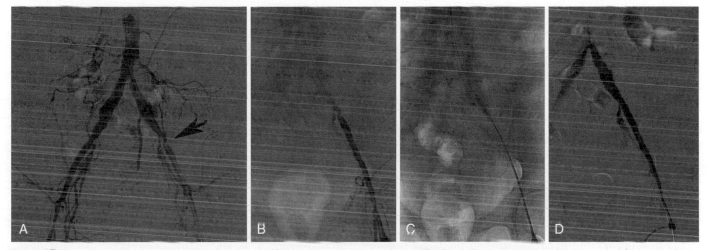

Figure 37-4 Left external iliac artery intervention. A. Abdominal aortogram with runoffs where the lesion is noted (arrow). B. Using an ipsilateral approach, the lesion is crossed with a guidewire. C. Angioplasty is done. D. Successful final result with resolution of the obstructive lesion and no flow-limiting dissection or significant elastic recoil.

was equivalence in outcomes between percutaneous transluminal angioplasty (PTA) and surgery.[13] In the iliac disease subgroup, the patency rate at one year was 90% in the PTA arm versus 94% in the surgical arm. Table 37-3 summarizes the strategy recommended by the Trans-Atlantic Inter-Society Consensus (TASC) working group for the revascularization of iliac lesions.

Techniques

ACCESS AND RECANALIZATION TECHNIQUES

In patients with unilateral stenotic iliac lesions that do not involve the common femoral artery (CFA), ipsilateral access through the CFA with retrograde PTA is usually preferred as it provides direct access to the diseased segment as well as a coaxial alignment of the equipment (Fig. 37-4A to D). Contralateral access with the use of a crossover sheath is reserved for patients with disease involving the ipsilateral CFA (Fig. 37-5A to D), if there are plans to intervene on more distal lesions in the same limb, or if there is concern about jeopardizing the flow to the

affected limb by placement of the sheath in the ipsilateral CFA. Various crossover sheaths are available; the ArrowFlex (Arrow International, Reading, PA) sheath is a more flexible sheath, which can be helpful in crossing over acute aortic bifurcation angles but provides less support as opposed to the RAABE and Balkin sheaths (both from Cook Inc., Bloomington, IN), which provide more support but are less compliant. If the iliac artery is occluded, either or both approaches may be needed. For lesions of the aortic bifurcation, the optimal approach is a bilateral retrograde one with the placement of kissing balloons and subsequently kissing stents.

In lesions distal to the aortic bifurcation (in the body of the common iliac artery or the external iliac artery), PTA is attempted and, if satisfactory results are achieved (less than 5 mm Hg residual gradient and less than 30% residual stenosis with no flow-limiting dissection), stenting may not be indicated. However, ostial lesions of the common iliac arteries (i.e., aortoiliac bifurcation lesions) are preferably stented with kissing stents. In general, 0.035-in. guidewires are used in PTA and stenting of the iliac arteries, but 0.018- or 0.014-inch guidewires may be used as well. In nonocclusive lesions regular nonhydrophilic

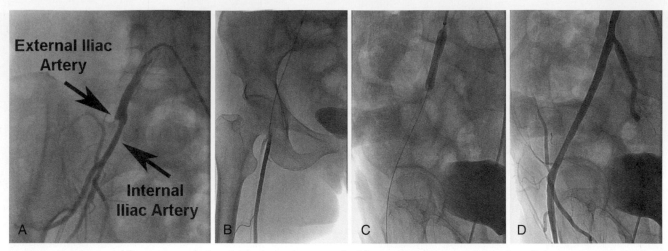

Figure 37-5 Ostial external iliac artery occlusion. A. The lesion is approached from a contralateral access point utilizing a crossover sheath. B. The lesion is crossed with a hydrophilic guidewire and a balloon is placed at the level of the noted distal external iliac artery lesion; angioplasty is then done. C. The first stent deployed and a second, more proximal stent is placed. D. Final result after stent placement.

guidewire can be used; however, if crossing such lesions is difficult, then the use of hydrophilic wires is indicated.

Stent Choice

Both balloon-expandable and self-expandable stents can be used in aortoiliac disease. The balloon-expandable stent is advantageous in the context of lesions of the aortic bifurcation, where kissing stents are usually placed. It is also superior to self-expandable stents when precision in stent placement is needed. The self-expanding stent will provide flexibility in flexion points, reducing the risk of stent deformity and fracture, and is ideal in the setting of lesions of the common iliac artery not involving the ostium and lesions of the external iliac artery.

Clinical Data

Percutaneous revascularization in the management of patients with IC secondary to iliofemoral disease (specifically PTA without stenting) has been compared with conservative management (specifically with exercise training, smoking cessation counseling, and antiplatelet therapy with aspirin). The results revealed two important findings: first that PTA can effectively alleviate patients' symptoms and improve treadmill distance and ABI during a short-term follow-up period, but these benefits are mostly lost by 2 years. The second observation was that although PTA improves perfusion to the feet, which may confer protection particularly for populations at higher risk for limb loss, such as diabetics, supervised exercise improves functional outcome and also enhances global conditioning. These two strategies should therefore be considered complementary because they address different but interrelated issues.[14-16] Overall, for iliofemoral lesions, the clinical results of percutaneous revascularization are generally comparable with those of surgical bypass or reconstruction. The Swedish trial randomized patients with threatened limb loss (40% with rest pain or gangrene) or claudication who had not improved with exercise training (60%) to either PTA or surgical revascularization.[17] The study population had a mean age of 70 years, a 26% prevalence of diabetes, and average symptom duration of 18 months. There were no differences between the PTA or surgery treatment groups with regard to 1-year primary and secondary patency rates, which were 61% and approximately 72%, respectively. The complications rates were not statistically different between treatment groups, although most of the adverse events involved patients who presented with rest pain or gangrene, highlighting the impact of baseline limb status on subsequent outcomes. Adverse events included a 1-year death rate of ~10% and a reocclusion rate of 5%

(both treatment groups), a major amputation rate of 5.7% versus 16%, and a hematoma rate of 7.5% versus 4.1% (PTA vs. surgery, respectively). The infection and embolization rates were 8.2% each and seen only in the surgical group and not with PTA. These findings were corroborated by the Veterans Administration (VA) Cooperative study, which randomized 255 male patients with iliac or femoropopliteal disease and claudication or rest pain. To be eligible, patients needed to be suitable for either PTA or surgery, which may have resulted in a case mix with less diffuse disease compared with the typical vascular surgery population.[18] The average age was 61.5 years, 29% had diabetes, 20% had a history of MI, more than a quarter had previous surgery or PTA for PAD, and 99% were current or previous smokers (~48 pack-years each). There were three study-related deaths, all in the surgery group ($n = 126$). There were no deaths among the 129 patients randomized to PTA but there were 20 (15.4%) procedural failures: inability to cross the lesion with wire in 7.8%, inability to dilate the lesion in 2.3%, thrombosis within 24 hours in 3.9%, and no hemodynamic improvement after PTA in 1.6%. No stents were available for this trial. Seventeen of the failed PTA patients subsequently underwent successful surgical revascularization. At a median follow-up of 2 years there was no statistically significant difference between the PTA and surgery groups with regard to death and major amputations. This pattern of equivalent outcome held true at 4 years' follow-up. However, the 2-year target-limb repeat revascularization rate was higher after PTA compared with surgery.[14] In a review of the available literature between 1989 and 1997, Bosch et al., in their metanalysis of 6 studies including 2,116 patients with IC secondary to aortoiliac disease, reported greater technical success with stenting, with no difference in complication rates and 30-day mortality rates.[19] The severity-adjusted primary patency rates were 65% for PTA versus 77% with stenting for stenotic lesions and 54% for PTA versus 61% with stenting for occlusions.

A strategy of primary stenting as opposed to provisional stenting is generally recommended for aorto-ostial lesions. While an equivalent outcome between primary versus provisional stenting was reported in the Dutch Iliac Stent Trial, only 57% of patients randomized to PTA did not require stenting.[20] In comparison, a strategy of routine implantation of the same stent (Palmaz balloon-expandable) gave results that were superior to PTA in a randomized controlled trial of 185 patients by Richter and colleagues.[21] The authors reported a 4-year patency rate of 94% in the stent arm versus 69% with PTA. Cumulative clinical success, defined as improvement of clinical stage of one level or more, was 89% for stenting and 67% PTA, respectively. Major periprocedural complications were noted in 4 patients in the stent group as opposed to 3 in the PTA group (3.7% overall). These findings were confirmed in the metanalysis by Bosch, as stenting offered a superior technical success rate and long-term patency compared with PTA in occluded arteries.[19] The use of two different self-expanding stents, the stainless steel WALLSTENT (Boston Scientific, Plymouth, MA) and the nitinol SMART stent (Cordis Endovascular, Warren, NJ) for the treatment of iliac artery lesions was compared in a multicenter prospective randomized trial.[22] The acute procedural success was higher with the SMART stent (98.2%, vs. 87.5% with the WALLSTENT; $P = 0.002$). The patency rate, at 1 year was similar for both stents (91.1% for the WALLSTENT and 94.7% with the SMART stent), with similar complication rates (5.9% vs. 5.9%, respectively; $P = NS$). Overall, it is fair to say that technical and clinical success rates of endovascular interventions for iliac artery stenosis exceed 90% (approaching almost 100% in focal iliac lesions), with a fairly comparable intermediate and long-term patency versus that of surgical revascularization. Factors that negatively affect the long-term patency for either modality are the quality of the distal runoff vessels, the severity of ischemia, and the length of the diseased segment.[23,24] Female gender has been associated with decreased patency following the placement of external iliac stents.[25] Technical success is commonly defined as <30% residual stenosis (anatomical success), a postintervention mean across the lesion gradient of ≤5 mm Hg, and an increase in the ABI of >0.1 and/or a decrease in symptoms by one category (hemodynamic success). Another criterion that has been suggested (clinical success) is an improvement of at least one category of symptoms.[26]

Complications and Their Management

Complications rates are generally low in aortoiliac interventions. These include access-site complications (such as groin hematoma, retroperitoneal bleed, pseudoaneurysm, and arteriovenous fistula formation), thrombosis at the site of PTA, arterial rupture, and distal embolization. These complications happen at a rate of <5% to 6% in most series.[27] Death, contrast-induced nephropathy, myocardial infarction, and cerebrovascular accident occurred at a rate of <0.5%. The need for urgent vascular repair is reported to be around 2%. With regard to serious complications, rupture (particularly of the external iliac artery) seems to be reported more frequently with the iliac arteries than with percutaneous interventions in other lower extremity arteries.[27,28]

When to Refer to Surgery

Surgery is usually reserved for patients with diffuse disease or those with long total occlusions. It is also the appropriate approach in those with associated infrarenal aortic aneurysms. Table 37-3 summarizes the recommendations of the TASC working group for the revascularization strategy of iliac lesions.

FEMOROPOPLITEAL INTERVENTION (OUTFLOW DISEASE)

While controversial, many believe that revascularization of the common femoral artery (CFA) should be done surgically. Concerns about elastic recoil and dissection following PTA and about the mechanical compression of stents and acute stent thrombosis have limited endovascular intervention to this territory. PTA has been used in case of severe fibrotic lesions following previous surgery.

The superficial femoral artery (SFA) and the proximal popliteal artery are the most common anatomical sites of stenosis and occlusion in patients with IC. It is estimated that slightly more than a quarter of diseased SFAs progress over a 3-year period and 17% may go on to occlusion. Predictors of progression are continued smoking, worsening symptoms, and the presence of an already occluded contralateral SFA.[25] For patients who have disease confined to the SFA, a supervised exercise program might offer a functional outcome that is equivalent or even superior to percutaneous revascularization. This could be due to preserved iliac inflow and profunda femoris artery, which is a common

and important source of collaterals for patients with SFA stenoses or occlusion. Surgery remains the gold standard when therapy is indicated, because primary femoropopliteal graft patency rates of about 80% at 5 years have been documented.[25] Continued improvements in technology, including metal alloys with shape memory and superelastic properties and stents coated with antiproliferative agents, are helping to surmount the problem of poor long-term durability, which is currently the main limitation of endovascular techniques. Femoropopliteal angioplasty can be considered for discrete single lesions <10 cm, <5 cm for calcified stenosis, or <3 cm for multiple lesions as long as the SFA origin or distal popliteal artery is not involved. Endovascular treatment of longer SFA lesions is more controversial. Factors that have been found to adversely affect long-term patency are critical limb ischemia (gangrene or rest pain), multiple stenoses, diffuse disease, and poor distal runoff.[29,30]

Indications

The low morbidity and mortality of endovascular intervention makes this strategy the preferred choice in patients with suitable lesions (Table 37-3). It is an appropriate option in the management of symptomatic patients with femoropopliteal lesions (1) that are <10 cm in length (unilateral or bilateral), (2) that involve multiple stenoses or occlusions <5 cm in size (excluding the trifurcation), (3) that involve a single stenosis <15 cm (excluding the trifurcation), and (4) with no continuous tibial runoffs in order to improve inflow for surgical bypass prior to surgery.

Techniques

Common Femoral Artery. Access to the common femoral artery (CFA) is usually obtained via the contralateral femoral artery (with a crossover sheath) or via the brachial artery. Lesions involving the bifurcation of the CFA represent a challenging problem; sometimes kissing balloons are needed to achieve a desirable angiographic outcome.

Stents have historically not been recommended, but now the use of self-expanding nitinol stents is gaining popularity among some interventionalists. Stents are routinely used in salvage situations, with the flexible self-expanding stent being the appropriate choice in this vessel. Stenting however, poses many concerns, as stent compression or fracture can occur and may render future surgical repair more complicated. It is important to point out that while restenosis rates are high in the CFA (>50%), restenosis may be associated with less limiting symptoms in patients who needed the PTA for persistent or critical symptoms.

Profunda Femoris Artery

Revascularization of the profunda femoris artery (PFA) may be needed in the setting of total occlusion of the SFA or of a femoropopliteal bypass graft, as this vessel plays an important role as a source of collaterals to the lower extremity. Surgery is the preferred strategy in this vessel; however, PTA may be tried in the setting of severe limb-threatening ischemia when surgery is contraindicated or if the disease involves the distal portion of the descending branch of the PFA, which is less accessible to the surgeons. Access via the contralateral femoral artery (with a crossover sheath) or from the brachial artery can be used. These interventions are usually done in the context of limb-threatening ischemia; thus it is important to emphasize that a rather conservative approach with regard to balloon sizing is used in this setting, especially with no available data regarding the placement of stents in the PFA. Stents are used provisionally in the context of flow-limiting dissections or severe residual lesions.

Superficial Femoral Artery

There are four possible approaches to accessing the superficial femoral artery (SFA). The lesion can be approached through a contralateral femoral artery (with a crossover sheath), an ipsilateral antegrade common femoral approach, a retrograde popliteal approach, or a brachial artery approach. By accessing the contralateral CFA and then

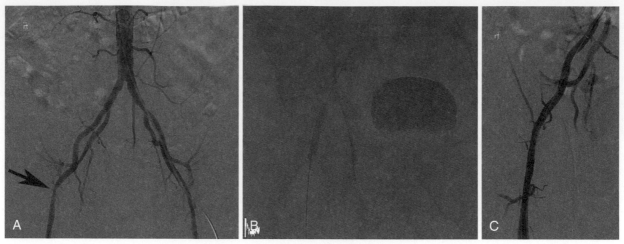

Figure 37-6   Right SFA intervention. A. Abdominal aortogram revealing the right SFA lesion (arrow). B. The lesion is crossed and angioplasty is done using a contralateral access point. C. Successful PTA result with no significant residual lesion or flow-limiting dissection.

using a curved catheter (such as the internal mammary [IM], Judkins right, Cobra, or a Simmons catheter) to engage the ostium of the common iliac artery of the diseased limb, a kink-resistant long sheath (the Balkin, RAABE, or ArrowFlex) is placed. The contralateral approach is more popular, as it provides excellent support and helps in accessing other segments (iliac or infrainguinal vessels) on the same limb. The antegrade CFA access, which is relatively more challenging than the retrograde approach, is also widely used. The antegrade brachial approach might be the only viable option in patients with bilateral iliofemoral disease. The popliteal approach is the least used, as it is associated with a higher risk of complications due to the smaller size of the popliteal artery and the nearby vital structures that may be injured and is uncomfortable for the patient. In general, familiarity with all different approaches is necessary, as the underlying anatomy of each patient will determine the most feasible vascular access point. Figure 37-6A to C shows an example of an SFA intervention.

Stent Choice. Stenting as a primary approach for femoropopliteal lesions is typically not indicated. Stenting is usually indicated as a salvage procedure following complicated PTA (flow-limiting dissection or thrombosis), as primary stenting has not been shown to be superior to PTA only with bailout stenting.[31] If stenting is indicated, self-expanding nitinol stents are generally used in SFA lesions in light of the high risk of stent compression and fracture. One small randomized study of 104 patients suggested that the treatment of SFA disease by primary implantation of a self-expanding nitinol stent yielded results superior to those with the currently recommended approach of balloon angioplasty with optional secondary stenting at 6 to 12 months.[32] Another study in 73 patients confirmed that primary stenting with a self-expanding nitinol stent for treatment of intermediate-length SFA disease resulted in morphologically and clinically superior midterm results compared with balloon angioplasty with optional secondary stenting.[33] However, in a metanalysis of 934 patients, Mwipatayi et al. concluded that stent placement in femoropopliteal occlusive disease does not increase the patency rate compared with PTA alone at 1 year.[34] The use of sirolimus-eluting SMART stents for SFA occlusion was evaluated in the SIROCCO II (Sirolimus-Eluting versus Bare Nitinol Stent for Obstructive Superficial Femoral Artery Disease) study; compared with bare metal stents, no significant differences in clinical outcome were found.[35] Stent/strut fractures were reported in about 8% of patients in both arms of the study. The coated stent proved to be safe and was not associated with any serious adverse events compared with noncoated stents. The IntraCoil Self-Expanding Peripheral Stent (Sulzer IntraTerapeutics, St. Paul, MN), LifeStent

FlexStar stent (Bard Peripheral Vascular, Inc., Tempe, AZ), and Zilver Vascular Stent (Cook, Medical, Bloomington, IN) are examples of FDA-approved stents for use in the femoral and peripheral arteries.

Specific Techniques (Laser, Atherectomy, Silver Hawk, etc.). While anecdotal experiences and reported case series have suggested some benefits, the use of directional atherectomy and laser angioplasty has not been shown to offer any clear advantage over PTA in femoropopliteal PAD.[36,37] A prospective database of 275 patients suggested that the SilverHawk device (Fox Hollow Technologies Inc., Redwood City, CA) was an effective endovascular therapy for peripheral arterial intervention with a low mortality, low complication rate, low amputation rate, and rare need for conversion to surgical bypass.[38] Atherectomy devices may be particularly useful for ostial SFA bifurcation lesions (Fig. 37-7A to D) and calcified lesions.

Clinical Data

Randomized controlled trials in patients with IC and femoropopliteal disease have compared medical therapy with PTA and have consistently revealed that PTA offers superior early symptomatic relief at 3 to 6 months; outcomes were similar at 2 years.[37,39] Clinical acute success rates of PTA of femoropopliteal disease in the contemporary era exceed 95%.[31] Contemporary endovascular approaches that include stenting offer acute technical success rates of up to 99%; short- to medium-term patency rates are superior to PTA alone.[32] The mid- to long-term data on endovascular interventions in patients with IC or critical limb ischemia and femoropopliteal disease are summarized in Tables 37-4 and 37-5.

The advantage of placing a sent in the SFA is that it limits elastic recoil, scaffolds flow-limiting dissection, and provides better acute technical support. However, these advantages are counterbalanced by a stent-induced enhanced endothelial hyperplasic response that may result in in-stent restenosis and negate the noted advantages of stenting on long-term follow up. Restenosis following endovascular interventions depends on the severity of the disease (total occlusion vs. patent vessel with a high-grade lesion), the status of the distal runoffs, and the length of the lesion. Whether different stent material and/or drug elution with antiproliferative agents can result in improved outcomes remains to be seen. Restenosis remains a limiting factor in achieving optimal intermediate- to long-term patency. The use of brachytherapy in treating in stent restenosis (ISR) resulted in a 50% reduction in the rate of restenosis with no noted increased risk in late thrombosis. The use of sirolimus-eluting stents was not associated with superior results when compared with bare metal stents.[35] Nitinol (an alloy of nickel

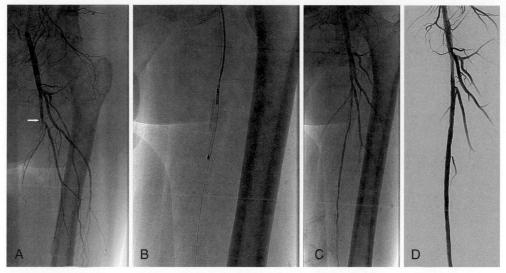

Figure 37-7 SFA ostial bifurcation lesion. A. Angiogram revealing the right SFA ostial occlusion (arrow). B. The lesion is crossed and atherectomy is done using a contralateral access point. C. PTA result with significant residual lesion. D. Stenting performed with no residual stenosis and normal flow noted in the profunda femoris.

TABLE 37-4	Estimated Pooled Primary Patency Rates following Balloon Dilatation and following Stent Implantation in Patients with Intermittent Claudication Secondary to Femoropopliteal Stenoses				
		Balloon Dilation		**Stent Implantation**	
Lesion Type	*Year after Treatment*	PATENCY (%)*	RANGE (%)	PATENCY (%)*	RANGE (%)
Stenosis	0	100 (1.0)	98–100	100 (1.2)	99–100
	1	77 (1.7)	78–80	75 (2.2)	73–79
	2	66 (2.0)	63–71	67 (2.4)	65–71
	3	61 (2.2)	55–68	66 (2.7)	64–70
	4	57 (2.5)	54–63	NA	NA
	5	55 (2.8)	52–62	NA	NA
Occlusion	0	88 (2.9)	81–94	99 (2.3)	92–100
	1	65 (3.0)	55–71	73 (2.8)	69–75
	2	54 (3.1)	45–61	66 (3.0)	61–68
	3	48 (3.3)	40–55	64 (3.2)	59–67
	4	44 (3.5)	36–53	NA	NA
	5	42 (3.7)	33–51	NA	NA

*Numbers in parentheses represent the standard error. NA, not available.
Ranges are derived from sensitivity analyses.
Reproduced with permission from Muradin GS et al., Balloon dilation and stent implantation for treatment of femoropopliteal arterial disease: meta-analysis. *Radiology.* 2001;221(1):137–145.

TABLE 37-5	Estimated Pooled Primary Patency Rates following Balloon Dilatation and following Stent Implantation in Patients with Critical Limb Ischemia Secondary to Femoropopliteal Stenoses				
		Balloon Dilation		**Stent Implantation**	
Lesion Type	*Year after Treatment*	PATENCY (%)*	RANGE (%)	PATENCY (%)*	RANGE (%)
Stenosis	0	83 (3.7)	69–88	100 (3.3)	94–100
	1	60 (4.0)	46–63	74 (3.8)	68–80
	2	49 (4.0)	35–54	66 (3.9)	59–72
	3	43 (4.1)	30–51	65 (4.1)	58–71
	4	40 (4.3)	26–46	NA	NA
	5	38 (4.5)	24–44	NA	NA
Occlusion	0	70 (3.5)	62–75	98 (3.2)	94–100
	1	47 (3.5)	41–51	73 (3.6)	68–75
	2	36 (3.6)	28–41	65 (3.7)	60–68
	3	30 (3.7)	20–37	63 (3.9)	58–68
	4	27 (3.9)	16–34	NA	NA
	5	25 (4.1)	13–32	NA	NA

*Numbers in parentheses represent the standard error. NA, not available.
Ranges are derived from sensitivity analyses.
Reproduced with permission from Muradin GS et al., Balloon dilation and stent implantation for treatment of femoropopliteal arterial disease: meta-analysis. *Radiology.* 2001;221(1):137–145.

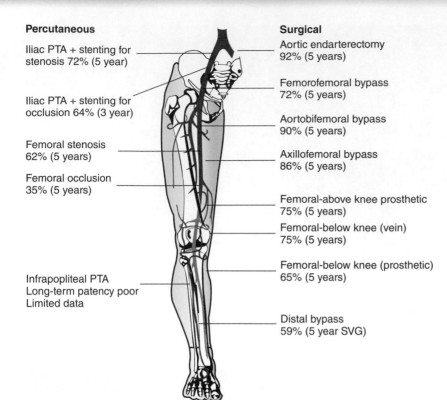

Percutaneous

Iliac PTA + stenting for
stenosis 72% (5 year)

Iliac PTA + stenting for
occlusion 64% (3 year)

Femoral stenosis
62% (5 years)

Femoral occlusion
35% (5 years)

Infrapopliteal PTA
Long-term patency poor
Limited data

Surgical

Aortic endarterectomy
92% (5 years)

Femorofemoral bypass
72% (5 years)

Aortobifemoral bypass
90% (5 years)

Axillofemoral bypass
86% (5 years)

Femoral-above knee prosthetic
75% (5 years)

Femoral-below knee (vein)
75% (5 years)

Femoral-below knee (prosthetic)
65% (5 years)

Distal bypass
59% (5 year SVG)

Figure 37-8   Patency rates for percutaneous and bypass procedures in intermittent claudication. *(Data adapted from TASC recommendation.)*

and titanium) is flexible and more likely to recover from being crushed as compared with stainless steel. A small single-center clinical trial compared the use of a self-expanding nitinol stent versus PTA with optional stenting (with 32% receiving stents in this arm) in symptomatic (severe IC or chronic limb ischemia) SFA disease. Here the use of stents was associated with a lower rate of angiographic restenosis at 6 months (24% vs. 43%, $P = 0.05$) and improved treadmill time at 6 to 12 months. This study is limited by its small size and short-term follow-up.[32] Figure 37-8 lists the overall success and patency rates of PTA (with and without stenting) versus surgery in all claudicants. There are limited randomized controlled trials comparing PTA versus surgery in the management of infrainguinal PAD. This is partly because the choice of revascularization modality will depend on the extent of disease in individual patients, with surgery being the most likely treatment in the setting of extensive long lesions and critical limb ischemia. In a multicenter randomized controlled trial of 263 men, Wolf et al. reported three operative deaths in the surgical arm ($n = 126$) and none in the PTA arm ($n = 129$). No difference in survival was noted, although there was a trend in favor of the PTA arm. While patients in both arms had sustained improvement in their hemodynamics and quality of life, there was higher reported success rate in the surgical arm and more limb salvage than in the PTA arm. No differences were reported in clinical outcome on median follow-up of 4 years.[14] In a small randomized trial, a 1-year patency rate of 43% in the PTA arm ($n = 30$) versus 82% in the surgical arm ($n = 24$) was reported.[40]

Complications and Their Management

Dissection, perforation, and distal embolization are the complications often encountered in femoropopliteal interventions. While the use of stenting is discouraged as a primary strategy, its use as a bailout strategy in the context of flow-limiting dissections and perforations is well established. The appropriate use of anticoagulation and antiplatelet therapy to safeguard against acute and subacute thrombosis may limit the incidence and the consequences of distal embolization.

When to Refer to Surgery

While somewhat controversial, surgery remains the preferred strategy for patients with common femoral and proximal profunda femoris obstructive PAD. It is also the preferred strategy for patients with heavily calcified or completely occluded common femoral arteries, femoropopliteal calcified stenosis, occlusions that are more than 15 cm in length, total occlusions (TOs) of the SFA that are more than 20 cm in length, and TOs of the popliteal artery or the proximal trifurcation.[1,7] It is important to point out that a strategy of initial PTA in lieu of surgery in selected patients is reasonable.[17]

INFRAPOPLITEAL PERIPHERAL ARTERIAL DISEASE (RUNOFF DISEASE)

Indications

Despite the fact that the first cases of endovascular interventions in the management of infrapopliteal PAD were reported in 1964 by Dotter and Judkins, endovascular therapy has had a limited role in the management of infrapopliteal PAD. In patients with IC secondary to infrapopliteal PAD, medical therapy is the most appropriate initial strategy.[7] Tibioperoneal angioplasty is limited by recurrence and also the need for highly skilled operators, since the need for emergency surgical bailout is associated with considerable risk that cannot be justified in patients with stable IC, especially when medical management is known to produce a similar outcome with limited risk.[1] However, in carefully selected patients and in the hands of experienced operators, an acute success rate of 95% (98% for stenoses, 86% for total occlusion [TO]) with a <1% rate of significant complications can be achieved.[24,41-43] The role of angioplasty in patients with critical leg ischemia (CLI) is more promising and justified since the results are comparable if not superior to those of infrapopliteal/tibial bypass surgery.[43] Endovascular techniques can thus be used as a primary therapy or as an adjunctive therapy to bypass surgery to improve inflow in diseased segments or to improve outflow. Up to a quarter of patients with CLI have lesions isolated to arteries below the knee, and they occur mostly in those with diabetes and other comorbid conditions. Historically the main concerns with regard to endovascular interventions of the infrapopliteal vessels were long-term patency, complications, or technical failure. With improved equipment, appropriate patient selection, and a meticulous technical approach, acute success rates >90% and 5-year limb salvage rates of close to 90% are now possible on a more consistent basis, particularly in the context of a comprehensive strategy that includes medical, endovascular. and surgical modalities as well as long-term lesion surveillance.[41]

Techniques

Access and Recanalization Techniques and Devices. Antegrade ipsilateral femoral access is usually used for infrapopliteal interventions. The advantages of such access include a straight-line approach to the lesion; it also allows a shorter length of catheter or balloon shaft, more torque control, and superior mechanical advantage and "pushability" for occlusions or lesions that are difficult to cross. This approach requires experience to minimize complications at the access site. If combined below- and above-knee PTA is necessary, angioplasty of the tibioperoneal arteries initially might lower the risk of peripheral embolization. In the Uppsala series, 6 of the initial 40 procedures had embolization that required either transcatheter embolectomy or local streptokinase infusion. After the practice was altered to performing distal prior to more proximal lower limb angioplasty, no embolization was seen in the subsequent 54 procedures. Because occlusion of these end arteries jeopardizes the foot and leaves no surgical bailout options, the characteristics of reported successful series must be carefully considered. In Dorros and colleagues' series, tibioperoneal lesions had to be less than 10 cm length, and distal vessels were visualized. Occlusions were less successfully opened than stenoses (73% vs. 98%). A residual stenosis of up to 50% was acceptable for these relatively small vessels. Complete multivessel revascularization may not be necessary, especially when a significant improvement in ABI is already documented. If angioplasty results in straight-line flow to the foot, clinical success rates of up to 80% at 24 months have been reported. Conversely, the lack of straight-line flow portends failure within 11 months. Vasospasm usually abates with intra-arterial nitroglycerin or verapamil.

Stent Choice. Stents are not recommended in the management of infrapopliteal disease; however, stent placement may be used as a bailout in the context of flow-limiting dissections. The PADI (Percutaneous transluminal Angioplasty and Drug eluting stents for Infrapopliteal lesions in critical limb ischemia) trial is a prospective, multicenter, randomized, controlled, double-arm study investigating the safety and efficacy of primary paclitaxel-eluting stent implantation versus PTA in infrapopliteal lesions in critical limb ischemia (CLI); it is expected to report results in mid 2012.[44]

Specific Techniques. Previous case series of the use of atherectomy in treatment of tibial lesions have had dismal results.[45] Zeller et al. reported that below-knee native vessel lesions with a diameter of at least 2.0 mm can be treated with the Silverhawk catheter with a high success rate and a low complication rate.[46] Orbital atherectomy was recently tested as a unique approach to infrapopliteal disease and provided predictable and safe luminal enlargement.[47] Short-term data demonstrated substantial symptomatic improvement and an infrequent need for further revascularization or amputation, but additional studies are needed.

Clinical Data. Despite advances in aggressive revascularization techniques, the mortality and morbidity rates for this cohort of patients have remained substantial, with 30-day mortality rates of around 4% to 10%, an amputation rate of 6% to 14%, and 90-day graft failure rates of close to 5%.[48] The 5-year patency rate for femoral below-knee bypass is about 75% (vein graft) to 60% (prosthetic grafts),

while for distal bypass it is about 50%.[1] An important contributor to these poor outcomes is the substantial disease burden in this cohort of patients, who have a preponderance of CAD, diabetes mellitus, and baseline tissue loss (foot ulcer, gangrene, or nonhealing wound).[1,48,49] There are no randomized controlled trials comparing strategies for the treatment of below-knee arterial occlusive disease. Dorros and colleagues reported the largest prospective series of infrapopliteal angioplasties on 284 limbs with critical limb ischemia (Fontaine stages III and IV) in 235 patients between 1983 and 1996.[49] The mean age was 67 years, 69% were males, half had diabetes, more than a quarter had previous myocardial infarction, a third had prior coronary artery bypass surgery, and 39% had prior peripheral vascular surgery. The overall acute technical success rate was 100% for inflow lesions and 92% for infrapopliteal lesions. The success rate was 98% for stenoses but only 73% for occlusions. Complications were infrequent: 0.7% in-hospital all-cause mortality, 0.7% emergency vascular surgery, 9% in-hospital major amputation, and 0.4%—or one case each—compartment syndrome, major infection, and transfusion. In a more contemporary series ($n = 60$) involving older (mean age 72 years) and sicker patients (more than three-fourths had diabetes, almost one-quarter had baseline renal insufficiency, 90% presented with minor [81%] or major [9.7%] tissue loss, the majority were not eligible for distal bypass surgery [no runoff in 70 limbs, single-vessel runoff in two limbs] and older cohort, Soder et al. reported a primary angiographic success rate of 84% (102 of 121) for stenosis and 61% (41 of 67) for occlusions with corresponding restenosis rates of 32% and 52% at follow-up angiography performed at a mean of 10 months after primary PTA. The rate of major complications was 2.8% (access-site pseudoaneurysms in two patients). The primary clinical success was 63% (45 of 72). A 48% cumulative primary patency rate, 56% secondary patency rate, and 80% cumulative limb salvage rate were reported at 18 months. Factors that independently correlated with continued lesion patency up to 12 months were angiographic improvement to the site of most severe ischemia (6-month primary patency of 68% vs. 16%; $P = 0.001$) and absence of renal insufficiency (patency of 63% vs. 24%; $P = 0.06$). Clinical success, defined as relief of claudication or avoidance of major amputation, was achieved in only 45 of 72 limbs (63%) acutely, but this is comparable with results from surgical series. No patient in this series had a subsequent surgical bypass operation, largely because of poor distal targets or pedal arteries.[41]

When to Refer to Surgery

In the management of infrapopliteal disease, bypass surgery has been associated with disappointing results. Just as with PTA, the patency rate of bypass grafts remains inferior to that of bypass grafts in more proximal PAD, as shown in Figure 37-7.[1] Success in achieving limb salvage with minimal periprocedual complications is dependent on the status of distal circulation and on the overall risk profile of the patient. Amputation (primary when no antecedent attempt is made on revascularization or secondary following failure of revascularization) may be necessary in patients with critical limb ischemia complicated by intractable infections or uncontrollable rest pain.

■ Acute Limb Ischemia

Acute limb ischemia (ALI) is defined as a sudden or rapidly developing loss of limb perfusion resulting in the development or worsening of symptoms and signs of an imminent threat to the limb viability. Acute limb ischemia may be the first manifestation of PAD in previously asymptomatic patients.[7] More commonly, patients with IC will experience progression of their disease with the development of rest pain, ischemic ulcers, and eventually gangrene. This progression, which may be gradual, is usually the result of recurrent acute ischemic events. Two mechanisms are implicated in ALI: embolism and in situ thrombosis. Differentiation based on history and clinical examination alone may be clinically impossible in 10% to 15% of cases. Although there is little information on the incidence of ALI in the general

TABLE 37-6	Classification of Acute Limb Ischemia		
Category	Description	Neuromuscular Findings	Doppler
I	Viable	No sensory or muscle weakness	Audible arterial and venous
IIa	Threatened (marginally)	Minimal	Often inaudible arterial, audible venous
IIb	Threatened (immediately)	Mild to moderate, associated with pain	Usually inaudible arterial, audible venous
III	Irreversible	Profound deficit	No signals

Reproduced with permission from Weaver FA et al. Surgical revascularization versus thrombolysis for nonembolic lower extremity native artery occlusions: results of a prospective randomized trial. The STILE Investigators. Surgery versus Thrombolysis for Ischemia of the Lower Extremity. *J Vasc Surg.* 1996;24(4):513–521; discussion 521–523.

TABLE 37-7	Recommended Doses of Antiplatelet, Antithrombotic Medications, and Thrombolytics for the Management of Acute Limb Ischemia		
Medication	Route	Dosage	Laboratory
Aspirin	PO/PR	325 mg	None
Clopidogrel	PO	300–600 mg loading dose, 75 mg maintainenance	None
Heparin	IV	600 U/kg bolus, then 12 U/kg per hour	aPTT, plts, Hct
Mannitol	IV	12.5–25 g	Creatinine
Plasminogen activator	IA	Depends on agent*	Hct, fibrinogen, FSP
Urokinase	IA	80–200,000 U/hr tapered infusion	Hct, fibrinogen, FSP

FSP, Fibrin split products; Hct, hematocrit; PO, orally; PR, rectally; IV, intravenous; IA, intraarterial; aPTT, activated partial thromboplastin time; plts, platelet count.

*Depends on thrombolytic (retaplase 0.25–1.0 U/hr; alteplase 0.2–1.0 mg/hr; tenecteplase 0.25–0.5 mg/hr).

Reproduced with permission from Rajagopalan S, Mukherjee D, Mohler E. *Manual of Vascular Diseases.* Philadelphia, PA: Lippincott Williams & Wilkins, 2004.

population, the rate is estimated to be about 14 per 100,000; it is the indication for 10% to 16% of all vascular procedures performed. Patients with embolic ALI are more likely to die than those with thrombosis, usually secondary to underlying cardiac disease, whereas patients with thrombotic ALI are more likely to lose their limbs when compared with embolic ALI. The natural history of ALI has remained largely unchanged despite advances in surgical, endovascular, and pharmacological therapies. Patients presenting with ALI continue to have a particularly poor short-term outlook both in terms of loss of the affected limb and mortality, with 30-day amputation rates of between 10% and 30% and a mortality rate of 15%. The fact that overall mortality rates after intervention for acute ischemia have not improved dramatically over the past 20 years reflects the severity of the underlying atherosclerotic burden in these high-risk patients.[1,7,50] Embolic events may be due to atrial fibrillation, myocardial infarction with left ventricular thrombus, or peripheral pseudoaneurysm. Thrombosis in situ is usually encountered in patients with PAD and tenuous collateral circulation or may be seen in patients with prior bypass surgery with an acute thrombosis of the graft. Also of importance are other mechanisms of ALI, such as septic or cardiac tumor emboli, trauma (such as popliteal artery disruption), and dissection of large vessels with distal progression (such as aortic dissection with iliac artery occlusion).

Table 37-6 shows a recommended classification of ALI that is useful in estimating the impact of this condition for the individual patient and determining the prognosis of the limb at the time of presentation.[51]

MANAGEMENT STRATEGIES FOR ACUTE LIMB ISCHEMIA

In approaching patients with suspected ALI, the history and physical examination should focus on attempting to establish the underlying mechanism of the ALI and categorizing the patient based on the underlying symptoms and signs; Doppler assessment of the peripheral pulses should also be done. Once the diagnosis of ALI is made, the objective should be to prevent thrombus propagation and worsening ischemia. Thus, anticoagulation (if not contraindicated) with heparin is the first step in management. Restoration of flow as soon as possible is the next step (for viable limbs in class I-II), utilizing either pharmacological or endovascular versus open catheter thromboembolectomy. If the patient has a true late nonviable limb (class III), amputation is the only option, as revascularization of such limbs is of no benefit but rather associated with a high risk of mortality. Table 37-7 has the recommended medications and doses of thrombolytic therapy. In general, patients with clear embolic etiologies and a discernible location of obstruction by physical exam are taken to surgery for open embolectomy. If there is no clear embolic etiology, an arteriogram

should be performed and a decision made, based on the findings, on endovascular versus surgical interventions.

INTERVENTIONAL TREATMENT

Pharmacological Thrombolysis

While systemic thrombolysis has no role in the management of ALI, catheter-directed thrombolytic therapy is effective in the management of patients with class I and IIa ischemia. This approach is clearly less invasive, has less morbidity and mortality when compared with open surgery, and may reduce the risk of reperfusion injury. The choice of lytic therapy will depend on location, anatomy, and patient comorbidities. Contraindication to thrombolysis should be observed.

Percutaneous Aspiration Thrombectomy

Percutaneous aspiration thrombectomy (PAT) is an alternative nonsurgical modality to treat ALI and uses large-lumen catheters and suction with a 50-mL syringe to remove embolus or thrombus from native vessels, bypass grafts, and runoff vessels. PAT devices such as the Amplatz "clot buster" (BARD-Microvena, White Bear Lake, MN) and the Straub Rotarex System (Straub Medical, Wangs, Switzerland) has been used with fibrinolysis to reduce the time and dose of the fibrinolytic agent or as a stand-alone procedure.

Percutaneous Mechanical Thrombectomy

The concept of creating a "hydrodynamic recirculation vortex" that would dissolve a thrombus and remove its fragment is the underlying theory behind most percutaneous mechanical thrombectomy (PMT) devices, such as the AngioJet (Possis Medical, Minneapolis, MN), Hydrolyser (Cordis, Warren, NJ), and Oasis (Boston Scientific/Meditech, Natick, MA). The efficacy of PMT depends on the age of the thrombus, since fresh thrombi can be efficiently removed, as opposed to old organized thrombi.

Surgery

The indications for surgery include a clear embolic etiology where an open embolectomy can be performed and patients with critical limb ischemia (class IIb and III). Surgery is associated with the risk of infections, hemorrhage, and periprocedural cardiovascular adverse events.

Critical Leg Ischemia

Critical leg (or limb) ischemia (CLI) is characterized by persistent rest pain with or without ongoing tissue loss, ischemic ulceration, or gangrene. The term CLI is traditionally used to describe patients with

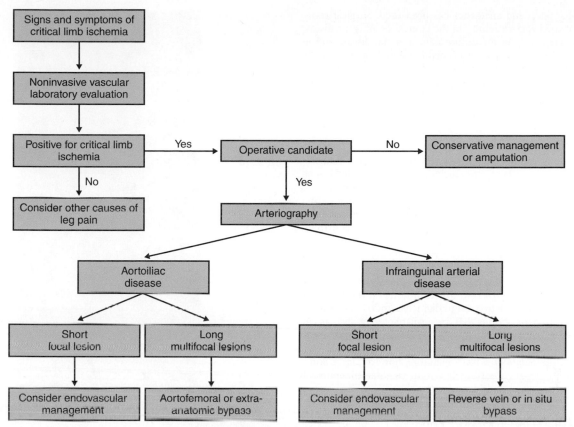

Figure 37-9 Treatment algorithm for patients with critical limb ischemia. *(Reproduced with permission from Rajagopalan S, Mukherjee D, Mohler E. Manual of Vascular Diseases. Philadelphia, PA: Lippincott Williams & Wilkins, 2004.)*

ischemic symptoms of more than 2 weeks' duration. Patients with CLI usually have an ankle systolic pressure <40 mm Hg and/or toe systolic pressure <30 and/or reduced transcutaneous oxygen concentration (TCP O$_2$) of <50 mm Hg. In general the underlying etiology is almost exclusively atherosclerosis; frequently it is a multivessel and multisegment disease. Smoking and diabetes are the most potent risk factors and are associated with a higher rate of amputation. The prognosis in patients with CLI is poor secondary to comorbid conditions, with mortality rates approaching 10% per year and amputation rates of 25% to 45% at 1 year.[1,7]

INTERVENTIONAL TREATMENT AND SURGERY

The decision regarding the management of patient with CLI depends on the patient's risk profile (expected operative mortality, underlying renal function, and the risk of contrast nephropathy, etc.) and his or her anatomical profile (multisegment or multivessel disease, number of runoffs, suitability of the disease to PTA versus surgery, etc). Figure 37-9 outlines a general approach to the management of CLI.

PERIPROCEDURAL ANTITHROMBOTIC THERAPY

PTA and stenting are usually conducted with weight-based heparinization to achieve an ACT of 200 to 250 seconds. A front load of aspirin and clopidogrel (300-600 mg) at least 12 hours prior to intervention is widely used. Glycoprotein IIb/IIIa inhibitors may be useful in the context of diabetes, evidence of angiographic thrombus, or ulceration and in patients with poor runoff (one vessel or none) to prevent distal embolization. After PTA and stenting, lifelong aspirin is recommended in the light of the high rate of cardiovascular events in patients with advanced PAD. Most clinicians prescribe adjunctive

clopidogrel for 1 to 12 months after a lower extremity percutaneous intervention.

SEQUELAE OF PERIPHERAL BYPASS SURGERY

Various types of vascular bypass grafts are used in the management of lower extremity PAD. A detailed discussion of this subject is beyond the scope of this chapter. However, interventionalists are likely to encounter graft-related complications, the most serious of which is ALI secondary to graft thrombosis. In general, acute thrombosis of bypass grafts is secondary to technical problems and usually presents in the early postoperative period; it requires an urgent intervention. In this setting, patients should be anticoagulated and then evaluated for balloon catheter thrombectomy. Mature graft thromboses occur at a rate of about 10% at 5 years and rarely present with ALI. Such patients are managed with thrombolytic therapy to clear the thrombotic burden. Thereafter, the underlying etiology should be addressed, either through an endovascular procedure or by open surgery.[52]

Miscellaneous Conditions

BURGER'S DISEASES (THROMBOANGIITIS)

Burger's disease is a nonatherosclerotic inflammatory vasculitis of the small and medium-sized arteries, veins, and nerves. It can affect upper and lower extremities and occurs most commonly in young male smokers. The etiology is uncertain, although there is a clear and a strong association with smoking and tobacco use. The mainstay of therapy is smoking cessation; in fact, without complete cessation of smoking and tobacco use, the prognosis for limb salvage is dismal.[53] Medical therapy with antiplatelets, immunosuppressant (cyclophosophamide), and analgesics has been used. Surgical revascularization of the lower extremity in the context of Burger's disease has a limited role owing to the diffuse nature of the disease and its tendency to involve distal small vessels before progressing proximally. Bypass surgery, when feasible, should be done with an autogenous vein that is not affected by the disease process. Percutaneous intervention has no clear role in the management of patients with Burger's disease.

PERIPHERAL ANEURYSM

The most common cause of peripheral aneurysm formation is atherosclerosis. Other predisposing factors include hypertension, inflammatory and infectious processes, trauma, connective tissue diseases, and familial tendencies. While most aneurysms are asymptomatic, they may become the source of distal embolization, become infected, compress surrounding tissues, or rupture. Aneurysms of the lower extremity have particular complications depending on their location: Iliac artery aneurysms are associated with atheroembolism, obstructive uropathies, iliac vein obstruction, and perineal or groin pain. The use of MRA or multidetector contrast CT is the preferred strategy for diagnosis. Traditionally surgical resection is indicated if the aneurysm is symptomatic or is more than 3 cm in diameter. Endovascular treatment (using a variety of options that are available today, such as coil embolization and stent-graft placement) may now be an alternative to surgery. Early experience indicates that endovascular treatment is safe and effective in the hands of skilled operators; however, large, long-term follow-up studies are needed to determine whether this approach is a practical alternative to open surgery.[54]

Femoral Artery Aneurysm

Femoral artery aneurysm is associated with atheroembolism and venous obstruction. This condition can be diagnosed with ultrasound and managed surgically if it is symptomatic. Case series of endovascular interventions have been reported but the data are limited and larger studies with long-term follow up are needed to help identify the role of this approach.[55]

POPLITEAL ARTERY ANEURYSM

Popliteal artery aneurysm is associated with thrombosis, atheroembolism, venous obstruction, popliteal neuropathy, and infection. Such aneurysms can be bilateral in 50% of patients. Ultrasound can be used to make the diagnosis, although contrast angiography is generally needed prior to surgery to assess the proximal and distal circulation (Fig. 37-10). Once diagnosed, popliteal artery aneurysm should be resected to prevent its potentially devastating thromboembolic complications. Endovascular repair of popliteal artery aneurysms is a new technique that has emerged as an alternative to open surgical bypass. The evidence to support its use is limited and long-term follow-up data are lacking; however, early results have been promising, with high rates of initial success.[55,56]

ATHEROEMBOLISM

Atheroembolism involves the occlusion of arteries secondary to the detachment and embolization of atheromatous debris, which includes cholesterol crystals, platelets, fibrin, and calcium. Atheroemboli can originate from any atherosclerotic segment although typically they originate from the aortic atheromas and aneurysms of the large and medium-size arteries. They tend to occlude small end arteries and arterioles, such as those of the kidneys, retina, brain, and extremities. Clinical features of this disorder are usually reflective of acute ischemic complications and vary with the affected organ. Atheroembolic events in the lower extremity would result in painful cyanotic toes (blue-toe syndrome) and are associated with digital and foot ulcerations in addition to multiorgan dysfunction, depending on the extent of the embolic

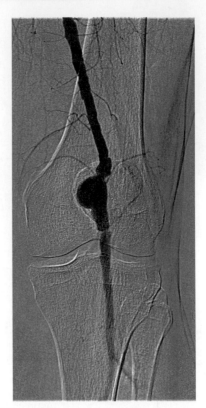

Figure 37-10 DSA of left popliteal artery showing aneurysm.

burden. Livido reticularis is commonly (up to 50%) encountered in patients with atheroembolism as well. It is important to point out that distal pulses will remain intact, unlike critical limb ischemia (CLI) and acute limb ischemia (ALI) secondary to thromboembolism, where pulses are usually abnormal because atheremboli occlude smaller more distal vessels. The differential diagnosis includes many conditions such as vasculitis and prothrombotic conditions like antiphospholipid syndrome and heparin-induced thrombocytopenia. Affected patients may have an elevated erythrocyte sedimentation rate, thrombocytopenia, eosinophilia, eosinophiluria, and hypocomplementemia. In biopsies of skin and muscle, the finding of cholesterol crystals in small arteries is a pathognomonic sign. Transesophageal echocardiography, CT scan, and MRA can be used to image the aorta (searching for shaggy mobile atheromas); assessment for aneurysms by ultrasound and angiography is part of the workup to identify the source of the emboli if possible. If the source cannot be identified, no definitive therapy exists, but antiplatelet therapy with aspirin has been advocated. If the source is identified, surgical removal or endovascular isolation of the source is the only definitive therapy.[57]

Conclusions and Future Directions

PAD of the lower extremity is a serious health problem associated with significant morbidity; it is a reflection of advanced atherosclerosis, which often affects other vascular trees. While the management of patients with IC is based on risk-factor modification and an integrated exercise program as well as pharmacological modification of the associated risk factors, percutaneous interventions have emerged as an alternative modality to surgical revascularization in patients who remain symptomatic or those who progress to critical limb ischemia. Advances in technology will likely continue to optimize the role of percutaneous interventions in the management of PAD. While such interventions are already very effective in the management of IC caused by iliofemoral disease, there remains room for improvement in the use of such interventions in the management of infrapopliteal disease and of acute and critical limb ischemia.

REFERENCES

1. Dormandy JA, Rutherford RB: Management of peripheral arterial disease (PAD). TASC Working Group. TransAtlantic Inter-Society Concensus (TASC). *J Vasc Surg* 31:S1–S296, 2000.
2. Management of peripheral arterial disease (PAD): TransAtlantic Inter-Society Consensus (TASC). Section D: chronic critical limb ischaemia. *Eur J Vasc Endovasc Surg* 19(Suppl A):S144–S243, 2000.
3. Hirsch AT, Halverson SL, Treat-Jacobson D, et al: The Minnesota Regional Peripheral Arterial Disease Screening Program: toward a definition of community standards of care. *Vasc Med* 6:87–96, 2001.
4. Selvin E, Erlinger TP: Prevalence of and risk factors for peripheral arterial disease in the United States: results from the National Health and Nutrition Examination Survey, 1999–2000. *Circulation* 110:738–743, 2004.
5. Fowkes FG, Housley E, Cawood EH, et al: Edinburgh Artery Study: prevalence of asymptomatic and symptomatic peripheral arterial disease in the general population. *Int J Epidemiol* 20:384–392, 1991.
6. Willigendael EM, Teijink JA, Bartelink ML, et al: Peripheral arterial disease: public and patient awareness in The Netherlands. *Eur J Vasc Endovasc Surg* 27:622–628, 2004.
7. Hirsch AT, Haskal ZJ, Hertzer NR, et al: ACC/AHA 2005 Practice Guidelines for the management of patients with peripheral arterial disease (lower extremity, renal, mesenteric, and abdominal aortic): a collaborative report from the American Association for Vascular Surgery/Society for Vascular Surgery, Society for Cardiovascular Angiography and Interventions, Society for Vascular Medicine and Biology, Society of Interventional Radiology, and the ACC/AHA Task Force on Practice Guidelines (Writing Committee to Develop Guidelines for the Management of Patients With Peripheral Arterial Disease): endorsed by the American Association of Cardiovascular and Pulmonary Rehabilitation; National Heart, Lung, and Blood Institute; Society for Vascular Nursing; TransAtlantic Inter-Society Consensus; and Vascular Disease Foundation. *Circulation* 113:e463–e654, 2006.
8. Criqui MH, Fronek A, Barrett-Connor E, et al: The prevalence of peripheral arterial disease in a defined population. *Circulation* 71:510–515, 1985.
9. Sherev DA, Shaw RE, Brent BN: Angiographic predictors of femoral access site complications: implication for planned percutaneous coronary intervention. *Catheter Cardiovasc Intervent* 65:196–202, 2005.
10. Met R, Bipat S, Legemate DA, et al: Diagnostic performance of computed tomography angiography in peripheral arterial disease: a systematic review and meta-analysis. *JAMA* 301:415–424, 2009.
11. Hausleiter J, Meyer T, Hadamitzky M, et al: Radiation dose estimates from cardiac multislice computed tomography in daily practice: impact of different scanning protocols on effective dose estimates. *Circulation* 113:1305–1310, 2006.
12. Whyman MR, Fowkes FG, Kerracher EM, et al: Randomised controlled trial of percutaneous transluminal angioplasty for intermittent claudication. *Eur J Vasc Endovasc Surg* 12:167–172, 1996.
13. Whyman MR, Fowkes FG, Kerracher EM, et al: Is intermittent claudication improved by percutaneous transluminal angioplasty? A randomized controlled trial. *J Vasc Surg* 26:551–557, 1997.
14. Wolf GL, Wilson SE, Cross AP, et al: Surgery or balloon angioplasty for peripheral vascular disease: a randomized clinical trial. Principal investigators and their Associates of Veterans Administration Cooperative Study Number 199. *J Vasc Intervent Radiol* 4:639–648, 1993.
15. Lundgren F, Dahllof AG, Lundholm K, et al: Intermittent claudication: surgical reconstruction or physical training? A prospective randomized trial of treatment efficiency. *Ann Surg* 209:346–355, 1989.
16. Perkins JM, Collin J, Creasy TS, et al: Exercise training versus angioplasty for stable claudication. Long and medium term results of a prospective, randomised trial. *Eur J Vasc Endovasc Surg* 11:409–413, 1996.
17. Holm J, Arfvidsson B, Jivegard L, et al: Chronic lower limb ischaemia. A prospective randomised controlled study comparing the 1-year results of vascular surgery and percutaneous transluminal angioplasty (PTA). *Eur J Vasc Surg* 5:517–522, 1991.
18. Wilson SE, Wolf GL, Cross AP: Percutaneous transluminal angioplasty versus operation for peripheral arteriosclerosis. Report of a prospective randomized trial in a selected group of patients. *J Vasc Surg* 9:1–9, 1989.
19. Bosch JL, Hunink MG: Meta-analysis of the results of percutaneous transluminal angioplasty and stent placement for aortoiliac occlusive disease. *Radiology* 204:87–96, 1997.
20. Tetteroo E, van der Graaf Y, Bosch JL, et al: Randomised comparison of primary stent placement versus primary angioplasty followed by selective stent placement in patients with iliac-artery occlusive disease. Dutch Iliac Stent Trial Study Group. *Lancet* 351:1153–1159, 1998.
21. Richter GM, Roeren T, Noeldge G, et al: [Initial long-term results of a randomized 5-year study: iliac stent implantation versus PTA]. *Vasa Suppl* 35:192–193, 1992.
22. Ponec D, Jaff MR, Swischuk J, et al: The Nitinol SMART stent vs Wallstent for suboptimal iliac artery angioplasty: CRISP-US trial results. *J Vasc Intervent Radiol* 15:911–918, 2004.
23. Sacks D, Marinelli DL, Martin LG, Spies JB: Reporting standards for clinical evaluation of new peripheral arterial revascularization devices. Technology Assessment Committee. *J Vasc Intervent Radiol* 8:137–149, 1997.
24. Management of peripheral arterial disease (PAD): TransAtlantic Inter-Society Consensus (TASC). *Int Angiol* 19:I–XXIV,1–304, 2000.
25. Taylor LM, Jr, Porter JM: Clinical and anatomic considerations for surgery in femoropopliteal disease and the results of surgery. *Circulation* 83:I63–I69, 1991.
26. Walsh DB, Gilbertson JJ, Zwolak RM, et al: The natural history of superficial femoral artery stenoses. *J Vasc Surg* 14:299–304, 1991.
27. Ballard JL, Sparks SR, Taylor FC, et al: Complications of iliac artery stent deployment. *J Vasc Surg* 24:545–553; discussion 553–545, 1996.
28. Creasy TS, McMillan PJ, Fletcher EW, et al: Is percutaneous transluminal angioplasty better than exercise for claudication? Preliminary results from a prospective randomised trial. *Eur J Vasc Surg* 4:135–140, 1990.
29. Matsi P: Percutaneous transluminal angioplasty in critical limb ischaemia. *Ann Chir Gynaecol* 84:359–362, 1995.
30. Ljungman C, Ulus AT, Almgren B, et al: A multivariate analysis of factors affecting patency of femoropopliteal and femorodistal bypass grafting. *Vasa* 29:215–220, 2000.
31. Muradin GS, Bosch JL, Stijnen T, Hunink MG: Balloon dilation and stent implantation for treatment of femoropopliteal arterial disease: meta-analysis. *Radiology* 221:137–145, 2001.
32. Schillinger M, Sabeti S, Loewe C, et al: Balloon angioplasty versus implantation of nitinol stents in the superficial femoral artery. *N Engl J Med* 354:1879–1888, 2006.
33. Dick P, Wallner H, Sabeti S, et al: Balloon angioplasty versus stenting with nitinol stents in intermediate length superficial femoral artery lesions. *Catheter Cardiovasc Intervent* 74:1090–1095, 2009.
34. Mwipatayi BP, Hockings A, Hofmann M, et al: Balloon angioplasty compared with stenting for treatment of femoropopliteal occlusive disease: a meta-analysis. *J Vasc Surg* 47:461–469, 2008.
35. Duda SH, Bosiers M, Lammer J, et al: Drug-eluting and bare nitinol stents for the treatment of atherosclerotic lesions in the superficial femoral artery: long-term results from the SIROCCO trial. *J Endovasc Ther* 13:701–710, 2006.
36. Nakamura S, Conroy RM, Gordon IL, et al: A randomized trial of transcutaneous extraction atherectomy in femoral arteries: intravascular ultrasound observations. *J Clin Ultrasound* 23:461–471, 1995.
37. Vroegindeweij D, Tielbeek AV, Buth J, et al: Directional atherectomy versus balloon angioplasty in segmental femoropopliteal artery disease: two-year follow-up with color-flow duplex scanning. *J Vasc Surg* 21:255–268; discussion 268–259, 1995.
38. McKinsey JF, Goldstein L, Khan HU, et al: Novel treatment of patients with lower extremity ischemia: use of percutaneous atherectomy in 579 lesions. *Ann Surg* 248:519–528, 2008
39. Vroegindeweij D, Vos LD, Tielbeek AV, et al: Balloon angioplasty combined with primary stenting versus balloon angioplasty alone in femoropopliteal obstructions: a comparative randomized study. *Cardiovasc Intervent Radiol* 20:420–425, 1997.
40. van der Zaag ES, Legemate DA, Prins MH, et al: Angioplasty or bypass for superficial femoral artery disease? A randomised controlled trial. *Eur J Vasc Endovasc Surg* 28:132–137, 2004.
41. Soder HK, Manninen HI, Jaakkola P, et al: Prospective trial of infrapopliteal artery balloon angioplasty for critical limb ischemia: angiographic and clinical results. *J Vasc Intervent Radiol* 11:1021–1031, 2000.
42. Matsi PJ, Manninen HI, Suhonen MT, et al: Chronic critical lower-limb ischemia: prospective trial of angioplasty with 1–36 months follow-up. *Radiology* 188:381–387, 1993.
43. Dorros G, Jaff MR, Murphy KJ, Mathiak L: The acute outcome of tibioperoneal vessel angioplasty in 417 cases with claudication and critical limb ischemia. *Catheter Cardiovasc Diagn* 45:251–256, 1998.
44. Martens JM, Knippenberg B, Vos JA, et al: Update on PADI trial: percutaneous transluminal angioplasty and drug-eluting stents for infrapopliteal lesions in critical limb ischemia. *J Vasc Surg* 50:687–689, 2009.
45. Grimm J, Muller-Hulsbeck S, Jahnke T, et al: Randomized study to compare PTA alone versus PTA with Palmaz stent placement for femoropopliteal lesions. *J Vasc Intervent Radiol* 12:935–942, 2001.
46. Zeller T, Rastan A, Schwarzwalder U, et al: Midterm results after atherectomy-assisted angioplasty of below knee arteries with use of the Silverhawk device. *J Vasc Intervent Radiol* 15:1391–1397, 2004.
47. Safian RD, Niazi K, Runyon JP, et al: Orbital atherectomy for infrapopliteal disease: device concept and outcome data for the OASIS trial. *Catheter Cardiovasc Intervent* 73:406–412, 2009.
48. Holdsworth RJ, McCollum PT: Results and resource implications of treating end-stage limb ischaemia. *Eur J Vasc Endovasc Surg* 13:164–173, 1997.
49. Dorros G, Jaff MR, Dorros AM, et al: Tibioperoneal (outflow lesion) angioplasty can be used as primary treatment in 235 patients with critical limb ischemia: five-year follow-up. *Circulation* 104:2057–2062, 2001.
50. Dormandy J, Heeck L, Vig S: Predictors of early disease in the lower limbs. *Semin Vasc Surg* 12:109–117, 1999.
51. Thrombolysis in the management of lower limb peripheral arterial occlusion: a consensus document. *J Vasc Intervent Radiol* 14:S337–S349, 2003.
52. Weaver FA, Comerota AJ, Youngblood M, et al: Surgical revascularization versus thrombolysis for nonembolic lower extremity native artery occlusions: results of a prospective randomized trial. The STILE investigators. Surgery versus Thrombolysis for Ischemia of the Lower Extremity. *J Vasc Surg* 24:513–521; discussion 521 513, 1996.
53. Olin JW, Shih A: Thromboangiitis obliterans (Buerger's disease). *Curr Opin Rheumatol* 18:18–24, 2006.
54. Sakamoto I, Sueyoshi E, Hazama S, et al: Endovascular treatment of iliac artery aneurysms. *Radiographics* 25(Suppl 1):S213–S227, 2005.
55. Saxon RR, Coffman JM, Gooding JM, Ponec DJ: Endograft use in the femoral and popliteal arteries. *Tech Vasc Intervent Radiol* 7:6–15, 2004.
56. Slauw R, Koh EH, Walker SR: Endovascular repair of popliteal artery aneurysms: techniques, current evidence and recent experience. *ANZ J Surg* 76:505–511, 2006.
57. Smyth JS, Scoble JE: Atheroembolism. *Curr Treat Options Cardiovasc Med* 4:255–265, 2002.

Upper Extremities and Aortic Arch

SAMUEL L. JOHNSTON | ROBERT S. DIETER

KEY POINTS

- Patients with peripheral artery disease are at extremely high risk for morbidity and mortality from myocardial infarction and stroke. They will derive their greatest benefit in terms of diminishing these complications with risk-factor reduction and best medical therapy.

- The differential diagnosis for arterial disease of the proximal arch and upper extremities is extensive.

- Significant anatomical variation in the proximal arch and upper extremity arteries occurs in 30% of the population.

- Subclavian steal syndrome occurs when there is retrograde vertebral artery blood flow away from the cerebral posterior circulation to accommodate demand for blood in the ipsilateral subclavian artery beyond a tight proximal stenosis.

- Coronary subclavian steal syndrome and other forms of iatrogenic steal phenomena are increasing in prevalence.

- Indications for intervention in patients with subclavian steal syndrome are predicated on the presence of symptoms.

- Percutaneous intervention for occlusive diseases of the aortic arch vessels and upper extremities has become a successful, safe, and durable alternative to surgical intervention and is reasonable as first-line therapy.

- Thoracic outlet syndrome occurs when there is a symptomatic compression of the neurovascular bundle as it exits the thorax. Most cases are primarily neurogenic rather than vascular.

- Thoracic outlet diagnostic maneuvers have a high false-positive rate.

- Most patients with thoracic outlet syndrome are adequately treated with conservative measures.

- The most common cause of axillary aneurysm is crutch syndrome.

- The most common source of emboli to the upper extremities is arterial aneurysm of the proximal arch or proximal vessels of the upper extremity.

Introduction

In the past decade we have seen the scope of interventional cardiology widen to encompass nearly the whole realm of vascular medicine, including arterial diseases of the proximal arch and upper extremity. The extension of cardiology to peripheral artery disease (PAD) has been a natural outgrowth for several reasons. First, the major risk factors for PAD are identical to those for coronary artery disease (CAD); hence there is considerable overlap in the affected patient populations. There is a high degree of correlation between the degree of atherosclerosis in the brachial, carotid, and coronary arteries.[1] The cardiologist will, therefore, invariably have initial exposure to these patients when they present for healthcare. Second, patients with PAD are at extremely high risk for morbidity and mortality from myocardial infarction (MI) and stroke and should arguably be regularly followed by a cardiologist for medical care.[2-5] Indeed, the majority of patients with PAD do not require surgical or catheter-based intervention and will derive their greatest benefits in terms of decreased morbidity and mortality simply from risk-factor reduction and best medical therapy.

Third, the tools and techniques that work for intervening in atherosclerosis of the coronary arteries are translatable to the large arteries of the peripheral vasculature. In most cases the same standard catheter skills that are used for coronary cases can be applied to noncoronary arch and upper extremity cases.[6] There is high primary success in treating proximal arch and upper extremity occlusive disease as well as reasonable long-term patency (Fig. 38-1). In some cases catheter-based therapies have become superior to traditional surgical techniques.[7] It has been estimated that atherosclerosis of the *upper* limbs accounts for 5% of PAD affecting the extremities.[8,9] Even so, when one considers that 25% to 40% of the patients seen in a typical cardiology clinic have significant PAD,[2,3,5] it becomes apparent that proximal arch and upper extremity arterial diseases constitute a significant disease burden. The PARTNERS trial revealed that PAD is underdiagnosed and undertreated[2]; this is especially true for arterial diseases of the proximal arch and upper extremities. Unlike PAD of the lower extremities, which is almost exclusively caused by atherosclerosis, the differential diagnosis for arterial disease of the proximal arch and upper extremities is extensive. While the relative infrequency of significant atherosclerosis in the proximal arch vessels and upper extremities (as opposed to the lower extremities) probably represents underlying differences in pathophysiology (e.g., turbulence, inflammation, oxidative stress, density of receptors), its low prevalence is likely also a result of our collective failure to diagnose it. The comparatively low prevalence of symptomatic arterial disease affecting the proximal arch and upper extremities combined with the complex differential diagnosis underlying these diseases make timely and accurate diagnosis problematic. Many of these patients, such as those with subclavian steal (coronary or vertebral artery) or thoracic outlet syndrome, are misdiagnosed and/or inappropriately treated. This is unfortunate because, when correctly diagnosed, these patients are highly treatable, and those with atherosclerotic PAD stand to benefit greatly in terms of decreased rates of cardiovascular events by receiving the appropriate medical therapy.

Objectives

In this chapter, we:
- Review the normal anatomy of the aortic arch, upper extremities, and the anatomical variants.
- Discuss the wide differential diagnosis that must be considered in evaluating a patient with suspected aortic arch or upper extremity arterial disease and show how tackling these problems frequently requires a multidisciplinary approach.
- Consider pertinent aspects of the patient's history, physical exam findings with special maneuvers, and initial laboratory workup.
- Introduce diagnostic modalities that are used in the peripheral vascular laboratory and review the application of several common imaging modalities as they are applied to PAD.
- Examine the application of catheter-based techniques for the diagnosis and treatment of arterial diseases of the proximal arch and upper extremities.
- Focus individually on the most common diseases: subclavian steal syndrome, coronary subclavian steal syndrome, arm claudication, thoracic outlet syndrome, axillary artery stenosis/crutch syndrome, and embolic diseases.
- Other vascular conditions—such as trauma, small-vessel vasculitis, hemodialysis access interventions, and venous and lymphatic disorders—are not emphasized.

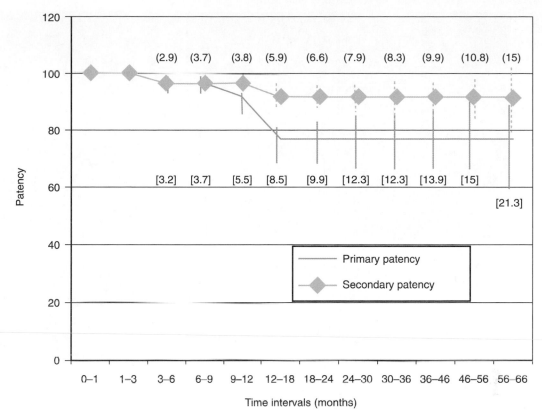

Figure 38-1 Long-term patency of subclavian artery stenting. *(From Brountzos EN et al. Primary stenting of subclavian and innominate artery occlusive disease: a single center's experience. Cardiovasc Intervent Radiol. 2004 27(6):616–623.)*

Normal Anatomy

The arterial system of the upper extremities (Fig. 38-2) is analogous to that of the lower extremities. In 70% of the population,[10] the arteries of the proximal arch are the brachiocephalic (innominate) artery on the right (which quickly divides into the right subclavian artery and the right common carotid artery), and the left common carotid artery and the left subclavian artery, which come off the arch separately, on the left. The subclavian artery becomes the axillary artery at the lateral border of the first rib. The axillary artery becomes the brachial artery, the first intrinsic artery of the upper extremity, in the shoulder girdle at the border of the teres major muscle. The brachial artery is superficial and should be palpable throughout its course. It first lies medial to the humerus and then courses anterior to it. Just below the antecubital fossa, the brachial artery divides into the ulnar artery, which courses medially, and the radial artery, which courses laterally. The ulnar and radial arteries are also superficial and normally palpable. In the wrist, the distal ulnar artery forms the superficial palmar arch and the distal radial artery forms the deep palmar arch. The palmar arches form extensive anastomoses before giving off the true digital arteries (medial and lateral).[11] There are extensive collaterals formed by lesser arteries around the shoulders and elbows and in the palms. These collaterals form a parallel arterial circuit that allows normal perfusion in the upper extremities even when there is a significant occlusion—with one major exception. In contrast to most other large vascular beds, each upper extremity is supplied by only one artery coming off of the aorta. Therefore all anastomoses in the extremities are distal to the aortic branch point, resulting in the potential for ischemic vulnerability and—as discussed further on in considering the upper extremities—for various steal phenomena.

Anatomical Variants

The presence of anomalous circulation in the arteries of the proximal arch and upper extremity (cumulatively in about 30% of the population)[10,12] can lead to misdiagnosis and confusion in the catheterization lab. Here we review some of the most prevalent anatomical variants. (Anatomical variants associated with thoracic outlet syndrome are described separately later in the chapter.)

Bovine Arch. The bovine arch is the most common anatomical variant of the aortic arch, occurring in 22% of the population and accounting for 73% of all arch vessel anomalies.[10,12] It consists of a common origin of the right brachiocephalic and left common carotid arteries (Fig. 38-3). It is not associated with any pathological significance.

Double Aortic Arch. The double aortic arch is a rare anomaly that is caused by persistence of the fetal double aortic arch system. It is rarely associated with congenital heart disease.

Right Aortic Arch. The right aortic arch is a rare anomaly that results from the persistence of the right fourth brachial arch—most commonly associated with an aberrant left subclavian artery (as below).

Left Vertebral Artery Originating from the Aorta. Normally the left vertebral artery comes off the left subclavian artery. In 4% to 6% of the population it originates directly from the aortic arch and accounts for 14% of arch vessel anomalies.[10,12] It is not associated with other anomalies and does not confer any pathological predilection, although it may predispose to more upper extremity symptoms in the presence of proximal left subclavian artery stenosis owing to the absence of a significant collateral pathway.

Aberrant Right Subclavian Artery. Aberrant right subclavian artery (ARSA, or arteria lusoria) is an example of a vascular ring with pathological significance (Fig. 38-4).[13–15] It is caused by the persistence of the posterior segment of the fourth aortic arch. It manifests as a right subclavian artery arising from the left aortic arch *distal* to the origin

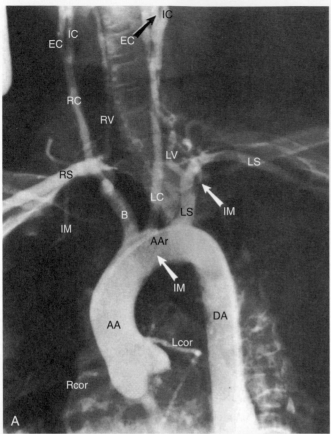

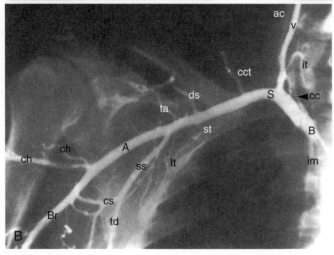

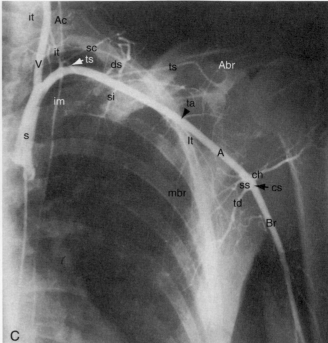

Figure 38-2 Normal anatomy. A. LAO arch aortogram. B. Right subclavian arteriogram. C. Left subclavian arteriogram. *(Reproduced with permission from Kadir S. Atlas of Normal and Variant Angiographic Anatomy. Philadelphia: Saunders; 1991.)*

of the left subclavian artery and follows a retroesophageal course. It occurs in less than 2% of the population and is associated with other anomalies of the arch vessels. The proximal section of an ARSA has a propensity for aneurysm (termed Kommerell's diverticulum) and may cause symptoms related to compression of nearby structures. The most common symptom is intermittent dysphagia (dysphagia lusoria) due to compression of the esophagus.[16] However, regardless of symptoms, the presence of Kommerell's diverticulum is an indication for surgical repair because of its significant risk of rupture.[17,18] Interestingly, surgical repair of ARSA by way of ligation of the anomalous origin has been described as an iatrogenic cause of the subclavian steal syndrome.[18]

Aberrant Left Subclavian Artery. An isolated left subclavian artery arises from a right aortic arch when there is interruption of the left fourth arch proximal to the seventh cervical intersegmental artery. This

anomaly is a rare cause of upper extremity ischemia and has been associated with subclavian steal syndrome (Fig. 38-5).[10,19] As above, its repair has also been associated with the development of the subclavian steal syndrome.[18]

Brachial, Radial, and Ulnar Arteries. In 20% of the population, the brachial artery is doubled during all or part of its course. Owing to extensive collateralization around the elbow, occlusion of one of these branches is generally well tolerated. In 15% to 20% of the population, the radial artery originates early on from the brachial artery or even as high as the axillary artery (Fig. 38-6).[10] It is relatively uncommon, however, for the ulnar artery to branch off prematurely (prevalence 1%-3%). The ulnar artery is congenitally absent in 2% to 3% of the population. These variants confer no intrinsic pathological significance.

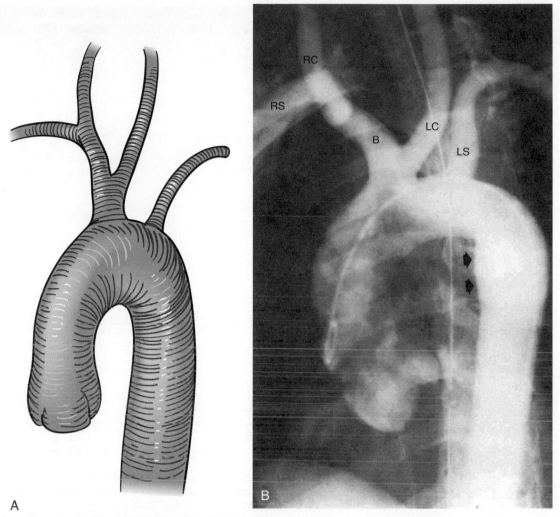

A

B

Figure 38-3 Common origin of left common carotid and brachiocephalic arteries (bovine arch). A. Schematic. B. LAO arch aortogram of a bovine arch. *(Reproduced with permission from Kadir S. Atlas of Normal and Variant Angiographic Anatomy. Philadelphia: Saunders; 1991.)*

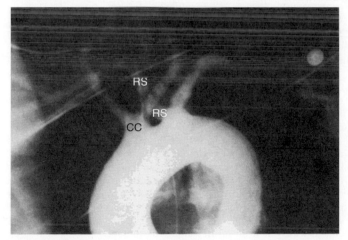

Figure 38-4 Aberrant right subclavian artery and a common carotid trunk. *(Reproduced with permission from Kadir S. Atlas of Normal and Variant Angiographic Anatomy. Philadelphia: Saunders; 1991.)*

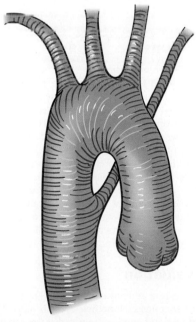

Figure 38-5 Right aortic arch with aberrant left subclavian artery (schematic). *(Reproduced with permission from Kadir S. Atlas of Normal and Variant Angiographic Anatomy. Philadelphia: Saunders; 1991.)*

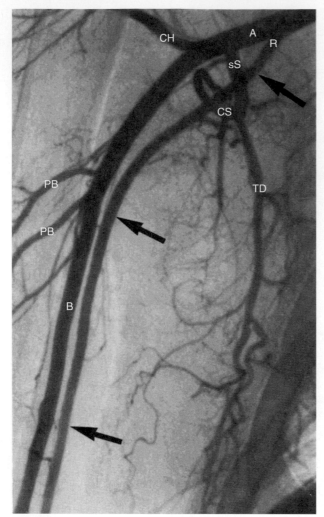

Figure 38-6   Radial artery originating from axillary artery. *(Reproduced with permission from Kadir S.* Atlas of Normal and Variant Angiographic Anatomy. *Philadelphia: Saunders; 1991.)*

TABLE 38-1	Diseases of the Large- and Medium-Size Arteries
	Site/Disease State
Atherosclerosis	Brachiocephalic artery Subclavian artery Axillary artery
Aneurysm	Thoracic outlet syndrome Trauma, crutch syndrome Vasculitis Fibromuscular dysplasia
Thromboembolism	Cardiac Aortic arch Proximal great vessels
Entrapment	Thoracic outlet syndrome Trauma Neoplasm
Vasculitis	Giant cell (temporal) arteritis Kawasaki's arteritis Takayasu's arteritis Radiation-induced arteritis

Adapted with permission from Rajagopalan S, Mukherjee D, Mohler E. *Manual of Vascular Diseases.* Baltimore: Lippincott Williams & Wilkins: 2004:464.

Classifications

Given the broad differential diagnoses that one must consider in approaching suspected arterial disease of the proximal arch vessel or upper extremity, it is useful to classify these diseases based on symptom acuity (time of onset) and size of the involved artery. The diseases involving large or medium-sized arteries, such as those proximal to the wrist, are most relevant to the cardiologist and are caused by one of five mechanisms (Table 38-1). The small-vessel diseases (i.e., those occurring distal to the wrist) are frequently rheumatological or hematological disorders and include blood dyscrasias, Buerger's disease, Henoch-Schönlein purpura, the various hypercoaguable states, and multiple small-vessel vasculitides. It can be clinically difficult to distinguish between large- and small-vessel disease. For example, although most think of Raynaud's phenomenon as a small-artery disease, it is a common feature of both large- and small-vessel disease.

Initial Evaluation

Unfortunately the history and physical exam will rarely suffice in establishing a definitive diagnosis. Nonetheless, the broad differential diagnosis of proximal arch and upper extremity diseases can be significantly narrowed with good history taking and a thorough exam. These fundamental skills remain essential to expediting a correct diagnosis, minimizing unnecessary testing, and making the necessary referrals.

HISTORY

Establishing the correct diagnosis in proximal arch and upper extremity disease is often facilitated by noting the company it keeps. Indeed, an awareness of the patient's comorbid illnesses usually provides important clues. For instance, complaints of chronic or recurrent headaches in a patient with tetralogy of Fallot and a history of the Blalock-Taussig procedure is highly suggestive of the subclavian steal syndrome. Most commonly, a patient will simply have a history of atherosclerosis or risk factors for it. Atherosclerosis is frequently a systemic process, so when a patient is known to already suffer from coronary or peripheral arterial disease, one's suspicion for ischemia of the proximal arch vessel or upper extremity should be raised. Likewise, a prior diagnosis of atrial fibrillation, severe left ventricular dysfunction, aortic plaquing, or arterial aneurysm increases the probability that thromboembolic disease is the culprit. Previously diagnosed hematological diseases, rheumatologic diseases, or malignancy all suggest vasospasm, vasculititis, or hypercoaguability. Vasculitides in general tend to be systemic diseases and patients usually present with constitutional symptoms such as fever, weight loss, and fatigue in the early phase of disease. The presence of arthralgias and myalgias is also suggestive of vasculitis. The vasculitides, particularly Takayasu's, are uncommon and affect women more often than men. Takayasu's arteritis is more common in the Asian races but not exclusive to them. Fibromuscular dysplasia may mimic Takayasu's arteritis but lacks the constitutional symptoms.

In terms of distinguishing the vasculitides, age is often the best initial discriminator. Kawasaki's disease is strictly a pediatric disease in onset; however, its sequelae, such as coronary and peripheral artery aneurysmal disease, can be significant in the adult population. Takayasu's arteritis generally occurs in patients below 40 years of age, whereas giant cell (temporal) arteritis is unlikely to affect patients below 65 years of age. Thoracic outlet syndrome (TOS) is, perhaps, most difficult to tease out from history alone. Its presence is suggested by an exacerbation of symptoms (e.g., pain or parasthesia) in the context of upper extremity movement, particularly abduction. Unfortunately this feature hardly distinguishes it from the upper extremity claudication that is characteristic of subclavian or axillary artery stenosis. Except in cases of trauma, symptom onset is usually vague and slowly progressive. During the initial evaluation, the clinician should inquire about timing of symptoms, symmetry, use of potentially vasospastic medications (Table 38-2), use of recreational drugs (including tobacco), prior

TABLE 38-2	Medication-Induced Vasospasm	
Class	*Example(s)*	*Common Uses*
5-HT agonists	Sumatriptan	Migraine headache
Ergot alkaloids	Methysergide Ergonovine	Migraine headache Post-partum bleeding
Dopamine agonists	Bromocriptine	Parkinson's disease Acromegaly Hyperprolactinemia
Immunomodulators	α-Interferon (α-IFN)	Hepatitis C virus Hepatitis B virus Hematological malignancies
Antiseizures	Phenytoin Carbamazepine	Seizure treatment and prevention
Antibiotics	Trimethoprim/ sulfamethoxazole Tetracycline, doxycycline	Antimicrobial
Xanthine oxidase inhibitors	Allopurinol	Gout prophylaxis Tumor lysis syndrome Nephrolithiasis prophylaxis (calcium oxalate)
Diuretics (thiazides)	Hydrochlorothiazide Chlorothiazide Chlorthalidone Metolazone	Congestive heart failure Edema Hypertension
Aldosterone receptor antagonists	Spironolactone	Congestive heart failure Edema Hypertension (systemic) Portal hypertension Hyperaldosteronism
Recreational	Nicotine Cocaine	Recreational

external beam radiation (as in the treatment of Hodgkin's disease, breast cancer, or lung cancer), and occupational exposures (Table 38-3). It is essential to know these details before prescribing further testing. The utility of gathering a comprehensive history from the patient with suspected proximal arch or upper extremity disease cannot be overstated. It is easy to be led astray by the large differential diagnosis that must be considered. Common sense dictates that common diseases occur commonly, and this line of thinking should be applied in approaching such patients. Nevertheless, one should be prepared to hunt for the occasional zebra. For instance, in the context of upper extremity symptoms, dysphagia may suggest a rheumatologic disorder, such as CREST (Calcinosis, Raynaud's syndrome, Esophageal dysmotility, Sclerodactyly, Telangiectasia) syndrome, or an anatomical variant, such as ARSA (Aberrant right subclavian artery) with dysphagia lusoria.

Physical Examination

Like a thorough history, careful attention to the physical exam will usually narrow the differential diagnosis and reveal the best next step in the patient's workup. For example, the absence of the brachial and radial pulses in a young Asian woman would be immediately suggestive

TABLE 38-3	Occupational Exposures Associated with Proximal Arch and Upper Extremity Disease	
Exposure	*Disease State*	
Vinyl chloride	Raynaud's phenomenon	
Vibratory tools	Raynaud's phenomenon Hypothenar hammer syndrome	
Repetitive palmar pressure/trauma	Raynaud's phenomenon Hypothenar hammer syndrome	
Sporting activities	TOS Hypothenar hammer syndrome	
Radiation	Atherosclerosis Vasculitis	

of Takayasu's arteritis. In the case of patients in whom proximal arch and upper extremity disease is already suspected, it is prudent to conduct a thorough (rather than focused) physical exam because the underlying pathology is so frequently a systemic process. But given the high prevalence of PAD, it is reasonable to at least perform office-based screening for upper extremity disease on all patients who present to the cardiology clinic by measuring the pulses and blood pressures in both arms. The physician should do this manually. A systolic gradient of more than 15 to 20 mm Hg is suspicious for significant proximal arch or upper extremity stenosis (although there may be no differential in patients with bilateral disease). The specificity of 10 and 20 mm Hg differentials in cuff pressures between arms is 85% and 94%, respectively.[20] The brachial, radial, and ulnar pulses should be palpable and symmetrical throughout their course. Multiple pulse deficits in a young patient (as in the example above) are suggestive of Takayasu's arteritis. TOS maneuvers, which typically entail palpation of the radial artery before and after a maneuver (usually involving arm abduction), are specifically discussed in the section on TOS (below). Allen's test and capillary refill (<5 seconds) should be compared in each hand. Bilateral findings indicate a systemic disease process. The carotid arteries and supraclavicular fossae should be palpated and auscultated. A supraclavicular pulsatile mass raises the possibility of a subclavian artery aneurysm or associated cervical rib. Fortunately the signs of acute and chronic arterial insufficiency are usually distinct. Signs of acute arterial insufficiency are neatly summarized by the five P's (pulselessness, pallor, poikilothermia, pain, parasthesia). Signs of chronic arterial insufficiency include muscle atrophy, skin bronzing, focal hair loss, and digital gangrene. Nonhealing skin ulcers are an exception to this rule, as they can result from either acute or chronic arterial insufficiency. The presence of skin ulceration should prompt consideration of atherosclerotic disease, embolic disease, Buerger's disease, or vasculitis. Patients with vasculitis or malignancy often look chronically ill and may present with fever, unintentional weight loss, or frank cachexia. The presence of synovitis, nail pitting, prominent nail-bed capillary loops, and skin lesions such as erythema nodosum, pyoderma gangrenosum, petechial rash, or palpable purpura are highly suggestive of a vasculitis or other rheumatological disease. However, the constellation of fever, rash, petechiae, and nail findings also warrants the consideration of infective endocarditis with embolization to the upper extremities. Splinter hemorrhages under the nail beds on the involved side indicate an atheroembolic process, such as one originating from the heart or the ipsilateral subclavian/axillary arteries, or from infective endocarditis.

LABORATORY

A few initial laboratory tests—such as a complete metabolic profile (CMP), a complete blood count (CBC), coagulation parameters, an erythrocyte sedimentation rate (ESR), and a lipid profile—are useful in narrowing the differential diagnosis. Table 38-4 gives a comprehensive list of laboratory tests organized according to a system-based differential diagnosis.

Vascular Laboratory

MEASURING SEGMENTAL LIMB PRESSURES

Segmental arm pressure measurement using a two-cuff system with continuous-wave Doppler (CWD) is available in most vascular laboratories. It is the most useful initial test to determine the level of obstruction, especially when symptoms are asymmetrical. Proximal blood pressure cuffs are placed on each arm to occlude the brachial arteries, and distal cuffs are placed on each forearm to occlude the radial and ulnar arteries. CWD is applied to detect arterial flow, measure pressures, and visualize the arterial waveforms. One can see waveforms and pressures in each upper extremity at the level of the subclavian, axillary, brachial, radial, and ulnar arteries. Arterial occlusion is indicated by flattened waveforms and decreased

TABLE 38-4	Laboratory Tests	
Cardiovascular	*Rheumatological*
Atherosclerotic	CBC with differential
BMP	Rheumatoid factor
Lipid profile	Antinuclear antibody
LP(a)	Anti-dsDNA antibodies
hsCRP	Extractable nuclear antigens
HgbA1c	ESR
Cardiac emboli	CRP
aPTT	Hepatitis virus screening
PT/INR	Cryoglobulins
Cholesterol emboli	
CBC with differential	*Hematological*
Urine eosinophils	Malignancy
	CMP
Infectious	CBC with differential
CBC with differential	SPEP with IFA
ESR	Serum free light chains
CRP	Hypercoagulability
Blood cultures	CBC
	aPTT, PT/INR
Neurological	Factor V Leiden
Vitamin B12	Prothrombin 20210 gene mutation
RPR	Antithrombin III
TSH	Antiphospholipid antibodies
HgbA1c	Protein C
hsCRP	Protein S
	Lupus anticoagulant

BMP, basic metabolic profile; LP(a), lipoprotein a; hsCRP, highly sensitive C-reactive protein; HbgA1, hemoglobin A1c; aPTT, activated partial thromboplastin time; PT/INR, prothrombin time/international normalized ratio; CBC, complete blood count; ESR, erythrocyte sedimentation rate; CRP, C-reactive protein; RPR, rapid plasma reagin; TSH, thryroid stimulating hormone; dsDNA, double-stranded deoxyribonucleic acid; CMP complete metabolic profile; SPEP with IFA, serum protein electrophoresis with immunofixation.

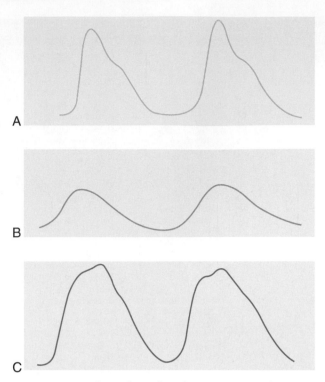

Figure 38-7   Arterial waveforms from finger pressure pulse contours.

amplitudes by CWD. The blood pressure differential between sides using this technique should be less than 10 mm Hg. The wrist-brachial index (WBI, analogous to the ankle-brachial index) and the finger-brachial index (FBI) can also be calculated. Either a WBI of less than 0.85 or an FBI of less than 0.70 is abnormal and suggests arterial insufficiency. Like the ABI, the WBI and FBI can be falsely elevated in the presence of arterial calcinosis and other forms of arterial incompressibility.

FINGER PRESSURE PULSE CONTOURS/ PHOTOPLETHYSMOGRAPHY WAVEFORMS

The measurement of finger pressure pulse contours with photoplethysmography is an excellent technique for discerning normal arterial flow from obstructive disease or from vasospastic disease (Fig. 38-7). The normal arterial waveform is characterized by a rapid systolic upstroke, a sharp systolic peak, and a dicrotic notch on the downstroke. Arterial obstruction is typified by a reduced waveform amplitude, increased time to peak systole (decreased slope), and loss of the dicrotic notch. Vasospasm, as in Raynaud's phenomenon, is characterized by a secondary ascending peak that results in a marked widening of the whole waveform (the "nipple sign"). Duplex ultrasonography is discussed below.

Imaging

Establishment of the patient's diagnosis is almost always facilitated by obtaining an imaging study. Choice of optimum therapy depends on precisely defining the patient's anatomy to guide interventions and for follow-up. The "gold standard" remains digital subtraction

angiography (DSA). But duplex ultrasonography remains the most popular initial imaging technique, and there is increasing application of computed tomography angiography (CTA) and magnetic resonance imaging/angiography (MRI/MRA).

Duplex Ultrasonography

Duplex ultrasonography (combined two-dimensional B-mode ultrasound, and pulsed-wave Doppler) is a noninvasive imaging technique that provides functional as well as anatomical detail based on the Doppler waveform and increases in peak systolic velocities (Fig. 38-8A). It is a relatively inexpensive test, is feasible for use in most patients, and can be performed in the clinic or at the bedside. Its primary disadvantage is that its results are highly operator-dependent.

The standard probe employs a 10-MHz transducer (as opposed to the 3- to 5-MHz transducers used for adult echocardiography). With the exception of a blind spot behind the clavicle, one can use duplex to visualize the course of the upper extremity's vasculature from the origin of the subclavian artery all the way to the palm (a >10-MHz transducer is needed to resolve the digital arteries). The sensitivity and specificity of duplex for detecting arterial stenosis is greater than 90%. However, its utility is not limited to detecting arterial stenoses. Duplex can detect the flow reversal characteristic of steal phenomena, iatrogenic trauma (such as pseudoaneurysm and arterial dissection), and deep venous thrombosis. It is often used to assess whether a lesion is amenable to angioplasty and then for the surveillance of patients after therapy.

Tomographic Imaging Techniques

Tomographic imaging techniques such as CT angiography (CTA) and magnetic resonance angiography (MRA) are excellent noninvasive high-resolution methods of imaging that are useful tools for establishing the diagnosis of proximal arch vessel and upper extremity disease. They are capable of defining complex anatomy (as in the case of a congenital abnormality or prior intervention), allow visualization of vasculature in multiple planes without the problem of overlap, and show extravascular structures. MR has the advantage over CTA (and

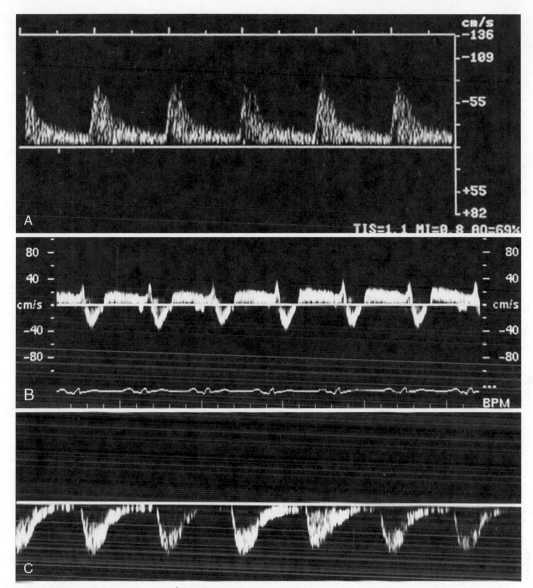

Figure 38-8 A Normal vertebral artery duplex waveform. B. Intermittant vertebral artery flow reversal, as seen with subclavian steal. C. Permanent vertebral artery flow reversal, as seen with subclavian steal.

catheter-based angiography), in that it does not use ionizing radiation or nephrotoxic contrast dye. Gadolinium contrast-enhanced (CE) MRA is the most useful MR technique for assessing peripheral vascular disease. Its sensitivity and specificity for detecting occlusive arterial disease is greater than 95% (compared to catheter-based DSA). It is also highly sensitive and specific for assessing vascular wall inflammation. Phase-contrast (PC) MRA is a separate technique that provides simultaneous anatomical and functional data, similar to duplex. PC-MRA can quantify flow across a stenosis or a shunt and can measure turbulence. It is not typically included in MR protocols at most institutions, so it must be specifically ordered. There are a number of disadvantages to MR. It is time-consuming, and imaging the vasculature within the thorax requires prolonged breath-holding. Patients who are susceptible to claustrophobia cannot tolerate MR or may require prior treatment with anxiolytics. It is highly operator-dependent and susceptible to artifact. The presence of permanent pacemakers, implantable cardiac defibrillators, Swan-Ganz catheters, and shrapnel are relative contraindications to MR in many institutions. However, contrary to the conventional wisdom, endovascular stents and most prosthetic cardiac valves are not contraindicated in MR scanners. CTA provides high-resolution multiplanar images that include perivascular structures, similar to MR, but it is more widely available, less operator-dependent, and less susceptible to artifact. Less patient cooperation is necessary as compared to MR, and claustrophobia and prolonged breath-holding are not as problematic. Ferric metal is not a contraindication to CTA, but its presence may impair image gathering and cause artifacts. Unfortunately, multidetector CTA requires relatively high doses of ionizing radiation as compared with catheter-based angiography and, like catheter-based angiography, CTA requires the use of iodinated contrast dye that has the potential to cause nephrotoxicity and/or an allergic reaction.

Angiography/Digital Subtraction Angiography

Catheter-based angiography, in particular digital subtraction angiography (DSA), remains the gold standard for imaging the peripheral vasculature, including the aortic arch, great vessels, and arteries of the upper extremities. It is the most definitive method of defining the vasculature and allows one to measure intra-arterial blood pressures, gradients, and waveforms. It can facilitate the use of intravascular ultrasound (IVUS, see below) or a pressure-sensing wire.[21] If a lesion is significant and amenable to intervention, it is accessible at the time of the diagnostic catheterization. The disadvantages of catheter-based angiography include its invasiveness, exposure to ionizing radiation, and potential for complications (vascular trauma, bleeding, infection, contrast-induced nephropathy, and contrast-induced allergic reaction).

It is usually feasible and preferable to obtain vascular access through the femoral artery for percutaneous catheter-based angiography and angioplasty of the aortic arch and upper extremities. In the case of a tight subclavian or axillary artery lesion, it may be necessary to obtain brachial artery access on the ipsilateral side. An array of diagnostic catheters is available for accessing and imaging the great arch vessels and upper extremities. The pigtail catheter in conjunction with an autoinjector is necessary to obtain good images of the aortic arch. Common projections are LAO 30 degrees for the origin of the great vessels and RAO 20 degrees for the brachiocephalic bifurcation. It is usually necessary to modify these angles to open up the arch. The arch vessels may be imaged with a variety of catheters, such as the Judkins Right no. 4 (JR4), internal mammary (IMA), Vitek (VTK), Simmons, or multipurpose. Injection rates for the arch are usually 30 to 40 mL over 2 seconds. The upper extremities may be selectively taken with hand injections.

Subclavian Steal Syndrome

DEFINITION, HISTORICAL BACKGROUND, AND CONTROVERSY

Subclavian steal is a result of the reversal of blood flow in vascular territories normally supplied by the subclavian artery. It is characterized by retrograde vertebral blood flow away from the cerebral posterior circulation to accommodate demand for blood in the ipsilateral subclavian artery beyond a tight proximal stenosis. The phenomenon was first described in 1960,[22] and it was quickly appreciated that such an occurrence could cause symptoms consequent to a paucity of arterial blood flow to the cerebral posterior circulation, extremity, or heart.[23–25] In the classic description, blood may flow up the right brachiocephalic artery to the right carotid artery or right vertebral artery, through the Circle of Willis, then down the left vertebral artery to the distal subclavian artery, where there is decreased arterial pressure (due to a proximal subclavian artery stenosis) and hence a gradient that results in the "stealing" of blood from the posterior cerebral vascular territory.[26] In the context of *symptoms,* the phenomenon is called the subclavian steal *syndrome* (SSS). More commonly, however, it is a phenomenon found incidentally (by way of vascular studies) in an asymptomatic patient. When this occurs, it is sometimes referred to as "radiologic" subclavian steal to distinguish it from clinically significant steal. The transient obstruction of the proximal segment of the subclavian artery with respiratory variation (Dieter's sign) that occurs in some individuals has been described (Fig. 38-9).[27] The concept of SSS has not been without controversy; some early papers suggested that the syndrome did not exist.[28,29] These authors pointed to evidence showing that even when there is reversal of blood flow in the vertebral

artery, there is no appreciable difference in total cerebral arterial flow.[28,29] That indeed may be the case for patients with an isolated severe proximal subclavian artery stenosis. Subsequent studies have shown that most patients affected by SSS have concurrent cerebrovascular lesions.[30] Upwards of 80% of patients who have SSS (i.e., symptomatic patients) also have concurrent stenosis in the contralateral carotid or vertebral artery. These patients presumably have inadequate cerebral arterial reserve in the context of increased demand from the affected extremity. The controversy has not ended with this discovery, however. There are many who speculate that these patients with symptoms of cerebral vascular ischemia in the context of both cerebrovascular lesions and a subclavian artery lesion are most likely to have symptoms intrinsic to the cerebrovascular lesions and that the subclavian lesion is merely incidental.

It is also important to note that some of the controversy surrounding the diagnosis of SSS is a result of the disparity in reports on its prevalence. Early literature reported a low prevalence of vertebral artery flow reversal in patients with severe subclavian artery stenosis (as assessed by contrast angiography),[30,31] while more recent literature reports a very high (although not necessarily clinically significant) incidence of vertebral artery flow reversal in the same patient population.[32] These differences are hard to reconcile but likely reflect an underdiagnosis of the phenomenon (but not necessarily syndrome) prior to the widespread use of duplex ultrasonography.

PRESENTATION

Most patients with the SSS come to the physician's attention because of symptoms or abnormal physical findings. Symptoms are due to vertebrobasilar insufficiency or ischemia of the upper extremity and may include syncope, dizziness, vertigo, ataxia, headache, visual disturbances, arm claudication, and parasthesia. These symptoms are generally worsened or precipitated by use of the extremity (as with exercise) or compression of the vertebral artery (as with head rotation). Since symptoms are usually related to a *transient* paucity of arterial blood flow to either the cerebral posterior circulation or the upper extremity, stroke and severe limb ischemia are uncommon presentations for SSS. A thorough physical exam (as described above), with particular attention to the upper extremities and a neurological exam are also often revealing.

ETIOLOGY

SSS is most commonly caused by an atherosclerotic narrowing of the proximal subclavian artery. The prevalence of significant subclavian artery atherosclerosis in patients with coronary artery disease (CAD) is 17% to 23%.[6,31] Of these patients, only 2.5% are estimated to be symptomatic (and many more have radiological steal). The left subclavian artery is affected three times more often than the brachiocephalic artery, possibly because of accelerated atherosclerosis caused by the more acute origin of the left subclavian artery and hence greater

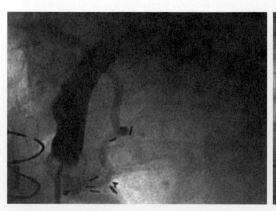
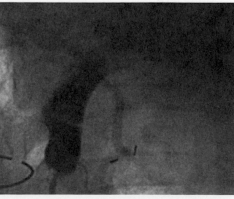

Figure 38-9 Dynamic left subclavian artery obstruction ("Dieter sign"). Exacerbation of proximal subclavian artery kink with expiration. Left subclavian arteriogram during inspiration (left) and expiration (right). (*Reproduced with permission from Dieter RS et al. Description of a new angiographic sign: dynamic left artery obstruction. Vasc Dis Management. 2006 3(5):298–299.*)

turbulence. The presence of SSS is twice as common in men as in women and reportedly has a peak incidence at 40 to 60 years of age.[33] SSS can also be caused by a vasculitis, such as Takayasu's. Vasculitides less commonly cause subclavian steal, however, because they typically involve a diffuse area of the artery. For example, if Takayasu's arteritis affects the subclavian artery, it is likely to involve a region both proximal and distal to the origin of the vertebral artery rather than the focal proximal stenosis that is the substrate for the subclavian steal phenomenon.

The thoracic outlet syndrome (TOS, described below) can also lead to the SSS by causing compression or kinking of the proximal subclavian artery. This phenomenon is most common in athletes, such as baseball pitchers, swimmers, golfers, or others who vigorously and repetitively abduct the upper extremity. Congenital heart and vascular abnormalities (as described under "Anatomical Variants," above) can predispose to SSS. A right aortic arch with isolation of the left subclavian artery or anomolies of the brachiocephalic arteries are the most common associations. Iatrogenic causes of SSS have been increasingly recognized. Prior vascular surgery is a significant risk factor for the development of SSS and should alert the physician to this and various other steal phenomena.[34] Classic examples include coronary artery bypass grafting (CABG) with a left internal mammary artery conduit (see "Coronary Subclavian Steal Syndrome," below), arteriovenous fistula creation for hemodialysis access,[35] repair of tetralogy of Fallot with a Blalock-Taussig anastomosis,[34,36] and surgical repair of coarctation of the aorta.[37] Numerous other inadvertent steal phenomena are created by various surgical techniques described previously.[18,26,34] External beam radiation—as for the treatment of Hodgkin's disease, breast cancer, and lung cancer—is another potential iatrogenic cause of SSS.[38] Intervention is generally warranted to correct iatrogenically created steal syndromes.[26,34]

ESTABLISHING THE DIAGNOSIS

The hallmark of the SSS is the presence of symptoms. When a patient is suspected of having SSS, an initial evaluation with a noninvasive study of the carotid and vertebral arteries (with particular attention to the direction of blood flow) is warranted.

Flow reversal in the vertebral artery is most readily seen by duplex.[39] There are three classifications of vertebral artery flow abnormalities. Stage I is used to describe reduced antegrade flow; stage II is used to describe intermittent flow reversal, as with exercise (Fig. 38-8B); and stage III is used to describe permanent retrograde flow through the vertebral artery (Fig. 38-8C). Depending on the results of noninvasive studies, one may decide to proceed with catheter-based angiography of the aortic arch and the brachiocephalic, subclavian, carotid, vertebral, and subclavian arteries. In patients who have had prior CABG using the left internal mammary artery as a conduit, the coronary arteries should also be evaluated (see "Coronary Subclavian Steal Syndrome," below). When the relative functional significance of a subclavian artery stenosis is unclear, as in the case of a concurrent ipsilateral vertebral artery stenosis, the use of a pressure-sensing wire can be helpful.[21] Noninvasive radionucleotide imaging of the upper extremities with thallium 201 to determine functional significance of subclavian artery stenosis after arm exercise (i.e., stress testing) has also been reported.[40] Finally, when there is a history of congenital heart disease or another complex anatomical variation, it may be helpful to obtain CTA or contrast-enhanced (CE) MRA prior to catheter-based angiography or in lieu of it.

PROGNOSIS

The long-term prognosis of the subclavian steal syndrome is generally favorable with regard to progression of neurological deficits and other associated symptoms.[32,41] However, when caused by atherosclerosis, the prognosis of SSS (as with all cases of PAD) is surprisingly dismal over the 5-year interval following its diagnosis.[2-5] For these patients (i.e., the majority of patients with SSS), the greatest benefit in terms

of decreasing morbidity and mortality will be derived from instituting best-medical therapy and cardiovascular risk factor modification.

The prognosis for patients with SSS caused by Takayasu's arteritis is considerably better than for those who have SSS caused by atherosclerosis. The 5 year survival for patients with Takayasu's arteritis is 80% to 90%.[42-44] The long-term prospects are excellent, even for patients who require surgical revascularization (mean survival is 19.8 years).[45] The favorable prognosis in these patients is contingent on lifelong surveillance and appropriate medical and surgical therapy.

THERAPY

Intervention for SSS should be reserved for symptomatic patients only. In the absence of symptoms (i.e., radiological SSS), the condition is generally benign. A relatively recent study reported the most common indications for subclavian artery revascularization in order of decreasing prevalence as SSS, arm claudication, coronary SSS (see below), and nonhealing wounds.[46]

Over the four decades since the SSS was first described, traditional surgical revascularization of the supra-aortic vessels has been largely supplanted by endovascular interventions. The impetus for the trend toward catheter-based therapy has been fewer complications and shorter recovery times. The first report on percutaneous transluminal angioplasty (PTA) for the SSS was published in 1980.[47] The past quarter-century has brought forth significant progress in this area, and recent studies demonstrate high primary success and reasonable long-term patency for PTA and stenting of the subclavian artery in patients with SSS (Fig. 38-1).[46,48] Primary success for subclavian artery stenting of subtotal occlusions is achieved in more than 98% of cases, with an incidence of major complications less than 1%.[46,48] Under conscious sedation and local anesthesia, subclavian stenoses can usually be approached using femoral access. In cases where there is complete or almost complete occlusion, access via a brachial or combined femorobrachial approach may be necessary to cross the lesion. The challenge posed by crossing a totally occluded subclavian artery proves insurmountable in nearly 50% of cases.[49] When the subclavian artery is selectively cannulated, a reference angiogram is obtained to visualize the lesion and size the balloon. Many interventionists advocate predilation, although primary stenting is gaining popularity. Balloon-expandable stents are used for lesions in the proximal subclavian artery. Self-expanding stents are used for subclavian artery lesions distal to the origin of the vertebral artery.[50] Positioning of the stent can be guided by angiography, calcification, and road mapping (Fig. 38-10).

Potential major complications of percutaneous intervention, albeit uncommon, include upper extremity embolization, transient ischemic attack and stroke, avulsion, perforation, dissection of the subclavian artery and aorta, and mycotic aneurysm.[46,48,49,51,52] Embolization to the vertebral artery or left internal mammary artery-left anterior descending artery (LIMA-LAD) graft can be catastrophic. However, given the rarity of major embolic complications, it has been suggested that there is persistent vertebral flow reversal for several seconds to minutes after PTA, thus providing some hemodynamic protection.[53] Nevertheless, some interventionalists prefer to use a distal protection device, such as a filter wire, in the vertebral artery via a radial/brachial approach.[54] The simplest method is balloon occlusion of the vertebral artery with a small compliant balloon that is deflated following the intervention— that is, after the subclavian balloon is deflated (i.e., any debris embolizes the arm rather than the brain).[55] Likewise, some have advocated that a double-balloon technique be used during subclavian artery interventions to protect a LIMA graft.[56] In most cases, the initial success of PTA with stent placement is equivalent to that of surgical revascularization, albeit with significantly lower morbidity and mortality. Furthermore, the long-term patency following PTA with stent placement (but not PTA alone) appears to be equivalent to the long-term patency with surgical revascularization.[7,46] Nevertheless, there has not been a randomized trial comparing the two techniques at the time of this writing. In complicated cases, such as the presence of a totally

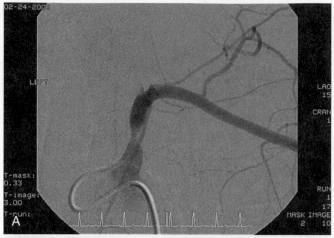

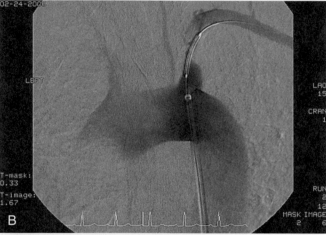

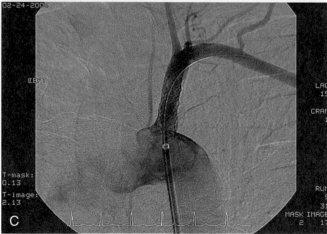

Figure 38-10 Proximal left subclavian artery stenosis (A), stent deployment (B), and poststent (C).

occluded subclavian artery, complex anatomy, or multiple lesions, a surgical or combined procedure may still be necessary. However, prior to undertaking a complex revascularization of the supra-aortic vessels, correction of a significant carotid stenosis (either by carotid endarterectomy or carotid stenting) should first be performed, as it will often be sufficient to resolve the patient's symptoms.[57] The risks of surgical revascularization of the supra-aortic vessels are significant and have been published extensively. The traditional transthoracic approach with median sternotomy is associated with a 10% to 20% risk of stroke and/or death.[58,59] Even so, this approach may be reasonable in cases where the patient also requires CABG or in cases of complex

brachiocephalic lesions. The potential for complications resulting from the transthoracic approach spurred the development of safer extrathoracic approaches. Extrathoracic revascularization is now the most popular form of surgical correction. Overall patency for extrathoracic revascularization has been reported as 95% at 1 year, 86% at 3 years, and 73% at 5 years.[60] Although it carries less perioperative mortality than the transthoracic approach, extrathoracic revascularization is technically challenging owing to the intrinsic friability of the subclavian arteries and their tendency to tear.[26,61] Risk of major complication with extrathoracic bypass is 13% overall, with 3% risk of stroke and 2% risk of death.[7] Medical therapy for SSS due to atherosclerosis is directed at cardiovascular event risk reduction rather than symptomatic relief. Unlike PAD of the lower extremities, there is no established role for phosphodiesterase III inhibitors (e.g., cilostazol). At least some data, by way of case reports, indicate that they are ineffective for SSS and upper extremity claudication.[40] Extrapolation of data for lower extremity PAD also suggests that there is no role for prostaglandin EI (PGE1) in the management of upper extremity ischemia.[62] Warfarin therapy should be reserved for the most severe and refractory cases and has been studied in neither a prospective nor randomized manner. If a large vessel vasculitis, such as Takayasu's or giant cell (temporal), is suspected, it is reasonable to initially treat with high-dose corticosteroids (prednisone 60 mg PO daily or equivalent). Early stages of vasculitis respond well to high-dose corticosteroids. Long-term therapy with a slow taper (e.g., a decrease in dose by 10% per week in responders) is necessary to prevent arterial stenosis. In the chronic stages of large-vessel vasculitis, the artery becomes irreversibly stenosed and may require PTA or surgical bypass. Intervention tends to be more difficult, since the artery may be friable, fibrotic, or inflamed. Since establishing a definitive diagnosis of vasculitis can be challenging and a large percentage of cases of Takayasu's arteritis do not respond to corticosteroid treatment, consultation with a rheumatologist is recommended.

Coronary Subclavian Steal Syndrome

A similar steal phenomenon can occur in patients who have undergone coronary artery bypass grafting (CABG) with an internal mammary artery (IMA) conduit and who also have proximal subclavian artery stenosis (or occlusion) (Fig. 38-11). In this variation, blood is shunted away from the coronary circulation retrograde through the IMA graft to supply the subclavian artery watershed. Classically, the patient experiences angina pectoris upon exercising the arm.[63,64] However, acute myocardial infarction in a patient with an IMA graft following occlusion of the subclavian artery has also been reported.[65] Coronary SSS has become increasingly relevant over the past two decades, as the use of the internal mammary artery has increased to 75% to 90% of all CABGs.[66] Given the prevalence of significant subclavian artery atherosclerosis (17%-23%) in patients with CAD,[6,31] one must consider coronary SSS in the differential diagnosis of post-CABG patients who present with chest pain. Citing the low risk and potential benefits, some cardiologists have made a strong argument for performing angiography of the left subclavian artery (with nonselective angiography of the LIMA) at the time of coronary angiography for all patients who are referred for CAGB.[6,67] In affected patients, it may be reasonable to perform subclavian artery stenting preoperatively to allow use of the LIMA or alternative conduits. As with SSS and other cases of symptomatic subclavian artery stenosis, it is preferable to approach coronary SSS with a catheter-based intervention as a first line of attack. The surgical approaches for coronary subclavian steal are similar to those for SSS.[68,69]

Thoracic Outlet Syndrome

DEFINITION

The thoracic outlet syndrome (TOS) encompasses a heterogeneous group of disorders that result in symptomatic compression of the

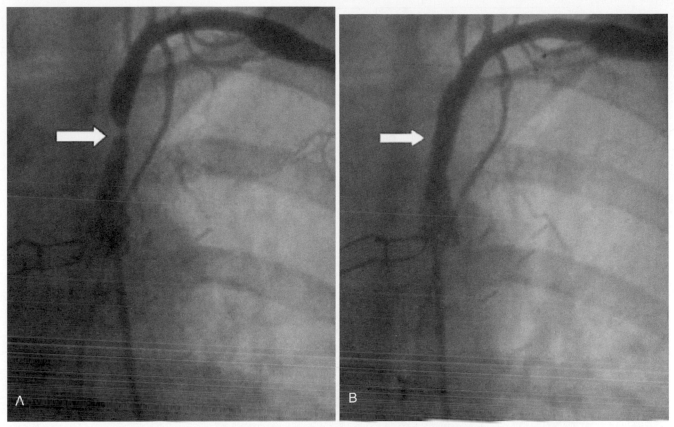

Figure 38-11 Coronary subclavian steal syndrome pre-intervention (A) and post intervention (B).[63]

neurovascular bundle at any of several points as it traverses the cervicoaxillary canal through the scalene triangle and costoclavicular space to enter the upper extremity (Fig. 38-12).[70] The neurovascular bundle principally comprises the five roots of the brachial plexus, the subclavian artery, and the subclavian vein (some anatomists would also include the phrenic nerve, long thoracic nerve, and sympathetic chain). The roots of the brachial plexus, along with the subclavian artery, pass through the scalene triangle, which is bounded by the anterior and middle scalene muscles on each side and the first rib at the base. The subclavian vein passes outside the scalene triangle in front of the anterior scalene muscle and behind the pectoralis major muscle. The components of the neurovascular bundle then pass through the costoclavicular space, which is bounded by the clavicle, first rib, costoclavicular ligament, and middle scalene muscle. In practice, one finds the anatomy of the thoracic outlet highly variable among individuals.[71] Nine separate types of congenital bands and ligaments have been described within the scalene triangle.[72] Cervical ribs, which have a tendency to impinge on the structures exiting the thoracic outlet, occur in 0.5% to 1.5% of the general population.

ETIOLOGY AND PREVALENCE

TOS is commonly classified as either neurogenic or vascular (Table 38-5). Neurogenic TOS, which refers to the symptomatic compression of the brachial plexus, is thought to account for 95% of cases. The site of compression is usually in the scalene triangle. 70% of neurogenic TOS cases occur in female patients. Vascular TOS comprises the remaining 5% of cases, with the majority of those affecting the subclavian artery and the minority affecting the subclavian vein. The site of compression in arterial TOS is most often an osseous narrowing in the costoclavicular space, as from a cervical rib. Compression of the

subclavian artery at this point commonly results in aneurysm formation and embolization (Fig. 38-13). Unlike neurogenic TOS, arterial TOS occurs equally among men and women. For unknown reasons, venous TOS occurs twice as often in men as it does in women. The overall prevalence of TOS is not known because it represents an assortment of various rare disorders that are collectively difficult to diagnose definitively. Age is a poor discriminator, but TOS tends to be most common in 20- to 40-year olds. Most of these patients have both an underlying anatomical predisposition for the disorder, such as a cervical rib or fibrous band, and an underlying mechanical feature, such as overuse or trauma. The chance of developing TOS is highest among those who have the susceptible anatomical substrate and engage in occupational or recreational activities that involve repetitive arm movements (e.g., painters, throwing athletes, rowers, and weight lifters).

PRESENTATION

The symptoms of TOS usually present with an insidious onset and become progressively worse. Patients are likely to describe bouts of pain or paresthesias of the upper limbs that occur in dermatomal patterns. The patient's dominant hand is most apt to be affected, although TOS occasionally presents bilaterally or in the nondominant hand. Various arm movements, especially those involving abduction, may precipitate or exacerbate the patient's symptoms. In time, weakness and muscle atrophy may arise. Raynaud's phenomenon and other discoloration or coldness in the hands can occur. Extreme hypersensitivity or causalgia may be present. Interestingly, headache is a common symptom and may represent referred pain to the occiput.[73] All of these symptoms can take hours to days to resolve following the precipitating arm movements. Since the symptoms of TOS are hardly

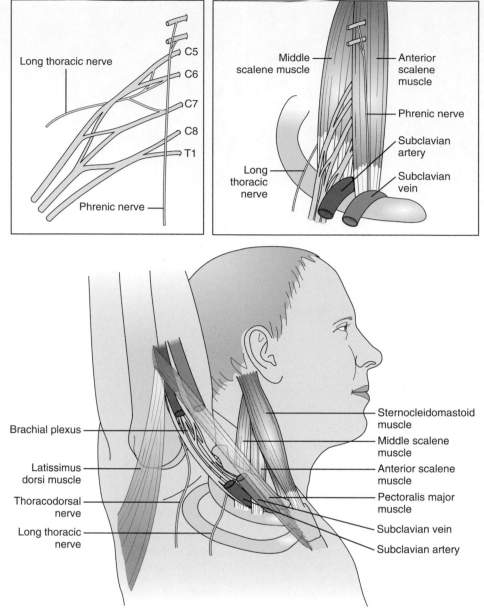

Figure 38-12 Anatomy of the thoracic outlet. (*Redrawn from* Ann Vasc Surg. *1997 11:315–323.*[70])

unique and the disorder is relatively uncommon, patients are usually initially misdiagnosed as having a pure musculoskeletal disorder or even PAD of the proximal arch or upper extremity. Establishing the diagnosis of TOS may be further delayed when patients are late in seeking medical attention. Late presentations can be attributed to the insidious and subtle onset of symptoms, adaptive modifications

TABLE 38-5	Causes of Thoracic Outlet Syndrome
Bony	Cervical rib
	First thoracic rib
	Enlarged C7 transverse process
	Dislocation of the head of the humerus
	Clavicle (fracture, exostosis, bifid)
	Cervical spondylosis
	Crushing injury to upper thorax
Soft tissue	Fibrous bands
	Scalene muscles
	Omohyoid muscle
	Large pendulous breasts

(adapted from Angiology)[74]

(conscious or subconscious) in the activities of daily living, and, in cases of arterial TOS, the presence of compensating arterial collaterals. The late presentation of vascular TOS occasionally leads to catastrophic results.

DIAGNOSIS

The diagnosis of TOS is often challenging owing to its lack of specific findings and its overall rarity. Indeed, there is no single test or pathognomonic finding to prove TOS. Most testing will either be negative or equivocal. Therefore the diagnosis must be based on clinical pattern recognition and the exclusion of other diagnoses (Table 38-6). Commonly the patient is seen by multiple specialists before the diagnosis is established. In addition to the components of the physical exam emphasized earlier in this chapter (see "Physical Examination," above), there are numerous diagnostic maneuvers that have been described especially for TOS (Table 38-7). The common denominator among most of these is some form of arm abduction while the examiner palpates the radial pulse and notes its disappearance (Fig. 38-14). The EAST (External rotation-abduction stress test) (see Table 38-7)

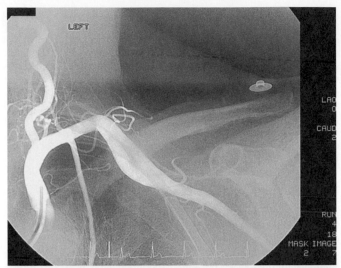

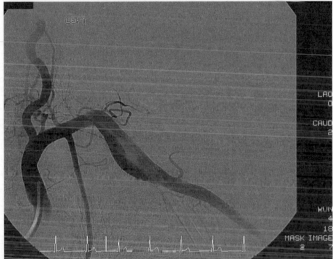

Figure 38-13 Arteriogram of the left subclavian artery showing a large subclavian aneurysm in a patient with a cervical rib and thoracic outlet syndrome.

TABLE 38-6	Differential Diagnosis for Thoracic Outlet Syndrome	
Arterial	Embolic disease
	Aneurysms
	Atherosclerosis
	Arterial dissection
	Aberrant anatomy
	Reflex, vasomotor
	Raynaud's syndrome
	Vasculitis
	Radiation injury
Venous	DVT
	SVC syndrome
	Other neoplastic compression
Cervical spine	Spinal cord tumor
	Ruptured intervertebral disk
	Degenerative joint disease/osteoarthritis
	Other neurological diseases
Compressive syndromes	Carpal tunnel syndrome
	Ulnar nerve entrapment
	Trauma (brachial plexus injury, compartment syndrome, hyperextension)
	Rotator cuff injury
	Pancoast's tumor
Referred pain, other	Coronary artery disease
	Esophageal spasm
Secondary gain	

DVT, deep venous thrombosis; SVC, superior vena cava.
(adapted from Angiology)[74]

However, it should be emphasized that there is no role for initial endovascular repair in cases of TOS (aside from thromboembolic complications). Barring an acute vascular syndrome, the best initial approach to the treatment of patients with TOS is a conservative one. Most patients derive considerable benefit from noninvasive therapies and have a favorable long-term outcome[74] (Table 38-8). Surgical intervention is reserved for severe or refractory cases of TOS and is directed at releasing the scalene muscles and/or removing any bony obstruction.

The relevance of TOS to the interventional cardiologist lies primarily in recognizing how this heterogeneous group of disorders can masquerade as PAD of the proximal arch and upper extremity. Since most cases of TOS are the result of nerve compression or related to musculoskeletal entrapment of the neurovascular bundle, many cardiologists will prefer to delegate the management of these patients to their respective medical and surgical colleagues.

Axillary Artery Disease

The incidence of atherosclerosis is much lower in the axillary artery than it is in the subclavian artery. The most common pathologies of the axillary arteries are aneurysm and vasculitis.

Axillary aneurysm in the United States is commonly a result of "crutch syndrome." As the name implies, long-term crutch use and compression of the axillary artery can lead to stenosis or aneurysm formation. Iatrogenic trauma to the axillary artery (as from catheter-based angiography, misdirected central line insertion, or pacemaker

maneuver is widely regarded as the most useful in diagnosing neurogenic TOS, while Adson's maneuver is most effective in identifying positional compression of the subclavian artery. All of the TOS maneuvers suffer from low specificity (a 15% false-positive rate overall). In terms of diagnostic testing, it is reasonable to begin with chest x-rays and possibly a cervical spine x-ray series (Fig. 38-15). When vascular TOS is suspected, the patient should be referred to the vascular laboratory for photoplethysmography and duplex ultrasound to measure arterial patterns during provocative TOS maneuvers. Tomographic imaging may be useful, especially MRI, as it can identify soft tissue abnormalities, such as congenital bands and ligaments in addition to bony abnormalities. If there is a high suspicion of vascular TOS, it is recommended to proceed with bilateral arteriography (and possibly venography), sometimes with provocative maneuvers during angiography.

THERAPY AND PROGNOSIS

In cases where TOS causes an acute vascular syndrome, therapy is directed at emergent surgical decompression of the subclavian artery and restoration of peripheral perfusion. Acute thromboembolism from a subclavian artery aneurysm can be treated by catheter-directed thrombolytic therapy (see "Embolic Disease," above) or embolectomy.

TABLE 38-7	Diagnostic Maneuvers for Thoracic Outlet Syndrome
Adson's maneuver	Patient sitting upright, takes a deep breath, looks upward, and turns his or her face *toward* the affected side.
EAST maneuver (external rotation-abduction stress test)	Arms extended, externally rotated, and behind the head. Patient repeatedly makes fists for 3 minutes while the radial pulses are palpated.
Hyperabduction maneuver	Patient hyperabducts the affected extremity (evaluates for compression).
Costoclavicular maneuver	Patient thrusts both shoulders maximally backward and downward.

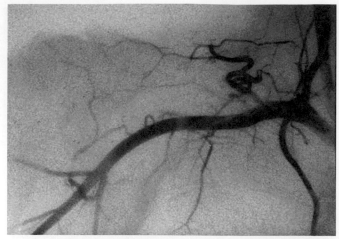

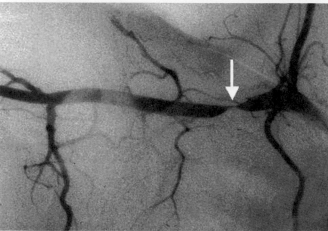

Figure 38-14 Right subclavian artery occlusion with arm abduction (lower frame) and absence of occlusion with arm relaxed (upper frame).

placement) can also result in vascular aneurysm formation. Large-vessel vasculitides commonly affect the axillary arteries and can acutely result in severe vasospasm and chronically result in stenosis or aneurysm. Kawasaki's disease, a pediatric cause of vasculitis, frequently leads to arterial aneurysms (including axillary artery aneurysms) that become symptomatic during adulthood. Aggressive therapy of Kawasaki's disease with immunosuppressive therapy, including gamma

TABLE 38-8	Therapies for Thoracic Outlet Syndrome	
Physiotherapy	
Lifestyle changes	
Psychiatric therapy	
Medication	Acetaminophen
	Non-steroidal anti-inflammatory drugs
	Muscle relaxants
	Opioids
	Anticoagulants
	Thrombolytics
Surgery	Rib resection
	Clavicle resection
	Scalenus transaction
	Breast reduction
	Thrombectomy/embolectomy
	Bypass graft
	Dorsal sympathectomy
	Neurolysis

(adapted from Angiology)[74]

globulin, minimizes the formation of aneurysm. Takayasu's arteritis, a rare autoimmune-mediated vasculitis of young adults, often affects the subclavian and axillary arteries. Giant cell (temporal) arteritis is a disease of older adults that can involve the axillary arteries (and occasionally affects arteries as distal as the radial). Axillary artery vasculitis may also be caused by external beam radiation used to treat cancer (especially of the lung or breast as well as Hodgkin's disease). Axillary artery aneurysm commonly results in thrombus formation and embolization to the distal arteries of the upper extremity. Large or symptomatic axillary artery aneurysms should be treated, either percutaneously with self-expanding stents or with surgical correction. Embolic complications are discussed below.

Embolic Disease

Thromboembolism to the upper extremities is a vascular emergency. Clinical manifestations depend on the arterial segment affected by thromboembolism but often manifest as acute unilateral digital ischemia (see "Initial Evaluation," above).[75] Raynaud's phenomenon is also a familiar finding. When the source of emboli is the heart or thoracic aorta, it is typical for the patient to present with multiple simultaneously involved arterial beds. Unlike atheroembolic disease in general, which is most often attributable to a cardiac source, embolism to the upper extremities is usually caused by aneurysmal disease of the proximal arch vessels. As previously discussed, the most widespread causes of proximal arch vessel aneurysm are crutch syndrome, TOS, and the large-vessel vasculitides. It should be noted that vasculitis-induced thromboembolic phenomena can occur in the absence of aneurysm. The distal arteries of the upper extremity can also be affected by aneurysmal disease. The most common mechanism for this pathology is the hypothenar hand syndrome, an occupationally related repeated compression of the ulnar artery against the hamate bone. Affected patients usually have a history of using the heel of the hand as a hammer or extensive handling of vibratory tools. Involvement in certain sporting activities, such as martial arts or mountain biking, has also been implicated. As with aneurysmal disease in the proximal arteries, thromboembolism is not an unusual complication. Cardiac emboli are a slightly less common source of embolism to the upper extremities. However, approximately 30% of cardiac emboli will travel to the upper extremities. Other potential sources of upper extremity emboli include atherosclerosis of the proximal arch vessels in the absence of aneurysm and atherosclerosis of the aortic arch. The occurrence of thromboembolism must be diagnosed and treated swiftly. Treatment can be dependent upon the source of embolism, so it is important to try establishing it before initiating an intervention. Often, a focused history and physical examination along with an electrocardiogram can delineate a proximal arch vessel source of embolization from a cardiogenic one. Duplex ultrasonography and/or transesophageal echocardiography may be useful adjuncts. Otherwise, procession to the catheterization laboratory to identify the occluded arterial segment should not be delayed. Endovascular treatment options for atheroembolism to the upper extremities include catheter-directed thrombolytic therapy, Fogarty catheter-facilitated removal of emboli, and PTA with or without placement of a self-expanding stent. It is wise to alert one's surgical colleagues early in the management of complex cases, such as patients with a large embolic burden or those who are late in seeking medical attention. Surgical options for these patients include use of the Fogarty catheter, bypass grafting, and limb/digit amputation. Following revascularization, it is often necessary for these patients to receive a prolonged course of anticoagulation.

Conclusion

Cardiologists continue to enlarge their scope of knowledge and apply their skills to a wider field of practice. The management of patients with arterial diseases of the proximal arch and upper extremity is one of the latest examples of this phenomenon. It represents a logical extension of our field of practice. However, diseases of the aortic arch

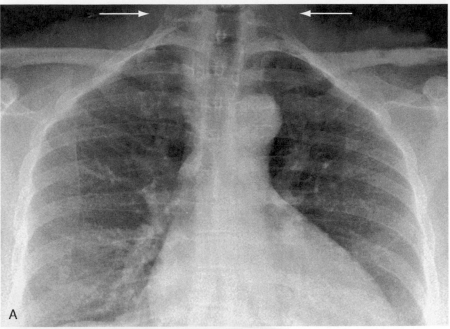

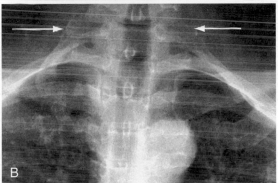

Figure 38-15 Chest x ray demonstrating cervical ribs. (*Courtesy Terrence Demos, MD, Loyola University Medical Center.*)

and upper extremity are uniquely challenging. For the interventional cardiologist who pursues this realm of vascular medicine, it is vital to have an awareness of the differences from coronary and lower extremity peripheral artery disease. The differential diagnosis for arterial diseases of the proximal arch and upper extremity is vast, and the potential for various (and often iatrogenic) steal phenomena exists. Nevertheless, when one understands these distinctions, the standard techniques for angiography and angioplasty that have been used on the lower extremity can be applied with great success to the upper extremity. Percutaneous intervention for occlusive diseases of the aortic arch

vessels and upper extremities has become a successful, safe, and durable alternative to surgical intervention and is reasonable as first line therapy. The optimal techniques regarding stent deployment, type of stent, use of distal protection devices, and when to refer for surgery remain unknown and await randomized clinical trials.

Acknowledgments

We give special thanks to Connie Hsu Swenson for her keen editing and final reading of this work.

REFERENCES

1. Sorensen KE, Kristensen IB, Celermajer DS: Atherosclerosis in the human brachial artery. *J Am Coll Cardiol* 29(2):318–322, 1997.
2. Hirsch AT, et al: Peripheral arterial disease detection, awareness, and treatment in primary care. *JAMA* 286(11):1317–1324, 2001.
3. Hirsch AT, et al: *NHLBI Workshop on Peripheral Arterial Disease (PAD): Developing A Public Awareness Campaign*, Bethesda, MD, 2003, National Heart, Lung and Blood Institute.
4. Weitz JI, et al: Diagnosis and treatment of chronic arterial insufficiency of the lower extremities: a critical review. *Circulation* 94(11):3026–3049, 1996.
5. Dieter RS, et al: Lower extremity peripheral arterial disease in hospitalized patients with coronary artery disease. *Vasc Med* 8(4):233–236, 2003.
6. Rigatelli G, Rigatelli G: Screening angiography of supraaortic vessels performed by invasive cardiologists at the time of cardiac catheterization: indications and results. *Int J Cardiovasc Imaging* 21(2–3):179–183, 2005.

7. Hadjipetrou P, et al: Percutaneous revascularization of atherosclerotic obstruction of aortic arch vessels. *J Am Coll Cardiol* 33(5):1238–1245, 1999.
8. Rajagopalan S, Mukherjee D, Mohler E: *Manual of Vascular Diseases*, Baltimore, 2004, Lippincott Williams & Wilkins, p 464.
9. Bogey WM, et al: Percutaneous transluminal angioplasty for subclavian artery stenosis. *Am Surg* 60(2):103–106, 1994.
10. Kadir S: *Atlas of Normal and Variant Angiographic Anatomy*, Philadelphia, 1991, Saunders, pp xi, 529.
11. Moore KL, Dalley AF, Agur AMR: *Clinically Oriented Anatomy*, ed 5, Philadelphia, 2006, Lippincott Williams & Wilkins, pp xxxiii, 1209.
12. Blake HA, Manion WC: Thoracic arterial arch anomalies. *Circulation* 26:251–265, 1962.
13. Grollman, JH Jr, Harris CH, Hamilton LC: Congenital diverticula of the aortic arch. *N Engl J Med* 276(21):1178–1182, 1967.

14. Klinkhamer AC: berrant right subclavian artery. Clinical and roentgenologic aspects. *Am J Roentgenol Radium Ther Nucl Med* 97(2):438–446, 1966.
15. Kommerell B: Verlagernung des *osophagus* durch eine abnorm verlaufende arteria subclavia Dextra (arteria lusoria). *Fortschr Geb Rontgenstr Nuklearmed Erganzungsband* 54:5905, 1936.
16. Brown DL, et al: Dysphagia lusoria: aberrant right subclavian artery with a Kommerell's diverticulum. *Am Surg* 59(9):582–586, 1993.
17. Verkroost MW, Hamerlijnck RP, Vermeulen FE: Surgical management of aneurysms at the origin of an aberrant right subclavian artery. *J Thorac Cardiovasc Surg* 107(6):1469–1471, 1994.
18. Pifarre R, Dieter RA Jr, Niedballa RG: Definitive surgical treatment of the aberrant retroesophageal right subclavian artery in the adult. *J Thorac Cardiovasc Surg* 61(1):154–159, 1971.

19. Tschirch E, et al: Perinatal management of right aortic arch with aberrant left subclavian artery associated with critical stenosis of the subclavian artery in a newborn. *Ultrasound Obstet Gynecol* 25(3):296–298, 2005.

20. English JA, et al: Angiographic prevalence and clinical predictors of left subclavian stenosis in patients undergoing diagnostic cardiac catheterization. *Catheter Cardiovasc Intervent* 54(1):8–11, 2001.

21. Liu CP, Ling YH, Kao HL: Use of a pressure-sensing wire to detect sequential pressure gradients for ipsilateral vertebral and subclavian artery stenoses. *AJNR Am J Neuroradiol* 26(7):1810–1812, 2005.

22. Contorni L. [The vertebro-vertebral collateral circulation in obliteration of the subclavian artery at its origin.]. *Minerva Chir* 15:268–271, 1960.

23. Reivich M, et al: Reversal of blood flow through the vertebral artery and its effect on cerebral circulation. *N Engl J Med* 265:878–885, 1961.

24. Fischer C: A new vascular syndrome: "the subclavian steal." *N Engl J Med* 265:912–913, 1961.

25. Mannick JA, Suter CG, Hume DM: The "subclavian steal" syndrome: further documentation. *JAMA* 182:134–139, 1962.

26. Dieter RA Jr, Maganini RO, Dieter R: Subclavian steal syndrome. In Chang JB, et al, editors: *Textbook of Angiology*, New York, 2000, Springer, pp 629–634.

27. Dieter RS, et al: Description of a new angiographic sign: dynamic left artery obstruction. *Vasc Dis Management* 3(5):298–299, 2006.

28. Eklof B, Schwartz SI: Effects of subclavian steal and compromised cephalic blood flow on cerebral circulation. *Surgery* 68(3):431–441, 1970.

29. Bornstein NM, Norris JW: Subclavian steal: a harmless haemodynamic phenomenon? *Lancet* 2(8502):303–305, 1986.

30. Lord RS, Adar R, Stein RL: Contribution of the circle of Willis to the subclavian steal syndrome. *Circulation* 40(6):871–878, 1969.

31. Fields WS, Lemak NA: Joint study of extracranial arterial occlusion. VII: Subclavian steal: a review of 168 cases. *JAMA* 222(9):1139–1143, 1972.

32. Hennerici M, Klemm C, Rautenberg W: The subclavian steal phenomenon: a common vascular disorder with rare neurologic deficits. *Neurology* 38(5):669–673, 1988.

33. Ackermann H, Diener HC, Dichgans J: Stenosis and occlusion of the subclavian artery: ultrasonographic and clinical findings. *J Neurol* 234(6):396–400, 1987.

34. Dieter RA Jr, Kuzycz GB: Iatrogenic steal syndromes. *Int Surg* 83(4):355–357, 1998.

35. Lee PY, Ng W, Chen WH: Concomitant coronary and subclavian steal caused by ipsilateral subclavian artery stenosis and arteriovenous fistula in a hemodialysis patient. *Catheter Cardiovasc Intervent* 62(2):244–248, 2004.

36. Kurlan R, Krall RL, Deweese JA: Vertebrobasilar ischemia after total repair of tetralogy of Fallot: significance of subclavian steal created by Blalock-Taussig anastomosis. Vertebrobasilar ischemia after correction of tetralogy of Fallot. *Stroke* 15(2):359–362, 1984.

37. Saalouke MG, et al: Cerebrovascular abnormalities in postoperative coarctation of aorta. Four cases demonstrating left subclavian steal on aortography. *Am J Cardiol* 42(1):97–101, 1978.

38. Cavendish JJ, et al: Concomitant coronary and multiple arch vessel stenoses in patients treated with external beam radiation: pathophysiological basis and endovascular treatment. *Catheter Cardiovasc Intervent* 62(3):385–390, 2004.

39. Kliewer MA, et al: Vertebral artery Doppler waveform changes indicating subclavian steal physiology. *AJR Am J Roentgenol* 174(3):815–819, 2000.

40. Wasson S, Bedi A, Singh A: Determining functional significance of subclavian artery stenosis using exercise thallium-201 stress imaging. *South Med J* 98(5):559–560, 2005.

41. Ackermann H, et al: Ultrasonographic follow-up of subclavian stenosis and occlusion: natural history and surgical treatment. *Stroke* 19(4):431–435, 1988.

42. Hall S, et al: Takayasu arteritis. A study of 32 North American patients. *Medicine (Baltimore)* 64(2):89–99, 1985.

43. Ishikawa K: Natural history and classification of occlusive thromboaortopathy (Takayasu's disease). *Circulation* 57(1):27–35, 1978.

44. Eichhorn J, et al: Anti-endothelial cell antibodies in Takayasu arteritis. *Circulation* 94(10):2396–2401, 1996.

45. Miyata T, et al: Long-term survival after surgical treatment of patients with Takayasu's arteritis. *Circulation* 108(12):1474–1480, 2003.

46. Bates MC, et al: Subclavian artery stenting: factors influencing long-term outcome. *Catheter Cardiovasc Intervent* 61(1):5–11, 2004.

47. Bachman DM, Kim RM: Transluminal dilatation for subclavian steal syndrome. *AJR Am J Roentgenol* 135(5):995–996, 1980.

48. De Vries JP, et al: Durability of percutaneous transluminal angioplasty for obstructive lesions of proximal subclavian artery: long-term results. *J Vasc Surg* 41(1):19–23, 2005.

49. Amor M, et al: Endovascular treatment of the subclavian artery: stent implantation with or without predilatation. *Catheter Cardiovasc Intervent* 63(3):364–370, 2004.

50. Brountzos EN, et al: Primary stenting of subclavian and innominate artery occlusive disease: a single center's experience. *Cardiovasc Intervent Radiol* 27(6):616–623, 2004.

51. Bates MC, Almehmi A: Fatal subclavian stent infection remote from implantation. *Catheter Cardiovasc Intervent* 65(4):535–539, 2005.

52. Salerno JL, Vitek J: Fatal cerebral hemorrhage early after subclavian artery endovascular therapy. *AJNR Am J Neuroradiol* 26(1):183–185, 2005.

53. Ringelstein EB, Zeumer H: Delayed reversal of vertebral artery blood flow following percutaneous transluminal angioplasty for subclavian steal syndrome. *Neuroradiology* 26(3):189–198, 1984.

54. Gimelli G, Tefera G, Turnipseed WD: Vertebral artery embolic protection via ipsilateral brachial approach during left subclavian artery angioplasty and stenting: a case report. *Vasc Endovascular Surg* 40(3):235–238, 2006.

55. Turi ZG: The way to a man's heart (or head) is through his shoulder. *Catheter Cardiovasc Intervent* 63(3):371–372, 2004.

56. Jones RD, Uberoi R: Subclavian artery angioplasty for the treatment of angina using a double balloon technique to protect a left internal mammary artery graft. *Eur Radiol* 12(4):908–910, 2002.

57. Smith JM, et al: Subclavian steal syndrome. A review of 59 consecutive cases. *J Cardiovasc Surg (Torino)*. 35(1):11–14, 1994.

58. Berguer R, Morasch MD, Kline RA: Transthoracic repair of innominate and common carotid artery disease: immediate and long-term outcome for 100 consecutive surgical reconstructions. *J Vasc Surg* 27(1):34–41; discussion 42, 1998.

59. Vogt DP, et al: Brachiocephalic arterial reconstruction. *Ann Surg* 196(5):541–552, 1982.

60. Salam TA, Lumsden AB, Smith RB III: Subclavian artery revascularization: a decade of experience with extrathoracic bypass procedures. *J Surg Res* 56(5):387–392, 1994.

61. Wittwer T, et al: Carotid-subclavian bypass for subclavian artery revascularization: long-term follow-up and effect of antiplatelet therapy. *Angiology* 49(4):279–287, 1998.

62. Prostanoids for chronic critical leg ischemia. A randomized, controlled, open-label trial with prostaglandin E1. The ICAI Study Group. *Ischemia Cronica degli Arti Inferiori. Ann Intern Med* 130(5):412–421, 1999.

63. Bilku RS, Khogali SS, Been M: Subclavian artery stenosis as a cause for recurrent angina after LIMA graft stenting. *Heart* 89(12):1429, 2003.

64. Fergus T, et al: *Coronary-Subclavian Steal: Presentation and Management*, Baltimore, MD, 2006, Loyola University Medical Center, p 6.

65. Barlis P, et al: Subclavian artery occlusion causing acute myocardial infarction in a patient with a left internal mammary artery graft. *Catheter Cardiovasc Intervent* 68(2):326–331, 2006.

66. Ferguson TB Jr, Coombs LP, Peterson ED: Internal thoracic artery grafting in the elderly patient undergoing coronary artery bypass grafting: room for process improvement? *J Thorac Cardiovasc Surg* 123(5):869–880, 2002.

67. Speciale G, et al: A uncommon cause of angina during upper limb exercise. *Ital Heart J* 5(7):548–550, 2004.

68. Norsa A, et al: The coronary subclavian steal syndrome: an uncommon sequel to internal mammary-coronary artery bypass surgery. *Thorac Cardiovasc Surg* 42(6):351–354, 1994.

69. Saydjari R, Upp JR, Wolma FJ: Coronary-subclavian steal syndrome following coronary artery bypass grafting. *Cardiology* 78(1):53–57, 1991.

70. Thompson RW, Petrinec D: Surgical treatment of thoracic outlet compression syndromes: diagnostic considerations and transaxillary first rib resection. *Ann Vasc Surg* 11(3):315–323, 1997.

71. Juvonen T, et al: Anomalies at the thoracic outlet are frequent in the general population. *Am J Surg* 170(1):33–37, 1995.

72. Roos DB: Congenital anomalies associated with thoracic outlet syndrome. Anatomy, symptoms, diagnosis, and treatment. *Am J Surg* 132(6):771–778, 1976.

73. Raskin NH, Howard MW, Ehrenfeld WK: Headache as the leading symptom of the thoracic outlet syndrome. *Headache* 25(4):208–210, 1985.

74. Dieter RA Jr, O'Brien T, Dieter RA III: Thoracic outlet syndrome. In Chang JB, et al, editors: *Textbook of Angiology*, New York, 2000, Springer, pp 635–643.

75. Bryan AJ, Hicks E, Lewis MH: Unilateral digital ischaemia secondary to embolisation from subclavian atheroma. *Ann R Coll Surg Engl* 71(2):140–142, 1989.

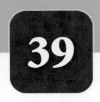

39

Carotid and Cerebrovascular Intervention

R. KEVIN ROGERS | IVAN P. CASSERLY

KEY POINTS

- Cerebrovascular intervention has largely evolved for the treatment of atherosclerotic disease. The potential for serious neurological complications during such procedures places a premium on careful studies documenting the overall clinical efficacy of intervention compared with medical therapy.

- Carotid bifurcation disease and intracranial atherosclerosis account for 15% to 20% of all ischemic strokes and represent an important target for stroke prevention.

- Contemporary carotid bifurcation intervention involves the use of self-expanding stents with embolic protection systems to reduce the risk of distal embolization. The technique has been proven equivalent to carotid endarterectomy in high-risk patients, and data from randomized controlled trials in low-risk populations are emerging.

- Proximal vertebral artery disease may account for up to 10% of posterior circulation ischemic events. Intervention at this site is straightforward and safe but has not been proven superior to medical therapy alone.

- Intracranial intervention, when practiced by skilled and experienced operators, is technically feasible and reasonably safe. Randomized studies documenting superiority over medical therapy are needed.

- Further refinements in technique, technology, and patient selection, together with dedicated randomized controlled trials, will allow cerebrovascular intervention to realize its true potential in stroke victims.

Introduction

Stroke is the leading cause of adult disability and the third leading cause of death in North America, Europe, South America, and Asia. The vast majority of strokes (~80%–85%) are ischemic in etiology. In the United States, atherosclerotic disease affecting the extra- and intracranial arterial circulation accounts for approximately 20% of ischemic strokes (Fig. 39-1) and thus is an important target for stroke prevention.[1] Cerebrovascular intervention has evolved largely for the treatment of atherosclerotic disease with the goal of stroke prevention. Based on dramatic technological advances and increased operator expertise, these procedures can now be performed with a high rate of technical success. However, because of the potential for serious neurological complications from endovascular intervention in the cerebrovascular circulation, clear documentation of the safety of these procedures and of the overall clinical efficacy is of paramount importance. These considerations have raised the bar for cerebrovascular intervention compared with other peripheral vascular procedures. In the field of cerebrovascular intervention, carotid bifurcation intervention is unique in that the natural history of carotid artery bifurcation disease has been well defined, and large randomized trials have previously documented the clinical effectiveness of surgical revascularization for this disease. There is already a large evidence base supporting carotid intervention in specific patient subgroups, and several randomized trials are ongoing in the remaining patient populations. With over 140,000 and 280,000 carotid endarterectomy (CEA) procedures performed each year in the United States and worldwide, respectively, the potential impact of percutaneous revascularization has captured the interest of endovascular specialists who are keen to offer an alternative to surgery. In contrast, endovascular intervention in the cerebrovascular circulation outside of the carotid bifurcation has been hampered by two important considerations: the natural history of noncarotid cerebrovascular disease is less well defined, and there is a notable absence of randomized data documenting the benefit of revascularization compared with medical therapy alone. Despite these obstacles, dramatic advances in the technical aspects of these interventions have been made, and there is an increased recognition of the need for well-designed clinical studies that address these deficiencies. What is often underappreciated is that noncarotid bifurcation cerebrovascular disease is responsible for at least the same number of ischemic strokes as carotid bifurcation disease and represents an equally important target for stroke prevention. This chapter summarizes the current status of carotid bifurcation intervention and the most frequently performed noncarotid bifurcation cerebrovascular interventions, notably proximal vertebral artery and intracranial intervention.

Carotid Bifurcation Intervention

CAROTID BIFURCATION ATHEROSCLEROSIS AND STROKE

The carotid bifurcation has a remarkable predilection for the development of atherosclerosis, which is typically located at the origin of the internal carotid artery (ICA) (Fig. 39-2). This plaque is similar to that found at other sites throughout the arterial system in that it contains a dense cap of connective tissue with embedded smooth muscle cells and an underlying core of lipid and necrotic debris.[2] Histological studies of plaque from the carotid bifurcation of symptomatic and asymptomatic individuals have revealed features associated with the development of symptoms that are similar to those associated with plaque vulnerability in the coronary circulation. i.e., reduced amounts of collagen, increased inflammation, thinning of the fibrous cap, and increased cholesterol in the necrotic core.[2,3] Based on our current understanding, these processes result in plaque fissuring or rupture at the carotid bifurcation, causing either occlusive or nonocclusive thrombus formation. The dominant mechanism of stroke is believed to result from distal thromboembolism to the anterior cerebral circulation. However, a number of considerations such as the size and composition of the embolus, the presence of contralateral disease, the anatomy of the circle of Willis, and the activity of fibrinolytic pathways may attenuate or accentuate the clinical consequence of the pathological event, such that the same pathological event may result in a reversible neurological deficit (i.e., transient ischemic attack), an irreversible neurological deficit (i.e., stroke), or no symptoms at all.

NATURAL HISTORY OF CAROTID ARTERY BIFURCATION DISEASE

In clinical practice, two dominant factors are used to determine the risk of ischemic complications from a lesion of the carotid artery bifurcation: the symptomatic status of the lesion and the severity of stenosis. Although many of these data are derived from the medical arm of the large randomized CEA trials performed between the late 1980s and early 2000s, these considerations continue to be used as the major criteria for choosing patients for endovascular procedures and for enrolling subjects in carotid endovascular trials. Symptomatic

513

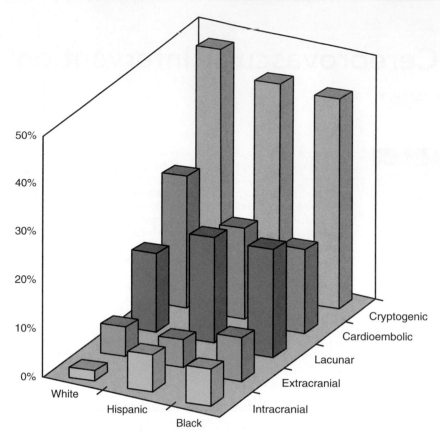

Ischemic stroke subtype

Figure 39-1 Proportion of ischemic stroke subtypes according to race in the Northern Manhattan Study. *(Adapted from White H et al. Circulation. 2005;111: 1327–1331.)*[1]

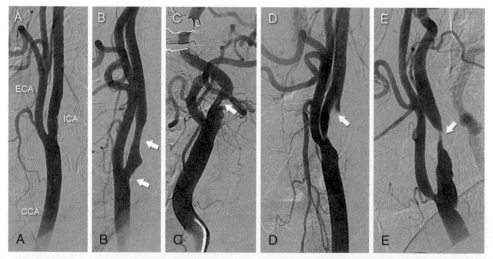

Figure 39-2 Angiographic images from the carotid bifurcation showing the spectrum of atherosclerotic disease at this site. A. Minimal disease at the origin of the internal carotid artery (ICA). B. Mild stenosis extending from the distal common carotid artery (CCA) into the proximal ICA. C. Moderate eccentric stenosis in the proximal portion of the ICA. D. A thrombotic lesion in the proximal portion of the ICA in a patient with recent stroke. E. High-grade stenosis in the proximal portion of the ICA. Note that atherosclerotic plaque tends to accumulate in the posterior aspect of the ICA. ECA, external carotid artery. Arrows indicate location of plaque.

lesions of the carotid bifurcation are associated with a high risk of recurrent ischemic stroke. Based on data from the NASCET (North American Symptomatic Carotid Endarterectomy Trial), the risk of any ipsilateral stroke at 2-year follow-up in medically treated patients with symptomatic stenoses of 70% to 99% was 26%.[4] Among patients with symptomatic stenoses of 50% to 69%, the 5-year risk of any ipsilateral stroke was 22.2%.[5] There is a close temporal relationship between these recurrent strokes and the index event, with a steep exponential decline in risk within the first months, followed by a more gradual decline and ultimate normalization of risk at 2 to 3 years (Fig. 39-3). By contrast, asymptomatic lesions of the carotid bifurcation are associated with a much lower risk of ischemic stroke. Over a 5-year period following the

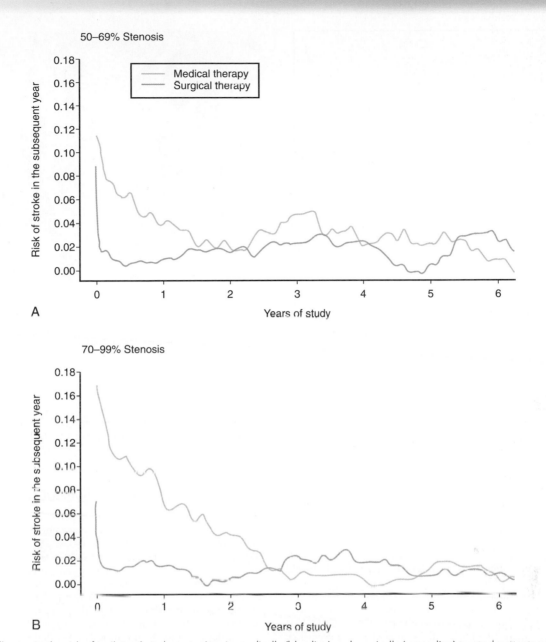

Figure 39-3 Change in the risk of ipsilateral stroke over time in medically (blue line) and surgically (green line) treated patients with symptomatic 50% to 69% stenosis (A) and 70% to 79% stenosis (B) in the NASCET trial (North American Symptomatic Carotid Endarterectomy Trial). *(Adapted from Barnett et al. N Engl J Med. 1998;339:1415–1425.)*[5]

diagnosis of an asymptomatic carotid stenosis, >60% by ultrasound, the risk of any stroke among medically treated patients in the ACST (Asymptomatic Carotid Surgery Trial) was 11%.[6] Not surprisingly, the risk of stroke was constant over the duration of the study. The implication from these findings is that carotid revascularization should be performed as expediently as possible following a neurological event caused by a culprit symptomatic stenosis, while intervention for an asymptomatic lesion may be approached in a more elective fashion.[7] Among symptomatic patients, a close relationship between the severity of stenosis as assessed by careful angiographic methods and subsequent risk of ipsilateral stroke has been demonstrated.[8] The relationship is nonlinear, with a steep increase in risk associated with the tightest degree of stenosis (Fig. 39-4). However, for symptomatic patients with "near occlusion" of the internal carotid artery, defined as a stenosis causing sufficient obstruction to flow as to result in a decrease in the ICA diameter beyond the lesion (Fig. 39-5), there are data to suggest that the risk of recurrent stroke is reduced compared with

patients with severe stenosis without features of near occlusion.[9] One potential explanation for this finding is the reduced likelihood of distal cerebral embolization caused by diminished flow distal to a critical stenosis. Among asymptomatic patients, the association between stenosis severity and risk of subsequent stroke has been inconsistent.[6,10] This finding likely underscores the heterogenous nature of carotid plaque histology in asymptomatic patients and suggests that assessments of plaque vulnerability may be a more potent predictor of recurrent events than severity of stenosis in this patient group. Today there are more sophisticated models to predict the risk of stroke in patients with carotid disease, particularly for symptomatic patients.[11,12] In addition to stenosis severity, these models incorporate variables such as age, sex, nature of the presenting symptomatic event, time from index event, plaque surface morphology, and transcranial Doppler findings to provide a more individualized estimate of risk. However, these models have yet to be incorporated into patient selection criteria of randomized trials to more fully establish their clinical relevance.

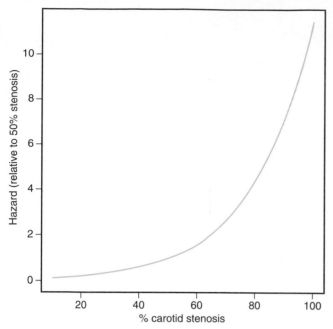

Figure 39-4 Hazard of ipsilateral ischemic stroke within 3 years of index transient ischemic attack or stroke as a function of percent carotid stenosis, determined using biplane angiographic views. *(Adapted from Cuffe RL et al. Stroke. 2006;37:1785–1791.)*[8]

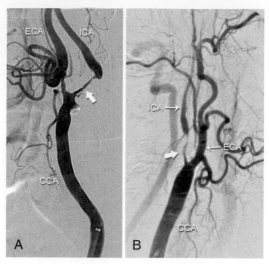

Figure 39-5 Angiographic appearance of "near occlusion" of the internal carotid artery (ICA). A. Reduction in diameter of the ICA compared with the external carotid artery (ECA) reflects a mild form of near occlusion of ICA (arrow). B. Major collapse of the ICA beyond critical stenosis (arrow) reflects a severe form of near occlusion of the ICA and is often referred to as a string sign.

BENEFIT OF CAROTID REVASCULARIZATION

The benefit of carotid revascularization in patients with carotid artery disease has been documented in several randomized controlled trials (RCTs) comparing medical therapy with surgical revascularization (i.e., CEA). These data are extremely important in any discussion of endovascular therapy for carotid bifurcation disease as they form the cornerstone justifying revascularization in certain subsets of patients. In a pooled analysis of data from the three major RCTs in symptomatic patients,[13] CEA as compared with medical therapy reduced the endpoint of stroke or operative death at 5 years in patients with carotid stenoses ≥50%, as assessed by carotid angiography using the NASCET criteria (Fig. 39-6). This benefit was more pronounced in patients with stenoses of 70% to 99% (absolute risk reduction [ARR] 15.3%, 95% CI 9.8-20.7) compared with those with stenoses of 50% to 69% (ARR 7.8%, 95% CI 3.1-12.5). In addition, the crossover of the event-free curves occurs very early in the patient cohort with 70% to 99% stenoses (1–2 months) compared with the patient cohort with 50% to 69% stenosis (1 year). The incidence of perioperative stroke and/or death in these studies was uniformly <6%; the benefits derived from CEA are predicated on the maintenance of similar procedural outcomes. No significant benefit was observed in patients with near occlusion of the carotid artery (ARR 0.1%, 95% CI -10.3-10.2), likely related to the lower risk of recurrent stroke with medical therapy in this group. These studies were performed in the late 1980s and early to mid-1990s; therefore the only stipulated medical therapy in the nonsurgical arm was aspirin. Contemporary medical therapy would likely attenuate the observed benefit associated with CEA. However, given the magnitude of the observed benefit associated with CEA in symptomatic patients, investigators have been reluctant to repeat randomized studies using contemporary medical therapy alone as a treatment arm. Compared with medical therapy, CEA has also been shown to significantly reduce the incidence of stroke or operative death at 5-year follow-up in asymptomatic patients with carotid stenoses ≥60%, as assessed by carotid ultrasound (11.8% vs. 6.4%, ARR 5.4%, 95% CI 3-7.8).[6] It is important to emphasize that in this asymptomatic population, the early hazard associated with revascularization persists up to 2 years from the time of CEA. If the life expectancy of a patient is less than 5 years, then significant benefit should not be anticipated. In addition, participation in these trials involving patient's with asymptomatic carotid stenoses required documentation of a perioperative stroke and death rate of <3% at the investigation site, and the generalization of these findings is predicated on reproducing similar procedural outcomes.

PERCUTANEOUS CAROTID REVASCULARIZATION

Initial animal experimentation with percutaneous carotid revascularization began in the late 1970s, followed by the first clinical reports of carotid angioplasty in the early 1980s. The first rigorous clinical testing of percutaneous carotid revascularization began in the mid-1990s. While these studies demonstrated feasibility, two subsequent pivotal developments have allowed percutaneous carotid revascularization to emerge as a viable alternative to CEA in the treatment of carotid disease: the ability to provide protection from distal embolization at the time of intervention, using a variety of embolic protection devices, and the use of self-expanding stents. Carotid artery stenting (CAS) using self-expanding stents in combination with distal embolic protection represents the contemporary approach to carotid revascularization.

CAROTID ARTERY STENTING: THE PROCEDURE[14]

Preprocedural Assessment

Prior to any CAS procedure, clinical assessment of the patient and anatomic assessment of the aortic arch and carotid/cerebral vasculature is essential. Advanced age (>80 years) has been associated with significantly worse outcomes with CAS and should be carefully considered for the appropriateness of intervention.[15,16] Decreased cerebral reserve, manifest by the presence of dementia or cognitive impairment, and a history of prior strokes or lacunar infarcts increase the likelihood that distal embolization will be clinically manifest and is a relative contraindication for the procedure.[17] Anatomical assessments can generally be made using noninvasive studies, notably computed tomography angiography (CTA) and magnetic resonance angiography (MRA). CTA offers higher spatial resolution and superior visualization of the aortic arch compared with MRA and allows an assessment of the degree of calcification of the aortic arch and carotid bifurcation lesion that is not possible with MRA. Table 39-1 lists the anatomical features

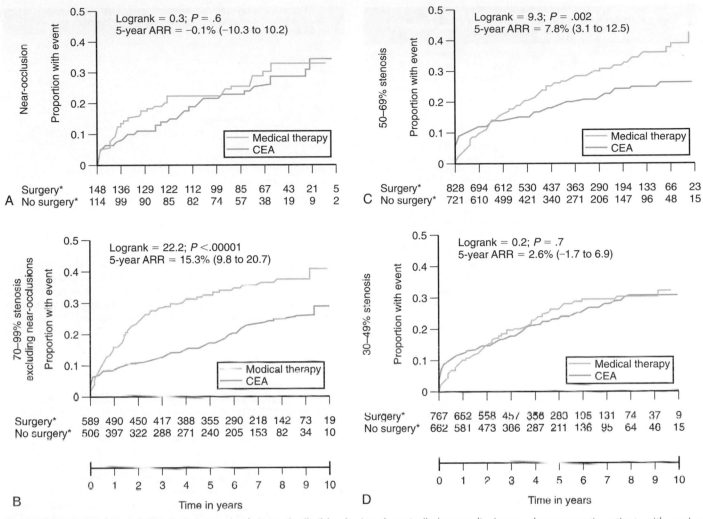

Figure 39-6   Risk of any stroke or operative death in medically (blue line) and surgically (orange line) treated symptomatic patients with varying degrees of carotid artery stenosis. (*Adapted from Rothwell PM. Lancet. 2003;361:107–116.*)[13]

that should be reviewed using these studies and highlights the importance of each. Overall, these anatomical features allow the operator to more accurately determine the procedural risk and facilitate the planning of appropriate technique for procedural success.

Baseline Angiography

In most circumstances, CAS procedures are performed using femoral artery access. While the extent of baseline angiography will vary depending on the preprocedural noninvasive assessment, high-quality angiography of the carotid bifurcation, ipsilateral internal carotid artery, and intracranial anterior circulation is essential. The authors administer a heparin bolus of 25 mg/kg prior to all diagnostic cerebrovascular procedures in an effort to minimize the risk of thrombotic complications. A variety of catheter types are used to perform angiography, depending on the personal preference of the operator and the anatomy of the aortic arch and great vessels. For patients with uncomplicated anatomy (i.e., type I aortic arch, no tortuosity of the great vessels), a Bernstein catheter functions well. For more complicated anatomies (i.e., type II or III arch, tortuosity of the great vessels, bovine origin of the left common carotid artery), Vitek or Simmons catheters are generally required.

Interventional Technique

The technique for CAS placement follows a number of well-defined steps. Prior to CAS placement, all patients should receive aspirin. In addition, it is the authors' practice to administer clopidogrel for at least 3 days prior to the procedure. During the procedure, anticoagulation using unfractionated heparin to achieve an activated coagulation time (ACT) of 275 to 300 seconds is standard.[18] For patients with a contraindication to heparin, a direct thrombin inhibitor such as bivalirudin is administered.[19] Currently there are limited data documenting the safety of bivalirudin for routine use during CAS. Most operators perform the procedure without the administration of sedatives, which enhances the ability to screen for any neurological change during the procedure.

Delivery of Sheath or Guide to the Common Carotid Artery. In order to deliver the range of contemporary equipment required for CAS, a 6-Fr sheath or 8-Fr guide must be delivered to the distal CCA. In patients with difficult aortic arch anatomy, bovine origin of the left CCA, occlusion of the external carotid artery (ECA), distal CCA lesions, and significant tortuosity of the great vessels, this can be one of the most technically challenging parts of the procedure. This portion of the procedure is "unprotected" in that there is no distal embolic protection device (EPD) to protect from distal embolization; therefore the safety of this step is heavily operator-dependent. The standard procedure for delivery of a 6-Fr sheath in the CCA is as follows: The CCA of interest is engaged with a diagnostic catheter. A stiff-angled glidewire is advanced into the ECA, over which the diagnostic catheter is advanced. The glidewire is exchanged for a superstiff

TABLE 39-1	Anatomic Assessments Recommended Prior to Carotid Artery Stenting Procedure and Their Impact on Interventional Planning	
Angiographic Assessment	*Impact on Interventional Procedure*	
Arch anatomy		
Type I, II, or III arch	Predict difficulty of percutaneous approach and influence strategy for delivery of guide or sheath to CCA	
Anomalies of origin of great vessels		
Tortuosity of proximal portion of great vessels		
Lesion characteristics		
Precise location of the lesion, with definition of the proximal and distal extent of lesion	Influences planned location for stent placement and stent length	
Lesion length	Influences strategy for delivery of guide/sheath to distal CCA	
Complex lesion ulceration	Influences choice of stent length	
Severity of stenosis	Predict difficulty of crossing lesion with filter device or wire	
Severity of lesion calcification	Predict need for predilation of lesion prior to filter delivery	
Diameter of vessel(s) proximal and distal to lesion	Predict ability to achieve adequate stent expansion	
	Influences choice of stent diameter	
ICA distal to lesion		
Assess cervical portion of the ICA for presence of disease and tortuosity	Influences the choice of landing zone for the filter or proximal occlusion EPD	
Diameter of cervical ICA	Increased tortuosity favors use of guide to provide support for delivery of filter	
	Influences choice of diameter of filter-type or proximal occlusion EPD	
Patency of external carotid artery	Influences strategy for delivery of guide/sheath to distal CCA	

CCA, common carotid artery; ICA, internal carotid artery; EPD, embolic protection device.

TABLE 39-2	Filter-Type Embolic Protection Devices Used during Carotid Intervention		
Filter	*Manufacturer*	*Diameter (mm)*	*Pore Size (μm)*
Interceptor	Medtronic	4.5, 5.5, 6.5	100
FilterWire EZ	Boston Scientific	3.5–5.5	80
Angioguard XP Angioguard RX	Cordis	4, 5, 6, 7, 8	100
Emboshield NAV[6]	Abbott Laboratories	2.5–4.8, 4–7	140
Spider	ev3	3, 4, 5, 6, 7	50–200
Accunet OTW Accunet RX	Abbott Laboratories	4.5, 5.5, 6.5, 7.5	120
FiberNet	Medtronic	3.5–5, 5–6, 6–7	40

RX, monorail; OTW, over the wire.

Amplatz or SupraCore wire, followed by removal of the diagnostic catheter. Over this stiff wire, the 6-Fr sheath and its dilator are delivered to the distal CCA, followed by removal of the dilator. While this standard approach is sufficient for ~70% of cases, a number of variations to the technique may be necessary, depending on the specific anatomical features of the individual patient. Much of the learning curve in CAS involves achieving experience with these variations and in learning how to predict which variation is appropriate for an individual patient's anatomy. One of the pivotal dogmas in CAS is that guidewires and catheters should never be placed across the carotid lesion in order to deliver the sheath or guide to the CCA. It is preferable to refer the patient for CEA than to persist in risky attempts to deliver the guide or sheath.

Delivery of Embolic Protection Device. The use of embolic protection devices (EPDs) is now considered the standard of care during CAS. Compelling observational data support this recommendation. Several studies demonstrate that distal embolization is ubiquitous during CAS,[20,21] and observational series have shown a significant association between decreased periprocedural rates of stroke and death and the use of EPDs.[16,22] Over the last decade, three different device systems that provide protection from distal embolization at the time of carotid intervention have been developed.[23,24] In clinical practice, the most popular and user-friendly of these systems is the filter-type EPD (Table 39-2, Fig. 39-7). These systems allow continued antegrade flow during carotid intervention, an important consideration for patients with compromised collateral flow to the ipsilateral carotid territory (e.g., patients with contralateral carotid artery disease or occlusion). Since filter-type EPDs have been used in most contemporary CAS registries and RCTs, more data exist to support their use in carotid intervention as compared with other EPDs. Based on the submission of these data

to the FDA, multiple filter-type EPDs have received FDA approval (i.e., Accunet, Emboshield, Spider, Angioguard, FilterWire, and FiberNet). Although there is some variation in the individual design of these devices, they typically contain a polyurethane membrane, with pores of fixed size ranging from 80 to 140 μm between devices, supported by a nitinol frame. The Spider and Interceptor EPDs are unique in that the filter pores are formed by a nitinol mesh. Each filter is designed such that it is integrated with a 0.014-in. guidewire with a 3- to 4-cm shapeable floppy tip. With the exception of the Emboshield and Spider devices, the filter is fixed to the wire.

The technique for delivery of the filter-type EPD varies according to the design of the system. In systems such as the Accunet, FilterWire EZ, and Angioguard, the filter is delivered in a collapsed form across the carotid lesion on the attached guidewire. With the Emboshield system, a unique 0.014-in. wire (BareWire) is used to cross the lesion first; the filter is then delivered in a collapsed form over this wire and deployed over the distal portion of the wire. The Spider system allows the lesion to be crossed using any 0.014-in. wire, followed by a 2.9-Fr delivery catheter. It allows delivery of the Spider filter, which is integrated with a dedicated 0.014-in. wire that allows a small range of independent motion of the wire and filter. Predilation of the carotid lesion prior to delivery of the filter-type EPD is required in <1% to 2% of cases. If required, a small-caliber coronary balloon (i.e., 2.0 mm diameter) that minimizes the risk of distal embolization should be used. Regardless of the filter-type EPD that is used, the filter should ideally be deployed in a straight and nondiseased portion of the cervical ICA, which is typically in the distal cervical portion of the vessel. The presence of tortuosity or disease in the cervical portion of the ICA may require an alternate placement, but there must be at least 3 to 4 cm of distance between the proximal margin of the filter and the distal margin of the ICA lesion to allow subsequent delivery of interventional equipment. Distal occlusion balloon EPDs were the first type of EPD used during a carotid intervention (circa 1998). The only remaining example of this type of system is the Percusurge GuardWire device (Medtronic Vascular, Minneapolis, MN), which consists of an 0.014-in. angioplasty wire with a hollow nitinol hypotube and a distal compliant balloon that is inflated and deflated through the hypotube. The GuardWire is advanced across the carotid lesion with the balloon deflated. Complete interruption of antegrade flow is then achieved by inflating the balloon. Following treatment of the carotid lesion, a monorail Export catheter is used to aspirate the column of blood proximal to the balloon, thus removing any debris that may have embolized from the treatment site. The balloon is then deflated and the GuardWire removed. There are no randomized comparisons of carotid intervention using filter-type and distal occlusion EPDs. A retrospective comparison of outcomes from a large CAS registry showed no significant difference in in-hospital death or stroke between these systems (2.3% for distal occlusion EPDs vs. 1.8% for filter-type EPDs, $P = 0.96$).[25] The most recent group of EPDs

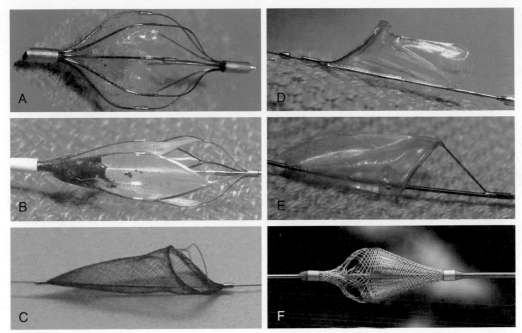

Figure 39-7 Examples of filter-type embolic protection devices used during carotid intervention. A. Angioguard XP (Cordis, Warren, NJ). B. Accunet (Abbott Vascular, Abbott Park, IL). C. Spider (ev3, Plymouth, MN). D. FilterWire EX (Boston Scientific, Natick, MA). E. FilterWire EZ (Boston Scientific, Natick, MA). F. Interceptor (Medtronic, Minneapolis, MN). *(Reproduced with permission.)*[14]

developed for carotid intervention comprises the proximal occlusion devices (e.g., the Parodi Anti-embolism System from Gore Medical, Flagstaff, AZ, and the MO.MA System from Medtronic). These systems attempt to protect the brain from distal embolization by eliminating antegrade flow in the ICA during the procedure and thus, essentially generating an endovascular clamp.[26] Compliant balloons are inflated in the distal CCA and ECA, interrupting antegrade carotid flow and theoretically eliminating the risk of distal embolization from debris liberated during angioplasty and stenting. The success of such systems is predicated on adequate collateral circulation from the circle of Willis to maintain cerebral perfusion. With the Parodi device, retrograde flow is generated in the internal carotid artery by connecting the lumen of the catheter, whose tip is in the CCA and distal to the occlusive balloon to a catheter in the femoral vein. Consequently blood flows down its pressure gradient from the common carotid, through the blood return system, and to the femoral vein. In contrast, the MO.MA device simply creates a static column of blood in the internal carotid artery without continuous flow reversal, and removal of this unfiltered column of blood is achieved by aspiration with a syringe. Proximal EPDs appear particularly useful for cases in which tortuosity or disease distal to the carotid bifurcation lesion would preclude the use of filter-type or distal balloon-occlusion EPDs. Data with proximal EPDs are more limited than those for distal EPDs, but they are emerging. An initial large registry using a proximal balloon-occlusion system (i.e., PRIAMUS, which enrolled 416 "real world" patients with carotid disease) reported a high rate of technical success (~99%) and acceptable clinical outcomes (4.5% incidence of in-hospital stroke, death, and myocardial infarction [MI]). Two recent prospective registries using the MO.MA system have also been reported. In the ARMOUR study, 262 high-risk patients undergoing carotid artery stenting with embolic protection were enrolled, with a reported 30-day rate of stroke, death, and MI of 2.7%.[27] In a larger, single-center registry of 1,300 patients who also underwent CAS with embolic protection from the MO.MA device, the 30-day rate of stroke and death was an impressive 1.4%, and the procedural success rate was 99.7%.[28] While these results are encouraging, a direct comparison of proximal versus distal embolic protection in a randomized trial is needed.

ANGIOPLASTY AND STENTING

See Figure 39-8.

Predilation

Following placement of the EPD system, the lesion is generally predilated to facilitate stent delivery. Low-profile coronary balloons with 3.0- to 4.0-mm diameters are generally used. Attempts to deliver the stent without predilation have been associated with a greater amount of atheroembolism,[17] likely related to increased trauma to the lesion with forcible passage of the stent across a tight stenosis.

Stent Selection and Placement

See Table 39-4. As is the case in other vascular territories, the ability to stent carotid lesions has allowed operators to achieve a predictable angiographic result, deal with procedural complications such as dissection and abrupt vessel closure, and improve long-term patency by eliminating vessel recoil. Initial attempts at carotid stenting using relatively inflexible stainless steel balloon-expandable stents (e.g., Palmaz, Cordis) were associated with acute technical success. However, their use was abandoned owing to the subsequent development of stent crushing, likely related to compression of the superficially located carotid stent from neck movements.[29] This complication led to the development and use of flexible self-expanding stents that could conform to the tortuous anatomy of the carotid bifurcation and changes in vessel shape associated with neck movements (Table 39-3). The functional properties of these stents are defined by their metal composition and design.[30] Nitinol, a nickel-titanium alloy, is the most widely used material for carotid self-expanding stents; because of its large elastic range, it confers an ability to withstand significant deformations. A variety of nitinol stents with either a closed- or open-cell design are available. The closed-cell design offers superior scaffolding at the cost of reduced flexibility. A single cobalt-based alloy stent with a closed-cell design is currently available (e.g., WALLSTENT, Boston Scientific, Natick, MA). Both the metal composition and design of this stent result in a more rigid stent with excellent scaffolding properties. Carotid stents come in a variety of sizes that match the typical diameter of the ICA and CCA (5 to 10 mm), and are generally 20 to 40 mm long.

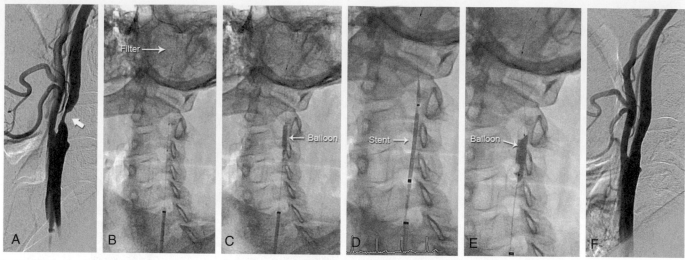

Figure 39-8 Angiographic images from carotid artery stent procedure. A. Baseline angiographic image showing severe internal carotid stenosis (arrow). B. Placement of filter-type embolic protection device (5.5-mm-diameter Accunet filter, Abbott Vascular, Abbott Park, IL). C. Predilation (4.0- by 20-mm Maverick balloon, Boston Scientific, Natick, MA). Placement of 6- to 8-mm-diameter (tapered) by 30-mm long self-expanding nitinol stent (Acculink, Abbott Vascular, Abbott Park, IL). E. Postdilation with 5.0- by 20-mm Aviator balloon (Cordis, Warren, NJ). F. Final angiographic appearance following removal of filter.

TABLE 39-3	Self-Expanding Carotid Artery Stents				
Stent	**Manufacturer**	**Metal Composition**	**Design**	**Tapered Version Available**	**FDA-Approved**
Carotid WALLSTENT	Boston Scientific	Cobalt chromium	Closed-cell	No	Yes
Exponent	Medtronic	Nitinol	Open-cell	No	Yes
Precise	Cordis	Nitinol	Open-cell	No	Yes
Protégé	ev3	Nitinol	Open-cell	No	Yes
AccuLink	Abbott	Nitinol	Open-cell	Yes	Yes
X-Act	Abbott	Nitinol	Closed-cell	Yes	Yes
Zilver	Cook	Nitinol	Open-cell	No	No
Cristallo Ideale	Invatec	Nitinol	Hybrid	Yes	No

The nominal diameter of the stent used should be 1 to 2 mm larger than the diameter of the largest treated vessel (usually the CCA). Stent lengths are chosen to provide complete lesion coverage. Initially, all carotid stents were cylindrical. However, tapered stents that conform to the size mismatch between the ICA and CCA and facilitate treatment across the carotid bifurcation are now commonly used. When tapered stents are used, the majority of cases are performed using 6- to 8-mm or 7- to 9-mm-diameter stents that are either 30 or 40 mm long. When cylindrical stents are used, the majority of cases are performed using 8-mm-diameter stents of similar length (i.e., 30 to 40 mm). For most cases, all of the available carotid stents will achieve similar technical success and clinical outcomes. In the remaining cases (~25%), assuming that all stents were available to the operator, the choice of stent should be individualized and is largely influenced by arterial anatomy and lesion morphology.[31] For example, stents with the greatest degree of flexibility (i.e., open-cell-design nitinol stents with large open-cell areas and highly flexible interconnecting bridges; e.g., Precise, Zilver) may be optimal for treating lesions in tortuous locations. Calcified lesions should be treated with stents with a high radial force and moderate outward expansive force, as provided by nitinol stents with a closed cell design (e.g., X-Act). Finally, lesions with the greatest risk for distal embolism should be treated with stents that provide greater vessel scaffolding (closed-cell nitinol or cobalt alloy stents; e.g., WALLSTENT, X-Act).

Postdilation

Postdilation of the self-expanding stent is generally performed using a 4.5–5.5 mm diameter non-compliant balloon (e.g., Aviator, Cordis, Warren, NJ; Sterling, Boston Scientific, Natick, MA). There is general agreement that postdilation is associated with the greatest propensity for plaque embolization; therefore experienced operators advocate a conservative approach to postdilation balloon sizing. A residual stenosis of <20% is generally accepted.

Following predilation, stent deployment, and postdilation, contrast angiography is performed to assess the angiographic result and detect any potential complications. When filter-type EPDs are being used, this practice allows the detection of "slow flow," which is an important finding that requires special management.[32] Slow flow is manifest by delayed antegrade flow in the ICA and may vary from complete cessation of antegrade flow to mild delay of ICA flow compared with the ECA (Fig. 39-9). Most likely this phenomenon is caused by excessive distal embolization of plaque elements that occlude the filter pores, compromising antegrade flow through the filter (Fig. 39-10). The phenomenon is frequent, occurring in 8% to 10% of cases,[32,33] and is most commonly observed following postdilation of the stent (~75% of cases) and stent deployment (~25% of cases). Predictors of this event include treatment of symptomatic lesions, increased patient age, and increased stent diameter.[32] In patients with slow flow, the column of blood proximal to the filter has not been appropriately cleared of debris embolized from the treatment site by the filter EPD. In an effort to prevent distal embolization of this debris at the time of filter retrieval, aspiration of 40 to 60 mL of blood from the column of blood proximal to the filter using an Export catheter, prior to retrieval of the filter EPD, is recommended. If slow flow is observed following stent deployment, poststent dilation is discouraged, as this would probably exacerbate the degree of embolization from the treatment site.

Removal of the Embolic Protection Device and Final Angiography

Removal of filter-type EPD devices is achieved by advancing a retrieval sheath over the interventional wire and collapsing the filter. The collapsed filter is then withdrawn carefully across the stent and removed.

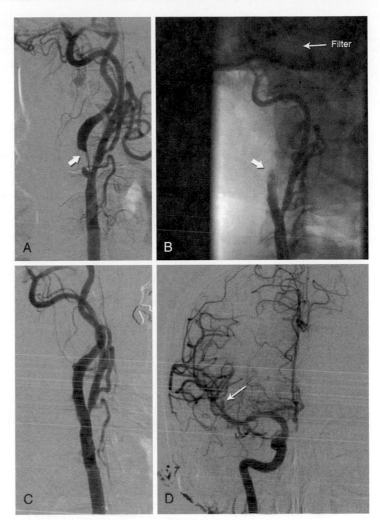

Figure 39-9 Angiographic appearance and complication of slow flow during carotid intervention. A. Baseline angiogram showing critical bulky stenosis at the origin of the right internal carotid artery in a symptomatic patient. B. Angiographic appearance following post-stent dilation showing cessation of flow in the internal carotid artery (arrow). Note complete filling of the external carotid artery. C. Angiographic appearance following aspiration of the column of blood proximal to the filter and subsequent retrieval of the filter. D. Angiogram of the middle cerebral artery following retrieval of the filter showing occlusion of a branch of middle cerebral artery (arrow).

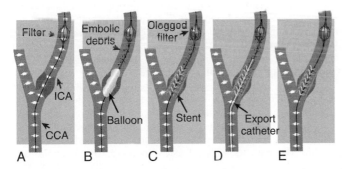

Figure 39-10 Schematic of proposed mechanism of slow flow and rationale for aspiration. A. Carotid bifurcation lesion with filter placed distally. B and C. Balloon angioplasty and stenting results in embolization of debris from atherosclerotic plaque toward filter, causing occlusion of filter pores and accumulation of debris in the column of blood proximal to the filter. D and E. Aspiration proximal to the filter removes debris from the column of blood without affecting the debris causing occlusion of filter. (*Reproduced with permission from Casserly I et al. J Am Coll Cardiol. 2005;46:1466–1472.*)[32]

Most retrieval sheaths are available in a straight or angled shape to allow the retrieval sheath to be advanced past the stent. Rarely, either the patient may have to turn his or her head or external compression may have to be applied to the carotid in order to facilitate this maneuver. Final angiography at the treatment site, the EPD landing zone, and the ipsilateral anterior cerebral circulation is performed to assess the procedural outcome and detect any procedural complication (e.g., distal embolization, spasm at the filter site).

POSTPROCEDURAL CARE AND FOLLOW-UP

At most centers, patients are admitted overnight to a step-down telemetry floor and typically discharged the following day. Neurological and hemodynamic monitoring are the most important components of care. All patients should receive lifelong aspirin therapy unless contraindicated, and clopidogrel is recommended for a minimum of 4 weeks following the procedure. Patients are seen at 1 month and 12 months following the procedure for clinical assessment and carotid ultrasound to screen for in-stent stenosis. Thereafter, yearly carotid ultrasound is recommended.[34]

▣ Complications of Carotid Intervention

STROKE

Stroke represents the most important complication of carotid artery stenting. Regardless of whether the patient is deemed at high or normal risk for CEA, the risk of periprocedural stroke is most strongly related to the patient's symptomatic status.[28] In studies of high-risk patients, the vast majority of them were asymptomatic. The 30-day incidence of stroke following CAS in multiple observational studies of high-risk patients has ranged from 2.3% to 6.9%,[27,33,35–40] with a majority of high-risk registry studies in recent years reporting stroke rates of 2.3% to 4.4% (Fig. 39-11).[27,33,35,37,38,40] These rates are comparable to the

30-day stroke rate of 3.1% observed in the sole randomized trial of high-risk patients.[41] Roughly 80% of these reported strokes were ipsilateral to the treatment site; of these, 25% to 33% were classified as major strokes (i.e., persistence of neurological deficit beyond 30 days with NIH Stroke Scale >3). The 30-day rate of stroke in the four contemporary trials of normal-risk, symptomatic patients has ranged from 5% to 9% (Table 39-4).[42-45] A lower 30-day stroke rate of 2.5% was reported in an asymptomatic subgroup from a trial of normal-risk patients (Table 39-4).[45]

Although poorly documented in most studies, based on the authors' experience, the majority of strokes occur at the time of the CAS procedure. This impression is corroborated by data from the CAVATAS trial (CArotid and Vertebral Artery Transluminal Angioplasty Study), in which 16 of the 22 ischemic strokes in the 30-day period following carotid intervention occurred within the first 24 hours of the procedure.[46] Beyond 30 days, the risk of ipsilateral stroke with CAS is extremely low. In the SAPPHIRE trial (Stenting and Angioplasty with Protection in Patients at High Risk for Endarterectomy), there were only two additional strokes (both minor) in the period between 30 days and 1 year following CAS among 167 patients, emphasizing the long-term safety of the procedure.[41] The majority of procedure-related strokes (>80%) are ischemic in nature, with the dominant mechanism being distal embolization of plaque from manipulation of catheters and wires in the aortic arch and CCA, and embolization of plaque elements associated with angioplasty and stent placement at the treatment site. Hemorrhagic strokes accounted for 15% to 20% of all strokes in larger high-risk stent registries.[35,36] The timing of these strokes is slightly later when compared with ischemic strokes, and the dominant mechanism is probably related to cerebral hyperperfusion following CAS. Neurological deficits during the CAS procedure should be assumed to be ischemic in nature, and immediate cerebral angiography should be performed. A normal angiogram is associated with an excellent clinical outcome, and no further treatment should be instituted. In contrast, occlusion of a large artery (≥2–2.5 mm diameter) is associated with a poor neurological outcome, and attempted recanalization using a combination of mechanical (i.e., angioplasty) and pharmacological therapies (i.e., thrombolytics, glycoprotein IIb/IIIa inhibitors) by qualified interventionalists with experience in intracranial intervention is reasonable.[47] Even in skilled hands, the outcome of such rescue maneuvers is unpredictable, since conventional therapies have largely been designed to treat thrombus, and the occlusive emboli in the setting of CAS are composed of atheromatous debris.

HEMODYNAMIC DEPRESSION

Baroreceptors located in the adventitia of the carotid sinus form part of the rapidly acting pressure control mechanism of the body and are activated by increases in blood pressure. Signals from these receptors are transmitted through the glossopharyngeal nerve (CN IX) toward the vasomotor center in the medulla, which in turn activates the vagus nerve (CN X) and reticulospinal tract, resulting in peripheral vasodilation, bradycardia, and decreased cardiac contractility (Fig. 39-12). Transient pressure from angioplasty and more prolonged pressure from self-expanding stents activates these baroreceptors, causing the hypotension and bradycardia that is frequently associated with CAS. In general, these hemodynamic effects are seen immediately at the time of intervention; in some patients, they persist into the postprocedural period for 24 to 48 hours.[48-50] It is uncommon for significant effects to be seen beyond 48 to 72 hours, as the baroreceptors gradually adapt to the pressure from the self-expanding stent.

In a retrospective analysis of 500 consecutive CAS cases from a single center, the frequency of procedural hemodynamic depression—defined as a systolic blood pressure <90 mm Hg or bradycardia <60 beats per minute—was 42%, with persistent hemodynamic depression after the procedure in 17% of cases.[50] Not surprisingly, the location of the lesion at the carotid bulb was a predictor of the event. Prior endarterectomy was associated with a reduced incidence of hemodynamic depression, likely due to denervation of the carotid sinus. The management of hemodynamic depression is usually straightforward. Prophylactic measures include withholding antihypertensive medications on the morning of the procedure and ensuring adequate hydration with intravenous fluids prior to and during the procedure. Some operators routinely administer atropine (0.25–0.5 mg IV) prior to the angioplasty and stenting portion of the procedure, whereas others restrict its use to patients who have critical aortic stenosis or critical coronary artery disease or who demonstrate an exaggerated hemodynamic response to angioplasty or stent deployment. In the presence of severe asymptomatic (i.e., systolic blood pressure <75 mm Hg) or any symptomatic hemodynamic depression, the use of intravenous pressors is indicated (e.g., phenylephrine, dopamine, epinephrine). For less severe, asymptomatic hemodynamic depression, oral pseudoephedrine (40–60 mg every 4–6 hours) may be used in an effort to avoid intravenous pressors. For patients with persistent postprocedural hemodyamic

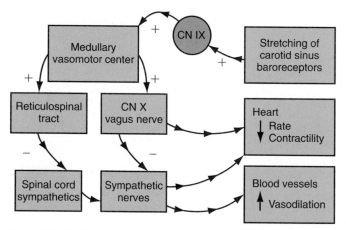

Figure 39-11 Diagrammatic representation of the effect of activation of mechanoreceptors in the carotid sinus during carotid intervention.

TABLE 39-4	Thirty-Day Outcomes from Randomized Trials of CAS in Normal-Risk Patients								
	Stroke (%)			MI (%)			Death (%)		
Trial	CAS	CEA	*P* VALUE	CAS	CEA	*P* VALUE	CAS	CEA	*P* VALUE
CREST									
Total	4.1	2.3	0.01	1.1	2.3	0.03	0.7	0.3	0.18
Symptomatic	5.5	3.2	0.04	1.0	2.3	0.08	3	0	NR
Asymptomatic	2.5	1.4	0.15	1.2	2.2	0.2	0	0	NA
ICSS	7.0	3.3	<0.01	0.4	0.5	NR	1.3	0.5	0.07
EVA 3S	8.8	2.7	<0.01	0.4	0.8	0.62	0.8	1.2	0.68
SPACE	7.5	6.2	NS	NR	NR	NR	0.7	0.9	NS

CREST, Carotid Revascularization Endarterectomy versus Stent Trial; CAS, Carotid artery stenting; EEVA-3S, Endarterctomy Versus Angioplasty in patients with Symptomatic Severe carotid Stenosis; ICCS, International Carotid Stenting Study; MI, myocardial infarction; NR, not reported; SPACE, Stent-Supported Percutaneous Angioplasty of the Carotid Artery versus Endarterectomy Trial; NS, not statistically significant, though specific *P* values were not reported; NA, not applicable.

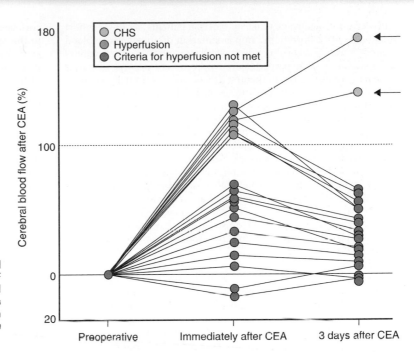

Figure 39-12 Graph showing the increase in cerebral blood flow (CBF) following carotid endarterectomy. Increase in CBF >100% from baseline defines the patient group with cerebral hyperperfusion (purple circles). Within this group, two patients (arrows) developed clinical signs and symptoms consistent with cerebral hyperperfusion syndrome (CHS). *(Reproduced with permission from van Mook W et al. Lancet. 2005;4:877–888.)*[51]

depression, it is important to withhold routine antihypertensive medications and to carefully titrate these medications as the patient's blood pressure returns to baseline. Providing the patient with an automated blood pressure cuff and ensuring daily contact between the patient and healthcare provider is advisable to optimize this management following hospital discharge.

HYPERPERFUSION SYNDROME

Cerebral hyperperfusion syndrome is a rare but potentially life-threatening complication of carotid and vertebral revascularization procedures that improve flow to a chronically ischemic cerebral territory.[51] The syndrome is thought to be caused by significant increases in cerebral blood flow (>100% of baseline) following revascularization,[52] which in combination with impaired cerebral autoregulation results in transudation of fluid into the brain's interstitium and cerebral edema (Fig. 39-13). While hypertension is always present in these patients, it is not a universal finding. Clinically, patients typically complain of a throbbing headache that is ipsilateral to the revascularization site, although the headache may be diffuse. Associated symptoms include nausea, vomiting, confusion, and visual disturbances. In the most severe cases, patients may develop focal neurological deficits and seizures. The feared complication of the hyperperfusion syndrome is intracerebral or subarachnoid hemorrhage, which is associated with a high mortality (40%–60%), and severe morbidity among survivors. In 12 observational studies published since 2003 reporting rates of hyperperfusion syndrome following carotid stenting, the incidence of hyperperfusion syndrome was 1.3% (73 of 5431 cases).[53–56] There is some variation in the timing of the syndrome, but in general most cases manifest within 24 hours of the procedure, and cases beyond 2 to 4 days are rare. Based on data following carotid revascularization with CEA, an increased risk of the syndrome likely persists up to 28 days following CAS. The rate of hemorrhagic complications of the syndrome following CAS appears to be high, with 25%–60% of cases being complicated by intraparenchymal or subarachnoid hemorrhage.[54,57,58] The low event rates for hyperperfusion syndrome in these reports preclude multivariate analyses of predictors of the syndrome following CAS. Several risk factors have been reported in the CEA literature; these probably also apply in patients undergoing CAS. They include preexisting hypertension, postprocedural hypertension, contralateral carotid

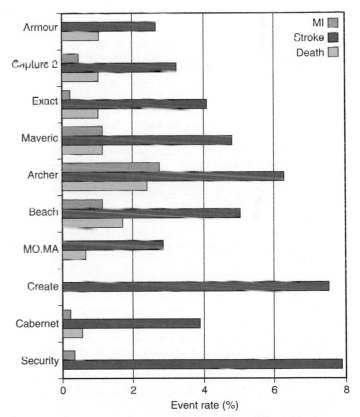

Figure 39-13 Incidence of death, stroke, and myocardial infarction (MI) at 30 days in high-risk carotid artery stent registries. The registries are ordered, with the most recently published at the top and the earliest published at the bottom.[27,33,35–40,100]

occlusion, critical ipsilateral carotid stenosis, and incomplete circle of Willis.[51] These risk factors permit the identification of patients at high risk for cerebral hyperperfusion after CAS. However, aggressive control of blood pressure following CAS is recommended in all patients to prevent it. One study has reported a rate of hyperperfusion syndrome of 0.5% (3 of 570 patients) among a cohort of 570 patients following the implementation of an aggressive blood pressure-lowering algorithm after carotid stenting.[59] The cornerstones of management of hyperperfusion syndrome are prompt diagnosis and emergent institution of therapy. The diagnosis is initially a clinical one, based on the patient's symptoms. While confirmatory studies are helpful, the clinical diagnosis of hyperperfusion syndrome mandates immediate medical therapy. Since blood flow is pressure-dependent in patients with cerebral hyperperfusion syndrome, the major focus of therapy is a reduction in systemic arterial pressure.[51] Several antihypertensive agents are associated with increased cerebral blood flow and are therefore contraindicated (e.g., glycerol trinitrate, nitroprusside, calcium channel antagonists, and angiotensin converting enzyme inhibitors). Recommended agents include beta blockers, labetalol (mixed alpha- and beta-adrenergic antagonist), and clonidine (central alpha$_2$-adrenergic antagonist), which have favorable effects on cerebral blood flow and cerebral perfusion pressure in this clinical situation. Patients should be cared for in an intensive care setting that facilitates meticulous control of systemic arterial pressure. Following institution of treatment, imaging studies (i.e., computed tomography and magnetic resonance imaging) are helpful to screen for hemorrhagic complications and assess for the presence of cerebral edema. In addition, transcranial Doppler documenting a significant increase in the ipsilateral middle cerebral artery flow velocity (>150%–300% compared with baseline) is useful in confirming the diagnosis.

ADVERSE CARDIAC EVENTS

MI (MI) was not included in the outcomes analysis of all RCTs of normal-risk patients (Table 39-4). However, the importance of MI as a component of the primary composite endpoint is underscored by the increased risk of death in patients who suffer MI in the perioperative period after vascular surgery.[60,61] For this reason, the incidence of MI, as determined by pre- and postprocedural electrocardiograms and serial CK/CK MB measurements, has been included in the endpoint of most high-risk CAS registries and trials. In this patient cohort, the 30-day incidence of MI is in the range of 0% to 2.4% (Fig. 39-11)[27,33,35–41] Over 80% of these are non-Q-wave in type. When compared with CEA in high-risk patients, there appears to be a significant and consistent reduction in MI with CAS versus CEA (2.4% versus 6.1%, $P = 0.04$) in the SAPPHIRE trial.[41] The risk of MI in normal-risk patients undergoing CAS is likely to be lower, a contention supported by data from the CREST trial, which reported 30-day rates of MI of 1.1% in the CAS arm and 2.3% in the CEA group ($P = 0.03$) (Table 39-4).[45]

RESTENOSIS

In-stent restenosis (ISR) is an important late complication of CAS. Based on the acceptable sensitivity, safety, and accessibility of duplex ultrasound in screening for carotid ISR,[62] estimates of the frequency of ISR have largely been based on assessments using this imaging modality. Using this method, the incidence of severe ISR (i.e., ≥80%) is 3% to 4% at ~18 month follow-up.[63,64] The rate of ISR at 2 years in a randomized trial of CAS and CEA was higher (11.1%) when a lower cutoff was used to define it (≥70%).[65] However, for less severe degrees of ISR, conventional ultrasound criteria for determination of the degree of stenosis in a nonstented carotid artery may overestimate the degree of stenosis after CAS because of alterations in the compliance of the stented artery.[66] Nonetheless, data suggest that ISR is associated with low rates of clinical events. In two large series, only 1 of 12 patients with severe ISR (i.e., >80%) was symptomatic[63,64] and only 2 of 54 patients with ISR of >70% were symptomatic.[65] Additionally, the rate of clinically driven target vessel revascularization was only 2.4% at 3 years in a randomized trial of high-risk patients.[41] A serial intravenous ultrasound (IVUS) study demonstrated that the immediate postprocedural minimal carotid stent area was negatively

correlated with the percentage of restenotic area at follow-up.[67] Prior to this study, it had been thought that such a relationship would not exist owing to the large caliber of the carotid artery. This finding emphasizes the need to balance the short-term procedural risk of distal embolization and stroke from aggressive poststent dilation versus the long-term risk of ISR. As in the case of restenosis following CEA, the clinical benefits of revascularization for ISR following CAS have not been demonstrated. Both of these pathologies appear to be associated with a relatively benign clinical outcome,[67] suggesting that a conservative approach is appropriate. Repeat revascularization is usually limited to patients with severe ISR and may be influenced by other considerations, such as the presence of contralateral disease or occlusion. A variety of interventional techniques have been reported for treating carotid ISR, including angioplasty, cutting-balloon angioplasty, repeat stenting, and brachytherapy, with recurrence rates of 0%–50%.[63,64,68,69]

▮ Carotid Artery Stenting—Clinical Data

While the benefits of CEA over medical therapy have been clearly demonstrated in RCTs, these trials systematically excluded patients with certain baseline comorbitities or high-risk anatomical features (Table 39-5). Subsequent "real world" assessments of clinical outcomes with CEA suggested that the conclusions of these trials might not be broadly applicable in clinical practice. For example, Wennberg et al. analyzed outcomes in 113,000 Medicare patients undergoing CEA between 1992 and 1993 and reported mortality rates at least three times greater than those reported in prior RCTs.[70] A single-center CEA registry of over 3,000 patients demonstrated that comorbidities such as severe coronary artery disease, chronic obstructive pulmonary disease, and renal insufficiency were associated with an incidence of perioperative death, stroke, or MI of 7.4%, versus 2.9% in a low-risk cohort of patients without these comorbidities.[71] Based on such data, initial attempts to demonstrate equipoise between contemporary percutaneous carotid revascularization and CEA focused on a high-risk patient cohort as the study population of interest. Accepting that carotid revascularization has not been proven in RCTs to be more efficacious than medical therapy in this study population, surgical CEA has been widely employed by vascular surgeons on the basis that a

TABLE 39-5	Criteria Used to Define a High-Risk Population in Carotid Artery Stent Studies
Clinical	
Age >75–80 years	
Congestive heart failure (class III/IV)	
Known severe left ventricular dysfunction, LVEF <30%–35%	
Planned CABG or heart valve surgery	
Recent MI (>24 hours and <4–6 weeks)	
Unstable angina (CCS class III/IV)	
Severe pulmonary disease*	
Contralateral cranial nerve injury	
Anatomical	
Previous CEA with recurrent stenosis	
Surgically inaccessible lesion	
High-cervical lesion (at or above C2)	
Below the clavicle	
Contralateral carotid occlusion	
Radiation therapy to neck	
Prior radical neck surgery	
Severe tandem lesions	
Spinal immobility of the neck	

CABG, coronary artery bypass surgery; CEA, carotid endarterectomy; CCS, Canadian Cardiovascular Society;
LVEF, left ventricular ejection fraction; MI, myocardial infarction.
*Defined as need for home oxygen, Po$_2$ < 60 mm Hg on room air, FEV$_1$ less than 30% to 50% of predicted.

TABLE 39-6	"High-Risk" Registries of Carotid Artery Stenting with Embolic Protection					
Study	*Sponsor*	*Sample Size*	*Stent*	*Embolic Protection Device*	*Status*
SAPPHIRE (CAS registry)	Cordis	409	Precise	Angioguard	3-year outcomes published
ARCHeR 2, 3	Guidant	ARCHeR 2 - 278 ARCHeR 3 - 145	Acculink (OTW & Rx)	Accunet	2-year outcomes published
SECuRITY	Abbott Vascular Devices	320	MedNova Xact	MedNova NeuroShield/ EmboShield	1-year outcomes presented
BEACH	Boston Scientifc	480	WALLSTENT	FilterWire EX and EZ	1-year outcomes published
CABERNET	EndoTex	380	NexStent	FilterWire EX	3-year outcomes published
MAVErIC International	Medtronic	51	Exponent	Interceptor	1-year outcomes published
MAVErIC II	Medtronic	Phase I – 99 Phase II - 399	Exponent	GuardWire	1-year outcomes published
PASCAL	Medtronic	115	Exponent	Any CE Mark-approved device	30-day outcomes presented
CREATE	ev3	400	Protégé	Spider	30-day outcomes published
MO.MA*	Invatec	157	Any carotid stent	MO.MA	30-day outcomes published
CAPTURE 2	Abbott	4,175	Acculink	Accunet	30-day outcomes published
EXACT	Abbott	2,145	Xact	Emboshield	30-day outcomes published
ARMOUR	Invatec	262	Any carotid stent	MO.MA	30-day outcomes published

ARCHeR, Acculinnk for Revascularization of Carotids in High-Risk Patients; BEACH, The Boston Scienfitic Scientific EPI: A Carotid Stenting Trial for High-Risk Surgical Patients Trial; CABERNET, Carotid Artery Revascularization Using the Boston Scientific EPI FilteRwire EX/EZ aNd the EndoTex NexStent; Carotid RX ACCULINK/RX ACCUNET Post-Approval Trial to Uncover Unanticipated or Rare Events; CAS, carotid artery stent; CREATE, The Carotid Revascularization with ev3 Arterial Technology Evolution Trial; Emboshield and Xact Post Approval Carotid Stent Trial; MAVErIC, Evaluation of the Medtronic AVE Self-Expanding Carotid Stent System with Distal Protection in the Treatment of Carotid Stenosis; MO.MA, A Prospective Multicenter Clinical Registry for Carotid Stenting with a New Neuro-Protection Device based on Endovascular Clamping; OTW, over-the-wire; PASCAL, Performance And Safety of the Medtronic AVE Self Expandable Stent in Treatment of Carotid Artery Lesions; Rx, monorail; sAPPHIRE, Stenting and Angioplasty with Protection in Patients and HIgh Risk for Endarterectomy Endarterectomy; SECuRITY, A Registry Study to Evaluate the Neuroshied Bare Wire Cerebral Protection System and X.act Stent in Patients at High RIsk for Carotid EndarterterecTomY.

*75% of patients were high-risk.

beneficial effect in high-risk patients could be extrapolated from trial data in normal-risk study populations.

Carotid Artery Stenting in High-Risk Patients

Among high-risk patients, outcomes of carotid artery stenting using contemporary techniques have been reported in the form of case series, industry-sponsored registries, and a single RCT. In general, studies of high-risk patients have grouped symptomatic and asymptomatic patients together, with the majority of patients being asymptomatic (~75%). The enrollment criteria have relied heavily on data from prior RCTs in normal-risk patients, with symptomatic patients with >50% carotid stenosis and asymptomatic patients with >70% to 80% carotid stenosis being eligible for inclusion. Case series were particularly helpful in the early stages of the development of CAS but in general suffer from a lack of stringent oversight. A large number of multicenter, industry-sponsored registries with stricter oversight have been performed (Table 39-6, Fig. 39-11). The largest and most recently published of these registries include the EXACT (Emboshield and Xact Post Approval Carotid Stent Trial, $N = 2,145$) and CAPTURE 2 (Carotid RX ACCULINK/RX ACCUNET Post-Approval Trial to Uncover Unanticipated or Rare Events, $N = 4,175$) studies. Importantly, in both of these studies there was independent adjudication of neurological outcomes. At 30 days, the rate of death was 0.9% in both trials; the rate

of stroke was 3.6% in EXACT and 2.8% in CAPTURE.[40] These event rates are somewhat lower than what was reported in smaller, earlier published registries of carotid stenting with distal EPD in which the study populations ranged from roughly 200 to 500 participants and the stroke rates were 3.4% to 6.9% (Table 39-6, Fig. 39-11).[35,37,39] This temporal trend suggests that increased operator experience has played a role in reducing adverse outcomes. Emerging data with the use of proximal EPDs also suggest that these devices may be associated with reduced rates of stroke. In a European multicenter registry of 157 high-risk patients treated with carotid stenting and proximal embolic protection with MO.MA, the 30-day rate of stroke was 2.5%. Similarly, in another multicenter registry of 263 subjects treated with CAS and MO.MA, the stroke rate was 2.3% (Table 39-6, Fig. 39-11).[27,33] The SAPPHIRE trial is the sole randomized trial comparing CEA with CAS in high-risk patients.[41] Enrollment in this study differed from the multicenter industry-sponsored registries in one important respect: the carotid lesion had to be deemed amenable to revascularization by both surgical and percutaneous methods. As a result, the overall risk of the cohort in the randomized portion of this trial was likely somewhat less than in registry-type studies. Given its randomized design, the SAPPHIRE trial provides the most robust data supporting the role of CAS with filter-type EPDs as compared with CEA in high-risk patients. At 30-day and 1-year follow-up, there was a trend toward a reduction in the incidence of death in the CAS group, a significant reduction in the incidence of MI in the CAS arm, but no significant difference in stoke

TABLE 39-7	Thirty-Day, 1-Year, and 3-Year Outcomes in the SAPPHIRE Trial (Based on Intention-to-Treat Analysis)	
	Randomized Trial	
	CAS (%)	CEA (%)
30-day outcomes		
Death	0.6	2.0
Stroke	3.1	3.3
MI	1.9	6.6
Death/stroke/MI	4.4	9.9
1-year outcomes		
Death	7.4	13.5
Stroke	6.2	7.9
MI	3.0	7.5
30-day death/stroke/MI plus death and ipsilateral stroke between 31 days and 1 year	12.2	20.1
3- year outcomes		
Death	18.6	21.0
Stroke	9.0	9.0
MI	5.4	8,4
30-day death/stroke/MI plus death and ipsilateral stroke between 1 and 3 years	24.6	26.9

CAS, carotid artery stenting; CEA, carotid endarterectomy; MI, myocardial infarction.

rates (Table 39-7). Target lesion revascularization (0.7% vs. 4.6%, $P = 0.04$) and cranial nerve palsies (0% vs. 5.3%, $P = 0.003$) were also significantly reduced in the CAS arm. At 3 years' follow-up in this RCT, event rates were comparable between CAS and CEA patients: death occurred in 19% of patients in the CEA arm and 21% of patients in the CAS arm ($P = 0.68$) and stroke occurred in 9% of patients in both arms. Overall, these data support the conclusion that CAS with embolic protection is not inferior to CEA in high-risk patients and provides equivalent long-term protection from stroke events.[72]

Carotid Artery Stenting in Normal-Risk Patients

Carotid intervention remains investigational in normal-risk patients. In contrast to high-risk CAS trials, studies in normal-risk patients have generally included symptomatic and asymptomatic patients seen in isolation, based on the clearly established differences in their natural history based on symptomatic status. Additionally, most major normal-risk studies have had a randomized design and in general have compared CAS with CEA. A total of five randomized trials of carotid intervention in normal-risk patients have been completed (Tables 39-4 and 39-8). The CAVATAS (Carotid and Vertebral Artery Transluminal Angioplasty Study) trial was the first of these and included a largely symptomatic patient cohort with carotid disease.[46] However, because this study enrolled patients between 1992 and 1997, the endovascular arm largely employed a strategy of angioplasty alone, since EPDs were not available and carotid stents became available only toward the end of the trial. Despite the lack of a contemporary CAS technique, the 30-day incidence of death or disabling stroke was identical in each arm (6%, $P = NS$). Not surprisingly, the low rate of stent usage was associated with a high rate of restenosis in the endovascular arm. Given the absence of EPD and carotid stent use in this trial, the relevance of the CAVATAS data to contemporary practice is limited. The SPACE (Stent-protected Percutaneous Angioplasty of the Carotid versus Endarterectomy) and EVA-3S (Endarterectomy Versus Angioplasty in patients with Symptomatic Severe carotid Stenosis) trials represented the first two RCTs comparing contemporary CAS technique (i.e., EPD and carotid stent use) with CEA.[43,73] Both were performed in Europe, and the 30-day and long-term outcomes (i.e., 2–4 years) of these studies have been published. In the EVA-3S trial, the 30-day incidence of stroke or death was 9.6% in the CAS arm versus 3.9% in the CEA arm ($p = 0.01$).[43] The SPACE trial reported an incidence of ipsilateral stroke and death at 30 days in the CAS arm of 6.8% versus 6.3% in the CEA arm.[73]

Based on predefined statistical rules to prove the equivalence of CAS versus CEA, the SPACE investigators concluded that CAS failed to demonstrate equivalence, and because enrollment would have had to be doubled to provide enough power to prove equivalence, they stopped further patient recruitment into the trial. For proponents of CAS, these results were disappointing and certainly raised concern regarding the safety of CAS in this patient subset. However, the results of both of these studies need to be interpreted in the context of several factors that challenge the validity of the findings. Neither study had a roll-in phase to ensure that operators were completely familiar with the equipment for CAS being used and to audit their clinical outcomes. This limitation was compounded by the fact that the threshold carotid interventional experience required for operators in both of these studies was suboptimal. For example, in the EVA-3S trial, an operator who had performed only five prior CAS procedures was eligible to treat randomized patients. Similarly, in the SPACE trial, eligible operators for the CAS arm need not have ever performed carotid stenting; rather, eligibility was set by a threshold of having performed 25 successful angioplasty procedures in any vascular bed. There were additional issues with regard to the interventional technique used in these studies. Despite the availability of EPDs, the EVA-3S study did not initially mandate their use. Only after an interim analysis demonstrated an increased incidence of strokes in patients in whom EPDs were not used was the protocol amended to mandate their use. In the SPACE trial, the use of EPDs was left to the discretion of the operator and they were ultimately used in only 27% of all patients. Predilation prior to stenting was performed in only 17% of patients in the EVA-3S trial, which is a definite deviation from accepted CAS technique in the United States. In a further deviation from accepted U.S. practice, 15% of patients in EVA-3S were not administered dual antiplatelet therapy following carotid stent placement. In summary, the data provided by the EVA-3S and SPACE trials did not support equivalency of CAS versus CEA in symptomatic patients at normal risk for CEA, but deficiencies in trial design and execution are felt by proponents of CAS to explain the signal of harm associated with CAS in these trials. The remaining two RCTs of CAS versus CEA in normal-risk symptomatic patients were the ICSS (International Carotid Stenting Study) and CREST (Carotid Revascularization Endarterectomy versus Stenting Trial) trials.[44,45] Over 1,700 patients from Europe, Australia, New Zealand, and Canada were enrolled in the ICSS trial. Unfortunately this study did not have a roll-in phase, and the minimum training requirement for CAS operators was set at 50 total stenting procedures, of which only 10 had to be in the carotid territory. In addition, the use of EPDs was not mandated; they appear to have been used in ~80% of cases. Considerable controversy has been generated by the finding that there was an increased incidence of new ischemic lesions on diffuse weighted MRI in patients treated at centers in which EPDs were used versus centers in which EPDs were not used. It is unclear whether this finding represents real harm due to EPD use or whether operators were inexperienced with their use. Accepting these limitations, the major finding of ICSS was that the incidence of stroke at 30 days was significantly lower with CEA compared with CAS (3.9% vs. 7.6%). This difference was driven largely by an excess of nondisabling strokes in the CAS group. At 120 days' follow-up, the rates of death and stroke were significantly lower with CEA compared with CAS (0.8% vs. 2.3%, and 4.1% vs. 7.7%, respectively). There was an extremely low rate of MI in both arms (0.4% for CAS and 0.5% for CEA).[44] The CREST trial was a U.S.-based trial sponsored by the NIH that enrolled over 2,500 patients. Unlike other RCTs in normal-risk populations, both symptomatic (53%) and asymptomatic patients were included, a decision that was driven by initial problems with patient recruitment. In contrast to other trials of normal-risk patients, there was a stringent lead-in phase to ensure that operators were familiar with the single carotid stent and filter system in the study and to audit clinical outcomes prior to approval for recruitment of patients into the randomized portion of the trial. The primary endpoint of the trial (periprocedural death, stroke, and MI plus ipsilateral stroke up to 4 years after carotid revascularization) occurred in 7.2% of the CAS group versus 6.8% of the CEA group

TABLE 39-8	"Normal-Risk" Carotid Artery Stent Trials							
Trial	Planned Sample Size	Sites of Enrollment	Funding	Clinical Enrollment Criteria	Lesion Enrollment Criteria	Endovascular Strategy	Primary Endpoints	Status of Trial
ICSS (CAVATAS-2)	1,500	Europe Australia Canada	Stroke Association Sanofi Synthelabo European Commission	TIA/stroke within 12 months	>50% by NASCET method or noninvasive equivalent	CAS + EPD	30-day death/ stroke/MI 3 year death/ disabling stroke	120-day outcomes published.
EVA-3S	900	France	National Research Organization	TIA/stroke within 4 months	>60% by NASCET or noninvasive equivalent	CAS + EPD	30-day death/stroke 30-day death/stroke + ipsilateral stroke at 2–4 years.	4-year outcomes published.
SPACE	1,900	Germany Austria Switzerland	Federal Ministry of Education and Research German Research Foundation Industry Funding	TIA/stroke within 6 months	>50% by NASCET or 70% by Doppler	CAS ± EPD	30-day death/ ipsilateral stroke	2-year outcomes published.
CREST	2,500	North America Europe	National Institute of Neurological Disorders and Stroke National Institute of Health Guidant Corooration	Symptomatic Asymptomatic	>50% by NASCET >70% by ultrasound >60% by NASCET >70% by ultrasound	CAS + EPD	30-day death/ stroke/MI ipsilateral stroke after 30 days	30-day outcomes published.
ACT 1	1,540	North America	Abbott Vascular	Asymptomatic		CAS + EPD	Stroke/death/MI within 30 days of procedure plus ipsilateral stroke between 30 days and 365 days postprocedure	Enrollment began April 2005
TACIT	3,700	North America Europe	NIH, Pharma, Device Industry	Asymptomatic	>60% by ultrasound	CAS + EDP	Stroke/death at 3- to 5-year follow-up	Held due to lack of funding
SPACE2	3,523	Germany Austria Switzerland	Federal Ministry of Education and Research German Research Foundation Industry Funding	Asymptomatic	>50% by ultrasound	CAS + EPD	30-day stroke/death Ipsilateral stroke at 5 years	Enrolling study participants.

ACT 1, Asymptomatic Carotid Stenosis, Stenting versus Endarterectomy Trial; CAS, Carotid artery stenting; CREST, Carotid Revascularization Endarterectomy versus Stent Trial; EPD, embolic protection device; EVA-3S, Endarterectomy Versus Angioplasty in patients with Symptomatic Severe carotid Stenosis; ICAS, International Carotid Stenting Study; MI, myocardial infarction; TIA, transient ischemic attack; SPACE, Stent-Supported Percutaneous Angioplasty of the Carotid Artery versus Endarterectomy Trial; TACIT, Transatlantic Asymptomatic Carotid Intervention Trial.

($P = 0.51$). There was an increased incidence of stroke at 30 days in the CAS group (4.1% vs. 2.3%, $P = 0.01$), driven by an increased incidence of minor rather than major stroke. There was a lower rate of periprocedural MI in the CAS group (1.1% vs. 2.3%, $P = 0.03$) and, not surprisingly, cranial nerve palsies were more frequent in the CEA group (4.8% vs. 0.3%, $P < 0.01$).[45] Proponents of CAS are likely to promote CREST as an example of a well-designed and executed U.S.-based trial where stroke rates with CAS are lower than in prior non-U.S.-based trials with recognized limitations. While debate is likely to continue, CREST appears to have restored confidence among the interventional community that CAS will ultimately become a viable alternative option for normal-risk symptomatic (and asymptomatic) patients. In summary, results from trials of CEA versus CAS in normal-risk symptomatic patients are mixed. The optimal method of carotid revascularization may depend on patient age, operator experience, and patient preference regarding the risks of periprocedural MI (higher with CEA), periprocedural stroke (higher with CAS, particularly if operators are inexperienced), and cranial nerve palsy (higher with CEA). Regarding asymptomatic patients at normal risk for CEA, further dissection of

the data from the asymptomatic arm of the CREST trial is required, and completion of the ACT-1 (Asymptomatic Carotid Trial) trial is awaited. A further RCT in asymptomatic patients that included a medical arm (the TACIT trial, or Transatlantic Asymptomatic Carotid Intervention Trial) was planned but appears to have run into difficulties with funding and may never be performed.[74] Data from the medical arm of such a trial would have made a significant contribution to the current body of literature, as such a design would have allowed an accurate determination of the true impact of carotid revascularization superimposed on optimal contemporary medical treatment.

Carotid Artery Stenting— Future Perspective

Realizing the potential of CAS will require further refinements in interventional tools and technique. Perhaps more dramatic may be a reevaluation of our current paradigm for choosing patients for carotid revascularization. We need to move beyond using symptomatic status and percent carotid stenosis as the sole determinants of the need for

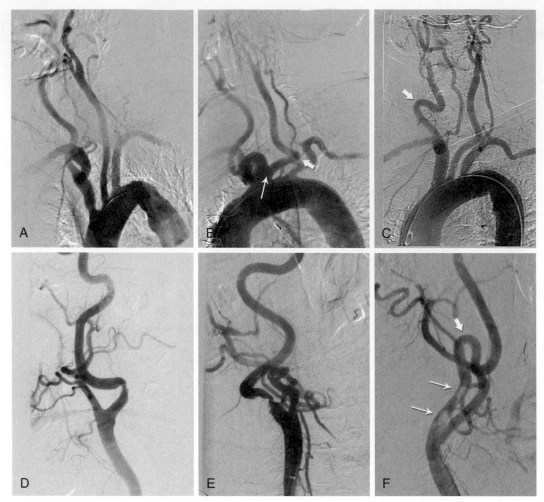

Figure 39-14 Examples of anatomical variations that increase procedural risk during carotid artery stenting. A. Type III aortic arch. B. Bovine origin of the left common carotid artery (narrow arrow) and severe tortuosity in the left common carotid artery (thick arrow). C. Severe tortuosity in the right common carotid artery (arrow). (D) Marked angulation in the internal carotid artery (ICA) at the site of stenosis. E. Tandem areas of angulation distal to stenosis of the ICA. F. Dense circumferential calcification at lesion site (narrow arrows) and severe tortuosity distal to the ICA stenosis.

revascularization. Combining more sophisticated prediction models that incorporate multiple clinical variables with advanced imaging studies of carotid plaque (e.g., tissue characterization with MRI or ultrasound) that allow a more accurate estimate of individuals' risk of recurrent neurological events is necessary. Combining the latter with an estimate of the individuals' procedural risk (for either CEA or CAS), based on clinical and anatomical assessments, will allow physicians to make a more valid judgment regarding the risk-benefit ratio for the individual patient (Fig. 39-14). Further, the current culture of viewing CAS and CEA as competitive strategies for carotid revascularization is counterproductive and reminiscent of the debate on percutaneous coronary intervention versus coronary artery bypass surgery. Instead, these strategies should be viewed as complementary. The mode of revascularization that is most likely to achieve the safest procedural outcome for an individual patient should be chosen. Close examination of outcomes from CAS versus CEA trials should help elucidate those variables that favor one mode of revascularization over the other.

Proximal Vertebral Artery Intervention

Atherosclerotic disease of the vertebral artery (VA) is most commonly located at the origin and proximal V1 extracranial segment of the vessel. Typically, disease at this location represents extension of plaque from the subclavian artery into the proximal VA. In a large prospective New England registry of patients with symptomatic ischemia of the posterior circulation, proximal VA disease was deemed the primary mechanism of stroke in 9%, underscoring the importance of atherosclerotic disease at this site.[75] The mechanism of stroke was attributed predominantly to either hemodynamic compromise or artery-to-artery embolism (i.e., VA to distal posterior circulation). Contemporary surgical revascularization of proximal VA disease typically involves transposition of the VA to the ipsilateral common or internal carotid artery. Other surgical options include VA endarterectomy and vein patch angioplasty.[76] While some centers have reported excellent procedural and long-term results,[77] these surgical techniques have now been almost completely replaced by endovascular therapies. Unfortunately, the lack of RCT data demonstrating a benefit of revascularization over medical therapy alone in patients with proximal VA disease makes clinical decision making problematic. Moreover, there is almost a complete absence of data regarding the natural history of asymptomatic patients with proximal VA disease and a relative paucity of data regarding the natural history in symptomatic patients. Given these uncertainties, most operators will restrict endovascular revascularization to symptomatic patients, especially those who fail medical therapy. Intervention in asymptomatic patients should be strictly limited to those deemed at high risk based on the appearance of the lesion, the presence of poor collateral flow from the carotid circulation, and the existence of contralateral VA disease.

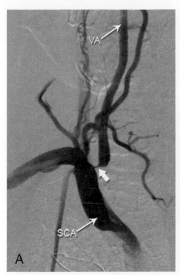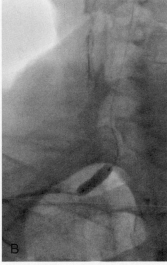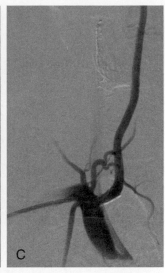

Figure 39-15 Vertebral artery intervention. A. Right subclavian artery (SCA) angiography showing severe stenosis at the origin of right vertebral artery (VA). Because of the takeoff angle of the right VA, it was decided to approach the lesion from the right brachial artery. B. Inflation of a 5.0- by 12-mm Palmaz Blue (Cordis) balloon-expandable cobalt-chromium stent at the ostium of the right VA. C. Final angiographic appearance.

TABLE 39-9 Clinical Outcomes in Selected Series of Proximal Vertebral Artery Stenting

	N	Technical Success	Procedural Complications	Improvement In Symptoms	Mean Follow-Up (Months)	Late Stroke	Restenosis
Mukherjee et al.	12	100%	None	12/12	6.4	0	1/12
Malek et al.	13	100%	1 TIA	11/13	20.7	0	N/A
Jenkins et al.	32	100%	1 TIA	31/32	10.6	0	1/32
Chastain et al.	50	98%	None	48/50	25	1	5/50
Qureshi et al.	12	92%*	None	N/R	1	0	N/R
Ogilvy et al.	50	100%	None	41/43	21	0	11/36
Jenkins et al.	105†	100%	1 TIA 1 dissection	95/105	29	5	14/105‡
Parkhutik et al.	29	100%	1 stroke	N/A	32	1	1/29

TIA, transient ischemic attack; N/A, not available.
*Technical success defined as successful deployment of distal protection device and final residual stenosis of <30%.
†97 cases involved proximal vertebral artery.
‡Target vessel revascularization.

TECHNIQUE[79]

Most proximal VA interventions are performed using femoral artery access, but the ipsilateral brachial artery may also be used, particularly if the VA origin has a retroflexed takeoff from the subclavian artery (Fig. 39-15). Radial access has also been described as a feasible alternative.[79] A 6-Fr guide or 8-Fr sheath is delivered to the proximal subclavian artery, and the lesion is crossed using a soft-tipped 0.014-in. coronary wire. This wire is advanced to the distal V2 segment of the VA to provide support for device delivery. Predilation with a coronary balloon is routinely performed to facilitate stent delivery. Stenting with a balloon-expandable stent is recommended to provide radial strength and reduce restenosis. For smaller-sized VAs (i.e., diameter <3.75 mm), the author typically uses a coronary stainless steel drug-eluting or bare metal stent. For larger sized VAs (>4 mm diameter), stainless steel or cobalt chromium peripheral balloon-expandable stents may be used. There is a lack of consensus regarding the need for embolic protection devices during proximal VA intervention. If the V2 segment of vessel is sufficiently large to accommodate current-generation filter-type EPDs (i.e., ≥4 mm) and the ostial lesion has a high-risk appearance (e.g., ulceration), the use of such devices is recommended.

ENDOVASCULAR OUTCOMES

Data regarding the endovascular treatment of proximal VA disease are largely derived from a number of single-institution cases series treating a symptomatic patient population.[78] Using contemporary stenting techniques, procedural success approaches 100% and periprocedural neurological complications are rare (Table 39-9). The high restenosis rates associated with angioplasty alone have been significantly improved with stenting, with most series reporting in-stent restenosis in 3% to 10% of patients. As expected, lesion length has been identified as an independent predictor of in-stent restenosis, which may have implications for the selection of drug-eluting rather than bare metal stents for longer lesions.[80] Long-term follow-up shows a late stroke rate of <1%, reinforcing the overall safety of the procedure. Coward et al. reported an analysis of a small subset of patients from the CAVATAS trial with proximal VA disease (mean stenosis ~75%).[81] From a cohort of 16 patients, 8 patients received endovascular therapy (angioplasty 6, stenting 2), and 8 patients received medical therapy. There were two procedure-related posterior circulation TIAs in the endovascular group and no neurological events in the medically treated group. While this trial subgroup involves a small number of patients and does not reflect contemporary endovascular techniques, it does reinforce the need for dedicated trials of endovascular revascularization versus medical therapy in patients with proximal VA disease to help define the benefit, if any, of endovascular revascularization in this patient cohort. Currently, the VAST (Vertebral Artery Stenting Trial) trial, comparing medical therapy with vertebral artery stenting for recently symptomatic vertebral artery stenoses >50%, is under way.[82]

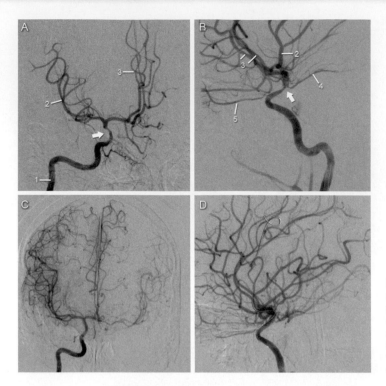

Figure 39-16 Intracranial intervention. A and B. Baseline cerebral angiography in PA cranial and lateral projections, respectively, showing severe stenosis in the supraclinoid portion of the internal carotid artery (arrows). C and D. Cerebral angiography in PA cranial and lateral projections, respectively, following placement of 3.0- by 8-mm balloon-expandable Multilink Vision stent (Guidant Corporation). 1. internal carotid artery, 2. middle cerebral artery, 3. anterior cerebral artery, 4. anterior choroidal branch, 5. ophthalmic branch.

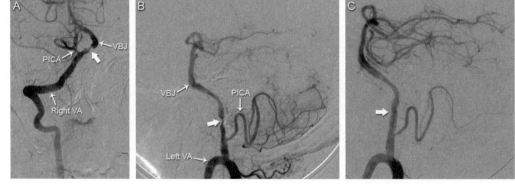

Figure 39-17 Intracranial intervention. A and B. Baseline angiography of right vertebral artery (VA) demonstrating severe stenosis in intracranial portion of vessel between origin of posterior inferior cerebellar artery (PICA) and vertebrobasilar junction (VBJ). C. Vertebral artery angiography following placement of 3.0- by 12-mm Multilink stent.

Intracranial Intervention

Intracranial large vessel atherosclerosis is estimated to account for 5% to 10% of all ischemic strokes in the United States. In Asian, Hispanic, and black populations, the incidence of intracranial atherosclerosis is significantly greater and accounts for a greater proportion of all ischemic strokes.[1,83] As in the extracranial circulation, atherosclerosis of the intracranial circulation has a predilection for specific anatomical sites: in the anterior cerebral circulation, these include the petrous, cavernous, and supraclinoid (Fig. 39-16) portions of the ICA and the main trunk of the MCA; in the posterior cerebral circulation, the distal VA (Fig. 39-17), vertebrobasilar junction, and midportion of the basilar artery are most commonly affected. Intracranial atherosclerosis may cause ischemic stroke by a variety of mechanisms including hypoperfusion, thrombotic occlusion at the site of disease, distal embolization from the site of disease, and occlusion of small penetrating arteries due to plaque extension. In identifying those patients most likely to benefit from revascularization therapy, it is important to develop an understanding of the likely mechanism of stroke in each individual patient based on clinical evaluation, noninvasive imaging, and contrast angiography.

The natural history of asymptomatic intracranial atherosclerosis is largely unknown, but limited data suggest a benign course.[84] By contrast, the WASID trial (Warfarin-Aspirin Symptomatic Intracranial Disease Trial) provides a reasonable estimate of the high risk of recurrent events in patients with a recent TIA or stroke due to angiographically verified 50% to 99% stenoses of a major intracranial vessel.[85] In this cohort, the 1-year risk of an ischemic stroke in the distribution of the diseased intracranial artery in medically treated patients was ~12%. Additional retrospective studies have suggested a variety of clinical and angiographic variables to further risk stratify patients with symptomatic intracranial atherosclerosis, including recurrent symptoms despite medical therapy,[86] lesion location (e.g., vertebral and ICA lesions proximal to major points of collateral supply have a lower risk than lesions involving the basilar artery or MCA), and severity of stenosis.[87] Surgical revascularization of intracranial ICA and MCA disease was first performed in 1967 and subsequently tested in a large RCT of nearly 1,400 patients, which was reported in 1985.[88] Patients were randomized to surgical revascularization (by anastomosing branches of the external carotid artery to the cortical branches of the MCA) versus medical therapy with aspirin (325 mg four times daily). Surgical therapy was associated with a 14% increase in the relative risk of nonfatal and fatal stroke and has subsequently been abandoned as a therapy for the treatment of intracranial carotid disease. Despite this finding, initial attempts at percutaneous revascularization of intracranial disease were made in the 1980s. The initial experience was disappointing, with limited technical success and prohibitively high complication rates. However, by the mid-1990s, a variety of technological advances, borrowed from coronary intervention, and improved operator expertise resulted in a renewed enthusiasm for the technique. Technological advances included the availability of 0.014-in. wires that could negotiate the tortuous intracranial anatomy and low-profile flexible balloon dilation catheters. As in other vascular territories, stents were used to address some of the shortcomings associated with angioplasty of intracranial vessels (i.e., vessel recoil, abrupt vessel closure, and restenosis). However, the tortuosity of the intracranial circulation presented a significantly greater challenge for stent delivery than that encountered in the coronary circulation, so it was not until the availability of third- and fourth-generation coronary stents with improved flexibility and lower crossing profiles that stenting of intracranial disease became more widespread. Today, a number of stents designed specifically for use in intracranial intervention, most notably the nitinol self-expanding Wingspan Stent (Boston Scientific, Natick, MA), the balloon-expandable stainless steel Apollo stent (MicroPort Medical [Shanghai], Shanghai, China), and the balloon-expandable Pharos device (Micrus Endovascular, Sunnyvale, CA) have been developed and tested in prospective studies.[89,90] Although stenting offers an effective treatment for arterial dissection and vessel recoil and improves restenosis rates, the use of stents in intracranial vessels raises a number of unique concerns. Intracranial arteries are particularly fragile owing to the sparse adventitia and elastic layers of the media and hence are prone to perforation. Depending on the lesion location, such perforations result in either subarachnoid or intraparenchymal hemorrhages, which are associated with high morbidity and mortality.[91] Given this consideration, intracranial stents are generally undersized and inflated to lower pressures (4–8 atm). However, several studies of stenting in the coronary circulation have shown that the use of stents that are appropriately sized to the reference vessel diameter and are inflated to high pressures (14–16 atm) is required for optimal stent deployment and apposition of stent struts to the vessel wall. The latter considerations are believed to minimize the risk of stent thrombosis and to reduce the rate of restenosis. Hence potentially serious consequences are associated with the current practice of intracranial stenting. Moreover, stenting is associated with significantly more plaque shifting than angioplasty alone. While the occlusion of small side branches in the coronary circulation is generally a benign event, compromise of critical side branches from intracranial vessels (e.g., lenticulostriate branches of the MCA and perforating branches of the basilar artery) can have severe neurological consequences.[92] Finally, significant complications may occur with attempts to deliver stents through the technically challenging vascular terrain of the intracranial circulation (e.g., stent dislodgement, vessel dissection, and distal embolization of plaque).

TECHNIQUE

Intracranial intervention is almost universally performed using femoral arterial access. Most operators use general anesthesia, in contrast to other cerebrovascular interventions, but the use of conscious sedation has been shown to be a viable alternative.[93] Preprocedural antiplatelet and procedural anticoagulation regimens mirror those practiced during carotid bifurcation intervention. The first task during anterior and posterior circulation intracranial intervention is the delivery of a guide or sheath to the distal CCA and proximal subclavian artery, respectively. Sheaths are most commonly used (e.g., Shuttle sheath, Cook, Bloomington, IN), and the inner luminal diameter of a 6-Fr sheath is adequate for delivery of standard interventional equipment. For normal-sized individuals, a 70-cm length sheath is optimal, as longer sheath lengths may restrict the ability to treat distal intracranial lesions owing to limitations in the length of current balloon and stent

delivery systems. Through this sheath, a 6-Fr Envoy guide is advanced over an 0.035-in. wire to the level of the distal cervical internal carotid artery for anterior circulation intracranial intervention, and distal V2 segment of the VA for posterior circulation intracranial intervention. Having achieved this platform, a variety of 0.010- to 0.014-in. wires (e.g., Synchro, Boston Scientific, Natick, MA) may be used to cross the intracranial lesion. In order to provide sufficient support for device delivery, the wire is generally advanced to the second- or third-order branches of the middle and posterior cerebral arteries for anterior and posterior circulation interventions respectively. Angioplasty is performed using coronary balloons (e.g., Maverick, Boston Scientific, Natick, MA), and the angioplasty technique is modified to minimize the risk of vessel perforation. These modifications include the use of balloon diameters that are 70% to 80% of the vessel diameter and performing slow prolonged inflation of the balloon to less than nominal pressures (4–8 atm), followed by slow deflation. In addition, the minimal balloon length required to treat the lesion is chosen to minimize the risk of compromising flow in side or perforating branches. While some operators adopt a practice of "provisional" stenting (i.e., stenting only if the angioplasty result is suboptimal), an increasing number practice a strategy of primary stenting (stent placement regardless of the initial angioplasty result). Currently, the most popular stents being used for intracranial intervention include the recent generation of cobalt-chromium balloon-expandable coronary stents (e.g., Multilink Vision, Abbott Vascular, Abbott Park, IL, and Driver, Medtronic, Minneapolis, MN), which have superior deliverability to stainless steel coronary stents. Balloon-expandable stents are sized 0.5 mm smaller than the estimated vessel diameter and are inflated to moderate pressures (6–8 atm). The minimal stent length is used to attenuate the risk of plaque shift into critical side or perforating branches. Final angiography of the lesion site and distal cerebral circulation is performed, and patients recover in a neurointensive care setting.

INTRACRANIAL INTERVENTION—CLINICAL OUTCOMES

The majority of initial data regarding intracranial intervention were derived from retrospective observational case series at a small number of institutions with highly experienced operators; as such, they had significant limitations in applicability to broad clinical settings. Case series from the late 1990s and early 2000s reported the experience with intracranial angioplasty. However, the availability of balloon-expandable coronary stents appears to have improved the technical success rate to >90%, without a significant increase in periprocedural complications. A recent systematic review of 31 studies, many of which were early case series, reported results from 1,177 intracranial stenting procedures. The median rate of technical success was 96% (interquartile range 90%–100%), while the median rate of stroke and death was 7.7% (interquartile range 4.4%–14.3%).[94] A number of multicenter prospective studies of intracranial stenting for symptomatic atherosclerotic lesions have been performed in the past decade.[95–99] Each of these studies reported procedural success rates of ≥90%, and 4 of these 5 studies reported procedural success of ≥95%. Early complications rates have ranged from 2% to 7% for ischemic stroke, 1% to 3% for intracerebral hemorrhage, and 0% to 5% for death (Table 39-10). The evidence for long-term complication rates, such as restenosis, are less robust, as there are fewer data, varying definitions of restenosis, and differing strategies for patient surveillance. Nonetheless, in the SSYLVIA (Stenting of SYmptomatic Atherosclerotic Lesions in the Vertebral or Intracranial Arteries) trial, between 30 days and 1 year of follow-up, there were two strokes, giving a cumulative 1 year stroke incidence of 14%. Repeat angiography at 6 months documented a restenosis rate of 32% in the intracranial cohort. In the overall group (intracranial and extracranial procedures), 39% of patients with restenosis were symptomatic (i.e., with TIAs or strokes).[95] In contrast to the SSYLVIA study, all patients in the WingSpan study with restenosis were asymptomatic. In this latter registry, the restenosis rate (>50% by angiography) at 6

TABLE 39-10	Multicenter Prospective Observational Studies of Intracranial Stenting										
				Lesion Location				Adverse Outcomes			
Study	Year	N	Lesions	ANT	POST	Technical Success (%)	FOLLOW-UP	ISCHEMIC STROKE	INTRACEREBRAL HEMORRHAGE	DEATH
SSYLVIA	2004	61*	61	20	23	95	30 days	3 (5%)	1 (2%)	0
WINGSPAN	2007	45	45	23	22	100	30 days	1 (2%)	1 (2%)	0
Fiorella et al.	2007	78	82	54	28	99	Peri-procedural	4 (5%)	1 (1%)	4[†] (5%)
Zaidat et al.	2008	129	129	76	53	97	30 days	6 (5%)	3 (2%)	4[‡] (3%)
INTRASTENT[§]	2010	372	388	223	165	90	Periprocedural	28 (7%)	12 (3%)	8 (2%)

*43 lesions were intracranial.
[†]Deaths were due to the 4 ischemic strokes.
[‡]3 deaths were due to either ischemic or hemorrhagic strokes.
[§]149 patients were enrolled prospectively. A study center could enter consecutive patients retrospectively if done completely (n=239).

months was 7.5%, and the incidence of ipsilateral stroke or death was 7.0%.[96] These prospective studies underscore the technical success of intracranial procedures, mirroring the rates reported in other observational series. However, the 6-month and 1-year rates of death and stroke in prospective cohort studies appear to be greater than in retrospective longitudinal studies, highlighting potential publication bias in the latter type of study design. Indeed, the 14% rate of stroke at 1 year in the SSYLVIA study is remarkably similar to the 1-year risk of stroke reported in the WASID trial in medically treated patients.[85,95] Therefore these prospective studies reinforce the urgent need for randomized studies of contemporary endovascular therapies versus optimal medical management for patients with stroke or TIA due to intracranial disease. Randomized trials are also needed to establish the preferred modality of endovascular therapy (e.g., balloon-expandable stents versus self-expanding stents and drug-eluting stents versus bare metal stents).

Conclusions

Cerebrovascular intervention has evolved dramatically over the last decade. It is clear that these procedures are feasible, and—when performed by experienced endovascular specialists using contemporary interventional equipment and techniques—are safe. The challenge for the future is to advance our understanding of the natural history of cerebrovascular atherosclerosis, more accurately predict those patients who will develop recurrent events, and refine the patient populations in whom endovascular revascularization provides meaningful clinical benefit.

REFERENCES

1. White H, Boden-Albala B, Wang C, et al: Ischemic stroke subtype incidence among whites, blacks, and Hispanics: the Northern Manhattan Study. *Circulation* 111:1327–1331, 2005.
2. Golledge J, Greenhalgh RM, Davies AH: The symptomatic carotid plaque. *Stroke* 31:774–781, 2000.
3. Redgrave JN, Lovett JK, Gallagher PJ, et al: Histological assessment of 526 symptomatic carotid plaques in relation to the nature and timing of ischemic symptoms: the Oxford plaque study. *Circulation* 113:2320–2328, 2006.
4. Beneficial effect of carotid endarterectomy in symptomatic patients with high-grade carotid stenosis. North American Symptomatic Carotid Endarterectomy Trial collaborators. *N Engl J Med* 325:445–453, 1991.
5. Barnett HJ, Taylor DW, Eliasziw M, et al: Benefit of carotid endarterectomy in patients with symptomatic moderate or severe stenosis. North American Symptomatic Carotid Endarterectomy trial collaborators. *N Engl J Med* 339:1415–1425, 1998.
6. Halliday A, Mansfield A, Marro J, et al: Prevention of disabling and fatal strokes by successful carotid endarterectomy in patients without recent neurological symptoms: randomised controlled trial. *Lancet* 363:1491–1502, 2004.
7. Naylor AR: ICSS and Exact/Capture: More questions than answers. *Eur J Vasc Endovasc Surg* 38:397–401, 2009.
8. Cuffe RL, Rothwell PM: Effect of nonoptimal imaging on the relationship between the measured degree of symptomatic carotid stenosis and risk of ischemic stroke. *Stroke* 37:1785–1791, 2006.
9. Fox AJ, Eliasziw M, Rothwell PM, et al: Identification, prognosis, and management of patients with carotid artery near occlusion. *AJNR Am J Neuroradiol* 26:2086–2094, 2005.
10. Inzitari D, Eliasziw M, Gates P, et al: The causes and risk of stroke in patients with asymptomatic internal-carotid-artery stenosis. North American Symptomatic Carotid Endarterectomy Trial collaborators. *N Engl J Med* 342:1693–1700, 2000.
11. Rothwell PM, Mehta Z, Howard SC, et al: Treating individuals 3: From subgroups to individuals: general principles and the example of carotid endarterectomy. *Lancet* 365:256–265, 2005.
12. Rothwell PM: Prediction and prevention of stroke in patients with symptomatic carotid stenosis: The high-risk period and the high-risk patient. *Eur J Vasc Endovasc Surg* 35:255–263, 2008.
13. Rothwell PM, Eliasziw M, Gutnikov SA, et al: Analysis of pooled data from the randomised controlled trials of endarterectomy for symptomatic carotid stenosis. *Lancet* 361:107–116, 2003.
14. Casserly IP: *Carotid Intervention*. Philadelphia, 2005, Lippincott Williams & Wilkins.
15. Hobson RW, II, Howard VJ, Roubin GS, et al: Carotid artery stenting is associated with increased complications in

octogenarians: 30-day stroke and death rates in the CREST lead-in phase. *J Vasc Surg* 40:1106–1111, 2004.
16. Roubin GS, New G, Iyer SS, et al: Immediate and late clinical outcomes of carotid artery stenting in patients with symptomatic and asymptomatic carotid stenosis: a 5-year prospective analysis. *Circulation* 103:532–537, 2001.
17. Roubin GS, Iyer S, Halkin A, et al: Realizing the potential of carotid artery stenting: Proposed paradigms for patient selection and procedural technique. *Circulation* 113:2021–2030, 2006.
18. Saw J, Bajzer C, Casserly IP, et al: Evaluating the optimal activated clotting time during carotid artery stenting. *Am J Cardiol* 97:1657–1660, 2006.
19. Katzen BT, Ardid MI, MacLean AA, et al: Bivalirudin as an anticoagulation agent: safety and efficacy in peripheral interventions. *J Vasc Intervent Radiol* 16:1183–1187; quiz 1187, 2005.
20. Al-Mubarak N, Roubin GS, Vitek JJ, et al: Microembolization during carotid stenting with the distal-balloon antiemboli system. *Int Angiol* 21:344–348, 2002.
21. Angelini A, Reimers B, Della Barbera M, et al: Cerebral protection during carotid artery stenting: Collection and histopathologic analysis of embolized debris. *Stroke* 33:456–461, 2002.
22. Zahn R, Mark B, Niedermaier N, et al: Embolic protection devices for carotid artery stenting: Better results than stenting without protection? *Eur Heart J* 25:1550–1558, 2004.
23. Gruberg L, Beyar R: Cerebral embolic protection devices and percutaneous carotid artery stenting. *Int J Cardiovasc Intervent* 7:117–121, 2005.
24. Kasirajan K, Schneider PA, Kent KC: Filter devices for cerebral protection during carotid angioplasty and stenting. *J Endovasc Ther* 10:1039–1045, 2003.
25. Zahn R, Ischinger T, Mark B, et al: Embolic protection devices for carotid artery stenting: is there a difference between filter and distal occlusive devices? *J Am Coll Cardiol* 45:1769–1774, 2005.
26. Bates MC, Dorros G, Parodi J, et al: Reversal of the direction of internal carotid artery blood flow by occlusion of the common and external carotid arteries in a swine model. *Catheter Cardiovasc Intervent* 60:270–275, 2003.
27. Ansel GM, Hopkins LN, Jaff MR, et al: Safety and effectiveness of the Invatec Mo.Ma proximal cerebral protection device during carotid artery stenting: Results from the Armour pivotal trial. *Catheter Cardiovasc Intervent* 76:1–8, 2010.
28. Stabile E, Salemme L, Sorropago G, et al: Proximal endovascular occlusion for carotid artery stenting: results from a prospective registry of 1,300 patients. *J Am Coll Cardiol* 55:1661–1667, 2010.
29. Mathur A, Dorros G, Iyer SS, et al: Palmaz stent compression in patients following carotid artery stenting. *Cathet Cardiovasc Diagn* 41:137–140, 1997.

30. Stoeckel D, Bonsignore C, Duda S: A survey of stent designs. *Min Invas Ther Allied Technol* 11:137–147, 2002.
31. Bosiers M, Deloose K, Verbist J, et al: Carotid artery stenting: which stent for which lesion? *Vascular* 13:205–210, 2005.
32. Casserly IP, Abou-Chebl A, Fathi RB, et al: Slow-flow phenomenon during carotid artery intervention with embolic protection devices: predictors and clinical outcome. *J Am Coll Cardiol* 46:1466–1472, 2005.
33. Reimers B, Sievert H, Schuler GC, et al: Proximal endovascular flow blockage for cerebral protection during carotid artery stenting: results from a prospective multicenter registry. *J Endovasc Ther* 12:156–165, 2005.
34. Bates ER, Babb JD, Casey DE, Jr, et al: ACCF/SCAI/SVMB/SIR/ASITN 2007 clinical expert consensus document on carotid stenting: a report of the American College Of Cardiology Foundation Task Force on clinical expert consensus documents (ACCF/SCAI/SVMB/SIR/ASITN Clinical Expert Consensus Document Committee on Carotid Stenting). *J Am Coll Cardiol* 49:126–170, 2007.
35. White CJ, Iyer SS, Hopkins LN, et al: Carotid stenting with distal protection in high surgical risk patients: The beach trial 30 day results. *Catheter Cardiovasc Intervent* 67:503–512, 2006.
36. Safian RD, Bresnahan JF, Jaff MR, et al: Protected carotid stenting in high-risk patients with severe carotid artery stenosis. *J Am Coll Cardiol* 47:2384–2389, 2006.
37. Hopkins LN, Myla S, Grube E, et al: Carotid artery revascularization in high surgical risk patients with the Nexstent and the FilterWire Ex/Ez: 1-year results in the Cabernet trial. *Catheter Cardiovasc Intervent* 71:950–960, 2008.
38. Higashida RT, Popma JJ, Apruzzese P, et al: Evaluation of the medtronic exponent self-expanding carotid stent system with the medtronic guardwire temporary occlusion and aspiration system in the treatment of carotid stenosis: Combined from the MAVERIC (Medtronic AVE self-expanding carotid stent system with distal protection in the treatment of carotid stenosis) I and MAVERIC II trials. *Stroke* 41:e102–e109, 2010.
39. Gray WA, Hopkins LN, Yadav S, et al: Protected carotid stenting in high-surgical-risk patients: the ARCHER results. *J Vasc Surg* 44:258–268, 2006.
40. Gray WA, Chaturvedi S, Verta P: Thirty-day outcomes for carotid artery stenting in 6320 patients from 2 prospective, multicenter, high-surgical-risk registries. *Circ Cardiovasc Intervent* 2:159–166, 2009.
41. Yadav JS, Wholey MH, Kuntz RE, et al: Protected carotid-artery stenting versus endarterectomy in high-risk patients. *N Engl J Med* 351:1493–1501, 2004.

42. Ringleb PA, Allenberg J, Bruckmann H, et al: 30 day results from the space trial of stent-protected angioplasty versus carotid endarterectomy in symptomatic patients: a randomised non-inferiority trial. *Lancet* 368;1239–1247, 2006.

43. Mas JL, Chatellier G, Beyssen B, et al: Endarterectomy versus stenting in patients with symptomatic severe carotid stenosis. *N Engl J Med* 355:1660–1671, 2006.

44. Ederle J, Dobson J, Featherstone RL, et al: Carotid artery stenting compared with endarterectomy in patients with symptomatic carotid stenosis (International Carotid Stenting Study): an interim analysis of a randomised controlled trial. *Lancet* 375:985–997, 2010.

45. Brott TG, Hobson RW, II, Howard G, et al: Stenting versus endarterectomy for treatment of carotid-artery stenosis. *N Engl J Med* 363:11–23, 2010.

46. Endovascular versus surgical treatment in patients with carotid stenosis in the carotid and vertebral artery transluminal angioplasty study (CAVATAS): A randomised trial. *Lancet* 357:1729–1737, 2001.

47. Wholey MH, Tan WA, Toursarkissian B, et al: Management of neurological complications of carotid artery stenting. *J Endovasc Ther* 8:341–353, 2001.

48. Trocciola SM, Chaer RA, Lin SC, et al: Analysis of parameters associated with hypotension requiring vasopressor support after carotid angioplasty and stenting. *J Vasc Surg* 43:714–720, 2006.

49. Qureshi AI, Luft AR, Sharma M, et al: Frequency and determinants of postprocedural hemodynamic instability after carotid angioplasty and stenting. *Stroke* 30:2086–2093, 1999.

50. Gupta R, Phatouros CC, Bajzer CT, et al: Rate, predictors, and consequences of hemodynamic depression after carotid artery stenting. *J Am Coll Cardiol* 47:1538–1543, 2006.

51. van Mook WN, Rennenberg RJ, Schurink GW, et al: Cerebral hyperperfusion syndrome. *Lancet Neurol* 4:877–888, 2005.

52. Ogasawara K, Yukawa H, Kobayashi M, et al: Prediction and monitoring of cerebral hyperperfusion after carotid endarterectomy by using single photon emission computerized tomography scanning. *J Neurosurg* 99:504–510, 2003.

53. Tan GS, Phatouros CC: Cerebral hyperperfusion syndrome post-carotid artery stenting. *J Med Imaging Radiat Oncol* 53:81–86, 2009.

54. Moulakakis KG, Mylonas SN, Sfyroeras GS, et al: Hyperperfusion syndrome after carotid revascularization. *J Vasc Surg* 49:1060–1068, 2009.

55. Karkos CD, Karamanos DG, Papazoglou KO, et al: Thirty-day outcome following carotid artery stenting: a 10-year experience from a single center. *Cardiovasc Intervent Radiol* 33:34–40, 2010.

56. Brantley HP, Kiessling JL, Milteer HB, Jr, et al: Hyperperfusion syndrome following carotid artery stenting: The largest single-operator series to date. *J Invas Cardiol* 21:27–30, 2009.

57. Meyers PM, Higashida RT, Phatouros CC, et al: Cerebral hyperperfusion syndrome after percutaneous transluminal stenting of the craniocervical arteries. *Neurosurgery* 47:335–343; discussion 343–335, 2000.

58. Abou-Chebl A, Yadav JS, Reginelli JP, et al: Intracranial hemorrhage and hyperperfusion syndrome following carotid artery stenting: risk factors, prevention, and treatment. *J Am Coll Cardiol* 43:1596–1601, 2004.

59. Abou-Chebl A, Reginelli J, Bajzer CT, et al: Intensive treatment of hypertension decreases the risk of hyperperfusion and intracerebral hemorrhage following carotid artery stenting. *Catheter Cardiovasc Intervent* 69:690–696, 2007.

60. Lopez-Jimenez F, Goldman L, Sacks DB, et al: Prognostic value of cardiac troponin T after noncardiac surgery: 6-month follow-up data. *J Am Coll Cardiol* 29:1241–1245, 1997.

61. Kim LJ, Martinez EA, Faraday N, et al: Cardiac troponin I predicts short-term mortality in vascular surgery patients. *Circulation* 106:2366–2371, 2002.

62. Goldman CK, Morshedi-Meibodi A, et al: Surveillance imaging for carotid in-stent restenosis. *Catheter Cardiovasc Intervent* 67:302–308, 2006.

63. Zhou W, Lin PH, Bush RL, et al: Management of in-stent restenosis after carotid artery stenting in high-risk patients. *J Vasc Surg* 43:305–312, 2006.

64. Lal BK, Hobson RW, II, Goldstein J, et al: In-stent recurrent stenosis after carotid artery stenting: life table analysis and clinical relevance. *J Vasc Surg* 38:1162–1168; discussion 1169, 2003.

65. Eckstein HH, Ringleb P, Allenberg JR, et al: Results of the Stent-Protected Angioplasty versus Carotid Endarterectomy (SPACE) study to treat symptomatic stenoses at 2 years: a multinational, prospective, randomised trial. *Lancet Neurol* 7:893–902, 2008.

66. Lal BK, Hobson RW, II, Goldstein J, et al: Carotid artery stenting: is there a need to revise ultrasound velocity criteria? *J Vasc Surg* 39:58–66, 2004.

67. Clark DJ, Lessio S, O'Donoghue M, et al: Mechanisms and predictors of carotid artery stent restenosis: a serial intravascular ultrasound study. *J Am Coll Cardiol* 47:2390–2396, 2006.

68. Setacci C, de Donato G, Setacci F, et al: In-stent restenosis after carotid angioplasty and stenting: a challenge for the vascular surgeon. *Eur J Vasc Endovasc Surg* 29:601–607, 2005.

69. Chan AW, Roffi M, Mukherjee D, et al: Carotid brachytherapy for in-stent restenosis. *Catheter Cardiovasc Intervent* 58:86–92, 2003.

70. Wennberg DE, Lucas FL, Birkmeyer JD, et al: Variation in carotid endarterectomy mortality in the medicare population: trial hospitals, volume, and patient characteristics. *JAMA* 279:1278–1281, 1998.

71. Ouriel K, Hertzer NR, Beven EG, et al: Preprocedural risk stratification: identifying an appropriate population for carotid stenting. *J Vasc Surg* 33:728–732, 2001.

72. Gurm HS, Yadav JS, Fayad P, et al: Long-term results of carotid stenting versus endarterectomy in high-risk patients. *N Engl J Med* 358:1572–1579, 2008.

73. Hacke W, Brown MM, Mas JL: Carotid endarterectomy versus stenting: an international perspective. *Stroke* 37:344; author reply, 344, 2006.

74. Katzen BT, for the TACIT Investigators: The Transatlantic Asymptomatic Carotid Intervention Trial. *Endovascular Today* 49–50, 2005.

75. Wityk RJ, Chang HM, Rosengart A, et al: Proximal extracranial vertebral artery disease in the New England Medical Center posterior circulation registry. *Arch Neurol* 55:470–478, 1998.

76. Jenkins JS, Patel SN, White CJ, et al: Endovascular stenting for vertebral artery stenosis. *J Am Coll Cardiol* 55:538–542, 2010.

77. Berguer R, Flynn LM, Kline RA, et al: Surgical reconstruction of the extracranial vertebral artery: management and outcome. *J Vasc Surg* 31:9–18, 2000.

78. Mukherjee D, Rosenfield K: *Vertebral Artery Disease*. Philadelphia, 2005. Lippincott Williams & Wilkins.

79. Patel T, Shah S, Malhotra H, et al: Transradial approach for stenting of vertebrobasilar stenosis: a feasibility study. *Catheter Cardiovasc Intervent* 74:925–931, 2009.

80. Lin YH, Liu YC, Tseng WY, et al: The impact of lesion length on angiographic restenosis after vertebral artery origin stenting. *Eur J Vasc Endovasc Surg* 32:379–385, 2006.

81. Coward LJ, Featherstone RL, Brown MM: Percutaneous transluminal angioplasty and stenting for vertebral artery stenosis. *Cochrane Database Syst Rev* 2005:CD000516.

82. Compter A, van der Worp HB, Schonewille WJ, et al: VAST: Vertebral Artery Stenting Trial. Protocol for a randomised safety and feasibility trial. *Trials* 9:65, 2008.

83. Wong KS, Huang YN, Gao S, et al: Intracranial stenosis in chinese patients with acute stroke. *Neurology* 50:812–813, 1998.

84. Kremer C, Schaettin T, Georgiadis D, et al: Prognosis of asymptomatic stenosis of the middle cerebral artery. *J Neurol Neurosurg Psychiatry* 75:1300–1303, 2004.

85. Chimowitz MI, Lynn MJ, Howlett-Smith H, et al: Comparison of warfarin and aspirin for symptomatic intracranial arterial stenosis. *N Engl J Med* 352:1305–1316, 2005.

86. Thijs VN, Albers GW: Symptomatic intracranial atherosclerosis: outcome of patients who fail antithrombotic therapy. *Neurology* 55:490–497, 2000.

87. Prognosis of patients with symptomatic vertebral or basilar artery stenosis. The Warfarin-Aspirin Symptomatic Intracranial Disease (WASID) study group. *Stroke* 29:1389–1392, 1998.

88. Failure of extracranial-intracranial arterial bypass to reduce the risk of ischemic stroke. Results of an international randomized trial. The EC/IC bypass study group. *N Engl J Med* 313:1191–1200, 1985.

89. Jiang WJ, Xu XT, Jin M, et al: Apollo stent for symptomatic atherosclerotic intracranial stenosis: Study results. *AJNR Am J Neuroradiol* 28:830–834, 2007.

90. Kurre W, Berkefeld J, Sitzer M, et al: Treatment of symptomatic high-grade intracranial stenoses with the balloon-expandable Ppharos stent: initial experience. *Neuroradiology* 50:701–708, 2008.

91. Terada T, Tsuura M, Matsumoto H, et al: Hemorrhagic complications after endovascular therapy for atherosclerotic intracranial arterial stenoses. *Neurosurgery* 59:310–318; discussion 310–318, 2006.

92. Levy EI, Chaturvedi S: Perforator stroke following intracranial stenting: a sacrifice for the greater good? *Neurology* 66:1803–1804, 2006.

93. Abou-Chebl A, Krieger DW, Bajzer CT, et al: Intracranial angioplasty and stenting in the awake patient. *J Neuroimaging* 16:216–223, 2006.

94. Groschel K, Schnaudigel S, Pilgram SM, et al: A systematic review on outcome after stenting for intracranial atherosclerosis. *Stroke* 40:e340–e347, 2009.

95. Stenting of symptomatic atherosclerotic lesions in the vertebral or intracranial arteries (SSYLVIA): study results. *Stroke* 35:1388–1392, 2004.

96. Bose A, Hartmann M, Henkes H, et al: A novel, self-expanding, nitinol stent in medically refractory intracranial atherosclerotic stenoses: the wingspan study. *Stroke* 29:1531–1537, 2007.

97. Fiorella D, Levy EI, Turk AS, et al: US multicenter experience with the wingspan stent system for the treatment of intracranial atheromatous disease: periprocedural results. *Stroke* 38:881–887, 2007.

98. Kurre W, Berkefeld J, Brassel F, et al: In-hospital complication rates after stent treatment of 388 symptomatic intracranial stenoses: results from the intrastent multicentric registry. *Stroke* 41:494–498, 2010.

99. Zaidat OO, Klucznik R, Alexander MJ, et al: The NIH registry on use of the wingspan stent for symptomatic 70–99% intracranial arterial stenosis. *Neurology* 70:1518–1524, 2008.

100. Iyer SS, White CJ, Hopkins LN, et al: Carotid artery revascularization in high-surgical risk patients using the carotid WALLSTENT and FilterWire Ex/Ez: 1-year outcomes in the beach pivotal group. *J Am Coll Cardiol* 51:427–434, 2008.

40

Chronic Mesenteric Ischemia: Diagnosis and Intervention

CHRISTOPHER J. WHITE

KEY POINTS

- Atherosclerotic stenoses commonly involve the major mesenteric arteries (celiac, superior mesenteric, and internal mammary) but rarely cause symptomatic mesenteric ischemia because of an excellent collateral circulation that interconnects the visceral vascular beds.

- The classic presentation is postprandial abdominal pain with weight loss. Patients with functional bowel complaints rarely have significant weight loss.

- Patients suspected of chronic mesenteric ischemia will commonly have atherosclerosis involving other vascular territories (i.e., coronary disease, stroke, renovascular disease, or lower extremity atherosclerotic disease).

- Single-vessel disease of the mesenteric circulation is a rare cause of symptomatic mesenteric ischemia but may occur after abdominal surgery that interrupts the collateral circulation.

- Noninvasive testing with ultrasound, computed tomographic angiography, or magnetic resonance angiography is an appropriate screening test in patients suspected of chronic mesenteric ischemia.

- Invasive digital subtraction angiography requires a lateral view to visualize the origins of the mesenteric vessels as they arise anteriorly from the aorta.

- Catheter-based therapy with stents has largely replaced conventional open surgery as the treatment of choice for this disease.

- The clinical recurrence rate appears to be about 1 in 5 patients, so that careful follow-up is warranted.

Introduction

Although the most common vascular disorder involving the intestines is ischemia, the clinical syndrome of chronic mesenteric ischemia (CMI) or chronic intestinal ischemia is very unusual. Other etiologies associated with this uncommon syndrome include fibromuscular dysplasia (FMD), Buerger's disease, and aortic dissection, but atherosclerosis is by far the most common etiology. Atherosclerotic disease of the aorta with associated aorto-ostial stenosis of the visceral vessels is a relatively common angiographic finding but an infrequent clinical problem. In a population-based prevalence study of mesenteric artery stenosis, 553 healthy Medicare beneficiaries were screened with abdominal ultrasound for evidence of mesenteric disease.[1] Significant (>50% diameter stenosis) narrowing of a mesenteric vessel, in by far the most instances (>97%) isolated celiac artery narrowing, was detected in 17.5% of the total cohort. There was no correlation with age, race, gender, or body mass index and the presence of mesenteric artery stenosis. Only 1.3% of the patients had involvement of more than one mesenteric vessel. Another natural history study reported on a group of 980 asymptomatic patients with mesenteric ischemia who were followed clinically.[2] Only three patients eventually developed symptoms, and in each three mesenteric vessels were severely affected. The most likely explanation for the infrequent occurrence of CMI in clinical practice is the redundancy of the visceral circulation, with multiple interconnections between the superior mesenteric artery (SMA) and the inferior mesenteric artery (IMA).

Clinical Presentation

Women are much more commonly affected (70%) than men. The classic presentation of this disease is postprandial abdominal discomfort with significant weight loss (Fig. 40-1). The abdominal discomfort associated with eating leads these patients to avoid food; therefore they lose weight. Patients with CMI typically avoid food and demonstrate significant weight loss. In addition, however, patients with ischemic gastropathy may manifest atypical symptoms such as vomiting, diarrhea, constipation, ischemic colitis, and lower gastrointestinal bleeding. Most patients will have evidence of atherosclerosis in other vascular beds and may have suffered prior myocardial infarction, stroke, or claudication. Patients with atypical symptoms may be very difficult to diagnose, but a high degree of suspicion for CMI in those with other manifestations of atherosclerosis and unexplained weight loss is appropriate. Often the diagnosis is delayed in patients who are being evaluated for a possible malignancy as an explanation for their weight loss. Patients with functional bowel complaints rarely experience significant weight loss, which helps to differentiate them from CMI patients. Evidence of significant obstruction of two or more of these vessels is often found when classic symptoms and endoscopy suggest bowel ischemia,[3] although single-vessel disease, usually of the SMA, has been described, particularly if collateral connections have been disrupted by prior abdominal surgery.

Diagnosis

The diagnosis of CMI is a clinical one, based upon symptoms and consistent anatomic findings. Where there is a high clinical suspicion for CMI, patients should undergo Doppler ultrasound (duplex) imaging or noninvasive angiography with computed tomographic angiography (CTA) and magnetic resonance angiography (MRA) to confirm their anatomy. The ability to visualize the mesenteric vessels with duplex ultrasound is technically challenging and requires a skilled, dedicated technologist. The reported accuracy for duplex imaging in identifying significant stenoses of the celiac and superior mesenteric arteries approaches 90%.[4,5] With the relatively common application of CTA and MRA imaging for abdominal pathology, it is now possible to make the "anatomic" diagnosis without performing an invasive procedure.[6] Invasive digital subtraction angiography is useful for diagnosis but requires a lateral aortogram to visualize the ostia of the mesenteric vessels (Fig. 40-2). Occasionally an enlarged collateral vessel connecting a branch of the IMA with the SMA (arc of Riolan) is seen on the anteroposterior aortogram; it is an indication of proximal mesenteric artery disease. When critical stenoses (≥70%) in multiple vessels are found in symptomatic patients, revascularization is appropriate. However, in patients with borderline lesions or questionable symptoms, there is no stress test to confirm mesenteric ischemia.

Treatment

Revascularization has traditionally involved open surgery with either endarterectomy or bypass grafting. However, this patient group has a

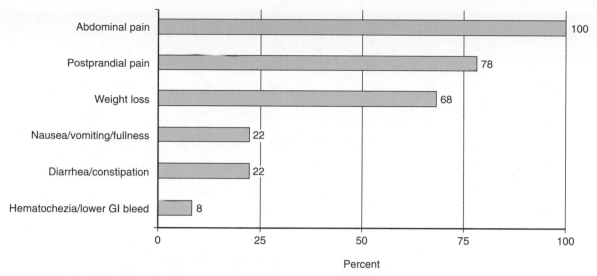

Figure 40-1 Initial clinical presentation of CMI patients. *(From Silva JA, White CJ, Collins TJ, et al. Endovascular therapy for chronic mesenteric ischemia. J Am Coll Cardiol. 2006;47:944–950.)*

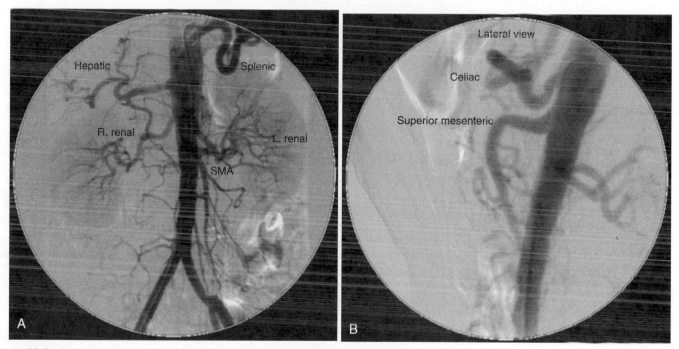

Figure 40-2 A. Anteroposterior view of an abdominal aortogram showing the branches of the celiac artery (hepatic and splenic), the renal arteries, and the superior mesenteric artery (SMA). B. Lateral view of an abdominal aortogram showing the origin of the celiac and superior mesenteric arteries.

high incidence of underlying coronary artery disease and the perioperative surgical mortality ranges from 3.5% to 15% (Table 40-1),[7-21] with the highest incidence of complications occurring in patients above age 70.[22] Atherosclerotic aorto-ostial obstructions of the visceral vessels are similar to those of the renal arteries, and the technical considerations for percutaneous transluminal angioplasty (PTA) with stent placement are similar to those for renal artery intervention (Fig. 40-3). As with renal interventions, stent placement offers a superior late patency compared to PTA alone.[23] The endovascular approach circumvents the need for general anesthesia and the operative trauma associated with open surgery and, it is believed, will result in a lower acute mortality and morbidity (Table 40-2).[3,17,23–34] Because of the relative infrequency of this disease, there are no randomized trials comparing surgery with endovascular treatment for CMI. The 20-year

(1977–1997) Cleveland Clinic experience in 85 patients with CMI treated with surgery demonstrated an 8% perioperative mortality and one-third of the patients had a major complication of surgery.[16] Advanced age, hypertension, coronary disease, and disease in other vascular beds correlated with surgical complications. At late follow-up, 23% ($n = 18$) had objective evidence of restenosis, 21% ($n = 16$) had recurrent CMI symptoms, and 12% ($n = 9$) underwent target vessel revascularization (TVR). Interestingly, the use of vein conduit as graft material was associated with poorer patency than Dacron as a graft material. The 5-year survival rate was 64% (95% confidence interval [CI] 53%–75%) and the 3-year symptom-free survival rate was 81% (95% CI 72%–90%). As a follow-up, a retrospective comparison of a 3-year percutaneous revascularization experience from the Cleveland Clinic with the surgical cohort reported by Mateo and colleagues[16]

TABLE 40-1	Surgical Outcomes for Chronic Mesenteric Ischemia						
Author	**Year**	**Patients (N)**	**Vessels (N)**	**Technical Success (%)**	**30-Day Mortality (%)**	**Symptom Relief (%)**	**Restenosis (%)**
Kieny[7]	1990	60	69	100	3.5	NA	25
Cormier[8]	1991	32	90	100	9	NA	9
Cunningham[9]	1991	74	194	100	12	86	NA
McAfee[10]	1992	58	119	100	10	90	10
Calderon[11]	1992	20	36	100	0	100	0
Christensen[12]	1994	90	109	100	13	NA	NA
Gentile[13]	1994	26	29	100	10	89	11
Johnston[14]	1995	21	43	100	0	NA	16
Moawad[15]	1997	24	38	100	4	78	23
Mateo[16]	1999	85	130	100	8	87	24
Sivamurthy[17]	2006	41	59	100	15	68	17
Atkins[37]	2007	49	88	100	4	88	20

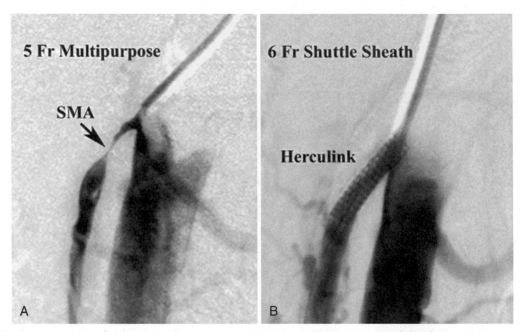

Figure 40-3   A. Baseline angiogram of tight proximal superior mesenteric artery (SMA) stenosis with brachial artery access. B. Final angiogram after deployment of balloon expandable stent.

failed to show an advantage for the percutaneous treatment group.[29] Their 8% perioperative surgical mortality was not different than the 11% (3 of 28 patients) mortality in the angioplasty and stent group. Two of the angioplasty and stent patients who died developed bowel gangrene. There was no difference in the length of hospital stay, suggesting that the angioplasty and stent group must have had severe comorbidities that perhaps made the cohorts not very comparable. At follow-up, the restenosis rate for patients treated with a balloon alone was 33%, but it fell to 11.5% in the stent-treated patients. Late patency and survival were not different between open surgery and the percutaneous group. The largest single series of CMI patients, from the Ochsner Medical Center, includes 59 patients and 79 vessels treated percutaneously.[32] The technical success rate was 96%, achieving symptom relief in 88% of the patients. There was one perioperative death (1.7%) and also two access site complications. At a mean follow-up of 38 ± 15 months, 17% of the patients had recurrence of their symptoms, but none developed acute mesenteric ischemia. All patients with recurrent symptoms underwent successful retreatment without complication. The in-stent restenosis rate at 14 ± 5 months with 90% of the vessels imaged with either CTA, invasive angiography, or duplex ultrasound was 29% (Table 40-2). The TVR was 17%. The 5-year cumulative freedom from death, symptom recurrence, or both

was 72%, 79%, and 57%, respectively. Several papers have summarized noncontemporaneous comparisons of surgical therapy compared with catheter-based therapies for CMI patients.[35–38] These trials emphasize that complete surgical revascularization has benefits in terms of midterm patency, but generally at a cost of significant morbidity and mortality for the patients. Endovascular approaches are preferred in patients at increased risk for surgery, including those with severe comorbidities, including severe cachexia and a hostile abdomen. For lower-risk patients, either procedure is a reasonable alternative and treatment selection should be governed by the patient's informed choice.

Conclusion

The infrequent occurrence of CMI has made randomized controlled trials comparing treatment outcomes very difficult to perform. Case series have shown that percutaneous therapy with stent placement offers the lowest morbidity and roughly equivalent long-term outcomes when compared with surgery. The current treatment recommendation is that patients who are candidates for either surgery or percutaneous therapy should receive percutaneous therapy with stent placement.

TABLE 40-2	Percutaneous Outcomes for Chronic Mesenteric Ischemia						
Author	Year	Patients (N)	Vessels (N)	Technical Success (%)	30-Day Mortality (%)	Symptom Relief (%)	Restenosis (%)
Matsumoto[3]	1995	19	20	79	0	52	NA
Hallisey[24]	1995	16	25	84	6	75	25
Allen[25]	1996	19	24	95	5	79	NA
Maspes[26]	1997	23	41	90	0	75	12
Nyman[27]	1998	5	6	100	0	80	60
Sheeran[28]	1999	12	13	92	8	75	16
Kasirajan[29]	2001	28	32	100	11	66	27
AbuRahma[30]	2003	22	24	95	0	67	30
Sharafuddin[31]	2003	25	26	96	4	85	8
Landis[23]	2005	29	33	97	6.9	90	16.3
Sivamurthy[17]	2006	21	29	95.3	16	27	32
Silva[32]	2006	59	79	96	1.7	83	29
Atkins[37]	2007	31	42	97	3	84	20

REFERENCES

1. Hansen KJ, Wilson DB, Craven TE, et al: Mesenteric artery disease in the elderly. J Vasc Surg 40:45–52, 2004.
2. Thomas JH, Blake K, Pierce GE, et al: The clinical course of asymptomatic mesenteric arterial stenosis. J Vasc Surg 27:840–844, 1998.
3. Matsumoto AH, Tegtmeyer CJ, Fitzcharles EK, et al: Percutaneous transluminal angioplasty of visceral arterial stenoses: results and long-term clinical follow-up. J Vasc Interv Radiol 6:165–174, 1995.
4. Bowersox JC, Zwolak RM, Walsh DB, et al: Duplex ultrasonography in the diagnosis of celiac and mesenteric artery occlusive disease. J Vasc Surg 14:780–786; discussion 6–8, 1991.
5. Zwolak RM, Fillinger MF, Walsh DB, et al: Mesenteric and celiac duplex scanning: a validation study. J Vasc Surg 27:1078–1087; discussion 88, 1998.
6. Chow LC, Chan FP, Li KCr: A comprehensive approach to MR imaging of mesenteric ischemia. Abdom Imaging 27:507–516, 2002.
7. Kieny R, Batellier J, Kretz JG: Aortic reimplantation of the superior mesenteric artery for atherosclerotic lesions of the visceral arteries: late results. Ann Vasc Surg 4:122–125, 1990.
8. Cormier JM, Fichelle JM, Vennin J, et al: Atherosclerotic occlusive disease of the superior mesenteric artery: late results of reconstructive surgery. Ann Vasc Surg 5:510–518, 1991.
9. Cunningham CG, Reilly LM, Rapp JH, et al: Chronic visceral ischemia. Three decades of progress. Ann Surg 214:276–287; discussion 87–88, 1991.
10. McAfee MK, Cherry KJ, Jr, Naessens JM, et al: Influence of complete revascularization on chronic mesenteric ischemia. Am J Surg 164:220–224, 1992.
11. Calderon M, Reul GJ, Gregoric ID, et al: Long-term results of the surgical management of symptomatic chronic intestinal ischemia. J Cardiovasc Surg (Torino) 33:723–728, 1992.
12. Christensen MG, Lorentzen JE, Schroeder TV: Revascularisation of atherosclerotic mesenteric arteries: experience in 90 consecutive patients. Eur J Vasc Surg 8:297–302, 1994.
13. Gentile AT, Moneta GL, Taylor LM, Jr, et al: Isolated bypass to the superior mesenteric artery for intestinal ischemia. Arch Surg 129:926–931; discussion 31–32, 1994.
14. Johnston KW, Lindsay TF, Walker PM, et al: Mesenteric arterial bypass grafts: early and late results and suggested surgical approach for chronic and acute mesenteric ischemia. Surgery 118:1–7, 1995.
15. Moawad J, Gewertz BL: Chronic mesenteric ischemia. Clinical presentation and diagnosis. Surg Clin North Am 77:357–369, 1997.
16. Mateo RB, O'Hara PJ, Hertzer NR, et al: Elective surgical treatment of symptomatic chronic mesenteric occlusive disease: early results and late outcomes. J Vasc Surg 29:821–831; discussion 32, 1999.
17. Sivamurthy N, Rhodes JM, Lee D, et al: Endovascular versus open mesenteric revascularization: immediate benefits do not equate with short-term functional outcomes. J Am Coll Surg 202:859–867, 2006.
18. Foley RN, Parfrey PS, Kent GM, et al: Serial change in echocardiographic parameters and cardiac failure in end-stage renal disease. J Am Soc Nephrol 11:912–916, 2000.
19. Jimenez JG, Huber TS, Ozaki CK, et al: Durability of antegrade synthetic aortomesenteric bypass for chronic mesenteric ischemia. J Vasc Surg 35:1078–1084, 2009.
20. Kihara TK, Blebea J, Anderson KM, et al: Risk factors and outcomes following revascularization for chronic mesenteric ischemia. Ann Vasc Surg 13:37–44, 1999.
21. Leke MA, Hood DB, Rowe VL, et al: Technical consideration in the management of chronic mesenteric ischemia. Am Surg 68:1088–1092, 2002.
22. Park WM, Cherry KJ, Jr, Chua HK, et al: Current results of open revascularization for chronic mesenteric ischemia: a standard for comparison. J Vasc Surg 35:853–859, 2002.
23. Landis MS, Rajan DK, Simons ME, et al: Percutaneous management of chronic mesenteric ischemia: outcomes after intervention. J Vasc Intervent Radiol 16:1319–1325, 2005.
24. Hallisey MJ, Deschaine J, Illescas FF, et al: Angioplasty for the treatment of visceral ischemia. J Vasc Intervent Radiol 6:785–791, 1995.
25. Allen RC, Martin GH, Rees CR, et al: Mesenteric angioplasty in the treatment of chronic intestinal ischemia. J Vasc Surg 24:415–421; discussion 21–23, 1996.
26. Maspes F, Mazzetti di Pietralata G, Gandini R, et al: Percutaneous transluminal angioplasty in the treatment of chronic mesenteric ischemia: results and 3 years of follow-up in 23 patients. Abdom Imaging 23:358–363, 1998.
27. Nyman U, Ivancev K, Lindh M, et al: Endovascular treatment of chronic mesenteric ischemia: report of five cases. Cardiovasc Intervent Radiol 21:305–313, 1998.
28. Sheeran SR, Murphy TP, Khwaja A, et al: Stent placement for treatment of mesenteric artery stenoses or occlusions. J Vasc Intervent Radiol 10:861–867, 1999.
29. Kasirajan K, O'Hara PJ, Gray BH, et al: Chronic mesenteric ischemia: open surgery versus percutaneous angioplasty and stenting. J Vasc Surg 33:63–71, 2001.
30. AbuRahma AF, Stone PA, Bates MC, et al: Angioplasty/stenting of the superior mesenteric artery and celiac trunk: early and late outcomes. J Endovasc Ther 10:1046–1053, 2003.
31. Sharafuddin MJ, Olson CH, Sun S, et al: Endovascular treatment of celiac and mesenteric arteries stenoses: applications and results. J Vasc Surg 38:692–698, 2003.
32. Silva JA, White CJ, Collins TJ, et al: Endovascular therapy for chronic mesenteric ischemia. J Am Coll Cardiol 47:944–950, 2006.
33. Cognet F, Ben Salem D, Dranssart M, et al: Chronic mesenteric ischemia: imaging and percutaneous treatment. Radiographics 22:863–879; discussion 79–80, 2002.
34. Matsumoto AH, Angle JF, Spinosa DJ, et al: Percutaneous transluminal angioplasty and stenting in the treatment of chronic mesenteric ischemia: results and long-term follow-up. J Am Coll Surg 194:S22–S31, 2002.
35. van Petersen AS, Kolkman JJ, Beuk RJ, et al: Open or percutaneous revascularization for chronic splanchnic syndrome. J Vasc Surg 51:1309–1316, 2010.
36. Davies RSM, Wall ML, Silverman SH, et al: Surgical versus endovascular reconstruction for chronic mesenteric ischemia: a contemporary UK series. Vasc Endovasc Surg 43:157–164, 2009.
37. Atkins MD, Kwolek CJ, LaMuraglia GM, et al: Surgical revascularization versus endovascular therapy for chronic mesenteric ischemia: A comparative experience. J Vasc Surg 45:1162–1171, 2007.
38. Dias NV, Acosta S, Resch T, et al: Mid-term outcome of endovascular revascularization for chronic mesenteric ischaemia. Br J Surg 97:195–201, 2010.

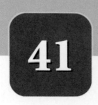

41

Renal Artery Stenosis

KRISHNA ROCHA-SINGH | NILESH J. GOSWANI |
RAGHU KOLLURI | JEFFREY GOLDSTEIN

KEY POINTS

- Renal artery stenosis is caused by a heterogeneous group of diseases with varying pathophysiology, clinical manifestations and courses, treatments, and outcomes. Atherosclerotic renal artery sclerosis and fibromuscular dysplasia are the most common causes of renal artery sclerosis.

- Patients in whom atherosclerosis is progressive may manifest signs and symptoms of chronic ischemic renal disease, resulting in renovascular hypertension and renal dysfunction. However, the causal relationship between renal artery stenosis, hypertension, and renal dysfunction is difficult to prove.

- Duplex Doppler ultrasonography, when performed noninvasively in a high-volume, experienced vascular lab, is an excellent diagnostic tool and ideal for surveillance. In terms of specificity and sensitivity, ultrasound is competitive with computed tomographic angiography and magnetic resonance angiography, but at a lower cost.

- Renal arteriography remains the "gold standard" for the diagnosis of atherosclerotic renal artery sclerosis, allowing for the full definition of the perirenal abdominal aorta and assessment of the diameter and contour of the renal artery and its branch vessels. However, angiographic evaluation of the severity of atherosclerosis (i.e., percent diameter stenosis) alone may be inadequate in establishing the cause and effect between atherosclerotic renal artery sclerosis and hypertension and/or renal dysfunction.

- Currently accepted "consensus" indications for renal artery revascularization include severe, refractory hypertension, recurrent/pulmonary edema, and progressive renal insufficiency despite optimal medical therapy. However, these recommendations are based on limited supporting clinical trial evidence.

- Percutaneous revascularization with bare metal stents represents the current endovascular standard of care in atherosclerotic patients with appropriate clinical indications. The clinical effectiveness and safety of adjunctive renal endovascular technologies (i.e., distal protection devices) and medications (i.e., glycoprotein IIb/IIIa inhibitors) have not been established in robust clinical trials.

- Percutaneous radiofrequency renal sympathetic denervation is a safe, effective, and durable method of reducing blood pressure in hypertensive patients who are resistant to medical therapy.

Introduction

Atherosclerotic renal artery stenosis (ARAS) is associated with chronic renal ischemia as well as increased cardiovascular morbidity and mortality. The primary aim of renal revascularization therapies is to improve blood pressure control, salvage renal function, and reduce cardiovascular risk. However, while technical advances in the endovascular treatment of ARAS have improved dramatically in the past decade, allowing patients with more extensive ARAS to be considered for revascularization, the indications for treating these patients remains controversial and highlights the major divergence in practice between physicians regarding the appropriate treatment for patients with ARAS.[1] Recent prospective randomized clinical trials, both small and large, from Europe have failed to demonstrate the clinical benefit of renal revascularization in reducing cardiovascular events and/or renal outcomes compared with medical therapy alone.[2-4] Determining the

essential role of renal revascularization and appropriate patient selection is now the central issue among physicians, as consensus regarding the general technical aspects of renal stent revascularization has reached a general level of acceptance among interventionalists. Finally, the recent emergence of percutaneous renal sympathetic denervation as a safe and effective technology in the management of drug-resistant hypertensive patients has highlighted the important role of the sympathetic nervous system in hypertension.[5] As such, ongoing large clinical trials in the treatment of hypertension and renal insufficiency in these patient populations, with and without ARAS, will ensure that renal interventional therapies for hypertension control will remain an exciting area of clinical research.

Epidemiology and Natural History

ARAS is the most common secondary cause of hypertension; left untreated, it may progress to renal dysfunction. The prevalence of end-stage renal disease in the United States is 372,407 patients per year, with approximately 100,000 new cases diagnosed each year;[6] 2.1% of these new cases are thought to be due to ARAS.[7] ARAS is reported in 0.5% to 5%[8] of all hypertensive patients and 45% of patients with severe or malignant hypertension.[9] The prevalence of ARAS increases with age, especially in patients with diabetes, hypertension, coronary artery disease, or aortoiliac occlusive disease.[10] A population-based study reported a prevalence of renal artery stenosis (RAS) (>60% stenosis) to be 6.8% in patients above age 65.[11] In a Mayo Clinic series, more than 19% of patients with coronary artery disease and hypertension were found to have >50% stenosis of the renal arteries.[12] As such, the risk factors for the development of ARAS are similar to those of coronary artery disease. Similarly, stroke and peripheral arterial disease are highly prevalent in patients with end-stage renal disease on hemodialysis. ARAS is progressive in 36% to 71% of patients with this condition, and 39% of patients with >75% ARAS progress to complete occlusion within 3-year follow-up.[13] In a prospective study of 84 patients with at least one abnormal renal artery, progression of RAS was reported to occur at a rate of approximately 20% per year.[14] Unfortunately, it is difficult to identify the subset of patients who will progress to renal failure. While 90% of renal artery lesions are atherosclerotic, the remaining 10% result from other etiologies. Fibromuscular dysplasia (FMD) is the second most common cause of RAS and results in fibrous thickening of the intima, media, or adventitia of the arterial wall. FMD is more common among women between the ages of 15 and 50 and is recognized by its beaded appearance on angiography.[15] Other less common causes include trauma, dissection, external compression with tumor or mass, thromboemboli, renal artery aneurysms, neurofibromatosis, vasculitis, retroperitoneal fibrosi, and radiation-induced stenosis.[16]

The Pathophysiology of Renovascular Hypertension and Ischemic Nephropathy

The renal vasculature is richly innervated by sympathetic afferent and efferent nerve fibers which controls renovascular resistance, and the resultant increase in renin release.[17] Several inputs control efferent renal nerve activity, such as aortic and carotid baroreflexes[18] and cardiac stretch receptors.[19] Renal nerves often receive greater

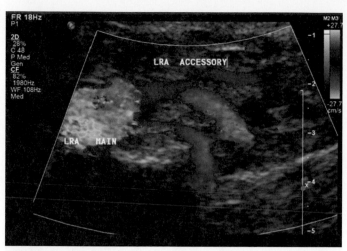

Figure 41-1 Main and accessory renal arteries as defined on duplex ultrasound.

sympathetic activation than others, especially in the presence of essential hypertension.[20] This disproportionate increase in renal sympathetic activity results in increased renovascular resistance and increased plasma renin activity; it also promotes the retention of sodium and water.[21] The afferent renal nerves contribute to the pathogenesis of renovascular hypertension by increasing activation of the sympathetic nervous system.[17] In unilateral ARAS, decreased blood flow through the affected kidney results in increased production of rennin, which, in turn, cleaves angiotensin to produce angiotensin I, which is converted to angiotensin II. Angiotensin II is a direct vasoconstrictor that stimulates aldosterone secretion and results in sodium reabsorption. The retained salt and water is then excreted by the unaffected kidney, producing a rennin-dependent hypertensive state. In bilateral ARAS or ARAS in a solitary functioning kidney where there is no ability to sense an elevated blood pressure, a pressure natriuresis does not occur, resulting in volume expansion. This, in turn, results in the suppression of renin activity. These patients become highly dependent on angiotensin II for glomerular filtration. Angiotensin II maintains the efferent arteriolar tone of the glomeruli. When angiotensin converting enzyme inhibitors (ACEIs) or angiotensin receptor blockers (ARBs) are administered, the efferent arteriolar tone is no longer maintained and glomerular filtration is decreased, resulting in renal insufficiency. Sodium restriction and diuresis convert bilateral RAS to a renin-mediated form of hypertension.[22]

Diagnostic Tests and Imaging

Duplex ultrasound, computed tomography angiography (CTA), and magnetic resonance angiography (MRA) are three contemporary noninvasive imaging modalities used to diagnose RAS. Other tests can be used to assess the potential physiological effect of RAS. Duplex ultrasonography is a useful noninvasive test to screen for RAS, with sensitivity between 75% and 98% and specificity between 87% and 100%.[23] Its sensitivity in identifying accessory renal arteries is 67% (Fig. 41-1). Duplex ultrasonography can produce images of the renal arteries, assess blood-flow velocity and pressure waveforms, and measure kidney size without contrast or radiation exposure (Figs. 41-2 and 41-3). Estimation of renal artery percent diameter stenosis is based on the renal artery velocity and renal artery to aortic velocity ratio (Table 41-3), and anti-hypertensive medications do not interfere with duplex imagining. It can also provide information regarding renal parenchymal disease, tumors, and calculi. It is less expensive than CTA or MRA, can be used for renal artery stenting surveillance, and can be easily performed at the patient's bedside. Unfortunately, early studies of this technology reported a 10 to 20% rate of failure due to operator inexperience, patient obesity, or bowel gas.[23] The test may be time consuming when done by inexperienced technologists.

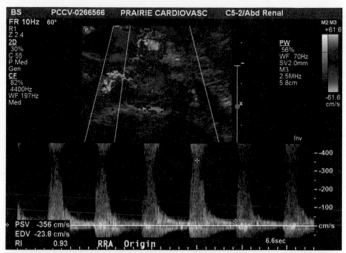

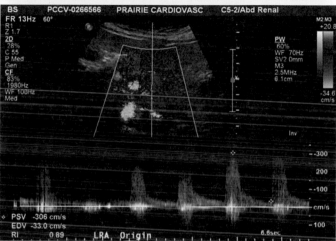

Figure 41-2 Bilateral renal artery stenosis of 60% to 99% on duplex ultrasonography in a 69-year old woman.

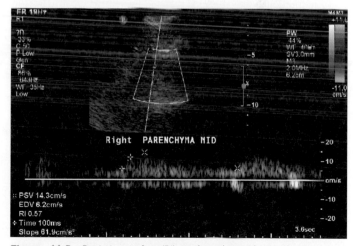

Figure 41-3 Resistive index (RI) and prolonged acceleration time (≥100 msecs, white arrow) in a patient with 60–99% RAS.

The renal resistive index (RI) is a commonly used measure of resistance to arterial flow within the renal vascular bed and is calculated during the duplex ultrasonography (Fig. 41-1).

Renal resistive index = peak systolic renal parenchymal velocity
− end diastolic renal parenchymal velocity

PEAK SYSTOLIC RENAL PARENCHYMAL VELOCITY

An elevated RI is considered to be an indicator of nephrosclerosis and intrinsic kidney disease. Radermacher et al. used an RI >0.8 as the sole screening tool to identify a patient subset that may have a less than optimal response of blood pressure control as well as improved renal function with renal artery stent revascularization.[24] However, these findings were refuted by other studies suggesting improved renal function and blood pressure control after successful renal artery stenting.[25,26] Therefore RI should not be considered the sole parameter in deciding whether a patient will have a clinically favorable response to percutaneous renal revascularization.

MAGNETIC RESONANCE ANGIOGRAPHY AND COMPUTED TOMOGRAPHY ANGIOGRAPHY

MRA and CTA, both excellent noninvasive techniques to evaluate patients for possible renal pathology, are now widely available. If duplex ultrasonography is nondiagnostic, these modalities can be used to confirm the findings of duplex ultrasound and used with patients whose anatomy is unfavorable for invasive angiography; however, CTA does require the use of iodinated contrast. Both CTA and MRI can provide additional visualization of the aorta, accessory renal arteries, and renal parenchymal anatomy. MRA requires no contrast but cannot be used in patients with ferromagnetic devices or those who are claustrophobic. Stented vessels cannot be adequately evaluated by MRA. Grobner and Marckmann postulated the causative role of gadolinium used in MRA in the development of nephrogenic fibrosing dermopathy.[27,28] Since then, the use of MRA has been restricted to patients with serum creatinine <1.5 to 2.0 mg/dL. The sensitivity and specificity of MRA are 62% and 84%, respectively.[29] The drawbacks of CTA include large contrast load and nephrotoxicity, along with the radiation exposure. The sensitivity and specificity of CTA are 64% and 92%, respectively.[29] CTA can also be used for stent surveillance if duplex ultrasonography is nondiagnostic (Fig. 41-4).

Functional Assessment of Renal Artery Stenosis

Brain naturetic peptide (BNP) is secreted by ventricular myocytes in response to increased myofibril stretch. Its production is also stimulated by angiotensin II, which is elevated in patients with RAS, and by hypertension. BNP, in turn, antagonizes plasma renin activity and promotes diuresis and sodium excretion. Silva et al. studied the role of BNP level in patients with RAS and hypertension.[30] In this small study, baseline BNP was elevated in patients with severe ARAS. A significant blood pressure response to renal stenting was seen in patients with elevated baseline BNP. Therefore this test may be useful in identifying patients with renovascular hypertension who would be likely to respond to stent revascularization; however, larger confirmatory studies are required to prove this. Radionuclide imaging has also been historically used to diagnose unilateral RAS. With this technique, a detector gamma camera is used to assess baseline renal flow by injecting a radionuclide tracer (^{99m}Tc diethylene triamine pentaacetic acid [DTPA]). Repeat scans are performed after administering the ACEI captopril, which decreases renal function on the ipsilateral side of RAS, while the uptake of the unaffected side is either normal or increased. The reported sensitivity and specificity are 90% and 93%, respectively.[31,32] The wide availability of duplex ultrasound, CTA, and MRA has resulted in the near elimination of this test to diagnose RAS. It is occasionally utilized for cortical functional assessment of the ipsilateral and contralateral kidney in the setting of renal atrophy and RAS or for cortical functional assessment of a horseshoe kidney with RAS. Plasma renin activity or plasma renin assay (PRA) has also been used as a screening test for renovascular hypertension. Plasma renin levels have a low specificity in the diagnosis of RAS; however, the concomitant use of an ACEI improves the specificity of PRA levels. PRA is measured at

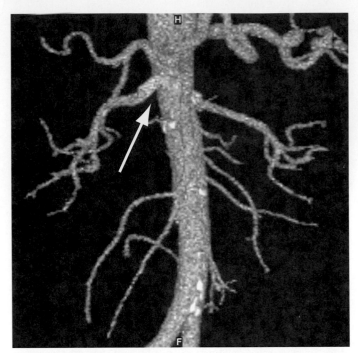

Figure 41-4 CTA images after right renal artery stenting demonstrating patency (white arrow).

baseline and 1 hour after oral administration of 50 mg of captopril. Unfortunately the sensitivity ranges widely, between 34% and 100%, and the specificity varies from 80% to 90%.[33,34] In patients with bilateral or unilateral RAS and a solitary kidney, the sensitivity and specificity is this assay is much lower because the resultant volume overload suppresses PRA levels. Assessment of renal vein renin level is another test for diagnosing renovascular hypertension. This is performed using a catheter to compare the renin levels of both kidneys. Although it may identify blood pressure responders to endovascular intervention or surgery, it has fallen out of favor owing to the invasive nature of the test. Therefore the measurement of plasma renin and renal vein renin activity is seldom needed in contemporary diagnosis and management of RAS because of the availability of noninvasive imaging modalities.

IDENTIFICATION OF AT-RISK PATIENTS AND INDICATIONS FOR RENAL ARTERY REVASCULARIZATION

The presence of ARAS should be suspected in patients with resistant hypertension and/or progressive renal insufficiency who have coronary artery disease (CAD) and/or peripheral arterial disease (PAD). Specific clinical clues are listed in Table 41-2. The preprocedural identification of the patient with poorly controlled hypertension who is likely to benefit from renal stent revascularization is challenging. The recommendations of the American College of Cardiology/American Heart Association (ACC/AHA) for the management of PAD in peripheral arterial disease, including revascularization in RAS, are as listed in Table 41-1.[35] Appropriate indications for renal revascularization include unilateral RAS, bilateral RAS, or RAS involving a solitary functioning kidney in patients in whom blood pressure cannot be adequately controlled with maximal tolerable doses of at least three antihypertensive medications of different classes or if side effects of the antihypertensive medication prohibit sufficient control.[36] In patients with unilateral RAS with normal renal function and well-controlled hypertension, revascularization may not be required; instead, close follow-up for potential loss of pharmacological control and accelerating hypertension and/or a potential decline in renal function may suffice. In these instances, a renal duplex ultrasound should be

TABLE 41-1	Duplex Ultrasound Criteria for a Diagnosis of Renal Artery Stenosis		
Indication		*Classification of Recommendation*	*Level of Evidence*
Asymptomatic bilateral or unilateral RAS to a solitary kidney		IIb	C
Accelerated hypertension		IIa	B
Resistant hypertension		IIa	B
Hypertension and unexplained unilateral small kidney		IIa	B
Hypertension with intolerance to antihypertensive medications		IIa	B
Progressive kidney disease and bilateral RAS or RAS to a solitary kidney		IIa	B
Chronic renal insufficiency and unilateral RAS		IIb	C
Recurrent, unexplained CHF or sudden unexplained pulmonary edema		I	B

CHF, congestive heart failure; RAS, renal artery stenosis.

TABLE 41-3	ACC/AHA Peripheral Arterial Guidelines for the Management of Renal Artery Stenosis
Degree of Stenosis	*Duplex Criteria*
0% to 59%	RAR <3.5 and renal artery PSV <200 cm/s
60% to 99%	RAR ≥3.5 or renal artery PSV >200 cm/s (and flow turbulence)
Occluded	Absence of arterial flow and low-amplitude signal

PSV, Peak Systolic Velocity; RAR, Renal-Aortic-Ratio

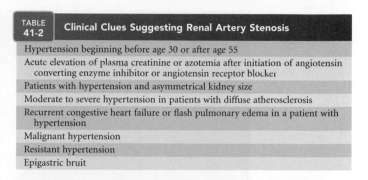

TABLE 41-2	Clinical Clues Suggesting Renal Artery Stenosis

Hypertension beginning before age 30 or after age 55

Acute elevation of plasma creatinine or azotemia after initiation of angiotensin converting enzyme inhibitor or angiotensin receptor blocker

Patients with hypertension and asymmetrical kidney size

Moderate to severe hypertension in patients with diffuse atherosclerosis

Recurrent congestive heart failure or flash pulmonary edema in a patient with hypertension

Malignant hypertension

Resistant hypertension

Epigastric bruit

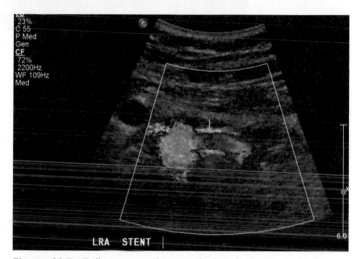

Figure 41-5 Follow-up renal artery duplex demonstrating a patent stent (green arrow).

considered. Patients who have undergone successful stent revascularization are often prescribed antiplatelet and statin therapies. The routine use of clopidogrel in combination with aspirin after successful stent revascularizaton has not been adequately evaluated; however, most investigators use this combination in light of other indications (i.e., drug-eluting coronary stent implantation). Statins (HMG-CoA reductase inhibitors) are frequently given to patients with ARAS; these agents may slow the progression of renal atherosclerosis after renal revascularization and in some instances induce plaque regression.[37] Cheung et al. found a reduction of ARAS progression from 30% to 6% in patients without and with statins, respectively. They also found 12 of 79 patients exhibited signs of disease regression.[37] Therefore statins should be considered in all patients with established dyslipidemia and ARAS.

CLINICAL FOLLOW-UP

It is imperative that patients be monitored closely after renal artery intervention for recurrent or worsening hypertension or renal dysfunction. Although no medical society has offered guidelines, surveillance duplex ultrasonography should be considered every 6 months after the placement of a renal artery stent (Figs. 41-5 and 41-6A and B). Four duplex ultrasound criteria have been reported for the diagnosis of in-stent restenosis (ISR) (Table 41-4). If ISR is identified in a patient with stable renal function and well-controlled hypertension, the original indication for renal artery intervention should be reviewed and close clinical monitoring should continue.

Renal Endovascular Interventions

INVASIVE ASSESSMENT OF RENAL ISCHEMIA

The first renal artery balloon angioplasty was reported by Andreas Grüntizig in Zurich, Switzerland in 1977.[42] The initial endovascular strategies consisted of balloon angioplasty alone and were associated with relatively poor acute procedural success and poor patency rates.

These outcomes were the direct result of heavy renal aorto-ostial plaque burden and calcification with resultant vessel recoil dissections. However, with the introduction of balloon-expandable metal stents, many of the mechanical limitations of primary balloon angioplasty were overcome, with resultant acute procedural success rates as high as 98% and 9-month duplex Doppler binary restenosis rates of approximately 20% to 25%.[43] Over the subsequent decade, the tools used for percutaneous renal artery intervention have evolved rapidly, from hand-crimped stents on 5- or 6-Fr balloons designed on 0.035-in wire systems to low-profile 6-Fr guiding-catheter-compatible premounted stent balloon combinations on 0.014- to 0.018-in. wire systems designed specifically for renal interventions. Despite these technical improvements, the enthusiasm for percutaneous renal artery stent revascularization has waxed and waned, in part owing to the lack of clinical evidence supporting the effectiveness of renal stenting in ARAS patients to improve blood pressure and renal function.[2,4,44-46] While the limitation of the trials (visual estimate of ARAS degree of stenosis, significant crossover to the intervention therapy, lack of standardized methodologies of blood pressure and microcirculation assessment, and the definition of clinical success) have been well enumerated, patients in these studies were all selected on the basis of angiographic lesion severity. This common inclusion criterion reflects the commonly held belief that angiographic lesion severity is proportional to renal ischemia and that stent revascularization will result in clinical benefit. However, this paradigm has been challenged by several investigators,[47,48] underscoring the fact that while quantitative angiography improves the accuracy of assessment compared with visual estimation, it does not improve the accuracy of diagnosing renal ischemia. Indeed, ARAS angiographic severity may often be overestimated as compared with other modalities that may reflect the presence of renal ischemia.[49] Among the other invasive modalities that can be used to assess ischemia is renal fractional flow reserve (FFR).[50] A series of reports by

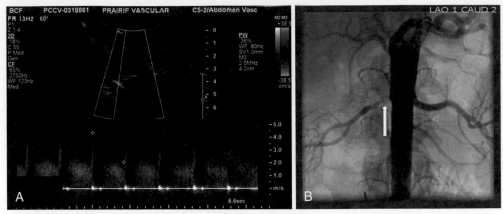

Figure 41-6 A. In-stent restenosis demonstrated by duplex ultrasound with very high peak systolic (440 cm/s) and end-diastolic (206 cm/sec) velocities. B. Right renal artery in-stent restenosis confirmed by contrast angiography.

TABLE 41-4	Ultrasound Criteria for the Diagnosis of In-Stent Restenosis	
Percent In-Stent Restenosis	**Criteria**	
>60% stenosis	PSV >200 cm/s or renal-to-aortic ratio >3.5[38]	
>60% stenosis	PSV >225 cm/s or renal-to-aortic ratio >3.5[39]	
>70% stenosis	PSV >395 cm/s or RAR >5.1[40]	
>60% stenosis	PSV >280 cm/s or renal-to-aortic ratio >4.5[41] (renal artery PTRAS following fenestrated and branched endovascular repair)	

Belgian investigators emphasized the importance, in preparation for renal revascularization, of the invasive physiological assessment of ARAS lesions in a well-selected group of patients. De Bruyne et al. demonstrated that the magnitude of the renal artery occlusion was proportional to the activation of the renin-angiotensin system and requires at least a 10% gradient (Fig. 41-7). Follow-up work by Mangiacapra et al. suggested that similar invasive translesional pressure gradient assessment after a bolus administration of intra-arterial dopamine might further improve the patient selection for renal stenting. In this small study ($n = 53$), a dopamine-induced mean pressure gradient ≥20 mmHg before revascularization was the sole independent predictor of blood pressure improvement at 3-month follow-up. However, the investigators noted an 18% nonresponder rate despite a dopamine-induced ≥20 mm Hg gradient, underscoring the heterogeneity of the potential pathophysiological mechanisms responsible for hypertension in this patient cohort.[1]

RENAL CONTRAST ANGIOGRAPHY

Abdominal aortography should be performed prior to renal stenting. This will assist in identifying the renal ostia, the presence and extent of ostial disease, accessory renal arteries, the degree of perirenal aortic calcification, angulation of the renal artery takeoff from the aorta, and the presence and degree of aneurysmal enlargement of the abdominal aorta. If indicated, subsequent selective renal angiography can be performed with a series of 4-, 5-, or 6-Fr diagnostic catheters. Typical catheter configurations include internal mammary, renal double curve, Sos, and Cobra catheters. Left anterior oblique (LAO)-angled views will often assist in the identification of both the right and left renal ostia.[51]

RENAL ARTERY STENTING

All patients should be pretreated with aspirin therapy; the efficacy of adjunctive use of clopidogrel (Plavix), although widely practiced, has not been adequately studied in renal stent patients. After sheath insertion, the patient should be fully anticoagulated with unfractionated

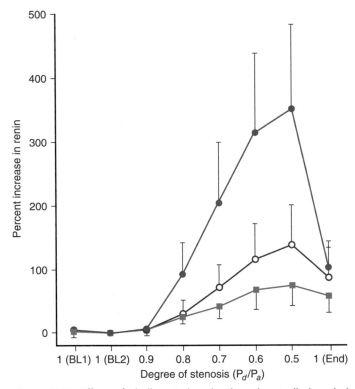

Figure 41-7 Effects of a balloon-induced unilateral controlled graded stenosis (expressed as Pd). *(Redrawn with permission from De Bruyne B, Manoharan G, Pijils M, et al. Assessment of renal artery stenosis severity by pressure gradient measurements. J Am Coll Cardiol 2006;48;48:1851–1855.)*

heparin to obtain an activated coagulation time (ACT) of at least 250 seconds. In most cases arterial access is acquired in a retrograde approach from either common femoral artery. However, in patients with severe bilateral aortoiliac disease and/or tortuosity or a sharply downward-angulated renal artery, an antegrade radial or brachial approach may be considered. In the majority of cases, renal artery revascularization will be performed using a 6-Fr guiding catheter. The guiding catheter should reflect the angle at which the renal artery arises off the aorta, the location of the stenosis, the anatomy of the perirenal aorta, and operator preference. The most commonly used guides are the internal mammary artery (IMA), renal standard curve, renal double curve, or hockey stick. The multipurpose guide is well suited

THE "NO-TOUCH" TECHNIQUE:
BASIC GUIDING CATHETER APPROACH

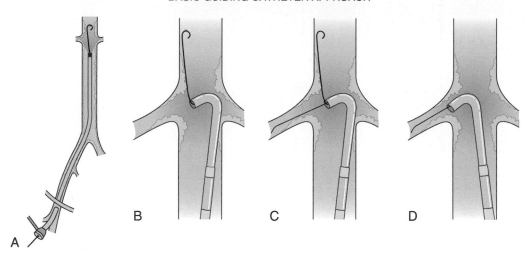

Figure 41-8 The "no-touch" technique: basic guiding catheter approach.

for a brachial or radial approach. For the common femoral arterial approach, a sheath 35-cm in length is preferable, as it minimizes guide catheter manipulation in a potentially heavily diseased perirenal aorta and can facilitate guiding catheter exchanges over smaller diagnostic catheters, if required. The goal of renal artery intervention is to achieve an optimal angiographic and hemodynamic result with minimal manipulation of the renal artery and to minimize potential atheroembolization and dissection of the renal artery or aortic wall. The "no-touch" technique can be used in an attempt to minimize distal atheroembolization (Fig. 41-8A–D). To use this technique, a 35-cm sheath is placed below the renal artery and a hand injection of contrast is performed to locate the renal ostium (Fig. 41-8A). A 0.035-in. J-tip guidewire is advanced in the abdominal aorta superior to the renal arteries. Over this wire, the guide catheter is advanced in proximity to the renal artery. The 0.035-in. wire is then retracted to the soft portion of the wire so that the guide catheter begins to assume its shape and approach the ostium of the renal artery. The "J" portion of the wire is left outside to guide, against the aortic wall (Fig. 41-8B). The ostium of the guiding catheter is gently rotated and aligned with the renal ostium with the J wire preventing guiding catheter intubation into the renal artery. From this position, a 0.014-in. wire is directed through the guide and into the distal renal artery (Fig. 41-8C). The 0.035-in. J wire is then removed and the guide catheter allowed to gently engage the ostium of the renal artery (Fig. 41-8D). Another method for safely engaging the renal ostium is the "exchange technique" (Fig. 41-9). Here too, a 35-cm sheath is placed below the renal artery and a hand injection of contrast is used to locate the renal ostium. A 4-Fr soft-tipped diagnostic catheter is used to gently locate and engage the renal ostium (Fig. 41-9B). Use of a small, soft catheter minimizes the possibility of atheroembolization and/or dissection, which could be caused by a larger, stiffer guide. Once engaged, a 0.014- or 0.018-in. guidewire is passed through the diagnostic catheter and into the main renal artery (Fig. 41-9C). The diagnostic catheter is then removed (Fig. 41-9D), leaving the guidewire in place. A 6- or 7-Fr guide is placed over the guidewire, maintaining the 35-cm sheath below the renal artery and facilitating placement the guide (Fig. 41-9E). The renal predilation balloon can then be safely passed into the renal artery (Fig. 41-9F). Another commonly used method for engaging the renal artery involves a dilator/guide system (Abbott Vascular Devices, Mountain View, CA, Veripath). With this technique, the renal artery is wired with a 0.014-in. wire through the softer selective diagnostic catheter. With the 0.014-in. wire in the renal artery, the diagnostic catheter is removed and the renal dilator/guide system is back-loaded onto the 0.014-in. wire. The dilator thus provides a smooth transition across the lesion and is gently withdrawn, allowing the guiding catheter to advance to the renal

ostium; however, "dottering" of the renal lesion occurs with this technique and the possibility of artheroembolization is a potential concern. The average diameter of a normal renal artery is approximately 5.0 to 6.0 mm. However, this may vary depending on the presence of accessory renal arteries and poststenotic dilaton. Pre-dilation of the renal lesion is highly recommended and should be performed with a balloon diameter slightly smaller than that of the renal reference vessel. Inflation is performed to full expansion of the balloon. Flank pain should be closely monitored, as it indicates stretching of the adventitia. If present, higher-pressure inflations should be avoided, as further dilation could result in perforation. Most atherosclerotic renal artery lesions demonstrate significant recoil after balloon angioplasty and will therefore require stent placement. Balloon-expandable stents should be positioned such that 1 to 2 mm of the stent protrudes into the aorta so as to ensure proper coverage of the arterial ostium. To achieve this, it is often necessary to place the stent in two views to assure proper placement. Use of the Ostial Pro stent positioning system (Ostial Solutions, Kalamazoo, MI) can assist in proper stent placement and adequate coverage of the ostium of the renal artery (Fig. 41-10). This is a disposable device compatible with 6-, 7-, and 8-Fr systems. It has opaque gold-plated feet that are used to identify the ostium and thus assist in placement of the stent to confirm coverage of the ostium. Once properly positioned, the stent should be deployed with the proper pressure to achieve a 1:1 ratio with the diameter of the reference vessel. After stent deployment to nominal balloon pressures, the deflated balloon is reduced to within the stent confines with the distal aspect of the balloon protruding into the aorta; the balloon is then taken to high pressures for postdilation. For this maneuver, as the balloon is being deflated, the guide can be advanced forward to reengage the renal artery. In this manner, the deflating balloon is used as a dilator to less traumatically advance the guide back into proper position if necessary. A final completion angiogram should be done to assess proper coverage of the renal ostium by the stent, the main renal artery, and its branches for signs of dissection or spasm and the renal parenchymal blush to exclude evidence of atheroembolization. Although there are no data to establish the routine use of aspirin and clopidogrel post-stenting, most operators continue the use of these agents for at least 30 days.

DISTAL PROTECTION DEVICES TO PREVENT ATHEROEMBOLIZATION

Despite successful renal artery revascularization, renal function may deteriorate in 8% to 32% of patients.[51] While this decline in renal function may reflect the continued effects of underlying disease

"EXCHANGE" TECHNIQUE

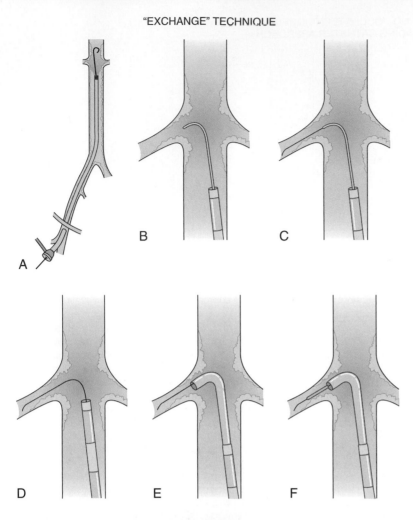

Figure 41-9 The "exchange" technique.

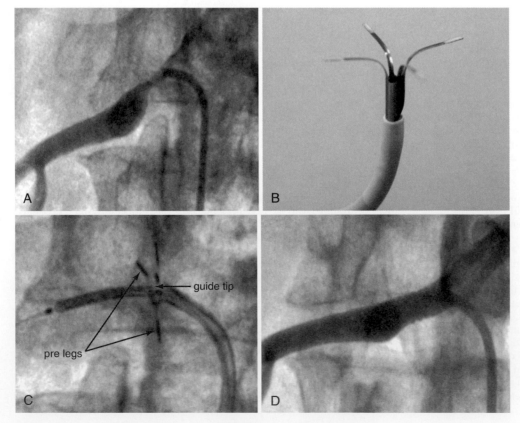

Figure 41-10 A, High grade renal lesion is identified using a 5F diagnostic catheter. **B,** The ostial Pro stent positioning (Ostial Solutions, Kalamazoo, MI) demonstrating the four gold-plated "feet" in the deployed position through a 6F guide catheter. **C,** The deployed radio-opaque "feet" are deployed against the aortic wall. These markers are aligned with the proximal balloon marker prior to stent deployment. **D,** Post stent completion angiogram demonstrating excellent renal stent deployment at the aorto-renal ostium.

processes (e.g., diabetes, hypertension) or "reperfusion injury," atheroembolization may also be a potential cause. Hiramoto et al. demonstrated, during a simulated renal stent procedure, that angioplasty and stenting of ex vivo aortorenal atheroma specimens can produce thousands of atheroemboli particles.[52] Intuitively, distal protection devices may provide beneficial results in selected patients by preventing distal atheroembolization; however, limited clinical studies have proven inconclusive. While several authors[53,54] have suggested an improvement in renal function or its stabilization associated with the use of distal protection devices, they are designed primarily for use in carotid artery stent procedures and coronary artery bypass grafts; which particular patient cohort may potentially benefit from the use of these devices has not been clearly established.

Insight into the potential mechanism of atheroembolic decline in renal function was provided by Cooper et al.[55] This study randomized 100 patients in a 2×2 factorial design to distal protection (filter type) versus no distal protection and the glycoprotein IIb/IIIa platelet receptor inhibitor abciximab or placebo. Notably, renal artery stenting, with either distal protection or abciximab alone, was associated with a decline in estimated glomerular filtration rate (GFR) at 30 days. However, the combination of distal protection and abciximab use was not associated with a decline in GFR. Furthermore, abciximab use was associated with lower incidence of platelet-rich emboli in the filter device. However, the use of distal protection in the renal arteries is not without risk; occlusive devices (e.g., PercuSurge) can predispose to renal ischemia, and filter devices not specifically designed for the renal vasculature may cause renal artery spasm; moreover, the distal filter wire may cause dissection of the distal renal vessel. Additionally, these filters are associated with varying filter efficiencies and may not trap all of the atheromatous debris generated by the renal intervention. Finally, the use of the filters is limited to renal arteries with sufficient "landing zones," thus excluding their use in patients with early renal artery bifurcations. Finally, they are associated with a learning curve, which may prolong the procedure and increase contrast use; in addition, filter retrieval may be problematic, as the recapture catheter can become entrapped within the newly deployed stent.

Management of In-Stent Restenosis

Duplex Doppler-defined restenosis rates after successful stenting vary depending on a variety of anatomical and patient-related factors. Smaller diameter vessels (<4 mm) can have restenosis rates as high as 40%, whereas larger vessels (>6 cm) generally have restenosis rates of less than 10%.[56] A history of tobacco use, diabetes, and time to restenosis evaluation also appear to be associated with higher restenosis rates.[57] While the endovascular options for ISR treatment are many — including repeat balloon angioplasty, repeat stenting deployment (bare metal or drug-eluting stent), or covered stent placement (iCAST, Atrium Medical, Hudson, NH)—there are few data to suggest the superiority of any one modality.[58] Because of the recoil in this vessel, balloon angioplasty for in-stent restenosis usually does not provide a durable result. Placement of more metal into the vessel often results in recurrent restenosis.[59] Techniques including brachytherapy,[60] atherectomy, cryoplasty,[61] and laser debulking[62] have been described.[60] While the efficacy of drug-eluting stents in the coronary vasculature is well established, their use in the renal revascularization is less clear. The GREAT trial was a randomized evaluation of bare metal stents versus drug-eluting stents in 105 patients with ARAS. At 6 months, no significant difference in stent patency between the two treatment arms was discerned (6.7% vs. 14.6%, $P = 0.30$). At 1 year, target lesion revascularization rates were 11.5% for bare metal stents and 1.9% for drug-eluting stents (sirolimus-eluting balloon expandable stent versus bare metal low-profile stent for renal artery treatment[63]). Although the rate of adverse events were lower in the treatment group, statistical significance was not demonstrated in this small patient cohort. Drug-eluting stents have been further compared to brachytherapy for the treatment of renal ISR. At 3 years, there were lower rates of major adverse clinical events and target lesion revascularization (TLR) with drug-eluting stents, but they did not reach

statistical significance.[64] One challenge for the use of drug-eluting stents in the renal arteries is sizing. Currently, the largest-diameter coronary artery drug-eluting stent is 4.0 mm, and overdilation of an undersized stent may reduce its radial strength. At this diameter, most small renal arteries can be safely treated; however, recoil at the renal ostium may be problematic, as the radial strength of these stents (designed for coronary arteries) is not comparable with that of bare metal stents designed specifically for the renal artery. Another option for treatment of ISR is placement of a balloon-expandable covered stent (iCast Covered Stent, Atrium Medical Corp., Hudson, NH). In theory, this strategy could reduce the risk of neointimal proliferation through the stent struts. Use of this stent has been reported in the renal and iliac beds for treatment of restenosis.[65]

COMPLICATIONS

The majority of complications associated with percutaneous renal artery revascularization are related to arterial access; they include groin hematomas, retroperitoneal hemorrhage, pseudoaneurysm, arteriovenous fistula, and infection. These should be treated as usual and are discussed in other sections of this textbook. Serious complications may arise secondary to atheroembolization to the kidneys, bowel, or lower extremities, resulting in renal failure, ischemic bowel, or digital ischemia, respectively. Renal artery dissection can usually be treated with stent placement. Distal wire perforation may resolve spontaneously with reversal of anticoagulation or may require coil embolization. Renal artery perforation may respond to prolonged balloon inflation with reversal of anticoagulation or may require the placement of a stent graft.

Percutaneous Renal Sympathetic Denervation to Treat Resistant Hypertension

The kidney plays an essential role in the regulation of blood pressure through sodium, volume, renin modulation, and renal sympathetic neuronal activation. Renal sympathetic drive, which contributes to the development and perpetuation of hypertension and sympathetic outflow to the kidney, is activated in patients with essential hypertension. Studies indicate that the renal nerves contribute to the development and maintenance of hypertension and all hypertensive processes. Efferent sympathetic outflow stimulates renin release, increases tubular sodium reabsorption, and reduces renal blood flow. Additionally, afferent signals from the kidney modulate central sympathetic outflow and directly contribute to neurogenic hypertension. Early studies in nonselective surgical sympathectomy have demonstrated effective control of severe hypertension. Recently developed catheter-based technologies now enable selective denervation of the human kidney with radiofrequency energy delivered to the renal artery lumen, ablating the renal nerves located in the adventitia of the renal arteries (Ardian Inc., Mountain View, CA). Krum et al., in a first study of this approach in humans, demonstrated successful renal denervation with resultant reduction of sympathetic activity, renin release, and central sympathetic outflow.[5] This feasibility trial demonstrated that percutaneous sympathetic renal denervation was both safe and effective in reducing blood pressure in patients with severe resistant hypertension. A subsequent case report has suggested renal denervation is also associated with a decrease in norepinephrine level "spill-over" and in muscle sympathetic activity.[66] Two-year follow-up in this patient cohort demonstrated a substantial reduction in blood pressure, averaging 33 mm Hg, which persisted without significant adverse events[67] (Fig. 41-11). More recently, the Simplicity HTN II trial has extended these original observations. The Sympathetic Hypertension II trial[68] was a multicenter, prospective, randomized, crossover trial of patients with baseline systolic hypertension of ≥160 mm Hg although they were taking three or more antihypertensive medications. The trial randomized 106 patients in a 1:1 ratio to undergo either renal denervation or previous

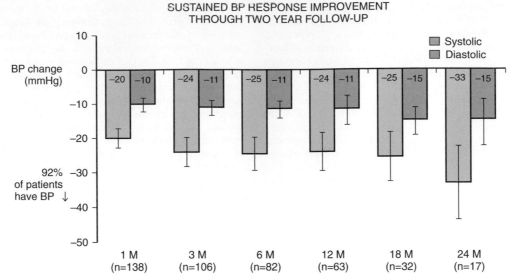

Figure 41-11 Sustained improvement in BP response through 2-year follow-up.

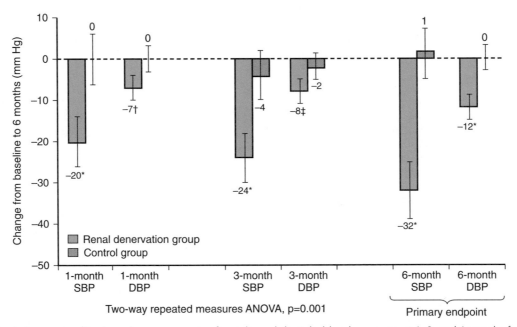

Figure 41-12 Paired changes in office-based measurements of systolic and diastolic blood pressures at 1, 3, and 6 months for renal denervation and control groups. Error bars are 95% CI. A multivariate stepwise regression analysis of baseline characteristics, drugs, and treatment assignment was examined for predictors of increased 6-month systolic blood pressure response; only variables with $P < 0.15$ on univariate screening were entered into the model, with variables with $P < 0.05$ remaining in the final model. Multivariate analysis of baseline characteristics showed that assignment to the renal denervation group ($P < 0.0001$), higher baseline systolic blood pressure ($P < 0.0001$), and slower heart rate ($P < 0.004$) predicted increased 6-month blood pressure reduction. SBP, systolic blood pressure; DBP, diastolic blood pressure. *$P < 0.0001$. †$P = 0.002$. ‡$P = 0.005$. *(Redrawn with permission from Renal sympathetic denervation in patients with treatment-resistant hypertension (The Symplicity HTN-2 Trial): a randomised controlled trial. Lancet. 2010;376(9756):1903–1909.)*

drug treatment alone with a primary endpoint of blood pressure control assessed at 6 months. 6 month office-based blood pressure assessment demonstrated a mean reduction of 31/12 mmHg below the pre-treatment baseline values in the renal denervation cohort. The blood pressure values in the control group were unchanged, while 84% of the patients who underwent renal denervation had a reduction of systolic blood pressure of at least 10 mmHg (Fig. 41-12). There were no serious procedure- or device-related complications or adverse events in the renal denervation group. Therefore these two trials demonstrated that catheter-based renal denervation can safely be used to substantially reduce blood pressure in patients with resistant

hypertension. Importantly, there may be additional benefits to renal sympathetic denervation; preliminary subgroup analyses from the Simplicity I and Simplicity II trials suggest that fasting blood sugar and hemoglobin A1C values drop significantly; additionally, the estimated glomerular filtration rate (eGFR) appeared to improve over time in the renal denervation group. This exciting new therapeutic innovation affirms the crucial relevance of renal nerves in the pathogenesis of resistant hypertension. The potential for renal sympathetic denervation in treating other clinical syndromes associated with hypersympathetic states—including diastolic heart failure, cardiorenal syndromes, and obstructive sleep apnea—remains to the explored.

REFERENCES

1. Textor S, Lerman L, McKusick M: The uncertain value of renal artery interventions. Where are we now? *J Am Coll Cardiol Intervent* 2:175–182, 2009.

2. Wheatley K, Ives N, Gray R, et al: Revascularization versus medical therapy for renal-artery stenosis. *N Engl J Med* 361:1953–1962, 2009.

3. Balk E, Raman G, Chung M, et al: Effectiveness of management strategies for renal artery stenosis: a systematic review. *Ann Intern Med* 145:901–912, 2006.

4. Bax L, Woittiez A, Kouwenberg H, et al: Stent placement in patients with atherosclerotic renal artery stenosis and impaired renal function: a randomized trial. *Ann Intern Med* 150:840–848, 2009.

5. Krum H, Schlaich M, Whitbourn R, et al: Catheter-based renal sympathetic denervation for resistant hypertension: a multicentre safety and proof-of-principle cohort study. *Lancet* 373:1275–1281, 2009.

6. McCullough PA: Cardiorenal risk: an important clinical intersection. *Rev Cardiovasc Med* 3(2):71–76, 2002.

7. Fatica RA, Port FK, Young EW: Incidence trends and mortality in end-stage renal disease attributed to renovascular disease in the United States. *Am J Kidney Dis* 37(6):1184–1190, 2001.

8. Derkx FH, Schalekamp MA: Renal artery stenosis and hypertension. *Lancet* 344(8917):237–239, 1994.

9. Mann SJ, Pickering TG: Detection of renovascular hypertension. State of the art: 1992. *Ann Intern Med* 117(10):845–853, 1992.

10. Crowley JJ, Santos RM, Peter RH, et al: Progression of renal artery stenosis in patients undergoing cardiac catheterization. *Am Heart J* 136(5):913–918, 1998.

11. Hansen KJ, Edwards MS, Craven TE, et al: Prevalence of renovascular disease in the elderly: a population-based study. *J Vasc Surg* 36(3):443–451, 2002.

12. Rihal CS, Textor SC, Breen JF, et al: Incidental renal artery stenosis among a prospective cohort of hypertensive patients undergoing coronary angiography. *Mayo Clin Proc* 77(4):309–316, 2002.

13. Leertouwer TC, Gussenhoven EJ, Bosch JL, et al: Stent placement for renal arterial stenosis: where do we stand? A meta-analysis. *Radiology* 216(1):8–85, 2000.

14. Zierler RE, Bergelin RO, Davidson RC, et al: A prospective study of disease progression in patients with atherosclerotic renal artery stenosis. *Am J Hypertens* 9(11):1055–1061, 1996.

15. Olin JW, Pierce M: Contemporary management of fibromuscular dysplasia. *Curr Opin Cardiol* 23(6):527–536, 2008.

16. Kolluri R, Goldstein JA, Rocha-Singh K: Percutaneous vascular interventions in renal artery diseases. *Minerva Cardioangiol* 54(1):95–107, 2006.

17. Katholi RE, Rocha-Singh KJ: The role of renal sympathetic nerves in hypertension: has percutaneous renal denervation refocused attention on their clinical significance? *Prog Cardiovasc Dis* 52(3):243–248, 2009.

18. Schultz HD, Li YL, Ding Y: Arterial chemoreceptors and sympathetic nerve activity: implications for hypertension and heart failure. *Hypertension* 50(1):6–13, 2007.

19. Zucker IH: Novel mechanisms of sympathetic regulation in chronic heart failure. *Hypertension* 48(6):1005–1011, 2006.

20. DiBona GF: Sympathetic nervous system and the kidney in hypertension. *Curr Opin Nephrol Hypertens* 11(2):197–200, 2002.

21. Kirchheim H, Ehmke H, Persson P: Sympathetic modulation of renal hemodynamics, renin release and sodium excretion. *Klin Wochenschr* 67(17):858–864, 1989.

22. White CJ, Olin JW: Diagnosis and management of atherosclerotic renal artery stenosis: improving patient selection and outcomes. *Nat Clin Pract Cardiovasc Med* 6(3):176–190, 2009.

23. Olin JW, Piedmonte MR, Young JR, et al: The utility of duplex ultrasound scanning of the renal arteries for diagnosing significant renal artery stenosis. *Ann Intern Med* 122(11):833–838, 1995.

24. Radermacher J, Chavan A, Bleck J, et al: Use of Doppler ultrasonography to predict the outcome of therapy for renal-artery stenosis. *N Engl J Med* 344(6):410–417, 2001.

25. Zeller T, Frank U, Muller C, et al: Predictors of improved renal function after percutaneous stent-supported angioplasty of severe atherosclerotic ostial renal artery stenosis. *Circulation* 108(18):2244–2249, 2003.

26. Zeller T, Muller C, Frank U, et al: Stent angioplasty of severe atherosclerotic ostial renal artery stenosis in patients with diabetes mellitus and nephrosclerosis. *Catheter Cardiovasc Intervent* 58(4):510–515, 2003.

27. Grobner T: Gadolinium—a specific trigger for the development of nephrogenic fibrosing dermopathy and nephrogenic systemic fibrosis? *Nephrol Dial Transplant* 21(4):1104–1108, 2006.

28. Marckmann P, Skov L, Rossen K, et al: Nephrogenic systemic fibrosis: suspected causative role of gadodiamide used for contrast-enhanced magnetic resonance imaging. *J Am Soc Nephrol* 17(9):2359–2362, 2006.

29. Vasbinder GB, Nelemans PJ, Kessels AG, et al: Accuracy of computed tomographic angiography and magnetic resonance angiography for diagnosing renal artery stenosis. *Ann Intern Med* 141(9):674–682; discussion 682, 2004.

30. Silva JA, Chan AW, White CJ, et al: Elevated brain natriuretic peptide predicts blood pressure response after stent revascularization in patients with renal artery stenosis. *Circulation* 111(3):328–333, 2005.

31. Mann SJ, Pickering TG, Sos TA, et al: Captopril renography in the diagnosis of renal artery stenosis: accuracy and limitations. *Am J Med* 90(1):30–40, 1991.

32. Nally JV, Jr, Black HR: State-of-the-art review: captopril renography—pathophysiological considerations and clinical observations. *Semin Nucl Med* 22(2):85–97, 1992.

33. Elliott WJ, Martin WB, Murphy MB: Comparison of two noninvasive screening tests for renovascular hypertension. *Arch Intern Med* 153(6):755–764, 1993.

34. Frederickson ED, Wilcox CS, Bucci M, et al: A prospective evaluation of a simplified captopril test for the detection of renovascular hypertension. *Arch Intern Med* 150(3):569–572, 1990.

35. Hirsch AT, Haskal ZJ, Hertzer NR: ACC/AHA guidelines for the management of patients with peripheral arterial disease (lower extremity, renal, mesenteric, and abdominal aortic). *J Am Coll Cardiol* 47:1239–1312, 2006.

36. Rosenfield K, Jaff MR: An 82-year-old woman with worsening hypertension: review of renal artery stenosis. *JAMA* 300(17):2036–2044, 2008.

37. Cheung CM, Patel A, Shaheen N, et al: The effects of statins on the progression of atherosclerotic renovascular disease. *Nephron Clin Pract* 107(2):c35–c42, 2007.

38. Nolan BW, Schermerhorn ML, Powell RJ, et al: Restenosis in gold-coated renal artery stents. *J Vasc Surg* 42(1):40–46, 2005.

39. Rocha-Singh K, Jaff MR, Lynne Kelley E: Renal artery stenting with noninvasive duplex ultrasound follow-up: 3-year results from the RENAISSANCE renal stent trial. *Catheter Cardiovasc Intervent* 72(6):853–862, 2008.

40. Chi YW, White CJ, Thornton S, et al: Ultrasound velocity criteria for renal in-stent restenosis. *J Vasc Surg* 50(1):119–123, 2009.

41. Mohabbat W, Greenberg RK, Mastracci TM, et al: Revised duplex criteria and outcomes for renal stents and stent grafts following endovascular repair of juxtarenal and thoracoabdominal aneurysm. *J Vasc Surg* 49(4):827–837; discussion 37, 2009.

42. Gruntzig A, Vetter W, Meier B, et al: Treatment of renovascular hypertension with percutaneous transluminal dilatation of a renal artery stenosis. *Lancet* 13:801–802, 1978.

43. Leertouwer TC, Gussenhoven EJ, Bosch JL, et al: Stent placement for renal arterial stenosis: where do we stand? A meta-analysis. *Radiology* 216:78–85, 2000.

44. Plouin PF, Chatellier G, Darne B, et al: Blood pressure outcome of angioplasty in atherosclerotic renal artery stenosis: a randomized trial. The EMMA Study Group. *Hypertension* 31:823–829, 1998.

45. Webster J, Marshall F, Abdalla M, et al: Randomized comparison of percutaneous angioplasty vs. continued medical therapy for hypertensive patients with atheromatous renal artery stenosis. *J Hum Hypertens* 12:329–335, 1998.

46. Van Jaarsveld BC, Krijnen P, Pieterman H, et al: For the Dutch Renal Artery Stenosis Intervention Cooperative Study Group. The effect of balloon angioplasty on hypertension in atherosclerotic renal-artery stenosis. *N Engl J Med* 342:1007–1014, 2000.

47. De Bruyne B, Manoharan G, Pijls M, et al: Assessment of renal artery stenosis severity by pressure gradient measurements. *J Am Coll Cardiol* 48(48):1851–1855, 2006.

48. Mangiacapra F, Trana C, Sarno G, et al: Translesional pressure gradients to predict blood pressure response after renal artery stenting in patients with renovascular hypertension. *Circ Cardiovasc Interv* 2010; DOI 10.1161.

49. Drieghe B, Madaric J, Sarno G, et al: Assessment of renal artery stenosis: side-by-side comparison of angiography and duplex ultrasound with pressure gradient measurements. *Eur Heart J* 29:517–524, 2008.

50. Submramanian R, White C, Rosenfield K, et al: Renal fractional flow reserve: a hemodynamic evaluation of moderate renal artery stenoses. *Catheter Cardiovasc Intervent* 64:480–486, 2005.

51. Bates MC, Crotty B, Kavasmaneck C, et al: Renal artery angiography: "the right ipsilateral oblique" myth. *Catheter Cardiovasc Intervent* 67(2):283–287, 2006.

52. Hiramoto J, Hansen KJ, Pan XM, et al: Atheroemboli during renal artery angioplasty: an ex-vivo study. *J Vasc Surg* 41:1026–1030, 2005.

53. Henry M, Klonaris C, Henry I, et al: Protected renal stenting with the PercuSurge GuardWire device: a pilot study. *J Endovasc Ther* 8:227–237, 2001.

54. Holden A, Hill A, Jaff MR, et al: Renal artery stenting revascularization with embolic protection in patients with ischemic nephropathy. *Kidney Int* 70:948–955, 2006.

55. Cooper CJ, Haller ST, Colyer W, et al: Embolic protection and platelet inhibition during renal artery stenting. *Circulation* 117:2752–2760, 2008.

56. Gray BH: Intervention for renal artery stenosis: endovascular and surgical roles. *J Hypertens* 23(Suppl 3):S23–S29, 2005.

57. Shammas NW, Kapalis MJ, Dippel EJ, et al: Clinical and angiographic predictors of restenosis following renal artery stenting. *J Invas Cardiol* 16(1):10–13, 2004.

58. Bax L, Mali WP, Van De Ven PJ, et al: Repeated intervention for in-stent restenosis of the renal arteries. *J Vasc Intervent Radiol* 13(12):1219–1224, 2002.

59. Zeller T, Rastan A, Schwarzwälder U, et al: Treatment of in-stent restenosis following stent-supported renal artery angioplasty. *Catheter Cardiovasc Intervent* 70(3):454–459, 2007.

60. Chrysant GS, Goldstein JA, Casserly IP, et al: Endovascular brachytherapy for treatment of bilateral renal artery in-stent restenosis. *Catheter Cardiovasc Intervent* 59(2):251–254, 2003.

61. Jeffries IL, Dougherty K, Krajcer Z: First use of cryoplasty to treat in-stent renal artery restenosis. *Texas Heart Inst J* 35(4):489–491, 2008.

62. Waheed A, Rajachandran M, Allin R, et al: An unusual case of renal artery stent restenosis: a case report. *Angiology* 58:249–254, 2007.

63. Zähringer M, Sapoval M, Pattynama P, et al: GREAT trial: angiographic follow-up after 6 months and clinical outcome up to 2 years. *Endovasc Ther* 14:460–468, 2007.

64. Holmes D, Teirstein P, Satler L, et al: 3-year follow-up of the SISR (Sirolimus Eluting Stents Versus Vascular Brachytherapy for In-Stent Restenosis) trial. *JACC Cardiovasc Intervent* 1(4):439–448, 2008.

65. Giles H, Lesar C, Erdoes L, et al: Balloon-expandable covered stent therapy of complex endovascular pathology. *Ann Vasc Surg* 22(6):762–768, Epub 2008 Oct 15, 2008.

66. Schlaich M, Sobotka P, Krum H, et al: Sympathetic nerve ablation for uncontrolled hypertension. *N Engl J Med* 361:932–934, 2009.

67. Symplicity HTN-1 Investigators: Catheter-based renal sympathetic denervation for resistant hypertension: durability of blood pressure reduction out to 24 months. *Hypertension* 57:911–917, 2011.

68. Symplicity HTN-2 Investigators: Renal sympathetic denervation in patients with treatment-resistant hypertension (The Symplicity HTN-2 Trial): a randomized controlled trial. *Lancet* 376:1903–1909, 2010.

Aortic Vascular Interventions (Thoracic and Abdominal)

CHRISTOPH A. NIENABER | IBRAHIM AKIN | HÜSEYIN INCE

KEY POINTS

- Acute aortic dissection is an uncommon but potentially catastrophic illness that occurs with an incidence of approximately 3.5/1000,000 per year, with at least 8,000 cases per year in the United States.

- The exact role of percutaneous stent grafting in the treatment of aortic dissection is not yet fully established.

- Aortic stent grafts are primarily used to reconstruct the compressed true lumen cranial to major aortic branches and to increase distal aortic flow. Therefore proximal communications should be sealed to direct flow into the true lumen, depressurize the false lumen, and induce thrombosis in the false lumen with fibrotic transformation and subsequent remodeling of the aortic wall.

- Recent reports suggest that percutaneous stent graft placement in the dissected aorta is safer and produces better results than surgery for type B dissection.

- The use of endovascular stent grafts for repair of thoracic aortic aneurysms is emerging as a promising, less invasive therapeutic alternative to conventional surgical treatment.

- The evaluation of a patient for repair of a thoracic aortic aneurysm considers the patient's overall risk profile, evidence of rapid enlargement of the aneurysm, diameter equal to or greater than 5.5 cm, and presence of symptoms. The suitability of the patient for endovascular repair is based on both clinical and anatomical considerations.

- Endoleaks are the most prevalent complications following stent graft treatment of thoracic aortic aneurysms. Treatment options include transcatheter coil or glue embolization, balloon angioplasty, placement of endovascular graft extensions, and open repair.

- The key features of endovascular repair of abdominal aortic aneurysms that determines procedural success and long-term outcome are proximal and distal fixation and sealing. Most of the devices use, throughout the graft, a metal skeleton made of stainless steel, nitinol, or Elgiloy.

Introduction

INTERVENTIONAL TREATMENT OF AORTIC DISSECTION

Acute aortic dissection is an uncommon but potentially catastrophic illness that occurs with an incidence of approximately 3.5/100,000 per year, with at least 8,000 cases per year in the United States.[1] Around 0.5% of patients with chest or back pain suffer from aortic dissection.[2] Within 14 days of onset, aortic dissection is considered acute, whereas it is chronic beyond a fortnight (Fig. 42-1). Men are twice as often affected as women by acute aortic dissection, with 60% classified as proximal (type A) and 40% as distal (type B) according to the Stanford classification.[1] Historical data of untreated aortic dissection of the ascending aorta show a mortality rate of 1% to 2% per hour within the first 24 hours, resulting in a mortality rate of up to 50% to 74% in the acute phase.[1] Acute type B dissection—when uncomplicated—is

less frequently lethal, with survival rates in medically treated patients of 89% at 1 month, 84% at 1 year, and up to 80% within 5 years.[1] Survival may be significantly improved by the timely institution of appropriate therapy; thus prompt clinical recognition and definitive diagnostic testing are therefore essential in the management of aortic dissection. Conventional treatment of Stanford type A (De Bakey types I and II) dissection (Fig. 42-1) consists of surgical reconstruction of the ascending aorta with complete or partial resection of the dissected aortic segment. Therefore, in type A dissections, interventional endovascular strategies have no clinical application except to relieve critical malperfusion before surgery of the ascending aorta. This is done by distal endovascular interventions in cases of thoracoabdominal extension of a proximal dissection (De Bakey type I) with distal ischemic complications. Conversely, stent graft placement aims at remodeling of the thoracic descending aorta, typically in Stanford type B dissection, by sealing one (or multiple) proximal entry tears with a Dacron-covered stent, thus initiating thrombosis of the false lumen.[3-6] In addition, reconstruction of a collapsed true lumen might result in re-establishment of side branch flow (Fig. 42-2). Various scenarios of malperfusion syndrome are amenable to endovascular management. These include static or dynamic (by intima invagination) collapse of the aortic true lumen (so-called pseudocoarctation (Fig. 42-3), static or dynamic occlusion of one or more vital side branches, and enlarging false aneurysm due to patent proximal entry tear. Although peripheral pulse deficits can be acutely reversed with surgical repair of the dissected thoracic aorta in many cases, patients with signs of mesenteric or renal ischemia do not fare well. Mortality of patients with renal ischemia is 50% to 70%, and as high as 87% with mesenteric ischemia.[7-9] Surgical mortality rates in patients with acute peripheral vascular ischemic complications are similar to those of patients with mesenteric ischemia, reaching an 89% in-hospital mortality rate.[10-13] Operative mortality of surgical fenestration varies from 21% to 61%, which has encouraged percutaneous interventional management by endovascular balloon fenestration of a dissecting aortic membrane to treat mesenteric ischemia, a concept discussed as a niche indication in such complicated cases of malperfusion.[12-14] Management of Stanford type B (De Bakey type III) dissection with the use of endovascular stent grafts is evolving slowly in anticipation of an unknown risk of paraplegia from spinal artery occlusion, as seen in up to 18% of cases after open surgery.[13,14] With further technical improvement, a large series of patients has now been successfully treated in various specialized centers by endovascular stent graft placement covering entry tears in the descending aorta and even in the aortic arch. Recent studies have demonstrated that closure of proximal entry tears is essential to reconstruct the aortic wall and reduce total aortic diameter. Entry tear closure promotes depressurization of the false lumen, thrombus formation in the false lumen (Fig. 42-4), and remodeling of the entire aorta.[4,5,14] In the near future, combined surgical and interventional procedures even for proximal dissection are likely to evolve.[15-17]

CURRENT INDICATIONS FOR ENDOVASCULAR AORTIC INTERVENTIONS

Significant perioperative morbidity and mortality in acute, complicated type B dissection has prompted alternative therapeutic concepts. Thoracic endovascular aortic repair (TEVAR), even though an

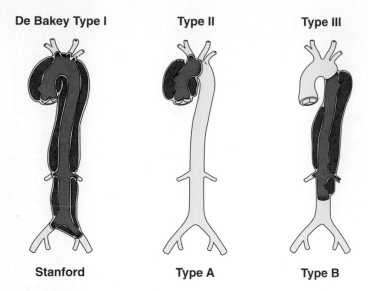

De Bakey Type I   **Type II**   **Type III**

Stanford   **Type A**   **Type B**

De Bakey

Type I   Originates in the ascending aorta, propagates at least to the
           aortic arch and often beyond it distally
Type II   Originates in and is confined to the ascending aorta
Type III   Originates in the descending aorta and extends distally down the
           aorta or, rarely, retrograde into the aortic arch and ascending
           aorta

Stanford

Type A   All dissections involving the ascending aorta,
           regardless of the site of origin
Type B   All dissections not involving the ascending aorta

Figure 42-1 The most common classifications of thoracic aortic dissection.

off-label indication for dissection, has been approved by the U. S. Food and Drug Administration for aneurysmal disease of the aorta. The natural course of aortic dissection is determined by two elements: early complication and late events. In the acute phase, TEVAR has been shown to abrogate impending rupture and relieve static and dynamic malperfusion. Later benefit appears to be false lumen thrombosis, mitigating the risk of aneurysmal dilation and subsequent rupture. Thus, in 2010 the role of interventional management of static or dynamic obstruction of aortic branch arteries in complicated and complex distal dissection is settled. Static obstruction of a branch can be overcome by placing endovascular stents in the ostium of a compromised side branch, and dynamic obstruction may benefit from stents in the aortic true lumen, sometimes combined with side branch stenting and preferentially without any additional balloon fenestration, because fenestration does not improve stress and tension on the thin aortic wall.[18] Sometimes bare stents deployed from the true lumen into side branches are useful to buttress the flap in a stable position.[19] In rare cases, fenestration may be helpful to create a reentry tear for the dead-end false lumen back into the true lumen, with the aim of preventing thrombosis of the false lumen and compromise of branches fed exclusively from the false lumen; however, this concept lacks clinical proof of benefit. Conversely, fenestration increases the long-term risk of aortic rupture, because a large reentry tear promotes flow in the false lumen and provides the basis for its aneurysmal expansion. There is also a risk of peripheral embolism from a patent but partly thrombosed false lumen.[19,20] The most effective method to avoid an enlarging false lumen is the scaling of proximal entry tears with a customized stent graft (Fig. 42-5); the absence of a distal reentry tear is desirable for optimal results but is not a prerequisite. Compression of the true aortic lumen cranial to the main abdominal branches with distal malperfusion (pseudocoarctation) is usually corrected by stent grafts that expand the compressed true lumen and improve distal aortic blood flow.[4,5,12,14] Depressurization and shrinking of the false lumen is the most beneficial result to be gained, ideally

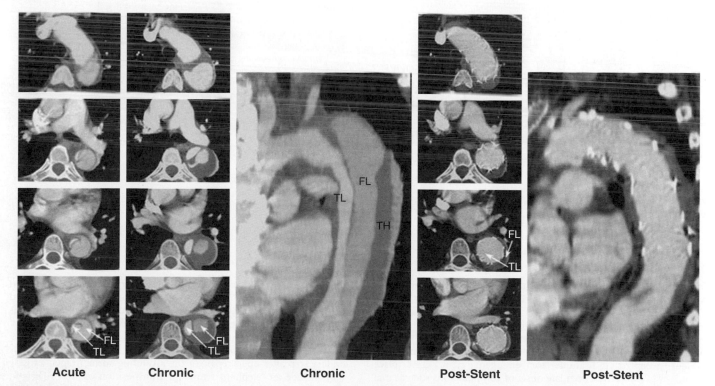

Acute   **Chronic**   **Chronic**   **Post-Stent**   **Post-Stent**

Figure 42-2 Type B aortic dissection in a 48-year-old man. Note the dynamic obstruction of the true lumen (TL) in the acute phase. After stent graft placement across the proximal thoracic entry, the entire true lumen of the thoracic vascular is reconstructed over time, with complete "healing" of the dissected aortic wall and shrinking of the completely thrombosed false lumen (FL). TH, thrombus.

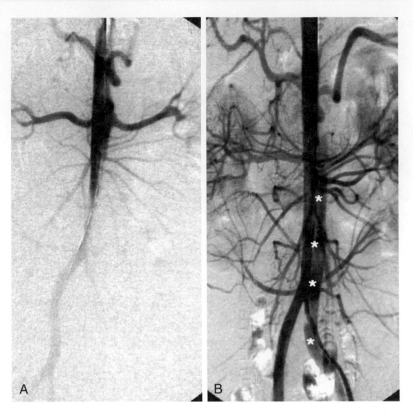

Figure 42-3 Digital subtraction angiography in a thoracoabdominal type B dissection. A. Dynamic obstruction of the true lumen distally to the renal arteries, causing malperfusion of the mesentery and both lower extremities. B. At follow-up (3 months after stent graft placement in the proximal descending aorta), the true lumen has widened as a consequence of aortic remodeling and the patient is asymptomatic. However, the false lumen (white stars) in the abdominal aorta is not completely thrombosed.

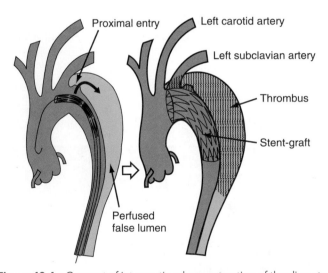

Figure 42-4 Concept of interventional reconstruction of the dissected aorta with sealing of the proximal entries, depressurization of the false lumen, and initiation of false lumen thrombosis.

TABLE 42-1	Distribution of Differential Therapeutic Strategies in Aortic Dissection
Surgery	
Type A aortic dissection	
Acute type B dissection complicated by the following:	
Retrograde extension into the ascending aorta	
Dissection in fibrilinopathies (e.g., Marfan's syndrome, Ehlers-Danlos syndrome)	
Rupture or impending rupture (historically classic indication)	
Progression with compromise of vital organs	
Medical therapy	
Uncomplicated type B dissection	
Stable, isolated arch dissection	
Uncomplicated chronic type B dissection	
Interventional therapy	
Unstable acute/chronic type B dissection	
Malperfusion	
Rapid expansion (>1 cm/year)	
Critical diameter (≥5.5 cm)	
Refractory pain	
Type B dissection with retrograde extension into the ascending aorta	
Hybrid procedure for extended type A aortic dissection	

followed by complete thrombosis of the false lumen and remodeling of the entire dissected aorta (see Fig. 42-2).[16] Like previously accepted indications for open surgical repair in complicated type B dissection, scenarios such as intractable pain with descending dissection, rapidly expanding false lumen diameter, extra-aortic blood collection as a sign of imminent rupture, and distal malperfusion syndrome are at present accepted indications for emergent stent graft placement.[16,17,19–21] Moreover, even late onset of complications such as malperfusion of vital aortic side branches is likely to justify endovascular stent grafting of an occlusive lamella to improve distal true lumen flow as a first option, with surgery employed only after an

unsuccessful attempt, considering that surgical repair has failed to prove superior to interventional treatment even in uncomplicated cases. In complicated cases, the concept of endoluminal treatment is currently replacing open surgery in advanced aortic centers.[3–5,19–22] Even in some cases of retrogradely extended type A dissections, TEVAR is feasible as a primary approach to seal the entry or as a secondary step after open repair of the ascending aorta.[16] Open surgery may include an "elephant trunk" or transposition of arch vessels to allow for optimal landing zones for endovascular completion in a hybrid approach.[23,24] A summary of potential treatment options is given in Table 42-1.

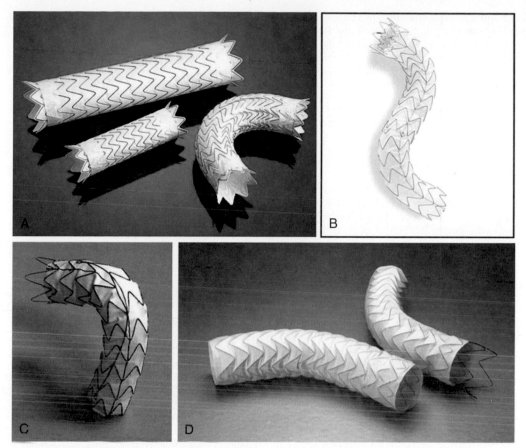

Figure 42-5   A selection of thoracic stent grafts from American manufacturers currently available in Europe: A, TAG (Gore; Flagstaff, AZ); B, Valiant (Medtronic AVE; Santa Rosa, CA), C, Relay Thoracic Stent graft (Bolton Medical, Sunrise, FL); D, EndoFit (LeMaitre Vascular, Burlington, MA).

TABLE 42-2	Initial Medical Treatment in Aortic Dissection		
Name	*Mechanism*	*Dose*	*Cautions/Contraindications*
Esmolol	Cardioselective beta-1 blocker	Load: 500 µg/kg IV Drip: 50 µg kg^{-1} min^{-1} IV. Increase by increments of 50 µg/min	Asthma or bronchospasm Bradycardia 2nd- or 3rd-degree AV block Cocaine or methamphetamine abuse
Labetalol	Nonselective beta 1,2 blocker Selective alpha-1 blocker	Load: 20 mg IV Drip: 2 mg/min IV	Asthma or bronchospasm Bradycardia 2nd- or 3rd-degree AV block Cocaine or methamphetamine abuse
Enalaprilat	ACE inhibitor	0.625–1.25 mg IV q 6 hours. Max dose: 5 mg q 6 hours.	Angioedema Pregnancy Renal artery stenosis Severe renal insufficiency
Nitroprusside	Direct arterial vasodilator	Begin at 0.3 µg kg^{-1} min^{-1} IV. Max dose 10 µg kg^{-1} min^{-1}	May cause reflex tachycardia Cyanide/thiocyanate toxicity, especially in renal or hepatic insufficiency
Nitroglycerin	Vascular smooth muscle relaxation	5 to 200 µg/min IV	Decreases preload; contraindicated in tamponade or other preload-dependent states Concomitant use of sildenafil or similar agents

STABLE ACUTE TYPE B AORTIC DISSECTION

Patients with suspected acute aortic dissection should be admitted to intensive care and subjected to immediate diagnostic evaluation. Reduction of systolic blood pressure to 100 to 120 mm Hg with an eye on renal function and pain relief are initial priorities and are usually achieved by morphine sulfate and intravenous beta-blocking agents with or without vasodilating drugs such as sodium nitroprusside at a dose of 0.3 µg/kg per min or angiotensin-converting enzyme inhibitors (Table 42-2). Additionally, heart rate should be kept low; a heart rate below 60 beats per minute significantly decreases secondary adverse events (aortic expansion, recurrent aortic dissection, aortic rupture and/or need for aortic surgery) in type B aortic dissection compared to a conventional rate of more than 60 beats per minute.[25] Once both stable blood pressure and symptom relief are manifested, a patient with uncomplicated type B aortic dissection can be discharged (usually within 14 days) on oral drugs; clinical and imaging follow-up should be advised at 3 and 6 months and annually thereafter. In 384 patients with type B dissections from the International Registry of Aortic Dissection (IRAD), 73% were managed medically with an in-hospital mortality of 10%.[1,26] Short-term survival rates were 91% at 1 month and 89% at 1 year. The reported long-term survival rate with medical therapy varies between 60% and 80% at 4 to 5 years and is around 40% to 45% at 10 years.[1,26] Potential beneficial effects of early stenting are being studied in the ongoing ADSORB (Acute Uncomplicated Aortic Dissection Type B: Evaluation Stent graft Placement or best medical Treatment Alone) trial.[27]

UNSTABLE ACUTE TYPE B AORTIC DISSECTION

About 30% to 42% of acute type B aortic dissections are complicated, as evidenced by hemodynamic instability or peripheral vascular ischemia, and have an unpredictable outcome.[26] Acute lower limb and visceral ischemia has been reported in 30% to 50%; malperfusion syndrome occurs frequently with extended dissections, with mortality between 50% and 85% if untreated.[28] However, operative mortality in patients with acute aortic dissection complicated by renal ischemia has been reported around 50% and even 88% with mesenteric malperfusion.[29] Conversely, of 571 patients with acute type B aortic dissection in IRAD, 390 were treated medically; among 125 complicated cases, 59 underwent standard open surgery and 66 were subjected to TEVAR. In this case, in-hospital mortality was significantly lower with TEVAR than after open surgery (10.2% vs. 33.9%; $P = 0.002$) (Fig. 42-6).[30] The PETTICOAT (Provisional Extension to Induce Complete Attachment) concept takes the idea of endothoracic reconstruction even further by extending the stent graft scaffold distally with open-cell bare metal stents until distal malperfusion is corrected.[31] With this concept, aortic fenestration maneuvers or branch vessel revascularization with side branch stents are usually not needed and almost obsolete. A metanalysis has summarized 942 patients from 29 studies showing an in-hospital mortality of 9% with reinterventions in 10.4%.[32] Emergency surgical conversion or periprocedural stroke was rare (0.6% and 3.1%, respectively), while the survival rate was 88% at mean follow-up of 20 months. A second metanalysis comprised 1,304 patients subjected to TEVAR for complicated acute type B aortic dissection, with technical success in 99% and a 30-day mortality of 2.6%.[33] At late follow-up, false lumen thrombosis was documented in 92.9% of patients and surgical conversion was required in 0.8%, with endovascular reintervention performed in 1.6%. Retrograde extension into the ascending aorta and neurological complications were reported in 0.4% and 0.6%,

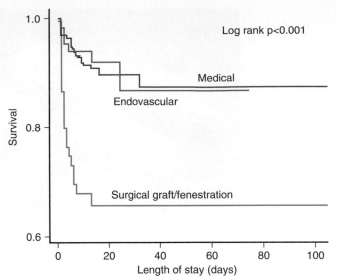

Figure 42-6 Comparison of medical, surgical, and endovascular treatment of complicated type B aortic dissection.[30]

respectively.[33] Further results are listed in Table 42-3. In patients deemed unsuitable candidates for conventional open surgical repair, 1- and 5-year survival rates were 74% and 31% with TEVAR compared with 93% and 78% ($P < 0.001$) survival in patients considered candidates for conventional open repair.[34] Interestingly, a comparison between endovascular treatment of complicated type B aortic dissection and medical therapy of uncomplicated type B dissections in 56 patients with a follow-up of 18.1 ± 16.9 months reported similar outcomes in both groups with a better midterm fate of the descending thoracic aorta in the stent graft group, with no associated paraplegia; there were no differences in the 5-year survival rate (86.3% in both groups).[35]

CHRONIC TYPE B AORTIC DISSECTION

The evolution of an acute dissection to a chronic dissection involves progressive thickening of the intimal flap due to fibrosis. Additionally, more intimal tears are reported in chronic type B aortic dissection

TABLE 42-3	Results of Endovascular Stent Graft Implantation in Different Clinical Conditions					
Author (Ref. No.)	*Year*	*N*	*Technical Success (%)*	*Paraplegia (%)*	*Mortality (%)*	*Follow-up (month)*
Acute Complicated Type B Dissection						
Bortone[22]	2004	43	100	0	7	21
Xu[151]	2006	63	95	0	10.6	48
Verhoye[152]	2008	16	100	0	27	36
Fattori[30]	2008	66	100	3.4	10.6	1
Szeto[153]	2008	35	97.1	2.8	2.8	18
Khoynezhad[154]	2009	28	90	n.a.	18 (1y) 22(5y)	36
Alves[155]	2009	106	99	1.8	18 (acute AD) 7 (chronic AD)	35.9
Parsa[156]	2010	55	100	2	37 (overall) 6 (aorta-related)	14.4
Chronic Type B Dissection						
Nienaber[4]	1999	12	100	0	0	12
Kato[47]	2001	15	100	0	0	24
Eggebrecht[45]	2005	28	100	0	13.6	12
Jing[46]	2008	35	100	0	7.6	48
Nienaber[36]	2009	72	95.7	2.8	11.1 (overall) 5.6 (aorta-related)	24

Ad, aortic dissection.

compared with acute dissection. The growth rate of the chronically dissected distal aorta is estimated to be between 0.10 and 0.74 cm per year depending on both initial aortic diameter and state of hypertension.[1,24] Unfortunately the long-term outcome of medical therapy alone is suboptimal, with a reported 50% mortality at 5 years and delayed expansion of the false lumen in 20% to 50% of patients at 4 years.[1,24] This expansion of the false lumen, for which an initial diameter beyond 4 cm and persistent perfusion of the false lumen were predictors, predisposes patients to aortic rupture or retrograde migration of the dissection toward the ascending aorta.[1,24] Thus TEVAR should be considered when the aortic diameter exceeds 55 mm, there is persisting thoracic pain, or in the presence of uncontrolled hypertension and rapid growth of the dissecting aneurysm (>1 cm per year). Our group prospectively evaluated elective TEVAR in 12 patients with chronic type B dissection and compared the results with 12 matched surgical controls. Proximal entry closure and complete thrombosis of the false lumen at 3 months were achieved in all patients. Stent graft treatment resulted in no morbidity or mortality, whereas surgical treatment resulted in 4 deaths (33%; $P = 0.04$) and 5 adverse events (42%; $P = 0.04$)[4]; this has been confirmed by similar observations (Table 42-3). Whether prophylactic use of TEVAR in patients with chronic type B aortic dissections is superior to medical treatment alone was evaluated in the prospective randomized controlled INSTEAD (Investigation of STEnt grafts in Aortic Dissection) trial.[36] A total of 140 patients in stable clinical condition at least 2 weeks after index dissection were randomly subjected to elective stent graft placement in addition to optimal medical therapy ($n = 72$) or to optimal medical therapy alone ($n = 68$). There was no difference in all-cause deaths and a 2-year cumulative survival rate of 95.5% ± 2.5% with optimal medical therapy versus 88.9% ± 3.7% with TEVAR ($P = 0.15$) (Fig. 42-7). Moreover, the aorta-related death rate was not different (2.9% vs. 5.6%; $P = 0.68$), and the risk for the combined endpoint of aorta-related death and progression was similar ($P = 0.65$). Aortic remodeling (with true lumen recovery and thoracic false lumen thrombosis) occurred in 91.3% of patients with TEVAR versus 19.4% of those who received medical treatment ($P < 0.001$), which suggests ongoing aortic remodeling. Initial (30-day) mortality is 10% or less with medical therapy in acute uncomplicated type B dissection,[1,24] and data from the INSTEAD trial suggest no prognostic advantage of TEVAR within 2 years compared with monitored medical therapy for uncomplicated chronic type B dissection; these observations indicate that TEVAR should be reserved for complicated cases of acute or chronic descending thoracic aortic dissection or for those in which medical management has failed.

TECHNIQUE OF AORTIC STENT GRAFT PLACEMENT

Aortic stent grafts are primarily used to reconstruct the compressed true lumen cranial to major aortic branches and to increase distal aortic flow. Therefore proximal communications should be sealed to direct flow into the true lumen, depressurize the false lumen, and induce thrombosis in the false lumen with fibrotic transformation and subsequent remodeling of the aortic wall. Stent graft placement across the origin of the celiac, superior mesenteric, and renal arteries may lead to fatal organ failure. Based on the measurements obtained during angiography, transesophageal echography (mandatory for the detection of small entries), contrast-enhanced spiral computed tomography angiography (CTA) (the best technique for unstable patients in an emergency situation), magnetic resonance angiography (MRA) (contraindicated for patients with pacemakers or implantable defibrillators), or intravascular ultrasound, customized stent grafts are available to both scaffold up to 20 cm of dissected aorta and cover major tears. The procedure is best performed in the catheterization and imaging laboratory using digital angiography and general anesthesia. The femoral artery is the most popular access site and can usually accommodate a 24-Fr stent graft system. In the Seldinger technique, a 260-cm stiff wire is placed over a pigtail catheter that is navigated with a soft wire in the true lumen under both fluoroscopic and transesophageal ultrasound guidance. In complex cases with multiple reentries in the abdominal aorta, the "embracement technique," using two pigtail catheters, is useful (Fig. 42-8). A pigtail catheter that has been installed in the true aortic lumen via the left brachial artery picks up the femoral pigtail catheter in the true lumen of the abdominal aorta and pulls it

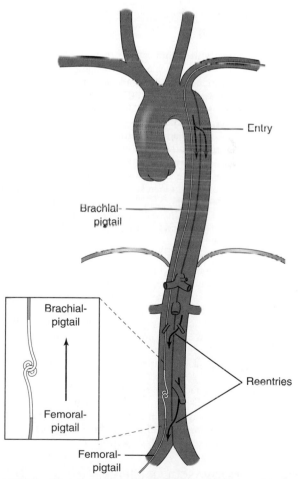

Figure 42-8 "Embracing pigtails" technique to ensure navigation of the guidewire in the true lumen before stent graft placement. See text for details.

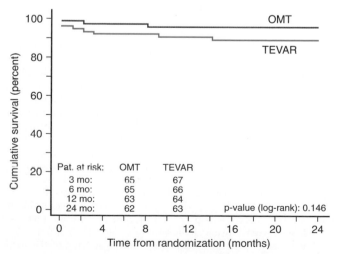

Figure 42-7 Cumulative survival of patients with chronic type B aortic dissection within 24 months after randomization.[36]

up into the aortic arch. This procedure ensures definite positioning of the stiff guidewire in the true lumen, which is essential for correct deployment of the stent graft. The stent is carefully advanced over the stiff wire, and the launching of the stent graft is performed with systolic blood pressure lowered to 50 to 60 mm Hg by infusion of sodium nitroprusside or by rapid right ventricular pacing to prevent dislodgement.[37,38] After deployment, short inflation of a latex balloon can improve apposition of the stent struts to the aortic wall, but only if proximal sealing of thoracic communications is incomplete. Paraplegia may occur after use of multiple stent grafts, but this still appears to be a rare phenomenon, especially when the stented segment does not exceed 16 cm. Both Doppler ultrasound and contrast fluoroscopy are instrumental for documenting the immediate result or initiating adjunctive maneuvers. For thoracic aortic aneurysms or ulcers, the navigation of wires and instruments is easier, but dual imaging using ultrasound and fluoroscopy simultaneously is equally important. A frequent anatomical consideration is the short distance between the origin of the left subclavian artery (LSA) and the primary tear in type B dissections. Coverage of the ostium to the LSA must sometimes be accepted in order to perform endovascular aortic repair in this aortic pathology adjacent to the LSA. According to observational evidence, prophylactic surgical maneuvers are not imperative or always required for safety reasons but may be relegated to an elective measure after an endovascular aortic intervention if intolerable signs or symptoms of ischemia occur.[39] However, before intentional LSA occlusion, careful attention must be paid to potential supra-aortic variants (e.g., presence of a lusorian artery, a nonintact vertebrobasilar system, dominant left vertebral artery) that originate directly from the aortic arch and other pathologies recognized during preinterventional vascular staging.

RETROGRADE TYPE A THORACIC AORTIC DISSECTION

TEVAR is associated with complications; new, formerly unexpected complications have emerged, such as endoleak, graft migration, device separation, and retrograde type A thoracic aortic dissection (rATAD). A European multicenter registry of 4,750 procedures estimated the incidence of rATAD at 1.33%, with 25% being asymptomatic cases[40]; one single center recently reported a 2.5% rate of rATAD ($n = 11$, among whom 3 patients had Marfan's syndrome).[41] Interestingly, rATAD developed intraoperatively in 2 patients, 2 hours after the procedure in one patient, at 1 week in 1 patient, and in 7 patients a month after TEVAR; of these cases, 8 were converted to open surgery while 2 received medical treatment.[41] Open surgery is the treatment of choice in an effort to tackle such potentially fatal complications; however, the procedure-related mortality following rATAD surgery was itself between 20% to 57%.[40,41] With the mechanisms of rATAD after TEVAR still unclear, observational evidence suggests that rATAD may be due to several causes (procedure-related, oversize ballooning, device-related, unfavorable aortic dissection anatomy, and natural progression of initial aortic dissection). As far as TEVAR-related factors are concerned, injury from proximal bare spring was suspected with outward pointing radial force. Lack of conformability of stent grafts when passively bent at the aortic arch may cause traumatic strain to the wall and create a tear. Balloon dilation after TEVAR can cause injury to the inner layers and retrograde extension. Indeed, additional balloon dilation was performed in 11 cases of rATAD (23%).[40] Oversizing of the stent graft by more than 20% in relation to the landing zone diameter is also considered a risk factor for rATAD. Finally, genuine fragility of the aortic wall may predispose to rATAD as a sign of natural disease progression. Even under medical management, newly developed type A dissections were observed in 4 of 180 and in 5 of 66 patients under medical treatment for acute type B dissection.[42,43]

TIMING OF ENDOVASCULAR REPAIR

The optimal timing for endovascular intervention in type B dissections remains controversial. Bortone et al. favor an early intervention within

2 weeks of the initial diagnosis; stent graft placement was successful in all patients referred for intervention within the first 2 weeks.[22] A high rate of reverse remodeling is likely when the patient is treated early after development of the dissection flap. With the passage of time, the dissection flap becomes more fibrosed, thickened, and matured—that is, less compliant to TEVAR. Shimono et al. reported that complete obliteration and resolution of the false lumen following endovascular stent graft treatment was more frequently achieved in cases of acute aortic dissection compared with those of chronic aortic dissection (70% vs. 38.5%).[44] Conversely, others have observed higher mortality rates in patients with acute type B aortic dissection.[45,46] Morphological changes of the initially fragile dissecting membrane to a more fibrotic and seemingly stable membrane in the chronic phase are critical for endovascular repair, suggesting TEVAR to be safer after a minimum of 4 weeks following the onset of aortic dissection but before the chronic stage.[47] Additionally, the more stable clinical status of patients in the chronic phase of aortic dissection may be an important determinant of better survival after TEVAR. Towing to the lack of prospective randomized data comparing immediate and delayed intervention in various clinical and anatomical constellations, no general recommendation has been issued with respect to the timing of endovascular treatment; observational evidence, however, may favor an early intervention in the window of aortic plasticity when justified by a low complication rate.

CONCLUSION

The emergence of endovascular stent grafting as an alternative therapy to the classic, formerly used open surgical repair of aortic dissection is an exciting new field. Although it is apparent that patients at high surgical risk will benefit from endovascular technology, the exact role of stent grafting remains to be defined as long-term data and experience continue to accumulate and as devices and techniques evolve. Instead of replacing conventional surgical treatment completely, endovascular repair will likely play a complementary role and offer a less invasive option in the treatment armamentarium. It is clear that the limitations of both approaches are distinct. Although what is considered high risk for surgery is defined by clinical parameters in terms of comorbidities, contraindications for endovascular stent graft treatment are defined by anatomical constraints. In this regard, both strategies will continue to coexist and may even merge to generate hybrid procedures.

Descending Thoracic Aortic Aneurysm

ENDOVASCULAR REPAIR BY STENT GRAFTS

Thoracic aortic aneurysms, classified according to Crawford and Safi (Fig. 42-9), occur predominantly in the elderly and therefore have been increasing in incidence as the population ages and diagnostic capabilities advance.[48] With an incidence of 6 to 10 per 100,000 person-years, thoracic aortic aneurysms (TAAs) are less common than abdominal aortic aneurysms (AAAs) but remain life-threatening.[48–50] The distribution of aortic segments was as follows: the ascending aorta was involved in 51%, the aortic arch in 11%, and the descending thoracic aorta in 38%. One-quarter of the patients had concomitant infrarenal aneurysmal aortic disease and up to 13% had multiple aneurysms, whereas the risk of having a TAA when AAA was diagnosed was between 3.5% and 12%.[50] The pathogenesis of aortic aneurysms has not been established to its full extent, but it is believed to be multifactorial and to include atherosclerosis, increased tissue protease activity, antiprotease deficiency, mechanical factors, inflammatory disorders, infection, and genetic collagen defects, such as Marfan's syndrome and Ehlers-Danlos syndrome. Up to 20% of patients with an aneurysm have a first-degree relative with the same disorder.[51] The natural history of TAAs is one of progressive expansion and weakening of the aortic wall, leading to eventual rupture.[52–54] Initial aneurysmal size can also be an important predictor of aneurysm growth; a study based on 721

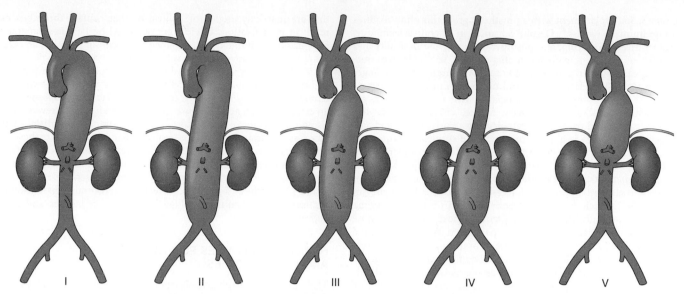

Figure 42-9 Classification of thoracoabdominal aortic aneurysm (TAA).

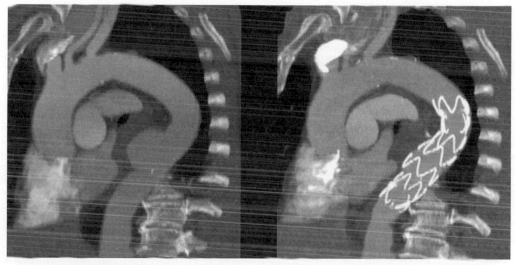

Figure 42-10 CTA showing a circumscribed aneurysm of the descending thoracic aorta in a middle-aged male selected for endografting (left side). One-year follow-up after successful endovascular exclusion of the aneurysm by stent graft placement demonstrates marked shrinkage of the periprosthetic aneurysm and optimal wall apposition of the stent graft (right side).

patients supported the fact that TAA size had a profound impact on risk for rupture, with an annual rate of 2% in aneurysms <5 cm, 3% in aneurysms 5 to 5.9 cm, and 7% for aneurysms beyond 6 cm. Therefore the risk appears to rise abruptly as thoracic aneurysms reach a size of 6 cm.[55] Beyond this dimensional view, nondimensional variables with an impact on expansion rate and risk of rupture should also be evaluated. In a multivariate regression analysis, the Mount Sinai group identified older age, the presence of even uncharacteristic pain, and a history of chronic obstructive pulmonary disease (COPD) as independent risk factors for rupture of TAA.[56] With an associated mortality rate of 94%, TAA rupture is usually a fatal event.[49,57] Olsson et al. showed in their survey that 22% of the patients with ruptured aortic aneurysms and dissection did not reach the hospital alive, with the diagnosis being made at autopsy.[58] The 5-year survival rate of unoperated TAA patients approximates 13%, whereas 70% to 79% of those who undergo elective surgical intervention are alive at 5 years.[59–61] The risk of rupture mandates consideration for surgical treatment in all patients who are suitable candidates for operation. The use of

endovascular stent grafts for the repair of TAAs is emerging as a promising, less invasive therapeutic alternative to conventional surgical treatment. Endovascular treatment of aortic aneurysms is achieved by transluminal placement of one or more stent graft devices across the longitudinal extent of the lesion. The prosthesis bridges the aneurysmal sac to exclude it from high-pressure aortic blood flow, thereby allowing for sac thrombosis around the endograft and possible remodeling of the aortic wall (Fig. 42-10). Although the advent and ensuing rapid evolution of endovascular aortic repair techniques occurred initially in cases of AAA, efforts to adapt this technology for the thoracic aorta are ongoing. As is the case for AAA, a less invasive approach to TAA repair is highly desirable because the patient population tends to be elderly and harbors multiple comorbidities.[54,61,62] Continued development of endovascular therapy for thoracic aneurysms is likely to provide greater benefits in terms of patient outcomes than those observed with AAAs. Conventional surgical treatment of TAA is physiologically more demanding and carries a greater operative risk. It mandates open thoracotomy, aortic cross-clamping, resection of the aneurysm, and replacement with a prosthetic graft; this often requires cardiopulmonary bypass.[63] Despite advances in operative technique, intraoperative monitoring, and postoperative care, the mortality and morbidity of surgery remain substantial and less favorable than outcomes for open AAA repair. Mortality for TAA surgical repair ranges from 5% to 20% in elective cases and up to 50% in emergent situations.[61,64–68] Major complications associated with surgical TAA treatment include renal and pulmonary failure, visceral and cardiac ischemia, stroke, and paraplegia. Paraplegia is a particularly devastating complication that is almost unique to the surgical treatment of thoracic aneurysms, occurring in 5% to 25% of cases, compared with less than 1% for AAAs.[59,61,67–70] For these reasons, a significant population of TAA patients are not candidates for open repair and have been without a treatment option until recently. Endovascular aneurysm repair of the thoracic aorta is currently focused on the descending portion. Anatomically, this aortic segment provides a substrate more amenable for endovascular stent graft repair, given its avoidance of the great vessels proximally and major visceral branches and aortic bifurcation distally. Despite these anatomical advantages and the ability to draw from early experiences with endovascular AAA repair, the development of stent grafting in the thoracic aorta has progressed more slowly than that involving its infrarenal counterpart. The thoracic aorta poses several unique challenges that have impeded simple adaptation of the endovascular devices and techniques developed for the abdominal aorta.[71] First, the hemodynamic forces of the thoracic aorta are significantly more aggressive and place greater mechanical demands on thoracic endografts. The potential for device migration, kinking, and late structural failure are important concerns. Second, greater flexibility is required of thoracic devices to conform to the natural curvature of the proximal descending aorta and to lesions with tortuous morphology. Third, because larger devices are necessary to accommodate the diameter of the thoracic aorta, arterial access is more problematic. This is an important concern because a greater proportion of TAA patients, compared with AAA patients, are women, and in women access vessels tend to be smaller. Fourth, as with conventional open TAA repair, paraplegia remains a potential complication in the endovascular approach despite the absence of aortic cross-clamping.[72,73] Last, TAAs often extend beyond the boundaries of the descending thoracic aorta and involve more proximal or distal aorta than desired. Management of the LSA, in particular, has gained considerable attention.[74–76]

With these challenges in mind, significant progress has been achieved, since the first stent graft was deployed for TAA exclusion in 1992.[39,72,77]

TECHNICAL ASPECTS OF ENDOVASCULAR REPAIR

Early clinical experience with stent grafting of the thoracic aorta was based on the use of first-generation homemade devices that were rigid and required large delivery systems (24 to 27 Fr).[77,78] Since then, several commercial manufacturers of abdominal endografts have created derivatives for the thoracic aorta with dramatic improvements over homemade devices. The endoprostheses are composed of a stent (nitinol or stainless steel) covered with fabric (polyester or polytetrafluoroethylene [PTFE]). The evaluation of a patient for repair of a TAA considers the patient's overall risk profile, evidence of rapid enlargement of the aneurysm, diameter ≥5.5 cm, and presence of symptoms. The suitability of the patient for endovascular repair is based on both clinical and anatomical considerations. Preprocedural imaging is essential to fully characterize the lesion and access route. Detailed imaging evaluation can be obtained with spiral CT or MRI. Measurements from imaging data are used to select the appropriate diameter and length of device. Determination of the aneurysm's location in relation to the LSA and celiac axis is of utmost importance. Successful TAA exclusion requires normal segments of native aorta at both ends of the lesion (the so-called landing zone or neck) of at least 15 to 25 mm to ensure adequate contact between the endoprosthesis and the aortic wall and formation of a tight circumferential seal. Landing zones

that are markedly angled or conical or that contain thrombus can result in poor fixation. Devices are oversized by 10% in diameter to provide sufficient radial force for adequate fixation. The vascular access route for device introduction and delivery to the pathological target must be of sufficient size and of suitable morphology. The preferred and most common site (41%–58%) of vascular access is the common femoral artery. Less frequently, access to the iliac artery (9%–44%) via an extraperitoneal approach is required.[78,79] Additionally, severe stenosis and tortuosity of the abdominal and thoracic aorta distal to the target are contraindications for endovascular repair. Despite these criteria, treatment failures can occur. However, the specific contributing factors and frequencies are currently unknown, particularly over the long term. Therefore follow-up surveillance with serial CT scans at 1, 6, and 12 months and annually thereafter is recommended to monitor changes in aneurysm morphology, identify device failures, and detect endoleaks.

HYBRID PROCEDURES FOR AORTIC ARCH PATHOLOGIES

The aortic arch morphology is challenging because of angulation and the proximity of the supra-aortic branches that need to be preserved. Traditionally open arch reconstruction using hypothermic cardiac arrest, extracorporeal circulation, and selective cerebral perfusion has been demonstrated to effectively manage aortic arch pathologies. However, this current standard procedure for any arch pathology carries significant mortality (2%–9%) and risk of paraplegia and cerebral stroke in 4% to 13% of cases.[80,81] Therefore open repair is often reserved for low-risk patients. Hybrid arch procedures are a combination of debranching bypass (supra-aortic vessel transposition) to establish cerebral perfusion and subsequent thoracic endografting to provide patient-centered solutions for complex aortic arch lesions. Hybrid arch procedures are performed without hypothermic circulatory arrest and extracorporal circulation; these could expand the treatment group to older patients with severe comorbidities as well as to those requiring redo surgery who are currently ineligible for open surgical intervention. The key to success is the quality of the unimpaired suitable ascending aorta as a donor site for the debranching bypass and proximal landing zone for the endografts (Fig. 42-11).

CLINICAL EXPERIENCE

The literature on thoracic stent grafting consists mostly of small to medium-sized case series with short- to medium-term follow-up (Table 42-4). Nevertheless, these studies illustrate a consensual pattern of outcomes when viewed in the aggregate. Overall, successful device deployment is achieved in 85% to 100% of cases, and periprocedural mortality ranges from 0% to 14%, falling within or below elective surgery mortality rates of 5% to 20%.[71,78–96] As expected, outcomes have improved over time with accumulated technical expertise, the use of commercially manufactured devices, and improved patient selection criteria. The recently published collective experiences of the EUROSTAR and United Kingdom Thoracic Endograft registries, the largest series to date ($N = 249$), demonstrate successful deployment in 87% of cases, a 30-day mortality rate of 5% for elective cases, and paraplegia and endoleak rates of 4% each.[96] The U.S. Food and Drug Administration (FDA) phase II trial data from exclusive deployment of the Gore TAG endograft in 142 patients with TAA revealed similar results: technical success in 98%, a 30-day mortality rate of 1.5%, paraplegia in 3.5%, and endoleak in 8.8%.[95] These results cannot be directly compared with the outcomes of contemporary surgical studies. The majority of patients with TAA repaired by the endovascular approach in these studies were older and sicker, having been deemed either high-risk or not suitable for open surgical repair. For example, 52% of patients in the combined EUROSTAR and United Kingdom registries were preoperatively classified as ASA 3 or above by the American Society of Anesthesiologists' physical status classification predicting procedural risk (1 to 2, low risk; 3, intermediate risk; 4 to 5, high risk;

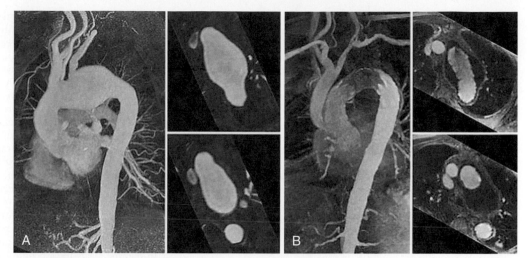

Figure 42-11 Contrast medium-enhanced MRA of the aorta in a case of an aortic aneurysm. A. Aneurysm of the aortic arch involving the supra-aortic branches. B. Postinterventional surgical result after hybrid procedure with debranching of the supra-aortic vessels and stent graft implantation in the aortic arch.

TABLE 42-4 Summary Data on Studies of Endovascular Repair of Thoracic Aortic Aneurysm

Author, Year (Ref. No.)	N	Mean Follow-Up (mo)	Devices	Technical Success	30-Day Mortality (%)	Long-Term Survival (%)	Paraplegia (%)	Endoleak (%)
Dake, 1998[78]	103	22	Homemade	83% complete thrombosis	9	73 (actuarial 2 yr)	3	24
Ehrlich, 1998[82]	10	NA	Talent	80% complete thrombosis	10	NA	0	20
Cartes-Zumelzu, 2000[83]	32	16	Excluder, Talent	90.6%	9.4	90.6 (32 mo)	3.1	15.4
Grabenwoger, 2000[81]	21	NA	Talent, Prograft	100%	9.5	NA	0	14.3
Greenberg, 2000[85]	25	15.4	Homemade	NA	20 (12.5 for elective, 33 for emergent)	NA	12	12
Temudom, 2000[86]	14	5.5	Homemade, Vanguard, Excluder	78.6%	14.3	NA	7.1	14.3
Najibi, 2002[87]	24	12	Excluder, Talent	94.7%	5.3	89.5 (1 yr)	0	0
Heijmen, 2002[88]	28	21	Talent, AneuRx, Excluder	96.4%	0	96.4 (mean, 21 mo)	0	28.6
Schoder, 2003[89]	28	22.7	Excluder	100%, 89.3% complete exclusion	0	96.1 (1 yr), 80.2 (3 yr)	0	0.25
Marin, 2003[90]	94	15.4	Excluder, Talent	85.1%	NA	NA	NA	24
Lepore, 2003[91]	21	12	Excluder, Talent	100%	9.5	76.2 (1 yr)	4.8	19
Sunder-Plassman, 2003[92]	45	21	Corvita, Stentord, Vanguard, AneuRx, Talent, Excluder	NA	6.7	NA	2.2	22.2
Ouriel, 2003[71]	31	6	Excluder, Talent, Other commercial	NA	12.9	81.6 (1 yr)	6.5	32.3
Bergeron, 2003[93]	33	24	Excluder, Talent	NA	9.1	75.8 (mean 24 mo)	0	0
Czerny, 2004[94]	54	38	Excluder, Talent	94.4%	9.3	63 (3 yr event free)	0	27.8
Makaroun, 2004[95]	142	29.6	TAG	97.9%	1.5	75 (2-yr freedom from death)	3.5	8.8
Leurs, 2004[96]	249	1-60	Excluder, Talent, Zenith, EndoFit	87%	10.4 (5.3 for elective, 27.9 for emergent)	80.3 (1 yr)	4	4.2
Greenberg, 2005[157]	100	14	Zenith	NA	NA	83 (1 year)	1	6
Wheatley, 2006[158]	156	21.5	Gore	98.7	3.8	76.6 (1 year)	0.6	11.5
Bavaria, 2007[159]	140	24	Gore	98	2.1	NA	2.9	10
Fairman, 2008[160]	195	12	Talent	99.5	2.1	83.9 (1 year, all cause) 96.9 (1 year, aneurysm-rel.)	1.5 (paraplegia) 3.6 (stroke)	NA
Hughes, 2010[161]	79	23	Zenith, Gore, Talent	98.7	5.1	77 (55 mo, overall) 86 (aorta-specific)	1.3 (paraplegia) 2.5 (stroke)	2.5

6, organ donor).[96] True comparisons between conventional therapy and the endovascular alternative can be made only after the completion of prospective randomized controlled trials. Although such trials are under way, a few studies have compared endovascular treatment with anatomically similar open-surgery historical controls. As part of the phase II Gore Excluder study, 19 TAA patients who were candidates for open repair received stent graft therapy and were compared with a nonrandomized cohort of 10 patients who had undergone open repair before the availability of thoracic stent grafts.[87] All aneurysms met the same inclusion/exclusion criteria for anatomical involvement. The 1-year survival rate was 89.5% in the endovascular group and 70% in the operative group. As expected, mean hospital stay (6.2 vs. 16.3 days) and length of intervention (155 vs. 256 minutes) were significantly less in those treated endovascularly. In a similar study, Ehrlich and colleagues found decreased 30-day mortality (10% vs. 31%), mean hospital stay (6 vs. 10 days), and mean intervention time (150 vs. 325 minutes) with endovascular repair; the paraplegia rate was also decreased (0% vs. 12%).[82]

COMPLICATIONS AND CURRENT CONCLUSIONS

With the avoidance of aortic cross-clamping and prolonged iatrogenic hypotension, endovascular TAA repair was expected to result in lower incidences of paraplegia relative to conventional treatment. Indeed, this has held true, with paraplegia rates generally ranging from 0% to 5% in endovascular studies,[71,78–96] compared with 5% to 25% in open repair cases.[59,61,67,68] Although low, these rates remain significant, especially because it is impossible to reimplant intercostal arteries in this setting. Some evidence suggests that the occurrence of paraplegia is associated with concomitant or prior surgical AAA repair and increased exclusion length due to the absence of lumbar and hypogastric collateral circulation.[85,97] Adjunctive measures to further reduce spinal cord ischemic complication rates in endovascular TAA repair are being investigated.[98]

Endoleaks are the most prevalent of TAA stent graft treatment complications. However, their observed frequency is substantially less than that reported for AAA endograft repair.[99] Interestingly, the distribution of endoleak types also differs. TAA endoleaks occur more commonly at the proximal or distal attachment site (type I endoleak), whereas most AAA endoleaks are type II.[100] It is generally accepted that type I endoleaks are more serious and require expeditious intervention, because they represent direct communications between the aneurysm sac and aortic blood flow.[101] Treatment options include transcatheter coil or glue embolization, balloon angioplasty, placement of endovascular graft extensions, and open repair.[102,103] Although current anatomical criteria limit thoracic stent graft exclusion to lesions located at least 15 to 25 mm away from the origin of the LSA and celiac trunk, it is common for descending TAAs to be located within the proximal or distal neck length necessary for adequate fixation. At the proximal end, the landing zone can be extended by prophylactic transposition of the LSA to the left carotid artery or by bypass graft placement.[72] Alternatively, the uncovered proximal portion of the Talent endograft can be placed across the LSA origin to achieve fixation without blocking flow. However, case reports of inadvertent coverage of the LSA origin found no resulting complications,[104] and subsequent studies determined that such maneuvers may not be necessary as long as there is no obstruction of the right vertebral or carotid artery and the left internal mammary artery is not used as a coronary bypass conduit.[74–76] Complications such as left arm ischemia were found to be rare, possibly owing to collateral blood supply via retrograde left vertebral flow. Most centers now intentionally cover the LSA origin if necessary and reserve secondary revascularization procedures for treatment of related symptoms if they develop.[39,72]

For even more proximal TAAs involving the aortic arch, branched and fenestrated stent grafts are being developed to accommodate perfusion through the great vessels.[105,106] Although feasibility has been demonstrated, it is already apparent that the required implantation techniques would be highly complex and would demand considerable technical expertise. Some centers have been investigating techniques to create fenestrations intraoperatively after device deployment and coverage of critical branches.[107] In contrast, there are no easy management strategies to deal with a short distal neck. In this setting as well, fenestrated and branched grafts have been used in isolated cases, but the overall experience is very limited. Intentional coverage of the celiac artery is not recommended given the risk of hepatic and visceral ischemia. Although a normal superior mesenteric artery may provide collateral flow, no methods exist to predetermine whether such collateral supply would be sufficient. Furthermore, the celiac trunk may serve as a prominent source of retrograde endoleak if the artery is covered without adjunctive transcatheter occlusion. In distal aneurysms that involve both the descending thoracic and the abdominal aorta, combined open AAA repair and endovascular TAA exclusion is a novel treatment approach under investigation. Stent grafts are also being used to treat patients with diffuse aneurysmal disease involving the entire thoracic aorta. In such patients, the traditional surgical treatment is a two-stage procedure called the "elephant trunk technique."[108] In the first stage, the ascending aorta and aortic arch are repaired via a median sternotomy and an extra long graft is used for reconstruction, which leaves the excess portion of the graft, the elephant trunk, dangling within the lumen of the remaining diseased aorta. In the second stage, the lesion in the descending aorta is repaired via a left thoracotomy, and the graft replacement is connected to the elephant trunk proximally. To bypass the need for thoracotomy, a few centers have successfully deployed thoracic stent grafts into the elephant trunk extension, altogether replacing the second stage of the traditional elephant trunk procedure.[109] Following closely on the heels of early clinical experiences with stent grafting for TAA repair, experimental application of this less invasive approach has been extended to a growing number of other pathologies of the thoracic aorta. Most noteworthy among these are aortic dissection,[5] traumatic aortic injury,[110] penetrating atherosclerotic ulcer,[111] and aortic rupture.[112] Some investigators believe that thoracic stent graft technology may eventually have the greatest impact on clinical care in the management of aortic dissections, because current treatment standards are far from optimal.

The emergence of endovascular stent grafting as an alternative therapy to open surgical repair of thoracic aneurysms is an exciting advance. But the exact role of stent grafting remains to be defined as long-term data and experience continue to accumulate and devices and techniques evolve.

Abdominal Aortic Aneurysm

THERAPEUTIC STRATEGIES FOR ABDOMINAL AORTIC ANEURYSM

Aneurysm of the abdominal aorta represents a potentially life-threatening scenario affecting an increasingly important segment of the aging patient population. With improved overall health care, many patients reach an advanced age despite severe cardiovascular, hypertensive, and/or pulmonary comorbidities, thus buying time for an AAA to enlarge to a critical diameter and qualify for open surgical or endovascular treatment. Although surgical resection and interposition of an abdominal aortic prosthesis (Dacron or Gore-Tex) have long been considered standard treatment, despite a well known perioperative mortality risk, endovascular strategies have evolved over the last decade to be perceived as an accepted standard of care in patients considered too sick or too old for open surgery. Advanced technology, ease of use, and the temptation of a fully percutaneous procedure have attracted a new breed of "endovascular surgeons" propelled by the prospect of both avoiding surgical risk and inducing reconstructive remodeling of the aneurysmatic aorta through depressurization and complete exclusion of the aneurysmal sac. Once deployed, the stent graft serves to bridge the region of the aneurysm, thereby excluding it from the circulation while allowing aortic blood flow to continue distally through the prosthetic stent graft lumen. Only 30% to 60% of AAAs are anatomically suitable for endovascular repair. When such repair is undertaken, the rate of successful stent graft implantation has ranged from 78% to 94%. One of the major technical difficulties associated with the stent graft technique that has yet to be overcome is endoleaks, which occur in 10% to 20% of cases[113] and are seen angiographically as persistent contrast flow into the aneurysmal sac owing to failure to completely exclude the aneurysm from the aortic circulation. If left untreated, these endoleaks can leave the patient at continued risk for aneurysmal expansion or rupture. Indeed, in a follow-up study of outcomes at 12 months or longer among more than 1,000 stent graft recipients, the EUROSTAR investigators reported that almost 10% of patients per year required secondary interventions, suggesting that there should be caution in the broad application of endovascular aneurysmal repair (EVAR).[114] Patients and physicians have embraced EVAR as the method of choice to treat AAAs in patients at high risk. EVAR has great appeal for this older population because it leads to faster recovery with fewer systemic complications than open repair.[115–120] Parodi and colleagues[121] reported the first endovascular repair of an AAA in a human in 1991; they used a graft fashioned from prosthetic vascular grafts and expandable stents. Current estimates are that more than 20,000 EVAR procedures take place each year in the United States, representing 36% of all AAA repairs. The estimate is that more than 12% of all procedures in Europe involve EVAR, and the expected annual growth is 15% at this time (Medtronic Marketing Department, personal communication, 2006). EVAR is the method of choice in high-risk older patients because of its minimal incisions, shorter operating time, and reduced blood loss.

INDICATIONS FOR TREATMENT

Most asymptomatic AAAs are discovered serendipitously, often on imaging examinations for other complaints. Increasing evidence indicates that there is value to screening patients for AAA, and it is likely that screening will be approved in the near future.[122] Once the diagnosis of AAA is made, two critical questions need to be answered: when to intervene and how to intervene. The availability of EVAR has made these decisions somewhat more complex while adding a significant treatment option. Recent studies have questioned whether aneurysms smaller than 5 cm should be treated.[123] However, in general, the clinical recommendation remains to offer treatment for aneurysms between 5 and 5.5 cm, depending on the results of clinical trials.[124] An exception to this guideline is that intervention should be offered despite the size of the aneurysm if symptoms develop or if the aneurysm increases in size by 1 cm per year.[125] In addition, if the patient is a woman with smaller native vessels, the relative size that represents aneurysmal disease may be less than the conventional 5- to 5.5-cm range. Patient selection has emerged as the most important factor related to successful EVAR. The assessment begins with consideration of the body habitus and gender of the patient; small body size and female gender have been associated with a higher risk of procedure abortion.[126,127] In addition, the comorbidities of the patient must be assessed, with careful attention to cardiac, pulmonary, and renal conditions. The use of risk stratification to analyze outcomes clearly indicates that survival for those at low to minimal risk is excellent over 10 years; those at highest risk succumb to cardiac disease or cancer, and survival is poorest for those patients.[128] EVAR has shown a reduction in 30-day mortality relative to that achieved with open repair (1.2% vs. 4.6%). Risk stratification determines survival in general and shows that both open surgery and EVAR decrease the risk of death from AAA rupture.[129] The characteristics of the aneurysm must be matched to the most suitable device; this has a direct impact on outcomes and the complication profile of the procedure. The aneurysm is evaluated from a three-dimensional reconstruction CT scan or aortography with a calibrated catheter. There are at least four important features that must be assessed before a patient's eligibility for EVAR can be determined, and this analysis leads to a list of contraindications[130] (Table 42-5). Experienced interventionists can deal with some of these challenges, but morphological features of the aneurysm and access vessels may preclude EVAR. The key features of endovascular repair of AAAs that

TABLE 42-5	Evaluation for Endovascular Aneurysm Repair
Computed tomographic scan assessment for EVAR eligibility
Proximal neck: diameter, length, angle, presence or absence of thrombus
Distal landing zone: diameter and length
Iliac arteries: presence of aneurysms and occlusive disease
Access arteries: diameter, presence of occlusive disease
Contraindications for EVAR
Short proximal neck
Thrombus presence in proximal landing zone
Conical proximal neck
Greater than 120-degree angulation of the proximal neck
Critical inferior mesenteric artery
Significant iliac occlusive disease
Tortuosity of iliac vessels

EVAR, endovascular aneurysm repair.

TABLE 42-6	Classification of Endoleaks
Type I: attachment-site leaks
Proximal end of endograft
Distal end of endograft
Iliac occluder (plug)
Type II: branch leaks (without attachment site connection)
Simple or to-and-fro (from only one patent branch)
Complex or flow-through (with two or more patent branches)
Type III: graft defect
Junctional leak or modular disconnect
Fabric disruption (midgraft hole)
Minor (≤2 mm; e.g., suture holes)
Major (≥2 mm)
Type IV: Graft wall (fabric) porosity (30 days after graft placement)

determine procedural success and long-term outcomes are proximal and distal fixation and sealing. Throughout the graft, most of the devices use a metal skeleton made of stainless steel, nitinol, or Elgiloy. Attachment is facilitated by the use of hooks or radial force. Once the graft is inserted through the sheath, it can be deployed by a self-expanding mechanism or by balloon expansion. Some grafts attach superior to the renal arteries (suprarenal attachment), whereas most of the devices require at least 15 mm of proximal neck to achieve fixation and sealing in the infrarenal position. The grafts also differ in their "profile" or the size of the delivery system. Low-profile devices permit access through smaller arteries. Most of the complications associated with EVAR are minor and can be watched carefully or treated easily with additional interventional procedures. Some complications occur during or soon after the procedure, whereas others may be noticed only during graft surveillance.[131] A study by Ohki and colleagues[132] analyzed complication and death rates within 30 days after EVAR and reported them to be 17.6% and 8.5%, respectively. This remains an active and important area of EVAR research, and standards have been developed to facilitate reporting of endovascular abdominal aortic repair complications.[133] Endoleaks can have substantial clinical significance, because they carry an increased risk of symptoms or aneurysmal rupture. The term *endoleak* describes the continuation of blood flow into the extragraft portion of the aneurysm; this flow increases the size of the aneurysmal sac.[134] Endoleaks occur in either the acute setting during graft implantation or during the postoperative surveillance period. The majority of procedural endoleaks disappear without intervention. Endoleaks are either graft related or non-graft related, and a classification system has been developed (Table 42-6).[135] Type I endoleaks occur when the attachment is not complete, either proximally or distally; blood is able to flow into the aneurysmal sac and is not completely occluded by endograft attachment to the arterial wall. Type II endoleaks result from continued backflow from aortic branches, such as the inferior mesenteric artery and lumbar arteries. This flow occurs retrograde into the aneurysmal sac around the endograft. Type III endoleaks are caused by defects in the endograft structure that lead to the leakage of blood flow from inside the endograft to the aneurysmal sac. Finally, type IV endoleaks are noted early after endograft placement and resolve when the fabric's porosity is decreased by clotted blood. Because endovascular repair uses a relatively new technology, graft surveillance for complications such as endoleaks is essential. Endoleaks are diagnosed by a variety of techniques: arteriography, pressure monitoring during or after the procedure, CT scanning, and duplex scanning. The preferred method of detecting endoleaks is by CT scanning. An analysis of 2,463 patients from the EUROSTAR registry revealed that 171 had an endoleak by the time of their 1-month postoperative evaluation and 317 developed an endoleak at a later date.[136] Of these, 7.8% had a type II endoleak and 12% had a type I, a type III, or a combination. There are many different ways to treat endoleaks, including coil embolization, placement of stent graft cuffs and extensions, laparoscopic ligation of inferior mesenteric and lumbar arteries, open surgical repair, and repeat EVAR procedures. Type I and III endoleaks require fairly urgent intervention because blood flow and sac pressure will continue to increase and lead to rupture. Type IV endoleaks usually resolve on their own. The management of type II endoleaks is more controversial because some of them will thrombose on their own whereas others will lead to sac enlargement. Endograft surveillance is important to document normal and abnormal morphological changes in the repair and in the involved vessels. This process is vital for the detection of endoleaks, increased aneurysm diameter, and possible device migration.[137] The recommended surveillance routine includes a CT scan at 1, 6, and 12 months and annually thereafter. If an endoleak is detected, the frequency of the scans increases to every 6 months until resolution of the endoleak is detected. The use of EVAR technology has led to a greater understanding of the basic science of aneurysmal disease. For example, Curci and Thompson[138] have been studying the relationship between the secretion of matrix metalloproteinases (MMPs) and AAAs. They have measured increased levels in the aneurysmal rather than the normal arterial wall.

RANDOMIZED DATA AND CURRENT CONCLUSIONS

The EVAR study group has provided the community with important revelations from randomized studies on the treatment of a "moving target" called AAA in the context of increasing age of patients, continuously refined technology, and improving operator skills. Whereas treatment of large AAAs with EVAR reduced the 30-day mortality rate to 1.7%, compared with 4.7% with open repair ($P < 0.009$) on an intention-to-treat basis, the authors were prudent to judge such early benefits only as a license to continue evaluation of EVAR by the use of longer follow-up.[139,140] However, no differences were seen in total mortality or aneurysm-related mortality in the long-term follow-up.[141] Similarly, in the DREAM trial 6 years after randomization, endovascular and open repair of abdominal aortic aneurysms resulted in similar rates of survival (68.9% vs. 69.9%; $P = 0.97$).[142] Scores for measures of quality of life and sexual functioning favored EVAR only in the early postoperative period but equalized after 6 months in comparison with open repair, in parallel with a continued need for reinterventions with EVAR. A closer look, however, revealed that many late complications after successful EVAR were of low prognostic impact, such as endoleak type II requiring reintervention in only 17 of 79 cases. Severe complications such as graft rupture ($n = 9$), graft migration ($n = 12$), endoleak type I ($n = 27$), and graft thrombosis ($n = 12$), which required reintervention in 35 of 60 cases, were likely to be attributed to technical or procedural problems with the stent graft or unsuitable anatomy, again reminding the medical community of the inherently immature nature of an emerging technology. Moreover, at least six different brands of endovascular devices were used by surgeons with different levels of experience. Endovascular repair of AAAs was associated with a significantly lower rate of aneurysm-related mortality than no repair in

patients who were ineligible for open repair (adjusted hazard ratio [HR] 0.53; 95% confidence interval [CI] 0.32–0.89; $P = 0.02$). The 30-day operative mortality was 7.3% in the endovascular repair group. The overall rate of aneurysmal rupture in the no-intervention group was 12.4 (95% CI 9.6–16.2) per 100 person-years. This advantage did not result in any benefit in terms of total mortality (adjusted HR 0.99; 95% CI 0.78–1.27; $P = 0.97$). A total of 48% of patients who survived endovascular repair had graft-related complications and 27% required reintervention within the first 6 years. During 8 years of follow-up, endovascular repair was considerably more expensive than no repair (cost difference, £9,826 [U.S. $14,867]; 95% CI 7,638 to 12,013 [11,556 to 18,176]).[143,144] The data presented by the EVAR trialists (both 30-day and midterm outcomes in EVAR-1 and data from EVAR-2 in patients unfit for open surgery) are not just sobering but also provocative and revealing. In accordance with the DREAM studies,[140,142,145,146] EVAR-1 showed significant early survival benefit after 30 days with endovascular repair owing to reduced peri-interventional risk, corroborating previous observational evidence.[147–149] Careful analysis of randomized data provides highly valuable information:

1. Health status—comprising age, comorbidities, and prognostic confounders—was the most important denominator of individual prognosis, followed by, to a lesser degree, the nonsurgical nature of EVAR (which can be performed percutaneously with local anesthesia). Therefore assessment of the general state of health of patients in the older and sicker population and serious attempts at improvement should precede EVAR; examples are cardiopulmonary workup, potentially including percutaneous coronary intervention, and respiratory improvement as an integral part of strategic planning. Under particular conditions, it appears justified to reject EVAR when conservative care is more appropriate.

2. The nature of complications requiring reinterventions after EVAR is often related to technical shortcomings with current-generation devices or to nonsuitable anatomy. Physicians and industry must recognize those limitations and develop both better devices and improved selection algorithms for treatment with EVAR.

3. Eventually, although the endovascular community should always embrace the "Nihil nocere" principle (a classic in medicine and surgery) and avoid well-intended but harmful treatment, it should also realize the moving-target nature of the problem. Some patients considered unfit for surgery can possibly improve and find themselves in a lower-risk category and eventually fit for surgery or EVAR. EVAR technology and interventional skills constantly improve with training, and the short-term differential advantage over open surgery is likely to increase. More elderly patients may express a personal preference for a less traumatic procedure such as EVAR (if performed by an expert) despite lack of a clear-cut midterm advantage and accept surveillance and interventions during follow-up. Finally, the higher costs for follow-up imaging with EVAR could be dramatically reduced with a smarter surveillance strategy based on clinical and ultrasound interrogation instead of serial CT or MRI.

All things considered—even though, at midterm, EVAR may not improve AAA prognosis compared with classic surgery, resulting at present in a draw after an early advantage—EVAR is here to stay. Better staging and selection of patients, constantly improving technology,[148] and the expertise of centers of excellence for aortic diseases will enhance matching of a given patient with one of a variety of therapeutic options, including EVAR or even conservative treatment. Thus, despite all the new technology, it is still wise to adhere to the old principles of responsible use of clinical judgment and to offer, especially to the growing segment of older patients with multiple comorbidities, a holistic approach with intelligent use of prognosticating tools and interdisciplinary cooperation. Whether the results of the EVAR trials and the cautious voice of Jonathan Michaels[150] will halt the trend of increasing use of EVAR instead of open surgery remains to be seen; it is certain, however, that the randomized data from EVAR-1 and EVAR-2 will refocus the debate on natural history and patient selection for a forward-moving technology.

REFERENCES

1. Hagan PG, Nienaber CA, Isselbacher EM, et al: The International Registry of Aortic Dissection (IRAD). *JAMA* 283:897–903, 2000.
2. Kodolitsch Y, Schwartz AG, Nienaber CA: Clinical prediction of acute aortic dissection. *Arch Intern Med* 160:2977–2982, 2000.
3. Ince H, Nienaber CA: The concept of interventional therapy in acute aortic syndrome. *J Card Surg* 17:135–142, 2002.
4. Nienaber CA, Fattori R, Lund G, et al: Nonsurgical reconstruction of thoracic aortic dissection by stent graft placement. *N Engl J Med* 340:1539–1545, 1999.
5. Dake MD, Kato N, Mitchell RS, et al: Endovascular stent graft placement for the treatment of acute aortic dissection. *N Engl J Med* 340:1546–1552, 1999.
6. Walkers PJ, Miller DC: Aneurysmal and ischemic complications of type B (type III) aortic dissections. *Semin Vasc Surg* 5:198–214, 1992.
7. Bossone E, Rampoldi V, Nienaber CA, et al: Usefulness of pulse deficit to predict in-hospital complications and mortality in patients with acute type A aortic dissection. *Am J Cardiol* 89:851–855, 2002.
8. Cambria RP, Brewster DC, Gertler J, et al: Vascular complications associated with spontaneous aortic dissection. *J Vasc Surg* 7:197–209, 1988.
9. Laas J, Heinemann M, Schaefers HJ, et al: Management of thoracoabdominal malperfusion in aortic dissection. *Circulation* 84:20–24, 1991.
10. Miller DC: The continuing dilemma concerning medical versus surgical management of patients with acute type B dissections. *Semin Thorac Cardiovasc Surg* 5:33–46, 1993.
11. Miller DC, Mitchell RS, Oyer PE, et al: Independent determinants of operative mortality for patients with aortic dissections. *Circulation* 70:153–164, 1984.
12. Elefteriades JA, Hartleroad J, Gusberg RJ, et al: Long-term experience with descending aortic dissection: the complication-specific approach. *Ann Thorac Surg* 53:11–20, 1992.
13. Walker PJ, Dake MD, Mitchell RS, et al: The use of endovascular techniques for the treatment of complications of aortic dissection. *J Vasc Surg* 18:1042–1051, 1993.
14. Fann JI, Sarris GE, Mitchell RS, et al: Treatment of patients with aortic dissection presenting with peripheral vascular complications. *Ann Surg* 212:705–713, 1990.
15. Yano H, Ishimaru S, Kawaguchi S, et al: Endovascular stent grafting of the descending thoracic aorta after arch repair in acute type A dissection. *Ann Thorac Surg* 73:288–291, 2002.
16. Kato N, Shimono T, Hirano T, et al: Transluminal placement of endovascular stent grafts for the treatment of type A aortic dissection with an entry tear in the descending thoracic aorta. *J Vasc Surg* 34:1023–1028, 2001.
17. Iannelli G, Piscione F, Di Tommaso L, et al: Thoracic aortic emergencies: Impact of endovascular surgery. *Ann Thorac Surg* 77:591–596, 2004.
18. Saito S, Arai H, Kim K, et al: Percutaneous fenestration of dissecting intima with a transseptal needle: A new therapeutic technique for visceral ischemia complicating acute aortic dissection. *Cathet Cardiovasc Diagn* 26:130–135, 1992.
19. Nienaber CA, Ince H, Petzsch M, et al: Endovascular treatment of thoracic aortic dissection and its variants. *Acta Chir Belg* 102:292–298, 2002.
20. Nienaber CA, Ince H, Weber F, et al: Emergency stent graft placement in thoracic aortic dissection and evolving rupture. *J Card Surg* 18:464–470, 2003.
21. Beregi JP, Haulon S, Otal P, et al: Endovascular treatment of acute complications associated with aortic dissection: midterm results from a multicenter study. *J Endovasc Ther* 10:486–493, 2003.
22. Bortone AS, Schena S, D'Agostino D, et al: Immediate versus delayed endovascular treatment of post-traumatic aortic pseudoaneurysms and type B dissections: retrospective analysis and premises to the upcoming European trial. *Circulation* 106:234–240, 2002.
23. Diethrich EB, Ghazoul M, Wheatley GH, et al: Surgical correction of ascending type a thoracic aortic dissection: simultaneous endoluminal exclusion of the arch and distal aorta. *J Endovasc Ther* 12:660–666, 2005.
24. Svensson LG, Kouchoukos NF, Miller DC, et al: Expert consensus document on the treatment of descending thoracic aortic disease using endovascular stent grafts. *Ann Thorac Surg* 85:S1-S41, 2008.
25. Kodama K, Nishigami K, Sakamoto T, et al: Tight heart rate control reduces secondary adverse events in patients with type B acute aortic dissection. *Circulation* 118(Suppl 1):S167-S170, 2008.
26. Tsai TT, Fattori R, Trimarchi S, et al: Long-term survival in patients with type B acute aortic dissection: insight from the International Registry of Acute Aortic Dissection. *Circulation* 114:2226–2231, 2006.
27. Tang DG, Dake MD: TEVAR for acute uncomplicated aortic dissection: immediate repair versus medical therapy. *Semin Vasc Surg* 22:145–151, 2009.
28. Estrera AL, Miller CC, Safi H, et al: Outcomes of medical management of acute type B aortic dissection. *Circulation* 114(Suppl 1):384–389, 2006.
29. Trimarchi S, Nienaber CA, Rampoldi V, et al: Role and results of surgery in acute type B aortic dissection: insights from the International Registry of Acute Aortic Dissection (IRAD). *Circulation* 114(Suppl I):I357–I364, 2006.
30. Fattori R, Tsai TT, Myrmel T, et al: Complicated acute type B dissection: is surgery still the best option? *J Am Coll Cardiol Intervent* 1:395–402, 2008.
31. Nienaber CA, Kische S, Zeller T, et al: Provisional extension to induce complete attachment after stent graft placement in type B aortic dissection: the PETTICOAT concept. *J Endovasc Ther* 13:738–746, 2006.
32. Parker JD, Golledge J: Outcome of endovascular treatment of acute type B aortic dissection. *Ann Thorac Surg* 86:1707–1712, 2008.
33. Xiong J, Jiang B, Guo W, et al: Endovascular stent graft placement in patients with type B aortic dissection: a meta-analysis in China. *J Thorac Cardiovasc Surg* 138:865–872, 2009.
34. Demers P, Miller DC, Mitchell RS, et al: Midterm results of endovascular repair of descending thoracic aortic aneurysms with first-generation stent grafts. *J Thorac Cardiovasc Surg* 127:664–673, 2004.
35. Dialetto G, Cocino FE, Scognamiglio G, et al: Treatment of type B aortic dissection: endoluminal repair or conventional medical therapy? *Eur J Cardiothorac Surg* 27:826–830, 2005.
36. Nienaber CA, Rousseau H, Eggebrecht H, et al: Randomized comparison of strategies for type B aortic dissection: the Investigation of STEnt grafts in Aortic Dissection (INSTEAD) trial. *Circulation* 120:2519–2528, 2009.
37. Nienaber CA, Kische S, Rehders TC, et al: Rapid pacing for better placing: comparison of techniques for precise deployment of endografts in the thoracic aorta. *J Endovasc Ther* 14:506–512, 2007.
38. Koschyk DH, Nienaber CA, Knap M, et al: How to guide stent graft implantation in type B aortic dissection? Comparison of angiography, transesophageal echocardiography, and intravascular ultrasound. *Circulation* 112(Suppl I):I-260–I-264, 2005.
39. Rehders TC, Petzsch M, Ince H, et al: Intentional occlusion of the left subclavian artery during endovascular stent graft implantation in the thoracic aorta: risk and relevance. *J Endovasc Ther* 11:659–666, 2004.
40. Eggebrecht H, Thompson M, Rousseau H, et al: European Registry on Endovascular Aortic Repair Complications. Retrograde ascending aortic dissection during or after thoracic aortic stent graft placement: insight from the European registry on endovascular aortic repair complications. *Circulation* 120(Suppl 11):S276–S281, 2009.
41. Dong ZH, Fu WG, Wang YQ, et al: Retrograde type A aortic dissection after endovascular stent graft placement of type B dissection. *Circulation* 119:735–741, 2009.
42. Hata M, Sezai A, Niino T, et al: Prognosis for patients with type B acute aortic dissection: risk analysis of early requirement for elective surgery. *Circ J* 71:1279–1282, 2007.
43. Winnerkvist A, Lockowandt U, Rasmussen E, et al: A prospective study of medically treated acute type B aortic dissection. *Eur J Vasc Endovasc Surg* 32:356–357, 2006.
44. Shimono T, Kato N, Yasuda F, et al: Transluminal stent graft placements for the treatment of acute onset and chronic aortic dissections. *Circulation* 106:1241–1247, 2002.
45. Eggebrecht H, Herold U, Kuhnt O, et al: Endovascular stent graft treatment of aortic dissection: determinants of postinterventional outcome. *Eur Heart J* 26:489–497, 2005.
46. Jing QM, Han YL, Wang XZ, et al: Endovascular stent grafts for acute and chronic type B aortic dissection: comparison of clinical outcomes. *Chin Med J* 121:2213–2217, 2008.
47. Kato N, Hirano T, Ishida M, et al: Acute and contained rupture of the descending thoracic aorta: treatment with endovascular stent grafts. *J Vasc Surg* 37:100–105, 2003.
48. Clouse WD, Hallett JW, Jr, Schaff HV, et al: Improved prognosis of thoracic aortic aneurysms: A population-based study. *JAMA* 280:1926–1929, 1998.
49. Bickerstaff LK, Pairolero PC, Hollier LH, et al: Thoracic aortic aneurysms: A population-based study. *Surgery* 92:1103–1108, 1982.
50. Gloviczki P, Pairolero P, Welch T, et al: Multiple aortic aneurysms: the results of surgical management. *J Vasc Surg* 11:19–27, 1990.
51. Thomson MM, Bell PR: ABC of arterial and venous disease: arterial aneurysms. *BMJ* 320:1193–1196, 2000.
52. Coady MA, Rizzo JA, Goldstein LJ, et al: Natural history, pathogenesis, and etiology of thoracic aortic aneurysms and dissections. *Cardiol Clin* 17:615–635, 1999.
53. Crawford ES, DeNatale RW: Thoracoabdominal aortic aneurysm: observations regarding the natural course of the disease. *J Vasc Surg* 3:578–582, 1986.
54. McNamara JJ, Pressler VM: Natural history of arteriosclerotic thoracic aortic aneurysms. *Ann Thorac Surg* 26:468–473, 1998.
55. Davies RR, Goldstein LJ, Coady MA, et al: Yearly rupture or dissection rate for thoracic aortic aneurysms: simple prediction based on size. *Ann Thorac Surg* 73:17–27, 2002.
56. Juvonen T, Ergin MA, Galla JD, et al: Prospective study of the natural history of thoracic aortic aneurysms. *Ann Thorac Surg* 63:1533–1545, 1997.
57. Johansson G, Markstrom U, Swedenborg J: Ruptured thoracic aortic aneurysms: a study of incidence and mortality rates. *J Vasc Surg* 21:985–988, 1995.
58. Olsson C, Thelin S, Ståhle E, et al: Thoracic aortic aneurysm and dissection: increasing prevalence and improved outcomes reported in a nationwide population-based study of more than 14,000 cases from 1987 to 2002. *Circulation* 114:2611–2618, 2006.
59. DeBakey ME, McCollum CH, Graham JM: Surgical treatment of aneurysms of the descending thoracic aorta: Long-term results in 500 patients. *J Cardiovasc Surg (Torino)* 19:571–576, 1998.
60. Hilgenberg AD, Rainer WG, Sadler TR, Jr: Aneurysm of the descending thoracic aorta: Replacement with the use of a shunt or bypass. *J Thorac Cardiovasc Surg* 81:818–824, 1981.
61. Moreno-Cabral CE, Miller DC, Mitchell RS, et al: Degenerative and atherosclerotic aneurysms of the thoracic aorta: determinants of early and late surgical outcome. *J Thorac Cardiovasc Surg* 88:1020–1032, 1984.
62. Pressler V, McNamara JJ: Thoracic aortic aneurysm: natural history and treatment. *J Thorac Cardiovasc Surg* 79:489–498, 1980.
63. Fann JI: Descending thoracic and thoracoabdominal aortic aneurysms. *Coron Artery Dis* 13:93–102, 2002.
64. Svensson LG, Crawford ES, Hess KR, et al: Variables predictive of outcome in 832 patients undergoing repairs of the descending thoracic aorta. *Chest* 104:1248–1253, 1993.
65. Borst HG, Jurmann M, Buhner B, et al: Risk of replacement of descending aorta with a standardized left heart bypass technique. *J Thorac Cardiovasc Surg* 105:126–132, 1994.
66. Pressler V, McNamara JJ: Aneurysm of the thoracic aorta: review of 260 cases. *J Thorac Cardiovasc Surg* 89:50–54, 1985.
67. Svensson LG, Crawford ES, Hess KR, et al: Experience with 1509 patients undergoing thoracoabdominal aortic operations. *J Vasc Surg* 17:357–368, 1993.
68. Livesay JJ, Cooley DA, Ventemiglia RA, et al: Surgical experience in descending thoracic aneurysmectomy with and without adjuncts to avoid ischemia. *Ann Thorac Surg* 39:37–46, 1985.
69. Berg P, Kaufmann D, van Marrewijk CJ, et al: Spinal cord ischaemia after stent graft treatment for infra-renal abdominal aortic aneurysms: analysis of the EUROSTAR database. *Eur J Vasc Endovasc Surg* 22:342–347, 2001.
70. Rosenthal D: Spinal cord ischemia after abdominal aortic operation: is it preventable? *J Vasc Surg* 30:391–397, 1999.
71. Ouriel K, Greenberg RK: Endovascular treatment of thoracic aortic aneurysms. *J Cardiol Surg* 18:455–463, 2003.
72. Dake MD: Endovascular stent graft management of thoracic aortic diseases. *Eur J Radiol* 39:42–49, 2001.
73. Gravereaux EC, Faries PL, Burks JA, et al: Risk of spinal cord ischemia after endograft repair of thoracic aortic aneurysms. *J Vasc Surg* 34:977–1003, 2001.
74. Burks JA, Jr, Faries PL, Gravereaux EC, et al: Endovascular repair of thoracic aortic aneurysms: stent graft fixation across the aortic arch vessels. *Ann Vasc Surg* 16:24–28, 2002.
75. Gorich J, Asquan Y, Seifarth H, et al: Initial experience with intentional stent graft coverage of the subclavian artery during endovascular thoracic aortic repairs. *J Endovasc Ther* 9(Suppl 2):II39–II43, 2002.
76. Tiesenhausen K, Hausegger KA, Oberwalder P, et al: Left subclavian artery management in endovascular repair of thoracic aortic aneurysms and aortic dissections. *J Card Surg* 18:429–435, 2003.
77. Dake MD, Miller DC, Semba CP, et al: Transluminal placement of endovascular stent grafts for the treatment of descending thoracic aortic aneurysms. *N Engl J Med* 331:1729–1734, 1994.
78. Dake MD, Miller DC, Mitchell RS, et al: The "first generation" of endovascular stent grafts for patients with aneurysms of the descending thoracic aorta. *J Thorac Cardiovasc Surg* 116:689–703, 1998.
79. Fann JI, Miller DC: Endovascular treatment of descending thoracic aortic aneurysms and dissections. *Surg Clin North Am* 79:551–574, 1999.
80. Kazui T, Washiyamoi N, Muhammod BA, et al: Improved results of atherosclerotic arch aneurysm operation with a refined technique. *J Thorac Cardiovasc Surg* 121:491–499, 2001.
81. Spielvogel D, Holstead JC, Meies M, et al: Aortic arch replacement using a trifurcated graft: simple, versatile and safe. *Ann Thorac Surg* 80:90–95, 2005.
82. Ehrlich M, Grabenwoeger M, Cartes-Zumelzu F, et al: Endovascular stent graft repair for aneurysms on the descending thoracic aorta. *Ann Thorac Surg* 66:19–24, 1998.
83. Cartes-Zumelzu F, Lammer J, Kretschmer G, et al: Endovascular repair of thoracic aortic aneurysms. *Semin Interv Cardiol* 5:53–57, 2000.
84. Grabenwoger M, Hutschala D, Ehrlich MP, et al: Thoracic aortic aneurysms: treatment with endovascular self-expandable stent grafts. *Ann Thorac Surg* 69:421–425, 2000.
85. Greenberg R, Resch T, Nyman U, et al: Endovascular repair of descending thoracic aortic aneurysms: an early experience with intermediate-term follow-up. *J Vasc Surg* 31:147–156, 2000.
86. Temudom T, D'Ayala M, Marin ML, et al: Endovascular grafts in the treatment of thoracic aortic aneurysms and pseudoaneurysms. *Ann Vasc Surg* 14:230–238, 2000.

87. Najibi S, Terramani TT, Weiss VJ, et al: Endoluminal versus open treatment of descending thoracic aortic aneurysms. *J Vasc Surg* 36:732–737, 2002.
88. Heijmen RH, Deblier IG, Moll FL, et al: Endovascular stent grafting for descending thoracic aortic aneurysms. *Eur J Cardiothorac Surg* 21:5–9, 2002.
89. Schoder M, Cartes-Zumelzu F, Grabenwoger M, et al: Elective endovascular stent graft repair of atherosclerotic thoracic aortic aneurysms: clinical results and midterm follow-up. *AJR Am J Roentgenol* 180:709–715, 2003.
90. Marin ML, Hollier LH, Ellozy SH, et al: Endovascular stent graft repair of abdominal and thoracic aortic aneurysms: a ten-year experience with 817 patients. *Ann Surg* 238:586–593, 2003.
91. Lepore V, Lonn L, Delle M, et al: Treatment of descending thoracic aneurysms by endovascular stent grafting. *J Card Surg* 18:416–423, 2003.
92. Sunder-Plassmann L, Scharrer-Pamler R, Liewald F, et al: Endovascular exclusion of thoracic aortic aneurysms: Mid-term results of elective treatment and in contained rupture. *J Card Surg* 18:367–374, 2003.
93. Bergeron P, De Chaumaray T, Gay J, et al: Endovascular treatment of thoracic aortic aneurysms. *J Cardiovasc Surg (Torino)* 42:349–361, 2003.
94. Czerny M, Cejna M, Hutschala D, et al: Stent graft placement in atherosclerotic descending thoracic aortic aneurysms: midterm results. *J Endovasc Ther* 11:26–32, 2004.
95. Makaroun MS, Dillavou ED, Kee ST, et al: Endovascular treatment of thoracic aortic aneurysms: results of the phase II multicenter trial of the GORE TAG thoracic endoprosthesis. *J Vasc Surg* 41:1–9, 2005.
96. Leurs LJ, Bell R, Degrieck Y, et al: Endovascular treatment of thoracic aortic diseases: Combined experience from the EUROSTAR and United Kingdom Thoracic Endograft registries. *J Vasc Surg* 40:670–679, 2004.
97. Mitchell RS, Miller DC, Dake MD: Stent graft repair of thoracic aortic aneurysms. *Semin Vasc Surg* 10:257–271, 1997.
98. Carroccio A, Marin ML, Ellozy S, et al: Pathophysiology of paraplegia following endovascular thoracic aortic aneurysm repair. *J Card Surg* 18:359–366, 2003.
99. Thurnher SA, Grabenwoger M: Endovascular treatment of thoracic aortic aneurysms: a review. *Eur Radiol* 12:1370–1387, 2002.
100. Resch T, Koul B, Dias NV, et al: Changes in aneurysm morphology and stent graft configuration after endovascular repair of aneurysms of the descending thoracic aorta. *J Thorac Cardiovasc Surg* 122:47–52, 2001.
101. Buth J, Harris PL, van Marrewijk C, et al: The significance and management of different types of endoleaks. *Semin Vasc Surg* 16:95–102, 2003.
102. Chuter TA, Faruqi RM, Sawhney R, et al: Endoleak after endovascular repair of abdominal aortic aneurysm. *J Vasc Surg* 34: 98–105, 2001.
103. Kato N, Semba CP, Dake MD: Embolization of perigraft leaks after endovascular stent graft treatment of aortic aneurysms. *J Vasc Intervent Radiol* 7:805–811, 1996.
104. Hausegger KA, Oberwalder P, Tiesenhausen K, et al: Intentional left subclavian artery occlusion by thoracic aortic stent grafts without surgical transposition. *J Endovasc Ther* 8:472–476, 2001.
105. Stanley BM, Semmens JB, Lawrence-Brown MM, et al: Fenestration in endovascular grafts for aortic aneurysm repair: new horizons for preserving blood flow in branch vessels. *J Endovasc Ther* 8:16–24, 2001.
106. Inoue K, Hosokawa H, Iwase T, et al: Aortic arch reconstruction by transluminally placed endovascular branched stent graft. *Circulation* 100(Suppl II):II-316–II-321, 1999.
107. McWilliams RG, Murphy M, Hartley D, et al: In situ stent graft fenestration to preserve the left subclavian artery. *J Endovasc Ther* 11:170–174, 2004.
108. Heinemann MK, Buehner B, Jurmann MJ, Borst HG: Use of the "elephant trunk technique" in aortic surgery. *Ann Thorac Surg* 60:2–6, 1995.
109. Fann JI, Dake MD, Semba CP, et al: Endovascular stent grafting after arch aneurysm repair using the "elephant trunk." *Ann Thorac Surg* 60:1102–1105, 1995.
110. Kato N, Dake MD, Miller DC, et al: Traumatic thoracic aortic aneurysm: treatment with endovascular stent grafts. *Radiology* 205:657–662, 1997.
111. Eggebrecht H, Baumgart D, Schmermund A, et al: Penetrating atherosclerotic ulcer of the aorta: treatment by endovascular stent graft placement. *Curr Opin Cardiol* 18:431–435, 2003.
112. Kato N, Hirano T, Ishida M, et al: Acute and contained rupture of the descending thoracic aorta: treatment with endovascular stent grafts. *J Vasc Surg* 37:100–105, 2003.
113. Brewster DC, Cronenwett JL, Hallett JW, Jr, et al: Joint Council of the American Association for Vascular Surgery and Society for Vascular Surgery: Guidelines for the treatment of abdominal aortic aneurysms: report of a subcommittee of the Joint Council of the American Association for Vascular Surgery and Society for Vascular Surgery. *J Vasc Surg* 37:1106–1117, 2003.
114. Laheij RJ, Buth J, Harris PL, et al: Need for secondary interventions after endovascular repair of abdominal aortic aneurysms: intermediate-term follow-up results of a European collaborative registry (EUROSTAR). *Br J Surg* 87:1666–1673, 2000.
115. Criado FJ, Fairman RM, Becker GJ: Talent LPS AAA stent graft: results of a pivotal clinical trial. *J Vasc Surg* 37:709–715, 2003.
116. Matsumura JS, Brewster DC, Makaroun MS, et al: A multicenter controlled clinical trial of open versus endovascular treatment of abdominal aortic aneurysm. *J Vasc Surg* 37:262–271, 2003.
117. Ouriel K, Clair DG, Greenberg RK, et al: Endovascular repair of abdominal aortic aneurysms: device-specific outcome. *J Vasc Surg* 37:971–978, 2003.
118. Moore WS: The Guidant Ancure bifurcation endograft: five-year follow-up. *Semin Vasc Surg* 16:139–143, 2003.
119. Zarins CK, White RA, Moll FL, et al: The AneuRx stent graft: four-year results and worldwide experience 2000. *J Vasc Surg* 33:S135-S145, 2001.
120. Greenberg RK, Chuter TA, Sternbergh WC III, et al: Zenith AAA endovascular graft: intermediate-term results of the US multicenter trial. *J Vasc Surg* 39:1209–1218, 2004.
121. Parodi JC, Palmaz JC, Barone HD: Transfemoral intraluminal graft implantation for abdominal aortic aneurysms. *Ann Vasc Surg* 5:491–497, 1991.
122. Kent KC, Zwolak RM, Jaff MR, et al: Screening for abdominal aortic aneurysm: a consensus statement. *J Vasc Surg* 39:267–269, 2004.
123. The UK Small Aneurysm Trial Participants: Mortality results for randomised controlled trial of early elective surgery or ultrasonographic surveillance for small abdominal aortic aneurysms. *Lancet* 352:1649–1655, 1998.
124. Powell JT, Greenhalgh RM: Clinical practice: small abdominal aortic aneurysms. *N Engl J Med* 348:1895–1901, 2003.
125. Scott RA, Tisi PV, Ashton HA, et al: Abdominal aortic aneurysm rupture rates: a 7-year follow-up of the entire abdominal aortic aneurysm population detected by screening. *J Vasc Surg* 28:124–128, 1998.
126. Mathison M, Becker GJ, Katzen BT, et al: The influence of female gender on the outcome of endovascular abdominal aortic aneurysm repair. *J Vasc Interv Radiol* 12:1047–1051, 2001.
127. Mathison MN, Becker GJ, Katzen BT, et al: Implications of problematic access in transluminal endografting of abdominal aortic aneurysm. *J Vasc Intervent Radiol* 14:33–39, 2003.
128. Becker GJ, Kovacs M, Mathison MN, et al: Risk stratification and outcomes of transluminal endografting for abdominal aortic aneurysm: 7-year experience and long-term follow-up. *J Vasc Intervent Radiol* 12:1033–1046, 2001.
129. Huber TS, Wang JG, Derrow AE, et al: Experience in the United States with intact abdominal aortic aneurysm repair. *J Vasc Surg* 33:304–310, 2001.
130. Ohki T, Veith FJ: Patient selection for endovascular repair of abdominal aortic aneurysms: changing the threshold for intervention. *Semin Vasc Surg* 12:226–234, 1999.
131. Elkouri S, Gloviczki P, McKusick MA, et al: Perioperative complications and early outcome after endovascular and open surgical repair of abdominal aortic aneurysms. *J Vasc Surg* 39:497–505, 2004.
132. Ohki T, Veith FJ, Shaw P, et al: Increasing incidence of midterm and long-term complications after endovascular graft repair of abdominal aortic aneurysms: a note of caution based on a 9-year experience. *Ann Surg* 234:323–334, 2001.
133. Chaikof EL, Blankensteijn JD, Harris PL, et al: Reporting standards for endovascular aortic aneurysm repair. *J Vasc Surg* 35:1048–1060, 2002.
134. White GH, Yu W, May J: Endoleak: a proposed new terminology to describe incomplete aneurysm exclusion by an endoluminal graft. *J Endovasc Surg* 3:124–125, 1996.
135. Veith FJ, Baum RA, Ohki T, et al: Nature and significance of endoleaks and endotension: summary of opinions expressed at an international conference. *J Vasc Surg* 35:1029–1035, 2002.
136. van Marrewijk C, Buth J, Harris PL, et al: Significance of endoleaks after endovascular repair of abdominal aortic aneurysms: the EUROSTAR experience. *J Vasc Surg* 35:461–473, 2002.
137. Corriere MA, Feurer ID, Becker SY, et al: Endoleak following endovascular abdominal aortic aneurysm repair: implications for duration of screening. *Ann Surg* 239:800–805, 2004.
138. Curci JA, Thompson RW: Adaptive cellular immunity in aortic aneurysms: cause, consequence, or context? *J Clin Invest* 114: 168–171, 2004.
139. Greenhalgh RM, Brown LC, Kwong GP, et al: Comparison of endovascular aneurysm repair with open repair in patients with abdominal aortic aneurysm (EVAR trial 1)—30-day operative mortality results: randomised controlled trial. *Lancet* 364:843–848, 2004.
140. EVAR trial participants. Endovascular aneurysm repair versus open repair in patients with abdominal aortic aneurysm (EVAR trial 1): randomised controlled trial. *Lancet* 365:2179–2186, 2005.
141. Greenhalgh RM, Brown LC, Powel JT, et al: for The United Kingdom EVAR Trial Investigators. Endovascular versus open repair of abdominal aortic aneurysm. *N Engl J Med* 362(20): 1863–1871, 2010.
142. DeBruin JL, Baas AF, Buth J, et al, for the DREAM Study Group: Long-term outcome of open or endovascular repair of abdominal aortic aneurysm. *N Engl J Med* 362(20):1881–1889, 2010.
143. EVAR Trial Participants: Endovascular aneurysm repair and outcome in patients unfit for open repair of abdominal aortic aneurysm (EVAR trial 2): randomised controlled trial. *Lancet* 365:2187–2192, 2005.
144. Greenhalgh RM, Brown LC, Powel JT, et al, for The United Kingdom EVAR Trial Investigators: Endovascular repair of aortic aneurysm in patients physically ineligible for open repair. *N Engl J Med* 362(20):1872–1880, 2010.
145. Prinssen M, Verhoeven ELG, Buth J, et al: A randomized trial comparing conventional and endovascular repair of abdominal aortic aneurysms. *N Engl J Med* 351:1607–1618, 2004.
146. Blankensteijn JD, de Jong SECA, Prinssen M, et al: Two-year outcomes after conventional or endovascular repair of abdominal aortic aneurysms. *N Engl J Med* 352:2398–2405, 2005.
147. Anderson PL, Arons RR, Moskowitz AJ, et al: A statewide experience with endovascular abdominal aortic aneurysm repair: rapid diffusion with excellent early results. *J Vasc Surg* 39:10–19, 2004.
148. Lee WA, Carter JW, Upchurch G, et al: Perioperative outcomes after open and endovascular repair of intact abdominal aortic aneurysms in the United States during 2001. *J Vasc Surg* 39:491–496, 2004.
149. Hua HT, Campria RP, Chuang SK, et al: Early outcomes of endovascular versus open abdominal aortic aneurysm repair in the National Surgical Quality Improvement Program-Private Sector (NS-QIP-PS). *J Vasc Surg* 41:382–389, 2005.
150. Michaels J: The future of endovascular aneurysm repair. *Eur J Vasc Endovasc Surg* 30:115–118, 2005.
151. Xu S, Hunag F, Yang J, et al: Endovascular repair of acute type B aortic dissection: early and mid-term results. *J Vasc Surg* 43(27):489–498, 2006.
152. Verhoye JP, Miller DC, Sze D, et al: Complicated acute type B aortic disection: midterm results of emergency endovascular stent grafting. *J Thorac Cardiovasc Surg* 136:424–430, 2008.
153. Szeto WY, McGarvey M, Pochettino A, et al: Endovascular repair of acute type B aortic dissection: early and mid-term results. *J Vasc Surg* 43:1090–1095, 2006.
154. Khoynezhad A, Donayre CE, Omari BO, et al: Midterm results of endovascular treatment of complicated acute type B aortic dissection. *J Thorac Cardiovasc Surg* 138:625–631, 2009.
155. Alves CMR, da Fonseca JHP, de Souza JAM, et al: Endovascular treatment of type B aortic dissection: the challenge of late success. *Ann Thorac Surg* 87:1360–1365, 2009.
156. Parsa CJ, Schroder JN, Danehmand MA, et al: Midterm results for endovascular repair of complicated acute and chronic type B aortic dissection. *Ann Thorac Surg* 89:97–104, 2010.
157. Greenberg RK, O'Neill S, Walker E, et al: Endovascular repair of thoracic aortic lesions with the Zenith TX1 and TX2 thoracic grafts: intermediate-term results. *J Vasc Surg* 41:589–596, 2005.
158. Wheatley GH III, Gurbuz AT, Rodriguez-Lopez JA, et al: Midterm outcome in 158 consecutive Gore TAG thoracic endoprostheses: single center experience. *Ann Thorac Surg* 81:1570–1577, 2006.
159. Bavaria JE, Appoo JJ, Makaroun MS, et al: Endovascular stent grafting versus open surgical repair of descending thoracic aortic aneurysms in low-risk patients: a multicenter comparative trial. *J Thorac Cardiovasc Surg* 1333:369–377, 2007.
160. Fairman RM, Criado F, Farber M, et al: Pivotal results of the Medtronic Vascular Talent Thoracic Stent Graft System: the VALOR Trial. *J Vasc Surg* 48(3):546–554, 2008.
161. Hughes CC, Lee SM, Daneshmand MA, et al: Endovascular repair of descending thoracic aneurysms: results with "on-label" application in the post Food and Drug Administration approval era. *Ann Thorac Surg* 90:83–89, 2010.

43

Venous Intervention

MITCHELL J. SILVER | GARY M. ANSEL

KEY POINTS

- Typical symptoms of superior vena cava syndrome include severe congestion and edema of the face, arms, and upper thorax; these may progress to dyspnea, cognitive dysfunction, and headache.

- Thrombolytic therapy prior to endovascular stenting of the superior vena cava has great utility. Once the acute thrombus has been resolved, it remains only to stent the rest of the stenosis, which in most cases is shorter than the occluded segment that had been occupied by thrombus.

- After successful treatment of an acute deep venous thrombosis of the upper extremity, it is imperative that some form of imaging be undertaken to look for possible venous compression.

- Patients with Paget-Schroetter syndrome develop spontaneous deep venous thrombosis of the upper extremity, usually in the dominant arm, after strenuous physical activity. Heavy repetitive exertion causes microtrauma to the vessels' intima and leads to activation of the coagulation cascade.

- Clinical pulmonary embolism occurs in 26% and 67% of patients with untreated proximal deep venous thrombosis and is associated with a mortality rate of 11% to 23% if not treated. Under treatment, the incidence of pulmonary embolism decreases to 5% and the mortality to less than 1%.

- Catheter-directed thrombolysis, or the delivery of thrombolytic agents directly into the thrombus, offers significant advantages over systemic therapy for deep venous thrombosis of the lower extremity, as systemic therapy may fail to reach and penetrate an occluded venous segment.

- With the advent of retrievable filters for the inferior vena cava, there is an expanding role for their prophylactic use during catheter-directed thrombolysis for deep venous thrombosis of the lower extremity, particularly in patients with "free-floating" iliac vein thrombi or in those whose cardiopulmonary reserve is already compromised.

- Percutaneous mechanical thrombectomy is an important adjunct to catheter-directed thrombolysis; it may result in a shorter time to vein patency, shorter length of hospitalization, reduced hemorrhagic risk, and overall cost savings.

Introduction

As interventional cardiologists with training in peripheral vascular disease have expanded their "skill set" from coronary interventions to the endovascular management of peripheral vascular disease, venous intervention has gradually become a natural extension to the "global cardiovascular interventionist." In fact, more and more interventional cardiologists have become interested in the management of venous disorders, which now include central venous stenosis and the endovascular treatment of upper and lower extremity deep venous thrombosis.

The Venous System: Basic Histology and Physiology

Veins are larger in caliber and more numerous than arteries. The venous system has a much greater volume capacity than the arterial system. The walls of veins are thinner and less elastic than the walls of arteries. Most anatomists distinguish three layers in the walls of veins: tunica intima, tunica media, and tunica adventitia. The distinctions between the layers are subtle. The internal elastic membrane is poorly defined, and the tunica media is not as developed as that of arteries. There are three categories of veins: venules and small veins, medium-size veins, and large veins. Only medium and large veins are discussed in this chapter. For a complete review of venous embryology and anatomy, an anatomic textbook should be consulted.

Medium-size veins range between 2 and 9 mm in diameter. These include veins from extremities distal to the axillary or inguinal crease and cutaneous veins. The intima consists of endothelium, basal lamina, and reticular fibers. The media consists of a very thin layer of circular smooth muscle and few collagen fibers. The adventitia is thickest of all the layers and consists of collagen and elastic fibers. The large veins consist of veins central to the axillary or inguinal crease, the superior vena cava (SVC), the inferior vena cava (IVC), renal veins, hepatic veins, and azygos veins. The intima is similar to the medium-size veins. A tunica media is lacking in most of the large veins with the exception of the gravid uterus and pulmonary veins. A thick adventitia makes up the greater part of the thickness of the wall. This layer is rich in elastic fibers and longitudinally oriented collagen. The IVC is exceptional in that its adventitia contains scattered longitudinal bundles of smooth muscle. Large veins get their blood supply from very small penetrating vessels called vasa vasorum.

VEIN VALVES

Valve leaflets comprise a thin fold of the intima, with a thin layer of collagen and a network of elastic fibers that extend toward the intima of the vessel wall. The space between the valve and the vessel wall is called the sinus of the valve. The wall of the vessel becomes thinner and slightly expanded just above the attachment of each valve cusp. Only the medium-size veins have valves. Their main function is to ensure the antegrade flow of blood, peripheral to central and superficial to deep, and to prevent the backflow of blood away from the heart. In general, the small and large veins have no valves. Valves have a bicuspid structure and are more numerous in the veins of the lower extremity, where the force of gravity is the greatest. Venous valves have cuplike endothelial flaps, which fill when there is retrograde flow of blood. When filled, the valves completely block the lumen, preventing flow reversal and transference of pressure.

PHYSIOLOGY

The venous system has a large capacity, accounting for approximately two-thirds of the systemic blood. Veins, because of their unique vascular structure, can undergo a large change in volume with minimal change in transmural pressure. This characteristic is called venous capacitance.

Because of their low elastic tissue content and prominent collagen-composed adventitia, the veins are actually stiffer than arteries when they are compared at the same distending pressure. A person in a resting upright position has significantly elevated venous pressures at the level of the feet and calves, accumulating a large volume of blood in the lower extremities. In similar cases, the calf muscles magnify the venous return by working as a pump system. During walking or exercise, calf muscle contraction pushes the accumulated blood toward the heart, decreasing the venous pressures close to zero. The venous pressure remains low even during calf muscle relaxation. At this time, the venous valves come into play, preventing the backflow of blood but allowing the inflow of blood to refill the system. It is imperative that the vein valves be competent for this pump system to work appropriately. The calf muscle pump works most efficiently when all venous valves are competent. A normal pump system reduces venous pressures and volume in the exercising muscle, increases venous return, and improves arterial perfusion.

VARICOSE VEINS

Incompetent valves in the saphenous system permit reflux of blood from the central veins to the peripheral veins. As the vein dilates because of an excessive volume of blood, each valve becomes incompetent. This valve incompetence occurs in the deep and superficial systems, creating a standing column of blood with a constant increase in pressure transmitted through the systems and resulting in varicose veins.

CHRONIC VENOUS DISEASE

Chronic venous insufficiency is a significant problem in the United States, affecting as much as a quarter of the population. Venous valve incompetence is central to the underlying venous hypertension that appears to underlie most or all signs of chronic venous disease. Chronic venous disease affects a younger segment of the population; the resulting morbidity of edema, leg pain, and ulceration may then lead to lifestyle alterations, loss of work, and frequent hospitalizations. The prevalence of venous ulcerations is not restricted to the elderly but certainly increases with age.[1] It has been estimated that venous ulcers have had a major negative economic impact, with the loss of approximately 2 million working days and treatment costs of approximately $3 billion per year in the United States.[2] The chief clinical manifestations of chronic venous disease are aching, leg pain, heaviness, a sensation of swelling, itching, cramps, and restless legs. Chronic venous disease can be graded according to the descriptive clinical, etiological, anatomical, and pathophysiological (CEAP) classification, which provides an orderly framework for communication and decision making[3] (Table 43-1). The pathophysiology of chronic venous disease in regard to its clinical expression has been well described, involving venous valve incompetence, structural changes in the vein wall (manifest as hypertrophy), and the role of elevated venous pressure and shear stress.[4] There has been much newer work in understanding the pathophysiology of the skin changes of chronic venous disease. These studies have emerged to validate that chronic inflammation has a key role in the skin changes of chronic venous disease. Support for the role of chronic inflammation in chronic venous disease has come to be known as the microvascular leukocyte-trapping hypothesis, where elegant studies have shown elevated numbers of macrophages, T lymphocytes, and mast cells in skin biopsy specimens from lower limbs affected by chronic venous disease.[5] The chronic inflammatory state in patients with chronic venous disease is related to the skin changes typical of the condition.[4] Increased expression and activity of metalloproteinase (MMP, especially MMP2) has been reported in lipodermatosclerosis,[6] venous leg ulcers,[7] and wound fluid from nonhealing ulcers.[8] The treatment of chronic venous disease is beyond the scope of this chapter but would be aimed at preventing venous hypertension, venous reflux, and chronic inflammation (Fig. 43-1). Compression stockings and devices are certainly the mainstay of controlling venous hypertension. New endovenous ablation procedures utilizing laser energy or radiofrequency are available to treat venous reflux. Clinical research is now being actively pursued seeking pharmacotherapy to alleviate the chronic inflammatory state of chronic venous disease, particularly targeting the interaction of leukocytes and endothelial cells.

◼ Central Venous Stenosis

Superior vena cava (SVC) syndrome is a serious disorder resulting from impeded venous return from the upper body; it is caused by obstruction of the SVC. The symptoms include severe congestion and edema of the face, arms, and upper thorax and may progress to dyspnea, cognitive dysfunction, and headache. A clinical classification system that helps to classify the severity of symptoms (Table 43-2) has

TABLE 43-1	Revised Clinical Classification of Chronic Venous Disease of the Leg*	
Class	**Definition**	**Comments**
C$_0$	No visible or palpable signs of venous disease	
C$_2$	Telangiectasis, reticular veins, malleolar flare	Telangiectasis defined by dilated intradermal venules <1 mm in diameter Reticular veins defined by dilated, nonpalpable, subdermal veins ≤3 mm in diameter
C$_2$	Varicose veins	Dilated, palpable subcutaneous veins generally >3 mm in diameter
C$_3$	Edema without skin changes	
C$_4$	Skin changes ascribed to venous disease	
C$_{4A}$		Pigmentation, venous eczema, or both
C$_{4B}$		Lipodermatosclerosis, atrophie blanche, or both
C$_5$	Skin changes with healed ulceration	
C$_6$	Skin changes with active ulceration	

*Chronic Venous Disease grading system based on descriptive clinical, etiological, anatomical, and pathophysiological classification scheme.

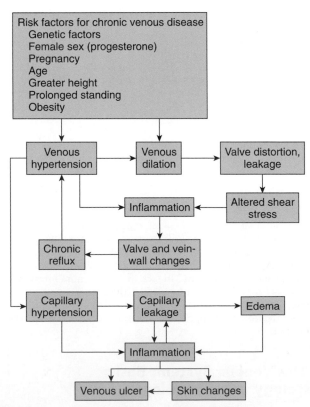

Figure 43-1 Venous hypertension as the hypothetical cause of the clinical manifestations of chronic venous disease, emphasizing the importance of inflammation.

TABLE 43-2	Clinical Scoring System for Central Venous Stenosis	
Signs and Symptoms		**Grade**
Neurologic symptoms		
Stupor, coma, blackout		4
Blurry vision, headache, dizziness, amnesia		3
Changes in mentation		2
Uneasiness		1
Laryngotracheal or thoracic symptoms		
Orthopnea, laryngeal edema		3
Stridor, hoarseness, dysphagia, shortness of breath		2
Cough, pleural effusion		1
Nasal and facial signs or symptoms		
Lip edema, nasal stiffness, epistaxis, rhinorrhea		2
Facial swelling		1
Venous dilation		
Neck vein or arm vein distension, upper extremity swelling or upper body plethora		1

Modified from Kish K, Sonomura T, Mitsuzane K, et al. Self expandable metallic stent therapy for superior vena cava syndrome: clinical observations. *Radiology.* 1993;189:531-535.

been used by several clinicians. The SVC syndrome is usually caused by obstruction, extrinsic or intrinsic, of the SVC, although bilateral obstruction of both brachiocephalic venous segments can result in a similar syndrome. Compression caused by mediastinal malignancy or lymphadenopathy is the most common cause of SVC syndrome.[9] The syndrome can also result from extension of central deep venous thrombosis (DVT) to the SVC, usually in the presence of bilateral subclavian vein stenosis. Other benign etiologies include (1) thrombosis caused by underlying stenosis from long-term indwelling central venous catheters or other transvenous instruments and (2) benign compressive or constrictive conditions of the mediastinum, such as adenopathy from earlier histoplasmosis, fibrosing mediastinitis, previous irradiation, tuberculosis, and histiocytosis.[10–14]

DIAGNOSIS OF CENTRAL VENOUS STENOSIS

The clinical presentation of SVC syndrome is relatively consistent and can be verified with multiple diagnostic modalities. Computed tomography (CT) is helpful for the workup of SVC syndrome and often gives enough information to proceed directly to an endovascular procedure.[15] An upper extremity venogram will reveal multiple collaterals if the obstruction is of long standing. With acute SVC obstruction, however, there are often surprisingly few collaterals. In most cases, the venogram will demonstrate the level of involvement, but it can still overestimate the length of involvement of the innominate veins and even the SVC because of the high resistance to flow. Magnetic resonance imaging (MRI) is helpful for the evaluation of SVC syndrome, and procedure planning can be based solely on MRI findings.[16] MRI will give good information regarding the extent of occlusion and collateral flow. Ultrasound, on the other hand, is not accurate in locating the central obstruction. The Doppler signal will raise a suspicion of obstruction because of the flattened character of the waveform, but the level of obstruction is difficult or impossible to estimate with ultrasound, especially in the central portion of the SVC. Ultrasound with Doppler can, however, be a useful tool for follow-up after endovascular repair. Obstructive changes in the waveform will raise suspicion of recurrent narrowing or occlusion of the recanalized vessel.

TECHNIQUE

Endovascular therapy has emerged as first-line treatment for central vein stenosis.[17] It is important to have a plan of approach before attempting SVC recanalization or stent placement. Taking into account the patient's clinical presentation and preprocedural noninvasive imaging is essential to a successful outcome. Many operators have used femoral vein access, but others have used jugular, subclavian,[18] and arm vein access or even transhepatic venous approaches for stent delivery.[19] One may use any combination of these approaches, but it is always paramount to have a guidewire "through and through," especially when stenoses are severe and difficult to pass.[20,21] It certainly adds to the safety of the procedure to have a guidewire passing the right atrium into the inferior vena cava (IVC) during stent delivery and dilation. This is particularly important in preventing stent migration. This guidewire position will prevent the stent from migrating into the right side of the heart or pulmonary artery. The stent is thus more likely to stay on the wire and can be more safely manipulated, removed, or moved to a different location. Accessing the SVC from the right internal jugular vein or upper extremity veins has several benefits. Manipulation is easier because of the limited space in the internal jugular vein compared with the right atrium, which one has to work through in coming from a femoral vein access. The distance from the access site to the obstruction is also shorter, which can make it easier to cross chronic total occlusions. An upper extremity access, as via the brachial or basilic vein, is also a viable option. The entire venous intervention can be performed from this access, including thrombolysis, angioplasty, and stent placement in most cases.[22] This is also comfortable and well tolerated by most patients. Hemostasis is not usually problematic, placing a pressure dressing for 20 minutes or holding pressure for 5 to 10 minutes is usually successful. If double-barrel stenting is required to treat the SVC, bilateral upper extremity access is ideal, with the stents each traversing the brachiocephalic veins. Several operators advocate using the common femoral vein for access, but it may be difficult to access an occluded or severely narrowed SVC from the femoral vein because of its anatomical relationship with the right atrium.[23,24] Some operators have therefore crossed the obstruction from the brachial veins, creating a through-and through access from the femoral vein by snaring the wire and pulling it through the femoral vein.[25] In addition, double-barrel stents into each of the brachiocephalic veins can be easily placed from a bilateral common femoral vein access

There is some experience in performing thrombolytic therapy prior to SVC stent placement as well as in conjunction with it. Isolated pharmacomechanical thrombolysis plus primary stenting is a combined procedure that opens an acutely thrombosed superior vena cava rapidly to alleviate symptoms in seriously ill patients with SVC syndrome. O'Sullivan[26] reported a case series where all patients received isolated pharmacomechanical thrombolysis with tissue plasminogen activator delivered in a Trellis Peripheral Infusion System (Bacchus Vascular, Santa Clara, CA) that removed obstructive clots in minutes versus the 24 to 48 hours required for traditional catheter-directed thrombolysis. In each patient, stents were deployed immediately following pharmacomechanical thrombolysis in a combined procedure lasting less than 1 hour. In the appropriate clinical setting, thrombolysis for SVC syndrome prior to endovascular therapy may have great utility. By resolving the acute thrombus, one need only stent the underlying stenosis, which most of the time is shorter than the occluded segment that was occupied by thrombus. Therefore a shorter segment of vessel has to be stented, thus reducing the number of stents utilized and ultimately also reducing the potential thrombogenic stent surface. Gray, et al.[27] reviewed the outcomes from thrombolysis of SVC thrombus in 16 patients; they had no major complications and complete success in 56% without stents. Thrombolysis was effective in 73%. Stents were not used in any of the patients, which may explain many of the poor clinical outcomes. Many patients with SVC syndrome have central venous catheters in place, on which they are dependent. Numerous reports describe pulling the catheters up from the SVC during the procedure and then placing the catheter down through the stent immediately after the procedure.[28]

STENT SELECTION

Early reports of SVC stenting described the use of Gianturco (Cook, Incorporated, Bloomington, IN) stents. This was the first

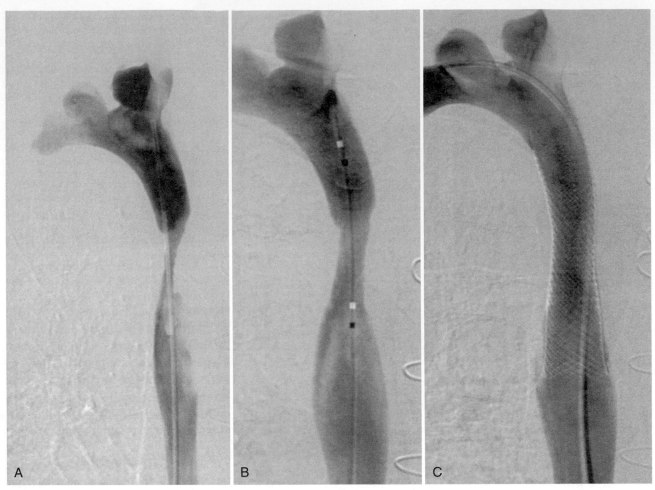

Figure 43-2 **A.** Venogram of significant SVC stenosis. **B.** Venogram of SVC after 12-mm PTA. **C.** Venogram after 14-mm WALLSTENT. *(Boston Scientific, Natick, MA.)*

self-expanding stent in wide use and had diameters that were acceptable. There were few complications reported, but large sheath introducers are required for this stent, and it is used only in cases where inflow vessels must be covered because of the large spaces between the stent's interstices. Next, the Palmaz stent (Cordis Corporation, Miami, FL) was released for use. This stent is balloon-expandable and is now rarely used in the SVC. It has a higher radial force than self-expanding stents and, on occasion, when extra radial force is needed, can be used either primarily or secondarily within a deployed self-expanding stent that cannot sustain the radial force of SVC recoil. In today's era of endovascular therapy, self-expanding stent delivery systems are used mainly for SVC stenting (Fig. 43-2).[29,30] The newer self-expanding stent delivery systems are easily deployed and come on a small 6- to 7-Fr delivery system. The WALLSTENT (Boston Scientific Corporation, Natick, MA) was one of the earlier versions of a self-expanding stent and is still widely used for SVC intervention. Its main shortcoming is that it foreshortens significantly on delivery, which makes precise placement difficult. Recent generations of self-expanding stents are made of nitinol and do not have this problem. A few examples of self-expanding nitinol stents include the Smart Stent (Cordis Corporation, Miami, FL), Luminex (Angiomed/Bard, Karlsruhe, Germany), and Zilver (Cook Incorporated, Bloomington, IN). For the SVC, a stent 12 to 16 mm in diameter is usually adequate.

COMPLICATIONS

In a group of 59 patients with malignant disease, Lanciego reported 6 reocclusions, all of which were treated successfully with restenting in

combination with thrombolysis.[31] One of the patients in this series had stent migration to the right atrium, which was successfully treated.

Hemopericardium has been reported by several operators in the literature. This complication most commonly occurs during the procedure itself or immediately after stent placement,[32] but delayed bleeding into the pericardium has also been described.[33] The pericardial reflection can extend very high in the mediastinum, and the position is unpredictable.[34] In this regard, it is advisable to place stents high in the SVC without compromising clinical results. If there is a high index of suspicion for hemopericardium, an echocardiogram or right heart catherization should be done immediately.

Deep Venous Thrombosis of the Upper Extremity

Upper extremity deep vein thrombosis (UEDVT) is an increasingly important clinical condition with potential consequenes of significant morbidity and mortality. Subclinical pulmonary embolism may be present in 33% of patients with a UEDVT, but clinical pulmonary embolysis is detected in only 4% of such patients undergoing ventilation/perfusion scanning.[35] The venous pathway of the upper limb is less likely to develop a DVT compared with the lower limb because of the relatively high rate of blood flow, gravitational effects, and lack of stasis.

Traditionally named after Paget and von Shroetter, UEDVT was typically regarded as a rare and benign condition. As available case reports and literature grew in the 1990s, UEDVT was increasingly seen as a more common and less benign disease potentially leading to serious complications, such as pulmonary embolism (PE), postthrombotic syndrome, and mortality.[36–38] This change of view regarding UEDVT can certainly be explained by a higher degree of clinical awareness and the increased effectiveness and availability of noninvasive diagnostic techniques.[39–41] Primary UEDVT is a rare disorder (2 per 100,000 persons per year)[42] that refers either to effort thrombosis (Paget-Schroetter syndrome) or idiopathic UEDVT. Patients with Paget-Schroetter syndrome develop spontaneous UEDVT, usually in the dominant arm, after strenuous activity such as rowing, wrestling, weight lifting, or baseball pitching, but they are otherwise young and healthy.[43] The heavy exertion causes microtrauma to the vessels' intima and leads to activation of the coagulation cascade. Significant thrombosis may occur with repeated insults to the vein wall, especially if mechanical compression of the vessel is also present.[44] Thoracic outlet syndrome involves compression of the neurovascular bundle (brachial plexus, subclavian artery, subclavian vein) as it exits the thoracic inlet.[45] Although this disorder may initially cause intermittent positional extrinsic vein compression, repeated trauma to the vessel can result in the formation of dense perivascular fibrous scar tissue that will persistently compress the vein.[45] Compression of the subclavian vein typically develops in young athletes with hypertrophied muscles who do heavy lifting or completely abduct their arms. Cervical ribs, long transverse processes of the cervical spine, musculofacial bands, and clavicular or first rib anomalies are sometimes found in these patients. Therefore plain films of the cervical spine and chest should be obtained in all patients undergoing evaluation for thoracic outlet syndrome.[45] Presenting signs and symptoms of UEDVT can be found in Table 43-3. Secondary UEDVT is associated with both exogenous and endogenous risk factors and usually develops in older, ill patients, with a slight preference for females.[46] Among exogenous risk factors, the positioning of central venous lines, malignancy, previous or actual episodes of lower extremity DVT, treatment with oral contraceptives, and trauma appear to have the highest impact on the development of UEDVT. Patients with indwelling central venous catheters constitute a particularly high-risk population, especially when undergoing chemotherapy, invasive hemodynamic monitoring, chronic parenteral nutrition, hemodialysis, or transvenous pacing, with a more than 60% prevalence of either symptomatic or asymptomatic UEDVT.[47–49] In fact, ipsilateral catheter-related UEDVT accounts for up to 70% of all cases of secondary UEDVT.[46] Malignancy, either overt or undiagnosed, is also frequently associated with UEDVT (more than 40% of cases).[50] Recent data indicate that occult malignancy, especially lung cancer and lymphomas, may be discovered during follow-up in up to 24% of patients with UEDVT, mostly during the first week of hospital admission.[51] A history of previous episodes or an ongoing deep venous thrombosis of the lower extremities is associated with UEDVT in up to 18% of cases.[46] In an ultrasound surveillance study, nearly 30% of high-risk trauma patients developed UEDVT during the course of hospitalization; this may be asymptomatic in up to 30% of such cases.[52] Treatment with oral contraceptives may also represent a significant risk factor in females (up to 14%), although the data are conflicting.[53] Infrequently, UEDVT arises in carriers of peripheral venous catheters, generally from a superficial phlebitis spreading to the deep venous system,[49] or is associated with intravenous drug abuse, especially of cocaine.[54] The prevalence of hypercoaguable states in patients with UEDVT is uncertain because observational studies report varying results.[55] Furthermore, screening for coagulation disorders is controversial and has never been shown to be cost-effective.[56] The yield of these tests is highest for patients with idiopathic UEDVT, a family history of DVT, a history of recurrent unexplained pregnancy loss, or a personal history of a prior DVT.

DIAGNOSTIC TESTING

The gold standard for the diagnosis of UEDVT, which involves direct imaging of the whole deep venous system of the arm, is contrast venography. This is balanced by its invasive nature, inconvenience for patients, and technical difficulty in performance and interpretation; it may also induce contrast dye-related allergic reactions and thrombosis. Several noninvasive methods are now available as alternatives to contrast venography; these are highlighted below.

Contrast Venography

Contrast venography is the standard reference for the diagnosis of UEDVT. Ideally, contrast injections should be made into medial antecubital veins or more distally (in the back of the hand, for instance). This will guarantee adequate opacification of the brachial, axillary, and subclavian veins. Hand injections should be used preferentially over power injection to reduce the risk of serious contrast extravasation. A common pitfall of contrast venography is nonfilling of the cephalic segment; isolated thrombosis of this venous segment could then go unnoticed. It is essential to perform one series of the SVC during a single breath-hold. Contrast venography may not be feasible in up to 20% of patients due to the inaccessibility of arm veins and contraindications for contrast agents, such as renal failure and hypersensitivity.

Despite some apparent disadvantages, venography may be required to confirm the diagnosis of UEDVT if suspicion for thrombosis remains high despite a negative noninvasive test. Venography is also required as a prelude to endovascular intervention and is used to assess response to these treatments, including thrombolytic therapy.

Duplex Ultrasonography

Duplex ultrasound has largely replaced invasive venography for the diagnosis of DVT. It has many positive features, which include no requirement for nephrotoxic contrast agents, noninvasiveness, and no need for ionizing radiation. In addition, it is widely available and can be performed at the bedside. Duplex ultrasonography has high sensitivity and specificity for peripheral (jugular, distal subclavian, axillary) UEDVT.[57] Acoustic shadowing from the clavicle, however, will limit visualization of a segment of subclavian vein and may result in a false-negative study.[58] Some technical recommendations regarding the use of duplex ultrasonography for the diagnosis of UEDVT would include employing a combination of real-time compression gray-scale ultrasonography, color Doppler, and flow measurements using duplex technique with a 7.5-MHz linear-array probe. In considering the diagnosis of UEDVT utilizing duplex ultrasonography, the definition of thrombosis is critical. It is widely accepted that noncompressibility of a venous segment with or without visible thrombus constitutes thrombosis. There is also a building body of evidence regarding isolated flow abnormalities which turn out to be crucial, as the entire venous system

TABLE 43-3	Signs and Symptoms of Deep Venous Thrombosis of the Upper Extremity*	
	Symptoms	*Signs*
Axillary or subclavian vein thrombosis	Vague shoulder or neck discomfort Arm or hand edema	Supraclavicular fullness Palpable cord Arm or hand edema Extremity cyanosis Diluted cutaneous veins Jugular venous distention Unable to access central venous catheter
Thoracic outlet syndrome	Pain radiating to arm/forearm Hand weakness	Brachial plexus tenderness Arm or hand atrophy Positive Adson's† or Wright's‡ maneuver

*These are nonspecific and may be recognized with provocative maneuvers.

†Adson's maneuver: The examiner extends the patient's arm on the affected side while the patient extends the neck and rotates the head toward the same side. The test is positive if there is weakening of the radial pulse with deep inspiration and suggests compression of the subclavian artery.

‡Wright's maneuver: The patient's shoulder is abducted and the humerus externally rotated. The test is positive if symptoms are reproduced and there is weakening of the radial pulse.

of the upper extremity cannot be followed beyond the clavicle.[58] These flow abnormalities seen on duplex ultrasound are only suggestive of thrombosis, and contrast venography should be considered if there is a high clinical index of suspicion. No studies have specifically addressed interobserver and intraobserver variability, but it is a widely known fact that ultrasonography is operator-dependent in clinical practice and that some patients may be more difficult to investigate, such as those who are obese or have very extensive edema.

Magnetic Resonance Imaging

Magnetic resonance venography is an accurate, noninvasive method of detecting thrombus in the central chest veins, such as the SVC and brachiocephalic veins. Magnetic resonance venography (MRV) will provide a complete evaluation of central collaterals, central veins, and blood-flow patterns. The correlation with traditional contrast venography is very good; therefore MRV is a valuable imaging modality for the diagnosis of UEDVT when contrast venography is contraindicated or impossible. The increased use of pacemakers and internal defibrillators does not make this imaging modality completely uniform, as these devices contra-indicate the use of MRI.

Computed Tomography Venography

As CT technology evolves with the recent use of multidetector CT equipment, where coronal and sagittal slice reformation and three-dimensional reconstruction are possible, this imaging modality will likely play an important role in managing patients with UEDVT. One major advantage of CT venography is the ability to assess for the presence of pulmonary emboli and other etiologies for upper extremity complaints during the same imaging session. Comparative studies that will evaluate the correlation of CT venography with digital subtraction venography are under way for the diagnosis of UEDVT.

TREATMENT OPTIONS

The optimal approach for the treatment of UEDVT remains unknown, but in general it has two goals: first, to prevent further propagation of thrombi and thus reduce the risk of secondary events, such as pulmonary embolus or disease recurrence, and second, to preserve the normal venous anatomy by recanalizing the existing thrombus in some way. It is quite likely that henceforth more patients with UEDVT will be approached with a multimodal effort. These treatment options will include either individually or in combination anticoagulant therapy, thrombolytic therapy, endovascular intervention, and/or vascular surgery.

Anticoagulation

Anticoagulation is the mainstay of therapy for UEDVT. Anticoagulation helps maintain the patency of venous collaterals and reduces thrombus propagation even if the clot does not completely resolve.[59] Unfortunately, anticoagulation rarely achieves recanalization, thus leading to permanent obstruction of the upper extremity's veins. Collateral veins often develop, but these are not accessible for the placement of intravenous lines. Typically, standard anticoagulation includes unfractionated heparin or low-molecular-weight heparin for 5 to 7 days, as a "bridge" to oral warfarin. Warfarin is typically continued for a minimum of 3 months, with a goal international normalized ratio (INR) of 2.0 to 3.0. A longer duration of warfarin anticoagulation may be indicated if some form of coagulation abnormality is detected.

Thrombolytic Therapy

Because many patients with UEDVT are young, active, and healthy, thrombolytic therapy rather than conservative anticoagulation should be considered strongly on a case-to-case basis. Certainly, a young, healthy patient with UEDVT may have significant long-term morbidity if treated with anticoagulation only.[60] In this regard, thrombolysis restores venous patency early, minimizes damage to the vessels' endothelium, and reduces the risk of long-term complications, especially the development of postthrombotic syndrome, with its disabling chronic aching and swelling of the arm and hand. The obvious disadvantage of thrombolytic therapy is the greater risk of a bleeding complication. The ideal candidate for thrombolytic therapy for UEDVT would be an otherwise healthy young patient with a primary UEDVT. In addition, those patients with indwelling central venous catheters that are essential to maintain patency for central venous access should also be considered for this intervention.

Results from a large series of patients with UEDVT who were treated with catheter-directed thrombolysis showed that treatment restored venous drainage, with a subsequent low frequency of mild postthrombotic syndrome at follow-up.[61] No intracerebral bleeding, clinical pulmonary embolism, or death occurred during treatment.[61] Thrombolysis has the best chance of success if used within 4 to 6 weeks of the onset of symptoms, as older, organized thrombus is more resistant to thrombolysis. In performing catheter-directed thrombolysis, the catheter should be placed directly within the entire length of thrombus; otherwise the potential for collateral circulation to divert drug distribution away from the thrombus may lead to an unsuccessful procedure. There are no randomized prospective controlled clinical trials comparing different thrombolytic agents for treating UEDVT. At our tertiary referral center, catheter-directed retavase (rPA) is usually administered at 0.25 to 0.5 U/hr for 8 hours. Clinical examination and serial venography are used to assess response to treatment. We often employ a percutaneous mechanical thrombectomy device in combination with thrombolytic therapy. This adjunctive catheter-based thrombectomy has the benefit of extracting thrombus before thrombolytic therapy, which often initiates some blood flow, thereby improving drug distribution and reducing both the dose of drug and the duration of thrombolytic therapy.[62] A complete description of percutaneous mechanical thrombectomy devices can be found below, in the discussion of lower extremity DVT. The time to achieve complete thrombolysis in subclavian vein thrombosis can take up to 72 hours. Oral anticoagulation, such as warfarin, should be utilized for 3 to 6 months following successful thrombolysis for UEDVT. Certainly the duration of warfarin therapy should be individualized on a case-by-case basis depending on the clinical situation.

Interventional Therapy

Catheter-based mechanical thrombectomy is an important adjunct to thrombolytic therapy, as stated above. It is theoretically advantageous, since instant debulking or removal of thrombus and thereby restoration of flow is highly beneficial prior to catheter-directed thrombolysis. As a result, drug distribution is improved and both dose of drug and duration of thrombolytic therapy are decreased. Adjunctive percutaneous transluminal angioplasty (PTA) or stenting of the subclavian vein has utility, especially for catheter-related stenosis, when there is a hemodynamically significant pressure gradient following thrombolytic therapy. A flexible self-expanding oversized stent is best suited for this location. Intravascular ultrasound has proven to be very useful in determining stent sizing in the treatment of subclavian vein stenosis. Figure 43-3 demonstrates catheter-directed thrombolysis for a left subclavian DVT followed by adjunctive PTA.

Surgical Therapy

Vein compression in patients with primary UEDVT represents an important cause of recurrent thrombosis and long-term morbidity.[63] It is paramount, after successful treatment of an acute UEDVT, that some form of imaging be undertaken to evaluate for the presence of vein compression. Following successful thrombolysis, venography in the neutral and shoulder abducted position can help demonstrate vein compression. Recent surgical series recommend surgical correction of extrinsic vein compression,[63] which typically requires resection of part of the first rib or clavicle. Lysis of adhesions around the subclavian vein may also be required if anatomical anomalies have caused chronic, repeated trauma to the subclavian vein. Today, surgical thrombectomy is rarely required owing to advancements in pharmacological and catheter-based therapies. However, in symptomatic patients who are refractory to other therapies, surgical thrombectomy can restore

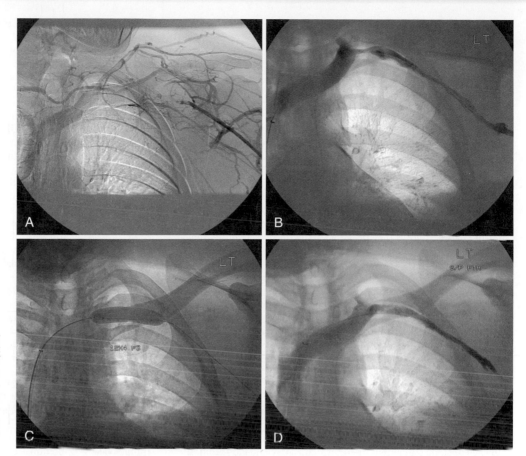

Figure 43-3 A. Left upper extremity venogram demonstrating acute left subclavian vein DVT. **B.** Placement of infusion catheter into left subclavian vein thrombus. **C.** Following thrombolysis, PTA of left subclavian vein with 12-mm balloon. **D.** Completion venogram of left subclavian vein following successful catheter directed thrombolysis with adjunctive PTA.

venous patency. Treatment of UEDVT is aimed at the preservation of venous anatomy, prevention of potentially fatal PE, and reduction of the risk of postphlebitic syndrome. Treatment is dependent on the cause and duration of thrombosis and the clinical circumstances. For the majority of patients with UEDVT, anticoagulation with an antithrombin agent followed by 3 to 6 months of oral anticoagulation is usually sufficient. However, there is a tendency to be more aggressive with thrombolytic therapy and catheter-based thrombectomy in individual cases, especially in younger patients who are at risk of chronic venous insufficiency or in an effort to minimize long-term morbidity and optimize functionality. A structured physical therapy program to loosen muscles compressing the subclavian vein and weight loss if indicated are other important adjuncts to complete therapy.

Deep Venous Thrombosis of the Lower Extremity

DVT is a process that can affect each one of the deep veins of the body, but it is more frequently present in the deep veins of the lower extremity. Venous thrombus formation is initiated by intravascular clotting and is increased in the presence of risk factors. These risk factors were postulated more than 100 years ago by Virchow and are summarized by his classic triad of coagulation abnormalities, endothelial damage, and stasis. The main conditions contributing to the formation of venous thrombus in the deep veins of the legs are related to these three basic risk factors; they include advanced age, prolonged bed rest, and major surgery. In particular, surgery that involves large abdominal operations (especially orthopedic surgery), previous venous thrombosis, malignancy, trauma, varicose veins, chronic venous insufficiency, pregnancy and the postpartum period, contraceptive pills, and hypercoagulable states, either primary or secondary. The main complications of lower extremity DVT are pulmonary embolism and postthrombotic syndrome (PTS). Clinical pulmonary embolism occurs in

26% to 67% of the cases of untreated proximal DVT and is associated with a mortality rate of 11% to 23% if not treated. Under treatment, the incidence of pulmonary embolism decreases to 5%, and the mortality to less than 1%. PTS, however, is a cause of increased morbidity and disability. Up to two-thirds of patients with ileofemoral DVT develop edema and pain, with 5% developing ulcers in spite of adequate anticoagulation.[6] Early diagnosis and treatment of DVT are essential to minimize the mortality and morbidity due to pulmonary embolism and PTS.

DIAGNOSIS OF ACUTE DEEP VENOUS THROMBOSIS OF THE LOWER EXTREMITY

Venous Duplex Ultrasound

The clinical diagnosis of lower extremity DVT (LEDVT) is notoriously inaccurate, with the classic signs and symptoms of DVT being as common in patients without DVT as they are in those with confirmed DVT. Objective confirmation of clinically suspected DVT is therefore required. Despite its many limitations, as noted earlier, ascending venography historically has been the "gold standard" for the diagnosis of acute DVT. It is invasive, not easily repeatable, impossible to perform or interpret in 9% to 14% of patients, fails to visualize all venous segments in 10% to 30% of studies, and may be associated with interobserver disagreements in 4% to 10% of studies. Therefore, not surprisingly, venography has been replaced by venous duplex ultrasound as the most widely used diagnostic test for acute DVT. In comparison with venography, duplex ultrasound has the advantages of being widely available, noninvasive, portable, and easily repeatable. A complete ultrasound evaluation of the lower extremities includes an assessment of venous compressibility, intraluminal echoes, venous flow characteristics, and luminal color filling. Venous incompressibility, or failure to completely coapt the venous walls with gentle probe compression, is the most widely used diagnostic criterion for acute

DVT. Adjunctive gray-scale findings include the appearance of echogenic thrombus within the venous lumen and dilation of an acutely thrombosed segment. Normal flow in the proximal veins should be spontaneous and vary with respiration, increasing during expiration and decreasing during inspiration.

Other noninvasive imaging techniques for the diagnosis of LEDVT include magnetic resonance venography and computed tomography angiography. These modalities are comparable to conventional venography, but are not able to be done at the bedside, carry the risk of contrast allergy, and are more expensive than venous duplex ultrasound.

Diagnostic Testing and Clinical Risk Stratification

D-dimer, which is formed as a by-product in the degradation of crosslinked fibrin by plasmin, reflects thrombus and has been proposed as an alternative or adjunct to initial diagnostic testing. Although D-dimer is sensitive for the diagnosis of DVT, such measurements are nonspecific, and elevated levels may be associated with preeclampsia, malignancy, infection, trauma, or recent surgery. The high sensitivity of D-dimer measurements makes it theoretically possible to exclude a diagnosis of DVT; however, the low specificity and positive predictive value necessitate confirmatory noninvasive testing for positive results. A combined strategy using an assessment of clinical probability, D-dimer testing, and venous duplex ultrasound may hold the greatest diagnostic promise. This approach relies on observations that its negative predictive value approaches 100% in outpatients with a low pretest clinical probability for DVT.[64]

GOALS OF THERAPY

There are generally four accepted goals for the treatment of LEDVT. These treatment goals have expanded as our understanding of the pathophysiology of venous thromboembolism has evolved, coupled with the constant refinement of endovascular devices and thrombotic therapy. Therapy for LEDVT is undertaken to (1) diminish the severity and duration of lower extremity symptoms, (2) prevent pulmonary embolism, (3) minimize the risk of recurrent venous thrombosis, and (4) prevent the postthrombotic syndrome.

Detailed monographs regarding the medical management of LEDVT are numerous and readily available. There is uniform agreement that adequate initial anticoagulant therapy is required to prevent thrombus growth and pulmonary embolism. Intravenous unfractionated heparin is being replaced by low-molecular-weight heparin as the anticoagulant of choice for the initial treatment of LEDVT. Both agents are relatively safe and effective in this context, with low-molecular-weight heparin being suitable for outpatient therapy because of its improved bioavailability and more predictable anticoagulant response. Serious potential complications of heparin therapy, such as heparin-induced thrombocytopenia and osteoporosis, seem less common with low-molecular-weight heparin. Although medical therapy with anticoagulation is the mainstay of the initial management of LEDVT, many patients, particularly those with large proximal ileofemoral DVTs, have persistent leg edema, pain, and difficulty ambulating. These symptoms arise from venous hypertension caused by outflow obstruction. As relief of outflow obstruction is one of the primary goals of therapy for LEDVT, this, unfortunately, is not accomplished by anticoagulation alone, as thrombus regression occurs in only 50% of patients.[65] Therefore, with the evolution of endovascular techniques—including catheter-directed thrombolysis, mechanical thrombectomy, and stenting—there are now very viable options in treating and restoring the pathways of thrombosed veins.[66,67] The details of endovascular venous intervention—which are targeted to restore venous patency, preserve valvular function, and minimize the risk of late postthrombotic complications—are discussed below.

CATHETER-DIRECTED THROMBOLYSIS

In the early 1990s, Semba and Dake[68] first reported the feasibility of catheter-directed thrombolysis (CDT) for iliofemoral thrombosis as an alternative to systemic anticoagulation, systemic thrombolysis, or surgical venous thrombectomy. CDT, or the delivery of thrombolytic agents directly into the thrombus, offers significant advantages over systemic therapy, which may fail to reach and penetrate an occluded venous segment. Because thrombolytic agents activate plasminogen within the thrombus, the delivery of the drug to that site enhances its effectiveness. By focusing the delivery of higher concentrations of the drug, lysis rates can be improved, the duration of treatment reduced, and complications associated with the exposure of the patient to systemic thrombolytic therapy minimized. Following successful CDT, the implication is that preservation of valvular function and removal of the obstructing thrombus will facilitate a lower incidence of postthrombotic syndrome. In addition, this endovascular approach will allow for the detection and correction of any underlying venous obstructive lesions with balloon angioplasty and/or stents. Currently there are no thrombolytic agents that are approved for CDT by the U.S. Food and Drug Administration. The use of thrombolytic agents in CDT for venous thrombosis constitutes an "off label" use. There are five thrombolytic agents available in the United States that can be used during CDT for venous thrombosis. Although the various agents have unique properties that might theoretically imply one being superior to another, there is no peer-reviewed consensus on a superior or "best choice" agent for CDT for venous thrombosis. The literature on CDT for venous thrombosis includes few prospective randomized comparative trials. Therefore the choice of thrombolytic agent is generally individualized to the physician's discretion. The largest published experience with CDT has come from the National Venous Thrombolysis Registry,[68] which included 287 patients treated with urokinase and followed up for 1 year. Overall, 71% of the patients were treated for iliofemoral DVT. Complete dissolution of thrombus was achieved in 31% and partial thrombus dissolution was reported in an additional 52%. Primary patency at 1 year was 60%. Preservation of valvular competence was demonstrated in 72% of patients with complete thrombolysis. Table 43-4 reviews the available clinical experience with CDT for the treatment of DVT. The decision to perform CDT for LEDVT must be individualized to each case and the associated risk-benefit analysis. The technique of CDT for LEDVT is not standardized; however, the primary goal is to deliver the lytic agent directly into the venous clot.

The location of the LEDVT and the patient's symptoms determine the access technique. For most cases of iliofemoral DVT, the ipsilateral popliteal vein is favored if the clinical situation allows. With the patient prone on the angiographic table, the venous access site should be accessed under ultrasound guidance with a small-gauge echogenic needle. Should the popliteal vein be thrombosed, the ipsilateral posterior tibial vein can be cannulated. Following popliteal vein cannulation, a 5-Fr short sheath is then introduced, through which all subsequent catheters can be exchanged. Next, a baseline venogram is obtained utilizing the venous sheath, and then a combination of

TABLE 43-4	Single-Center Case Studies Supporting Catheter-Directed Thrombolysis for Deep Venous Thrombosis*			
Author	N	*Agent*	*Outcome*	Hemorrhage, %
Molina et al.	12	UK	95% lysis	0%
Comerota et al.	7	UK	71% lysis	0%
Semba and Dake	27	UK	92% lysis	0%
Bjarnason et al.	87	UK	86% lysis	6.9% major/14.9 % minor
Patel et al.	10	UK	100% lysis	0%
Ouriel et al.	11	r-PA	73% lysis	0%
Castenada et al.	25	r-PA	92% lysis	4%
Chang et al.	10	t-PA	90% lysis	0%
Horne et al.	10	t-PA	90% lysis	30% minor
Razavi et al.	36	TNK	83%	2.7 % major 8.3% minor

N, number of patients; UK, urokinase; R-PA, reteplase; t-PA, alteplase; TNK, tenecteplase.

*Series evaluating catheter-directed thrombolysis for deep venous thrombosis.

0.035-in. straight and curved glide wires are used to cross the occluded venous segment. Following wire and then catheter traversal of the occluded venous segment, venography is repeated to confirm the intraluminal position of the catheter. The catheter is then exchanged for a 5-Fr infusing coaxial system consisting of a proximal multiside-hole catheter and a distal infusion wire. It is essential to position the system directly into the thrombus in order to maximize plasminogen activation at the site of obstruction. Figure 43-4 illustrates the endovascular management of an acute DVT of the left common iliac vein. Patients are then monitored in the interventional recovery unit as the thrombolytic agent is infused. It is quite common, particularly with an extensive thrombus burden, for the duration of therapy to exceed 24 hours. Follow-up venography should be performed every 12 hours to assess and/or reposition the infusion catheter directly into any remaining thrombus. Weighing the risk versus the benefit of lytic therapy, the infusion should be continued until complete lysis is achieved.

In patients where venous patency has been restored and there is no underlying stenotic/occlusive lesion, thrombolysis is discontinued and anticoagulation initiated. Hemodynamically significant lesions that are uncovered in the iliac veins should be considered for endovascular stenting, although the long-term benefits of venous stenting are not known. However, if left untreated, a significant iliac vein stenosis appears to pose a significant risk for early rethrombosis. Indications for placement of an IVC filter during CDT for LEDVT fall within the same spectrum as indications for routine prophylactic IVC filters. The use of IVC filters during lower extremity venous thrombolysis has always been controversial because of the low incidence of complications that is seen when lysis is performed without filter protection. Since retrievable IVC filters have become available, we have been implementing them routinely in performing CDT for iliofemoral DVT (Fig. 43-5). This seems particularly reasonable in patients in whom the venogram defines a true "free-floating" iliac vein thrombus or in a patient with a documented pulmonary embolus and limited cardiopulmonary reserve for additional emboli. If an underlying stenosis following successful CDT is felt to be secondary to iliac vein compression, this typically does not respond to stand-alone angioplasty and stent deployment will be required. This iliac vein compression, or May-Thurner syndrome, involves extrinsic compression of the common iliac vein by the crossing iliac artery, generally on the left, at the iliocaval junction. Self-expanding stents are generally preferred because of their longitudinal flexibility and ability to conform to various venous configurations. Care should be exercised to avoid

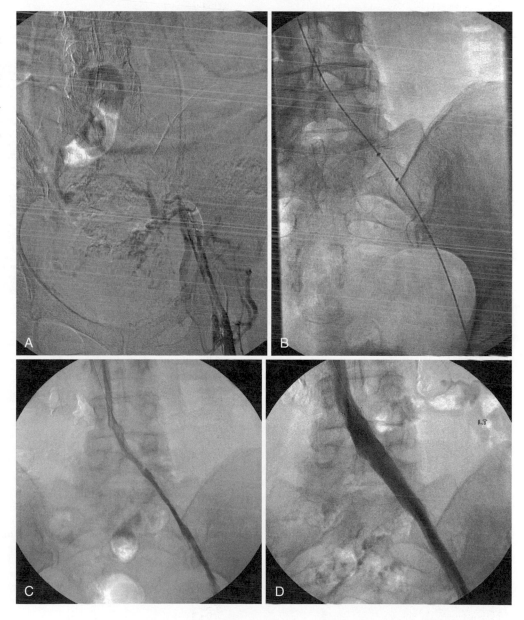

Figure 43-4 **A.** Thrombotic occlusion of left common and external iliac veins. **B.** Angiojet Expedior Catheter in left common iliac vein performing "pulse-spray" pharmacomechanical thrombolysis. MedRad, Inc. **C.** Venogram of left common and external iliac veins after 20-minute dwell time following pulse-spray technique. **D.** Final venogram of left common and external iliac vein status after deployment of 14 × 60 smart-control nitinol self-expanding stent. (*Cordis Corp., Miami, FL.*)

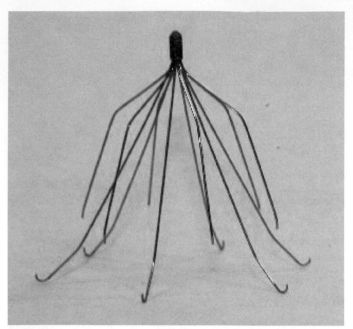

Figure 43-5   G2-X retrievable IVC filter, which has nitinol construction, utilized in IVCs of up to 28 mm. It is delivered via a 7-Fr delivery sheath. *(Bard Peripheral Vascular, Inc, Tempe, AZ.)*

stenting across the common femoral vein, particularly at the sapheno-femoral junction.

PERCUTANEOUS MECHANICAL THROMBECTOMY

Several issues surrounding CDT for LEDVT include the time to lysis, need for intensive care monitoring, hemorrhagic risks, cost, and lack of prospective randomized clinical trials. With these issues in mind, percutaneous mechanical thrombectomy (PMT) is conceptually attractive because such a technique may result in a shorter time to vein patency, shorter length of stay, reduction in hemorrhagic risk, and overall cost savings because of reduced hospitalization and the elimination or reduction in thrombolytic drugs. From a mechanistic standpoint, PMT devices can be categorized as rotational, hydrodynamic, or ultrasound-facilitated. Table 43-5 outlines current mechanical thrombectomy devices. In addition, the use of some of these PMT devices can incorporate the simultaneous administration of thrombolytic therapy, also know as pharmacomechanical thrombectomy. Rotational thrombectomy devices employ a high-speed rotating basket or impeller to pulverize or fragment the thrombus. Preclinical evaluation of these devices has focused on clot removal and assessment of potential valve injury. In one such study, the Arrow-Trerotola (Arrow, Research Triangle Park, NC) percutaneous thrombectomy device did not cause physiologically significant damage to valves 7 mm or larger in diameter.[69] However, because these rotational thrombectomy devices all have the potential to damage the endothelial lining of the vein, the Bacchus Fino device (Bacchus Vascular, Santa Clara, CA) uses a rotating Archimedes screw that is protected from vessel wall contact by a helically oriented nitinol framework. The screw fragments the thrombus, extracting much of it into a sheath through rotational motion. Hydrodynamic or "rheolytic" recirculation devices have become a common treatment modality for LEDVT. One of the PMT devices that have been shown to be effective in removal of acute thrombus is the AngioJet (MedRad, Inc., Pittsburgh, PA) system. The principle of this device is based on the venturi effect, which creates rapidly flowing saline jets that are directed backward from the tip of the device to outflow channels in a coaxial fashion. This generates a vacuum force that draws the thrombus into the catheter (Fig. 43-6). One major advantage of this PMT device is that the thrombectomy catheter can

TABLE 43-5	Mechanical Thrombectomy Devices
Wall-Contact Devices	
Arrow percutaneous thrombectomy device (PTD, Arrow International, Reading, PA)	
Solera (Bacchus Vascular, Santa Clara, CA)	
Cleaner (Rex Medical, Forth Worth, TX)	
MTI_Castaneda Brush (Microtherapeutics, San Clemente, CA)	
Fino (Bacchus Vascular, Santa Clara, CA)	
Cragg Brush (Microtherapeutics, San Clemente, CA)	
Prolumen (Datascope, Maheah, NJ)	
Hydrodynamic Thrombectomy Fragmentation Devices	
Amplatz thrombectomy device (ATD/Helix, Microvena, White Bear Lake, MN)	
Rotarex catheter (Straub Medical, Wangs, Switzerland)	
Thrombex PMT (Edwards Lifesciences, Irvine, CA)	
Rheolytic (Flow-Based) Thrombectomy	
AngioJet (Possis Medical, Minneapolis, MN)	
Oasis (Boston Scientific, Natick, MA)	
Hydrolyzer (Cordis, Warren, NJ)	

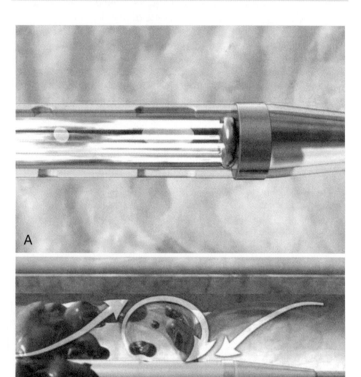

Figure 43-6   A. The AngioJet System emits high-velocity saline jets directed backward from the tip of the device to outflow channels in a coaxial function. **B.** This generates a vacuum force that draws the thrombus into the catheter. *(Possis Medical, Inc., Minneapolis, MN.)*

be delivered through a 6-Fr introducer sheath, which reduces access-site complications. Devices based on rheolytic recirculation might possibly produce less valvular or endothelial damage than PMT devices that employ rotational thrombectomy. A head-to-head comparative trial has not yet been performed comparing these two different mechanisms of thrombus removal. Examples of other rheolytic recirculation devices include the Hydrolyser (Cordis Corporation, Bridgewater, NJ) and the Oasis Thrombectomy System (Boston Scientific, Natick, MA). The hydrolyzer system utilizes a conventional contrast power injector to inject saline solution through an injection lumen. This resultant pressure reduction at the nozzle tip creates a 360-degree vortex that fragments and aspirates thrombus into an exhaust lumen. The thrombotic material is then discharged through the exhaust lumen into a collection bag. The Oasis Thrombectomy System operates in a similar fashion to the AngioJet, utilizing a venturi effect with thrombus fragmentation. However, the AngioJet System now has a "large vessel" catheter (DVX) that can extract a large amount of thrombus. Using "wall contact" mechanical thrombectomy devices in patients with symptomatic lower extremity DVT, Shi et al.[67] demonstrated an 89% technical success rate, with high patency rates during a mean follow-up period of 13 months. Despite great advances in PMT technologies, complete thrombus resolution rarely occurs; this often requires adjunctive thrombolytic therapy. In an effort to improve on complete thrombus resolution, an ultrasound-based infusion system, Lysus Infusion System (EKOS Corporation, Bothell, WA), has been developed. It combines high-frequency low-power ultrasound with simultaneous catheter-directed thrombolytics to accelerate clot dissolution. The exposure of nonfragmenting ultrasound to thrombus has no lytic effect on it own. However, the combination of directed ultrasound with local lytic infusion accelerates the thrombolytic process.[70] The mechanism for accelerated thrombolysis is that the delivery of high-frequency low-power ultrasound loosens the fibrin matrix to increase clot permeability and drive the thrombolytic agent deep into the thrombus for better drug distribution. In addition, the ultrasound energy will penetrate venous valves and facilitate clearing of thrombus associated with them. The EKOS System consists of a 5.2-Fr multilumen drug-delivery catheter with one central lumen and three separate infusion ports (Fig. 43-7). Each catheter has a matched ultrasound core wire that is placed in the central lumen to deliver the ultrasound energy evenly along the entire infusion pathway. After the catheter is positioned in the thrombus, an infusion of lytic agent is started, along with saline to serve as a coolant. Ultrasound is then started and delivered simultaneously with the infusion of lytic agent. In a multicenter series of 53 patients, ultrasound-accelerated thrombolysis was shown to be a safe and effective treatment for DVT with a high incidence of complete lysis and a reduction in bleeding rates.[71] Pharmacomechanical thrombectomy, or the simultaneous administration of thrombolytics during PMT, represents true combination therapy. This form of PMT has been reported with the AngioJet (MedRad, Inc.) and Trellis (Bacchus Vascular) devices. In a small series, Uppot et al.[72] reported a technique mixing the thrombolytic drug in the AngioJet Saline Infusion Bag for direct administration during PMT. In 24 patients, complete or substantial thrombus removal was achieved. With more experience, this technique was refined to develop the Power Pulse Technique, which has become very user-friendly with the new Angiojet catheter console (MedRad, Inc.) (Fig. 43-8). After delivery of the lytic

agent throughout the thrombus, up to 30 to 45 minutes are allowed to elapse, permitting maximal lytic time. After this period, the AngioJet is activated in a normal fashion, with the outflow port open to promote aspiration of thrombus. Two contemporary series utilizing pharmacomechanical thrombectomy or pulse-spray techniques both report high technical success rates with acceptable safety and long-term improved functional outcomes.[73,74] The Bacchus Trellis (Bacchus Vascular, Santa Clara, CA) consists of a catheter with proximal and distal occlusion balloons (Fig. 43-9), and a sheath designed to aspirate

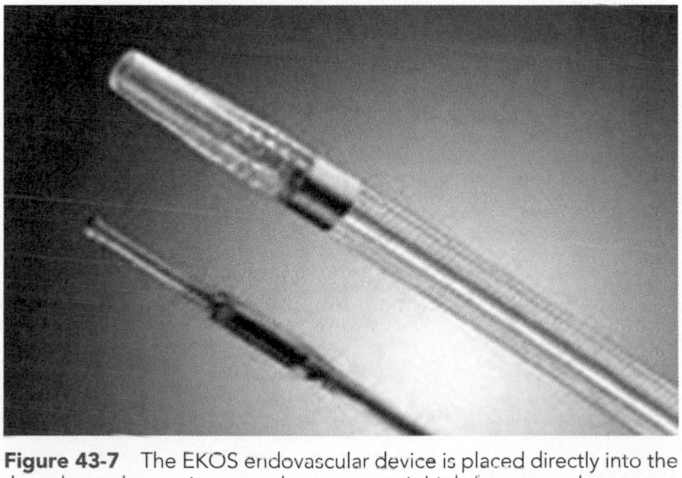

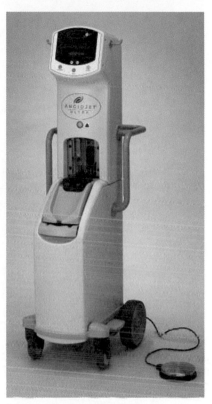

Figure 43-8 AngioJet Console with "pulse-spray" option and simplified setup process. *(MedRad, Inc, Warrendale, PA.)*

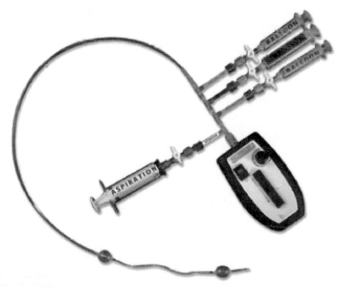

Figure 43-9 The Trellis 8 System consists of proximal and distal balloons with balloon inflation syringes, a thrombolysis infusion port, the thrombus aspiration syringe, and a drive unit for mechanical dispersion of the thrombolytic agent. *(Bacchus Vascular, Santa Clara, CA.)*

Figure 43-7 The EKOS endovascular device is placed directly into the thrombus, where microtransducers transmit high-frequency, low-power sound waves.

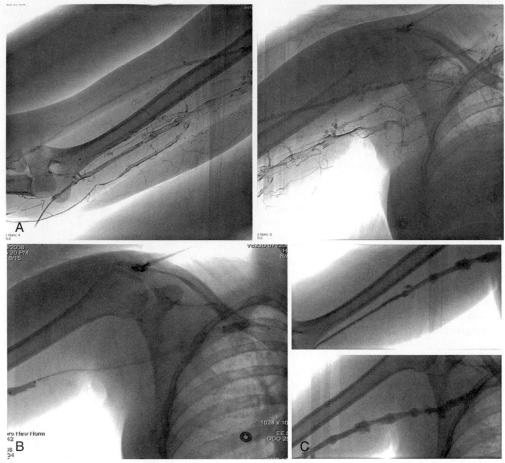

Figure 43-10 **A.** Acute right upper extremity DVT with classic intraluminal filling defects in the right brachial and axillary veins. **B.** The Trellis 8 system deployed in the right brachial and axillary vein utilizing a 30-cm treatment zone. **C.** Completion venogram demonstrating complete resolution of thrombus in right brachial and axillary veins following pharmacomechanical thrombectomy utilizing the Trellis-8 thrombolysis catheter. *(Bachus Vascular, Santa Clara, CA.)*

contents between the balloons. A sinusoidal nitinol wire placed within the catheter is rotated to mix the blood between the balloons. The Trellis device, which combines a high concentration of thrombolytic medication with mechanical disruption of thrombus, has been used with success to treat patients with DVT.[75] The occlusive balloons limit leakage of thrombolytic agent into the systemic circulation, potentially reducing the risk of bleeding complications, whereas the central balloon is intended to reduce embolization of particulate matter to the pulmonary circulation. Figure 43-10 illustrates the use of the Trellis 8 system in treating a right brachial and axillary DVT. One limitation with this catheter system is that it cannot be used in large veins such as the common iliac or SVC. These exciting combination strategies continue to be developed and investigated; with further follow-up, they will be better defined for their efficacy and role in PMT for DVT.

REFERENCES

1. Moffatt CJ, Franks PJ, Doherty DC, et al: Prevalence of leg ulceration in a London population. *QJM* 97:431–437, 2004.
2. McGuckin M, Waterman R, Brooks J, et al: Validation of venous leg ulcer guidelines in the United States and United Kingdom. *Am J Surg* 183:132–137, 2002.
3. Eklof B, Rutherford RB, Bergan JJ, et al: Revision of the CEAP classification for chronic venous disorders: consensus statement. *J Vasc Surg* 40:1248–1252, 2004.
4. Bergan JJ, Schmid-Schonbein GW, Cooleridge Smith PD, et al: Chronic venous disease. *N Engl J Med* 355:488–498, 2006.
5. Wilkinson LS, Bunker C, Edwards JC, et al: Leukocytes: their role in the etiopathogenesis of skin damage in venous disease. *J Vasc Surg* 17:669–675, 1993.
6. Herouy Y, May AE, Pornschlegel G, et al: Lipodermatosclerosis is characterized by elevated expression and activation of matrix metalloproteinases: implications for venous ulcer formation. *J Invest Dermatol* 111:822–827, 1998.
7. Norgauer J, Hildenbrand T, Idzko M, et al: Elevated expression of extracellular atrix metalloproteinase inducer (CD147) and membrane-type matrix metalloproteinases in venous leg ulcers. *Br J Dermatol* 147:1180–1186, 2002.
8. Mwaura B, Mahendran B, Hynes N, et al: The impace of differential expression of extracellular matrix metalloproteinase inducer, matrix metalloproteinase-2, tissue inhibitor of matrix

metalloproteinase-2 and PDGF-AA on the chronicity of venous leg ulcers. *Eur J Vasc Endovasc Surg* 31:306–310, 2006.
9. Kee ST, Kinoshita L, Razavi MK, et al: Superior vena cava syndrome: treatment with catheter-directed thrombolysis and endovascular stent placement. *Radiology* 206:187–193, 1998.
10. Chamorro H, Rao G, Wholey M: Superior vena cava syndrome: a complication of transvenous pacemaker implantation. *Radiology* 126:377–378, 1978.
11. Mocherla S, Wheat LJ: Treatment of histoplasmosis. *Semin Respir Infect* 16:141–148, 2001.
12. Christenson ML, Franks TJ, Galvin JR: Fibrosing mediastinitis. *Radiographics* 21:737–757, 2001.
13. Mahajan V, Strimlan V, Ordstrand HS, et al: Benign superior vena cava syndrome. *Chest* 68:32–35, 1975.
14. Connell J, Muhm J: Radiographic manifestations of pulmonary histoplasmosis: a 10-year review. *Radiology* 121:281–285 1976.
15. Qanadli SD, El Hajjam M, Bruckert F, et al: Helical CT phlebography of the superior vena cava: diagnosis and evaluation of venous obstruction. *AJR Am J Roentgenol* 172(5):1327–1333, 1999.
16. Hartnell GG, Hughes LA, Finn JP, et al: Magnetic resonance angiography of the central chest veins. A new gold standard? *Chest* 107(4):1053–1057, 1995.

17. Rizvi AZ, Kalra M, Bjarnason H, et al: Benign superior vena cava syndrome: stenting is now the first line of treatment. *J Vasc Surg* 47(2):372–380, 2008.
18. Miller JH, McBride K, Little F, et al: Malignant superior vena cava obstruction: stent placement via the subclavian route. *Cardiovasc Intervent Radiol* 23(2):155–158, 2000.
19. Petersen BD, Uchida B: Long-term results of treatment of benign central venous obstructions unrelated to dialysis with expandable Z stents. *J Vasc Intervent Radiol* 10:757–766, 1999.
20. Link J, Brossmann J, Muller-Hulsbeck S, et al: Venous stent application with a simultaneous cubitofemoral approach [German]. *Rofo* 163:81–83, 1995.
21. Dondelinger RF, Gofette P, Kurdziel JC, et al: Expandable metal stents for stenosis of the vena cava and large veins. *Semin Intervent Radiol* 8:252–263, 1991.
22. Smayra T, Otal P, Chabbert V, et al: Longer-term results of endovascular stent placement in the superior caval venous system. *Cardiovasc Intervent Radiol* 24:388–394, 2001.
23. Chatziioannou A, Alexopoulos TH, Mourikis D, et al: Stent therapy for malignant superior vena cava syndrome: should be first line therapy or simple adjunct to radiotherapy. *Eur J Radiol* 47:247–250, 2003.
24. Courtheoux P, Alkofer B, Al Refai M, et al: Stent placement in superior vena cava syndrome. *Ann Thorac Surg* 75:158–161, 2003.

25. Hennequin L, Fade O, Fays JG, et al: Superior vena cava stent placement: results with Wallstent endoprosthesis. *Radiology* 196:353–361, 1995.

26. O'Sullivan GJ, Mhyircheartaigh JN, Ferguson D, et al: Isolated Pharmacomechanical thrombolysis plus primary stenting in a single procedure to treat acute thrombotic superior vena cava syndrome. *J Endovasc Ther* 2010 Feb;17(1):124–125.

27. Gray BH, Olin JW, Graor RA, et al: Safety and efficiency of thrombolytic therapy for superior vena cava syndrome. *Chest* 99(1):54–59, 1991.

28. Perno J, Putnam SG, III, Cohen GS, et al: Endovascular treatment of superior vena cava syndrome without removing a central venous catheter. *J Vasc Intervent Radiol* 10:917–918, 1999.

29. Ganeshan A, Hon LQ, Warakaulle DR, et al: Superior vena caval stenting for SVC obstruction: current status. *Eur J Radiol* 71(2):343–349, 2009.

30. Cheng S: Superior vena cava syndrome: a contemporary review of a historic disease. *Cardiol Rev* 17(1):16–23, 2009.

31. Lanciego C, Chacon JL, Julian A, et al: Stenting as first option for endovascular treatment of malignant superior vena cava syndrome. *AJR Am J Roentgenol* 177:585–593, 2001.

32. Daines D, Chabrot P, Motreff P, et al: Cardiac Tamponade after malignant superior vena cava stenting: two case reports and brief review of the literature. *Acta Radiol* 51(3):256–259, 2010.

33. Smith SL, Manhire AR, Clark DM: Delayed spontaneous superior vena cava perforation associated with a SVC wallstent. *Cardiovasc Intervent Radiol* 24:286–287, 2001.

34. Choe YH, Im JG, Park JH, et al: The anatomy of the pericardial space: a study in cadavers and patients. *AJR Am Roentgenol* 149:693–697, 1987.

35. Sajid M, Ahmed N, Desai M, et al: Upper limb deep vein thrombosis: a literature review to streamline the protocol for management. *Acta Haematol* 117:10–18, 2007.

36. Prandoni P, Polistena P, Bernardi E, et al: Upper extremity deep-vein thrombosis risk factors, diagnosis, and complications. *Arch Intern Med* 157:57–62, 1997.

37. Hingorani A, Ascher E, Lorenson E, et al: Upper extremity deep venous thrombosis and its impact on morbidity and mortality rates in a hospital-based population. *J Vasc Surg* 26:853–860, 1997.

38. Becker DM, Philbrick JT, Walker FB: Axillary and subclavian venous thrombosis. Prognosis and treatment. *Arch Intern Med* 151:1934–1943, 1991.

39. Knudson GJ, Wiedmeyer DA, Erickson SJ, et al: Color Doppler sonographic imaging in the assessment of upper extremity deep venous thrombosis. *AJR Am J Roentgenol* 154:399–403, 1990.

40. Fraser JD, Anderson DR: Deep venous thrombosis: recent advances and optimal investigation with US. *Radiology* 211:9–24, 1999.

41. Fielding JR, Nagel JS, Pomery O: Upper extremity DVT: correlation of MR and nuclear medicine flow imaging. *Clin Imaging* 21:260–263, 1997.

42. Lindbald B, Tengborn L, Bergqvist D: Deep vein thrombosis of the axillary-subclavian veins: epidemiologic data, effects of differ-

ent types of treatment and late sequelae. *Eur J Vasc Surg* 2:161–165, 1988.

43. Zell L, Kindermann W, Marschall F, et al: Paget-Schroetter syndrome in sports activities: case study and literature review. *Angiology* 52:337–342, 2001.

44. Thompson RW, Schneider PA, Nelken NA, et al: Circumferential venolysis and paraclavacular thoracic outlet decompression for "effort thrombosis" of the subclavian vein. *J Vasc Surg* 16:723–732, 1992.

45. Parziale JR, Akelman E, Weiss AP, et al: Thoracic outlet syndrome. *Am J Orthop* 29:353–360, 2000.

46. Marinella MA, Kathula SK, Markert RJ: Spectrum of upper-extremity deep venous thrombosis in a community teaching hospital. *Heart Lung* 29:113–117, 2000.

47. Lokich JJ, Becker B: Subclavian vein thrombosis in patients treated with infusion chemotherapy for advanced malignancy. *Cancer* 52:1586–1589, 1983.

48. Monreal M, Raventos A, Lerma R, et al: Pulmonary embolism in patients with upper extremity DVT associated to venous central lines: a prospective study. *Thromb Haemost* 72:548–550, 1994.

49. Timsit JF, Farkas JC, Boyer JM, et al: Central vein catheter-related thrombosis in intensive care patients: incidence, risks factors, and relationship with catheter-related sepsis. *Chest* 114:207–213, 1998.

50. Girolami A, Prandoni P, Zanon E, et al: Venous thromboses of upper limbs are more frequently associated with occult cancer as compared with those of lower limbs. *Blood Coagul Fibrinol* 10:455–457, 1999.

51. Martinelli I, Cattaneo M, Panzeri D, et al: Risk factors for deep vein thrombosis of the upper extremities. *Ann Intern Med* 126:707–711, 1997.

52. Hammers LW, Cohn SM, Brown JM, et al: Doppler color flow imaging surveillance of deep vein thrombosis in high-risk trauma patients. *J Ultrasound Med* 15:19–24, 1996.

53. Heron E, Lozinguez O, Alhenc-Gelas M, et al: Hypercoagulable states in primary upper-extremity deep vein thrombosis. *Arch Intern Med* 160:382–386, 2000.

54. Lisse JR, Davis CP, Thurmond-Anderle M: Cocaine abuse and deep venous thrombosis. *Ann Intern Med* 110:571–572, 1989.

55. Leebeek FW, Stadhouders NA, van Stein D, et al: Hypercoagulability states in upper-extremity deep venous thrombosis. *Am J Hematol* 67:15–19, 2001.

56. Ruggeri M, Castaman G, Tosetto A, et al: Low prevalence of thrombophilic coagulation defects in patients with deep vein thrombosis of the upper limbs. *Blood Coagul Fibrinolysis* 8:191–194, 1997.

57. Baarslag HJ, van Beek EJR, Koopman MMW, et al: Prospective study of color duplex ultrasonography compared with contrast venography in patients suspected of having deep venous thrombosis of the upper extremities. *Ann Intern Med* 136:865–872, 2002.

58. Haire WD, Lynch TG, Lund GB, et al: Limitations of magnetic resonance imaging and ultrasound-directed (duplex) scanning in the diagnosis of subclavian vein thrombosis. *J Vasc Surg* 13:391–397, 1991.

59. Urschel HC, Razzuk MA: Paget-Schroetter syndrome: what is the best management? *Ann Thorac Surg* 69:1663–1669, 2000.

60. Strandness DE, Langlois Y, Cromor M, et al: Long-term sequelae of acute venous thrombosis. *JAMA* 250:1289–1292, 1983.

61. Vik A, Holme PA, Singh K, et al: Catheter-directed thrombolysis for treatment of deep venous thrombosis in the upper extremities. *Cardiovasc Intervent Radiol* 32(5): 980–987, 2009.

62. Kasirajan K, Gray B, Ouriel K: Percutaneous AngioJet thrombectomy in the management of extensive deep venous thrombosis. *J Vasc Intervent Radiol* 12:179–185, 2001.

63. Lee MC, Grassi CJ, Belkin M, et al: Early operative intervention after thrombolytic therapy for primary subclavian vein thrombosis, an effective treatment approach. *J Vasc Surg* 27:1101–1108, 1998.

64. Shields GP, Turnipseed S, Panacek EA, et al: Validation of the Canadian clinical probability model for acute venous thrombosis. *Acad Emerg Med* 9:561–566, 2002.

65. Breddin HK, Hach-Wunderle V, Nakov R, et al: Effects of a low molecular-weight heparin on thrombus regression and recurrent thromboembolism in patients with deep-vein thrombosis. *N Engl J Med* 344:626–631, 2001.

66. Nazir SA, Ganeshan A, Nazir S, et al: Endovascular treatment options in the management of lower limb deep venous thrombosis. *Cardiovasc Intervent Radiol* 32:861–876, 2009.

67. Shi HJ, Huang YH, Shen T, et al: percutaneous mechanical thrombectomy combined with catheter directed thrombolysis in the treatment of symptomatic lower extremity deep venous thrombosis. *Eur J Radiol* 71:350–355, 2009.

68. Semba CP, Dake M: Iliofemoral deep vein thrombosis: aggressive therapy using catheter-directed thrombolysis. *Radiology* 191:487–494, 1994.

69. McClennan G, Trerotola S, Davidson D, et al: The effects of a mechanical thrombolytic device on normal canine vein valves. *J Vasc Intervent Radiol* 12:89–94, 2001.

70. Braaten JV, Goss RA, Francis CW: Ultrasound reversibly disaggregates fibrin fibers. *Thromb Haemost* 78:1063–1068, 1997.

71. Parikh S, Motarjeme A, McNamara T, et al: Ultrasound-accelerated thrombolysis for the treatment of deep vein thrombosis: initial clinical experience. *J Vasc Intervent Radiol* 19:521–528, 2008.

72. Uppot RN, Garcia MJ, Roe C, et al: Management of deep venous thrombosis using the AngioJet rheolytic thrombectomy system. *J Vasc Intervent Radiol* 13(S):S116, 2002.

73. Gasparis AP, Labropoulos, N, Tassiopoulos AK, et al: Midterm follow-up after pharmacomechanical thrombolysis for lower extremity deep vein thrombosis. *Vasc Endovasc Surg* 43(1):61–68, 2009.

74. Rao AS, Konig G, Leers SA, et al: Pharmacomechanical thrombectomy for iliofemoral deep vein thrombosis: an alternative in patients with contraindications to thrombolysis. *J Vasc Surg* 50:1092–1098, 2009.

75. Hilleman DE, Razaui MK: Clinical and economic evaluation of the Trellis-8 infusion catheter for deep vein thrombosis. *J Vasc Intervent Radiol* 19(3):377–383, 2008.

Stroke Centers and Interventional Cardiology

CHRISTOPHER J. WHITE

KEY POINTS

- There are three broad categories of stroke, including (1) hemorrhagic, (2) thrombotic, and (3) embolic (artery to artery and chamber to artery).

- Carotid plaque, unlike coronary lesions, most often results in symptoms caused by atheroembolization, rather than thrombotic occlusion.

- The size of a brain infarction is determined by the time it takes for reperfusion to occur, the patency of the circle of Willis as a collateral source, and the viability of the surrounding penumbra of ischemic tissue.

- The only approved treatment for acute ischemic stroke is intravenous thrombolysis for patients presenting within 3 hours of the onset and without contraindications.

- The risk of intracranial hemorrhage complicating intravenous thrombolytic therapy for stroke is increased in direct relation to the size of the stroke, time to treatment (>3 hours), patient age (>85 years), and uncontrolled hypertension.

- Catheter-based therapy for stroke is reasonable in patients in whom systemic thrombolysis is contraindicated and in patients with larger strokes and greater disabilities.

- Catheter-based therapy for stroke differs from catheter-based therapy for myocardial infarction (MI) in that the occlusion is often embolic in origin and the thrombus may be older, more organized, and thus more resistant to thrombolysis.

- Interventional cardiologists (ICs) with carotid stent and angiography experience will make excellent additions to a multidisciplinary acute stroke team to provide round-the-clock interventional treatment to patients who are not candidates for intravenous thrombolysis.

Stroke will affect approximately three quarters of a million Americans each year and result in nearly 150,000 deaths.[1] Stroke is the third leading cause of death in the United States after heart disease and cancer and the number one cause of disability and the number one reason for rehabilitation. Over three million stroke survivors are estimated to be in the United States, a third of these being young adults with long-term disability.[2] The etiologies of stroke include (1) hemorrhagic, (2) thrombotic, and (3) embolic. Embolic strokes may be from an artery to an artery or from a heart chamber (left atrium or ventricle) to an artery, particularly in patients with atrial fibrillation (AF). One of the major tenets of treatment of ischemic stroke is that "time is brain." Variables that impact on the extent of ischemic brain injury are (1) the time from the onset of symptoms to reperfusion; (2) the presence of collateral circulation, including an intact circle of Willis; and (3) the "penumbra of viability" surrounding the infarcted brain tissue. The penumbra is the region of brain surrounding the infarct area, where the blood supply is significantly reduced but energy metabolism is maintained because of collateral flow. The viability of this area is dependent on both the severity and the duration of ischemia. If blood flow is rapidly restored, some ischemic brain tissue will be saved. For both ischemic stroke and hemorrhagic stroke, there are opportunities to minimize injury early after the onset of the stroke. This puts a premium on the rapid assessment of patients presenting with stroke (Table 44-1).[3] The goals of treatment include preventing or limiting the mortality and morbidity of the acute event and preventing recurrent events. The great majority (>80%) of strokes are ischemic.[4] Ischemic stroke therapy, designed to achieve reperfusion as quickly as possible and minimize further damage, consists of either intravenous (IV) thrombolysis or catheter-based reperfusion therapy, which can include intra-arterial (IA) thrombolysis, mechanical thrombectomy, or balloon angioplasty with or without stent placement.

New Imaging Strategies

The American Heart Association (AHA)/American Stroke Association (ASA) class I recommendation is to perform noncontrast computed tomography (CT) or magnetic resonance imaging (MRI) in patients who present within 3 hours of stroke symptom onset to exclude intracranial bleeding.[2] Imaging is the cornerstone for triaging candidates for stroke therapy. The purpose of the baseline CT is to detect conditions that make the patient ineligible for thrombolysis such as subdural, subarachnoid, or parenchymal intracranial hemorrhage (ICH). CT may also detect mass lesions or hemorrhagic infarctions. There are four major goals of brain imaging in the setting of an acute stroke: (1) Most importantly, ICH must be excluded. If ICH is present, then the patient has a neurosurgical emergency, and neurosurgery needs to be involved immediately. (2) Both CT and MRI can be used to noninvasively identify intravascular thrombus. Data regarding the geographic distribution and the size of the thrombus burden can assist in deciding on IV thrombolysis, IA thrombolysis, or endovascular thrombectomy. (3) The volume of the nonviable, irreversibly infarcted brain predicts the patient's potential for recovery. (4) The size of the penumbra—the peri-infarct zone of viable but ischemic brain tissue—can be assessed and compared with the volume of infarcted brain tissue.

Management of Physiologic Variables

The cornerstone of managing an acute stroke patient is reducing the risk of recurrent events and minimizing disability secondary to the established stroke. Acute therapy involves management of physiologic variables, reperfusion of ischemic tissue, and reduction of the risk of intracerebral hemorrhage. The patient's level of consciousness, airway, and oxygenation must be determined immediately. An electrocardiogram (ECG) must be performed to rule out a concomitant MI.

HYPERTENSION

Arterial hypertension is present in the majority of patients presenting with a stroke and is associated with a poorer outcome; however, lower blood pressure may result in decreased perfusion to the ischemic penumbra, thus extending the size of the infarction. There is a great deal of uncertainty regarding the treatment of hypertension during acute stroke. Current recommendations include lowering blood pressure to 220 mm Hg or more of systolic and 120 mm Hg or more of diastolic.[5]

TABLE 44-1	The Seven "D's" of Stroke Care

- Detection
- Dispatch
- Delivery
- Door-to-treatment time
- Data
- Decision
- Drug or Device administration

HYPOGLYCEMIA

Severe hypoglycemia may mimic a stroke and can be detected by fingerstick glucose. Immediate reversal is warranted with intravenous solutions, oral glucose solutions, or both.

HYPERGLYCEMIA

Elevated blood sugars are associated with worse outcomes in patients who have suffered acute stroke. This may be related to increased lactate production, which increases infarct size, reduces the effectiveness of thrombolytic therapy, and may increase the risk of hemorrhagic transformation of infarcted brain tissue. Hyperglycemia can increase the extent of infarction in cerebral ischemia, so blood glucose above 200 should be controlled and brought as close to the normal range as possible with insulin, if necessary.

FEVER

Fever is associated with poorer stroke outcomes possibly because of a detrimental effect on brain metabolism, increased free radical production, or deterioration of the blood–brain barrier function. If bacterial endocarditis is suspected, blood cultures and echocardiogram should be performed before starting interventional management. Current recommendations are to use antipyretics to maintain normothermia.

▪ Reperfusion Strategies

INTRAVENOUS THROMBOLYSIS

IV administration of the thrombolytic agent—recombinant tissue-plasminogen activator (rt-PA)—is the only therapy approved by the U.S. Food and Drug Administration (FDA) for the treatment of acute ischemic stroke (Table 44-2).[6] This has been shown to be an effective therapy for stroke by a recent meta-analysis of 2,775 patients treated within 6 hours of onset of stroke.[7] Patients treated within 90 minutes of onset had almost a threefold increase in beneficial outcomes, dropping to 1.6-fold increase in the odds for improved outcome if patients were treated between 91 and 180 minutes. For those treated between 180 and 270 minutes, the odds ratio (OR) for benefit was 1.4 times

greater compared with those given placebo. The risk of intracerebral hemorrhage was greater for the thrombolytic group (5.9%) compared with the placebo group (1.1%). The risk-to-benefit ratio for IV thrombolysis in ischemic stroke is narrow. About 11% more patients will benefit at 3 months from IV lysis, whereas 6.4% will experience ICH. Unfortunately, fewer than 10% of eligible patients with acute ischemic stroke receive reperfusion treatment in the United States.[8] Seven patients are the number needed to treat (NNT) with IV lysis to achieve an excellent outcome and avoid one stroke death or dependency. For every 100 stroke patients treated with IV thrombolysis within 3 hours, 32 will have a better outcome despite the 3 who will suffer a significant intracerebral hemorrhage. At 1 year after treatment, those treated with IV lysis have a 30% increased likelihood of minimal or no disability compared with those given placebo; however, there was no difference in the mortality rate and in the rate of recurrent strokes.[9] The risk of hemorrhage is increased in older patients and in patients with larger strokes, diabetes mellitus, a history of prior stroke, and thrombocytopenia. The European Cooperative Acute Stroke Study-3 (ECASS-3) tested the efficacy of extending the treatment window for intravenous thrombolysis to between 3 and 4.5 hours after stroke symptom onset. A favorable outcome occurred in 52.4% of patients assigned to rt-PA compared with 45.2% of the placebo group (OR 1.34; 95% confidence interval [CI] 1.02–1.76, $P = 0.04$). However, the incidence of ICH was higher in the rt-PA group (27%) compared with the placebo group (17.6%, $P = 0.001$). There was no difference in mortality rates between the two groups. Important exclusion criteria in this trial included a history of both stroke and diabetes mellitus, oral anticoagulation therapy regardless of international normalized ratio (INR), an NIHSS (National Institute of Health Stroke Scale) score of greater than 25, and age greater than 80 years.[10] The AHA/ASA has published a science advisory with a class 1, evidence level B recommendation for the administration of rt-PA to patients with ischemic stroke who present within 3 to 4.5 hours of symptom onset and meet the ECASS-3 inclusion criteria (Table 44-3).[11] Management with IV thrombolysis includes admission to an intensive care unit and frequent monitoring of vital signs and neurologic status. Arterial, central venous, and bladder catheters should not be placed until at least 2 hours after infusion of the thrombolytic agent. An elevated blood pressure should be lowered very cautiously. A head CT should be done if ICH is suspected. All anticoagulants (anti-thrombotic and anti-platelet therapies) should be withheld for at least 24 hours.

INTRA-ARTERIAL THROMBOLYSIS

Intra-arterial thrombolysis involves the selective placement of a catheter into cerebral vessels and is analogous, in many ways, to the treatment of an acute MI. There are also major differences between catheter-based treatments of acute stroke and acute MI. The benefit of catheter-based intra-cranial therapy is the ability to use smaller doses of lytic agents and to employ mechanical clot disruption and extraction with guidewires, balloons, and thrombectomy devices. The effectiveness of intra-arterial thrombolysis has been established in several trials. The Prolyse in Acute Cerebral Thromboembolism II (PROACT

TABLE 44-2	Randomized Trials of Thrombolytic Therapy for Acute Ischemic Stroke				
Name of Study	*Treatment Window*	*Medications Tested*	*Delivery*	*Dose of Agent*	*No. of Patients*
NINDS t-PA Stroke Trial (Parts 1 and 2)	3 h, 1/2 90 min	t-PA	IV	0.9 mg/kg over 1 h	624
ECASS I	6 h	t-PA	IV	1.1 mg/kg over 1 h	620
ECASS II	6 h	t-PA	IV	0.9 mg/kg over 1 h	800
Atlantis A62,63	6 h	t-PA	IV	0.9 mg/kg over 1 h	142
Atlantis B	0 to 5 h	t-PA	IV	0.9 mg/kg over 1 h	613 (31 3 h)
ASK	4 h	Streptokinase	IV	1.5 million units over 1 h	340
MAST I	6 h	Streptokinase	IV	1.5 million units over 1 h	622
MAST E	6 h	Streptokinase	IV	1.5 million units over 1 h	310
PROACT II	6 h	Prourokinase plus IV heparin	IA	9 mg over 2 h	180

TABLE 44-3	Eligibility for Thrombolysis in Stroke

- Indication: Ischemic stroke within 3 hours of onset of symptoms
- Clinical contraindications:
  - Any history of intracranial hemorrhage (ICH)
  - Systolic blood pressure (SBP) >185 mm Hg; diastolic blood pressure (DBP) >110 mm Hg
  - Rapid improvement in neurologic status
  - Mild neurologic impairment
  - Symptoms of subarachnoid bleeding
  - Stroke or head trauma within the last 3 months
  - Gastrointestinal or genitourinary (GI/GU) hemorrhage within 3 weeks
  - Major surgery within 3 weeks
  - Recent heart attack
  - Seizure with stroke
  - Taking oral anticoagulants
  - Received heparin within 48 hours
- Radiologic contraindications:
  - Evidence of ICH
- Laboratory contraindications:
  - International normalized ratio (INR) >1.7
  - Platelet count <100,000
  - Elevated activated partial thromboplastin time (aPTT)
  - Blood glucose <50 mg/dL

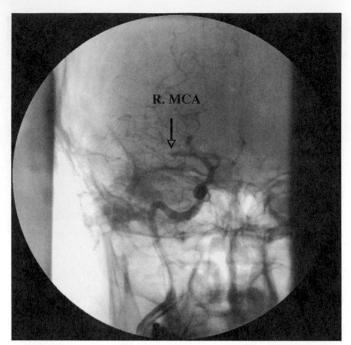

Figure 44-1 Patient with atrial fibrillation and an acute right middle cerebral artery occlusion.

II) trial randomized patients presenting within 6 hours of stroke onset and angiographically documented the occlusion of the middle cerebral artery (MCA) to 9 mg of intra-arterial pro-urokinase (pro-UK) plus unfractionated heparin (UFH) versus UFH alone.[12] Successful reperfusion was achieved in 66% of the IC-proUK group compared with only 18% of the control group ($P < 0.001$). The clinical benefit was that 40% of the pro-UK group had slight or no neurologic disability (modified Rankin scale [mRs] ≤2) at 90 days compared with only 25% of the control group ($P = 0.04$).

The incidence of symptomatic ICH was higher in the thrombolytic group (11% vs. 3%, $P = 0.03$). The NNT to make 1 patient independent was 7. This trial extended the efficacy of stroke treatment to 6 hours from onset of symptoms; however, only a small minority (2%) of all screened patients was enrolled. Contraindications to catheter-directed thrombolysis include recent brain surgery, unknown time of onset of the deficit, uncontrolled hypertension, and CT evidence of hemorrhage or tumor.

MECHANICAL THROMBECTOMY

An alternative strategy for reperfusion in patients with stroke who are not candidates for thrombolysis is mechanical clot removal or thrombectomy (Figs. 44-1 to 44-5). There are two approved devices (MERCI, Concentric Medical, Mountain View, CA; and PENUMBRA, Penumbra Inc, San Leandro, CA) for mechanical thrombectomy during acute stroke intervention. Compared with historical controls, both these devices have demonstrated superior outcomes with intracranial thrombus removal.[13,14]

ANGIOPLASTY AND STENT PLACEMENT

Balloon angioplasty is commonly performed for residual stenoses following IA lysis or mechanical thrombectomy.[14a] Balloons are commonly undersized to avoid arterial dissection and perforation. Often, lesions manifest acute recoil or flow-limiting dissections, necessitating the use of off-label stents. There has been recent interest in a strategy of immediate stent placement as in the treatment for acute MI. This technique of immediate direct stenting of the culprit lesion can minimize the time for reperfusion of the infarct zone.[15-22] Three stent systems are currently approved by the FDA for treatment of intracranial stroke (but not acute stroke) in the United States—Neuroform (Boston

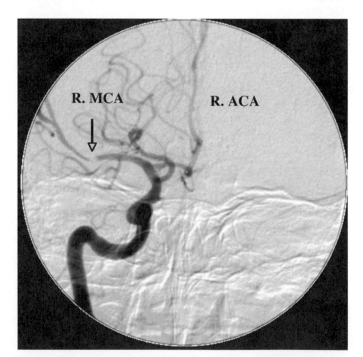

Figure 44-2 Intracranial administration of 2 mg recombinant tissue–plasminogen activator (rt-PA) with partial recanalization (*arrow*) of right middle cerebral artery (MCA).

Scientific, Natick, MA), Wingspan (Boston Scientific, Natick, MA) and Enterprise (Codman Neurovascular/Cordis, Raynham, MA). These devices are all self-expanding stents with extremely deliverable catheters to navigate the tortuous intracranial circulation. The Stent-Assisted Recanalization in Acute Ischemic Stroke (SARIS) trial was a prospective, FDA-approved, single-site registry designed to test the efficacy of direct stent placement in acute stroke. The trial included twenty patients with severe impairment (NIHSS = 14 ± 3.8) with a duration of 313 ± 114 minutes from symptom onset to intervention. On baseline

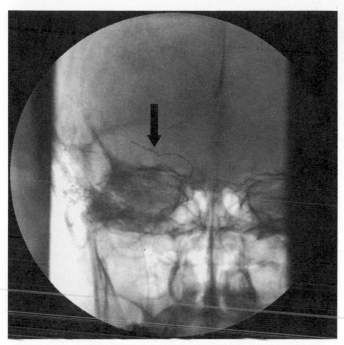

Figure 44-3 Placement of the MERCI thrombectomy catheter (arrow) in the right middle cerebral artery (MCA).

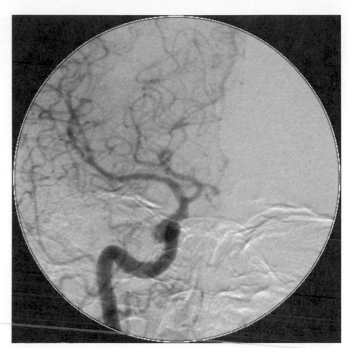

Figure 44-5 Final result with recanalization of right middle cerebral artery (MCA).

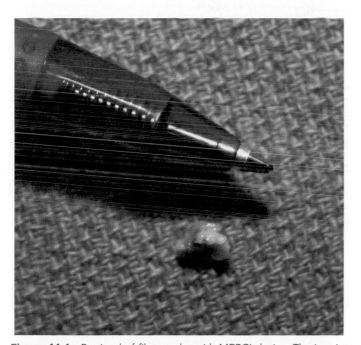

Figure 44-4 Retrieval of fibrous clot with MERCI device. The imprint from the left atrial appendage can be seen.

angiography, 17 patients had thrombolysis in MI (TIMI) grade 0 flow and 3 patients had TIMI grade 1 flow. All patients were successfully recanalized (TIMI 3 = 60%; TIMI 2 = 40%). Serious complications included ICH in three patients, of which one was symptomatic; the 1-month mortality rate was 25%. This rapid reperfusion strategy demonstrated a marked improvement in discharge NIHSS (7.4), and at 1 month, almost 50% of these patients were functioning independently, with a modified Rankin score of 1.[23] This type of registry data suggest

a potential role for early endovascular therapy in select patients, but larger randomized trials will be needed to quantify the risk-and-benefit ratio and for better patient selection criteria.

NEUROPROTECTION

Although many drugs and devices are under investigation to prolong the life of the penumbra, maintain the blood–brain barrier, and reduce hemorrhage and reperfusion injury, none have been proven effective in humans. The latest *AHA/ASA Guidelines for the Early Management of Adults with Ischemic Stroke*, published in 2007, conclude that "no intervention with putative neuroprotective actions has been established as effective in improving outcomes after stroke, and therefore none currently can be recommended," thus assigning a class III recommendation for neuroprotection.[2] Despite this pessimism, there is growing enthusiasm among investigators with regard to systemic hypothermia as an emerging therapy for stroke. Hypothermia functions as a neuroprotectant by decreasing cellular metabolism, limiting cytotoxicity, reducing free radical formation, and preventing blood–brain barrier breakdown. Mechanisms of cooling include invasive central venous catheters as well as surface methods. There is much data to support the neuroprotective effects of hypothermia in animal models but no comparative data for humans are available. The benefits of hypothermia are facilitated by early initiation.[24,25]

Stroke Centers

Stroke centers are a key component of building a successful stroke program. The relatively new concept of stroke centers was outlined by the Brain Attack Coalition (BAC) in 2000.[26] Stroke centers are modeled after streamlined trauma care and acute MI care in that these modalities require rapid identification and triage of patients to provide timely provision of care.

This systems-based approach requires community-wide coordination and planning. This includes empowering ambulances to bypass hospitals to bring patients to facilities with specialized stroke treatment capabilities. Primary Stroke Centers (PSC) provide basic acute stroke care, including initial assessment and treatment of patients by stroke

TABLE 44-4	Comparison of "Real-World" Catheter-Based Therapy in the Ochsner Clinic Series and Intravenous and Intra-arterial Thrombolysis for Stroke Treatment Trials					
Study	*Patients* (n)	*Age; Males%*	*NIHSS Baseline*	*Symptomatic ICH*	*Mortality at Follow-Up*	*Good Outcome at Follow-Up*
NINDS	168	69 years; 57%	14	6.4%	17% at 3 months	39%
STARS	389	69 years; 55%	13	3.3%	13% at 1 month	35%
PROACT II	121	64 years; 58%	17	10%	25% at 3 months	26%
Ochsner Clinic	42	64 years; 44%	16	12%	9.5% at 1 month	45%

ICH, intracranial hemorrhage; *NIHSS*, National Institute of Health Stroke Scale; *NINDS*, National Institute of Neurologic Disorders and Stroke; *PROACT II*, PROlyse in Acute Cerebral Thromboembolism II; *STARS*, Standard Treatment with Alteplase to Reverse Stroke Study.

teams, and have stroke units and 24-hour access to CT scans available. Comprehensive Stroke Centers (CSC) are intended for complicated or high-risk patients and offer (1) specialized stroke personnel, including specialized neurologic intensive care unit; (2) advanced neuroimaging capabilities; (3) on-demand neurosurgical and endovascular interventional capabilities; and (4) the infrastructure to support the above activities.[27] The CSC has an endovascular specialist as well as a neurosurgeon available round the clock for consultation and immediate procedural support, including aneurysm clipping, ventriculostomy placement, intracranial pressure transducer placement, and percutaneous, catheter-based therapy for stroke. Dedicated stroke units allow for close monitoring by providers accustomed to treating these patients and familiar with their unique needs. Part of the infrastructure of the CSC includes rigorous data collection and outcomes assessment to advance the field of stroke care. Additionally, community education about recognition of stroke risk factors, in conjunction with ambulance bypass systems, is a crucial component to building successful stroke systems.

THE ROLE OF CARDIOLOGY IN A STROKE PROGRAM

There are similarities in the treatments of acute stroke and acute MI. In both, a strong emphasis is placed on achieving early reperfusion, which is driven by early patient recognition, early hospital presentation, and early treatment initiation. However, there are significant differences between the treatments of stroke and heart attack, for example, stroke thrombi are usually of embolic origin, which makes them older, more organized, and more resistant to lysis compared with thrombi in acute MI. Also, the volume of the clot is larger in stroke, and cerebral vessel tortuosity can make CBT more difficult compared with the treatment for acute MI.

The author's center has reported its experience with a multidisciplinary team, including interventional cardiologists (ICs) to provide emergent endovascular therapy to patients with acute ischemic stroke who are ineligible for intravenous thrombolysis (Table 44-4).[28,29] Following consultation with an IC or a neuroradiologist, a stroke neurologist, is called to assess the patient and determine the need for intervention. In the authors' center, stroke patients are considered eligible for intervention if they present less than 8 hours from symptom onset. No specific cut-off or lower limit for the NIHSS score is used to exclude patients from intervention; rather, patients are eligible if they have a serious deficit, even if the corresponding NIHSS score is comparatively low (e.g., monocular blindness).

The most important problem facing stroke therapy today is a lack of on-demand interventional therapy for the majority of patients who are not candidates for lysis. Unlike the national standard of care for heart attacks, for which an army of ICs have been mobilized in a national effort to minimize "door-to-balloon time" for early reperfusion, endovascular therapy for stroke is uncommon because of the paucity of neurointerventional physicians to provide this service round the clock in most communities.[30] Quite simply, this can be attributed to the relatively few neuroradiologists who are available to provide continuous coverage in every hospital that accepts patients for treatment of stroke. One way to expand this service is to take advantage of the abundant manpower available in interventional cardiology (Fig. 44-6).[31] ICs are currently providing round-the-clock interventional care for acute MI. With training and formation of a multi-disciplinary stroke treatment group that includes neurology, radiology, and surgical specialties, the stroke treatment capability that is so badly needed in many communities can be significantly extended. The other fortuitous factor is that many ICs are currently performing carotid stent placement, including intracerebral angiography. It is a reasonable and achievable step to enable a competent carotid interventionalist who has cerebral angiography experience to perform acute stroke intervention (Table 44-5). A significant manpower shortage exists for the management of stroke, and ICs are in a position to meet the demand for round-the-clock stroke intervention service. In their roles as skilled angiographers, skilled interventionalists, and productive members of a multi-disciplinary team, they can help meet the challenge of bringing reperfusion therapy to patients with this devastating disease.

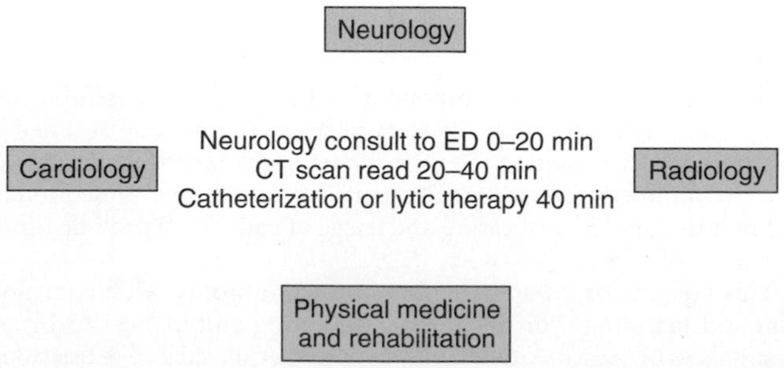

Figure 44-6 Ochsner Acute Stroke Intervention Service (OASIS). Multi-disciplinary service led and coordinated by Stroke Neurology.

TABLE 44-5	Strengths and Weaknesses of Cardiologists on the Stroke Intervention Team
Strengths	
• Excellent catheter skills	
• Experience with carotid stent placement and cerebral angiography	
• Ability to manage atherosclerotic risk factors for stroke	
• Round-the-clock rapid response to assist and relieve interventional neuroradiology	
• Ability to manage coexistent cardiac disease (atrial fibrillation [AF])	
Weaknesses	
• Limited knowledge of:	
• Cerebral anatomy	
• Computed tomography (CT) and magnetic resonance imaging (MRI) interpretation	
• Localization of deficit	
• National Institute of Health Stroke Scale (NIHSS) and neurologic examination	
• Management of stroke complications (intracerebral hemorrhage [ICH]).	

REFERENCES

1. Lloyd-Jones D, Adams RJ, Brown TM, et al: Heart disease and stroke statistics—2010 update: A report from the american heart association. *Circulation* 121:e46–e215, 2010.
2. Adams HP, Jr, del Zoppo G, Alberts MJ, et al: Guidelines for the early management of adults with ischemic stroke: A guideline from the American Heart Association/American Stroke Association Stroke Council, Clinical Cardiology Council, Cardiovascular Radiology and Intervention Council, and the Atherosclerotic Peripheral Vascular Disease and Quality of Care Outcomes in Research Interdisciplinary Working Groups: The American Academy of Neurology affirms the value of this guideline as an educational tool for neurologists. *Circulation* 115:e478–e534, 2007.
3. Adams HP, Jr, Adams RJ, Brott T, et al: Guidelines for the early management of patients with ischemic stroke: A scientific statement from the Stroke Council of the American Stroke Association. *Stroke* 34:1056–1083, 2003.
4. Pencina MJ, D'Agostino RB, Sr, Larson MG, et al: Predicting the 30-year risk of cardiovascular disease: The framingham heart study. *Circulation* 119:3078–3084, 2009.
5. Dawson J, Walters M: New and emerging treatments for stroke. *Br Med Bull* 77–78, 87–102, 2006.
6. The National Institute of Neurological Disorders and Stroke rt-PA Stroke Study Group: Tissue plasminogen activator for acute ischemic stroke. *N Engl J Med* 333:1581–1587, 1995.
7. Hacke W, Donnan G, Fieschi C, et al: Association of outcome with early stroke treatment: Pooled analysis of ATLANTIS, ECASS, and NINDS rt-PA stroke trials. *Lancet* 363:768–774, 2004.
8. Reeves MJ, Arora S, Broderick JP, et al: Acute stroke care in the US: Results from 4 pilot prototypes of the Paul Coverdell National Acute Stroke Registry. *Stroke* 36:1232–1240, 2005.
9. Kwiatkowski TG, Libman RB, Frankel M, et al: Effects of tissue plasminogen activator for acute ischemic stroke at one year. National Institute of Neurological Disorders and Stroke Recombinant Tissue Plasminogen Activator Stroke Study Group. *N Engl J Med* 340:1781–1787, 1999.
10. Hacke W, Kaste M, Bluhmki E, et al: Thrombolysis with alteplase 3 to 4.5 hours after acute ischemic stroke. *N Engl J Med* 359:1317–1329, 2008.
11. Del Zoppo GJ, Saver JL, Jauch EC, et al: Expansion of the time window for treatment of acute ischemic stroke with intravenous tissue plasminogen activator: A science advisory from the American Heart Association/American Stroke Association. *Stroke* 40:2945–2948, 2009.
12. Furlan A, Higashida R, Wechsler L, et al: Intra-arterial prourokinase for acute ischemic stroke. The PROACT II study: a randomized controlled trial. Prolyse in Acute Cerebral Thromboembolism. *JAMA* 282:2003–2011, 1999.
13. Clark W, Lutsep H, Barnwell S, et al: The Penumbra Stroke Trial: Safety and effectiveness f a new generation of mechanical device for clot removal in acute ischemic stroke. *Stroke* 40(8):2761–2768, 2009; abstract LB4, 2008.
14. Nogueira RG, Liebeskind DS, Sung G, et al: Predictors of good clinical outcomes, mortality, and successful revascularization in patients with acute ischemic stroke undergoing thrombectomy: Pooled analysis of the Mechanical Embolus Removal in Cerebral Ischemia (MERCI) and Multi MERCI Trials. *Stroke* 40:3777–3783, 2009.
14a. White CJ, Abou-Chebl A, Cates CU, et al: Stroke intervention catheter-based therapy for acute ischemic stoke. *J Am Coll Cardiol* 58:101–116, 2011.
15. Fiorella DJ, Levy EI, Turk AS, et al: Target lesion revascularization after wingspan: Assessment of safety and durability. *Stroke* 40:106–110, 2009.
16. Levy EI, Mehta R, Gupta R, et al: Self-expanding stents for recanalization of acute cerebrovascular occlusions. *AJNR Am J Neuroradiol* 28:816–822, 2007.
17. Turk AS, Levy EI, Albuquerque FC, et al: Influence of patient age and stenosis location on wingspan in-stent restenosis. *AJNR Am J Neuroradiol* 29:23–27, 2008.
18. Brekenfeld C, Schroth G, Mattle HP, et al: Stent placement in acute cerebral artery occlusion: Use of a self-expandable intracranial stent for acute stroke treatment. *Stroke* 40:847–852, 2009.
19. Levy EI, Turk AS, Albuquerque FC, et al: Wingspan in-stent restenosis and thrombosis: Incidence, clinical presentation, and management. *Neurosurgery* 61:644–650; discussion 650–641, 2007.
20. Zaidat OO, Wolfe T, Hussain SI, et al: Interventional acute ischemic stroke therapy with intracranial self-expanding stent. *Stroke* 39:2392–2395, 2008.
21. Mocco J, Hanel RA, Sharma J, et al: Use of a vascular reconstruction device to salvage acute ischemic occlusions refractory to traditional endovascular recanalization methods. *J Neurosurg* 112(3):557–562, 2010.
22. Mathews MS, Sharma J, Snyder KV, et al: Safety, effectiveness, and practicality of endovascular therapy within the first 3 hours of acute ischemic stroke onset. *Neurosurgery* 65:860–865; discussion 865, 2009.
23. Levy EI, Siddiqui AH, Crumlish A, et al: First Food and Drug Administration-approved prospective trial of primary intracranial stenting for acute stroke: SARIS (stent-assisted recanalization in acute ischemic stroke). *Stroke* 40:3552–3556, 2009.
24. Berger C, Schramm P, Schwab S: Reduction of diffusion-weighted MRI lesion volume after early moderate hypothermia in ischemic stroke. *Stroke* 36:e56–e58, 2005.
25. Holzer M: Devices for rapid induction of hypothermia. *Eur J Anaesthesiol Suppl* 42:31–38, 2008.
26. Alberts MJ, Hademenos G, Latchaw RE, et al, for the Brain Attack Coalition: Recommendations for the establishment of primary stroke centers. *JAMA* 283:3102–3109, 2000.
27. Alberts MJ, Latchaw RE, Selman WR, et al, for the Brain Attack Coalition: Recommendations for comprehensive stroke centers: A consensus statement from the Brain Attack Coalition. *Stroke* 36:1597–1616, 2005.
28. Ramee SR, Subramanian R, Felberg RA, et al: Catheter-based treatment for patients with acute ischemic stroke ineligible for intravenous thrombolysis. *Stroke* 35:e109–e111, 2004.
29. DeVries JT, White CJ, Collins TJ, et al: Acute stroke intervention by interventional cardiologists. *Catheter Cardiovasc Interv* 73:692–698, 2009.
30. Suzuki S, Saver JL, Scott P, et al: Access to intra-arterial therapies for acute ischemic stroke: An analysis of the US population. *AJNR Am J Neuroradiol* 25:1802–1806, 2004.
31. White CJ, Cates CU, Cowley MJ, et al: Interventional stroke therapy: Current state of the art and needs assessment. *Catheter Cardiovasc Interv* 70:471–476, 2007.

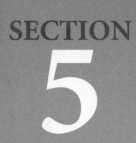

SECTION
5

Intracardiac Intervention

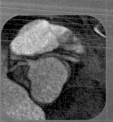

Imaging for Intracardiac Interventions

MEHDI H. SHISHEHBOR | SAMIR R. KAPADIA

KEY POINTS

- Interventions for structural heart disease require multi-modality imaging in the cardiac catheterization laboratory (cath lab), including fluoroscopy, three-dimensional rotational imaging, and echocardiography.

- Fluoroscopy allows the operator to monitor the manipulation of radiopaque devices and visualize intracardiac structures with contrast injection, as necessary. Echocardiography shows nonradiopaque cardiac structures in greater detail and helps with the safety and precision of the procedures.

- Fluoroscopy visualizes a large area of the heart with excellent temporal and spatial resolution and projects this three-dimensional information on a two-dimensional screen. Therefore, multiple projections (commonly biplane imaging) may be needed to determine the precise location of devices and structures in a three-dimensional space.

- Availability to acquire three-dimensional dataset with rotational imaging in the cardiac cath lab has revolutionized imaging and fusion possibilities. Faster rotational capabilities of the gantry and electrocardiographic gating options will make this field grow even faster.

- Three-dimensional and biplane echocardiography helps localize structures and devices in a significant way. Live three dimensional color imaging is expected to further advance this field in the near future.

- Echocardiography can be performed by an intracardiac echocardiography (ICE) or a trans-esophageal echocardiography (TEE) probe in the cath lab. ICE is currently used for septal interventions (trans-septal puncture, patent foramen ovale [PFO], and atrial septal defect [ASD] closures); however, its use for other interventions is increasing. Mitral valve interventions are primarily done under TEE guidance at the present time.

- Synthesis of fluoroscopic, computed tomographic (CT), and echocardiographic images in the cath lab is becoming increasingly important with expanding percutaneous interventions for structural heart disease.

Introduction

Interventional cardiac procedures rely on various imaging modalities for their safety and efficacy. Traditionally, x-ray fluoroscopy and cine-angiography have been used to guide coronary angioplasty procedures, and they remain an integral part of intracardiac interventions. Fluoroscopy creates a two-dimensional view of a three-dimensional object by superimposing images. Accurate position of an object in a three-dimensional space can be determined by viewing multiple different projections or by observing motion of an object that is moving in a known direction (e.g., catheter). The major limitation of fluoroscopy is that only radiopaque objects are visible; therefore, to visualize soft tissue structures such as the myocardium, the inter-atrial and inter-ventricular septa, and cardiac valves, radiopaque dye has to be injected. Fusion of CT images with intra-procedural three-dimensional CT and fluoroscopy can improve fluoroscopic guidance tremendously.[1,2] Ultrasound-based imaging is another imaging modality that is used to guide intracardiac interventions. Both TEE and ICE depict a two-dimensional image from a two-dimensional plane. Ultrasound imaging

allows visualization of soft tissue without injection of contrast material; this allows for real-time imaging during device manipulation. Although the spatial resolution of ultrasound is not as good as cine-angiography, it is adequate for visualization of most intracardiac structures. The precise location of an object in a three-dimensional space can be obtained by capturing the image of an object in multiple planes or by manipulating the ultrasound probe in a known direction. A particular limitation of ICE and TEE imaging is the difficulty of recognizing the specific aspect of a device; for instance, the tip of a catheter may appear indistinguishable from the shaft just a few millimeters proximal to the tip. However, three-dimensional TEE has helped overcome this limitation in a major way. Other limitations include restricted areas where the probe can be placed (esophagus or cardiac chambers), limiting imaging at times because of shadowing caused by metallic objects, calcium, and air. The most comprehensive approach to intracardiac imaging is the complementary use of fluoroscopy along with ultrasound imaging; this allows for combining the strengths of these imaging modalities while compensating for their weaknesses. This chapter will discuss how the structural anatomy is highlighted by using each of these imaging techniques and how imaging pearls for different intracardiac procedures are synthesized.

Fluoroscopy

LEFT VENTRICULOGRAM

The left ventricle is typically divided into inflow and outflow segments.[3] The inflow consists of the mitral valve apparatus, and the outflow portion includes the apex, the left ventricular outflow tract (LVOT), and the aortic valve. The angle between the inflow and outflow tract is around 30 degrees in young age and increases with "unfolding of the aorta." Since the interventricular septum maintains its position while the aorta is transposed anteriorly and more horizontally, there can be "bulging" of the septum. Most commonly, this location is in the inflow portion of the left ventricular midcavity away from the septum as seen in the left anterior oblique (LAO) projection. Left ventriculogram is typically performed in the 30-degree right anterior oblique (RAO) projection; however, different views should be considered, according to the purpose of the procedure. The RAO projection delineates the separation of atria from ventricles. Various structures seen on the RAO projection are delineated in Fig. 45-1. Anterior and inferior walls and the apex are seen without overlap in this view. The lateral wall and the septum are overlapped, and their motion is perpendicular to the x-ray beam, which makes it difficult to assess them. Anterior and posterior mitral valve leaflets are seen from the side in a longitudinal plane along with the inflow portion of the ventricle. This relationship is critical and must be recognized when performing mitral valve intervention, in which devices have to be advanced coaxially in the inflow (e.g., Inoue balloon). Anterolateral and posteromedial commissures superimpose in this view; therefore, there is significant overlap between the various segments of the anterior and posterior leaflets of the mitral valve. The aortic valve and the coronary sinus can be appreciated in this view. Typically, the right coronary sinus is well separated from the posteriorly superimposed noncoronary and left sinuses. The noncoronary sinus is typically lower than the left sinus in this projection. Different structures seen on the LAO view are outlined in Fig. 45-2. To align the mitral inflow to the apex of the ventricle, some caudal angulation can be added to the LAO projection, depending on patient habitus.

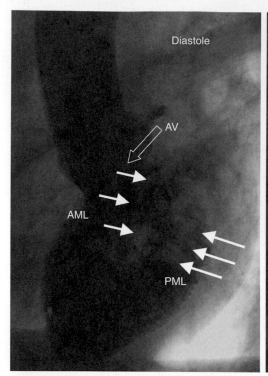

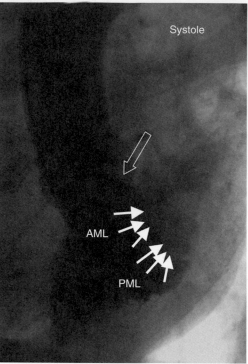

Figure 45-1 Right anterior oblique (RAO) 30-degree view of the left ventricle in diastole and systole. The aortic valve *(open arrow)*, the mitral valve *(solid white arrow)*, and papillary muscles *(solid black arrows)* are shown. In diastole, mitral valve is open, and there is clearance of contrast as blood enters the left ventricle from the left atrium. Anterior and posterior leaflets are separate in diastole *(left panel)*. In systole, the mitral valve is closed, and the aortic valve is open *(right panel)*. In this view, the anterior, apex, and inferior walls can be assessed. *Ant PM*, anterolateral papillary muscle; *AML*, anterior mitral leaflet; *AV*, aortic valve; *PML*, posterior mitral leaflet; *Post PM*, posterolateral papillary muscle.

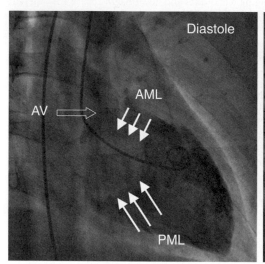

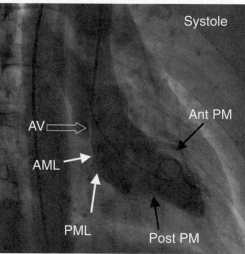

Figure 45-2 Left anterior oblique (LAO) 60-degree view of the left ventricle in diastole and systole. The aortic valve *(open arrow)*, the mitral valve *(solid white arrow)*, and papillary muscles *(solid black arrows)* are shown. In diastole, the mitral valve is open, and there is clearance of contrast as blood without contrast enters the left ventricle from the left atrium. Anterior and posterior leaflets are separate in diastole *(left panel)*. In this view, the lateral and septal walls can be assessed. *Ant PM*, anterolateral papillary muscle; *AML*, anterior mitral leaflet; *AV*, aortic valve; *PML*, posterior mitral leaflet; *Post PM*, posterolateral papillary muscle.

This allows visualization of the left ventricle in the end-on projection, where papillary muscles as well as anterior and posterior leaflets can be clearly identified. Note that the inflow and outflow of the ventricle are typically well separated in this view. (See Fig. 45-2.) The left coronary sinus is seen clearly, but the right and the noncoronary sinuses typically overlap in this projection. Unconventional views allow better delineation of certain parts of the left ventricle. The LAO cranial projection provides a better view to assess LVOT. The purpose of this projection is to visualize the anterior leaflet of the mitral valve in a longitudinal view when it does not overlap the interventricular septum. It is also the view of choice to visualize the interventricular septum in the muscular portion for the assessment of ventricular septal defect (VSD). LAO caudal projection allows the end-on view of the mitral valve. One important fluoroscopic landmark that helps "coronary interventionalists" identify mitral commissures is the coronary artery. The anterolateral commissure is located close to the division of the left

main trunk (LMT) in the left anterior descending (LAD) artery and the left circumflex (LCx) artery, and the posterolateral commissure is close to the origin of the posterior descending artery.

RIGHT VENTRICULOGRAM

The right ventricle is a trabeculated ventricle with the inflow and outflow tracts at right angles to each other. Most typically, right ventriculogram is performed in anteroposterior and lateral projections, with the catheter positioned in midcavity to prevent ventricular ectopy. The pigtail catheter or the National Institute of Health (NIH) catheter can be used to perform a right ventriculogram. The rate of injection has to be higher to identify the details (>25 cc/second). A right ventriculogram can be used to assess the pulmonary valve, the tricuspid valve, and right ventricular outflow tract (RVOT) obstruction (Fig. 45-3).

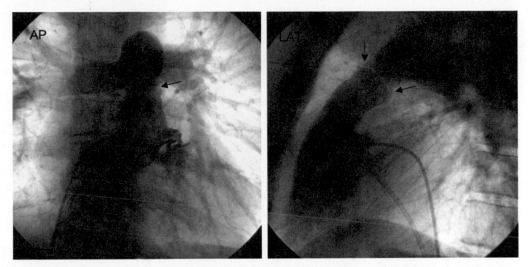

Figure 45-3 Anteroposterior and lateral views of the right ventricle with the pigtail catheter in the right ventricular outflow tract. Note the doming of the pulmonary valve (*black arrows*).

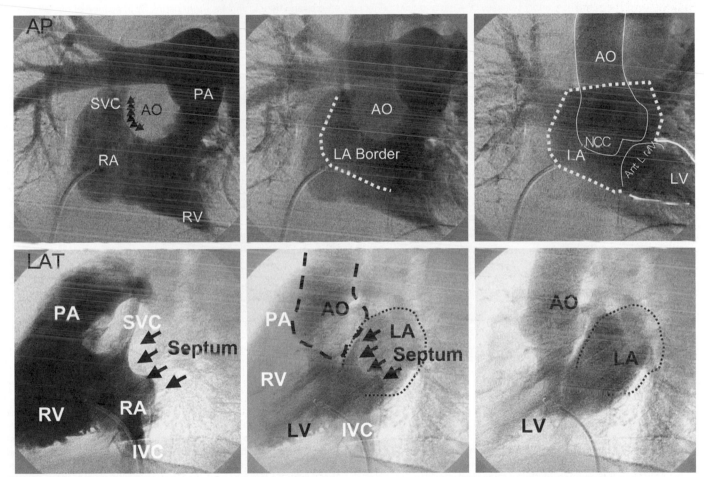

Figure 45-4 Anteroposterior (*top panel*) and lateral (*bottom panel*) view of a right atrial angiogram is shown. Dextro phase (*left panel*), levo phase (*right panel*), and two phases superimposed on each other (*middle panel*) are presented. *ant LMV*, anterior leaflet of the mitral valve; *AO*, aorta; *IVC*, inferior vena cava; *RA*, right atrium; *LA*, left atrium; *NCC*, non-coronary cusp; *PA*, pulmonary artery; *RV*, right ventricle; *SVC*, superior vena cava.

RIGHT ATRIAL ANGIOGRAM

A right atrial angiogram is performed to visualize the inter-atrial septum by using the pigtail catheter or the NIH catheter with a rapid injection rate. Various anatomic structures are shown in Figure 45-4. This procedure can be used for trans-septal puncture and for the closure of patent foreman ovale (PFO) or atrial septal defect (ASD). The right atrial angiogram is performed after ASD closure to determine the relationship of the device to surrounding structures such as the aorta and left atrial walls.

LEFT ATRIAL ANGIOGRAM

A left atrial angiogram is rarely performed by direct injection but the left atrium (LA) is frequently seen on the levo phase of the right-sided

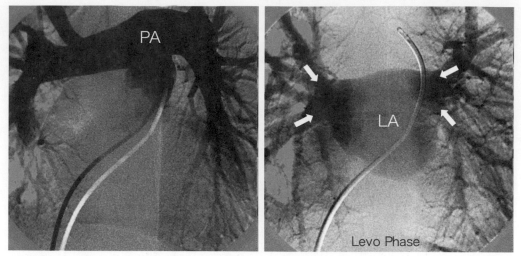

Figure 45-5   Normal pulmonary angiogram in the anteroposterior view. Large volume of dye (40 cc/second) is rapidly injected using an NIH catheter. *Left panel,* The pulmonary artery trunk and the left and right pulmonary arteries and their branches. *Right panel,* Opacification of the left atrium in the levo phase. Digital subtraction is used to visualize the pulmonary veins *(solid white arrows). LA,* left atrium; *NIH,* National Institute of Health; *PA,* pulmonary artery.

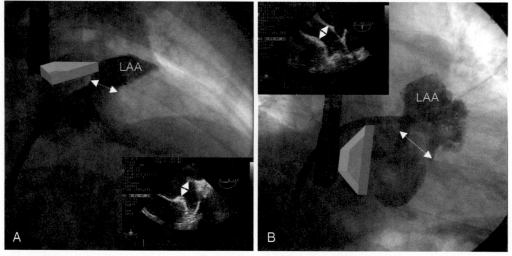

Figure 45-6   *Panel A,* Right anterior oblique (RAO) cranial view of left atrial appendage (LAA) injection. The "width" of the LAA opening is shown (dotted arrows), which is also depicted by horizontal view in TEE (insert). *Panel B,* RAO caudal view of the LAA in the same subject, showing the "height" of the opening, which corresponds to the vertical view by trans-esophageal echocardiography (TEE) *(insert).*

angiogram. Frequently, pulmonary artery angiogram is performed in the anteroposterior and lateral views to visualize the LA and assess pulmonary vein drainage before ASD closure (Fig. 45-5). Direct injection in the left atrial appendage (LAA) is performed to evaluate the anatomy before percutaneous closure (Fig. 45-6). The RAO cranial view shows the LAA opening in the mediolateral diameter, and the RAO caudal view delineates the superoinferior opening diameter (see Fig. 45-6). These views are also important to study the shape of the LAA, which is critical to planning percutaneous closure.

AORTOGRAM

An ascending aortogram is performed to examine the aortic valve and root, aortic aneurysms, and, rarely, aortic dissections. It is performed in the RAO (30 degrees) and LAO (40 degrees) projections. High rate of injection (20 cc/second for 2–3 seconds) and proper catheter positioning allow for assessment of different aortic cusps. The aortogram is usually performed with a multi-side-hole pigtail catheter positioned

just 2 to 3 cm above the sinus of Valsalva (Fig. 45-7). Various anatomic relationships must be recognized on fluoroscopy, including the relationship of the noncoronary cusp to the inter-atrial septum for transseptal puncture, to the superior vena cava (SVC) for ICE imaging, and to the anterior leaflet of the mitral valve for antegrade interventions. These relationships are well demonstrated in a posteroanterior view on the right atrial angiogram (see Fig. 45-4).

PULMONARY ANGIOGRAM

Pulmonary angiography is the gold standard technique for diagnosing a pulmonary embolism.[4] In addition, it is used to assess a variety of other conditions such as pulmonary valve stenosis, pulmonary artery stenosis, anomalous pulmonary venous return, and pulmonary arteriovenous malformation. Most commonly, multi-side-hole pigtail or NIH catheter are used with a high injection rate (40 cc/second) to visualize pulmonary veins. The dextro and levo phases of the injections are shown in Figure 45-5.

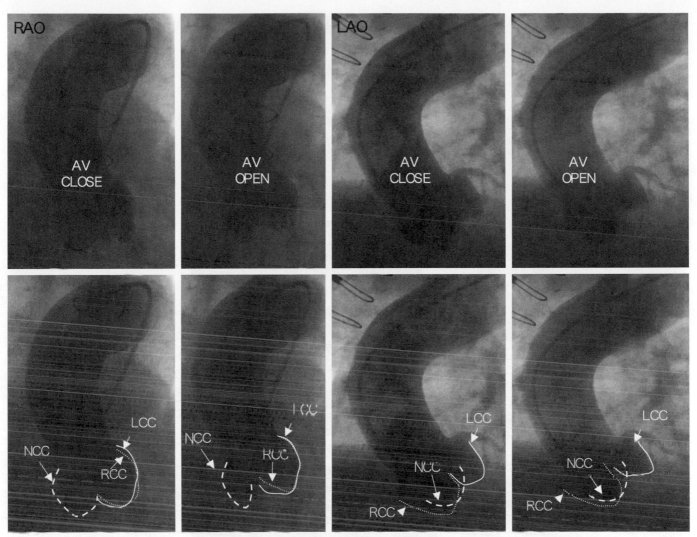

Figure 45-7 Shallow Right anterior oblique (RAO) and left anterior oblique (LAO) aortograms in a subject with aortic stenosis and restricted leaflet motion. *Bottom,* Different structures are delineated by dashed lines and arrows. For each view, the aortic valve is shown in closed and open positions. Note the overlap of the left and right coronary cusps in the right anterior oblique (RAO) projection and the right and noncoronary cusps in the left anterior oblique (LAO) projection. *AV,* aortic valve; *LCC,* left coronary cusp; *NCC,* non coronary cusp; *RCC,* right coronary cusp

Trans-Esophageal Echocardiography

TEE has become an integral part of invasive cardiac procedures, including ASD and PFO closures, mitral valvuloplasty, aortic valvuloplasty, percutaneous aortic valve replacement, and mitral valve E-clip.[5] TEE is a relatively safe procedure; however, in rare cases, esophageal tearing has been reported. Most patients in the cath lab are able to tolerate this procedure in the supine position without endotracheal intubation. Judicious use of short-acting sedatives such as midazolam and good suction of the posterior pharynx are critical for patient comfort. The TEE probe contains a 3- to 7.5-MHz (megahertz) ultrasound transducer at its tip and can be advanced to the esophagus or the stomach for proper visualization of cardiac structures.[6] The tip of the probe can be anteflexed, retroflexed, or moved side to side, as needed. The currently available TEE transducers are multi-plane and consist of a single array of crystals that can be rotated from 0 degrees to 180 degrees. The common views include the 0, 40 to 60, 90, and 120 degrees. The common positions for the TEE transducer are the upper mid-esophagus, mid-esophagus, and trans-gastric positions. Three important planes can be visualized at 0 degrees from the upper esophagus to the lower esophagus (Fig. 45-8). From the upper mid-esophagus

in the horizontal (0 degree) view or the basal short-axis view, the aortic arch, the pulmonary artery, the LAA, pulmonary veins, and the aortic valve can be visualized by scanning from left to right. At 0 to 20 degrees, in the mid-esophageal view or the four-chamber view, the LA, the left ventricle, the right atrium (RA), the right ventricle, the mitral valve, the tricuspid valve, and the inter-atrial septum can all be seen (see Fig. 45-8). The 0-degree trans-gastric view shows a cross-section of the left ventricle and the mitral valve (see Fig. 45-8). At 40 to 60 degrees, in the upper to mid-esophageal view, two important planes can be seen (Fig. 45-9). From the 40- to 60-degree view, the aortic valve, RVOT, the RA, the inter-atrial septum, and the LA can all be seen (see Fig. 45-9). From the 60-degree mid-esophageal level (the mitral commissural view) the mitral valve, the left ventricle, and the LA can be seen (see Fig. 45-9). In this view, the posterior mitral leaflet is to the left of the image display, and the anterior leaflet is to the right (see Fig. 45-9). Typically, A2 is located in the middle of the left ventricular inflow tract, with P1 and P3 on each side (see Fig. 45-9). At 80 to 100 degrees, with the view from the upper esophagus to the lower esophagus, three important planes can be visualized (Fig. 45-10). From the 90-degree upper-to-mid-esophageal view (the bicaval view), the SVC, the RA, the inferior vena cava (IVC), the inter-atrial septum, and the LA can all be

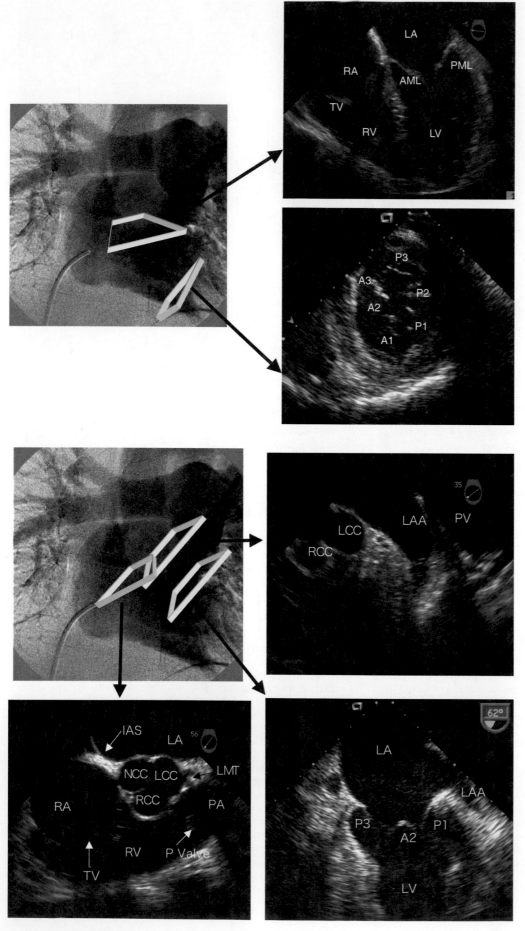

Figure 45-8 *Right panels*, Trans-esophageal echocardiography shows "0-degree" (horizontal) mid-esophageal and trans-gastric views. *Left panel*, The heart in the anteroposterior view (refer to Figure 46-4 for orientation). *Upper right panel*, The four-chamber view. *Lower right panel*, Short-axis view of the mitral valve with the corresponding leaflet segments. The posterior leaflet is divided into P1 to P3, and the anterior leaflet is divided into A1 to A3 from lateral to medial. *AML*, anterior mitral leaflet; *LA*, left atrium; *LV*, left ventricle; *PML*, posterior mitral leaflet; *RA*, right atrium; *RV*, right ventricle; *TV*, tricuspid valve.

Figure 45-9 Trans-esophageal echocardiography "40- to 60-degree" views in the upper to mid-esophagus with probe turned to the left *(right upper panel)*, upper to mid-esophageal junction with probe directed anteriorly *(left lower panel)*, and mid-esophageal commissural view *(right lower panel)*. *Left panel*, The heart in the anteroposterior view (refer to Figure 46-4 for orientation). *IAS*, inter-atrial septum; *LA*, left atrium; *LAA*, left atrial appendage; *LCC*, left coronary cusp; *LMT*, left main trunk; *LV*, left ventricle; *NCC*, non-coronary cusp; *PV*, pulmonary vein; *RA*, right atrium; *RCC*, right coronary cusp; *RV*, right ventricle; *TV*, tricuspid valve.

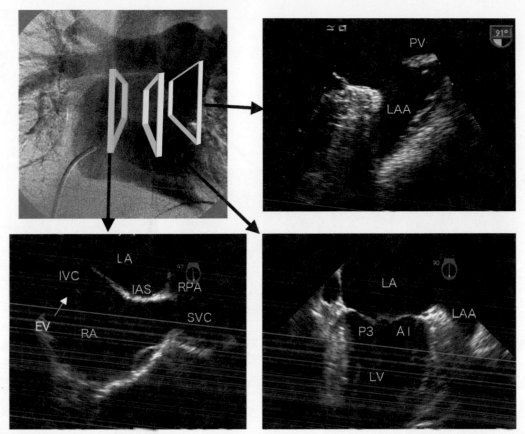

Figure 45-10 Trans-esophageal echocardiography shows "90-degree" mid-esophageal view of the left atrial appendage *(upper right panel)*, bicaval *(lower left panel)*, and the two-chamber *(lower right panel)* views as the probe is directed from left to right. *Left panel*, The heart in the anteroposterior view (refer to Figure 46-4 for orientation). *EV*, Eustachian valve; *IAS*, inter-atrial septum; *IVC*, inferior vena cava; *LA*, left atrium; *LAA*, left atrial appendage; *LV*, left ventricle; *PV*, pulmonary vein; *RA*, right atrium; *RPA*, right pulmonary artery; *RV*, right ventricle; *SVC*, superior vena cava.

Figure 45-11 *Right panel*, Trans-esophageal echocardiography shows "130-degree" mid-esophageal long-axis view of the ascending aorta. *Left panel*, The heart in the anteroposterior view (refer to Figure 46-4 for orientation). *AO*, aorta; *LA*, left atrium; *LV*, left ventricle; *RV*, right ventricle. P2 and A2 refer to the posterior and anterior middle scallops of mitral leaflets.

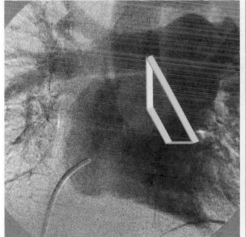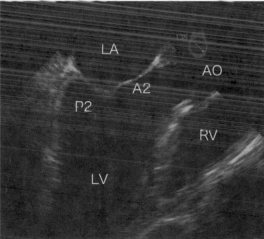

seen (see Fig. 45-10). From the 80- to 100-degree mid-esophagus (two chamber) view, the anterior and inferior left ventricular walls, the LAA, the mitral valve, and the coronary sinus can be visualized (see Fig. 45-10). In this view, the LAA can be examined for the presence of thrombi. Similarly, in this view, P3 is to the left of the image display, and A1 is to the right (see Fig. 45-10).

In the 120- to 160-degree mid-esophagus (long axis) view, the left ventricle, the LA, the aortic valve, the LVOT, the mitral valve, and the ascending aorta can be seen (Fig. 45-11). The most import TEE views are the four-chamber, long-axis, and two-chamber views as described above.

Intracardiac Echocardiography

ICE provides excellent images of intracardiac structures without the associated patient discomfort and airway issues that are present with other modalities such as TEE.[7] In addition, ICE can produce a clearer, well-defined image compared with TEE in certain situations,

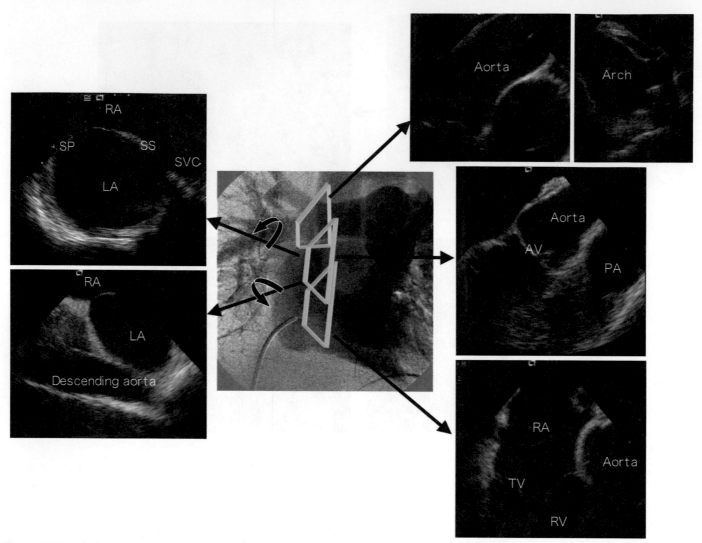

Figure 45-12 The basic views obtained by intracardiac echocardiography (ICE) in the neutral position (*right panel*) and with progressive clockwise rotation (*left panel*). The corresponding planes are shown on the fluoroscopy (*center panel*). Refer to Figure 46-4 for the orientation of the fluoroscopic image. In the neutral position from the superior vena cava (*top panel*), mid-right atrium (*right middle panel*) and at the level of tricuspid valve (*right bottom panel*), the above structures can be seen. The panel on the left is obtained by turning the probe clockwise from the mid-right atrium to visualize the entire inter-atrial septum from the anterior to the posterior aspect. *AV*, aortic valve; *PA*, pulmonary artery; *RA*, right atrium; *SP*, septum primum; *SS*, septum secundum; *SVC*, superior vena cava; *TV*, tricuspid valve.

including: assessment of the posterior part of the inter-atrial septum, where a TEE probe is too close to the area of interest, the pulmonary valve, because of its anterior position; during assessment of the aortic arch for dissection because of air shadowing from the bronchus; and in some cases of mechanical aortic valve because of shadowing. ICE is less optimal for evaluating mitral regurgitation (MR), the LAA, and left ventricular wall motion (e.g., contrast distribution for alcohol ablation). The two main ICE transducer systems are mechanical or rotational systems and phased-array systems. The mechanical transducer typically operates at 9 MHz or higher and produces a circular scan path perpendicular to the catheter. Mechanical catheters are imaging catheters without color or Doppler capabilities and are less useful than the phased-array systems, which allow complete evaluation comparable with TEE. In the authors' cath lab, phased array systems are used exclusively to guide structural heart disease interventions. The phased-array system (Acuson) uses 64 piezoelectric elements with frequencies of 5.5, 7.5, 8.5, and 10 MHz to produce a single-sector scan that is perpendicular to the long axis of the catheter. The probe is available as an 8 French (F) or 11F catheter with "monoplane" imaging. Each device has two handles, which allow the

operator to move the probe tip in anterior, posterior, and side-to-side directions. Maximum tissue penetration with ICE is around 10 to 12 cm. ICE is currently being used for assessment of the inter-atrial septum, pulmonary veins, the crista terminalis, the eustachian valve, the tricuspid annulus, the coronary sinus ostium, the aortic valve, the ascending aorta, and the aortic arch and for the assessment of the mitral valve in some cases. In general, there are three standard views; however, modification of these views by clocking or counterclocking may be necessary. One can start from the SVC and pull the probe back caudally for visualization of different structures. The initial view is from the SVC when the transducer is in the neutral position (Fig. 45-12). Subsequent counterclockwise rotation will rotate the transducer anteriorly, and the ascending aorta, the aortic valve, part of the pulmonary trunk, and the tricuspid valve can be seen (see Fig. 45-12). Clockwise rotation from this neutral position will rotate the transducer posteriorly, and the inter-atrial septum, the right pulmonary artery, and the descending aorta may be seen (see Fig. 45-12). The next view is typically obtained from the RA at the level of the tricuspid valve (see Fig. 45-12). This view shows the tricuspid valve and the ascending aorta. Further clockwise rotation delineates part of

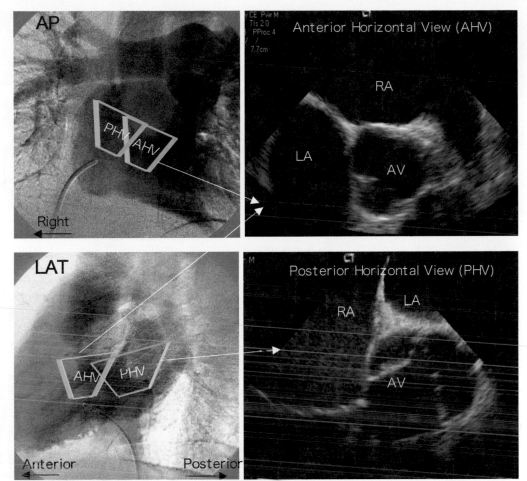

Figure 45-13 Intracardiac echocardiography (ICE) in the anterior and posterior horizontal views (*right panel*). The corresponding planes are shown in the anteroposterior (*left upper panel*) and lateral views (*left lower panel*) on fluoroscopy (see the text for details). *AP*, anteroposterior; *AV*, aortic valve; *LAT*, lateral view; *LA*, left atrium; *RA*, right atrium.

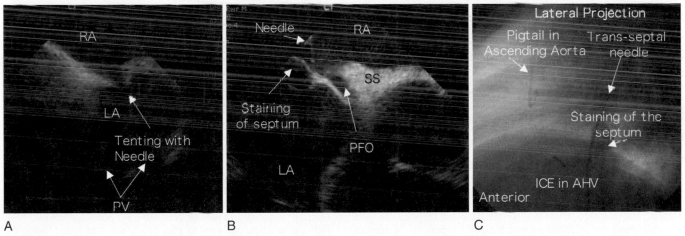

Figure 45-14 **A,** Intracardiac echocardiography (ICE) shows a good location of puncture demonstrated by needle tenting opposite to the pulmonary veins. **B and C,** A trans-septal puncture in a patient with patent foramen ovale with a long tunnel. Panel B shows the needle with stained septum. Note that the puncture site is close to the end of septum secundum (SS). Panel C shows the position of the ICE probe and septal staining in the lateral projection for the same patient shown in panel B. Note that ascending aorta is anterior, whereas the Brockenbrough needle is pointing posteriorly (C). *AHV*, anterior horizontal view; *LA*, left atrium; *PFO*, patent foramen ovale; *PV*, pulmonary vein; *RA*, right atrium.

the inter-atrial septum. To visualize the entire inter-atrial septum, posterior flexion is applied to the probe. This will allow enough depth so the entire inter-atrial septum can be visualized (Fig. 45-13). The third standard view (anterior horizontal view) is obtained by flexing the probe in the mid-RA with some clockwise rotation (Fig. 45-14). This generates a short-axis view of the aortic valve and allows

for better visualization of the anteroposterior section of the septum. Further clockwise rotation will demonstrate the mitral valve and its apparatus. It is possible to see the aortic valve in cross-section by rotating the probe clockwise and posteriorly; however, this view is less reproducible compared with the anterior horizontal view described above (see Fig. 45-12). Occasionally, the mitral valve can

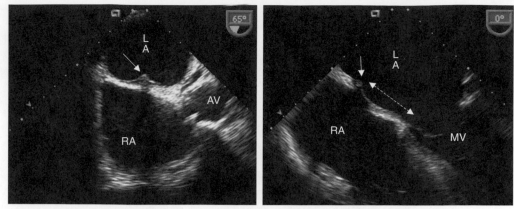

Figure 45-15   Trans-esophageal echocardiography shows "65-degree" (mid-esophagus) and "0-degree" (four-chamber) location of the puncture site. The distance between the puncture site and the aortic (*left panel*) and the mitral valve (*right panel*) can be determined on these views. Presence of tenting (*white arrow*) confirms the location and position of the needle. *AV*, aortic valve; *LA*, left atrium; *MV*, mitral valve; *RA*, right atrium.

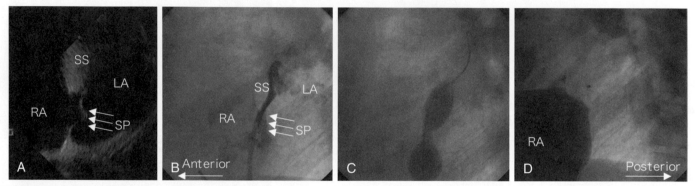

Figure 45-16   *Panel A*, Patent foramen ovale (PFO) with the septum primum (SP) and the septum secundum (SS) on intracardiac echocardiography. *Panel B*, The image is rotated to match the fluoroscopic image. The septum primum is flimsy (atrial septal aneurysm). Lateral view on fluoroscopy shows a patent PFO (*B*), "feeling" of PFO with sizing balloon (*C*), and proper positioning of the device with a right atrial angiogram before detachment (*D*).

be visualized from the coronary sinus, the right ventricle, or the superior aspect of the RA.

Specific Procedural Uses for Intracardiac Imaging

TRANS-SEPTAL PUNCTURE

The trans-septal puncture has become an integral part of many intracardiac procedures, including percutaneous mitral valvuloplasty, mitral valve repair, LAA closure, some cases of PFO closure, and AF ablation.[8] The goal is to cross the inter-atrial septum through the fossa ovalis, an area 2-cm in diameter that is bound superiorly by septum secundum and is called *limbus*. It is located posterior and inferior to the aortic root in the mid-portion of the inter-atrial septum. The procedure is performed using the Brockenbrough needle (USCI, Billerica, MA), which is introduced through a combination of an 8F Mullins sheath and a dilator. The procedure is performed primarily by fluoroscopic guidance, with ultrasound imaging as an important supplement. The most important fluoroscopic landmarks are the position of the aorta (determined by placing a catheter in the aortic root) and the margins of the RA and the LA. This can be determined by a right atrial angiogram in the anteroposterior and lateral projections (see Fig. 45-4). The needle is withdrawn caudally in the anteroposterior projection from the SVC; three medial drops, which correspond to the SVC-RA junction, the noncoronary sinus of aorta, and the limbus of

the fossa ovalis, are identified. The needle position is then checked in the lateral projection to ensure a posterior direction in relation to the aorta (see Fig. 45-14). The needle is advanced to the LA with close monitoring to ensure that there is no drop in pressure as the needle traverses the inter-atrial septum. Staining of the septum can be very helpful if there is any doubt about the location of the puncture site (see Fig. 45-14). TEE can also help determine the appropriate location of the puncture site. The vertical distance from the mitral valve and the aorta can be determined by four-chamber and 45- to 60-degree views, respectively (Fig. 45-15). TEE also helps rule out thrombi in the LA and the LAA and monitor the pericardium for the presence of effusion. The puncture site must be identified through recognition of tenting, as it indicates the correct needle tip position (see Fig. 45-15). ICE is now frequently used for this procedure, and it can clearly identify the inter-atrial septum, pulmonary veins, and the aorta. The ICE probe is kept in neutral view with retroflexion, as necessary, to stay away from the septum and is rotated clockwise to identify left pulmonary veins through the inter-atrial septum. The presence of left pulmonary veins opposite the ICE probe confirms posterior entry into the LA (see Figure 45-14, *A*). The appropriate site can also be confirmed in the anterior horizontal view (Fig. 45-16).[9]

PATENT FORAMEN OVALE

Closure of the PFO is discussed in more detail in another chapter in this text. In the normal embryologic process, the septum primum and the septum secundum (two independent crescent-shaped membranes)

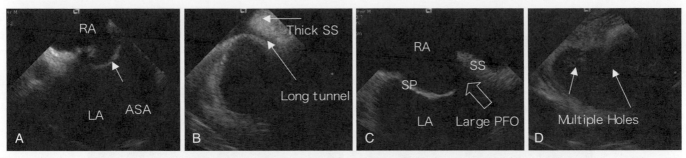

Figure 45-17 Intracardiac echocardiography shows presence of atrial septal aneurysm (A), the overlap of the septum primum and the septum secundum showing the "tunnel" (B), the thickness of the septum secundum (B), the size of the patent foreman ovale (C), and the presence of additional openings (D). ASA, atrial septal aneurysm; LA, left atrium; RA, right atrium; SP, septum primum; SS, septum secundum.

Figure 45-18 Intracardiac echocardiography shows the inferior and superior rims of the secundum atrial septal defect (left panel). Note the presence of small anterior rim (right panel). AV, aortic valve; LA, left atrium; RA, right atrium; TV, tricuspid valve.

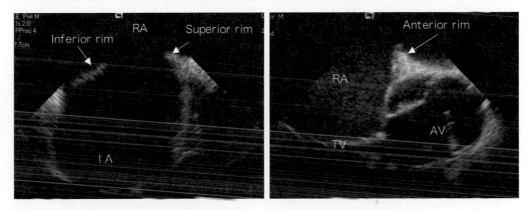

make up the inter-atrial septum. During fetal life, the mobile septum primum allows right-to-left shunting to maintain life. However, after birth, the left atrial pressure increases and helps fuse these two membranes. In about 15% to 20% of individuals, this fusion does not occur, causing occasional right-to-left shunting; this is called *patent foramen ovale*. Fluoroscopy is used in conjunction with ICE for percutaneous PFO closure. The most common view is the shallow LAO (10-degree) cranial (10 degree) view or the lateral (or 60-degree LAO) view, which allows better appreciation of the PFO orientation. A catheter is used to cross the PFO, and while the catheter is being pulled back, injection of the contrast material is performed to visualize the PFO on fluoroscopy (see Fig. 45-16). This allows visualization of the length of the tunnel (the overlap between the septum primum and the septum secundum) and the thickness of the septum secundum. Additionally, balloon inflation in the PFO not only helps determine the size of the PFO but also helps delineate the shape and size of the tunnel and allows one to "feel" the quality of the tissue around the PFO (see Fig. 45-16). Deployment of the device is usually done in the shallow LAO cranial view (10–10 degree), which allows perpendicular visualization of the inter-atrial septum. Lastly, injection of the contrast material under fluoroscopy from the guiding catheter before release confirms good apposition (see Fig. 45-16). ICE is commonly used to first assess the inter-atrial septum in the longitudinal plane, from top to bottom, in the anteroposterior direction. This is done by turning the probe in clockwise and counterclockwise directions at various heights in the RA (see Fig. 45-12). Next, the probe is flexed anteriorly, and the ultrasound beam is directed superiorly and posteriorly to visualize the anteroposterior length of the inter-atrial septum (see Fig. 45-13). ICE should be performed carefully keeping the following points in mind: (1) the presence or absence of an atrial septal aneurysm (Fig. 45-17, A), (2) the relationship of the septum primum to the septum secundum to determine the length of the "tunnel" (Fig. 45-17, B), (3) the thickness of the septum secundum (see Fig. 45-17, B), (4) the size of the PFO (see Fig. 45-17, C), (5) the presence of additional openings (see Fig. 45-17, D), (6) the degree of the shunt, (7) the presence of a

prominent Chiari network, and (8) the presence of other pathologies such as an ascending aortic atheroma. ICE can also show whether the wire has crossed the PFO when other holes are present. Similarly, ICE can be very useful when a trans-septal puncture for a tunneled PFO is necessary (see Fig. 45-16). The puncture has to be made fairly anteriorly near the PFO to adequately cover the PFO with the device. Device deployment is performed under ICE and fluoroscopy guidance. Proper tension in device deployment can make the device sit well without the risk of deploying both disks in the LA. Once the device is deployed, correct interrogation of all the margins ensures that the device will not embolize. The "push and pull" maneuver is then performed, and simultaneous imaging with ICE confirms that the atrial tissue is between the disks. Once the operator is satisfied, the device is released, and bubbles are injected to document any residual shunt. In the authors' institution almost all PFOs are closed under fluoroscopic and ICE guidance; however, TEE can also be used for this procedure. TEE is associated with greater patient discomfort and requires an additional operator. Two views are most helpful when using TEE: (1) the (30- to 40-degree) mid-esophageal short-axis view of the aortic valve and the inter-atrial septum, and (2) the (90- to 100-degree) mid-esophageal bicaval view, which shows the IVC and the SVC, the RA, and the inter-atrial septum. However, every patient is anatomically different, and subtle changes in these views and angles may be necessary for better visualization.

SECUNDUM ATRIAL SEPTAL DEFECT

Secundum atrial septal defect (ASD) results from an underdeveloped septum secundum that results in a true opening in the inter-atrial septum. The key elements in the assessment of ASD with echocardiography for percutaneous closure include (1) identification of the location of the defect in the septum secundum (superior, inferior, anterior, or posterior), (2) determination of the adequacy of the rims (Fig. 45-18), (3) identification of multiple defects, and (4) determination of the size of the defect. Pulmonary angiography is the most

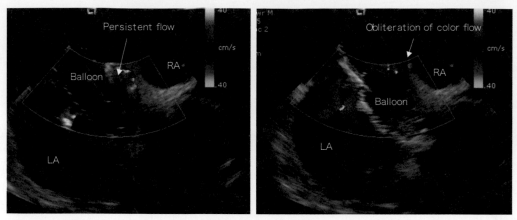

Figure 45-19 Intracardiac echocardiography shows the process of atrial septal defect (ASD) sizing. Balloon is inflated with color interrogation of the ASD. Initially, there is persistent flow around the ASD balloon (*left panel*). The balloon is inflated further to barely obliterate the flow across the ASD, and the size is measured. This allows choosing the proper size of ASD closure device without oversizing. *LA*, left atrium; *RA*, right atrium.

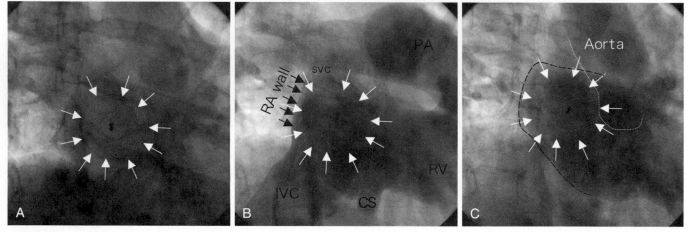

Figure 45-20 **A**, Right anterior oblique (RAO) caudal view of a right atrial angiogram shows atrial septal defect (ASD) device "end on." **B and C,** Surrounding structures in the dextro and levo phases of contrast injection. Note the relation of the device with the right atrial walls, the left atrial walls, and the aorta. White arrows show the margin of the left atrial device disk. Black arrows point to the right atrial wall. The aortic silhouette is traced with dashed white line. The left atrial border is shown by the dashed black line. *CS*, coronary sinus; *IVC*, inferior vena cava; *LA*, left atrium; *PA*, pulmonary artery; *RA*, right atrium; *RV*, right ventricle; *SVC*, superior vena cava.

helpful modality to identify anomalous venous drainage in the cath lab (see Fig. 45-5). ICE is the preferred imaging method for this procedure.[10] In general, the two views described above for PFO visualization are adequate for visualizing ASD and its structural details as well. Individualization of views should be considered because ASD occurs in many different sizes and shapes. Obliteration of color flow with balloon inflation allows proper sizing and avoids oversizing, which commonly happens when only the waist of the balloon is used with fluoroscopy (Fig. 45-19). Device deployment is guided by ICE, and proper gripping can be tested with the "push and pull" maneuver. Impingement of surrounding structures (e.g., mitral valve, SVC, roof of the LA, aorta, and coronary sinus) should be carefully assessed before releasing the device. Right atrial angiography with the end-on view of the device allows clear visualization of device margins and the relationship of the device to the left atrial walls and the aorta (Fig. 45-20).

MITRAL VALVULOPLASTY

Proper guidance with imaging can make percutaneous mitral valvuloplasty (PMV) safer and more effective, especially in countries where the patient population is mostly older in age and valves are less optimal for balloon valvuloplasty.[11,12] TEE is most helpful in guiding PMV (Fig.

45-21). It helps with (1) guidance for trans-septal puncture, (2) ruling out clots in the LAA before PMV, (3) monitoring the degree and the mechanism of mitral regurgitation (MR) with each balloon inflation, and (4) documenting the size of hole at the site of inter-atrial puncture after removal of the balloon. The authors prefer to use TEE in the cardiac cath lab for this procedure.[13] This can be safely accomplished in the supine position without endotracheal intubation if proper sedation and suction of posterior pharynx is performed. Careful interrogation of the mitral valve with TEE in the esophageal and trans-gastric views is helpful for determining the mechanism and severity of MR. Currently, ICE is not very helpful for mitral valve interrogation and assessment.

Fluoroscopy is also an important component of this procedure. Left ventricular angiography can assess the severity of MR; however, an adequate volume of dye should be injected in patients with mitral stenosis and a large LA. Fluoroscopy is also used to ensure that the balloon is in proper position and that it is not entangled with the mitral subvalvular apparatus. The RAO projection on fluoroscopy is helpful to ensure coaxial entry of the balloon through the mitral valve without going through the chordae. Before engagement and inflation, partial inflation of the Inoue balloon and advancement of the balloon to the cardiac apex in this view can ensure that the balloon is not entangled with the chordae.

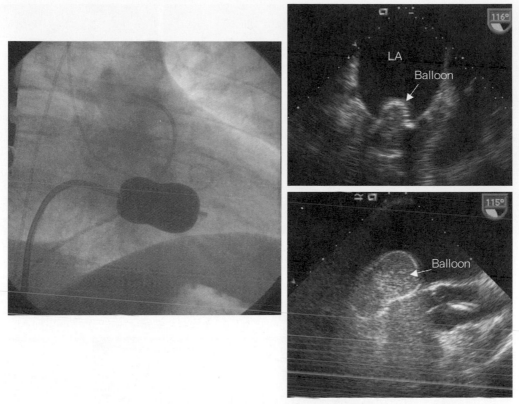

Figure 45-21 Mitral valvuloplasty using the Inoue balloon in the right anterior oblique (RAO) projection under fluoroscopy (*left panel*). Upper and lower right panels show a stepwise balloon inflation in the 110- to 120-degree long-axis view under trans-esophageal echocardiography guidance.

AORTIC VALVULOPLASTY

Fluoroscopy plays a significant role in visualizing the aortic valve and its orifice. Using fluoroscopy in the LAO and RAO projections can help determine which leaflet has the most motion (see Fig. 45-7). The AL-1 catheter should be pointed under the moving leaflet to cross the valve with a straight wire. If the right coronary cusp (RCC) is moving, this motion is best appreciated in the RAO projection. If the left coronary cusp (LCC) or the noncoronary cusp (NCC) has the most motion, then the LAO projection is helpful. The LAO view is the safest view to cross the aortic valve to prevent inadvertent entry into coronary ostia with a straight wire. This procedure is done with fluoroscopy only.[14,15] Hemodynamic measurements are important to determine the aggressiveness of balloon valvuloplasty. In the event of complications, TEE or ICE can help determine the exact cause, for example, the severity and mechanism of aortic insufficiency.

PULMONARY VALVULOPLASTY

Pulmonary valve stenosis is a common congenital abnormality. Many patients with this condition undergo pulmonary valvuloplasty in adulthood. Cine-angiography, trans-thoracic echocardiography (TTE), TEE, and ICE are helpful modalities used for this procedure.[16] Pulmonary artery angiography in the anteroposterior and lateral views is helpful to visualize the size of a pulmonary annulus and pre-existing pulmonary insufficiency (Fig. 45-22). Occasionally, right ventriculography in the same views may be performed to assess the RVOT (Fig. 45-23). Severe subpulmonary hypertrophy may be associated with significant dynamic RVOT obstruction following pulmonary valvuloplasty. Both TTE and TEE can be helpful in assessing the size of a pulmonary valve annulus. ICE provides useful assessment of

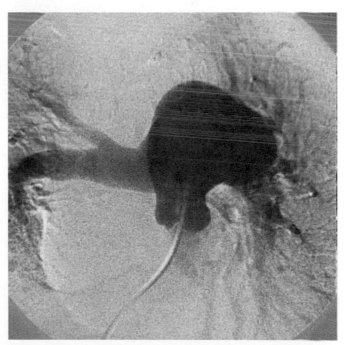

Figure 45-22 Pulmonary angiography assessment of the pulmonary valve using the National Institute of Health (NIH) catheter. Note the presence of mild pulmonary insufficiency and post-stenotic pulmonary artery dilatation. Digital subtraction was used for better visualization.

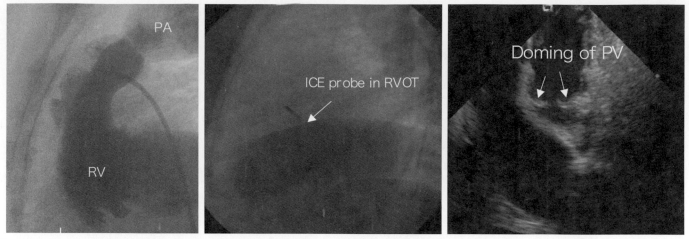

Figure 45-23 Right ventriculogram showing pulmonary stenosis in the lateral view (*left panel*). Intracardiac echocardiogram (ICE) probe in the right ventricular outflow tract in the lateral view (*middle panel*, same projection as the left panel). Pulmonary valve doming in the corresponding ICE view (*right panel*). *PA*, pulmonary artery; *PV*, pulmonary valve; *RV*, right ventricle.

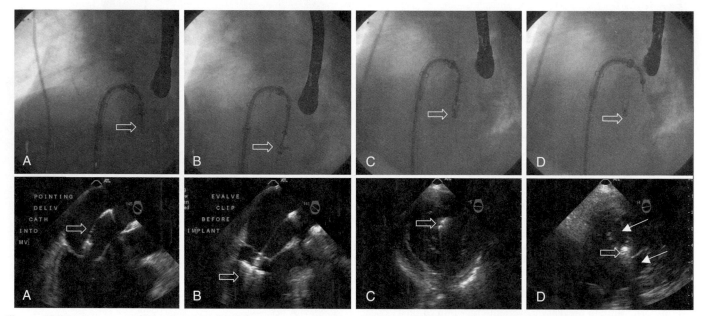

Figure 45-24 *Upper panel*, The device in the left atrium pointing toward the mitral valve (*A*), the opening of the clip and advancing across MV (*B*), grabbing the leaflet tips (*C*), and releasing the clip (*D*). *Lower panel*, Trans-esophageal echocardiography images of the device in the left atrium pointing toward the mitral valve (*A*), the opening of the clip and advancing across MV (*B*), perpendicular orientation of the clip to the mitral valve coaptation line in trans-gastric view (*C*), and final result with double orifice (*two white arrows*) (*D*).

pulmonary insufficiency and allows measurement of an annulus. The ICE probe can be placed in the RVOT for assessment of the pulmonary valve (see Fig. 45-23).

PERCUTANEOUS MITRAL VALVE REPAIR

The mitral valve apparatus consists of the annulus, the leaflet, chordae, and papillary muscles. The mitral annulus is saddle shaped, with a trigonal part and lateral commissures as the highest points. Some have suggested that the shape of the annulus changes when the LA and the left ventricle dilate. The anterior leaflet is longer but covers only one third of the circumference of the annulus. The posterior leaflet is

shorter but covers two thirds of the annulus. For edge-to-edge percutaneous mitral valve repair, TEE is used to guide the trans-septal puncture and to assess proper mediolateral, axial, and anteroposterior adjustments of the mitral system (Fig. 45-24). In addition, TEE can guide the perpendicular alignment of the clip arms to the line of coaptation. It is also useful for the assessment of MR with each attempt at treatment. The most common views include the mid-esophageal short-axis view (typically for trans-septal puncture and to guide catheter manipulation), the mid-esophageal commissural or "two-chamber" view, the mid-esophageal long-axis view (LVOT) (multi-plane angle of approximately 120 to 150 degrees), and the trans-gastric short-axis view (multi-plane angle 0 to 30 degrees) at the mitral valve

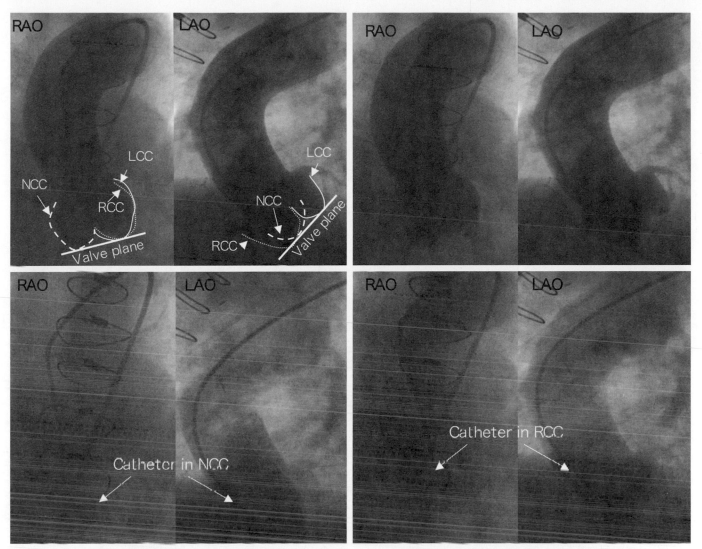

Figure 45-25 Left anterior oblique (LAO) cranial "40/20 degree" and right anterior oblique (RAO) caudal "20/20 degree" views of the aortic valve and its plane. The proper angulation of the camera has to be customized for each patient so that all the cusps are superimposed. Note that catheter is in different sinuses in different phases of injection. *LCC,* left coronary cusp; *NCC,* noncoronary cusp; *RCC,* right coronary cusp.

level. For coronary sinus–related procedures, fluoroscopy and TEE are helpful for the proper positioning of the device and for evaluating the effectiveness of the intervention. Angiography helps determine the relationship to the LCx artery and the coronary sinus. CT can help patient selection by defining the relationship among the coronary sinus, the mitral annulus, and the LCx coronary artery.[17]

PERCUTANEOUS AORTIC VALVE REPLACEMENT

Percutaneous aortic valve replacement is becoming a reality in the twenty-first century.[19] Different approaches with balloon-expandable or self-expanding, stented or unstented valves are being investigated. Accurate positioning of the valve is critical for both balloon-expandable and self-expanding valves; therefore, proper imaging in the cath lab is of paramount importance. Several elements are important to making this procedure accurate and reproducible. The aortic valve plane has to be accurately defined (see Fig. 45-7). Fluoroscopy with minimal contrast injection can, at times, determine the appropriate angles so that the aortic valve plane is seen without any overlap of the sinuses (Fig. 45-25). Usually, the LAO cranial and

the RAO caudal views are used. It is also important to identify the leaflets and commissures that are calcified and restricted. Accurate definition of leaflet morphology may help identify patients in whom compromise of coronary ostia is likely at the time of valve deployment. Injection of dye at the time of balloon valvuloplasty may also help predict this relationship. The ascending aortic slope (horizontal versus vertical in the LAO projection) may determine the ease or difficulty in delivering the valve. Angiography is important in determining the size, the calcification, and the degree of tortuosity of the iliac and femoral vessels. TEE is also important for valve assessment (calcification, annulus size, and severity), accurate positioning of the valve, and assessing the results of valve replacement (valvular or perivalvular leak and function). Again, complementary use of these imaging modalities is critical for the success of this procedure (Fig. 45-26).

Four-dimensional cardiac CT may allow better visualization of the aortic valve and its relation to coronary ostia and the morphology and extent of leaflet calcification (Fig. 45-27). Additionally, CT is critically helpful in the assessment of iliac and femoral arteries for size, tortuosity, and extent of calcification.

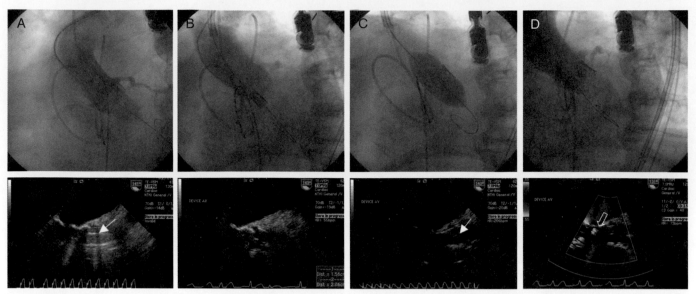

Figure 45-26 Percutaneous aortic valve replacement. *Panel A,* Valvuloplasty balloon in the aortic position with contrast injection depicting the distance from aortic cusp tips to coronary ostia. *Panel B,* Positioning of the stent-valve in proper position. *Panel C,* Once appropriately positioned, the valve is deployed with rapid pacing. *Panel D,* Final aortogram shows good position of aortic valve with mild regurgitation (*open arrow*). Upper panels are in left anterior oblique (LAO) cranial projection, and lower panels show TEE pictures in the aortic long-axis view (130 degrees).

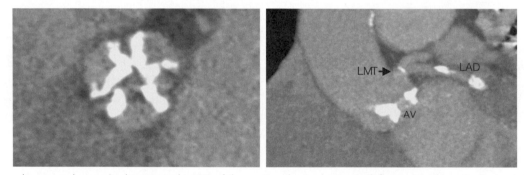

Figure 45-27 Four-dimensional computed tomography (CT) of the aortic valve in short axis (*left panel*) and longitudinal cuts (*right panel*). Note the significant calcification on the aortic valve and left anterior descending artery. CT can also help to determine the distance between aortic valve and left main trunk. *AV,* aortic valve; *LAD,* left anterior descending; *LMT,* left main trunk.

MECHANICAL PROSTHETIC VALVE ASSESSMENT

Occasionally, mechanical valves require full assessment for the presence of dehiscence, vegetations, or obstruction secondary to thrombus or pannus formation. While TTE and TEE can provide valuable information, some limitations persist. These include shadowing, pressure recovery phenomenon, and difficulty in visualizing the aortic valve caused by its anterior location. Fluoroscopy has been helpful in measuring the opening and closing angles of the mechanical aortic valve. To determine this, fluoroscopy cameras should be positioned such that tangential views of the leaflets can be obtained (Fig. 45-28). Since the rotational orientation during the placement of the prosthetic aortic valve can vary from patient to patient, there is no single view that can correctly visualize this valve. Therefore, the authors recommend a systematic approach starting with the 20- to 30-degree RAO caudal view and gradually increasing this angle toward an LAO

cranial projection (see Fig. 45-28). Occasionally, ventriculography may be helpful to visualize subvalvular pathology such as a pannus. In patients with a low-profile tilting disk (i.e., Bjork-Shiley, St. Jude, Medtronic-Hall valve), trans-septal puncture and pressure measurements with or without ventriculography may be necessary for better assessment of the prosthetic valve. Although the prosthetic aortic valve can be crossed with a 0.014 pressure wire, the safety of such a procedure is unclear. In situations where both the mitral and aortic valves have mechanical prostheses, an apical puncture or crossing of the aortic or mitral valve with a pressure wire can be considered (see Fig. 45-28). Cardiac CT also allows assessment of the opening and closing angles of the mechanical prosthetic valves. ICE can be used to assess prosthetic aortic valve function as well. It is possible to visualize the LVOT just below the mechanical aortic valve from the RA using ICE.

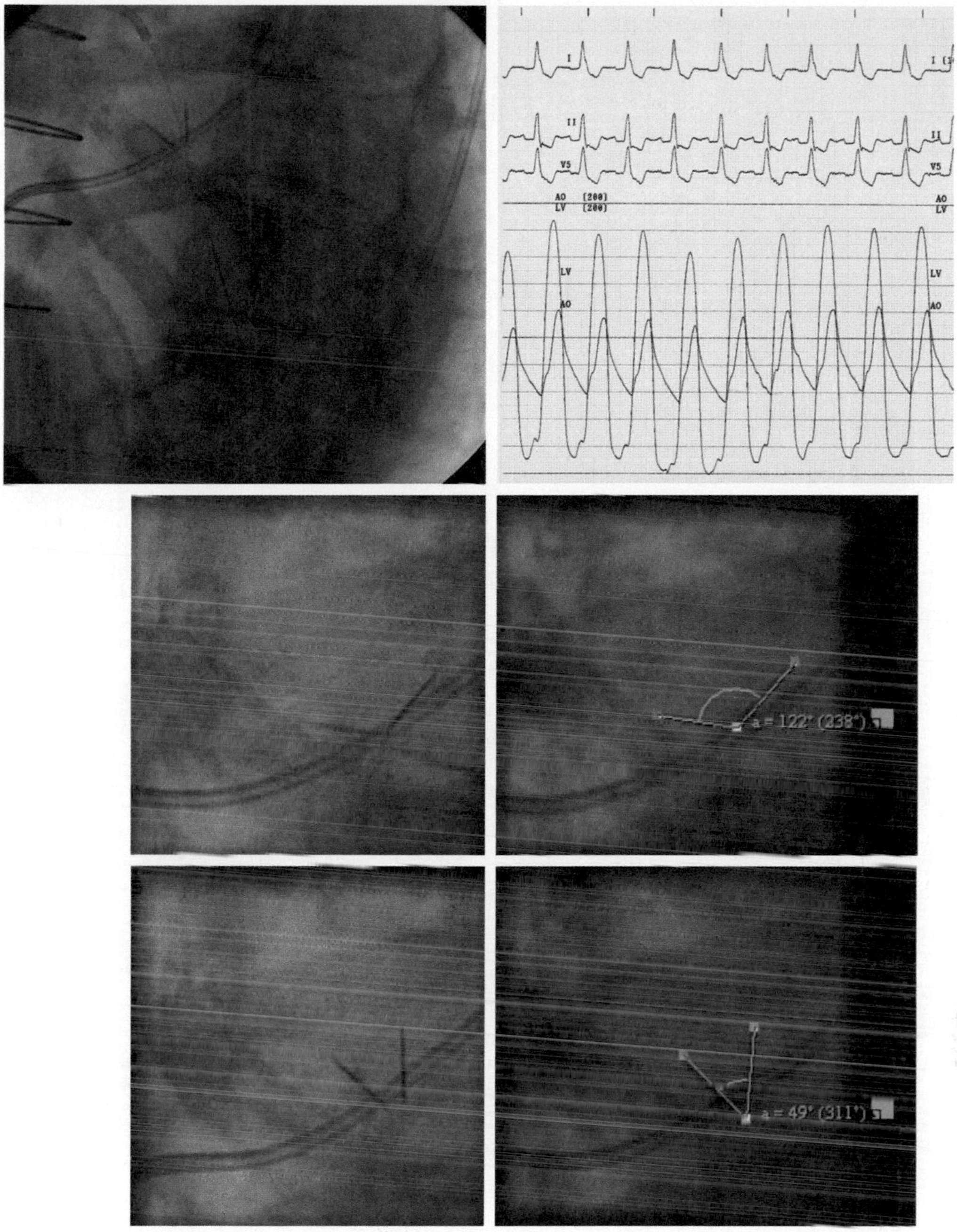

Figure 45-28 Prosthetic aortic valve assessment using fluoroscopy. This valve was crossed with 0.014″ pressure wire. Hemodynamic tracings show significant gradient across AV. Opening and closing angles are measured in the lower panel. Note that valve is imaged so that the leaflets are seen end on.

REFERENCES

1. Schoenhagen P, Numburi U, Halliburton SS, et al: Three-dimensional imaging in the context of minimally invasive and transcatheter cardiovascular interventions using multi-detector computed tomography. From pre-operative planning to intra-operative guidance. *Eur Heart J* 31(22):2727–2740, 2010.

2. Tuzcu EM, Kapadia SR, Schoenhagen P: Multimodality quantitative imaging of aortic root for transcatheter aortic valve implantation: More complex than it appears. *J Am Coll Cardiol* 55(3):195–197, 2010.

3. Hildner FJ, Furst A, Krieger R, et al: New principles for optimum left ventriculography. *Cathet Cardiovasc Diagn* 12(4):266–273, 1986.

4. Grollman JH, Jr: Pulmonary arteriography. *Cardiovasc Interv Radiol* 15(3):166–170, 1992.

5. Shanewise JS, Cheung AT, Aronson S, et al: ASE/SCA guidelines for performing a comprehensive intraoperative multiplane transesophageal echocardiography examination: Recommendations of the American Society of Echocardiography Council for Intraoperative Echocardiography and the Society of Cardiovascular Anesthesiologists Task Force for Certification in Perioperative Transesophageal Echocardiography. *J Am Soc Echocardiogr* 12(10):884–900, 1999.

6. Shanewise JS, Cheung AT, Aronson S, et al: ASE/SCA guidelines for performing a comprehensive intraoperative multiplane transesophageal echocardiography examination: Recommendations of the American Society of Echocardiography Council for Intraoperative Echocardiography and the Society of Cardiovascular Anesthesiologists Task Force for Certification in Perioperative

Transesophageal Echocardiography. *Anesth Analg* 89(4):870–884, 1999.

7. Kort S: Intracardiac echocardiography: Evolution, recent advances, and current applications. *J Am Soc Echocardiogr* 19(9):1197–1201, 2006.

8. Solomon SB: The future of interventional cardiology lies in the left atrium. *Int J Cardiovasc Intervent* 6(3–4):101–106, 2004.

9. Cafri C, de la Guardia B, Barasch E, et al: Transseptal puncture guided by intracardiac echocardiography during percutaneous transvenous mitral commissurotomy in patients with distorted anatomy of the fossa ovalis. *Catheter Cardiovasc Interv* 50(4):463–467, 2000.

10. Salome N, Braga P, Goncalves M, et al: Transcatheter device occlusion of atrial septal defects and patent foramen ovale

under intracardiac echocardiographic guidance. *Rev Port Cardiol* 23(5):709–717, 2004.

11. Guerios EE, Bueno R, Nercolini D, et al: Mitral stenosis and percutaneous mitral valvuloplasty (part 1). *J Invasive Cardiol* 17(7):382–386, 2005.

12. Guerios EE, Bueno R, Nercolini D, et al: Mitral stenosis and percutaneous mitral valvuloplasty (part 2). *J Invasive Cardiol.* 17(8):440–444, 2005.

13. Roberts JW, Lima JA: Role of echocardiography in mitral commissurotomy with the Inoue balloon. *Cathet Cardiovasc Diagn* (Suppl 2):69–75, 1994.

14. Feldman T: Transseptal antegrade access for aortic valvuloplasty. *Catheter Cardiovasc Interv* 50(4):492–494, 2000.

15. Vahanian A: Balloon valvuloplasty. *Heart* 85(2):223–228, 2001.

16. Shively BK: Transesophageal echocardiographic (TEE) evaluation of the aortic valve, left ventricular outflow tract, and pulmonic valve. *Cardiol Clin* 18(4):711–729, 2000.

17. Feldman T, Wasserman HS, Herrmann HC, et al: Percutaneous mitral valve repair using the edge-to-edge technique: Six-month results of the EVEREST Phase I Clinical Trial. *J Am Coll Cardiol* 46(11):2134–2140, 2005.

18. Choure AJ, Garcia MJ, Hesse B, et al: In vivo analysis of the anatomical relationship of coronary sinus to mitral annulus and left circumflex coronary artery using cardiac multidetector computed tomography: Implications for percutaneous coronary sinus mitral annuloplasty. *J Am Coll Cardiol* 48(10):1938–1945, 2006.

19. Cribier A, Eltchaninoff H, Tron C, et al: Percutaneous implantation of aortic valve prosthesis in patients with calcific aortic stenosis: Technical advances, clinical results and future strategies. *J Interv Cardiol* 19(5 Suppl):S87–S96, 2006.

46

Percutaneous Closure of Patent Foramen Ovale and Atrial Septal Defect

ALAN ZAJARIAS | DAVID T. BALZER | JOHN LASALA

KEY POINTS

- Although patent foramen ovale (PFO) and atrial septal defect (ASD) both involve an abnormal communication across the inter-atrial septum (IAS), their etiologic mechanisms are markedly different. PFO results from lack of fusion between the septum primum and the septum secundum, whereas a secundum ASD is caused by the absence of a segment of the atrial septum.

- PFO has been associated with paradoxical embolization, cryptogenic stroke, migraine headache, decompression sickness (DCS), and platypnea orthodeoxia syndrome.

- Until the results of ongoing clinical trials and registries become available, the routine closure of PFOs can be recommended only for patients who participate in clinical trials or who have had a recurrent cerebrovascular event while being therapeutically anticoagulated.

- Percutaneous closure of a PFO or a secundum ASD is a simple, safe, and effective treatment option for the appropriate candidates.

Introduction

The advent of cardiopulmonary bypass support revolutionized the management of many structural cardiac abnormalities. Ever since the first surgical repair of an ASD in 1952, surgical techniques were refined steadily, which conferred excellent short-term as well as long-term outcomes. Until recently, the management of ASD was primarily surgical. The last two decades witnessed the growth of percutaneous techniques for the management of coronary and other vascular pathologies. The refinements in percutaneous interventional technology and recent advances in the cardiac imaging techniques permitted percutaneous treatment of selected structural cardiac defects. ASD, one of the most common congenital cardiac anomalies, was one of the earliest to be approached percutaneously. King and Mills first reported ASD closure in five patients in 1976 using a double umbrella device.[1] They have since reported a 27-year follow-up on these five patients.[2] This device required a very large delivery system, which limited its use. These early successes were followed by the Rashkind device and subsequently the Lock Clamshell Occluder in the late 1980's.[3,4] Improvements in the technology paved the way for a newer generation of devices that made percutaneous closure of a secundum ASD not only acceptable but also preferable to the surgical approach. The closely related entity patent foramen ovale (PFO), which, until now, was rarely treated surgically despite its known association with paradoxical embolism, also became accessible to percutaneous closure. The last 9 years since the U.S. Food and Drug Administration (FDA) approval of selected devices for closure of ASDs and PFOs have seen a paradigm shift in the management of these two entities. ASD and PFO shifted away from the surgical arena and into the catheterization laboratory (cath lab); because of this, patient recovery time was shortened, complications were decreased, and treatment efficacy was maintained. The association of PFO with other disease processes such as migraine was identified, and this opened the door to new treatment options for a large portion of patients. This chapter provides an introduction to the percutaneous closure of ASDs and PFOs. It includes an overview of their embryology, pathophysiology, and clinical associations, followed by a description of the available devices for closure. The procedure, its indications, and complications are also detailed.

Embryology

By the eighteenth day of gestation, the primordium of the heart becomes evident. At the end of the fourth week, the endocardial cushions fuse to form the right and left atrioventricular (AV) canals. The endocardial cushions will serve as the primordium of the AV valves and the inferior wall of the atrium. At this time, the common atrium undergoes a complicated process of septation. The *septum primum* grows in a caudal direction toward the endocardial cushions, thus closing the inter-atrial communication (*ostium primum*). As the septum primum reaches its destination, the cells in its superior portion undergo apoptosis and coalesce to form the *ostium secundum*. A muscular *septum secundum* forms to the right of the septum primum and extends to reach the caudal border of the ostium secundum, forming a "flap-like valve" between both atria (Fig. 46-1; see Video 46-1).[5] Oxygenated placental blood enters the right atrium from the inferior vena cava (IVC) and is directed toward the IAS by the eustachian valve. The low left atrial pressure, the lack of blood flow through the pulmonary veins, and the preferential flow of the IVC to the IAS allows oxygenated blood to cross the foramen ovale and enter the systemic circulation. Blood entering the right atrium from the SVC is directed away from the IAS by the *crista interveniens*, preventing the mixture of nonoxygenated blood in this chamber. The right horn of the *sinus venosus* incorporates the SVC and the IVC into the right atrium (see Video 46-2) At birth, the pulmonary vascular resistances and the right cardiac pressures fall, and the left atrial pressure increases, forcing the *septum primum* against the *septum secundum* and occluding the "valve-like" foramen ovale. Complete occlusion occurs in the majority of the population, but in approximately 25% of the population, the fusion is incomplete, giving rise to a PFO.[6]

Patent Foramen Ovale

By echocardiography, the incidence of a PFO in the adult population is estimated to be approximately 25%.[6] Autopsy studies revealed the presence of a probe-patent PFO of 0.2 to 0.5 cm in 29%.[7] The frequency of PFO decreases with age and increases in size with each decade of life.[8] Spontaneous PFO closure may occur during adulthood, although recent data suggest that PFOs may recanalize over time.[9] The incidence rate of PFO is equal in both genders and among all ethnic groups; however, the PFOs in whites and Hispanics are larger and are associated with a greater degree of shunting.[10] The presence of a PFO was thought to be inconsequential until 1877 when Cohnheim postulated that a venous thrombosis may paradoxically traverse a foramen ovale and give rise to a systemic embolism.[11] Since that time, PFOs have been associated with varying disease processes, including cryptogenic stroke and paradoxical embolization, platypnea orthodeoxia syndrome, hypoxemia with normal pulmonary pressures, DCS in divers and high-altitude pilots, and migraine headaches.[12–17]

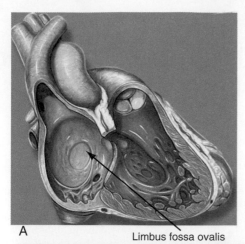

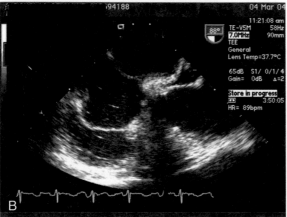

Limbus fossa ovalis

Figure 46-1 Diagram and photograph of the inter-atrial septum depicting the limbus of the fossa ovalis and the anatomic location of the patent foramen ovale (PFO). *(Modified from Patrick J. Lynch., Director of Yale University's ITS Web Services.)*

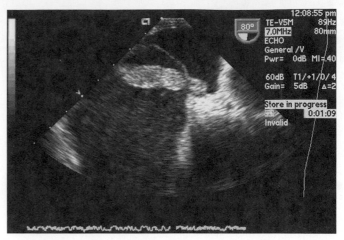

Figure 46-2 Thrombus in transit from the right atrium through a patent foramen ovale into the left atrium, illustrating the concept of paradoxical embolization.

PATENT FORAMEN OVALE AND CRYPTOGENIC STROKE

Depending on the age group, the etiology of a cerebrovascular accident (CVA) may vary. Atrial fibrillation (AF) and small vessel disease contribute to the majority of the strokes in patients older than 50 years of age. In patients younger than 35 years, the most common causes include nonatherosclerotic arteriopathies, arterial dissection, and thromboembolism.[9] However, in 35% to 40% of patients who suffer CVAs, the etiologies remain unknown even after a thorough evaluation, and the CVAs are classified as *cryptogenic*. Under this classification, different etiologies that remain unidentified by current diagnostic modalities may be included. The search for the probable etiologies of cryptogenic strokes has generated conflicting information. In a retrospective case-control study, PFOs were seen to be four times more prevalent among young adults who experienced a stroke without an identifiable cause compared with others with known causes.[13] In a meta-analysis, PFOs were found to occur up to six times more frequently among patients younger than 55 years who suffered a cryptogenic stroke compared with those who had identifiable causes of CVAs.[18] Others have noted a higher frequency of PFOs in patients with cryptogenic strokes irrespective of age (<55 years 48% vs. 4%; >55 years 38% vs. 8%, $P < 0.001$), although this observation is not generally accepted.[14] Among patients with cryptogenic strokes, patients with PFOs were less likely to have traditional cardiovascular risk factors such as hypertension, hypercholesterolemia, and tobacco use, which suggests a different mechanism for CVAs in this population subset.[19] The mechanism by which a PFO may participate in the generation of

a cryptogenic stroke is unclear. In situ thrombosis, paradoxical embolization, and predisposition to atrial arrhythmias have been proposed as mechanisms for PFO-associated cryptogenic strokes.[20] Paradoxical embolization—the passage of a venous thrombus into the systemic circulation through a PFO—has been the predominant theory (see Video 46-3 ; Fig. 46-2). Evidence that supports the role of PFOs in cryptogenic strokes includes case reports of the transit of thrombi across PFOs; cerebral distribution of cryptogenic CVAs, which suggests an embolic nature; and the increased frequency of deep venous thrombosis (DVT) in patients who had cryptogenic CVAs.[21–23] The Paradoxical Embolism from Large Veins in Ischemic Stroke (PELVIS) trial noted an increased frequency of positive magnetic resonance venography (MRV) testing for pelvic thrombus in patients with PFOs and cryptogenic CVAs compared with patients with known causes (20% vs. 4%, $P < 0.03$).[24] The corollary that patients with pulmonary emboli have a significantly higher stroke rate in the presence of PFOs (13% vs. 2%, $P = 0.02$) is also true.[25] In a prospective trial of 503 patients, Handke et al have shown that PFOs were more frequent in patients experiencing cryptogenic strokes irrespective of age (in patients younger than 55 years 43.9% vs. 14.3%; odds ratio [OR] 4.70, $P < 0.001$; and in patients older than 55 years 28.3% vs. 11.9%; OR 2.92, $P < 0.001$).[26] These data underline the causative role of paradoxical embolization in patients who had cryptogenic strokes. However, this association is still being debated. The majority of the information available on the association of PFOs and cryptogenic strokes originates from small case-control or retrospective studies, which places constraints on drawing a definitive conclusion. A large population-based case-control study that included 1072 participants (random controls, patients who had suffered noncryptogenic strokes, and patients who had suffered cryptogenic strokes) failed to show an association between cryptogenic strokes and PFOs.[27] The lack of association may have been related to the study design, since case selection included patients who did not have recurrent CVAs. Data from the SPARC trial, a prospective trial that questioned the veracity of a causal relationship between PFOs and strokes of unknown etiology, have been published.[28] The trial included 588 healthy volunteers in Olmstead County, who underwent multimodality testing and follow-up for stroke risk assessment. Over a period of 5 years, 41 of the subjects experienced a stroke. After adjusting for age and other cardiovascular comorbidities, PFOs were not found to be an independent predictor of stroke (hazard ratio [HR] 1.28; 95% confidence interval [CI] 0.65–2.50). The Kaplan Meier estimate of survival free of CVA was 91% and 93% in patients with and without PFOs, respectively. The trial confirms that the presence of a PFO does not pose an increased risk of stroke in asymptomatic patients. Unfortunately, this trial included an older population (66.9 ±

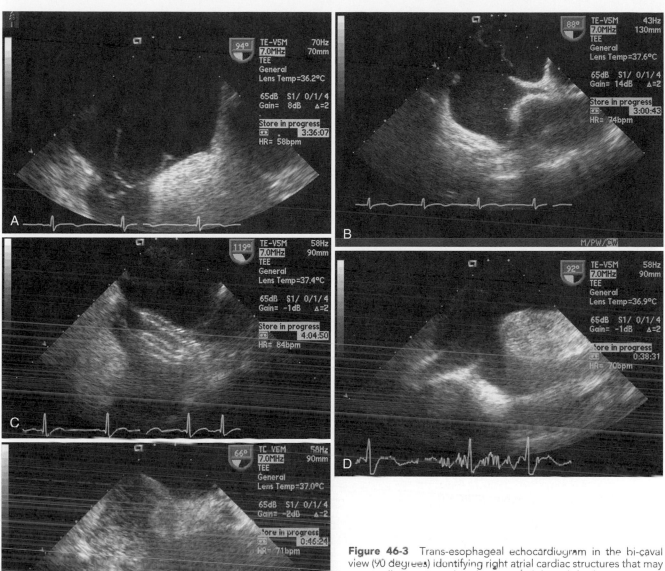

Figure 46-3 Trans-esophageal echocardiogram in the bi-caval view (90 degrees) identifying right atrial cardiac structures that may potentially increase the degree of right-to-left shunt across a patent foramen ovale (PFO) or may complicate the closure procedure. **A,** Prominent eustachian valve. **B,** Atrial septal aneurysm. **C,** A 25-mm AGA Foramen Occluder successfully captures the septum secundum and primum closing the PFO. **D and E,** Lipomatous hypertrophy of the atrial septum also creates a challenge in placing the closure device. Immediately after device deployment (*arrow*), the saline contrast study is mildly positive.

13 years) even though most other trials recognize the association between cryptogenic stroke and age in patients younger than 55 years; and this trial had a low prevalence of CVAs, which limited its ability to detect a statistically significant hazard. The hazard ratio may be as low as 0.65 or as high as 2.5 and still be consistent with the study's findings.

STROKE RECURRENCE AND RISK IDENTIFICATION

Prospective data from an observational study presented in abstract form have documented the incidence of CVAs in patients with PFOs as 1.10 per 100 person-years and in patients without PFOs as 0.97 per 100 person-years.[29] The low incidence does not make primary prevention cost effective. Additional risk factors that may detect people at risk need to be identified. The reported recurrence rate of cryptogenic stroke varies from 1.2% to greater than 16% but is generally around 2%.[30,31] In retrospective studies, the risk of recurrence has been found to be related to PFO size, patency at rest, shunt severity, and the presence of atrial septal aneurysm (ASA).[32–34] A prominent eustachian valve has been associated with increased patency of the foramen ovale and the risk of stroke recurrence, as it preferentially directs blood flow to the IAS (see Video 46-4 ; Fig. 46-3).[35] It has been postulated that a mobile IAS may increase the size of the foramen ovale facilitating the passage of thrombi. Recurrences of cryptogenic CVAs have been found to be associated with the degree of septal protrusion: patients with septum excursion greater than 6.5 mm had a risk of recurrence of 12.3% versus 4.3% at 3 years.[30] The combination of ASA and PFO was associated with an increased risk of recurrence in the French PFO/ASA study (HR 4.17; 95% CI 1.47–11.84).[36] However, this finding was not supported by the PICSS (PFO in Cryptogenic Stroke Study) trial.[37]

The PICSS trial was designed to define the rate of recurrent stroke or death in patients with and without PFOs, who were randomly treated with aspirin or warfarin over a period of 2 years. The multi-center, double-blind study included 265 patients who had cryptogenic strokes and 365 who had noncryptogenic strokes. PFOs were more frequently found in the cryptogenic stroke group (48% vs. 38%, $P < 0.02$), and larger PFOs were more frequently associated with the same stroke subtype (20% vs. 9.7%, $P < 0.001$). There was no statistically significant difference in the time to recurrent stroke or death in the cryptogenic stroke group when categorized by PFO status (14.3% vs. 12%). In all these patients, there was no difference in stroke recurrence when categorized by the presence of PFOs and ASAs. However, this study has significant limitations that may alter the generalization of its results. The subjects were older, had higher prevalence of CVA risk factors (diabetes and hypertension), and only 42% of the enrolled patients had had cryptogenic strokes. Because of this, the subgroup analysis of patients who had cryptogenic stroke may be underpowered for treatment assumptions. Because of the inherent limitations of the study design, the small patient population, and the differences in control groups, the association between PFOs and CVAs cannot be established at the present time. Larger randomized trials are required to answer this question.

Diagnosis of a Paradoxical Embolic Stroke

The diagnosis of a cryptogenic stroke is a diagnosis of exclusion. A complete evaluation to rule out other causes must be performed before assigning this diagnosis and should include a hypercoagulable evaluation, echocardiogram, heart rhythm evaluation, and carotid Doppler, as detailed in Table 46-1. If the working diagnosis of paradoxical embolization is still feasible, then a right-to-left shunt should be evaluated with an echocardiogram with bubble study or a trans-cranial Doppler.

TREATMENT FOR CRYPTOGENIC STROKE

Medical Treatment

Controversy exists regarding the best method for the prevention of recurrent events in patients who have experienced cryptogenic strokes. Medical treatment with aspirin or oral anticoagulants has been reported. In the PFO–ASA study, 267 patients who experienced cryptogenic strokes and had PFOs only or PFOs with ASA were treated with aspirin or with aspirin and warfarin if they had a venous thrombosis.[36] After 4 years of follow-up, there were 12 episodes of recurrent strokes and 9 recurrent transient ischemic attacks (TIAs). All episodes occurred in patients treated with aspirin. In the Lausanne Study, the 140 patients with the same characteristics were followed up for 36 months.

TABLE 46-1	Evaluation of Cryptogenic Stroke
Condition	**Diagnostic Test**
Cerebrovascular disease	Carotid Doppler
	Magnetic resonance angiography
Cardiac source of embolism	
Left atrial appendage thrombus	Trans-esophageal echocardiogram
Left ventricular aneurysm	Trans-thoracic or trans-esophageal echocardiogram
Ascending aorta atheroma	Trans-esophageal echocardiogram
Paroxysmal atrial fibrillation	Holter monitor
Hypercoagulable state	Protein C and S activity
	Anti-thrombin III level
	Lupus anticoagulant
	Anticardiolipin antibody
	Factor V Leiden
	Prothrombin 20210A mutation

Treatment was assigned on the basis of number of risk factors and included surgical PFO closure (8%), oral anticoagulation with target international normalized ratio (INR) of 3 to 4 (26%), or aspirin (66%). There was 1.9% yearly event rate for CVAs and 3.8% for the combination of CVAs and TIAs.[38] A meta-analysis, which included 895 patients in the medical therapy arm, evaluated the benefit of medical therapy versus trans-catheter closure of PFOs in patients with presumed paradoxical embolization; the analysis yielded a 1-year recurrence rate between 3.8% and 12%.[39] The PICSS trial was the only prospective, blinded, randomized trial that compared the efficacy of aspirin versus oral anticoagulation in patients with CVAs.[38] It found no statistically significant difference in stroke recurrence between patients with PFOs treated with aspirin and those treated with warfarin (17.9% vs. 9.5%; HR 0.52; 95% CI 0.16–1.67, $P = 0.28$). The high recurrence rate suggests other (non-PFO) mechanisms for CVAs in the older population. As expected, there was a slight increase in the rate of minor hemorrhage in patients on the warfarin arm. Currently, there is no consensus on the superiority of anti-platelet or oral anticoagulation therapy in patients with cryptogenic strokes and PFOs.[40]

Surgical Treatment

Surgical closure of PFOs in patients who had cryptogenic strokes has been reported. The largest series included 91 consecutive patients with a mean age of 44 years and one prior CVA. Surgery was evaluated with intraoperative trans-esophageal echocardiography (TEE), and suture or patch closure was employed. Closure was achieved in 98% of cases, and the actuarial freedom from recurrence was 93% at 1 year and 83% at 4 years. The surgical procedure was associated with significant morbidity in 21%.[41] Other smaller series reflected similar closure rates and significant morbidity.

Percutaneous Treatment

Percutaneous closure of PFOs has been available for the last decade. There have been no completed randomized trials to evaluate the superiority of percutaneous closure over medical treatment. The available data reflect single-operator or multiple-center experiences with moderate follow-up. Procedural success has been greater than 90% and may depend on the closure device used and associated anatomic variants. The presence of an ASA may decrease the rate of successful closure. Device modifications as well as growing experience and familiarity with the technique have greatly reduced the complication rate while maintaining appropriate closure rates. Windeker et al reported on 80 patients with a procedural success of 98% and a 2.5% recurrent TIA rate at 5 years.[42] Residual shunting has been identified as a risk for recurrent CVAs; overall percutaneous closure has a recurrent rate similar to that of medical therapy.[43,44] The only series that compared medical therapy to percutaneous closure in patients with PFOs and cryptogenic strokes was published by Windeker.[45] Patients were non-randomly assigned to percutaneous closure ($n = 150$) or medical treatment with aspirin ($n = 78$) or oral anticoagulation ($n = 78$) with an INR of 2 to 3. They were followed for 2.3 ± 1.7 years. Groups were comparable in terms of age, gender, and cardiovascular risk factors. Percutaneous closure led to a lower risk of the combined endpoint of death, recurrent stroke, or TIA (8.5% vs. 24%; RR = 0.48; 95% CI 0.23–1.01, $P = 0.05$) Patients with more than one event at baseline and those with complete occlusion of the foramen ovale were at lower risk of recurrent stroke or TIA after percutaneous treatment compared with those receiving medical therapy (7.3% vs. 33.2%; 95% CI 0.008–0.81, $P = 0.01$; and 6.5% vs. 22%4; 95% CI 0.14–0.99, $P = 0.0$). With its inherent limitations, this study demonstrated an advantage of percutaneous treatment in high-risk patients (recurrent CVAs), and hence the trials evaluating PFO closure have been developed as superiority trials and not as noninferior trials. Percutaneous closure of PFOs in patients who experienced recurrent CVAs despite being on medical therapy carries a class IIb indication by the American Heart Association (AHA) guidelines on stroke prevention.[46] Data to support PFO closure after a first stroke are insufficient. The FDA has permitted the use of the Amplatzer and Cardioseal septal occluder device under humanitarian device exemption (HDE) only in patients who have experienced recurrent CVAs while on conventional medical therapy (oral anticoagulation with a therapeutic INR). Currently, two prospective trials that are aimed at comparing medical treatment with percutaneous closure of foramen ovale in patients with recurrent cryptogenic strokes are under way in the United States. Both CLOSURE-1 (Evaluation of the STARFlex Septal Closure system in patients with strokes or TIAs caused by the possible passage of clot of unknown origin through a patent foramen ovale), and RESPECT (Randomized evaluation of recurrent stroke comparing PFO closure with treatments with established current standard of care) are facing slow enrollment because of the widespread use of the HDE clause and placement of an ASD occluder or other devices in an off-label manner. It is strongly recommended that physicians refer their patients who may be eligible for enrollment in the trial so that the appropriate questions are answered. This HDE has been replaced with a registry for patients who do not meet the criteria for the RESPECT trial.

Migraine Headache

Migraine headaches affect 12% of the U.S. population and generate significant morbidity and economic burden. The etiology of migraine headache with aura has remained elusive. People with migraine headaches have a twofold increase in the risk of stroke, and the risk increases to 3.5 in patients younger than 35 years of age.[47] Observational studies have also revealed that patients who experience migraines have increased frequency of silent, deep, white-matter lesions.[48] Migraine headaches are more frequently seen in patients younger than 45 years of age who had experienced an infarct in the posterior cerebral circulation.[49] These facts, and the growing information obtained from the evaluation of PFOs and cryptogenic strokes, prompted researchers to assess the frequency of right-to-left shunting in migraineurs. Anzola evaluated the presence of right-to-left shunting by trans-cranial Doppler (TCD) in 113 patients with migraine with aura and compared these patients with 53 patients with migraine without aura and 25 healthy age-matched controls. The presence of a PFO was significantly higher in the migraineurs with aura compared with the migraineurs without aura or the controls (48% vs. 23% vs. 20%).[50] Retrospective analysis of patients who underwent PFO closure for cryptogenic strokes revealed a decrease in the frequency of attacks of migraine with aura in 80% or even complete resolution in 56%.[51,52] Unfortunately, these studies may have been influenced by recall bias; the therapeutic effect of aspirin or clopidogrel, which may have been used for migraine prophylaxis; a high placebo effect; and the fact that migraine frequency decreases with age. In addition, retrospective studies do not demonstrate a causal association. The high frequencies of both PFOs and migraine headaches in the general population may favor a spurious association. Anzola et al prospectively compared patients with PFOs and cryptogenic strokes who underwent PFO closure ($n = 23$) with patients who had migraines, peripheral embolic events, or TIAs who underwent PFO closure ($n = 27$), and patients with migraines and PFOs who were treated medically ($n = 27$). After a 12-month follow-up, the frequency and intensity of the migraine attacks were significantly decreased in patients who underwent PFO closure.[53] Nonrandomized registries of patients suffering from migraines with aura have shown a 70% to 90% improvement or symptom resolution after successful PFO closure.[54,56] The association between migraine headache with aura and PFOs has generated new hypotheses on the etiology of migraines. It is now postulated that migraines may be related to microembolic events or the presence of high concentrations of circulating vasoactive substances that are not filtered by the lung, since they cross to the systemic circulation through PFOs. The MIST (Migraine Intervention With STARFlex Technology) trial attempted to test the association between PFOs and migraine headaches with aura. It was a multi-center, blinded study that randomized 432 patients with migraine to PFO closure with a STARFlex Septal Repair (NMT Medical, Boston, MA) implant or a sham procedure. The primary endpoint of cessation of migraines was not met. However, reduction in headache days in at least 50% occurred more frequently in the PFO closure group (42% vs. 23%, $P =$

0.038).[57] The discrepancy between the results from the MIST trial and other registries may be related to the exclusion of patients with previous CVAs or TIAs and the lack of complete PFO closure in the MIST trial. The exclusion of patients with previous TIAs or CVAs potentially filtered out those most likely to experience paradoxical embolization and clinical benefit. There is an ongoing attempt to study such patients in a randomized fashion. The U.S.-based MIST II trial (NMT Medical, Boston, MA) and the ESCAPE (St. Jude Medical, Fullerton, CA) trial have been discontinued because of slow enrollment. The PREMIUM trial (AGA Medical, Golden Valley, MN) has been enrolling since 2006, will have longer follow-up, and will attempt to answer questions left unanswered on previous attempts. Until these results are available, PFO closure should not be considered for the treatment of migraine headache with aura. The Gore Helex PFO closure device may be evaluated in patients with migraine who have had CVAs or TIAs (Personal communication, Mark Reisman, MD, April 2010).

Platypnea–Orthodeoxia and Hypoxia

PFO has also been associated with the rare platypnea–orthodeoxia syndrome. *Platypnea* refers to the feeling of dyspnea when in an upright posture, and *orthodeoxia* is arterial desaturation that occurs on standing. It is postulated that right-to-left shunting occurs across a patent foramen, particularly if an ASA is present. This entity is seen primarily in the very old and is associated with an event that alters the geometry of intra-thoracic organs, such as a pneumonectomy or an enlarged ascending aorta. Extrinsic compression of the right atrium or decreased compliance of the right ventricle may also predispose to shunting at the atrial level in these patients.[58] It is postulated that in patients with an elongated aorta, the heart is shifted laterally so that the IVC drains directly toward the atrial septum, although this is not fully understood as yet. This anatomic shift maintains the PFO open throughout the cardiac cycle and generates the physical findings.[59] Diagnosis is made by using saline contrast echocardiography with the patient in the supine and seated positions.[11] Surgical or percutaneous closure has been done successfully, leading to marked improvement in the patient's symptoms.[60,61] Hypoxia related to PFOs may also be observed in patients with severe pulmonary hypertension (PH) or obstructive sleep apnea.[62] The mechanism involves transient or persistent elevation of the right atrial pressure in relation to the left atrial pressure or re-direction of the IVC blood flow toward the IAS. Hypoxia related to right-to-left shunting at the atrial level has been associated with pulmonary arteriovenous malformations (AVMs), liver disease, amiodarone toxicity, pulmonary emboli with transient pulmonary hypertension, positive pressure ventilation, hypovolemia, aortic aneurysm, right ventricular infarction, Ebstein's anomaly, and carcinoid valve disease, among others. Making the diagnosis may be challenging, as it requires documentation of right-to-left shunting while the patient is hypoxic, and frank improvement occurs after closure. In patients with severe PH with decreased right ventricular function, the PFO serves as an escape valve, which aids the emptying of the right atrium into a lower pressure circuit (left atrium). In these patients, PFO closure may be fatal.

Decompression Sickness

DCS is caused by the presence of nitrogen bubbles that come out of solution in blood as the ambient pressure decreases when a person ascends from a dive. The amount of nitrogen bubbles generated will depend on the total time spent in the dive, the speed of ascent, compliance with decompression stops, and individual factors such as cardiac output. Generally, the nitrogen bubbles stay in the venous circulation and make it to the lungs, where they are rapidly diffused. It has been postulated that in the presence of a PFO, the nitrogen bubbles may enter the systemic circulation and travel superiorly toward the brain, occluding a small arterial branch. DCS in patients with PFOs is associated with early onset of cerebral or vestibular symptoms that occur within 30 minutes after a dive, even after the person has performed all the appropriate rest stops.[63] The association of PFOs and DCS is relatively new. In a case control study, Germonpre noted an OR of 2.25 for the development of DCS in divers with PFOs.[64] In a small case control study, patients with PFOs had an OR to develop DCS and were more likely to have silent ischemic lesions as shown on brain MRI.[65] Torti noted that divers with PFOs had a higher risk of developing DCS, required treatment for DCS, and had DCS that lasted more than 24 hours.[66] Currently, PFO closure to prevent DCS is not indicated because of low overall incidence and ease of avoidance of DCS.

DIAGNOSIS

Echocardiography plays an important role in the diagnosis of abnormalities of the atrial septum. Traditionally, TEE has been considered the gold standard to diagnose a PFO. The advantage of TEE is that it can identify all portions of the IAS, allowing for the diagnosis of all subtypes of ASDs, a fenestrated atrial septum, and PFOs. TEE also allows for the detailed identification of lipomatous hypertrophy of the septum, atrial septal aneurysms, a prominent eustachian valve, or a long PFO tunnel that may alter a planned closing procedure (see Fig. 46-3; see Video 46-5 ▣). TEE can identify other potential sources of embolization (i.e., left atrial appendage thrombus, cardiac tumors, aortic atheroma, etc.) as well. An ASA is defined as a redundance of the atrial septum with excursion greater than 10 mm into either of the atria and a 15-mm base. The degree and direction of the inter-atrial shunt will depend on the net pressure difference between both atria. The inter-atrial shunt direction will change with the phase of respiration and the cardiac cycle. It can be documented by color Doppler interrogation of the IAS (Fig. 46-4). Color interrogation along the fossa ovalis may cause erroneous identification of a PFO because of color cross-contamination when lowering the Nyquist limit. TEE's diagnostic sensitivity is significantly lower than that of a saline-contrasted study; the addition of saline contrast improves TEE's diagnostic sensitivity.[67] The injection of saline contrast through the femoral vein has been shown to be superior for the diagnosis of PFOs by TEE and for the appropriate sizing of ASDs.[68] Appropriate provocative measures that transiently increase the right atrial pressure (Valsalva maneuver), may be difficult to perform during a TEE because of the patient's sedation, relative hypovolemia from a fasting state, and the inability to close the glottis against the echo probe (Fig. 46-5; see Videos 46-6 through 46-8 ▣). Fundamental imaging trans-thoracic echocardiography (TTE) has been considered inferior for the diagnosis of PFOs. However, the advent of second harmonic imaging has improved the sensitivity of TTE to 90%.[69] An easier and more effective performance of a provocative maneuver (no sedation, euvolemia, complete glottic closure) during TTE may improve the image quality and is associated with a higher sensitivity than that of TEE for the diagnosis of PFOs.[70] In addition, the lack of invasiveness makes TTE a more attractive screening tool for PFOs (Fig. 46-6).

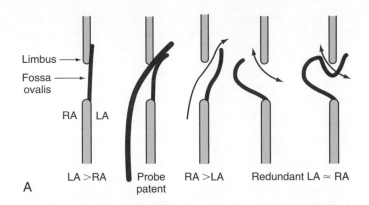

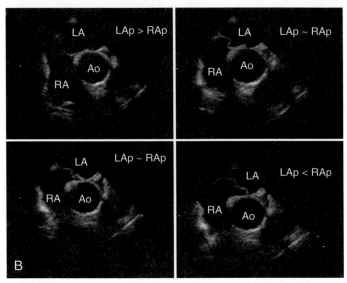

Figure 46-4   A, Association of inter-atrial septal anatomy and direction of inter-atrial shunt. **B,** Trans-esophageal echocardiogram depicting inter-atrial septal mobility related to left and right atrial pressures. *RA,* right atrium; *LA,* left atrium; *Ao,* aorta; *Lap,* left atrial pressure; *Rap,* right atrial pressure. *(Modified from Amplatz K:* Radiology of congenital heart disease, *St Louis, 1993, Mosby.)*

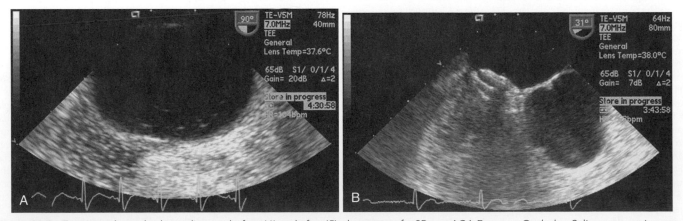

Figure 46-5   Trans-esophageal echocardiogram before (*A*) and after (*B*) placement of a 25-mm AGA Foramen Occluder. Saline contrast is present in the left atrium before device placement. After device placement, the saline contrast study is negative.

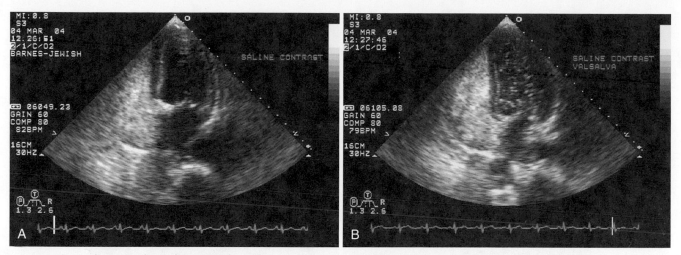

Figure 46-6 Trans-thoracic echocardiogram with a saline contrast study at rest (A) and during Valsalva maneuver (B). Transient increase in the right atrial pressure during the release phase of the Valsalva maneuver demonstrates a large right-to-left shunt at the atrial level secondary to a patent foramen ovale (PFO).

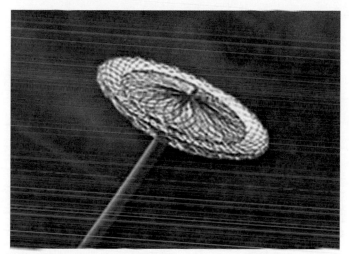

Figure 46-7 Frontal view of the AGA Amplatzer patent foramen ovale (PFO) occluder.

TABLE 46-2	Measurement for Device Selection for AGA Patent Foramen Ovale Occluder		
Distance from Defect to SVC or Aorta (mm)	*Suggested Device*		*Delivery Sheath*
>17.5	35 mm		9F
12.5–17.4	25 mm		8F
9–12.4	18 mm		8F
<9	None		

F, French; *mm*, millimeters; *SVC*, superior vena cava.

Trans-cranial Doppler (TCD) also has a role in the detection and quantification of right-to-left shunt. TCD insonates the middle cerebral artery and detects the presence of high-intensity transient signals when injected through a vein. Its sensitivity is similar to that of TEE, but its major limitation is its inability to detect the origin of the shunt. The number of transient signals has been shown to correlate with PFO size and postprocedure PFO patency.[67,71]

DEVICES

Currently, the two PFO septal occluder devices—(1) the Amplatzer PFO occluder (AGA Medical, Golden Valley, MN, USA) and (2) the STARFlex septal closure (NMT Medical, Inc. Boston, MA, USA)— have been approved by the FDA in the United States, under a registry and trial basis only, for the treatment of recurrent paradoxical embolization in the presence of a therapeutic INR. The Premere PFO closure device by St Jude Medical is no longer under investigation for migraine treatment.

Amplatzer Patent Foramen Ovale Occluder

The Amplatzer PFO occluder is a self-expanding, double-disk device made from 0.005-inch nitinol wire, with a polyester fabric sewn into both disks (Fig. 46-7). There are three device sizes based on the right

atrial disk diameter—18 mm, 25 mm, and 35 mm. In contrast to the ASD occluder, the stem is thin and mobile. The right atrial arm is larger than the left arm in the 25 mm and 35 mm sizes, whereas both are equal in the 18 mm. The right atrial disk stabilizes the device, thus preventing embolization from right to left. The thin stem allows varying degrees of disk mobility that permits the PFO occluder to seat appropriately in a long tunnel or around a hypertrophied septum. The left atrial disk dimensions are designed to decrease interference with pulmonary venous drainage or with the mitral valve and to minimize the presence of thrombogenic material in the systemic circulation. Device sizing will depend on the measurement from the foramen ovale to the SVC and from the foramen ovale to the aorta. The right disk radius should not exceed the shortest distance obtained (Table 46-2). The 25-mm device is used in the vast majority of the cases. The Amplatzer PFO occluder has the advantage of being self-expanding, has a simple deployment, and is placed through a small venous sheath (8F for 18 mm and 25 mm, and 9F for 35 mm). It is fully retractable until it is released. Its major disadvantage is that it is bulky within the atrial septum.

STARFlex Septal Occluder

The STARFlex septal occluder is characterized by a self-centering mechanism made from a single nitinol microspring, which attaches each arm to the corresponding arm of the opposing umbrella (Fig. 46-8). Available sizes are 23 mm, 28 mm, and 33 mm and the use of each is determined by PFO balloon sizing. Its major advantage is its low profile. Although modifications in the delivery system have been made, device retrieval may be cumbersome. It was used in the CLOSURE-I trial, which has completed enrollment.

Premere Patent Foramen Ovale Closure System

The Premere PFO closure system was available to patients participating in the PFO/Migraine trial sponsored by St Jude's Medical (Fig. 46-9),

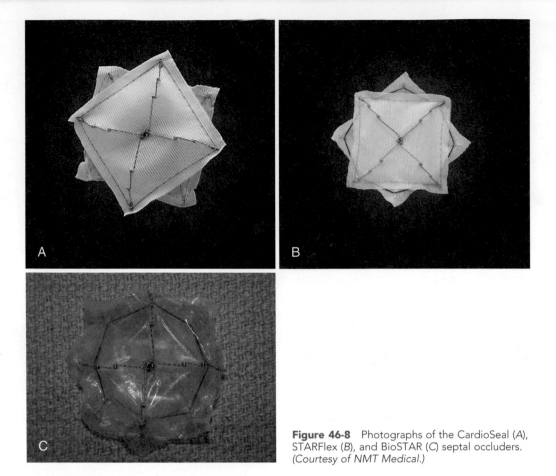

Figure 46-8 Photographs of the CardioSeal (*A*), STARFlex (*B*), and BioSTAR (*C*) septal occluders. (*Courtesy of NMT Medical.*)

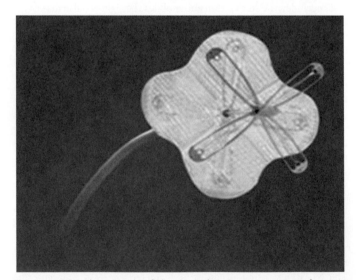

Figure 46-9 Photograph of the St Jude's Premere patent foramen ovale (PFO) occluding system. (*Courtesy of St. Jude's Medical.*)

which has now been discontinued. The Premere system has a very small profile and may be difficult to detect with echocardiography. Placement requires balloon sizing. Its unique design allows the operator to increase tension between the left and right atrial components by pulling the suture linking the two components together until locked, allowing it to conform to various tunnel lengths. Its major disadvantage is that larger venous sheaths (11F) and many steps are required

for closure. The operator has to be extremely careful not to excessively tighten the knot that holds the two disks together, since excessively tightened knots cannot be loosened subsequently and may lead to device fracture or malapposition.

Future Devices

The next generation of devices will be aimed at reducing the material that persists within the atria after closure. Initial trials using a bioabsorbable device, BioSTAR by NMT Medical, have been completed, and the device is currently available in Europe (see Fig. 46-8). Alternative methods of closure are also being developed and include suture closure (Sutura Inc.) or tissue cauterization with radiofrequency (Coaptus RF (CoAptus Medical Inc.) and PFx (Cierra Inc.) (Fig. 46-10); these methods have been evaluated with inconsistent results. The Coherex device (Coherex Medical, Salt Lake, UT, USA) (Fig. 46-11), which uses technology to selectively close the PFO tunnel without leaving significant material in the atrial chambers has been approved for commercial use in Europe. The Gore Helex (Gore Medical, AZ, USA) (Fig. 46-12) device is approved for ASD closure and, along with the Cribriform (Amplatzer, MN USA) device, has been used off label for PFO closure (Figs. 46-13 and 46-14).

INDICATIONS FOR PATENT FORAMEN OVALE CLOSURE

There is no FDA-approved indication for PFO closure in patients with PFOs for primary prevention of cryptogenic strokes. The AHA and the American Academy of Neurology (AAN) guidelines identify PFO closure after one CVA as a class IIb indication.[46] Currently, PFO closure for cryptogenic stroke is FDA approved in patients who experience recurrent strokes presumed to be paradoxical in nature and who have

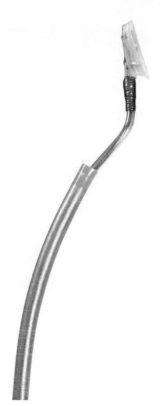

Figure 46-10 Photograph of the PFx closure catheter with radiofrequency ablation. *(Courtesy of Cierra, Inc.)*

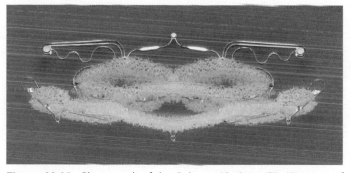

Figure 46-11 Photograph of the Coherex FlatStent EF. *(Courtesy of Coherex Medical.)*

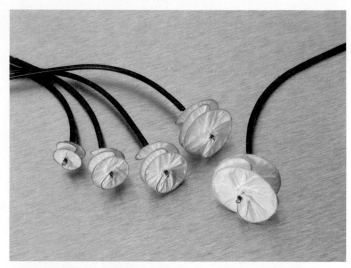

Figure 46-12 Photograph of the Helex septal occluder. *(Courtesy of Gore Medical.)*

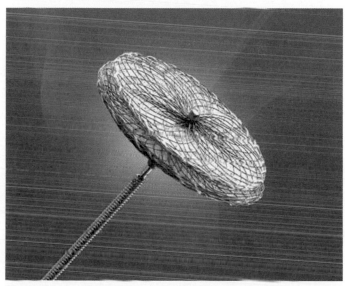

Figure 46-13 Photograph of the Cribriform Septal Occluder. *(Courtesy of AGA Medical.)*

failed conventional drug therapy or have had complications from drug therapy. Conventional drug therapy requires a therapeutic INR on oral anticoagulants.[72] On October 31, 2006, the HDE label given to the CardioSEAL septal occluder and the Amplatzer PFO occluder for PFO closure expired. PFO closure is only performed in patients enrolled in ongoing research protocols or registries, with the exception of "off label" use of ASD closure devices used for PFO treatment. Currently, there is no indication for PFO closure in patients who have migraine with aura and PFOs. There were three trials in the United States (ESCAPE, MIST II, and PREMIUM) evaluating the efficacy of PFO closure for the treatment of migraines. The MIST II and ESCAPE trials were halted early because of slow enrollment. The PREMIUM trial is still enrolling patients. Percutaneous treatment for refractory hypoxemia related to right-to-left shunting across a PFO is still available under humanitarian device exemption or by off-label application of the cribriform (AGA Medical) or Helex (Gore) occluders.

TECHNIQUE

Percutaneous closure of PFOs is done in the cardiac cath lab. It is a procedure that is performed under ultrasound (either TEE or intracardiac echocardiography [ICE]) and fluoroscopic guidance and requires the operator's familiarity with both sets of images. Ideally, patients scheduled for PFO closure have the diagnosis confirmed before their arrival at the cath lab. The procedure begins with an explanation of the risks and benefits of the procedure, and then patient consent to treatment is obtained.

Infection Prophylaxis

PFO occluder devices require the placement of prosthetic material in the IAS. To decrease the risk of prosthetic-related infection, infection prevention measures are followed. Procedures are postponed until indolent infections (urinary tract infections, upper respiratory infections) are cleared. Patients are given intravenous antibiotics (cefazolin or vancomycin) on call to the cath lab. Indwelling urinary catheters

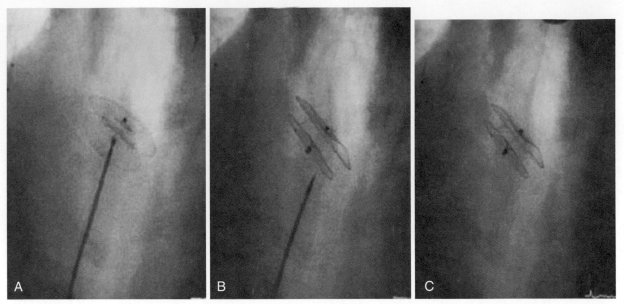

Figure 46-14 Deployment of an AGA Septal Occluder. **A,** Once in place, the device is "wiggled" to ensure stability. **B,** After stability is confirmed, the device is released by rotating the delivery cable. **C,** Once released, the cable is withdrawn into the delivery sheath to avoid trauma.

are not recommended to avoid transient bacteremia or nidus for infection.

Venous Access

Femoral venous access is obtained with an 8F sheath. If an ICE is planned, a second sheath (8F) is placed in the ipsilateral or contralateral femoral vein. If the contralateral vein is punctured, a 25-mm sheath is preferred for ease of catheter manipulation.

Crossing the Inter-atrial Septum

An end-hole multi-purpose catheter (MPA) is advanced over a stiff 0.035-inch or 0.038-inch 1.5-mm "J-" tipped guidewire (Amplatzer wire). On arrival to the right atrium–inferior vena cava (RA-IVC) junction, the wire is advanced toward the IAS at the level of the aortic valve. The catheter may be advanced or rotated medially to direct the wire across the PFO. If the guidewire does not cross easily, a Judkins right coronary catheter may be used instead. If the wire still cannot be threaded through the PFO, a hydrophilic coated wire (Glidewire, Terumo Medical Corporation, Tokyo, Japan) may be used to negotiate through the tunnel. If the crossing cannot be achieved after a significant amount of time or effort, it is important to confirm or refute the diagnosis of a PFO by repeating a bubble study from the femoral vein. If a PFO is present, intracardiac shunting will occur within the first five beats; the presence of late bubble passage into the left atrium implies an intra-pulmonary shunt. If significant passage of contrast is seen, a septal puncture and closing the opening of the PFO with a device instead of inserting the device through the tunnel itself may be considered. Once into the left atria, the guidewire is advanced to the left upper pulmonary vein, extending beyond the left main stem bronchus. It is important to remember that the passage of the guidewire should occur without resistance. The wire tip should be kept in the pulmonary vein to avoid perforation of the left atrium or stimulation of a cough reflex. Placing the guidewire in the left atrial appendage is not recommended, since it may lead to perforation. Recognizing incorrect localization of the wire is done by visualization of the wire coiling within the cardiac silhouette or the presence of premature atrial depolarizations.

Anticoagulation

Once across the foramen ovale, systemic anticoagulation with heparin to yield an activated clotting time 200 seconds or greater is done by administering heparin at 40 units of heparin per kilogram. Aspirin 325 mg should be administered before the procedure and clopidogrel after the procedure.

Device Selection

Echocardiographic measurements are made to aid in device selection (see Table 46-2). Some operators prefer to measure the PFO diameter with a sizing balloon to select the appropriate device (as with the St Jude and Cardioseal devices) or identify a long PFO tunnel. Balloon inflation must be done carefully to avoid tearing of the septum primum. With the use of the Amplatzer occluder, greater than 95% of the cases are done with the 25-mm or 30-mm device. The use of a sizing balloon is controversial with this device.

Delivery Sheath Insertion and Device Preparation

Once the device is selected, the short sheath is removed and replaced with a long delivery sheath. The sheath is advanced until the dilator has crossed the IAS. At this time, the dilator is separated, and the sheath is advanced slowly into the mid-left atrium. The dilator and the guidewire are removed, and the sheath is connected to the manifold, ensuring that air bubbles are cleared meticulously. The occluder devices are loaded according to the manufacturers' instructions. Generally, the device is attached to its delivery cable and retracted into the delivery catheter. Special care must be exercised on flushing the delivery catheter and device meticulously to remove all air bubbles from the device and system. Once flushed, the delivery catheter is introduced into the delivery sheath.

Device Positioning and Release

The device is pushed through the delivery sheath under fluoroscopy, and the presence of any air bubbles is noted. If air bubbles are present, the device is removed and re-prepped while the sheath is allowed to bleed back. Once the device reaches the tip of the delivery sheath, the sheath is withdrawn slowly until the entire left atrial disk is exposed. Echocardiographic confirmation of left disk deployment is required to ensure that the left atrial disk is not in the PFO tunnel. Once exposed, traction is applied on both the device and the delivery sheath to ensure that the left atrial disk abuts the atrial septum. Once the left disk is in place, the delivery sheath is withdrawn until the right atrial disk is expanded. As this is confirmed by fluoroscopy and echocardiography, the device is "wiggled" back and forth to ensure appropriate seating.

Echocardiographic evaluation of pulmonary veins and the mitral valve is performed to avoid device obstruction by these structures. It is normal to see color flow across the center but not around the newly placed and anticoagulated Amplatzer PFO occluder device, particularly those positioned in patients with ASAs. If no obstruction exists and the device appears stable, in appropriate position, and fully expanded, then release can be done according to the manufacturer's recommendations. It is important to retract the delivery cable back into the delivery sheath to avoid cardiac perforation. After the device is released, its conformation changes slightly as a result of released tension. Rotation of up to 45 degrees is not unusual. A saline contrast study is then performed to assess shunt severity. Generally, shunting may be absent, or at least significantly decreased, after the device is released. The bubble study becomes progressively negative as the device reaches its normal conformation and becomes endothelialized (see Videos 46-9 through 46-11 ▶).

Postprocedure Care

The authors' preference is to hospitalize patients overnight in a telemetry unit and administer two more doses of antibiotics. Chest x-ray to confirm correct device position is done the day after the procedure. A TTE with bubble study to quantify residual shunting is done 24 hours and 6 months after the procedure. Patients are prescribed 75 mg of clopidogrel daily for 1 to 3 months and daily aspirin for 6 months. For patients with histories of CVAs or TIAs, aspirin therapy may be continued indefinitely. Standard precautionary measures against subacute bacterial endocarditis should be followed for 6 months.

SPECIAL CONSIDERATIONS

Trans-septal Puncture

Trans-septal puncture is only rarely required to close a PFO. It is favored in two instances: (1) when the PFO tunnel is long, and passage with a guidewire or delivery sheath is unsuccessful; and (2) when the inferior border of an appropriately measured device interferes with the mitral valve.

Multiple Shunts

If an ASD is seen in association to a PFO, a single cribriform septal occluder may be used to minimize the shunt. If there is persistent shunting, then a second device may be placed, as long as there is no interaction with the mitral valve or pulmonary veins.

Atrial Septal Aneurysms

The presence of an ASA generally does not require a larger device. Closure of such PFOs is as successful with a standard technique at 6 months (see Fig. 46-3).[73] It is imperative to capture the septum secundum with the device to ensure a stable position, closure, and prevent device embolization or slippage.

Lipomatous Hypertrophy of the Atrial Septum

When closing a PFO in patients with lipomatous hypertrophy of the atrial septum, the device needs to straddle the septum secundum, giving the appearance of a "Pacman sign," where the disks are not parallel but divergent to each other at the septum secundum. This will ensure device stability and PFO closure. The off-label use of an ASD or VSD occluder (if the hypertrophy is >2 cm) may be required in these conditions.

COMPLICATIONS

Percutaneous closure of PFOs is a safe procedure. Procedural complications occur in 4% to 7% of patients but are usually mild.[45,74,75] A short procedural learning curve and significant device modifications have transformed PFO closure into an effective and safe procedure. Peri-procedural complications include air embolism, device migration, cardiac rupture and device erosion, vascular complications, and peri-procedural atrial arrhythmias. Complications occurring after discharge include endocarditis, device fracture, and device thrombosis.

Procedure-Related Complications

Air Embolism. Air embolus is a potentially devastating complication, but it can be easily recognized and avoided. Air embolus is caused by air entering the delivery sheath as the dilator is removed or during its preparation. It may also be associated with incomplete flushing of the device when introducing it to the delivery catheter or delivery sheath. Air bubbles in the delivery catheter can be easily recognized as the device is being pushed through the delivery sheath if done under fluoroscopy. It can manifest as sudden onset of hypotension, heart block, ventricular tachycardia, inferior ST segment elevation (as the right coronary artery is anterior), and transient neurologic decline. If air is seen within the delivery sheath, it is important to remove the device slowly to reduce the ensuing vacuum and to let the delivery sheath bleed back. If, however, the air bubble has entered the circulation, hypotension or ensuing arrhythmias should be treated with standard advanced cardiac life support (ACLS) protocol. Supplemental oxygen may aid in bubble resolution. The placement of patients in the Trendelenburg position may decrease the risk of cerebral embolization. Direct aspiration of the right coronary artery may be warranted if an airlock is present. Transfer to a hyperbaric chamber may be considered, if warranted.

Device-Related Complications

Device migration: Device migration is characterized by the loss of the correct position of the device. It may be related to incomplete device exit from the tunnel or placement of a smaller device in a large PFO or in an unrecognized ASD. If migration occurs, devices may be removed percutaneously with a snare. If this cannot be done, surgical removal is recommended.

Device arm fracture: This complication was mostly seen with the use of the earlier generation PFO STAR device but now is rarely encountered.

Device erosion: Although not seen in PFOs, recent data support that erosion is seen in patients with closures of large ASDs that lack an appropriate aortic rim of tissue.

Device thrombosis: Thrombosis has been seen in patients with concomitant hypercoagulable states who undergo PFO closure. It was also seen in up to 2% of the patients who received STARFlex devices, but newer generations of the device have addressed this limitation.[45] A device thrombus requires surgical removal. It is recommended that a hypercoagulability workup be performed for every patient who undergoes PFO closure for paradoxical embolization. If the workup is positive for hypercoagulability, therapeutic anticoagulation is warranted. Thrombus formation associated with AGA PFO closure devices has not been reported.

Transient arrhythmias: Atrial arrhythmias may be spontaneously seen in the first 6 weeks after the procedure and do not usually require treatment.

Nickel allergy: Brief case reports have noted an increase of headaches after device placement in a patient allergic to nickel. Although this has been difficult to prove, nickel desensitization should, nevertheless, be performed before elective PFO closure.

Endocarditis: Bacterial device infection or colonization may prove catastrophic. Strict sterile technique should be followed throughout the procedure and antibiotic prophylaxis for subacute bacterial endocarditis continued for 6 months. Surgical excision is warranted if endocarditis occurs.

CONCLUSION

Percutaneous closure of PFOs is an effective procedure that can be performed safely for the right indications. Its future will depend on generation of data that support its use. Interventional cardiologists should inform their patients and referring physicians about ongoing trials and registries that will generate the required information to determine who benefits the most from PFO closure and under what circumstances PFO closure is indicated. Once these questions are answered, this procedure has the potential to positively influence treatment for a large number of patients with PFOs.

Atrial Septal Defect

Among the various congenital cardiac anomalies encountered in the adult population, ASD is one of the most commonly seen; it is easily treated and has excellent long-term prognosis. Less than a decade ago, surgical repair was considered the standard of care and provided durable long-term results. Ever since the FDA approved a device for percutaneous ASD closure in December 2001, there has been a dramatic shift toward catheter-based closure of ASDs, which provides durable results paralleling surgical techniques, with remarkably less morbidity and extremely short recovery time and hospitalization. Patients and physicians alike prefer the less invasive percutaneous approach, although there are no studies, to date, that directly compare the surgical and percutaneous techniques for efficacy and safety. The preceding section provided an in-depth discussion on the PFO with regard to its embryology, physiology, clinical pathophysiology, and diagnosis, as well as its catheter-based management. Since there is a considerable overlap between the PFO and the ASD, the following discussion will highlight salient characteristics that are specific to ASD.

EMBRYOLOGY

Unlike a PFO, an ASD occurs when a portion of the inter-atrial septum is absent. Incomplete caudal growth of the septum secundum or excessive resorption of the septum primum gives rise to a *secundum ASD*. If the septum primum fails to reach the endocardial cushions, then a *primum ASD* occurs with its associated abnormalities (cleft mitral valve, inlet ventricular septal defect). A sinus venosus ASD occurs when there is abnormal resorption of atrial septal tissue adjacent to the caval–atrial junction. An "unroofed" coronary sinus or the absence of atrial tissue adjacent to the site of coronary sinus drainage into the right atrium results in a coronary sinus ASD (Table 46-3; Fig. 46-15).[76]

ANATOMIC AND MORPHOLOGIC CONSIDERATIONS

The secundum defect is located at the center of the atrial septum involving the fossa ovalis. This is a true tissue defect compared with a PFO. This is the only type of ASD that is amenable to trans-catheter

closure techniques. To permit percutaneous closure, there should be adequate tissue margins of the defect for securing the closure device to the tissue. Lack of adequate tissue margin predisposes to device prolapse or potential embolization. Furthermore, large defects also predispose the device to encroaching on the adjacent aortic root and the mitral valve, which can result in major complications. A thorough assessment of the atrial septum using echocardiography is a prerequisite for optimal closure. The choice of imaging depends on the operator's experience and preferences. The sinus venosus–type defects are

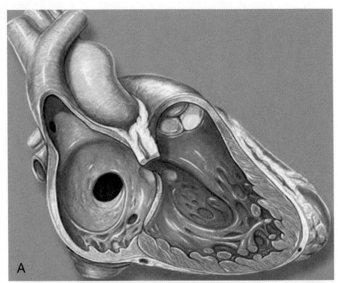

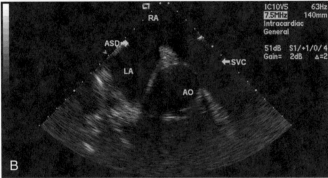

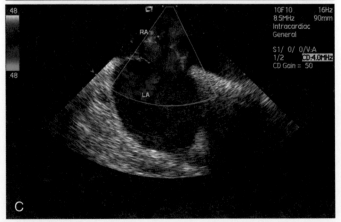

Figure 46-15 A, Diagram of a secundum atrial septal defect (ASD) depicted in cartoon form. **B,** ASD as seen by intracardiac echocardiogram. **C,** With color Doppler interrogation, a left-to-right shunt is identified. *(Modified from Patrick J. Lynch., Director of Yale University's ITS Web Services.)*

TABLE 46-3	**Characteristics of Atrial Septal Defects and Patent Foramen Ovale**	
	Patent Foramen Ovale	*Atrial Septal Defect*
Embryology	• Failure of the septum primum and the septum secundum to fuse completely	• Failure of the septum primum, the septum secundum, or both to develop normally
	• Pathway or channel between tissue flaps	• Tissue defect
Direction of Shunt	• Right atrial (RA) pressure greater than left atrial (LA) pressure; shunts right to left.	• Usually RA pressure equal to LA pressure, but shunts left to right, since RV is more compliant
	• LA pressure greater than RA pressure; may stay closed or shunt left to right	• Shunt reverses with Eisenmenger physiology
	• Shunt is dynamic and bi-directional in both atrial septal defect (ASD) and patent foramen ovale (PFO)	
	• Shunt direction depends on RA–LA pressure difference, right ventricular end-diastolic pressure (RVEDP)–left ventricular end-diastolic pressure (LVEDP) difference, phase of respiration, and volume status	

located in the perimeter of the atrial septum near the entry of the SVC. This defect prevents the normal separation of pulmonary veins from the right lung, the SVC, and the right atrium, as a result of which there is anomalous drainage of one or more pulmonary veins.[77] Typically, defects located close to the IVC are very rare and are termed *caval defects*. These can be associated with anomalous pulmonary venous drainage as well. Ostium primum atrial septal defects, also known as *endocardial cushion defects* or *common atrioventricular canal defects*, are accompanied by ventricular septal defects and a cleft mitral valve. With the exception of secundum defects, management of other types of atrial septal defects require surgical repair and will not be detailed here.

CLINICAL PRESENTATION

Usually, patients with ASDs remain asymptomatic during their childhood. Typically, the pulmonary outflow murmur or a fixed split of the second heart sound detected during routine physical examination prompts further evaluation, which finally results in the diagnosis. Some patients may experience recurrent heart failure and a predilection for recurrent respiratory infection during their childhood and may also present with easy fatigability and exertional dyspnea.[78] In adults, a longstanding ASD with significant shunting may manifest itself with atrial arrhythmias, pulmonary arterial hypertension, and heart failure.

HEMODYNAMICS

The direction and magnitude of the shunt across an ASD depends on the size of the defect, right and left atrial pressures, right and left ventricular compliance and end-diastolic pressures, vascular resistance in the pulmonary and systemic circuits, the phase of respiration, intra-thoracic pressure, and intravascular volume status.[79] In most patients who present with moderate- to large-sized ASDs, both atria are in open communication, and the mean atrial pressure is equal. The shunt is directed left to right, since the compliance of the right atrium and the right ventricle is higher than that of the left atrium and the left ventricle. In those with very small ASDs, without equalization of atrial pressures, the gradient across the atria will also play a role in the direction of shunt.

A close review of the Doppler performed across the defect shows that the flow is present during the entire cardiac cycle. Left-to-right shunting occurs mostly during late systole and early diastole, but atrial contraction also provides additional flow augmentation. The shunt results in diastolic overloading of the right ventricle and increased pulmonary blood flow. Depending on the size of the defect, pulmonary blood flow may be as high as five times the systemic flow. In those with longstanding and untreated ASDs, PH may ensue, which can result in reversal of the shunt's direction, depending on the status of the right ventricle. It should be noted that even in an uncomplicated ASD, a transient and small right-to-left shunt occurs during the early phase of ventricular systole and is further accentuated by respiration that decreases intra-thoracic pressure. This is the rationale behind performing a saline contrast study during echocardiography for the detection of ASDs (see Video 46-12).

DIAGNOSIS

As noted earlier, physical examination findings usually initiate the evaluation for suspected ASDs. This includes a hyperdynamic precordium, a fixed split of the second heart sound without respiratory variation, a loud pulmonic component of the second heart sound, and pulmonary outflow tract murmur. Primum-type defects may have associated tricuspid and mitral regurgitation murmurs. The electrocardiogram (ECG) further supports the clinical findings. Right-axis deviation, right ventricular hypertrophy, rSR', or rsR' pattern in the right precordial leads with normal QRS duration are common electrocardiographic findings in ostium secundum defects. Inverted P wave in lead III is seen in sinus venosus defects, whereas left-axis deviation

may denote an ostium primum defect. Lengthening of the P–R interval secondary to atrial enlargement and conduction delay can be seen in all three types of ASD.[80] Chest x-ray findings include right atrial and ventricular enlargement, prominent pulmonary artery, and increased pulmonary vascular markings.

Echocardiography

Echocardiography has replaced cardiac catheterization techniques for the diagnosis of ASDs.[81,82] Even shunt fraction can be reliably calculated using an echocardiogram. A TTE with saline contrast study should be done first. The defect may be visualized directly by TTE imaging, particularly from a subcostal view of the inter-atrial septum, but a TEE will provide much better anatomic characterization of the septum and the adjoining structures.[83,84] Typical echocardiographic findings include right atrial and right ventricular enlargement, increased pulmonary artery pressures, and Doppler demonstrating the presence of continuous flow across the atrial septum.[85] Recently, three-dimensional echocardiography with image reconstruction has been used to plan closure procedural details. ICE can also be used, but its use is mostly restricted to provide imaging guidance for percutaneous closure (see Video 46-13).

Cardiac Catheterization

In current clinical practice, cardiac catheterization primarily for diagnostic purposes is uncommon but is reserved for use when there is discrepancy between clinical and echocardiographic findings. In general, invasive hemodynamic assessment (cardiac catheterization) is performed during a planned percutaneous closure. The presence of a defect in the atrial septum is usually obvious when the guidewire or the catheter crosses the midline (atrial septum) into the left atrium. The site at which the catheter crosses provides diagnostic clues about the defects. In secundum defects, the site of crossing is midseptal, whereas in the case of sinus venosus and primum defects, the catheter crosses the IAS at a high level and a low level, respectively. Angiograms will further demonstrate the presence of shunting and other associated anomalies.[86] In the past, an injection in the right upper pulmonary vein was recommended, however, in clinical practice, this is rarely performed any longer. The authors do recommend performance of a pulmonary arteriogram in a straight pulmonary artery projection to rule out associated partial anomalous pulmonary venous return (PAPVR). A right heart catheterization with measurement of oxygen saturations in the innominate vein, the SVC, the right atrium, the right ventricle, and pulmonary arteries is also important to assess the size of the shunt and rule out associated problems such as PH and PAPVR. In addition, it is important to measure left atrial pressure, left ventricular pressure, or both, especially in older adults, as discussed below.

INDICATION FOR CLOSURE

Unrepaired ASDs that result in right heart volume overload can lead to progressive exertional dyspnea and exercise intolerance, atrial arrhythmias, and pulmonary hypertension. Therefore, right atrial or right ventricular enlargement as documented by echocardiography is accepted as an indication for percutaneous ASD closure. Previously a Qp/Qs ratio of 1.5:1 or greater was used to indicate closure, but this is no longer the case. Other indications, including paradoxical embolus, decompression sickness, and migraine headaches, are controversial and have been discussed above.

DEVICES FOR PERCUTANEOUS CLOSURE OF A SECUNDUM ATRIAL SEPTAL DEFECT

Percutaneous closure of ASD has proven to be reliable, safe, and effective as indicated by the recent available data, but choosing defects with appropriate anatomic characteristics is critical for successful closure. At the present time, only two devices are approved by the FDA for percutaneous closure of secundum ASD. The Amplatzer Septal

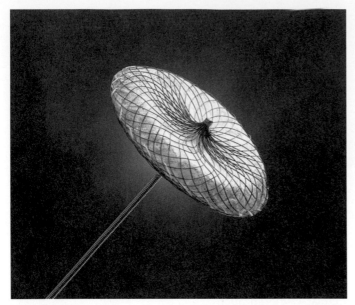

Figure 46-16 Amplatzer Septal Occluder. *(Courtesy AGA Medical Corporation.)*

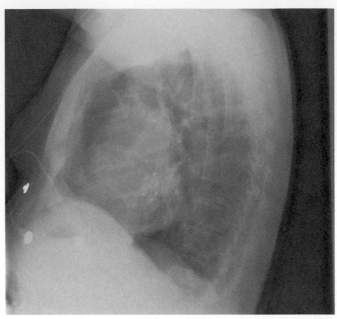

Figure 46-17 Chest x-ray after deployment of two AGA Septal Occluders.

Occluder (ASO) received FDA approval in December 2001, and the Gore Helex Occluder received approval in August 2006.

Amplatzer Occlusion Device

The AMPLATZER Septal Occluder (ASO, AGA Medical, Plymouth, MN) is a self-expandable, double-disk device made from a Nitinol wire mesh (Fig. 46-16). The two disks are linked together by a connecting waist, which corresponds to the balloon size of the ASD. To increase its closing ability, the disks and the waist are filled with polyester fabric. The polyester fabric is securely sewn to each disk by a polyester thread. The device is available in various sizes ranging from 4 mm to 38 mm (4 to 20 mm at 1-mm increments, 22 to 38 mm at 2-mm increments), and the size refers to the diameter of the waist. Device selection is based on the stretched diameter of the defect (i.e., a 10-mm stretched defect will require a 10-mm device). Devices are generally chosen to be the same size as or 1 mm larger than the balloon-stretched diameter to ensure an appropriate fit and to avoid oversizing. The pivotal study reported technical success rates of 95.7%.[87] Technical success was defined as successful deployment of a device. Twelve-month closure success rates were 98.5%, with closure success being defined as a shunt of less than 2 mm in those patients in whom a device was successfully placed. Patient selection and optimal imaging are key to success. Multiple ASDs in a patient may be closed with more than one device (Fig. 46-17). A cribriform device that is approved for closure of multi-fenestrated ASDs is also available. This device is available in four sizes: in 18-mm, 25-mm, 30-mm, and 35-mm diameters. Modifications to the basic technique may be needed to close very large ASDs; these will be discussed separately. The reported advantages of the Amplatzer device include ease of use, delivery possible with smaller-diameter catheters, and facility to retrieve and reposition before complete deployment. Furthermore, the device design permits it to self-center across the defect.

Gore Helex Occluder

The Gore Helex Septal Occluder (WL Gore, Flagstaff, AZ) consists of a device and special delivery system (Fig. 46-18). The device is a non–self-centering double-disk device that consists of a nitinol wire frame covered by an expanded polytetrafluoroethylene (ePTFE) membrane. The ePTFE is treated with a hydrophilic coating to facilitate

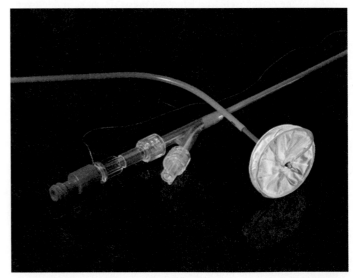

Figure 46-18 Gore Helex Septal Occluder and delivery system. *(Courtesy W.L. Gore & Associates.)*

echocardiographic imaging during device implantation. This device is approved for closure of ASDs with greater than 18 mm diameter. The device is currently available in 5-mm increments, from a 15-mm device up to a 35-mm device. Since the device is not self-centering, a device to balloon-stretched defect ratio of at least 2:1 is required to prevent residual shunting or device embolization. In the pivotal study and the continued-access trial, technical success rates of 88.1% and 85.6% were achieved, respectively, with "technical success" being defined as successful delivery of a device in patients in whom it was attempted.[88] Clinical closure success in patients who had technical success was 98.1% in the pivotal study and 98% in the continued-access trial at 12 months from implantation. "Clinical closure success" was defined as a completely occluded defect or one with a clinically insignificant leak. Theoretical advantages to the Helex occluder compared with the ASO is that it is a lower-profile device, has less Nitinol and therefore less nickel exposure, and may have a lower risk of erosions. Disadvantages include the larger and more complicated delivery system, the lower overall success rate, and the inability to close defects with larger than 18 mm diameter.

PROCEDURAL DETAILS

Patients receive 2 days of aspirin therapy before the procedure. Antibiotics are given on achieving access. Patients should be adequately anticoagulated with unfractionated heparin during the entire procedure and the ACT maintained above 250 seconds before device placement. Typically, femoral venous access is used, and the size of the sheath will be based on the size and type of the device and delivery sheath system chosen. TEE or ICE is used for imaging guidance during the procedure. If ICE is used, a second venous sheath is required during the procedure. As mentioned above, the authors recommend performing a right heart catheterization with every ASD closure. This includes measurements of oxygen saturations and pressures in the innominate vein, the SVC, the right atrium, and pulmonary arteries, as well as performance of pulmonary arteriography. This information is important to assess for the presence of partial anomalous pulmonary venous return (PAPVR) and pulmonary hypertension. If PAPVR is documented in the presence of a secundum ASD, it is important to decide how much of the total lung parenchyma is draining anomalously. If a single segmental vein is anomalous in the presence of a moderate-sized or larger ASD, then device closure of the ASD is still indicated, and the anomalous vein can be left in situ. It is also very important to measure left atrial pressure, left ventricular end-diastolic pressure, or both, especially in older adults, since left ventricular diastolic dysfunction can complicate trans-catheter ASD closure and precipitate left heart failure. Once the right heart catheterization has been completed, a 0.035-inch "J-" tipped guidewire, guided through a 6F multi purpose catheter, serves as the best tool to cross the defect. The wire is positioned in the left upper pulmonary vein. After crossing the defect, its size is measured using special sizing balloons. Sizing of the defect is very important for appropriate selection of the occlusion device. The ASD diameter is measured with a balloon specifically designed for sizing atrial communications such as the AMPLATZER (AGA Medical, Plymouth, MN) or the NuMed (NuMed Inc, Hopkinton, NY) sizing balloon. Under fluoroscopic and echocardiographic guidance, the balloon catheter is placed across the defect and gently inflated with diluted contrast medium until the left-to-right shunt ceases, as observed with echocardiography. The maximum stretched diameter of the balloon waist, while occluding flow across the IAS, is measured. This is the stop-flow diameter. It is critical not to overinflate the balloon, since this can lead to selection of an inappropriately large device and potentially increase the risk of erosion. The stretched diameter of the balloon is measured both fluoroscopically and with echocardiography and should be in close agreement (<1 mm difference). If an ASO is chosen, the sizing balloon is removed, and the appropriately sized sheath for delivery is advanced into the right atrium. The dilator is removed and the sheath is de-aired and then advanced over the wire into the left atrium. Alternatively, the sheath and the dilator can be advanced over the guidewire into the left upper pulmonary vein, and the wire and the dilator can then be removed. It is very important to de-air the sheath completely if this latter approach is taken, since otherwise an air embolus can result. The device is loaded and advanced into the delivery sheath under fluoroscopic and echo guidance (see Fig. 46-14 and Videos 46-9 through 46-11 ▮). Meticulous attention should be paid to avoid suction of air into the system, which occurs particularly when using large-caliber delivery sheaths. If the Helex occluder is chosen, its size will need to be at least two times the stop-flow diameter of the defect. The device can be delivered in two ways: (1) by removing the sizing balloon and guidewire and advancing the chosen device and delivery system through a 10F sheath across the defect under echocardiographic guidance or (2) by removing the sizing balloon and leaving the guidewire in place and sliding the guidewire through the tip of the catheter.

The catheter is then advanced across the defect and into the left atrium, where the guidewire is removed.

COMPLICATIONS

Complications are frequent with closure of ASDs. The vast majority of these are minor. The Amplatzer pivotal trial described a major adverse cardiac event (MACE) rate of 1.6% (7 of 442 patients). This included 2 arrhythmias requiring treatment, 3 device embolizations with surgical removal, 1 embolization with percutaneous removal, and 1 delivery system failure. This compares with an MACE rate of 5.2% (8 of 154) in the surgical control group in this study. Minor adverse cardiac events occurred in 6.1% of patients (27 of 442) compared with a rate of 18.8% (29 of 154) in the surgical group. Erosions associated with the use of the ASO are the most life-threatening complication. These are reported to occur with a frequency of approximately 1 per 1000 implants (0.1%); however, the true incidence is unknown, since the number of device implants is unknown. Amin et al reported on erosions associated with the use of the ASO and, based on a panel of physicians, developed recommendations to avoid this complication.[89] They recommended using the "stop-flow" method of balloon sizing. They also recommended only a gentle to-and-fro motion on the device once it is implanted. Patients at high risk for erosions were felt to be those needing an ASO greater than 1.5 times the unstretched diameter of the defect and those with deficient superior or aortic rims. It was also felt that devices that were deformed at the level of the aortic root (splayed around the aorta) were at higher risk of erosion. It should be noted that these recommendations are based on a panel of expert implanters and have not been verified in a prospective manner. Nevertheless, these recommendations have led to a general change in clinical practice. They are not without controversy, however. El-Said and Moore reported a survey of members of the Congenital Cardiovascular Interventional Study Consortium (CCISC), in which 71.7% felt that a device in which the disks approximated each other and touched the aorta without splaying were felt to be at highest risk of an erosion.[90] Embolization can occur with the ASO, and the implanters need to be familiar with retrieval techniques. Levi and Moore reported a survey of AGA Medical proctors, which demonstrated an embolization rate of 0.55% (21 of 3,824 device implants).[91] DiBardino et al reported an estimated embolization rate of 0.62% using data from the FDA's Maude database (Manufacturer and User Facility Device Experience).[92] In this latter study, two deaths were associated with embolization. Device embolization can occur to either the right heart or the left heart or to the aorta. Most device embolizations occur at the time of or shortly after implantation, although late embolization has been reported. Percutaneous device retrieval is possible in a significant number of cases. The device should initially be stabilized with a bioptome or a snare such that it does not cause hemodynamic compromise. This may require a second venous line from an inferior or superior approach; one site of access is used to hold the device, and the second is used to snare and subsequently retrieve the device. A long, relatively stiff sheath can be advanced adjacent to the device. The tip of the sheath can be beveled by cutting it at a 30- to 45-degree angle. This will facilitate pulling the device into the sheath. The right atrial microscrew can then be snared using a gooseneck snare delivered through a 6F cut pigtail catheter or other angled guiding catheter delivered through the retrieval sheath. The pigtail can be cut such that the distal end assumes a 90-degree angle in relation to the shaft of the catheter. This allows turning of the snare so that it may be steered to the microscrew. Once the microscrew is snared, the device is pulled back into the sheath. This may require rotation of the delivery sheath, the snare, or traction placed on the device from the bioptome to allow the microscrew to enter the beveled portion of the sheath. Once the microscrew enters the sheath, the entire device may be withdrawn. A fully deployed device should not be pulled across the mitral or tricuspid valves in view of the risk of valve damage. Instead, the long delivery sheath should be placed next to the device for retrieval if the device lies within the ventricle. In the case of devices that embolize to the atria, they may be snared and pulled into the IVC. Traction using a bioptome from above may then be applied to the superior portion of the device to facilitate entry into the retrieval sheath. Devices may also be retrieved from the pulmonary artery or aorta using modifications of this technique. If the device cannot be percutaneously removed, surgical removal will be necessary. The Helex pivotal trial and the continued-access trial reported MACE rates of 5.9% (7 of 119) and 3.9% (3 of 77), respectively.[88] This included a total of 4 cases of device embolization requiring percutaneous removal, 1 device removal secondary to wire fractures, 1 skin allergy, 2 patients with migraines, 1 with paresthesia, 1 hemorrhage requiring treatment, 1 allergic reaction, which was felt to be device related, and 2 possibly inappropriately sized devices. This compares with an MACE rate of 10.9% (14/128) for the surgical patients in the pivotal trial. Minor adverse cardiac events occurred in 28.6% (34 of 119) of patients in the pivotal study and 27.3% (21 of 77) of patients in the continued-access study. Wire fractures were reported in 5% (6 of 119) of patients in the pivotal group and 6.5% (5 of 77) in the continued-access group. Minor adverse cardiac events were reported in 28.1% (36 of 128) of patients in the surgical arm of the pivotal study. No erosions related to the Helex device have been reported. As noted previously, wire frame fractures are a relatively common problem associated with the use of the Helex device. Fagan et al reported data on wire frame fractures for every Helex device implanted in the United States over a 5-year period from April 2000 to April 2005.[93] During this time frame, there were 298 implants of which 19 (6.4%) developed wire frame fractures. Two devices fractured by 1 month, 10 by 6 months and 7 between 12 and 18 months. Eight of the devices had multiple fractures. Multivariate analysis found large device size to be an independent predictor for wire frame fracture. The 30-mm and 35-mm devices accounted for 84% of all fractures. There were no clinical problems such as embolization or increase in shunting related to the wire frame fractures in this study; however, Qureshi et al subsequently reported a case of wire frame fracture that resulted in an increase in shunting and a perforation of the mitral valve resulting in severe mitral regurgitation requiring surgical repair.[94] Close follow-up of any patient experiencing a wire frame fracture is therefore required. Embolization of the Helex occluder appears to be more frequent than that associated with the ASO; fortunately, the Helex device is relatively easy to retrieve. Latson et al reported a postprocedural embolization rate of 2.3% (6 of 260 implants) in patients with 12-month follow-up data.[95] Five of the embolizations occurred within 24 hours of the implantation procedure. In all 6 patients, the devices were removed by using trans-catheter retrieval techniques, but these procedures were not explained further. The authors have used both a vascular retrieval forceps and a gooseneck snare on separate occasions to grasp the device and pull it into a delivery sheath. Latson, as related by Tan, has suggested snaring the locking loop and pulling the device into the delivery sheath.[96] There is one case report detailing failure of percutaneous retrieval attempts of a Helex device that had embolized to the pulmonary artery in a small child.[97]

CLOSURE OF LARGE ATRIAL SEPTAL DEFECTS

Closure of large ASDs or those with very deficient rims can be difficult. Since the Helex device cannot be used to close large ASDs, the focus of this discussion will be on techniques that have been described for use with the ASO in this situation. In patients with a deficient SVC, superior or anterosuperior rims (retroaortic), it is very easy for the left atrial disk to prolapse through the defect on initial deployment. This can also occur with deficient posteroinferior rims. If multiple rims are deficient, the likelihood of successful closure decreases further. The operator's familiarity with advanced techniques of deployment greatly improves the chances of procedural success; therefore, it is imperative that the implanter become comfortable with several of these techniques.

In right upper pulmonary vein deployment, the delivery sheath is positioned with the tip in the right upper pulmonary vein (RUPV).[98] The left atrial disk is partially deployed in the os of the RUPV or near the roof of the left atrium, and the remainder of the device is then rapidly deployed by pulling down on the delivery sheath while fixing the delivery cable. Once the device is fully exposed, the cable can be pushed forward to reorient the device, if necessary. The unsheathing of the device in this technique must be performed rapidly to be successful.

In the left upper pulmonary vein (LUPV) deployment, the delivery sheath is placed in the LUPV, and the LA disc is deployed.[99] The left atrial disk is held in place in the LUPV and assumes an oblong shape. The remainder of the device is unsheathed by retracting the delivery sheath over the cable. Tension on the cable is then released, allowing the right atrial disc to reconfigure against the septum. This results in the left atrial disk being released from the LUPV and orienting correctly against the atrial septum. The unsheathing maneuver and the release of tension on the delivery cable must be performed sequentially and rapidly for the procedure to be successful. Proper deployment of the left atrial disk in the LUPV is paramount; if the left atrial disk is deployed too far into the LUPV, it will not be released from the vein; conversely, if the left atrial disk is not deployed far enough in the LUPV, it will be released prematurely, and thus the technique will not be successful. The left bronchus is a useful fluoroscopic landmark for the ostium of the LUPV and should be used as a guide for placement.

Alternative sheath uses are described below. The Hausdorf sheath (Cook, Bloomington, IN) has a double curve at the distal end, which facilitates appropriate alignment of the left atrial disk against the septum. This sheath is available in 10F, 11F, and 12F sizes. Use of this sheath is particularly helpful in patients with deficient superior or anterosuperior rims. A Mullins sheath may also be used. This sheath has more of a curve compared with the standard 45-degree TorqVue delivery sheath and may help align the left atrial disk appropriately. Kutty et al described the use of a Mullins sheath, in which the sheath is modified by cutting off the distal curved portion of the sheath parallel to the shaft. This results in what they termed *a straight side-hole sheath*.[100] The very sharp distal end of the modified sheath is then cut off to reduce the risk of perforation. This modification of the Mullins sheath results in the device exiting the tip of the delivery sheath at an angle that makes deployment of the left atrial disk parallel to the septum much easier.

With regard to the balloon-assisted technique (Fig. 46-19; see Videos 46-13 through 46-16 ▶), Dalvi et al reported a technique that uses a balloon as a buttress to prevent prolapse of the left atrial disk through the ASD during deployment. This technique is easy to learn and quite successful in the authors' experience. To perform this procedure, a second venous line is inserted. The ASD is crossed in a standard fashion, and the defect is sized using stop-flow. The appropriate device and delivery sheath are chosen and placed in the left atrium in the standard fashion. Through the second venous sheath, a catheter is placed in the LUPV and a 0.035-inch guidewire is placed. Over this guidewire, the sizing balloon or a Meditech occlusion balloon can be placed. The balloon is inflated in the right atrium and placed against the right side of the atrial septum. The left atrial disk of the device is then deployed and pulled against the left side of the septum. The balloon helps prevent prolapse of the device at this time. The remainder of the device is deployed while the balloon remains in place against the septum. Once the entire device is deployed, the sizing balloon is deflated. TEE or ICE is used to assess the results; if the device has been correctly placed, the deflated balloon and guidewire are removed from across the septum. One disadvantage of this technique is that a second or third (if ICE is used) venous access is required.

Miscellaneous Techniques

Several other techniques have been described to assist in closure of large ASDs or those with deficient rims. These include the use of the dilator as a buttress similar to that described for the balloon-assisted technique, use of a right coronary guiding catheter, and use of a deflectable electrophysiology sheath.[101-103]

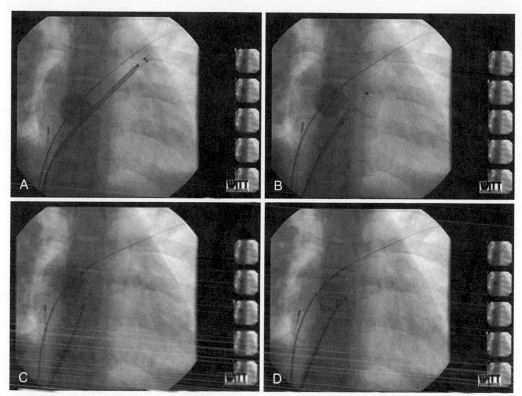

Figure 46-19 Steps in balloon assisted technique. **A,** Inflation of occlusion balloon against the right atrial side of the atrial septum with the Amplatzer delivery sheath in place. **B,** Deployment of left atrial disk using an occlusion balloon as buttress to prevent prolapse of the disk. **C,** Deployment of right atrial disk with the occlusion balloon still in place. **D,** Deflation of the occlusion balloon and reconfiguration of the Amplatzer device without prolapse of disk. (See corresponding Videos 46-13 through 46-16.)

Multi-Fenestrated Atrial Septal Defects

Fenestrations are frequently encountered with secundum ASDs. These additional defects are often found along the posteroinferior portion of the atrial septum. In many situations, closure of the primary defect within the fossa ovalis is enough to provide closure of the secondary defects as well. If the secondary fenestrated portion of the septum is fairly remote from the primary defect, then closure using multiple devices may be required (see discussion later). If the fossa ovalis itself has multiple fenestrations, then use of a non–self-centering device such as the Helex device or the Amplatzer cribriform device is appropriate. The procedural details for closure of fenestrated ASDs differ from a standard secundum ASD in that the defect is *not* balloon sized. Instead, the distance from the central-most defect to the furthest reaches of the outer-most defect is measured under TEE or ICE guidance. It is important to measure this in multiple views and to use the largest diameter measured to choose a device. This measured dimension represents the radius of the device to be chosen. The chosen device must have a diameter at least twice the measured radius to ensure that all the holes will be covered with device material.

Once the device is chosen, the central-most defect is crossed under ultrasound guidance. It is very important to make sure that the central defect is crossed and not one of the satellite lesions. This may be difficult, especially in the setting of a septal aneurysm. A variety of catheters may be used for this purpose, but the authors have found that a multi-purpose or Judkins right coronary catheter is often successful. Since the fenestrations are often small the use of a non–"J-" tipped wire such as a Wholey wire or Terumo wire is necessary. The presence of the wire within the catheter makes identification of the catheter on ultrasound easier. In the presence of a very thin floppy septum, as the catheter or wire crosses the septum, the tissue is often moved out of plane on the echocardiogram, and therefore it is important to look in

several views to decide if the appropriate hole has been crossed. Once the correct hole has been crossed, the guidewire is placed in the LUPV. If the Amplatzer cribriform device is chosen, the appropriate delivery sheath is advanced across the septum and the device deployed as previously described. If a Gore Helex device is chosen, then the sheath should be advanced over the guidewire, as mentioned in the procedural section above. Once the Helex sheath is across the defect, the guidewire is removed and the device deployed in the standard fashion. A full TEE or ICE study should be repeated after device deployment to make certain that all the defects have been covered with the device.

Multiple Atrial Septal Defects

Multiple ASDs have been reported to occur in up to 7.3% of cases.[104] They can often be treated with a single device. If the secondary defect is not covered appropriately by a single device, then deployment of a second device will be necessary if the secondary defect is felt to be hemodynamically significant. Use of a second device may be anticipated if an Amplatzer septal occluder is chosen to close the primary defect and if the distance between the edges of the primary and secondary defects is 7 mm or more. Several techniques have been used to close multiple defects, including simultaneous defect sizing and device deployment and sequential sizing and closure. It is the authors' opinion that either approach is acceptable. They typically now perform sequential defect sizing and closure, in which one of the defects is crossed, sized, and then closed with an appropriate device; this is followed by crossing the secondary defect, sizing it, and closing it. It is the authors' opinion that it does not matter if the smaller defect is addressed first and then the larger defect, or vice versa. The relationship of the two devices to each other is likewise not critical. On some occasions, the larger device will sandwich the smaller device; at other times, the devices, disks will be intercalated. Either approach is acceptable. Often, the smaller defects are at the posteroinferior portion of the septum, as described above, and once these are closed, the two devices may orient themselves at almost 90 degrees to each other. This is to be expected, since the atrial septum is a three-dimensional structure. On rare occasions, more than two devices are necessary to close additional defects. Meticulous attention to echocardiographic images is required to make certain that there is enough room in the left atrium to accommodate additional devices without impingement on adjacent structures.

Atrial Septal Defect Closure and Pulmonary Hypertension

PH (pulmonary artery systolic pressures > 40 mm Hg) is reported to occur in 6% to 50% of adults with ASDs.[105-110] This is, therefore, a frequently encountered phenomenon when considering trans-catheter ASD closure. Until recently, there has been a relative paucity of data to guide the decision to perform trans-catheter ASD closure in these patients. The availability of pulmonary vasodilator therapy such as sildenafil, bosentan, or prostacyclin has further clouded the issue. Most studies use pulmonary artery systolic pressure (PASP) or right ventricular systolic pressure, as assessed by echocardiography, to divide patients into mild (PASP 40–49 mm Hg), moderate (PASP 50–59 mm Hg), or severe (PASP >60 mm Hg). Pressure estimates are based on the modified Bernoulli equation using the tricuspid regurgitant velocity (v, $4v^2$ + right atrial pressure). Yong et al reported on 215 consecutive adult patients undergoing trans-catheter ASD closure with the ASO.[107] Of these patients, 108 (50.2%) had some elevation of pulmonary artery pressure, as assessed on baseline echocardiography. Mild PH was seen in 62 (28.8%), moderate in 27 (12.6%), and severe in 19 (8.8%). ASD closure was successful in 194 patients, and they were followed up at a median duration of 15 months. A decrease in PASP of at least 5 mm Hg, as assessed by echocardiography, was noted on follow-up in 33.7%, 73.9%, 79.2%, and 100% of patients with no, mild, moderate, or severe pulmonary hypertension, respectively. For those patients with moderate or severe PH, the median reduction in PASP was 18 mm Hg. PASP normalized in 141 patients (75.8%), which included 48.8% of those with moderate or severe PH. Functional deterioration occurred in 2 patients who had a baseline PASP of 50 mm Hg or more and were New York Heart Association (NYHA) functional class II before ASD closure. Multivariate analysis demonstrated that a higher baseline PASP, younger age, and smaller body size were independent factors associated with a reduction in PASP following trans-catheter ASD closure. It should be noted that in this study, at the time of the cardiac catheterization, all but three patients had a pulmonary artery to systemic pressure ratio of 0.67 or less.

Balint et al reviewed their experience with trans-catheter closure of ASDs in patients with moderate or severe PH undergoing closure between April 1999 and November 2004.[109] Of patients referred for ASD closure, 11% (54 of 484) had moderate or severe PH. There were 34 patients with moderate (63%) and 20 (37%) with severe PH. Early follow-up was performed a mean of 2.3 months from device closure, and the RVSP decreased from 57 to 51 mm Hg. The RVSP normalized in 26% (14 of 54) of patients, including 13 with moderate and 1 with severe PH; however, 5 patients had an increase in RVSP greater than 10 mm Hg compared with baseline. Late follow-up was obtained in 45 patients (83%) an average of 31 months from implantation. Two patients died during follow-up, one from bowel obstruction and one from pulmonary thromboembolism. Two patients had pulmonary vasodilators started after closure and one patient was receiving prostacyclin therapy before closure and bosentan therapy after closure. Late follow-up echocardiograms were available for 39 patients. In this group, the RVSP decreased from 58 mm Hg baseline to 44 mm Hg. RVSP increased by greater than 10 mm Hg in three patients. In patients with moderate PH, the RVSP decreased from 51 mm Hg to 38 mm Hg, and in those with severe PH, the RVSP decreased from 70 mm Hg to 48 mm Hg. Overall 17 of 39 (44%) patients on late follow-up had normalization of RVSP, including 15 with moderate and 2 with severe PH. De Lezo et al reviewed their experience with adults with PH and

trans-catheter ASD closure.[110] Twenty-nine patients out of a total of 101 (28.7%) patients undergoing percutaneous closure had echocardiographic evidence of PH. At cardiac catheterization, PASP ranged from 41 mm Hg to 147 mm Hg with a mean of 64 mm Hg. The pulmonary to systemic pressure ratio averaged 0.66 and the mean Qp/Qs ratio was 1:8. Three patients had systemic PASP and bi-directional shunts. These patients had further assessment with hyperoxia, balloon test occlusion of the ASD, or both and underwent closure after a favorable test result. Immediately after the procedure, the mean PASP decreased to 54 mm Hg, and the pulmonary to systemic pressure ratio decreased to 0.54. All symptomatic patients improved, including those with systemic-level PH. After a mean follow-up period of 21 months, the mean PASP, as assessed by Doppler, had decreased further to 34 mm Hg, and no clinical deterioration was noted. On the basis of the results of these studies, the authors recommend ASD closure in patients with any level of PH and a left-to-right shunt. If a bi-directional shunt is present and there is systemic desaturation (aortic saturation <92%), the patient should undergo pulmonary vasodilator testing with test occlusion of the ASD. If the response is favorable, percutaneous ASD closure may be performed. A favorable response is considered to have occurred if there is a fall in the mean pulmonary arterial pressures with oxygen and test occlusion, with no decrease in the cardiac output and no increase in the right atrial pressure. If the response is unfavorable, the patient should be started on pulmonary vasodilator therapy and a cardiac catheterization repeated after several months to reassess the hemodynamics. If there has been a favorable change, the ASD may be closed at that time.

Diastolic Left Ventricular Dysfunction and Atrial Septal Defect Closure

An increasing number of older patients (>60 years) are being referred for trans-catheter closure of ASDs. Up to 25% of these patients may have left ventricular restrictive physiology.[111] Closure of the ASD in this situation may result in an acute increase in left atrial pressure and precipitation of pulmonary edema and left heart failure.[112] Anticipation of this is very important, and proper evaluation of the patient before ASD closure is necessary. Ewert et al describe a group of 18 patients over 60 years of age in whom trans-catheter ASD closure was planned.[113] These patients underwent a baseline hemodynamic assessment as well as TEE to assess the mitral valve inflow pattern. In addition, the ASD was test-occluded for 10 minutes with a sizing balloon, following which the left atrial pressure measurement was repeated as well as the assessment of the mitral inflow Doppler. Eleven of the patients had no significant change in the left atrial pressure or the mitral Doppler, and of these, 10 underwent uneventful trans-catheter ASD closure. In one patient, the defect was too large to be closed in the cath lab. The remaining 7 patients had a marked increase in the mean left atrial pressure from 14 mm Hg to 23 mm Hg with an increase in the a wave from 18 mm Hg to 26 mm Hg and the v wave from 24 mm Hg to 41 mm Hg. The mitral valve E/A ratio also increased dramatically in this group of patients. Two patients in this group had trans-catheter ASD closure; one subsequently developed atrial flutter and biventricular heart failure, and the second developed pulmonary edema shortly after the procedure. In this study, all patients who had a mean left atrial pressure greater than 10 mm Hg before test occlusion developed significantly elevated left atrial pressure after occlusion. Schubert et al reported on a group of 59 consecutive patients older than 60 years admitted for trans-catheter ASD closure.[111] They performed balloon test occlusion in all patients and considered a patient to have restrictive left ventricular physiology if the mean left atrial pressure increased greater than 10 mm Hg with test occlusion. Patients were divided into two groups based on whether the mean left atrial pressure increase was less than 10 mm Hg (group A) or greater than 10 mm Hg (group B) with test occlusion. Patients in group B underwent conditioning with dopamine, milrinone, and lasix infusions for 48 to 60 hours before ASD closure, followed by stepwise discontinuation of the IV infusions and a change to oral lasix 24 to 36 hours after the procedure. Forty-four of 59 patients were in group A and 15 patients (25%) were in group B. All patients in group A had an uncomplicated recovery after ASD closure. In group B, the mean left atrial pressure increased from 10 mm Hg to 21 mm Hg with test occlusion before medical conditioning of the left ventricle. Following 48 to 72 hours of conditioning, the mean left atrial pressure increased from 5 mm Hg to only 7 mm Hg with test occlusion. The ASD was successfully closed in 11 of 13 patients. In 2 patients, there was no reduction in left atrial pressure with medical conditioning, and these patients underwent ASD closure with fenestrated Amplatzer devices. Two other patients in group B had ASD closure, but this was performed without medical conditioning; one of these patients developed pulmonary edema and required mechanical ventilation, and the second developed pleural effusion 4 weeks after the procedure. Both these patients were managed medically. It is apparent from these and other studies that older adults are at high risk for restrictive physiology of the left heart, which may be unmasked by trans-catheter ASD closure, and therefore recognition of this phenomenon is important. The authors recommend a protocol similar to that described above by Schubert, in which patients have their left atrial pressure assessed with and without balloon occlusion.[111] If the left atrial pressure increases significantly (>10 mm Hg) with test occlusion, the patient should undergo medical conditioning with diuretics and a drug such as milrinone or nesiritide. It can be helpful to place a swan Ganz catheter in these patients and monitor their wedge pressures. After 48 to 72 hours of medical therapy, the patient can then undergo a repeat catheterization, and if the left atrial pressure does not increase to greater than 10 mm Hg, the ASD can then be closed and the patient weaned from the medications over the next 48 hours. Diuretics are usually necessary on discharge.

Conclusion

Percutaneous closure of the secundum ASDs has changed the approach to congenital heart disease. Trans-catheter secundum ASD closure is now considered the procedure of choice. This technique has moved beyond just the spectrum of the simple secundum ASD and is now applicable to increasingly complex defects such as large, multiple, or multi-fenestrated defects or to increasingly complex patients such as those with PH or restrictive left ventricular physiology. Multiple other devices are currently in development for ASD closure, and these may further expand the spectrum of defects that can be closed or may further improve the safety of the procedure.

REFERENCE

1. King TD, Thompson SL, Steiner C, et al: Secundum atrial septal defect: Non-operative closure during cardiac catheterization. *JAMA* 235:2506–2509, 1976.
2. Mills NL, King TD: Late follow-up of nonoperative closure of secundum atrial septal defects using the King-Mills double umbrella device. *Am J Cardiol* 92:353–355, 2003.
3. Rashkind WJ: Transcatheter treatment of congenital heart disease. *Circulation* 67:711–716, 1983.
4. Rome JJ, Perry SB, Spevak PJ, et al: Double umbrella closure of atrial defects. Initial clinical applications. *Circulation* 82:751–758, 1990.
5. Moore KL, Persaud TUN: *Developing human: Clinically oriented embryology*. Philadelphia, 1998, Saunders.
6. Meissner I, Whissant JP, Khandheria BK, et al: Prevalence of potential risk factors for stroke assessed by TEE and carotid ultrasonography: The SPARC Study. Stroke Prevention assessment of risk in a community. *Mayo Clin Proc* 74:862–869, 1999.
7. Thompson T, Evans W: Paradoxical embolism. *Q J Med* 23:135–152, 1930.
8. Wu LA, Malouf JF, Dearani JA, et al: Patent foramen ovale in cryptogenic stroke. Current understanding and management options. *Arch Intern Med* 164:950–956, 2004.
9. Germonpre P, Hastir F, Dendale P, et al: Evidence for increasing patency of foramen ovale in divers. *Am J Cardiol* 95:912–915, 2005.
10. Rodriguez CJ, Homma S, Sacco RL, et al: Race ethnic differences in patent foramen ovale, atrial septal aneurysm, and right atrial anatomy among ischemic stroke patients. *Stroke* 34:2097–2102, 2003.
11. Cohnheim J: *Thrombose und embolie: Vorlesung uber allgemeine pathologie*. Berlin, 134, 1877.
12. Lechat PH, Mas MD, Lascault G, et al: Prevalence of patent foramen ovale in patients with stroke. *N Eng J Med* 318:1148–1152, 1988.
13. Di Tullio M, Sacco RL, Gopal A, et al: Patent foramen ovale as a risk factor for cryptogenic stroke. *Ann Intern Med* 117:461–465, 1992.
14. Seward JB, Hayes DL, Smith HC, et al: Platypnea orthodeoxia: Clinical profile, diagnostic work up, management, and report of seven cases. *Mayo Clin Proc* 59:221–231, 1984.
15. Godart F, Rey C, Prat A, et al: Atrial right to left shunting causing severe hypoxemia despite normal right sided pressures. *Eur Hear J* 21:483–489, 2000.
16. Bason R, Yacavone D: Decompression sickness: US navy altitude chamber experience 1 October 1981 to 30 September 1988. *Aviat Space Environ Med* 62:1180–1184, 1991.
17. Scherzmann M, Wiher S, Nedeltchev K, et al: Percutaneous closure of patent foramen ovale reduces the frequency of migraine attacks. *Neurology* 62:1399–1401, 2004.
18. Overell JR, Bone I, Lees KR: Interatrial septal abnormalities and stroke. A meta-analysis of case control studies. *Neurology* 55:1172–1179, 2000.
19. Lamy C, Giannesini C, Zuber M, et al: Clinical and imaging findings in cryptogenic stroke patients with and without patent foramen ovale. The PFO- ASA study. *Stroke* 33:706–711, 2002.
20. Berthet K, Lavergne T, Cohen A, et al: Significant association of atrial vulnerability with atrial septal abnormalities in young patients with ischemic stroke of unknown cause. *Stroke* 31:298–403, 2000.
21. Thanigaraj S, Zajarias A, Lasala J, et al: Caught in the act: Serial real time images of a thrombus traversing from the right to left atrium across a patent foramen ovale. *Eur J Echo* 7:179–181, 2006.
22. Sacco RL, Ellenberg JH, Mohr JP, et al: Infarcts of undetermined cause: The NINCDS Stroke Data Bank. *Ann Neurol* 25:382–390, 1989.
23. Cramer SC: Patent foramen ovale and its relationship to stroke. *Cardiol Clin* 23:7–11, 2005.
24. Cramer SC, Rordorf G, Maki JH, et al: Increased pelvic vein thrombi in cryptogenic stroke: Results of the paradoxical emboli from large veins in ischemic stroke (PELVIS) study. *Stroke* 35:46–50, 2004.
25. Konstantinides S, Geibel A, Kapser W, et al: Patent foramen ovale is an important predictor of adverse outcome in patients with major pulmonary embolism. *Circulation* 97:1946–1951, 1998.
26. Handke M, Harloff A, Olschewski M, et al. Patent foramen ovale and cryptogenic stroke in older patients. *N Engl J Med* 357:2262–2268, 2007.
27. Petty GW, KMayo, Khandreia B, et al: Population based study of the relationship between patent foramen ovale and cerebrovascular ischemic events. *Mayo Clin Proc* 81:602–608, 2006.
28. Meissner I, Khandeira B, Heit JA, et al: Patent foramen ovale: Innocent or guilty? *J Am Coll Cardiol* 47;440–445, 2006.
29. Di Tullio MR, Sacco R, Sciacca RR, et al: Patent foramen ovale and risk of ischemic stroke in a community—the northern Manhattan study. *Stroke* 34 (abstract), 2003.
30. Mas JL, Zuber M: Recurrent cerebrovascular events in patients with patent foramen ovale, atrial septal aneurysm or both and cryptogenic stroke or transient ischemic attack. *Am Heart J* 130:1083–1088, 1995.
31. De Castro S, Cartón D, Fiorelli M, et al: Morphological and functional characteristics of patent foramen ovale and their embolic complications. *Stroke* 31:2407–2413, 2000.
32. Cabanes L, Mas JL, Cohen A, et al: Atrial septal aneurysm and patent foramen ovale as risk factors for cryptogenic stroke in patients less than 55 years of age. *Stroke* 24:1865–1873, 1993.
33. Natanzon A, Goldman ME: Patent foramen ovale. Anatomy versus pathophysiology—which determines stroke risk. *J Am Soc Echo* 16:71–76, 2003.
34. Homma S, Di Tullio MR, Sacco RL, et al: Characteristics of patent foramen ovale associated with cryptogenic stroke. A biplane transesophageal echocardiographic study. *Stroke* 25:582–586, 1994.
35. Schuchlenz HW, Saurer G, Wehis W, et al: Persisting Eustachian valve in adults: Relation to patent foramen ovale and cerebrovascular events. *J Am Soc Echocardiogr* 17:231–233, 2004.
36. Mas JL, Aruquizan C, Lamy C, et al:. Recurrent cerebrovascular events associated with patent foramen ovale, atrial septal aneurysm or both. *N Engl J Med* 345:1740–1746, 2001.
37. Homma S, Sacco RL, Di Tullio MR, et al: Effect of medical therapy in stroke patients with patent foramen ovale. Patent foramen ovale in cryptogenic stroke study. *Circulation* 105:2625–2631, 2002.
38. Bogousslavsky J, Garazi S, Jeanrenaud X, et al: Stroke recurrence in patients with patent foramen ovale. *Neurology* 46:1301–1305, 1996.
39. Khairy P, O'Donnell CP, Landzbergb MJ: Transcatheter closure versus medical therapy of patent foramen ovale and presumed paradoxical emboli. *Ann Intern Med* 139:753–760, 2003.
40. Messe SR, Silverman IE, Kizer JR, et al: Practice parameter: recurrent stroke with patent foramen ovale and atrial septal aneurysm. Report of the quality standards subcommittee of the American Academy of Neurology. *Neurology* 62:1042–1050, 2004.
41. Dearani JA, Ugurlu BS, Danielson GK, et al: Surgical patent foramen ovale closure for prevention of paradoxical embolism-related cerebrovascular ischemic events. *Circulation* 100:II171–II175, 1999.
42. Windeker S, Wahl A, Chatterjee T, et al: Percutaneous closure of patent foramen ovale in patients with paradoxical embolism: Long term risk of recurrent thromboembolic events. *Circulation* 101:893–898, 2000.
43. Wahl A, Meier B, Haxel B, et al: Prognosis after percutaneous closure of patent foramen ovale for paradoxical embolism. *Neurology* 57:1330–1332, 2001.
44. Braun M, Fassbender D, Schoen S, et al: Transcatheter closure of patent foramen ovale in patients with cerebral ischemia. *J Am Coll Cardiol* 39:2019–2025, 2002.
45. Windeker S, Wahl A, Nedeltchev K: Comparison of medical treatment with percutaneous closure of patent foramen ovale in patients with cryptogenic stroke. *J Am Coll Cardiol* 44:750–758, 2004.
46. Sacco RL, Adams R, Albers G, et al: Guidelines for the prevention of stroke in patients with ischemic stroke or transient ischemic attack: A statement for healthcare professionals from the American Heart Association/American Stroke Association Council on Stroke: Co-sponsored by the council on Cardiovascular Radiology and Intervention: The American Academy of Neurology affirms the value of this guideline. *Stroke* 37:577–617, 2006.
47. Piechowski-Jozwiack A, Devuyst G, Bogousslavsky J: Migraine and patent foramen ovale: A residual coincidence or pathophysiological intrigue. *Cerebrovasc Dis* 22:91–100, 2006.
48. Kruit MC, van Buchem MA, Hofman PA, et al: Migraine as a risk factor for subclinical brain lesions. *JAMA* 291:427–434, 2004.
49. Milhaud D, Bogousslavsky J, van Melle G, et al: Ischemic stroke and active migraine. *Neurology* 57:1805–1811, 2001.
50. Anzola GP, Majuni M, Guindani M: Potential source of cerebral embolism in migraine with aura. A transcranial Doppler study. *Neurology* 52:1622–1625, 1999.
51. Scwerzmann M, Wiher S, Nedeltchev K, et al: Percutaneous closure of patent foramen ovale reduces the frequency of migraine attacks. *Neurology* 62:1399–1401, 2004.
52. Resiman M, Christofferson RD, Jesrum J, et al: Migraine headache relief after transcatheter closure of patent foramen ovale. *J Am Coll Cardiol* 45:233–299, 2005.
53. Anzola GP, Morad E, Casilli F, Onorato E: Shunt associated migraine responds favorable to atrial septal repair. A case control study. *Stroke* 37:430–434, 2006.
54. Reisman M, Christofferson RD, Jesrum J, et al: Migraine headache relief after transcatheter closure of patent foramen ovale. *J Am Coll Cardiol* 45:493–495, 2005.
55. Arzabal B, Tobis J, Suh W, et al: Association of interatrial shunts and migraine headaches: Impact of transcatheter closure. *J Am Coll Cardiol* 45:489–492, 2005.
56. Giardini A, Donti A, Formigari R, et al: Transcatheter patent foramen ovale closure mitigates aura migraine headaches abolishing spontaneous right to left shunting. *Am Heart J* 151:922, E1–E5, 2006.
57. Dowson A, Mullen MJ, Peatfield R, et al: Migraine intervention with STARFlex technology (MIST) trial: A prospective multicenter, double blind, sham-controlled trial to evaluate the effectiveness of patent foramen ovale closure with STARFlex septal

repair implant to resolve refractory migraine headaches. *Circulation* 117:197–1404, 2008.

58. Chen GPW, Goldberg S, Gill EA: Patent foramen ovale and the platypnea orthodeoxia syndrome. *Cardiol Clin* 2:85–89, 2005.

59. Ilkhanoff L, Naidu S, Rohatgi S, et al: Transcatheter device closure of interatrial septal defects in patients with hypoxia. *J Interven Cardiol* 18:227–232, 2005.

60. Waight DJ, Cao QL, Hijazi ZM: Closure of patent foramen oval in patients with orthodeoxia-platypnea using the Amplatzer devices. *Catheter Cardiovasc Interv* 50:195–198, 2000.

61. Roxas Timonera M, Larracas C, Gersony D, et al: Patent foramen ovale presenting as platypnea orthodeoxia: Diagnosis by transesophageal echocardiography. *J Am Soc Echocardiogr* 14:1039–1041, 2001.

62. Shanoudy H, Soliman A, Raggi P, et al: Prevalence of patent foramen ovale and its contribution to hypoxemia in patients with obstructive sleep apnea. *Chest* 113:91–96, 1998.

63. Germonpre P: Patent foramen ovale and diving. *Cardiol Clin* 23:97–104, 2005.

64. Germonpre P, Dendle P, Unger P, et al: Patent foramen ovale and decompression illness in sport divers. *J Appl Physiol* 84:1622–1626, 1998.

65. Scherzmann M, Siller C, Lipp E, et al: Relation between directly detected patent foramen ovale and ischemic brain lesions in sport divers. *Ann Intern Med* 134:21–28, 2001.

66. Torti SR, Billager M, Schwerzmann M, et al: Risk of decompression among 230 divers in relation to the presence and size of PFO. *Eur Heart J* 25:1014–1020, 2004.

67. Kerut EK, Norfleet WT, Plotnick GD, et al: Patent foramen ovale: A review of associated condition and the impact of physiological size. *J Am Coll Cardiol* 38:613–623, 2001.

68. Hamman GF, Schatzer-Klotz D, Frohliq G, et al: Femoral infection of echo contrast medium may increase the sensitivity of testing for a patent foramen ovale. *Neurology* 50:1423–1428, 1998.

69. Daniels C, Weytjens C, Cosyns B, et al: Second harmonic transthoracic echocardiography: The new reference screening method for the detection of patent foramen ovale. *Eur J Echocardiogr* 5:449–452, 2004.

70. Thanigaraj S, Valika A, Zajarias A, et al: Comparison of transthoracic versus transesophageal echocardiography for the detection of right to left atrial shunting using agitated saline contrast. *Am J Cardiol* 96:1007–1010, 2005.

71. Anzola GP, Mornadi E, Casilli F, et al: Does transcatheter closure of patent foramen ovale really "shut the door?" A prospective study with transcranial Doppler. *Stroke* 35:2140–2144, 2004.

72. USA Food and Drug Administration: *HDE #H990011*. Washington, D.C., 2000, FDA.

73. Zajarias A, Thanigaraj S, Lasala J: Predictors and clinical outcomes of residual shunt in patients undergoing percutaneous transcatheter closure of patent foramen ovale. *J Inv Cardiol* 18(11):533–537, 2006.

74. Alameddine F, Block PC: Transcatheter patent foramen ovale closure for secondary prevention of paradoxical embolic events: Acute results from the FORECAST Registry. *Catheter Cardiovasc Interv* 62:512–516, 2004.

75. Braun M, Gliech V, Boscheri A, et al: Transcatheter closure of patent foramen ovale (PFO) in patients with paradoxical embolism. Periprocedural safety and mid-term follow up results of three different device occluder systems. *Eur Heart J* 25:424–420, 2004.

76. Perloff JK: *Clinical recognition of congenital heart disease*, 493–495, Philadelphia, 2003, Saunders.

77. Van Praagh S, Carrera ME, Sanders SP, et al: Sinus venosus defects: Unroofing of the right pulmonary veins—anatomic and echocardiographic findings and surgical treatment [abstract]. *Am Heart J* 128:365, 1994.

78. Hunt CE, Lucas RV, Jr: Symptomatic atrial septal defect in infancy. *Circulation* 42:1042, 1973.

79. Levin AR, Spach MS, Boineau JP, et al: Atrial pressure flow dynamics and atrial septal defects (secundum type). *Circulation* 37:476, 1968.

80. Clark EB, Kugler JD: Preoperative secundum atrial septal defect with coexisting sinus node and atrioventricular node dysfunction. *Circulation* 65:976, 1982.

81. Shub C, Tajik, AJ, Seward JB, et al: Surgical repair of uncomplicated atrial septal defect without "routine" preoperative cardiac catheterization. *J Am Coll Cardiol* 6:49, 1985.

82. Freed MD, Nadas AS, Norwood WI, et al: Is routine preoperative cardiac catheterization necessary before repair of secundum and sinus venosus atrial septal defects? *J Am Coll Cardiol* 4:333, 1984.

83. Konstantinides S, Kasper W, Geibel A, et al: Detection of left-to-right shunt in atrial septal defect by negative contrast echocardiography: A comparison of transthoracic and transesophageal approach. *Am Heart J* 126:909–917, 1993.

84. Ishii M, Kato H, Inoue O, et al: Biplane transesophageal echo-Doppler studies of atrial septal defects: Quantitative evaluation and monitoring for transcatheter closure [abstract]. *Am Heart J* 125:1363, 1993.

85. Silverman NH, Schmidt KG: The current role of Doppler echocardiography in the diagnosis of heart disease in children. *Cardiol Clin* 7:265, 1989.

86. Taketa RM, Sahn DJ, Simon AL, et al: Catheter positions in congenital cardiac malformations. *Circulation* 51:749, 1975.

87. Du ZD, Hijazi ZM, Kleinman CS, et al: Comparison between transcatheter and surgical closure of secundum atrial septal defect in children and adults: Results of a multicenter nonrandomized trial. *J Am Coll Cardiol* 39(11):1836–1844, 2002.

88. Jones TK, Latson LA, Zahn E, et al: Results of the US multicenter pivotal study of the Helex septal occluder for percutaneous closure of secundum atrial septal defects. *J Am Coll Cardiol* 49:2215–2221, 2007.

89. Amin Z, Hijazi ZM, Bass JL, et al: Erosion of Amplatzer septal occluder device after closure of secundum atrial septal defects: review of registry of complications and recommendations to minimize future risk. *Catheter Cardiovasc Interv* 63:496–502, 2004.

90. El-Said HG, Moore JW: Erosion of the Amplatzer septal occluder: Experienced operator opinions at odds with manufacturer recommendations? *Catheter Cardiovasc Interv* 73:925–930, 2009.

91. Levi DS, Moore JW: Embolization and retrieval of the Amplatzer septal occluder. *Catheter Cardiovasc Interv* 61:543–547, 2004.

92. Dibardino SJ, McElhinney DB, Kaza AK, et al: Analysis of the US food and drug administration manufacturer and user facility device experience database for adverse events involving Amplatzer septal occluder devices and comparison with the society of thoracic surgery congenital cardiac surgery database. *J Thor Cardiovasc Surg* 137(6):1334–1339, 2009.

93. Fagan T, Dreher D, Cutright W, et al: Fracture of the Gore Helex septal occluder: Associated factors and clinical outcomes. *Catheter Cardiovasc Interv* 73:941–948, 2009.

94. Quershi AM, Mumtaz MA, Latson LA: Partial prolapse of a Helex device associated with early frame fracture and mitral valve perforation. *Catheter Cardiovasc Interv* 74:777–782, 2009.

95. Latson LA, Jones TK, Jacobson J, et al: Analysis of factors related to successful transcatheter closure of secundum atrial septal defects using the Helex septal occluder. *Am Heart J* 151(5): 1129.e7–1129.e11, 2006.

96. Tan CA, Levi DS, Moore JW: Embolization and transcatheter retrieval of coils and devices. *Pediatr Cardiol* 26:267–274, 2005.

97. Peuster M, Reckers J, Fink C: Secondary embolization of a Helex occluder implanted into a secundum atrial septal defect. *Catheter Cardivasc Interv* 59:77–82, 2003.

98. Kannan BR, Francis E, Sivakumar K, et al: Transcatheter closure of very large (>25 mm) atrial septal defects using the Amplatzer septal occluder. *Catheter Cardiovasc Interv* 59:522–527, 2003.

99. Varma C, Benson LN, Silversides C, et al: Outcomes and alternative techniques for device closure of the large secundum atrial septal defect. *Catheter Cardiovasc Interv* 61:131–139, 2004.

100. Kutty S, Asnes JD, Srinath G, et al: Use of a straight, side-hole delivery sheath for improved delivery of Amplatzer ASD occluder. *Catheter Cardiovasc Interv* 69:15–20, 2007.

101. Dalvi BV, Pinto RJ, Gupta A: New technique for device closure of large atrial septal defects. *Catheter Cardiovasc Interv* 64:102–107, 2005.

102. Wahab HA, Bairam AR, Cao QL, et al: Novel Technique to prevent prolapse of the Amplatzer septal occluder through large atrial septal defect. *Catheter Cardiovasc Interv* 60:543–545, 2003.

103. Hijazi AM, Cao QL: Transcatheter closure of secundum atrial septal defect associated with deficient posterior rim in a child under echocardiographic guidance. *Appl Cardiac Imag* Nov:7–10, 2002.

104. Podnar T, Martanovic P, Gavora P, et al: Morphological variations of secundum-type atrial septal defects: Feasibility for percutaneous closure using Amplatzer septal occluders. *Catheter Cardiovasc Interv* 53:386–391, 2001.

105. Engelfriet PM, Duffels MG, Moller T, et al: Pulmonary arterial hypertension in adults born with a heart septal defect: The Euro Heart Survey on adult congenital heart disease. *Heart* 93:682–687, 2007.

106. Vogel M, Berger F, Kramer A, et al: Incidence of secondary pulmonary hypertension in adults with atrial septal or sinus venosus defects. *Heart* 82:30–33, 1999.

107. Yong G, Khairy P, De Guise P, et al: Pulmonary arterial hypertension in patients with transcatheter closure of secundum atrial septal defects: A longitudinal study. *Catheter Cardiovasc Interv* 2:455–462, 2009.

108. Steele PM, Fuster V, Cohen M, et al: Isolated atrial septal defect with pulmonary vascular obstructive disease-long-term follow-up and prediction of outcome after surgical correction. *Circulation* 76:1037–1042, 1987.

109. Balint OH, Samman A, Heberer K, et al: Outcomes in patients with pulmonary hypertension undergoing percutaneous atrial septal defect closure. *Heart* 94:1189–1193, 2008.

110. De Lezo JS, Medina A, Romero M, et al: Effectiveness of percutaneous device occlusion for atrial septal defect in adult patients with pulmonary hypertension. *Am Heart J* 144:877–880, 2002.

111. Schubert S, Peters B, Abdul-Khaliq H, et al: Left ventricular conditioning in the elderly patient to prevent congestive heart failure after transcatheter closure of atrial septal defect. *Catheter Cardiovasc Interv* 64:333–337, 2005.

112. Ewert P, Berger F, Nagdyman N, et al: Acute left heart failure after interventional occlusion of an atrial septal defect. *Z Kardiol* 90:362–366, 2001.

113. Ewert P, Berger F, Nagdyman N, et al: Masked left ventricular restriction in elderly patients with atrial septal defects: A contraindication for closure? *Catheter Cardiovasc Interv* 52:177–180, 2001.

47

Left Atrial Appendage Closure and Stroke: Local Device Therapy for Cardioembolic Stroke Protection

ROBERT S. SCHWARTZ | ROBERT A. VAN TASSEL |
HIDEHIKO HARA | DAVID R. HOLMES, JR.

KEY POINTS

- The left atrial appendage (LAA) has traditionally been considered a structure without activity or apparent purpose. Yet, evolving evidence suggests quite the contrary. It has a shape and a three-dimensional configuration much like bellows, and it appears to function as a left atrial pressure.

- The LAA is distinct from the left atrium (LA). It is a separate chamber with volume as much as one third or one half that of the atrium. Moreover, it originates embryologically from pulmonary veins rather than the LA. These facts suggest that it is a biologic structure that is fundamentally different from the atrium.

- The volume and shape of the LAA make it a chamber with low blood flow, promoting hemostasis, which, in turn, promotes thrombus formation. More than 20% of all strokes are thought to be related to atrial fibrillation (AF) and the LA, principally from thrombus embolization, and more than 90% of all emboli originating from the heart are from the LAA. The LAA is the principal source of morbidity and mortality in AF.

- Older patients have a high rate of stroke from AF but also a high rate of major bleeds while taking warfarin. Mechanical ablation of the LAA is therefore an attractive therapy. Several implanted devices are under study and are used to close the mouth of this structure at the entrance to the atrium. This permits long-term elimination of warfarin therapy, even in patients with chronic AF. Interventional ablation of the LAA in early clinical trials has shown promise to change the clinical approach to patients with chronic AF while limiting embolic episodes.

Modern interventional cardiology is rapidly moving toward local device therapy for local anatomic and physiologic problems. This paradigm shift represents an exciting departure from systemic therapies that are typically pharmacologically based, with the medications administered either orally or parenterally. An evolving application of this principle is reducing or eliminating cardioembolic stroke originating in the LAA in patients who have AF. This chapter discusses AF and its role in strokes, the role of the LAA, and how percutaneous occlusion of the LAA will likely change the clinical approach to stroke prevention in the patient with AF.

Atrial Fibrillation and Stroke

AF is the most prevalent significant cardiac arrhythmia in the world. It affects more than two million people age 40 years or more (2.3% of the U.S. population).[1-5] The median age of patients with AF is 75 years. Accordingly, as the population ages, the number of patients will increase drastically, and by the year 2020, more than 3,300,000 patients will have been affected. AF prevalence increases with age, 1.5% of those aged 50 to 59 years are affected; and nearly 24% of people aged 80 to 89 years have this arrhythmia.[6] Roughly 500,000 ischemic strokes occur each year in the United States. AF is responsible for 20% of these strokes; among patients aged 50 to 59 years, 10% of ischemic strokes are caused by AF, whereas among patients aged 80 to 89 years, this number dramatically rises to 32%.[6-8] Stroke is the number one cause of long-term disability and the third leading cause of death in patients with AF.[4,9] Patients with AF have a fivefold increased stroke risk compared with the general population. Nearly 87% of ischemic strokes are thromboembolic, and of these, nearly 90% of emboli originate in the LAA. In nonvalvular AF, strokes can be catastrophic events.[10] Henricksson examined stroke survival, and in 31,000 patients with AF in the Swedish Stroke Registry, the AF diagnosis carried a much higher death risk, even after adjustment for age and gender.[11] Thirty-one percent of strokes in nonvalvular AF are fatal, 28% are seriously disabling, and 11% are moderately disabling[10] (Fig. 47-1). Strokes in AF differ from those caused by vascular atheroemboli (e.g., atheroma in the carotid, the aorta, and vertebral arteries). Emboli originating from within the heart are more clinically serious; they carry higher mortality and often cause worse disability, possibly because intracardiac thrombi (from the LAA) are larger than embolic atheromatous vascular debris.[9,12-14] Strokes from AF affect the brain parenchyma 25 times more often compared with strokes from carotid artery disease.[15] Clinical symptoms involving the retina likely originate from carotid artery disease rather than from AF or cardioemboli. Patients presenting with retinal symptoms are, thus, far more likely to have a cerebrovascular cause rather than a cardioembolic cause.[15] AF is associated with more subclinical brain infarcts, as shown in the VA SPINAF (Veterans Administration Stroke Prevention in Atrial Fibrillation) trial, in which 15% of patients with AF had subclinical strokes occurring at 1.3% per year. Interestingly, comparable subclinical stroke and transient ischemic attack (TIA) rates occur even in patients taking both aspirin and warfarin.[16,17]

Warfarin

STATE OF THE ART FOR STROKE PROPHYLAXIS IN ATRIAL FIBRILLATION

Warfarin is the best medical therapy for stroke prevention in nonvalvular AF. Stroke risk in AF is assessed by the CHADS-2 score (See Table 47-1 for CHADS-2 score definition, and Table 47-2 for stroke risk with and without warfarin). Many well known, large trials agree on the benefits of warfarin, including the Stroke Prevention in Atrial Fibrillation (SPAF)- I, II, and III; the Canadian Atrial Fibrillation Anticoagulation (CAFA); the Boston Area Anticoagulation Trial for Atrial Fibrillation (BAATAF); and the SPINAF trials.[18-23] Meta-analyses of these trials compare stroke prevention in nonvalvular AF using warfarin, aspirin, and placebo (see Table 47-3 for therapy recommendations based on these trials). The collective message is that warfarin is effective in reducing stroke and death compared with aspirin and placebo. When given in appropriate, therapeutic doses with therapeutic international normalized ratio (INR) values, warfarin reduces stroke risk by 60% to 70% compared with no treatment and by 30% to 40% compared with aspirin alone.[15] Although warfarin is a therapeutic

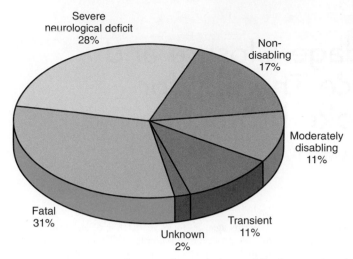

Figure 47-1 Functional impact of nonvalvular atrial fibrillation–related strokes. Cardioembolic stroke in atrial fibrillation has major clinical consequences, showing here that 59% of such strokes are either fatal or result in severe disability. *(Redrawn from Fisher CM: Reducing risks of cerebral embolism, Geriatrics 34(2):59–61, 65–56, 1979.)*

TABLE 47-2	Annual Stroke Risk (percent/year) by CHADS-2 Score, with and without Warfarin Therapy	
CHADS	*Warfarin*	*No Warfarin*
0	0.25	0.49
1	0.72	1.50
2	1.27	2.50
3	2.20	5.27
4	2.35	6.02
5 or 6	4.60	6.88

TABLE 47-3	Prophylaxis Recommendations based on Age and Clinical Status	
Age	*Clinical Condition*	*Therapy*
>60 years	Coronary artery disease (CAD) or diabetes	Warfarin
>75 years	All patients	Warfarin
All	Heart failure	Warfarin
All	Hypertension	Warfarin
All	Prior embolism	Warfarin
All	Thrombus present by transesophageal echocardiography (TEE)	Warfarin

TABLE 47-1	CHADS-2 Score Calculation	
Condition		*Points*
Prior stroke		2
Congestive heart failure		1
Hypertension		1
Age >75 years		1
Diabetes		1

cornerstone, it has major limitations and has serious adverse effects. For example, in one large meta-analysis, the authors calculated that if 51 ischemic strokes occur per 1000 patient-years without warfarin treatment, appropriately dosed warfarin would be expected to prevent 28 strokes but at the expense of 11 fatal bleeds. Aspirin therapy alone would prevent 16 strokes at the expense of 6 fatal bleeds.[24,25] Patients with AF taking neither warfarin nor aspirin have a stroke risk of 5% per year.

Warfarin is often difficult to control from the perspectives of both safety and efficacy. Bungard examined INR values in a population of AF patients taking warfarin in the emergency department. The mean age was 73 years, and 45% of these patients had subtherapeutic INR values, 37% had therapeutic values, and 19% had supratherapeutic values. Thus, even in warfarin-treated patients, 63% were out of the prescribed INR range.[26] Another study examined combined patients from the Stroke Prevention using ORal Thrombin Inhibitor in atrial Fibrillation (SPORTIF) III and V trials, who were taking warfarin, and divided their INR control into groups rated as poor, moderate, or good (therapeutic INR <60%, 60% to 75%, or >75% of the time, respectively). Only 60% of patients taking warfarin were within a therapeutic INR range (2–3.0), 29% had INR levels below 2, and 15% had levels above 3. Patients with poorly controlled disease (INR too high) compared with those with moderate or good control have much higher mortality (4.2% vs. 1.8% and 1.7% per year, respectively) and major bleeding (3.9% vs. 2% and 1.6%). Patients with poorly controlled disease have significantly higher strokes and systemic embolization compared with those with good control (2.1% vs. 1.1%).[27] Warfarin effectiveness is impacted by its interactions with food, other medications, and ill-defined genetically determined responses. It has a long half-life and is a problem in patients undergoing percutaneous coronary interventions (PCIs), since triple therapy—with acetyl salicylic

acid (ASA), clopidogrel, and warfarin—is mandated in this situation, even though it is associated with a rate of bleeds as high as 9% per year. Perhaps because of all these considerations, as well as patient intolerance, noncompliance, or other management difficulties, less than 50% of patients who need warfarin and are eligible to take it are treated at therapeutic INR levels. Safety is a clear concern, since hemorrhagic stroke in patients taking warfarin is very often fatal. These concerns may underlie warfarin under-utilization in AF. For example, one study found that only 55% of patients with AF and no contraindications actually took the drug within 3 months preceding the study; other studies cite even lower warfarin use in these patients, ranging between 17% and 50%.[28] Older patients have the highest absolute stroke risk in AF and yet are the least likely to take warfarin, as contraindications to warfarin are present in 30% to 40% of them.

HEMORRHAGE IN PATIENTS TAKING WARFARIN

While warfarin is better at stroke prevention compared with placebo or aspirin, intracerebral hemorrhage is a substantial risk in warfarin-anticoagulated patients.[28a,28b] Warfarin was evaluated using a meta-analysis of 28,044 patients with AF (from 29 centers) who were followed up for a mean of 1.5 years.[29] Though warfarin limited stroke by 64% (aspirin by 22%), the rate of intracranial hemorrhage doubled in the warfarin group compared with the aspirin group. Another study also examined major hemorrhage during the first year of warfarin therapy in older patients with AF.[30] In 492 of these patients (>65 years old), major bleeding (including intracranial) during the first year of treatment was 7%.[29] The risk of intracranial bleeding increases with age.[31]

Other Pharmacologic Therapies for Stroke Prevention

Combined anti-platelet (aspirin plus clopidogrel) therapy is not as effective as warfarin for preventing stroke. The Atrial Fibrillation Clopidogrel Trial with Irbesartan for Prevention of Vascular Events (ACTIVE) W trial reported on AF and stroke in patients randomized to warfarin or aspirin plus clopidogrel.[32] Warfarin was substantially superior to anti-platelet therapy, and the trial was terminated before its planned follow-up. New therapies under consideration for stroke

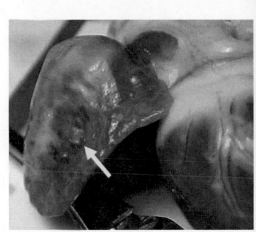
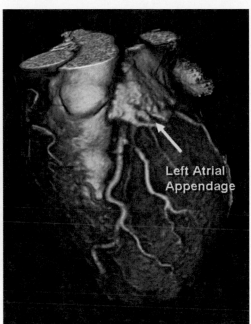

Figure 47-2 The left atrial appendage. This autopsy specimen image is from a normal canine heart (*left*). Cardiac computed tomographic angiography (CCTA) shows the left atrial appendage sits on top of the left main, left anterior descending, and left circumflex coronary artery origins (*right*). (*Modified with permission, Schwartz et al: JACC Cardiovascular Interventions 3(8):870–877, 2010.*)

prophylaxis in AF include direct oral thrombin or Factor Xa inhibitors.[33] Dabigatran is one such oral thrombin inhibitor recently approved by the U.S. Food and Drug Administration (FDA). In the Randomised Evaluation of Long-term Anticoagulation Therapy (RE-LY) trial, 18,113 randomized patients with nonvalvular AF were followed for primary outcomes defined as stroke or systemic embolism.[34] Two doses of dabigatran (110 mg or 150 mg orally twice daily) were given to patients and compared with standard-care warfarin after a 2-year follow-up. Primary outcomes occurred at 1.7% per year in the warfarin group versus 1.5% per year in the dabigatran 110 mg and 1.1% per year in the dabigatran 150 mg groups. Major bleeds occurred in 3.4% per year with warfarin versus 2.7% per year and 3.1% per year in the dabigatran 110 mg and 150 mg groups, respectively. Warfarin caused hemorrhagic stroke in 0.38% per year versus 0.1% in both dabigatran groups, whereas mortality was 4.1% per year for warfarin versus 3.4% and 3.6% per year in the dabigatran 110 mg and 150 mg groups. The study may be summarized as follows: oral dabigatran 110 mg twice daily has stroke and embolism rates similar to those with warfarin but less probability of bleeds, whereas dabigatran 150 twice daily has lower stroke and systemic embolism rates but similar hemorrhage rates. Also, more myocardial infarctions (MIs) occurred in the dabigatran 150 group compared with the warfarin group (0.74% vs. 0.53%, P = NS), a finding of unclear safety significance. It will be difficult to determine the optimal dose, as the ability to predict stroke is limited despite using predictive scores. A new bleeding risk score (HAS-BLED) may assist in this capacity:[34a] Hypertension, Abnormal renal/liver function, Stroke, Bleeding history or predisposition, Labile INR, Elderly (>65), Drugs and alcohol concomitantly.[36] Based on many of these considerations, an alternative technology for stroke prevention in AF that is both safe and effective is clearly needed. The oral anticoagulant strategy amounts to a systemic treatment for what is a local problem, namely, thrombus formation within the LAA.

Left Atrial Appendage

EMBRYOLOGY, STRUCTURE, AND FUNCTION

The LAA is a small epicardial chamber (see Fig. 47-1). It sits directly over the origins of the left main, left anterior descending (LAD), and left circumflex (LCx) coronary arteries. The right atrial appendage

(RAA) is more tubular in shape, is longer, and generally covers the origin of the right coronary artery (Figs. 47-2 and 47-3). Hara reviewed the embryology, structure, and function of the LAA.[35] The LAA originates from primordial atrial tissue, and the primordial left atrial wall becomes the tubular LAA. It is attached to the left atrial chamber, which suggests that the LAA may be an independent structure and perhaps not simply an appendage of the atrial wall. The rough, trabeculated cavitary surface of the LAA makes it a potential site for thrombus formation (Fig. 47-4).[35] Plastic casts of the human LAA show substantial variations of anatomic shape and volume.[36] Shape analysis shows that the LAA's principal axis is angulated less than 100 degrees in about 56% of adults, and the remaining 46% are more severely bent. The volume of the LAA ranges from 770 to 19,270 mm³. Fifty-four percent of patients have two lobes, and the numbers range from one to four lobes (Figs. 47-5 and 47-6). There is no apparent relation to age or gender for any of these features of the LAA.

Although the pump function of the LAA is not key to cardiac output, the LAA is not simply an "appendage" without purpose. It probably measures and provides systemic feedback for left atrial wall stretch and intracavitary atrial and left ventricular end-diastolic pressure. The normal LAA undergoes contraction in its normal state, though normal sinus rhythm does not mean that the LAA is contracting (Fig. 47-7). Atrial natriuretic peptide (ANP) and brain natriuretic peptide (BNP) are produced and stored in the walls of the LAA in large quantities; their secretion varies in response to changes in hemodynamic and neuroendocrinologic balance.[37] The LAA and the left atrium (LA) are major BNP sources in the body.[38] Dysfunction of the LA results in elevated BNP levels in patients with nonvalvular AF, and elevated BNP occurs in prothrombotic states.[39] The diuretic effects of ANP and BNP arise from left atrial distension. The walls of the LAA are packed densely with myocardial stretch receptors, and the bellows-like shape of the LAA makes it an ideal configuration for sensing left atrial pressure and, by extension, LVEDP. Increased pressures in the LA and the LAA distend the bellows early, before the remainder of the atrial muscle stretches, and the large radius-of-curvature shape to the LAA maximizes wall tension for pressure transduction. Tabata found that the stretch of the walls of the LAA, rather than left atrial pressure elevation or distension of the body of the LA, predicts the plasma ANP level, suggesting the known distribution of ANP-secreting cardiocytes.[40] As noted below, no clinical and physiologic consequences to the occlusion

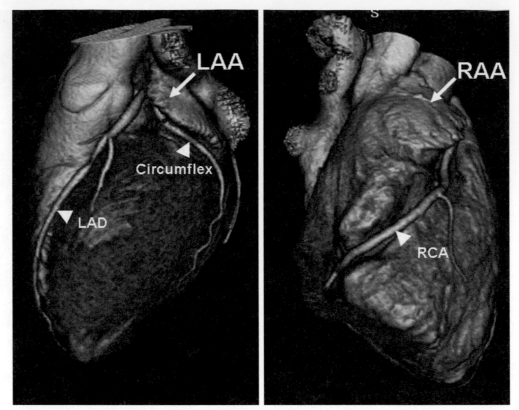

Figure 47-3   The right and left atrial appendages. Cardiac computed tomographic angiography (CCTA) shows the left atrial appendage and its relationship to the left anterior descending (LAD) and left circumflex (LCx) arteries. This structure is of variable size and shape (*left*). The right atrial appendage is more tubular in shape, is longer, and generally covers the right coronary artery origin (*right*).

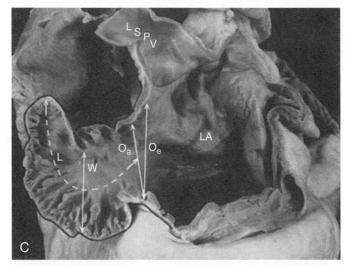

Figure 47-4   The left atrial appendage (LAA) has a highly trabeculated interior. Trabeculation makes the LAA susceptible to thrombus formation. *(Reprinted with permission.)*[40a]

of the LAA and dilatation and stunning of the LA seem to occur in the setting of chronic persistent AF.

LEFT ATRIAL APPENDAGE AS THE PRINCIPAL SOURCE OF CARDIOEMBOLI

Virchow's criteria for the formation of thrombi and emboli are met by the LAA. Three elements of Virchow's Triad are found in patients with

AF: (1) structural or vessel wall abnormalities, (2) abnormal blood flow patterns, and (3) abnormal constituents in blood; these have been summarized recently.[41] Goldsmith identified endocardial changes in the muscular wall of the LAA, and echocardiographic studies have long documented spontaneous echo contrast or "smoke" that indicates stasis of intracavitary blood.[42] Pollick and Taylor studied two-dimensional echocardiographic and Doppler LAA patterns in 82 patients and found them to be associated with dilation and poor contraction of the LAA, whether or not the patient was in AF.[43] Blackshear and Odel reviewed 23 studies that included patients with rheumatic and nonrheumatic AF and found distinct differences in the frequency and distribution of thrombi from the LAA.[13] In nonrheumatic AF, 91% of left atrial thrombi were isolated to or had originated in the LAA.

OCCLUSION OF THE LEFT ATRIAL APPENDAGE: A VIABLE STROKE PREVENTION STRATEGY IN ATRIAL FIBRILLATION

Mechanical occlusion of the LAA is a novel strategy to limit or eliminate cardioemboli, as the LAA is the major site of origin of such emboli. LAA occlusion is a local therapy for a local problem, and its advantage is that no adjunct pharmacology is required in the long term.

The occlusion or exclusion of the LAA is recommended in the American College of Cardiology and American Heart Association (ACC/AHA) guidelines for patients undergoing open-chest mitral valve surgery; it is performed during surgical approaches for ablation of AF, as in the maze procedure.[44] A pilot randomized trial of ligation of the LAA during coronary artery bypass grafting (CABG) studied 77 randomized patients. In 52 patients ligation of the LAA was attempted, and 25 were controls.[45] During surgery, 9 patients experienced laceration of the LAA. Full occlusion was achieved in 45% of patients, whose wounds were closed with suture compared with success in 72% of

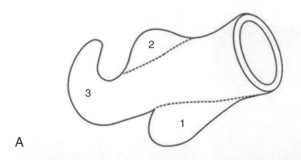

A

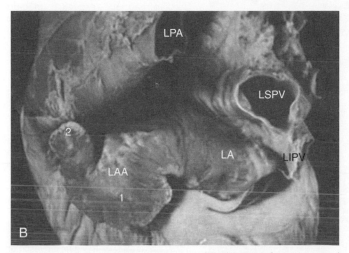

B

Figure 47-5 Lobar definition: anatomy of the human left atrial appendage (LAA). Veinot described methods for characterizing lobes of the LAA, an important consideration if device-based occlusion is considered. (Modified with permission from Veinot JP, Harrity PJ, Gentile F, et al: Anatomy of the normal left atrial appendage: a quantitative study of age-related changes in 500 autopsy hearts: Implications for echocardiographic examination, Circulation 96(9):3112–3115, 1997; and Schwartz et al: JACC Cardiovascular Interventions 3(8):870–877, 2010.)

patients in whom surgical stapling was employed. During a mean follow-up of 13 ± 7 months, 2.6% of patients had embolic events; both occurred in the perioperative period. Continued technological improvements are being made to make these open surgical approaches easier, more reliable, and safer. Blackshear and colleagues performed a meta-analysis of 23 published studies of surgical occlusion of the LAA in 3504 patients and summarized the results.[13] Thirteen percent of patients with rheumatic AF and 17% of patients with nonrheumatic AF had proven thrombi in the LAA, sometimes extending into the left atrial chamber. They suggested that occlusion of the LAA might reduce stroke in nonrheumatic AF, though an early, retrospective surgical review found no effect of surgical ligation of the LAA.[46] Subsequently, when results were carefully reviewed, it was shown that surgical ligation may not be as simple as originally thought, with significant early (33%) and late (40%) postoperative failure rates.[47] Several considerations are important with regard to percutaneous occlusion of the LAA. The thin walls of the LAA (typically 0.4–1.5 mm) are easily perforated if undue or excessive force is applied. The shape of the orifice of the LAA is elliptical, and it sometimes has a three-dimensional spiral shape (Fig. 47-8). Pectinate muscles are frequent in the LAA and may be close to the ostium (Fig. 47-9), and the posterior wall of the LAA is of variable distance from the ostium.

PERCUTANEOUS, CATHETER-BASED OCCLUSION OF THE LEFT ATRIAL APPENDAGE

Transcatheter occlusion of the LAA is now feasible.[48–52] The first such device was the *percutaneous left atrial appendage trans-catheter occlusion* (PLAATO) system. It was a self expanding nitinol cage that was covered with an impermeable PTFE membrane (Fig. 47-10) and used anchors to prevent device embolization. The device was implanted percutaneously via a transseptal approach. The device fit into the LAA and the anchors attached to the LAA wall to lessen the likelihood of device embolization. Several reports of clinical studies using PLAATO in nonvalvular AF have been published.[53–55] In one report, patients had at least one stroke risk factor beyond AF, and all had clinical contraindications for warfarin therapy.[51] The primary endpoint was a

Figure 47-6 Variations in the anatomy of the left atrial appendage (LAA), as shown by cardiac computer tomographic angiography (CCTA). Sample CCTA from six different normal subjects showing great variability of size, shape, and angulation

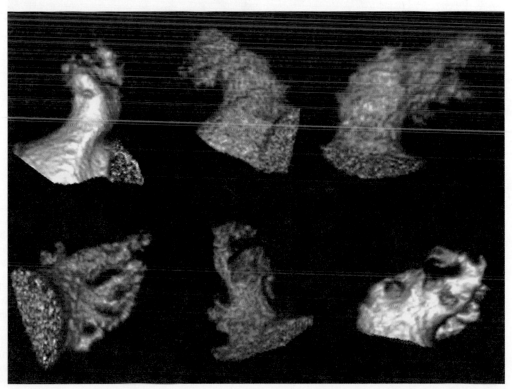

Atrial Diastole   Atrial Systole

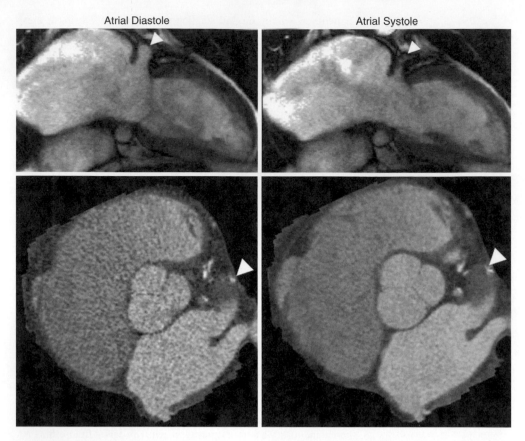

Figure 47-7 Contraction and paralysis of the left atrial appendage (LAA). Cardiac magnetic resonance imaging (MRI) (*top panels*) scans showing freeze-frames (systole and diastole) from a normally contracting LAA in normal sinus rhythm. The ejection fraction of the LAA is quite high from visual estimation. Conversely, the bottom images (cardiac computer tomographic angiography [CCTA]) show a different patient, cardioverted to normal sinus rhythm (NSR) within 3 days before the scan. There is little to no visible contraction and, importantly, severe hemostasis within the appendage, as seen by lack of contrast flow into the distal recesses of the appendage. Such hemostasis likely predisposes to thrombus formation in the body of the LAA. White arrowheads show the apices of the LAA. (*Modified with permission, Schwartz et al: JACC Cardiovascular Interventions 3(8):870–877, 2010.*)

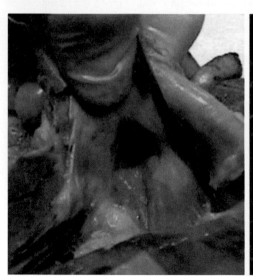
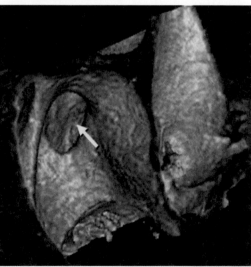

Figure 47-8 Ostium of the left atrial appendage (LAA). The shape of the orifice of the LAA has a variable size, can be elliptical, and may have a three-dimensional spiral shape. *Left*, Actual LAA ostium, normal human heart. *Right*, cardiac computer tomographic angiography (CCTA) showing an ostium of the LAA with a spiral configuration. (*Modified with permission, Schwartz et al: JACC Cardiovascular Interventions 3(8):870–877, 2010.*)

composite of stroke, cardiac or neurologic death, myocardial infarction, or requirement for procedure-related cardiovascular surgery within 30 days. The patients had a mean CHADS-2 score of 2.5. Of 111 patients, 38% had prior stroke or TIA. Occlusion of the LAA was successful in 97% of patients. After device placement, 93% of patients received aspirin, and 75.9% received clopidogrel. Of the 111 enrolled patients, two experienced stroke, one at 173 days and one at 215 days (1.8%; 95% confidence interval [CI] 0.2%–6.4%). Additionally, three transient ischemic attacks occurred in two patients. Six deaths occurred, four of which had cardiac or neurologic etiology. The annual stroke rate was 2.2%. Patient populations with a similar CHADS-2 score would be expected to have a stroke rate of 6.3%. PLAATO thus reduced stroke by 65% compared with aspirin-only therapy. The

nonrandomized study design and short follow-up limited firm conclusions about efficacy, but these results were promising. Five-year follow-up results were published for a 64-patient subset, and they included 7 deaths, 5 major strokes, 3 minor strokes, 1 cardiac tamponade requiring surgery, 1 MI, and 1 probable cerebral hemorrhage causing death. Only the cardiac tamponade was considered to result from the PLAATO device. At 5-year follow-up, the rate of stroke or TIA was 3.8%, still 42% lower than the expected rate (6.6% per year) predicted by the CHADS-2 score.[54] A newer percutaneous technology is the WATCHMAN device for occlusion of the LAA. It has a self-expanding nitinol frame with fixation barbs (Fig. 47-11), a permeable polyethylene filter membrane, and comes in different sizes for the variable anatomy of the LAA. It seals the ostium of the LAA, resulting in

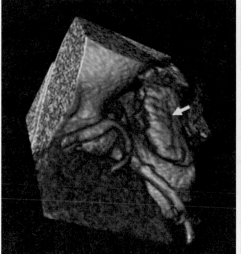

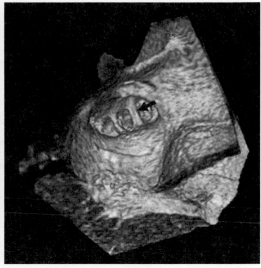

Figure 47-9 Pectinate muscles of the left atrial appendage (LAA). Pectinate muscles are frequent in the LAA and may be close to the ostium as shown in this cardiac computer tomographic angiography (CCTA) image from a normal subject. The posterior appendage wall may be close to the ostium, depending on angulation of the appendage. *(Modified with permission, Schwartz et al: JACC Cardiovascular Interventions 3(8):870–877, 2010.)*

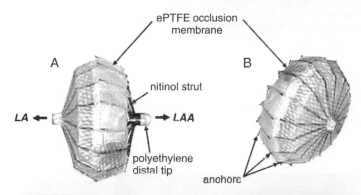

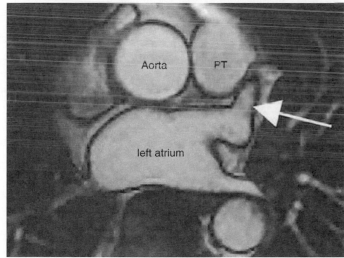

Figure 47-10 The percutaneous left atrial appendage trans-catheter occlusion (PLAATO) device. The PLAATO device was never used in large clinical trials but showed promising results for preventing stroke using occlusion of the left atrial appendage (LAA). *(Reprinted with permission from Mohrs, OK, Shraeder R, et al: Percutaneous left atrial appendage transcatheter occlusion (PLAATO): planning and follow-up using contrast-enhanced MRI. AJR AM J Roentgenol 186(2):361–364, 2006.)*

a smooth endocardial lining chronically (Figs. 47-12 and 47-13). This device was extensively evaluated over time by histopathologic methods. A study in canine and human hearts (none of the subjects died from device-related problems) after device placement showed excellent ostial closure. At early time points, in dogs, the atrial surface was covered by fibrin, which sealed the gaps between the left atrial wall and the device and filled the LAA cavity (Figs. 47-14 through 47-16). At 45 days, endothelial cells covered the endocardial surface with underlying smooth muscle cells, which sealed the device–LA interface. Regions with prior thrombi were replaced by endocardium surrounding the device membrane. Disorganized thrombus remained in the body of the LAA and at the periphery near the appendage walls, and mild inflammation was observed as the thrombi resorbed. By 90 days, a complete endocardial lining covered the former ostium of the LAA. Organizing thrombi had become connective tissue, with no residual inflammation.

The human hearts showed similar findings at necropsy. In the four hearts (139, 200, 480, and 852 days after implant) studied, the ostial fabric membrane was covered with endocardium. The surface of the LAA contained organizing thrombi with minimal inflammation. Organizing fibrous tissue was inside the LAA cavity, prominent near the atrial wall. The interior of the LAA contained organizing thrombi. This study showed that device integration in the LAA happens in several healing stages: early thrombus deposition, thrombus organization, inflammation and granulation of tissue, and final healing by connective tissue endothelialization without inflammation. The need for warfarin therapy remains unclear.

■ Clinical Trial: PROTECT-AF

The WATCHMAN® was tested in the PROTECT AF (Embolic Protection in Patients with Atrial Fibrillation) trial.[56] This trial randomized patients with nonvalvular AF in a 2:1 (device:control) scheme to the device or to control (conventional warfarin treatment). The primary efficacy endpoint was a composite of freedom from all stroke, cardiovascular death, and systemic embolization (Fig. 47-17). Safety endpoints were major bleeding, pericardial effusion, and device embolization. Patients randomized to the device received warfarin for 45 days until follow-up by trans-esophageal echocardiography (TEE). If the device was well seated and the LAA was sealed without significant leak, warfarin was discontinued. All-cause stroke and all-cause mortality proved noninferior to warfarin. Results on an intention-to-treat basis, with 900 patient-year follow-up, showed the primary efficacy rate (combined stroke, cardiovascular death, and systemic embolism) was 3% in the WATCHMAN group compared with 5% in the control (warfarin) group. For the primary safety endpoint (major

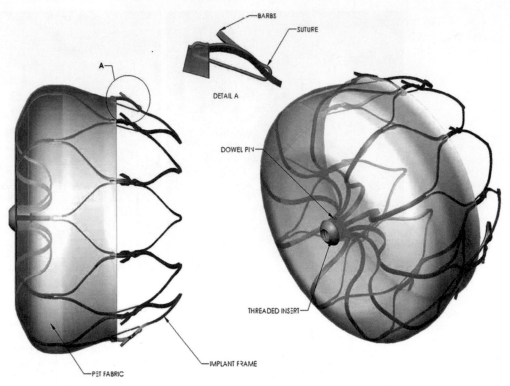

Figure 47-11   The WATCHMAN® device. The WATCHMAN device is designed to obliterate the left atrial appendage (LAA). The nitinol frame is self-expanding and has barbs for fixation. The surface contacting the left atrial chamber is permeable polyethylene filter. The device seals the ostium, resulting in a smooth endocardial lining chronically. (See Figures 47-12 and 47-13.)

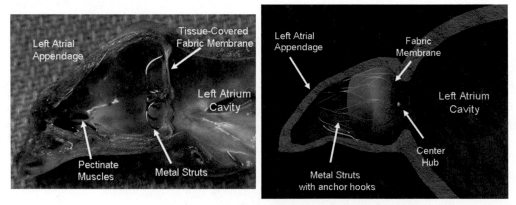

Figure 47-12   Occlusion of the left atrial appendage (LAA) by the WATCHMAN device. *Left,* Canine autopsy specimen 28 days after WATCHMAN implantation, showing a cross-sectional cutaway view of the device. The fabric membrane is covered with a fine layer of endocardium, and the metal struts are shown holding the device in place. Pectinate muscles internal to the LAA cavity are labeled. *Right,* Diagrammatic view of the WATCHMAN occlusion method. Metal struts with anchoring hooks secure the device within the body of the cavity of the LAA. A fabric membrane filter covers the atrial surface of the device, preventing thrombi from escaping into the left atrial chamber. A center hub is used to connect the device to the catheter delivery system. *(Adapted from Schwartz et al: JACC Cardiovascular Intervention 3(8):870–877, 2010.)*

bleeds, pericardial effusion, and device embolization), event rates were higher in the device group than in the control group (8.7% vs. 4.2%) because of pericardial effusion. These high rates, 4.8% of which were classified as "serious" were related to peri-procedural events, which decreased with operator experience. Fifteen of these events were successfully treated by percutaneous pericardiocentesis. None resulted in death. The most serious safety-related event in the control group was stroke, both ischemic and hemorrhagic. Hemorrhagic stroke markedly increased the risk of death. Conversely, data from the 1350 patient-year time point showed that adverse events in the device group had no late sequelae. A majority of patients (87%) successfully discontinued warfarin. The WATCHMAN device showed good results compared with warfarin for both primary efficacy as a function of age and stroke or mortality and was noninferior to warfarin.[56,57] The summary was that the WATCHMAN technology offers a safe and effective alternative to warfarin in patients with nonvalvular AF, who are at risk for stroke and are eligible for warfarin therapy. Pericardial effusion was the most frequent safety-related event in the device group (implant-related), while stroke was the most serious fraction of safety in the control group. Bleeding was more frequent in the control

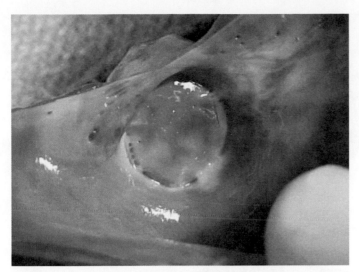

Figure 47-13 The WATCHMAN device. Canine necropsy specimen showing a view of the former ostium of the left atrial appendage (LAA), now completely obliterated by the endocardium-covered fabric membrane. This view is from the left atrial cavity, where it is clear that thrombi potentially residing in the body of the LAA could no longer escape into the left atrium and systemic circulation. (*Adapted from Schwartz et al: JACC Cardiovascular Intervention 3(8):870–877, 2010.*)

group and was often serious. An ongoing registry study called CAP (Continued-Access PROTECT AF) found improved safety; in 379 patients, the procedural stroke rate was 0% vs. 1% in the trial population, and the pericardial effusion rate of 2.4% was less than half the original 5.8% in the trial population. Importantly, the risk–benefit ratio is not affected by the CHADS-2 score. For the primary efficacy endpoint, patients with a CHADS-2 score of 1 had a relative risk of 0.50, whereas patients with a CHADS-2 score greater than 1 had a relative risk of 0.68. The CHADS-2 score is rendered largely irrelevant because thrombi typically originate in the LAA. This is characteristic of site-specific therapy to prevent cardiothromboembolism, and the results strongly suggest that many strokes originate from the LAA in patients with AF.[57] Concerns have been raised about the potential complications of occlusion of the LAA.[58,59] These principally relate to hypothesized effects on hemodynamics and fluid regulation in hypertension, AF, coronary heart disease, and valvular heart disease. Other hypothetical concerns include interference with thirst in hypovolemia and exacerbation of heart failure. Fortunately, large patient experience has shown that virtually none of these complications has been seen in percutaneous occlusion of the LAA. In retrospect, such results are entirely consistent with the large surgical experience of occlusion of the LAA, where no such complications have materialized despite many years of study and literally thousands of patients studied. These concerns can therefore be discounted now on the basis of clinical experience.

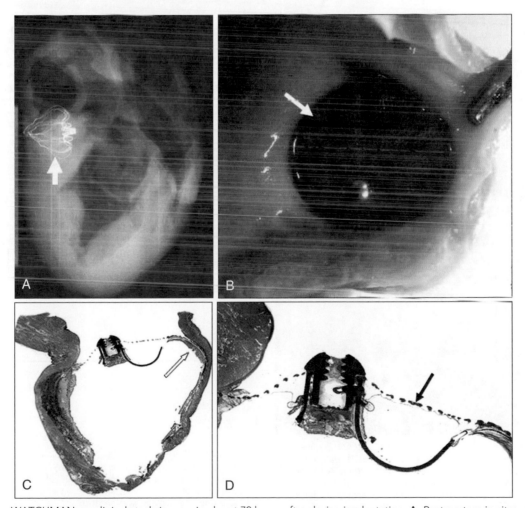

Figure 47-14 The WATCHMAN preclinical study in a canine heart 72 hours after device implantation. **A,** Postmortem in vitro x-ray showing position of the left atrial appendage (LAA) occlusion device (*arrow*) **B,** Gross photograph showing that the device membrane (*arrow*) is coated with a thin layer of fibrin. **C and D,** Methyl methacrylate embedded sections showing thin fibrin coating on the membrane (*closed arrow*) and fibrinous sealing of the membrane to the left atrial wall (*open arrow*). (*Reprinted from Schwartz et al: JACC Cardiovascular Intervention 3(8):870–877, 2010.*)

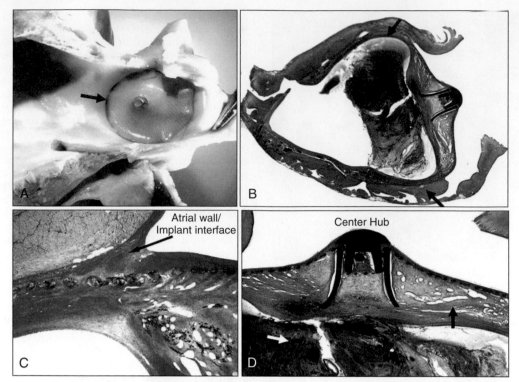

Figure 47-15 **Human** heart 200 days after implant of the WATCHMAN device. **A,** Opened left atrium showing the device seated within the appendage orifice. There are small linear gaps between the concave surface of the device fabric and the edge of the ostial margin of the left atrial appendage (LAA) (*arrow*), though the appendage cavity behind the covered membrane was healing with endocardium, so no thrombi could form nor exit this appendage (see Figure 47-4b). **B,** Sagittal section through the center of the LAA and the device. The section shows tight apposition of the device to the wall of the LAA and sealing of the device–LAA wall interface. Inside the device, the reddish-pink areas indicate fibrous organization. Toluidine blue and basic fuchsin stain. **C,** Close-up view through the center of the device, showing neointimal coverage over the surface. Toluidine blue and basic fuchsin stain, 1.25×. **D,** Close-up view of the device surface showing effective sealing of the atrial wall–device interface (*arrow*). Brown areas represent hemosiderin resulting from red cell breakdown. Toluidine blue and basic fuchsin stain, 4×. (*Adapted from Schwartz et al: JACC Cardiovascular Intervention 3(8):870–877, 2010.*)

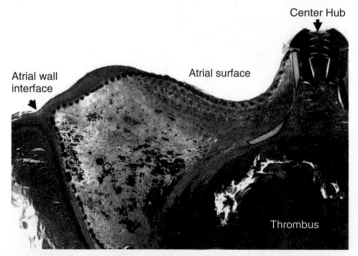

Figure 47-16 Atrial wall interface of the WATCHMAN device. This image shows that the device seals against the atrial wall, with the covered filter membrane becoming fused at the margins. Additionally, the atrial surface develops a thin endocardial lining that covers the membrane. (*Adapted from Schwartz et al: JACC Cardiovascular Intervention 3(8):870–877, 2010.*)

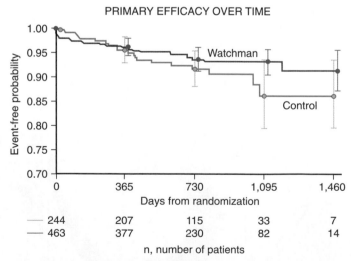

PRIMARY EFFICACY OVER TIME

| — | 244 | 207 | 115 | 33 | 7 |
| — | 463 | 377 | 230 | 82 | 14 |

n, number of patients

Figure 47-17 The WATCHMAN® device's primary efficacy over time. This graph shows that the primary efficacy of device-based therapy may continue to improve over time, though difficult to state with certainty at the time of this writing, since few patients have yet reached the 1460th day after device implantation.

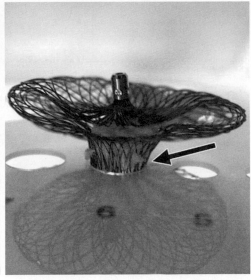

Figure 47-18   AMPLATZER® device. The Amplatzer device used for occlusion of the left atrial appendage (LAA) is a self-expanding, two-disk system consisting of a Nitinol wire mesh. The double disks are connected by a connecting waist. The disks and the waist may be filled with polyester fabric in some iterations of this device. *(Reproduced from Lee T, Tsai IC, Fu YC, et al: MDCT evaluation after closure of atrial septal defect with an Amplatzer septal occluder, AJR Am J Roentgenol 188(5):W431–439, 2007.)*

Additional Occlusion Technologies

Other technologies for occlusion of the LAA include the Amplatzer device (Fig. 47-18), which has been used previously for atrial septal defect (ASD) closure. To date, the number of patients receiving this therapy is small but growing; substantive data for commentary are not available at this time.[49,60–62] Early data suggest that procedure-related and device-related risks peak early in the course of treatment with occlusion, in comparison with the risks associated with anticoagulation, which continue to increase over the time a patient is anticoagulated. This continued incremental risk with anticoagulant therapy will likely be true for both conventional warfarin or for new agents under development.

Conclusion

Data are continuing to accumulate, and several tentative conclusions can be proposed in support for trans-catheter occlusion of the LAA:

1. AF is increasing in incidence and prevalence as the population ages. The relationships among age, AF, and stroke have been studied extensively. AF, embolic stroke, and complications from warfarin anticoagulation are progressively more frequent and dangerous with increasing age.
2. Cardiac emboli in patients with nonvalvular AF originate in the LAA in the majority of cases (90%), as suggested by prior data.
3. Warfarin anticoagulation reduces embolic stroke in AF but is under-used, difficult to maintain within a therapeutic range, and associated with increased bleeding; all these disadvantages continue to increase over time.
4. Novel methods of trans-catheter occlusion of the LAA are under evaluation and may find clinical use if they effectively reduce stroke and mortality without warfarin use. While these new approaches have early peri-procedural risks, late complications appear minimal and outweigh the long-term risks of anticoagulation.

REFERENCES

1. Miyasaka Y, Barnes ME, Gersh BJ, et al: Secular trends in incidence of atrial fibrillation in Olmsted County, Minnesota, 1980 to 2000, and implications on the projections for future prevalence. *Circulation* 114(2):119–125, 2006.
2. Go AS, Hylek EM, Phillips KA, et al: Prevalence of diagnosed atrial fibrillation in adults: national implications for rhythm management and stroke prevention: The AnTicoagulation and Risk Factors in Atrial Fibrillation (ATRIA) Study. *JAMA* 285(18):2370–2375, 2001.
3. Go AS: The epidemiology of atrial fibrillation in elderly persons: The tip of the iceberg. *Am J Geriatr Cardiol* 14(2):56–61, 2005.
4. Benjamin EJ, Wolf PA, D'Agostino RB, et al: Impact of atrial fibrillation on the risk of death: The Framingham Heart Study. *Circulation* 98(10):946–952, 1998.
5. Page RL, Tilsch TW, Connolly SJ, et al: Asymptomatic or "silent" atrial fibrillation: Frequency in untreated patients and patients receiving azimilide. *Circulation* 107(8):1141–1145, 2003.
6. Wolf PA, Abbott RD, Kannel WB: Atrial fibrillation as an independent risk factor for stroke: The Framingham Study. *Stroke* 22(8):983–988, 1991.
7. Wolf PA, Abbott RD, Kannel WB: Atrial fibrillation: A major contributor to stroke in the elderly. The Framingham Study. *Arch Intern Med* 147(9):1561–1564, 1987.

8. Wolf PA, D'Agostino RB, Belanger AJ, et al: Probability of stroke: A risk profile from the Framingham Study. *Stroke* 22(3):312–318, 1991.
9. Lamassa M, Di Carlo A, Pracucci G, et al: Characteristics, outcome, and care of stroke associated with atrial fibrillation in Europe: Data from a multicenter multinational hospital-based registry (The European Community Stroke Project). *Stroke* 32(2):392–398, 2001.
10. Fisher CM: Reducing risks of cerebral embolism. *Geriatrics* 34(2):59–61, 65–56, 1979.
11. Henriksson KM, Farahmand B, Johansson S, et al: Survival after stroke—The impact of CHADS(2) score and atrial fibrillation. *Int J Cardiol* 141(1):18–23, 2010.
12. Di Carlo A, Lamassa M, Baldereschi M, et al: Risk factors and outcome of subtypes of ischemic stroke. Data from a multicenter multinational hospital based registry. The European Community Stroke Project. *J Neurol Sci* 244(1–2):143–150, 2006.
13. Blackshear JL, Odell JA: Appendage obliteration to reduce stroke in cardiac surgical patients with atrial fibrillation. *Ann Thorac Surg* 61(2):755–759, 1996.
14. Jorgensen HS, Nakayama H, Reith J, et al: Acute stroke with atrial fibrillation. The Copenhagen Stroke Study. *Stroke* 27(10):1765–1769, 1996.

15. Anderson DC, Kappelle LJ, Eliasziw M, et al: Occurrence of hemispheric and retinal ischemia in atrial fibrillation compared with carotid stenosis. *Stroke* 33(8):1963–1967, 2002.
16. Morley J, Marinchak R, Rials SJ, et al: Atrial fibrillation, anticoagulation, and stroke. *Am J Cardiol* 77(3):38A–44A, 1996.
17. Nademanee K, Kosar EM: Long-term antithrombotic treatment for atrial fibrillation. *Am J Cardiol* 82(8A):37N–42N, 1998.
18. The effect of low-dose warfarin on the risk of stroke in patients with nonrheumatic atrial fibrillation. The Boston Area Anticoagulation Trial for Atrial Fibrillation Investigators. *N Engl J Med* 323(22):1505–1511, 1990.
19. Warfarin versus aspirin for prevention of thromboembolism in atrial fibrillation: Stroke Prevention in Atrial Fibrillation II Study. *Lancet* 343(8899):687–691, 1994.
20. Stroke Prevention in Atrial Fibrillation Study: Final results. *Circulation* 84(2):527–539, 1991.
21. Petersen P, Boysen G, Godtfredsen J, et al: Placebo-controlled, randomised trial of warfarin and aspirin for prevention of thromboembolic complications in chronic atrial fibrillation. The Copenhagen AFASAK study. *Lancet* 1(8631):175–179, 1989.
22. Connolly SJ, Laupacis A, Gent M, et al: Canadian Atrial Fibrillation Anticoagulation (CAFA) Study. *J Am Coll Cardiol* 18(2):349–355, 1991.

23. Ezekowitz MD, Bridgers SL, James KE, et al: Warfarin in the prevention of stroke associated with nonrheumatic atrial fibrillation. Veterans Affairs Stroke Prevention in Nonrheumatic Atrial Fibrillation Investigators. *N Engl J Med* 327(20):1406–1412, 1992.

24. Cooper NJ, Sutton AJ, Lu G, et al: Mixed comparison of stroke prevention treatments in individuals with nonrheumatic atrial fibrillation. *Arch Intern Med* 166(12):1269–1275, 2006.

25. Lip GY, Edwards SJ: Stroke prevention with aspirin, warfarin and ximelagatran in patients with non-valvular atrial fibrillation: A systematic review and meta-analysis. *Thromb Res* 118(3):321–333, 2006.

26. Bungard TJ, Ackman ML, Ho G, et al: Adequacy of anticoagulation in patients with atrial fibrillation coming to a hospital. *Pharmacotherapy* 20(9):1060–1065, 2000.

27. White HD, Gruber M, Feyzi J, et al: Comparison of outcomes among patients randomized to warfarin therapy according to anticoagulant control: Results from SPORTIF III and V. *Arch Intern Med* 167(3):239–245, 2007.

28. Go AS, Hylek EM, Borowsky LH, et al: Warfarin use among ambulatory patients with nonvalvular atrial fibrillation: The anticoagulation and risk factors in atrial fibrillation (ATRIA) study. *Ann Intern Med* 131(12):927–934, 1999.

29. Hart RG, Pearce LA, Aguilar MI: Meta-analysis: antithrombotic therapy to prevent stroke in patients who have nonvalvular atrial fibrillation. *Ann Intern Med* 146(12):857–867, 2007.

30. Hylek EM, Evans-Molina C, Shea C, et al: Major hemorrhage and tolerability of warfarin in the first year of therapy among elderly patients with atrial fibrillation. *Circulation* 115(21):2689–2696, 2007.

31. Fang MC, Go AS, Hylek EM, et al: Age and the risk of warfarin-associated hemorrhage: The anticoagulation and risk factors in atrial fibrillation study. *J Am Geriatr Soc* 54(8):1231–1236, 2006.

32. Connolly S, Pogue J, Hart R, et al: Clopidogrel plus aspirin versus oral anticoagulation for atrial fibrillation in the Atrial fibrillation Clopidogrel Trial with Irbesartan for prevention of Vascular Events (ACTIVE W): A randomised controlled trial. *Lancet* 367(9526):1903–1912, 2006.

33. Albers GW, Diener HC, Frison L, et al: Ximelagatran vs warfarin for stroke prevention in patients with nonvalvular atrial fibrillation: A randomized trial. *JAMA* 293(6):690–698, 2005.

34. Connolly SJ, Ezekowitz MD, Yusuf S, et al: Dabigatran versus warfarin in patients with atrial fibrillation. *N Engl J Med* 361(12):1139–1151, 2009.

35. Hara H, Virmani R, Holmes DR, Jr., et al: Is the left atrial appendage more than a simple appendage? *Catheter Cardiovasc Interv* 74(2):234–242, 2009.

36. Ernst G, Stollberger C, Abzieher F, et al: Morphology of the left atrial appendage. *Anat Rec* 242(4):553–561, 1995.

37. de Bold AJ, Bruneau BG, Kuroski de Bold ML: Mechanical and neuroendocrine regulation of the endocrine heart. *Cardiovasc Res* 31(1):7–18, 1996.

38. Inoue S, Murakami Y, Sano K, et al: Atrium as a source of brain natriuretic polypeptide in patients with atrial fibrillation. *J Card Fail* 6(2):92–96, 2000.

39. Igarashi Y, Kashimura K, Makiyama Y, et al: Left atrial appendage dysfunction in chronic nonvalvular atrial fibrillation is significantly associated with an elevated level of brain natriuretic peptide and a prothrombotic state. *Jpn Circ J* 65(9):788–792, 2001.

40. Tabata T, Oki T, Yamada H, et al: Relationship between left atrial appendage function and plasma concentration of atrial natriuretic peptide. *Eur J Echocardiogr* 1(2):130–137, 2000.

41. Watson T, Shantsila E, Lip GY: Mechanisms of thrombogenesis in atrial fibrillation: Virchow's triad revisited. *Lancet* 373(9658):155–166, 2009.

42. Goldsmith I, Kumar P, Carter P, et al: Atrial endocardial changes in mitral valve disease: A scanning electron microscopy study. *Am Heart J* 140(5):777–784, 2000.

43. Pollick C, Taylor D: Assessment of left atrial appendage function by transesophageal echocardiography. Implications for the development of thrombus. *Circulation* 84(1):223–231, 1991.

44. Bonow RO, Carabello BA, Kanu C, et al: ACC/AHA 2006 guidelines for the management of patients with valvular heart disease: A report of the American College of Cardiology/American Heart Association Task Force on Practice Guidelines (writing committee to revise the 1998 Guidelines for the Management of Patients With Valvular Heart Disease): Developed in collaboration with the Society of Cardiovascular Anesthesiologists: Endorsed by the Society for Cardiovascular Angiography and Interventions and the Society of Thoracic Surgeons. *Circulation* 114(5):e84–e231, 2006.

45. Healey JS, Crystal E, Lamy A, et al: Left Atrial Appendage Occlusion Study (LAAOS): Results of a randomized controlled pilot study of left atrial appendage occlusion during coronary bypass surgery in patients at risk for stroke. *Am Heart J* 150(2):288–293, 2005.

46. Coulshed N, Epstein EJ, McKendrick CS, et al: Systemic embolism in mitral valve disease. *Br Heart J* 32(1):26–34, 1970.

47. Katz ES, Tsiamtsiouris T, Applebaum RM, et al: Surgical left atrial appendage ligation is frequently incomplete: A transesophageal echocardiorahic study. *J Am Coll Cardiol* 36(2):468–471, 2000.

48. Bayard YL, Ostermayer SH, Hein R, et al: Percutaneous devices for stroke prevention. *Cardiovasc Revasc Med* 8(3):216–225, 2007.

49. Bayard YL, Ostermayer SH, Sievert H: Transcatheter occlusion of the left atrial appendage for stroke prevention. *Expert Rev Cardiovasc Ther* 3(6):1003–1008, 2005.

50. Ostermayer S, Reschke M, Billinger K, et al: Percutaneous closure of the left atrial appendage. *J Interv Cardiol* 16(6):553–556, 2003.

51. Ostermayer SH, Reisman M, Kramer PH, et al: Percutaneous left atrial appendage transcatheter occlusion (PLAATO system) to prevent stroke in high-risk patients with non-rheumatic atrial fibrillation: Results from the international multi-center feasibility trials. *J Am Coll Cardiol* 46(1):9–14, 2005.

52. Meier B, Palacios I, Windecker S, et al: Transcatheter left atrial appendage occlusion with Amplatzer devices to obviate anticoagulation in patients with atrial fibrillation. *Catheter Cardiovasc Interv* 60(3):417–422, 2003.

53. Ussia GP, Mule M, Cammalleri V, et al: Percutaneous closure of left atrial appendage to prevent embolic events in high-risk patients with chronic atrial fibrillation. *Catheter Cardiovasc Interv* 74(2):217–222, 2009.

54. Block PC, Burstein S, Casale PN, et al: Percutaneous left atrial appendage occlusion for patients in atrial fibrillation suboptimal for warfarin therapy: 5-year results of the PLAATO (Percutaneous Left Atrial Appendage Transcatheter Occlusion) Study. *JACC Cardiovasc Interv* 2(7):594–600, 2009.

55. El-Chami MF, Grow P, Eilen D, et al: Clinical outcomes three years after PLAATO implantation. *Catheter Cardiovasc Interv* 69(5):704–707, 2007.

56. Holmes DR, Reddy VY, Turi ZG, et al: Percutaneous closure of the left atrial appendage versus warfarin therapy for prevention of stroke in patients with atrial fibrillation: A randomised non-inferiority trial. *Lancet* 374(9689):534–542, 2009.

57. Holmes DR, Jr: *The PROTECT AF trial: Intermediate-term outcome.* Presented at: American College of Cardiology Annual Scientific Session/i2 Summit; March 15, 2010; Atlanta, GA. 2010.

58. Stollberger C, Finsterer J, Ernst G, et al: Is left atrial appendage occlusion useful for prevention of stroke or embolism in atrial fibrillation? *Z Kardiol* 91(5):376–379, 2002.

59. Stollberger C, Finsterer J, Schneider B: Arguments against left atrial appendage occlusion for stroke prevention. *Stroke* 38(9):e77, 2007.

60. Crowley DI, Donnelly JP: Use of Amplatzer occlusion devices to occlude Fontan baffle leaks during fenestration closure procedures. *Catheter Cardiovasc Interv* 71(2):244–249, 2008.

61. Cruz-Gonzalez I, Cubeddu RJ, Sanchez-Ledesma M, et al: Left atrial appendage exclusion using an Amplatzer device. *Int J Cardiol* 134(1):e1–e3, 2009.

62. Cruz-Gonzalez I, Yan BP, Lam YY: Left atrial appendage exclusion: State-of-the-art. *Catheter Cardiovasc Interv* 75(5):806–813, 2010.

48

Mitral Valvuloplasty

ALEC VAHANIAN | DOMINIQUE HIMBERT |
ERIC BROCHET | BERNARD IUNG

KEY POINTS

- The efficacy, safety, and applicability of the Inoue balloon technique are clearly established worldwide, and this technique is currently the point of reference for percutaneous mitral commissurotomy (PMC).

- Trans-esophageal echocardiography (TEE) is essential for monitoring the procedure and for the assessment of immediate results.

- The importance of experience cannot be stressed enough for the safety of the procedure and for the selection of patients.

- PMC shows good immediate and long-term clinical results and carries a low risk when performed by experienced teams.

- The prediction of results is multi-factorial; therefore, patient selection must be based on patient anatomy as well as other characteristics.

- PMC is the treatment of choice in patients with favorable characteristics.

- For other patients, the decision must be individualized, and PMC and valve replacement should be considered complementary techniques.

■ Introduction

Until the first publication by Inoue and coworkers describing percutaneous mitral commissurotomy (PMC) in 1984, surgery was the only treatment for patients with mitral stenosis.[1] Since then, the technique has evolved considerably. A large number of patients with a wide range of clinical conditions have now been treated, enabling efficacy and risk to be assessed; long-term results are now available, so it is possible to select the most appropriate candidates for treatment by this method.[2] As expected from the earlier experience with closed surgical commissurotomy, the positive immediate as well as long term results obtained during this period have led to increased worldwide use of the technique. We begin this chapter with a report of our own experience and then review the data available in the literature.

■ Personal Experience

PATIENTS

We have attempted PMC in 2773 patients, whose mean age was 47 ± 15 years (range, 9–86 years).[3] Altogether, 71% were in class III or IV, according to the classification system of the New York Heart Association (NYHA), and 31% were in atrial fibrillation (AF). After fluoroscopic examination and echocardiography, the patients were divided into the following anatomic groups for selection of the most adequate treatments:

- The first group (11%) had flexible valves and mild subvalvular disease.
- The second group (62%) had flexible valves but extensive subvalvular disease (length of chordae <1 cm).
- The third group (27%) had calcified valves, as determined by echocardiography and confirmed by fluoroscopy.

Mild mitral regurgitation (grade 1 or 4) was present in 39% of patients. Regurgitation was moderate (grade 2 or 4) in only 2%.

PROCEDURE

The antegrade approach was used in all cases. Trans-septal catheterization was performed via the right femoral vein, using a standard Brockenbrough needle and a dilator (Cook). The atrial puncture was carried out using anteroposterior and 30-degree right anterior oblique (RAO) views under continuous pressure monitoring. At this stage, heparin was given (3000 to 4000 Units when using the Inoue technique). In the early cases, we used a single-balloon technique (n = 30). We have also used a combination of the trefoil and the conventional balloon (n = 586). Since 1990, we have used the stepwise Inoue technique (n = 2125). No left heart catheterization was performed in the last 500 cases. Patients were usually discharged 1 to 2 days after the procedure. Oral anticoagulation was continued in cases of AF or previous embolism.

RESULTS

Immediate Hemodynamic and Echocardiographic Results

Successful PMC brought immediate hemodynamic improvement, as shown in Table 48-1. Echocardiographic techniques confirmed the results obtained by hemodynamics. The valve area increased from 1.0 ± 0.2 to 1.9 ± 0.3 cm^2, as assessed by two-dimensional echocardiography. Poor results, as defined by a valve area less than 1.5 cm^2 or mitral regurgitation greater than 2 or 4 (or both), occurred in 11.5% of patients.

Technical Failures and Complications

We attempted PMC in 2773 patients, but the procedure was discontinued in 32 patients (1.2%) because of complications that occurred before PMC or technical failure. The major adverse cardiac events (MACEs) were in-hospital death in 11 patients (0.4%), tamponade in 6 (0.2%), embolism with sequelae in 11 (0.4%), and severe mitral regurgitation (≥3 or 4) in 113 (4.1%). Among the last group of patients, 84% were operated on. Other MACEs included local complications leading to urgent surgery in 17 patients (0.7%). Finally, 5% of patients had one or more major complications, and 130 (4.7%) underwent surgery within 1 month.

Long-Term Results

The mid-term results were obtained from a series of 1024 consecutive patients residing in France who underwent PMC. Altogether, 96% of these patients were monitored for a mean of 52 months (range, 1–132 months). The follow-up evaluation consisted of a clinical examination with three major endpoints: (1) survival, (2) need for secondary surgery, and (3) quality of the functional results. At 10 years, the mid-term results were good: 85% ± 4% of patients were alive, 61% ± 4% were free from reoperation, and 56% ± 4% were in good functional condition (i.e., NYHA class I or II). Of the patients with poor initial results (n = 112) because of severe mitral regurgitation or insufficient initial opening, 16 died (cardiac causes in 12), 74 were operated on (valve replacement in 60, conservative surgery in 14), and 6 were in NYHA class III or IV but were not operated on because of contra-indications to surgery. In the remaining patients, the moderate

TABLE 48-1	Immediate Results of Percutaneous Mitral Commissurotomy				
Mean Pulmonary Artery Condition	Mean Left Atrial Pressure (mm Hg)	Cardiac Index (mm Hg)	Gradient (mm Hg)	Valve Area (cm²)	Mean Pressure (mm Hg)
Before PMC	35 ± 13	22 ± 7	2.9 ± 0.7	1.04 ± 0.23	10.8 ± 4.8
After PMC	26 ± 10	13 ± 5	3.1 ± 5 1	92 ± 0.31	4.8 ± 2.1

PMC, percutaneous mitral commissurotomy.

improvement in valve function, nevertheless, provided transient symptomatic improvement. In the group of patients with initially successful PMC (*n* = 912), the mid-term results were good. The 10-year actuarial rates for (1) global survival (i.e., survival with no cardiac-related death), (2) survival with no cardiac-related death and no need for surgery or repeat dilation, and (3) the composite endpoint of good functional results were, respectively, 87% ± 4%, 67% ± 4%, and 61% ± 5%. A total of 46 patients died during follow-up (23 of cardiac-related causes). A repeat mitral valve procedure was required in 109 patients: repeat dilation in 21, open-heart commissurotomy in 13, and mitral valve replacement in 75. Surgical findings during the operations were re-stenosis in 97% of patients.

Devices and Techniques

PMC acts in the same way as surgical commissurotomy, by opening the fused commissures (Fig. 48-1). PMC is of little or no help in cases of restricted valvular mobility caused by valve fibrosis or severe sub-valvular disease. The techniques and devices used for PMC have varied over time and from group to group. At the present time, there are two approaches—trans-arterial and trans-venous—and two main techniques—the double-balloon technique and the Inoue technique.

TRANS-ARTERIAL OR RETROGRADE APPROACH

The trans-arterial, or retrograde, approach has the advantage of minimizing or eliminating the risk of atrial septal defect (ASD) and the disadvantage of potential arterial damage. This technique has now been abandoned because of its complexity. The retrograde technique without trans-septal catheterization has been used with good results and no serious complications, but its use is not widespread.[4]

TRANS-VENOUS OR ANTEGRADE APPROACH

The trans-venous, or antegrade, approach is more widely used. It is performed through the femoral vein or, exceptionally, through the jugular vein. Trans-septal catheterization is the first and one of the most crucial steps of the procedure. The conditions necessary for safe and successful trans-septal catheterization are (1) knowledge of the anatomy, which may be modified in patients with mitral stenosis, in whom normal geometry has been lost because both atria are enlarged and the convexity of the septum is exaggerated; (2) knowledge of contraindications; and (3) experience of the operators acquired by performance of the technique on a regular basis. Usually, trans-septal catheterization is performed under fluoroscopic guidance, ideally with use of several views. Continuous pressure monitoring is recommended. Echocardiography is not systematic during trans-septal catheterization; however, it has the potential to enhance its safety, especially in the early part of the operator's experience. This has been done primarily with TEE, which is superior to trans-thoracic echocardiography (TTE) for imaging the inter-atrial septum (IAS). Nevertheless, the trans-esophageal approach is not easy in the catheterization laboratory (cath lab) and should probably be restricted to cases in which technical difficulties are encountered (e.g., severe anatomic distortion) (see Video 48-1). Intracardiac echocardiography (ICE) is currently considered the imaging tool of choice in several catheterization centers to guide trans-septal puncture because it may be used without additional operators or general anesthesia, although the price of the device seriously limits its use in most places.[5] Recent data suggest that the

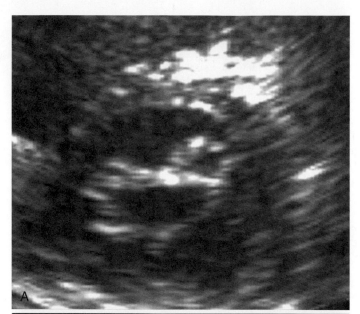
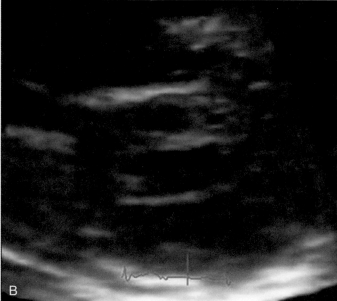

Figure 48-1 Trans-thoracic echocardiography before (*upper part,* two-dimensional echocardiography) and after (*lower part,* three-dimensional echocardiography) percutaneous mitral commissurotomy (PMC). The arrows show the bilateral commissural opening after PMC.

real-time three-dimensional trans-esophageal technique (RT 3DTEE) may further improve visualization of the septum and assessment of tenting during septal puncture.[6]

DOUBLE-BALLOON TECHNIQUE

The double-balloon technique is one of the two main balloon techniques in current use; it has been described extensively.[7] Briefly, the

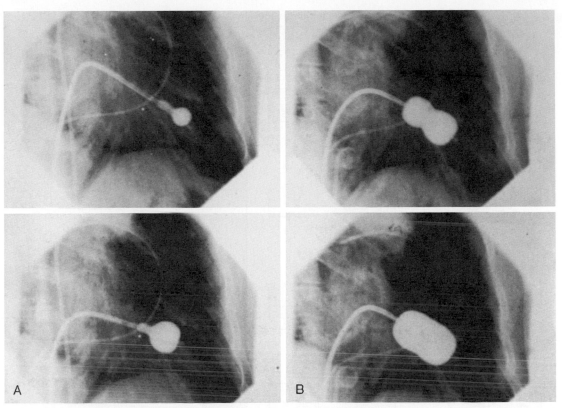

Figure 48-2 Inoue's percutaneous mitral commissurotomy technique. **A,** Inflation of the distal portion of the balloon, which is thereafter pulled back and anchored at the mitral valve. **B,** Subsequent inflation of the proximal and middle portions of the balloon. At full inflation, the waist of the balloon in its mid-portion has disappeared.

technique is as follows: After trans-septal catheterization, the left ventricle is catheterized with the use of a floating balloon catheter. One or two long exchange guidewires are positioned in the apex of the left ventricle or, less frequently, in the ascending aorta. The IAS is dilated with the use of a peripheral angioplasty balloon (8 or 6 mm in diameter). Finally, the balloons (15 to 20 mm in diameter) are positioned across the mitral valve. The multi-track system is a more recent refinement of the double-balloon technique that uses a monorail system, requiring the presence of only one guidewire and easing the performance of the dilation compared with the standard double balloon technique. Clinical experience with this device is, however, limited.[8]

INOUE TECHNIQUE

The Inoue technique was the first to be described, and wide experience has now been acquired by a number of groups worldwide.[1,3,9] The Inoue balloon, composed of nylon and rubber micromesh, is self-positioning and pressure extensible. It is large (24 to 30 mm in diameter) and has a low profile (4.5 mm). The balloon has three distinct parts, each with a specific elasticity, enabling them to be inflated sequentially. This sequence allows fast, stable positioning across the valve. There are four sizes of the Inoue balloon (24 mm, 26 mm, 28 mm, and 30 mm); each is pressure dependent, so its diameter can be varied by up to 4 mm, as required by circumstances. The main steps are as follows: After trans-septal catheterization, a stiff guidewire is introduced into the left atrium. The femoral entry site and the atrial septum are dilated with a rigid dilator (14 French [F]), and the balloon is introduced into the left atrium. Inoue recommended the use of a stepwise dilation technique under echocardiographic guidance. Balloon size is chosen in accordance with the patient's height (26 mm in very small patients or infants, 28 mm in patients shorter than 1.60 m, and 30 mm in patients taller than 1.60 m). The balloon is inflated sequentially. First, the distal portion is inflated with 1 or 2 mL

of a diluted contrast medium; it acts as a floating balloon catheter when crossing the mitral valve. Second, the distal part is further inflated, and the balloon is pulled back into the mitral orifice. Inflation then occurs at the level of the proximal part and finally in the central portion, with the disappearance of the central waist at full inflation (Fig. 48-2; see Videos 48-2 and 48-3 📹).

The first inflation is performed 4 mm below the maximal balloon size, and the balloon size is increased in steps of 1 mm each. The balloon is then deflated and withdrawn into the left atrium. If mitral regurgitation (assessed by color Doppler echocardiography) has not increased by more than ¼ and the valve area is less than 1 cm²/m² of body surface area, the balloon is re-advanced across the valve, and PMC is repeated with a balloon diameter increased by 1 mm (Fig. 48-3).[5] The criteria for ending are an adequate valve area or an increase in the degree of mitral regurgitation. Data currently available comparing the double-balloon and Inoue techniques suggest that the Inoue technique eases the procedure and has equivalent efficacy and lower risk.[9] In fact, the Inoue technique has already become the most popular in the world, having been used in more than 10,000 patients. Finally, even though randomized studies are lacking and intra-procedural echocardiography lacks practicality, the stepwise technique under echocardiographic guidance certainly allows the best use of the mechanical properties of the Inoue balloon and therefore optimizes the results.

METALLIC COMMISSUROTOME

During the late 1990s, Cribier and colleagues introduced the metallic commissurotome, which uses a device similar to the Tubb dilator used during closed commissurotomy.[10] Experience with this device comprises about 1000 cases, mainly from developing countries. The initial results suggest that the technique has efficacy similar to that of balloon commissurotomy, but the risk of hemopericardium seems higher

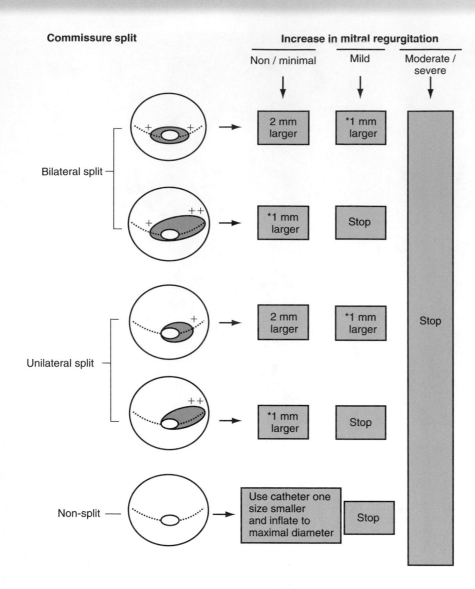

Figure 48-3   Decision making during the stepwise dilation technique based on echocardiographic findings after each balloon dilation. +, incomplete split; ++, complete split; *, stop in cases of severely diseased valve or age older than 65 years.

owing to the presence of a stiff guidewire in the left ventricle. In addition, this technique is more demanding on the operator compared with the Inoue technique. The potential advantage is that the dilator is reusable, which reduces the cost of the procedure. Its use is currently very limited, if any.

■ Monitoring of the Procedure and Evaluation of Immediate Results

There are two ways to monitor the procedure and assess immediate results in the cath lab: hemodynamics and echocardiography. Although echocardiography may be difficult to perform in the cath lab for logistic reasons, it provides essential information. Besides its usefulness for the guidance of trans-septal catheterization, echocardiography provides information on the course of the mitral opening, which is of utmost importance when using the stepwise Inoue technique. Echocardiography enables detection of early complications such as pericardial hemorrhage or severe mitral regurgitation.

MONITORING OF THE PROCEDURE

Trans-thoracic echocardiography (TTE) is the preferred technique for echocardiographic monitoring in most centers. Trans-esophageal guidance under general anesthesia, although performed systematically

in some centers, is restricted in others to cases in which difficulty is encountered or in pregnant patients to reduce radiation exposure. TEE provides excellent views of the position of the balloon as it is advanced into the mitral orifice. TEE may also better assess the severity and mechanism of mitral regurgitation and residual shunting. The recently introduced real-time three-dimensional technique has the added advantage of providing an "en face" view of the mitral valve, allowing better visualization of the trajectory and positioning of the balloon before inflation.[6] ICE is another alternative that helps monitor balloon positioning and inflation. Although the visualization of the mitral orifice is less optimal with ICE than with TEE, adequate views may be obtained from the right ventricle.[5] The following guidelines have been suggested for monitoring the procedure: First, use of the mean left atrial pressure and mean valve gradient can be criticized because of variations that may occur, particularly with respect to changes in heart rate or cardiac output. Second, repeated evaluation of the valve area during the procedure by hemodynamic measurements lacks practicality and may be subject to error because of the instability of the patient's condition and the inaccuracy of Gorlin's formula in the presence of atrial shunts or mitral regurgitation. The accuracy of Doppler measurements during valvuloplasty is low, so planimetry from two-dimensional echocardiography appears to be the method of choice if it is technically feasible. Color Doppler assessment is the method of choice for sequential evaluation of the changes in the degree of regurgitation. The commissural opening, which is the main parameter, is usually assessed in the parasternal short-axis view during TTE. Real-time three-dimensional echocardiography is the most accurate method for assessing the degree of opening using short-axis views or real-time three-dimensional TEE en face views, which may provide further information regarding the extent of the commissural opening (Video 48-4 [image]).[6,11] The following criteria have been proposed for the desired endpoint of the procedure: (1) mitral valve area of more than 1 cm^2/m^2 of the body surface area; (2) complete opening of at least one commissure; or (3) appearance or increment of regurgitation greater than ¼. It is vital that the strategy be tailored to individual circumstances, taking into account clinical as well as anatomic factors and the cumulative data of peri-procedural monitoring. For example, balloon size, increments of size, and expected final valve area are smaller in certain clinical subsets such as older or pregnant patients, in whom the need for emergency surgery is of concern, and in the presence of tight mitral stenosis, extensive valve or subvalvular disease, and nodular commissural calcification. After the procedure, the most accurate evaluation of the valve area is achieved by echocardiography. To allow for the slight loss during the first 24 hours, this should be performed 1 to 2 days after mitral valvuloplasty, when the valve area may be calculated by planimetry or by the half-pressure time or continuity equation method. The degree of regurgitation may be finally assessed by angiography or color Doppler flow. The most sensitive method for assessing shunting is color Doppler flow, especially when TEE is used; In current practice, the use of postvalvuloplasty TEE is restricted to patients with severe mitral regurgitation to evaluate the mechanisms. In experienced centers, the procedure can be performed using a single venous approach and noninvasive monitoring, which reduces the risk, discomfort, and costs.

IMMEDIATE RESULTS

Failures

The failure rate ranges from 1% to 17%.[3,4,7–10,12–14] Failure is often caused by an inability to puncture the atrial septum or position the balloon correctly across the valve. Most failures occur early in the operator's experience. Failures can also result from unfavorable anatomy such as severe atrial stenosis or predominant subvalvular stenosis.

Hemodynamics

Our results, like those of others, demonstrate the efficacy of PMC, which usually provides an increase of more than 100% in the valve area (Table 48-2). The improvement in valve function results in an immediate decrease in left atrial pressure (Fig. 48-4) and a slight increase in cardiac index. A gradual decrease in pulmonary arterial pressure and pulmonary vascular resistance is seen. High pulmonary vascular

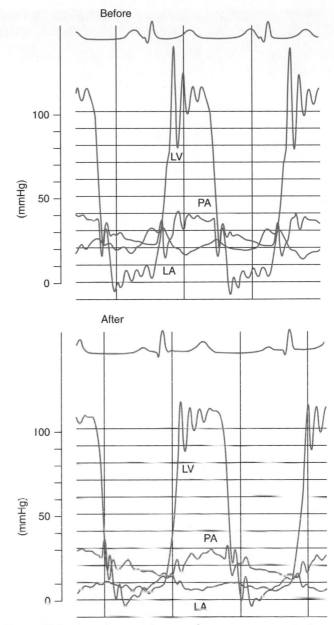

Figure 48-4 Hemodynamic changes after percutaneous mitral commissurotomy. *LA,* left atrium; *LV,* left ventricle; *PAP,* pulmonary artery pressure.

TABLE 48-2	Immediate Results of Percutaneous Commissurotomy (PMC): Increase in Mitral Valve Area				
Author (Ref. No.)	*N*	*Age (Yr)*	*Mitral Valve Area (cm^2) Before PMC*	*Mitral Valve Area (cm^2) After PMC*	*Technique*
Chen et al.* (14)	4832	37	1.1	2.1	Inoue balloon
Stefanadis et al. (4)	441	44	1.0	2.1	Modified single-, double-, or Inoue balloon (retrograde)
Bonhoeffer et al. (8)	100	31	0.8	2.0	Multi-track balloon
Cribier et al. (10)	500	34	0.9	2.1	Metallic commissurotome
Kang et al. (9)	152	42	0.9	1.8	Inoue balloon
Randomized comparison	150	40	0.9	1.9	Double-balloon
Ben Farhat et al. (12)	654	33	1.0	2.1	Inoue or double-balloon
Arora et al. (13)	4850	27	0.7	1.9	Inoue or double-balloon or metallic commissurotome
Palacios et al. (7)	879	55	0.9	1.9	Inoue or double-balloon
Iung et al. (3)	2773	47	1.0	1.9	Inoue, single-, or double-balloon

*Multicenter series.

TABLE 48-3	Severe Complications of Percutaneous Mitral Commissurotomy					
Author (Ref. No.)	*N*	*Age (Yr)*	*In-Hospital Death (%)*	*Tamponade (%)*	*Embolic Events (%)*	*Severe Mitral Regurgitation (%)*
Chen et al.* (14)	4832	37	0.1	0.8	0.5	1.4
Stefanadis et al.* (4)	441	44	0.2	0	0	3.4
Ben Farhat et al. (12)	654	33	0.5	0.6	1.5	4.6
Arora et al. (13)	4850	27	0.2	0.2	0.1	1.4
Palacios et al. (7)	879	55	0.6	1.0	1.8	9.4
Iung et al. (3)	2773	47	0.4	0.2	0.4	4.1

*Multicenter series.

resistance continues to decrease in the absence of re-stenosis. PMC has a beneficial effect on exercise capacity. In addition, studies have shown that this technique improves the pump function of the left atrium and the LAA and decreases left atrial stiffness. It also results in a decrease in the intensity of spontaneous echocardiographic contrast in the left atrium.

Complications

Large series have enabled assessment of the risks in the technique (Table 48-3).[3,4,7–10,12–14] Procedural mortality has ranged from 0% to 3% in most series. The main causes of death are left ventricular perforation and poor general condition of the patient. The incidence of hemopericardium has varied from 0.5% to 12%. Pericardial hemorrhage may be related to trans-septal catheterization or to apex perforation by guidewires or the balloon itself when exaggerated movement occurs with the over-the-wire techniques; however, this complication is virtually eliminated with the Inoue balloon technique. If hypotension occurs during PMC, hemopericardium must be suspected and echocardiography immediately performed. Pericardiocentesis in the cath lab, ideally under echocardiographic guidance, usually allows stabilization of the patient's condition and secondary transfer for cardiac surgery.

Embolism is encountered in 0.5% to 5% of cases. It is seldom the cause of permanent incapacitation and even more seldom the cause of death. It can be caused by gas if it occurs immediately after balloon rupture, by fibrinothrombotic material, or, on occasion, by calcium accumulation. Although the incidence of embolism is low, its potential consequences are severe, and all possible precautions must be taken to prevent it. The treatment of cerebral embolism should be provided in collaboration with a stroke center. In most cases, the degree of mitral regurgitation remains stable or, more often, slightly increases after PMC. Conversely, in a few cases, the degree of mitral regurgitation decreases, probably because of the increased mobility of the leaflets. Severe mitral regurgitation is rare, its frequency ranging from 2% to 19%.[3,4,7–10] The occurrence of severe mitral regurgitation remains largely unpredictable for a given patient. Surgical findings have shown that it is related to noncommissural tearing of the posterior or anterior leaflet (Fig. 48-5).[15,16] In these cases, one or both commissures are too tightly fused to be split. It may also be caused by excessive commissural splitting or, in rare cases, by rupture of a papillary muscle. In our experience, anatomic findings on surgery showed that severe mitral regurgitation occurred almost exclusively in patients with unfavorable anatomy; all had extensive subvalvular disease, and half had valve calcification. It has been suggested that the development of severe regurgitation depends more on the distribution of morphologic changes than on their severity. Severe mitral regurgitation may be well tolerated; more often, in our experience, it is not, and surgery must be scheduled. In most cases, valve replacement is necessary because of the severity of the underlying valve disease.[17,18] Conservative surgery, combining suture of the tear and commissurotomy, has been performed successfully in young patients with a less severe valve deformity. In groups with positive outcomes of mitral valve reconstruction, the need for valve replacement is more closely related to the extent of valve disease than to the tear itself. The frequency of ASD after PMC varies from 10% to 90%, according to the

technique used for its detection (Fig. 48-6; Video 48-5 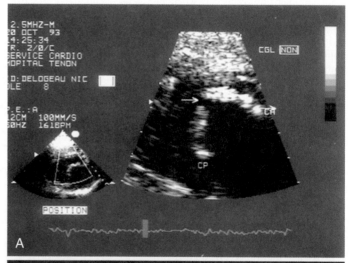).[19] These shunts are usually small and restrictive, with high-velocity flow. Right-to-left shunts occur on rare occasion in patients with elevated right-sided heart pressures and pulmonary hypertension. The incidence of transient, complete heart block is 1.5%, and it seldom requires a permanent pacemaker. After the trans-venous approach, vascular complications are the exception. Urgent surgery (within 24 hours) is

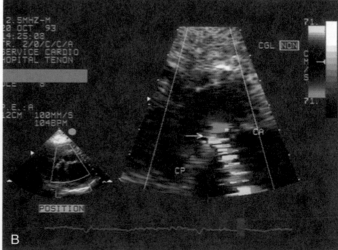

Figure 48-5 Severe mitral regurgitation after percutaneous mitral commissurotomy (PMC). Trans-thoracic echocardiography. *Left*, Tear of the anterior leaflet (A2). *Right*, Doppler color flow, showing a severe regurgitation at the level of the leaflet tear. *CA*, anterior commissure; *CP*, posterior commissure.

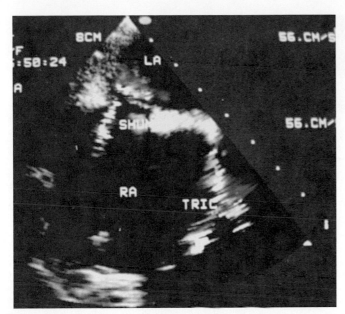

Figure 48-6 Trans-esophageal echocardiographic view of the atrial septum showing a small left-to-right shunt across the foramen ovale. *LA,* left atrium; *RA,* right atrium; *TRIC,* tricuspid valve.

TABLE 48-4	Late Results after Percutaneous Mitral Commissurotomy			
Author (Ref. No.)	*N*	*Age (Yr)*	*Follow-Up (Yr)*	*Event-Free Survival (%)*
Stefanadis et al. (4)	441	44	9	75*
Iung et al. (20)	1024	49	10	56*
Ben Farhat et al. (12)	654	34	10	72*
Palacios et al. (7)	879	55	12	33*
Song et al. (23)	329	44	9	90†
Fawzy et al. (27)	493	31	13	74*

*Survival without intervention and in New York Heart Association class I or II.
†After successful procedure.

seldom needed for complications resulting from PMC. It may be required, however, for massive hemopericardium resulting from left ventricular perforation unresponsive to pericardiocentesis or, less frequently, for severe mitral regurgitation leading to hemodynamic collapse or refractory pulmonary edema.

Overall, the incidence of failures and serious complications such as tamponade is clearly related to experience. When performed by experienced teams on properly selected patients, PMC is a relatively low-risk procedure.

Predictors of Immediate Results

Evaluation of immediate results is mainly based on hemodynamic criteria. The definition of good immediate results varies from series to series. The two definitions frequently employed are (1) a final valve area larger than 1.5 cm² and an increase of at least 25% in the valve area or (2) a final valve area larger than 1.5 cm² without mitral regurgitation greater than ¾. Many studies using different techniques of valvuloplasty have identified anatomy as a predictive factor of the mitral valve area after the procedure. It was initially thought to be the main predictor of results, but it later appeared to be only a relative predictor. In fact, prediction of results is multi-factorial.[7,20,21] Several studies have shown that, in addition to morphologic factors, preoperative variables such as age, history of surgical commissurotomy, functional class, small mitral valve area, presence of mitral regurgitation before valvuloplasty, sinus rhythm, pulmonary artery pressure, and presence of severe tricuspid regurgitation, as well as procedural factors such as balloon size, are all independent predictors of the immediate results.[22]

Identification of these variables linked to outcome has enabled models to be developed with a high sensitivity of prediction. Nevertheless, the specificity is low, indicating insufficient prediction of poor immediate results. This low specificity is particularly true in regard to the lack of accurate prediction of severe mitral regurgitation.

LONG-TERM RESULTS

Follow-up data up to 17 years, representing long-term results, can now be analyzed.[4,7,20–27] However, these data cover a relatively short period compared with surgical results (Table 48-4). In clinical terms, which

are the most widely used, the overall mid-term results of valvuloplasty are encouraging, with event-free survival rates ranging from 35% to 70% after 10 to 15 years, as shown in Table 48-4. Prediction of long-term results is also multi-factorial, based on clinical variables such as age, valve anatomy as assessed by echocardiography scores, factors related to the evolutionary stage of the disease (i.e., higher NYHA class before valvuloplasty), history of previous commissurotomy, severe tricuspid regurgitation, cardiomegaly, AF, high pulmonary vascular resistance, the results of the procedure in terms of final valve area and quality of commissural opening, and the presence of mitral regurgitation.[20–24] The quality of the late results is generally considered to be independent of the technique used.[9] Identification of these predictors provides important information for patient selection and is relevant to follow-up: Patients who have favorable immediate results but who are at high risk for further events must be carefully monitored to detect deterioration and institute timely intervention. Awareness of these predictors explains the discrepancies in follow-up results from reports that included patients with different characteristics; late results are clearly less satisfactory in North American and European series, in which patients are older and frequently have severe valve deformities, compared with studies from developing countries, in which the patients studied have more favorable characteristics. Interpretation of the results must also take into account the inclusion of patients with poor immediate results in several series. If PMC is initially successful, survival rates are excellent, the need for secondary surgery is infrequent, and functional improvement occurs in most cases. Ultrasound techniques are ideally suited for serially assessing the results of the procedure, whereas serial hemodynamic data are more difficult to obtain and less satisfactory because of overestimation of the valve area immediately after the procedure. With two-dimensional echocardiography or the Doppler technique, the improvement in valve function is stable in most cases (Fig. 48-7). Determining the incidence of re-stenosis is compromised by lack of a uniform definition. Re-stenosis after PMC has generally been defined as a loss of more than 50% of the initial gain, with a valve area less than 1.5 cm². After successful PMC, the incidence of re-stenosis is usually low, between 2% and 40%, at time intervals ranging from 3 to 10 years.[7,20,21,23–28] Age, mitral valve area after PMC, and anatomy are considered to be predictors of re-stenosis, but the small number of series reporting patients with re-stenosis and the limited duration of follow-up preclude any definite conclusion in this regard. The ability to perform repeat valvuloplasty in cases of recurrent mitral stenosis is one of the potentials of this nonsurgical procedure. Repeat valvuloplasty can be proposed if recurrent stenosis leads to symptoms, if it occurs several years after an initially successful procedure, and if the predominant mechanism of re-stenosis is commissural refusion. Currently, despite the fact that repeat PMC represents 10% to 30% of the total number of balloon commissurotomies, only a few series are available on revalvuloplasty; they report positive immediate and mid-term outcomes in patients with favorable characteristics. In our personal experience of 53 patients with favorable presenting characteristics who underwent repeat PMC, the 5-year rates of continuing positive functional results were 69%

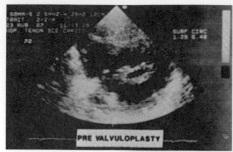
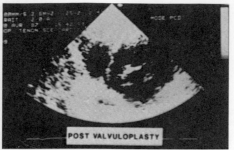
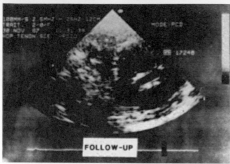

Figure 48-7 Trans-thoracic echocardiography (parasternal short-axis view) showing stable improvement in valve area after percutaneous mitral commissurotomy with a persistent bicommissural opening on follow-up.

for the total population and 76% after a successful procedure.[29-31] Although the results are less favorable in patients presenting with worse characteristics, repeat valvuloplasty has a palliative role in patients who are at high risk for surgery.[31] These preliminary results are encouraging, but definition of the exact role of re-valvuloplasty must await larger series with longer follow-up periods.

If the immediate results are unsatisfactory, mid-term functional results are usually poor. The prognosis of patients with severe mitral regurgitation after surgical commissurotomy or PMC is usually poor, with a lack of symptom alleviation and secondary objective deterioration. Surgical treatment is usually necessary in the following months.[17,18] In cases of an insufficient initial opening, delayed surgery is usually performed when extracardiac conditions allow it. Here, valve replacement is necessary in almost all cases because of the unfavorable valve anatomy that was responsible for the poor initial results. Follow-up studies using sequential TEE have shown that despite numerous individual variations, the degree of mitral regurgitation, on the whole, remains stable or slightly decreases during follow-up. ASDs are likely to close later in most cases because of a reduced inter-atrial pressure gradient. The persistence of shunts is related to their magnitude (diameter of the defect ≥0.5 cm or QP [pulmonary blood flow] or QS [systemic blood flow] ratio >1.5) or to unsatisfactory relief of the valve obstruction. These defects very seldom require individual treatment. The low incidence of embolism during follow-up, the progressive decrease in intensity or disappearance of spontaneous echocardiographic contrast, and the improved left atrial function after PMC suggest a beneficial effect of the procedure on left atrial blood stasis, from which a lower risk of thromboembolism may be expected.[32] There is no direct evidence that PMC reduces the incidence of AF, even though it has a favorable influence on the predictors of AF (e.g., atrial size, degree of obstruction).[33] It is recommended that electric countershock cardioversion be performed early after successful PMC if the AF is of recent onset and in the absence of severe enlargement of the left atrium.

Finally, several studies have compared surgical commissurotomy with PMC, mostly in patients with favorable characteristics.[34] They have shown that valvuloplasty is at least comparable with surgical commissurotomy with regard to short-term and mid-term follow-up up to 7 years. There is no randomized comparison between percutaneous commissurotomy and surgical commissurotomy in patients with less favorable anatomy, and the results of observational series are somewhat contradictory.[35,36]

Particular Applications of Percutaneous Mitral Commissurotomy

PERCUTANEOUS MITRAL COMMISSUROTOMY AFTER SURGICAL COMMISSUROTOMY

Several series have reported the results of PMC in patients with previous surgical commissurotomy.[37,38] This category of patients is of interest because in Western countries recurrent mitral stenosis is becoming more frequent than primary mitral stenosis. Reoperation in this context is associated with a higher risk of morbidity and mortality and requires valve replacement in most cases. All of the series reported to date show that PMC is feasible in this setting, although the procedure may be technically difficult in the case of "funnel-shaped" stenosis, which is frequent in these circumstances. PMC significantly improves valve function. The risks appear to be low, on a par with those of initial procedures. Mid-term results are also satisfactory. As illustrated in our series of 232 patients who underwent PMC a mean of 16 years after surgical commissurotomy, the 8-year survival rate without intervention and without symptoms was 48% for the total series and 58% after positive initial results.[37] On the whole, the results are favorable, even if slightly less satisfactory than those obtained in patients without previous commissurotomy; this probably can be attributed to less favorable characteristics observed in patients previously subjected to operation. These encouraging preliminary data suggest that PMC may well postpone reoperation in selected patients with re-stenosis after commissurotomy. The indications for PMC in this subgroup of patients are similar to those for "primary PMC," but echocardiographic examination must be conducted with great care to exclude any patients in whom re-stenosis is mainly caused by valve rigidity without significant commissural refusion. The latter mechanism should not be overlooked in the rare cases of mitral stenosis that develop in patients who have undergone mitral ring annuloplasty for correction of mitral regurgitation. In such cases, PMC can be proposed to postpone surgery, which will always be valve replacement in patients with rheumatic disease, especially if acute rheumatic fever attacks occurred after the initial PMC.

PERCUTANEOUS MITRAL COMMISSUROTOMY IN PATIENTS WITH HIGH SURGICAL RISK

Valvuloplasty is the only solution when surgery is contraindicated. It is also preferable to surgery, at least as the first attempt, in patients for whom surgery, especially cardiac surgery, poses a high risk, as in the following situations: Preliminary reports have suggested that valvuloplasty can be performed safely and effectively in patients with severe pulmonary hypertension.[39] These results are encouraging, even though they concern a limited number of patients. In such cases, even if the valve opening is suboptimal, it may allow the decrease of pulmonary pressures and thus the operative risk. In Western countries, many patients with mitral stenosis have concomitant noncardiac diseases, which may also increase the risks in surgery. Valvuloplasty can be performed as a life-saving procedure in critically ill patients, as the sole treatment when there is an absolute contraindication to surgery, or as a "bridge" to surgery in other cases.[40] In this context, dramatic improvement has been observed in young patients; conversely, the outcome is very bad in older patients presenting with "end-stage" disease, who would probably be better treated conservatively. In older patients, valvuloplasty results in a moderate but significant improvement in valve function at an acceptable risk, although subsequent functional deterioration is frequent.[28] Therefore, when surgery is high risk or even contraindicated but life expectancy is still acceptable, PMC, even if only palliative, is a useful option. In patients who still have favorable anatomy, PMC can be attempted first, and surgery resorted to if the results are unsatisfactory. In other patients, surgery is preferable as the first option. During pregnancy, surgery carries a substantial risk of fetal mortality and morbidity, especially if extracorporeal circulation is required. The experience of PMC during pregnancy reported in the literature is still limited, as represented by several hundreds of cases.[41,42] However, the following points are suggested by these data. From a technical point of view, during the last weeks of pregnancy (which was the time of PMC in most cases), the procedure may be challenging and should be performed only by experienced operators. The Inoue technique seems to be a particularly attractive option in this setting because fluoroscopy time is reduced and the short inflation-deflation cycle probably decreases hemodynamic compromise. The procedure is effective and allows for normal delivery in most cases. With regard to radiation exposure, PMC is safe for the fetus, provided that protection is provided by a shield that completely surrounds the patient's abdomen and the procedure is performed after the twentieth week. In addition to radiation, PMC carries the potential risk of related hypotension and the ever-present risk of complications that require urgent surgery. These data suggest that PMC can be a useful technique in the treatment of pregnant patients with mitral stenosis and refractory heart failure despite medical treatment.

PERCUTANEOUS MITRAL COMMISSUROTOMY AND LEFT ATRIAL THROMBOSIS

Left atrial thrombosis is generally considered a contraindication to PMC.[43,44] However, a few limited series have shown that PMC using the Inoue balloon is feasible and is not a cause of systemic embolization.[45] In cases of left atrial thrombosis, the clinical condition of the patient may require urgent treatment; the limited number of patients in these series, however, makes it difficult to recommend PMC if the patient is a candidate for surgery. This recommendation is self-evident if the thrombus is a free-floating one or is situated in the left atrial cavity; it also applies when the thrombus is located on the IAS. If the thrombus is located in the LAA, it has not been shown satisfactorily that the Inoue technique under TEE guidance precludes any risk of embolism. If the patient is clinically stable, as in the case of most patients with mitral stenosis, anticoagulant therapy can be given for 2 to 6 months; then, if a new trans-esophageal examination shows that the thrombus has disappeared, PMC can be attempted.[46]

Selection of Patients

The application of PMC depends on four major factors: (1) the patient's clinical condition; (2) the valve anatomy; (3) the experience of the medical and surgical teams of the institution concerned; and (4) the financial aspect.

EVALUATION OF THE PATIENT'S CLINICAL CONDITION

Evaluation of the patient must take into account the degree of functional disability, the presence of contraindications to trans-septal catheterization, and the risks involved in surgery as a function of the underlying cardiac and noncardiac status. Because of the small but definite risk inherent in the technique, truly asymptomatic patients with severe mitral stenosis (i.e., patients with normal physical working capacity on exercise testing) are not usually candidates for PMC, except in cases of urgent need for extracardiac surgery, to allow continuation of pregnancy in young women, or in patients with an increased risk of embolism, such as those with a previous history of embolism, heavy spontaneous contrast in the left atrium, or recurrent atrial arrhythmias. Finally, PMC can be proposed in patients who are declared to be asymptomatic but who have pulmonary hypertension either at rest (systolic pulmonary pressure >50 mm Hg) or on exercise (>60 mm Hg), the thresholds of which should be refined by the increasing experience gained in exercise echocardiography.[44,45] Under these conditions, PMC should be performed only by experienced interventionalists when the anatomy is suitable, leading to a safe, effective procedure. Contraindications to trans-septal catheterization include suspected left atrial thrombosis (see Video 48-6 📹), severe hemorrhagic disorder, and severe cardiothoracic deformity. Increased surgical risks related to cardiac factors (previous surgical commissurotomy or aortic valve replacement) or extracardiac factors (respiratory insufficiency, old age) make balloon valvuloplasty preferable to surgery, at least as the first attempt, or even as the only solution in case of a strict contraindication to surgery. The coexistence of moderate aortic valve disease and severe mitral stenosis is another situation in which PMC is preferable so that the inevitable later surgical treatment of both valves can be postponed.

VALVE ANATOMY

The assessment of anatomy has several aims when establishing indications and prognostic considerations. It is critical to ensure that there are no anatomic contraindications to the technique (Table 48-5). The first of these is the presence of left atrial thrombosis, which must be excluded by systematic performance of TEE a few days before the procedure. The second is more-than-mild mitral regurgitation. PMC can, however, be carried out in selected patients with mitral regurgitation of 2 or more if the risks related to surgery are high, such as in pregnant patients. Third, in cases of combined mitral stenosis and severe aortic disease, the indication for surgery is obvious in the

TABLE 48-5	Anatomic Classification of the Mitral Valve (Bichat Hospital, Paris)
Echocardiographic Group	**Mitral Valve Anatomy**
1	Pliable noncalcified anterior mitral leaflet and mild subvalvular disease (i.e., thin chordae ≥10 mm long)
2	Pliable noncalcified anterior mitral leaflet and severe subvalvular disease (i.e., thickened chordae <10 mm long)
3	Calcification of mitral valve of any extent, as assessed by fluoroscopy, whatever the state of subvalvular apparatus

Adapted from Iung B, Cormier B, Ducimetiere P, et al: Immediate results of percutaneous mitral commissurotomy, *Circulation* 94:2124–2130, 1996.

TABLE 48-6	**Contraindications to Mitral Valvuloplasty**

- Left atrial thrombosis
- Mitral regurgitation greater than ¼
- Massive or bicommissural calcification
- Severe aortic valve disease, or severe tricuspid stenosis plus regurgitation, associated with mitral stenosis
- Severe concomitant coronary artery disease requiring bypass surgery

TABLE 48-7	**Anatomic Classification of the Mitral Valve (Massachusetts General Hospital, Boston)**

Leaflet Mobility (1 to 4)
1. Highly mobile valve with restriction of only the leaflet tips
2. Mid-portion and base of leaflets have reduced mobility
3. Valve leaflets move forward during diastole, mainly at the base
4. No or minimal forward movement of the leaflets during diastole

Valvular Thickening (1 to 4)
1. Leaflets near normal (4–5 mm)
2. Mid-leaflet thickening, marked thickening of the margins
3. Thickening extends through the entire leaflets (5–8 mm)
4. Marked thickening of all leaflet tissue (>8–10 mm)

Subvalvular Thickening (1 to 4)
1. Minimal thickening of chordal structures just below the valve
2. Thickening of chordae extending up to one third of chordal length
3. Thickening extending to the distal third of the chordae
4. Extensive thickening and shortening of all chordae extending down to the papillary muscle

Valvular Calcification (1 to 4)
1. Single area of increased echocardiographic brightness
2. Scattered areas of brightness confined to leaflet margins
3. Brightness extending into the mid-portion of leaflets
4. Extensive brightness through most of the leaflet tissue

The total score is calculated by adding each of its components. A total score <8 is considered favorable anatomy.

Adapted from Abascal V, Wilkins GT, O'Shea JP, et al: Prediction of successful outcome in 130 patients undergoing percutaneous balloon mitral valvotomy, *Circulation* 82:448–456, 1990.

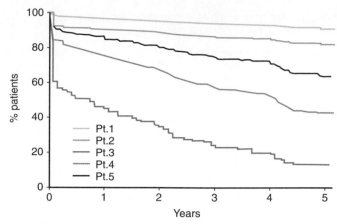

Figure 48-8 Predicted probability of positive immediate results (valve area ≥1.5 cm² without regurgitation, Sellers' grade >2) and positive late functional results (survival with no intervention and in New York Heart Association [NYHA] class I or II) according to patient characteristics. Values are given for a procedure using an Inoue balloon with an effective balloon dilating area of 5.5 cm² or more (i.e., final diameter ≥27 mm). *Pt. 1:* Age <50 years, NYHA class II, sinus rhythm, calcium grade 1, valve area 1.25–1.50 cm². *Pt. 2:* Age <50 years, class II, sinus rhythm, grade 2, area 1.00–1.25 cm². *Pt. 3:* Age 50–70 years, class III, sinus rhythm, grade 2, area 1.25–1.50 cm². *Pt. 4:* Age 50–70 years, class III, atrial fibrillation, grade 2, area 1.25–1.50 cm². *Pt. 5:* Age ≥70 years, class III, atrial fibrillation, grade 3, area 0.75–1.00 cm². *(From Iung B, Garbarz E, Doutrelant L, et al: Late results of percutaneous mitral commissurotomy for calcific mitral stenosis, Am J Cardiol 85:1308–1314, 2000.)*

absence of contraindications. Fourth, the presence of combined severe tricuspid stenosis and tricuspid regurgitation with clinical signs of heart failure is an indication for surgery on both valves. Conversely, the existence of tricuspid regurgitation is not, in itself, a contraindication to the procedure, even though it represents a negative prognostic factor, especially when it is associated with severe enlargement of the right atrium and AF.[47] The definition of a threshold of valve area above which PMC should not be performed is somewhat arbitrary. Besides measuring the valve area and the mean gradient, one must also take into account the stature of the patient, his or her functional disability, and pulmonary pressures at rest and on exercise in case of doubt. Our view on the performance of PMC in patients with mitral valve area greater than 1.5 cm² is that the risks probably outweigh the benefits, and these patients are usually well managed by medical treatment.[43,44] For prognostic considerations, echocardiographic assessment allows the classification of patients into anatomic groups with a view to predicting the results. Most investigators use the Wilkins score (Table 48-6), in which a total score under 8 is considered to represent favorable anatomy for PMC.[7] Others use a more general assessment of valve anatomy (Table 48-7) based on the potential surgical alternatives: grade 1 being ideal anatomy for PMC, or grade 2 being intermediate anatomy that could have been treated by commissurotomy or valve replacement, and grade 3 being unfavorable anatomy for which the only option is valve replacement.[3] Controversy exists regarding the most effective echocardiography scoring system in the prediction of

results of mitral valvuloplasty. In fact, none of the scores available today has been shown to be superior to the others, and all echocardiographic classifications have the same limitations: (1) Reproducibility is difficult because the scores are only semi-quantitative; (2) lesions may be underestimated, especially with regard to the assessment of subvalvular disease; and (3) the use of scores describing the degree of overall valve deformity may not identify localized changes in specific portions of the valve apparatus (leaflets, and especially commissures), which may increase the risk of severe mitral regurgitation. Therefore, we can only recommend the use of the system with which one is most familiar and at ease. More recently, scores that take into account the uneven distribution of the anatomic deformities of the leaflets or the commissural area have been developed; their preliminary results are promising but disputed, so further studies are needed to determine their exact value.

EXPERIENCE OF THE MEDICAL AND SURGICAL TEAMS

The importance of training for PMC is demonstrated by the comparison of early and late experiences within the same groups or by comparison of reports from large-volume centers, including centers with variable experience, and multi-center studies. The incidence of technical failures and complications, particularly those related to trans-septal catheterization, is clearly related to the operator's experience.[3] Even though the considerable simplification of the technique with the use of the Inoue balloon may lead to a false sense of security, PMC clearly should be restricted to teams that have extensive experience with trans-septal catheterization and are able to perform an adequate number of procedures. The interventionalists who perform PMC must also be able to perform emergency pericardiocentesis. The exact arrangement for surgical backup varies from institution to institution, according to the severity of the condition being treated, and the experience of the cardiologic and surgical teams. Because of the low prevalence of mitral stenosis in developed countries, ongoing experience will be difficult to keep up. It seems appropriate to concentrate the performance of the procedure in experienced centers so that the management of the interventional procedure is made more effective by improving the selection of patients through clinical evaluation and echocardiographic assessment and by decreasing risks.

POTENTIAL INDICATIONS

The selection of an individual candidate for PMC must be based on both clinical and anatomic variables, bearing in mind that anatomy is a simple, practical way to select patients for PMC, even though it should not be the sole criterion. The indication for PMC is clear in when surgery is contraindicated and in "ideal candidates" such as young adults with good anatomy: pliable valves and only moderate subvalvular disease (echocardiography score <8 [see Table 48-6]).[48] Randomized studies comparing valvuloplasty with surgical commissurotomy showed that valvuloplasty is at least comparable with surgical commissurotomy in terms of efficacy and is, no doubt, more comfortable for the patient. In practice, in Europe, PMC has virtually replaced surgical commissurotomy.[49] Hence, PMC appears to be the procedure of choice for patients with favorable anatomy, provided that it is affordable. In addition, if re-stenosis occurs, patients treated with valvuloplasty can undergo repeat balloon catheterization or surgery without the difficulties and inherent risks resulting from pericardial adhesions and chest wall scarring. Much remains to be done to

refine the indications for other patients, especially those with unfavorable anatomy, who are more common in Western countries. For this group, some advocate immediate surgery because of the less satisfying results of valvuloplasty, whereas others prefer valvuloplasty as an initial treatment for selected candidates, reserving surgery for cases of failure or late deterioration.[49] Unfortunately, data from randomized studies on these patients are not available, and a comparison of the results of balloon commissurotomy with those of surgical series is difficult because of differences in the patients involved and because the surgical alternative is valve replacement in most cases (since open commissurotomy is now seldom performed). Valve replacement has its drawbacks: (1) operative mortality, particularly in older adults; and (2) prosthesis-related complications, which have a cumulative incidence that compromises the late outcome, particularly in young patients who are most susceptible to the risk of long-term deterioration. The indications in this subgroup must take into account its heterogeneity with respect to anatomy, especially the extent and location of calcification. Clinical status is even more vital because this group includes patients in good clinical condition as well as others who are not surgical candidates because of comorbidities. In this group of patients, we favor an individualistic approach that allows for the multi-factorial nature of prediction. It is not possible to exclude the possibility of positive results in poor candidates; consequently, we are led to propose wider indications for valvuloplasty as an initial treatment in selected patients.

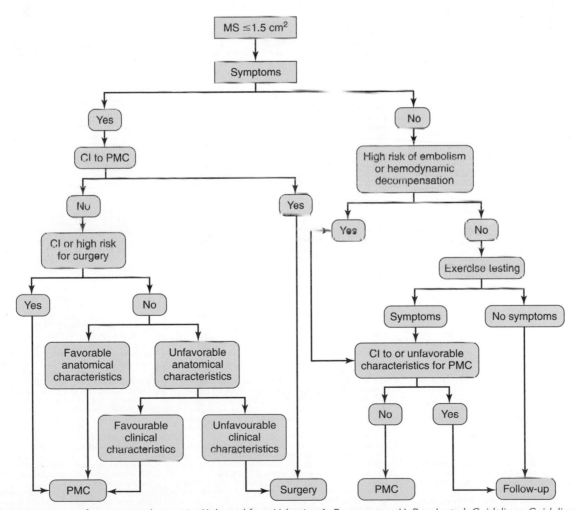

Figure 48-9 Management of severe mitral stenosis. (*Adapted from Vahanian A, Baumgartner H, Bax J, et al: Guidelines: Guidelines on the management of valvular heart disease: The Task Force on the Management of Valvular Heart Disease of the European Society of Cardiology, Eur Heart J 28:230–268, 2007.*)

As an illustration of what can be obtained by PMC in this setting, we analyzed the outcome of 432 patients who underwent PMC for mitral stenosis with mild to moderate calcification. At 8 years, the rate of continuing favorable functional results was 36%. The predictors were young age, low NYHA class, and sinus rhythm. With other presenting characteristics, the 5-year rate of favorable functional results varied from 15% to 90% (Fig. 48-8).[50] Current opinion is that surgery can be considered the treatment of choice in patients with bicommissural or heavy calcification. Conversely, in our opinion, balloon valvuloplasty can be attempted as a first approach in patients with extensive lesions of the subvalvular apparatus or moderate or unicommissural calcification, the more so because their clinical status argues in favor of it. Surgery should be considered reasonably early if the results are unsatisfactory or if there is secondary deterioration. The option of PMC for patients who are candidates for surgical commissurotomy depends on the results previously obtained by surgery and PMC in the given institution. In our experience, candidates for PMC have become older and have less favorable anatomy; however, they undergo the procedure at an earlier functional stage. The stability of the results, despite the less favorable characteristics, may be related to the role of experience in improving the technique and patient selection (Fig. 48-9).[3]

Future Prospects

Large-scale use of the technique would be beneficial in developing countries, where mitral stenosis occurs frequently in patients with anatomy favorable for PMC. However, this fundamentally depends on the solution of logistic and economic problems. In developed countries, the problems are different because most candidates are older, with somewhat less favorable anatomy. Careful evaluation of immediate and long-term results in this population is still needed to clearly define the respective indications for PMC and valve replacement. This process will be improved through better imaging, especially three-dimensional echocardiography. Further improvement may be achieved through combining PMC with other interventional procedures such as closure of the LAA, ablation of the pulmonary veins, or, perhaps in a more distant future, percutaneous mitral valve replacement in case of failure or deterioration after PMC. The positive results that have been obtained with PMC enable us to say that, currently, this technique has an important place in the treatment of mitral stenosis and has virtually replaced surgical commissurotomy. Finally, in our opinion, when treating mitral stenosis, PMC and valve replacement must be considered complementary, not opposing, techniques, each applicable at the appropriate stage of the disease.

REFERENCES

1. Inoue K, Owaki T, Nakamura T, et al: Clinical application of transvenous mitral commissurotomy by a new balloon catheter. *J Thorac Cardiovasc Surg* 87:394–402, 1984.
2. Marijon E, Iung B, Mocumbi AO, et al: What are the differences in presentation of candidates for percutaneous mitral commissurotomy across the world and do they influence the results of the procedure? *Arch Cardiovasc Dis* 10:611–617, 2008.
3. Iung B, Nicoud-Houel A, Fondard O, et al: Temporal trends in percutaneous mitral commissurotomy over a 15-year period. *Eur Heart J* 25:701–707, 2004.
4. Stefanadis C, Stratos C, Lambrou S, et al: Retrograde nontransseptal balloon mitral valvuloplasty: Immediate results and intermediate long-term outcome in 441 cases. A multi-center experience. *J Am Coll Cardiol* 32:1009–1016, 1998.
5. Perk G, Lang RM, Garcia-Fernandez MA, et al: Use of real time three dimensional transesophageal echocardiography in intracardiac catheter based interventions. *J Am Soc Echocardiogr* 22:865–882, 2009.
6. Silvestry FE, Kerber RE, Brook MM, et al: Echocardiography-guided interventions. *J Am Soc Echocardiogr* 22:213–231, 2009.
7. Palacios IF, Sanchez PL, Harrell LC, et al: Which patients benefit from percutaneous mitral balloon valvuloplasty? Prevalvuloplasty and postvalvuloplasty variables that predict long-term outcome. *Circulation* 105:1465–1471, 2002.
8. Bonhoeffer P, Hausse A, Yonga G, et al: Technique and results of percutaneous mitral valvuloplasty with the multi-track system. *J Interv Cardiol* 13:263–269, 2000.
9. Kang DH, Park SW, Song JK, et al: Long-term clinical and echocardiographic outcome of percutaneous mitral valvuloplasty: Randomized comparison of Inoue and double-balloon techniques. *J Am Coll Cardiol* 35:169–175, 2000.
10. Cribier A, Eltchaninoff H, Carlot R: Percutaneous mechanical mitral commissurotomy with the metallic valvotome: Detailed technical aspect and overview of the results of the multi-center registry 882 patients. *J Interv Cardiol* 13:255–256, 2000.
11. Messika–Zeitoun D, Brochet E, Holmin C, et al: Three-dimensional evaluation of the mitral valve area and commissural opening before and after percutaneous mitral commissurotomy in patients with mitral stenosis. *Eur Heart J* 28:72–79, 2007.
12. Ben Farhat M, Betbout F, Gamra H, et al: Predictors of long-term event-free survival and of freedom from restenosis after percutaneous balloon mitral commissurotomy. *Am Heart J* 142:1072–1079, 2001.
13. Arora R, Kalra GS, Sing S, et al: Percutaneous transvenous mitral commissurotomy: immediate and long-term follow-up results. *Catheter Cardiovasc Interv* 55:450–456, 2002.
14. Chen CR, Cheng TO: Percutaneous balloon mitral valvuloplasty by the Inoue technique: A multicenter study of 4832 patients in China. *Am Heart J* 129:1197–1202, 1995.
15. Varma PK, Theodore S, Neema PK, et al: Emergency surgery after percutaneous transmitral commissurotomy: Operative versus echocardiographic findings, mechanisms of complications, and outcomes. *J Thorac Cardiovasc Surg* 130:772–776, 2005.
16. Zimet AD, Almeida AA, Harper RW, et al: Predictors of surgery after percutaneous mitral valvuloplasty. *Ann Thorac Surg* 82:828–833, 2006.
17. Jneid H, Cruz-Gonzalez I, Sanchez-Ledesma M, et al: Impact of pre- and postprocedural mitral regurgitation on outcomes after percutaneous mitral valvuloplasty for mitral stenosis. *Am J Cardiol* 104:1122–1127, 2009.
18. Kim M-J, Song J-K, Song J-M, et al: Long-term outcomes of significant mitral regurgitation after percutaneous mitral valvuloplasty. *Circulation* 114:2815–2822, 2006.
19. Cequier A, Bonan R, Dyrda I, et al: Atrial shunting after percutaneous mitral valvuloplasty. *Circulation* 81:1190–1197, 1990.
20. Iung B, Garbarz E, Michaud P, et al: Late results of percutaneous mitral commissurotomy in a series of 1024 patients: Analysis of late clinical deterioration—Frequency, anatomic findings, and predictive factors. *Circulation* 99:3272–3278, 1999.
21. Cruz-Gonzalez I, Sanchez-Ledesma M, Martin-Moreiras J, et al: Predicting success and long-term outcomes of percutaneous mitral valvuloplasty: A multifactorial score. *Am J Med* 122:581.e9–581.e11, 2009.
22. Ramondo A, Napodano M, Fraccaro C, et al: Relation of patient age to outcome of percutaneous mitral valvuloplasty. *Am J Cardiol* 98(11):1493–1500, 2006.
23. Song J-K, Song J-M, Kang D-H, et al: Restenosis and adverse clinical events after successful percutaneous mitral valvuloplasty: Immediate post-procedural mitral valve area as an important prognosticator. *Eur Heart J* 30:1254–1262, 2009.
24. Messika-Zeitoun D, Blanc J, Iung B, et al: Impact of degree of commissural opening after percutaneous mitral commissurotomy on long-term outcome. *JACC Cardiovasc Imag* 2:1–7, 2009.
25. Wang A, Krasuski RA, Warner JJ, et al: Serial echocardiographic evaluation of restenosis after successful percutaneous mitral commissurotomy. *J Am Coll Cardiol* 39:328–334, 2002.
26. Hernandez R, Bañuelos C, Alfonso F, et al: Long-term clinical and echocardiographic follow-up after percutaneous mitral valvuloplasty with the Inoue balloon. *Circulation* 99:1580–1586, 1999.
27. Fawzy ME, Shoukri M, Al Buraiki J, et al: Seventeen years clinical and echocardiographic follow up of mitral balloon valvuloplasty in 520 patients, and predictors of long-term outcome. *J Heart Valve Dis* 16:454–460, 2007.
28. Hildick-Smith DJR, Taylor GJ, Shapiro LN: Inoue balloon mitral valvuloplasty: Long-term clinical and echocardiographic follow-up of a predominantly unfavorable population. *Eur Heart J* 21:1691–1698, 2000.
29. Iung B, Garbarz E, Michaud P, et al: Immediate and mid-term results of repeat percutaneous mitral commissurotomy for restenosis following earlier percutaneous mitral commissurotomy. *Eur Heart J* 21:1683–1690, 2000.
30. Turgeman Y, Atar S, Suleiman K, et al: Feasibility, safety, and morphologic predictors of outcome of repeat percutaneous balloon mitral commissurotomy. *Am J Cardiol* 95:989–991, 2005.
31. Kim JB, Ha JW, Kim JS, et al: Comparison of long-term outcome after mitral valve replacement or repeated balloon mitral valvotomy in patients with restenosis after previous balloon valvotomy. Does atrial fibrillation persist? *Europace* 5:47–53, 2003.
32. Chiang C-W, Lo S-K, Ko Y-S, et al: Predictors of systemic embolism in patients with mitral stenosis: A prospective study. *Ann Intern Med* 128:885–889, 1998.
33. Krasuski RA, Assar MD, Wang A, et al: Usefulness of percutaneous balloon mitral commissurotomy in preventing the development of atrial fibrillation in patients with mitral stenosis. *Am J Cardiol* 93:936–939, 2004.
34. Ben Fahrat M, Ayari M, Maatouk F: Percutaneous balloon versus surgical closed and open mitral commissurotomy: Seven-year follow-up results of a randomized trial. *Circulation* 97:245–250, 1998.
35. Cardoso LF, Grinberg M, Pomerantzeff PM, et al: Comparison of open commissurotomy and balloon valvuloplasty in mitral stenosis: A five-year follow-up. *Arq Bras Cardiol* 83:248–252, 2004.
36. Song JK, Kim MJ, Yun SC, et al: Long-term outcomes of percutaneous mitral balloon valvuloplasty versus open cardiac surgery. *J Thorac Cardiovasc Surg* 139:103–110, 2010.
37. Iung B, Garbarz E, Michaud P: Percutaneous mitral commissurotomy for restenosis after surgical commissurotomy. *J Am Coll Cardiol* 35:1295–1302, 2000.
38. Fawzy ME, Hassan W, Shoukri M, et al: Immediate and long-term results of mitral balloon valvotomy for restenosis following previous surgical or balloon mitral commissurotomy. *Am J Cardiol* 96:971–975, 2005.
39. Maoqin S, Guoxiang H, Zhiyuan S, et al: The clinical and hemodynamic results of mitral balloon valvuloplasty for patients with mitral stenosis complicated by severe pulmonary hypertension. *Eur J Intern Med* 16:413–418, 2005.
40. Vahanian A, Ducrocq G: Emergencies in valve disease. *Curr Opin Crit Care* 14:555–560, 2008.
41. Sivadasanpillai H, Srinivasan A, Sivasubramoniam S, et al: Long-term outcome of patients undergoing balloon mitral valvotomy in pregnancy. *Am J Cardiol* 95:1504–1506, 2005.
42. Esteves C, Munoz J, Braga S, et al: Immediate and long-term follow-up of percutaneous balloon mitral valvuloplasty in pregnant patients with rheumatic mitral stenosis. *Am J Cardiol* 98:812–816, 2006.
43. Bonow RO, Carabello BA, Chatterjee K, et al: ACC/AHA 2006 guidelines for the management of patients with valvular heart disease: A report of the American College of Cardiology/American Heart Association Task Force on Practice Guidelines. *J Am Coll Cardiol* 48:e1–e148, 2006.
44. Vahanian A, Baumgartner H, Bax J, et al: Guidelines: Guidelines on the management of valvular heart disease: The Task Force on the Management of Valvular Heart Disease of the European Society of Cardiology. *Eur Heart J* 28:230–268, 2007.
45. Shaw TRD, Northridge DB, Sutaria N: Mitral balloon valvotomy and left atrial thrombus. *Heart* 91:1088–1089, 2005.
46. Silaruks S, Thinkhamrop B, Kiatchoosakun S, et al: Resolution of left atrial thrombus after 6 months of anticoagulation in candidates for percutaneous transvenous mitral commissurotomy. *Ann Intern Med* 140:101–105, 2004.
47. Song H, Kang DH, Kim JH, et al: Percutaneous mitral valvuloplasty versus surgical treatment in mitral stenosis with severe tricuspid regurgitation. *Circulation* 116(Suppl):I246–1250, 2007.
48. Gamra H, Betbout F, Ben Hamda K, et al: Balloon mitral commissurotomy in juvenile rheumatic mitral stenosis: A ten-year clinical and echocardiographic actuarial results. *Eur Heart J* 24:1349–1356, 2003.
49. Iung B, Baron G, Butchart EG, et al: A prospective survey of patients with valvular heart disease in Europe: The Euro Heart Survey on valvular heart disease. *Eur Heart J* 13:1231–1243, 2003.
50. Iung B, Garbarz E, Doutrelant L, et al: Late results of percutaneous mitral commissurotomy for calcific mitral stenosis. *Am J Cardiol* 85:1308–1314, 2000.

49

Percutaneous Mitral Valve Repair

AMAR KRISHNASWAMY | SAMIR R. KAPADIA

KEY POINTS

- Mitral regurgitation (MR) is a significant problem, and the number of patients with MR is growing with an increase in the number of patients with congestive heart failure (CHF). Surgical correction of MR with repair techniques yields better results than valve replacement; however, a significant number of patients undergo valve replacement even in the current era.

- Various percutaneous approaches to mitral valve repair are under preclinical and clinical investigation and show great promise for the future. These approaches are predominantly based on established surgical strategies.

- Different percutaneous techniques provide specific advantages, depending on the anatomic and functional characteristics of MR. Selection of the appropriate technique or techniques for each patient will ultimately determine the success of these emerging technologies.

- Integration of established imaging modalities both in and out of the catheterization laboratory (cath lab) is critical for the safety and efficacy of percutaneous repair technologies. The development of emerging imaging modalities will likely play a role in the future of percutaneous technologies.

- Evaluation of new percutaneous devices poses a significant challenge because these devices have to be compared with surgical options that may have different criteria in the overall management of the patient. It is likely that percutaneous techniques will play a complementary role to surgery.

Introduction

Chronic MR poses a significant public health burden, with more than three million people in the United States alone suffering from moderate or severe MR.[1] Left untreated, chronic MR results in heart failure symptoms, left ventricular cavity dilation and systolic dysfunction, left atrial enlargement, atrial fibrillation (AF), and pulmonary hypertension. Medical therapy may provide some relief from symptoms and is necessary to treat ischemic heart disease and heart failure in patients with MR and these underlying disease states. However, there has been no proven benefit to these treatments with regard to MR itself.[2] Therefore, surgical correction with mitral valve repair (MVRe) or replacement (MVR) remains the mainstay of therapy for chronic MR. However, because of the invasive nature of open-heart surgery (OHS) and the frequent presence of comorbidities in this group, up to 50% of patients with severe MR may not be offered surgery.[3] This is especially true for older patients and those with impaired left ventricular function. As a result, percutaneous technology is poised to significantly alter the treatment paradigm for chronic MR. Percutaneous MVRe offers the potential benefit of decreased morbidity, improved recovery time, and shorter hospital stays compared with OHS. Current percutaneous options are loosely based on surgical repair techniques, with four primary methods to accomplish a reduction in MR: (1) edge-to-edge leaflet repair, (2) indirect coronary sinus annuloplasty, (3) direct annuloplasty, and (4) septal–lateral annular cinching. Percutaneous MVR is also being developed, although, at this time, it is in its infancy. Overall, the field is very exciting with promising initial studies highlighting the need for a better understanding of patient selection for appropriate management of MR.

Mitral Valve Disease

MITRAL VALVE ANATOMY

The mitral valve complex is composed of the mitral annulus, anterior and posterior leaflets, chordae tendineae, and papillary muscles.[4] The mitral annulus is the elliptical area of attachment of the mitral valve to the base of the left atrium (LA) (Fig. 49-1). The posterior leaflet has three lobes or "scallops": the lateral (P1), central (P2), and medial scallops (P3); the anterior leaflet segments are named A1, A2, and A3, respectively, corresponding to the posterior scallops. The anatomic position of the valve is such that the two leaflets meet at the anterolateral and posteromedial commissures. Chordae connect the leaflets to both the anterolateral and the posteromedial papillary muscles. The primary chordae connect to the free edge of the leaflet; the secondary chordae ("strut" chords) are thicker and connect to the rough zone of the leaflet; and the tertiary chordae are short and connect the basal zone of the leaflet to the ventricular free wall.

ETIOLOGY AND MECHANISM OF MITRAL REGURGITATION

Anatomic or functional abnormalities of any of the structures in the mitral valve apparatus may lead to MR.[5,6] The disease process leading to MR may be primary mitral valve disease, secondary regurgitation resulting from another cardiac disease, or mitral valve involvement in a systemic inflammatory disease (Table 49-1). Various terminologies are used to characterize the mechanisms of MR. The morphologic description, proposed by Carpentier, classifies the mechanism of regurgitation according to leaflet pathophysiology (Fig. 49-2).[7] Type I regurgitation occurs in the presence of normal leaflet motion and is usually caused by annular dilatation or leaflet perforation. Type II is caused by leaflet prolapse, which is commonly the result of degenerative (myxomatous) disease, chordal elongation or rupture, or papillary muscle elongation or rupture. Type III is caused by restricted leaflet motion, which may arise from posterior wall motion abnormality or papillary muscle dysfunction due to ischemic cardiac disease. The restricted leaflet motion may also be caused by commissural fusion, leaflet or chordal thickening from rheumatic heart disease, or both. This simplification has usefulness in terms of both the surgical approach and the percutaneous approach, as the goal of therapy is to restore normal leaflet function but not necessarily normal valve anatomy. Another common method of categorizing MR is based on the etiology and mechanism of MR. This classification is commonly used in the literature to study the clinical outcomes of patients (Table 49-2). In this classification scheme, MR is loosely categorized on the basis of an abnormal ("primary") or normal ("secondary") mitral valve as degenerative or rheumatic disease (primary MR) and functional or ischemic disease (secondary MR), respectively. Of note, the terms *functional MR*, *ischemic MR*, and *secondary MR* are often used interchangeably and may represent many different mechanisms and morphologic variants. Degenerative disease includes Barlow's disease (myxomatous degeneration) and fibroelastic deficiency, both of which can result in mitral valve leaflet prolapse and MR. Fibroelastic deficiency is the most common etiology in those presenting for surgical MVRe, representing approximately 70% of the surgical population in the United States. MR in rheumatic disease is a result of leaflet deformity caused by severe calcification and apical leaflet doming. Although this is a common cause of MR worldwide, it is less frequently

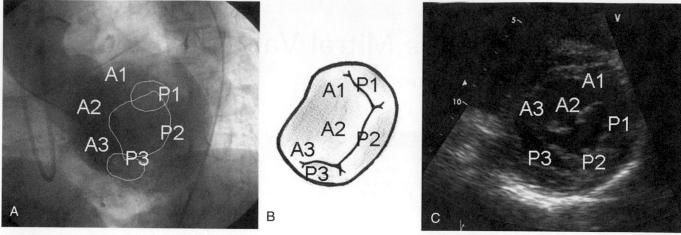

Figure 49-1 Mitral valve anatomy. **A,** Left ventriculogram in the left anterior oblique projection showing the mitral valve in short axis, with labeled leaflet segments. **B,** A schematic of the mitral valve in short axis. **C,** A trans-thoracic echocardiographic image of the mitral valve in the parasternal short-axis projection.

TABLE 49-1	Causes of Chronic Mitral Regurgitation

- Primary mitral valve disorder
  - Degenerative valve disease
  - Myxomatous degeneration
  - Fibroelastic deficiency
  - Rheumatic valve disease
  - Infective endocarditis
  - Chordal rupture
  - Idiopathic causes
  - Traumatic causes
  - Congenital lesions
  - Cleft anterior mitral leaflet or fenestration
  - Parachute mitral valve abnormality
  - Prosthetic valve disorder
  - Paravalvular regurgitation
  - Prosthetic valve degeneration
  - Prosthetic valve endocarditis
- Secondary mitral valve disorder (cardiac cause)
  - Ischemic mitral regurgitation (coronary artery disease)
  - Papillary muscle dysfunction or rupture
  - Mitral valve annular dilation
  - Global or regional ventricular dysfunction
  - Left ventricular dilation
  - Dilated (nonischemic) cardiomyopathy
  - Hypertrophic cardiomyopathy
- Systemic or inflammatory disease
  - Systemic lupus erythematosus
  - Amyloidosis
  - Connective tissue disorder
  - Rheumatoid arthritis

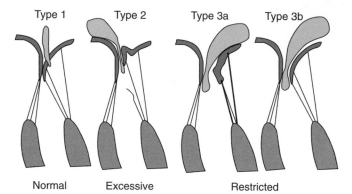

Figure 49-2 Carpentier classification of mitral regurgitation according to function leaflet mobility. Type 1 exhibits normal leaflet mobility as with endocarditis. Type 2 exhibits excessive leaflet mobility as in degenerative disease or mitral valve prolapse. Type 3a exhibits restricted leaflet motion caused by chordal and leaflet thickening from rheumatic heart disease. Type 3b exhibits restricted leaflet motion caused by ventricular wall motion abnormality from dilated or ischemic cardiomyopathy.

is involved in the generation, perpetuation, and progression of "functional" MR (Fig. 49-3).

NATURAL HISTORY

The natural history of patients with chronic MR depends on the degree of regurgitation, the cause of the underlying disorder, and the degree of left ventricular dysfunction.[13-15] Available data on the natural history of the disease are limited by small sample size, selection bias, inconsistent measures of MR severity, and the inclusion of disparate etiologies of regurgitation. However, it appears that many patients with chronic MR remain asymptomatic for many years.[16] Among patients with mild MR, there is an inconsistent rate of progression to severe MR, which appears to be independent of medical treatment.[17] When chronic severe MR is present, approximately 5% to 10% of patients per year develop significant symptoms, clinical indication for surgery, death, or all of these.[16,18] Whether there is a small risk of sudden cardiac death (SCD) in patients with severe asymptomatic MR remains controversial, and the data are not compelling enough to subject patients to intervention in the absence of other indications for MVRe.[18] The importance of symptoms on long-term prognosis is demonstrated by

encountered in the United States. Functional MR occurs in the setting of left ventricular dysfunction and is seen in patients with coronary artery disease (ischemic MR) or in patients with dilated cardiomyopathy from other causes. Ischemic MR results from decreased closing force and increased tethering force on the leaflets.[8] Various factors can lessen the closing force, including diminished left ventricular ejection fraction (LVEF), left ventricular dyssynchrony, and decreased annular contraction; similarly, many factors increase the tethering force, such as papillary muscle displacement, left ventricle (LV) remodeling, annular dilatation, and so on.[9-12] It is becoming increasingly clear that significant interaction among ventricular, valvular, and annular factors

TABLE 49-2	Mechanisms and Classification of Mitral Regurgitation

Carpentier's morphologic classification with mechanisms of MR
- Type I: Normal leaflet motion
  - Annular dilation
  - Dilated cardiomyopathy "Functional MR"*
  - Leaflet perforation
  - Annular calcification
- Type II: Leaflet prolapse
  - Chordal rupture or flail leaflet
  - Chordal elongation "degenerative MR"
  - Papillary muscle elongation
  - Papillary muscle rupture
- Type III: Restricted leaflet motion
  - IIIA: Fibrosis of the subvalvular apparatus "rheumatic MR"
  - IIIB: Regional LV remodeling or wall motion abnormality "ischemic MR"

*Functional mitral regurgitation (MR) sometimes used to describe ischemic and nonischemic MR as both share some common characteristics of left ventricular geometric remodeling and annular dilatation with normal leaflet morphology.

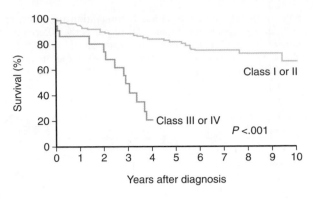

Figure 49-4 Long-term survival of patients with flail leaflet according to New York Heart Association functional class. Survival is significantly less in patients with class III or IV heart failure. (*From Ling LH, Enriquez-Sarano M, Seward JB, et al: Clinical outcome of mitral regurgitation due to flail leaflet,* N Engl Med 335:1417–1423, 1996.)

No. at risk

Class I or II	162	117	102	95	80	69	50	33	20	12	7
Class III or IV	66	15	12	7	3						

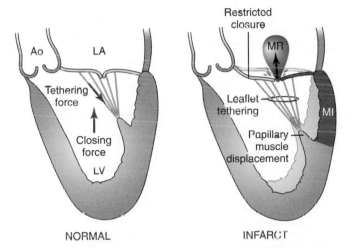

Figure 49-3 *Left,* Balance of forces acting on mitral leaflets in systole. *AO, aorta; LA, left atrium. Right,* Infarction causes LV cavity dilation and PM displacement, which together result in anular dilation, leaflet tethering, and restricted loaflet motion. Both factors contribute to functional MR. Dark shading indicates inferobasal myocardial infarction (MI); light hatching indicates normal baseline. (*Modified and used with permission from Liel-Cohen N, Guerrero JL, Otsuji Y, et al: Design of a new surgical approach for ventricular remodeling to relieve ischemic mitral regurgitation: Insights from 3-dimensional echocardiography, Circulation 101. 2756 –2763, 2000.*)

the high mortality rate reported for patients with New York Heart Association class III or IV symptoms, even in degenerative mitral valve disease (Fig. 49-4). LVEF is also an important independent predictor of outcome in patients with functional MR.[15] Patients with degenerative valve disease have a favorable long-term prognosis, whether they are treated conservatively or when indicated, surgically. However, patients with degenerative valve disease and coronary disease are fundamentally different from those with degenerative disease alone and have a worse prognosis that is dominated by the contribution of coronary disease.[14] Conversely, in the absence of degenerative disease, the presence and degree of MR after myocardial infarction (MI) is an independent predictor of mortality, emphasizing the need for accurate quantification; further studies to investigate whether treatment of MR in these patients will modify outcomes.[19,20]

IMAGING: ECHOCARDIOGRAPHY

Echocardiography is the dominant modality for imaging the mitral valve and for the assessment of MR severity. Two-dimensional

trans-thoracic echocardiography (TTE) is useful to evaluate the valvular anatomy, the structure and function of the LV, and assess the origin and degree of regurgitation. Therefore, TTE provides an understanding of MR severity as well as an insight into the primary or secondary nature of the disease. Furthermore, the anatomic assessment of the mitral valve and the LV also allows determination of whether surgical or percutaneous MVRe may be feasible or whether valve replacement will be necessary. Longitudinal data collected using serial echocardiography may be used to determine the timing of intervention and to follow up the results. If trans-thoracic images are not adequate, transesophageal echocardiography (TEE) provides an excellent assessment of mitral valve anatomy and severity of regurgitation. This can be particularly useful to determine if valve repair is feasible. Evaluating the severity of valvular regurgitation with echocardiography relies heavily on Doppler methods, including color, pulsed-wave (PW), and continuous-wave (CW) Doppler. The American Society of Echocardiography has determined the qualitative and quantitative echocardiographic parameters that are useful in grading MR (Table 49-3).[21] The assessment of severity should rely on the integration of both quantitative and qualitative measures obtained by Doppler techniques.[22] In addition, structural findings such as a flail leaflet or an enlarged left atrium (LA) can add useful information with regard to regurgitation severity. Color Doppler provides a number of qualitative and quantitative means to determine MR severity. A proximal flow convergence on color Doppler is present in severe regurgitation. The proximal isovelocity surface area (PISA) of this flow convergence can be used to accurately quantitate the effective regurgitant orifice (ERO) area.[23] The width of the regurgitant jet at or just downstream from the regurgitant orifice is known as the *vena contracta* and is slightly smaller than the anatomic regurgitant orifice.[24] This distinction is particularly relevant in some patients with functional MR, in which the regurgitant orifice has a slit-like rather than oval shape. The area of the MR jet occupying the LA can provide a rapid semi-quantitative assessment of regurgitation severity. However, this is influenced by instrument factors (such as gain) as well as jet orientation (a central jet may appear more severe than an equally large jet that adheres to the atrial wall). In addition, the color jet area is influenced by the driving pressure across the valve and can be enhanced by elevated blood pressure. Color Doppler imaging is also important in the parasternal short-axis view to determine the origin of the MR jet as percutaneous approaches (especially the MitraClip) are more effective in centrally originating jets than in medial or lateral ones. Regurgitant volume can be assessed using continuous-wave Doppler data. Regurgitant volume is calculated by applying the continuity equation (conservation of mass), in which left-sided regurgitation volume is calculated as the difference between Doppler-derived flows across the aortic and mitral valves.[25] The stroke volume equals the cross-sectional area of the valve annulus, multiplied by the velocity-time integral of flow across the annulus. The regurgitant volume at the mitral valve is calculated as the difference between stroke volumes across the mitral valve and the aortic valve. This can also be expressed as a regurgitant fraction.

Pulsed-wave Doppler is useful to assess the effect of regurgitation on the pulmonary venous flow. If the pulmonary venous flow is blunted or reversed in systole, this can indicate severe regurgitation.[26,27] The contour and density of the regurgitant envelope on continuous-wave Doppler is also useful, as a dense, early-peaking, or triangular envelope is most consistent with severe regurgitation. In addition, the mitral inflow pattern is typically E-wave dominant (>1.2 m per second) in severe regurgitation, reflecting increased flow across the valve.

ALTERNATIVE IMAGING MODALITIES

Although historically echocardiography has been the dominant imaging modality in the assessment of MR, cardiac computed tomography (CT), cardiac magnetic resonance imaging (MRI), and three-dimensional echocardiography are beginning to play more important roles.[22,28-30] As coronary sinus devices that indirectly alter annular geometry are under development, the relationship of the coronary sinus to the mitral annulus is becoming increasingly important (Fig. 49-5). In addition, the coronary sinus and left circumflex (LCx) arteries are close to each other and may overlap in more than 90% of patients, creating the potential for cinching devices to hinder coronary blood flow.[31] Cardiac CT, therefore, has the potential to provide significant anatomic details in the screening of patients and procedural planning. With cardiac MRI, it is possible to obtain significant structural information regarding the geometry of the left ventricle (LV), the mitral annulus and leaflets, and quantitative regurgitant volumes (Fig. 49-6).[30] It is likely that the regurgitant volumes calculated using cardiac MRI may be more accurate and operator or reader independent compared with TTE. However, limited experience with this modality currently limits its usefulness for research purposes. Three-dimensional echocardiography is a developing imaging modality that provides a more in-depth understanding of the anatomy of the mitral valve apparatus and the changes of MR. Because the position of the mitral valve apparatus in the LV can be disrupted in all directions, three-dimensional echocardiography is more likely to define the exact mechanism of MR in ischemic disease and to detect multiple jets of MR that may affect the treatment approach.[32] Furthermore, with recent advances, the ability to acquire real-time three-dimensional images allows use of the procedure to gauge safety and efficacy during both percutaneous and traditional surgical repairs.

TABLE 49-3	Qualitative and Quantitative Parameters Useful in Grading Mitral Regurgitation Severity		
	Mild	*Moderate*	*Severe*
Structural parameters			
LA size	Normal	Normal or dilated	Usually dilated
LV size	Normal	Normal or dilated	Usually dilated
Mitral leaflets or support apparatus	Normal or abnormal	Normal or abnormal	Abnormal/flail leaflet/ruptured papillary muscle
Doppler parameters			
Color flow jet area	Small, central jet (usually <4 cm² or <20% of LA area)	Variable	Large central jet (usually >10 cm² or >40% of LA area) or variable size wall-impinging jet swirling in LA
Mitral inflow—PW	A wave dominant	Variable	E wave dominant
Jet density—CW	Incomplete or faint	Dense	Dense
Jet contour—CW	Parabolic	Usually parabolic	Early peaking—triangular
Pulmonary vein flow	Systolic dominance	Systolic blunting	Systolic flow reversal
Quantitative parameters			
Vena contracta width (cm)	<0.3	0.3–0.69	≥0.7
Regurgitant volume (mL/beat)	<30	30–59	≥60
Regurgitant fraction (%)	<30	30–49	≥50
EROA (cm²)	<0.20	0.20–0.39	≥0.40

CW, Continuous wave; *EROA,* effective regurgitant orifice area; *LA,* left atrium; *LV,* left ventricle; *PW,* Pulse wave.

From Zoghbi WA, Enriquez-Sarano M, Foster E, et al: Recommendations for evaluation of the severity of native valvular regurgitation with two-dimensional and Doppler echocardiography, *J Am Soc Echocardiogr* 16(7):777, 2003.

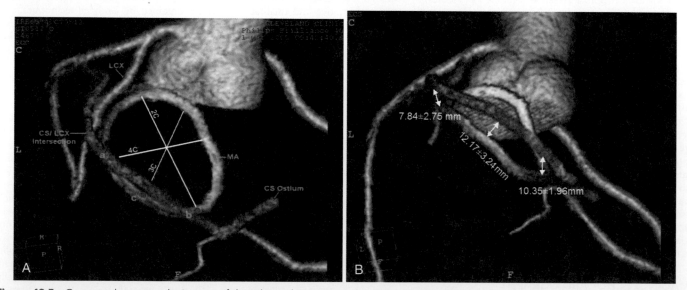

Figure 49-5 Computed tomography images of the relationships among the mitral annulus (MA), the coronary sinus (CS), and the left circumflex (LCx) coronary artery. *Panel A,* The coronary sinus traveling along the posterior mitral annulus and crossing over the left circumflex artery. *Panel B,* The distance between the annulus and the coronary sinus varies, depending on the location along the annulus.

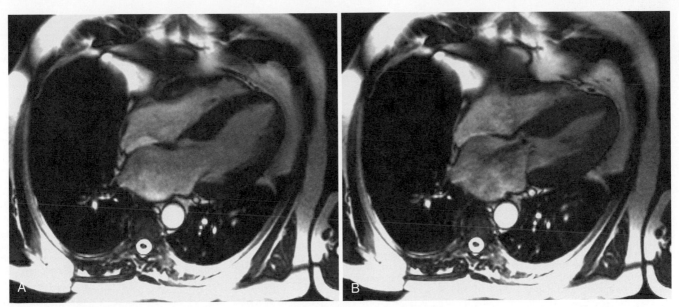

Figure 49-6 Magnetic resonance images of the mitral valve in systole (*Panel A*) and diastole (*Panel B*), demonstrating significant mitral regurgitation as a result of hypertrophic cardiomyopathy and systolic anterior motion of the mitral leaflet. (*Images courtesy of Dr. Sri Sola*).

Surgical Mitral Valve Repair

The American College of Cardiology and American Heart Association (ACC/AHA) guidelines provide a framework for patient selection and timing of mitral valve surgery.[33] Any patient with acute severe MR should undergo valve surgery. Valve surgery is recommended for patients with chronic severe MR in the presence of symptoms and for patients without symptoms in the presence of left ventricular systolic dysfunction or left ventricular cavity dilation (end-systolic dimension >40 mm), and results in the preservation of left ventricular function and improved survival.[34,35] The onset of AF or the development of significant pulmonary hypertension (pulmonary artery systolic pressure >50 mm Hg at rest or >60 mm Hg with exercise) in an asymptomatic patient with normal left ventricular size and systolic function is a reasonable indication for surgery. Management of asymptomatic patients with severe MR remains controversial, but surgery can be offered at centers where the repair likely (>90% chance) has a low operative risk.[36,37] MVRe is the preferred method of surgical management of MR to restore normal leaflet function and annular size.[33] When compared with MVR, the major advantages of MVRe are improved survival, preservation of left ventricular function, freedom from anticoagulation, and fewer complications.[38,39] Despite the advantages of MVRe, this technique appears to be under-utilized, as less than 50% of the patients undergoing mitral valve surgery currently receive a repair procedure, even though about 90% are suitable.[40,41]

SURGICAL APPROACH

Mitral valve surgery can be performed by using median sternotomy, a minimally invasive approach that uses partial upper sternotomy or small right thoracotomy, or it can be performed robotically through multiple "ports." Median sternotomy is required if concomitant coronary bypass is undertaken. Cardioplegic arrest and cardiopulmonary bypass are necessary regardless of the type of chest wall incision, although typically less than 1 hour is required for a valve repair.[7] Techniques of repair address the annulus (annuloplasty with or without a rigid or flexible ring, decalcification, débridement), the leaflets (triangular or quadrangular resection, sliding annuloplasty, patch enlargement, decalcification, edge-to-edge repair), the chordae (resection or elongation of chords), the myocardium itself (remodeling through the

Dor procedure, plication of scar, pericardial cushions, trans-ventricular slings, etc.), the papillary muscle (realignment), or some combination of all these.

ISOLATED ANNULOPLASTY

Available annuloplasty techniques include suture alone, suture with buttressing material, or prosthetic annuloplasty devices. The choice of annuloplasty technique is still being debated among surgeons. A prosthetic annuloplasty band or ring is placed to correct annular dilatation, increase leaflet coaptation by reducing the anteroposterior dimension of the annulus, and prevent future annular dilatation. Of these, the Cosgrove–Edwards annuloplasty band and the Carpentier–Edwards annuloplasty ring are the most commonly used. The Cosgrove–Edwards device is placed along the posterior annulus, which has been shown to be the area of greatest annular dilatation in degenerative and functional MR. The location and flexibility of this band may allow preservation of normal annular motion, although this has not been demonstrated to influence clinical outcome.[42] Functionally, the annuloplasty ring has the effect of transforming the mitral valve into a monocuspid valve, as the posterior leaflet motion is frequently restricted after the repair. More rigid and undersized rings are used in the treatment of functional MR, although the exact type of ring remains controversial. Annuloplasty for functional MR results in significant improvement in NYHA class, decreased hospital admissions for heart failure, and modest survival rates of 71% to 82% at 2 years and 58% at 5 years. Although favorable changes in left ventricular size, shape, and function have been demonstrated after successful mitral valve repair, a propensity analysis failed to demonstrate any mortality benefit compared with matched patients not undergoing valve surgery.[37,43] The recurrence rate of functional MR after isolated annuloplasty is disappointing (28% at 1 year) and remains a limitation to widespread use of the procedure.[44]

ANNULOPLASTY WITH LEAFLET REPAIR

The combination of annuloplasty and leaflet repair, referred to as *Carpentier's techniques*, is most frequently performed for degenerative mitral valve disease. Of the surgical methods of mitral leaflet repair, correction of posterior leaflet or bi-leaflet prolapse is the most common. Posterior leaflet prolapse occurs in the majority of cases of

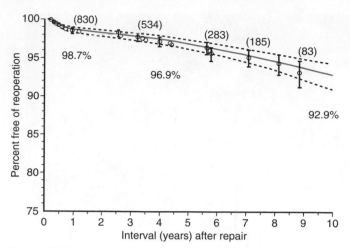

Figure 49-7 Freedom from reoperation after standard Carpentier repair for degenerative disease. *(From Gillinov AM, Cosgrove DM, Blackstone EH, et al: Durability of mitral valve repair for degenerative disease, J Thorac Cardiovasc Surg 116:734, 1998.)*

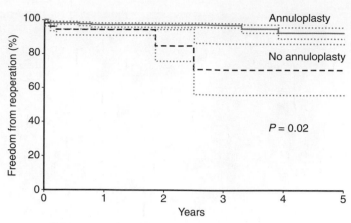

Figure 49-8 Long-term mortality results from the initial surgical edge-to-edge repair cohort from Milan, Italy. *(From Alfieri O, Maisano F, De Bonis M, et al: The double-orifice technique in mitral valve repair: a simple solution for complex problems, J Thorac Cardiovasc Surg 122:674–681, 2001.)*

degenerative mitral valve disease and is the primary cause of regurgitation in approximately 50% of patients. Prolapse is a result of chordal elongation or rupture and affects the P2 segment most frequently. This type of problem is most frequently corrected by posterior leaflet quadrangular resection and plication of the valve annulus.[7] It is generally accompanied by the placement of a prosthetic annuloplasty ring, except in cases of severe calcification of the annulus. Anterior leaflet prolapse, although less common than posterior leaflet prolapse, is a more challenging problem and was commonly treated with initial valve replacement. However, several methods have been developed to treat anterior leaflet prolapse with leaflet repair. The most common are chordal transfer, artificial chordae creation, and the Alfieri edge-to-edge repair. Chordal transfer is performed by resection of a segment of the posterior leaflet, which is then transferred and sewn to the prolapsing segment of the anterior leaflet. A quadrangular repair of the anterior leaflet completes this procedure. Another method of anterior leaflet repair involves the creation of artificial chordae from Gore-Tex sutures. These artificial chordae are attached to the prolapsing leaflet and the papillary muscle by pledgeted sutures. The long-term results for mortality, recurrent MR, and reoperation with MVRe in experienced centers are outstanding and are far superior compared with MVR, and the mortality rate is similar to that of the general population (86%–93% survival at 5 years).[42,45–47] The Cleveland Clinic has achieved excellent results, including a 0.3% operative mortality rate, and 10-year freedom-from-reoperation rate of 93% in a reported series of 1000 consecutive patients (Fig. 49-7).[46]

ISOLATED LEAFLET REPAIR WITH EDGE-TO-EDGE TECHNIQUE

Alfieri has pioneered a creative repair initially developed for anterior leaflet prolapse, where the free edge of the anterior and the posterior leaflets are sewn together in an attempt to increase leaflet contact and coaptation and reduce regurgitation.[48] This technique also works for repair of posterior leaflet and bi-leaflet prolapse. It is useful in preventing systolic anterior motion of the anterior mitral leaflet following traditional MVRe techniques.[49] The resulting double-orifice mitral valve does not generally cause stenosis, even when combined with an annuloplasty ring. The first report of this technique was published in 1998 by Dr. Alfieri's group in Milan, Italy.[48] Of a total of 432 patients undergoing valve repair at their institution between January 1991 to September 1997, 121 patients underwent edge-to-edge correction. The indication was anterior prolapse in 61% of patients. The majority of

patients had a double-orifice repair (60%), with the remainder undergoing paracommissural repair. There was a low rate of in-hospital mortality (1.6%), and overall survival was remarkable (92% at 6 years), with 95% freedom from reoperation (Fig. 49-8). The majority of patients (>80%) were NYHA class I or II.

Following Dr. Alfieri's lead, the technique was adopted into practice at many prominent institutions performing MVRe, although generally as a specialized technique and not as a primary method. The introduction of percutaneous edge-to-edge repair has fueled interest in the surgical outcomes of this procedure, leading to the publication of a number of single-center case series (Table 49-4).[49–54] The procedure has been applied to both degenerative and ischemic MR with favorable results. Although the surgical double-orifice MVRe has been shown to be effective as a treatment for structural or functional mitral valve disease, the surgical literature is limited by a lack of data on isolated edge-to-edge repair.[55]

PERCUTANEOUS MITRAL VALVE REPAIR

The aim of percutaneous strategies for MVRe is to provide relief from severe MR to patients who would otherwise not be candidates for surgical correction or to those who prefer a less-invasive approach without the need for cardiopulmonary bypass. The latter is a more difficult proposition, especially in patients with primary (degenerative) MR, given the historical success of surgical MVRe in treating this problem. These new technologies have shown promise in their various stages of evolution from preclinical to randomized trials. There are currently four major approaches to percutaneous repair. The best-studied approach is the edge-to-edge repair, based loosely on the surgical repair championed by Dr. Alfieri. The second approach uses the proximity of the coronary sinus to the mitral annulus to accomplish favorable changes in annular geometry, bringing the posterior leaflet toward the anterior leaflet, thus improving coaptation. In the third approach, left ventricular reshaping, which accomplishes a reduction in septal-to-lateral diameter and improves leaflet coaptation, can reduce MR. In the fourth approach, the trans-ventricular (direct) approach, mitral annuloplasty is performed by using different methods, including a suture-based annular cinching device, a radiofrequency (RF) ablation catheter to shrink the annulus, and shape-modifying annular devices that can be subsequently adjusted percutaneously. This chapter will focus on the description of the procedure, preclinical and clinical results, and the advantages and disadvantages of each approach (Table 49-5).

TABLE 49-4 Published Reports of Surgical Edge-to-Edge Repair for Mitral Insufficiency*

Study	Alfieri 2001	Lorusso 2001	Kherani 2004	Bhudia 2004	De Bonis 2005	Kuduvalli 2006
Number of Patients	260	75	71	224	54	41
Pathology						
– Degenerative	81%	49%	N/R	14%	—	73%
– Ischemic	2%	3%	N/R	64%	66%	12%
– Rheumatic	10%	24%	N/R	—	—	5%
– Endocarditis	6%	21%	N/R	3%	—	2%
– Other	1%	3%	N/R	19%	33%	8%
Associated annuloplasty	80%	82%	56%	84%	100%	80%
In-hospital mortality	0.7%	3.7%	4.2%†	2%	4.3%	4.8%
Long-term outcome						
– Follow-up	5 yr	8 yr	5 yr	5 yr	2.7 yr	5 yr
– Survival	94.4%	92%	58.3%	65%	90.7%	95.1%
– Freedom from reoperation	90%	80%	‡	#	§	86%
– Mitral regurgitation (MR) ≥3+	N/R	14%	NR	24%	9%	0%

*Indicating the etiology of regurgitation, the prevalence of associated annuloplasty and immediate and long-term outcomes for this procedure.
†= 30-day mortality.
‡3 reoperations.
#= 21 reoperations, including 7 transplantations.
§– 2 reoperations.
N/R = not reported.

TABLE 49-5 Percutaneous or Minimally Invasive Mitral Valve Repair Devices under Development

Device Design	Developmental Phase
Edge-to-edge leaflet repair (edge-to-edge)	
MitraClip™ (Evalve, Menlo Park, CA)	Phase II trial
Indirect annuloplasty via coronary sinus	
Viacor PTMA (Viacor, Wilmington, MA)	Phase II trial enrolling
CARILLON™ Mitral Contour System (Cardiac Dimensions, Kirkland, WA)	Phase II trial enrolling CE mark of approval
MONARC™ (Edwards Lifesciences, Irvine, CA)	Phase I trial completed
Cardiac chamber remodeling	
iCoapsys™ (Myocor, Maple Grove, MN)	First-in-human implants Development halted
PS3 System (Ample Medical Inc, Foster City, CA)	First-in-human implants Development halted
Trans-ventricular (retrograde) direct annuloplasty	
Mitralign Direct Annuloplasty System (Mitralign, Salem, NH)	First-in-man implants
GDS Accucinch Annuloplasty system (GDS)	First-in-man
Other	
QuantumCor RF Annuloplasty (Quantumcor, Lake Forest, CA)	Preclinical phase
Micardia Dynaplasty Dynamic Annuloplasty Ring (Micardia)	First-in-human

Phase I trial, feasibility and safety; *Phase II trial*, pivotal clinical trial; *Preclinical*, animal models or bench testing; *PTMA*, percutaneous trans-venous mitral annuloplasty.

EDGE-TO-EDGE (DOUBLE-ORIFICE) LEAFLET REPAIR WITH THE MITRACLIP™ SYSTEM

The MitraClip™ system (Evalve Inc, Menlo Park, CA) is the best-studied of the options for percutaneous MVRe, and results of a randomized trial of its use were recently reported.[56] The device uses a 24 French (F) steerable delivery guide catheter and a trans-septal approach to place a v-shaped clip (MitraClip™) on the mitral leaflets, effectively achieving a double-orifice repair similar to the Alfieri stitch (Fig. 49-9).[57] The procedure is performed primarily under TEE guidance. The clip is introduced via the guiding catheter into the LA, where the arms of the clip are opened when the clip is aligned with the long axis of the heart. The arms of the clip are rotated until they are perpendicular to the line of coaptation of the valve leaflets. The open clip is advanced into the LV and retracted during systole to grasp the middle scallops of the anterior and posterior valve leaflets in the gripper arms. Positioning is confirmed with TEE, and the clip is locked into position. If needed, the clip is reopened, detached from the leaflets, and withdrawn into the LA, and the process can be repeated until a satisfactory functional double orifice is created. When the positioning is considered adequate, the clip is released and remains attached to the mitral valve leaflets. Eventually, fibrosis and scarring occur in the bridging segment, similar to that seen with surgical edge-to-edge repair (Fig. 49-10).[58] Initial results from 27 patients in the phase I prospective, multi-center safety and feasibility trial EVEREST I (Endovascular Valve Edge-to-Edge Repair Study I) were published in 2005.[59] All patients had moderate to severe MR (3+ or 4+), the majority of whom had primary MR (93%) and a small percentage had ischemic MR (7%). Patients with rheumatic disease, severe mitral annular calcification, severe left ventricular systolic dysfunction, or severe left ventricular cavity dilation were excluded. The clip was successfully deployed initially in 24 (89%) patients, and 3 patients went on to successful surgical repair or replacement.[4] Subsequently, there was partial clip detachment in 3 patients (13%), all of whom went on to successful elective repair. At 30-day follow-up, 6 patients (25%) had MR severity of 3+ or more, 2 of whom went on to successful repair[4] or replacement.[4] Of the 27 original patients, 13 patients (48%) received a clip successfully and remained with MR severity 2+ or less at 6-month follow-up. The 2-year results of the first human implantation have also been reported, showing only mild regurgitation and positive ventricular remodeling.[60] The primary endpoint of EVEREST I was acute safety at 30 days, defined as freedom from death, MI, cardiac tamponade, cardiac surgery for failed clip, clip detachment, stroke, or septicemia. Ultimately, only 15% of patients had experienced a major adverse cardiac event (MACE)—3 clip detachments and 1 permanent stroke—less than the 34.4% required, based on comparison with surgical event rates. Subsequent to this initial report, the EVEREST investigators provided 12-month follow-up on the 55 patients enrolled in EVEREST I and the first 52 roll-in patients from the pivotal EVEREST II phase II trial (discussed further below).[61] In this group, 79% had primary MR, and 21% had functional MR. Acute procedural success (APS; defined as clip implantation with MR ≤2+) was achieved in 79 patients (74%), some of whom required two clips. Of these patients, 77% were discharged with less than or equal to 2+ MR, and at 12 months of follow-up, 50 of 76 patients (66%) still had less than or equal to 2+ MR. The primary efficacy endpoint (MR ≤2+, freedom from mitral valve surgery, and freedom

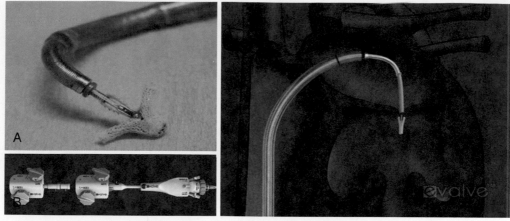

Figure 49-9   The Evalve MitraClip and delivery system. *Panel A*, The device with gripper arms open, attached to the delivery catheter. *Panel B*, The device delivery manipulation system. *Panel C*, A schematic of the delivery catheter and device across the septum and in place on the mitral valve, before device release.

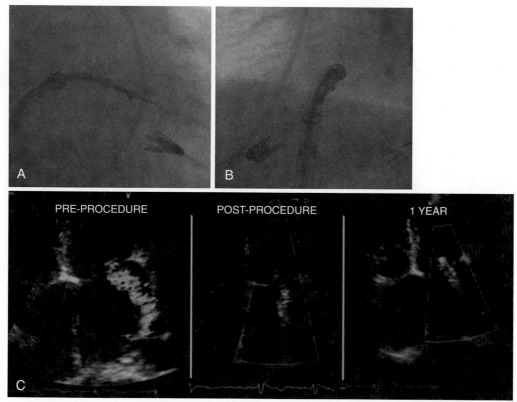

Figure 49-10   Angiographic view of the MitraClip and echocardiographic images before and after deployment. **A**, Right anterior oblique projection showing the two clips and a single delivery catheter after the second clip has been released. **B**, Left anterior oblique projection. **C**, Transthoracic echocardiography images of a patient before, immediately after, and 1 year after percutaneous mitral valve repair with the Evalve MitraClip.

from death) at 12 months was achieved in 66% of patients. These encouraging results were slightly tempered by the need for mitral valve surgery in a total of 32 patients, 23 of whom had clip placement. In those patients with a device, surgery was needed for partial clip detachment in 10 and for greater than 2+ MR in 9 patients. Importantly, of the 25 patients planned for MVRe, only 4 required conversion to valve replacement, demonstrating the feasibility of surgical repair up to 18 months after MitraClip placement.[62] Results of the pivotal phase II trial, EVEREST II, comparing the MitraClip with standard cardiac surgery were recently reported.[56] The study was a prospective, multi-center, randomized, controlled trial with a 2:1 randomization to the

study and control arms, respectively. A total of 279 patients with severe MR were randomized (184 to MitraClip and 85 to surgery), 73% of whom had degenerative MR and 27% had functional MR. Of the 184 patients assigned to the MitraClip, 178 underwent treatment, and APS was achieved in 137 (77%). One primary endpoint was a safety endpoint (MACEs consisting of death, stroke, MI, reoperation, transfusion, and others), designed to demonstrate the superiority of the endovascular strategy. At 30 days, the primary safety endpoint was experienced by 9.6% of the percutaneous group and 57% of the "control" surgical group, though it should be noted that much of this difference was accounted for by the need for transfusions of more than two units in the surgical group (53.2% vs. 8.8%). Also notable, however, was the lack of death, major stroke, urgent or emergent surgery, or repeat mitral valve surgery in any of the 136 patients with MitraClip who achieved APS. The second primary endpoint was for efficacy and was designed to demonstrate noninferiority to cardiac surgery with respect to a composite endpoint of freedom from surgery for valve dysfunction, death, and greater than or equal to 2+ MR. An analysis of clinical effectiveness showed the MitraClip to be "noninferior" to surgery (72.4% vs. 87.8%; prespecified margin for noninferiority 31%). Echocardiographic analysis also showed significant positive ventricular remodeling (decrease in left ventricular end-diastolic dimension) in the percutaneous and surgical groups at 12 months. There was also a durable reduction in MR: of the 137 patients with APS, follow-up echocardiograms were available in 119 patients, 81.5% of whom had less than or equal to 2+ MR. Furthermore, 97.6% of the patients in the MitraClip group were class I or II NYHA status, compared with 87.9% of those in the surgery group. Ultimately, 21% of patients who received the MitraClip crossed over to the surgery group. The safety and efficacy of the MitraClip system in more than 1500 patients, thus far, has been encouraging and, as discussed above, does not preclude future surgical MVRe in most patients. While initial studies concentrated on patients with degenerative disease, EVEREST II and the experience in Europe have shown efficacy in functional MR as well. Ultimately, the device is probably best suited for patients with a centrally originating jet of MR with anatomic features that are conducive to clip placement. Interesting data are also available from a registry of high-risk patients. In this registry, 78 patients with symptomatic moderate to severe MR and an estimated surgical risk of greater than 12% were enrolled. A control group of 36 patients was derived from patients screened but not enrolled in the registry. The mean age of patients in both groups was 77 years and greater than 50% of both groups had had previous cardiac surgery. MitraClips were successfully placed in 96% of the treated group, and 78% had at least one grade improvement in MR by core lab analysis. One-month mortality was 7.7% in the registry and 8.3% in the control group, with predicted surgical mortality of 18.2% and 17.4%, respectively. One-year survival was 76.4% in the treated group versus 55.3% in the control group ($P = 0.037$). At 1 year, 74% of the treated group had grade less than or equal to 2+ MR. NYHA functional class improved to 1 to 2 in 74% of patients, and the annual rate of hospitalizations for CHF decreased by 45%, comparing the year before and the year after treatment. The ongoing REALISM (Real World ExpAnded Multicenter Study of the MitraClip System) continued-access registry (high-risk and non–high-risk patients), as well as use of the device in Europe under the CE (Certification Experts) mark of approval, will provide more experience until approval is [likely] granted in the United States.

INDIRECT ANNULOPLASTY VIA CORONARY SINUS

Annuloplasty is the integral part of MVRe in the majority of surgical approaches to improve mitral valve leaflet coaptation and to reduce MR, and it usually achieves a reduction in mitral annulus diameter of 25% or more. The coronary sinus covers about 50% of the mitral annulus perimeter and 80% of the posterior inter-trigonal distance.[63] Indirect annuloplasty uses the anatomic proximity of the coronary sinus to the mitral annulus for modulating annular size and shape. However, there are several challenges to exploiting this relationship. The proximity and location of the coronary sinus to the annulus is variable (see Fig. 49-5).[64] Furthermore, the LCx artery crosses between the myocardium and the CS in nearly 50% of patients, increasing the risk of arterial compromise.[63,64] Proper definition of these relationships with different imaging techniques, including cardiac CT, angiography, and echocardiography may be helpful in matching the appropriate approach to the anatomy. The ultimate success of this approach will also depend on the long-term safety of instrumenting the coronary sinus (e.g., displacement of device or forces, thrombosis, perforation) and the need for other devices in the coronary sinus (e.g., bi-ventricular pacing).

PERCUTANEOUS TRANS-VENOUS MITRAL ANNULOPLASTY SYSTEM

Developed by Viacor, Inc. (Wilmington, MA), the percutaneous transvenous mitral annuloplasty (PTMA) system uses the relationship between the coronary sinus and the mitral annulus to decrease the septal–lateral mitral annular diameter. The device is made of a composite nitinol and stainless steel construct coated with teflon and plastic, and is available in lengths ranging from 35 mm to 85 mm. The device has a rigid distal element, connected to a flexible push rod to facilitate delivery. When passed through the lumen of the guiding catheter in the coronary sinus, the straight shape of the distal portion of the device causes a conformational change in the mitral annulus, bringing the posterior annulus toward the anterior annulus (Fig. 49-11). Access is obtained in the right internal jugular vein, and a balloon-tipped catheter is advanced to the ostium of the coronary sinus. The balloon is inflated, and a coronary venogram is obtained to identify the anterior interventricular branch of the great cardiac vein. This vein is then engaged by a standard hydrophilic wire, after which a custom 9F delivery catheter (Viacor, Inc.) is introduced into the coronary sinus and advanced up to the ostium of the anterior interventricular branch. The annuloplasty device is introduced into the lumen of the delivery catheter and advanced to the distal portion of the guiding catheter at the ostium of the anterior interventricular branch. Under fluoroscopic and echocardiographic guidance, devices of increasing length of the rigid, straight distal segment are introduced into the delivery catheter until the optimal size is determined. Although the first iteration of the device had only one rod implanted into the coronary sinus delivery catheter during the procedure, now up to three devices can be implanted, and the stiffness and length of each device can be modified until the optimal combination can be determined. The delivery catheter is exchanged for a proprietary multi-lumen implant catheter, which is filled with the optimal combination of device rods, after which it is capped and implanted subcutaneously. The device can be subsequently modified, and the number and stiffness of rods can be revised, if needed, which is an advantage of the PTMA device.

Human feasibility trials were initiated, and results of the experience in the first 27 patients were recently summarized and reported.[65] All of the patients had moderate or severe functional MR, and the procedure was performed under general anesthesia. A "diagnostic" PTMA device was initially placed to determine efficacy and safety; if a benefit to treatment was noted, the device was exchanged for the more permanent "implant" device. Of the 27 patients enrolled, the diagnostic procedure was performed in 19 (70%) and was successful in reducing MR by at least 1 grade in 13 (48%). The diagnostic device was successfully exchanged for the implant PTMA device in 9 patients (33%). Subsequent to the procedure, 1 patient had device fracture at day 7; 3 patients went on to surgical annuloplasty (at days 84, 197, and 216); and 1 patient died at 6 months from progressive heart failure (which was unrelated to the device). Evaluation of the mitral annulus in 5 patients, with follow-up between 3 months and 1 year, demonstrated a sustained reduction in the septal–lateral dimension, although the effect was described as "modest" by the investigators, as was the late reduction in MR. Procedural MACEs included 1 pericardial effusion (without tamponade), 1 device fracture, and 1 occurrence of circumflex impingement (which required stenting but was not complicated by MI). Although the outcomes and safety of the device are encouraging thus far, future trials will require a greater demonstration of long-term safety and efficacy for the device to be clinically relevant. The PTOLEMY (Percutaneous TransvenOus Mitral AnnuloplastY) trial is under way to further evaluate this device.

CARILLON™ Mitral Contour System

The CARILLON™ Mitral Contour System developed by Cardiac Dimensions (Kirkland, WA) is a fixed-length, double-anchor device (Fig. 49-12), which is advanced through a catheter and positioned in the coronary sinus. After the device is deployed and locked into position, tension applied to the anchors of the device results in tissue

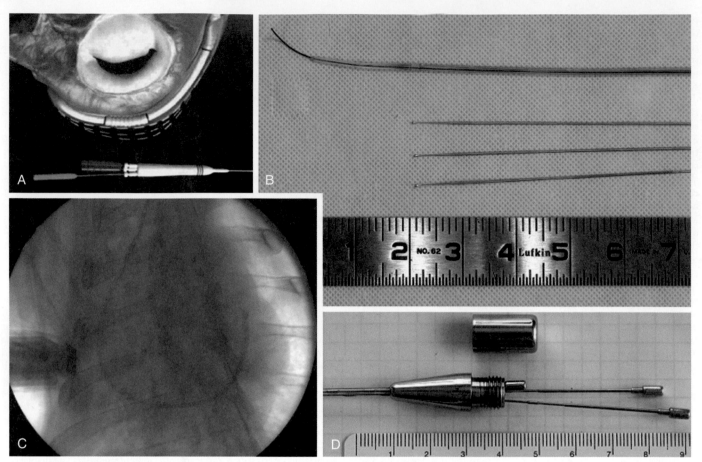

Figure 49-11 The Viacor Percutaneous Transvenous Mitral Annuloplasty (PTMA) device (used with permission from Viacor, Inc). *Panel A*, A representation of the device concept, with the multi-lumen delivery catheter in the coronary sinus. The dashed lines represent progressive remodeling of the coronary sinus, with each device placed in the multi-lumen catheter. *Panel B*, The custom PTMA devices, and the multi-lumen delivery catheter. The custom devices come in various lengths and stiffness. *Panel C*, A fluoroscopic image of the device in the coronary sinus. *Panel D*, A close-up view of the multi-lumen delivery catheter hub, which is implanted subcutaneously after the procedure.

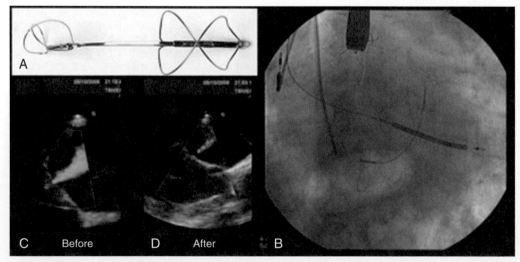

Figure 49-12 The CARILLON device from Cardiac Dimensions (used with permission from Cardiac Dimensions, Inc). *Panel A*, The device with proximal and distal anchors, with tension element. *Panel B*, A fluoroscopic image of the device in place in the coronary sinus. *Panel C*, An echocardiographic image mitral regurgitation before device placement. *Panel D*, The same view after device placement, with a significant reduction in the color jet of mitral regurgitation.

plication and reduces the mitral valve annular diameter and MR. The procedure is performed percutaneously via internal jugular vein access, followed by distal coronary sinus cannulation with a 9F catheter. A measuring catheter is used to determine the optimal positioning of the distal anchor in the coronary sinus. The nitinol annuloplasty device is advanced down the catheter to the target position in the coronary sinus. The distal anchor of the device is deployed by passive expansion and is locked into the fully expanded position by use of the delivery catheter. Tension is placed on the delivery system, bringing the proximal anchor toward the coronary sinus ostium. The amount of tension can be manipulated, as needed, to optimize reduction in annular dimension (approximately 25%) and reduction in MR, which is verified by real-time echocardiography. If the device position is considered to be optimal, the proximal anchor is deployed and locked into position in a similar fashion to the distal anchor. Importantly, if there is a concern about safety or efficacy, the device can be recaptured by advancing the delivery catheter over the device to collapse the anchors, and the apparatus can be adjusted or removed, as necessary. Clinical feasibility was evaluated in the prospective AMADEUS trial (CARILLON Mitral Annuloplasty Device European Union Study) using the next-generation CARILLON XE device in 48 patients with functional MR and left ventricular systolic dysfunction.[66] The device was successfully implanted in 30 patients. At the 6-month follow-up, there was a durable and significant decrease in mitral annulus diameter (4.2–3.78 cm, 10%), MR (average reduction 23%), and NYHA class (2.9–1.8), as well as improvement in the quality-of-life score and 6 minute walk testing (307–403 meters). Of the remaining 18 patients, 5 did not receive implantation because of coronary sinus–related complications ($n = 3$) or fluoroscopic equipment failure ($n = 2$), and 13 patients had retrieval of the device after implantation because of either inadequate MR reduction or coronary compromise. With respect to safety, 6 patients (13%) experienced a total of 7 complications within 30 days of the procedure: 1 patient died of multi-organ failure, 3 patients experienced MI, though none required percutaneous coronary intervention (PCI), and 3 patients experienced coronary sinus

dissection or perforation. The complications were clustered early in the experience and resulted in changes to the implantation procedure, with the appearance of improvement in safety later in the study. On the basis of this early work, the CARILLON system has been granted the CE mark of approval for use in Europe. Improvements to the device were evaluated in the follow-up TITAN (Tighten the Annulus Now) study, which enrolled 53 patients at eight centers across Europe. An interim report at 6 months revealed successful implantation in 68% of patients; 15% did not receive implants because of transient coronary impingement. There was a 1.9% rate of MACEs, which resulted from the death of a patient who did not receive an implant. At the 6-month follow-up, reduction in MR was 35%; there was a 1 grade reduction in NYHA class and 100-meter improvement in the 6-minute walk distance.[67]

MONARC™ Percutaneous Trans-venous Mitral Annuloplasty System

Originally developed as the VIKING system (Edwards Lifesciences Inc., Irvine, CA), the first iteration of this device consisted of a distal self-expanding anchor, a spring-like "bridge" segment, and a proximal self-expanding anchor. The bridge segment was designed with shape-memory properties that lead to shortening of the device at body temperature. The current MONARC™ system (Fig. 49-13) replaces the previous bridging segment with a "delayed-release system" of nitinol and biodegradable spacers, which slowly dissolve over 3 to 6 weeks. This shortening is intended to induce a conformational change in the coronary sinus, extending to the mitral annulus, further reducing any postprocedural MR. Implantation is performed by internal jugular venous access with a large diameter sheath. The coronary sinus is cannulated and a hydrophilic wire advanced into the distal great cardiac vein. A measurement catheter is used to select the proper device size. A 9F device delivery catheter is advanced over the guidewire into the coronary venous system. Left coronary injections are used to verify proper device positioning, and the distal anchor is released by retracting the outer restraining sheath. The intended location of the distal

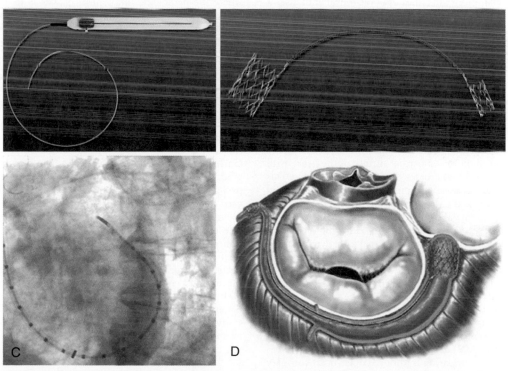

Figure 49-13 The Edwards MONARC™ annuloplasty system (used with permission from Edwards, Inc). *Panel A,* The delivery catheter. *Panel B,* The device, with proximal (smaller) and distal (larger) anchoring elements, as well as the bridge element, that shortens over time after the procedure. *Panel C,* A fluoroscopic image of the measuring device used to size the device. *Panel D,* A schematic of the device within the coronary sinus.

anchor of the device is on the inner curve of the coronary sinus. Slack is removed from the bridge element by placing tension on the delivery catheter, and the proximal anchor is released just within the proximal edge of the coronary sinus by further retraction of the outer restraining sheath of the delivery catheter. In contrast to the devices mentioned previously, this device cannot be recaptured after the anchor has been deployed.

The EVOLUTION trial (clinical EValuation of the Edwards Lifesciences PercUTaneous mItral annulOplasty system for the treatment of mitral regurgitatioN) was a multi-center feasibility and safety study conducted in Europe and Canada to evaluate the MONARC™ device. Interim 2-year follow-up on 72 patients was presented.[68] All patients had 2 to 4+ functional MR, and important exclusion criteria included severe left ventricular dysfunction (EF <25%), organic mitral valve disease, severe mitral annular calcification, or coronary sinus pacing leads. Device implantation was performed in 59 of the 72 patients (82%); 13 patients were not included because of significant venous tortuosity or unfavorable size. With regard to safety, freedom from the cumulative secondary endpoint was realized in 83% at 6 months, 81% at 1 year, and 72% at 2 years. NYHA class was available at the 2-year follow-up in 24 patients, who demonstrated an average decrease from 2.7 to 2.0 ($P = 0.002$). At 2 years, MR severity data were available for 21 patients and showed a trend toward improvement in the overall group (mean MR grade decreased from 2.3 to 1.9, $P = 0.11$) and significant improvement in the patients with baseline MR grade 3 to 4+ (3.3–1.9, $P = 0.001$). There were also sustained trends toward decreases in mitral annulus diameter and left ventricular volume at 2 years. Interestingly, patients with worse NYHA class at enrollment were more likely to respond to the procedure (defined as ≥1 grade reduction in MR). At 2 years, there was response in 75% of the patients with NYHA III or IV, in 50% with NYHA II to IV, and in 44% with NYHA II.[69] Overall, the device is moderately effective, but some safety concerns remain.

CARDIAC CHAMBER REMODELING DEVICES

Functional MR caused by dilated cardiomyopathy and ischemic MR caused by geometric alterations affect not only the mitral annulus but also the LA and the LV and their relationships to the annulus. One potential limitation of the typical ring annuloplasty is that it does not address these alterations in paravalvular geometry. Two devices have, therefore, been engineered with this consideration in mind. Unfortunately, while preliminary results have been encouraging, development of both these devices has been halted because of recent financial hardship.

Coapsys™ and iCoapsys™

The Coapsys™ (Myocor, Maple Grove, MN) annuloplasty system involves the surgical placement of pericardial implants off pump. These implants are placed on the epicardial surface of the heart, with a tethering subvalvular cord that crosses the ventricle internally. This cord is then cinched to decrease the mitral annulus diameter and eliminate MR. Advantages of the Coapsys system include the ability to treat functional MR off pump, allowing the combination of off-pump bypass and MVRe. Conceptually, the device provides a more comprehensive mechanism of action by preserving normal valve dynamics and addressing the mitral annulus as well as the subvalvular space and abnormal left ventricular geometry. In the initial clinical feasibility trial, the device was successfully implanted in 34 patients with functional MR at the time of bypass surgery. Data on the first 11 patients completing 1-year follow-up have been published and confirm the durability of MR decrease (grade 2.9–1.1; jet area 7.4 cm²–3.0 cm²) and NYHA class improvement (2.5–1.2) at 12 months.[70] A U.S. randomized trial (RESTORE-MV) enrolled patients with coronary artery disease and ischemic MR, comparing traditional open-heart coronary artery bypass grafting (CABG) with MVRe to CABG with Coapsys device placement. Intraoperative results from this trial have been reported in the first 19 patients receiving the implant, showing a

reduction in MR grade from 2.7 ± 0.8 to 0.4 ± 0.7 after implantation ($P < 0.0001$).[71] Because of funding issues, the trial was prematurely terminated after randomization of 165 patients (77 treated with MVRe and 87 with Coapsys); the results of this trial have not yet been published. A percutaneous version of the system, the iCoapsys™, is implanted through a pericardial access sheath. The ingeniously designed device was tried in two patients, but the VIVID trial (Valvular and Ventricular Improvement Via iCoapsys Delivery) of clinical feasibility was prematurely discontinued because of financial constraints.[72]

Percutaneous Septal Sinus Shortening (PS3) System

The percutaneous septal sinus shortening (PS3) system (Ample Medical Inc, Foster City, CA) differs from the Coapsys system in that it creates a trans-atrial bridge as opposed to a trans-ventricular bridge. This device uses the coronary sinus and a septal closure device to place a cord across the atrium, create tension on the annulus, and remodel the mitral annulus and the LA. Septal–lateral annular cinching (SLAC) occurs because of traction applied between the inter-atrial septum and the coronary sinus at the level of the P2 mitral segment. Palacios and colleagues published the first human use of the PS3 in two patients with functional MR. Both patients received implants before planned OHS (at which time the device was removed). The results are encouraging, with a reduction in MR grade from 2 to 1 in one patient and from 3 to 1 in the other. A substantial reduction in mitral annulus diameter was achieved (31% reduction in one patient and 29% in the other), comparable with surgical annuloplasty and greater than that achieved by other percutaneous coronary sinus–based indirect annuloplasty devices. No further testing is ongoing because of financial constraints.

TRANS-VENTRICULAR (RETROGRADE) DIRECT ANNULOPLASTY

Percutaneous direct annuloplasty via a retrograde trans-ventricular approach is an exciting area of development. The obvious advantage to this approach is the ability to apply a repair directly to the annulus, where the pathologic mechanism of MR is frequently located. This approach eliminates the anatomic uncertainty about the LCx artery anatomy and the proximity of the coronary sinus to the mitral annulus, which plagues coronary sinus approaches; it also addresses the pathologic basis of functional MR, which may be missed with leaflet-only techniques.

Mitralign Direct Annuloplasty System

Based on the concept of direct suture annuloplasty, the Mitralign Direct Annuloplasty System (Mitralign, Tewksbury, MA) uses a device composed of three metal anchors connected by standard suture material. The anchors are placed in the mitral annulus, and the suture is cinched to perform the annuloplasty. The device is placed via retrograde ventricular access by using a unique translation catheter with a two-pronged "bi-dent" design for device delivery. The initial design used a magnetic guiding catheter placed in the coronary sinus, but in the most recent iteration, the anchors are placed from the ventricular side using standard imaging techniques. The two anchors are positioned below the valve at the level of each posterior leaflet scallop and then deployed directly through the mitral annulus and remain connected by suture material. The suture is then cinched, directly plicating the annulus, emulating the results of a surgical, suture-based annuloplasty. Successful implantation in 1 patient in South America and 2 patients in Europe were reported in 2008 as part of the pilot clinical study.[73] Several device iterations have been incorporated, and clinical testing has continued, albeit slowly.

GDS AccuCinch Annuloplasty System

Another device currently under development is the GDS Accucinch Annuloplasty System (Guided Delivery Systems, Santa Clara, CA). Similar to the Mitralign, it provides a catheter-based trans-ventricular approach to place anchors in the myocardium directly beneath the mitral annulus, yielding a plication annuloplasty. On the basis of encouraging studies in animal models, a first-in-human study was initiated in Europe, and implantation has been successful in several patients thus far.

OTHER ANNULOPLASTY DEVICES

The application of subablative RF energy to remodel the mitral annulus is under development by QuantumCor (Lake Forest, CA).[74] The concept, termed *trans-ventricular annulus remodeling*, relies on scarring and shrinkage of the mitral annulus after application of RF energy directly to the annulus. The device is intended both for surgical and trans-catheter (trans-septal) uses; it has a malleable tip with seven electrodes to deliver RF energy. The catheter is connected to a pulse generator that is modulated by temperature sensors in the electrodes to regulate the amount and duration of energy delivery. The catheter can be manipulated to deliver energy to specific locations on the annulus, allowing for adjustment of the procedure to individual anatomy. Human data are not available. Another device developed by Micardia, the Dynaplasty ring, uses an adjustable annuloplasty ring, implanted surgically during conventional repair procedures. The ring responds to electrical stimulation by RF wires placed directly against the ring in the activation zones of the ring. In vivo activation of the ring by direct RF application causes the ring to change configuration, allowing the ring to take a favorable shape to eliminate MR. The ring may be reshaped intraoperatively or subsequently via the trans-septal approach if MR recurs. This device is in the early phases of development and has not yet been used in humans.

▆ Trans-Catheter Mitral Valve Implantation

Trans-catheter aortic valve implantation (TAVI) has made significant progress, and there have been thousands of successful implantations performed to date. Conversely, trans-catheter mitral valve implantation (TMVI) has not yet been applied clinically. In large part, this is because radial force, which is used to secure aortic prostheses in a calcified aortic root, cannot be applied in the mitral position. CardiAQ Valve Technologies and EndoValve are currently engaged in the development of devices for this purpose, but at this time there are no human trials.

PATIENT SELECTION

The current data on the use of percutaneous mitral valve therapy is derived from experience with less than 2000 patients, and much less patient-reported data are available. Therefore, at this time, it is impossible to precisely define the subgroups of patients who will benefit from these. However, some clinical pearls can be summarized from the experience gathered from large numbers of referrals for this problem. Indications for percutaneous intervention for MR remain very similar to those for surgical intervention.[33] Although there has been some interest in lowering the threshold for the severity of MR for percutaneous therapies, with the contention that they are less invasive and safer, there are no data to implement such liberalization. The major excitement in the field is derived from the ability to provide options for patients with higher surgical risk who are symptomatic with severe MR and who do not have any other options (including coronary revascularization or cardiac resynchronization therapy). The surgical risk assessment should take into consideration not just the estimated mortality but also the morbidity and the risk of compromising quality of life. With this in mind, the most common target for these therapies, at least initially, will be older patients (irrespective of the etiology of MR) with poor left ventricular function and patients with severe functional MR, as identified in the Euro Survey, who are not undergoing surgical intervention.[75] It is difficult to justify the use of these techniques in young

patients with degenerative mitral valve disease who are otherwise appropriate candidates for surgical MVRe. However, the fact that some of these therapies usually do not impair future surgical options is encouraging.

In many ways, percutaneous mitral valve therapies fit the mold of "personalized medicine," which has been cast in the world of pharmacotherapy. Identifying the mechanisms of MR and then defining the anatomy to predict whether a certain device will work is critical to the clinical application of these procedures. A clear understanding of the specific pathology causing MR is necessary to determine whether a percutaneous edge-to-edge repair is required or whether annular dilation needs to be addressed with a direct or indirect annuloplasty device. Furthermore, it should be carefully determined whether the relationship between the coronary sinus and the mitral annulus and that between the coronary sinus and the LCx artery or other anatomic predictors are conducive to a safe and effective coronary sinus–based approach in a specific patient. A comprehensive understanding of imaging technologies and parameters will be key to success. Currently, in the United States, all of the percutaneous MVRe devices are available only as investigational devices, and as such, patients will need to meet inclusion criteria for individual device studies. With the availability of some of these devices in Europe under the CE mark of approval, clinical data are accumulating to shed more light on the proper selection of patients.

▆ Future Directions

Percutaneous MVRe is an exciting new field with many devices at early stages of preclinical and clinical evaluation. The majority of strategies are based on principles learned from surgical MVRe techniques. The most advanced technique, to date, is the edge-to-edge repair, with recently reported results of the pivotal trial comparing the percutaneous technique to surgical repair. As the majority of percutaneous MVRe devices are at early developmental stages, many issues still need to be resolved before widespread application of this technology. Percutaneous MVRe has the potential to be a "preventive" technology, as it may be applied early in the disease course to alter the natural history of MR by disrupting the pathologic feedback loop of MR and left ventricular dysfunction. However, it is unclear whether percutaneous devices will need to eliminate all of the MR to be effective. If a percutaneous repair can achieve a significant and durable reduction, even though not complete elimination, of MR, it may still remain a worthy goal if it prevents clinical events. However, it is important that percutaneous devices preserve future surgical options. If the procedure is safe, is relatively free of complications, and preserves surgical options, then the "nothing to lose" standard may be applied to these devices. The need to determine which patients should be targeted in clinical trials is still present. Trials may have to address specific populations and progressively expand the role of these therapies to lower-risk surgical populations. Further, surgical techniques are beginning to be tailored to the specific valve anatomy, but the percutaneous techniques, in their investigational stages, continue to be limited to one type of device per patient. It seems likely that the future of percutaneous repair will be a combination of techniques. However, this poses significant limitations to the device development process with current regulations, and the use of multiple devices in the same patient is unlikely at the present time in the United States. As percutaneous devices become more specifically tailored to the etiology of MR and the anatomy of the individual patient, the proper imaging and patient selection criteria for each device will have to be learned by interventionalists. Improvements in imaging techniques and the interpretation of these techniques with regard to percutaneous repair will be necessary in pre-procedural planning, in assessing intra-procedural efficacy and complications, and in postprocedural follow-up. Finally, it will be critical to develop collegial interaction between the specialties of cardiac imaging, interventional cardiology, and cardiothoracic surgery to achieve proper patient selection and clinical advancement in this burgeoning field.

REFERENCES

1. Nkomo VT, Gardin JM, Skelton TN, et al: Burden of valvular heart diseases: A population-based study. *Lancet 16* 368(9540):1005–1011, 2006.
2. Carabello BA: The current therapy for mitral regurgitation. *J Am Coll Cardiol* 52(5):319–326, 2008.
3. Mirabel M, Iung B, Baron G, et al: What are the characteristics of patients with severe, symptomatic, mitral regurgitation who are denied surgery? *Eur Heart J* 28(11):1358–1365, 2007.
4. Ho SY: Anatomy of the mitral valve. *Heart* 88(Suppl 4):iv5–iv10, 2002.
5. Roberts WC, Perloff JK: Mitral valvular disease. A clinicopathologic survey of the conditions causing the mitral valve to function abnormally. *Ann Intern Med* 77:939–975, 1972.
6. Braunwald E: Valvular heart disease. In: Zipes DP, Braunwald E, editors: *Braunwald's heart disease: A textbook of cardiovascular medicine*, ed 7, Philadelphia, 2005, Saunders.
7. Carpentier A: Cardiac valve surgery—the "French correction." *J Thorac Cardiovasc Surg* 86:323–337, 1983.
8. Levine RA, Schwammenthal E: Ischemic mitral regurgitation on the threshold of a solution: From paradoxes to unifying concepts. *Circulation* 112(5): 745–758, 2005.
9. Filsoufi F, Salzberg SP, Adams DH: Current management of ischemic mitral regurgitation. *Mt Sinai J Med* 72(2):105–115, 2005.
10. Paparella D, Malvindi PG, Romito R, et al: Ischemic mitral regurgitation: Pathophysiology, diagnosis and surgical treatment. *Expert Rev Cardiovasc Ther* 4(6):827–838, 2006.
11. Timek TA, Lai DT, Tibayan F, et al: Annular versus subvalvular approaches to acute ischemic mitral regurgitation. *Circulation* 106;I-27–I-32, 2002.
12. Dent JM, Spotnitz WD, Nolan SP, et al: Mechanism of mitral leaflet excursion. *Am J Physiol* 269:H2100–H2108, 1995.
13. Enriquez-Sarano M, Avierinos JF, Messika-Zeitoun D, et al: Quantitative determinants of the outcome of asymptomatic mitral regurgitation. *N Engl J Med* 352:875–883, 2005.
14. Gillinov AM, Blackstone EH, Rajeswaran J, et al: Ischemic versus degenerative mitral regurgitation: Does etiology affect survival? *Ann Thorac Surg* 80:811–819; discussion 809, 2005.
15. Ling LH, Enriquez-Sarano M, Seward JB, et al: Clinical outcome of mitral regurgitation due to flail leaflet. *N Engl J Med* 335:1417–1423, 1996.
16. Rosenhek R, Rader F, Klaar U, et al: Outcome of watchful waiting in asymptomatic severe mitral regurgitation. *Circulation* 113:2238–2244, 2006.
17. Enriquez-Sarano M, Basmadjian AJ, Rossi A, et al: Progression of mitral regurgitation: A prospective Doppler echocardiographic study. *J Am Coll Cardiol* 34:1137–1144, 1999.
18. Rosen SE, Borer JS, Hochreiter C, et al: Natural history of the asymptomatic/minimally symptomatic patient with severe mitral regurgitation secondary to mitral valve prolapse and normal right and left ventricular performance. *Am J Cardiol* 74:374–380, 1994.
19. Grigioni F, Enriquez-Sarano M, Zehr KJ, et al: Ischemic mitral regurgitation: Long-term outcome and prognostic implications with quantitative Doppler assessment. *Circulation* 103:1759–1764, 2001.
20. Mihaljevic T, Lam BK, Rajeswaran J, et al: Impact of mitral valve annuloplasty combined with revascularization in patients with functional ischemic mitral regurgitation. *J Am Coll Cardiol* 49(22): 2191–2201, 2007.
21. Zoghbi WA, Enriquez-Sarano M, Foster E, et al: Recommendations for evaluation of the severity of native valvular regurgitation with two-dimensional and Doppler echocardiography. *J Am Soc Echocardiogr* 16:777–802, 2003.
22. Khanna D, Miller AP, Nanda NC, et al: Transthoracic and transesophageal echocardiographic assessment of mitral regurgitation severity: Usefulness of qualitative and semiquantitative techniques. *Echocardiography* 22:748–769, 2005.
23. Enriquez-Sarano M, Miller FA, Jr, Hayes SN, et al: Effective mitral regurgitant orifice area: Clinical use and pitfalls of the proximal isovelocity surface area method. *J Am Coll Cardiol* 25:703–709, 1995.
24. Fehske W, Omran H, Manz M, et al: Color-coded Doppler imaging of the vena contracta as a basis for quantification of pure mitral regurgitation. *Am J Cardiol* 73:268–274, 1994.
25. Enriquez-Sarano M, Seward JB, Bailey KR, et al: Effective regurgitant orifice area: A noninvasive Doppler development of an old hemodynamic concept. *J Am Coll Cardiol* 23:443–451, 1994.
26. Klein AL, Stewart WJ, Bartlett J, et al: Effects of mitral regurgitation on pulmonary venous flow and left atrial pressure: An intraoperative transesophageal echocardiographic study. *J Am Coll Cardiol* 20:1345–1352, 1992.
27. Pu M, Griffin BP, Vandervoort PM, et al: The value of assessing pulmonary venous flow velocity for predicting severity of mitral regurgitation: A quantitative assessment integrating left ventricular function. *J Am Soc Echocardiogr* 12:736–743, 1999.
28. Alkadhi H, Bettex D, Wildermuth S, et al: Dynamic cine imaging of the mitral valve with 16-MDCT: A feasibility study. *Am J Roentgenol* 185:636–646, 2005.
29. Delgado V, Tops LF, Schuijf JD, et al: Assessment of mitral valve anatomy and geometry with multislice computed tomography. *JACC Cardiovasc Imaging* 2(5):556–565, 2009.
30. Fujita N, Chazouilleres AF, Hartiala JJ, et al: Quantification of mitral regurgitation by velocity-encoded cine nuclear magnetic resonance imaging, *J Am Coll Cardiol* 23:951–958, 1994.
31. Gopal A, Shah A, Shareghi S, et al: The role of cardiovascular computed tomographic angiography for coronary sinus mitral annuloplasty. *J Invasive Cardiol* 22:67–73, 2010.
32. Daimon M, Saracino G, Gillinov AM, et al: Local dysfunction and asymmetrical deformation of mitral annular geometry in ischemic mitral regurgitation: A novel computerized 3D echocardiographic analysis. *Echocardiography* 25(4):414–423, 2008.
33. Bonow RO, Carabello BA, Chatterjee K, et al: ACC/AHA 2006 guidelines for the management of patients with valvular heart disease: A report of the American College of Cardiology/American Heart Association Task Force on Practice Guidelines (writing Committee to Revise the 1998 guidelines for the management of patients with valvular heart disease) developed in collaboration with the Society of Cardiovascular Anesthesiologists endorsed by the Society for Cardiovascular Angiography and Interventions and the Society of Thoracic Surgeons. *J Am Coll Cardiol* 48:e1–e148, 2006.
34. Dare AJ, Veinot JP, Edwards WD, et al: new observations on the etiology of aortic valve disease: A surgical pathologic study of 236 cases from 1990. *Hum Pathol* 1993;24:1330–1338
35. Rozich JD, Carabello BA, Usher BW, et al: Mitral valve replacement with and without chordal preservation in patients with chronic mitral regurgitation: Mechanisms for differences in post-operative ejection performance. *Circulation* 86:1718–1726, 1992.
36. Griffin BP: Timing of surgical intervention in chronic mitral regurgitation: is vigilance enough? *Circulation* 113:2169–2172, 2006.
37. Bishay ES, McCarthy PM, Cosgrove DM, et al: Mitral valve surgery in patients with severe left ventricular dysfunction. *Eur J Cardiothorac Surg* 17:213–221, 2000.
38. Enriquez-Sarano M, Schaff HV, Orszulak TA, et al: Valve repair improves the outcome of surgery for mitral regurgitation. A multivariate analysis. *Circulation* 91:1022–1028, 1995.
39. Grossi EA, Goldberg JD, LaPietra A, et al: Ischemic mitral valve reconstruction and replacement: Comparison of long-term survival and complications. *J Thorac Cardiovasc Surg* 122:1107–1124, 2001.
40. Savage EB, Ferguson TB, Jr, DiSesa VJ: Use of mitral valve repair: Analysis of contemporary United States experience reported to the Society of Thoracic Surgeons National Cardiac Database. *Ann Thorac Surg* 75:820–825, 2003.
41. Oliveira JM, Antunes MJ: Mitral valve repair: Better than replacement. *Heart* 92:275–281, 2006.
42. Braunberger E, Deloche A, Berrebi A, et al: Very long-term results (more than 20 years) of valve repair with Carpentier's techniques in nonrheumatic mitral valve insufficiency. *Circulation* 104:I8–I11, 2001.
43. Wu AH, Aaronson KD, Bolling SF, et al: Impact of mitral valve annuloplasty on mortality risk in patients with mitral regurgitation and left ventricular systolic dysfunction. *J Am Coll Cardiol* 45:381–387, 2005.
44. McGee EC, Gillinov AM, Blackstone EH, et al: Recurrent mitral regurgitation after annuloplasty for functional ischemic mitral regurgitation. *J Thorac Cardiovasc Surg* 128:916–924, 2004.
45. Mohty D, Orszulak TA, Schaff HV, et al: Very long-term survival and durability of mitral valve repair for mitral valve prolapse. *Circulation* 104:I-1–I-7, 2001.
46. Gillinov AM, Cosgrove DM, Blackstone EH, et al: Durability of mitral valve repair for degenerative disease. *J Thorac Cardiovasc Surg* 116:734–743, 1998.
47. Flameng W, Herijgers P, Bogaerts K: Recurrence of mitral valve regurgitation after mitral valve repair in degenerative valve disease. *Circulation* 107:1609–1613, 2003.
48. Maisano F, Torracca L, Oppizzi M, et al: The edge-to-edge technique: A simplified method to correct mitral insufficiency. *Eur J Cardiothorac Surg* 13:240–245; discussion 245–246, 1998.
49. Bhudia SK, McCarthy PM, Smedira NG, et al: Edge-to-edge (Alfieri) mitral repair: Results in diverse clinical settings. *Ann Thorac Surg* 77:1598–1606, 2004.
50. Alfieri O, Maisano F, De Bonis M, et al: The double-orifice technique in mitral valve repair: A simple solution for complex problems. *J Thorac Cardiovasc Surg* 122:674–681, 2001.
51. Lorusso R, Borghetti V, Totaro P, et al: The double-orifice technique for mitral valve reconstruction: Predictors of postoperative outcome. *Eur J Cardiothorac Surg* 20:583–589, 2001.
52. Kherani AR, Cheema FH, Casher J, et al: Edge-to-edge mitral valve repair: The Columbia Presbyterian experience. *Ann Thorac Surg* 78:73–76, 2004.
53. De Bonis M, Lapenna E, La Canna G, et al: Mitral valve repair for functional mitral regurgitation in end-stage dilated cardiomyopathy: Role of the "edge-to-edge" technique. *Circulation* 112:I402–I408, 2005.
54. Kuduvalli M, Ghotkar SV, Grayson AD, et al: Edge-to-edge technique for mitral valve repair: Medium-term results with echocardiographic follow-up. *Ann Thorac Surg* 82:1356–1361, 2006.
55. Maisano F, Vigano G, Blasio A, et al: Surgical isolated edge-to-edge mitral valve repair without annuloplasty: Clinical proof of the principle for an endovascular approach. *EuroIntervention* 2:181–186, 2006.
56. Feldman T: on behalf of the EVEREST II investigators: Endovascular valve edge-to-edge repair study (EVEREST II) randomized clinical trial: Primary safety and efficacy endpoints. Atlanta, GA, March 14, 2010, American College of Cardiology/i2 Late Breaking Clinical Trials session.
57. St Goar FG, Fann JI, Komtebedde J, et al: Endovascular edge-to-edge mitral valve repair: Short-term results in a porcine model. *Circulation* 108:1990–1993, 2003.
58. Fann JI, St Goar FG, Komtebedde J, et al: Beating heart catheter-based edge-to-edge mitral valve procedure in a porcine model: Efficacy and healing response. *Circulation* 110:988–993, 2004.
59. Feldman T, Wasserman HS, Herrmann HC, et al: Percutaneous mitral valve repair using the edge-to-edge technique: Six-month results of the EVEREST Phase I Clinical Trial. *J Am Coll Cardiol* 46:2134–2140, 2005.
60. Condado JA, Acquatella H, Rodriguez L, et al: Percutaneous edge-to-edge mitral valve repair: 2-year follow-up in the first human case. *Catheter Cardiovasc Interv* 67:323–325, 2006.
61. Feldman T, Kar S, Rinaldi M, et al; EVEREST Investigators: Percutaneous mitral repair with the MitraClip system: Safety and midterm durability in the initial EVEREST (Endovascular Valve Edge-to-Edge REpair Study) cohort. *J Am Coll Cardiol* 54(8):686–694, 2009.
62. Argenziano M, Skipper E, Heimansohn D, et al; EVEREST Investigators: Surgical revision after percutaneous mitral repair with the MitraClip device. *Ann Thorac Surg* 89(1):72–80, 2010.
63. Iansac E, Di Centa I, Al Attar N, et al: Percutaneous mitral annuloplasty through the coronary sinus: An anatomical point of view. *Circulation* 114:II-565, 2006.
64. Choure AJ, Garcia MJ, Hesse B, et al: In vivo analysis of the anatomical relationship of coronary sinus to mitral annulus and left circumflex coronary artery using cardiac multidetector computed tomography: Implications for percutaneous coronary sinus annuloplasty. *J Am Coll Cardiol* 48:1938–1945, 2006.
65. Sack S, Kahlert P, Bilodeau L, et al: Percutaneous transvenous mitral annuloplasty: Initial human experience with a novel coronary sinus implant device. *Circ Cardiovasc Interv* 2(4):277–284, 2009.
66. Schofer J, Siminiak T, Haude M, et al: Percutaneous mitral annuloplasty for functional mitral regurgitation: Results of the CARILLON Mitral Annuloplasty Device European Union Study. *Circulation.* 120(4):326–333, 2009.
67. Cardiac Dimensions announces presentation of 12-month follow-up data on Titan Trial at European Society of Cardiology Meeting: Available at http://www.cardiacdimensions.com/usa/press-release-20100818: Accessed September 8, 2010.
68. Harnek J, Webb J, Kuck KH, et al: Percutaneous treatment of functional mitral repair. 2-years results from the Evolution 1 study. *Eurointervention* 5(Supplement 1):E24, 2009.
69. Webb JG, Kuck K, Stone G, et al: Percutaneous mitral annuloplasty with the MONARC system: Preliminary results from the EVOLUTION trial. *Am J Cardiol* 98:49M, 2006.
70. Mishra YK, Mittal S, Jaguri P, et al: Coapsys mitral annuloplasty for chronic functional ischemic mitral regurgitation: 1-year results. *Ann Thorac Surg* 81:42–46, 2006.
71. Grossi EA, Saunders PC, Woo YJ, et al: Intraoperative effects of the coapsys annuloplasty system in a randomized evaluation (RESTOR-MV) of functional ischemic mitral regurgitation. *Ann Thorac Surg* 80:1706–1711, 2005.
72. Pedersen WR, Block P, Leon M, et al: iCoapsys mitral valve repair system: Percutaneous implantation in an animal model. *Catheter Cardiovasc Interv* 72(1):125–131, 2008.
73. Mitralign News & Information: Available at http://www.mitralign.com/eurostudy.shtml: Accessed April 19, 2010.
74. Heuser RR, Witzel T, Dickens D, et al: Percutaneous treatment for mitral regurgitation: The QuantumCor system. *J Interv Cardiol* 21(2):178–182, 2008.
75. Mirabel M, Iung B, Baron G, et al. What are the characteristics of patients with severe, symptomatic, mitral regurgitation who are denied surgery? *Eur Heart J* 28(11): 1358–1365, 2007.

50

Trans-catheter Aortic Valve Interventions: From Balloon Aortic Valvuloplasty to Trans-catheter Aortic Valve Implantation

ALAIN CRIBIER | ALAN ZAJARIAS | HELENE ELTCHANINOFF |
CHRISTOPHE TRON | ROGER LAHAM | JEFFREY POPMA

KEY POINTS

- Aortic stenosis is the most common form of adult valvular heart disease, and it has become more prevalent in the aging population. Surgical aortic valve replacement is the treatment of choice, and it is the only definitive treatment to relieve symptoms and improve survival. Despite guidelines and recommendations, one third of patients are not referred to surgery, often because of old age, left ventricular dysfunction, and comorbidities.

- Balloon aortic valvuloplasty (BAV) is a palliative procedure that can provide immediate relief of symptoms. Advanced technologies have made the procedure safer, faster, and more efficient. However, the possibility of improved survival is limited to patients who can be bridged to surgery or can undergo serial dilations. With the aging population, there is a renewed interest in BAV, which offers the only therapeutic option to palliate the symptoms of inoperable or high-surgical-risk patients until approval is granted for percutaneous valve implantation techniques.

- Percutaneous aortic valve implantation is a promising new technique, still under investigation, with ongoing technical improvements in devices, materials, and protocols for delivery. It offers durable improvement in valve area associated with improved left ventricular function and long-lasting (up to 3 years) alleviation of symptoms. Valve implantation has been restricted to patients who have been determined to be inoperable or for whom surgery is considered inappropriate because of age, poor left ventricular function, cardiac or noncardiac comorbidities, or all of these causes

- The percutaneous aortic valve was initially implanted using the antegrade trans-septal approach. The retrograde approach, using an advanced technology, is less demanding and is currently receiving the most interest. Clinical trials on the trans-apical approach (through the apex of the left ventricle after a small chest opening) are in the early stages. In the future, these various methods for valve implantation should be considered according to the patient's clinical status and the quality of vascular access.

- With the onset of nonsurgically implantable heart valves, a multidisciplinary approach is required. It is time for close collaboration among noninvasive and interventional cardiologists, cardiac and vascular surgeons, and internists and geriatricians, along with engineers and representatives from industry and government to bring the potential of this new treatment modality into reality.

Aortic stenosis (AS) remains the most common form of adult acquired valvular heart disease in developed countries, increasing in prevalence with age.[1] As noted earlier by Ross and Braunwald, the natural history of symptomatic aortic stenosis carries a poor prognosis.[2] Medically treated patients with symptomatic AS have 1-year and 5-year survival rates of 60% and 32%, respectively.[3] Aortic valve replacement (AVR) is the only effective treatment that alleviates symptoms and improves survival in patients symptomatic AS. In the ideal candidate, surgical AVR has an estimated operative mortality of 4%.[4] However, the rates

of operative mortality and postoperative complications increase with age and become significantly higher when surgery is done urgently and when pre-existent comorbidities such as coronary artery disease, poor left ventricular function, renal insufficiency, pulmonary disease, and diabetes are present.[5,6] These factors are considered some of the major reasons for one third of patients with valve disease not being referred for surgery.[7] Trans-catheter aortic valve implantation (TAVI) has opened the possibility for treating patients who, until now, had been left untreated as it was believed that their operative mortality outweighed the benefits offered by traditional AVR.

Before the onset of BAV in 1986, AVR was the only recommended therapy for patients with symptomatic severe AS or was the expectant observation if patients were thought to be "too old" or "high risk."[8,9] The concept of "old age" has continued to be redefined and has resulted in a moving target for comparison as these techniques have been evolving and the population has been aging. Currently, age is no longer considered a surgical contraindication, and very old patients (octogenarians and nonagenarians) are offered the option if they do not have significant physical or psychological comorbidities.[10-12] The percentage of patients 90 years of age and over undergoing heart surgery has doubled from 1994 to 2001.[11] Patients with poor left ventricular function are also more aggressively managed surgically.[13-15] In Europe and the United States, a large number of patients with severe AS are still not offered valve replacement.[7,16] In the 1990s, the early enthusiasm for BAV as a possible alternative to surgical aortic valve replacement in adult patients disappeared following the recognition of the problem of re-stenosis. The procedure appeared to provide only temporary benefit in symptoms and, at best, a modest survival benefit with a relatively high complication rate.[17,18] As more experience was reported, there were discrepancies in reported results and complication rates. Whereas there is agreement with regard to the benefit of the procedure in neonates, infants, and young patients, the role of BAV in adults remains controversial as reflected in the updated American College of Cardiology (ACC) guidelines.[19] For the high-risk older adult with severe calcific AS, the response from the cardiologist has been to limit the recommendation for BAV and for the cardiac surgeon to continue to broaden the inclusion of patients for surgery, regardless of age or left ventricular function. A large number of patients with severe AS and comorbidities that render them inoperable or very high risk still remain untreated, particularly when the risk assessment by the Parsonnet score or the EuroSCORE appears unfavorable.[17] In spite of some patients being determined to be too sick for surgery, BAV is not offered to them in most centers because of its perceived limitations.[7] TAVI was introduced in a subset of patients with severe AS who were not surgical candidates, and over the last 8 years, the technique has been refined dramatically.[21] The results of early registry data show significant hemodynamic improvement without re-stenosis and have allowed its commercialization in Europe, but randomized control trials are still ongoing in the United States. On the basis of current results, TAVI carries the potential of offering a therapeutic option to patients who until recently have been left untreated and also revolutionizes the treatment of severe AS and prosthetic dysfunction. BAV plays an integral role in TAVI, and as a result, there has been increased interest in interventional cardiologists and surgeons in learning this technique.

The objectives of this chapter are to:

1. Describe the current technique of BAV, highlighting the modifications in the technique and materials.
2. Review current BAV results and discuss its current role in the era of TAVI.
3. Review the development of TAVI for calcific AS in adults, describe the implantation technique, review the short and mid-term follow-up of patients who have received this therapy, and provide insight into the future advances and clinical applications.

Balloon Aortic Valvuloplasty

Since the first reported cases, we have published their continuing experience, which now exceeds 1000 cases.[22–28] Like others, immediate improvement in symptoms, hemodynamics, and left ventricular function could be obtained but the mid-term and long-term results were disappointing.[17,18] In our hands, BAV remains a valuable palliative procedure for frail patients who are extremely old, often with compromised clinical status from concomitant coronary artery disease (CAD) and other extracardiac comorbidities. Most of the referred patients have been turned down by surgeons, and BAV is attempted as a "bridge to surgery" in about one third of the cases. The technique used now allows us to obtain improved hemodynamic results and reduced complications in this high-risk subset of patients.[28]

The goal of the procedure is to achieve a 100% increase in the aortic valve area. This requires attention to obtaining the maximum pressure exerted on the valve leaflets during balloon inflation, proper balloon sizing, and optimal contact with the valve structures. Improper techniques may explain the disparity of the results in the literature. The final valve area is a determinant of the prognosis, and in some reported series, the increase in the aortic valve area after the procedure was very modest.[17,29,30] The results of BAV are limited by the pathology involved in the disease. Degenerative AS is its most common etiology and appears to be associated to a chronic inflammatory process.[31–34] Unlike rheumatic mitral stenosis, commissural fusion is not the predominant feature in the majority of older patients with calcific AS, and as a result, commissural splitting is not the major mechanism of action in balloon dilatation of adult calcific AS.[35] The primary mechanism of the balloon action in AS is fracture of nodular calcium deposits, thereby improving leaflet mobility, which allows increased valve opening and blood flow during left ventricular contraction.[36] At full inflation, the rigid balloon can stretch the elastic component of the valve structures and the annulus. These elastic properties can result in immediate or early recoil, which are associated with an unsuccessful or suboptimal procedure result. Overstretching can result in tearing or rupture of the elastic and fibrocalcific components of the leaflets, the annulus, or the adjacent myocardium, leading to aortic insufficiency.[37] Despite improvement in technique and materials, re-stenosis continues to plague BAV.[18,38–40] Early re-stenosis occurring within hours or days is caused by early recoil and could be related to the pathology of the valve components, or inappropriate balloon diameter (because of size or insufficient inflation). The causes of re-stenosis occurring after several months may be multi-factorial, including the original degenerative process and an altered healing process with fibrosis and ossification.[41,42] When patients develop recurrent symptoms, BAV can be repeated, usually after an interval of 12 to 24 months, and the dilations can be done serially.[26–28,43,44] In some cases, the patient may be "bridged" to AVR or TAVI.[19] Despite its limitations, BAV can provide symptomatic relief and modest survival benefit in selected patients who are very old or have comorbidities and who currently may have no other options.[17–19,29] BAV can be done using either the retrograde approach or the antegrade approach. The retrograde approach was first described by Lababidi in infants and children, and then by our group in adults.[8,45] The antegrade approach was reported by Block, and comparisons

between the techniques have been reported.[46–48] There is no significant benefit to the antegrade approach compared with the retrograde approach except in patients with peripheral vascular disease or small vessel size.[49] For both approaches, we typically perform the baseline hemodynamic study to confirm the presence of severe AS at the same setting as the planned BAV intervention.

THE RETROGRADE APPROACH

Using our current technique for the retrograde approach, the procedure is usually performed in less than 1 hour with few complications. Technical "pearls" that we have learned are helpful to make the procedure fast and safe in this critically ill, fragile, older adult population.

Patient Preparation

We use mild sedation with intravenous (IV) midazolam, and local anesthesia. Unfractionated heparin is given intravenously (3000–5000 international units [IU]) at the start of the procedure. All of the anticipated supplies are brought to the catheterization laboratory (cath lab) table to reduce procedure time. Femoral arterial and venous accesses are obtained with 8 French (8F) sheaths. Coronary angiography is obtained, and if indicated, coronary intervention is performed in the same setting but usually after the BAV has been completed. Right heart catheterization is performed using a Swan-Ganz thermodilution catheter. If the patient is being considered for TAVI, then a supra-aortic angiography is obtained in a shallow left anterior oblique (LAO) projection, followed by abdominal aortic and pelvic vessel angiography.

Technique for Retrograde Crossing of the Native Aortic Valve

When using the appropriate technique, the stenotic aortic valve can be crossed within a few minutes in most cases. An Amplatz left coronary catheter 2 (AL-2) is commonly used for this task. A straight-tip, fixed-core, 0.035-inch guidewire is positioned at the tip of the catheter. In the 40-degree LAO projection, the catheter tip is positioned at the rim of the valve. The catheter is slowly pulled back, while a firm clockwise rotation is maintained to direct the catheter tip toward the center of the valve plane (Fig. 50-1, A). The guidewire is carefully moved in and out of the catheter tip, sequentially mapping the valve surface and exploring for the valve orifice. Once the wire crosses the valve, the catheter is advanced over the wire and positioned in the middle of the left ventricle (LV). The trans-valvular gradient is obtained using the side arm of the femoral sheath to record the aortic pressure. A dual-lumen multi-purpose or pigtail catheter may be used to reduce the peripheral augmentation of the systemic pressure. Cardiac output is then measured. The aortic valve area is calculated using Gorlin's formula.[50]

EQUIPMENT REQUIRED FOR BALLOON AORTIC VALVULOPLASTY

Guidewire

An extra-stiff Amplatz 0.035-inch, 270-cm length guidewire (Cook, Bjaeverskov, Denmark) is used to perform all catheter exchanges and to assist in stabilizing the valvuloplasty balloon during inflation, deflation, and withdrawal. Before inserting the wire, a large pigtail-shaped curve is formed at the distal end of the wire with a dull instrument (Fig. 50-2, A) to prevent ventricular perforation and to decrease ectopy.

Sheaths

The 8F arterial sheath is replaced over the extra-stiff wire with a 10F, 12F, or 14F sheath (Cook, Bjaeverskov, Denmark), depending on the balloon catheter required. The evolution of the technique has seen a reduction in the profile of the devices, reducing local complications at the femoral artery puncture site, which was previously the most common complication reported.[51] Until recently, we have been using 12F to 14F sheaths, facilitating hemostasis by "preclosing" with a 10F

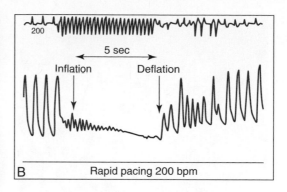

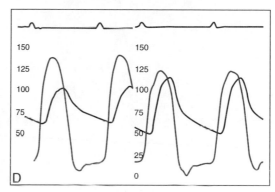

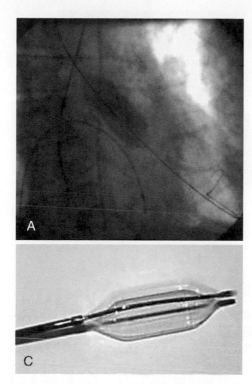

Figure 50-1 Balloon aortic valvuloplasty (*A*) is performed under rapid ventricular pacing (*B*) which decreases the effective cardiac output by inducing ventricular tachycardia. The balloon catheter (*C*) must be sized to the aortic annulus to avoid severe aortic insufficiency. Doubling of the valve area or decreasing the trans-valvular gradient by greater than 50% is considered a successful procedure (*D*).

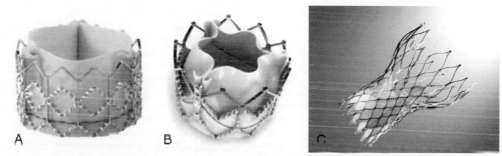

Figure 50-2 **A,** The Edwards-SAPIEN valve is a tri-leaflet bovine pericardial valve mounted on a balloon-expandable stainless steel stent that is placed in the subcoronary position. A PET skirt is placed around the ventricular third of the valve to decrease perivalvular insufficiency. **B,** The second-generation Edwards-SAPIEN XT valve has a new bovine pericardial leaflet design, is mounted on a cobalt chromium stent reducing its profile, and has a longer skirt to minimize perivalvular insufficiency. **C,** The CoreValve Revalving system consists of a tri-leaflet porcine pericardial valve that is mounted on a self-expanding nitinol frame.

Prostar device (Prostar, Abbott Vascular, Redwood City, Ca). Currently, since a 10F sheath is generally required, we are able to close the arteriotomy site using an 8F Angioseal device (Angioseal Vascular Closure Device, St. Jude Medical, Belgium) at the end of the procedure.

Balloon Catheters

The majority of our experience was obtained with specifically designed balloon catheters for BAV, the double-sized Cribier-Letac catheters. When the production of those catheters was discontinued, we chose the Z-Med II balloon catheter (Numed Inc., Hopkinton NY, USA), compatible with a 12F or 14F sheath. Currently, we use the lower-profile Cristal balloons (Balt Extrusion, Montmorency, France), which are compatible with a 10F sheath. The 20-mm and 23-mm diameter balloons are 45 mm in length, and the 25-mm diameter balloon is 50 mm in length. In general, we start with a 23-mm balloon. A 20-mm balloon is used if the valve is densely calcified or the aortic annulus is small (<19 mm by echocardiography). In up to 25% of the cases, the

25-mm diameter balloon size can be used if the aortic annulus diameter is larger than 24 mm.

RAPID VENTRICULAR PACING

A 6F temporary bipolar pacing lead is positioned in the right ventricular posterior wall and connected to a pulse generator capable of pacing at up to 220 beats per minute (beats/min). Pacing and sensing parameters are determined and then the blood pressure response to pacing at 200 to 220 beats/min is evaluated. The rapid ventricular pacing (RVP) causes a precipitous fall of blood pressure to at least 50 mm Hg to be effective (Fig. 50-3). If this is not achieved at a rate of 200 beats/min, then the response is checked again at 220 beats/min. If 2:1 conduction block is seen, then the rate will need to be reduced to 180 beats/min or the lead position modified. The pacer is set on demand mode at 80 beats/min, serving as a backup in the event of a vagal episode or an interruption of AV conduction resulting in bradycardia

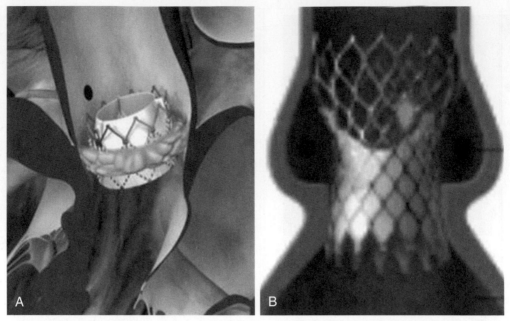

Figure 50-3   A, The Edwards-SAPIEN prosthesis is placed in the subcoronary position without interfering with flow across the coronary arteries. **B,** The CoreValve Revalving system is placed from the left ventricular outflow tract to the ascending aorta. The concavity of the frame allows coronary perfusion.

or asystole in response to balloon inflations. The diagnostic catheter is removed from the LV over the extra-stiff wire, while the looped flexible segment of wire is carefully maintained in the LV cavity (see Fig. 50-1, *B*). The 8F sheath is replaced by the 10F sheath over the extra-stiff wire (see Fig. 50-2, *B*). A short extension tubing with a three-way stopcock attached is connected to a hand-held 30-mL luer-lock syringe filled with diluted contrast. The contrast is diluted at 15% contrast to 85% saline to reduce viscosity and thus facilitate the inflation–deflation cycles. After flushing the distal lumen and applying negative pressure on the balloon port, the balloon catheter is mounted on the extra-stiff wire and advanced into the aorta and allowed to rest above the aortic valve. At this time, the balloon is partially inflated and then completely deflated one or more times to completely purge it of air bubbles. De-airing the balloon in the ascending aorta has the advantage of maintaining the lowest balloon profile while crossing the aortic arch, thus decreasing the risk of atheromatous plaque dislodgement and embolization. The balloon catheter is advanced across the aortic valve, centering the valve between the two markers. In the past, before using RVP, it was always challenging to maintain the balloon in the optimal position during balloon inflation. The inflated balloon would tend to "pop" into the LV abruptly, striking the apex, or would "eject" itself back into the aorta with the possibility of disrupting atheromatous plaque, which could embolize.

BALLOON INFLATION

RVP and simultaneous forward pressure on the balloon catheter and forward pressure on the extra-stiff wire help stabilize the balloon during inflation. Traction on the guidewire causes forward movement on the balloon. Pushing the guidewire displaces the balloon in an aortic direction allowing for better positioning. There must be clear communication between the operators manipulating the balloon catheter and the pacing device. RVP is turned on, and balloon inflation is started quickly and with enough pressure to rapidly inflate the balloon (see Fig. 50-1, *C*) as soon as the blood pressure falls. RVP is continued for a few seconds after the balloon reaches maximal inflation. The balloon is rapidly deflated, the pacer is turned off, and the balloon is withdrawn from the valve. This step requires the coordination of the two operators to quickly allow restoration of antegrade flow while

maintaining safe wire position in the LV. Rapid balloon deflation and restoration of blood flow are important to minimize the time of hypotension and hypoperfusion. We allow time for heart rate and blood pressure to return to preinflation parameters before proceeding to inflate the balloon again. Since the pressure gradient cannot be measured through the current generation of balloon catheters, it is important to assess the effects of the balloon dilation and the hemodynamic consequences by observing the wave form of the aortic pressure tracing as well as the heart rate response and rhythm and blood pressure recovery. A sudden change in waveform with loss of the dicrotic notch or falling diastolic blood pressure could indicate the presence of severe aortic regurgitation. An improvement in the pressure slope is suggestive of a successful procedure. If the balloon does not appear to be fully expanded, or there is no hemodynamic improvement, then repeat inflations are usually carried out before measuring the trans-aortic gradient again. The balloon catheter is removed while applying negative pressure on the balloon port, maintaining guidewire position in the LV. Particular care must be taken as the deflated balloon is drawn through the sheath. If resistance is encountered, it may be necessary to remove the catheter and the sheath together as a single unit. The residual gradient is then obtained by simultaneous measurement of pressures in the LV and in the aorta (Fig. 50-4). If there is a significant gradient, the next larger size balloon may be chosen, and the sequence is repeated. A pullback gradient is also obtained after the final balloon inflation. For the final results, the pacemaker is removed, the cardiac output is measured, and the final aortic valve area is calculated. An optimal result is considered to be doubling of the valve area or decreasing the gradient by 50% compared with the baseline value. Supra-aortic angiography to determine the presence and the severity of aortic regurgitation may be performed (see Fig. 50-1, *D*). If contrast cannot be used, assessment of the presence of aortic insufficiency and its severity may be performed by trans-thoracic echocardiography (TTE).

IMMEDIATE MANAGEMENT AFTER BALLOON AORTIC VALVULOPLASTY

Manual compression is used for hemostasis at the venous entry site. Arterial hemostasis is achieved with the closure device as specified earlier. If a technical failure occurs, a pneumatic pressure device is used

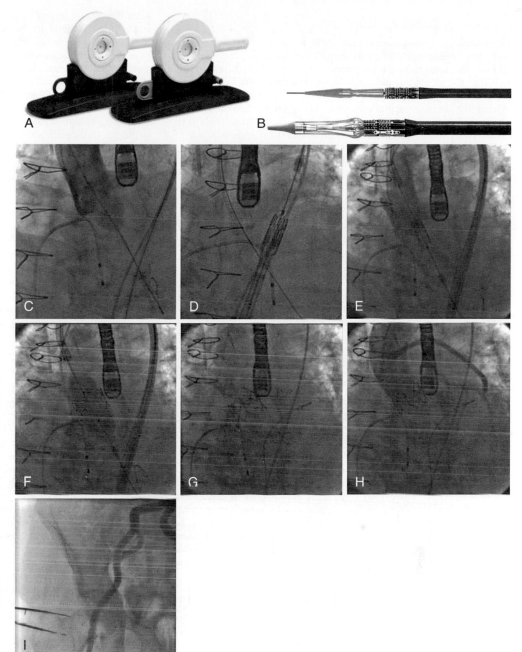

Figure 50-4 For the trans-femoral trans-catheter aortic valve implantation (TAVI), the SAPIEN valve (A) is crimped over the delivery catheter (B). Supra-aortic angiogram is performed in a view that places all three coronary cusps in the same plane. A balloon aortic valvuloplasty is performed (C) to facilitate valve positioning. The delivery catheter is advanced through the descending aorta (D). The retroflex catheter is activated to allow the passage of the valve through the aortic arch. Correct valve position is confirmed by echocardiography and angiography (E), and the valve is deployed under rapid ventricular pacing (F). Aortic angiography confirms the valve position, lack of aortic insufficiency, and unrestricted flow through native coronary arteries and bypass grafts (G and H). The delivery sheath is removed, and ilio-femoral angiogram (I) is performed to confirm the absence of vascular complications.

(FemoStop II Plus, Radi Medical Systems AB, Uppsala, Sweden). When the case is uncomplicated, the patient is usually discharged within 2 days. However, when BAV is performed in patients with severely impaired left ventricular function or after rescuing a patient from cardiogenic shock, hemodynamic monitoring with inotropic support is usually required in the intensive care unit (ICU). Vagal reactions are the most common cause of hypotension associated with BAV. There must be a low threshold for ruling out the occurrence of pericardial tamponade or retroperitoneal bleed when evaluating the patient with hypotension after BAV.

THE ANTEGRADE TRANS-SEPTAL APPROACH

We reserve the use of this approach for BAV for those patients who have severe peripheral vascular disease, which precludes femoral arterial access or would increase complications if the retrograde approach is used.

Patient Preparation

The patient is given mild IV sedation and local anesthesia at the access sites. Femoral venous access is obtained bilaterally with an 8F sheath in the right femoral vein and with a 6F sheath in the left femoral vein. Through a 6F sheath in the femoral artery, if possible, or in the brachial (or radial) artery, coronary angiography is performed when indicated, and a pigtail catheter is placed above the aortic valve. Right heart catheterization and baseline hemodynamic measurements are recorded. Using the left femoral vein access, a bipolar pacing catheter is positioned in the right ventricular apex, pacing parameters are determined, and RVP is assessed as described previously.

Trans-septal Catheterization

Trans-septal catheterization is performed using an 8F Mullins sheath and a Brockenbrough needle via the right femoral vein. In our method, we cross the septum in the left lateral view. A pigtail catheter is positioned in the ascending aorta throughout the procedure for monitoring blood pressure and at this stage of the procedure as a reference marker for the trans-septal puncture. The puncture is made in the middle third of a virtual line connecting the distal tip of the pigtail catheter adjacent to the aortic calcification and the posterior border of the heart. When entry into the LA is confirmed, heparin, 5000 IU, is administered intravenously. The Mullins sheath is then used to direct a 7F Swan-Ganz catheter which has an inner lumen compatible with a 0.035-inch guidewire (Edwards LifeSciences, Irvine, CA, USA) across the mitral valve into the LV under fluoroscopic guidance in the 40-degree right anterior oblique (RAO) projection. The trans-aortic gradient is determined with the Swan-Ganz catheter in the LV and with the pigtail catheter in the aorta. The aortic valve area is calculated using Gorlin's formula.

Crossing the Aortic Valve

The Mullins sheath is advanced approximately 2 cm beyond the mitral valve. The balloon of the Swan-Ganz catheter is inflated and directed into the left ventricular outflow approaching the native aortic valve. A 0.035-inch straight wire may facilitate crossing the aortic valve with the balloon deflated, as the catheter is pushed over the wire into the ascending aorta. The wire is removed, and the balloon is re-inflated. The catheter is advanced into the descending aorta and positioned at the level of the distal aortic bifurcation with an Amplatz 0.035-inch, 360-cm long extra-stiff guidewire (Cook, Bloomington, Indiana). The balloon is deflated, and the Swan-Ganz catheter is removed.

The "Essential" Guidewire Loop in the Left Ventricle

We have learned that during this step of the procedure, it is very important to keep a large loop in the guidewire within the LV. Straightening of the guidewire between the mitral valve and the aortic valve can keep the mitral valve open, resulting in severe mitral regurgitation with hemodynamic deterioration. The loop within the LV is maintained with continuous monitoring at each step of the procedure. The 8F venous sheath is replaced with a 10F sheath for the subsequent balloon dilations using the Cristal balloon catheter (12F or 14F if NuMed balloons are used).

Atrial Septostomy

The atrial septum is dilated with an 8-mm diameter balloon septostomy catheter through the 10F sheath in the right femoral vein. Diluted solution of contrast media : saline (15 : 85) is used with a 10-mL syringe for at least two balloon inflations of 30 seconds each.

Antegrade Balloon Aortic Valvuloplasty

The same balloon catheters are used as for the retrograde approach. Dilation of the aortic valve is done preferentially with the 23-mm diameter balloon, which is advanced through the 10F sheath and positioned across the aortic valve, while the loop in the LV is maintained carefully. The balloon has been purged of air before use. BAV is then performed, as described above, using RVP for stabilization during balloon inflations. Again, the loop in the LV must be carefully monitored during this step, particularly as the balloon is withdrawn from the valve quickly during balloon deflation. It is not feasible to measure the gradient after inflations of each diameter of balloon with this technique. After the initial balloon inflations are completed, the hemodynamic result is assessed by observing the aortic pressure waveform. If a significant fall of the diastolic pressure does not occur, then the next larger balloon size can be chosen. When two to three inflations using the largest selected balloon size are completed, the balloon catheter is removed. A 6F pigtail catheter is advanced over the extra-stiff wire and positioned over the arch so that the wire can be removed shielded by the catheter, thus avoiding injury to the aorta or the mitral valve. The final gradient is obtained with the pigtail catheter in the LV and another catheter in the aorta. Supra-aortic angiograms may be obtained. If there is no AV conduction defect, the pacing catheter is removed and replaced with the Swan-Ganz catheter for final hemodynamic measurements. Hemostasis is obtained with manual compression of the femoral artery and vein after sheath removal. Bed rest is recommended for 24 hours. Observation in the ICU with inotropic support and prolonged hemodynamic monitoring is required, on rare occasions, for hemodynamically unstable patients, typically those presenting in cardiogenic shock.

RESULTS USING CONTEMPORARY BALLOON AORTIC VALVULOPLASTY TECHNIQUES

The results of our series of 141 consecutive patients with severe AS who underwent BAV (with the exception of patients undergoing percutaneous heart valve implantation) between January 2002 and April 2005 have been published.[28] In this group of patients, the average age was 80.3 ± 10 years, 45% were women, and they were high risk for surgery or were inoperable. Eighty percent were in New York Heart Association (NYHA) functional class IV, with 28% of patients having poor left ventricular function (ejection fraction [EF] <30%). The procedure was done emergently for patients in cardiogenic shock in 5.6% of cases. BAV was done using the retrograde approach in 95% of the cases. The largest balloon was 23 mm in 84% of the procedures. The immediate results showed an increase in aortic valve area from 0.59 ± 0.19 to 1.02 ± 0.34 cm^2 ($P < 0.001$) and a decrease in trans-valvular gradient from 49.3 ± 21.2 to 22.2 ± 11.8 mm Hg ($P < 0.001$). Post-BAV aortic regurgitation was grade 2 in 14%, grade 3 in 3.5%, and grade 4 in 1.4% of the cases. Six patients (4%) died. Nonfatal severe complications occurred in 9 patients (6%): 2 transient strokes, 5 episodes of complete atrioventricular (AV) block, and 2 severe aortic regurgitation. There were 8 vascular complications that did not require surgical repair. Discharge from the hospital was at 5.6 ± 3 days. In our series, the frequency of clinically apparent neurologic events was less than 2%. This compares favorably with the reported incidence of cerebrovascular events in a series of retrograde catheterizations of the aortic valve without intervention.[52] We give heparin before crossing and then use a technique that minimizes trauma to the aortic valve structure during the attempted crossing. Although feared as a potentially fatal and disabling complication, embolization of atheromatous debris, which could break loose during the balloon's impact on the valve, is, in fact, quite rare. Since many of these patients have concomitant cerebrovascular disease, hypotension and hypoperfusion during balloon inflation can also result in a neurologic event. Minimizing the duration of rapid ventricular pacing and balloon inflation is an important technical issue, and maintaining optimal heart rate and blood pressure during the procedure is crucial. Preventing, recognizing, and treating vagal reactions expeditiously are also important to avoid the possible neurologic consequences of hypotension. Improvements in procedures such as RVP and in vascular closure devices as well as continued experience have resulted in decreased complications despite an increasingly older and sicker population of patients. The large registries reported higher complication rates, possibly related to multiple participating centers, many of whose operators were reporting their first experience.[18,51] The reduction of complications in our series, compared with the results of an early registry, is notable as shown in Table 50-1.

CURRENT PERSPECTIVES OF BALLOON AORTIC VALVULOPLASTY

The recently updated ACC/AHA guidelines for the management of patients with valvular heart disease continue to regard the role of BAV as controversial.[19] There are no class I or IIa recommendations for BAV. The class IIb indications for adult patients with severe AS are (1) for patients who are at high risk for AVR because they are hemodynamically unstable and would be candidates for "a bridge to surgery" or (2) as a palliative procedure for patients with a serious comorbid condition

TABLE 50-1 Comparisons of Complication Rates in the Rouen Series and in the Mansfield Registry		
Complications	Mansfield Scientific Aortic Valvuloplasty Registry 1986–1988 (N = 492)	Rouen Series 2002–2005 (N = 141)
Procedural death	2 (4.9%)	3 (2.1%)
Postprocedural death (<7 days)	12 (2.6%)	3 (2.1%)
Cerebral embolic events	11 (2.2%)	2 (1.4%)
Transient ischemic attacks	5 (1.1%)	0 (0%)
Ventricular perforation with tamponade	11 (2.2%)	0 (0%)
Severe aortic insufficiency	5 (1.1%)	2 (1.4%)
Vascular complications (surgical repair)	27 (5.5%)	0 (0%)
Nonfatal arrhythmias	5 (1.1%)	5 (3.5%)
Other: myocardial infarction, sepsis, renal failure	8 (1.6%)	1 (1%)

which would preclude AVR. Because of improvements in the surgical technique, all older patients who are suitable candidates should receive surgical AVR.[10,11,53,54] However, in the frail older patient with comorbidities, the risk for perioperative complications, individual patient preferences, and ethical and economical factors should be taken into consideration when considering AVR or a less invasive option. Other potential indications for BAV are:

1. For the management of patients who present with critical symptomatic AS in need for emergent noncardiac surgery. The hemodynamic improvement achieved by BAV is immediate and may decrease the risk from general anesthesia. In these situations, BAV should be reserved only for those patients with severe AS and who face the risk for hemodynamic compromise.

2. To determine the contributing role of AS to dyspnea in patients with concomitant severe lung disease to gauge the potential for improvement as well as the risks in undergoing AVR or TAVI.

3. To assess the myocardial contractile reserve in patients with low-gradient or low EF, in whom associated cardiomyopathy is doubtful. Perioperative mortality can be as high as 62% in patients with no demonstrated contractile reserve.[55] The indication of AVR or TAVI in these patients can be clarified 2 to 3 weeks after BAV if a marked improvement in the left ventricular ejection fraction (LVEF) occurs.

At present, BAV remains a viable alternative for the management of selected patients with severe AS. BAV continues to play an important role in the management of AS, particularly as a palliative modality for the increasing population of older adults, in whom the risk of surgery is too high or not appropriate.[27,28,44,56,57] Interventional cardiologists and surgeons should become familiar with this technique, particularly if they are interested in the trans-femoral or trans-apical TAVI, as it plays a crucial role in patient selection and valve implantation.

Trans-Catheter Aortic Valve Implantation

Percutaneous catheter-based systems for the treatment of patients with valvular disease has been an exciting area for research since the mid-1960s. The initial animal investigations were performed by Davies in 1965, followed by Moulopoulos in 1971, Phillips in 1976, and Matsubara in 1992.[58–61] These investigators reported on various catheter-based systems for temporary relief of aortic insufficiency, but no further human application was possible because of unsolved major limitations. A new era of investigations started with the development of endovascular stents, giving rise to the concept of balloon expandable valvular prosthesis. In 1992, Andersen et al reported their work in a porcine model, in which they evaluated a trans-luminal stented heart valve.[62] Here again, despite encouraging experimental results, there was

no development of human application. Subsequently, in 2000, Bonhoeffer and coworkers using a valve from a bovine jugular vein mounted within an expandable stent reported the feasibility of delivering such a device inside the native pulmonary valve of lambs; thereafter, they were able to perform the first successful human percutaneous replacement of a pulmonary valve in an RV–PA (right ventricle–to–pulmonary artery) prosthetic conduit with valve dysfunction.[63,64] Our team in Rouen has been working since the early 1990s on the development of a catheter-based treatment for nonsurgical patients with severe calcific AS that could overcome the high re-stenosis rate seen after BAV. Early cadaver work in 1994 provided information on the ability to deploy a Palmaz stent in the aortic position and contributed to appropriate stent dimensions. In 1999, under the auspices of PVT (Percutaneous Valve Technologies, Fort Lee, NJ), an original catheter valve was developed and tested in the sheep model.[65] In vitro testing confirmed the valve's hemodynamic profile and durability. An original animal model of chronic aortic regurgitation, which allowed long-term evaluation of the catheter valve in the systemic circulation, was developed for in vivo testing.[66] The first TAVI in a human was performed by our group in April 2002,[21] and this was followed by an initial series of human implantations for compassionate use.[67–69] Following the acquisition of PVT by Edwards LifeSciences in 2003, further modifications of the device (Cribier–Edwards and the Edwards-SAPIEN Heart Valve) preceded multi-center clinical trials. Results from other centers were published, confirming the feasibility of TAVI.[70,71] The first series of patients with severe AS treated with the self-expanding CoreValve Revalving system was reported by Grube et al subsequently.[72] Eight years after the first valve implantation, and after multiple device modifications, TAVI has been made commercially available in Europe, and the first multicenter randomized trial has been completed in the United States. To date, more than 50 TAVI procedures occur weekly, and the number continues to grow. TAVI is the most exciting advancement in the field of interventional cardiology, as it has provided innovative therapy and created a strong interaction among cardiac surgeons. This section will provide a review of patient selection, procedural techniques, results, and future strategies with balloon-expandable Edwards-SAPIEN valves and the Medtronic CoreValve. In addition, other valve prostheses in different stages of development will be mentioned (see Fig. 50-1).

RISK STRATIFICATION

Currently, TAVI is being offered to patients who are at high risk for surgical complications because of their age or comorbidities. Patients are considered to have a high operative risk when their scores are in the upper decile for mortality or have a 30-day mortality greater than 15%. Surgical risk is most commonly estimated by the Society of Thoracic Surgery Predicted Risk of Mortality (STS-PROM) and the European System for Cardiac Operative Risk Evaluation (EuroSCORE). The EuroSCORE has been validated in patients undergoing valvular surgery.[73] Since the prevalence of high-risk patients was low in the initial population that generated this tool, the logistic EuroSCORE was then developed to more accurately predict the mortality rate in this patient population.[74] However, this algorithm has been shown to persistently overestimate the mortality rate.[75,76] The STS-PROM score is derived from the Society of Thoracic Surgeons (STS) database, a voluntary registry of practice outcomes, which estimates the risks of mortality, morbidity, renal failure, and length of stay after valvular and nonvalvular cardiac surgeries.[77] This score has been shown to underestimate the true mortality rate after cardiac surgery, but it more closely reflects the operative and 30-day mortality for the highest-risk patients undergoing aortic valve replacement.[78] The STS-PROM and the EuroSCORE provide an objective way to quantify risk. Although thorough, these risk scores do not include certain characteristics that would complicate surgery and increase operative mortality, such as: previous mediastinal irradiation, the presence of severe calcification in the thoracic aorta (porcelain aorta), anatomic abnormality of the chest wall, history of mediastinitis, liver cirrhosis, or the patient's frailty. In addition, the algorithms were calculated from patients who underwent surgery, thus limiting their applicability to patients who were not considered surgical candidates. Clinical judgment and the patient's level of independent functioning are subjective parameters that influence outcomes after cardiac surgery but are difficult to measure. The information from the PARTNER (Placement of AoRTic traNscathetER valves) trial will likely aid in the development of risk calculators that will more precisely estimate the risk for patients selected for TAVI.

PATIENT SCREENING

In the United States, no indications for TAVI have been established, as the devices are still under investigation. Inclusion in the PARTNER trial required patients to have severe symptomatic AS, be considered high risk for surgical complications (STS risk score >10%), have a greater than 1 year survival with regard to their comorbidities, and might benefit from valve replacement. In the European Union countries, where TAVI is commercially available, the procedure is limited to patients with severe AS (valve area <0.8 cm^2) and who have high surgical risk (Logistic EuroScore >20%) or a contraindication to AVR.

All patients considered for TAVI need to undergo:

1. Screening echocardiography to document the severity of AS, the absence of other severe valvular disease, describe the valve anatomy and calcium distribution, and determine aortic annular diameter and left ventricular function.
2. Right and left catheterization to determine the presence of pulmonary hypertension and concomitant CAD, which may need to be treated before valve implantation.
3. Aortic angiography to identify the correct orientation of the image intensifier during valve positioning and to determine potential complicating factors in the aortic arch that may interfere with the procedure.
4. Thoraco-abdominal computed tomographic angiography (CTA) with ilio-femoral runoff to determine the anatomy of the aorta, vessel diameter, calcification, and tortuosity.

VASCULAR SCREENING

After the screening process has been completed and the patients have been deemed eligible for TAVI, then the route of implantation needs to be determined. The CoreValve Revalving system may be delivered by the femoral or subclavian approach.[79,80] With the Edwards-SAPIEN valve, two implantation routes are available: trans-apical and transfemoral. Both delivery methods are comparable in success and complication rates. Selection depends on the tortuosity, calcification, and internal diameter of the femoral, external iliac, and common iliac arteries. The presence of abdominal aortic aneurysms or history of their repair would favor the use of the trans-apical approach or the subclavian approach. Vascular complications have been associated with significant mortality and may be prevented with appropriate screening.[81] Safety should not be sacrificed if both approaches are available and patients are considered good candidates. Contrast angiography provides an appropriate screening tool for route selection.[82] However, it does not provide a detailed determination of the vascular anatomy. By inserting a guidewire across the iliac arteries, the degree that the vessels will straighten can be evaluated; if the arteries persist with significant tortuosities after insertion of a stiff guidewire, a TA or subclavian approach is preferred. CTA allows for precise determination of the degree, extent, and localization of vascular calcification. In addition, three-dimensional vessel reconstruction and cross-section imaging allow for the precise determination of vessel luminal diameter. The minimal luminal diameter and the length of the segment with the minimal luminal diameter are the main considerations for selecting the delivery approach. Contrasted CT scans are preferred; however, if chronic renal insufficiency precludes the use of a fully contrasted study, then intra-arterial administration of a small contrast bolus or a non-contrasted CT may provide appropriate images for the necessary

TABLE 50-2	Minimal Vessel Diameter Requirements for Arterial Trans-catheter Aortic Valve Implantation		
Valve Size	Sheath Size	Minimal Arterial Diameter
Edwards-SAPIEN		
23 mm	22 French (F)	7 mm
26 mm	24F	8 mm
Edwards-SAPIEN XT		
23 mm	18F	6 mm
26 mm	19F	6.5 mm
CoreValve	18F	6 mm

measurements.[83] The use of intravascular ultrasound (IVU) is an invasive way of measuring the arterial diameter; however, it may provide unreliable dimensions because of image obliquity. The Edwards-SAPIEN valve requires minimal luminal diameters of 7 mm and 8 mm to allow for the 22F and 24F sheaths, respectively, which are required for valve delivery. The new Edwards-SAPIEN XT valve allows for the vessels of 6 mm and 6.5 mm, requiring an 18F and a 19F sheath, respectively. The CoreValve Revalving System allows for a vessel diameter of 6 mm for the insertion of an 18F sheath. Special attention needs to be paid at the level of the aorto-iliac and internal–external iliac artery bifurcations, as these areas tend to be involved in vascular complications (Table 50-2).

THE EDWARDS-SAPIEN VALVE

The Edwards-SAPIEN valve (Edwards LifeSciences, Irvine, CA) consists of a bioprosthetic valve, the balloon catheter on which it is mounted, the Retroflex catheter (Edwards LifeSciences, Irvine, CA), and the crimping tool.

The Edwards-SAPIEN valve (Fig. 50-5) is a tri-leaflet bioprosthesis made of bovine pericardium mounted on a balloon-expandable stainless steel stent. It has been pre-treated to decrease calcification and functional deterioration. The stent has a fabric cuff on the ventricular side, which covers one half of the frame, limiting stent expansion and decreasing perivalvular insufficiency. Because of the lack of a sewing ring, the valve is oversized to the aortic annulus to ensure post-deployment stability and is currently available in two sizes: a 23-mm valve, with a stent height of 14.5 mm; and a 26-mm valve, with a stent height of 16 mm. In bench-top testing its durability is greater than 10 years. The Edwards-SAPIEN valve provides a larger effective orifice area and a lower hemodynamic profile compared with corresponding surgically implanted valves but has a higher incidence of perivalvular insufficiency.[84] The new-generation device, Edwards-SAPIEN XT, currently commercially available in Europe, is made of a cobalt–chromium alloy, which provides the same radial strength while reducing the valve profile. This valve is currently approved for the trans-femoral approach and is under investigation for the trans-apical approach. In the future, 21-mm and 29-mm valves will be available.

The Balloon Catheter

The valve is mounted on a custom-made balloon that is 30 mm in length, with balloon diameters corresponding to the sizes of prostheses, and ends in a nose cone that facilitates crossing the native valve (see Fig. 50-2). Its inflation profile decreases movement during inflation.

The Crimping Tool

An original crimping tool (see Fig. 50-2) is used to manually and symmetrically compress the overall diameter of the percutaneous heart valve (PHV) from its expanded size to its minimal delivery profile. A cylindrical gauge is used to confirm the collapsed profile of the delivery system to ensure that it will move smoothly through the introducer sheath. A measuring ring is used to calibrate the balloon inflation to

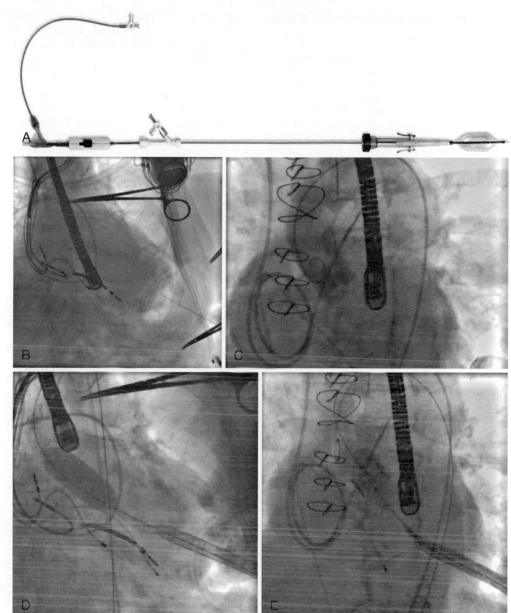

Figure 50-5 Trans-apical delivery of the Edwards-SAPIEN valve requires the Ascendra delivery system (*A*). The procedure starts with a lateral thoracotomy. After the heart is exposed and a purse-string suture is placed around the puncture site, a needle is placed in the left ventricular apex (*B*) to mark the trajectory. An aortic angiogram (*C*) is performed to align the aortic cusps in the same plane, and the delivery sheath is inserted into the left ventricular cavity. A balloon valvuloplasty is performed through the delivery sheath under rapid ventricular pacing (*D*). The valve is then advanced to its appropriate position and deployed under rapid ventricular pacing.

its desired size and to determine the amount of saline–contrast mixture in the syringe necessary for the proper inflation at the time of deployment.

The RetroFlex Guiding Catheter and the Ascendra Delivery System

The Retroflex catheter (Edwards LifeSciences Inc., Irvine, CA), an innovation to facilitate the PHV passage across the aortic arch from the retrograde approach, was initially evaluated by Webb (see Fig. 50-2).[85] This catheter has a deflectable tip that changes direction when activated by the rotation of an actuator incorporated in the handle. The catheter is then used to direct the valve delivery system through the arterial system, around the aortic arch, and across the aortic valve, providing a less traumatic passage. The Retroflex catheter assists in centering and supporting the valve as it crosses the calcified and stenotic native valve. This system also provides precise positioning at the aortic annulus. The Novoflex catheter (Edwards LifeScience Inc. Irvine, CA), is a newer-generation catheter that allows loading the

Edwards-SAPIEN XT prosthesis onto the balloon while in the body, decreasing the sheath size dramatically.

The Ascendra Delivery System (Edwards LifeSciences Inc., Irvine, CA) is the delivery catheter used for the trans-apical route (see Fig. 50-3). This catheter allows for easy valve manipulation to improve the orientation of the prosthesis.

Delivery Sheath

The PHV assembly and deflecting guiding catheter are introduced through a 25-cm-long, hydrophilic-coated sheath that extends into the abdominal aorta to decrease vascular complications. The trans-femoral delivery system requires 22F and 24F sheaths for the 23-mm and 26-mm valves, respectively. With the introduction of Edwards-SAPIEN XT and Novoflex, the insertion sheath has decreased to 18F and 19F, respectively. The sheaths are equipped with a hemostatic mechanism to decrease blood loss. The trans-apical delivery sheath is 26F in diameter, is shorter, and has a flexible tip to decrease trauma when placed in the LV.

TRANS-FEMORAL VALVE IMPLANTATION

Room Requirements

The trans-femoral TAVI can be performed in the cardiac cath lab or in the hybrid operating room. The room must be equipped with a fixed fluoroscopy unit that provides high image quality and the ability to store reference images for roadmapping. The room needs to be large enough to allow all operators to work comfortably and the circulators to move freely. A cardiopulmonary bypass machine should be accessible if complications arise. Equipment to treat vascular or coronary complications should be stocked in the room and available on demand.

Anesthesia

The procedure can be done under general anesthesia or conscious sedation.[85] General anesthesia is preferred if trans-esophageal echocardiography (TEE) is performed simultaneously during the procedure. If not, conscious sedation and local anesthesia may provide enough relief during the procedure. Continuous invasive hemodynamic monitoring should be used throughout the procedure. Vasopressor support should be used judiciously, as vasoconstrictors may interfere with the insertion and removal of the arterial sheath and predispose to vascular complications.

Infection and Anti-thrombotic Prophylaxis

To decrease the risk of infection of the prosthesis, measures to reduce infections are followed. Patients are given intravenous antibiotics (vancomycin or cefazolin) on call to the procedure room, and the medications are continued for 48 hours. Aspirin (160–325 mg) and clopidogrel (300 mg) are administered at least 24 hours before the procedure. After the procedure, clopidogrel 75 mg daily is continued for 1 to 6 months and daily aspirin (75 mg) indefinitely.

Venous and Arterial Accesses

In the ipsilateral leg, femoral arterial access is obtained for aortic angiography with a 5F or 6F pigtail catheter, and a venous sheath is inserted for RVP. The contralateral artery is cannulated percutaneously or by surgical cut-down. If accessed percutaneously, the contralateral artery can be preclosed with two suture-mediated devices (10F Prostar, Abbott Vascular, Illinois, USA).[86] If a surgical cut-down is performed, the common femoral artery should not be completely dissected in the posterior aspect, as sheath insertion is easier when the vessel is partially anchored. With the new-generation Edwards-SAPIEN XT device, preclosing with a single 10F device is regularly performed (see Fig. 50-2).

Aortic Angiography

Ascending aortic angiography is performed in a projection that places all of the aortic cusps in line and perpendicular to the image intensifier. Ideally, the projection is previously determined to minimize radiation and contrast exposures.

Temporary Pacemaker Placement

A ventricular stimulation lead such as the 6F Soloist lead (Medtronic, Minneapolis, MN, USA) is placed in the right ventricle. After testing for appropriate capture, a rapid ventricular pacing test is performed at a rate of 180 to 220 beats/min, as detailed in the section on BAV.

Crossing the Aortic Valve

Once the patient is anticoagulated with heparin and a therapeutic activated clotting time (ACT) is confirmed, the native aortic valve is crossed (as described earlier in the section on BAV) using an Amplatz AL-2 catheter and a straight guidewire. The previously shaped extra-stiff IA is then exchanged through the AL-2, and the catheter is withdrawn while the distal wire position is maintained in the LV. A pigtail catheter is advanced, and the valve gradient is then obtained.

Delivery Sheath Insertion

With the guidewire in the apex of the LA, the previously inserted 8F sheath is removed. Serial dilation of the femoral and iliac arteries are performed with arterial dilators of increasing size (16F–25F) (Edwards LifeSciences, Irvine, CA). The delivery sheath is then inserted and positioned in the descending aorta.

Balloon Aortic Valvuloplasty

Balloon aortic valvuloplasty is performed under RVP before TAVI with the same technique described previously. A 20-mm or 23-mm Retroflex balloon (Edwards LifeSciences, Irvine, CA) is used for placement of a 23-mm or 26-mm Edwards-SAPIEN prosthesis (Edwards LifeScience, Irvine, CA). The valve prosthesis should be ready to be inserted before the completion of the BAV in case severe aortic insufficiency and hemodynamic instability develop.

Valve Insertion and Deployment

The Edwards-SAPIEN prosthesis and the delivery system are then inserted in the sheath over the extra-stiff wire. Once the delivery system reaches the aortic arch, the Retroflex catheter is activated, allowing the safe passage of the delivery system across the aortic arch. The system is then advanced until it reaches the ascending aorta. In the pre-determined reference projection (aortic annulus perpendicular to the screen, the valve is positioned in the aortic position, maintaining a 60%:40% ratio of ventricular:aortic positioning. After confirmation of the appropriate location with angiography (and TEE, if available), the valve is deployed under RVP. The valve is deployed after the confirmation that the systemic blood pressure has reached and maintained its nadir. Balloon inflation is held 3 to 5 seconds before deflation, and RVP is then stopped to avoid traction on the prosthesis while the balloon catheter is being withdrawn. The RVP run generally does not last longer than 15 seconds. The delivery system is straightened and withdrawn. The trans-valvular gradient is measured, and paravalvular leaks are evaluated by angiography and echocardiography.

Sheath Removal and Arteriotomy Closure

The sheath is withdrawn with careful monitoring of blood pressure and simultaneous contrast administration through the pigtail catheter placed at the level of the iliac bifurcation. A precipitous drop in blood pressure or extravasation of contrast media indicates vascular rupture. This complication should be treated appropriately and expeditiously by using a covered stent or by surgical repair. Immediate tamponade of the ruptured vessel with the large sheath, closure of the iliac artery or abdominal aorta with a large size balloon, or both can be emergently performed before arterial repair. The arteriotomy site is then closed surgically or percutaneously with the previously placed preclosure device.

TRANS-APICAL APPROACH

The procedural steps of valve deployment are relatively similar to the trans-femoral route, so only the differences will be discussed here (see Fig. 50-3).[87] Femoral arterial and venous accesses are obtained for aortic root angiography and RVP, as previously described. A small left lateral thoracotomy is performed. The planes are dissected until the left ventricular apex is visualized. A purse string suture is placed in a muscular segment of the apico-lateral wall. Once the patient is anticoagulated and the ACT is therapeutic, a direct puncture of the LV is performed and a 7F or 8F sheath is inserted into the LV. A 0.035-inch J-tipped wire is then advanced through the valve into the descending aorta while being guided with a Judkins right (JR) curve catheter. The wire must be free of the papillary muscles or mitral chordal structures to avoid complications with the insertion of the delivery sheath. Once in the descending aorta, the wire is exchanged for an extra-stiff wire, the Amplatz 0.035-inch, 270-cm long guidewire (Cook, Bloomington, IA) and the JR catheter is removed. The sheath is exchanged for a 26F delivery sheath that is inserted 3 to 4 cm into the left ventricular cavity. Under RVP, a BAV is performed with a 20-mm Retroflex balloon. The Ascendra delivery system (Edwards LifeSciences, Irvine, CA) is advanced into the sheath and de-aired. The valve–catheter ensemble is advanced into the aortic position, maintaining a ratio of 50:50

aortic: ventricular positioning. After confirmation of the appropriate position with TEE and angiography, RVP and a patient breath-hold are initiated. The valve is deployed as blood pressure is at its nadir, and the balloon is deflated and withdrawn. Once the degree of aortal insufficiency is assessed and the valve position is confirmed with TEE, the ventricular sheath can be removed. If needed, the valve may be dilated thereafter. If no further intervention is needed, then the delivery sheath is removed, the puncture site repaired, and the anticoagulation reversed.[102] The thoracotomy is closed over a drain.

Results

The initial report of a successful percutaneous implantation of an aortic bioprosthesis in a patient with severe symptomatic AS who presented in cardiogenic shock in April 2002 was greeted with enthusiasm.[21] From 2003 to 2004, single-center registries were started under the names of Initial Registry of Endovascular Implantation of Valves in Europe (I-REVIVE) and Registry of Endovascular Critical Aortic Stenosis Treatment (RECAST) to document the feasibility of performing the procedure on a compassionate basis.[69] These registries used a 23-mm bioprosthesis made of equine pericardium mounted on a stainless steel balloon-expandable stent, and valve placement was primarily done via the antegrade (trans-septal) approach. Procedural success was achieved in 75%. The aortic valve area increased consistently from 0.6 cm^2 to 1.6 cm^2, and this was accompanied by a fall in mean trans-valvular gradient (37 mm Hg to 9 mm Hg), and an increase in left LVEF (45%+18% to 53%+14%). The 30-day mortality rate was 23%, and the 30-day major adverse cardiovascular and cerebrovascular event (MACCE) rate was 26%.[69] Patient survival was 63% by 6 months and was limited by the severity of patients' comorbidities. Moderate to severe perivalvular aortic insufficiency (63%) and valve embolization were procedural limitations caused by the availability of a single valve size. Because of venous distensibility, sheath insertion was not limited by vessel size, tortuosity, or the presence of peripheral vascular disease. Valve placement was simple, as the device crossed the smooth aspect of the aortic valve. However, the technique was challenging because of the need of a trans-septal puncture, the navigation of the catheter–valve ensemble across the mitral and aortic valves, and the guidewire interaction with the mitral valve and the subvalvular apparatus, contributing to poorly tolerated acute mitral insufficiency. All these problems limited the widespread use of this approach,

prompted technical improvements in the delivery system, and promoted the resurgence of the retrograde approach. This was followed by significant technical and prosthetic modifications to solve the previously encountered limitations. To reduce the degree of perivalvular regurgitation, valves were oversized in relation to the aortic annulus, and a second prosthesis size, 26 mm, became available. The transverse diameter of the aortic annulus at the level of the aortic leaflet insertion was identified for appropriate valve sizing. In addition, the necessary landmarks for valve positioning were recognized, decreasing the risk of valve embolization. A catheter with a manually activated deflectable tip (Retroflex™ catheter) aided in the atraumatic passage across the aortic arch and in the centering of the guidewire through the aortic commissures and facilitated valve delivery through the retrograde approach. Modifications in the delivery sheath also reduced vascular complications. Sheath length was increased to deliver the catheter–valve ensemble directly in the descending aorta, decreasing the risk of vascular injury.[72] Minimal arterial diameter, vessel tortuosity, and vessel calcification were still the major limiting factors. Multi-center registries from the United States (REVIVAL [TRanscatheter EndoVascular Implantation of VALves] II), European Union (REVIVE [Randomized Multicenter Evaluation of Intravenous Levosimendan Efficacy] II), and Canada (Canadian Special Access) included patients with a valve area less than 0.8 cm^2 and a high predicted operative mortality (logistic EuroSCORE >20%) to continue to evaluate procedural safety and efficacy. New valve modifications were added to improve long-term function. These included use of bovine pericardium, elongation of the skirt to decrease perivalvular insufficiency, and the addition of an anticalcification treatment, culminating in the prosthesis that is currently used. The series of retrograde implantation published by Webb showed initial procedural success of 78%, which increased to 96% after the first 25 cases, reflecting an important learning curve.[72,89] Observed 30-day mortality was 12%, whereas the expected 30-day mortality was 28%. At median follow-up, there was no evidence of valve deterioration, migration, re-stenosis, or valvular insufficiency. Moderate perivalvular leaks were seen in 3 cases at 1 month. Perivalvular aortic insufficiency was mild, clinically inconsequential, and stable during follow-up in the majority of patients. This information led to the approval and valve commercialization in Europe in the fall of 2007 (Tables 50-3 and 50-4). The trans-apical approach is the most recently developed form of trans-catheter AVR. Initial

TABLE 50-3	**Baseline and Follow-up Characteristics of Patients Undergoing Trans-catheter Aortic Valve Implantation with the Edwards-SAPIEN Valve**													
Study	Patients	Age (years)	Logistic Euroscore (%)	STS Score (%)	Procedural Success (%)	AVA Pre (cm^2)	AVA Post (cm^2)	Mean gradient Pre (mmHg)	Mean gradient Post (mmHg)	NYHA III/IV, Pre (%)	NYHA III/IV Post (%)	LVEF Pre (%)	LVEF Post (%)	Survival 1 year (%)
Canada[193]	339	81 + 8	NR	9.8	93.3%	0.63 + 0.17	1.55 + 0.41	46 + 17	10 + 4	90.9	NR	55+14	NR	76
SOURCE[94]	1038	81.2	27.4	NR	93.8	0.59	1.7	53.5	3.95	79.2	10	NR	NR	NR
PARTNER[99]	358	83.1 + 8	26.4 + 17.2	11.6 + 6	96.6	0.6 + 0.2	1.5 + 0.5	44.5 + 15.7	11 + 6.9	92%	16.7%	53.9	57.2	69.3

AVA, aortic valve area; *LVEF*, left ventricular ejection fraction; *NR*, not reported; *NYHA*, New York Heart Association classification.

TABLE 50-4	**Procedural Characteristics and Complications of Patients Undergoing Trans-catheter Aortic Valve Implantation with the Edwards-SAPIEN Valve**											
Study	Procedural Mortality (%)	30-Day Mortality (%)	Valve in Valve (%)	Conversion to open AVR (%)	AI > 2 + (%)	Major CVA/ TIA (%)	Major Vascular Complications (%)	MI (%)	Acute Kidney Injury (%)	Pacemaker (%)	Major Bleeding (%)
Canada TF[193]	1.8	9.5	2.4	1.2	6	0.6	13.1	0.6	1.8	3.6	NR
Canada TA[193]	1.7	11.3	2.8	2.3	6	0.6	13	1.7	3.4	6.2	NR
SOURCE[94] TA	NR	10.3	0.03	3.5	2.3	2.6	2.4	0.6	7.1	7	9.9
SOURCE[94] TF	NR	6.3	0.006	1.7	1.5	2.4	10.6	0.6	1.3	7	8.9
PARTNER[9]	1.1	5.0	1.7	0	12	5/0	16.2	0	1.1	3.4	16.8

AI, aortic insufficiency; *CVA*, cerebrovascular accident; *MI*, myocardial infarction; *NR*, not reported; *TIA*, transient ischemic attack; *TA*, trans-apical; *TF*, trans-femoral.

experience in an animal model has been able to be extrapolated to early human experience with promising results.[90,91] The first published data from Lichtenstein, consisted of 7 high-risk patients with AS.[90] Valve implantation was successful in all of them, and there were no procedural deaths. Improvement in the trans-valvular gradient and in the aortic valve area was seen in all patients, and the results were consistent with those found after retrograde implantation. Observed 30-day mortality was lower than the expected mortality (14% vs. 35%).[87,90] Published multi-center experience using this innovative approach has been growing. Walther et al reported on 93.2% successful implantations with a conversion rate to traditional AVR of 6.8%.[92] These high-risk patients had a median ICU stay of 20 hours. Trace to mild aortic insufficiency was seen in 23 patients. The 30-day mortality was 13.6%, whereas the predicted operative mortality was 26.8%. Use of extracorporeal circulatory support was frequent (47%) during the initial procedures; however, after familiarization of the technique, the rate of use dropped. Currently, prophylactic insertion of venous guidewires is operator dependent, but the use of extracorporeal circulation is rare. A recently published U.S.-based feasibility study noted a rate of 90% successful valve placements accompanied by persistent improvement in symptoms, valve area, mean gradient, aortic insufficiency, and quality of life (QoL).[93] Forty-seven percent of the patients were considered inoperable, and their mean STS score was 13.4%. Patient survival was 81.8% at 1 month, 71.7% at 3 months, and 58.7% at 6 months. MACCEs were seen in 65% and included 5% incidence of stroke, 2.5% need for emergent cardiac surgery, and 17.5% myocardial infarction (MI).

PARTNER European Registry

So far, the majority of short-term and mid-term TAVI data have come from European and Canadian registries. The PARTNER European Registry is one of three major registries of experience "outside the United States," using the Edwards-SAPIEN valve. Its primary safety endpoint was freedom from death from the index procedure to 30 days and 6 months. The primary efficacy endpoint was "hemodynamic status of the valve, QoL, and NYHA class improvement at 12 months after implantation." To be included in the registry, patients had to meet strict criteria for high surgical risk: a logistic EuroScore of greater than 20%, an STS score of 10% or more if the EuroScore was less than 20%, or both; and comorbidities such as porcelain aorta or chest deformities that precluded open-chest surgery. All patients had senile degenerative aortic valve stenosis with a documented aortic valve area less than 0.8 cm^2, a mean valve gradient of greater than 40 mm Hg, jet velocity by ultrasound greater than 4.0 m/sec, or all of them. Mean patient age was 82 years, and 84% and 85% of the trans-femoral and trans-apical groups, respectively, had NYHA class III and class IV heart failure. The EuroScore was 26 and 34 for the trans-femoral and trans-apical groups, respectively. Not surprisingly, the trans-apical cohort had greater comorbidities. After valve implantation, the mean aortic gradient fell to 10 mm Hg, and the aortic valve area rose to 1.6 cm^2. These values remained the same at 6-month and 1-year follow-up. The mean LVEF, reasonably well preserved at 54% before implantation, remained unchanged. Patients who survived to 1-year follow-up had a dramatic improvement of NYHA class (60% class I or II). To support this, quality-of-life (QOL) scores improved at 1 year by 23 points. At the 18-month follow-up, patients in the trans-femoral group had a 71% survival rate, whereas those in the trans-apical group had a 44% survival. It must be emphasized that comparisons between the trans-femoral and trans-apical groups are not appropriate because of the major differences in comorbidities between the two groups, especially the presence of peripheral vascular disease (a marker of more severe atherosclerotic disease and hence poorer outcomes) in the trans-apical group.

SOURCE Registry

The Source Registry (The Edwards-SAPIEN Aortic Bioprosthesis European Outcome), which included 1123 consecutive patients who underwent TAVI in 32 centers across Europe, was created for postmarketing surveillance. Seventy-two of the enrolling centers had no prior experience with the Edwards-SAPIEN valve and underwent structured training and proctoring. Procedural success was 93.8% with a 30-day mortality of 6.3%.[94] Single-center experience has noted a 30-day mortality of 3.6%.[95] At 30 days, functional improvement was dramatic (NYHA class I or II at baseline 19% vs. 86% at 30 days, $P < 0.001$), with mean survival of 74% at 224 days.[94] The symptomatic improvement persisted during follow-up. The mean trans-aortic gradient decreased from 46.1+ 6.7 mm Hg to 11.2 + 4.9 mm Hg at 1 year. The majority of patient mortality and hospital re-admission was not valve related. In addition, perivalvular aortic insufficiency remained constant during follow-up, and there was no structural deterioration of the valve. Overall complication rates have decreased since the original experience. Most recent data report major vascular complications in 8% of the trans-femoral implantations, need for hemodynamic support 0.9%, tamponade in 4%, permanent pacemaker in 4.4%, infection in 2.4%, and stroke in 5.3%.[94] (Table 50-4). Results from the SOURCE registry confirm a similar procedural success (92.7%) with conversion to open AVR in 3.5%.[94] Other complications included vascular injury in 3.6%, need for circulatory bypass in 3.6%, stroke in 1.8%, atrial fibrillation (AF) in 12% (see Table 50-4). Although vascular injury was less common in the trans-apical group, when present, it was associated with a higher mortality rate. Thirty-day and 1-year mortality rates are higher in the trans-apical group when compared with the trans-femoral group; however, this is likely caused by selection bias. Patients who undergo the trans-apical implantation are generally older, have a higher degree of comorbidities, and have a higher Euro-SCORE. In addition, the procedure is more invasive and has a steeper learning curve. To date, trans-femoral valve implantation is the default strategy and trans-apical implantation is only offered to those who do not qualify for the trans-femoral approach. Nonrandomized comparisons of patients undergoing surgical AVR versus trans-apical TAVI in high-risk patients show a similar operative mortality, similar 1-year survival, shorter ICU stay, and shorter duration of mechanical ventilation.[96,97] In general, the trans-apical approach is complementary to the trans-femoral approach, as a number of patients are not candidates for the trans-femoral approach because of the presence of peripheral vascular disease and would remain untreated, as up to 70% are not considered surgical candidates.[98]

Canadian Edwards-SAPIEN Registry

The Canadian registry of the Edwards-SAPIEN valve from 2005 to 2009 in six centers also had very encouraging results.[98] There were 339 high-risk patients (STS 9.8 ± 6.4) enrolled with 49.6% in the trans-femoral group and 50.4% in the trans-apical group. The procedural success was 93.3% with a 30-day mortality of 10.4%. Mortality was 22% at a mean follow-up of 8 months with peri-procedural sepsis, need for hemodynamic support, chronic kidney disease, and chronic obstructive pulmonary disease (COPD) as independent predictors of late mortality regardless of the approach. Patients with porcelain aorta and frailty had acute outcomes similar to the overall cohort, and patients with porcelain aorta had as good or better survival at 1-year follow-up.

FRANCE Registry

In November, 2009 the results of the FRANCE (French Aortic National CoreValve and Edwards) Registry were released from 19 sites. Patients in this registry had baseline demographics similar to the European PARTNER Registry, but patients in this registry received either the Edwards-SAPIEN valve or the Medtronic CoreValve.[146] Patients had severe aortic stenosis with valve areas less than 0.6 cm^2/m^2, NHYA class greater than 2, high surgical risk with Euroscore greater than 20% (STS >10%) or a contraindication for surgery. The primary endpoint was 30-day mortality, and secondary endpoints were up to 3-year mortality, major adverse cardiac events (MACEs), hemodynamics, and QoL analysis. The patients in this registry received either the Edwards-SAPIEN valve (trans-femoral 39%, trans-apical 29%) or the CoreValve (27% trans-femoral, 5% subclavian). Placement of the devices was accomplished in 97% of patients. Major complications of death at 30 days, stroke, vascular complications, and transfusions of greater than 1 unit occurred in 13%, 4%, 7%, and 21%, respectively. There were little differences in mortality, stroke, or vascular complications between the groups. However, the need for a new permanent pacemaker was considerably higher in the CoreValve group compared with the Edwards-SAPIEN group. At 6 months, 76.5% of the registry patients were alive, with mean valvular gradients of approximately 10 mm Hg. Eighty-six percent were in NHYA class 1 and 2.

PARTNER US

A US and Canadian multi-center randomized trial, Placement of AoRTic traNscathetER (PARTNER) US, whose primary endpoint is 1-year mortality, has completed patient enrollment, and data are being analyzed.[99] The trial, which includes patients with severe symptomatic AS who are poor surgical candidates, has two treatment arms. An arm powered for noninferiority analysis randomized 700 patients with an elevated surgical risk (STS score >10%) to traditional AVR or TAVI (trans-apical or trans-femoral); a second arm powered for superiority analysis randomized 358 patients with severe AS who were deemed inoperable to optimal medical treatment (including BAV) or TAVI. The results of the inoperable arm have been reported.[99] All-cause mortality (30.7% vs. 50.7%, $P < 0.001$), cardiovascular mortality (19.6% vs. 41.9%, $P < 0.001$), repeat hospitalization (22.3% vs. 44.1%, $P < 0.001$), and the composite endpoint of death or repeat hospitalization (42.5% vs.71.6%, $P < 0.001$) were seen less frequently in patients randomized to TAVI. During follow-up, there was no evidence of degeneration of the valvular prosthesis or of re-stenosis. Heart failure symptoms were less severe in patients treated with TAVI. Patients treated with TAVI had a higher incidence of major vascular complications (16.2% vs. 1.1%, $P < 0.001$), major bleeding (22.3% vs. 11.2%, $P < 0.001$), and major strokes (5.0% vs.1.1%, $P = 0.06$). In patients with severe AS who are not suitable for AVR, TAVI should be the new standard of care (see Table 50-4 and Table 50-5). The results of the high risk operative cohort are expected in 2011.

COMPLICATIONS

Stroke

The general incidence of clinically significant stroke is 2.5% to 4.2%.[90-95] It was originally postulated that the rate of cerebrovascular accident was going to be lower with the trans-apical approach, as the aortic arch was not manipulated; however, the incidence appears to be similar. Recent studies suggest a higher incidence of subclinical

perfusion abnormalities documented by magnetic resonance imaging (MRI).[100] Cerebral embolization can occur during the passage of the valve across the aortic arch during the attempt to traverse the aortic valve to gain access into the LA, during BAV and valve implantation. The use of cerebral embolic protection devices during TAVI is currently being evaluated.

Heart Block and Arrhythmias

Conduction abnormalities are commonly seen in patients undergoing TAVI. It is estimated that AF is seen in approximately 12% after transapical implantation. The incidence of conduction abnormalities in patients undergoing TAVI with the Edwards-SAPIEN prosthesis are complete heart block that requires a pacemaker (5.7%), left bundle branch block (12%), and first-degree AV block (15%).[101] The presence of a pre-existing right bundle branch block (RBBB) is a predisposing factor to pacemaker dependency. Conduction defects are transient when related to trauma to the conduction tissue; however, if there is myocyte necrosis in the interventricular septum, then new AV block will likely develop. With the CoreValve revalving system, the insertion depth into the left ventricular cavity and a smaller aortic annulus is associated with complete heart block.[102]

Renal dysfunction

Acute kidney injury after TAVI is not uncommon; it has an incidence of 12% to 28% and may progress to the need for renal replacement therapy in 1.4%. The presence of hypertension (odds ratio [OR] 4.66), COPD (OR = 2.64), and transfusion requirement (OR = 3.47) are important risk factors for its development. The presence of acute kidney injury is associated with mortality (28% vs. 7%).[103,104] When compared with surgery, acute kidney injury (9.2% vs. 25%) and the need for dialysis (2.5% vs. 8.7%) are less common in patients undergoing TAVI.[103]

Severe Aortic Insufficiency

Severe aortic insufficiency is a rare event. It may be categorized according to its etiology as valvular or perivalvular. The valvular (central) type is most commonly caused by the guidewire and disappears once the wire is removed. It is rarely caused by prosthetic malfunction or when the native leaflets interfere with prosthetic function. This is treated with placement of a new valve inside the previously placed valve. Perivalvular insufficiency is caused by (1) inappropriate sizing, (2) malposition, (3) stent underexpansion, or all. Valve dilatation after the procedure may be performed cautiously by adding 1 or 2 mL to the same balloon catheter, which must be centered within the valve. Since the stent has a skirt that does not allow further expansion,

TABLE 50-5	CoreValve Clinical Trials and National Registries								
Study	Number Patients	Number Centers	Age, years	Women, %	Logistic Euroscore, %	NYHA Class III/IV, %	LVEF %	Mean Gradient, mmHg	AVA, cm²
Feasibility study									
18F Safety/Efficacy[40]	126	9	81.9	57.1	23.4	74.6	51.6	46.8	0.72
Single center series									
Siegburg[107]	102	Single	81.8	52	24.5	95.1	51.0	41.6	0.64
Munich*[141]	137	Single	81.4	57	24.3	—	—	—	—
Catania[142]	129	Single	81	59	26	61.6	50.8	56.9	0.6
Bern Registry[189]	98	Single	82.1	56	24	—	—	—	0.7
National registries									
Australian[143]	62	9	83.7	48.4	18.7	80.7	58.7	46.4	0.8
Italian Registry[144]	772	14	82	56	22.9	70.6	51	52	NR
Belgian Registry[151]	141	6	82	56	25	78	59	49	0.63
Spanish Registry[145]	108	3	78.6	54.6	16	58.4	NR	55	0.63
French Registry[146]	78	16	82.5	51.5	24.7	NR	51	46	0.71
UK Registry*[147]	460	25	83	48	20.3	74	NR	NR	0.71
German Registry*[152]	588	22	81.4	55.8	20.8	88.2	52.1	48.7	0.64

AVA, aortic valve area; LVEF, left ventricular ejection fraction; NR, not reported; NYHA, New York Heart Association.
*Combined SAPIEN and CoreValve

postprocedure dilatation with a larger balloon will cause flaring of the aortic portion of the stent, changing the conformation of the ventricular portion worsening the aortic insufficiency.

Valve Embolization

Valve embolization is generally caused by malposition, undersizing of the prosthesis, or inappropriate capture during RVP. Valvular embolization to the left ventricular cavity is uniformly fatal. If aortic embolization occurs, it is imperative not to remove the guidewire from across the prosthetic valve until it is anchored in the distal aorta, as this prevents it from turning. A balloon catheter is placed in the proximal end of the valve, and the valve is then pulled until it can be deployed or fully expanded distal to the left subclavian artery. After the embolized valve is fixed, then a new valve can be placed in the aortic position when correcting the original cause of the complication. If the guidewire is removed before fixing the valve in place, the valve may become inverted, not allowing the passage of blood through it. Unless the valve can be opened with a stent or surgically, this complication is also uniformly fatal. Aortic angiography is recommended after valve manipulation, as the manipulation can cause aortic dissection.

Vascular Complications

Vascular complications occur in 6.6% of the cases. They more commonly occur with the trans-femoral approach (8% vs. 3.6%), but are more likely to be fatal with the trans-apical approach.[94] Vascular complications include small dissection, vascular perforation, and vessel avulsion. Prevention is important, hence the importance of vascular screening and the determination of the appropriate luminal diameter and absence of luminal calcification. Although previously associated with higher mortality, with increasing experience, vascular complications are easy to anticipate, which decreases mortality. They may arise from difficult sheath insertion, or prolonged sheath time, as the adluminal surface adheres to the endothelium. They are easily recognized by sudden onset of hypotension. Aortic occlusion balloons should be accessible to minimize bleeding when stabilizing the patient. Aortic root dissections may occur if the native valve is not appropriately predilated and the passage of the prosthesis is vigorous or may occur after attempts to capture an embolized valve. Aortic annular tear is seen in patients with a heavily calcified aortic root and can be avoided by limiting the degree of prosthesis oversizing.

Coronary obstruction

The Edwards-SAPIEN prosthesis is placed in the subcoronary position and should not interfere with the coronary ostia or future attempts at percutaneous revascularization.[105] Coronary obstruction occurs in 0.6% of the cases and is seen in patients with effacement of the sinotubular junction, which causes the coronary ostia to migrate.[95] The distance of the ostia to the aortic annulus is routinely determined by using CTA during patient screening. Coronary obstruction may be inconsequential if patients have functioning coronary artery bypass grafts. If occlusion occurs, emergency revascularization can be performed.

▦ CoreValve

Although surgical aortic valve replacement (AVR) is the preferred treatment for patients with symptomatic aortic stenosis, the surgical risk is substantial (13.3%) in patients with the highest decile of STS risk, and another 33% of patients are felt to have excessive surgical risk and are deemed "inoperable" by their primary care providers.[19,78,106] The CoreValve Revalving System has also been developed to address these high-risk and inoperable patients with aortic stenosis.[72,79,107–114]

THE COREVALVE REVALVING SYSTEM

Three generations of the CoreValve Revalving System (CRS) have been developed. The first-generation CoreValve comprised a 25F delivery catheter that housed a self-expanding Nitinol frame supporting a bovine pericardial valve.[107,115] The second-generation 21F delivery catheter used lower-profile porcine pericardial tissue and scalloped the inflow portion of the valve to provide better flow hemodynamics.[107,116–118] The current third-generation 18F CoreValve percutaneous aortic valve achieved its lower profile by cutting the skirt and leaflet into six independent sections and sewed these sections onto the Nitinol frame. The third-generation CoreValve device received Conformiteé Européenne (CE Mark) approval in March 2007 and has been used in over 10,000 implantations worldwide. The CRS comprises three components: (1) a self-expanding Nitinol support frame with cells configured in a diamond cell design, which anchors a tri-leaflet porcine pericardial tissue valve; (2) an 18F delivery catheter; and (3) a disposable loading system. CoreValve frames are currently available in 26-mm (for use with an aortic annular diameter between 20 mm and 23 mm) and 29 mm (for use with aortic annular diameters between 24 mm and 27 mm) sizes. The Nitinol frame was specifically designed for optimal functionality, stability, and durability (see Fig. 50-4) and has three levels of radial and hoop strength. The frame inflow exerts high radial expansive force to secure the frame within the aortic annular location. The strength of this portion of the frame prevents annular recoil and allows the frame to partially conform to the noncircular shape of the aortic annulus. In addition, it prevents frame migration and minimizes the occurrence of paravalvular leaks. The "constrained" center portion of the frame has high hoop strength that resists size and shape deformation, which is critical, as this portion of the frame contains the "supra-annular" valve leaflets. The frame is concave at this location to avoid the coronary ostium with the native valve and allows coronary cannulation after the implantation. The outflow portion of the frame exerts low radial forces and serves to orient the frame to the aorta parallel to flow through the valve. The porcine pericardium was selected for its lower profile (compared with the bovine pericardium) and its durability. The three leaflet elements that are constructed with long commissures, similar to a "suspension bridge," that more uniformly distribute the aortic pressure load to the valve leaflets and the commissural posts. An angled take-off of the posts further reduces stress and optimizes leaflet motion. The ability to maintain functionality in a nonround shape at the inflow is a critical feature of the CRS, as the constrained portion of the frame that supports the valve remains in a circular configuration. In a series of 30 patients in whom multislice CTA was performed after CoreValve placement, the difference between the smallest and the largest orthogonal diameters at the ventricular end was 4.4 mm but decreased progressively toward the outflow.[118] There was incomplete and nonuniform expansion of the CoreValve frame at the inflow, but the functionally important midsegment was well expanded and almost symmetrical (see Fig. 50-5).[119]

ANATOMIC–PATHOLOGIC FINDINGS AFTER COREVALVE IMPLANTATION

Histologic changes within the CoreValve frame have been documented in four patients with macroscopic and microscopic analyses, and 350 days after CoreValve implantation.[3,13,104,120] Fibrin deposition and inflammation occur early after CoreValve implantation, which is followed by neointimal coverage with progressive regression of the inflammatory response over time. Gross examination of the valve at 350 days showed neointimal tissue covering most of the frame struts in contact with the aortic wall, but areas of high velocity blood flow were bare. There was no excessive pannus formation occurring over the valve leaflet. No fractures of the nitinol frame struts have been found with angiographic imaging up to 2 years after the procedure.[121]

PATIENT SELECTION

Patients deemed "high risk" or "inoperable" for conventional AVR are ideally suited for TAVI, although, once screened, only a modest percentage of patients are actual candidates for percutaneous treatment.[122–124] A multi-disciplinary team generally reviews the clinical, anatomic, and vascular information for the individual patient before determining the candidacy for CoreValve placement. The following factors should be considered when selecting patients for CoreValve TAVI.

Clinical Criteria

Symptomatic patients with severe degenerative aortic stenosis who have substantial comorbidities that would impart a prohibitive risk to AVR would generally be acceptable candidates for CoreValve TAVI. Clinical contraindications to CoreValve placement include sepsis, including active endocarditis, recent MI or CVA, left ventricular or atrial thrombus, uncontrolled AF, or severe mitral, pulmonary, or tricuspid regurgitation. Patients with pre-terminal comorbidities that would shorten the life expectancy to less than 1 year would also not be candidates for TAVI. Relative precautions would include active gastritis or peptic ulcer disease, severe renal insufficiency (creatinine clearance <20 mL/min), uncontrolled bleeding diathesis, symptomatic carotid artery disease, or abdominal or thoracic aortic aneurysm. In the absence of demonstrable contractile reserve, an LVEF of less than 20% would also be a relative precaution to CoreValve placement.

Anatomic Criteria

The design of the CoreValve frame requires that there is careful evaluation of the aortoannular complex with imaging studies before the procedure. These anatomic factors are included in the CoreValve selection matrix (Fig. 50-6). TTE and TEE have been the primary noninvasive tools used to measure the aortic annular diameter before TAVI, but CTA is being used more frequently because of its ability to assess the true aortic annular area.[175-127]

Vascular Criteria

The 18F CoreValve Revalving System is advanced through an 18F sheath, requiring that the access vessel diameter is more than 6 mm. In the presence of severe calcification and vessel tortuosity, the access vessel diameter should be at least 7 mm. Although initial studies used aortography to select patients for CoreValve placement, more recent screening procedures have included CTA of the torso, including the ascending aorta and the descending aorta and the subclavian, iliac, and femoral vessels.[128] If there is focal iliac disease, percutaneous intervention may allow placement of the 18F sheath.[129]

PROCEDURE DESCRIPTION

The patient is pretreated with aspirin, clopidogrel, and antibiotic coverage, the last performed at least 1 hour before the procedure. Depending on the clinical status of the patient, either general anesthesia or conscious sedation is used. A temporary 5F pacing wire is positioned within the right ventricle. Arterial access is then obtained on the side contralateral to the planned 18F sheath for the CRS. As cannulation of the anterior common femoral artery is essential for successful percutaneous closure, both angiographically guided and ultrasound-guided methods have been used for arterial puncture (Fig. 50-7).[130] Once access has been obtained, anticoagulation is administered to achieve an ACT of 250 seconds or more. A graduated pigtail catheter is advanced to the ascending aorta, and the distal tip of the catheter is positioned in the noncoronary aortic cusp. The gantry position is optimized to allow visualization of all three coronary sinuses in the same plane, preferably in the LAO projection. An angiographic catheter is then advanced over a standard, J-tip guidewire through the primary access sheath and advanced to the ascending aorta. The J-tip guidewire is exchanged for a 0.035-inch straight-tip guidewire, which is used to cross the aortic valve. Once the guidewire is across the aortic valve, the catheter is advanced into the ventricle. A 0.035-inch superstiff or extra-stiff guidewire is advanced through the angiographic catheter and positioned in the apex of the left ventricle. Careful shaping of the distal portion of the wire prevents inadvertent perforation. Balloon valvuloplasty is then performed using an appropriately sized balloon under RVP. Balloon sizing should be directed to 1:1 sizing of the minimal annular diameter by CTA or echocardiography with maximum 25 mm balloon. After the valvuloplasty, the CoreValve device is advanced over the 0.035-inch guidewire and positioned across the native valve (see Fig. 50-7). Aortography is used to identify the most inferior aspect of the valvular plane. The CoreValve bioprosthesis is then positioned with the inflow portion within the aortic annulus (<6 mm below the annulus). The CoreValve device deployment then begins. As the inflow aspect of the device begins to flare outward, aortography is performed sequentially, and the final positioning is obtained. Once the CoreValve frame has been deployed, aortography is performed to assess the degree of residual stenosis within the frame and the degree of aortic regurgitation. The vascular sheath is then removed, and percutaneous or open closure is performed. The patient should be observed with temporary pacemaker placement in a cardiovascular ICU for up to 48 hours to monitor for conduction system disturbances. If these not are observed, the patient is monitored for an additional 72 hours and discharged. The patient is continued on the combination of aspirin and clopidogrel for 3 months after the procedure.

ALTERNATIVE VASCULAR ACCESS SITES

In patients whose peripheral vascular anatomy is unsuitable for the trans-femoral approach, the subclavian (or axillary) or trans-aortic access may be a useful alternative.[131-133] In a series of 54 cases treated

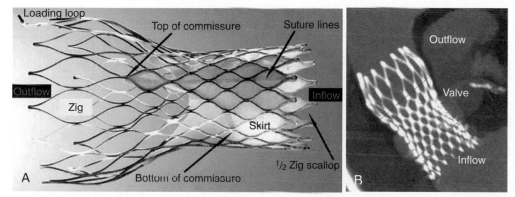

Figure 50-6 **A,** The components of the CoreValve frame. Reproduced with permission from Michiels R: Corevalve revalving systems for percutaneous aortic valve replacement. In Serruys PW, Piazza N, Cribier A, Webb JG, Laborde JC, de Jaegere P, editors: *Transcatheter aortic valve implantation: Tips and tricks to avoid failure,* New York, 2010, Informa Healthcase. **B,** Multi-detector computed tomographic angiography (CTA) imaging of the placement of the CoreValve frame in the aortic annulus and left ventricular outflow tract (*Inflow*), the constrained portion of the frame containing the supra-annular porcine pericardial valve (*Valve*) at the level of the origin of the coronary arteries, and the expanded portion of the frame in the aortic root (*Outflow*).

Diagnostic findings	Non-invasive		Angiography				Selection criteria	
	Echo	CT/MRI	LV	Ao Root	CAG	Vascular	Recommended	Not recommended
Atrialor ventricular thrombus	X						Not present	Present
Sub aortic stenosis	X	X	X				Not present	Present
LV ejection fraction	X		X				≥20%	<20% without contractile reserve
Mitral regurgitation	X						≤Grade 2	>Grade 2 organic reason
Vascular access diameter		X				X	≥6 mm diameter	<6 mm diameter
Aortic and vascular disease		X				X	None to moderate	Sever vascular disease
Indications for 26 mm CoreValve device								
Annulus diameter	X	X					20-23 mm	<20 mm or >23 mm
Ascending aorta diameter		X		X			≤40 mm	≥40 mm
Indications for 29 mm CoreValve device								
Annulus diameter	X	X					24-27 mm	<24 mm or >27 mm
Ascending aorta diameter		X		X			≤43 mm	>43 mm

General medical guidance for use CoreValve*

Diagnostic findings	Non-invasive		Angiography				Selection criteria	
	Echo	CT/MRI	LV	Ao Root	CAG	Vascular	Recommended	Moderate-high risk
LV hypertrophy	X	X					Normal to moderate 0.6-1.6 cm	Severe ≥1.7 cm
Coronary artery disease		X			X		None, mid. or distal >70%	Proximal lesions >70%
Aortic arch angulation		X				X	Large radial turn	Sharp turn
Aortic root angulation		X				X	<30 degrees	30-45 degrees
Aortic and vascular disease		X				X	No or light vascular disease	Moderate vascular disease
Vascular access diameter		X				X	>6 mm	Calcified and elongated >7 mm
Anatomic considerations for 26 mm CoreValve device								
Sinus of valsalva width	X	X		X			≥27 mm	<27 mm
Sinus of valsalva height	X	X		X			≥15 mm	<15 mm
Anatomic considerations for 29 mm CoreValve device								
Sinus of valsalva width	X	X		X			≥29 mm	<29 mm
Sinus of valsalva height	X	X		X			>15 mm	<15 mm

Figure 50-7   Anatomic criteria for recommended CoreValve placement.

via the subclavian approach in the Italian National Registry, procedural success was obtained in 100% of CoreValve cases.[134] There were no specific complications associated with the subclavian access, such as vessel rupture and vertebral or internal mammary ischemia, and there were no deaths at 30 days in this series. The 6-month mortality rate was 9.4%, not different from the rate for the trans-femoral approach. Caution must be exercised when selecting cases to ensure adequate vessel caliber, as the subclavian artery dissection and transient left arm paralysis have been reported by some.[135]

VALVE-IN-VALVE AND OTHER ANATOMIC CIRCUMSTANCES

The CoreValve Revalving System has also been used to treat degenerative bioprosthetic valves.[136–138] In the first-reported valve-in-valve procedure, the CoreValve Revalving System was used to treated a stenotic 21-mm aortic bioprosthesis.[137] The CoreValve has been successfully implanted in patients with prior mechanical mitral valve prostheses.[139]

CLINICAL SERIES

A number of single and multi-center registries have been reported following CoreValve implantation (see Table 50-6).[107,140–147] The feasibility and safety of the 18F CoreValve Revalving System was first evaluated in a prospective, multi-center Registry of implants at nine centers in Europe and Canada.[140] Inclusion criteria included age 75 years or above, surgical risk with logistic EuroSCORE 15% or more, or one or two high-risk comorbidities. Technical success (functionality with

absence of valve malfunction) at implantation was 83%. The 30-day mortality rate was 15.1%, and the 1-year mortality rate was 28.1%. No emergent cardiac re-interventions or nonstructural valve dysfunctions occurred after the 30-day visit. The 30-day mortality rate was 15.1% in this series. The Siegburg Heart Center reported its experience with the first-generation ($N = 10$), second-generation ($N = 24$), and third-generation ($N = 102$) CoreValve prostheses.[107] Patients were all deemed "high risk" for surgery (logistic EuroScore 23.1 ± 15%) with severe symptomatic aortic valve stenosis. The mean trans-valvular pressure gradient was 41.5 ± 16.7 mm Hg. The procedural success rate increased from generation 1 (25F) and 2 (21F) to 3 (18F) from 70% and 70.8% to 91.2%, respectively ($P = 0.003$). The 30-day combined rate of death, stroke, or MI was 40%, 20.8%, and 14.7%, respectively, for 25F, 21F, and 18F. There were no procedural deaths with the 18F device. Similar favorable findings following CoreValve implantation were reported by others.[141,148,149] In an expansion to the Siegburg series, which included patients treated in Bern, Switzerland, a total of 168 consecutive patients with symptomatic aortic valve stenosis were treated with CRS.[150] Patients were highly symptomatic with a NYHA class III or IV (93%) and a mean aortic valve area of 0.66 ± 0.21 cm². Acute and in-hospital procedural success rates were 90.5% and 83.9%, respectively, with an in-hospital mortality, MI, and stroke rate of 11.9%, 1.8%, and 3.6%, respectively. The pre-procedural Karnofsky (frailty) index was the only independent predictor of procedural success (OR 1.04, $P = 0.032$). A multi-center, expanded evaluation registry (EER) was established 1 year after the Certification of Experts (CE) mark of approval for marketing of the CoreValve TAVI in Europe.[79] A total of 646 patients with symptomatic severe aortic stenosis and logistic Euroscore 15% or more, or age 75 years or more, or age 65 years or more associated with

TABLE 50-6	Comorbidities in Patients Undergoing CoreValve Implantation											
Study	Diabetes, %	Prior MI, %	PVD, %	Porcelain Aorta, %	CRI, %	COPD, %	Liver/ Cirrhosis, %	Prior Stroke, %	Prior CABG, %	Prior PPM, %	CAD-Prior PCI, %
Feasibility study												
18F Safety/Efficacy[140]	26.2	24	19	10	55	29	—	28	26.2	7.9	65.9
Single center series												
Siegburg[107]	—	26.5	22.5	—	33.3	—	—	9.8	33.3	11.8	63.7
Munich*[141]	25	—	26	7	21.0	1.5	4	8	27	—	48
Catania[142]	—	21.3	7.9	16.5	24.4	20.5	1.6	6.0 (7.1)	9.7	10.2	30.8
National registries												
Australian[143]	21	30.6	14.5	—	19.4	19.4	—	19.4	27.4	16.1	24.2
Italian Registry[144]	27.5	20.7	20.7	—	—	—	—	7.5	15.2	9.1	48.2
Spanish Registry[145]	23.1	—	—	—	16.7	—	—	—	8.3	—	33.3
French Registry†[146]	33.3	21.2	4.5	—	—	—	—	12.1	22.7	—	42.4
UK Registry*[147]	23	—	23	—	—	—	—	—	—	23	44

CABG, coronary artery bypass graft surgery; CAD, coronary artery disease; COPD, chronic obstruction pulmonary disease; CRI, chronic renal insufficiency; MI, myocardial infarction; PCI, percutaneous coronary intervention; PPP, permanent pacemaker placement; PVD, peripheral vascular disease.
*Combined Edwards-SAPIEN and CoreValve.
†Trans-femoral groups only.

TABLE 50-7	Clinical Outcomes after CoreValve Implantation										
Study	Number Patients	Procedure Success, %	30-day Mortality, %	MI, %	Stroke, %	PPM, %	AR > 2+	Vascular Complications, %	Renal Failure, %	1-Year Survival, %
Feasibility study											
18F Safety/Efficacy[140]	126	83.1	15.1	—	9.6	28	6	9.5	—	71.9
Single center series											
Siegburg[107]	102	91.2	10.8	2	2.9	33.3	1.7	—	—	84
Munich*[141]	137	98.5	12.4	—	5.1	19.7	—	—	—	—
Catania[142]	129	96.2	6.9	0	3.9 (2.3)	25.6	—	13.9	—	—
Bern Registry[189]	98	98	7.1	1.4	—	30	—	—	—	—
National registries											
Australian Registry[143]	62	96.8	3.2	3	0	39	—	—	0	—
Italian Registry[144]	772	98.1	7.2	—	1.7	18.5	—	6.7	4.4	78.8
Belgian Registry[151]	141	98.0	9.0	—	4.0 (1.0)	23	—	—	7	79.0
Spanish Registry[145]	108	98.1	7.4	—	—	35.2	0	—	—	—
French Registry[146]	66	97.0	15.1	—	3.6*	26.9	0.5†	7.5	—	NR
UK Registry[147]	460	99.0	5.5	1.2†	4.0†	36	NR	3.9	—	81.6
German Registry[152]	588	98.7	12.4	—	2.5	42.5	2.5	16.9	—	—

AR, aortic regurgitation; MI, myocardial infarction; PPP, permanent pacemaker placement.
*Combined Edwards-SAPIEN and CoreValve.
†Transfemoral group only.

predefined risk factors, were included. The mean age was 81 ± 6.6 years, the mean aortic valve area was 0.6 ± 0.2 cm^2, and logistic EuroSCORE was 23.1 ± 13.8%. After valve implantation, the mean trans-aortic valve gradient decreased from 49.4 ± 13.9 to 3 ± 2 mm Hg. All patients had paravalvular aortic regurgitation less than or equal to grade 2. The rate of procedural success was 97%. At 30 days, the all-cause mortality rate (i.e., including procedural) was 8%, and the combined rate of death, stroke, and MI was 9.3%. A series of national registries have reported marked improvements in 30-day mortality rates compared with the initial 18F Safety and Efficacy Studies (Table 50-7).[143–147,151–152] These improvements can be attributed to both improved operator experience and better case selection.

VALVE PERFORMANCE AFTER COREVALVE IMPLANTATION

Sustained reduction in aortic valve gradients and improvements in effective orifice areas have been reported after CoreValve implantation (Fig. 50-8).[153] Improvement in aortic valve areas and reductions in mean aortic valve gradients have been sustained at 1-year and 2-year follow-up.[140,142] One series has shown an improvement in left ventricular function after CoreValve implantation.[154] In patients with an LVEF less than 50%, the LVEF improved from 37.3 ± 7.6 at baseline to

46 ± 11.3 after the procedure and to 51.4 ± 11 at late follow-up (P < 0.001). No worsening of mitral valve function has been reported after CoreValve implantation.[155] Regression of left ventricular hypertrophy has also been demonstrated after CoreValve implantation. In a series of 15 patients undergoing CoreValve implantation, there was a reduction in peak aortic gradient (76.6 ± 28.1 mm Hg to 16.3 ± 7.5 mm Hg; P < 0.001), mean aortic gradient (45.3 ± 18.4 mm Hg to 8.2 ± 3.7 mm Hg; P = 0.001), and septal wall thickness (1.54 ± 0.30 cm at baseline to 1.35 ± 0.27 cm at 1 month (P = 0.002).[156] Patient–prosthetic mismatch is an important predictor of outcome after traditional surgical AVR.[157] The indexed effective orifice area (EOA) was measured after CoreValve implantation in 74 patients with symptomatic severe aortic stenosis.[158] Patient–prosthetic mismatch was defined as severe (indexed EOA <0.65 cm^2/m^2) or moderate (indexed EOA 0.65–0.85 cm^2/m^2). The indexed EOA increased from 0.35 ± 0.13 to 0.97 ± 0.34 cm^2/m^2 after trans-catheter aortic valve implantation (P < 0.001) and was accompanied by significant clinical improvement. Severe and moderate patient–prosthetic mismatch were found in 16% and 23% of patients, respectively. Patients with severe patient–prosthetic mismatch were more symptomatic and had a smaller indexed EOA at baseline compared with those with moderate or no patient–prosthetic mismatch (0.28 ± 0.09 vs 0.36 ± 0.12 cm^2/m^2, P < 0.05). Functional status and mortality at 30 days and 6 months were not significantly different

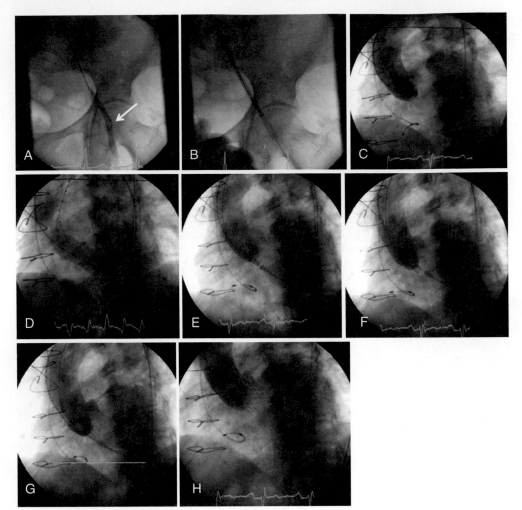

Figure 50-8 CoreValve aortic valve placement. A 5F pigtail catheter is advanced to the contralateral artery (*arrow*) to delineate the precise site of arterial puncture performed under fluoroscopy in the common femoral artery (*Panel A*). Using a "preclose" technique, the retraction of the four needles of the ProStar XL (Abbott Vascular, Santa Clara, CA) are visualized under fluoroscopy (*Panel B*). An arch aortogram is obtained preferably in the left anterior oblique (LAO) projection to demonstrate the simultaneous visualization of all three coronary sinuses in the same axial plane (*Panel C*). Balloon aortic valvuloplasty is then performed using rapid ventricular pacing (*Panel D*). The CoreValve device is then advanced across the aortic valve with careful positioning of the inflow portion of the frame just below the coronary sinuses (*Panel E*). The delivery sheath is then slowly withdrawn allowing the inflow portion of the frame to open and fixing in the aortic annulus (*Panel F*). The CoreValve is fully functioning once the sheath is withdrawn approximately two thirds of its length (*Panel G*). The CoreValve frame is then released. Final aortography shows a well-positioned frame and no paravalvular regurgitation (*Panel H*).

between the patients with severe patient–prosthetic mismatch and those with moderate or no patient–prosthetic mismatch.

IMPROVEMENTS IN QUALITY OF LIFE

A sustained improvement in NYHA classification has been shown after 12 to 24 months following CoreValve implantation.[140,142] In the 18F Safety and Efficacy Registry, the NYHA class improved at least by one class in 72% of subjects, and 18% had no change 2 years after the procedure ($P < 0.001$) (Fig. 50-9).[140] In a single-center series of 126 patients, improvement of QoL scores were demonstrated at 5 months and were sustained to 24 months after the procedure.[142] In a series of 30 patients with CoreValve implantation, QoL assessments and scales for physical and mental health 5 months after the CoreValve procedure.[159] There was an improvement in NYHA class at discharge and after 5 months. Pre-procedural evaluation showed a severe impairment of perceived QoL compared with the general population older than 75 years both for physical and mental scores, with a striking improvement in both scores after 5 months.[159]

MID-TERM AND LATE MORTALITY RATES

One-year survival rates after CoreValve placement range from 71.9% to 84% (see Table 50-6).[107,144,149,151] The majority of deaths occurred after 30 days, and most had noncardiovascular reasons.[151] Although the year survival rates were 59.7% in the 18 Fr Safety and Efficacy Registry,[149] survival rates were substantially improved (77.6%) in a more contemporary national registry.[149,160] A number of predictors of early

and later survival have been identified after TAVI.[161] Multivariable predictors of late survival include early (versus later) experience, no prior coronary bypass surgery, COPD, impaired renal function, cardiac decompensation, male gender, high American Society of Anesthesiologists (ASA) class, and a high logistic EuroScore.[142,162–164]

COMPLICATIONS

A unique series of complications has been reported after TAVI (see Table 50-6) and a refinement of traditional endpoints used for surgical aortic valve replacement was needed.[165,166] The Valve Academic Research Consortium (VARC) has developed standardized definitions for outcomes after TAVI, and these criteria will form the evidence base for studies in the future.

Strokes and Transient Ischemic Attacks

Stroke has been reported in approximately 5% of patients after traditional surgical AVR; similar stroke rates have been reported after CoreValve placement.[139] The etiology of CVAs after TAVI likely relates to the embolization of atherothrombotic material during advancement of the device to and across the aortic valve.[167] Microembolization demonstrated by MRI is common after TAVI, but clinical strokes are infrequent (2.9%–5.1%).[107,141,167–169] A more inclusive definition of stroke that includes transient ischemic attacks (TIAs) (<24 hours) with new structural defects on imaging studies may increase the reporting of this complication in contemporary series.[169,170] Novel embolic protection devices to protect the cerebral circulation are under development.

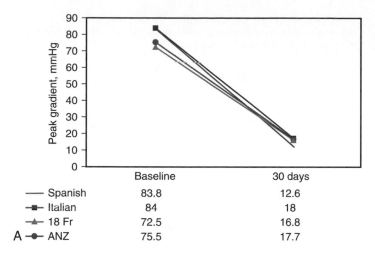

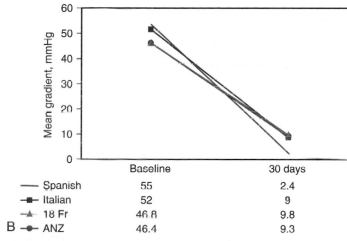

Figure 50-9 Improvements in mean (*Panel A*) and peak (*Panel B*) aortic valve gradients before and after CoreValve placement. (*Adapted from the Spanish Registry, the Italian Registry, the 18 Fr Safety and Efficacy Registry, and the Australian–New Zealand Registry.*[140,143–145])

Aortic Regurgitation

Determination of the etiology of aortic regurgitation after CoreValve placement is an important factor in determining both its significance and its treatment.[171] Significant aortic regurgitation caused by paravalvular leaks is uncommon after CoreValve TAVI and primarily relates to low positioning of the CoreValve frame, incomplete expansion of the frame into the eccentrically shaped annulus, rigidity of the underlying aortic annulus caused by calcification, or undersizing of the valve relative to the aortic annular size. When the CoreValve frame is underexpanded, post-deployment valvuloplasty may useful, and when the CoreValve frame is positioned too low after deployment, retraction of the frame loops using a retrieval snare may allow appropriate positioning within the annulus.[172–174] Higher degrees of post-implantation aortic regurgitation (≥2+) has been associated with a worse clinical outcome and include low cardiac output, respiratory failure, delirium, new left bundle branch block (LBBB), and in-hospital death.[125] Surgical aortic valve replacement has been successfully performed 4 months after CoreValve placement in one case with persistent aortic regurgitation.[175]

Vascular Access Complications

Because of the relatively large (18F)–caliber sheath required, vascular complications may occur during and after CoreValve placement. In a series of 91 consecutive patients who were treated with TAVI using the 18F Medtronic CoreValve System, vascular events were encountered in 13 patients (13%), and 7 of these (54%) were related to incomplete arteriotomy closure with the Prostar device.[176] Depending on how the major vascular complications were defined, the incidence varied from 4% to 13%.[176] Meticulous pre-procedural screening using CTA, the use of vascular ultrasound guidance for arterial access, and the use of alternative (e.g., subclavian) access have provided better case selection to avoid vascular complications.

Conduction System Disturbances

Aortic stenosis is commonly associated with latent and manifest conduction disease in the bundle of His and the tri-fascicular conduction system.[177,178] Conduction disease is more extensive with calcified valves and greater valve obstruction.[177] Owing to the location of the AV node and origin of the left bundle adjacent to the junction of the right coronary and noncoronary cusps, irritation of the membranous septum can affect AV conduction. Paired electrophysiologic studies in patients undergoing BAV showed that a new intraventricular conduction defect (QRS complex duration >100 milliseconds [ms]) or bundle branch block occurred in 5 of 13 patients who had normal QRS duration before the procedure.[179] In 4 patients, the newly acquired intraventricular conduction defect was still present on follow-up electrocardiogram (ECG) tracing.[179] Similarly, surgical AVR is associated with a nearly sixfold increased risk for permanent pacemaker placement compared with other cardiac operations.[180] In a series of 354 patients undergoing surgical AVR, 29 (8.5%) required early permanent pacemaker placement.[181] Preoperative conduction system disease was the only independent predictor of patient–prosthesis mismatch (P < 0.01); the relative risk (RR) of patient–prosthesis mismatch in this group was 2.88 (95% confidence interval [CI] 1.31–6.33).[181] Conduction disturbances and heart block occur in some patients after percutaneous aortic valve replacement (PAVR) with CoreValve.[182] In an initial series of 30 patients undergoing CoreValve placement, the incidence of new, postoperative conduction system disturbances diagnosed by 12-hour or 24-hour Holter monitoring was 68%.[103] LBBB occurred in 45.8% to 55%, and complete AV block requiring permanent pacemaker placement (PPP) occurred in approximately 20% of patients.[104] In another series of 30 patients who underwent CoreValve PAVR, 10 underwent permanent pacemaker implantation during the same admission (33.3%).[184] PPP was performed for prolonged high-grade AV block in 4 cases, episodic high-grade AV block in 5, and sinus node disease in 1.[184] The need for pacemaker was correlated to left axis deviation at baseline, and LBBB with left axis deviation (P = 0.002).[184] Baseline RBBB is an important predictor of the need for PPP.[182] It was also related to diastolic interventricular septal dimension on TTE greater than 17 mm (P = .045, r = 0.39) and the baseline thickness of the native noncoronary cusp (P = .002, r = 0.655).[184] Current attention to avoiding septal trauma during balloon valvuloplasty before CoreValve implantation and higher CoreValve placements (<6 mm below the sinus) may reduce the need for PPP after CoreValve PAVR.

Coronary Artery Occlusion

Coronary occlusion after CoreValve TAVI is a rare (<1%) occurrence. Multi-detector CTA has shown that the distance between the aortic annulus and the coronary arteries is reduced in patients with aortic stenosis, likely because of longitudinal remodeling of the aortic root in patients with degenerative aortic stenosis.[185] As the degenerative native aortic valve is not removed but is circumferentially displaced after TAVI, patients with a narrow sinus of Valsalva and low origin of the native coronary arteries may be predisposed to coronary occlusion from the displacement of the native valve during TAVI.[186] Coupled with the constrained CoreValve frame diameter in the region of the coronary ostia and better pre-procedural screening using aortography and CTA to ensure an adequate sinus of Valsalva width and height, the frequency of coronary occlusion is now rare. However, when it does occur on the rare occasion, rescue percutaneous coronary intervention (PCI) can be performed to re-establish coronary perfusion.[187]

Acute Renal Failure

Contrast aortography is required for CoreValve positioning, and post-contrast nephropathy may occur is some patients. In a series of 161 patients who underwent TAVI, postprocedural acute renal failure (ARF) was defined as an increase of greater than or equal to 25%, 0.5 mg/dL or more, or both in baseline serum creatinine within 48 hours after the procedure.[188] Baseline estimated glomerular filtration rate (eGFR) was 46.1 (43.5–48.7) mL/min/1.73 m^2 and chronic kidney disease (eGFR ≤60 mL/min/1.73 m^2) at baseline was present in 54% of patients. Postprocedural ARF occurred in 57 patients (35%), requiring dialysis in 23 of them. Multivariable analysis identified the use of the balloon-expandable prosthesis, trans-apical access, a prolonged procedure time, and pre-existing chronic kidney disease as independent predictors of postprocedural ARF. Compared with patients without ARF, those with ARF had a markedly higher 30-day mortality (25% vs. 8%, $P = 0.004$).[188]

PLANNED INVESTIGATIONS

USA CoreValve Pivotal Trial

The planned USA CoreValve Pivotal Trial will examine the safety and efficacy of the CoreValve Revalving System in two cohorts of patients. The first cohort comprised those deemed "extreme risk" or "inoperable" for sAVR, based on an estimated 30-day risk for mortality or substantial morbidity greater than 50%. A total of 487 patients designated "extreme risk" for surgery will be evaluated against a prospectively defined performance goal using the primary endpoint of 12-month all-cause mortality or major stroke. A second cohort of 790 patients will be assessed for the noninferiority of CoreValve treatment compared with traditional surgical AVR in patients with "high risk" for sAVR as determined by an estimated risk of 30-day mortality greater than 15%. "High-risk" patients will be randomized in a 1:1 fashion to CoreValve placement or conventional AVR. The primary endpoint will be 12-month all-cause mortality. An additional registry of up to 100 "extreme-risk" patients who are treated using a subclavian–axillary or trans-aortic access will also be evaluated.

SURTAVI

SURTAVI (Surgical Replacement And Transcatheter Aortic Valve Implantation), a multi-center randomized clinical study primarily based in Europe, will evaluate the safety and efficacy of CoreValve TAVI compared with surgical AVR in a broader patient population, including those patients with "intermediate" risk for surgical AVR. This study will use a "heart team" approach, where the interventional cardiologist and surgeon will collaborate to determine patient eligibility and inclusion and will randomize patients to TAVI or AVR.

ADVANCE

The CoreValve ADVANCE trial will study long-term and real world impact of TAVI therapy on a broad population basis. The ADVANCE Registry is a prospective, observational international postmarket study to evaluate clinical outcomes of patients with severe AS who are treated with CoreValve implantation. Approximately 1000 patients with severe AS will be enrolled in the study at up to 90 clinical trial sites in countries where the CoreValve system is commercially available. Patients will be followed up for at least 5 years after the implantation. The primary endpoint is MACCEs at 30 days after the procedure.

ADVANCE-II

The ADVANCE II will enroll just over 100 patients in 7 to 10 experienced CoreValve European sites in an effort to characterize implantation procedures at the best European practices. Enrollment will start in early fall 2010. The Registry will focus on documenting the intermediate-term outcomes in these high-risk patients and define "best practice" event rates, including 30-day and 1-year mortality, stroke, vascular complications, aortic regurgitation, and the development of conduction disturbance requiring PPP.

Other Prostheses

Second-generation trans-catheter aortic valve prototypes such as the Lotus117 (Sadra Medical, Saratoga, CA), AorTx (Palo Alto CA), Jenna Valve, Direct Flow (Santa Rosa, CA), and Paniagua valves have been used in first-in-human implantations.[190,191] Their availability will depend on the result of initial feasibility registries and how they perform against the older-generation devices.

Future Directions

The use of a catheter-based valve implantation to treat bioprosthetic valve dysfunction is an attractive procedure, as it would simplify the surgical procedure, reduce the need for cardiopulmonary bypass, and potentially decrease surgical risk and the need for long-term oral anticoagulation. With the ease of trans-femoral and trans-apical accesses, valve-in-valve procedures can be performed on any position as long as the catheter valves can be sized appropriately and valve positioning can be done without interference from the valvular struts. Initial data have provided encouraging results and may modify our approach to these patients if appropriate prosthetic function is seen in long-term follow-up.[192] Future modification of the prosthetic material and design will generate catheter-based valve implantation systems that are fully repositionable, require smaller delivery systems, and eradicate the presence of perivalvular insufficiency. New stent anchoring systems may be developed to treat aortic insufficiency as well. Work is currently in progress in the development of embolic protection devices to decrease the risk of peri-procedural embolic events generated by the passage of the catheter valve or guidewire across the aortic arch. As longer follow-up data are accrued in patients treated with TAVI, the questions of in vivo prosthetic durability and clinical consequences of chronic perivalvular insufficiency will be answered. The results of the PARTNER trial are anxiously awaited, as this may lead to future trials aimed at lower-risk patients or patients with low-gradient AS. TAVI has the potential of changing our approach to valvular surgery and prosthetic selection.

Conclusion

Catheter-based treatment of aortic stenosis is improving. With the development of TAVI, re-stenosis after valvuloplasty has been overcome. Mid-term and long-term follow-up of patients treated with TAVI is slowly becoming available, and as more patients reach significant milestones and valve durability is confirmed, indications for TAVI may be expanded. Successful TAVI will depend on patient selection, and cooperation among cardiac surgeons, interventional cardiologists, anesthesiologists, and all the individuals who participate in the care of these frail patients. Centers interested in performing TAVI will need specific training in this procedure in addition to a commitment to have on hand appropriate imaging equipment and personnel required to perform the procedures safely. A concerted effort from industry, physicians, and the governing medical bodies must take place to facilitate diffusion in a safe and effective manner. Patient selection for AVR, TAVI, BAV, or palliative care is becoming more complex. Special attention must be paid to the patient's best interests, safety, and treatment durability. Surgical AVR still is the treatment of choice for patients with severe symptomatic AS; however, in the inoperable or high-risk patient, TAVI may become a reality.

Disclosures

Dr. Cribier is a consultant for Edwards LifeScience. Dr. Popma receives research grants from Medtronic.

REFERENCES

1. Lindroos M, Kupari M, Heikkila J, et al: Prevalence of aortic valve abnormalities in the elderly: An echocardiographic study of a random population sample. *J Am Coll Cardiol* 21:1220–1225, 1993.
2. Ross JR, Braunwald E: Aortic stenosis. *Circulation* 38(1Suppl):61–67, 1968.
3. Varadarajan P, Kapoor N, Bansal RC, et al: Clinical profile and natural history of 453 nonsurgically managed patients with severe aortic stenosis. *Ann Thorac Surg* 82:2111–2115, 2006.
4. Edwards FH, Peterson ED, Coombs LP, et al: Prediction of operative mortality after valve replacement surgery. *J Am Coll Cardiol* 37:885–892, 2001.
5. Society of Thoracic Surgeons: STS national database: STS U.S. Cardiac Surgery Database: 1997. Aortic valve replacement patients: Preoperative risk variables: Chicago: Society of Thoracic Surgeons, 2000: Available at http://www.ctsnet.org/doc/3031: Accessed September 16, 2011.
6. Otto C: Valvular aortic stenosis: Disease severity and timing of intervention. *J Am Coll Cardiol* 47:2141–2151, 2006.
7. Iung B, Baron G, Butchart EG, et al: A prospective survey of patients with valvular heart disease in Europe: The Euro Heart Survey on Valvular Heart Disease. *Euro Heart J* 24:1231–1243, 2003.
8. Cribier A, Savin T, Saoudi N, et al: Percutaneous transluminal valvuloplasty in acquired aortic stenosis in elderly patients: An alternative to valve replacement? *Lancet* 1:63–67, 1986.
9. Schwarz F, Baumann P, Manthey J, et al: The effect of aortic valve replacement on survival. *Circulation* 66:1105–1110, 1982.
10. Kohl P, Kerzman A, Lahaye L: Cardiac surgery in octogenarians. Peri-operative outcome and long-term results. *Eur Heart J* 22:1235–1243, 2001.
11. Bridges CR, Edwards FH, Peterson ED: Cardiac surgery in nonagenarians and centenarians. *J Am Coll Surg* 197:347–357, 2003.
12. Chukwuemeka A, Borger MA, Ivanov J, et al: Valve surgery in octogenarians: A safe option with good medium term results. *J Heart Valve Dis* 15:191–196, 2006.
13. Connolly HM, Oh JK, Schaff HV, et al: Severe aortic stenosis with low transvalvular gradient and severe left ventricular dysfunction: Result of aortic valve replacement in 52 patients. *Circulation* 101:1940–1946, 2000.
14. Tarantini G, Buja P, Scognamiglio R, et al: Aortic valve replacement in severe aortic stenosis with left ventricular dysfunction. Determinants of cardiac mortality and ventricular function recovery. *Eur J Cardio-Thorac Surg* 24:879–885, 2003.
15. Vaquette B, Corbineau H, Laurent M, et al: Valve replacement in patients with critical aortic stenosis and depressed left ventricular function: Predictors of operative risk, left ventricular function recovery, and long term outcome. *Heart* 91:1324–1329, 2005.
16. Kapoor N, Varadajan P, Pai R: Survival patterns in conservatively treated patients with severe aortic stenosis: Prognostic variables in 457 patients. *Circulation* 110(Suppl III):548, 2004.
17. O'Neill WW: Predictors of long term survival after percutaneous aortic valvuloplasty: Report of the Mansfield scientific balloon aortic valvuloplasty registry. *J Am Coll Cardiol* 17:193–198, 1991.
18. NHLBI Balloon Valvuloplasty Registry: Percutaneous balloon aortic valvuloplasty: Acute and 30-day follow-up results in 674 patients from the NHLBI Balloon Valvuloplasty Registry. *Circulation* 84:2383–2397, 1991.
19. Bonow RO, Carabello BA, Chatterjee K, et al. ACC/AHA 2006 guidelines for the management of patients with valvular heart disease: A report of the American College of Cardiology/American Heart Association Task Force on Practice Guidelines (Writing Committee to Develop Guidelines for the Management of Patients with Valvular Heart Disease). American College of Cardiology Web Site: Available at http//www.acc.org/clinical/guidelines/valvular.index.pdf: Accessed September 16, 2010.
20. Kawachi Y, Nakashima A, Toshima Y, et al: Risk stratification analysis of operative mortality in heart and thoracic aorta surgery: Comparison between Parsonnet and EuroSCORE additive model. *Eur J Cardiothorac Surg* 20:961–966, 2001
21. Cribier A, Eltchaninoff H, Bash A, et al: Percutaneous transcatheter implantation of an aortic valve prosthesis for calcific aortic stenosis: First human case description. *Circulation* 106:3006–3008, 2002.
22. Letac B, Cribier A, Koning R, et al: Results of percutaneous transluminal valvuloplasty in 218 patients with valvular aortic stenosis. *Am J Cardiol* 62.1241–1247, 1988.
23. Letac B, Cribier A, Koning R, et al: Aortic stenosis in elderly patients aged 80 or older: Treatment by percutaneous balloon valvuloplasty in a series of 92 cases. *Circulation* 80:1514–1520, 1989.
24. Berland J, Cribier A, Savin T, et al: Percutaneous balloon valvuloplasty in patients with severe aortic stenosis and low ejection fraction: Immediate results and 1-year follow-up. *Circulation* 79:1189–1196, 1989.
25. Letac B, Cribier A, Eltchaninoff H, et al: Evaluation of restenosis after balloon dilation in adult aortic stenosis by repeat catheterization. *Am Heart J* 122:55–60, 1991.
26. Koning R, Cribier A, Asselin C, et al: Repeat balloon aortic valvuloplasty. *Catheter Cardiovasc Diagn* 26:249–254, 1992.
27. Eltchaninoff H, Cribier A, Tron C, et al: Balloon aortic valvuloplasty in elderly patients at high risk for surgery, or inoperable: Immediate and mid-term results. *Eur Heart J* 16:1079–1084, 1995.
28. Agatiello C, Eltchaninoff H, Tron C, et al: Balloon aortic valvuloplasty in the adult. Immediate results and in-hospital complications in the latest series of 141 consecutive patients at the University Hospital of Rouen (2002–2005). *Arch Mal Coeur* 99:195–200, 2006.
29. Litvack F, Jakubowski AT, Butchbinder NA, et al: Lack of sustained clinical improvement in an elderly population after percutaneous aortic valvuloplasty. *Am J Cardiol* 62:270–275, 1988.
30. Lieberman EB, Bashore TM, Hermiller JB, et al: Balloon aortic valvuloplasty in adults: Failure of procedure to improve long term survival. *J Am Coll Cardiol* 26:1522–1528, 1995.
31. Dare AJ, Veinot JP, Edwards WD, et al: New observations on the etiology of aortic valve disease: a surgical pathologic study of 236 cases from 1990. *Hum Path* 24:1330–1338, 1993.
32. Roberts WC, Ko JM: Frequency by decades of unicuspid, bicuspid, and tricuspid aortic valves in adults having isolated aortic valve replacement for aortic stenosis, with or without associated aortic regurgitation. *Circulation* 111:920–925, 2005.
33. Freeman R, Otto C. Spectrum of calcific aortic valve disease: Pathogenesis, disease progression, and treatment strategies. *Circulation* 111:3316–3326, 2005.
34. O'Brien KD: Pathogenesis of calcific aortic valve disease. A disease process comes of age (and a good del more). *Arterioscler Thromb Vasc Biol* 26:1721–1728, 2006.
35. Inoue K, Owaki T, Nakamura T, et al: Clinical application of transvenous mitral commissurotomy by a new balloon catheter. *J Thorac Cardiovasc Surg* 87:394–402, 1984.
36. Letac B, Gerber L, Koning R: Insight in the mechanism of balloon aortic valvuloplasty of aortic stenosis. *Am J Cardiol* 62:1241–1247, 1988.
37. Lembo NJ, King SB, Roubin GS: Fatal aortic rupture during percutaneous balloon valvuloplasty for valvular aortic stenosis. *Am J Cardiol* 60:733–737, 1987.
38. Letac B, Cribier A, Eltchaninoff H, et al: Evaluation of restenosis after balloon dilation in adult aortic stenosis by repeat catheterization. *Am Heart J* 122:55–60, 1991.
39. Bashore TM, Davidson CJ, and the Mansfield Scientific Aortic Valvuloplasty Registry Investigators: Follow-up recatheterization after balloon aortic valvuloplasty. *J Am Coll Cardiol* 17:1181–1195, 1991.
40. Feldman T, Glagov S, Caroll J: Restenosis following successful balloon valvuloplasty: Bone formation in aortic valve leaflets. *Catheter Cardiovasc Interv* 29:1–7, 1993.
41. Feldman T, Glagov S, Caroll J: Restenosis following successful balloon valvuloplasty: Bone formation in aortic valve leaflets. *Catheter Cardiovasc Interv* 29:1–7, 1993.
42. van den Brand M, Essed CE, Di Mario C, et al: Histological changes in the aortic valve after balloon dilation: Evidence for a delayed healing process. *Br Heart J* 67:445–449, 1992.
43. Soyer R, Bouchart F, Bessou JP, et al: Aortic valve replacement after aortic valvuloplasty for calcified aortic stenosis. *Eur J Cardio-Thorac Surg* 10.977–982, 1996.
44. Agarwal A, Kini AS, Attani S, et al: Results of repeat balloon valvuloplasty for treatment of aortic stenosis in patients aged 59 to 104 years. *Am J Cardiol* 95:43–47, 2005.
45. Lababidi Z, Wu JR, Walls JT: Percutaneous balloon aortic valvuloplasty: Results in 23 patients. *Am J Cardiol* 53:194–197, 1984.
46. Block PC, Palacios IF: Comparison of hemodynamic results of antegrade versus retrograde percutaneous balloon aortic valvuloplasty. *Am J Cardiol* 60:659–662, 1987.
47. Orme EC, Wray RB, Barry WH, et al: Comparison of three techniques for percutaneous balloon aortic valvuloplasty of aortic stenosis in adults. *Am Heart J* 117:11–17, 1989.
48. Sakata,Y, Syed Z, Salinger M, et al: Percutaneous balloon aortic valvuloplasty : antegrade transseptal vs conventional retrograde transarterial approach. *Catheter Cardiovasc Interv* 64:314–321, 2005.
49. Rutgers D, Bots ML, Hofman A, et al: Peripheral arterial disease in the elderly, the Rotterdam study. *Aterioscler Thromb Vasc Biol* 18:185–192, 1998.
50. Gorlin R. Gorlin SG: Hydraulic formula for calculations of the area of the stenotic mitral valve, other cardiac valves, and central circulatory shunts. *Am Heart J* 41:1–29, 1951.
51. McKay RG: The Mansfield Scientific Aortic Valvuloplasty Registry: Overview of acute hemodynamic results and procedural complications. *J Am Coll Cardiol* 17:485–491, 1991.
52. Omram H, Schmidt H, Hackenbroch M, et al: Silent and apparent cerebral embolism after retrograde catheterization of the aortic valve in valvular stenosis: A prospective, randomized study. *Lancet* 361:1241–1244, 2003.
53. Rosengart TK, Finnin EB, Kim DY, et al: Open heart surgery in the elderly: Results from a consecutive series of 100 patients aged 85 years or older. *Am J Med* 112:143–147, 2002.
54. Conti V, Lick S: Cardiac surgery in the elderly: Indications and management options to optimize outcomes. *Clin Geriatr Med* 22:559–574, 2006.
55. Monin JL, Quere JPM, Monchi M, et al: Low-gradient aortic stenosis: Operative risk stratification and predictors for long-term outcome: A multicenter study using dobutamine stress hemodynamics. *Circulation* 108:319–324, 2003.
56. Dauterman KW, Michaels AD, Ports TA: Is there any indication for aortic valvuloplasty in the elderly? *Am J Geriatr Cardiol* 12:190–196, 2003.
57. Feldman T: Proceedings of the TCT: Balloon aortic valvuloplasty appropriate for elderly valve patients. *J Interv Cardiol* 19:276–279, 2006 .
58. Davies H: Catheter mounted valve for temporary relief of aortic insufficiency. *Lancet* 1:250, 1965.
59. Moulopoulos SD, Anthopoulos L, Stamatelopoulos S, et al: Catheter mounted aortic valves. *Ann Thorac Surg* 11:423–430, 1971.
60. Phillips SJ, Ciborski M, Freed PS, et al: A temporary catheter-tip aortic valve: Hemodynamic effects for experimental relief of acute aortic insufficiency. *Ann Thorac Surg* 21:134–137, 1976.
61. Matsubara T, Yamazoe M, Tamura Y, et al: Balloon catheter with check valves for experimental relief of acute aortic regurgitation. *Am Heart J* 124:134–137, 1992.
62. Andersen HR, Knudsen LL, Hasenkam JM: Transluminal implantation of artificial heart valves. Description of a new expandable aortic valve and initial results with implantation by catheter technique in closed chest pigs. *Eur Heart J* 13:704–708, 1992.
63. Bonhoeffer P, Boudjemline Y, Saliba Z, et al: Transcatheter implantation of a bovine valve in a pulmonary position: A lamb study. *Circulation* 102:813–816, 2000.
64. Bonhoeffer P, Boudjemline Y, Saliba Z, et al: Percutaneous replacement of pulmonary valve in a right-ventricle to pulmonary-artery conduit with valve dysfunction. *Lancet* 356:1403–1405, 2000.
65. Cribier A, Eltchaninoff H, Letac B: Advances in percutaneous techniques for the treatment of aortic and mitral stenosis. In Topol EJ, editor: *Textbook of Interventional cardiology*, ed 4, Philadelphia, 2003, Saunders.
66. Eltchaninoff H, Nusimovici-Avadis D, Babaliaros V, et al: Five month study of percutaneous heart valves in the systemic circulation of sheep using a novel model of aortic insufficiency. *EuroIntervention* 1:438–444, 2006.
67. Cribier A, Eltchaninoff H, Tron C, et al: Early experience with percutaneous transcatheter implantation of heart valve prosthesis for the treatment of end-stage inoperable patients with calcific aortic stenosis. *J Am Coll Cardiol* 43:698–703, 2004.
68. Bauer F, Eltchaninoff H, Tron C, et al: Acute improvement in global and regional left ventricular systolic function after percutaneous heart valve implantation in patients with symptomatic aortic stenosis. *Circulation* 110:1473–1476, 2004.
69. Cribier A, Eltchaninoff H, Tron C, et al. Treatment of calcific aortic stenosis with the percutaneous heart valve. Mid-term follow up from the initial feasibility studies. *The French experience* 47(6):1214–1223, 2006.
70. Hanzel GS, Harrity PJ, Schreiber TL, et al: Retrograde percutaneous aortic valve implantation for critical aortic stenosis. *Catheter Cardiovasc Interv* 64:322–326, 2005.
71. Webb GW, Chandavimol M, Thompson CR, et al: Percutaneous aortic valve implantation retrograde from the femoral artery. *Circulation* 113:842–850, 2006.
72. Grube E, Laborde JC, Gerckens U, et al: Percutaneous implantation of the CoreValve self expanding valve prosthesis in high risk patients with aortic valve disease. *Circulation* 114:1616–1624, 2006.
73. Collart F, Feier H, Kerbaul F, et al: Valvular surgery in octogenarians: Operative risk factors, evaluation of Euroscore and long term results. *Eur J Cardiothorac Surg* 27:276–280, 2005.
74. Roques F, Michel P, Goldstone AR, et al: The logistic Euroscore. *Eur Heart J* 24:882–883, 2003.
75. Pinna-Pintor P, Bobbio M, Colangelo S, et al: Inaccuracy of four coronary risk adjusted models to predict mortality in individual patients. *Euro J Cardio Thorac Surg* 21:199–204, 2002.
76. Gossi EA, Schwartz CF, Yu PJ, et al: High risk aortic valve replacement: Are the outcomes as bad as predicted? *Ann Thorac Surg* 85:102–107, 2008.
77. Shroyer AL, Coombs LP, Peterson E, et al: The Society of Thoracic Surgeons. 30-day operative mortality and morbidity risk models. *Ann Thorac Surg* 75:1856–1865, 2003.
78. Dewey TM, Brown D, Ryan W, et al: Reliability of risk algorithms in predicting early and late operative outcomes in high risk patients undergoing aortic valve replacement. *J Thorac Cardiovasc Surg* 135:180–187, 2008.
79. Piazza N, Grube E, Greckens U, et al: Procedural and 30 day outcomes following transcatheter aortic valve implantation using the third generation (18Fr) CoreValve revalving system: Results from the multicenter, expanded evaluation registry 1-year following CE mark approval. *EuroIntervention* 4:242–249, 2008.
80. Fraccaro C, Napodano M, Tarantini G, et al: Expanding the eligibility for transcatheter aortic valve implantation the trans-subclavian retrograde approach using the III generation CoreValve revalving system. *JACC Cardiovasc Interv* 2:828–833, 2009.
81. Masson JB, Kovac J, Schuler G, et al: Transcatheter aortic valve implantation: A review of the nature, management, and avoidance of procedural complications. *JACC Cardiovasc Interv* 2:811–820, 2009.

82. Eltchaninoff E, Kerkeni M, Zajarias A, et al: Aorto-iliac angiography as a screening tool in selecting patients for transfemoral aortic valve implantation with Edwards SAPIEN bioprosthesis, *EuroIntervention* 5:438–442, 2009.
83. Joshi SB, Mendoza DD, Steinberg DH, et al: Ultra-low-dose intra-arterial contrast injection for iliofemoral computed tomographic angiography. *JACC Cardiovasc Imaging 2009.* 2:1404, 2009.
84. Clavel MA, Webb JG, Pibarot P, et al: Comparison of the hemodynamic performance of percutaneous and surgical bioprosthesis for the treatment of severe aortic stenosis. *J Am Coll Cardiol* 53:1883–1891, 2009.
85. Covello RD, Ruggeri L, Landoni G, et al: Transcatheter implantation of an aortic valve: Anesthesiological management. *Minerva Anestesiol* 76:100–108, 2010.
86. Sharp AS, Michev F, Taramasso M, et al: A new technique for vascular access management in transcatheter aortic valve implantation. *Catheter Cardiovasc Interv* 75:784–793, 2010.
87. Ye J, Cheung A, Lichtenstein AV, et al: Six month outcome of transapical aortic valve implantation in the initial seven patients. *Euro J Cardiothorac Surg* 31:16–21, 2007.
88. Dumont E, Rodes-Cabau J, De La Rochelliere R, et al: Rapid pacing technique for preventing ventricular tears during transapical aortic valve implantation. *J Card Surg* 24:295–298, 2009.
89. Webb JG, Pasupati S, Humphries K, et al: Percutaneous aortic valve replacement in selected high risk patients with aortic stenosis. *Circulation* 116:755–763, 2007.
90. Lichtenstein SV, Cheung A, Ye J, et al: Transapical transcatheter aortic valve implantation in humans: Initial clinical experience. *Circulation* 114:591–596, 2006.
91. Dewey TM, Walther T, Doss M, et al: Transapical aortic valve implantation: an animal feasibility study. *Ann Thorac Surg* 82:110–116, 2006.
92. Walther T, Simon P, Dewey T, et al: Transapical minimally invasive aortic valve implantation. Multicenter experience. *Circulation* 116(Suppl I):I-240–I-24, 2007.
93. Svensson LG, Dewey T, Kapadia S, et al. United States feasibility study of transcatheter insertion of a stented aortic valve by the left ventricular apex. *Ann Thorac Surg* 86:46–55, 2008.
94. Thomas M, Schymik G, Walther T, et al: Thirty day results of the SAPIEN aortic bioprosthesis European Outcome (SOURCE) Registry: A European registry of transcatheter aortic valve implantation using the Edwards SAPIEN valve. *Circulation.* 122:62–69, 2010.
95. Webb JG, Altwegg L, Boone RH, et al: Transcatheter aortic valve implantation: Impact on clinical and valve-related outcomes. *Circulation* 119:3009–3016, 2009.
96. Walther T, Schuler G, Borger MA, et al: Transapical aortic valve implantation in 100 consecutive patients: Comparison to propensity-matched conventional aortic valve replacement. *Euro Heart J* 31:1398–1403, 2010.
97. Zierer A, Wimmer-Greinecer G, Martens S, et al: Is transapical aortic valve implantation really less invasive than minimally invasive aortic valve replacement? *J Thorac Cardiovasc Surg* 138:1067–1072, 2009.
98. Rodes-Cabau J, Dumont E, Dela Rochelliere R, et al: Feasibility and initial results of Percutaneous aortic valve implantation including selection of the transfemoral or transapical approach in patients with severe aortic stenosis. *Am J Cardiol* 102:1240–1246, 2008.
99. Leon MB, Smith CR, Mack MM, et al: Transcatheter aortic valve implantation for aortic stenosis in patients who cannot undergo surgery. *N Engl J Med* 363(17):1597–1607, commentary 10.1056/NEJMoa1008232, 2010.
100. Ghanem W, Muller A, Nahle CP, et al: Risk and fate of cerebral embolism after transfemoral aortic valve implantation. *J Am Coll Cardiol* 55:1427–1432, 2010.
101. Sinhal A, Altwegg L, Pasupati S, et al: Atrioventricular block after transcatheter balloon expandable aortic valve implantation. *J Am Coll Cardiol Interv* 1:305–309, 2008.
102. Bleiziffer S, Ruge H, Horer J, et al: Predictors for new onset complete heart block afer transcatheter aortic valve implantation. *J Am Coll Cardiol Interv* 5:524–530, 2010.
103. Bagur R, Webb JG, Nietlispach F, et al: Acute kidney injury following transcatheter aortic valve implantation: Predictive factors, prognostic value, and comparison with surgical aortic valve replacement. *Eur Heart J* 31:865–874, 2010.
104. Arregger F, Wenaweser P, Hellige GJ, et al: Risk of acute kidney injury in patients with severe aortic valve stenosis undergoing transcatheter valve replacement. *Nephrol Dial Transplant* 24:2175–2179, 2009.
105. Zajarias A, Eltchaninoff H, Cribier A: Successful coronary intervention after percutaneous aortic valve replacement. *Catheter Cardiovasc Interv* 69:522–524, 2007.
106. Iung B, Cachier A, Baron G, et al: Decision-making in elderly patients with severe aortic stenosis: Why are so many denied surgery? *Eur Heart J* 26(24):2714–2720, 2005.
107. Grube E, Buellesfeld L, Mueller R, et al: Progress and current status of percutaneous aortic valve replacement: Results of three device generations of the CoreValve Revalving system. *Circ Cardiovasc Interv* 1(3):167–175, 2008.
108. Chiam PT, Ruiz CE: Percutaneous transcatheter aortic valve implantation: Evolution of the technology. *Am Heart J* 157(2):229–242, 2009.
109. De Jaegere P, Kappetein AP, Knook M, et al: Percutaneous aortic valve replacement in a patient who could not undergo surgical treatment. A case report with the Core Valve aortic valve prosthesis. *Eurointervention* 1(4):475–479, 2006.
110. Grube E, Laborde JC, Zickmann B, et al: First report on a human percutaneous transluminal implantation of a self-expanding valve prosthesis for interventional treatment of aortic valve stenosis. *Catheter Cardiovasc Interv* 66(4):465–469, 2005.
111. Grube E, Schuler G, Buellesfeld L, et al: Percutaneous aortic valve replacement for severe aortic stenosis in high-risk patients using the second- and current third-generation self-expanding CoreValve prosthesis: Device success and 30-day clinical outcome. *J Am Coll Cardiol* 50:69–76, 2007.
112. Laborde JC, Borenstein N, Behr L, et al: Percutaneous implantation of an aortic valve prosthesis. *Catheter Cardiovasc Interv* 65(2):171–174, discussion 175, 2005.
113. Laborde JC, Borenstein N, Behr L, et al: Percutaneous implantation of the CoreValve aortic valve prosthesis for patients presenting high risk for surgical valve replacement. *Eurointervention* 1:472–474, 2006.
114. Lamarche Y, Cartier R, Denault AY, et al: Implantation of the CoreValve percutaneous aortic valve. *Ann Thorac Surg* 83(1):284–287, 2007.
115. Ruiz CE, Laborde JC, Condado JF, et al: First percutaneous transcatheter aortic valve-in-valve implant with three year follow-up. *Catheter Cardiovasc Interv* 72(2):143–148, 2008.
116. Berry C, Asgar A, Lamarche Y, et al: Novel therapeutic aspects of percutaneous aortic valve replacement with the 21F CoreValve Revalving System. *Catheter Cardiovasc Interv* 70(4):610–616, 2007.
117. Buellesfeld L, Gerckens U, Grube E: Percutaneous implantation of the first repositionable aortic valve prosthesis in a patient with severe aortic stenosis. *Catheter Cardiovasc Interv* 71:579–584, 2008.
118. Berry C, Basmadjuan A, Bonan R: First case of combined percutaneous aortic valve replacement and coronary artery revascularization. *Eurointervention* 2:257–261, 2006.
119. Schultz CJ, Weustink A, Piazza N, et al: Geometry and degree of apposition of the CoreValve Revalving system with multislice computed tomography after implantation in patients with aortic stenosis. *J Am Coll Cardiol* 54(10):911–918, 2009.
120. Noble S, Asgar A, Cartier R, et al: Anatomo-pathological analysis after CoreValve Revalving system implantation. *EuroIntervention* 5(1):78–85, 2009.
121. Piazza N, Grube E, Gerckens U, et al: A clinical protocol for analysis of the structural integrity of the Medtronic CoreValve System frame and its application in patients with 1-year minimum follow-up. *EuroIntervention* 5(6):680–686, 2010.
122. Dewey TM, Brown DL, Das TS, et al: High-risk patients referred for transcatheter aortic valve implantation: management and outcomes. *Ann Thorac Surg* 86(5):1450–1456, discussion 1456–1457, 2008.
123. Kapadia SR, Goel SS, Svensson L, et al: Characterization and outcome of patients with severe symptomatic aortic stenosis referred for percutaneous aortic valve replacement. *J Thorac Cardiovasc Surg* 137(6):1430–1435, 2009.
124. Otten AM, van Domburg RT, van Gameren M, et al: Population characteristics, treatment assignment and survival of patients with aortic stenosis referred for percutaneous valve replacement. *EuroIntervention* 4(2):250–255, 2008.
125. Abdel-Wahab M, Zahn R, Sheri M, et al: In-hospital outcome of aortic regurgitation after transcatheter aortic valve implantation: Results from the prospective multicentre German TAVI registry [abstract]. *Eur Heart J* 31(Suppl):160, 2010.
126. Tops LF, Wood DA, Delgado V, et al: Noninvasive evaluation of the aortic root with multislice computed tomography implications for transcatheter aortic valve replacement. *JACC Cardiovasc Imaging* 1(3):321–330, 2008.
127. Wood DA, Tops LF, Mayo JR, et al: Role of multislice computed tomography in transcatheter aortic valve replacement. *Am J Cardiol* 103(9):1295–1301, 2009.
128. Leipsic J, Wood D, Manders D, et al: The evolving role of MDCT in transcatheter aortic valve replacement: A radiologists' perspective. *AJR Am J Roentgenol* 193(3):W214–W219, 2009.
129. Jilaihawi H, Spyt T, Chin D, et al: Percutaneous aortic valve replacement in patients with challenging aortoiliofemoral access. *Catheter Cardiovasc Interv* 72(6):885–890, 2008.
130. de Jaegere P, van Dijk L, Laborde J, et al: True percutaneous implantation of the CoreValve aortic valve prosthesis by the combined use of ultrasound guided vascular access, Prostar XL, and the TandemHeart, *EuroIntervention* 2:500–505, 2007.
131. Fraccaro C, Napodano M, Tarantini G, et al: Expanding the eligibility for transcatheter aortic valve implantation the trans-subclavian retrograde approach using: The III generation CoreValve revalving system. *JACC Cardiovasc Interv* 2(9):828–833, 2009.
132. Bojara W, Mumme A, Gerckens U, et al: Implantation of the CoreValve self-expanding valve prosthesis via a subclavian artery approach: A case report. *Clin Res Cardiol* 98(3):201–204, 2009.
133. Ruge H, Lange R, Bleiziffer S, et al: First successful aortic valve implantation with the CoreValve revalving trade mark system via right subclavian artery access: A case report. *Heart Surg Forum* 11(5):E323–E324, 2008.
134. Petronio AS, De Carlo M, Bedogni F, et al: Safety and efficacy of the subclavian approach for transcatheter aortic valve implantation with the CoreValve revalving system. *Circ Cardiovasc Interv* 3(4):359–366, 2010.
135. Vavuranakis M, Vrachatis DA, Filis K, et al: Trans-catheter aortic-valve implantation by the subclavian approach complicated with vessel dissection and transient left-arm paralysis. *Eur J Cardiothorac Surg* 39(1):127–129, 2011.
136. Wenaweser P, Buellesfeld L, Gerckens U, et al: Percutaneous aortic valve replacement for severe aortic regurgitation in degenerated bioprosthesis: The first valve in valve procedure using the CoreValve revalving system. *Catheter Cardiovasc Interv* 70(5):760–764, 2007.
137. Giannini C, De Carlo M, Guarracino F, et al: Dysfunction of a 21-mm aortic bioprosthesis treated with percutaneous implantation of a CoreValve prosthesis. *J Cardiovasc Med (Hagerstown)* Apr 17 (epublication ahead of print), 2010.
138. Khawaja MZ, Haworth P, Ghuran A, et al: Transcatheter aortic valve implantation for stenosed and regurgitant aortic valve bioprostheses CoreValve for failed bioprosthetic aortic valve replacements. *J Am Coll Cardiol* 55(2):97–101, 2010.
139. Bruschi G, De Marco F, Oreglia J, et al: Percutaneous implantation of CoreValve aortic prostheses in patients with a mechanical mitral valve. *Ann Thorac Surg* 88(5):e50–e52, 2009.
140. Schuler G, Bonan R, Kovac J, et al: Effectiveness and durability at two years with CoreValve transcatheter aortic valve [abstract]. *Eur Heart J* 31(Suppl):159–160, 2010.
141. Bleiziffer S, Ruge H, Mazzitelli D, et al: Results of percutaneous and transapical transcatheter aortic valve implantation performed by a surgical team. *Eur J Cardiothorac Surg* 35(4):615–620, 2009.
142. Barbanti M: *Two-year outcomes of transcatheter aortic valve implantation: A single center experience*, Paris, France, May 26, 2010, EuroPCR.
143. Meredith I: *A snapshot from the ongoing Australia-New Zealand Medtronic CoreValve(r) Registry. Transcatheter cardiovascular therapeutics, September 21–25, 2009*, San Francisco, 2009, CA.
144. Petronio AS: *The Italian CoreValve Registry*, Paris, France, May 25, 2010, EuroPCR.
145 Avanzas P, Munoz-Garcia A, Segura J: Percutaneous implantation of the CoreValve(r) self-expanding aortic valve prosthesis in patients with severe aortic stenosis: Early experience in Spain. *Rev Esp Cardiol* 63:141–148, 2010.
146. Eltchaninoff H: *FRANCE Registry: FRench Aortic National Corevalve and Edwards Registry*. Paris, France, May 25 ,2010, EuroPCR.
147. Ludman P: *UK TAVI Registry*, Paris, France, May 25, 2010, EuroPCR.
148. Tamburino C, Capodanno D, Mule M, et al: Procedural success and 30-day clinical outcomes after percutaneous aortic valve replacement using current third-generation self-expanding CoreValve prosthesis. *J Invasive Cardiol* 21(3):93–98, 2009.
149. Buellesfeld L, Gerckens U, Schuler G, et al: 2-year follow-up of patients undergoing transcatheter aortic valve implantation using a self-expanding valve prosthesis. *J Am Coll Cardiol* 57: 1650–1657, 2011.
150. Buellesfeld L, Wenaweser P, Gerckens U, et al: Transcatheter aortic valve implantation: Predictors of procedural success—the Siegburg-Bern experience. *Eur Heart J* 31(8):984–991, 2010.
151 Bosmans J: *The Belgian TAVI Registry*. Paris, France, May 25, 2010, EuroPCR.
152. Zahn R: *The German TAVI Registry*, Paris, France, May 25, 2010, EuroPCR.
153 deJaegere PP, Piazza N, Galema TW, et al: Early echocardiographic evaluation following percutaneous implantation with the self-expanding CoreValve Revalving System aortic valve bioprosthesis. *EuroIntervention* 4(3):351–357, 2008.
154. Ewe S, Ajmone-Marsan N, Delgado V, et al: Clinical and echocardiographic outcomes after transcatheter aortic valve implantation: Comparison between patients with normal and impaired left ventricular systolic function [abstract]. *Eur Heart J* 31(Suppl):957–958, 2010.
155 Tzikas A, Piazza N, van Dalen BM, et al: Changes in mitral regurgitation after transcatheter aortic valve implantation. *Catheter Cardiovasc Interv* 75(1):43–49, 2010.
156. Jilaihawi H, Jeilan M, Spyt T, et al: Early regression of left ventricular wall thickness following percutaneous aortic valve replacement with the CoreValve bioprosthesis. *J Invasive Cardiol* 21(4):151–155; discussion 156–158, 2009.
157. Yap CH, Mohajeri M, Yii M: Prosthesis-patient mismatch is associated with higher operative mortality following aortic valve replacement. *Heart Lung Circ* 16(4):260–264, 2007.
158. Tzikas A, Piazza N, Geleijnse ML, et al: Prosthesis-patient mismatch after transcatheter aortic valve implantation with the Medtronic CoreValve system in patients with aortic stenosis. *Am J Cardiol* 106(2):255–260, 2010.
159. Ussia GP, Mule M, Barbanti M, et al: Quality of life assessment after percutaneous aortic valve implantation. *Eur Heart J* 30(14):1790–1796, 2009.
160. Ludman UK, Registry TAVI: *Facts, Figures and National Registries*, Paris, France, 2010, EuroPCR.
161. Dewey TM, Brown DL, Herbert MA, et al: Effect of concomitant coronary artery disease on procedural and late outcomes of transcatheter aortic valve implantation. *Ann Thorac Surg* 89(3):758–767; discussion 767, 2010.
162. Himbert D, Iung B, Attias D, et al: Predictive factors of mid-term mortality after transcatheter aortic valve implantation [abstract]. *Eur Heart J* 31(Suppl):956–957, 2010.
163. Sinning J-H, Ghanem A, Steinhaeuser H, et al: Renal function as predictor of mortality in patients after percutaneous transcatheter aortic valve implantation. *Eur Heart J* 31(Suppl):957, 2010.
164. Zahn R, Gerckens U, Schuler G, et al: Predictors of hospital mortality in patients with severe symptomatic aortic stenosis undergoing trans-catheter aortic valve implantation. Results of a prospective multi-centre registry. *Eur Heart J* 31(Suppl):956, 2010.

165. Masson JB, Kovac J, Schuler G, et al: Transcatheter aortic valve implantation: Review of the nature, management, and avoidance of procedural complications. *JACC Cardiovasc Interv* 2(9):811–820, 2009.

166. Akins CW, Miller DC, Turina MI, et al: Guidelines for reporting mortality and morbidity after cardiac valve interventions. *J Thorac Cardiovasc Surg* 135(4):732–738, 2008.

167. Berry C, Cartier R, Bonan R: Fatal ischemic stroke related to nonpermissive peripheral artery access for percutaneous aortic valve replacement. *Catheter Cardiovasc Interv* 69(1):56–63, 2007.

168. Kahlert P, Knipp SC, Schlamann M, et al: Silent and apparent cerebral ischemia after percutaneous transfemoral aortic valve implantation: A diffusion-weighted magnetic resonance imaging study. *Circulation* 121(7):870–878, 2010.

169. Blazek S, Vollmann R, Simbrunner J, et al: Cerebral magnetic resonance imaging unmasks microembolic cerebral lesions after transcatheter aortic valve implantation. *Eur Heart J* 31(Suppl): 145–146, 2010.

170. Easton JD, Saver JL, Albers GW, et al: Definition and evaluation of transient ischemic attack: A scientific statement for healthcare professionals from the American Heart Association/American Stroke Association Stroke Council; Council on Cardiovascular Surgery and Anesthesia; Council on Cardiovascular Radiology and Intervention; Council on Cardiovascular Nursing; and the Interdisciplinary Council on Peripheral Vascular Disease. The American Academy of Neurology affirms the value of this statement as an educational tool for neurologists. *Stroke*. 40(6):2276–2293, 2009.

171. Zahn R, Schiele R, Kilkowski C, et al: Severe aortic regurgitation after percutaneous transcatheter aortic valve implantation: On the importance to clarify the underlying pathophysiology. *Clin Res Cardiol* 99(3):193–197, 2009.

172. Hoffmann R, Rieck B, Dohmen G: Correction of CoreValve position using snare traction from a right brachial artery access. *J Invasive Cardiol* 22(4):E59–E60, 2010.

173. Vavuranakis M, Vrachatis D, Stefanadis C: CoreValve aortic bioprosthesis: Repositioning techniques. *JACC Cardiovasc Interv* 3(5):565; author reply 566, 2010.

174. Vavouranakis M, Vrachatis DA, Toutouzas KP, et al: "Bail out" procedures for malpositioning of aortic valve prosthesis (CoreValve). *Int J Cardiol* 145(1):154–155, 2009.

175. Thyregod HG, Lund JT, Engstrom T, et al: Transcatheter aortic valve prosthesis surgically replaced 4 months after implantation. *Eur J Cardiothorac Surg* 37(2):494–496, 2010.

176. Van Mieghem NM, Nuis RJ, Piazza N, et al: Vascular complications with transcatheter aortic valve implantation using the 18 Fr Medtronic CoreValve System: The Rotterdam experience. *EuroIntervention* 5(6):673–679, 2010.

177. Dhingra RC, Amat-y-Leon F, Pietras RJ, et al: Sites of conduction disease in aortic stenosis: Significance of valve gradient and calcification. *Ann Intern Med* 87(3):275–280, 1977.

178. Friedman HS, Zaman Q, Haft JI, et al: Assessment of atrioventricular conduction in aortic valve disease. *Br Heart J* 40(8):911–917, 1978.

179. Carlson MD, Palacios I, Thomas JD, et al: Cardiac conduction abnormalities during percutaneous balloon mitral or aortic valvotomy, *Circulation* 79(6):1197–1203, 1989.

180. Gordon RS, Ivanov J, Cohen G, et al: Permanent cardiac pacing after a cardiac operation: Predicting the use of permanent pacemakers. *Ann Thorac Surg* 66(5):1698–1704, 1998.

181. Dawkins S, Hobson AR, Kalra PR, et al: Permanent pacemaker implantation after isolated aortic valve replacement: Incidence, indications, and predictors. *Ann Thorac Surg (Netherlands)* 85:108–112, 2008.

182. Piazza N, Onuma Y, Jesserun E, et al: Early and persistent intraventricular conduction abnormalities and requirements for pacemaking after percutaneous replacement of the aortic valve. *JACC Cardiovasc Interv.*1(3):310–316, 2008.

183. Calvi V, Puzzangara E, Pruiti GP, et al: Early conduction disorders following percutaneous aortic valve replacement. *Pacing Clin Electrophysiol* 32(Suppl)1:S126–S130, 2009.

184. Jalaihawi H, Chin D, Vasa-Nicotera M, et al: Predictors for permanent pacemaker requirement after transcatheter aortic valve implantation with the CoreValve bioprosthesis. *Am Heart J* 157:860, 2009.

185. Akhtar M, Tuzcu EM, Kapadia SR, et al: Aortic root morphology in patients undergoing percutaneous aortic valve replacement: Evidence of aortic root remodeling. *J Thorac Cardiovasc Surg* 137(4):950–956, 2009.

186. Bombien R, Humme T, Schunke M, et al: Percutaneous aortic valve replacement: Computed tomography scan after valved stent implantation in human cadaver hearts. *Eur J Cardiothorac Surg* 36(3):592–594, 2009.

187. Gerckens U, Latsios G, Mueller R, et al: Left main PCI after trans-subclavian CoreValve implantation. Successful outcome of a combined procedure for management of a rare complication. *Clin Res Cardiol* 98(10):687–690, 2009.

188. Kahlert P, Al-Rashid F, Frahm U, et al: Acute renal failure after transcatheter aortic valve implantation [abstract]. *Eur Heart J* 31(Suppl):957, 2010.

189. Wenaweser P, Pilgrim T, Kadner A, et al: Procedural and long-term clinical outcome of elderly patients with severe aortic stenosis undergoing transcatheter aortic valve implantation [abstract]. *Eur Heart J* 31(Suppl):665–666, 2010.

190. Low R, Bolling S, Yeo KK, et al: Direct Flow Medical percutaneous aortic valve: Proof of concept. *Eurointervention* 4:256–261, 2008.

191. Paniagua D, Condado JA, Besso J, et al: First human case of retrograde transcatheter implantation of an aortic valve prosthesis. *Tex Heart Inst J* 32:393–398, 2005.

192. Webb JG, Wood DA, Ye J, et al: Transcatheter valve in valve implantation for failed bioprosthetic heart valves. *Circulation* 121:1848–1857, 2010.

193. Rodes-Cahau J, Webb JG, Cheung A, et al: Transcatheter aortic valve implantation for the treatment of severe symptomatic aortic stenosis in patients at very high or prohibitive surgical risk. *J Am Coll Cardiol* 55:1080–1090, 2010.

51

Pulmonary and Tricuspid Valve Interventions

LOUISE COATS | PHILIPP BONHOEFFER

KEY POINTS

- Transcatheter pulmonary valve implantation is suitable for patients with dysfunctional right ventricle-to-pulmonary artery conduits that are less than 22 mm in diameter.

- It is performed under general anesthesia from a femoral approach.

- It results in an early symptomatic improvement and reduction in right ventricular volumes.

- It can be complicated by device displacement, homograft rupture, or coronary artery compression at the time of implantation.

- It requires careful radiographic and echocardiographic follow-up for the early detection and treatment of stent fractures.

- It is less invasive than surgery and compares well in terms of safety.

- It prolongs conduit life and may reduce the number of operations required by patients with congenital heart disease during their lifetimes.

- It has become part of routine clinical practice in the last few years.

- Percutaneous tricuspid valve replacement is mainly experimental, but early clinical applications are being reported.

Introduction

Acquired pulmonary and tricuspid valve disease in the adult population is unusual and mostly relates to rarities such as carcinoid disease, rheumatic fever, and infective endocarditis, typically in the context of intravenous drug use. For those with congenital heart disease, however, dysfunction of these valves is both a primary component of many conditions and, in the case of the pulmonary valve, also a common consequence of several early repair strategies. With growing information regarding the harmful effects of chronic pulmonary regurgitation, surgical revision of the right ventricular outflow tract (RVOT) is now a commonly performed operation in this population, with some patients requiring several reoperations during a lifetime to maintain valvar function. Transcatheter pulmonary valve implantation (TPVI) was first proposed and tested experimentally by one of the authors in the year 2000.[1] The procedure is now gaining widespread clinical acceptance, as its potential to reduce surgical reintervention in adults with repaired congenital heart disease is increasingly recognized. The Melody transcatheter valve now has both European and American regulatory approval, while other devices are under investigation for use in this position. Percutaneous tricuspid valve replacement, on the other hand, remains at a much earlier stage of development with initial clinical applications just beginning to emerge.[2] In this chapter, we reflect on the progression of this revolutionary technology since the last edition of this textbook, discuss current indications and patient selection, report updated clinical results, and contemplate future directions.

Transcatheter Pulmonary Valve Implantation

BACKGROUND AND CLINICAL INDICATIONS

Progress in surgery for congenital heart disease over the last 60 years has led to a considerable improvement in survival, with over 85% of babies now reaching adulthood.[3] As a result, the prevalence of complex congenital heart disease in the adult population more than doubled between 1985 and the year 2000 and will continue to rise for the foreseeable future.[4] Focus has therefore shifted toward the management of late morbidity in this growing population, with repeated surgery or catheter intervention often employed to treat various residual lesions or complications. Pulmonary regurgitation, which is common after transannular patch repair of tetralogy of Fallot, is a major cause of morbidity and may cause right ventricular dysfunction, impaired exercise capacity, and an increased risk of ventricular arrhythmia and sudden death.[5-7] RVOT obstruction may also cause symptoms in patients with conduits or following the arterial switch operation.[8-10] Surgical pulmonary valve replacement can halt and may reverse these detrimental outcomes.[11-13] Severe pulmonary regurgitation with symptoms or reduced exercise tolerance is a class I indication for surgery. Valve replacement is also considered reasonable if severe pulmonary regurgitation is accompanied by moderate to severe right ventricular dysfunction or enlargement, symptomatic or sustained atrial and/or ventricular arrhythmias, or moderate to severe tricuspid regurgitation. For those with RVOT obstruction, surgery is considered in the presence of a peak Doppler gradient >50 mm Hg, a right-to-left ventricular pressure ratio >0.7, progressive and/or severe right ventricular dilation with dysfunction, or if there are associated lesions requiring surgical repair. In conduit dysfunction, percutaneous intervention may be useful where the diameter narrowing of the prosthesis is >50%.[14] It has been suggested, however, that intervention is being performed too late, as the ability of the right ventricle to remodel following surgery may be limited.[15] Implanted biological valves, however, have a limited life span, and the desire to avoid progressive right ventricular dysfunction has been moderated by the risks associated with redo surgery and cardiopulmonary bypass.[16,17] Additionally, placement of bare stents for RVOT obstruction has been complicated by inevitable pulmonary regurgitation.[18] TPVI is a transcatheter approach that can treat both pulmonary regurgitation and stenosis in patients with suitable RVOT anatomy. Traditional criteria for surgery have provided the baseline clinical indications for this new technique. Inclusion criteria in the U.S. Melody Trans-catheter Pulmonary Valve trial required a mean Doppler gradient ≥35 mm Hg or at least moderate pulmonary regurgitation in symptomatic patients or a mean Doppler gradient ≥40 mmHg or severe pulmonary regurgitation with an associated tricuspid valve annulus z-score ≥2 or right ventricular fractional shortening <40% in asymptomatic patients.[19] Because of technical feasibility relating to the dimensions of the delivery system, the procedure is also restricted to patients over the age of 5 years with a weight above 30 kg. Once established, the less invasive nature of TPVI will support the current inclination for earlier intervention and offer a treatment option to those who are not surgical candidates.[20] Importantly, TPVI does not affect subsequent suitability for surgery. Careful investigation will be required to redefine the indications clearly and determine the optimal timing for

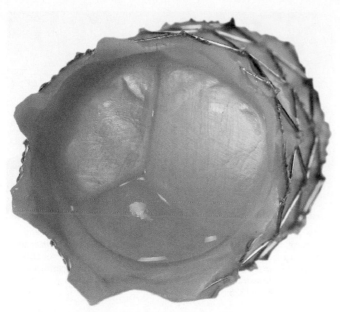

Figure 51-1 Melody transcatheter pulmonary valve device. (*Medtronic, Minneapolis, MN.*)

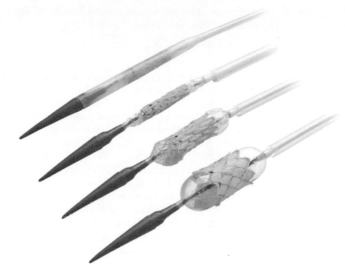

Figure 51-2 A. Melody transcatheter pulmonary valve mounted on the balloon-in-balloon delivery system. B. Ensemble device. From left to right: sheathed, unsheathed, inner balloon inflation, outer balloon inflation. (*Medtronic, Minneapolis, MN.*)

treatment in this growing patient population. In some rare cases of acquired pulmonary valvular disease (e.g., carcinoid disease), TPVI may also be considered as a treatment option.

THE DEVICE

The Medtronic transcatheter pulmonary valve (Melody, Medtronic, Minneapolis, MN) is composed of a segment of bovine jugular vein with a thinned down wall and a central valve (Fig. 51-1). The vein is sutured inside an expanded platinum-iridium stent (length, 28 mm; diameter, 18 mm) that can be crimped to a size of 6 mm and reexpanded up to 22 mm. The current stent design, which has an eight-crown zig pattern with six segments along its length, is reinforced at each strut intersection with gold weld. The venous segment is attached to the stent by continuous 5-0 polypropylene sutures around the entire circumference at the inflow and outflow and also discretely at each strut intersection. The suture is clear for all points except the outflow line, which is blue to signify the outflow end of the device. The venous segment is fixed in a buffered glutaraldehyde solution in a concentration low enough to preserve the flexibility of the venous valve leaflets. A final sterilization step is performed on the combined device using a proprietary sterilant containing glutaraldehyde and isopropyl alcohol, in which it is then packaged.

THE DELIVERY SYSTEM

The delivery system, also manufactured by Medtronic (Ensemble, Medtronic, Minneapolis, MN), comprises a balloon in balloon (BiB) deployment design at its distal end onto which the valved stent is front-loaded and crimped (Fig. 51-2). The system is available with three outer balloon diameters: 18, 20, and 22 mm. The tip of the system is blue to correspond with the outflow suture of the device and encourage correct orientation. The body of the system is composed of a one-piece Teflon sheath containing a braided wire-reinforced elastomer lumen. This design minimizes the risk of kinking while optimizing flexibility and retaining the necessary pushability required for the procedure. There is a retractable sheath that covers the stented valve during delivery and is pulled back just prior to deployment. Contrast can be delivered via the retracted sheath from a side port to confirm positioning of the device prior to deployment. Proximally, there are three ports, one for the guidewire (green), one to deploy the inner balloon (indigo), and one to deploy the outer balloon (orange).

ANIMAL STUDIES

The feasibility of TPVI was first demonstrated in lambs using a device that combined commercially available products (Contegra, Medtronic, Minneapolis, MN) and CP (Cheatham Platinum) stent (NuMed Inc., Hopkinton, NY) and was a precursor of that described above.[21,22] Bench testing had already confirmed that crimping and reexpansion of the device by balloon catheter would not affect valvar competence. Devices were delivered from a right internal jugular approach under fluoroscopic guidance. The valved stents were deployed in the native pulmonary artery of 7 of 11 lambs, with the procedure failing in 4 owing to an inability to cross the tricuspid valve. In humans, the femoral vessel, which is relatively larger, can be utilized and promotes a straighter catheter course, thus overcoming this technical difficulty. Of 7 valved stents, 5 were implanted in an optimal position impinging on the function of the native valve. No complications occurred during the procedure or follow-up. Two of the animals developed a mild fever, but this disappeared in 48 hours without intervention. During the subsequent 2 months, all animals were asymptomatic and nearly doubled their body weight. At the end of the protocol, hemodynamic evaluation showed normal pulmonary pressures in all lambs. One stent was mildly stenotic with a gradient of 15 mm Hg across it. At autopsy, fibrosis of the valve leaflets occurred in the two devices that had not been implanted in the desired position. Subsequently, valved stent designs have been implanted in the pulmonary position in other trials employing animal models, with positive results.[23–25] Histological investigation has also shown that calcification of valved stents in this position occurs in the wall portions without affecting the cusps and that cardiac structures in the vicinity have normal histology without inflammation.[26]

CLINICAL STUDIES

The first human application of transcatheter pulmonary valve implantation was reported in the year 2000. A 12-year-old boy with an original diagnosis of pulmonary atresia and ventricular septal defect underwent TPVI to treat stenosis and insufficiency of an 18-mm Carpentier-Edwards conduit that had been placed between the right ventricle and pulmonary artery when he was 4.[27] The procedure was uncomplicated and resulted in complete relief of the insufficiency and partial relief of the stenosis. Since then, the procedure has been performed in over 1,200 patients and more than 90 centers worldwide. The London/Paris experience (155 patients) and the U.S. experience

(136 patients) currently comprise the largest reported series in the literature.[28,29] The results are described below.

PATIENT COHORT

Dysfunctional circumferential conduits provide the most suitable environment for implantation of a transcatheter valve. Most patients in both series had undergone at least one surgical RVOT revision with conduit placement, usually following transannular patch repair of tetralogy of Fallot. Some, however, had had their conduits placed as part of the primary repair strategy (e.g., truncus arteriosus, Rastelli repair for transposition of the great arteries, or Ross operation for aortic valve disease). In the London/Paris series, TPVI was attempted in a few patients with native outflow tracts or transannular patches, but these were exceptional and in some cases complicated. Acceptance for TPVI in the London/Paris series was based on traditional surgical criteria with humanitarian exemption sought on an individual patient basis. The U.S. Trans-catheter Pulmonary Valve trial was a multicenter, industry-sponsored safety and efficacy trial with inclusion and exclusion criteria referred to earlier in this chapter.

THE PROCEDURE

Under general anesthesia with invasive blood pressure monitoring, TPVI is performed predominantly via a right femoral venous approach. A full aseptic technique to surgical standards is used and a single dose of broad-spectrum intravenous antibiotics is given for endocarditis prophylaxis. Heparin is administered routinely at the beginning of the procedure and repeated hourly thereafter as required to maintain an activated clotting time >250 seconds. Right heart catheterization is performed according to standard techniques to assess pressures and saturations. Routinely, measurements are made in the right ventricle, pulmonary artery, and aorta with additional measurements (e.g., in the branch pulmonary arteries) made as appropriate. A stiff guidewire (0.035 Amplatz Ultrastiff, Cook Inc., Bloomington, IN) is then positioned into a distal branch pulmonary artery to provide an anchor from which to advance the delivery system. First, biplane angiography is performed using a Multi-Track catheter (NuMed Inc., Hopkinton, NY) with the tip placed just beyond the expected position of the pulmonary valve to allow assessment of the proposed site for device implantation and quantification of pulmonary regurgitation. Angiography is also performed in the aortic root. If there is suspicion that a coronary artery is at risk of compression from valve implantation, coronary angiography is performed with an angioplasty balloon (18–20 mm Mullins balloon, NuMed Inc., Hopkinton, NY) simultaneously inflated in the conduit. If there is a risk of coronary compression, implantation should not be attempted and the patient referred for surgery (Fig. 51-3). Conduit predilation should also be performed using a balloon 2 mm larger than the narrowest diameter of the conduit and less than 110% the original conduit diameter (PTS sizing balloon, NuMed Inc., Hopkinton, NY). If the balloon waist measures between 14 and 20 mm on subsequent low-pressure (≤8 atm) balloon sizing, the conduit can be considered anatomically suitable and the procedure can continue. To minimize the risk of conduit rupture, the diameter of the predilation balloon or the delivery system balloon used should not exceed 110% of the nominal diameter (original implant size) of the conduit. Concurrently, the valved stent is prepared in three sequential saline baths (5 minutes in each) to wash off the glutaraldehyde in which it is stored. The size of the valved stent is reduced by crimping it on mandrels of increasingly smaller sizes prior to front loading onto the delivery system. It is recommended to use a 2.5-mL syringe for crimping to an intermediate size prior to final crimping onto the balloon catheter. The blue stitching on the distal portion of the device is matched to the blue portion of the delivery system and verified by an independent observer to guarantee correct orientation. Further hand crimping of the device onto the balloon is performed, following which the sheath is retracted over the device while a saline flush is administered via the side port to exclude air bubbles from the

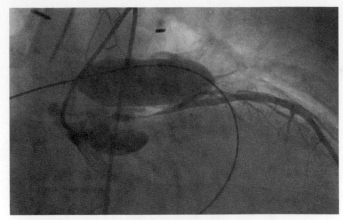

Figure 51-3 Angiogram: left anterior oblique projection with 20 degrees of cranial angulation showing compression of the left anterior descending coronary artery during balloon inflation in the conduit. *(From Sridharan S, Coats L, Khambadkone S, et al. Transcatheter right ventricular outflow tract intervention: the risk to the coronary circulation. Circulation. 2006;11325:e934–e935.)*

system. Following removal of the Multi-Track catheter, the femoral vein is dilated to 24 Fr and the front-loaded delivery system is advanced into the RVOT under fluoroscopic guidance. The sheath is then retracted from the valved stent and contrast is injected via the side port to confirm position. Partial deployment is achieved by hand inflation of the inner balloon and, after final confirmation of the position, the outer balloon is also hand-inflated to complete deployment. The balloons are then deflated and the delivery system is withdrawn. Repeat angiography and pressure measurements are made to confirm a positive outcome. Post-dilation of the valve may be performed at the discretion of the operator.

Modification of the Technique

The nature and position of right ventricular to pulmonary artery conduits is heterogeneous; cannulation with a large delivery system can therefore be challenging. Predilation (Mullins balloon and indeflator, NuMed Inc., Hopkinton, NY) and in some cases bare stenting (Max LD, EV3, Plymouth, MN) conduits that are heavily calcified or tortuous can facilitate passage of the system in addition to optimizing the final result. This may also have the additional benefit of reducing the risk of future stent fractures.[30] Further maneuvers that can be used to advance the delivery system when it is at the entrance to the conduit include looping the system within the right atrium, partial retraction of the sheath, and repositioning of the guidewire in the contralateral branch pulmonary artery. The first two actions generate a forward force often overcoming any resistance the system is experiencing and aid passage into the conduit. Once deflated, the delivery system is withdrawn. If further dilation of the valved stent is required, this is performed using a high-pressure Mullins balloon and indeflator (NuMed Inc., Hopkinton, NY). Care is taken not to dilate conduits beyond their original documented size to minimize the risk of rupture. Postdilation of the device has not been observed to cause any damage to valve leaflets or affect valve competency. Although the preferred approach is via the right femoral vein, mainly for practical and logistical reasons, successful valve implantation has also been achieved via left femoral, right and left internal jugular, and left subclavian veins. A transhepatic route is neither used nor recommended in view of the size of the delivery system.

RESULTS

Procedural

A total of 155 patients underwent TPVI in London and Paris between September 2000 and February 2007 and 136 underwent TPVI at five centers in the United States between January 2007 and August 2009.

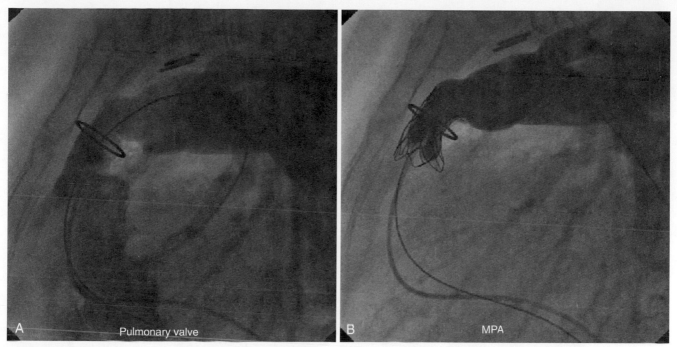

Figure 51-4 Lateral angiogram demonstrating complete relief of pulmonary regurgitation following transcatheter pulmonary valve implantation into a Hancock conduit.

In the American series, which circumvented the effects of the learning curve, mean procedural time was 174 ± 67 minutes and fluoroscopy time was 46 ± 25 minutes. The majority of patients, however, underwent additional percutaneous procedures ranging from bare stenting of the pulmonary artery and its branches to the closure of atrial septal defects. In the London/Paris series, ventricular septal defect closure, paravalvular leak closure, and coarctation stenting were also performed. TPVI was not performed in <10% of both cohorts catheterized. The main reasons for this were unfavorable RVOT morphology on final testing and the presence of coronary artery anatomy at risk of compression.

Hemodynamics

Following TPVI, angiography showed a significant improvement in regurgitation, with no one in either cohort having more than trivial to mild regurgitation (Fig. 51-4). RVOT gradient and RV pressures fell significantly in patients with stenotic lesions as well as those with predominant regurgitation, albeit to a lesser extent. In this group, pulmonary artery diastolic pressure increased, reflecting the restoration of a competent pulmonary valve. All patients experienced a small rise in systemic pressure, which might reflect improved cardiac output but could also indicate lightening of the anaesthesia toward the end of the procedure. Subsequent investigation has suggested that different patterns of hemodynamic change can be expected depending on the nature of the RVOT dysfunction being treated.[31,32]

Procedural Complications

In the London/Paris series, 7 patients experienced major procedural complications that necessitated conversion to surgery. These included device instability in dilated regurgitant outflow tracts (2), homograft rupture (3), compression of the left coronary artery (1), and obstruction of the origin of the right pulmonary artery (1). Other less serious complications included guidewire injury to a distal branch pulmonary artery (2); damage to the tricuspid valve, probably due to entrapment of the delivery system in the chordae (2); and a limited homograft rupture (1). All responded to conservative management. It should be remembered that these patients represent the first cohort ever to undergo this procedure, and it was this experience that led to the refinement of device design, patient selection, and procedural approach.

In the subsequent U.S. series there were eight significant procedural complications including coronary artery dissection, conduit rupture (one requiring surgery, one managed with a covered stent), broad complex tachycardia, hypercarbia and elevated left ventricular filling pressure, femoral vein thrombosis, and two guidewire perforations of a distal pulmonary artery branch. The patient who developed coronary artery dissection had preexisting severe biventricular failure and, despite stenting of the coronary artery and TPVI, subsequently suffered an intracranial hemorrhage and died.

Follow-up and Clinical Consequences

Follow-up ranged from 0 to 83.7 months (median 28.4) in the London/Paris series. In the U.S. series, 99 patients reached the 1-year follow-up and 24 had completed the 2-year evaluation. Patients were subjected to clinical review, electrocardiography, anteroposterior and lateral chest x-ray, and transthoracic echocardiography at 1, 3, and 6 months and 1 year following the procedure and at yearly intervals thereafter. Magnetic resonance imaging was performed early and late after valve implantation unless contraindicated and computed tomography pulmonary angiography was incorporated into the follow-up of the initial U.S. cohort to assess the risk of thromboembolic phenomenon following device implantation.

Patients in both cohorts reported an early symptomatic improvement with sustained abolition of pulmonary regurgitation at latest follow-up. In the London/Paris series, there was an early improvement in objective exercise capacity (VO_2max and anaerobic threshold) in the overall group, which appeared more prominent in those being treated for RVOT obstruction as opposed to pulmonary regurgitation.[31,32] While these findings were not replicated in the U.S. cohort, this study included a large number of submaximal exercise tests. Subsequent analysis has found that reduction in RVOT gradient, and not restoration of pulmonary valve competence, is an independent predictor of improved peak oxygen uptake.[33] Early assessment with magnetic resonance imaging showed a reduction in right ventricular volumes though no change in ejection fraction. More detailed investigation suggests that effective increases in stroke volume and cardiac output and that the mechanism may again be different in pressure and volume overload right ventricles.[31-33] Valvar competency was well maintained, with only two of the London/Paris patients having more than moderate

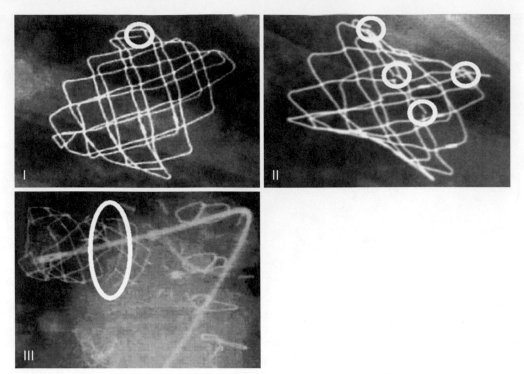

Figure 51-5 A. The probability of stent fracture free survival following transcatheter pulmonary valve implantation. B. Stent fracture classification. *(Adapted from Nordmeyer J, Khambadkone S, Coats L, et al. Risk stratification, systematic classification, and anticipatory management strategies for stent fracture after percutaneous pulmonary valve implantation. Circulation. 2007;11511:1392–1397.)*

pulmonary regurgitation during follow-up, both in the context of infective endocarditis. In the U.S. series, over 90% of patients had no more than trivial regurgitation following TPVI. Device-related complications presented instead with RVOT obstruction.

Device-Related Complications

The "Hammock" Effect. The hammock effect became apparent in the early cohort of patients undergoing valve implantation, when a high incidence of in-stent stenosis was noted (7/22 patients, 31.8%). Originally, the venous segment of the bovine valve was sutured to the stent only at its distal extremities. This permitted passage of blood between the wall of the vein and the recipient outflow tract, resulting in an effective stenosis. Recognition of this problem led to additional sutures being placed at all strut intersections, which resolved the issue with no further cases being seen. In theory the hammock effect could still occur in the context of stent or suture rupture where adherence of the venous wall to the stent became disrupted.

Stent Fractures. Stent fractures are well-recognized sequelae of stent implantation for all cardiovascular applications. The etiology is likely to be multifactorial and depends both on the nature of the stent as well as the characteristics of the implantation site. The prevalence of stent fracture in bare stenting of the RVOT has been reported to be as high as 43%, with embolization occurring in 11%, though without death or acute hemodynamic compromise.[34] Following TPVI, the prevalence of stent fracture has been reported as 21.1%, with a stent fracture-free survival at 1 year of 85.1% and at 3 years of 69.2%.[35] Implantation into a "native" RVOT, absence of RVOT calcification, and qualitative recoil of the valved stent just after implantation are predictive of stent fracture. Substernal location, high pressure of the valved stent postdilatation, initial RVOT gradient, and other indicators of compression or asymmetry do not pose increased risk. A classification that can guide management has been formulated whereby type I fractures (minor: no loss of stent integrity) can be managed conservatively, type II (major: loss of integrity with restenosis on echocardiography) should be considered for repeat TPVI or surgery, and type III (major: separation of

fragments or embolization), of which only one case has been reported, inevitably necessitates surgery (Fig. 51-5). Serial radiographic and echocardiographic follow-up is therefore essential to detect stent fractures and allow early treatment in those with hemodynamic consequences before device embolization occurs. Fluoroscopy provides a useful adjunct to assess stent stability in this situation and aid decisions regarding the need for reintervention.

Hemolysis. Hemolysis has occurred in one patient in the London/Paris series in whom sequential balloon dilatation and TPVI failed to adequately relieve RVOT obstruction in a small conduit (15-mm homograft). On the first day postprocedure, the patient developed dark urine, containing free hemoglobin on dipstick, and his serum hemoglobin dropped from 13 to 9 g/dL. Following transfusion, the patient went forward to surgery at 21 days and made an uneventful recovery. While hemolysis should be considered a potential device-related adverse event, it is rare and routine screening is not performed.

Endocarditis. Endocarditis of the valved stent has been seen in five patients from the London/Paris series (at a median of 4.9 months, range 1.9–23.2) but not in the U.S. cohort. It can occur either on the venous wall or the valve itself and has led to pulmonary regurgitation in 3 patients, RVOT obstruction in 1, and was without consequence for valvar function in 1. The organisms were *Staphylococcus aureus,* *Streptococcus aurelius,* and *Candida albicans* in a patient with known immunocompromise. Endocarditis led to explantation of the device in 3 patients; 2 patients were successfully treated medically.

Thromboembolism. Thromboembolism or valve thrombosis has not been documented following TPVI. Concern about the potential for pulmonary thromboembolism was raised on the basis of lung histopathology from in vivo animal experiments, submitted as part of the original FDA application, where microemboli (<0.6 mm) were identified in animals implanted with a Melody valve (Medtronic, Minneapolis, MN). In the U.S. clinical study, no new pulmonary emboli were identified among 63 patients who underwent 6-month follow-up computed tomography pulmonary angiograms or in the 32 subjects who underwent computed tomography scans at 1 year. It is recommended that these patients take aspirin 75 mg daily for life.

Treatment of Device-Related Complications.

Experience with bare stenting[18] has shown that repeat intervention using a stent-in-stent technique is both a feasible and effective treatment for suboptimal results. Repeat TPVI (and in a few cases a third TPVI) has been performed for the hammock effect, stent fracture, and residual stenosis. Repeat TPVI was feasible in all patients, with no procedural complications. Procedural technique is unchanged for stent-in-stent TPVI; hemodynamic results have been both excellent and sustained. Repeat TPVI leads to improved freedom from reintervention.[36] In the future, issues like the hammock effect will become irrelevant and indications may shift toward the treatment of late valvar degeneration. Repeat TPVI is, however, not suitable for all suboptimal or complicated outcomes. Clearly infection, external conduit compression, and conduit outgrowth will still require surgical revision of the pulmonary valve. Nevertheless, where appropriate, this approach should be considered before proceeding to surgery, as adopting such a management strategy could defer the need for surgical reintervention indefinitely.

MIDTERM FOLLOW-UP AND MORTALITY

Actuarial freedom from reintervention following TPVI was 95.4% at 1 year (number at risk 70) and 87.6% at 2 years (number at risk 24) in the U.S. study. The likelihood of valve dysfunction was greater in those with a primary indication for obstruction or a mixed lesion as opposed to pulmonary regurgitation (Fig. 51 6). Ten-year follow-up is available in the London/Paris cohort; however, actuarial survival and freedom from reintervention is strongly influenced by the impact of the learning curve on procedural results and thus should be interpreted cautiously.[28] Procedural and device-related mortality following TPVI is <1%. In the London/Paris series, 2 patients died early after technically successful TPVI (at 24 hours and 6 weeks); both were in cardiogenic shock at presentation and underwent TPVI as a palliative procedure. There were also two late deaths (at 8 and 35 months), which

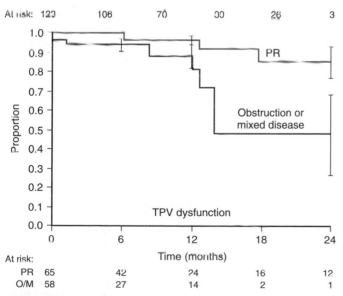

At risk:

PR	65	42	24	16	12
O/M	58	27	14	2	1

Figure 51-6 Kaplan-Meier curve depicting freedom from Melody valve dysfunction according to primary implantation indication. *(From McElhinney DB, Hellenbrand WE, Zahn EM et al. Short- and medium-term outcomes after transcatheter pulmonary valve placement in the expanded multicenter U.S. Melody valve trial. Circulation. 2010;1225: 507–516.)*

were presumed to be arrhythmic in origin, although one of these patients had type II stent fractures. In the U.S. cohort, there was one death at 20 days in a patient who suffered coronary artery dissection.

COMPARISON WITH SURGERY

At present, TPVI cannot be directly compared with surgery as it is not available to the same patient population. In addition, surgery permits resection of patch aneurysms or hypertrophied muscle bundles and remodeling of the RVOT. Nevertheless, early safety and efficacy data are encouraging and the technique should be regarded as an important complementary therapy in the lifetime management of congenital heart disease.[37] Treatment of residual lesions such as ventricular septal defects can also now be carried out by catheter techniques. The aim of TPVI should be to prolong conduit life without the complication of pulmonary regurgitation associated with bare stenting and to reduce the number of surgical interventions a patient will require. Perhaps in the future, with evolving device design and procedural technique, direct comparison will be possible.

PATIENT SELECTION

The main limitation of the currently available transcatheter valve device is the maximum diameter to which it can be deployed (22 mm) before compromising valvular competence. Selection of patients with suitable anatomy for TPVI is therefore critical to ensure procedural success and optimize long-term outcome. The RVOT morphology in this patient group is heterogeneous and detailed assessment with three-dimensional noninvasive imaging is invaluable.[38] In the first instance, the surgical history and nature of the right ventricular outflow tract must be clearly understood before a patient is accepted for further assessment. Homografts or other circumferential conduits provide the optimal implantation targets because of their tendency to deform in a predictable manner. TPVI into bioprosthetic conduits, can be achieved successfully with sustained results, but it should be noted that these valves have rigid, nondilatable sewing rings; thus while there may be an initial hemodynamic improvement, further reduction in the original orifice diameter will be obligatory owing to the added thickness of the valved stent. Thus in a growing child, although acute recovery from right ventricular pressure or volume overload can be achieved, long-lasting hemodynamic improvement should not be anticipated.[39] Those patients with transannular patches or native outflow tracts are rarely suitable, as they deform asymmetrically and thus risk device stability. An exception to this is following the arterial switch operation when the obstructed native RVOT does offer a safe environment for TPVI. The presence of a limited RVOT patch may also permit safe and effective TPVI.[40] However, when the predominant indication for intervention is pulmonary regurgitation, the presence of some level of obstruction or at least calcification of the conduit is essential to achieve device stability. Anteroposterior and lateral chest x-rays should be used to identify conduit calcification and transthoracic echocardiography to assess the gradient across the RVOT. The absence of calcification or a measurable gradient should raise concern, particularly in larger homografts or conduits.

It is often difficult to establish the precise morphology of the proposed implantation site by echocardiography because of limited echo windows and two-dimensional imaging planes. Assessment of these patients with magnetic resonance imaging (MRI)—or computed tomography if MRI is contraindicated—is therefore extremely valuable. Measurement of the RVOT dimensions is best made on two perpendicular gradient echo cine images (Fig. 51-7A and B), as this permits measurement of the maximum (systolic) diameter at the potential site of implantation. Reliance on "black-blood" spin echo (usually acquired in mid- to late diastole) or angiography images (non-gated image acquisition) may underestimate the maximum size of the RVOT. Gadolinium contrast-enhanced angiography, while it should not be used for measurements, allows three-dimensional reconstruction of the entire RVOT and a more complete appreciation of the

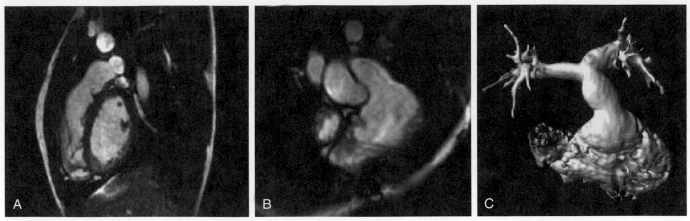

Figure 51-7 A and B. Perpendicular planes through the right ventricular outflow tract; gradient echo cine sequences. C. Three-dimensional reconstruction of the right ventricular outflow tract from gadolinium contrast-enhanced angiography. *(Courtesy of Dr Andrew Taylor, Cardiac Magnetic Resonance Unit, UCL Institute of Child Health, London.)*

overall morphology (Fig. 51-7C). MRI is also useful to quantify the pulmonary regurgitation, assess right and left ventricular dimensions and function, and determine the presence of distal pulmonary artery stenoses or other intracardiac defects.[41] Finally, there are two important considerations at the time of catheterization; the protocol for these has been outlined earlier. First, those patients who have borderline RVOT dimensions on MRI (20–24 mm) should undergo balloon sizing prior to proceeding to TPVI. In addition to further measurement, this permits assessment of the distensibility of the conduit wall and the likelihood of device stability. Second, the course of the coronary circulation with respect to the RVOT should be defined if it is not already known. An aortogram, with or without simultaneous injection into the RVOT depending on the degree of conduit calcification, is usually sufficient to resolve uncertainty. If concern remains with regard to the proximity of these structures, selective coronary angiography with simultaneous balloon inflation in the RVOT designed to mimic TPVI should be carried out. Potential compression of the coronary artery can thus be identified prospectively, allowing safe termination of the procedure and referral for surgery.

EXTENDING THE INDICATIONS

Many patients, particularly those who have undergone transannular patch repair of tetralogy of Fallot, have RVOTs >30 mm in diameter. TPVI is therefore technically impossible with the current device. To broaden the application of TPVI to all RVOT morphologies, a number of strategies have been proposed.

Stent Design

The limiting factor of the current commercially available device is the bovine jugular venous valve, which is available only up to 22 mm. The Edwards SAPIEN valve (Edwards Lifesciences, Irvine, CA), a bovine pericardial valve mounted inside a balloon-expandable stainless steel stent, has been proposed for use in the pulmonary position as it is currently available in diameters of 23 and 26 mm. Prototypes with 20- and 29-mm diameters are also under development. Early feasibility data are encouraging, with the outcome of the COMPASSION (COngenital Multicenter trial of Pulmonic valve regurgitation Studying the SAPIEN InterventIONal trans-catheter heart valve) safety and efficacy trial awaited.[42] One further benefit of this device is the lower incidence of stent fractures in the stainless steel frame; however, because of its balloon-expandable nature, it cannot be retrieved once deployed, and a degree of obstruction is still required for anchorage, making it unsuitable for patients with transannular patches. To implant valves into dilated unobstructed outflow tracts, new types of technology are required. Various experimental models have been proposed and can broadly be categorized into two groups. First, those intended for the

two-step procedure whereby implantation of a conventional device is facilitated by placement of a stent that downsizes the RVOT, and, second, the novel stand-alone device, which can be anchored within the dilated RVOT.[43–46] Use of computer modeling with finite element analysis and the development of rapid prototype models from MRI datasets highlights the heterogeneous RVOT morphology present in this patient population but also offers an opportunity to tailor device construction to patient anatomy.[47,48] It is this approach, rather than the conventional animal experimental model, that has resulted in successful clinical application.[49,50]

Hybrid Procedures

One limitation of animal experiments, already alluded to, is the uniform RVOT morphology that is encountered. In fact, pulmonary anatomy is commonly tortuous following repair of complex congenital heart disease. The deployment of self-expandable valved stents, as described above, could therefore be problematic. Insertion of the present device into a dilated outflow tract may, however, be facilitated by a simple surgical modification. Experimental work has demonstrated the feasibility of a hybrid procedure that combines banding of the RVOT via a left thoracotomy with subsequent valve implantation.[51] Recently, implantation of the Shelhigh Injectable Stented Pulmonic Valve has been reported in humans.[52] The device consists of a porcine pulmonic valve mounted inside a self-expandable stent and covered by No-React-treated pericardium. It is available in sizes 17 to 29 mm and is delivered, via a standard median sternotomy, with a trocar that is introduced through a small incision in the distal RVOT. After deployment, the valve is secured in position with several transmural sutures placed at the proximal and distal rim. While this approach avoids cardiopulmonary bypass and its adverse effects, it still requires resternotomy, which is itself associated with substantial risk. Although not strictly in the realm of interventional cardiology, the development of such procedures underlines the impact that advances in percutaneous valve technology are having on conventional surgical practice.

Rethinking the Substrate

The deleterious effects of pulmonary regurgitation on right ventricular function are now well documented. As a consequence, surgeons have moved toward placing smaller transannular patches and, where possible, valved conduits as part of the primary repair to try and minimize this complication. The development of percutaneous valve technology places an additional responsibility on the surgeon, who must now try to prepare the patient for percutaneous rather than surgical intervention in the future. Additionally, the availability of TPVI may influence the popularity of operations such as the Ross procedure.[53] At present, the size of the delivery system precludes TPVI in those less than 5 years of age or 20 kg in weight, although a smaller, tailor-made device that can be implanted on a 16-Fr system has been described.[54] Implantation was, however, technically difficult, and this procedure would not address the impact of somatic growth on conduit function. A novel concept that has been tested in the experimental setting is the insertion of an expandable valved conduit for reconstruction of the RVOT.[55] The principle of this approach is that the conduit could be balloon-dilated alongside somatic growth and, when valve failure occurred, percutaneous valve implantation could be safely performed.

FUTURE DIRECTIONS

Despite the potential for repeat percutaneous valve implantation with the currently available device, the endurance of biological valves remains an important issue for both surgeons and interventionalists. The mechanisms of degradation are multifactorial and include immunological rejection, mechanical deterioration, calcification, and enzymatic digestion. There is much interest in developing valves with infinite durability but comparable function and no need for anticoagulation. In the percutaneous field, low-profile biodegradable pulmonary valves made of small intestinal submucosa have been tested experimentally.[56] These valves provide a decellularized matrix that is repopulated following implantation by the adjacent host tissue and does not invoke significant immunological rejection. The development of progressive leaflet thickening in the animal model, however, currently precludes human application. An alternative approach is preimplantation seeding of the matrix by means of tissue engineering. Experimental transcatheter implantation of such valves in the pulmonary position has recently been reported.[57,58]

Transcatheter Tricuspid Valve Implantation

BACKGROUND AND CLINICAL INDICATIONS

Disease of the tricuspid valve is often regarded as of lesser clinical consequence than that of the other heart valves. Despite this, dysfunction is common, particularly in the setting of congestive heart failure, and can lead to atrial arrhythmias, hepatic congestion, ascites, and peripheral edema. Other etiologies include rheumatic heart disease, pulmonary hypertension, infective endocarditis, and congenital conditions such as Ebstein's anomaly.[59] In the context of mitral valve disease, repair of concomitant tricuspid regurgitation has clearly been shown to improve both symptoms and survival and is the surgical standard of care.[60] With rapidly evolving percutaneous mitral valve repair techniques, a transcatheter approach to tricuspid valve disease is fundamental if optimal care is to continue to be delivered. Surgical tricuspid valve replacement at present represents the last treatment option for patients with tricuspid regurgitation or stenosis in whom medical management has failed and repair of the valve is not feasible. Mortality and morbidity from the procedure is high, reflecting the poor preoperative condition of these patients; the decision to intervene requires the presence of symptoms or an indication for mitral valve surgery.[61,62] A percutaneous approach to replacing the tricuspid valve may therefore also have significant benefits for this high-risk population.

ANIMAL STUDIES

To date, there are two published studies examining the experimental feasibility of percutaneous valve implantation into a native tricuspid valve.[63,64] These studies report new types of devices designed to address the complex challenges of the tricuspid valve. The first device, a self-expandable nitinol stent with two flat disks (diameter 40 mm) and a tubular portion (diameter 18 mm) supporting a bovine jugular venous valve, was successfully implanted into 7 of 8 ewes via a right internal jugular approach. The device was deployed in a similar manner to an atrial septal defect closure device with the ventricular disk covered with polytetrafluoroethylene (PTFE) to ensure sealing (Fig. 51-8). There

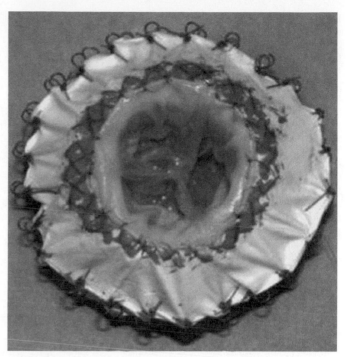

Figure 51-8 Percutaneous tricuspid valve device. (Adapted from Boudjemline Y, Agnoletti G, Bonnet D, et al. Steps toward the percutaneous replacement of atrioventricular valves: an experimental study. J Am Coll Cardiol. 2005;462:360–365.)

was no sustained arrhythmia or early or late stent migrations in the series, and at autopsy the devices had become integrated into the walls of the right atrial and ventricular cavities. The native tricuspid valves were completely inactivated by the stent and partially retracted. The second device consisted of three semilunar leaflets of porcine pericardium sutured onto a nitinol ring designed to imitate the shape of the native tricuspid annulus. The formed valve was then inserted inside a double-edge nitinol stent. This device was implanted successfully into 8 of 10 healthy sheep. Two sheep died during the procedure owing to stent migration and fatal arrhythmia; otherwise sustained results were achieved with no elevation of right ventricular pressure. The pathological tricuspid valve is likely to present a number of difficulties for this technique; these are not addressed here. In Ebstein's anomaly, for example, the deployment of these devices would be problematic because of the lack of an identifiable annulus. Further, the dynamic nature of the tricuspid annulus raises major concerns regarding the long-term stability of such devices, the risk of stent fractures, and the potential for myocardial trauma. An indication that does provide hope for clinical applicability in the near future is the treatment of the failing bioprosthesis. While this is relevant to only a small patient group, it provides a safe environment for valve implantation in the tricuspid position and should lay the foundations for progression to the treatment of native valve disease. Experimental feasibility has been demonstrated.[65] A novel transcatheter approach to the management of tricuspid regurgitation that comprises valved stent implantation into the superior vena cava and inferior vena cava has also been trialled.[66]

CLINICAL STUDIES

A few cases have recently been reported whereby the Melody valve (Medtronic, Minneapolis, MN) has been implanted into patients who have undergone the Bjork modification of the Fontan operation (originally described as anastomosis of the right atrial appendage to the right ventricle with the aid of a pericardial patch but also including conduit placement between the right atrium and ventricle).[67–69]

Percutaneous creation of a functioning tricuspid valve in this highly selected patient group appears to provide a good alternative to redo open heart surgery, improving symptoms and functional class. A further multicenter series describing successful implantation of the Melody valve into 15 patients with failed tricuspid prostheses has recently been published;[70] 5 cases involved implantation into dysfunctional conduits forming part of a Fontan palliation (as described above) and 10 involved implantation into various failing bioprosthetic valves. Median New York Heart Association (NYHA) class was III and all patients were considered at too high a risk for conventional surgery. The primary lesion was predominantly stenosis, although a few had significant regurgitation. Procedural success was achieved in all. Mean tricuspid gradient fell from 12.9 to 3.9 mm Hg and tricuspid regurgitation was reduced to no more than mild. NYHA functional class improved in 12 patients. There was 1 case of atrioventricular block requiring a pacemaker and 1 case of endocarditis 2 months postimplant. One patient with preexisting multiorgan failure died 17 days after the procedure. The remaining patients were well, with sustained results 9 months after implantation.

FUTURE DIRECTIONS

Percutaneous repair strategies have demonstrated much promise for the treatment of mitral valve disease. In particular the edge-to-edge repair, which opposes the valve leaflets with a stitch or clip to reduce valve excursion and thus regurgitation, could be applied in the right heart. This repair technique, which has been used surgically for tricuspid valve repair, may overcome some of the problems encountered when trying to replace the valve by catheter.[71]

▤ Summary

Percutaneous valve therapies are currently among the most exciting areas of interventional cardiology. Their application in the right heart covers the spectrum from clinically applicable devices to pure experimental models. Recent times have seen rapid progress in the evolution of these devices from bench to bedside. Further creative thought regarding device design and cooperation between cardiologists and surgeons should see wider clinical application in coming years.

REFERENCES

1. Bonhoeffer P, Boudjemline Y, Saliba Z, et al: Transcatheter implantation of a bovine valve in pulmonary position: a lamb study. *Circulation* 102(7):813–816, 2000.
2. Eicken A, Fratz S, Hager A, et al: Transcutaneous Melody valve implantation in "tricuspid position" after a Fontan Björk (RA-RV homograft) operation results in biventricular circulation. *Int J Cardiol* 142(3):e45–e47, 2010.
3. Warnes CA, Liberthson R, Danielson GK, et al: Task force 1: the changing profile of congenital heart disease in adult life. *J Am Coll Cardiol* 37:1170–1175 2001.
4. Marelli AJ, Mackie AS, Ionescu-Ittu R, et al: Congenital heart disease in the general population: changing prevalence and age distribution. *Circulation* 115(2):163–172, 2007.
5. Frigiola A, Redington AN, Cullen S, et al: Pulmonary regurgitation is an important determinant of right ventricular contractile dysfunction in patients with surgically repaired tetralogy of Fallot. *Circulation* 110(suppl I):II-153–II-157, 2004.
6. Carvalho JS, Shinebourne EA, Busst C, et al: Exercise capacity after complete repair of tetralogy of Fallot: deleterious effects of residual pulmonary regurgitation. *Br Heart J* 67(6):470–473, 1992.
7. Gatzoulis MA, Balaji S, Webber SA, et al: Risk factors for arrhythmia and sudden cardiac death late after repair of tetralogy of Fallot: a multicentre study. *Lancet* 356(9234):975–981, 2000.
8. Cleveland DC, Williams WG, Razzouk AJ, et al: Failure of cryopreserved homograft valved conduits in the pulmonary circulation. *Circulation* 86(5 Suppl):II150–II153, 1992.
9. Bando K, Danielson GK, Schaff HV, et al: Outcome of pulmonary and aortic homografts for right ventricular outflow tract reconstruction. *J Thorac Cardiovasc Surg* 109(3):509–517, 1995.
10. Williams WG, Quaegebeur JM, Kirklin JW, et al: Outflow obstruction after the arterial switch operation: a multiinstitutional study. *J Thorac Cardiovasc Surg* 114(6):975–987, 1997.
11. Eyskens B, Reybrouck T, Bogaert J, et al: Homograft insertion for pulmonary regurgitation after repair of tetralogy of Fallot improves cardio-respiratory exercise performance. *Am J Cardiol* 85:221–225, 2000.
12. Therrien J, Siu SC, Harris L, et al: Impact of pulmonary valve replacement on arrhythmia propensity late after repair of tetralogy of Fallot. *Circulation* 103(20):2489–2494, 2001.
13. Doughan AR, McConnell ME, Lyle TA, et al: Effects of pulmonary valve replacement on QRS duration and right ventricular cavity size late after repair of right ventricular outflow tract obstruction. *Am J Cardiol* 95(12):1511–1514, 2005.
14. Warnes CA, Williams RG, Bashore TM, et al: ACC/AHA 2008 Guidelines for the Management of Adults with Congenital Heart Disease: executive summary: a report of the American College of Cardiology/American Heart Association Task Force on Practice Guidelines (writing committee to develop guidelines for the management of adults with congenital heart disease). *Circulation* 118(23):2395–2451, 2008.
15. Therrien J, Siu SC, McLaughlin PR, et al: Pulmonary valve replacement in adults late after repair of tetralogy of Fallot: are we operating too late? *J Am Coll Cardiol* 36(5):1670–1675, 2000.
16. Stark J, Bull C, Stajevic M, et al: Fate of subpulmonary homograft conduits: determinants of late homograft failure. *J Thorac Cardiovasc Surg* 115(3):506–516, 1998.
17. Meyns B, Jashari R, Gewillig M, et al: Factors influencing the survival of cryopreserved homografts. The second homograft performs as well as the first. *Eur J Cardiothorac Surg* 28(2):211–216, 2005.

18. Sugiyama H, Williams W, Benson LN: Implantation of endovascular stents for the obstructive right ventricular outflow tract. *Heart* 91(8):1058–1063, 2005.
19. Zahn EM, Hellenbrand WE, Lock JE, et al: Implantation of the melody transcatheter pulmonary valve in patients with a dysfunctional right ventricular outflow tract conduit early results from the U.S. clinical trial. *J Am Coll Cardiol* 54(18):1722–1729, 2009.
20. Lurz P, Nordmeyer J, Coats L, et al: Immediate clinical and haemodynamic benefits of restoration of pulmonary valvar competence in patients with pulmonary hypertension. *Heart* 95(8):646–650, 2009.
21. Boethig D, Thies WR, Hecker H, et al: Mid term course after pediatric right ventricular outflow tract reconstruction: a comparison of homografts, porcine xenografts and Contegras. *Eur J Cardiothorac Surg* 27(1):58–66, 2005.
22. Ewert P, Schubert S, Peters B, et al: The CP stent—short, long, covered—for the treatment of aortic coarctation, stenosis of pulmonary arteries and caval veins, and Fontan anastomosis in children and adults: an evaluation of 60 stents in 53 patients. *Heart* 91(7):948–953, 2005.
23. Webb JG, Munt B, Makkar RR, et al: Percutaneous stent-mounted valve for treatment of aortic or pulmonary valve disease. *Catheter Cardiovasc Intervent* 63:89–93, 2004.
24. Attmann T, Quaden R, Jahnke T, et al: Percutaneous pulmonary valve replacement: 3-month evaluation of self-expanding valved stents. *Ann Thorac Surg* 82(2):708–713, 2006.
25. Metzner A, Iino K, Steinseifer U, et al: Percutaneous pulmonary polyurethane valved stent implantation. *J Thorac Cardiovasc Surg* 139(3):748–752, 2010.
26. Attmann T, Quaden R, Freistedt A, et al: Percutaneous heart valve replacement: histology and calcification characteristics of biological valved stents in juvenile sheep. *Cardiovasc Pathol* 16(3):165–170, 2007.
27. Bonhoeffer P, Boudjemline Y, Saliba Z, et al: Percutaneous replacement of pulmonary valve in a right-ventricle to pulmonary-artery prosthetic conduit with valve dysfunction. *Lancet* 356:1403–1405, 2000.
28. Lurz P, Coats L, Khambadkone S, et al: Percutaneous pulmonary valve implantation: impact of evolving technology and learning curve on clinical outcome. *Circulation* 117(15):1964–1972, 2008.
29. McElhinney DB, Hellenbrand WE, Zahn EM, et al: Short- and medium-term outcomes after transcatheter pulmonary valve placement in the expanded multicenter US Melody Valve Trial. *Circulation* 122(5):507–516, 2010.
30. Nordmeyer J, Lurz P, Khambadkone S, Schievano S: Pre-stenting with a bare metal stent before percutaneous pulmonary valve implantation: acute and 1-year outcomes. *Heart* 97(2):118–123, 2011.
31. Coats L, Khambadkone S, Derrick G, et al: Physiological and clinical consequences of relief of right ventricular outflow tract obstruction late after repair of congenital heart defects. *Circulation* 113:2037–2044, 2006.
32. Coats L, Khambadkone S, Derrick G, et al: Physiological consequences of percutaneous pulmonary valve implantation: the different behaviour of volume- and pressure-overloaded ventricles. *Eur Heart J* 28(15):1886–1893, 2007.
33. Lurz P, Giardini A, Taylor AM, et al: Effect of altering pathologic right ventricular loading conditions by percutaneous pulmonary valve implantation on exercise capacity. *Am J Cardiol* 105(5):721–726, 2010.

34. Peng LF, McElhinney DB, Nugent AW, et al: Endovascular stenting of obstructed right ventricle-to-pulmonary artery conduits: a 15-year experience. *Circulation* 113(22):2598–2605, 2006.
35. Nordmeyer J, Khambadkone S, Coats L, et al: Risk stratification, systematic classification, and anticipatory management strategies for stent fracture after percutaneous pulmonary valve implantation. *Circulation* 115(11):1392–1397 2007.
36. Nordmeyer J, Coats L, Lurz P, et al: Percutaneous pulmonary valve-in-valve implantation: a successful treatment concept for early device failure. *Eur Heart J* 29(6):810–815, 2008.
37. Coats L, Tsang V, Khambadkone S, et al: The potential impact of percutaneous pulmonary valve stent implantation on right ventricular outflow tract re-intervention. *Eur J Cardiothorac Surg* 27(4):536–543, 2005.
38. Schievano S, Coats L, Migliavacca F, et al: Variations in right ventricular outflow tract morphology following repair of congenital heart disease: implications for percutaneous pulmonary valve implantation. *J Cardiovasc Magn Reson* 9(4):687–695, 2007.
39. Asoh K, Walsh M, Hickey E, et al: Percutaneous pulmonary valve implantation within bioprosthetic valves. *Eur Heart J* 31(11):1404–1409, 2010.
40. Momenah TS, El Oakley R, Al Najashi K, et al: Extended application of percutaneous pulmonary valve implantation. *J Am Coll Cardiol* 53(20):1859–1863, 2009.
41. Taylor AM: Assessment of the pulmonary valve with magnetic resonance imaging. In Hijazi ZM, Bonhoeffer P, Feldman T, et al, editors: *Transcatheter Valve Repair*, London, 2006, Taylor and Francis, pp 25–44.
42. Boone RH, Webb JG, Horlick E, et al: Transcatheter pulmonary valve implantation using the Edwards SAPIEN transcatheter heart valve. *Catheter Cardiovasc Intervent* 75(2):286–294, 2010.
43. Boudjemline Y, Agnoletti G, Bonnet D, et al: Percutaneous pulmonary valve replacement in a large right ventricular outflow tract: an experimental study. *J Am Coll Cardiol* 43(6):1082–1087, 2004.
44. Mollet A, Basquin A, Stos B, et al: Off-pump replacement of the pulmonary valve in large right ventricular outflow tracts: a transcatheter approach using an intravascular infundibulum reducer. *Pediatr Res* 62(4):428–433, 2007.
45. Zong GJ, Bai Y, Jiang HB, et al: Use of a novel valve stent for transcatheter pulmonary valve replacement: an animal study. *J Thorac Cardiovasc Surg* 137(6):1363–1369, 2009.
46. Amahzoune B, Szymansky C, Fabiani JN, et al: A new endovascular size reducer for large pulmonary outflow tract. *Eur J Cardiothorac Surg* 37(3):730–732, 2010.
47. Schievano S, Petrini L, Migliavacca F, et al: Finite element analysis of stent deployment: understanding stent fracture in percutaneous pulmonary valve implantation. *J Intervent Cardiol* 20(6):546–554, 2007.
48. Schievano S, Migliavacca F, Coats L, et al: Percutaneous pulmonary valve implantation based on rapid prototyping of right ventricular outflow tract and pulmonary trunk from MR data. *Radiology* 242(2):490–497, 2007.
49. Schievano S, Taylor AM, Capelli C, et al: First-in-man implantation of a novel percutaneous valve: a new approach to medical device development. *EuroIntervention* 5(6):745–750, 2010.
50. Capelli C, Taylor AM, Migliavacca F, et al: Patient-specific reconstructed anatomies and computer simulations are fundamental for selecting medical device treatment: application to a new

percutaneous pulmonary valve. *Philos Transact A Math Phys Eng Sci* 368(1921):3027–3038, 2010.

51. Boudjemline Y, Schievano S, Bonnet C, et al: Off-pump replacement of the pulmonary valve in large right ventricular outflow tracts: a hybrid approach. *J Thorac Cardiovasc Surg* 129(4):831–837, 2005.

52. Schreiber C, Hörer J, Vogt M, et al: A new treatment option for pulmonary valvar insufficiency: first experiences with implantation of a self-expanding stented valve without use of cardiopulmonary bypass. *Eur J Cardiothorac Surg* 31(1):26–30, 2007.

53. Nordmeyer J, Lurz P, Tsang VT, et al: Effective transcatheter valve implantation after pulmonary homograft failure: a new perspective on the Ross operation. *J Thorac Cardiovasc Surg* 138(1):84–88, 2009.

54. Feinstein JA, Kim N, Reddy VM, et al: Percutaneous pulmonary valve placement in a 10-month-old patient using a hand crafted stent-mounted porcine valve. *Catheter Cardiovasc Intervent* 67(4):644–649, 2006.

55. Boudjemline Y, Laborde F, Pineau E, et al: Expandable right ventricular-to-pulmonary artery conduit: an animal study. *Pediatr Res* 59(6):773–777, 2006.

56. Ruiz CE, Iemura M, Medie S, et al: Transcatheter placement of a low-profile biodegradable pulmonary valve made of small intestinal submucosa: a long-term study in a swine model. *J Thorac Cardiovasc Surg* 130(2):477–484, 2005.

57. Lutter G, Metzner A, Jahnke T, et al: Percutaneous tissue-engineered pulmonary valved stent implantation. *Ann Thorac Surg* 89(1):259–263, 2010.

58. Metzner A, Stock UA, Iino K, et al: Percutaneous pulmonary valve replacement: autologous tissue-engineered valved stents. *Cardiovasc Res* 8(3):453–461, 2010.

59. Hauck AJ, Freeman DP, Ackermann DM, et al: Surgical pathology of the tricuspid valve: a study of 363 cases spanning 25 years. *Mayo Clin Proc* 63(9):851–863, 1988.

60. Tang GH, David TE, Singh SK, et al: Tricuspid valve repair with an annuloplasty ring results in improved long-term outcomes. *Circulation* 114(1 Suppl):I577–I581, 2006.

61. Carrier M, Hébert Y, Pellerin M, et al: Tricuspid valve replacement: an analysis of 25 years of experience at a single center. *Ann Thorac Surg* 75:47–50, 2003.

62. Bonow RO, Carabello BA, Kanu C, et al: ACC/AHA 2006 guidelines for the management of patients with valvular heart disease: a report of the American College of Cardiology/American Heart Association Task Force on Practice Guidelines (writing committee to revise the 1998 Guidelines for the Management of Patients With Valvular Heart Disease): developed in collaboration with the Society of Cardiovascular Anesthesiologists: endorsed by the Society for Cardiovascular Angiography and Interventions and the Society of Thoracic Surgeons. *Circulation* 114(5):e84–e231, 2006 Aug 1.

63. Boudjemline Y, Agnoletti G, Bonnet D, et al: Steps toward the percutaneous replacement of atrioventricular valves an experimental study. *J Am Coll Cardiol* 46(2):360–365, 2005.

64. Bai Y, Zong GJ, Wang HR, et al: An integrated pericardial valved stent special for percutaneous tricuspid implantation: an animal feasibility study. *J Surg Res* 160(2):215–221, 2010.

65. Zegdi R, Khabbaz Z, Borenstein N, et al: A repositionable valved stent for endovascular treatment of deteriorated bioprostheses. *J Am Coll Cardiol* 48(7):1365–1368, 2006.

66. Lauten A, Figulla HR, Willich C, et al: Percutaneous caval stent valve implantation: investigation of an interventional approach for treatment of tricuspid regurgitation. *Eur Heart J* 31(10):1274–1281, 2010.

67. Butcher CJ, Plymen CM, Walker F: A novel and unique treatment of right ventricular inflow obstruction in a patient with a Bjork modification of the Fontan palliation before pregnancy. *Cardiology* 29:1–2, 2010.

68. Tanous D, Nadeem SN, Mason X, et al: Creation of a functional tricuspid valve: novel use of percutaneously implanted valve in right atrial to right ventricular conduit in a patient with tricuspid atresia. *Int J Cardiol* 144:e8–e10, 2010.

69. Eicken A, Fratz S, Hager A, et al: Transcutaneous Melody valve implantation in "tricuspid position" after a Fontan Björk (RA-RV homograft) operation results in biventricular circulation. *Int J Cardiol* 142(3):e45–e47, 2010.

70. Roberts PA, Boudjemline Y, Cheatham J, et al: Percutaneous tricuspid valve replacement in congenital and acquired heart disease. *J Am Coll Cardiol* 58:117–122, 2011.

71. De Bonis M, Lapenna E, La Canna G, et al: A novel technique for correction of severe tricuspid valve regurgitation due to complex lesions. *Eur J Cardiothorac Surg* 25(5):760–765, 2004.

Hypertrophic Cardiomyopathy

GUS THEODOS | SAMIR R. KAPADIA

Introduction

By virtue of the broad variability in its phenotypic expression, hypertrophic cardiomyopathy (HCM) is a unique cardiovascular condition with a potential for the development of clinical symptoms during any phase of life, from infancy to greater than 90 years of age.[1-7] The genetic foundation of HCM has been directly related to abnormalities of the genes encoding the cardiac sarcomere unit and may result in a complex disease phenotype that encompasses a spectrum of clinical and pathological presentations. In the past, the nomenclature regarding HCM has often been noted to be misleading. *Idiopathic hypertrophic subaortic stenosis* or *hypertrophic obstructive cardiomyopathy* (HOCM) typically described only a subset of patients with this disorder. With an improved understanding of the clinical heterogeneity of this process, *hypertrophic cardiomyopathy* appears to be a more appropriate descriptive term. The rapid demystification of the genetic underpinnings of HCM has greatly expanded our understanding of this entity. HCM is inherited in an autosomal dominant fashion with over 12 genes identified as being involved in the phenotypic manifestation.[1,7-10] Three of those genes account for over 50% of the known cases of HCM.[1,9,58] Traditionally, the diagnosis of HCM has been primarily clinical, involving the use of echocardiography to evaluate for certain characteristic features such as asymmetrical septal hypertrophy or systolic anterior motion of the mitral valve (SAM) with left ventricular outflow tract (LVOT) obstruction. While there have been dramatic advances in the understanding of the genetic predisposition for this disease state, the utility of genetic study for the absolute diagnosis remains preliminary at the present. However, the future holds promise that genetics will become a more reliable tool for establishing and confirming this diagnosis. The use of genotyping in risk stratification is also evolving.

Given the heterogeneity of the disease process, even within the same family, its clinical course and long-term outcomes differ significantly. Therefore management strategies span the range from close outpatient follow-up to surgical remodeling of the myocardium. HCM appears to be an evolving process in some patients, with a change in the phenotype with age. This presents a challenging dilemma in terms of grasping the clinical course of this disorder. Consequently therapeutic strategies need to be individualized for each patient.

Epidemiology

The prevalence of this genetic disorder is on the order of 1:500 in the general adult population and it is one of the more common cardiac genetic disorders known.[1,6,9] While is not routinely accounted for in general practice, it is not uncommon to see these patients in tertiary referral centers. The clinical heterogeneity of this disorder plays into the difficulty in establishing a diagnosis. Often the presentation lacks the classic features noted on echocardiography. HCM is a disease process that is known to evolve with age, and the development of left ventricular hypertrophy has been observed to occur in children after full growth is attained.[52,53,60] This can make diagnosis of HCM challenging and suggests that repeat evaluation in patients may be required to establish a diagnosis.

Natural History of the Disease

The heterogeneity of HCM lies not only in its varied presentations but also in the natural history of disease in the patient population. Attempts to understand the links between genotype, phenotype, and natural history have as yet yielded only limited clinical associations. One of the most interesting aspects of the study of the natural history of patients with HCM is how selection bias has played a significant role in initial attempts to characterize patient outcomes. Earlier studies from tertiary referral centers implied ominously high annual mortality rates of 3% to 6%; however, this work was limited by a significant referral bias.[1] More recent data from regional and community-based centers suggest an annual mortality of approximately 1%.[3,4] However, in select populations, the annual mortality rate may be as high as 5% to 6%, particularly in those symptomatic patients who are eventually referred to larger centers.[1,11,12] The clinical course of the HCM population is often difficult to predict and poses a challenge to clinicians. However, the options in terms of disease progression remain limited. The most feared and least predictable of the entities is sudden cardiac death, particularly in the younger population. More commonly, patients develop symptoms such as angina, syncope, or exertional dyspnea. These symptoms can become progressively worse over time, and such patients can progress toward end-stage heart failure with left ventricular failure. HCM patients also develop atrial fibrillation and are at risk for embolic strokes. A certain percentage of HCM patients remain asymptomatic and have a comparably normal life expectancy. However, at some point even they are at risk for the development of sudden cardiac death or atrial fibrillation. The challenge for clinicians is to closely follow those who eventually develop symptoms and to offer timely therapy when it is indicated.

Clinical Presentation

While the spectrum of clinical presentation in HCM is large, most patients are actually asymptomatic and diagnosed as the result of a murmur on exam, abnormal electrocardiogram (ECG), or unexplained left ventricular hypertrophy (LVH) discovered by echocardiography. The complex pathophysiological interplay between left ventricular outflow tract (LVOT) obstruction, diastolic dysfunction, myocardial ischemia, and mitral regurgitation generally results in the presenting complaints of exertional dyspnea, chest discomfort, syncope or near syncope, and sudden cardiac death. Symptomatic patients who will have an adverse clinical course will typically follow along one of several pathways: (1) those at high risk for sudden cardiac death; (2) progressive symptoms of exertional dyspnea and chest pain associated with presyncope or syncope in the setting of preserved LV function; (3) development of progressive congestive heart failure due to severe LV remodelling, resulting in systolic dysfunction; and (4) consequences of supraventricular or ventricular arrhythmias such as atrial fibrillation (AF) or ventricular tachycardia (VT).[1,7,13–15] Sudden cardiac death is the most common presentation and source of mortality in HCM.[1,7,14,16,17] In addition, sudden cardiac death (SCD) is the single leading cause of cardiovascular death among young people as well as the most common cause of mortality in competitive athletes.[1,18] Most commonly observed in asymptomatic children and young adults, it appears that there is no advanced age at which the risk of SCD becomes negligible.[19] While SCD is obviously the most fearsome and dramatic complication of HCM, those at high risk for SCD actually constitute only a small fraction of the disease spectrum,[1,6,7,20,21] and much effort has been devoted to the premorbid identification of this subset of patients. Currently identified risk factors for SCD include prior cardiac arrest, family history of SCD, unexplained syncope or near syncope, left ventricular thickness greater than 30 mm, a high-risk genetic mutation (e.g., beta myosin heavy chain mutations Arg403Gln and Arg719Gln), hypotensive response during exercise stress testing, and nonsustained VT on Holter monitoring (Table 52-1).[1,7,14,20,22–27] In addition, an LVOT gradient greater than 30 mm Hg has been associated with an increased risk of SCD, progression to heart failure, and morbidity related to arrhythmia, including stroke.[28,29] However, an incremental increase in the subaortic gradient above 30 mm Hg has not been demonstrated to impart any additional risk. It is uncommon for HCM patients to suffer SCD without at least one of the aforementioned risk factors (<3%).[20] It has been suggested that the etiology of SCD in this population is related to the development of complex ventricular tachyarrhythmia,[7,30,31] often during mild to moderate physical exertion and with a circadian predilection for the early morning hours.[32] Chest pain, both typical and atypical in character, is a common feature in HCM and has been reported in up to 80% of patients in this population.[33] In many cases, angiography reveals normal coronary arteries. Despite this finding, numerous studies incorporating nuclear single photon emission computed tomography (SPECT), positron emission tomography (PET), and magnetic resonance imaging (MRI) technologies have demonstrated significant reversible and nonreversible myocardial perfusion defects in this subset of patients, including autopsy data reporting findings of myocardial infarction in up to 15% of such patients.[1,7,33–37] Collectively, these data have led to a mounting body of evidence suggesting that microvascular dysfunction may have a pivotal role in the development of myocardial ischemia and infarction in this group. The etiology of microvascular dysfunction is probably multifactorial and due in part to arteriolar medial hypertrophy, resulting in reduced luminal diameter, impaired coronary vasodilatory response, and a supply : demand mismatch due to an abnormally thickened ventricle.[1,7,34,38] In addition, early work has suggested that evidence of microvascular dysfunction, as demonstrated by PET, is an independent predictor of increased mortality and may portend a worse prognosis years prior to the development of clinical deterioration.[39] Syncope in patients with HCM is not an uncommon phenomenon and has a diverse array of possible etiologies, making the exact determination of mechanism challenging. While regarded as an ominous prognostic sign and known risk factor for SCD in the younger population, syncope in the adult population has not been independently associated with premature demise, and recurrent episodes are rarely reported in patients who have suffered SCD.[40–42] Arrhythmic sources of syncope may be supraventricular, such as atrial fibrillation or flutter, or ventricular, such as ventricular tachycardia or fibrillation. Hemodynamic mechanisms of syncope all result in a sudden and severe reduction in cardiac output that may involve ischemia, outflow tract obstruction, or severe diastolic dysfunction. Additionally, it has been suggested that activation of left ventricular baroreceptors due to elevated intracavity pressures may induce reflex hypotension and a consequent syncopal episode in a select subgroup of patients.[43] Heart failure—as manifested by a symptom complex of exertional dyspnea, orthopnea, and progressive fatigue—is most commonly encountered in adult patients with HCM, but it has been described in the juvenile population as well.[1] Usually, in the setting of preserved systolic function, symptoms are most commonly the consequence of diastolic dysfunction due to an abnormally thickened and noncompliant ventricle.[7] The combined influence of other variables such as ischemia, AF, and mitral regurgitation may also play a significant role in the development of hemodynamic decompensation in this population. A smaller number of patients with HCM and heart failure may have significantly reduced left ventricular systolic function and chamber enlargement. It is important to recognize this subset of patients, given the potential alteration in therapeutic strategy.[41] Atrial fibrillation complicates the course of approximately 20% of patients with HCM and is associated with an increased risk of heart failure-related death.[17,24] The risk seems to be substantially greater in the subset of patients with outflow tract obstruction or an earlier onset of arrhythmia (<50 years of age). Advancing age, left atrial enlargement, and congestive symptoms are independently linked with the development of atrial fibrillation. While strongly associated with an increased risk of fatal and nonfatal stroke, atrial fibrillation does not appear to be a risk factor for the development of SCD, and approximately one-third of patients have no long-term sequelae from this arrhythmia.[24] Severe functional deterioration due to dyspnea, chest pain, palpitations, or pulmonary edema may complicate the course of the chronically affected. This is most likely due to the loss of atrial contraction, reduction in diastolic filling time, and exacerbation of underlying ischemia.[7,24] The nature of the clinical presentation may also be affected by a particular patient's age or gender. In contrast to their younger counterparts, elderly patients with HCM often develop marked symptomatology at an advanced age (>55 years), have lesser degrees of left ventricular hypertrophy usually confined to the septum, and a dynamic subaortic gradient due to restricted

TABLE 52-1	Risk Factors for Sudden Cardiac Death
Spontaneous sustained VT	
Nonsustained VT (>3 beats at rate of >120 beats per minute) on ambulatory monitoring	
Family history of cardiac arrest or SCD	
Prior personal history of cardiac arrest	
Unexplained syncope (especially if exertional)	
Abnormal response to exercise stress testing (especially hypotension)	
LV thickness greater than 30 mm	
Early onset of disease	
Nuclear stress testing demonstrating ischemia (even if related to microvascular disease)	
High-risk genetic mutation (see Table 52-2)	
Concomitant CHF or severe aortic stenosis	
Other comorbidities, such as pulmonary embolus and malignancy	
LVOT gradient >30 mm Hg	
Atrial fibrillation*	
Near syncope*	

LVOT, left ventricular outflow tract; SCD, sudden cardiac death; VT, ventricular tachycardia.

*Direct relationship with SCD less well established.

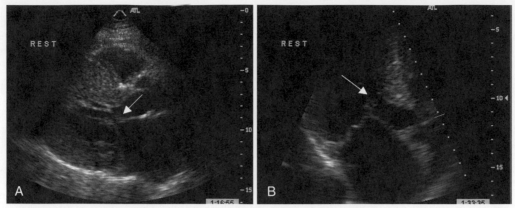

Figure 52-1 Echocardiographic parasternal long (A) and apical three chamber (B) views demonstrating systolic anterior motion (SAM) (arrow) at rest, resulting in severe LVOT obstruction in a patient with severe symptomatic hypertrophic obstructive cardiomyopathy (HOCM).

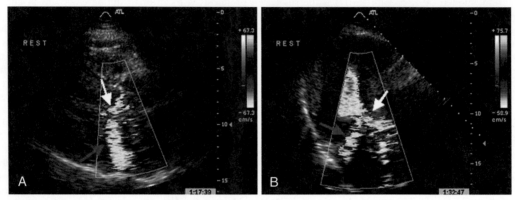

Figure 52-2 Color Doppler images displaying flow acceleration in LVOT (white arrow) and resulting in posteriorly directed mitral regurgitation (orange arrow) in the parasternal long (A) and apical three-chamber (B) views.

excursion of the often anteriorly displaced mitral leaflets and posteriorly directed septal motion.[44] While HCM seems to have a male predominance, female patients often present at a later age, are more symptomatic, and are at a greater risk of death due to heart failure or stroke.[45]

Diagnosis

ECHOCARDIOGRAPHY

Given its safety and ubiquity, two-dimensional echocardiography is the most common method for establishing the clinical diagnosis of HCM via the identification of a thickened, nondilated left ventricle in the absence of comorbidities known to cause such a degree of left ventricular hypertrophy (i.e., hypertension or aortic stenosis).[1,7,46] Classically thought to involve primarily the ventricular septum, the morphological expression of left ventricular hypertrophy is extremely heterogeneous and virtually any pattern of thickening may be observed.[1,7,47] In addition, there are significant differences in the pattern of hypertrophy between young and elderly patients. Elderly patients are often found to have an *elliptical* ventricular cavity with hypertrophy predominantly of the basal septum. In contrast, young patients (<55 years) often have a crescent-shaped ventricular cavity associated with diffuse hypertrophy of the interventricular septum.[48] While a maximal wall thickness greater than 15 mm is the traditional echocardiographic benchmark for HCM, the degree of hypertrophy may demonstrate considerable variability (with a mean thickness of

approximately 22 mm).[47] It is important to realize, however, that the paucity of characteristic LVH (>15 mm) on echocardiographic exam *does not* exclude the presence of a HCM gene mutation.[7,9,49–51] Thus, serial echocardiographic assessment may be necessary for adequate identification of suspected carriers, especially in the younger population, in whom the development of LVH may be delayed until after puberty.[1,14,51]

LVOT is observed in approximately 20% of patients with HCM and is usually dynamic in nature.[17,28] Subaortic obstruction is due to systolic anterior motion (SAM) of the anterior mitral leaflet, resulting in mitral-septal contact during midsystole[7] (Fig. 52-1). Obstruction may not be present under resting conditions but can be provoked by pharmacological (i.e., amyl nitrite) or physiological maneuvers (i.e., Valsalva). Significant mitral regurgitation frequently accompanies SAM owing to distortion of the valvular apparatus and malcoaptation of the anterior and posterior leaflets (Fig. 52-2). Mitral regurgitation is also observed in up to 30% of patients who do not demonstrate obstructive physiology primarily due to leaflet prolapse, chordal rupture, or trauma resulting in calcification or fibrosis.[52] Less commonly, a mid-cavity gradient is formed because of the anomalous insertion of the anterolateral papillary muscle directly onto the anterior mitral leaflet or an exaggerated proliferation of midventricular papillary musculature coming into apposition with the ventricular septum.[7,53,54] While the threshold for therapeutic intervention has traditionally been a gradient >50 mm Hg, it has been demonstrated that the presence of a resting LVOT obstruction >30 mm Hg is an independent predictor of death from heart failure or stroke, progression of heart failure symptoms, and reduced functional capacity as well as SCD.[28] It is important not to misinterpret the Doppler spectral display of mitral regurgitation for LVOT gradient given its frequent presence in the setting of obstruction and its close spatial orientation to the LVOT. In the setting of SAM, mitral regurgitation is usually posteriorly directed into the left atrium and is often difficult to distinguish from LVOT flow. It is most useful to sweep anterior to posterior with continuous Doppler to distinguish these two flows. Given the magnitude of left ventricular hypertrophy consummate with HCM, it is not surprising that more than 80% of patients have evidence of diastolic dysfunction by echocardiogram. This is manifested by reduced maximal flow velocity in early diastole, an increase in isovolumic relaxation time, and increased atrial contribution to ventricular filling.[46,55] These findings are similar in patients both with and without an LVOT gradient or cardiac symptoms, suggesting that diastolic dysfunction may be an earlier clinical manifestation in the spectrum of this disease process. Several studies have suggested that the presence of significant diastolic dysfunction by transthoracic or tissue Doppler echocardiography may imply an increased risk of cardiac arrest, VT, or progression to significant cardiac symptoms.[56]

ELECTROCARDIOGRAPHY

ECG findings in HCM are extremely heterogeneous and the vast majority (>90%) of patients will have demonstrable abnormalities.[1,7,57,58] However, no pattern is highly specific for the condition and the presence of a normal tracing does not imply absence of the disease state.[58,59] Increased voltages consistent with LVH and early repolarization abnormalities are most commonly encountered, while left axis deviation, left atrial enlargement, T-wave inversion, and nonspecific ST-segment abnormalities are also frequently noted. The degree of LVH by ECG does not appear to correlate with the magnitude of hypertrophy when assessed by echocardiography.[60] In a subset of Japanese patients with hypertrophy primarily limited to the ventricular apex, giant T-wave inversions are frequently noted in the anterior leads, these are often termed Yamaguchi's disease.[61] Pathological Q waves, often in the inferolateral leads, may be observed in up to 50% of patients with known HCM. While not apparent on the surface ECG, approximately one third of patients have delayed His-Purkinje conduction on formal electrophysiological studies, possibly owing to strain on the anterior fasciculus, which overlies the hypertrophied ventricle.[37]

MAGNETIC RESONANCE IMAGING

In comparison with traditional echocardiography, cardiac magnetic resonance imaging (CMRI) offers the advantages of superior resolution with precise morphological characterization, enhanced tissue contrast capability, and production of three-dimensional images.[62] These advantages result in the ability of CMRI to better detect areas of hypertrophy that are not well visualized or missed by traditional echocardiography. Particularly in patients with atypical hypertrophy of the anterolateral free wall, CMRI is a powerful adjunctive tool in the diagnosis of HCM.[62]

Through delayed hyperenhancement techniques, CMRI has demonstrated that asymptomatic patients with HCM frequently have patchy foci of myocardial scarring at the junction of the interventricular septum and the right ventricular free wall. Furthermore, scarring was limited to the areas of abnormal hypertrophy and the degree of scarring was proportional to the magnitude of hypertrophy, while wall thickening was inversely related.[35] In addition, a greater extent of hyperenhancement has been positively associated with patients at high risk for SCD and in those with progressive disease.[63] CMRI also allows for better characterization of papillary muscle insertion and orientation. It is not uncommon to see hypertrophic, displaced, or distorted papillary muscles contributing to the obstruction and/or mitral valve dysfunction. Considering all these, CMRI is a valuable adjunctive imaging modality for the diagnosis of HCM.

CATHETERIZATION AND HEMODYNAMICS

Given the wealth of hemodynamic and anatomical data that can be derived noninvasively by echocardiography, cardiac catheterization is not required for the diagnosis of HCM. Catheterization is often employed, however, if noninvasive imaging is of insufficient quality to quantify the degree or location of obstruction, to evaluate for coronary disease prior to a planned surgical therapy (i.e., myectomy or pacemaker), or if anginal symptoms that may be attributable to ischemia are present in older patients. The coronary arteries in patients with HCM are usually normal and typically of large caliber. Quite different from intramyocardial "bridging," compression of the left anterior descending artery (LAD) may be observed during systole due to contraction of the hypertrophied ventricle, resulting in a "sawfish" appearance.[64] Ventriculography may demonstrate systolic cavity obliteration, varying degrees of mitral regurgitation, and occasionally the hypertrophied septum prolapsing into the LVOT. Direct measurement and localization of the gradient is easily obtained by passing a multipurpose catheter into the apical portion of the left ventricle and slowly withdrawing it while continuously monitoring the pressure waveform. Use of a wire via a guide catheter often results in increased control during the pullback and a more accurate determination of the level of obstruction. As opposed to what is observed in aortic stenosis (AS), the gradient is reduced prior to crossing the aortic valve. This same technique can be performed using simultaneous aortic and LV pressure waveforms to allow side-by-side comparison. The gradient in HCM is characteristically labile and various pharmacological and physiological maneuvers similar to echocardiography may be employed to accentuate the obstruction while in the catheterization laboratory. The term *postextrasystolic potentiation*[64a] refers to the augmentation of LV pressure with a concomitant decrement in the aortic systolic and pulse pressures as a result of increased LVOT obstruction in the cardiac cycle that follows a premature ventricular contraction (PVC). Postextrasystolic increase in gradient between LV and aorta is seen even with aortic stenosis but, unlike the case in HCM, pulse pressure (stroke volume) does not decrease. This is because in aortic stenosis, the larger stroke volume of the postextrasystolic beat leads to a higher gradient with no change in the severity of obstruction (Fig. 52-3).

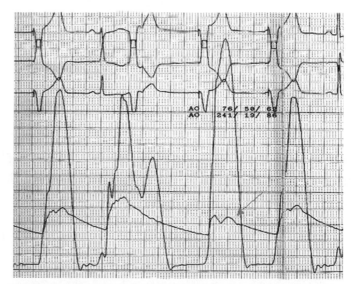

Figure 52-3 Brockenbrough-Braunwald-Morrow sign (postextrasystolic potentiation): simultaneous LV and aortic pressure tracing demonstrating the augmentation in LV pressure with concomitant decrement in the aortic systolic and pulse pressures as a result of increased LVOT obstruction following premature ventricular contraction (arrow).

GENETIC OVERVIEW

HCM is the result of mutations to genes primarily encoding sarcomeric proteins that regulate contractile, regulatory, and structural functions; they are inherited in an autosomal dominant manner.[1,7–10] To date, more than 400 mutations have been described involving 12 genes, the most common of which include cardiac troponins T, C, and I, cardiac myosin-binding protein C, cardiac beta- and alpha-myosin heavy chains, myosin ventricular essential and regulatory light chains, cardiac alpha actin, and titin.[8,10] While most of these mutations are missense with resultant substitution of the correct amino acid for another, deletions, insertions, and splice-site mutations are also well described.[65] Several nonsarcomeric mutations that produce phenotypes similar to HCM have been identified. *PRKAG2* affects the regulatory subunit of the AMP-activated protein kinase and may result in preexcitation, progressive conduction system abnormalities, and mild ventricular hypertrophy due to aberrant accumulation of glycogen within the myocyte.[65–67] Mutations of 2 alpha-galactosidase or acid alpha-1, 4-glucosidase (both lysosome-associated membrane proteins) frequently result in multisystem glycogen storage disease and may also present with extreme LVH associated with ventricular preexcitation and mental retardation.[65,66,68] There is great phenotypical heterogeneity among carriers of the same mutations, in part due to the effect of modifier genes and environmental factors.[7,69] While it has been known that many young carriers may not demonstrate the morphological characteristics of the disease state until after adolescence, it has now been demonstrated that phenotypical expression of LVH can be delayed into late adulthood owing to incomplete penetrance of mutations involving cardiac myosin-binding protein C or troponin T.[7,49,50,59,70] While the majority of studied HCM cases involve familial mutations, sporadic cases are also well described and may constitute a significant proportion of the population. Recent work involving the systematic molecular screening of known HCM cases has demonstrated that two mutations (*MYBPC3* and *MYH7*) may account for 82% of familial cases and that mutations were detected in up to 60% of "sporadic cases."[10] These data would imply that a relatively limited screening process may be sufficient to identify the culprit gene in most familial cases and that identifiable mutations are responsible for the majority of sporadic cases. Given the fact that a number of studies have identified specific genetic mutations (Table 52-2) seemingly associated with a worse clinical prognosis and higher rates of SCD, there has been initial enthusiasm that genetic testing could prospectively identify patients at higher risk for premature demise.[1,9,14,27,49,50,71] However, significant limitations including selection bias, the small number of included familial cohorts, low frequency of specific gene mutations, and variability of the phenotypical product have hindered most of these genotype-phenotype correlation studies.[71,72] Thus, because of the numerous genetic and environmental influences affecting the phenotypical product, there remains a great deal of clinical heterogeneity associated with specific mutations, making accurate risk stratification based on genetic analysis alone impractical at this time.

TABLE 52-2	Sarcomeric Gene Mutations of Hypertrophic Cardiomyopathy
Beta myosin heavy chain 14q12 *MYH7* 30-40	
Myosin binding protein C 11q1 MYBPC3 30-40	
Cardiac troponin T 1q32 *TNNTT2* 15-20	
Cardiac troponin I 19q13.4 *TNNI3* 1-5	
Alpha tropomyosin 15q22.1 *TPM1* 1-5	
Myosin essential light chain 3p21 *MYL3* <1	
Myosin regulatory light chain 12q24.3 *MYL2* <1	
Cardiac troponin C 3p *TNNC1* rare	
Alpha myosin heavy chain 14q12 *MYHH6* rare	
Actin 15q14 *ACTC* rare	
Titin 2q24.3 *TTN* rare	

Modified from Tsoutsman et al.[73] and Ho et al.[8]

■ Treatment

MEDICAL THERAPY

Medical therapy should be considered the initial therapeutic approach for the treatment of symptoms arising from the numerous pathophysiological processes constituting HCM. Because of the relatively small number of cases, pharmacological therapy for HCM is largely based on expert opinion, clinical experience, and retrospective observational analyses. While patients with LVOT obstruction make up the greatest proportion of the symptomatic population, a significant number of *nonobstructing* patients may also suffer the consequences of diastolic dysfunction, such as heart failure, angina, and atrial fibrillation.[1,7,14] Given the increasing utilization of early genetic and echocardiographic screening of athletes and affected families, it has become apparent that a significant percentage of phenotypically affected patients are entirely asymptomatic for an extended time and, while somewhat controversial, available data suggest that this population does not warrant empirical therapy until and if symptoms develop.[1,5,7,17] Historically, the pharmacological treatment of HCM has been limited to beta blockers, verapamil, and disopyramide.

Pharmacotherapy

Beta-Adrenergic Receptor Blocking Agents. Beta blockers have traditionally been the drugs of choice for the treatment of HCM. This may stem from the fact that the physiological effects of these agents are well suited to address much of the problematic pathophysiology encountered in this population. Their negative chronotropic effect results in increased diastolic filling time, which reduces left atrial pressure and may improve congestive symptoms related to diastolic dysfunction. This is especially true in cases complicated by supraventricular arrhythmias such as atrial fibrillation. The negative inotropic effect of these agents results in reduced myocardial oxygen consumption with a resultant decrease in anginal symptoms. While there is no convincing evidence that beta blockers effectively reduce *resting* LVOT gradients, prior work and a large amount of clinical experience suggest that these agents reduce provocable gradients as well as substantially improving disabling symptoms related to exertion.[1,2,7,74] This is supported by data demonstrating an inverse relationship between peak oxygen consumption (VO_2) and degree of LVOT obstruction during cardiopulmonary exercise testing.[7,75] As a result, beta blockers as a class are the favored agents for patients with *latent* outflow tract obstruction. The first agent initially used for the treatment of HCM, propranolol, has largely been replaced by newer-generation, longer-acting, nonselective beta-blocking agents including atenolol and metoprolol.[7,12,74] Given the significant heterogeneity in clinical symptomatology, even within the same patient at different times in the disease course, it is important to individualize the titration of therapy based on current symptoms, resting heart rate (goal of 60 bpm), exertional capacity, and the presence of untoward side effects.

Verapamil. Functioning both as a negative inotrope and chronotrope by blocking the intracellular migration of calcium ions, the nondihydropyridine calcium channel blocking agent verapamil results in symptomatic improvement in patients with HCM owing to increased diastolic filling time and enhanced diastolic ventricular relaxation without negatively affecting systolic function as well as ensuring reduced myocardial oxygen consumption.[7,76,77] In addition, verapamil has been shown to increase absolute myocardial blood flow during pharmacological stress testing while also reducing ischemic burden and improving exercise tolerance in the asymptomatic patient population.[78,79] These effects may be due to verapamil's enhanced vasodilatory properties, which are more pronounced than those seen with beta blockade and may well explain this agent's superior efficacy in patients with chest pain. While verapamil has classically been used in both obstructing and nonobstructing disease, caution should be exercised in initiating this agent in symptomatic patients with large resting gradients owing to well-documented reports of severe hemodynamic decompensation resulting in cardiogenic shock and pulmonary edema.[7] In addition, verapamil should not be used in infants with HCM because of a well established increased risk of SCD when it is administered in the intravenous formulation.[7] Approximately 5% of patients with HCM will progress to an end stage characterized by impaired systolic function and symptoms of heart failure. Standard therapy for congestive heart failure (CHF)—including diuretics, cautious use of vasodilators, beta blockers, avoidance of calcium channel blockers, and possibly digoxin—should constitute the pharmacological regimen in these patients.[1] In symptomatic patients, it is common clinical practice to initiate therapy using beta blockers rather than verapamil. Should the patient be intolerant of side effects (i.e., fatigue, depression, or impotence) or if symptoms persist despite adequate titration of the medication, consideration should be given to changing (or adding) therapy to verapamil.[1,7,41] At present, there are no data to suggest that combination therapy is more effective than either a beta blocker or verapamil alone.

Disopyramide. Disopyramide, a class IA antiarrhythmic agent, has a side-effect profile that includes a negative inotropic effect with reduced contractility and a reflexive increase in systemic vascular resistance, both of which have made it an attractive agent for the treatment of HCM for over 30 years. While it appears to have little or no effect on diastolic function, disopyramide has been shown to effectively reduce the outflow obstruction due to SAM with improved symptomatic control in patients with resting gradients who have failed other forms of therapy.[7,80-82] Owing to the possible potentiation of supraventricular arrhythmias such as AF and case reports of QT prolongation leading to torsades de pointes, close supervision and monitoring are essential during the initiation of this therapy.[83] Other side effects of disopyramide are primarily related to its anticholinergic properties; they include dry mouth (32%), urinary retention (14%), constipation (11%), and rarely hypoglycemia.

Amiodarone. While current data are somewhat conflicting and conclusive evidence is lacking, it has been suggested that amiodarone may reduce the risk of SCD and improve survival in selected high-risk patients noted to have nonsustained VT (NSVT) on Holter monitoring.[84] However, some reports suggest that amiodarone may improve a patient's symptom score and functional status but that it may also be proarrhythmic and thus lead to an *increased risk* of SCD due to ventricular arrhythmia.[85,86] In contrast, more recent data indicate that lower-dose amiodarone (200 mg/day) in high-risk patients with recurrent NSVT is not associated with any increase in cardiovascular mortality.[25] Amiodarone has been demonstrated to be effective therapy for the treatment and prevention of ventricular arrhythmias in patients with HCM.[87] Selection of which patients are appropriate for chronic, long-term empirical therapy with this agent, especially considering its attendant side-effect profile, may be impossible until more definitive trial data become available.

Dual-Chamber Pacing

Dual-chamber pacing, as a less invasive alternative to the surgical septal myectomy, was met with initial enthusiasm in the early 1990s, when several observational and uncontrolled studies demonstrated a significant decrease in outflow gradient, reduced symptomatology with improved quality of life, and homogenous redistribution of myocardial perfusion reserve.[88,89] While the exact mechanism is unclear, it has been proposed that activation of the right ventricular apex results in a dyssynchronous contraction of the septum with a reduction in outflow tract obstruction in the short term and a positive ventricular remodeling effect in the long term.[88,90] However, subsequent randomized controlled cross-over trials comparing DDD- to AAI-mode pacing demonstrated a significant placebo effect in regard to sustained symptomatic relief and quality-of-life assessment, little improvement in functional capacity, and a more modest reduction in outflow gradient in most patients as compared with the earlier uncontrolled trials.[1,7,90–92] Of importance, a subpopulation of elderly patients (age >65 years) was objectively measured to have both symptomatic and clinical benefit as a result of DDD pacing.[91] However, during the same period, a randomized trial did demonstrate a significant improvement in exercise tolerance, symptom score, and LVOT gradient in patients with symptoms refractory to drug therapy and with resting gradients >30 mm Hg.[92] Thus there may be subsets of patients in whom dual-chamber pacing may be of some symptomatic or clinical benefit. There are, however, no data to suggest that dual-chamber pacing effectively reduces the risk of SCD in this patient population.[7,88,91] Further work suggests that the reduction in LVOT gradient depends on optimal timing of the atrioventricular interval (AVI), with too short an interval interfering with diastolic filling and left atrial emptying while too long an interval results in ineffective reduction of outflow obstruction.[93] Taking this into account, recent nonrandomized, observational data have demonstrated a significant reduction in symptoms, improved functional capacity, and consistent reduction in LVOT gradient when serial echocardiographic assessment was used to optimize the AVI, pacing rate, and mode settings in the treatment of patients using DDD pacemakers.[94] This may constitute the foundation for further randomized trials in this area. While data comparing dual-chamber pacing with surgical septal myectomy have demonstrated improvement in both groups in regard to functional status, a significantly greater reduction in LVOT gradient, improved subjective symptom status, and increased overall exercise duration was reported in patients who underwent myectomy.[95] Thus, while not considered a primary therapeutic modality for most patients with symptomatic HCM, it has been suggested that the use of dual-chamber pacemakers may be reasonable in certain subsets of patients, including elderly patients averse to more invasive therapies as well as patients in whom pharmacotherapy is limited owing to bradycardia.[7]

ICD Implantation

Ventricular fibrillation or tachycardia is the primary mode of SCD in patients with HOCM. Given the success of the implantable cardioverter defibrillator (ICD) in reducing arrhythmic mortality in patients with coronary artery disease and a reduced ejection fraction, there has been an increasing interest in utilizing the ICD for the prevention and treatment of HOCM-related arrhythmic death.[96] While randomized data are lacking, a multicenter, retrospective trial demonstrated that implantation of an ICD in patients classically considered at high risk for SCD resulted in appropriate device intervention and aborted SCD in almost 25% of the enrolled patients over a 3-year period.[31] Patients in whom the device was implanted for primary prevention purposes experienced appropriate intervention at a rate of 5% annually as compared with patients who received the device after cardiac arrest or sustained VT, in whom appropriate intervention was noted at a rate of 11% annually.[1,7,31,97] Based on these results, it has been suggested that ICD implantation is reasonable and should be considered in patients with one or more risk factors for SCD and is warranted in patients with a prior history of cardiac arrest or sustained VT.[1,7] Device selection should be based primarily on individual patient preference and characteristics. Dual-chamber devices have the advantage of atrial sensing and pacing functions, as well as the ability to discriminate supraventricular from ventricular arrhythmias, thus resulting in a reduction in the number of inappropriate interventions. Unfortunately the dual-chamber devices have a higher potential for complications (usually related to the transvenous lead systems) than do single-chamber devices.[97] The 2002 American College of Cardiology/American Heart Association/North American Society of Pacing and Electrophysiology (ACC/AHA/NASPE) consensus guidelines designate implantation of an ICD as a prophylactic measure in selected high-risk patients as a class IIb intervention (i.e., usefulness and/or efficacy is less well established), while implantation of an ICD for secondary prevention was designated a class I intervention (i.e., evidence or consensus that given procedure or treatment is useful and effective).[98]

SURGERY

Patients with resting or provocable gradients >50 mm Hg who continue to experience significant functional limitation (i.e., NYHA class

III-IV) due to limiting symptoms of exertional dyspnea, chest pain, or recurrent syncope despite maximal medical therapy may be considered candidates for surgical therapy.[1,7,14] Surgical therapy is not currently recommended for patients *without* significant outflow tract obstruction, in those with relatively *mild* symptoms with obstruction, or to treat associated complications of this condition, such as atrial fibrillation or syncope, alone.[7] There has been a significant evolution in the spectrum of surgical therapy for HOCM designed to effectively reduce outflow tract obstruction, from the original isolated septal myotomy performed by Cleland[98a] in the 1960s to the more modern and widely employed Morrow myectomy[99] in combination with mitral valve repair or even replacement in selected patients.[100, 101] The "gold standard" septal myectomy, described by Morrow, is performed via an aortotomy so that the proximal septum is approachable via the aortic valve and 5 to 15 g of myocardial tissue is resected from the base of the aortic valve to a region distal to the mitral leaflets such that the area of mitral:septal contact that results in SAM is removed and the LVOT is enlarged.[7,99,100] Because it is of critical importance to correctly identify the involved portion of the ventricular septum and resect enough myocardium to relieve the outflow tract gradient, most experienced centers employ transesophageal echocardiography (TEE) to assist in localizing the desired region for resection as well as to monitor the effect of resection on the gradient intraoperatively.[100] Despite its more aggressive nature, an alteration in the classic Morrow procedure has been described in which an extended myectomy is combined with partial excision and mobilization of the papillary muscles, which results in amelioration of the outflow tract obstruction, reduced tethering of the subvalvular mitral structures, and a more individualized surgical resection depending on the extent and location of the patient's LVH.[100–102] In patients with specific comorbidities, such as atrial fibrillation or coronary artery disease, myectomy may be combined with adjunctive surgical procedures such as the MAZE procedure atrial fibrillation, or coronary bypass grafting in a single efficient procedure. Mitral valvular abnormalities, such as elongated and flexible leaflets, may substantially contribute to the degree of outflow tract obstruction in an important minority of patients. These patients often benefit from mitral valve plication at the time of myectomy to more effectively reduce the degree of outflow tract obstruction that results from SAM and to reduce the associated mitral regurgitation.[52,100,103,104] Mitral valve replacement is generally reserved for patients with significant primary valvular abnormalities such as myxomatous degeneration leading to mitral valve prolapse or regurgitation.[7,105] The modern-day septal myectomy procedure carries a relatively low operative risk due to continued technical refinement with a cumulative operative mortality rate of approximately 1% to 3% overall; more recent data report <1% in very experienced centers.[1,7,41,106,107] Left bundle branch block following myectomy is understandably very common because of the location of the procedure. Complete heart block requiring implantation of a permanent pacemaker is more recently a rare complication, as is iatrogenic formation of a ventricular septal defect.[7,105,108] A conclusive reduction in the long-term mortality following myectomy has yet to be demonstrated in a randomized controlled fashion. However, nonrandomized multicenter observational data (as well as a wealth of clinical experience) suggest that this procedure results in significant improvement in a patient's functional capacity, heart failure symptoms, quality of life, and possibly even life expectancy.[1,7,14,100] In addition to this, reduction of the outflow tract gradient usually results in amelioration of SAM of the mitral apparatus and the resultant mitral regurgitation.[7,100,109,110] In fact, a recent clinical surgical series suggests that patients treated with surgical myectomy have an excellent prognosis, with a life expectancy similar to that of the general population, which may be partly due to a reduction in the rate of SCD.[111]

SEPTAL ABLATION

In an effort to provide an alternative treatment strategy to relieve outflow tract obstruction in symptomatic patients who do not wish to undergo the more invasive surgical myectomy, are suboptimal surgical

TABLE 52-3	Patient Selection Criteria for Alcohol Septal Ablation
Severe heart failure symptoms (i.e., NYHA class III-IV) despite maximal medical therapy
Septal thickness >18 mm
Subaortic gradient >50 mm Hg (resting or with provocation) due to mitral-septal contact
Absence of papillary muscle or mitral valvular anomalies (i.e., anomalous papillary muscle insertion)
Absence of significant coronary arterial disease
Compatible septal perforator branch arterial anatomy
Relative contraindications to surgical myectomy (i.e., age, comorbidity) *

NYHA, New York Heart Association.
*Relative contraindication to surgical myectomy is a controversial selection criteria not uniformly followed.

candidates due to comorbidities, or are located in areas without sufficient surgical expertise, percutaneous septal ablation was introduced by Sigwart in 1995.[112] Through the selective infusion of 100% ethanol into either the first or second septal perforator arteries, the septal ablation technique attempts to mimic the effect of the more traditional Morrow myectomy by inducing a controlled infarct in the basal portion of the hypertrophied septum, resulting in scarring, thinning, and akinesis and leading to a significant reduction in the LVOT gradient and SAM of the mitral valvular apparatus.[1,7,41,112–115] Despite the paucity of large-scale randomized controlled trials documenting the long-term outcome of these patients, short-term observational studies have demonstrated a significant reduction in LVOT gradient, often a rapid reduction in limiting symptoms, and improved exercise tolerance following ablation, with a reported mortality equal to or less than that of surgery at 1% to 4%.[7,113–118] Thus, the short-term success of this procedure combined with its obviously less invasive nature has led to a dramatic increase in its utilization over the past 10 years, with ablation estimated to be 15 to 20 times more common than surgical myectomy. In fact, more than 5,000 ablations have been performed worldwide to date.[7,119,120,134] It is very important to carefully screen all patients being considered for septal ablation and to select for patients who will realize maximum benefit from the intervention (Table 52-3). As in the case of patients recommended for the traditional myectomy, the updated American College of Cardiology/European Society of Cardiology (ACC/ESC) consensus statement recommends that selection criteria include patients with septal hypertrophy >18 mm, dynamic LVOT obstruction with gradient >50 mm Hg (either at rest or with provocation), and severely limiting heart failure symptoms (i.e., NYHA functional class III-IV) despite maximal medical therapy.[7,121] A thorough search for abnormalities that are better addressed surgically is essential prior to proceeding with catheter-based septal ablation. Such abnormalities would include anomalous papillary muscle insertion into the mitral valve, anatomically abnormal mitral valve with a long anteroposterior leaflet, coexistent coronary artery disease, primary valvular disease (aortic or mitral), or subaortic membrane or pannus, all of which would not be adequately addressed by septal ablation.[7,121] In addition, abnormally elongated and flexible anterior mitral leaflets resulting in an anterior location of the coaptation line and outflow tract obstruction will not be correctable via catheter-based techniques and require surgical myectomy with plication.[52] In addition, many experienced centers refer patients with a septal thickness greater than 2.5 cm for surgical correction.

Procedural Technique

Given the fact that most patients with HOCM are diagnosed noninvasively with echocardiography and many have not had invasive hemodynamic studies performed prior to presenting for ablation, many operators will reconfirm the presence of significant LVOT obstruction by positioning an end-hole catheter in the ventricular apex and recording a slow pullback under fluoroscopy. Alternatively, simultaneous measurement of the ascending aortic and intracavity pressures may be obtained via the placement of an ascending aortic catheter as well as an end-hole catheter as described above. If an LVOT gradient is not confirmed under basal/resting conditions, provocation with amyl nitrate or the Valsalva maneuver may be attempted.[121] Failure to confirm a significant gradient following these maneuvers should prompt the operator to further pursue alternative etiologies for the patient's symptom complex.

Standard diagnostic coronary cineangiography is performed as a first step in order to clearly define the patient's anatomy as well as to evaluate for concomitant atherosclerotic disease. Once this is completed, attention is turned to selection of the appropriate septal perforator branch through which to perform the ablation. To best view the anatomical course of the septal branches as they course through the basal interventricular septum, the camera should be positioned in the right anterior oblique (RAO) posteroanterior (PA) cranial view or PA cranial view. It is also important to determine the septal vessel's course along the septum (i.e., on the right or left side) utilizing the LAO projection. At times, septal anatomy may vary such that one subdivision runs along the left side of the septum while another runs along the right. Selection of the left-sided subdivision is optimal for the ablation, as there is a reduced likelihood of inducing complete heart block (CHB) during ethanol infusion. While the vast majority of septal perforators arise from the left anterior descending (LAD), substantial anatomical variation has been described in which the vessels may arise from the left main trunk (LMT), ramus intermedius (RI), left circumflex (LCx), diagonal branches, or even from a branch of the right coronary artery (RCA).[121] A temporary transvenous pacemaker is placed in advance as a prophylactic measure in case of the development of complete heart block during, or in days following, the ablation. Since heparin will be utilized for anticoagulation during the procedure, care should be taken to minimize the risk of bleeding during pacemaker insertion. Following successful placement of *both* the temporary pacemaker and the arterial sheath, heparin is administered to achieve an activated clotting time of 250 to 300 in order to prevent thrombosis in guide catheters and on wires.

Following the angiographic identification of the septal arteries, close attention must be given to vessel size, angulation, and the distribution of myocardial territories served by the given vessel. Angulation of the septal vessels, either at the origin from the primary vessel (such as the LAD) or the bifurcation of a larger septal artery, is an important consideration in vessel selection. Vessels with angulations greater than 90 degrees are often technically challenging and result in difficulty passing the balloon into the selected vessel, with frequent prolapse of the wire into the mid-LAD.[121] Specialized techniques using catheters that allow control of the distal angle (Venture Catheter, St. Jude Medical, St Paul, MN) may be useful in these circumstances. There is substantial variation in the distribution of blood flow supplied by the septal perforators in patients with HOCM as compared with the unaffected population. In both autopsy and angiography studies, it has been demonstrated that the first septal artery may provide blood flow to regions other than the targeted basal septum (including the right ventricle); it may supply the basal septum incompletely and share this responsibility with a second septal branch, or it may subtend a substantially larger distribution of myocardium than would be expected.[121,122] Thus, an intimate knowledge of the myocardial distribution of blood flow supplied by the selected septal branch is essential to accurately target the correct area for ablation and to avoid infarction of an unanticipated region or an oversized infarction of the septum itself. This is most commonly accomplished during the procedure by the selective injection of dye under cine and the concomitant use of transthoracic echocardiography (TTE) utilizing injectable contrast material (see below).

Following angiographic assessment of the septal anatomy, a guide catheter providing extra support (such as a 6- or 7-Fr XB catheter) is used to engage the left main trunk (LMT). Subsequently, a 0.014-in. extra support wire with a soft tip is passed into the selected septal perforator branch, most commonly the first septal perforator (Fig. 52-4). A short angioplasty balloon, usually 1.5 to 2 mm in diameter and 10 mm in length, is passed over the guidewire and into the septal branch. Difficulty in passing the balloon may be resolved by using a

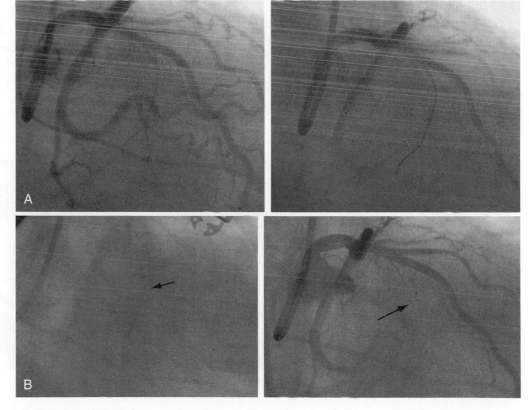

Figure 52-4 A. Coronary angiogram (DSA) demonstrating the introduction of a 0.014-in. guidewire into a septal perforator branch with anatomical characteristics ideal for septal ablation. DSA, digital subtraction angiography. B. Coronary angiogram demonstrating the introduction of a 1.5- by 10-mm balloon (arrow) into the selected septal vessel. Injection of contrast into the balloon and LAD subsequently confirms correct positioning.

stiffer guidewire to provide greater support for balloon placement.[121] Care must be taken that the balloon is seated deeply enough into the septal artery and fully expanded to ensure that the injected ethanol is not refluxed in to the LAD. Conversely, if the balloon is placed too deeply into the septal vessel, the injected ethanol may spare the basal-most portion of the septum, resulting in an unsuccessful procedure (Fig. 52-5). Following successful placement, the balloon is inflated to occlude the perforator (typically to 10–12 atm). As noted above, it is essential at this point in the procedure to verify the distribution of myocardium being supplied by the selected vessel, given the substantial degree of variability in the anatomy of this patient population. This is accomplished by both traditional angiography as well as transesophageal echocardiography (TEE), often with the aid of echo contrast. After correct positioning of the balloon, as noted above, the operator will inflate the balloon and 1 to 2 mL of contrast will be injected to assess the full extent of myocardium supplied by the chosen vessel. Contrast should be injected slowly so as to mimic the anticipated alcohol infusion. Extreme caution should be taken to verify that the infused contrast does not reflux into the LAD or into other coronary arteries (e.g., the posterior descending artery [PDA]), thus possibly exposing a large amount of unintended myocardium to damage when the ethanol is infused. Aggressive contrast infusion may overwhelm collateral vessels and create an inferior left ventricular wall infarction.

Following angiographic confirmation of septal occlusion, further assessment of the septal distribution is obtained via contrast echocardiography (Fig. 52-6). After carefully inspecting the septum in the apical long axis, four-chamber, and parasternal long-axis views, 1 to 2 mL of Albunex contrast is injected into the septal branch through a tuberculin-type syringe. Since Albumex, a first-generation echocardiographic contrast agent, is no longer available in many countries, second- and third-generation agents are currently employed. These agents have proven to be suboptimal because they traverse the capillary beds rapidly and produce a large amount of echocardiographic "shadowing" from the opacified ventricles. Thus it is important to dilute these agents prior to injection. In our laboratory, the contrast vials are typically opened 10 to 15 minutes prior to the time of expected use so as to decrease their potency. The contrast is then further diluted with sterile saline in a 1:5 or 1:10 mixture at the time of injection. Pulsed-wave Doppler is the imaging method of choice in using the diluted contrast so as to avoid destruction of the microbubbles with the higher-frequency continuous-wave ultrasound. This procedure will allow the operator to verify that the chosen vessel primarily supplies the proximal interventricular septum and not portions of the inferior wall, left ventricular papillary musculature, or right ventricular free wall via the moderator band.[121,123] Ideally, this will result in the appearance of contrast material in the basal portion of septum responsible for the greatest extent of septal:mitral contact. Appearance of contrast in the distal septum or other regions of myocardium is a contraindication to ethanol infusion, as this can result in infarction of an undesired territory or of unanticipated size. As a final method of ensuring that the desired area of myocardium has been selected, it is recommended that the operator document a >30% reduction in the LVOT gradient during balloon inflation. A rather rapid reduction in gradient can be observed with prolonged balloon occlusion of a septal perforator branch. Such an observation suggests that the correct septal distribution has been targeted for ablation.[121,124] Prior to proceeding with ethanol injection, it is essential to confirm that the balloon has not migrated during this process and that the previously placed temporary pacemaker continues to have a suitable pacing threshold. This is easily done by fluoroscopic verification and injection of another 1 to 2 mL of contrast through the guide catheter. With confirmation of proper balloon positioning, the operator may proceed with ethanol injection. While most experienced centers use between 1 to 3 mL of desiccated ethanol, this volume may be adjusted based upon the appearance of the septal anatomy and the degree of contrast washout.[7,114,121,125–127] Recent work has documented similar midterm hemodynamic outcomes with reduced complication rates, especially permanent pacemaker requirement, when smaller amounts of ethanol (1–2 mL) are utilized.[128] In situations where there is rapid contrast washout due to collateralization of the septal branch, the rate and volume of ethanol infusion should be reduced to prevent the alcohol from escaping to undesirable areas of myocardium via the collaterals.[113,114,121] At this point, the ethanol is injected into the vessel over a 1- to 5-minute

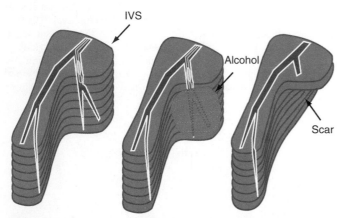

Figure 52-5 Schematic overview of the alcohol septal ablation procedure depicting the resultant basal septal scar and enlargement of the LVOT. If the balloon is placed distally, the anterior septum is not ablated, which can result in a suboptimal result. IVS, interventricular septum.

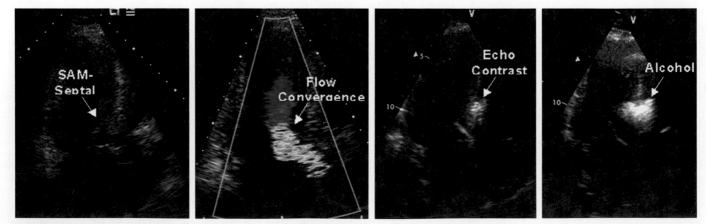

Figure 52-6 Contrast echocardiography (apical three-chamber view) confirming the desired distribution of myocardial blood flow through the injection of an appropriately selected septal perforator artery prior to ethanol infusion.

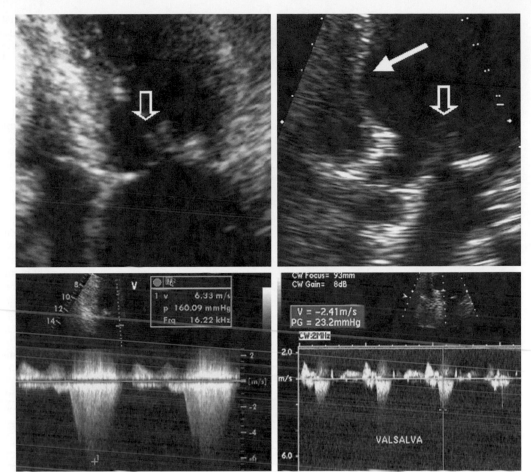

Figure 52-7 Contrast echocardiography. The images on the left were taken prior to alcohol ablation. The images on the right were acquired from the same patient 6 months following successful ablation and clearly demonstrate scarring (white arrow) in the basal septum with a resultant increase in the LVOT area and decrease in the outflow tract obstruction. Systolic anterior motion (open arrow) is present at baseline and is absent on follow-up

period with the balloon remaining inflated. During the initial infusion, continued monitoring of the resting gradient is essential in order to judge the efficacy of the procedure. In general, a reduction in the LVOT gradient to <30 mm Hg in the setting of a resting gradient >50 mm Hg or a >50% reduction of a provocable gradient is considered indicative of a successful procedure in the catheterization laboratory[114,121] (Fig. 52-7). Prior to disengaging the balloon from the septal vessel, it is recommended that the guidewire be replaced into the septal branch for smooth removal of the balloon and maintenance of access across the LMT and LAD. As a final step, angiography of the LAD and septal vessels is performed to verify the integrity of the coronary circulation. Phasic flow may be observed in the injected septal branch immediately following the ablation, although total occlusion is frequently observed. Postprocedural care should take place in a coronary intensive care unit for 48 hours following ablation to allow for the rapid identification and treatment of possible complications. The amount of induced myocardial tissue destruction will often result in elevation of the creatinine phosphokinase (CPK) to levels between 800 and 1,200 U/L, although this is variable depending upon the amount of alcohol injected, vessel size, and method of enzyme measurement.[7,113,120,127,128] The transvenous pacing wire may be discontinued 48 hours after the procedure if there is an absence of bradyarrhythmia or heart block that would require continued observation or a permanent pacemaker. In most centers, the patient is transferred to a regular nursing floor for another 48 to 72 hours to observe for postprocedural complications prior to discharge. The complication rate following septal ablation is relatively low and comparable to that of septal myectomy. As opposed to the left bundle branch block so commonly observed after septal myectomy, a right bundle branch block is observed in up to 80% of patients following ablation.[7,114,121] The incidence of complete heart block has decreased in recent years and ranges from 5% to 40%, with an average value of 12% to 15% at experienced centers.[7,107,114,115,121,129] The presence of a

preexisting left bundle branch block and a rapid bolus injection of ethanol during ablation have both been positively correlated with an increased incidence of high degree atrioventricular block requiring permanent pacemaker implantation.[129] Extravasation of alcohol into the LAD during infusion is a rare but catastrophic complication that often results in a large infarction of the mid- to distal anterior wall and is clearly associated with an increased mortality. Coronary dissection from either the extra support guidewire or the catheter has been reported in rare instances. Tamponade due to perforation of the right ventricular apex during insertion of a transvenous pacing wire or during interatrial septal puncture for periprocedural hemodynamic monitoring have also been reported. Overly extensive infarction of the interventricular septum as a result of too generous a quantity of infused alcohol or from too rapid an infusion rate during ablation can result in a ventricular septal rupture.[121] Ventricular arrhythmias can be seen both during and up to 48 hours after the procedure, but this is rare and usually does not require prolonged therapy. Unlike myectomy, septal ablation results in the formation of a large intramyocardial scar that may serve as substrate for future malignant ventricular arrhythmias. There has been some conjecture that this could result in an increased risk of late arrhythmic mortality, especially in younger patients undergoing ablation.[7,31,114,126] However, this hypothesis has yet to garner substantial evidentiary support. Patients should be followed closely for recurrence of symptoms or any arrhythmia. ICD implantation should be considered if there is evidence of nonsustained ventricular tachycardia, but this is extremely rare. Objective assessment of functional capacity using exercise testing is appropriate for monitoring these patients. Repeat alcohol ablation can be considered if symptoms recur and an appropriate septal perforator is available for injection. If repeat ablation is not feasible, surgical myectomy may need to be considered in this group[130] (Fig. 52-8). Despite the increase in the number of septal ablation procedures performed worldwide, there

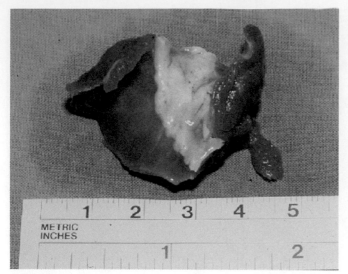

Figure 52-8 Pathology specimen of the basal interventricular septum in a patient with HCM several years following an ethanol ablation demonstrating fibrosis and scarring.

remains a paucity of randomized controlled trials. Existing data would suggest that septal ablation and surgical myectomy both have a similar success rate in the short and longer term.[135] In the immediate postprocedural period (3–72 hours), both modalities of septal reduction resulted in similar degrees of LVOT gradient reduction, and this improvement appears to be maintained up to 1 year after either procedure.[1,7,107,114,118,127,130–132] In fact, a recent metanalysis has demonstrated that, after adjusting for preprocedural gradient, the reduction in gradient postprocedure is similar between the two modalities[136] (Fig. 52-9). In addition to improvements in the NYHA functional class and the Canadian Cardiovascular angina class (CCS), the number of syncopal and presyncopal events were significantly reduced to a similar degree in both groups at 6- and 12-month follow up.[107,118,131] Both procedures have advantages as well as associated complications, which underscores the importance of careful patient selection and consideration of comorbidities prior to choosing an intervention. Complete heart block requiring permanent pacemaker has been reported in up to 25% of patients undergoing alcohol ablation, as compared with only 5% to 10% following myectomy.[107,131] Given that ablation commonly produces a pattern of right bundle branch block (RBBB), patients with a preexisting left bundle branch block (LBBB) are at very high risk of complete heart block (CHB) following the procedure.[136] In addition, it has been suggested that female gender, first-degree atrioventricular block (AVB), and an increased volume of injected alcohol are also risk factors for postprocedural CHB.[133] In contrast, myectomy produces a LBBB and less commonly requires permanent pacing. Myectomy can result in mild to moderate aortic insufficiency in up to 10% to 20% of

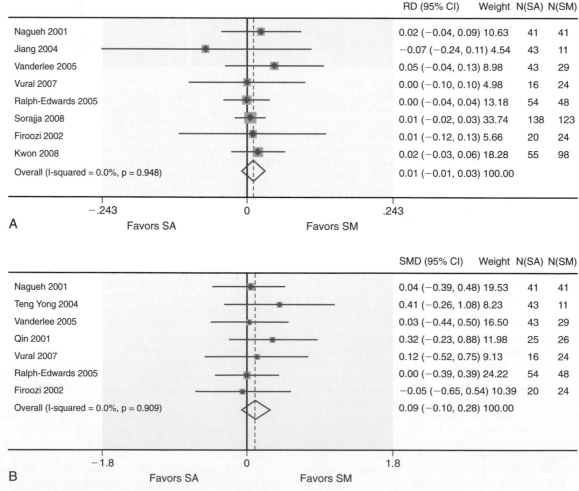

Figure 52-9 A. Short-term mortality risk difference estimates between the septal ablation and septal myectomy groups. B. Postprocedure reduction in LVOT gradient from preprocedure value; standardized mean difference between the septal ablation and septal myectomy groups.

patients but rarely leads to an adverse outcome.[131] By the nature of the procedure, ablation results in a permanent scar in the interventricular septum, and there remains some concern that this may serve as substrate for future ventricular arrhythmia, although this has not as yet been objectively documented. Expectedly, ablation results in a reduced length of stay as compared with myectomy and substantially contributes to an overall reduction in cost. Mortality is relatively low with both interventions and approaches approximately 1% in experienced centers.[7,41,107,131] Several recent metanalyses have also shown similar postprocedural outcomes, with no difference in long-term mortality between ablation and myectomy.[136,137,138] In summary, either surgical myectomy or alcohol ablation may be selected as a viable treatment option in symptomatic patients with LVOT obstruction. Which therapy should be selected is a complex decision that must be made only after taking into consideration the patient's clinical situation.

Acknowledgments

The authors would like to thank Dr. Matthew "Casey" Becker for his contributions to earlier versions of this chapter.

REFERENCES

1. Maron BJ: Hypertrophic cardiomyopathy: a systematic review. *JAMA* 287(10):1308–1320, 2002.
2. Braunwald E, Lambrew CT, Rockoff SD, et al: Idiopathic hypertrophic subaortic stenosis. I. A description of the disease based upon an analysis of 64 patients. *Circulation* 30(Suppl 4):3–119, 1964.
3. Maron BJ, Spirito P: Impact of patient selection biases on the perception of hypertrophic cardiomyopathy and its natural history. *Am J Cardiol* 72(12):970–972, 1993.
4. Maron BJ, Casey SA, Poliac LC, et al: Clinical course of hypertrophic cardiomyopathy in a regional United States cohort. *JAMA* 281(7):650–655, 1999.
5. Spirito P, Chiarella F, Carratino L, et al: Clinical course and prognosis of hypertrophic cardiomyopathy in an outpatient population. *N Engl J Med* 320(12):749–755, 1989.
6. Elliott P: Relation between the severity of left ventricular hypertrophy and prognosis in patients with hypertrophic cardiomyopathy. *Lancet* 357:420–424, 2001
7. Maron BJ, McKenna WJ, Danielson GK, et al: ACC/ESC Expert Consensus Document on Hypertrophic Cardiomyopathy. *J Am Coll Cardiol* 42(9):1687–1713, 2003.
8. Ho CY, Seidman CE: A contemporary approach to hypertrophic cardiomyopathy. *Circulation* 113(24):e858–e862, 2006.
9. Maron BJ, Moller JH, Seidman CE, et al: Impact of laboratory molecular diagnosis on contemporary diagnostic criteria for genetically transmitted cardiovascular diseases: hypertrophic cardiomyopathy, long-QT syndrome, and Marfan syndrome. A statement for healthcare professionals from the Councils on Clinical Cardiology, Cardiovascular Disease in the Young, and Basic Science, American Heart Association]. *Circulation* 98(14):1460–1471, 1998.
10. Richard P, Charron P, Carrier L, et al: Hypertrophic cardiomyopathy: distribution of disease genes, spectrum of mutations, and implications for a molecular diagnosis strategy. *Circulation* 107(17):2227–2232, 2003.
11. McKenna WJ, Deanfield JE: Hypertrophic cardiomyopathy: an important cause of sudden death. *Arch Dis Child* 59(10):971–975, 1984.
12. Shah PM, Adelman AG, Wigle ED, et al: The natural (and unnatural) history of hypertrophic obstructive cardiomyopathy. *Circ Res* 35(Suppl 2):II179–II195, 1974.
13. Maron BJ: Hypertrophic cardiomyopathy. *Lancet* 350:127–133, 1997.
14. Spirito P: The management of hypertrophic cardiomyopathy. *N Engl J Med* 336:775–785, 1997.
15. Maron BJ: Clinical profile of stroke in 900 patients with hypertrophic cardiomyopathy. *J Am Coll Cardiol* 39:301–307, 2002.
16. Elliott P, McKenna WJ: Hypertrophic cardiomyopathy. *Lancet* 363(9424):1881–1891, 2004.
17. Spirito P, Autore C: Management of hypertrophic cardiomyopathy. *BMJ* 332(7552):1251–1255, 2006.
18. Maron BJ, Shirani J, Poliac LC, et al: Sudden death in young competitive athletes. Clinical, demographic, and pathological profiles. *JAMA* 276(3):199–204, 1996.
19. Maron BJ, Olivotto I, Spirito P, et al: Epidemiology of hypertrophic cardiomyopathy-related death: revisited in a large non-referral-based patient population. *Circulation* 102(8):858–864, 2000.
20. Elliott PM, Poloniecki J, Dickie S, et al: Sudden death in hypertrophic cardiomyopathy: identification of high risk patients. *J Am Coll Cardiol* 36(7):2212–2218, 2000.
21. Spirito P, Bellone P, Harris KM, et al: Magnitude of left ventricular hypertrophy and risk of sudden death in hypertrophic cardiomyopathy. *N Engl J Med* 342(24):1778–1785, 2000.
22. Monserrat L, Elliott PM, Gimeno JR, et al: Non-sustained ventricular tachycardia in hypertrophic cardiomyopathy: an independent marker of sudden death risk in young patients. *J Am Coll Cardiol* 42(5):873–879, 2003
23. Yoshida N, Ikeda H, Wada T, et al: Exercise-induced abnormal blood pressure responses are related to subendocardial ischemia in hypertrophic cardiomyopathy. *J Am Coll Cardiol* 32(7):1938–1942, 1998.
24. Olivotto I, Cecchi F, Casey SA, et al: Impact of atrial fibrillation on the clinical course of hypertrophic cardiomyopathy. *Circulation* 104(21):2517–2524, 2001.
25. Cecchi F, Olivotto I, Montereggi A, et al: Prognostic value of non-sustained ventricular tachycardia and the potential role of amiodarone treatment in hypertrophic cardiomyopathy: assessment in an unselected non-referral based patient population. *Heart* 79(4):331–336, 1998.
26. Moolman JC, Corfield VA, Posen B, et al: Sudden death due to troponin T mutations. *J Am Coll Cardiol* 29(3):549–555, 1997.
27. Watkins H: Sudden death in hypertrophic cardiomyopathy. *N Engl J Med* 342(6):422–424, 2000.
28. Maron MS, Olivotto I, Betocchi S, et al: Effect of left ventricular outflow tract obstruction on clinical outcome in hypertrophic cardiomyopathy. *N Engl J Med* 348(4):295–303, 2003.
29. Kofflard MJ, Ten Cate FJ, van der Lee C, et al: Hypertrophic cardiomyopathy in a large community-based population: clinical outcome and identification of risk factors for sudden cardiac death and clinical deterioration. *J Am Coll Cardiol* 41(6):987–993, 2003.
30. Elliott PM, Sharma S, Varnava A, et al: Survival after cardiac arrest or sustained ventricular tachycardia in patients with hypertrophic cardiomyopathy. *J Am Coll Cardiol* 33(6):1596–1601, 1999.
31. Maron BJ, Shen WK, Link MS, et al: Efficacy of implantable cardioverter-defibrillators for the prevention of sudden death in patients with hypertrophic cardiomyopathy. *N Engl J Med* 342(6):365–373, 2000.
32. Maron BJ, Kogan J, Proschan MA, et al: Circadian variability in the occurrence of sudden cardiac death in patients with hypertrophic cardiomyopathy. *J Am Coll Cardiol* 23(6):1405–1409, 1994.
33. Maron BJ, Epstein SE, Roberts WC: Hypertrophic cardiomyopathy and transmural myocardial infarction without significant atherosclerosis of the extramural coronary arteries. *Am J Cardiol* 43(6):1086–1102, 1979.
34. Dilsizian V, Bonow RO, Epstein SE, et al: Myocardial ischemia detected by thallium scintigraphy is frequently related to cardiac arrest and syncope in young patients with hypertrophic cardiomyopathy. *J Am Coll Cardiol* 22(3):796–804, Sep 1993.
35. Choudhury L, Mahrholdt H, Wagner A, et al: Myocardial scarring in asymptomatic or mildly symptomatic patients with hypertrophic cardiomyopathy. *J Am Coll Cardiol* 40(12):2156–2164, 2002.
36. Basso C, Thiene G, Corrado D, et al: Hypertrophic cardiomyopathy and sudden death in the young: pathologic evidence of myocardial ischemia. *Hum Pathol* 31(8):988–998, 2000.
37. Schwartzkopff B, Mundhenke M, Strauer BE: Alterations of the architecture of subendocardial arterioles in patients with hypertrophic cardiomyopathy and impaired coronary vasodilator reserve: a possible cause for myocardial ischemia. *J Am Coll Cardiol* 31(5):1089–1096, 1998.
38. Schwartzkopff B, Mundhenke M, Strauer BE: Remodelling of intramyocardial arterioles and extracellular matrix in patients with arterial hypertension and impaired coronary reserve. *Eur Heart J* 16(Suppl I):82–86, 1995.
39. Cecchi F, Olivotto I, Gistri R, et al: Coronary microvascular dysfunction and prognosis in hypertrophic cardiomyopathy. *N Engl J Med* 349(11):1027–1035, 2003.
40. Maron BJ, Roberts WC, Epstein SE: Sudden death in hypertrophic cardiomyopathy: a profile of 78 patients. *Circulation* 65(7):1388–1394, 1982.
41. Spirito P, Seidman CE, McKenna WJ, et al: The management of hypertrophic cardiomyopathy. *N Engl J Med* 336(11):775–785, 1997.
42. Nienaber CA, Hiller S, Spielmann RP, et al: [Risk of syncope in hypertrophic cardiomyopathy: a multivariate analysis of prognostic variables]. *Z Kardiol* 79(4):286–296, 1990.
43. Gilligan D: Investigation of a hemodynamic basis for syncope in hypertrophic cardiomyopathy. Use of a head-up tilt test. *Circulation* 85:2140–2148, 1992.
44. Lewis JF, Maron BJ: Clinical and morphologic expression of hypertrophic cardiomyopathy in patients > or = 65 years of age. *Am J Cardiol* 73(15):1105–1111, 1994.
45. Olivotto I, Maron MS, Adabag AS, et al: Gender-related differences in the clinical presentation and outcome of hypertrophic cardiomyopathy. *J Am Coll Cardiol* 46(3):480–487, 2005.
46. Poliac LC, Barron ME, Maron BJ. Hypertrophic cardiomyopathy. *Anesthesiology* 104(1):183–192, 2006.
47. Klues HG, Schiffers A, Maron BJ: Phenotypic spectrum and patterns of left ventricular hypertrophy in hypertrophic cardiomyopathy: morphologic observations and significance as assessed by two-dimensional echocardiography in 600 patients. *J Am Coll Cardiol* 26(7):1699–1708, 1995.
48. Lever HM, Karam RF, Currie PJ, et al: Hypertrophic cardiomyopathy in the elderly. Distinctions from the young based on cardiac shape. *Circulation* 79(3):580–589, 1989.
49. Watkins H, McKenna WJ, Thierfelder L, et al: Mutations in the genes for cardiac troponin T and alpha tropomyosin in hypertrophic cardiomyopathy. *N Engl J Med* 332(16):1058–1064, 1995.
50. Niimura H, Bachinski LL, Sangwatanaroj S, et al: Mutations in the gene for cardiac myosin-binding protein C and late-onset familial hypertrophic cardiomyopathy. *N Engl J Med* 338(18): 1248–1257, 1998.
51. Spirito P, Maron BJ: Absence of progression of left ventricular hypertrophy in adult patients with hypertrophic cardiomyopathy. *J Am Coll Cardiol* 9(5):1013–1017, 1987.
52. Klues HG, Maron BJ, Dollar AL, et al: Diversity of structural mitral valve alterations in hypertrophic cardiomyopathy. *Circulation* 85(5):1651–1660, 1992.
53. Wigle ED, Sasson Z, Henderson MA, et al: Hypertrophic cardiomyopathy. The importance of the site and the extent of hypertrophy. A review. *Prog Cardiovasc Dis* 28(1):1–83, 1985.
54. Klues HG, Roberts WC, Maron BJ: Anomalous insertion of papillary muscle directly into anterior mitral leaflet in hypertrophic cardiomyopathy. Significance in producing left ventricular outflow obstruction. *Circulation* 84(3):1188–1197, 1991.
55. Maron BJ, Spirito P, Green KJ, et al: Noninvasive assessment of left ventricular diastolic function by pulsed Doppler echocardiography in patients with hypertrophic cardiomyopathy. *J Am Coll Cardiol* 10(4):733–742, Oct 1987.
56. Chikamori T, Dickie S, Poloniecki JD, et al: Prognostic significance of radionuclide-assessed diastolic function in hypertrophic cardiomyopathy. *Am J Cardiol* 65(7):478–482, 1990.
57. Fananapazir L, Tracy CM, Leon MB, et al: Electrophysiologic abnormalities in patients with hypertrophic cardiomyopathy. A consecutive analysis in 155 patients. *Circulation* 80(5):1259–1268, 1989.
58. Maron BJ: The electrocardiogram as a diagnostic tool for hypertrophic cardiomyopathy: revisited. *Ann Noninvasive Electrocardiol* 6(4):277–279, 2001
59. Maron BJ, Niimura H, Casey SA, et al: Development of left ventricular hypertrophy in adults in hypertrophic cardiomyopathy caused by cardiac myosin-binding protein C gene mutations. *J Am Coll Cardiol* 38(2):315–321, 2001.
60. Maron BJ, Wolfson JK, Ciro E, et al: Relation of electrocardiographic abnormalities and patterns of left ventricular hypertrophy identified by 2-dimensional echocardiography in patients with hypertrophic cardiomyopathy. *Am J Cardiol* 51(1):189–194, 1983.
61. Yamaguchi H, Ishimura T, Nishiyama S, et al: Hypertrophic nonobstructive cardiomyopathy with giant negative T waves (apical hypertrophy): ventriculographic and echocardiographic features in 30 patients. *Am J Cardiol* 44(3):401–412, 1979.
62. Rickers C, Wilke NM, Jerosch-Herold M, et al: Utility of cardiac magnetic resonance imaging in the diagnosis of hypertrophic cardiomyopathy. *Circulation* 112(6):855–861, 2005.
63. Moon JC, McKenna WJ, McCrohon JA, et al: Toward clinical risk assessment in hypertrophic cardiomyopathy with gadolinium cardiovascular magnetic resonance. *J Am Coll Cardiol* 41(9): 1561–1567, 2003.
64. Brugada P, Bar FW, de Zwaan C, et al: "Sawfish" systolic narrowing of the left anterior descending artery: an angiographic sign of hypertrophic cardiomyopathy. *Circulation* 66:800–803, 1982.
64a. Brockenbrough EC, Braunwald E, Morrow AG: A hemodynamic technic for the detection of hypertrophic subaortic stenosis. *Circul* 23:189–194, 1961.
65. Maron BJ, Seidman JG, Seidman CE: Proposal for contemporary screening strategies in families with hypertrophic cardiomyopathy. *J Am Coll Cardiol* 44(11):2125–2132, 2004.
66. Arad M, Benson DW, Perez-Atayde AR, et al: Constitutively active AMP kinase mutations cause glycogen storage disease mimicking hypertrophic cardiomyopathy. *J Clin Invest* 109(3): 357–362, 2002.
67. Gollob MH, Green MS, Tang AS, et al: Identification of a gene responsible for familial Wolff-Parkinson-White syndrome. *N Engl J Med* 344(24):1823–1831, 2001.
68. Arad M, Maron BJ, Gorham JM, et al: Glycogen storage diseases presenting as hypertrophic cardiomyopathy. *N Engl J Med* 352(4):362–372, 2005.

69. Osterop AP, Kofflard MJ, Sandkuijl LA, et al: AT1 receptor A/C1166 polymorphism contributes to cardiac hypertrophy in subjects with hypertrophic cardiomyopathy. *Hypertension* 32(5):825–830, 1998.

70. Erdmann J, Raible J, Maki-Abadi J, et al: Spectrum of clinical phenotypes and gene variants in cardiac myosin-binding protein C mutation carriers with hypertrophic cardiomyopathy. *J Am Coll Cardiol* 38(2):322–330, 2001.

71. Anan R, Shono H, Kisanuki A, et al: Patients with familial hypertrophic cardiomyopathy caused by a Phe110Ile missense mutation in the cardiac troponin T gene have variable cardiac morphologies and a favorable prognosis. *Circulation* 98(5):391–397, 1998.

72. Marian AJ: On genetic and phenotypic variability of hypertrophic cardiomyopathy: nature versus nurture. *J Am Coll Cardiol* 38(2):331–334, 2001.

73. Tsoutsman T, Lam L, Semsarian C: Genes, calcium and modifying factors in hypertrophic cardiomyopathy. *Clin Exp Pharmacol Physiol* 33(1-2):139–145, 2006.

74. Flamm MD, Harrison DC, Hancock EW: Muscular subaortic stenosis. Prevention of outflow obstruction with propranolol. *Circulation* 38(5):846–858, 1968.

75. Sharma S, Elliott P, Whyte G, et al: Utility of cardiopulmonary exercise in the assessment of clinical determinants of functional capacity in hypertrophic cardiomyopathy. *Am J Cardiol* 86(2):162–168, 2000.

76. Bonow RO, Dilsizian V, Rosing DR, et al: Verapamil-induced improvement in left ventricular diastolic filling and increased exercise tolerance in patients with hypertrophic cardiomyopathy: short- and long-term effects. *Circulation* 72(4):853–864, 1985.

77. Bonow RO, Rosing DR, Bacharach SL, et al: Effects of verapamil on left ventricular systolic function and diastolic filling in patients with hypertrophic cardiomyopathy. *Circulation* 64(4):787–796, 1981.

78. Gistri R, Cecchi F, Choudhury L, et al: Effect of verapamil on absolute myocardial blood flow in hypertrophic cardiomyopathy. *Am J Cardiol* 74(4):363–368, 1994.

79. Udelson JE, Bonow RO, O'Gara PT, et al: Verapamil prevents silent myocardial perfusion abnormalities during exercise in asymptomatic patients with hypertrophic cardiomyopathy. *Circulation* 79(5):1052–1060, 1989.

80. Pollick C: Muscular subaortic stenosis: hemodynamic and clinical improvement after disopyramide. *N Engl J Med* 307(16):997–999, 1982.

81. Matsubara H, Nakatani S, Nagata S, et al: Salutary effect of disopyramide on left ventricular diastolic function in hypertrophic obstructive cardiomyopathy. *J Am Coll Cardiol* 26(3):768–775, 1995.

82. Sherrid M, Delia E, Dwyer E: Oral disopyramide therapy for obstructive hypertrophic cardiomyopathy. *Am J Cardiol* 62(16):1085–1088, 1988.

83. Podrid PJ, Lampert S, Graboys TB, et al: Aggravation of arrhythmia by antiarrhythmic drugs—incidence and predictors. *Am J Cardiol* 59(11):38E–44E, 1987.

84. McKenna WJ, Oakley CM, Krikler DM, et al: Improved survival with amiodarone in patients with hypertrophic cardiomyopathy and ventricular tachycardia. *Br Heart J* 53(4):412–416, 1985.

85. Fananapazir L, Leon MB, Bonow RO, et al: Sudden death during empiric amiodarone therapy in symptomatic hypertrophic cardiomyopathy. *Am J Cardiol* 67(2):169–174, 1991.

86. Prasad K, Frenneaux MP: Hypertrophic cardiomyopathy: is there a role for amiodarone? *Heart* 79(4):317–318, 1998.

87. Almendral JM, Ormaetxe J, Martinez-Alday JD, et al: Treatment of ventricular arrhythmias in patients with hypertrophic cardiomyopathy. *Eur Heart J* 14(Suppl):J71–J72, 1993.

88. Fananapazir L, Epstein ND, Curiel RV, et al: Long-term results of dual-chamber (DDD) pacing in obstructive hypertrophic cardiomyopathy. Evidence for progressive symptomatic and hemodynamic improvement and reduction of left ventricular hypertrophy. *Circulation* 90(6):2731–2742, 1994.

89. Posma JL, Blanksma PK, Van Der Wall EE, et al: Effects of permanent dual chamber pacing on myocardial perfusion in symptomatic hypertrophic cardiomyopathy. *Heart* 76(4):358–362, 1996.

90. Nishimura RA, Trusty JM, Hayes DL, et al: Dual-chamber pacing for hypertrophic cardiomyopathy: a randomized, double-blind, crossover trial. *J Am Coll Cardiol* 29(2):435–441, 1997.

91. Maron BJ, Nishimura RA, McKenna WJ, et al: Assessment of permanent dual-chamber pacing as a treatment for drug-refractory symptomatic patients with obstructive hypertrophic cardiomyopathy. A randomized, double-blind, crossover study (M-PATHY). *Circulation* 99(22):2927–2933, 1999.

92. Kappenberger L, Linde C, Daubert C, et al: Pacing in hypertrophic obstructive cardiomyopathy. A randomized crossover study. PIC Study Group. *Eur Heart J* 18(8):1249–1256, 1997.

93. Betocchi S, Elliott PM, Briguori C, et al: Dual chamber pacing in hypertrophic cardiomyopathy: long-term effects on diastolic function. *Pacing Clin Electrophysiol* 25(10):1433–1440, 2002.

94. Topilski I, Sherez J, Keren G, et al: Long-term effects of dual-chamber pacing with periodic echocardiographic evaluation of optimal atrioventricular delay in patients with hypertrophic cardiomyopathy >50 years of age. *Am J Cardiol* 97(12):1769–1775, 2006.

95. Ommen SR, Nishimura RA, Squires RW, et al: Comparison of dual-chamber pacing versus septal myectomy for the treatment of patients with hypertropic obstructive cardiomyopathy: a comparison of objective hemodynamic and exercise end points. *J Am Coll Cardiol* 34(1):191–196, 1999.

96. Moss AJ, Zareba W, Hall WJ, et al: Prophylactic implantation of a defibrillator in patients with myocardial infarction and reduced ejection fraction. *N Engl J Med* 346(12):877–883, 2002.

97. Boriani G, Maron BJ, Shen WK, et al: Prevention of sudden death in hypertrophic cardiomyopathy: but which defibrillator for which patient? *Circulation* 110(15):e438–e442, 2004.

98. Gregoratos G, Abrams J, Epstein AE, et al: ACC/AHA/NASPE 2002 Guideline Update for Implantation of Cardiac Pacemakers and Antiarrhythmia Devices—summary article: a report of the American College of Cardiology/American Heart Association Task Force on Practice Guidelines (ACC/AHA/NASPE Committee to Update the 1998 Pacemaker Guidelines). *J Am Coll Cardiol* 40(9):1703–1719, 2002.

98a. Goodwin JF, Hollman A, Cleland WP, et al: Obstructive cardiomyopathy simulating aortic stenosis. *Br Heart J* 22:403–414, 1960.

99. Morrow AG: Hypertrophic subaortic stenosis. Operative methods utilized to relieve left ventricular outflow obstruction. *J Thorac Cardiovasc Surg* 76(4):423–430, 1978.

100. Maron BJ, Dearani JA, Ommen SR, et al: The case for surgery in obstructive hypertrophic cardiomyopathy. *J Am Coll Cardiol* 44(10):2044–2053, 2004.

101. Schoendube FA, Klues HG, Reith S, et al: Long-term clinical and echocardiographic follow-up after surgical correction of hypertrophic obstructive cardiomyopathy with extended myectomy and reconstruction of the subvalvular mitral apparatus. *Circulation* 92(9 Suppl):II122–II127, 1995.

102. Maron BJ, Nishimura RA, Danielson GK: Pitfalls in clinical recognition and a novel operative approach for hypertrophic cardiomyopathy with severe outflow obstruction due to anomalous papillary muscle. *Circulation* 98(23):2505–2508, 1998.

103. McIntosh CL, Maron BJ, Cannon RO, III, et al: Initial results of combined anterior mitral leaflet plication and ventricular septal myotomy-myectomy for relief of left ventricular outflow tract obstruction in patients with hypertrophic cardiomyopathy. *Circulation* 86(5 Suppl):II60–II67, 1992.

104. van der Lee C, Kofflard MJ, van Herwerden LA, et al: Sustained improvement after combined anterior mitral leaflet extension and myectomy in hypertrophic obstructive cardiomyopathy. *Circulation* 108(17):2088–2092, 2003.

105. Krajcer Z, Leachman RD, Cooley DA, et al: Mitral valve replacement and septal myomectomy in hypertrophic cardiomyopathy. Ten-year follow-up in 80 patients. *Circulation* 78(3 Pt 2):I35–143, 1988.

106. Merrill WH, Friesinger GC, Graham TP, Jr, et al: Long-lasting improvement after septal myectomy for hypertrophic obstructive cardiomyopathy. *Ann Thorac Surg* 69(6):1732–1735; discussion 1735–1736, 2000.

107. Qin JX, Shiota T, Lever HM, et al: Outcome of patients with hypertrophic obstructive cardiomyopathy after percutaneous transluminal septal myocardial ablation and septal myectomy surgery. *J Am Coll Cardiol* 38(7):1994–2000, 2001.

108. McCully RB, Nishimura RA, Tajik AJ, et al: Extent of clinical improvement after surgical treatment of hypertrophic obstructive cardiomyopathy. *Circulation* 94(3):467–471, 1996.

109. Sherrid MV, Chaudhry FA, Swistel DG: Obstructive hypertrophic cardiomyopathy: echocardiography, pathophysiology, and the continuing evolution of surgery for obstruction. *Ann Thorac Surg* 75(2):620–632, 2003.

110. Nishimura RA, Holmes DR, Jr: Clinical practice. Hypertrophic obstructive cardiomyopathy. *N Engl J Med* 350(13):1320–1327, 2004.

111. Ommen. The effect of surgical myectomy on survival in patients with hypertrophic cardiomyopathy. *J Am Coll Cardiol* 43(Suppl A):215A, 2004.

112. Sigwart U: Non-surgical myocardial reduction for hypertrophic obstructive cardiomyopathy. *Lancet* 346(8969):211–214, 1995.

113. Faber L, Meissner A, Ziemssen P, et al: Percutaneous transluminal septal myocardial ablation for hypertrophic obstructive cardiomyopathy: long term follow up of the first series of 25 patients. *Heart* 83(3):326–331, 2000.

114. Gietzen FH, Leuner CJ, Raute-Kreinsen U, et al: Acute and long-term results after transcoronary ablation of septal hypertrophy (TASH). Catheter interventional treatment for hypertrophic obstructive cardiomyopathy. *Eur Heart J* 20(18):1342–1354, 1999.

115. Lakkis NM, Nagueh SF, Dunn JK, et al: Nonsurgical septal reduction therapy for hypertrophic obstructive cardiomyopathy: one-year follow-up. *J Am Coll Cardiol* 36(3):852–855, 2000.

116. Knight C, Kurbaan AS, Seggewiss H, et al: Nonsurgical septal reduction for hypertrophic obstructive cardiomyopathy: outcome in the first series of patients. *Circulation* 95(8):2075–2081, 1997.

117. Ruzyllo W, Chojnowska L, Demkow M, et al: Left ventricular outflow tract gradient decrease with non-surgical myocardial reduction improves exercise capacity in patients with hypertrophic obstructive cardiomyopathy. *Eur Heart J* 21(9):770–777, 2000.

118. Firoozi S, Elliott PM, Sharma S, et al: Septal myotomy-myectomy and transcoronary septal alcohol ablation in hypertrophic obstructive cardiomyopathy. A comparison of clinical, haemodynamic and exercise outcomes. *Eur Heart J* 23(20):1617–1624, 2002.

119. Maron BJ: Role of alcohol septal ablation in treatment of obstructive hypertrophic cardiomyopathy. *Lancet* 355(9202):425–426, 2000.

120. Roberts R, Sigwart U: Current concepts of the pathogenesis and treatment of hypertrophic cardiomyopathy. *Circulation* 112(2):293–296, 2005.

121. Holmes DR, Jr, Valeti US, Nishimura RA: Alcohol septal ablation for hypertrophic cardiomyopathy: indications and technique. *Catheter Cardiovasc Intervent* 66(3):375–389, 2005.

122. Singh M, Edwards WD, Holmes DR, Jr, et al: Anatomy of the first septal perforating artery: a study with implications for ablation therapy for hypertrophic cardiomyopathy. *Mayo Clin Proc* 76(8):799–802, 2001..

123. Nagueh SF, Lakkis NM, He ZX, et al: Role of myocardial contrast echocardiography during nonsurgical septal reduction therapy for hypertrophic obstructive cardiomyopathy. *J Am Coll Cardiol* 32(1):225–229, 1998.

124. Bhagwandeen R, Woo A, Ross J, et al: Septal ethanol ablation for hypertrophic obstructive cardiomyopathy: early and intermediate results of a Canadian referral centre. *Can J Cardiol* 19(8):912–917, 2003.

125. Faber L, Seggewiss H, Gleichmann U: Percutaneous transluminal septal myocardial ablation in hypertrophic obstructive cardiomyopathy: results with respect to intraprocedural myocardial contrast echocardiography. *Circulation* 98(22):2415–2421, 1998.

126. Kuhn H, Gietzen FH, Leuner C, et al: Transcoronary ablation of septal hypertrophy (TASH): a new treatment option for hypertrophic obstructive cardiomyopathy. *Z Kardiol* 89(Suppl 4):IV41–IV54, 2000.

127. Boekstegers P, Steinbigler P, Molnar A, et al: Pressure-guided nonsurgical myocardial reduction induced by small septal infarctions in hypertrophic obstructive cardiomyopathy. *J Am Coll Cardiol* 38(3):846–853, 2001.

128. Veselka J, Duchonova R, Prochazkova S, et al: Effects of varying ethanol dosing in percutaneous septal ablation for obstructive hypertrophic cardiomyopathy on early hemodynamic changes. *Am J Cardiol* 95(5):675–678, 2005.

129. Chang SM, Nagueh SF, Spencer WH, III, et al: Complete heart block: determinants and clinical impact in patients with hypertrophic obstructive cardiomyopathy undergoing nonsurgical septal reduction therapy. *J Am Coll Cardiol* 42(2):296–300, 2003.

130. Ralph-Edwards A, Woo A, McCrindle BW, et al: Hypertrophic obstructive cardiomyopathy: comparison of outcomes after myectomy or alcohol ablation adjusted by propensity score. *J Thorac Cardiovasc Surg* 129(2):351–358, 2005.

131. Nagueh SF, Ommen SR, Lakkis NM, et al: Comparison of ethanol septal reduction therapy with surgical myectomy for the treatment of hypertrophic obstructive cardiomyopathy. *J Am Coll Cardiol* 38(6):1701–1706, 2001.

132. van Dockum WG, Beek AM, ten Cate FJ, et al: Early onset and progression of left ventricular remodeling after alcohol septal ablation in hypertrophic obstructive cardiomyopathy. *Circulation* 111(19):2503–2508, 2005.

133. Talreja DR, Nishimura RA, Edwards WD, et al: Alcohol septal ablation versus surgical septal myectomy: comparison of effects on atrioventricular conduction tissue. *J Am Coll Cardiol* 44(12):2329–2332, 2004.

134. Sigwart U: Catheter treatment for hypertrophic obstructive cardiomyopathy: for seniors only? *Circulation* 118:107–108 2008.

135. Smedira NG, Lytle BW, Lever HM, et al: Current effectiveness and risks of isolated septal myectomy for hypertrophic obstructive cardiomyopathy. *Ann Thorac Surg* 85:127–133, 2008.

136. Agarwal S, Tuzcu EM, Desai MY, et al: Updated meta-analysis of septal alcohol ablation versus myectomy for hypertrophic cardiomyopathy. *J Am Coll Cardiol* 55:823–834, 2010.

137. Alam M, Dokainish H, Lakkis NM: Hypertrophic obstructive cardiomyopathy-alcohol septal ablation vs. myectomy: a meta-analysis. *Eur Heart J* 30, 1080–1087, 2009.

138. Leonardi RA, Kransdorf EP, Simel DL, et al: Meta-analyses of septal reduction therapies for obstructive hypertrophic cardiomyopathy. *Circ Cardiovasc Intervent* 3(2):97–104, epub Mar 2010.

53

Percutaneous Balloon Pericardiotomy for Patients with Pericardial Effusion and Tamponade

HANI JNEID | ANDREW A. ZISKIND | IGOR PALACIOS

KEY POINTS

- Pericardiocentesis is the technique of catheter-based aspiration of pericardial fluid. It serves as a diagnostic and therapeutic modality in patients with pericarditis with pericardial effusion, pericardial effusion with pericardial tamponade, and effusive-constrictive pericarditis.

- The pericardial space can be safely entered with a blunt-tipped needle via a subxiphoid approach under fluoroscopic guidance, even in the absence of significant pericardial effusion.

- Percutaneous balloon pericardiotomy is an effective therapy for recurrent, free-flowing and hemodynamically significant pericardial effusions, especially if associated with neoplastic disease.

- It consists of creating a parietal pericardial window with a balloon dilating catheter under fluoroscopic guidance in the cardiac catheterization laboratory.

- It is a less invasive alternative to surgical pericardial window and avoids its perioperative risks.

- It should be avoided if possible in patients with large pleural effusions or marginal pulmonary reserve to avoid further pulmonary compromise.

- Catheter-based diagnostic and interventional techniques in the pericardial space have become increasingly common and include epicardial mapping and ablation, intrapericardial delivery of therapies, intrapericardial echocardiography, pericardioscopy-guided biopsy, and potentially other advanced techniques.

Introduction

The clinical presentation of patients with pericardial effusion is variable, with some being completely asymptomatic while others develop pericardial tamponade and cardiovascular collapse. Pericardiocentesis is a catheter-based technique that uses a needle to aspirate the pericardial fluid, usually under fluoroscopic and/or echocardiographic guidance. Percutaneous balloon pericardiotomy (PBP) is a relatively novel catheter-based technique that is gradually replacing the more invasive surgical pericardial window procedure. The improvement in techniques for percutaneous access to the pericardial space and the adjunctive use of pericardioscopy provides additional opportunities for the use of this space in diagnostic and interventional techniques. Novel pericardial interventions—such as epicardial mapping and ablation, percutaneous pericardial biopsy, and intrapericardial echocardiography—are therefore rapidly evolving.

Pericardial Effusion and Tamponade

The normal pericardium is a fibroelastic sac composed of visceral and parietal layers separated by a thin layer (20–50 mL) of straw-colored fluid.[1] The normal pericardium has a steep pressure-volume curve: it is distensible when the intrapericardial volume is small but becomes gradually inextensible when the volume increases.[1] In the presence of pericardial effusion, the intrapericardial pressure depends on the relationship between the absolute volume of the effusion, speed of fluid accumulation, and pericardial elasticity. The clinical presentation is thus related not only to the size of the effusion but also and more importantly to the rapidity of fluid accumulation. Pericardial effusion may result from a variety of clinical conditions (Table 53-1). Among medical patients, malignant disease is the most common cause of pericardial effusion with tamponade.[1,2] Pericardial tamponade is a clinical syndrome with defined hemodynamic and echocardiographic abnormalities that result from the accumulation of intrapericardial fluid and impairment of ventricular diastolic filling.[1,3] The ultimate mechanism of hemodynamic compromise is the compression of cardiac chambers secondary to increased intrapericardial pressure. In all cases of cardiac tamponade, the initial treatment consists of removing pericardial fluid by prompt pericardiocentesis and drainage. Reaccumulation of fluid with recurrence of cardiac tamponade may be an indication for a surgical intervention.[1] Autopsy and surgical studies have shown that myocardial or pericardial metastases are found in approximately 50% of patients who present with cardiac tamponade due to malignancy.[3–7] Although the short-term survival of patients with cardiac tamponade depends primarily on its early diagnosis and relief, long-term survival depends on the prognosis of the primary illness regardless of the intervention performed.[4,5,8]

Pericardiocentesis

INDICATIONS

Pericardiocentesis is the technique of catheter-based aspiration of pericardial fluid.[1,3] It serves as a diagnostic and therapeutic modality in patients with pericarditis with pericardial effusion, pericardial effusion with pericardial tamponade, and effusive-constrictive pericarditis. Many asymptomatic patients with large effusions do not require pericardiocentesis if they have no hemodynamic compromise, unless there is a diagnostic need for fluid analysis. In a prospective long-term follow-up of patients with large idiopathic chronic pericardial effusion, Sagrista-Sauleda and colleagues[9] concluded that large idiopathic chronic pericardial effusions were usually well tolerated for long periods in most patients with severe tamponade; however, they could develop unexpectedly at any time. Although pericardiocentesis was effective in resolving these effusions, recurrences were common, prompting the authors to recommend referral of these patients for pericardiectomy when recurrence occurs.[10] When cardiac tamponade occurs, the emergency drainage of pericardial fluid by pericardiocentesis is a lifesaving therapy in a patient who would otherwise develop pulseless electrical activity and cardiac arrest. When performed, pericardiocentesis should (1) relieve tamponade when present, (2) obtain fluid for appropriate analyses, and (3) assess hemodynamics before and after pericardial fluid evacuation to exclude effusive-constrictive pericardial effusion. Elective pericardiocentesis is contraindicated in patients receiving anticoagulation, in those with bleeding disorders or thrombocytopenia with platelet counts <50,000/μL, and in those with hemorrhagic pericardial tamponade complicating aortic dissection. Pericardiocentesis is also ill advised when the effusion is very small or loculated.[1,3]

TABLE 53-1	Etiology of Pericardial Effusion and/or Tamponade
Idiopathic	
Infectious	
Viral	
Bacterial	
Fungal	
Others	
Metabolic	
Uremia	
Myxedema	
Collagen and other autoimmune disorders	
Systemic lupus erythematosus	
Rheumatoid arthritis	
Rheumatic fever	
Dressler syndrome	
Others	
Neoplastic	
Primary	
Pericardial metastasis	
Local invasion	
Volume overload	
Chronic heart failure	
Miscellaneous	
Chest wall irradiation	
Cardiotomy or thoracic surgery	
Adverse drug reaction	
Aortic dissection	
Post-myocardial infarction	
Trauma	

From Jneid H, Maree AO, Palacios IF. Pericardial tamponade: clinical presentation, diagnosis and catheter-based therapies. In: J Parillo, PR Dellinger, eds. *Critical Care Medicine.* 3rd ed. St. Louis: Mosby; 2008.

TECHNIQUE

Pericardiocentesis is most commonly performed via a subxiphoid approach under ECG and fluoroscopic guidance (Fig. 53-1A).[3] Traditionally, pericardiocentesis has been performed in the cardiac catheterization laboratory with arterial and right heart pressure monitoring.[3] Today, however, the procedure is also performed in the noninvasive laboratory, intensive care unit, or even at bedside under echocardiographic guidance. Whichever modality is utilized, it is a safe procedure when performed by appropriately trained personnel. Pericardiocentesis is a procedure based on the Seldinger technique of percutaneous catheter insertion. After the administration of local anesthesia to the skin and deeper tissues of the left xiphocostal area, the pericardial needle is connected to an ECG lead. The needle is advanced from the left of the subxiphoid area while aiming toward the left shoulder (usually under fluoroscopic or echocardiographic guidance; however, blinded procedures can be undertaken during emergency procedures). Often, a discrete pop is felt as the needle enters the pericardial space. When ST-segment elevation is observed on the ECG lead tracing, it signifies that the needle has touched the epicardium and should be withdrawn slightly until the ST-segment elevation disappears (Fig. 53-1B). Once the pericardial space is entered, a stiff guidewire is introduced into the pericardial space through the needle, which is thereafter removed; then a catheter is inserted into the pericardial sac over the guidewire (Fig. 53-1C). The drainage catheter utilized usually has an end hole and multiple side holes. Intrapericardial pressure is measured by connecting a pressure transducer system to the intrapericardial catheter. Pericardial fluid is then removed, and samples of pericardial fluid are sent for appropriate biochemical, cytological, bacteriological, and immunological analyses for diagnostic purposes (the first sample is usually reserved for microbiological studies). In the presence of pericardial tamponade, aspiration of fluid should be continued until clinical and hemodynamic improvement occurs. The catheter is frequently left in place for continuous drainage and as a route to instill sclerosing or chemotherapeutic agents when needed. The catheter is secured to the skin using sterile sutures and covered with a sterile dressing. The success rate of pericardiocentesis is greater and the incidence of complications improves with the increasing size of the effusion.

COMPLICATIONS

The potential complications of pericardiocentesis include heart or a coronary vessel laceration, sometimes causing fatal consequences. Puncture of the right atrium or ventricle with hemopericardial fluid accumulation, arrhythmias, air embolism, pneumothorax, and puncture of the peritoneal cavity or abdominal viscera have all been reported. Acute pulmonary edema may infrequently occur when the pericardial tamponade is decompressed too rapidly. Other approaches of pericardiocentesis include the right xiphocostal, apical, right-sided, and parasternal approaches. Although these may be useful under certain circumstances, they are associated with a greater incidence of complications. The right xiphocostal approach is associated with higher incidence of right atrial and inferior vena cava injury. Puncture of the left pleura and the lingula is more frequent with the apical approach, while puncture of the left anterior descending and the internal mammary artery is more frequent with the parasternal approach. Echocardiographically-guided pericardiocentesis is a safe and effective technique. In a cohort of 1127 therapeutic echocardiography-guided pericardiocenteses performed in 977 patients at the Mayo Clinic (1979–1998), procedural success rate was 97% overall with a total complication rate of 4.7%.[10] Echocardiography may be especially useful in patients with loculated effusions and unlike pericardiocenteses performed in the cardiac catheterization laboratory the left chest wall is often utilized with echocardiographically-guided pericardiocenteses.

POSTPERICARDIOCENTESIS MANAGEMENT

Pericardiocentesis may not completely evacuate the effusion in most cases, given particularly that active secretion and bleeding into the pericardial space may continue.[1,3] The pericardial catheter should therefore be left in place for 24 to 72 hours after the initial fluid evacuation until total daily drainage is ≤75 to 100 mL. The patient is admitted for continuous ECG monitoring and assessment of the rate of pericardial drainage. The pericardial space should be drained every 8 hours and the catheter flushed with heparinized saline and systemic antibiotics (usually first-generation cephalosporin for empirical coverage of gram-positive bacteria) are administered for the duration of the catheter stay. Based on the etiology of the effusion, the patient's clinical and hemodynamic condition, and the amount drained, the pericardial catheter is usually removed within 72 hours and/or decisions for additional therapy are contemplated. Follow-up echocardiography is useful to monitor the resolution of the pericardial effusion and for signs of cardiac compression prior to catheter removal. Patients who continue to drain more than 75 to 100 mL/24 hr 3 days after standard catheter drainage should be considered for more aggressive therapy. Reaccumulation of the pericardial fluid is particularly common in patients with malignant pericardial effusions. Additional therapeutic approaches are available to prevent pericardial fluid reaccumulation. They include intrapericardial instillation of sclerosing agents, use of chemotherapy, radiotherapy, PBP, and surgical pericardial window. Reaccumulation of fluid with recurrence of cardiac tamponade is considered a definitive indication for a pericardial window.

Percutaneous Balloon Pericardiotomy

The management of cardiac tamponade or large pericardial effusions at risk for progression to tamponade remains controversial and is dictated to a large extent by local institutional practices. Life-threatening cardiac tamponade requires immediate removal of

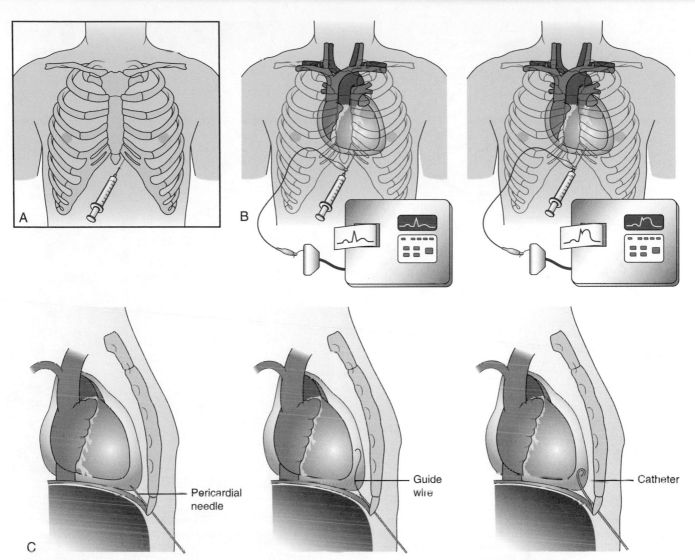

Figure 53-1 A. Diagrammatic representation of a pericardiocentesis procedure using the subxiphoid approach. B. The pericardial needle is connected to an ECG lead. The needle is advanced from the left of the subxiphoid area aiming toward the left shoulder. ST segment elevation is seen on the ECG lead tracing when the needle touches the epicardium. The needle should be retracted slightly until the ST-segment elevation disappears. C. Once the pericardial space is entered with the pericardial needle, a guidewire is introduced in the pericardial space through the needle. The needle is removed and a catheter is inserted in the pericardial sac over the guidewire (either anteriorly or inferiorly in the pericardial sac). (Redrawn from Jneid H, Maree AO, Palacios IF. Pericardial tamponade: clinical presentation, diagnosis and catheter-based therapies. In: J Parillo, PR Dellinger, eds. Critical Care Medicine. 3rd ed. St. Louis: Mosby; 2008.)

pericardial fluid to relieve the hemodynamic compromise. Furthermore, it is desirable to prevent recurrence. For many patients with a pericardial effusion and tamponade, standard percutaneous pericardial drainage with an indwelling pericardial catheter is sufficient to avoid recurrence. Recurrences after catheter drainage have been reported in 14% to 50% of patients with pericardial effusion and tamponade.[5,11–13] Patients who continue to drain more than 75 to 100 mL/24 hr 3 days after standard catheter drainage have been considered for more aggressive therapy. Several approaches are available to prevent reaccumulation of pericardial fluid, including intrapericardial instillation of sclerosing agents, use of chemotherapy, and radiation therapy.[14,15] A surgically created pericardial window may provide an alternative for the treatment of pericardial effusions,[16,17] but morbidity and late recurrence are not uncommon.[8,18,19] The use of a subxiphoid surgical pericardial window has been advocated as primary therapy for malignant pericardial tamponade based on the high initial success in relieving tamponade[18–23] and an acceptable recurrence rate.[19] However, it is associated with high morbidity rates.[8,16–23] Patients with advanced malignancy and cardiac tamponade are often poor

candidates for surgical therapy. Because their life expectancy is already limited, the increased length of hospital stay associated with a surgical procedure may compromise the quality of their remaining lives. In addition, the malnutrition and chemotherapy associated with advanced malignancy increase the risk of infection and other perioperative complications. Therefore it is preferable to offer a less invasive alternative.

Palacios and colleagues[24] proposed the technique of percutaneous balloon pericardiotomy (PBP) as a less invasive alternative to the surgical pericardial window procedure. With this technique, a pericardial window and adequate drainage of pericardial effusion can be done percutaneously with a balloon dilating catheter (Fig. 53-2). Since their initial report on 8 patients, the multicenter PBP registry investigators have reported data on >130 patients.[25]

TECHNIQUE

The PBP technique is relatively simple and safe. It is performed in the catheterization laboratory with the patient under local anesthesia and

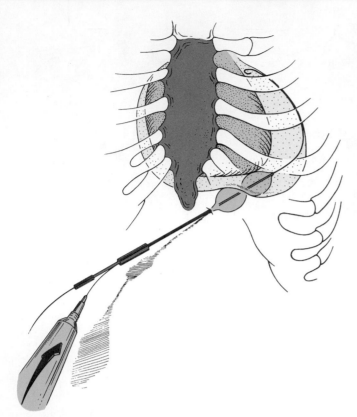

Figure 53-2 Percutaneous balloon pericardiotomy technique. *(From Ziskind AA, Pearce AC, Lemmon CC, et al. Percutaneous balloon pericardiotomy for the treatment of cardiac tamponade and large pericardial effusions: description of technique and report of the first fifty cases. J Am Coll Cardiol. 1993;21:1–5.)*

mild sedation with intravenous narcotics and a short-acting benzodiazepine. There is minimal discomfort. Patients may be candidates for PBP if they have undergone prior pericardiocentesis and have persistent catheter drainage. Alternatively, PBP may be done as a primary therapy at the time of initial pericardiocentesis. For those who have previously undergone standard pericardiocentesis using the subxiphoid approach, a pigtail catheter has typically been left in the pericardial space for drainage. For patients who, after 3 days, continue to drain more than 75 to 100 mL/24 hr, PBP is offered as an alternative to a surgical procedure. The subxiphoid area around the indwelling pigtail pericardial catheter is infiltrated with 1% lidocaine. A 0.038-in. guidewire with a preshaped curve at the tip is advanced through the pigtail catheter into the pericardial space (Fig. 53-3A). The catheter is then removed, leaving the guidewire in the pericardial space. The location of the wire should be confirmed by its looping within the pericardium. After predilation along the track of the wire with a 10-Fr dilator, a 20-mm-diameter 3-cm-long balloon dilating catheter (Boston Scientific, Natick, MA) is advanced over the guidewire and positioned to straddle the parietal pericardium. Care should be taken to advance the proximal end of the balloon beyond the skin and subcutaneous tissue. Precise localization of the balloon is accomplished by gentle inflation to identify the waist at the pericardial margin. The balloon is inflated manually until the waist produced by the parietal pericardium disappears (Fig. 53-3B and C). If the pericardium is opposed to the chest wall, as indicated by failure of the proximal portion of the balloon to expand, a countertraction technique should be used in which the catheter is withdrawn slightly, then gently advanced while the skin and soft tissues are pulled manually in the opposite direction. This maneuver isolates the pericardium for dilation (Fig. 53-4). Fluoroscopic imaging using multiple views (preferably biplane fluoroscopy) is helpful to ensure correct positioning of the balloon, which should be

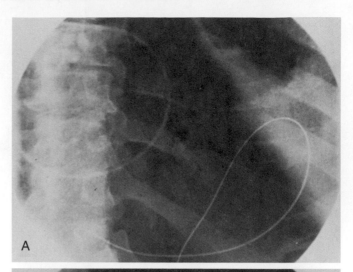

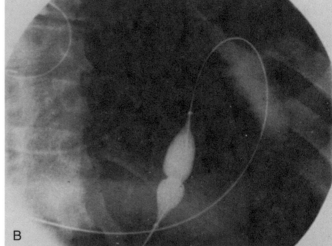

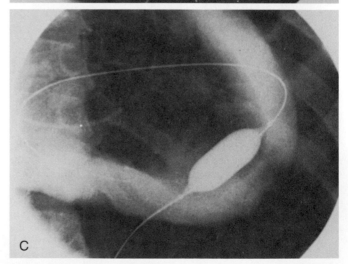

Figure 53-3 Anteroposterior fluoroscopic images. A. The guidewire (0.038-in.) has been advanced through the pigtail catheter and can be seen looping freely in the pericardial space. B. As the balloon is inflated manually, a waist is seen at the pericardial margin. C. The waist disappears with full inflation of the balloon as the pericardial window is created.

straddling the parietal pericardium (Fig. 53-5). At the operator's discretion, 5 to 10 mL of radiographic contrast material may be instilled into the pericardial space to help identify the pericardial margin. Two or three balloon inflations are then performed to ensure the creation of an adequate opening of the pericardium. Although transthoracic and transesophageal echocardiography may provide additional guidance to some aspects of the procedure, it is our experience that the balloon cannot be imaged adequately with echocardiography to identify the waist at the site of the pericardial margin.[26] The balloon dilating catheter is then removed, leaving the 0.038-in. guidewire in the pericardial space. A new pigtail catheter is then advanced over this guidewire and placed in the pericardial space. If PBP is being performed at the time of primary pericardiocentesis, the pericardium is entered by

a standard subxiphoid approach and a drainage catheter is inserted into the pericardial space. After the pericardial pressure has been measured, most of the pericardial fluid should be withdrawn, which reduces the volume remaining to pass into the pleural space. Technical variations of the subxiphoid technique have included dilation of two adjacent pericardial sites, use of the apical approach,[27] use of an Inoue balloon catheter,[27–29] use of double balloons,[30] use of a combination of one long and one short balloon,[31] and use of an 18-mm dilating balloon to facilitate introduction of a 16-Fr chest tube into the pericardial space.[32] Other investigators have attempted laparoscopic pericardial fenestration,[33,34] used a cutting pericardiotome,[35] or implanted a pericardioperitoneal shunt.[36] Thoracoscopic techniques have been developed to create a larger pericardial window with low morbidity compared with open surgical techniques.[37] With this technique, adequate long-term drainage may be provided and specimens for pathologic study obtained.[33,38]

POSTPROCEDURAL MANAGEMENT

Following the PBP procedure, the patient is returned to a telemetry floor. The pericardial catheter should be aspirated every 6 hours and flushed with heparinized saline (5 mL, 100 U/mL). Pericardial drainage volumes should be recorded, and the catheter removed after there is no significant pericardial drainage (≤75–100 mL) for 24 hours. Frequently, at the time of the catheter removal, there is evidence on the chest radiograph of a new or increasing pleural effusion. Follow-up two-dimensional transthoracic echocardiography is performed approximately 48 hours after removal of the pericardial catheter. Data are being collected on immediate removal of the pericardial catheter after PBP to facilitate early discharge. However, leaving the pericardial catheter in place may provide a measure of safety by allowing monitoring to determine whether the window is effective and whether bleeding is occurring. Periodic postprocedural echocardiography can be used to check for reaccumulation of pericardial fluid. Chest radiography should be performed to monitor the possible development of a pleural effusion (usually left) caused by drainage of the pericardial fluid.

MECHANISM OF PERCUTANEOUS BALLOON PERICARDIOTOMY

The precise mechanism by which PBP works remains unclear. We assume that balloon inflation results in localized tearing of the parietal pericardial tissues, leading to a communication of the pericardial space with the pleural space and possibly with the abdominal cavity.[19,40] The use of a flexible fiberoptic pericardioscope introduced over the guidewire after PBP has demonstrated a pericardial window freely

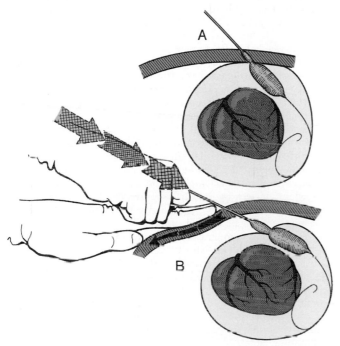

Figure 53-4 Countertraction technique to separate the pericardium from the adjacent chest wall (transverse view from below). A. Initial trial inflation of the balloon demonstrates trapping of the proximal portion of the balloon in the chest wall structures. B. Simultaneous traction on the skin and pushing of the balloon catheter results in displacement of the pericardium away from the chest wall, allowing proper inflation to occur. *(Redrawn from Ziskind AA, Burstein S. Echocardiography vs. fluoroscopic imaging [letter]. Catheter Cardiovasc Diagn. 1992;27:86.)*

Figure 53-5 Lateral fluoroscopic image of balloon inflation. A waist is seen at the pericardial margin (A); it disappears with full inflation (B).

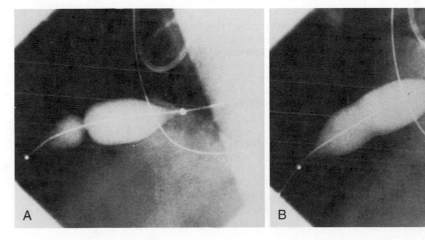

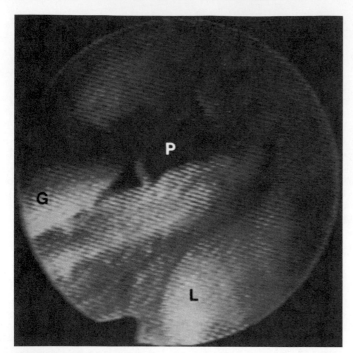

Figure 53-6 Pericardioscopic view of the balloon pericardiotomy site. The scope has been withdrawn over a guidewire to visualize the external pericardial surface. This figure demonstrates direct communication of the pericardial window with the left pleural space. G, guidewire; L, lung in left pleural space immediately outside the pericardium; P, pericardial window created by balloon dilation.

communicating with the left pleural space[41] (Fig. 53-6). Chow and colleagues supported this finding with their postmortem studies of balloon dilation, in which they used an Inoue balloon inflated to a maximum diameter of 23 mm.[42] Balloon dilation produced, without tearing, a smooth, oval pericardial window measuring 18.8 ± 16.4 mm. Histological analysis revealed fragmentation and breakage of the elastic and collagenous fibers in the connective tissue bordering the pericardial sites.[42] We have also demonstrated passage of pericardial fluid from the pericardial space to the pleural space in some patients after PBP by manually injecting 10 mL of radiographic contrast material through the pericardial catheter. However, the ability to visualize free exit of contrast from the pericardial space does not appear to correlate with procedural success. Based on experience with the subxiphoid surgical pericardial window procedure, it is unlikely that a long-term communication persists between the pericardium and the pleural cavity or subcutaneous tissues. Sugimoto and colleagues studied 28 patients who underwent surgical subxiphoid pericardial window procedures followed by tube decompression, of whom 93% experienced permanent relief.[43] Postoperative echocardiograms demonstrated thickening of the pericardium-epicardium with obliteration of the pericardial space. Autopsy data that confirmed this fusion were available for 4 patients. The authors concluded that the success of the subxiphoid pericardial window procedure depends on the inflammatory fusion of the epicardium to the pericardium, not on maintenance of a window.[43] Based on this surgical experience, it is unlikely that the PBP window remains open indefinitely. It is also possible that PBP, by leading to more effective pericardial drainage and maintaining a fluid-free pericardial space for a prolonged time, may permit autosclerosis to occur.

EVIDENCE-BASED LITERATURE

Palacios and coworkers reported the initial results of PBP in 8 patients with malignant pericardial effusion and tamponade.[24] The technique was successful in all patients. There were no immediate or late complications related to the procedure. The mean time to radiologic development of a new or a significantly increased pleural effusion was 2.9 ± 0.4 days (range 2–5 days). The mean follow-up in this initial report was 6 ± 2 months (range 1–11 months). No patients had recurrence of pericardial tamponade or pericardial effusion. Death occurred in 5 patients at 1, 4, 9, 10, and 11 months after PBP. In all cases, the cause of death was the patient's primary malignant disease. The remaining 3 patients were alive and free of cardiac symptoms at the time of the report. Following this initial favorable experience, the multicenter PBP registry was developed to collect additional data in a larger group of patients.

The Multicenter Registry Experience

The PBP technique has been studied in a multicenter registry to evaluate its therapeutic effectiveness and risks systematically. Data on 130 patients undergoing PBP from 1987 to 1994 in 16 centers have been presented.[25,41] In this cohort of 130 patients, the mean age was 59 ± 13 years, 52% were men; 69% presented with cardiac tamponade and 58% had prior pericardiocentesis procedure performed. Of these patients, 85% had known malignancy (mostly lung cancer), and only 15% had nonmalignant pericardial effusion (predominantly idiopathic or HIV-related). PBP was defined as successful if there was no recurrence of pericardial effusion on echocardiographic follow-up and if no complications occurred that required surgical exploration or a surgical pericardial window. PBP was successful in 111 (85%) of 130 patients, with no recurrences of pericardial effusion and/or tamponade during a mean follow-up of 5.0 ± 5.8 months. Five cases were considered failures because of pericardial bleeding, and those patients underwent surgical windowing. Thirteen patients had recurrence of pericardial effusion (mean time to recurrence, 53 ± 65 days). Of those 13 patients, 12 underwent surgical pericardial procedures, but 6 had a subsequent recurrence. Minor complications occurred in 11 patients (13%), the most frequent being fever. No patient had documented bacteremia or positive pericardial fluid cultures. After PBP, thoracentesis or chest tube placement was required in 15% of patients with preexisting pleural effusions, compared with 9% of patients without preexisting pleural effusions. Of the 104 patients with a history of malignancy, 86 died, compared with 2 of 16 patients with nonmalignant disease. The mean survival time for patients with a history of malignancy was 3.8 ± 3.3 months. No procedure-related variables were found to influence survival or freedom from recurrence (e.g., number of sites dilated, visualization of free fluid exit, duration of catheter placement). There was no significant difference in recurrence rate if PBP was performed as a primary treatment or after failed pericardiocentesis.

PERCUTANEOUS BALLOON PERICARDIOTOMY: TECHNICAL CONSIDERATIONS

Echocardiographic and Chest Radiographic Qualifications

Echocardiography should be performed before PBP to rule out the presence of loculated pericardial fluid. If pericardial fluid is not free-flowing, a surgical approach should be considered. If the chest radiograph reveals evidence of a large pleural effusion before PBP, this issue is less clear. If a left effusion is moderate or large before PBP, the chance of needing thoracentesis is high, and PBP should be performed only if the cardiac benefits outweigh the risks of thoracentesis or chest tube placement. Patients with marginal pulmonary mechanics, such as those who have undergone pneumonectomy, should be evaluated with caution, because the development of a left pleural effusion may compromise their remaining lung function.

Prophylactic Antibiotic Administration

Febrile episodes have been documented six times in the first 37 patients, although no patient had documented bacteremia or positive pericardial drainage cultures. Beginning with the 38th patient, prophylactic antibiotic therapy was initiated and continued until the catheter was removed. No febrile episodes were seen in 49 subsequent patients. It is unclear whether this was related to prophylactic antibiotics, a random effect, or more extensive operator experience, with a concomitant decrease in procedural time and catheter manipulation.

Patients with Bleeding Risk

The risk of bleeding from the pericardiotomy site appears to be increased in patients with platelet or coagulation abnormalities. For this reason, we do not recommend performing PBP on patients with uremic pericardial effusions or when coagulation parameters cannot be normalized (refractory coagulopathy or thrombocytopenia). In those patients at high risk for bleeding, a surgical procedure under direct visualization may be safer.

Fluoroscopic Guidance

Attempts to guide balloon placement by transthoracic or transesophageal echocardiography have been disappointing. Although the dilating balloon can be visualized, it is not possible to distinguish proper placement (with a discrete waist) from entrapment of the proximal balloon in the soft tissues and ineffective pericardial dilation. We have found fluoroscopic guidance to be particularly essential to the countertraction technique and believe it to be mandatory for PBP.[26]

Risks of Cardiac and Pulmonary Injury

Because PBP is not performed until successful access to the pericardial space is obtained and the guidewire is seen to be freely looping within the pericardium, the risks of cardiac injury are usually small. If the right ventricle is inadvertently entered and the balloon advanced, the results may be catastrophic. For this reason, PBP should be performed only by operators who have extensive experience with pericardiocentesis. In the emergency setting, it may be prudent to stabilize the patient with pericardiocentesis and leave a catheter in place for elective PBP under more controlled conditions.

Pleural Effusion

The development of a large pleural effusion following PBP is a significant concern. A left pleural effusion develops in most patients within 24 to 48 hours of the procedure (Fig. 53-7). In most cases, the pleural effusion resolves, presumably because of the greater resorptive capacity of the pleural surfaces. As noted earlier, thoracentesis or chest tube placement was required in 15% of patients with preexisting pleural effusions, compared with 9% of those without preexisting pleural effusions in the multicenter PBP registry. It is likely that some patients have a large volume of fluid flow from the pericardial to the pleural space;

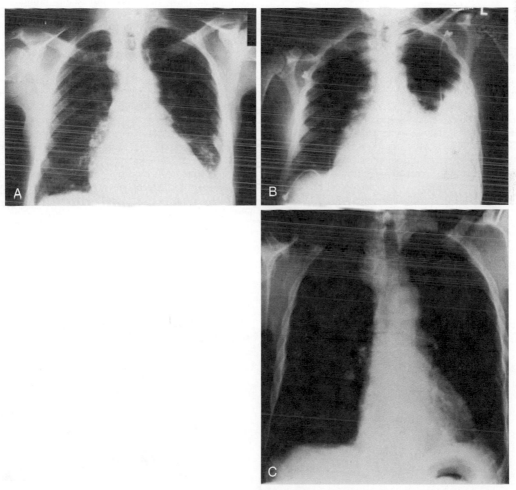

Figure 53-7   Posteroanterior chest radiographs. A. At admission, showing enlarged cardiac silhouette. B. At 24 hours after percutaneous balloon pericardiotomy, a new left pleural effusion is seen. C. One month later, complete resolution of the left pleural effusion is apparent. *(From Palacios IF, Tuzcu EM, Ziskind AA, et al. Percutaneous balloon pericardial window for patients with malignant pericardial effusion and tamponade. Catheter Cardiovasc Diagn. 1991;22:244–249.)*

however, in many cases it is difficult to determine whether the effusion results from drainage of fluid from the pericardial space or from the progression of concomitant pleural disease. For this reason it is desirable to remove most of the pericardial fluid before creating the PBP window so as to limit the potential volume of fluid that can immediately move to the pleural space.

Duration of Catheter Placement

Most patients have had a drainage catheter left in the pericardial space to monitor fluid output after the procedure. This is typically removed when pericardial drainage is ≤75 to 100 mL/24 hr. It may be possible to perform PBP without leaving a pericardial catheter in place, thus permitting an even shorter hospital stay and further decreasing the risk of infection.

Management of Balloon Rupture

Balloon rupture at the time of PBP can occur as a result of the combination of a large balloon, excessive inflation pressure, and an inelastic pericardium. Uncommonly, balloon rupture may be accompanied by catheter fracture because excessive resistance limits withdrawal. Our experience suggests that the frequency of balloon rupture can be minimized with proper technique, particularly the use of countertraction to isolate the pericardium, thereby avoiding dilation of the adjacent nonpericardial tissues.[26] Hemiballoon dislodgement sometimes occurs, and Block and Wilson have described a technique to retrieve it by placing a second pericardial catheter, snaring the guidewire, and using a second catheter to pull the balloon fragment back.[44]

Adjunctive Diagnostic Approaches

Although patients with pericardial effusion may have a history of malignancy, in only 50% of such patients is malignancy the cause of the effusion.[1,4] Although cytological analysis of the pericardial fluid may aid in the diagnosis, pericardial tissue is not routinely obtained by PBP for pathological analysis (as is the case during a surgical pericardial window procedure). To address this need, a percutaneously introduced pericardial bioptome has been successful in providing diagnostic-quality tissue.[25] With the use of an aggressive serrated-jaw bioptome (Boston Scientific, Natick, MA) (Fig. 53-8A) that is advanced though an 8-Fr vascular introducer, multiple samples can be obtained from the posterolateral aspect of the parietal pericardium (Fig. 53-8B). This technique remains investigational.

PERCUTANEOUS BALLOON PERICARDIOTOMY: SUMMARY

PBP offers a nonsurgical alternative for the management of pericardial effusion. PBP is particularly useful for critically ill patients with advanced malignancy and limited survival in whom it is desirable to avoid the risks and discomfort of anesthesia and surgery. For such patients, PBP appears to palliate malignant pericardial disease successfully for the duration of their survival. The decision to perform PBP, rather than pericardiocentesis with or without sclerotherapy, may depend on patient and institutional variables. PBP should be considered if pericardial fluid recurs after primary pericardiocentesis. In institutions with an aggressive surgical approach toward malignant pericardial disease, this "less invasive" alternative to a surgical pericardial window may be considered for the primary treatment of malignant cardiac tamponade. In contrast, pericardiocentesis alone, without PBP at that time, is preferred if the cause of the pericardial fluid is unknown. Samples of pericardial fluid should be sent for cell counts, cytological analysis, culture, and special stains to assist with the diagnosis. Simple pericardiocentesis is also preferred if uremic platelet dysfunction or other coagulation abnormalities are present or if there is the possibility of bacterial or fungal infection that could be spread to the pleural space. The immediate and late results of PBP for patients with malignant pericardial effusion appear to be similar to those of surgical pericardiotomy. The role of PBP in the management of nonmalignant pericardial disease remains, however, unclear. It is possible that PBP could be used for the treatment of pericardial effusions caused by viral infection, human immunodeficiency virus (HIV)-related disease, hypothyroidism, collagen vascular disease, and idiopathic effusions. PBP was reported with favorable results in a series of pediatric patients with nonmalignant effusions.[45] Additional long-term follow-up is needed on larger numbers of patients to clarify more fully the role of this procedure in nonmalignant pericardial disease. The application of PBP to patients with malignant pericardial disease is likely to increase in the future. It may potentially expand to the treatment of patients without malignancy,[45] especially those with limited survival time (e.g., advanced HIV infection). PBP procedures need not be limited to tertiary care hospitals, although they should be performed in centers that routinely perform pericardiocentesis procedures. The infrequency of effusive pericardial disease and the larger number of patients required limit the feasibility of randomized studies to compare the effectiveness of various treatment strategies. Vaitkus

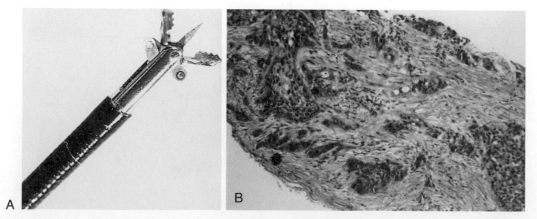

Figure 53-8   A. Pericardial bioptome with center needle and aggressive serrated-jaw configuration. B. Percutaneous pericardial biopsy specimen from a patient with newly diagnosed lung cancer. It contains sheets of squamous cell carcinoma. Malignant cells are seen trapped in the fibrin of the inflammatory exudate. (*From Ziskind AA, Rodriguez S, Lemmon C, Burstein S. Percutaneous pericardial biopsy as an adjunctive technique for the diagnosis of pericardial disease. Am J Cardiol. 1994;74:288–291.*)

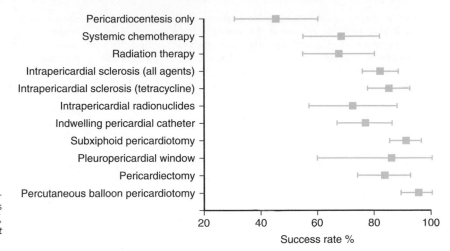

Figure 53-9 Success rates with 95% confidence intervals (indicated by bars) for various treatment modalities of malignant pericardial effusions. *(From Vaitkus PT, Herrmann HC, Le Winter MM. Treatment of malignant pericardial effusion. JAMA. 1994;272:272.)*

and colleagues performed a metanalysis of prior studies in which treatment of malignant pericardial effusions was defined as successful if the patient survived the procedure, the symptoms did not recur, and no other interventions directed at the pericardium were required regardless of the length of survival.[46] Success rates for the various treatments are shown in Figure 53-9. Because no randomized data are available comparing the efficacy of PBP with that of a surgical or thoracoscopic pericardial window or with catheter drainage and sclerotherapy, the combined use of PBP with sclerotherapy has not been done.

Novel Catheter-Based Intervention Techniques in the Pericardial Space

The use of percutaneous intervention techniques in the pericardial space has been progressively increasing and now encompasses multiple disciplines in cardiology. Many reasons contributed to the emergence of these techniques. On one hand, epicardial catheter mapping and ablation in the electrophysiology laboratory have opened a new horizon in cardiac electrophysiology, which was previously limited largely to the operating room. On the other hand, the pericardial space is recognized as a natural drug receptacle that can restrict drug delivery to the heart, with many investigators attempting to exploit it as a reservoir to deliver therapeutic substances.[47] In addition, there has been increasing need to replace the standard pericardiocentesis procedure with a safer technique, particularly in patients with small pericardial effusions who are at high risk for complications.

EPICARDIAL MAPPING AND ABLATION

Epicardial scar-related reentry has been recognized as an important cause of ventricular tachycardia, especially in patients with nonischemic cardiomyopathy. Other infrequent but clinically significant arrhythmias, such as supraventricular tachycardias and idiopathic ventricular tachycardia, were also found to possess epicardial foci that cannot be ablated but from the epicardium. Catheter-based intervention techniques in the pericardial space gained momentum after invasive cardiologists realized that the presence of pericardial fluid is not a prerequisite for a safe percutaneous entry into the pericardial space. Sosa and colleagues[48] were the first to show that the pericardial space can be safely entered with a blunt-tipped needle via a subxiphoid approach under fluoroscopic guidance. In their seminal work in 1996 in patients with Chagas' disease,[48] they advanced an epidural needle toward the right ventricular apex until a slight negative pressure was felt and confirmed the needle position by small injections of contrast medium to delineate the cardiac silhouette. They thus established the feasibility and safety of epicardial mapping in patients with Chagas'

disease and recurrent ventricular tachycardia, one of whom underwent a successful epicardial circuit ablation.[48] Epicardial mapping and ablation were subsequently adopted by several interventional electrophysiologists.[49] Sosa and colleagues[50] performed epicardial mapping to guide endocardial and epicardial ablation in a series of 10 consecutive patients with ventricular tachycardia and Chagas' disease. Epicardial mapping in that study enabled the detection of an epicardial circuit in 14 of 18 mappable ventricular tachycardias and helped guide endocardial ablation in 4 patients and epicardial ablation in 6. The same approach was also attempted successfully in patients with recurrent ventricular tachycardia after myocardial infarction, demonstrating that postinfarction pericardial adherence does not preclude epicardial mapping and ablation.[51] It has since become clear that failure of endocardial ablation can reflect the presence of an epicardial arrhythmic substrate, which can be safely treated by epicardial mapping and ablation using the percutaneous pericardial technique. In one series of 48 patients with prior unsuccessful endocardial ablation, for example, Schweikert et al.[52] showed that epicardial instrumentation and ablation was a safe and effective alternative strategy.

Laham and colleagues[53] subsequently confirmed the safety of subxiphoid access of the normal pericardium in a large animal model, using, in addition to fluoroscopy, continuous positive pressure of 20 to 30 mm Hg (achieved by saline infusion using an intraflow system) to push the right ventricle away from the needle's path. Access of the pericardial space was achieved in all 49 Yorkshire pigs with no adverse events, and histological examination in 15 animals 1 month after the procedure showed no evidence of myocardial damage.[53] Many invasive cardiologists argue that needle advancement under continuous positive pressure by saline infusion may not be necessary for a successful technique. In addition to the subxiphoid approach for pericardial puncture (i.e., from the epicardial surface of the heart), other investigational approaches have been studied. Mickelsen and colleagues examined transvenous access to the pericardial space for epicardial lead implantation for cardiac resynchronization therapy.[54] This approach was feasible in 8 pigs, which underwent puncture of the terminal anterior superior vena cava or the right atrial appendage to access the pericardial space; however, it resulted in a hemodynamically significant pericardial effusion in 4 of the 8 animals.[54]

INTRAPERICARDIAL ECHOCARDIOGRAPHY

Intrapericardial echocardiography is currently being investigated at the Massachusetts General Hospital[55] and represents yet another example of a promising catheter-based technique in the pericardial space. Rodrigues and coworkers[55] introduced phased-array ultrasound transducers into the pericardial space of 7 goats (using 10-Fr steerable catheters advanced via the transthoracic subxiphoid approach) and obtained detailed imaging of cardiac structures. This promising approach may help establish the relative positions of the ablation catheters and may facilitate epicardial ablation in the electrophysiology laboratory. Several devices are currently under study for safe and effective percutaneous access of the pericardial space. An example is the PerDUCER (Comedicus Inc., Columbia Heights, MN), which was proven to provide efficient, safe, and effective pericardial access in the normal or minimally abnormal pericardial space.[56,57]

PERCUTANEOUS PERICARDIAL BIOPSY

Percutaneous pericardial biopsy (PPB) was described in 1988 by Endrys and colleagues,[58] who reported a series of 18 patients undergoing pericardial biopsy using an endomyocardial bioptome inserted through an 8-Fr 4 0-cm Teflon sheath with a curved tip and multiple side holes.[58] Endrys and colleagues allowed air to enter the pericardium to delineate the visceral and parietal pericardial layers and obtained an average of 8 samples per patient with no complications; they therefore showed that PPB can be safely performed using conventional invasive cardiology techniques.[58] As the floppy nature of the bioptome made it difficult to direct it to the appropriate site in the pericardial cavity, a modified technique using the distal portion of a 9-Fr right Judkins coronary guiding catheter was adopted to target pericardial biopsy sites.[59] Ziskind and colleagues subsequently used a special pericardial bioptome with a central needle and serrated jaws to perform pericardial biopsy.[25] They also maintained separation of the visceral-pericardial layer by avoiding complete evacuation of pericardial fluid at the beginning of the procedure and therefore avoided instilling air into the pericardial cavity.[25] Selig and colleagues described a modified PPB technique using echocardiographic guidance without fluoroscopy.[60] Furthermore, Palacios and colleagues have reported their case series of 7 patients with pericardial effusion undergoing PPB.[61] Following complete drainage of the pericardial fluid under fluoroscopic and ECG guidance and using the subxiphoid approach, Palacios and colleagues exchanged the 5-Fr drainage pigtail for an 8-Fr 23-cm Arrow braided sheath and subsequently passed a 7-Fr BiPal biopsy forceps (Cordis, Johnson and Johnson, Bridgewater, NJ) through the sheath and away from the cardiac shadow to the lateral pericardial wall (Fig. 53-10). They obtained a total of five biopsy specimens per patient with no complications and demonstrated that pericardial biopsy adds incremental diagnostic value to the analysis of pericardial fluid alone. In their case series, PPB confirmed the absence of malignant invasion in 4 patients with neoplastic disease as well as the presence of lymphocytic and organizing effusive pericarditis in 1 and 2 patients, respectively.[61] In summary, the PPB technique is safe and feasible in the cardiac catheterization laboratory. It is less invasive than surgical biopsy, can be easily modified to obtain tissue samples from pericardial masses, and has also been shown to increase the diagnostic yield of pericardiocentesis and pericardial fluid analysis. For example, one clinical scenario where PPB may prove to be of particular importance is in the setting of tuberculous pericardial effusion, because *Mycobacterium tuberculosis* is rarely cultured and a positive acid-fast stain is infrequently obtained from the pericardial fluid (which makes tuberculosis, unlike malignant pericarditis, a commonly missed diagnosis without the technique of PPB).

PERICARDIOSCOPY

Seferovic and associates[62] reported their experience on the use of pericardioscopy to assist pericardial biopsy and demonstrated the diagnostic value of pericardial biopsy to be significantly improved by pericardioscopy-guided extensive sampling. Their study included 49 patients with large pericardial effusions undergoing parietal pericardial biopsy. In 12 patients (group 1), pericardial biopsy was guided by fluoroscopy (three to six samples per patient). In 22 patients (group 2), four to six pericardial biopsies per patient were obtained by pericardioscopic guidance using a 16-Fr flexible endoscope. In group 3, extensive pericardial sampling (18 to 20 samples per patient) was performed, guided by pericardioscopy in 15 patients. Sampling efficiency was better with pericardioscopy (group 2, 84.9%; group 3, 84.2%) compared with fluoroscopic guidance (group 1, 43.7%; $P < 0.01$). Pericardial biopsy in group 3 had higher diagnostic value than in group 1 for revealing a new diagnosis (40% vs. 8.3%, $P < 0.05$) or establishing the etiology (53.3% vs. 8.3%, $P < 0.05$). In group 2, pericardial biopsy had a higher yield in establishing etiology than in group 1 (40.9% vs. 8.3%; $P < 0.05$). No major complications were observed in their study.

▣ Other Pericardial Interventions

Adequate visualization of the space and the epicardial surface allows identification of scarred areas in the ventricles that can be treated by intramyocardial administration of vascular growth factors and/or cultured myocardial cells. Furthermore, techniques such as exclusion of the left atrial appendage can be attempted using this approach and imaging. We also anticipate the use of this space for successful percutaneous treatment of valvular heart disease, alone or in combination with endovascular techniques.

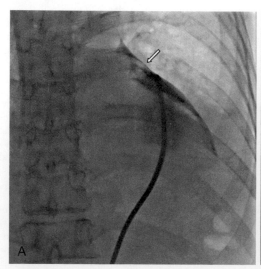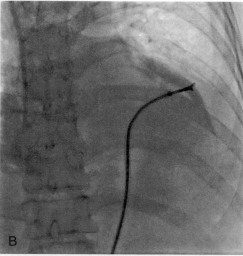

Figure 53-10   A. Contrast injection through an Arrow braided sheath confirms intrapericardial location; B. A biopsy is obtained through a 7-Fr BiPal catheter passed through the sheath and away from the cardiac shadow into the lateral pericardial wall.

REFERENCES

1. Jneid H, Maree AO, Palacios IF: Pericardial tamponade: clinical presentation, diagnosis and catheter-based therapies. In Parillo J, Dellinger PR, editors: *Critical Care Medicine*, ed 3, St. Louis, 2008, Mosby.
2. Guberman BA, Fowler NO, Engel PJ, et al: Cardiac tamponade in medical patients. *Circulation* 64(3):633–640, 1981.
3. Jneid H, Maree AO, Palacios IF: Acute pericardial disease: pericardiocentesis and percutaneous pericardiotomy. In Mebazaa A GM, Zannad FM, Parillo J, editors: *Acute Heart Failure*, London, 2008, Springer.
4. Mills SA, Julian S, Holliday RH, et al: Subxiphoid pericardial window for pericardial effusive disease. *J Cardiovasc Surg (Torino)* 30(5):768–773, 1989.
5. Markiewicz W, Borovik R, Ecker S: Cardiac tamponade in medical patients: treatment and prognosis in the echocardiographic era. *Am Heart J* 111(6):1138–1142, 1986.
6. Bisel HF, Wroblewski F, Ladue JS: Incidence and clinical manifestations of cardiac metastases. *JAMA* 153(8):712–715, 1953.
7. Goldman BS, Pearson FG: Malignant pericardial effusion. Review of hospital experience and report of a case successfully treated by talc poudrage. *Can J Surg* 8:157–161, 1965.
8. Piehler JM, Pluth JR, Schaff HV, et al: Surgical management of effusive pericardial disease. Influence of extent of pericardial resection on clinical course. *J Thorac Cardiovasc Surg* 90(4):506–516, 1985.
9. Sagrista-Sauleda J, Angel J, Permanyer-Miralda G, et al: Long-term follow-up of idiopathic chronic pericardial effusion. *N Engl J Med* 341(27):2054–2059, 1999.
10. Tsang TS, Enriquez-Sarano M, Freeman WK, et al: Consecutive 1127 therapeutic echocardiographically guided pericardiocenteses: clinical profile, practice patterns, and outcomes spanning 21 years. *Mayo Clin Proc* 77(5):429–436, 2002.
11. Flannery EP, Gregoratos G, Corder MP: Pericardial effusions in patients with malignant diseases. *Arch Intern Med* 135(7):976–977, 1975.
12. Kopecky SL, Callahan JA, Tajik AJ, et al: Percutaneous pericardial catheter drainage: report of 42 consecutive cases. *Am J Cardiol* 58(7):633–635, 1986.
13. Patel AK, Kosolcharoen PK, Nallasivan M, et al: Catheter drainage of the pericardium. Practical method to maintain long-term patency. *Chest* 92(6):1018–1021, 1987.
14. Shepherd FA, Morgan C, Evans WK, et al: Medical management of malignant pericardial effusion by tetracycline sclerosis. *Am J Cardiol* 60(14):1161–1166, 1987.
15. Davis S, Sharma SM, Blumberg ED, et al: Intrapericardial tetracycline for the management of cardiac tamponade secondary to malignant pericardial effusion. *N Engl J Med* 299(20):1113–1114, 1978.
16. Fontenelle LJ, Cuello L, Dooley BN: Subxiphoid pericardial window. A simple and safe method for diagnosing and treating acute and chronic pericardial effusions. *J Thorac Cardiovasc Surg* 62(1):95–97, 1971.
17. Santos GH, Frater RW: The subxiphoid approach in the treatment of pericardial effusion. *Ann Thorac Surg* 23(5):467–470, 1977.
18. Palatianos GM, Thurer RJ, Kaiser GA: Comparison of effectiveness and safety of operations on the pericardium. *Chest* 88(1):30–33, 1985.
19. Palatianos GM, Thurer RJ, Pompeo MQ, et al: Clinical experience with subxiphoid drainage of pericardial effusions. *Ann Thorac Surg* 48(3):381–385, 1989.
20. Hankins JR, Satterfield JR, Aisner J, et al: Pericardial window for malignant pericardial effusion. *Ann Thorac Surg* 30(5):465–471, 1980.
21. Levin BH, Aaron BL: The subxiphoid pericardial window. *Surg Gynecol Obstet* 155(6):804–806, 1982.

22. Alcan KE, Zabetakis PM, Marino ND, et al: Management of acute cardiac tamponade by subxiphoid pericardiotomy. *JAMA* 247(8):1143–1148, 1982.
23. Little AG, Kremser PC, Wade JL, et al: Operation for diagnosis and treatment of pericardial effusions. *Surgery* 96(4):738–744, 1984.
24. Palacios IF, Tuzcu EM, Ziskind AA, et al: Percutaneous balloon pericardial window for patients with malignant pericardial effusion and tamponade. *Cathet Cardiovasc Diagn* 22(4):244–249, 1991.
25. Ziskind AA, Rodriguez S, Lemmon C, et al: Percutaneous pericardial biopsy as an adjunctive technique for the diagnosis of pericardial disease. *Am J Cardiol* 74(3):288–291, 1994.
26. Ziskind AA, Burstein S: Echocardiography vs. fluoroscopic imaging. *Cathet Cardiovasc Diagn* 27(1):86–87, 1992.
27. Chow WH, Chow TC, Cheung KL: Nonsurgical creation of a pericardial window using the Inoue balloon catheter. *Am Heart J* 124(4):1100–1102, 1992.
28. Chow WH, Chow TC, Yip AS, et al: Inoue balloon pericardiotomy for patients with recurrent pericardial effusion. *Angiology* 47(1):57–60, 1996.
29. Ohke M, Bessho A, Haraoka K, et al: Percutaneous balloon pericardiotomy by use of Inoue balloon for the management of recurrent cardiac tamponade in a patient with lung cancer. *Intern Med* 39(12):1071–1074, 2000.
30. Iaffaldano RA, Jones P, Lewis BE, et al: Percutaneous balloon pericardiotomy: a double-balloon technique. *Catheter Cardiovasc Diagn* 36(1):79–81, 1995.
31. Hsu KL, Tsai CH, Chiang FT, et al: Percutaneous balloon pericardiotomy for patients with recurrent pericardial effusion: using a novel double-balloon technique with one long and one short balloon. *Am J Cardiol* 80(12):1635–1637, 1997.
32. Hajduczok ZD, Ferguson DW: Percutaneous balloon pericardiostomy for non-surgical management of recurrent pericardial tamponade: a case report. *Intens Care Med* 17(5):299–301, 1991.
33. Ready A, Black J, Lewis R, et al: Laparoscopic pericardial fenestration for malignant pericardial effusion. *Lancet* 339(8809):1609, 1992.
34. Hartnell GG: Laparoscopic pericardial fenestration. *Lancet* 340(8821):737, 1992.
35. Sochman J, Peregrin J, Pavenik D: The cutting pericardiotome: another option for pericardiopleural draining in recurrent pericardial effusion. Initial experience. *Int J Cardiol* 77(1):69–74, 2001.
36. Wang K, Fulton JR, Mogensen T, et al: Pericardioperitoneal shunt: an alternative treatment for malignant pericardial effusion. *Ann Thorac Surg* 57(2):289–292, 1994.
37. Ozuner G, Davidson PG, Isenberg JS, et al: Creation of a pericardial window using thoracoscopic techniques. *Surg Gynecol Obstet* 175(1):69–71, 1992.
38. Krasna MJ, Fiocco M: Thoracoscopic pericardiectomy. *Surg Laparosc Endosc* 5(3):202–204, 1995.
39. Bertrand O, Legrand V, Kulbertus H: Percutaneous balloon pericardiotomy: a case report and analysis of mechanism of action. *Catheter Cardiovasc Diagn* 38(2):180–182, 1996.
40. Block PC: Whither pericardial fluid? *Catheter Cardiovasc Diagn* 38(2):183, 1996.
41. Ziskind AA, Pearce AC, Lemmon CC, et al: Percutaneous balloon pericardiotomy for the treatment of cardiac tamponade and large pericardial effusions: description of technique and report of the first 50 cases. *J Am Coll Cardiol* 21(1):1–5, 1993.
42. Chow LT, Chow WH: Mechanism of pericardial window creation by balloon pericardiotomy. *Am J Cardiol* 72(17):1321–1322, 1993.
43. Sugimoto JT, Little AG, Ferguson MK, et al: Pericardial window: mechanisms of efficacy. *Ann Thorac Surg* 50(3):442–445, 1990.

44. Block PC, Wilson MA: Hemi-balloon dislodgement during a percutaneous balloon pericardial window procedure: removal using a second pericardial catheter. *Catheter Cardiovasc Diagn* 29(4):289–291, 1993.
45. Thanopoulos BD, Georgakopoulos D, Tsaousis GS, et al: Percutaneous balloon pericardiotomy for the treatment of large, nonmalignant pericardial effusions in children: immediate and medium-term results. *Catheter Cardiovasc Diagn* 40(1):97–100, 1997.
46. Vaitkus PT, Herrmann HC, LeWinter MM: Treatment of malignant pericardial effusion. *JAMA* 272(1):59–64, 1994.
47. Stoll HP, Carlson K, Keefer LK, et al: Pharmacokinetics and consistency of pericardial delivery directed to coronary arteries: direct comparison with endoluminal delivery. *Clin Cardiol* 22(1 Suppl 1):I10–I16, 1999.
48. Sosa E, Scanavacca M, D'Avila A, et al: A new technique to perform epicardial mapping in the electrophysiology laboratory. *J Cardiovasc Electrophysiol* 7(6):531–536, 1996.
49. Strickberger SA: Pericardial space exploration for ventricular tachycardia mapping: should the countdown begin? *J Cardiovasc Electrophysiol* 7(6):537–538, 1996.
50. Sosa E, Scanavacca M, D'Avila A, et al: Endocardial and epicardial ablation guided by nonsurgical transthoracic epicardial mapping to treat recurrent ventricular tachycardia. *J Cardiovasc Electrophysiol* 9(3):229–239, 1998.
51. Sosa E, Scanavacca M, d'Avila A, et al: Nonsurgical transthoracic epicardial catheter ablation to treat recurrent ventricular tachycardia occurring late after myocardial infarction. *J Am Coll Cardiol* 35(6):1442–1449, 2000.
52. Schweikert RA, Saliba WI, Tomassoni G, et al: Percutaneous pericardial instrumentation for endo-epicardial mapping of previously failed ablations. *Circulation* 108(11):1329–1335, 2003.
53. Laham RJ, Simons M, Hung D: Subxyphoid access of the normal pericardium: a novel drug delivery technique. *Catheter Cardiovasc Intervent* 47(1):109–111, 1999.
54. Mickelsen SR, Ashikaga H, DeSilva R, et al: Transvenous access to the pericardial space: an approach to epicardial lead implantation for cardiac resynchronization therapy. *Pacing Clin Electrophysiol* 28(10):1018–1024, 2005.
55. Rodrigues AC, d'Avila A, Houghtaling C, et al: Intrapericardial echocardiography: a novel catheter-based approach to cardiac imaging. *J Am Soc Echocardiogr* 17(3):269–274, 2004.
56. Macris MP, Igo SR: Minimally invasive access of the normal pericardium: initial clinical experience with a novel device. *Clin Cardiol* 22(1 Suppl 1):I36–I39, 1999.
57. Hou D, March KL: A novel percutaneous technique for accessing the normal pericardium: a single-center successful experience of 53 porcine procedures. *J Invas Cardiol* 15(1):13–17, 2003.
58. Endrys J, Simo M, Shafie MZ, et al: New nonsurgical technique for multiple pericardial biopsies. *Catheter Cardiovasc Diagn* 15(2):92–94, 1988.
59. Mehan VK, Dalvi BV, Lokhandwala YY, et al: Use of guiding catheters to target pericardial and endomyocardial biopsy sites. *Am Heart J* 122(3 Pt 1):882–883, 1991.
60. Selig MB: Percutaneous pericardial biopsy under echocardiographic guidance. *Am Heart J* 122(3 Pt 1):879–882, 1991.
61. Margey R, Suh W, Witzke C, et al: Percutaneous pericardial biopsy, a novel interventional technique to aid diagnosis and management of pericardial disease. Paper presented at Transcatheter Cardiovascular Therapeutics (TCT) 2010; September 2010; Washington DC.
62. Seferovic PM, Ristic AD, Maksimovic R, et al: Diagnostic value of pericardial biopsy: improvement with extensive sampling enabled by pericardioscopy. *Circulation* 107(7):978–983, 2003.

54

Transcatheter Therapies for Congenital Heart Disease

ROBERT H. BEEKMAN III | RUSSEL HIRSCH |
MATTHEW ZUSSMAN | THOMAS R. LLOYD

KEY POINTS

- Catheter-based therapies are available for a wide variety of congenital cardiovascular defects.

- Balloon dilation provides effective relief of obstruction for patients with congenital pulmonary or aortic valve stenosis. This therapy may not be adequate if the valve is hypoplastic or calcified.

- Congenital pulmonary artery stenosis can be very effectively relieved with balloon-expandable stents; late stent redilation may be necessary in a growing child.

- Coarctation of the aorta can be treated with balloon-expandable stenting; covered stents may provide important safety for older patients with a fragile aorta.

- Transcatheter occlusion devices are available to safely and effectively treat patients with a secundum type arterial septal defect or a patent ductus arteriosus.

- Transcatheter pulmonary valve replacement is now routine in patients with a failing right ventricle to pulmonary artery conduit, as in tetralogy of Fallot.

Introduction

This chapter summarizes the current state of the art of transcatheter therapy for congenital heart disease. It discusses catheter-based therapies available for some of the more common congenital defects, including semilunar valve stenosis, pulmonary artery stenosis, coarctation of the aorta, secundum atrial septal defect, and patent ductus arteriosus. The much newer development of transcatheter pulmonary valve replacement is also reviewed. Percutaneous balloon valvuloplasty provides effective treatment in patients with congenital pulmonary or aortic valve stenosis. For patients of all ages, surgical valvotomy for congenital semilunar valve stenosis has been replaced by these interventional catheterization techniques. Balloon-expandable stenting is currently regarded as standard therapy for most patients with pulmonary artery stenosis. These lesions are often elastic in nature—a characteristic that makes balloon angioplasty alone a less successful intervention. Coarctation stenting is recognized as an effective therapeutic intervention for selected patients with coarctation of the aorta. Transcatheter occlusion devices provide a safe, highly effective therapy for patients with a secundum atrial septal defect or a patent ductus arteriosus and constitute the treatment of choice for these defects. Last, transcatheter pulmonary valve replacement is now available for select patients with a failing right-ventricle-to-pulmonary-artery (RV-PA) conduit; this remarkable new intervention can replace reoperation and is therefore an important new option for many patients.

Pulmonary Balloon Valvuloplasty

Pulmonary valve stenosis is a common disorder, accounting for approximately 8% of all congenital heart disease.[1] Except for neonates with critical pulmonary stenosis, untreated patients often survive well into adulthood.[2] However, when more than mild obstruction to right ventricular outflow is present, pulmonary valve stenosis should be relieved to prevent progression of obstruction,[3] progressive right ventricular hypertrophy, and right ventricular myocardial fibrosis and dysfunction. If left untreated, significant pulmonary valve stenosis eventually produces clinical symptoms such as fatigue, dyspnea, and exercise intolerance. These long-term sequelae are more likely to be avoided if pulmonary valve stenosis is treated in childhood. Nevertheless, treatment is indicated at any age if hemodynamically significant pulmonary stenosis is documented. Since its introduction in 1982 by Kan et al.,[4] percutaneous balloon valvuloplasty has been shown to provide substantial relief of right ventricular outflow tract (RVOT) obstruction in patients with valvar pulmonary stenosis. Balloon pulmonary valvuloplasty can be performed safely and is obviously much less invasive than a surgical procedure. It is therefore regarded as the treatment of choice for patients with moderate to severe isolated pulmonary valve stenosis. In congenital pulmonary valve stenosis, the valve leaflets are thickened and the commissures fused to varying degree. The lines of commissural fusion may appear as two or three raphes extending from the valve annulus to a small central orifice.[5] During childhood and young adulthood, the pulmonary valve leaflets are typically supple, doming upward during systole (Fig. 54-1). In older adults, pulmonary valve calcification may occur and may lead to diminished leaflet mobility. A much less common form of pulmonary stenosis has been referred to as "pulmonary valve dysplasia."[5,6] It often occurs as a familial trait or as part of Noonan's syndrome. A dysplastic pulmonary valve is characterized by thick, cartilaginous valve leaflets with poor mobility (Fig. 54-2). The pulmonary valve annulus is often hypoplastic, and there may be little or no commissural fusion. In isolated pulmonary valve stenosis, balloon dilation reduces the degree of valvar obstruction by separating fused commissures or by tearing the valve leaflets themselves.[7,8] Patients with severe pulmonary valve dysplasia with marked hypoplasia of the annulus and absence of commissural fusion may have minimal improvement after balloon valvuloplasty.[9] However, because a spectrum of pulmonary valve dysplasia exists, some patients with this disorder may derive substantial benefit from the balloon valvuloplasty procedure.[10]

TECHNIQUE

Balloon pulmonary valvuloplasty is technically less challenging than balloon mitral or aortic valvuloplasty procedures. It is performed entirely transvenously and without the need for a transseptal left heart catheterization. The procedure also differs from aortic valvuloplasty in that the use of an oversized balloon, approximately 25% larger than the valve annulus diameter, is required for the most effective relief of obstruction. In general, we believe that pulmonary valvuloplasty is indicated for isolated pulmonary valve stenosis if the resting peak systolic pressure gradient exceeds 40 mm Hg in the presence of a normal cardiac output. In an infant with critical pulmonary stenosis, a right-to-left atrial shunt, and a patent ductus arteriosus, valvuloplasty is indicated even though the measured transvalvar gradient may be less than 40 mm Hg. Balloon pulmonary valvuloplasty is usually performed using a percutaneous transfemoral approach. Right heart catheterization documents the severity of the lesion. Right ventricular angiocardiography is performed to confirm the nature of the lesion and measure the diameter of the pulmonary valve annulus. Typically, the lateral projection is best suited to this purpose. Once the decision is made to proceed with valvuloplasty, an end-hole catheter is advanced to the left pulmonary artery. The left pulmonary artery provides better

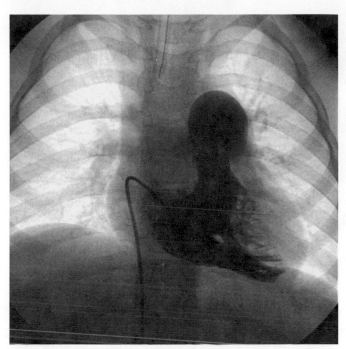

Figure 54-1 Lateral RV angiogram in a child with congenital pulmonary valve stenosis. The valve is thickened and domes in systole. There is poststenotic dilation of the main pulmonary artery.

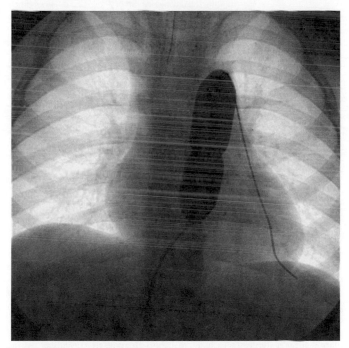

Figure 54-2 Lateral RV angiogram in an infant with severe pulmonary valve stenosis. The valve is thickened and dysplastic, and there is considerable myocardial hypertrophy evident.

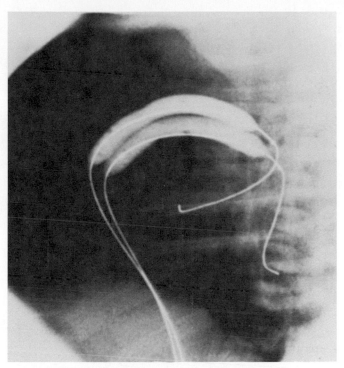

Figure 54-3 Lateral view during pulmonary balloon valvuloplasty in the same infant whose valve is demonstrated in Figure 54-2. The dilation balloon is inflated across the valve, and the impression of the valve annulus is clearly evident near the middle of the balloon.

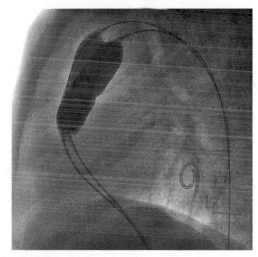

Figure 54-4 Double-balloon pulmonary valve dilation in a child with pulmonary valve stenosis. Two balloons may be used if a single balloon catheter requires a sheath thought too large for a child's femoral vein.

wire and balloon stability than a right pulmonary artery position. An exchange-length guidewire is advanced to the distal left pulmonary artery and the end-hole catheter is removed. The balloon valvuloplasty catheter is then inserted over the exchange wire. A balloon valvuloplasty catheter is used whose inflated balloon diameter is approximately 15% to 25% larger than the pulmonary valve annulus diameter (Fig. 54-3). Balloon oversizing improves valvuloplasty effectiveness, and injury to the pulmonary valve annulus is unlikely when balloons smaller than 140% of the annulus's diameter are used.[11,12] If the

pulmonary valve annulus exceeds 20 mm or if the single balloon catheter required is too large for safe introduction into a patient's femoral vein (Fig. 54-4), we recommend a double-balloon technique, with two balloons positioned across the valve and inflated simultaneously. The effective dilating diameter of two equal-sized balloons can be calculated based on cross-sectional area or on circumference. The sum of the balloon diameters by the circumference and area methods is 120% and 130% of the equivalent single–balloon diameters, respectively. Thus the operator first selects the optimal single-balloon size, multiplies this diameter by 1.2 or 1.3, and then selects two balloons whose diameters are half of that product. Once inserted, the balloon valvuloplasty catheter is advanced across the valve and positioned with the valve at the midportion of the balloon. Partial balloon inflation, with

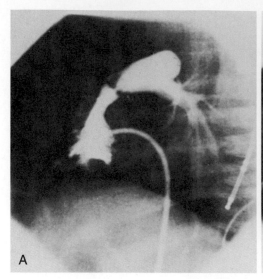
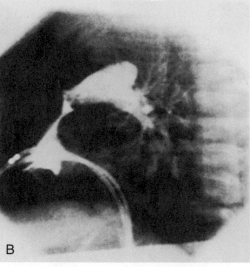

Figure 54-5 Lateral right ventricular angiogram before (A) and immediately after (B) valvuloplasty in an infant with pulmonary stenosis. There is marked systolic narrowing of the right ventricular infundibulum after valvuloplasty that was not present before the procedure. Such dynamic infundibular narrowing may account for some residual gradient that may be measured immediately after the procedure and typically improves with time.

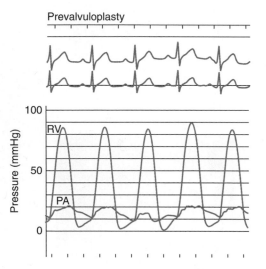
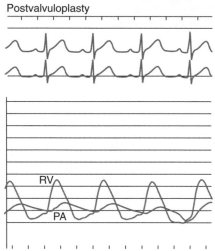

Figure 54-6 Simultaneous right ventricular and pulmonary artery pressure recordings before and immediately after pulmonary valve dilation in a 15-month-old boy with severe pulmonary stenosis. The right ventricular systolic pressure was reduced from 86 mm Hg to 36 mm Hg. The pulmonary valve systolic gradient decreased from 66 mm Hg to 20 mm Hg (pressure recordings were made on the same scale).

a mixture of saline and contrast, is helpful to determine the precise location of the valve on the balloon. The valvuloplasty balloon (or balloons) is then inflated by hand until the waist produced by the valve on the balloon disappears. The period of balloon inflation is kept as brief as possible to minimize the obstruction to right ventricular outflow. Typically three or four balloon inflations are performed with minor adjustments in balloon position to ensure adequate dilation of the pulmonary valve. After the dilation is completed, the valvuloplasty catheter is withdrawn and replaced with a diagnostic catheter. The residual RVOT gradient and cardiac output are measured to document the effectiveness of the procedure. A repeat right ventricular angiogram may be performed if necessary to document the degree of subvalvar infundibular narrowing (which may be increased immediately after valvuloplasty) present at this point (Fig. 54-5).

ACUTE RESULTS

In patients with isolated pulmonary valve stenosis, percutaneous balloon valvuloplasty can be expected to provide excellent relief of RVOT obstruction (Fig. 54-6). Numerous studies have clearly documented significant acute reduction in the peak systolic pulmonary valve gradient to 30 mm Hg or less (i.e., mild residual stenosis). In their landmark article, Kan and colleagues reported the acute effects of valvuloplasty in an 8-year-old child with pulmonary stenosis.[4] The

procedure decreased the peak transvalvar gradient from 48 to 14 mm Hg and was performed without significant complications. Other studies have subsequently confirmed Kan and associates' initial observation that valvuloplasty provides impressive gradient relief acutely.[11,13–19] The largest published clinical series of balloon pulmonary valvuloplasty was reported by the Pediatric Valvuloplasty Registry.[13] This registry reported the acute results of pulmonary valvuloplasty performed in 784 patients between 1981 and 1986. Overall, balloon dilation resulted in an acute decrease in the peak systolic pressure gradient from 71 to 28 mm Hg. The residual pressure gradients immediately after valvuloplasty were ascribed in part to subvalvar infundibular obstruction related to right ventricular hypertrophy. Effectiveness of the procedure was not related to age (the series included 35 adults older than age 21 years), but a larger residual gradient was observed in patients with a dysplastic pulmonary valve. The Pediatric Valvuloplasty Registry described five major complications (0.6%), primarily confined to infancy. There were two procedure-related deaths (0.2%) in 2 infants and 1 neonate in whom RVOT perforation and tamponade occurred. In 2 children, severe tricuspid regurgitation developed related to injury to the tricuspid valve apparatus. Minor complications reported included femoral venous thrombosis, hemorrhage, and transient arrhythmias. The authors' experience with percutaneous balloon pulmonary valvuloplasty is consistent with that reported from other centers. During our first 10-year experience,

TABLE 54-1	Pertinent Data before and after Balloon Pulmonary Valvuloplasty in 90 Patients	
Parameter		**Result**
Age (years)		
Mean ± SD		4.2 ± 5.2
Range		1 d to 34 yr
Weight (kg)		
Mean ± SD		18.4 ± 17.2
Range		3.2–89
Systolic gradient (mm Hg)		
Before		70 ± 24
Immediately after		30 ± 17
Right ventricle systolic pressure (mm Hg)		
Before		91 + 24
Immediately after		50 ± 17
Cardiac index (L/min/m²)		
Before		3.55 ± 0.91
Immediately after		3.69 ± 0.81

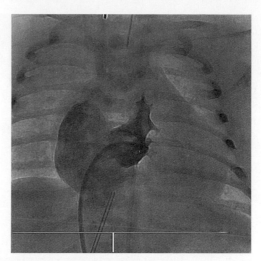

Figure 54-7 Anteroposterior right ventricular angiogram in a newborn with membranous pulmonary valve atresia and right ventricular hypoplasia. The right ventricle is small, and its outflow tract is evident immediately beneath the imperforate pulmonary valve. There was significant tricuspid regurgitation.

from 1982 to 1992, balloon valvuloplasty was performed in 90 patients with isolated pulmonary valve stenosis (Table 54-1). These patients ranged in age from 1 day to 34 years (4.2 ± 5.2 years [mean ± SD]) and in weight from 3.2 to 89 kg (18.4 ± 17.2 kg). Valvuloplasty was performed with balloons ranging in diameter from 5 to 20 mm, and the double-balloon technique was used in 16 instances. Overall, valvuloplasty decreased the peak systolic valve gradient acutely by 57%. The peak pulmonary stenosis gradient decreased from 70 + 24 to 30 ± 17 mm Hg after valvuloplasty ($P < 0.0001$). Right ventricular systolic pressure decreased from 91 ± 24 to 50 ± 17 mm Hg ($P < 0.0001$), and right ventricular end-diastolic pressure decreased from 9.8 ± 3.2 to 8.5 ± 2.5 mm Hg ($P < 0.01$). There was no significant change in heart rate or cardiac output after the procedure. In our experience, there has been no relationship between patient age or size and the residual pulmonary valve gradient after valvuloplasty.

Infants

Newborns and infants with critical pulmonary stenosis or atresia are frequently critically ill and hypoxemic (because of a right-to-left atrial shunt) and may have associated hypoplasia of the right ventricle and tricuspid valve (Fig. 54-7). Because of these factors, in addition to the presence of severe RVOT obstruction, it is a technical challenge to successfully catheterize the pulmonary artery and properly position a valvuloplasty balloon across the RVOT in these infants.[16,17,19–21] In infants with critical pulmonary stenosis, we prefer to perform the procedure with the child receiving prostaglandin E₁ infusion— for three reasons: first, the infant is in a more stable hemodynamic state during the procedure. Second, a left-to-right ductal shunt maintains pulmonary blood flow during balloon occlusion of the RVOT. Finally, the presence of a patent ductus arteriosus permits the exchange guidewire to be positioned across the pulmonary valve and into the descending aorta, a course that facilitates catheter exchanges and subsequent valve dilation. The authors have reported the results of balloon valvuloplasty attempted in 12 infants with critical pulmonary stenosis ($n = 10$) or membranous pulmonary atresia with intact ventricular septum ($n = 2$).[20] These infants ranged in age from 1 to 38 days and in weight from 2.9 to 4.5 kg. Nine were receiving a prostaglandin E₁ infusion. In one child with critical pulmonary stenosis and a diminutive right ventricle, the RVOT was perforated during an attempt to cross the valve. This child was taken to the operating room, where the perforation was oversewn and a Blalock-Taussig shunt performed. In the remaining 11 infants, balloon valvuloplasty was successfully performed using balloons ranging in diameter from 2.5 to 12 mm. In patients with membranous pulmonary atresia, the membrane can be perforated with a guidewire or a radiofrequency wire followed by balloon dilation (Fig. 54-8). If the infant remains significantly hypoxemic, additional

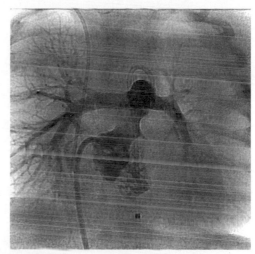

Figure 54-8 Anteroposterior right ventricular angiogram in the same infant as Figure 54-7, after radiofrequency perforation and dilation of membranous pulmonary valve atresia. The patent RV outflow tract is now evident, with good-size distal pulmonary arteries.

pulmonary blood flow can be provided by percutaneous stenting of the ductus arteriosus (Fig. 54-9).

Adults

Several reports have described the successful application of percutaneous balloon valvuloplasty for treatment of adults with pulmonary valve stenosis.[14,18,22–32] Table 54-2 summarizes the pertinent clinical and hemodynamic data from 14 publications (including this report) describing the acute results of pulmonary valvuloplasty in adolescents and adults. Pulmonary valvuloplasty has been performed successfully in patients as old as 84 years. In most published cases, a single-balloon technique has been used. When a 20-mm-diameter balloon is insufficient, however, the double-balloon technique has usually been necessary. In these reports, balloon valvuloplasty acutely reduced the peak systolic gradient by an average of 60% to 65%, from a range of 53 to 260 mm Hg before the procedure to 2 to 90 mm Hg after valvuloplasty. In most cases, the peak systolic gradient immediately after

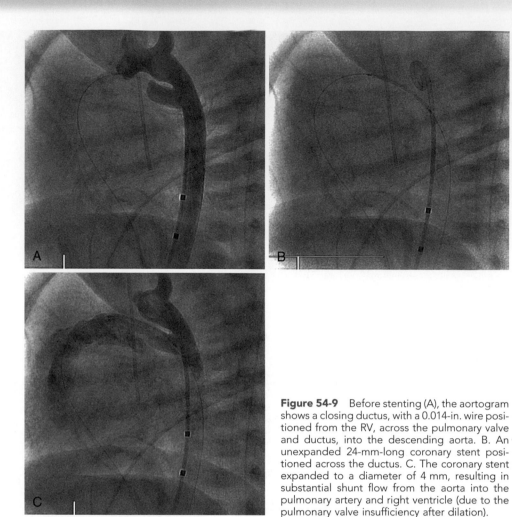

Figure 54-9 Before stenting (A), the aortogram shows a closing ductus, with a 0.014-in. wire positioned from the RV, across the pulmonary valve and ductus, into the descending aorta. B. An unexpanded 24-mm-long coronary stent positioned across the ductus. C. The coronary stent expanded to a diameter of 4 mm, resulting in substantial shunt flow from the aorta into the pulmonary artery and right ventricle (due to the pulmonary valve insufficiency after dilation).

TABLE 54-2	Summary of Published Reports of Pulmonary Valvuloplasty in Adults					
					Peak Systolic Gradient (mm Hg)	
Study Patients (years)	*No. of*	*Age Range*	*Balloon Technique*		BEFORE	AFTER
Beekman*	4	21–35	Double		53	15
Tentolouris[22]	1	84	Double		70	34
Herrmann[23]	8	23–66	Single		66	22
Sherman[24]	4	48–67	Single (3) Double (1)		109	38
Al Kasab[18]	12	21–37	Double		86	28
Fawzy[25]	8	21–45	Double		107	36
Flugelman[26]	1	62	Single		260	90
Presbitero[27]	3	21–45	Single		130	29
Park[28]	3	24–40	Double		108	51
Cooke[29]	1	61	Single		105	13
Leisch[30]	6	21–59	Single		78	38
Shuck[31]	1	23	Single		30	2
Pepine[14]	1	59	Single		130	30
Chen[32]	53	13–55	Single		191	38

*This report

valvuloplasty was in the mild range (20 to 40 mm Hg). For example, Al Kasab and colleagues[18] reported the effects of valvuloplasty in 12 adults, ranging in age from 21 to 37 years, with valvar pulmonary stenosis. In these patients, valvuloplasty acutely reduced the peak systolic gradient from 86 to 28 mm Hg. Transient ventricular arrhythmias were noted in 30% of patients, but no serious complications were described. Similarly, Fawzy and colleagues[25] described 8 adult patients with valvar pulmonary stenosis in whom percutaneous balloon valvuloplasty reduced the peak systolic gradient from 107 to 36 mm Hg. Thus, available data clearly indicate that percutaneous balloon valvuloplasty provides effective therapy in adults as well as in children with congenital pulmonary valve stenosis. Balloon valvuloplasty appears to be effective even in the oldest patients, in whom valve calcification may be present.[22]

LONG-TERM STUDIES

Long-term studies of balloon pulmonary valvuloplasty have confirmed that the benefits of this procedure are durable and comparable to the results of surgical valvotomy. McCrindle and Kan[33] reported the long-term results of balloon valvuloplasty performed between 1981 and 1986 in 42 patients (median age 4.6 years), for whom follow-up data beyond 2 years were available. Balloon valvuloplasty acutely reduced the peak systolic gradient from 70 to 23 mm Hg; at long-term follow-up more than 2 years after the procedure, the Doppler-predicted gradient was 20 mm Hg. Doppler peak instantaneous gradients were less than 36 mm Hg at long-term follow-up in 86% of patients. The authors found age younger than 2 years at the time of balloon valvuloplasty to be a risk factor for late follow-up gradients exceeding 36 mm Hg. Long-term data from the Pediatric Valvuloplasty Registry were reported on 533 patients up to 8.7 years after balloon pulmonary valvuloplasty.[34] A total of 84 patients (16%) required either a surgical valvotomy or a repeat balloon dilation. Of the 449 patients who had not undergone a repeat procedure, 399 had mild residual stenosis (<36 mm Hg), 36 had residual stenosis >36 mm Hg, and the late gradient was unknown in 14. Independent risk factors for a suboptimal late outcome included small valve annulus diameter, higher early residual gradient, smaller balloon-annulus diameter ratio, and earlier year at initial intervention. We assessed the long-term (4 to 5 years) outcome after balloon pulmonary valvuloplasty in childhood and compared the results to a matched surgical control group.[35] Follow-up data obtained in 20 children 4 to 7.8 years after balloon valvuloplasty documented excellent late results without significant restenosis. The peak systolic gradient measured at cardiac catheterization in these children averaged 76 mm Hg before and 35 mm Hg immediately after balloon valvuloplasty. At long-term follow-up, the Doppler peak instantaneous gradient was 24 mm Hg, or significantly less than that measured by catheterization immediately after the procedure (Fig. 54-10). Pulmonary valve insufficiency was mild in 9 of 20 patients and absent in the remainder. Twenty-four-hour Holter monitoring documented only grade 1 ventricular ectopic activity in one patient and none in the remaining 19 patients. Comparison to the matched surgical control group demonstrated that, although the residual gradient was slightly less after surgery (16 vs. 24 mm Hg; P = 0.01), the surgical group had significantly more pulmonary valve insufficiency and late ventricular arrhythmias. Late follow-up data, therefore, document excellent long-term results after percutaneous pulmonary balloon valvuloplasty and support the use of this procedure as treatment of choice for patients with isolated valvar pulmonary stenosis. A recent study of exercise capacity in 41 patients a median of 13.1 years after pulmonary balloon valvuloplasty showed that peak oxygen consumption was mildly below the expected value in this group (92 ± 17% of predicted, P = 0.006).[36] Cardiac magnetic resonance imaging in these patients showed pulmonary regurgitation fractions of 1% to 45%, with a median of 10%. Moderate regurgitation (fraction 31% to 49%) was present in 7 patients (17%), with mild regurgitation (fraction 16% to 30%) in 7 more patients. The 14 patients with mild or moderate pulmonary regurgitation had significantly lower peak oxygen consumption than those with lesser amounts of regurgitation (85 ± 17% vs. 96 ± 16% of predicted, P = 0.03). Right ventricular dilation (end-diastolic volume z-score >2) was present in 40% of the study group, and indexed end-diastolic volume of the right ventricle correlated with pulmonary regurgitation fraction (R = 0.79, P < 0.001). These results suggest that relatively modest amounts of pulmonary regurgitation may result in long-term right ventricular dilation and reduced exercise tolerance. Alternatively, these results may simply reflect the severe nature of the pulmonary stenosis in these patients prior to intervention and the aggressive balloon dilation procedures required (median age at intervention 0.2 years, median right-ventricle-to-aorta pressure ratio 110% before valvuloplasty, median balloon-to-annulus diameter ratio 1.3, range 1.0 to 2.0).

COMPLICATIONS

Beyond infancy, percutaneous balloon pulmonary valvuloplasty is a very safe procedure. In the Pediatric Valvuloplasty Registry, the only two deaths occurred in infants with critical pulmonary stenosis, and the single case of perforation and tamponade occurred in an 8-day-old neonate.[13] Minor complications were primarily related to vascular injury or hemorrhage and were also much more common during the first 12 months of life. Overall, the Pediatric Valvuloplasty Registry noted a 1.2% to 1.8% frequency of major complications and a 4.8% frequency of minor complications in 168 infants. In contrast, in 656 children and adults, the frequency of major complication was 0.8% and the frequency of minor complication was 1.7%. Premature ventricular beats and right-bundle-branch block occur commonly during the procedure owing to catheter and wire manipulation within the right ventricle, but there have been no reports of long-term arrhythmias after valvuloplasty. Valvuloplasty may cause injury to the femoral vein, especially when the procedure is performed in infancy. Finally, the mild pulmonary valve insufficiency commonly seen after pulmonary valvuloplasty, while perhaps not entirely benign,[36] is rarely of clinical importance and may be less severe than after surgical valvotomy.[35]

CONCLUSIONS AND RECOMMENDATIONS

Percutaneous balloon pulmonary valvuloplasty is the treatment of choice for children and adults with isolated congenital valvar pulmonary stenosis. Valvuloplasty successfully reduces significant RVOT obstruction, with a residual gradient that is usually in the trivial to mild range (i.e., <30 mm Hg). Follow-up studies have documented long-term effectiveness, with little restenosis as late as 9 years after the procedure. In our opinion, pulmonary valvuloplasty is indicated in patients with isolated pulmonary valve stenosis whose resting peak systolic pressure gradient exceeds 40 mm Hg in the presence of a normal cardiac output. The procedure is effective in neonates, children, and adults as old as 84 years.[22] Unless the valve annulus is severely hypoplastic, patients with a calcified or dysplastic pulmonary valve may also derive significant hemodynamic benefit from balloon valvuloplasty.

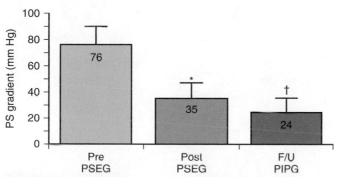

Figure 54-10 Serial pulmonary stenosis (PS) gradients in 20 children before and immediately after valvuloplasty and at follow-up (F/U) an average of 5.4 years later. PIPG, peak instantaneous pressure gradient; PSEG, peak systolic ejection gradient. (*Reproduced with permission from O'Connor EK, Beekman RH, Lindauer A, Rocchini A. Intermediate-term outcome after pulmonary balloon valvuloplasty: comparison to a matched surgical control group. J Am Coll Cardiol. 1992;20:169–173.*)

▪ Aortic Balloon Valvuloplasty

Aortic valve stenosis accounts for 4% to 6% of all cases of congenital heart disease.[37] Left ventricular outflow tract (LVOT) obstruction elicits left ventricular hypertrophy and myocardial fibrosis, which may eventually lead to left ventricular dysfunction and congestive heart failure. Unlike most cases of congenital pulmonary valve stenosis, congenital aortic stenosis tends to progress over time.[38] Nevertheless, intervention usually is not indicated unless the degree of LVOT obstruction is severe (catheter gradient >65 mm Hg) or there is associated left ventricular dysfunction, heart failure, ischemia, or symptoms of angina, syncope, or presyncope. This recommendation is based on the fact that all current forms of therapy for aortic valve stenosis are palliative in nature. Surgical valvotomy, widely regarded in the past as the initial treatment of choice for congenital aortic valve stenosis, is associated with a high incidence of late (5 to 20 years) restenosis.[39] Prosthetic aortic valve replacement is associated with risks of thromboembolic complications and risks associated with anticoagulation therapy that may be considerable in young, active patients. Thus, because current treatment options are not curative, intervention for congenital aortic valve stenosis is usually delayed until clear indications exist. Percutaneous balloon valvuloplasty for the treatment of congenital valvar aortic stenosis in children was first described in 1984.[40] Balloon valvuloplasty typically reduces the LVOT obstruction to the mild range and is the treatment of choice for children with congenital aortic stenosis who require intervention. The effectiveness of balloon dilation relates to the underlying morphological substrate. Most congenitally stenotic aortic valves are bicuspid, involving a single central or eccentric commissure with a variable degree of fusion of its edges. The valve leaflets themselves are thickened but are rarely calcified in childhood (Fig. 54-11). In older patients and in children with prior valve surgery, the leaflets may calcify, becoming less mobile and less amenable to balloon dilation. In congenital aortic valve stenosis as in pulmonary valve stenosis, balloon valvuloplasty reduces the degree of stenosis by separating valve leaflets along the lines of commissural fusion (Fig. 54-12). Because the valve leaflets are typically supple in younger patients and the obstruction to ventricular outflow relates primarily to incomplete cusp separation during systole, balloon dilation provides substantial hemodynamic improvement in these cases. This is in marked contrast to older patients with calcific aortic stenosis, in whom balloon valvuloplasty has proven to be much less successful.[41] In these patients the aortic valve stenosis is acquired, primarily as a result of calcium deposition within the leaflets, and little or no commissural fusion is present.[42,43] Therefore differences in valve morphology, and thus in the mechanism by which balloon dilation improves valve function, explain the observation that balloon valvuloplasty is effective in younger patients with congenital aortic stenosis but typically ineffective in adults with calcific aortic stenosis.

Successful percutaneous balloon valvuloplasty in children with congenital aortic valve stenosis was first reported in 1984 by Lababidi and colleagues.[40,44] Since then the effectiveness of balloon valvuloplasty in children and adolescents with congenital aortic valve stenosis has been clearly demonstrated.[45–53] The procedure usually reduces the peak systolic gradient by approximately 60%, and severe aortic regurgitation is uncommon. Vascular complications have been limited primarily to neonates and young infants and have diminished in recent years with the development of smaller-profile valvuloplasty catheters.

TECHNIQUE

Percutaneous aortic valvuloplasty is usually performed from a retrograde transarterial approach, although the antegrade transseptal approach can also be used. We prefer the retrograde approach, using a transseptal catheter for continuous left ventricular pressure monitoring throughout the procedure. After the transseptal puncture is accomplished, heparin is administered to increase the activated clotting time (ACT) to approximately 250 to 300 seconds. The aortic stenosis gradient is measured before angiography from simultaneous ventricular and aortic pressure recordings. In our center, the criteria for performing aortic balloon dilation include (1) a peak systolic pressure gradient at rest of 65 mm Hg or more, (2) a peak systolic gradient of 50 to

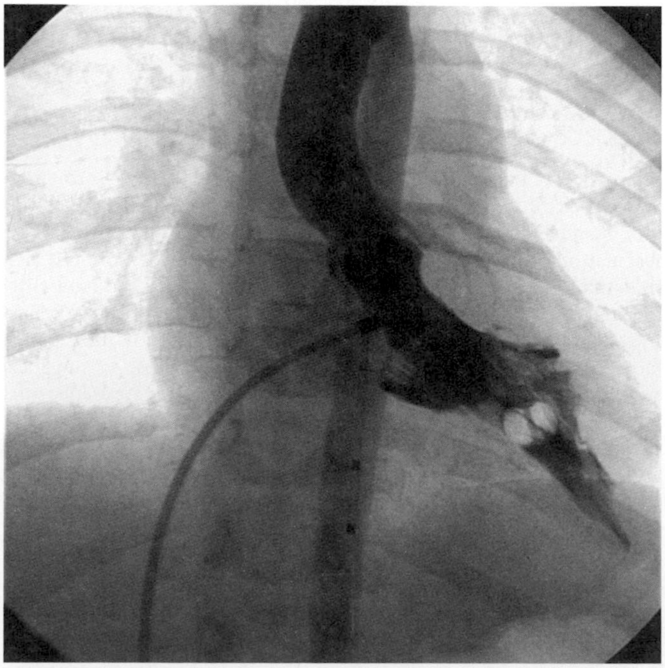

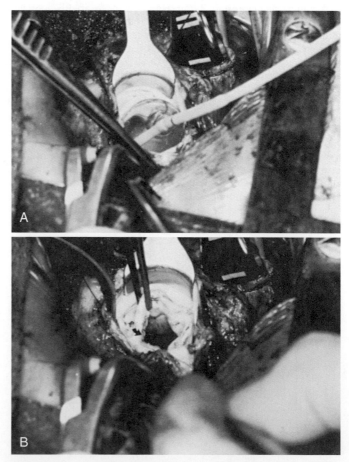

Figure 54-12 The mechanism of balloon aortic valvuloplasty is demonstrated during surgery in an 18-year-old woman with congenital aortic valve stenosis. A 20-mm balloon had been inflated across the valve (A), producing a 3- to 4-mm tear across the line of commissural fusion (arrowhead) (B). The valve leaflets are thick and dysplastic.

Figure 54-11 Anteroposterior left ventricular angiogram in a child with severe valvar aortic stenosis. The valve is thickened and domes in systole. There is left ventricular hypertrophy.

64 mm Hg in association with symptoms or ischemic changes on electrocardiography, or (3) patients with low cardiac output regardless of measured pressure gradient. A modest aortic stenosis gradient is typical in infants with critically severe aortic stenosis in whom left ventricular failure and shock are present. Once the decision to proceed with balloon valvuloplasty has been made, the correct balloon diameter must be selected. Proper balloon size depends on aortic valve annulus diameter, which can be measured by echocardiography or by angiography. If a single-balloon technique is used, a balloon is chosen whose diameter is equal to or 1 mm smaller than 90% to 100% of the diameter of the aortic valve annulus. If a double-balloon technique is used, we use two balloons of similar diameter whose sum is 1.2 to 1.3 times the diameter of the single-balloon diameter thought to be optimal for the patient.[46] We prefer the double-balloon technique in patients whose aortic valve annulus exceeds 25 mm or in those whose aortic valve annulus is large for their body size so as to minimize the size of the balloon catheter and arterial sheath required for the procedure. Unlike the case in pulmonary balloon valvuloplasty, oversized balloons are not used for aortic valvuloplasty because these have been shown to increase the risk of injury to the aortic valve and annulus.[47] The balloon or balloons are inflated by hand (i.e., a manometer is not used) until the waist produced on the balloon by the valve is relieved (Fig. 54-13). Balloon inflation is kept as brief as possible to minimize arterial hypotension during the procedure. Because the inflated balloon may be ejected across the aortic valve, several balloon inflations may be required, with minor adjustments in position to ensure that the valve is adequately dilated. Repeat simultaneous measurements of left ventricular and aortic pressures are made to quantify the residual aortic stenosis gradient. An aortic root angiogram is performed to detect any aortic insufficiency that may have been produced by the procedure.

ACUTE RESULTS

In most patients with congenital aortic valve stenosis, balloon valvuloplasty provides relief of LVOT obstruction (Fig. 54-14) comparable to the results of surgical valvotomy.[38,51] The expected peak systolic ejection gradient across the aortic valve after the procedure is approximately 20 to 40 mm Hg.[45-52] If a technically adequate balloon dilation fails to achieve a satisfactory hemodynamic result in a patient with congenital aortic valve stenosis, a more complex diagnosis is suggested; such patients may be found to have annular hypoplasia or valve

leaflet calcification. The largest series of balloon aortic valvuloplasty procedures for congenital aortic stenosis was reported by the Pediatric Valvuloplasty Registry.[45,52] The acute results of 630 balloon valvuloplasty procedures were reported in 606 children ranging in age from 1 day to 18 years who underwent the procedure at 23 institutions between 1984 and 1992. Overall, the procedure resulted in an immediate decrease in peak systolic pressure gradient across the aortic valve by 60%. In the initial registry report of 204 children,[45] most of the acute complications and deaths occurred in newborns. Five deaths were reported (mortality rate, 2.4%), four of which occurred in

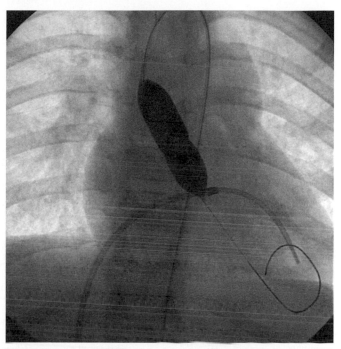

Figure 54-13 Balloon dilation in a child with severe aortic valve stenosis. The waist produced by the valve annulus on the balloon is evident. Ventricular pressure was monitored throughout the procedure by a catheter placed in the left ventricle through a transseptal puncture.

Figure 54-14 Aortic and left ventricular pressure tracings in an 11-day-old infant with critical aortic stenosis, measured before and immediately after balloon dilation. The peak systolic gradient decreased from 96 to 29 mm Hg. Note the improved aortic pulse pressure after valvuloplasty indicative of an improved cardiac output. *(Reproduced with permission from Beekman RH, Rocchini AP, Andes A. Balloon valvuloplasty for critical aortic stenosis in the newborn: influence of new catheter technology. J Am Coll Cardiol. 1991;17:1172–1176.)*

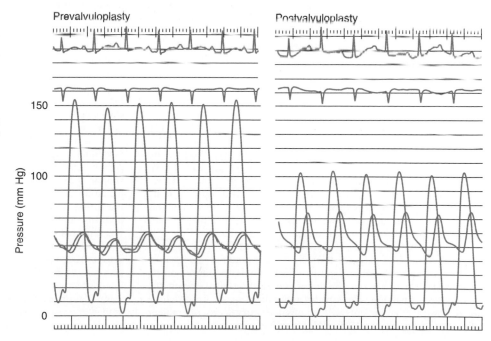

TABLE 54-3	Pertinent Data before and after Balloon Aortic Valvuloplasty in 68 Patients
Number	68
Age (years)	
Mean ± SD	8.7 ± 6.9
Range	1 d–24 yr
Weight (kg)	
Mean ± SD	35.7 ± 27.7
Range	2.1–120
Systolic gradient (mm Hg)	
Before	77 ± 21
Immediately after	34 ± 16
Left ventricle systolic pressure (mm Hg)	
Before	171 ± 31
Immediately after	133 ± 25
Cardiac index (L/min/m²)	
Before	3.64 ± 0.95
Immediately after	3.35 ± 0.80

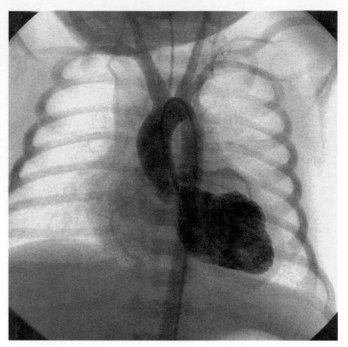

Figure 54-15 Anteroposterior left ventricular angiogram in a newborn with critical aortic valve stenosis. The aortic valve leaflets are thickened, and there was severe left ventricular dysfunction.

newborns and one in a 3-month-old child. Two deaths were related to aortic rupture, two due to aortic valve trauma, and one occurred as a result of a torn iliofemoral artery. There was no mortality in patients older than 3 months of age. The larger report[52] evaluated predictors of a suboptimal outcome, which was defined as failure to perform the valvuloplasty (which occurred in 4.1%), an immediate residual gradient of 60 mm Hg or more, a left ventricular systolic pressure exceeding aortic systolic by 60% or more, mortality, or major morbidity. Overall, a suboptimal outcome was reported for 17% of the 630 valvuloplasty procedures. The identified independent predictors for a suboptimal outcome included age younger than 3 months, a greater predilation systolic gradient, a balloon-annulus diameter ratio under 0.9, the coexistence of an unrepaired coarctation, and an earlier date of procedure. Three months appeared to be a significant threshold below which the procedural outcome was adversely affected. Patients younger than 3 months were more likely to experience failure to perform the procedure (15.7% vs. 1.7%), suboptimal residual stenosis (17.8% vs. 7.5%), major morbidity (16.7% vs. 4.1%), and mortality (8.3% vs. 0.6%). The effect of the balloon-annulus diameter ratio was thoroughly evaluated, and the optimal ratio was found to be between 0.90 and 0.99. Smaller ratios were associated with an increased risk of suboptimal gradient relief. Larger-diameter ratios were associated with a greater risk of aortic insufficiency after valvuloplasty. The authors' experience with percutaneous balloon aortic valvuloplasty was similar. Between 1985 and 1992, balloon aortic dilation was performed in 68 children, adolescents, and young adults with congenital aortic valve stenosis (Table 54-3). Patients ranged in age from 1 day to 24 years (8.7 ± 6.9 years) and in weight from 2.1 to 120 kg (35.7 ± 27.7 kg). The valvuloplasty procedure was performed with balloon diameters ranging from 5 to 20 mm, and the double-balloon technique was used in 36 patients. Percutaneous balloon valvuloplasty acutely decreased the peak systolic aortic stenosis gradient by 56%, from 77 ± 22 to 34 ± 16 mm Hg. Left ventricular systolic pressure decreased acutely from 171 ± 31 to 133 ± 25 mm Hg, and left ventricular end-diastolic pressure decreased slightly from 14.5 ± 4.3 to 11.9 ± 5.7 mm Hg. There was no change in cardiac output or heart rate after the dilation procedure. In 52 of 68 patients (76%), there was no increase in the degree of aortic insufficiency from that present before balloon valvuloplasty. An increase of 1 grade (on a scale of 0 to 4+) occurred acutely in 10 patients (15%), and an increase of 2 grades occurred in 6 patients (9%). No patient required emergent or urgent surgical intervention because of valvuloplasty-induced aortic insufficiency. In our series, we found no relationship between the effectiveness of balloon valvuloplasty and patient age or size. We have noted, however, that patients with an unsatisfactory degree of gradient relief (residual gradient >45 mm Hg) have had more complex disease, including annular hypoplasia or valve leaflet calcification. In this series, there has been no patient with unsatisfactory gradient relief from balloon valvuloplasty who subsequently underwent a successful surgical valvotomy. Such patients, instead, have required more complex surgical intervention, including prosthetic aortic valve replacement or the Konno operation.

Infants

Infants with critical aortic stenosis typically present in severe congestive heart failure and shock, with profound left ventricular dysfunction (Fig. 54-15). At times it can be difficult to distinguish neonatal critical aortic stenosis from hypoplastic left heart syndrome, as the aortic valve annulus, mitral valve annulus, and even the left ventricular length can be undersized. In addition, the aortic valve leaflets (or leaflet) often exhibit a markedly dysplastic appearance on echocardiography, which in an older child would indicate a low likelihood of successful balloon valvuloplasty. Despite these real or apparent obstacles to success, balloon aortic valvuloplasty has proved to be remarkably successful, with results comparable to surgical intervention at several premier institutions.[55–58] The clinical status of these patients generally leaves little room for doubt that urgent intervention is required, but the choice between relief of aortic stenosis and univentricular palliation is not always obvious. Unlike critical pulmonary stenosis, where placement of a systemic to pulmonary artery shunt can compensate for inadequate support of the pulmonary circulation by hypoplasia of right heart structures, patients with left heart structures inadequate to support the systemic circulation face death unless a successful Norwood palliation can be performed. Several systems have been developed for predicting which neonates have the potential for adequate systemic perfusion after relief of aortic valve stenosis, the most popular of which was reported by Rhodes and colleagues.[59] The child should be stabilized with prostaglandin E₁ infusion and intravenous inotropic support prior to the procedure, with extracorporeal life support if necessary. If possible, we use the transumbilical approach (Fig. 54-16) to spare the infant's femoral artery (which may be required for future percutaneous valve dilation procedures). The carotid artery[60] and transvenous antegrade[61] approaches have also been reported as means to avoid femoral artery injury in newborn infants. We have tended to employ a single

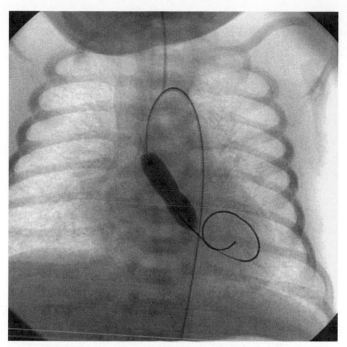

Figure 54-16 Balloon dilation in a newborn with critical aortic stenosis (same patient as in Fig. 54-15). The catheter was introduced through the umbilical artery, thereby avoiding potential femoral artery injury in a newborn with low cardiac output.

balloon, typically 6 to 7 mm in diameter, aiming for a single inflation. In contrast, McElhinney and colleagues[57] begin with smaller balloons and perform serial dilations with progressively larger balloons until the desired degree of relief is obtained. The Congenital Heart Surgeons Society reported the results of intervention in 110 neonates with critical aortic stenosis from 18 institutions.[56] Balloon aortic valvuloplasty was the initial procedure in 82 patients and surgical valvotomy in the remaining 28. Relief of aortic stenosis was significantly better in the balloon valvuloplasty group (gradient reduction of 65 ± 17%, median residual gradient 20 mm Hg, vs. 41 ± 32%, median residual gradient 36 mm Hg), although there was also a trend toward more aortic insufficiency in this group. Early mortality was 18%, with no difference between groups. In our own study,[55] 30 neonates were assigned to balloon valvuloplasty and 17 to surgical intervention on an intent-to-treat basis; early mortality was 13% in both groups. Early mortality was 14% in a series of 113 neonates treated with balloon aortic valvuloplasty, with about one-third of survivors requiring repeat intervention within 1 year.[57] Echocardiographic estimates of valve thickness or mobility have not correlated with valvuloplasty success in neonates.

Fetal Intervention

Balloon valvuloplasty has been proposed for fetuses with aortic stenosis for the purpose of preventing them from developing hypoplastic left heart syndrome. Research has focused on accurately identifying fetuses at risk for this progression, developing techniques for in utero intervention, reducing the risks of technical failure and of fetal demise, and on predicting which fetuses are most likely to benefit from intervention. The Harvard group has reported its experience with 70 fetuses from March 2000 through October 2008.[62] Valvuloplasty was attempted in midgestational fetuses who met criteria for aortic stenosis with evolving hypoplastic left heart syndrome, and all were thought to have a potentially salvageable left ventricle. Technical success was achieved in 52 procedures (74%), and 61 pregnancies resulted in live birth at a viable gestational age (87%). Of the 47 infants born alive at a viable gestational age after a technically successful midgestational valvuloplasty, 20 (43%) have achieved a biventricular circulation and 27 progressed to hypoplastic left heart syndrome despite intervention. Based

on this experience, the group has modified its selection criteria to require unequivocal demonstration of aortic stenosis (i.e., elimination of any candidates with possible aortic atresia) and a minimum left ventricular long-axis z-score of −2. In addition, candidates must qualify under at least four of the following five criteria: left ventricular long-axis z-score >0; left ventricular short-axis z-score >0; aortic valve annulus z-score >−3.5; mitral valve annulus z-score >−2; Doppler-estimated mitral regurgitation or aortic stenosis maximum systolic gradient ≥20 mm Hg. Of the fetuses who met these criteria in retrospect, technical success was achieved in 87%, with biventricular circulation in 50% of those born alive at a viable gestational age after successful valvuloplasty. These results warrant further investigation.

Young Adults

Balloon aortic valvuloplasty in young adults with congenital aortic valve stenosis yields results similar to those in children with the same disease and in patients with rheumatic aortic stenosis, all of whom exhibit commissural fusion to a significant degree. In contrast, balloon valvuloplasty is of limited utility in patients with degenerative or calcific aortic stenosis.[41,63-65] We have reported our experience with balloon valvuloplasty in 15 young adult patients, aged 15 to 24 years, with congenital aortic valve stenosis.[53] All were judged to have severe disease. The valve annulus ranged from 18.5 to 30 mm in diameter. Balloons were used ranging in diameter from 10 to 20 mm, and the double-balloon technique was used in 12 patients. In one patient with access to only one femoral artery available, the double-balloon technique was performed using a single retrograde balloon together with a balloon placed anterograde through a transseptal puncture. In these 15 young adults, balloon valvuloplasty acutely reduced the peak systolic aortic valve gradient from 73 to 35 mm Hg. Left ventricular systolic pressure decreased from 179 to 147 mm Hg without an associated change in cardiac output. Aortic insufficiency was unchanged by the procedure in 9 patients, increased by one grade in 4, and increased by two grades in 2. An unsatisfactory result was obtained in 3 patients, in whom the residual systolic gradient was 70 mm Hg or more. Two of these patients had mild annular hypoplasia (18.5 and 19 mm), and the third had moderate valve leaflet calcification (related to prior surgical valvotomy in childhood). All three of these patients have required prosthetic aortic valve replacement. The remaining 12 patients have done well during intermediate-term follow-up. Eight underwent elective follow-up cardiac catheterization 1 to 2.5 years after balloon valvuloplasty, which documented no restenosis. In these patients, the follow-up peak systolic gradient at cardiac catheterization was 30 mm Hg, and there was no change in the degree of aortic regurgitation. Although this is a small series, the data lead us to believe that percutaneous balloon valvuloplasty should be attempted in young adults with congenital aortic valve stenosis unless the valve annulus is hypoplastic or the valve is calcified.

LONG-TERM STUDIES

Percutaneous balloon valvuloplasty for congenital aortic stenosis should be regarded as a palliative therapeutic procedure. As is the case after surgical aortic valvotomy,[39] late restenosis (5 to 20 years) should be expected after a successful balloon dilation procedure. We would warn, however, against comparing follow-up peak instantaneous gradients determined by Doppler echocardiography against catheter-based measurements of peak systolic gradient obtained immediately after valvuloplasty.[66] Because Doppler peak instantaneous and catheter peak systolic gradients may differ substantially, particularly in patients with aortic insufficiency, a false impression of restenosis may be obtained in comparing Doppler with catheter gradient measurements. The intermediate-term effectiveness of balloon valvuloplasty in children with congenital aortic stenosis was prospectively evaluated in our center.[67] A follow-up cardiac catheterization was performed in 27 of the first 30 children to undergo successful percutaneous balloon dilation at our institution between 1985 and 1988 an average of 1.7 years (0.8 to 3.8 years) after balloon valvuloplasty. No restenosis

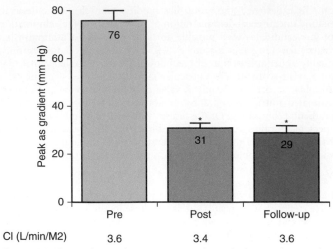

CI (L/min/M2)   3.6   3.4   3.6

Figure 54-17 Peak systolic pressure gradient determined at cardiac catheterization before (pre) and immediately after (post) valvuloplasty and at follow-up catheterization 1.7 years later in 27 children who underwent balloon dilation for congenital aortic stenosis. *(Reproduced with permission from O'Connor BK, Beekman RH, Rocchini AP, Rosenthal A. Intermediate-term effectiveness of balloon valvuloplasty for congenital aortic stenosis: a prospective follow-up study. Circulation. 1991;84:732–738.)*

was documented in these patients, with the greatest increase in peak systolic gradient at recatheterization being 14 mm Hg. In this group of 27 children (mean age, 8.6 years), balloon valvuloplasty acutely decreased the peak systolic gradient from 76 to 31 mm Hg. At follow-up 1.7 years later, the peak systolic gradient remained 29 mm Hg (Fig. 54-17). At the follow-up cardiac catheterization, 20 of 27 patients (74%) had no increase in the degree of aortic insufficiency that had been present before balloon valvuloplasty. In the 7 patients in whom balloon dilation resulted in increased valve insufficiency, 5 had a 2+ increase in aortic insufficiency and 2 had a 1+ increase in aortic insufficiency at the follow-up study (compared with prevalvuloplasty insufficiency). The degree of the aortic insufficiency after valvuloplasty remained stable during the follow-up period in 4 of these 7 patients and increased 1 to 2 grades in the remaining three patients. Galal and colleagues reported the 3- to 9-year follow-up of 26 patients who had balloon aortic valvuloplasty at ages ranging from 6 weeks to 20 years.[61] Restenosis requiring reintervention occurred within 2 years in 23% of the group, and actuarial reintervention-free survival was 76% at 3 to 9 years postvalvuloplasty. Neonates with critical aortic stenosis appear to have a substantially higher risk of restenosis and progressive aortic insufficiency following balloon valvuloplasty: reintervention-free survival has been approximately 50% at 5 years,[55–57] with aortic valve replacement or surgical repair of aortic insufficiency in approximately 50% at 10 years.[55,57] Kipps and coworkers reported results of exercise testing in 30 patients a median of 13.1 years after balloon aortic valvuloplasty performed in the first 6 months of life.[68] All patients were asymptomatic and most had mild residual aortic stenosis (median Doppler-estimated mean systolic gradient 20 mm Hg, range 0 to 42 mm Hg). Moderate (9 patients) or severe (2 patients) aortic regurgitation was present in 37%. Peak oxygen consumption was significantly reduced for the group as a whole (87 ± 18% predicted, $P <$ 0.001), and 7 patients (23%) had severely depressed (≤70% predicted) peak oxygen consumption. There was a significant inverse correlation between peak oxygen consumption and age at testing, with an estimated loss of 2% of predicted peak oxygen consumption each year (R^2 = 0.30, P = 0.002). The typical deficit in patients with severely reduced peak oxygen consumption was an inability to increase stroke volume. These results in asymptomatic patients serve to emphasize the importance of a report from the same institution presenting 4 patients who, following successful neonatal aortic balloon valvuloplasty, presented

in adolescence with diastolic left ventricular heart failure and evidence of endocardial fibroelastosis on magnetic resonance imaging (confirmed by histopathology in 2 patients).[69] These reports underscore the importance of ongoing medical supervision of aortic valvuloplasty patients, particularly those requiring intervention early in life.

COMPLICATIONS

Percutaneous balloon aortic valvuloplasty is a relatively safe procedure, with rare mortality outside of early infancy. The Pediatric Valvuloplasty Registry[45] described 5 deaths, 4 in the neonatal period and 1 in a critically ill 3-month-old. Early mortality after balloon valvuloplasty in neonates has ranged from 13% to 18%; appreciable late mortality has been observed in these series, with 5-year survival rates of 72% to 83%.[55–57] These data compare favorably with the surgical experience, where morbidity and mortality rates have been relatively high in neonates with critical aortic stenosis. Other complications reported in the Pediatric Valvuloplasty Registry have included potentially life-threatening arrhythmias in 3 infants, perforation of the left ventricle requiring surgery, and a mitral valve tear also requiring surgical repair. Valvuloplasty-induced aortic valve insufficiency may be the most significant complication of the procedure. In our experience, valve insufficiency occurs in approximately 24% of patients and is mild in most. Moderate to severe aortic insufficiency may be induced by balloon valvuloplasty in approximately 3% to 6% of patients and is more common if the balloon-to-annulus diameter ratio exceeds 1.0. Surgical techniques allowing repair rather than replacement of balloon-damaged valves have been a welcome development.[70] Femoral artery injury, thrombosis, and occlusion have been relatively common in the past, particularly in infants. In the Pediatric Valvuloplasty Registry, femoral artery injury was reported in 12% of children, most of whom were younger than 12 months of age.[45] In our follow-up evaluation,[67] femoral artery occlusion or stenosis was observed in 3 of 5 children younger than 12 months of age compared with only 1 of 22 children older than 12 months of age at the time of the valvuloplasty procedure (P = 0.01). Since 1988, when lower-profile catheters became available, femoral artery injury has become much less common.[71] We prefer not to exceed a 4-Fr exit profile in neonatal femoral arteries and to use the transumbilical approach for neonatal critical aortic stenosis if possible. Because future transfemoral valvuloplasty procedures (for restenosis) are likely to be necessary in these patients, femoral artery access should be preserved if at all possible. A newly recognized complication of neonatal aortic balloon valvuloplasty is aortic wall injury, in particular the creation of an intimal flap.[72] This diagnosis was made by angiography, echocardiography, or direct observation by the surgeon or pathologist. This complication was found in 28 of 187 procedures performed over a 23-year period (15%), with no change in frequency over the study period. The injury was recognized at the time of the procedure in only 57% of cases and usually occurred in the distal ascending aorta or aortic arch. In one instance, a flap in the proximal ascending aorta extended into a coronary artery ostium, causing death, and another patient died suddenly at home. No other clinical adverse events were noted. Multivariate analysis showed that aortic wall injury was more likely in patients with severe ventricular dysfunction at the time of the procedure, in procedures with greater numbers of balloon dilation attempts, and in procedures supervised by less experienced interventional staff.

CONCLUSIONS AND RECOMMENDATIONS

Percutaneous balloon aortic valvuloplasty provides effective palliative treatment for children and young adults with congenital valvar aortic stenosis. Valvuloplasty successfully reduces the peak systolic aortic stenosis gradient to the 20- to 40-mm Hg range, which compares favorably with open surgical valvotomy. Aortic insufficiency is not increased from its prevalvuloplasty status in most patients. Aortic insufficiency is produced in approximately 20% to 25% of patients but is mild in most of these. Mortality has been limited to critically ill neonates and young infants. Follow-up studies have documented early restenosis to be uncommon, but long-term investigations are lacking. Balloon valvuloplasty is an excellent therapeutic option for most patients with congenital aortic valve stenosis. At most pediatric cardiology centers, it is the treatment of choice. We recommend balloon valvuloplasty for patients whose resting peak systolic pressure gradient exceeds 65 mm Hg, for those with a resting peak gradient of 50 to 65 mm Hg in association with ischemic changes or symptoms, or in patients with heart failure and low cardiac output regardless of gradient. Balloon valvuloplasty is effective in neonates, children, and young adults with congenital aortic valve stenosis in whom commissural fusion is the primary anatomical cause of outflow obstruction. The procedure is less likely to be effective in patients with a hypoplastic valve annulus or with valve leaflet calcification. In utero balloon valvuloplasty in carefully selected fetuses with aortic stenosis by experienced centers shows promise in arresting the development of hypoplastic left heart syndrome.

Balloon-Expandable Stenting for Pulmonary Artery Stenosis

Pulmonary artery stenosis occurs commonly in patients with congenital heart disease. It is encountered as an isolated lesion in patients with the Williams or Alagille syndromes or as a feature of complex congenital heart disease such as tetralogy of Fallot pre- and postoperatively. Balloon angioplasty of pulmonary artery stenosis or hypoplasia has yielded mixed results. Numerous reports document an immediate success rate of only 50% to 60% after balloon angioplasty of this lesion,[73,74] and follow-up studies demonstrate a long-term success rate that is even lower.[75] Failure of angioplasty alone is often related to elastic recoil of the pulmonary artery. These observations have led to the application of stent therapy to treat pulmonary artery stenosis or hypoplasia. Transcatheter stenting is now the initial treatment of choice for many patients with pulmonary artery stenosis and has demonstrated excellent early and intermediate-term effectiveness.

ANIMAL STUDIES

Balloon-expandable stents were initially evaluated in several experimental models of pulmonary artery stenosis.[76–78] Benson and coworkers implanted a balloon-expandable stent into the left pulmonary artery of 9 pigs with a surgically created pulmonary artery stenosis. The diameter of the stenosis more than doubled, and follow-up studies 3 weeks and 3.5 months later documented no restenosis and no thrombosis, aneurysm formation, or obstruction of arterial side-branch vessels. Histological evaluation (approximately 3 months after implantation) documented virtually complete stent coverage with a neointima composed of fibroblasts as well as medial compression with mild fibrosis beneath the stent wires. Scanning electron microscopy disclosed the presence of a thin layer of neoendothelial cells covering the stent arms with the exception of areas overlying arterial side branches, where stents remain uncovered and side-branch vessels patent. Our program reported data supporting the feasibility and effectiveness of stent redilation in an experimental model of left pulmonary artery stenosis.[79] Six 3- to 4-month-old puppies underwent stent implantation (Palmaz P308), using an 8- to 10-mm balloon, at the site of a surgically created stenosis in the left pulmonary artery. The vessel diameter at the stenosis increased from 4.8 to 7.4 mm, and the diameter of the proximal stented left pulmonary artery increased from 7.3 to 9.6 mm. Four months after stent implantation, when the puppies had increased in weight by 54%, each stent was redilated to a larger diameter using a 12-mm angioplasty balloon. Redilation was effective, with the stenosis diameter increasing from 7.4 to 9.2 mm, and the proximal stented portion of the vessel enlarging from 9.2 to 11.5 mm. Redilation caused the stents to shorten from 27.4 to 25.7 mm (initial preimplantation length was 30 mm). Acute examination of two redilated stents documented small 1- to 3-mm linear tears in the neointima. Gross examination of specimens 1 month after redilation in

the 4 remaining animals revealed an intact neointima without restenosis, intimal tears, aneurysm formation, or obstruction of side-branch arteries. In one specimen, a small organized thrombus was found on the proximal portion of a stent that protruded freely into the main pulmonary artery.

CLINICAL STUDIES

Most clinical studies of pulmonary artery stenting have used the Palmaz or Palmaz-Genesis (Cordis, Bridgewater, NJ) stainless steel balloon-expandable stent.[80–84] (Figs. 54-18 and 54-19). In their 1991 landmark study, O'Laughlin and colleagues reported the acute and short-term follow-up results of 31 stent implantations in 23 patients with pulmonary artery stenosis.[80] A multi-institutional study of percutaneous stenting in the pediatric population was reported by the same investigators in 1993.[83] A total of 121 Palmaz stents, 80 for branch pulmonary artery stenosis, were implanted in 85 patients, most of whom had undergone repair of tetralogy of Fallot. In this series, stenting resulted in an increase in pulmonary artery diameter from 4.6 to 11.3 mm, with an immediate decrease in right ventricular systolic pressure. A follow-up cardiac catheterization was performed in 25 patients 8 months after stenting, and restenosis was identified in only one patient. These data indicated that pulmonary artery stenting was more effective than balloon angioplasty alone for treating most patients with pulmonary artery stenosis or hypoplasia. In 1995, Fogelman and colleagues[84] demonstrated the clinical benefits derived from pulmonary artery stenting in children with pulmonary artery stenosis. In this large single-institution series, pulmonary artery stenting was shown to result in important hemodynamic improvement, alleviation of symptoms, and deferral of surgical reintervention in many patients. A large series of pulmonary artery stenting in children was reported by McMahon and colleagues in 2002.[85] Over a 12-year period, 664 Palmaz stents were implanted in 338 patients, the majority with repaired tetralogy of Fallot. The mean systolic pressure gradient across the stenosis decreased from 41 to 9 mm Hg, and the mean diameter of the stented vessels more than doubled. At a follow-up of 5.6 years, the pulmonary artery systolic gradient averaged 20 mm Hg and the vessel diameter was 9.3 mm. With improved techniques and increased experience, morbidity and mortality decreased significantly during the second half of this series. The longest follow-up series was reported by Law in 2009,[86] who described the long-term outcome of children who were originally enrolled in the IDE (investigational device exemption) pulmonary artery stent trial approved by the U.S. Food and Drug Administration (FDA) between 1989 and 1992. Their data confirmed the long-term hemodynamic benefits in these children and documented the feasibility of late stent redilation if necessary to accommodate somatic growth. It is important that stents implanted into the pulmonary arteries of children can be safely and effectively redilated to a larger diameter when the child has grown. Reports from several institutions confirm the experimental observations that pulmonary artery stents can be safely redilated to a larger diameter.[83,84,86–89] In 2003, Duke and colleagues,[89] for example, reported safe and effective stent redilation in 12 children with pulmonary artery stenosis. Redilation was required because of a combination of patient growth and neointimal ingrowth within the stents. Redilation increased pulmonary artery stent diameter from 6.9 to 8.8 mm, with an associated decrease in systolic gradient from 24 to 12 mm Hg. The authors concluded that redilation of pulmonary artery stents is effective and relatively safe, as has been confirmed in numerous other series.

CONCLUSIONS AND RECOMMENDATIONS

Experimental and clinical data from several centers indicate that balloon-expandable stenting provides an effective form of therapy for many patients with pulmonary artery stenosis or hypoplasia. Because balloon angioplasty alone is unsuccessful in as many as 50% to 60% of patients, stenting is now considered standard first-line therapy for most children with pulmonary artery stenosis. If at all possible,

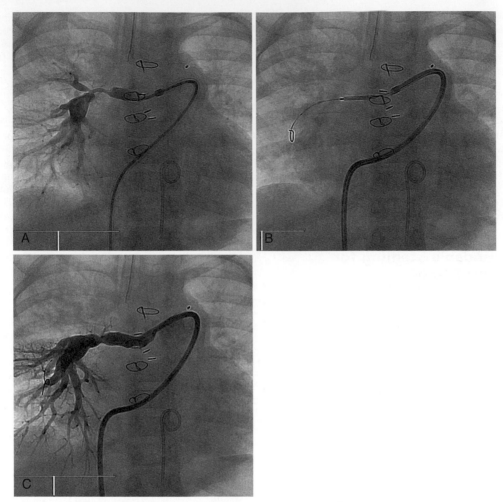

Figure 54-18 Anteroposterior pulmonary artery angiograms before (A), during (B), and after (C) right pulmonary artery stenting in a 5-month-old infant after repair of pulmonary atresia and ventricular septal defect. There is severe proximal right pulmonary artery stenosis prior to stenting. After stent implantation, there is improvement in the stenosis, but a small upper lobe branch has been jailed.

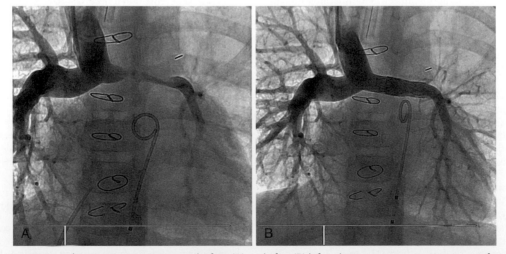

Figure 54-19 Anteroposterior pulmonary artery angiogram before (A) and after (B) left pulmonary artery stenting in an infant with hypoplastic left heart syndrome and left pulmonary artery hypoplasia. Angiography prior to stenting (A) demonstrates diffuse hypoplasia of the proximal left and central pulmonary artery. Following stenting with two balloon-expandable stents (B), there is significant improvement in the pulmonary artery diameter and flow. The patient has a bidirectional Glenn shunt (SVC-to-PA anastomosis).

implanted stents should have the capacity for later redilation when the child has grown. In infants and small children in whom larger stents may be difficult to implant, angioplasty alone may be preferable in an attempt to avoid implanting smaller stents which have a limited potential to expand with growth.

Balloon-Expandable Stenting for Coarctation of the Aorta

Coarctation of the aorta accounts for 8% to 10% of all congenital heart disease. Since the 1940s, surgical repair has been a conventional therapy for patients with a native (unoperated) or recurrent postoperative coarctation. Coarctation balloon angioplasty has been available since the mid-1980s, but its effectiveness has been diminished by restenosis (15%–20% of patients) and aneurysm formation (approximately 5% of patients). Therefore balloon-expandable stenting has emerged as the newest transcatheter therapy for coarctation. A stent's radial strength opposes elastic aortic wall recoil and may improve vessel integrity, thereby decreasing the risk of aneurysm formation at the dilation site. The availability of covered stents may provide an even safer therapy for coarctation in patients with a vulnerable aortic wall, such as in Turner's syndrome, or in older adults.

ANIMAL STUDIES

Our lab and others have reported acute effectiveness of balloon-expandable stenting in experimental models of coarctation.[90,91] A follow-up study in 6 dogs 1 to 1.5 months after stent implantation documented an excellent early result without restenosis, stent thrombosis, aneurysm formation, or stent migration.[90] Evaluation of explanted segments of the stented aorta demonstrated that the stents were thoroughly covered by a neointima composed of intimal cells with fibrosis and an endothelial cell surface (Fig. 54-20). Neointimal

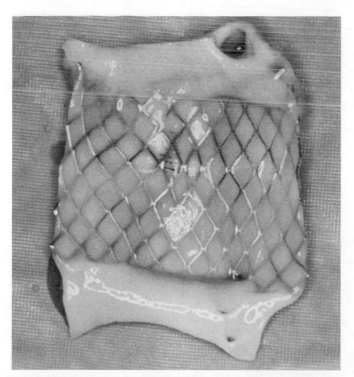

Figure 54-20 Aortic stent explanted 6 weeks after stenting of an experimental coarctation in a canine model. The Palmaz P-308 stainless steel stent is nearly completely covered with a thin layer of neointima. The sutures used to create the experimental coarctation are evident.

coverage was absent only where side-branch arteries, such as intercostals, arose from the aorta. As is the case with stent implantation in pulmonary arteries of children, stents implanted in the aorta of growing children may require redilation after a period of somatic growth. Limited animal data document the effectiveness and safety of coarctation stent redilation. In 1996, our group[79] reported data in a small experimental study of coarctation stent redilation. An experimental coarctation was surgically created in 8 puppies, and stent implantation (Palmaz P308) was performed at 2 to 3 months. Stent redilation was subsequently performed after 6 to 10 months in 7 animals, increasing the stenosis diameter from 9.8 to 13.5 mm. Redilation was effective in 5 animals, but aortic rupture through the stent resulted in the deaths of 2. In contrast, Morrow and colleagues reported data on aortic stent redilation in two experimental studies with relative safety and no acute animal deaths.[91,92]

CLINICAL STUDIES

Numerous clinical studies in the past decade have documented the effectiveness and relative safety of transcatheter stenting of coarctation of the aorta.[93-103] Stent therapy can benefit patients with a native unoperated coarctation or with a recurrent postoperative coarctation with equal effectiveness (Figs. 54-21 and 54-22). Most interventionalists attempt to limit stenting to older children and adolescents so as to maximize initial implant diameter and minimize the need for later stent redilation after somatic growth has occurred. In most reported series, balloon-expandable bare metal stents have been utilized. More recently, use of the covered CP platinum stent (Fig. 54-23) (currently available in the United States only in clinical trials or under compassionate use approval) has been reported; it may be particularly effective for stenting of complex coarctation anatomy or in patients in whom the aortic wall may be more fragile, as with advancing age.[104] In 1999, Suarez deLezo and colleagues reported one of the larger early clinical series of coarctation stenting.[94] Stainless steel balloon-expandable stents were implanted in 48 patients (mean age 14 years) with coarctation of the aorta. Follow-up cardiac catheterization performed in 30 patients 2 years following stent implantation documented excellent relief of stenosis, with a residual systolic coarctation gradient of 3 mm Hg. Angiography identified a mild degree of neointimal ingrowth within the stent in 27% of patients. A small aneurysm at the stent site was identified in 2 patients (7%), and both aneurysms were occluded by coil implantation through the stent. Harrison and colleagues[97] reported outcomes following coarctation stenting in 27 adolescent and adult patients. At follow-up evaluation 1.8 years later, the residual systolic gradient was 4 mm Hg, and 9 patients had been weaned from antihypertension medications. In this series, stenting complications included a cerebrovascular accident in 1 patient and an aortic aneurysm at the stent site in 3 patients (11%). The largest reported series of coarctation stenting to date was reported in 2007 by Forbes for the Congenital Cardiovascular Interventional Study Consortium of 17 institutions.[100,101] In this report, 555 patients underwent stenting for native (52.3%) or recurrent postoperative coarctation. A successful treatment outcome was achieved in 97.9% of cases, with the systolic pressure gradient decreasing from 32 to 3 mm Hg acutely. Complications included aortic wall injury (dissection or rupture) in 1.6% of procedures, stent migration in 5%, and cerebral vascular accident in 0.7%. There were 2 mortalities after emergent surgery for severe aortic wall injury (1 a coarctation stent and 1 an interposition graft stent). The authors identified an increased risk of aortic wall pathology in follow-up if the balloon : coarctation diameter ratio exceeded 3.5. Advanced patient age has also been found to increase the risk of aortic dissection during coarctation stenting.[105] In these patients, the primary use of a covered stent may prove to be beneficial. Transcatheter stent therapy may provide a reasonable treatment strategy for anatomical variations of coarctation that pose difficult surgical dilemmas. For example, hypoplasia of the transverse aortic arch is responsible for residual obstruction in a small proportion of patients after surgical coarctation repair. These lesions may be difficult to manage

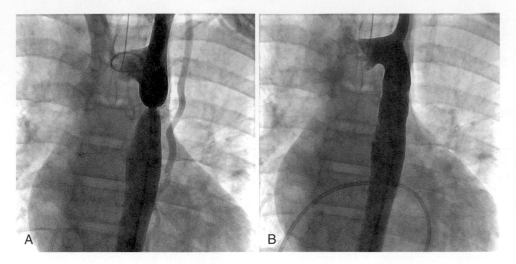

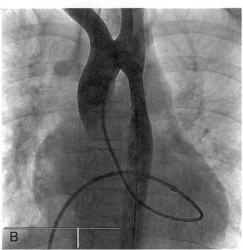

Figure 54-21 Anteroposterior aortogram before (A) and after stenting (B) in a 14-year-old teenager with a discrete native (unoperated) coarctation of the aorta. Prior to stenting (A) there is a severe stenosis and a systolic gradient of 41 mm Hg was measured. After stenting (B) with a balloon-expandable stainless steel stent dilated to a diameter of 16 mm, the pressure gradient was entirely eliminated.

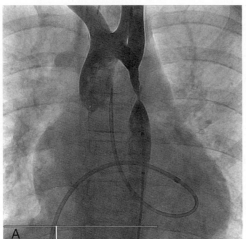

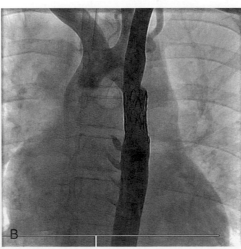

Figure 54-22 Anteroposterior aortogram before (A) and after stenting (B) in an 11-year-old teenager with a severe native coarctation of the aorta. Prior to stenting (A) there is a severe stenosis that measured approximately 2 mm in diameter. The coarctation was stented (B) with a bare metal stainless steel stent intentionally dilated to a subtherapeutic diameter (8 mm) in an attempt to avoid undue aortic wall trauma. The gradient decreased from 31 to 10 mm Hg.

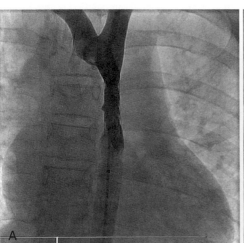

Figure 54-23 Anteroposterior aortogram, 10 months after bare metal stenting of a severe coarctation, in the same patient as in Figure 54-22. The initial angiogram (A) demonstrates a small saccular aneurysm on the medial aspect of the stented area. After stenting with a covered Cheatham platinum stent (B), under compassionate use approval, the aneurysm is excluded and the residual coarctation stenosis is relieved. Contrast reflux into several intercostal arteries is evident.

surgically, as the operative procedure often requires a period of hypothermic circulatory arrest. Pihkala and colleagues[106] reported the successful use of stent therapy in 4 children with transverse arch hypoplasia. The procedure was successful in all of these cases, with anatomical and hemodynamic relief of arch obstruction. We have also utilized stenting in several infants with complex aortic arch obstruction after the Norwood operation for hypoplastic left heart syndrome. In these infants a relatively large stent (Palmaz P188, P308, or Palmaz-Genesis 1910) was implanted via a right carotid cutdown and successfully relieved important arch obstruction. The carotid cutdown approach was utilized to avoid potential femoral artery injury associated with the relatively large sheath (8 Fr) required to deliver such stents. Mild coarctation (i.e., resting systolic gradient <20 mm Hg) has also posed a therapeutic dilemma in the past because it was often thought that the benefits did not outweigh the risks of surgery, which may require partial bypass due to poorly developed collateral circulation with mild coarctation. Nevertheless, more recent data suggest that mild coarctation may be associated with long-term rest and exercise hypertension and perhaps left ventricular hypertrophy and diastolic dysfunction. Marshall and colleagues[95] have reported the results of stent treatment in 33 patients, many of whom had a mild coarctation by traditional criteria. Stent implantation decreased the systolic gradient from 25 to 5 mm Hg. At follow-up catheterization, left ventricular end-diastolic pressure had decreased from 17 to 14 mm Hg, suggesting an improvement in diastolic function. These data suggest that nonsurgical intervention for even mild degrees of coarctation may have beneficial effects on cardiovascular function. Larger clinical studies, with longer follow-up and more sensitive measures of ventricular function are required to determine the true benefit of coarctation stenting for such patients.

CONCLUSIONS AND RECOMMENDATIONS

Coarctation stenting is an effective, relatively new approach to native and postoperative recurrent coarctation of the aorta. Most pediatric interventionalists limit stent implantation for coarctation to large children and adolescents in order to avoid the need for aortic stent redilation when a smaller child has grown. Stent implantation is a promising intervention for more difficult variations on coarctation anatomy, particularly transverse arch hypoplasia, arch obstruction after the Norwood operation, and mild degrees of coarctation that have not warranted surgery in the past. In older adults where the aortic wall is friable, covered stents may provide a safer alternative because of the increased risk of aortic dissection with coarctation dilation. Longer term follow-up studies are necessary to more precisely define the late risks of stent restenosis, aortic aneurysm formation, the safety of late stent redilation after somatic growth in children, and blood pressure response to exercise in the face of a rigid, stented aortic segment.

Transcatheter Closure of the Secundum Atrial Septal Defect

Atrial septal defects (ASDs) result from deficient development of the intra-atrial septum. The exact position of the defect is determined by the specific area of the septum that fails to develop. Sinus venosus defects result from abnormal development of either the superior or inferior horns of the sinus venosus and are located superiorly or inferiorly along the posterior margin of the atrial septum. Superior sinus venosus defects frequently have associated anomalous drainage of the right upper pulmonary vein. Primum ASDs result from deficiencies of the septum secundum, frequently as part of the complex of maldevelopment of the endocardial cushions (atrioventricular canal [AVC] defects). In the most severe form (complete AVC), the primum defect is part of a complex that also includes an inlet ventricular septal defect (VSD) and a common atrioventricular valve. In the least severe form, the primum ASD defect is associated with a cleft in the anterior mitral valve leaflet. Secundum ASDs result from deficiencies of the central portion of the atrial septum, the septum primum. These defects, usually in the region of the fossa ovalis, may be extensive in size, varied in shape, and often multiple in number (fenestrated atrial septum). It is only the secundum type of defect that is suitable for percutaneous device closure. Further discussion in this section focuses on secundum ASDs.

PHYSIOLOGY

Atrial septal defects represent one of the most common forms of acyanotic congenital heart disease.[107] The direction and magnitude of shunt flow across the atrial septum is determined in large part by the end-diastolic pressure within each ventricle, which in turn is reflective of relative ventricular compliance. The net size of the atrial-level shunt is thus only in part dependent on the size of the ASD. It is also important to realize that abnormal elevation of either left or right ventricular systolic pressure in the face of ventricular outflow tract obstruction will not affect atrial-level shunting unless ventricular relaxation is adversely affected. With persistence of atrial level shunting, the right atrial and right ventricular (RV) end-diastolic volumes are increased.[107] Augmented RV volume will result in delayed pulmonary valve closure compared with the aortic valve (causing the clinical sign of a fixed, split second heart sound) and also a flow murmur across a normal pulmonary valve (identical to that of pathological pulmonary valve stenosis but never with a thrill or an ejection click).[108] The increased pulmonary blood flow is well tolerated in most cases but can lead to RV dysfunction and/or pulmonary hypertension in some cases. In these patients Eisenmenger-type physiology will prevail, at which point shunt flow becomes right to left and the patient becomes cyanotic.[109,110]

CLINICAL PRESENTATION AND DIAGNOSIS

ASDs are typically asymptomatic during the first two decades of life. Diagnosis is most often made after detection of a murmur, similar to that of pulmonary valve stenosis, or a fixed split second heart sound.[108] Infrequently, infants or children may present with failure to thrive or recurrent lower respiratory tract infections. Later, if left untreated, in the third and fourth decades of life, symptoms may include fatigue, dyspnea on exertion, and a frequent sensation of palpitations.[107,110] The electrocardiogram (ECG) may be normal early in childhood or at any age if right atrial enlargement (RAE) or right ventricular dilation (RVD) have not yet occurred. As those changes progress over time, typical ECG changes of right axis deviation, RAE, and RVD become more clearly apparent. Echocardiography (transthoracic [TTE] or transesophageal [TEE]) remains the mainstay of diagnosis.[11] The first evidence that an ASD is present is often the detection of RV dilation in the short-axis and four-chamber views. However, the ASD itself is best imaged and evaluated from subcostal views in both long and short axis. These views allow for complete evaluation of the total septal length and provide excellent visualization of the defect margins. Color-flow mapping is of great importance. It allows determination of the direction of flow across the defect (left to right versus right to left) and provides further assessment to exclude the possibility of multiple defects (Fig. 54-24). If transthoracic images are poor, a TEE should be performed to confirm the diagnosis of an ASD and prior to further discussion regarding possible defect closure and repair.[112] Echocardiography is also invaluable in achieving a noninvasive measure of RV and pulmonary artery pressures and excluding the presence of associated defects such as partial anomalous pulmonary venous return.

TREATMENT AND OUTCOME

Surgical repair has long been the mainstay of treatment for ASDs of all types.[109,110,113] However, major advances have been made with percutaneous closure devices. Currently, percutaneous closure of secundum ASDs is clearly the standard of care for most defects.[114-116] In the United States, two devices are approved for use by the FDA: (1) The Amplatzer Septal Occluder (AGA Medical, Golden Valley MN) and (2)

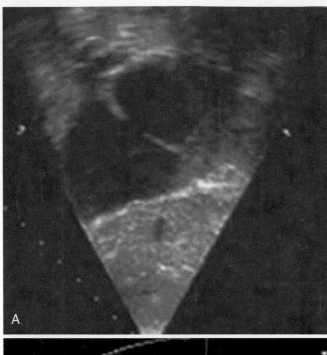

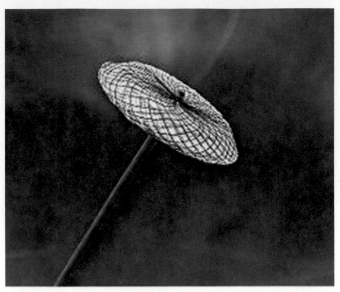

Figure 54-25 Amplatzer septal occluder. The device is constructed from an alloy of nickel and titanium. The two atrial discs are separated by the central waist. In this photograph, the tethering cable, covered by the delivery sheath, remains attached to the device. *(Image courtesy of AGA Medical, Golden Valley, MN.)*

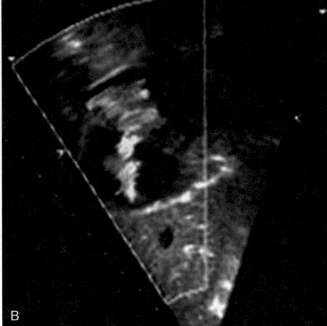

Figure 54-24 Subcostal short axis transthoracic echocardiographic images showing a secundum atrial septal defect in two dimensions (A) and with color-flow mapping (B). The defect is central in the septum and has excellent margins for device support.

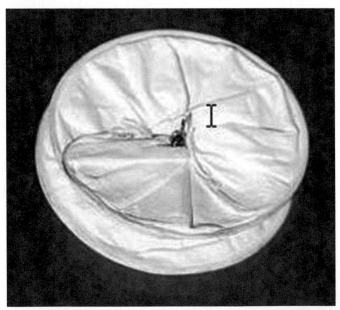

Figure 54-26 The Helix septal occluder. The device is composed of a nickel-titanium wire with a patch of microporous expanded polytetra-fluoroethylene attached along its length. The elastic properties of the wire form the device into two equal-sized opposing disks that reside on either side of the atrial septum after deployment, thus occluding the defect. *(Image courtesy of W. L. Gore and Associates, Flagstaff, AZ.)*

the Helex Septal Occluder (W. L. Gore and Associates, Flagstaff, AZ).[117,118] While different in design, the principles of function, deployment, and follow-up are similar for the two devices (Figs. 54-25 and 54-26). After deployment, both devices are designed to have two disks connected by a central core or waist. One disk is positioned on the left atrial side of the ASD, with the core or waist straddling the defect, and the other is opposed to the atrial septum from the right atrial side of the defect. The devices have intrinsic recoil that pulls both disks together, holding the devices securely in place on the atrial septum. Regardless of the device used, defect sizing is required prior to deployment. Reliance may be placed on the echocardiographic measurements

with an empirical adjustment (e.g., 115% of the TTE measurement). However, most operators continue to rely on balloon sizing of the defect before choosing a particular-sized device.[115,116] Balloon sizing is accomplished using a large, compliant balloon inflated across the atrial septum, with the narrowest area ("stretched diameter" or "waist") measured with angiographic calibration (Fig. 54-27). A device size is then chosen accordingly. Irrespective of the measurements, it is imperative that the device be sized to ensure that the margins of both

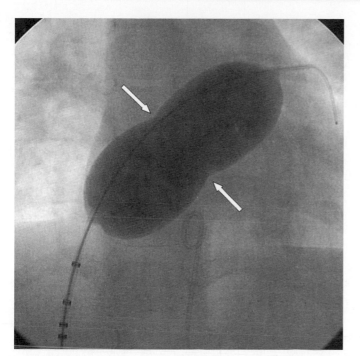

Figure 54-27 Still-frame of an angiogram demonstrating inflation of the balloon sizing catheter across the atrial septum. The indentations on the balloon (white arrows) indicate the stretched margin of the atrial septal defect. That diameter is measured, and an appropriate-sized septal occluder is chosen accordingly.

the left and right atrial disks are sufficiently large that, once deployed, the device remains stable on the atrial septum; however, it should not be so large that other cardiac structures (such as pulmonary veins, coronary sinus, or atrioventricular valves) are impinged upon. Both devices are deployed though a delivery sheath that is typically introduced percutaneously through a femoral vein, although other access sites have been utilized. The left atrial disk is initially deployed and the device then pulled back onto the atrial septum. The remainder of the device is then deployed within the right atrium, so that the waist or core of the device straddles the defect. The delivery cable remains attached to the device until the time of release and can be used to withdraw the device if positioning is not acceptable (Fig. 54-28). Even after release, the devices can be retrieved with various intravascular snares if that should become necessary. To ensure adequate device deployment, echocardiographic imaging is utilized in addition to fluoroscopy.[111] The majority of pediatric institutions continue to utilize TEE, but intracardiac echocardiography (ICE) is also commonly employed. This avoids the necessity of general anesthesia in most patients, but an additional 8-Fr femoral venous access site is required for insertion of the ICE probe. Deployment of the devices using echocardiography alone has also been described.[112] Three-dimensional echocardiographic imaging is increasingly used to guide device placement.[119] This modality provides an en face view of the septum and may offer the interventionalist a better understanding of the true shape and size and location of the defect. Percutaneous device closure has proven effective in repairing ASDs with minimal morbidity and effectively no mortality. Closure rates are comparable to those following surgical repair (97%-99% at 12 months), but procedural morbidity is considerably lower.[114,120] Percutaneous closure avoids the necessity of a sternotomy, cardiopulmonary bypass, and mediastinal and chest-tube drainage, but it does have the disadvantage of exposure to ionizing radiation. The risk of device embolization is small and in most cases related to operator inexperience. The incidence of this complication is in the region of 0.1%.[115,116] The majority of acute complications have been related to rhythm disturbances, in most cases atrial flutter or

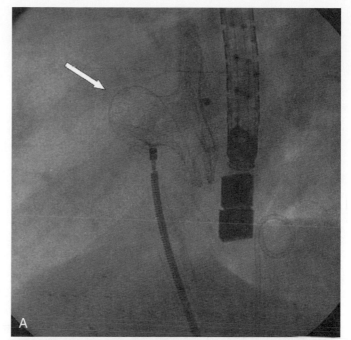

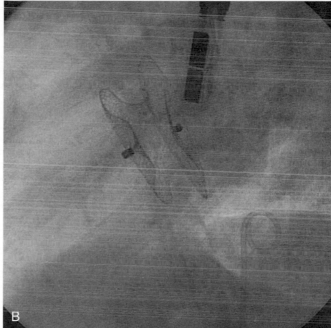

Figure 54-28 Still-frame lateral image (A) demonstrating full deployment of an Amplatzer Septal Occluder with the cable still attached. Distortion of the superior margin of the right atrial disk of the device (solid white arrow), resulting from downward tension by the delivery cable, is typical at this point of deployment. Retraction and redeployment of the device is easily achieved while still attached to the delivery cable. A transesophageal echo probe is noted in the image. (B) Still-frame lateral image after release of the Amplatzer Septal Occluder from the delivery cable. The septal occluder immediately assumes the typical position, with both the right and left atrial disks parallel to each other.

intermittent supraventricular tachycardia. However, these complications are also rare, occurring less than 1% of the time. Thrombus formation on the device, with distal embolization, is of great concern, justifying the recommendation for aspirin therapy until device endothelialization has occurred.[121] Collective review of this potential problem, including evaluation of various generations of early septal occluder devices, reveals a low incidence of thrombotic complications (54 patients over a 14-year period). Cardiac erosion with possible hemodynamic compromise, particularly by the Amplatzer septal occluder, is the most significant short- and long-term complication of percutaneous ASD closure.[122,123] The incidence appears to be low (<0.11%), according to both the manufacturer and published data, and in the majority of cases may be related to device oversizing.[122] The recognition of this rare complication has altered follow-up, with the general recommendation to obtain an echocardiogram within 24 hours of implantation to rule out the presence of a new pericardial effusion that could signal the presence of an erosion.

FOLLOW-UP

After device implantation, patients remain on aspirin for at least 6 months, during which time device endothelialization occurs. Antibiotic prophylaxis against bacterial endocarditis is also recommended during that period and should be continued if residual atrial-level shunting is apparent on the echocardiogram at 6 months. After that, follow-up should be at least on an annual basis, with echocardiography obtained during those visits. The right atrial and ventricular dimensions return to normal within 6 months if no significant atrial level shunting remains.[124]

Transcatheter Closure of the Patent Ductus Arteriosus

The ductus arteriosus is a muscular artery that extends from the roof of the main pulmonary artery to the undersurface of the aortic arch. While some degree of anatomical variation does occur (as with a right aortic arch, when the ductus passes from the main pulmonary artery to the base of the left innominate artery), the anatomical position is generally consistent. The ductus provides a vital function during fetal life, allowing blood ejected by the right ventricle to bypass the lungs and instead be redirected into the descending aorta. Shortly after birth, with an increase in arterial oxygen content and a decrease in circulating prostaglandins, the ductus arteriosus spasms, closes, and later becomes fibrotic with permanent closure. Persistence of the ductus arteriosus beyond the newborn period occurs in 1 in 2,500 to 5,000 live births.[125] After closure, the ductus arteriosus has no further significance unless a right aortic arch with an aberrant left subclavian artery is present; a vascular ring could then prove clinically significant.

PHYSIOLOGY

Discussion regarding the influence of the patent ductus arteriosus (PDA) on the physiology of the neonate, particularly with regard to prematurity and hyaline membrane disease, is beyond the scope of this text. This discussion is therefore confined to the effect of the PDA on older children and adults, where the impact is similar. The main factors contributing to the effects of a PDA are the size of the ductus and relative resistances of the systemic and pulmonary vascular beds. When these beds are anatomically small, the hemodynamic effect of a PDA is negligible, with flow occurring only during systole and limited by the resistance to flow through the narrow ductus itself. With a large PDA, flow through the ductus will be left to right as long as the pulmonary vascular resistance is lower than the systemic resistance, even in the presence of a completely unrestrictive PDA. Under these circumstances, pulmonary artery pressures are equal to aortic, and the flow is left to right during both systole and diastole. With a large left-to-right ductal shunt, the left atrium and ventricle become volume-loaded and dilated. Further, owing to this increased runoff into a lower-resistance pulmonary vascular bed, the aortic pulse pressure (difference between the aortic systolic and diastolic pressures) will widen considerably. With continued LV dilation, wall stress and end-diastolic pressures will continue to increase, in turn increasing the myocardial oxygen requirement. With the decrease in aortic diastolic pressure, coronary perfusion pressure can sometimes become

diminished substantially. Like other shunt lesions that expose the pulmonary vascular bed to persistently high pressure and flow, untreated large PDAs will ultimately result in the development of pulmonary vascular occlusive disease.[126] At that time, flow direction across the PDA will reverse, and Eisenmenger physiology will prevail.[127] Development of those changes will depend on the ductal size and duration of its presence, resistance to flow across the vessel, and individual patient susceptibility.

CLINICAL PRESENTATION AND DIAGNOSIS

In infancy and childhood, the clinical presentation of PDA may vary from a completely asymptomatic child to the full spectrum of congestive heart failure. Symptoms may thus be absent, but with larger shunts they can include failure to thrive, dyspnea, poor feeding, and excessive perspiration. In older children, adolescents, and adults, congestive symptoms are less likely. It is not uncommon for the diagnosis to be suspected when a murmur is heard during a well-child examination. Rarely, patients who have not been diagnosed in infancy may present with symptoms of endocarditis or pulmonary vascular occlusive disease if the PDA is sufficiently unrestrictive. Clinical signs may be absent if the PDA is small and hemodynamically insignificant. However, with increasing size of the PDA, more typical clinical features become apparent. The pulse pressure may be wide (by palpation and blood pressure measurement) and a murmur, of variable grade and duration, may be heard. If the PDA is small, flow may occur only during systole and a systolic murmur will be present. With a larger PDA, flow will occur throughout the entire cardiac cycle and the classic harsh, continuous machinery murmur will be present. If shunt flow is substantial, a middiastolic mitral flow murmur may also be audible. If a large PDA is present for years, the continuous murmur may disappear as pulmonary vascular resistance increases and pulmonary vascular obstructive disease develops. If the shunt reverses (to right to left), Eisenmenger physiology occurs, and oxygen saturations measured in the lower extremities will be lower than those in the upper extremities.[128] Confirmation of the diagnosis relies on echocardiography. The PDA is well seen in many different views, but the parasternal short-axis view, immediately above the level of the pulmonary valve, is ideal. If the PDA is small, two-dimensional imaging may not be helpful; in these cases color-flow mapping in the main pulmonary artery reveals a high-velocity jet occurring in an opposite direction to the antegrade flow of the pulmonary artery. Caution should be used to avoid confusing a pulmonary insufficiency color jet from that of the PDA. Doppler interrogation of the ductal flow can also help in determining the degree of stenosis across the PDA, and therefore in estimating the pulmonary artery pressure.

TREATMENT AND OUTCOME

During the past two decades, percutaneous therapy for the patient with an isolated PDA has become the standard of care at most pediatric institutions in the United States.[129] The exception to this is in the premature neonate or those patients in early infancy with particularly large, hemodynamically important lesions. In these cases, surgical therapy is still routine. Surgical PDA repair is performed via the left lateral thoracotomy approach. Usually, the PDA is identified and ligated. A chest tube drain remains in place for a brief period after surgery, and hospitalization lasts for 3 to 4 days. The most significant but fortunately very rare complication involves inadvertent ligation of the left pulmonary artery or descending aorta in a small infant, often with catastrophic outcomes. More commonly, there is low morbidity related to recurrent laryngeal nerve injury, pleural effusions, and wound and skin infections. Pain and discomfort are not insignificant, and in most cases opioid analgesics are required in the first 24 hours. There is also a low incidence of ductal recanalization with ligation (as opposed to ductal division). Transcatheter device closure of the PDA has now been available for close to 30 years. Different methods have been available during this time, but with the evolution of improved device technology and operator technique, two categories of devices

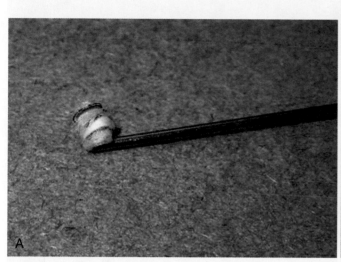
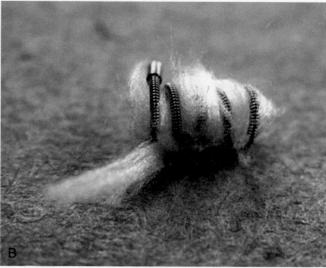

Figure 54-29 Partial (A) and full (B) extrusion of a Gianturco coil from its delivery sleeve. The coil has polyester fibers attached that promote thrombosis once deployed.

are currently in use: coils and occluder devices. Given the differences in their design and delivery, these are discussed separately below.

Coils

Stainless steel Gianturco coils (Cook, Bloomington, IN) of various thicknesses, lengths, and loop diameters were initially available and approved for general vascular occlusion (Fig. 54-29). The use of these coils for small PDA closure[130–132] began in the early 1990s; since then, different techniques for their safe delivery and variations on the initial design and delivery have been reported. Generally, after diagnostic angiography of the PDA is complete, a coil of the appropriate size is chosen. The PDA deemed ideal for coil closure should narrow significantly along its course (to <2 mm), be sufficiently long to accommodate the multiple loops of the coil, and have a sufficient aortic ductal diverticulum. In that way, once deployed, the loops of the coil on the aortic end of the PDA will not cause flow disturbance in the proximal descending aorta. Gianturco coils are delivered in a retrograde manner from the aortic end of the duct. Once the delivery catheter (often a Judkins right coronary catheter) has crossed the PDA, approximately two-thirds of a coil loop is extruded beyond the catheter tip (within the main pulmonary artery) using pusher wire of the appropriate diameter. The entire catheter-coil complex is then slowly withdrawn until the partially extruded coil is seen to "catch" on the narrow PA orifice of the duct. At that point, the delivery catheter is withdrawn back over the pusher wire into the aorta, with the coil held statically in place. As the catheter is withdrawn, the body of the coil straddles the length of the PDA until it is completely extruded from the delivery catheter when it springs back into the aortic ductal ampulla and coils appropriately (Fig. 54-30). With correct delivery, approximately two-thirds of a coil loop should remain on the pulmonary end of the PDA, a portion of the coil straddles the narrow section, and the remaining loops of coil are tightly looped within the aortic ampulla. Repeat aortic angiography is performed to confirm appropriate coil placement and complete closure. Adverse events related to PDA coil embolization have led to modifications, both of coil design and the delivery method. Detachable coils (Cook, Bloomington, IN) utilize a screw mechanism on a modified Gianturco coil that allows repositioning and retrieval if initial coil positioning is incorrect.[133,134] However, that modification has not completely alleviated the risk of coil embolization after deployment. Snare techniques to control coil delivery have also been described.[135] Once the initial loop of coil is advanced into the main pulmonary artery and prior to retraction of the delivery catheter back into the aorta, a goose neck-type snare is positioned on the coil to maintain control at the time of delivery. While this procedure may be

successful in experienced hands, greater coordination between the primary catheterizer and the assistant is necessary. Some difficulty in releasing the snare from the coil after complete delivery may also cause coil displacement after an initial apparently successful coil delivery. Multiple simultaneous coil deployment has also been used to close large PDAs.[136] However, with the advent of the larger duct occluder devices, this has become largely unnecessary. Generally, coil occlusion has been successful in occluding small PDAs, with closure rates between 95% and 100% at 2 years.[137,138] Ductal size has been shown to be the single most important factor in predicting complete early and late closure with coils. Small high-velocity residual shunts through ductal coils may cause hemolysis with resulting anemia.[139] In most cases, this resolves within 72 hours; if not, a repeat catheterization with additional coil placement may be necessary. Early experience with coil occlusion was also associated with rare mild stenosis of the left pulmonary artery or descending aorta.[140] However, with refinement of techniques and appropriate patient selection for coil placement, this is of less clinical concern in the current era of PDA closure. Two further modifications of PDA coil closure devices bear mention. The first is the Gianturco-Grifka Vascular Occlusion Device (GGVOD) (Cook, Bloomington, IN).[141] It allows delivery of a large Gianturco coil into a previously extruded bag. This is of use in selected instances, as when the PDA is unusually large or tubular, with no stenotic areas. The GGVOD has the theoretical advantage of conforming to the shape of the vessel; it can also be retracted and repositioned if necessary. The second device is the Nit-Occlud PDA occluder (pfm AG, Köln, Germany).[142] This is a preloaded nitinol coil that is positioned across the PDA. It is designed for larger vessel occlusion and will conform to different PDA shapes. As it is deployed, it assumes a tight, conical shape that straddles the PDA and results in obstruction to flow. Closure rates with this device have been similar to those of the other coil and device closure options.[143]

Ductal Occluder Devices

Currently, the only noncoil device approved by the FDA is the Amplatzer ductal occluder (AGA Medical, Golden Valley, MN).[144,145] This is a mushroom-shaped nitinol device that tapers from an edge ("cap") of larger circumference to conform to the ductal ampulla (Fig. 54-31). The device is delivered through a sheath via an antegrade transvenous approach and has a delivery cable that remains attached until release. The cable can be used for retraction and repositioning of the device if necessary. Once the delivery sheath has been placed across the PDA with its tip in the proximal descending aorta, the ductal occluder is advanced until its larger aortic cap opens in the aorta. The device-sheath complex is then pulled back until the cap is

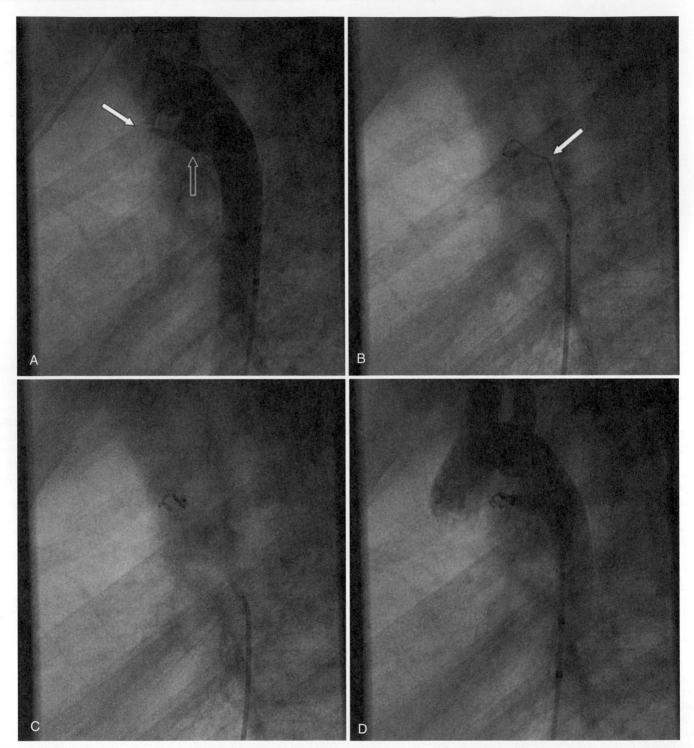

Figure 54-30   A. Still-frame lateral aortogram showing a small patent ductus arteriosus. The narrowed pulmonary artery end (solid white arrow) and the aortic ductal diverticulum are clearly shown. B. The coil has been partially deployed, with the initial loop placed within the pulmonary artery end. The body of the coil (solid white arrow) elongates as the delivery catheter is retracted back into the proximal descending aorta. C. The entire coil has been released. The body of the coil has sprung back and looped within the aortic ductal diverticulum. D. Still-frame lateral aortogram after coil occlusion of the PDA. No further shunting is seen across the coiled PDA.

positioned in the ductal ampulla. At that point, the delivery cable and device remain in place as the sheath is pulled back to deploy the remainder of the device within the body of the PDA. Repeat angiography is then performed to ensure adequate positioning of the device prior to final release of the device from its delivery cable (Fig. 54-32). This Amplatzer ductal occluder has proven to be highly

effective in closing moderate- and large-sized PDAs, with complete closure rates exceeding 98% at 6 to 12 months.[145] This device has also shown a very low rate of complications, with few serious adverse events. Similar concerns regarding left pulmonary artery or aortic coarctation apply, particularly in small infants, but in practice this has not been of particularly great concern.[144,145] Hemolysis occurring

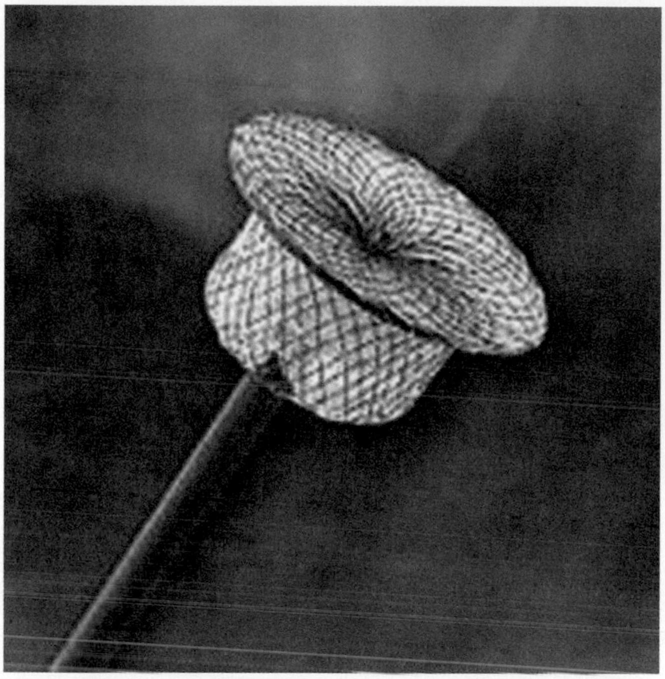

Figure 54-31 Amplatzer duct occluder. The device is constructed from an alloy of nickel and titanium. The larger end with the cap is designed to be placed on the aortic end of the PDA within the ductal diverticulum. The other end tapers slightly and houses the screw thread for placement of the delivery cable. This image shows the device attached to the delivery cable and the delivery sheath. (Image courtesy of AGA Medical, Golden Valley, MN.)

immediately after delivery of Amplatzer occluder devices has also been described only rarely, but it has either been self-limiting or has resolved with coil placement within the device.[146] Modifications of the Amplatzer ductal occluder device (ADO II) are currently being evaluated in clinical trials in the United States but are approved for use in many European countries. The design modifications theoretically allow for improved conformation of the device to the aortic and pulmonary ends of the ductus and enable the device to be delivered through guiding catheters without requiring the use of long sheaths.[147–149]

FOLLOW-UP

Anticoagulation is not required after PDA occlusion with coils or other devices. SBE prophylaxis remains indicated for at least the first 6 months and as long as residual PDA shunting is present through the device. Follow-up echocardiography should be performed at least 6 months after PDA closure; thereafter, if no murmur is present, further testing may not be necessary.

■ Transcatheter Pulmonary Valve Replacement (within Existing RV-PA Conduits)

Placement of an RVOT valved conduit is common in surgical palliation of congenital heart disease such as tetralogy of Fallot (TOF), truncus arteriosus, some forms of transposition, and aortic valve disease requiring the Ross procedure. Common long-term limitations to these conduits include recurrent stenosis and valve regurgitation. There is strong evidence that such conduit dysfunction can be associated with exercise intolerance, arrhythmias, and an increased risk of late sudden death.[150,151] There is also evidence to show that intervention on a dysfunctional RVOT conduit can stop or even reverse the risk of these adverse outcomes.[152–154] The long-established standard of care for

clinically important conduit stenosis or regurgitation is reoperation involving cardiopulmonary bypass and its attendant risks. Such patients face a lifetime of repeat operations to replace or repair their RVOT conduits.[155,156]

Percutaneous pulmonary valve replacement within an existing dysfunctional RVOT conduit is one of the newest transcatheter interventions for structural heart disease. The goal of this novel therapy is to prolong the interval between surgical conduit replacements with the intention to reduce the total number of open heart operations required over the lifetime of a patient. Percutaneous pulmonary valve implantation was introduced in the year 2000 by Bonhoeffer and colleagues.[157,158] This technology was subsequently acquired by Medtronic (Minneapolis, MN) and marketed as the Melody Transcatheter Pulmonary Valve and the Ensemble Delivery System (Figs. 54-33 and 54-34). In 2010, Medtronic received HDE (humanitarian device exemption) approval from the FDA to market the device in the United States. It has been used in other countries since approximately 2006; as of June 2011, approximately 2500 patients in over 170 centers worldwide have been treated with the Melody valve.

PHYSIOLOGY

RVOT obstruction is common in native as well as repaired congenital heart disease. Patients who undergo surgical repair that involves the placement of an RV-PA valved conduit require long-term monitoring (including echocardiography and cardiac magnetic resonance imaging [MRI]) to detect conduit dysfunction, specifically stenosis and/or regurgitation, which eventually occurs in the majority. Conduit stenosis has similar physiology to native pulmonary valve stenosis. There is an increase in RV systolic pressure directly related to the severity of the stenosis and the RV stroke volume. This elevated RV systolic pressure stimulates myocardial hypertrophy and, over time, also fibrosis. Eventually, if it is not relieved, severe stenosis will result in RV systolic and diastolic dysfunction and failure. If there is an associated atrial-level communication, the patient will become increasingly cyanotic as a right-to-left atrial shunt develops in response to the decreased RV compliance associated with progressive myocardial hypertrophy and fibrosis. Similarly, the physiology of conduit valve insufficiency can be compared with that of native pulmonary valve insufficiency. It results in an increased volume load on the RV that causes dilation and can eventually lead to the development of myocardial systolic and diastolic dysfunction. If left untreated, RV-PA conduit stenosis and insufficiency can also lead to LV dysfunction secondary to septal shift and adverse ventricular/ventricular interactions.[159]

CLINICAL PRESENTATION AND DIAGNOSIS

Patients with RV-PA conduit stenosis and/or insufficiency may be detected early by the presence of a systolic and/or diastolic murmur respectively, often without symptoms. As conduit dysfunction progresses in severity or duration, patients may report exercise intolerance and shortness of breath with modest aerobic exercise.[150] Eventually, with progressive severe RV-PA conduit dysfunction, for the reasons outlined above, patients may present with right-sided heart failure. As the RV dilates and myocardial dysfunction progresses, RV end-diastolic and RA pressures increase and may manifest clinically as hepatomegaly or lower extremity edema. RV dysfunction is well known to increase the risk of late arrhythmia and sudden death.[151] Echocardiography and cardiac MRI are the noninvasive diagnostic studies of choice for assessment of the degree of conduit regurgitation or stenosis. For conduit stenosis, Doppler echocardiography can make a quantitative assessment of severity by estimating the pressure gradient of the conduit. In general, peak systolic gradients below 30 mm Hg are mild and between 30 and 50 mm Hg are moderate (in the face of normal RV systolic function). For conduit insufficiency, the echocardiographic assessment is limited to the qualitative appraisal of the RV diastolic dimension and the size of the conduit regurgitant jet by color-flow Doppler. Echocardiography is of limited value in quantifying RV volumes and function.

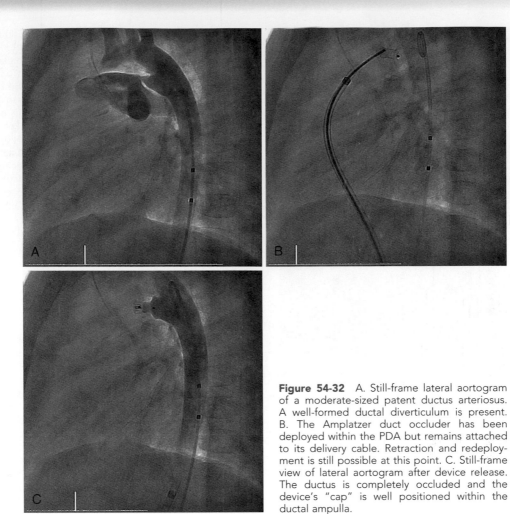

Figure 54-32 A. Still-frame lateral aortogram of a moderate-sized patent ductus arteriosus. A well-formed ductal diverticulum is present. B. The Amplatzer duct occluder has been deployed within the PDA but remains attached to its delivery cable. Retraction and redeployment is still possible at this point. C. Still-frame view of lateral aortogram after device release. The ductus is completely occluded and the device's "cap" is well positioned within the ductal ampulla.

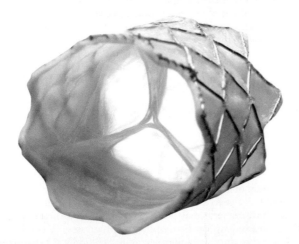

Figure 54-33 The Medtronic Melody transcatheter pulmonary valve consists of a bovine jugular venous valve sutured onto a 28-mm balloon-expandable stent. *(Image courtesy of Medtronic, Minneapolis, MN.)*

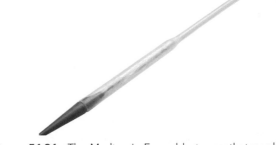

Figure 54-34 The Medtronic Ensemble transcatheter valve delivery system is designed to percutaneously deliver the Melody valve. It consists of a 16-Fr delivery catheter with a 22-Fr distal pod that encloses the crimped Melody valve. *(Image courtesy of Medtronic, Minneapolis, MN.)*

For these measures, cardiac MRI is the imaging modality of choice. Studies with cardiac MRI show that RV size and function can predict which patients may benefit from intervention for a dysfunctional RV-PA conduit.[160,161] Intervention is probably indicated for RV-PA conduits with stenosis and/or regurgitation if the RV ejection fraction is diminished or if the RV diastolic volume exceeds 160 to 180 mL/m². Geva and colleagues showed that all patients who had an RV end-systolic volume greater than 95 mL/m² had evidence of RV dysfunction by MRI.[159] Studies of patients with repaired tetralogy of Fallot have found that elevation of B-type natriuretic peptide correlates with RV size, ejection fraction, diastolic function, and exercise capacity.[162] Once the decision is made that a dysfunctional RV-PA conduit warrants intervention, the feasibility of percutaneous pulmonary valve placement must be evaluated. Currently, percutaneous pulmonary valve replacement with the Melody device is recommended only for RV-PA conduits that were ≥16 mm in diameter at surgical implantation and that have clinically important stenosis or insufficiency. Valved

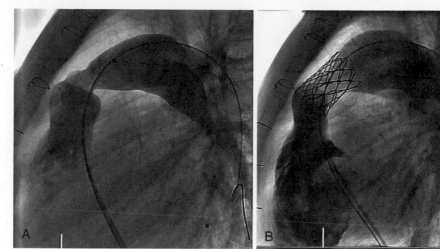

Figure 54-35 Lateral angiograms in a 10-year-old boy 8 years after a Ross procedure following aortic valve endocarditis. Prior to Melody valve implantation (A), there is significant stenosis and regurgitation of the RV-PA homograft. After Melody valve implantation (B), there is relief of the stenosis and Doppler echo documentsd only trace valve regurgitation.

homograft or heterograft conduits are equally suitable for Melody valve implantation. Precatheterization evaluation typically includes MRI with cine imaging to evaluate the RV-PA conduit's anatomical dimensions,[163,164] the more distal pulmonary artery's anatomy, as well as the RV's size and function. Cardiac MRI also can provide valuable information regarding the proximity of the RV-PA conduit to underlying coronary arteries. This is critical information, as high-pressure conduit dilation during valve implantation can rarely cause coronary artery compression. Patients with significant RVOT stenosis or insufficiency after repair of tetralogy of Fallot using a transannular outflow patch (rather than a conduit) are not candidates for Melody valve implantation at present.

TREATMENT AND OUTCOMES

The treatment options for significant RV-PA conduit dysfunction include surgical intervention with conduit replacement, bare metal stenting, and now percutaneous pulmonary valve placement within the existing conduit. In the United States, the only FDA-approved option for transcatheter pulmonary valve implantation is the Medtronic Melody valve (Medtronic, Minneapolis, MN). The valve is a trileaflet bovine jugular venous valve treated and preserved with glutaraldehyde and sutured into a 28-mm-long platinum/iridium stent (Fig 54-33). The device is delivered through a 22-Fr delivery system on an 18-, 20-, or 22-mm outer balloon catheter with a balloon-in-balloon design to minimize valve movement during balloon inflation (Fig. 54-34).

TECHNIQUE

The percutaneous deployment of the Melody pulmonary valve utilizes interventional cardiology techniques that are commonly employed in labs proficient in catheter-based therapies for structural heart disease. Percutaneous pulmonary valve implantation most commonly utilizes a femoral venous approach, but the internal jugular venous approach has also been used successfully. After baseline hemodynamic measurements are obtained, RV angiography is performed to assess RV function, the anatomy of the RV-PA conduit and its stenosis, and the branch pulmonary arteries; all are important for determining the valve implantation site. It is important to ensure that there will be no coronary artery compression with high-pressure balloon dilation of the existing RV-PA conduit. Using biplane angiography, the spatial relationship of the conduit and coronary arteries is assessed. This can be accomplished by performing coronary angiography during simultaneous inflation of a high-pressure balloon to the desired final diameter within the RV-PA conduit.[165] Once the possibility of coronary compression is ruled out, an ultrastiff exchange wire is positioned in a distal pulmonary artery, preferably the left pulmonary artery. The Melody valve is rinsed in normal saline baths to remove the gluteraldehyde

solution. The stent is hand-crimped and loaded onto the balloon (18, 20, or 22 mm) of the Ensemble delivery system. It is of vital importance to be certain that the Melody valve is oriented properly on the delivery balloon (implanting the valve "upside down" will cause complete RVOT obstruction that would be immediately fatal). In addition to visual confirmation, the operator must ensure that the blue sutures on the distal end of the Melody stent are facing the blue tip of the delivery system; this assures proper valve orientation so that the valve will open in systole. A formal "time out" at this step is recommended to ensure and document that the Melody valve is properly oriented on the delivery system prior to implantation. At this point, venous access is dilated with a 22-Fr dilator (Cook, Inc, Bloomington, IN). The delivery system is then advanced over the ultrastiff guidewire into the existing RV-PA conduit. Once the Melody valve is in the desired position, the delivery sheath is retracted to uncover the stent. Contrast can be injected through the side port of the sheath to help ensure proper valve positioning. The Melody valve is then implanted by first inflating the inner balloon and then the outer balloon of the Ensemble delivery system. The dilation balloons are then deflated and the delivery system withdrawn over the guidewire. Repeat hemodynamics and angiography are then performed to document the immediate outcome (Figs. 54-35 and 54-36). If significant residual stenosis is present, a high-pressure balloon can be used to further expand the Melody valve stent. It is recommended that the patient be heparinized throughout the procedure, maintaining an ACT above 250 seconds. Variations on the technique described above, particularly pre-stenting of a stenotic conduit prior to Melody implant, have become fairly widespread; currently, however, they are not endorsed by Medtronic or the FDA. Early evidence suggests that high-pressure predilation and pre-stenting of the RV-PA conduit with a bare metal stent, followed by Melody implantation within that stent, may improve the hemodynamic outcome and decrease the incidence of late Melody stent fracture.[166] Predilation of a stenotic RV-PA conduit may improve Melody valve function and durability by relieving some stress from the valve stent itself. As experience with this procedure grows, new techniques and changes in the device will undoubtedly occur to make this treatment option safer and more successful.

RESULTS

The early U.S. experience was reported by Zahn and colleagues from a multicenter prospective study performed over an 8-month period.[167] This study evaluated the safety, procedural success, and short-term effectiveness of the Melody valve in patients with dysfunctional RV-PA conduits. Data from 34 patients were reported, with attempted Melody valve placement in 30 of these patients. Procedural success occurred in 93% of cases (using a composite measure defined as valve fixed in desired location, postimplant RV-PA systolic gradient <35 mm Hg,

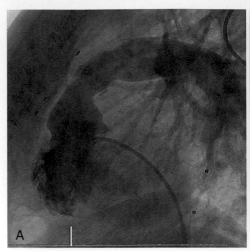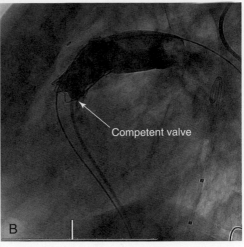

Competent valve

Figure 54-36 Lateral angiograms in a 14-year-old girl who had undergone a Rastelli procedure for complex transposition. Two years prior, she had undergone bare metal stenting of the RV-PA homograft for stenosis, but was left with free regurgitation (A). After Melody valve implantation (B), there is no residual conduit stenosis or regurgitation (white arrow).

angiographic evidence of trivial or no pulmonary regurgitation (PR), and 24-hour freedom from valve explant). Short-term effectiveness (defined as 6-month findings of PR fraction <20% by MRI and RVOT gradient <30 mm Hg) was achieved in 83% of the patients. There is a far more extensive international experience with percutaneous pulmonary valve placement, as it received a CE Mark in the European Union and a Canadian Medical Device License in 2006. One review by Lurz and colleagues reported results in 155 consecutive patients, with median follow-up of 28 months.[168] The procedure resulted in an immediate decrease in the RVOT gradient from 37 mm Hg to 17 mm Hg ($P < 0.001$) with no more than mild angiographic PR in any patient. Freedom from reintervention was achieved in 95% of these patients at 10 months postimplant.

COMPLICATIONS

Percutaneous pulmonary valve placement has proven to be safe, with a procedural mortality of less than 0.2%.[169] One procedural death, due to coronary occlusion after device placement, has been reported worldwide. The most common complication in follow-up is Melody stent fracture. In the U.S. experience reported by Zahn, nearly 30% of patients demonstrated stent fractures by 6 months postimplantation.[167] The European experience described by Lurz reported a 21% incidence of late stent fracture.[168] Most patients with a Melody stent fracture do well, but some fractures are associated with significant restenosis within the stent. In the Zahn and Lurz reports,[167,168] about one-third of patients with stent fracture had significant restenosis that was treated with a second percutaneous pulmonary valve implant. This "stent in stent" (i.e., "valve-in-valve") procedure appears to provide a safe and effective treatment for recurrent conduit stenosis secondary to stent fracture in some patients.[170] As mentioned above, some recent data suggest that pre-stenting the RV-PA conduit prior to placement

of the Melody valve may reduce the incidence of late stent fracture.[166] Other rare procedural complications that have been reported include RV-PA homograft rupture, dislodgement of the stent valve device, wide complex tachycardia, obstruction of the orifice of the right PA (the Melody valve is, in fact, a covered stent), and distal PA perforation from guidewire trauma. The availability of covered stents that can be dilated to a diameter of 20 to 23 mm improves the safety profile of this procedure, as a covered stent can often be used successfully to treat a tear or rupture of an RVOT conduit. Postcatheterization fever seems to be a relatively common occurrence, having been seen in up to 40% to 80% of patients in some studies.[171] It is important to exclude infection in a febrile patient, but there were no documented infections in any reported cases of transient postimplant fever.

Conclusion

Percutaneous interventions with bare metal valveless stents have been used for years to treat stenosis of a surgically placed RV-PA conduit. The goal has been to delay repeat surgical intervention, but the cost has been the creation of free conduit valve regurgitation. The recent availability of the Medtronic Melody pulmonary valve system is a remarkable advance for many patients. This technology provides a percutaneous intervention for the dysfunctional RV-PA conduit that has the ability to correct both stenosis and regurgitation. Studies have shown that transcatheter pulmonary valve placement improves RV hemodynamics and prolongs the life span of existing surgical conduits. Although early data are promising, with excellent effectiveness and low complication rates, percutaneous PA implantation is a work in progress. The ultimate goal is to prolong the life span of existing conduits and expose patients to fewer conduit replacement surgeries over their lifetimes. This technology is new, and it will be years before we know its long-term impact.

REFERENCES

1. Emmanouilides GC, Baylen BG: Pulmonary stenosis. In Adams FH, Emmanouilides GC, editors: *Heart Disease in Infants, Children, and Adolescents*, ed 3, Baltimore, 1983, Williams & Wilkins, pp 234.
2. Perloff JK: Postpediatric congenital heart disease: natural survival patterns. In Roberts WC, editor: *Congenital Heart Disease in Adults*, Philadelphia, 1979, Davis, pp 27–51.
3. Nugent EW, Freedom RM, Nora JJ, et al: Clinical course in pulmonary stenosis. *Circulation* 56(Suppl I):I-38–I-47, 1977.
4. Kan JS, White RI, Mitchell SE, et al: Percutaneous balloon valvuloplasty: a new method for treatment of congenital pulmonary-valve stenosis. *N Engl J Med* 307:540, 1982.
5. Becker AE, Anderson AH: Anomalies of the ventricular outflow tracts. In Becker AE, Anderson AH, editors: *Cardiac Pathology*, New York, 1983, Raven Press, pp 13.1–13.22.
6. Jeffery RF, Moller JH, Amplatz K: The dysplastic pulmonary valve: a new roentgenographic entity. *Am J Roentgenol Ther Radium Nucl Med* 114:322, 1972.
7. Lababidi Z, Wu JR: Percutaneous balloon pulmonary valvuloplasty. *Am J Cardiol* 52:560-562, 1983.
8. Walls JT, Lababidi Z, Curtis JJ: Morphologic effects of percutaneous balloon pulmonary valvuloplasty. *South Med J* 80:475–477, 1987.
9. DiSessa TG, Alpert BS, Chase NA, et al: Balloon valvuloplasty in children with dysplastic pulmonary valves. *Am J Cardiol* 60:405–407, 1987.
10. Rocchini AP, Beekman RH: Balloon angioplasty in the treatment of pulmonary valve stenosis and coarctation of the aorta. *Tex Heart Inst J* 13:377–385, 1986.
11. Radtke W, Keane JF, Fellows KE, et al: Percutaneous balloon valvotomy of congenital pulmonary stenosis using oversized balloons. *J Am Coll Cardiol* 8:909–915, 1986.
12. Ring JC, Kulik TJ, Burke BA, et al: Morphologic changes induced by dilation of the pulmonary valve annulus with overlarge balloons in normal newborn lambs. *Am J Cardiol* 55:210–214, 1985.
13. Stanger P, Cassidy SC, Girod DA, et al: Balloon pulmonary valvuloplasty: results of the Valvuloplasty and Angioplasty of Congenital Anomalies Registry. *Am J Cardiol* 65:775–783, 1990.
14. Pepine CJ, Gessner IH, Feldman RL: Percutaneous balloon valvuloplasty for pulmonary valve stenosis in the adult. *Am J Cardiol* 50:1442–1445, 1982.
15. Rocchini AP, Kveselis DA, Crowley D, et al: Percutaneous balloon valvuloplasty for treatment of congenital pulmonary valvular stenosis in children. *J Am Coll Cardiol* 3:1005–1012, 1984.
16. Zeevi B, Keane JF, Fellows K, et al: Balloon dilation of critical pulmonary stenosis in the first week of life. *J Am Coll Cardiol* 11:821–824, 1988.
17. Rey C, Marache P, Francart C, et al: Percutaneous transluminal balloon valvuloplasty of congenital pulmonary valve stenosis, with a special report on infants and neonates. *J Am Coll Cardiol* 11:815–820, 1988.

18. Al Kasab S, Ribeiro PA, al Raibag M, et al: Percutaneous double balloon pulmonary valvotomy in adults. *Am J Cardiol* 62: 822–824, 1988.
19. Khan MAA, Al-Yousef S, Huhta JC, et al: Critical pulmonary valve stenosis in patients less than 1 year of age: treatment with percutaneous gradational balloon pulmonary valvuloplasty. *Am Heart J* 117:1008–1014, 1989.
20. Fedderly RT, Lloyd TR, Mendelsohn AM, et al: Determinants of successful balloon valvotomy in infants with critical pulmonary stenosis or membranous pulmonary atresia with intact ventricular septum. *J Am Coll Cardiol* 25:460–465, 1995.
21. Colli AM, Perry SB, Lock JE, et al: Balloon dilation of critical valvar pulmonary stenosis in the first month of life. *Catheter Cardiovasc Diagn* 34:23–28, 1995.
22. Tentolouris CA, Kyriakidis MK, Gaualiatsis IP, et al: Percutaneous pulmonary valvuloplasty in an octogenarian with calcific pulmonary stenosis. *Chest* 101:1456–1458, 1992.
23. Herrmann HC, Hill JA, Krol J, et al: Effectiveness of percutaneous balloon valvuloplasty in adults with pulmonic valve stenosis. *Am J Cardiol* 68:1111–1113, 1991.
24. Sherman W, Hershman R, Alexopoulos D, et al: Pulmonic balloon valvuloplasty in adults. *Am Heart J* 119:186–190, 1990.
25. Fawzy ME, Mercer EN, Dunn B: Late results of pulmonary balloon valvuloplasty in adults using double balloon technique. *J Intervent Cardiol* 1:35–42, 1998.
26. Flugelman MY, Halon DA, Lewis BS: Pulmonary balloon valvuloplasty in the seventh decade of life. *Isr J Med Sci* 24:112–113, 1998.
27. Presbitero P, Orzan F, Defilippi G, et al: Percutaneous pulmonary valvuloplasty in adults. *G Ital Cardiol* 18:155–159, 1988.
28. Park JH, Yoon YS, Yeon KM, et al: Percutaneous pulmonary valvuloplasty with a double-balloon technique. *Radiology* 164:715–718, 1987.
29. Cooke JP, Seward JB, Holmes DR: Transluminal balloon valvotomy for pulmonic stenosis in an adult. *Mayo Clin Proc* 62:306–311, 1987.
30. Leisch F, Schutzenberger W, Kerschner K, et al: Percutaneous pulmonary valvuloplasty in adults. *Z Kardiol* 75:426–430, 1986.
31. Shuck JW, McCormick DJ, Cohen IS, et al: Percutaneous balloon valvuloplasty of the pulmonary valve: role of right to left shunting through a patent foramen ovale. *J Am Coll Cardiol* 4:132–135, 1984.
32. Chen CR, Cheng TO, Huang T, et al: Percutaneous balloon valvuloplasty for pulmonary stenosis in adolescents and adults. *N Engl J Med* 335:21–25, 1996.
33. McCrindle BW, Kan JS: Long term results after balloon pulmonary valvuloplasty. *Circulation* 83:1915–1922, 1991.
34. McCrindle BW: Independent predictors of long-term results after balloon pulmonary valvuloplasty. *Circulation* 89:1751–1759, 1994.
35. O'Connor BK, Beekman RH, Lindauer A, et al. Intermediate-term outcome after pulmonary balloon valvuloplasty: comparison to a matched surgical control group. *J Am Coll Cardiol* 20:169–173, 1992.
36. Harrild DM, Powell AJ, Trang TX, et al. Long-term pulmonary regurgitation following balloon valvuloplasty for pulmonary stenosis. *J Am Coll Cardiol* 55:1041–1047, 2010.
37. Friedman WF: Aortic stenosis. In Adams FH, Emmanouilides GC, editors: *Heart Disease in Infants, Children, and Adolescents*, ed 3, Baltimore, 1983, Williams & Wilkins, pp 224.
38. Wagner HR, Ellison RC, Keane JF, et al: Clinical course in aortic stenosis. *Circulation* 56(Suppl I):I-47–I-56, 1977.
39. Hsieh K, Keane JF, Nadas AS, et al: Long-term follow-up of valvotomy before 1968 for congenital aortic stenosis. *Am J Cardiol* 58:338–341, 1986.
40. Lababidi Z, Wu J, Walls JT. Percutaneous balloon aortic valvuloplasty: results in 23 patients. *Am J Cardiol* 53:194–197, 1984.
41. NHLBI Balloon Valvuloplasty Registry Participants: Percutaneous balloon aortic valvuloplasty: acute and 30-day follow-up results in 674 patients from NHLBI Balloon Valvuloplasty Registry. *Circulation* 84:2383–2397, 1991.
42. McKay RG, Safian RD, Lock JE, et al: Balloon dilation of calcific aortic stenosis in elderly patients: postmortem, intraoperative, and percutaneous valvuloplasty studies. *Circulation* 74:119–125, 1986.
43. Berdoff RL, Strain J, Crandall C, et al. Pathology of aortic valvuloplasty: findings after postmortem successful and failed dilatations. *Am Heart J* 117:688–690, 1989.
44. Walls JT, Lababidi Z, Curtis JJ, et al: Assessment of percutaneous balloon pulmonary and aortic valvuloplasty. *J Thorac Cardiovasc Surg* 88:352–356, 1984.
45. Rocchini AP, Beekman RH, Ben Shachar G, et al: Balloon aortic valvuloplasty: results of the valvuloplasty and angioplasty of congenital anomalies registry. *Am J Cardiol* 65:784–789, 1990.
46. Beekman RH, Rocchini AP, Crowley DC, et al: Aortic balloon valvuloplasty: two balloons are better than one. *Circulation* 76:266, 1987.
47. Helgason H, Keane JF, Fellows KE, et al: Balloon dilation of the aortic valve: studies in normal lambs and in children with aortic stenosis. *J Am Coll Cardiol* 9:816–822, 1987.
48. Sholler GF, Keane JF, Perry SB, et al: Balloon dilation of congenital aortic valve stenosis: results and influences of technical and morphological features on outcome. *Circulation* 78:351–360, 1988.
49. Meliones JN, Beekman RH, Rocchini AP, et al: Balloon valvuloplasty for recurrent aortic stenosis after surgical valvotomy in childhood: immediate and follow-up studies. *J Am Coll Cardiol* 13:1106–1110, 1989.
50. Vogel M, Benson LN, Burrows P, et al: Balloon dilatation of congenital aortic valve stenosis in infants and children: short and intermediate term results. *Br Heart J* 62:148–153, 1989.
51. Keane JF, Perry SB, Lock JE: Balloon dilation of congenital valvular aortic stenosis. *J Am Coll Cardiol* 16:457–458, 1990.
52. McCrindle BW: Independent predictors of immediate results of percutaneous balloon aortic valvotomy in childhood. *Am J Cardiol* 77:286–293, 1996.
53. Sandhu SK, Lloyd TR, Crowley DC, et al: Effectiveness of balloon valvuloplasty in the young adult with congenital aortic stenosis. *Catheter Cardiovasc Diagn* 36:122–127, 1995.
54. Jones M, Barnhart GR, Morrow AG: Late results after operations for left ventricular outflow tract obstruction. *Am J Cardiol* 50:569–579, 1982.
55. Cowley CG, Dietrich M, Mosca RS, et al: Balloon valvuloplasty versus transventricular dilation for neonatal critical aortic stenosis. *Am J Cardiol* 87:1125–1127, 2001.
56. McCrindle BW, Blackstone EH, Williams WG, et al: Are outcomes of surgical versus transcatheter balloon valvotomy equivalent in neonatal critical aortic stenosis? *Circulation* 104(suppl I):I-152–I-158, 2001.
57. McElhinney DB, Lock JE, Keane JF, et al: Left heart growth, function, and reintervention after balloon aortic valvuloplasty for neonatal aortic stenosis. *Circulation* 111:451–458, 2005.
58. Magee AG, Nykanen D, McCrindle BW, et al: Balloon dilation of severe aortic stenosis in the neonate: comparison of anterograde and retrograde catheter approaches. *J Am Coll Cardiol* 30: 1061–1066, 1997.
59. Rhodes LA, Colan SD, Perry SB, et al: Predictors of survival in neonates with critical aortic stenosis. *Circulation* 84:2325–2335, 1991.
60. Fischer DR, Ettedgui JA, Park SC, et al: Carotid artery approach for balloon dilation of aortic valve stenosis in the neonate: a preliminary report. *J Am Coll Cardiol* 15:1633–1636, 1990.
61. Galal O, Rao PS, Al-Fadley F, et al: Follow-up results of balloon aortic valvuloplasty in children with special reference to causes of late aortic insufficiency. *Am Heart J* 133:418–427, 1997.
62. McElhinney DB, Marshall AC, Wilkins-Haug LE, et al: Preditors of technical success and postnatal biventricular outcome after in utero aortic valvuloplasty for aortic stenosis with evolving hypoplastic left heart syndrome. *Circulation* 120:1482–1490, 2009.
63. Safian RD, Berman AD, Diver DJ, et al: Balloon aortic valvuloplasty in 170 consecutive patients. *N Engl J Med* 319:125–130, 1988.
64. Block PC, Palacios IF: Clinical and hemodynamic follow-up after percutaneous aortic valvuloplasty in the elderly. *Am J Cardiol* 62:760–763, 1988.
65. Del Core MG, Nair CK, Peetz D, Jr, et al: Early restenosis following successful percutaneous balloon valvuloplasty for calcific valvular aortic stenosis. *Am Heart J* 118:118–182, 1989.
66. Beekman RH, Rocchini AP, Gillon JH, et al: Hemodynamic determinants of the peak systolic pressure gradient in children with valvar aortic stenosis. *Am J Cardiol* 69:813–815, 1992.
67. O'Connor BK, Beekman RH, Rocchini AP, et al: Intermediate-term effectiveness of balloon valvuloplasty for congenital aortic stenosis: a prospective follow-up study. *Circulation* 84:732–738, 1991.
68. Kipps AK, McElhinney DB, Kane J, et al: Exercise function of children with congenital aortic stenosis following aortic valvuloplasty during early infancy. *Congen Heart Dis* 4:258–264, 2009.
69. Robinson JD, del Nido PJ, Geggel RL, et al: Left ventricular diastolic heart failure in teenagers who underwent balloon aortic valvuloplasty in early infancy. *Am J Cardiol* 106:426–429, 2010.
70. Bacha EA, Satou GM, Moran AM, et al: Valve sparing operation for balloon-induced aortic regurgitation in congenital aortic stenosis. *J Thorac Cardiovasc Surg* 122:162–168, 2001.
71. Beekman RH, Rocchini AP, Andes A: Balloon valvuloplasty for critical aortic stenosis in the newborn: influence of new catheter technology. *J Am Coll Cardiol* 17:1172–1176, 1991.
72. Brown DW, Chong EC, Gauvreau K, et al: Aortic wall injury as a complication of neonatal aortic valvuloplasty. Incidence and risk factors. *Circ Cardiovasc Intervent* 1:53–59, 2008.
73. Kan JS, Marvin WJ, Bass JL, et al: Balloon angioplasty for branch pulmonary artery stenosis: results from the valvuloplasty and angioplasty of congenital anomalies registry. *Am J Cardiol* 65:798–801, 1990.
74. Lock JE, Castaneda-Zuniga WR, Fuhrman BP, et al: Balloon dilation angioplasty of hypoplastic and stenotic pulmonary arteries. *Circulation* 67:962–967, 1983.
75. Rothman A, Perry SB, Keane JF, et al: Early results and follow-up of balloon angioplasty for branch pulmonary artery stenoses. *J Am Coll Cardiol* 15:1109–1117, 1990.
76. Benson LN, Hamilton F, Dasmahapatra HK, et al: Implantable stent dilation of the pulmonary artery: Early experience (abstract). *Circulation* 78(Suppl II):II-100, 1988.
77. Benson LN, Hamilton F, Dasmahapatra HK, et al: Percutaneous implantations of a balloon-expandable endoprosthesis for pulmonary artery stenosis: an experimental study. *J Am Coll Cardiol* 18:1303–1308, 1991.
78. Rocchini AP, Meliones JP, Beekman RH, et al: Use of balloon-expandable stents to treat experimental pulmonary artery and superior vena caval stenosis: preliminary experience. *Pediatr Cardiol* 13:92–96, 1992.
79. Mendelsohn AM, Dorostkar PC, Moorehead CP, et al: Stent redilation in models of congenital heart disease: pulmonary artery stenosis and coarctation. *Catheter Cardiovasc Diagn* 38:430–440, 1996.
80. O'Laughlin MP, Perry SB, Lock JE, et al: Use of endovascular stents in congenital heart disease. *Circulation* 83:1923–1939, 1991.
81. Hosking MC, Benson LN, Nakanishi T, et al: Intravascular stent prosthesis for right ventricular outflow obstruction. *J Am Coll Cardiol* 20:373–380, 1992.
82. Mendelsohn AM, Bove EL, Lupinetti FM, et al: Intraoperative and percutaneous stenting of congenital pulmonary artery and vein stenosis. *Circulation* 88:210–217, 1993.
83. O'Laughlin MP, Slack MC, Grifka RG, et al: Implantation and intermediate term follow-up of stents in congenital heart disease. *Circulation* 88:605–614, 1993.
84. Fogelman R, Nykanen D, Smallhorn JF, et al: Endovascular stents in the pulmonary circulation: clinical impact on management and medium-term follow-up. *Circulation* 92:881–885, 1995.
85. McMahon CJ, El Said HG, Vincent JA, et al: Refinements in the implementation of pulmonary arterial stents. *Cardiol Young* 12:445–452, 2002.
86. Law MA, Shamszad P, Nugent AW, et al: Pulmonary artery stents: long-term follow-up. *Catheter Cardiovasc Intervent* 75:757–764, 2010.
87. Shaffer KM, Mullins CE, Grifka RG, et al: Intravascular stents in congenital heart disease: short and long-term results from a large single-center experience. *J Am Coll Cardiol* 31:661–667, 1998.
88. Ing FF, Grifka RG, Nihill MR, et al: Repeat dilation of intravascular stents in congenital heart defects. *Circulation* 92:893–897, 1995.
89. Duke C, Rosenthal E, Qureshi SA: The efficacy and safety of stent redilation in congenital heart disease. *Heart* 89:905–912, 2003.
90. Beekman RH, Muller DW, Reynolds PI, et al: Balloon-expandable stent treatment of experimental coarctation of the aorta: early hemodynamic and pathological evaluation. *J Intervent Cardiol* 6:113–123, 1993.
91. Morrow WR, Smith VC, Ehler WJ, et al: Balloon angioplasty with stent implantation in experimental coarctation of the aorta. *Circulation* 89:2677–2683, 1994.
92. Morrow WR, Palmaz JC, Tio FO, et al. Re-expansion of balloon-expandable stents after growth. *J Am Coll Cardiol* 22:2007–2013, 1993.
93. Ebeid MR, Prieto LR, Latson LA: Use of balloon expandable stents for coarctation of the aorta. *J Am Coll Cardiol* 30: 1847–1852, 1997.
94. Suarez de Lezo J, Pan M, Romero M, et al: Immediate and follow-up findings after stent treatment for severe coarctation of the aorta. *Am J Cardiol* 83:400–406, 1999.
95. Marshall AC, Perry SB, Keane JF, et al: Early results and medium-term follow-up of stent implantation for residual aortic coarctation. *Am Heart J* 139:1054–1060, 2000.
96. Transpoulous BD, Hadjinikolaou L, Konstadopoulou GN, et al: Stent treatment for coarctation of the aorta: intermediate term follow-up and technical considerations. *Heart* 84:65–70, 2000.
97. Harrison DA, McLaughlin PR, Lazzam C, et al: Endovascular stents in the management of coarctation of the aorta in the adolescent and adult: one year follow-up. *Heart* 85:561–566, 2001.
98. Johnston TA, Grifka RG, Jones TK: Endovascular stents for treatment of coarctation of the aorta: acute results and follow-up experience. *Catheter Cardiovasc Intervent* 62:499–505, 2004.
99. Shah L, Hijazi Z, Sandhu S, et al: Use of endovascular stents for the treatment of coarctation of the aorta in children and adults: immediate and midterm results. *J Invas Cardiol* 17:614–618, 2005.
100. Forbes TJ, Garekar S, Amin Z, et al: Procedural results and acute complications in stenting native and recurrent coarctation of the aorta in patients over 4 years of age: a multi-institutional study. *Catheter Cardiovasc Intervent* 70:276–285, 2007.
101. Forbes TJ, Moore P, Pedra CAC, et al: Intermediate follow-up following intravascular stenting for treatment of coarctation of the aorta. *Catheter Cardiovasc Intervent* 70:569–577, 2007.
102. Mohan UR, Danon S, Levi D, et al: Stent implantation for coarctation of the aorta in children <30 kg. *J Am Coll Cardiol Cardiovasc Intervent* 2:877–883, 2009.
103. Wheatley GH, Koullias GJ, Rodriguez-Lopez JA, et al. Is endovascular repair the new gold standard for primary adult coarctation? *Eur J Cardiothorac Surg* 38(3):305–310, 2010.
104. Tzifa A, Ewert T, Brzezinska-Rajszys G, et al: Covered Cheatham-platinum stents for aortic coarctation. *J Am Coll Cardiol* 47:1457–1463, 2006.
105. Varma C, Benson LN, Butany J, et al: Aortic dissection after stent dilatation for coarctation of the aorta: a case report and literature review. *Catheter Cardiovasc Intervent* 59:528–535, 2003.
106. Pihkala J, Pedra CA, Nykanen D, et al: Implantation of endovascular stents for hypoplasia of the transverse arch. *Cardiol Young* 10:3–7, 2000.
107. Brassard M, Fouron JC, van Doesburg NH, et al: Outcome of children with atrial septal defect considered too small for surgical closure. *Am J Cardiol* 83:1552–1555, 1999.
108. Tabery S, Daniels O: How classical are the clinical features of the "ostium secundum" atrial septal defect? *Cardiol Young* 7:294–301, 1997.
109. Shah D, Azhar M, Oakley CM, et al: Natural history of secundum atrial septal defect in adults after medical or surgical treatment: a historical prospective study. *Br Heart J* 71:224–228, 1994.

110. Konstantinides S, Geibel A, Olschewski M, et al: A comparison of surgical and medical therapy for atrial septal defect in adults. *N Engl J Med* 333(8):469–514, 1995.
111. Salaymeh K, Taeed R, Michelfelder EC, et al: Unique echocardiographic features associated with deployment of the Amplatzer atrial septal defect device. *J Am Soc Echocardiogr* 14(2):128–137, 2001.
112. Ewert P, Daehnert I, Berger F, et al: Transcatheter closure of atrial septal defects under echocardiographic guidance without x-ray: initial experiences. *Cardiol Young* 9:136–140, 1999.
113. Formigari R, Di Donato RM, Mazzera E, et al: Minimally invasive or interventional repair of atrial septal defects in children: experience in 171 cases and comparison with conventional strategies. *J Am Coll Cardiol* 37(6):1707–1712, 2001.
114. Cowley CG, Lloyd TR, Bove EL, et al: Comparison of results of closure of secundum atrial septal defect by surgery versus Amplatzer septal occluder. *Am J Cardiol* 88:589–591, 2001.
115. Berger F, Ewett P, Björnstad PG, et al: transcatheter closure as standard treatment for most interatrial defects: experience in 200 patients treated with the Amplatzer septal occluder. *Cardiol Young* 9:468–473, 1999.
116. Bilkis AA, Alwi M, Hasri S, et al: The Amplatzer duct occluder: experience in 209 patients. *J Am Coll Cardiol* 37(1):258–261, 2001.
117. Chan KC, Godman MJ, Walsh K, et al: Transcatheter closure of atrial septal defect and interatrial communications with a new self expanding nitinol double disc device (Amplatzer septal occluder): multicentre UK experience. *Heart* 82:300–306, 1999.
118. Zahn EM, Wilson N, Cutright W, et al: development and testing of the Helex septal occluder, a new expanded polytetrafluoroethylene atrial septal defect occlusion system. *Circulation* 104:711–716, 2001.
119. Perk G, Lang RM, Garcia-Fernandez MA, et al: Use of real time three-dimensional transesophageal echocardiography in intracardiac catheter based interventions. *J Am Soc Echocardiogr* 22(8):865–882, 2009.
120. Berger F, Vogel M, Alexi-Meskishvili V, et al: comparison of results and complications of surgical and Amplatzer device closure of atrial septal defects. *J Thorac Cardiovasc Surg* 118(4): 674–680, 1999.
121. Sherman JM, Hagler DJ, Cetta F: Thrombosis after septal closure device placement: a review of the current literature. *Catheter Cardiovasc Intervent* 63:486–489, 2004.
122. Amin Z, Hijazi ZM, Bass JL, et al: Erosion of Amplatzer septal occluder device after closure of secundum atrial septal defects: review of registry of complications and recommendations to minimize future risk. *Catheter Cardiovasc Intervent* 63:496–502, 2004.
123. Divekar A, Gaamangwe T, Shaikh N, et al: Cardiac perforation after device closure of atrial septal defects with the Amplatzer septal occluder. *J Am Coll Cardiol* 45(8):1213–1218, 2005.
124. Veldtman GR, Razack V, Siu S, et al: Right ventricular form and function after percutaneous atrial septal defect device closure. *J Am Coll Cardiol* 37(8):2108–2113, 2001.
125. Jan SL, Hwang B, Fu YC, et al: Prediction of ductus arteriosus closure by neonatal screening echocardiography. *Int J Cardiovasc Imaging* 20(5):349–356, 2004.
126. Waddell TK, Bennett L, Kennedy R, et al: Heart-lung or lung transplantation for Eisenmenger syndrome. *J Heart Lung Transplant* 21(7):731–737, 2002.
127. Sahn DW, Kim YJ, ZO JH, et al: The value of contrast echocardiography in the diagnosis of patent ductus arteriosus with Eisenmenger's syndrome. *J Am Soc Echocardiogr* 14(1):57–59, 2001.
128. Panetta G, Schiller N: Evidence of patent ductus arteriosus and right-to-left shunt by finger pulse oximetry and Doppler signals of agitated saline in abdominal aorta. *J Am Soc Echocardiogr* 12(9):763–765, 1999.
129. Moore JW, Levi DS, Moore SD, et al: Interventional treatment of patent ductus arteriosus in 2004. *Catheter Cardiovasc Intervent* 64:91–101, 2005.
130. Lloyd TR, Fedderly R, Mendelsohn AM, et al: Transcatheter occlusion of patent ductus arteriosus with Gianturco coils. *Circulation* 88:1412–1420, 1993.
131. Rothman A, Lucas VW, Sklansky MS, et al: Percutaneous coil occlusion of patent ductus arteriosus. *J Pediatr* 130:447–454, 1997.
132. Wang, J-K, Liau C-S, Huang J-J, et al: Transcatheter closure of patent ductus arteriosus using Gianturco coils in adolescents and adults. *Catheter Cardiovasc Intervent* 55:513–518, 2002.
133. Uzun O, Hancock S, Parsons JM, et al: Transcatheter occlusion of the arterial duct with cook detachable coils: early experience. *Heart* 76:269–273, 1996.
134. Bermudez-Canete R, Santoro G, Bialkowsky J, et al: Patent ductus arteriosus occlusion using detachable coils. *Am J Cardiol* 82:1547–1549, 1998.
135. Ing FF, Sommer RJ: The snare-assisted technique for transcatheter coil occlusion of moderate to large patent ductus arteriosus: immediate and intermediate results. *J Am Coll Cardiol* 33: 1710–1718, 1999.
136. Hijazi ZM, Lloyd TR, Beekman RH, III, et al: Transcatheter closure with single or multiple gianturco coils of patent ductus arteriosus in infants weighing ≤8 kg: retrograde versus antegrade approach. *Am Heart J* 132:827–835, 1996.
137. Goyal VS, Fulwant MC, Ramakantan R, et al: Follow-up after coil closure of patent ductus arteriosus. *Am J Cardiol* 83:463–466, 1999.
138. Shim, D, Fedderly RT, Beekman RH, III, et al: Follow-up of coil occlusion of patent ductus arteriosus. *J Am Coll Cardiol* 28(1):207–211, 1996.
139. Radha S, Sivakumar K, Philip AK, et al: Clinical course and management strategies for hemolysis after transcatheter closure of patent arterial ducts. *Catheter Cardiovasc Intervent* 59: 538–543, 2003.
140. Carey LM, Vermilion RKP, Shim D, et al: Pulmonary artery size and flow disturbances after patent ductus arteriosus coil occlusion. *Am J Cardiol* 78:1307–1309, 1996.
141. Grifka RG, Vincent JA, Nihill MR, et al: Transcatheter patent ductus arteriosus closure in an infant using the Gianturco-Grifka vascular occlusion device. *Am J Cardiol* 78:721–723, 1996.
142. Tometzki A, Chan K, De Giovanni J, et al: Total UK multi-centre experience with a novel arterial occlusion device (duct occlud pfm). *Heart* 76:520–524, 1996.
143. Ghasemi A, Pandya S, Reddy SV, et al: Trans-catheter closure of patent ductus arteriosus: what is the best device? *Catheter Cardiovasc Intervent* 76(5):703–704, 2010.
144. Masura J, Tittel P, Gavora P, et al: Long-term outcome of transcatheter patent ductus arteriosus closure using Amplatzer duct occluders. *Am Heart J* 151(3):755.e7–755.e10, 2006.
145. Pass RH, Hijazi Z, Hsu DT, et al: Multicenter USA Amplatzer patent ductus arteriosus occlusion device trial: initial and one-year results. *J Am Coll Cardiol* 44(3):513–519, 2004.
146. Joseph G, Mandalay A, Zacharias TU, et al: Severe intravascular hemolysis after transcatheter closure of a large patent ductus arteriosus using the Amplatzer duct occluder: successful resolution by intradevice coil deployment. *Catheter Cardiovasc Intervent* 55:245–249, 2002.
147. Thanopoulos BV, Eleftherakis N, Tzannos K, et al: Further experience with catheter closure of patent ductus arteriosus using the new Amplatzer duct occluder in children. *Am J Cardiol* 105(7):1005–1009, 2010.
148. Saliba Z, El-Rassi I, Abi-Warde MT, et al: The Amplatzer Duct Occluder II: a new device for percutaneous ductus arteriosus closure. *J Intervent Cardiol* 22(6):496–502, 2009.
149. Bhole V, Miller P, Mehta C, et al: Clinical evaluation of the new Amplatzer duct occluder II for patent arterial duct occlusion. *Catheter Cardiovasc Intervent* 74(5):762–769, 2009.
150. Carvalho JS, Shinebourne EA, Busst C, et al: Exercise capacity after complete repair of tetralogy of Fallot: deleterious effects of residual pulmonary regurgitation. *Br Heart J* 67(6):470–473, 1992.
151. Gatzoulis MA, Balaji S, Webber SA, et al: Risk factors for arrhythmia and sudden cardiac death late after repair of tetralogy of Fallot: a multicentre study. *Lancet* 356(9234):975–981, 2000.
152. Bove EL, Kavey RE, Byrum CJ, et al: Improved right ventricular function following late pulmonary valve replacement for residual pulmonary insufficiency or stenosis. *J Thorac Cardiovasc Surg* 90(1):50–55, 1985.
153. Eyskens B, Reybrouck T, Bogaert J, et al: Homograft insertion for pulmonary regurgitation after repair of tetralogy of Fallot improves cardiorespiratory exercise performance. *Am J Cardiol* 85(2):221–225, 2000.
154. Therrien J, Siu SC, Harris L, et al: Impact of pulmonary valve replacement on arrhythmia propensity late after repair of tetralogy of Fallot. *Circulation* 103(20):2489–2494, 2001.
155. Bielefeld MR, Bishop DA, Campbell DN, et al: Reoperative homograft right ventricular outflow tract reconstruction. *Ann Thorac Surg* 71(2):482–487, 2001; discussion 487–488.
156. Stark J, Bull C, Stajevic M, et al: Fate of subpulmonary homograft conduits: determinants of late homograft failure. *J Thorac Cardiovasc Surg* 115(3):506–514, 1998; discussion 514–506.
157. Bonhoeffer P, Boudjemline Y, Saliba Z, et al: Percutaneous replacement of pulmonary valve in a right-ventricle to pulmonary-artery prosthetic conduit with valve dysfunction. *Lancet* 356(9239):1403–1405, 2000.
158. Bonhoeffer P, Boudjemline Y, Saliba Z, et al: Transcatheter implantation of a bovine valve in pulmonary position: a lamb study. *Circulation* 102(7):813–816, 2000.
159. Geva T, Sandweiss BM, Gauvreau K, et al: Factors associated with impaired clinical status in long-term survivors of tetralogy of Fallot repair evaluated by magnetic resonance imaging. *J Am Coll Cardiol* 43(6):1068–1074, 2004.
160. Karamlou T, Silber I, Lao R, et al: Outcomes after late reoperation in patients with repaired tetralogy of Fallot: the impact of arrhythmia and arrhythmia surgery. *Ann Thorac Surg* 81(5):1786–1793, 2006; discussion 1793.
161. Therrien J, Provost Y, Merchant N, et al: Optimal timing for pulmonary valve replacement in adults after tetralogy of Fallot repair. *Am J Cardiol* 95(6):779–782, 2005.
162. Norozi K, Buchhorn R, Bartmus D, et al: Elevated brain natriuretic peptide and reduced exercise capacity in adult patients operated on for tetralogy of Fallot is due to biventricular dysfunction as determined by the myocardial performance index. *Am J Cardiol* 97(9):1377–1382, 2006.
163. Schievano S, Coats L, Migliavacca F, et al: Variations in right ventricular outflow tract morphology following repair of congenital heart disease: implications for percutaneous pulmonary valve implantation. *J Cardiovasc Magn Reson* 9(4):687–695, 2007.
164. Schievano S, Migliavacca F, Coats L, et al: Percutaneous pulmonary valve implantation based on rapid prototyping of right ventricular outflow tract and pulmonary trunk from MR data. *Radiology* 242(2):490–497, 2007.
165. Sridharan S, Coats L, Khambadkone S, et al: Images in cardiovascular medicine. Transcatheter right ventricular outflow tract intervention: the risk to the coronary circulation. *Circulation* 113(25):e934–e935, 2006.
166. Nordmeyer J, Lurz P, Khambadkone S, et al: Pre-stenting with a bare metal stent before percutaneous pulmonary valve implantation: acute and 1-year outcomes. *Heart* 97(2):118–123, 2011.
167. Zahn EM, Hellenbrand WE, Lock JE, et al: Implantation of the melody transcatheter pulmonary valve in patients with a dysfunctional right ventricular outflow tract conduit early results from the U.S. clinical trial. *J Am Coll Cardiol* 54(18):1722–1729, 2009.
168. Lurz P, Coats L, Khambadkone S, et al: Percutaneous pulmonary valve implantation: impact of evolving technology and learning curve on clinical outcome. *Circulation* 117(15):1964–1972, 2008.
169. Lurz P, Gaudin R, Taylor AM, et al: Percutaneous pulmonary valve implantation. *Semin Thorac Cardiovasc Surg Pediatr Card Surg Annu* 112–117, 2009.
170. Nordmeyer J, Coats L, Lurz P, et al: Percutaneous pulmonary valve-in-valve implantation: a successful treatment concept for early device failure. *Eur Heart J* 29(6):810–815, 2008.
171. Bonhoeffer P, Boudjemline Y, Qureshi SA, et al: Percutaneous insertion of the pulmonary valve. *J Am Coll Cardiol* 39(10): 1664–1669, 2002.

Stem Cell Therapy for Ischemic Heart Disease

MARC S. PENN | SAIF ANWARUDDIN

KEY POINTS

- Advances in reperfusion therapy have led to the development of a large population of patients with chronic heart failure who need new therapies like stem cell therapy in order to experience improved outcomes.

- Several different stem cell populations have entered the clinical arena demonstrating varied benefits in acute myocardial infarction, with cell type and delivery strategies having significant effects on outcomes.

- Improvement in cardiac function with cell therapy does not necessarily imply improvement in electrical conduction or arrhythmogenic risk.

- Advances are still needed to optimize regenerative therapies for chronic heart failure.

- Recent advances in the generation of cardiac myocytes from induced pluripotent stem cells suggest that autologous cardiac myocyte regeneration may become possible.

Introduction

The many efforts to maximize therapy for the treatment of patients with acute myocardial infarction (AMI) have yielded significant benefits. Beginning first with thrombolytic therapy for AMI and more recently with the availability of primary percutaneous coronary intervention (PCI) for ST-segment elevation MI, the mortality rates of this devastating ischemic event have decreased from almost 15% in clinical trials in the late 1980s[1] to under 5% in recent primary PCI trials.[2] Prior to these advances, ischemic heart disease was the leading cause of chronic heart failure. While further improvements in reperfusion are needed, the current advances have led to the growing epidemic of heart disease, with many patients surviving what in the past might have been fatal events. With these advances, the prevalence of chronic heart failure (CHF) has increased dramatically over the preceding decade, with now more than 10% of the U.S. population over 65 years of age carrying this diagnosis. While the mechanisms are still under investigation,[3,4] the development of chronic heart failure following MI is more than just the loss of contractile tissue but also partly determined by the ventricular remodeling that occurs in response to myocardial necrosis.[5] The inflammatory response to myocardial necrosis leads to infarct expansion, dilation of the left ventricular (LV) cavity, and replacement of cardiomyocytes with fibrous tissue.[3,5] Currently available therapies to alter the remodeling process and the progression to chronic heart failure remain limited, and death rates from this condition continue to rise. Based on current trends the problem is predicted to increase to greater than 6 million people by the year 2030. The increasing burden of chronic heart failure has been addressed with pharmacological therapy, which in some can delay and improve the morbidity and mortality of heart disease; electrical therapy, including cardiac resynchronization therapy; LV remodeling surgery; and, with the approval of the first LV assist device for destination therapy, mechanical therapy. Given the shortcomings of each of these strategies and the fact that none of them address the underlying problem—loss of cardiac myocytes due to ischemic death—many have turned to molecular therapy, and more specifically stem cell-based therapy, as the hope for the future.

Approaches to Cell Therapy

The field of cell transplantation for the treatment of left ventricular dysfunction following ischemic injury continues to make significant progress, with dozens of studies now completed and metanalyses suggesting overall benefit to those patients who are treated compared with controls.[6,7] Theoretically, optimal cell therapy will use cell types that possess the capacity to incorporate themselves into the recipient myocardium and that will be able to survive, mature, and couple electromechanically with each other and native cardiac myocytes. The field began with differentiated cell transplantation (Fig. 55-1A), the goal of which was to functionally achieve myoplasty through the transplantation of autologous skeletal myoblasts that would engraft into injured myocardium in patients with chronic ischemic heart failure.[8] Another strategy that has been implemented clinically is stem cell mobilization (Fig. 55-1B), which involves the pharmacological mobilization of a patient's own bone marrow cells into the bloodstream, the idea being that these cells would engraft into areas of myocardial damage and then direct the engrafted stem cells to differentiate into cardiac myocytes and vascular structures that would fully integrate themselves with the native myocardium. By far the most comprehensively studied strategy to date that has shown some benefits is stem cell transplantation (Fig. 55-1C), which involves the removal of stem cells from the patient's bone marrow (autologous cells) or a well-screened donor (allogeneic cells) and then injecting the whole bone marrow or a selected population of bone marrow-derived stem cells into the infarct zone. Questions abound as to how these strategies will move forward and lead to clinical benefit in preventing (treatment in patients in the peri-infarct period) or treating (treatment in patients with chronic heart failure) cardiac dysfunction. Below we summarize the current state of knowledge and studies that are ongoing while also considering what their findings may mean and where the field may be moving.

DIFFERENTIATED CELL TRANSPLANTATION

The goal of differentiated cell transplantation is to replace scarred myocardium with living viable cells, ultimately leading to an overall improvement of myocardial function. A number of cell types, including smooth muscle cells and skeletal myoblasts, have been studied as potential candidates for differentiated cell transplantation. The value of these cell types is due to their accessibility and ability to be expanded in vitro prior to transplantation. Arguably the first strategy of cell therapy for chronic heart failure was cardiac myoplasty (cardiomyoplasty). During this procedure, the heart was wrapped in skeletal muscle that was then paced to increase the contractility of the weakened heart.[9–11] It was recognized that there was engraftment of skeletal muscle in the epicardial layers of the heart,[12,13] which we now recognize was the ingrowth and engraftment of skeletal myoblasts.[14] Following these observations, the early preclinical and clinical studies with skeletal myoblasts set the stage for the potential benefits associated with the delivery and engraftment of exogenous cells into the heart to prevent and treat cardiac dysfunction. We learned that exogenous cells could engraft into the heart and that the engraftment of skeletal

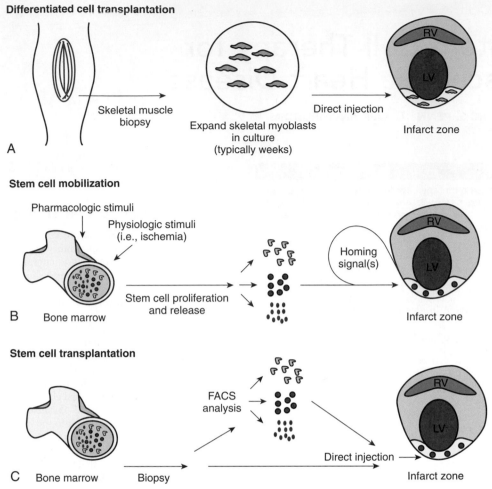

Figure 55-1   Schematic diagram of (A) differentiated cell transplantation, (B) stem cell mobilization, and (C) stem cell transplantation strategies of cell therapy for the treatment of cardiac dysfunction. FACS, fluorescence-activated cell sorting.

myoblasts could lead to clinical benefit, including inducing reverse LV remodeling.[15–17] We further learned the importance of the mechanical coupling of exogenous cells to the cellular milieu of the heart.[18] Skeletal myoblasts (SKMBs) do not integrate into the electrical syncytium of the myocardium and have been shown in animal studies to induce slow conduction,[19] increased risk of reentrant rhythm,[20] and increased premature ventricular contractions and ventricular tachycardia in patients.[8] It takes at least 2 to 3 weeks between skeletal muscle biopsy and the availability of a sufficient number of SKMBs for transplantation in humans. Thus, while SKMBs have some desirable properties for cell therapy, the timing of delivering SKMB treatment compared with the stem cell approaches is problematic. This timing issue, the lack of vascular growth induced by SKMBs alone,[21] and the proarrhythmogenic effect of SKMBs makes debatable the issue of whether SKMB transplantation alone will offer significant clinical benefit.

MYOCARDIAL REGENERATION

Since the turn of the century, a significant body of literature has rewritten the once strongly held belief that the heart cannot repair itself. We have learned that following MI in humans there is a transient mobilization of stem cells and expression of stem cell homing factors that recruit these cells to the heart.[22,23] Human female hearts transplanted into males were found to have cardiac myocytes and vascular structures that stained positive for the Y chromosome, suggesting that these cells originated from the stem cells of the transplant recipient.[24] Unfortunately these studies demonstrate that stem cell engraftment and

differentiation into cardiac myocytes is an infrequent event (0.02% cardiac myocytes, 3.3% endothelial cells). However, these studies do suggest that the normal physiological response to myocardial injury is mobilization of stem cells, "homing" of these cells to the damaged myocardium, and differentiation of at least some of them into cardiac myocytes. Furthermore, if this natural repair mechanism can be potentiated, clinically meaningful myocardial regeneration may be achievable. The excitement surrounding the use of stem cells is based on the unique biological properties of these cells and their capacity to self-renew and regenerate tissue and organ systems. Figure 55-2 groups different stem cell populations of interest in myocardial regeneration based on their cardiogenic potential. While it was once believed that all stem cell populations listed in Figure 55-2 could differentiate into cardiac myocytes,[25,26] it is now clear that while many of these cell populations may lead to improved cardiac function,[25,27] following transplantation, only a limited number of them become cardiac myocytes.[28,29] Importantly, recent studies using mesenchymal stem cells derived from the amniotic membrane demonstrate that the delivery of cardiogenic stem cells results in significant improvements in cardiac function despite the lack of significant regeneration of structural myocardium.[30,31]

BONE MARROW-DERIVED MONONUCLEAR CELLS

The transplantation of bone marrow-derived mononuclear cell preparations to the infarct-related vessel has progressed to the point where data from randomized controlled trials are now becoming available for

STEM CELL POPULATIONS OF INTEREST FOR CARDIAC REPAIR

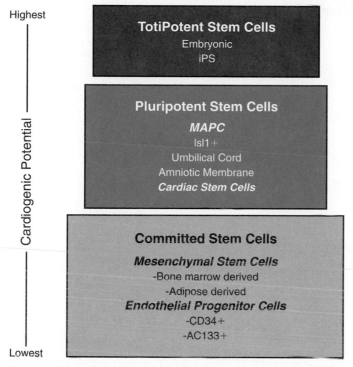

Figure 55-2 Different stem cell populations of interest for myocardial repair stratified by the differentiation capacity of the given populations.

patients with AMI (Table 55-1) and CHF (Table 55-2). The first randomized stem cell trial for patients with AMI was the BOOST trial.[32] These trials can be summarized as follows:

- Patient populations of interest includ patients with a first ST-segment elevation MI (STEMI) and presumed normal LV function at baseline.
- All patients underwent primary PCI with restoration of antegrade flow.
- Bone marrow harvest was done on the day of stem cell infusion, 3 to 7 days after AMI.
- The cell population of interest was isolated by Ficoll gradient or other methods, with cell dosing based on CD34+ cell number.
- Cells were infused down the infarct-related vessel either by direct infusion or using a stop-flow technique leading to the cessation of coronary blood flow during infusion.
- Baseline and follow-up measurements of LV function consisted of LV angiogram, cardiac magnetic resonance imaging (MRI), and/or echocardiography.

As seen in Table 55-1, while this strategy has not always resulted in improved cardiac function, most trials have demonstrated a significant increase in cardiac function ranging from 2% to 6%. Importantly, in some trials the early benefits seen with cell therapy were lost with subsequent follow-up, suggesting that the infusion of bone marrow mononuclear cells accelerates healing of the heart but may not further improve it.[33] In contrast, serial follow-up from the largest bone marrow infusion trial to date, the REPAIR-AMI study,[34] found continued improvement in cardiac function as well as continued trends in benefit in clinical parameters including hospitalization for heart failure, reinfarction, and survival. At the 4-month time point, the treated population had an increase in ejection fraction of 6% compared with baseline versus the control population, which exhibited only a 2.5% increase. In more recent follow-up studies, these benefits and evidence of decreased clinical events have been maintained out to 2 and 5 years

				TABLE 55-1	Stem Cell Transplantation in Acute Myocardial infarction	

Study	Number of Patients/ Placebo Control	Cell Type	Delivery Method	Time after Infarct	Baseline LV Function	Comments
Chen[75]	69/yes	BM-derived MSC	Intra-coronary	18.4 ± 1.5 days	49%–53%	Improvement in perfusion, cardiac function and decreased LV dilation. No increase in restenosis noted.
BOOST[32,76]	60/yes	BM-derived mononuclear cells	Intra-coronary	4.8 days	50%–51%	Six months after MI, increase in EF (6.7%) in patients that received BM cells compared to 0.6% in optimal medical management. Controls caught up, but benefit not lost at 18 months.
ASTAMI[77]	100/yes	BM-derived mononuclear cells	Intra-coronary	5–8 days	46%	Noted chest pain and/or ECG changes with infusion. No improvement 6 months after stem cell infusion.
REPAIR-AMI[34]	204/yes	BM-derived mononuclear cells	Intra-coronary	4 days	47%–48%	Modest improvement in EF 4 months after stem cell infusion 5.5% with stem cells vs. 3.0% for placebo. For EF < 49% at baseline, improvement was 7.5% with stem cells vs. 2.5% for placebo
Janssens[49]	66/yes	BM-derived mononuclear cells	Intra-coronary	4 days	46%–49%	First randomized, placebo controlled blinded study for cell therapy at the time of AMI. No benefit seen.
Yousef[78]	62/no	BM-derived mononuclear cells	Intra-coronary	7 days	51%	Registry control group. Improved LV function and quality of life and mortality out to 5 years.
Hare[47]	53/yes	MSC (allogeneic)	Intra-venous	1–10 days	53%	Trend towards improvement in LV function in AWMI. Evidence of decreased arrhythmia in treated patients.
Penn	28	MAPC (allogeneic)	Adventitial	2–5 days	43%	Registry control. Significant improvement at 50 M dose.
TIME Trial[79]	120/yes	BM-derived mononuclear cells	Intra-coronary	3 or 7 days		Ongoing NIH CCTRN trial, randomizing between 3 and 7 days after AMI.
LATETIME[80]	87/yes	BM-derived mononuclear cells	Intra-coronary	14–21 days		Ongoing NIH CCTRN trial, randomizing between placebo and late after AMI.

AWMI, anterior wall myocardial infarction; *BM,* bone marrow; *CCTRN,* cardiovascular cell therapy research network; *MSC,* mesenchymal stem cell; *MAPC,* multipotent adult progenitor cell; *SDF-1,* stromal cell derived factor-1.

TABLE 55-2	Stem Cell Transplantation in Congestive Heart Failure					
Study	*Number of Patients/ Placebo Cotrol*	*Cell Type*	*Delivery Method*	*Time after Infarct*	*Baseline LV Function*	*Comments*
Tse[81]	8/no	BM-derived mononuclear cells	Stem cell transplantation (NOGA-guided catheter-based intramyocardial injection)	Severe ischemic heart disease	Unchanged	Despite no change in EF, an improvement in target wall thickening and wall motion was seen by MRI. No acute procedure-related complications were seen.
Seiler[82]	21/yYes	Stem cells mobilized from the BM	GM-CSF, first dose intracoronary then SC for 2 weeks	Chronic ischemia	Unchanged, but decreased ischemia	Stem cell mobilization to induce angiogenesis as assessed by improved coronary collateral blood flow following 2 weeks of daily GM-CSF administration.
Assmus[83]	75/yes with crossover	Circulating progenitor cells (CPC) or BM-derived mononuclear cells (BMC)	Intracoronary infusion	Ischemic cardiomyopathy	Improved with BMC only	Baseline EF ~40% 2.9% improvement with BMC -1.2% without therapy -0.4% with CPC
Perin[84]	21/yes, nonrandomized	BM-derived mononuclear cells	NOGA-guided intramyocardial injection	Severe ischemic cardiomyopathy	Improved	
Fuchs[33]	10/no	BM-derived mononuclear cells	Catheter-based intramyocardial delivery	Chronic ischemia	Unchanged, but decreased ischemia	Decreased stress -induced ischemia and CCS angina score
FOCUS[85]	87/yes	BM-derived mononuclear cells	NOGA-guided intramyocardial injection	Ischemic cardiomyopathy		Ongoing NIH CCTRN trial

EF, ejection fraction; *NIH,* National Institutes of Health; *BMC,* bone marrow cells; *CPC,* cardiac progenitor cells.

after treatment.[35] There are several ongoing clinical studies using bone marrow-derived mononuclear cells in the peri-MI period that will address important questions. The Cardiovascular Cell Therapy Research Network, an NIH-funded network of clinical sites, is running the TIME and LateTIME studies. These are addressing the important question of the optimal timing for cell therapy. The TIME study is randomizing patients between cells and placebo and treatment 3 or 7 days after primary PCI. The LateTIME study is randomizing between cells and placebo at 2 to 3 weeks after primary PCI. These studies will further suggest optimal timing of bone marrow mononuclear cell treatment as well as beginning to define when is too late for treatment.

Novel Autologous Stem Cell Indications and Types

Two recent studies have demonstrated the potential of two specific autologous cell populations that significantly advance the field of cardiovascular cell therapy. The first is the ACT-34 study. This study, a randomized double-blind placebo-controlled trial, focused on patients with chronic myocardial ischemia. In this population, a placebo-controlled blinded study was performed in which patients received granulocyte-colony stimulating factor (G-CSF) mobilization followed by apheresis and isolation of CD34+ cells. These cells were injected via an endoventricular approach using the NOGA catheter. The recent release of the 1-year follow-up data for this patient population revealed a decrease of 5.6 angina events per week and a doubling of exercise treadmill time versus baseline. These data verify in the clinical setting the preclinical findings that stem cell-based cardiac repair results in a significant and sustained increase in vascular density, leading to improved perfusion of the myocardium. A second trial focused on the effects of cardiac stem cells in patients with ischemic cardiomyopathy. Based on the relative dosing of stem cells in preclinical trials, it would appear that cardiac stem cells may be the most potent of all the adult stem cells.[36] If true, then cardiac stem cells may be the best cells to use for stem cell transplantation (Fig. 55-1) as an adjunct to open heart surgery in the setting of coronary grafting, valve surgery, or left ventricular assist device implantation. Just as adipose-derived stem cells can be rapidly harvested from adipose tissue,[37,38] it may become possible to rapidly isolate cardiac stem cells from the left atrial appendage

in the operating room or from endomyocardial biopsies in sufficient number to allow for meaningful myocardial support. In the SCIPIO (Stem Cell Infusion in Patients with Ischemic cardiOmyopathy) trial (Clinicaltrials.org; NCT00474461), cardiac stem cells were isolated from atrial tissue obtained at the time of coronary artery bypass surgery. These cardiac stem cells were cultured and, after sufficient propagation, were injected into injured myocardium through a percutaneous approach Thus far, data from this trial have demonstrated varied results but, on average, a ~9% increase in cardiac function. While preliminary, this trial is a good example of the novel approaches being undertaken to investigate and optimize adult stem cell therapy.

MESENCHYMAL STEM CELLS AND MULTIPOTENT ADULT PROGENITOR CELLS

Perhaps the greatest recent advance in cardiovascular cell therapy has been the successful implementation of allogeneic stem cell sources in the treatment of patients with AMI. Stromal progenitor cells comprise less than 0.05% of the adult bone marrow. Mesenchymal stem cells (MSCs) and multipotent adult progenitor cells (MAPCs) from subpopulations of bone marrow stromal progenitor cells maintain the ability to differentiate along multiple lineages.[26,39] MSCs can be immunoselected via cell-surface CD45 negativity and cultured through as many as 40 population doublings before attaining senescence. In general the benefits observed with MSCs following cell transplantation at the time of MI may have little to do with the cell itself but more with how factors secreted by the MSCs alter the tissue microenvironment. This so-called paracrine effect of MSCs has been demonstrated,[40] showing that injection of the supernatant of MSC cell cultures at the time of MI results in benefits similar to those that have been associated with MSC cell transplantation. More recently we have demonstrated that stromal cell-derived factor 1 (SDF-1) released by MSCs results in the recruitment of cardiac stem cells to the infarct border zone while also inhibiting cardiac myocyte death through the binding of SDF-1 to CXCR4-expressing cardiac myocytes in the infarct border zone. Recent preclinical studies have demonstrated that modulation of wnt/b-catenin signaling through TGF-β pretreatment or more precisely by modulating disabled-2 induce MSCs to increase expression of proteins in vitro that are normally expressed by cardiac myocytes, leading to an improved functional response.[41] MAPCs are

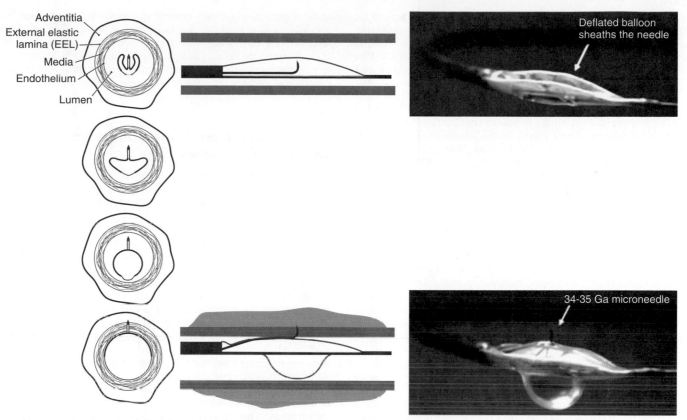

Figure 55-3 Schematic representation of microneedle catheter-mediated delivery to the coronary adventitia and photographs of the deflated and inflated Mercatormed Cricket Catheter. *(Mercator MedSystems, Inc, San Francisco, CA.)*

stromal cells derived from the bone marrow; they are able to differentiate into endothelial, epithelial, and mesenchymal cell types.[42] They can be expanded in culture for more than 80 population doublings and still maintain their pluripotency by differentiating into most somatic cell types.[42] Whether these multipotent stem cells exist in vivo or are the result of serial cell passages in culture remains to be determined. However, the demonstration that multipotent cells can be significantly expanded as well as the benefit they have shown in early animal studies[43] bode well for the development of future therapies. Both MSCs and MAPCs have been shown to lead to decreased cardiac myocyte cell death, decreased infarct size, improved cardiac remodeling, and improved function in rodent[44] and porcine models[45] of AMI. Each of these cell types has now entered the clinical realm and phase I clinical trials are now complete. Interestingly, while each has shown promise in preclinical studies, their effects in early trials are different. Understanding whether these differences are a result of the cell type, the accompanying delivery strategy, or the patient population will be critical for future clinical development. The phase I clinical trial for MSCs-studied patients with AMI diagnosed by a positive troponin; thus this is one of the first trials that enrolled individuals with NSTEMI. In order to take advantage of stem cell homing signaling in the peri-infarct period,[22,46] allogeneic MSCs were delivered intravenously between 1 and 10 days after AMI. The phase I study was a dose-escalating study. Importantly, no toxicities were observed in response to the intravenous infusion of allogeneic MSCs.[47] With respect to efficacy, two important observations were made: in the patients with STEMI AWMI (anterior wall myocardial infarction), there was a significant improvement in cardiac function. Also observed, as predicted by preclinical studies with MSCs, there was a significant decrease in premature ventricular contractions (PVCs) and arrhythmias.[47] These findings are consistent with the concept that cell therapy can be used to modulate the electrical and mechanical sizes of the infarct.[16] The MAPC phase I trial was similarly a dose-ranging study in which 20, 50, and 100 million MAPCs were delivered to patients with first-time STEMI MI with a postprimary PCI

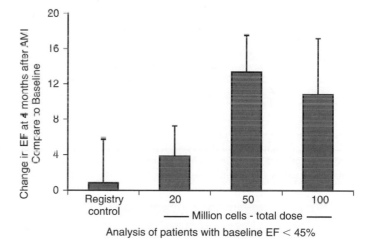

Figure 55-4 Analysis of patients with baseline EF <45%.

ejection fraction of 45% or less. In contrast to the MSC phase I trial, the MAPC phase I trial used catheter-mediated adventitial delivery of the MAPCs, using the Mercatormed Systems Cricket Catheter (Mercator MedSystems, Inc, San Francisco, CA), 2 to 5 days after primary PCI. As shown in Figure 55-3, as the balloon is inflated on this catheter, a single needle is deployed that goes through the medial layer of the infarct-related artery to deliver the MAPCs to the adventitia. Once in the adventitia, preclinical studies have demonstrated that the MAPCs distribute through the infarct zone. The delivery of MAPCs resulted, on average, in an absolute increase in ejection fraction of >12% in those patients with baseline ejection fractions <45% (Fig. 55-4). As in other studies, no significant improvement was observed in such patients.[48,49] It is quite possible that these allogeneic stem cell studies point to the future of cardiovascular stem cell therapy, in which "off-the-shelf" allogeneic stem cells will be available for delivery to the patient immediately following primary PCI. Both of these cell types have been shown to have some efficacy in preventing and treating graft-versus-host disease and thus have anti-inflammatory effects. That is, there may be real benefit to the delivery of these stem cells soon after reperfusion in order to minimize neutrophil infiltration and cardiac myocyte cell death and to optimize ventricular remodeling.[44] It is interesting to compare the loss of efficacy in the translation of MSCs and MAPCs from preclinical studies to human studies. The efficacy of the intravenous delivery of MSCs went from a relative increase of ~80% in rats to 10% at the high dose of MSCs in the phase I trial. For MAPCs, the improvement in ejection fraction in a porcine AMI model was ~38%, whereas it was ~35% in the phase I trial. While the consistency in effect in the MAPC trial could be because of the cells, it is more likely that the difference in translation was due to the delivery method. In the MAPC trial, the cells were delivered to the adventitia in similar fashions, avoiding the atherosclerotic intima of the diseased coronaries. In contrast, the efficiency of delivery of MSCs to the myocardium in patients with coronary artery disease could have been inhibited compared with that observed in rodents, which have nondiseased arteries. Future studies are needed to define optimal delivery strategies for stem cell delivery to the heart. The Cricket catheter offers an intriguing strategy for the delivery of stem cells to the infarct region immediately following primary PCI, thus obviating the need for complex delivery systems or additional procedures at a later date in the catheterization laboratory.

CARDIAC REGENERATION

As discussed above, there is little evidence that adult stem cells result in myocardial regeneration. It is likely that regeneration of cardiac myocytes and myocardial structures will require embryonic stem cells (ESs) or cardiac myocytes generated from induced pluripotent stem cells (iPSs). ESs are continuously replicating cell lines derived from an embryonic origin isolated from the blastocyst's inner cell mass.[50,51] The properties of ESs include derivation from the pre- or peri-implantation embryo, prolonged undifferentiated proliferation with conditional constraints, and the ability to form tissues derived from all three germ layers. When they are properly cultured, ESs expand at a rapid rate and group to form embryoid bodies that have the ability to differentiate into a wide variety of specialized cells, including cardiomyocytes. Adult somatic cells have recently been shown capable of being differentiated into cardiac myocytes through the intermediate step of generating induced pluripotent stem cells or by direct differentiation of somatic cells.[52-56] Transplantation of these cells leads to engraftment of cardiac myocytes in the infarct zone and improvement in cardiac function and remodeling. How these cells will ultimately translate into the clinic is

as yet unclear. Undoubtedly optimal translation will require scaffolds and biologicals to optimize the vascularization, integration, and workload of these contractile networks. To date there are no published clinical data on the delivery of significant numbers of cardiac myocytes to treat patients with chronic heart failure. Perhaps the closest ongoing clinical trial involves the delivery of autologous cardiospheres to such patients (Clinicaltrials.gov; NCT00893360).

■ Stem Cell-Based Chemokine and Cytokine Strategies

An early focus of clinical trials for stem cell-based repair of the myocardium was based on cytokine-mediated mobilization of the marrow space using G-CSF and granulocyte-macrophage colony-stimulating factor (GM-CSF).[57] While the results are somewhat mixed (Table 55-3), there is overall little evidence that stem cell mobilization of the marrow space in the peri-infarct period with G-CSF leads to a significant change in cardiac function or remodeling. Several things could explain the lack of efficacy of this approach to date. The first is the timing of stem cell mobilization relative to the heart's ability to recruit circulating stem cells. The only trial that has shown sustained improvement involved the administration of G-CSF within 1 hour of PCI.[58] A recent clinical study that varied the timing of G-CSF following primary PCI did not find any benefit.[60] Our group has demonstrated that stromal cell-derived factor 1 (SDF-1) expression is sufficient to induce stem cell homing to the heart in models of ischemic cardiomyopathy and that transiently reestablishing expression of SDF-1 in the remodeled heart at a time remote from MI is sufficient to induce neovascularization and significant restoration of cardiac contractility.[22,59] Our data further showed that by 7 days following MI, myocardial expression of SDF-1 has ceased. Thus timing is of the essence if we are to mobilize hematopoietic stem cells and expect them to engraft in the heart. Another reason this strategy may have failed is that G-CSF-mobilized hematopoietic stem cells are unable to home due to dysfunctional CXCR4 (the SDF-1 receptor) expression. G-CSF mobilizes stem cells via the degradation of CXCR4, thus releasing the stem cell from its anchor in the bone marrow. There is increasing evidence that the stem cell-mobilizing agent AMD3100—an antagonist to the CXCR4 receptor—induces stem cell mobilization, which leads to improvement in cardiac function in preclinical models.[61] Interestingly, early use of AMD3100 leads to stem cell mobilization but does not lead to persistent inhibition of CXCR4 binding in the myocardium,[61] whereas persistent AMD3100 administration leads to mobilization of stem cells but no improvement in cardiac function. These data suggest a potentially important role for cardiac CXCR4 expression in myocardial response to stem cell-mediated repair. The bone marrow naturally

TABLE 55-3	G-CSF Stem Cell Mobilization in Acute Myocardial Infarction				
Study	*Number of Patients/Placebo*	*Cell Type*	*Time after Infarct*	*LV Function*	*Comments*
Kang[86]	27/yes	Stem cells mobilized from the BM	3–270 days	Improved	Increased incidence of restenosis with G-CSF. Improved myocardial perfusion. Similar improvements seen with intracoronary infusion of peripheral blood stem cells.
Valgimigli[87]	20/yes	Stem cells mobilized from the BM		Trend towards improvement	No increase in restenosis with G-CSF. No improvement in myocardial perfusion.
Ellis[88]	18/yes	Stem cells mobilized from the BM	First dose ≤48 hours from onset of symptoms	No change	No benefit or harm with 5 or 10 mcg/kg per day within 48 hours after AMI.
Ince[58]	30/yes	Stem cell mobilized from the BM	1 hour	Improved	Control: EF 53-> 46%. Treated: EF 52 > 56%
Ripa[89]	78/yes	Stem cell mobilized from the BM		No change	No significant changes in wall thickening or EF by echo or MRI.
Zohlnhofer[90]	114/yes	Stem cell mobilized from the BM	5 days	No change	No evidence of increased rate of restenosis with G-CSF.
Overgaard[91]	54/yes	Stem cell mobilized from the BM	Variable	No change	No evidence of benefit by MRI LV assessment when G-CSF given between 17 and 65 h after PCI.

PCI, percutaneous coronary intervention; *BM*, bone marrow, *EF*, ejection fraction.

releases stem cells into the bloodstream on a daily basis. The concept of cytokine-based stem cell mobilization is to increase the number of circulating stem cells at the time the heart is signaling to recruit them. Thus, while G-CSF and AMD3100 induce stem cells to enter the bloodstream, if the heart is not signaling to recruit them to the injured myocardium, no benefit will be realized.[22,62] Initially we and now others have taken the opposite approach—to prolong the period of time that the heart signals to recruit stem cells to the injured myocardium and take advantage of the fact that there are always circulating stem cells present in the bloodstream. Several years ago we defined stromal cell-derived factor as a stem cell homing factor to injured tissues.[22] We have demonstrated that if one prolongs SDF-1 signaling in the myocardium—either via the delivery of mesenchymal stem cells, which express SDF-1 at baseline, or enhanced SDF-1 expressing mesenchymal stem cells—there is significant preservation of cardiac myocytes and cardiac function.[63] We have recently demonstrated that the reestablishment of SDF-1 expression through the delivery of SDF-1 plasmid to a model of ischemic cardiomyopathy leads to remodeling of the scar and improvement in ejection fraction.[64] Based on these data and those from porcine models, SDF-1 gene transfer is now the focus of a phase I clinical trial in patients with NYHA class III CHF. In this open-label dose-escalation study, SDF-1 plasmid is being delivered using a helical catheter retrograde through the aortic valve to the endocardial surface. Fifteen injections of 1 ml per injection to the infarct and infarct border zone are being performed. The trial is now fully enrolled, with 4-month primary endpoint data released in May, 2011.

Electrical Effects of Cell Therapy

While the field is moving forward in trying to identify strategies that either preserve or improve cardiac function in patients at the time of AMI or with CHF, it is becoming clear that the mechanical and electrical effects of cell therapy are independent.[59,65] We have previously demonstrated in animal models that the delivery of SKMBs or mesenchymal stem cells (1 million of each cell type) in the peri-infarct period to the myocardium results in similar improvements in cardiac function; however, when these hearts undergo an electrophysiology study with the introduction of extra systoles, the rate at which ventricular tachycardia is induced is significantly different depending on the cell type the animal received.[20] Animals that received SKMBs were always inducible for ventricular tachycardia. As noted in Table 55-1, multiple studies have suggested an increased incidence of ventricular tachycardia in patients who received SKMBs. This could be a spurious result because all the patients in these trials had a history of MI, however, while SKMBs do express connexin 43 in culture, they do not express connexin 43 after transplantation, and SKMBs do not electrically couple with the native myocardium.[65] The establishment of connexin 43 expression in SKMBs has been shown to decrease the arrhythmogenic risk of SKMBs. These data, coupled with the clinical data to date demonstrating a decrease in clinical measures of arrhythmia in patients who received intravenous MSC following AMI,[47] suggest that stem cell therapy could expand its potential clinical indications from simply improving cardiac function to decreasing reentry. Therefore it would be possible to contemplate a trial where instead of inducing further LV injury to interrupt a reentrant circuit, specific stem cells could be injected into the mapped circuit to reverse the area of slow conduction or remodel the size of the scar. Cell therapy has sufficiently advanced that novel indications and trial designs should be pursued.

Future Directions and Controversies

The field of stem cell therapy for the treatment of cardiovascular disease is continuing to make significant strides both at the molecular level and the clinical setting. The field has sufficiently matured that it is now stratified into distinct focuses: relevant basic science and clinical science. Within each focus there are clear critical issues that need to be addressed in order to advance the field to prevent or treat cardiac dysfunction and improve outcomes in patients with heart disease.

BENCH INVESTIGATION

Questions in the setting of basic science can generally be divided into two general areas. The first focuses on defining the molecular mechanisms associated with adult stem cell-based repair of the heart. As we have shown with SDF-1 over the past decade, defining the molecular mechanisms associated with stem cell-based repair can lead to novel targets for therapy and insights into the biology of tissue healing[46,66,67]; it can also offer clinical scientists novel agents for investigation. The second area involves the issue of whether we can truly achieve cardiogenesis. There are few data indicating that unmanipulated cardiac myocytes will divide and regenerate following myocardial injury. However, genetic manipulation of cardiac myocytes using engineered murine models indicates that cardiac myocytes can be induced to divide and regress infarct size.[68,69] Whether pharmacological strategies will be developed to allow these pathways to be activated following MI remains to be seen. The discovery of iPSs[70,71] clearly offers the potential for the generation of autologous cardiac myocytes that can be transplanted into the myocardium of patients with chronic heart failure.[55,72] Many hurdles remain, including the safety of iPSs, how best to generate cardiac myocytes from adult cells, how to integrate the cardiac myocytes into a functional contractile unit, and then how to integrate these units into the injured myocardium. It is important to recognize that all the work being done on adult stem cell therapy would still be highly relevant and clinically important even if these autologous cardiac myocytes were available today. Given the likely cost and complexities associated with generating, maintaining, delivering, and integrating these contractile units, adult stem cell therapy will still have a role in minimizing cardiac damage and optimizing ventricular remodeling following acute ischemic events in the hope of minimizing or delaying the need for cardiac myocyte replacement with iPSs.

CLINICAL INVESTIGATION

There are several important questions that remain to be addressed in the clinical realm. Perhaps the first should consider stem cell type and mode of delivery. To date the mode of delivery has been thought of as a separate question from cell type; however, mode of delivery should be tightly coupled with the cell of interest and the clinical indication. For example, both MSCs and MAPCs have been shown to have anti-inflammatory effects. Thus, delivery of these cells early after primary PCI could lead to a decrease in neutrophil infiltration and improved cardiac remodeling.[73,74] Therefore the optimal delivery system for allogeneic "off-the-shelf" cells should be a catheter that allows for rapid delivery of the stem cells of interest to the infarct-related vessel without the need for additional vascular access. At the opposite extreme, for patients with ischemic cardiomyopathy, the mode of access and time for such a scheduled procedure is not as important an issue. In this situation, if electromechanical mapping proves to be important for defining areas of delivery, it should be used; similarly if generalized delivery of stem cells to the myocardium is important, perhaps retrograde delivery of stem cells via the coronary sinus would be optimal. Given the data at hand, the field will soon progress to the point where clinical studies comparing modes of delivery will be necessary. An important question that needs to be addressed in the clinical realm is whether stem cell therapy will have significant benefit in patients with NSTEMI. Most trials to date have focused on patients with first STEMI with normal cardiac function prior to their ischemic event. The MSC trial, which did allow NSTEMI, still required the index event to be the person's first AMI or it required at least documented normal LV function if there was a prior event. While this study population has been critical to demonstrate proof of concept and biological effect, it is not the clinical population that is most at risk for adverse cardiac events. Furthermore, as many in the field are well aware, the number of STEMIs continues to decline. Ultimately, if adult stem cell therapy is going to have a significant impact on patient outcomes, the therapy must be transitioned to patients with ischemic cardiomyopathy prior to their index event and who present with NSTEMI. There are multiple potential mechanisms where stem cells could lead to improved outcomes in these patients, including limiting the infarct size, remodeling the scar, quieting vulnerable plaque in the coronary tree, optimizing LV remodeling, and decreasing arrhythmogenic risk. Multiple issues will need to be addressed for this therapy to successfully transition to NSTEMI, including where to inject the cells, how much damage is needed before the therapy will be useful, and what clinical measures can be used to assess efficacy. This transition will be challenging but will be an important milestone if adult stem cells are to have significant clinical impact on patients at risk.

Conclusions

The field of adult stem cell therapy for the prevention and treatment of cardiac dysfunction continues to make progress. The data suggest that there is a therapeutic effect; the issue is what the therapy will look like when it is optimized, which indications will receive approval, and how widely available the therapies will be. Given the growing prevalence of patients with congestive heart failure and MI combined with the economic burden of congestive heart failure, the potential human and societal benefits continue to be great.

REFERENCES

1. Randomized factorial trial of high-dose intravenous streptokinase, of oral aspirin and of intravenous heparin in acute myocardial infarction. ISIS (International Studies of Infarct Survival) pilot study. *Eur Heart J* 8:634–642, 1987.
2. Stone GW, Grines CL, Cox DA, et al: Comparison of angioplasty with stenting, with or without abciximab, in acute myocardial infarction. *N Engl J Med* 346:957–966, 2002.
3. Askari A, Brennan ML, Zhou X, et al: Myeloperoxidase and plasminogen activator inhibitor-1 play a central role in ventricular remodeling after myocardial infarction. *J Exp Med* 197:615–624, 2003.
4. Heymans S, Luttun A, Nuyens D, et al: Inhibition of plasminogen activators or matrix metalloproteinases prevents cardiac rupture but impairs therapeutic angiogenesis and causes cardiac failure. *Nat Med* 5:1135–1142, 1999.
5. Vasilyev N, Williams T, Brennan ML, et al: Myeloperoxidase-generated oxidants modulate left ventricular remodeling but not infarct size after myocardial infarction. *Circulation* 112:2812–2820, 2005.
6. Abdel-Latif A, Bolli R, Tleyjeh IM, et al: Adult bone marrow-derived cells for cardiac repair: a systematic review and meta-analysis. *Arch Intern Med* 167:989–997, 2007.
7. Jiang M, He B, Zhang Q, et al: Randomized controlled trials on the therapeutic effects of adult progenitor cells for myocardial infarction: meta-analysis. *Expert Opin Biol Ther* 10:667–680, 2010.
8. Menasche P, Alfieri O, Janssens S, et al: The Myoblast Autologous Grafting in Ischemic Cardiomyopathy (MAGIC) trial: first randomized placebo-controlled study of myoblast transplantation. *Circulation* 117:1189–1200, 2008.
9. Moreira LF, Bocchi EA, Stolf NA, et al: Dynamic cardiomyoplasty in the treatment of dilated cardiomyopathy: current results and perspectives. *J Card Surg* 11:207–216, 1996.
10. Bocchi EA, Moreira LF, de Moraes AV, et al: Effects of dynamic cardiomyoplasty on regional wall motion ejection fraction and geometry of left ventricle. *Circulation* 86:II231–II235, 1992.
11. Jatene AD, Moreira LF, Stolf NA, et al: Left ventricular function changes after cardiomyoplasty in patients with dilated cardiomyopathy. *J Thorac Cardiovasc Surg* 102:132–138, 1991.
12. Chiu RC, Kochamba G, Walsh G, et al: Biochemical and functional correlates of myocardium-like transformed skeletal muscle as a power source for cardiac assist devices. *J Card Surg* 4:171–179, 1989.
13. Misawa Y, Mott BD, Lough JO, et al: Pathologic findings of latissimus dorsi muscle graft in dynamic cardiomyoplasty: clinical implications. *J Heart Lung Transplant* 16:585–595, 1997.
14. Menasche P, Hagege AA, Vilquin JT, et al: Autologous skeletal myoblast transplantation for severe postinfarction left ventricular dysfunction. *J Am Coll Cardiol* 41:1078–1083, 2003.
15. Askari A, Goldman CK, Forudi F, et al: VEGF-expressing skeletal myoblast transplantation induces angiogenesis and improves left ventricular function late after myocardial infarction. *Mol Ther* 5:S162, 2002.
16. Deglurkar I, Mal N, Mills WR, et al: Mechanical and electrical effects of cell-based gene therapy for ischemic cardiomyopathy are independent. *Hum Gene Ther* 17:1144–1151, 2006.
17. Dowell JD, Rubart M, Pasumarthi KB, et al: Myocyte and myogenic stem cell transplantation in the heart. *Cardiovasc Res* 58:336–350, 2003.
18. Reinecke H, MacDonald GH, Hauschka SD, et al: Electromechanical coupling between skeletal and cardiac muscle. Implications for infarct repair. *J Cell Biol* 149:731–740, 2000.
19. Fouts K, Fernandes B, Mal N, et al: Electrophysiological consequence of skeletal myoblast transplantation in normal and infarcted canine myocardium. *Heart Rhythm* 3:452–461, 2006.
20. Mills WR, Mal N, Kiedrowski MJ, et al: Stem cell therapy enhances electrical viability in myocardial infarction. *J Mol Cell Cardiol* 42:314, 2007.
21. Askari A, Unzek S, Goldman CK, et al: Cellular but not direct adenoviral delivery of VEGF results in improved LV function and neovascularization in dilated ischemic cardiomyopathy. *J Am Coll Cardiol* 43:1908–1914, 2004.
22. Askari A, Unzek S, Popovic ZB, et al: Effect of stromal-cell-derived factor-1 on stem cell homing and tissue regeneration in ischemic cardiomyopathy. *Lancet* 362:697–703, 2003.
23. Hofmann M, Wollert KC, Meyer GP, et al: Monitoring of bone marrow cell homing into the infarcted human myocardium. *Circulation* 111:2198–2202, 2005.
24. Muller P, Pfeiffer P, Koglin J, et al: Cardiomyocytes of noncardiac origin in myocardial biopsies of human transplanted hearts. *Circulation* 106:31–35, 2002.
25. Orlic D, Kajstura J, Chimenti S, et al: Bone marrow cells regenerate infarcted myocardium. *Nature* 410:701–705, 2001.
26. Mangi AA, Noiseux N, Kong D, et al: Mesenchymal stem cells modified with Akt prevent remodeling and restore performance of infarcted hearts. *Nat Med* 9:1195–1201, 2003.
27. Kocher AA, Schuster MD, Szabolcs MJ, et al:Neovascularization of ischemic myocardium by human bone-marrow-derived angioblasts prevents cardiomyocyte apoptosis reduces remodeling and improves cardiac function. *Nat Med* 7:430–436, 2001.
28. Murry CE, Soonpaa MH, Reinecke H, et al: Haematopoietic stem cells do not transdifferentiate into cardiac myocytes in myocardial infarcts. *Nature* 428:664–668, 2004.
29. Schenk S, Mal N, Finan A, et al: MCP-3 is a myocardial mesenchymal stem cell homing factor. *Stem Cells* 25:245–251, 2007.
30. Tsuji H, Miyoshi S, Ikegami Y, et al: Xenografted human amniotic membrane-derived mesenchymal stem cells are immunologically tolerated and transdifferentiated into cardiomyocytes. *Circ Res* 106:1613–1623, 2010.
31. Penn MS, Mayorga ME: Searching for understanding with the cellular lining of life. *Circ Res* 106:1554–1556, 2010.
32. Wollert KC, Meyer GP, Lotz J, et al: Intracoronary autologous bone-marrow cell transfer after myocardial infarction: the BOOST randomised controlled clinical trial. *Lancet* 364:141–148, 2004.
33. Schaefer A, Meyer GP, Fuchs M, et al: Impact of intracoronary bone marrow cell transfer on diastolic function in patients after acute myocardial infarction: results from the BOOST trial. *Eur Heart J* 27:929–935, 2006.
34. Schachinger V, Erbs S, Elsasser A, et al: Intracoronary bone marrow-derived progenitor cells in acute myocardial infarction. *N Engl J Med* 355:1210–1221, 2006.
35. Assmus B, Rolf A, Erbs S, et al: Clinical outcome 2 years after intracoronary administration of bone marrow-derived progenitor cells in acute myocardial infarction. *Circ Heart Fail* 3:89–96, 2010.
36. Bearzi C, Rota M, Hosoda T, et al: Human cardiac stem cells. *Proc Natl Acad Sci USA* 104:14068–14073, 2007.
37. Cai L, Johnstone BH, Cook TG, et al: IFATS collection: Human adipose tissue-derived stem cells induce angiogenesis and nerve sprouting following myocardial infarction in conjunction with potent preservation of cardiac function. *Stem Cells* 27:230–237, 2009.
38. Hong SJ, Traktuev DO, March KL: Therapeutic potential of adipose-derived stem cells in vascular growth and tissue repair. *Curr Opin Organ Transplant* 15:86–91, 2010.
39. Toma C, Pittenger MF, Cahill KS, et al: Human mesenchymal stem cells differentiate to a cardiomyocyte phenotype in the adult murine heart. *Circulation* 105:93–98, 2002.
40. Gnecchi M, He H, Noiseux N, et al: Evidence supporting paracrine hypothesis for Akt-modified mesenchymal stem cell-mediated cardiac protection and functional improvement. *FASEB J* 20:661–669, 2006.
41. Mayorga M, Dong F, Mal N, et al: Inverse relationship between paracrine and cell associated effects of cardiovascular stem cell therapy. *Stem Cells Dev* 20:681–693, 2011.
42. Jiang Y, Jahagirdar BN, Reinhardt RL, et al: Pluripotency of mesenchymal stem cells derived from adult marrow. *Nature* 418:41–49, 2002.
43. Yoon YS, Wecker A, Heyd L, et al: Clonally expanded novel multipotent stem cells from human bone marrow regenerate myocardium after myocardial infarction. *J Clin. Invest* 115:326–338, 2005.
44. Van't HW, Mal N, Huang Y, et al: Direct delivery of syngeneic and allogeneic large-scale expanded multipotent adult progenitor cells improves cardiac function after myocardial infarct. *Cytotherapy* 9:477–487, 2007.
45. Medicetty S, Wiktor D, Lehman N, et al: Percutaneous adventitial delivery of allogeneic bone marrow derived stem cells via infarct related artery improves long-term ventricular function in acute myocardial infarction. *Cell Transplant* 2011. In press.
46. Penn MS: Importance of the SDF-1:CXCR4 axis in myocardial repair. *Circ Res* 104:1133–1135, 2009.
47. Hare J, Traverse J, Henry T, et al: A randomized double-blind placebo-controlled dose-escalation study of intravenous adult human mesenchymal stem cells (Prochymal) following acute myocardial infarction. *J Am Coll Cardiol* 54:2277–2286, 2009.
48. Penn MS: Stem-cell therapy after acute myocardial infarction: the focus should be on those at risk. *Lancet* 367:87–88, 2006.
49. Janssens S, Dubois C, Bogaert J, et al: Autologous bone marrow-derived stem-cell transfer in patients with ST-segment elevation myocardial infarction: double-blind randomised controlled trial. *Lancet* 367:113–121, 2006.
50. Thomson JA, Itskovitz-Eldor J, Shapiro SS, et al: Embryonic stem cell lines derived from human blastocysts. *Science* 282:1145–1147, 1998.
51. Reubinoff BE, Pera MF, Fong CY, et al: Embryonic stem cell lines from human blastocysts: somatic differentiation in vitro. *Nat Biotechnol* 18:399–404, 2000.
52. van Laake LW, Qian L, Cheng P, et al: Reporter-based isolation of induced pluripotent stem cell- and embryonic stem cell-derived cardiac progenitors reveals limited gene expression variance. *Circ Res* 107:340–347, 2010.
53. Ieda M, Fu JD, Delgado-Olguin P, et al: Direct reprogramming of fibroblasts into functional cardiomyocytes by defined factors. *Cell* 142:375–386, 2010.
54. Kuzmenkin A, Liang H, Xu G, et al: Functional characterization of cardiomyocytes derived from murine induced pluripotent stem cells in vitro. *FASEB J* 23:4168–4180, 2009.
55. Nelson TJ, Martinez-Fernandez A, Yamada S, et al: Induced pluripotent reprogramming from promiscuous human stemness related factors. *Clin Transl Sci* 2:118–126, 2009.
56. Moretti A, Bellin M, Jung CB, et al: Mouse and human induced pluripotent stem cells as a source for multipotent Isl1+ cardiovascular progenitors. *FASEB J* 24:700–711, 2010.
57. Orlic D, Kajstura J, Chimenti S, et al: Mobilized bone marrow cells repair the infarcted heart improving function and survival. *Proc Natl Acad Sci USA* 98:10344–10349, 2001.
58. Ince H, Petzsch M, Kleine HD, et al: Prevention of left ventricular remodeling with granulocyte colony-stimulating factor after acute myocardial infarction: final 1-year results of the Front-Integrated Revascularization and Stem Cell Liberation in Evolving Acute Myocardial Infarction by Granulocyte Colony-Stimulating Factor (FIRSTLINE-AMI) trial. *Circulation* 112:I73–I80, 2005.
59. Deglurkar I, Mal N, Mills WR, et al: Mechanical and electrical effects of cell based gene therapy for ischemic cardiomyopathy are independent (abstract). *Hum Gene Ther* 17:1144–1151, 2006.
60. Honold J, Lehmann R, Heeschen C, et al: Effects of granulocyte colony simulating factor on functional activities of endothelial progenitor cells in patients with chronic ischemic heart disease. *Arterioscler Thromb Vasc Biol* 26:2238–2243, 2006.
61. Jujo K, Hamada H, Iwakura A, et al: CXCR4 blockade augments bone marrow progenitor cell recruitment to the neovasculature and reduces mortality after myocardial infarction. *Proc Natl Acad Sci USA* 107:11008–11013, 2010.
62. Schenk S, Mal N, Finan A, et al: Monocyte chemotactic protein-3 is a myocardial mesenchymal stem cell homing factor. *Stem Cells* 25:245–251, 2007.
63. Zhang M, Mal N, Kiedrowski M, et al: SDF-1 expression by mesenchymal stem cells results in trophic support of cardiac myocytes after myocardial infarction. *FASEB J* 21:3197–3207, 2007.
64. Sundararaman S, Miller TJ, Pastore J, et al: Plasmid based transient human stromal cell-derived factor-1 gene transfer improves cardiac function in chronic heart failure. *Gene Ther* 2011. In press.
65. Mills WR, Mal N, Kiedrowski M, et al: Stem cell therapy enhances electrical viability in myocardial infarction (abstract). *J Mol. Cell Cardiol* 42:304–314, 2007.
66. Rabbany SY, Pastore J, Yamamoto M, et al: Continuous delivery of stromal cell-derived factor-1 from alginate scaffolds accelerates wound healing. *Cell Transplant* 19:399–408, 2010.
67. Penn MS: SDF-1:CXCR4 axis is fundamental for tissue preservation and repair. *Am J Pathol* 177:2166–2168, 2010.
68. Pasumarthi KB, Nakajima H, Nakajima HO, et al: Targeted expression of cyclin D2 results in cardiomyocyte DNA synthesis and infarct regression in transgenic mice. *Circ Res* 96:110–118, 2005.
69. Nakajima H, Nakajima HO, Tsai SC, et al: Expression of mutant p193 and p53 permits cardiomyocyte cell cycle reentry after myocardial infarction in transgenic mice. *Circ Res* 94:1606–1614, 2004.
70. Okita K, Ichisaka T, Yamanaka S: Generation of germline-competent induced pluripotent stem cells. *Nature* 448:313–317, 2007.

71. Nakagawa M, Koyanagi M, Tanabe K, et al: Generation of induced pluripotent stem cells without Myc from mouse and human fibroblasts. *Nat Biotechnol* 26:101–106, 2008.

72. Narazaki G, Uosaki H, Teranishi M, et al: Directed and systematic differentiation of cardiovascular cells from mouse induced pluripotent stem cells. *Circulation* 118:498–506, 2008.

73. Dong F, Khalil M, Kiedrowski M, et al: Critical role for leukocyte hypoxia inducible factor-1alpha expression in post-myocardial infarction left ventricular remodeling. *Circ Res* 106:601–610, 2010.

74. Agarwal U, Zhou X, Weber K, et al: Critical role for white blood cell NAD(P)H oxidase-mediated plasminogen activator inhibitor-1 oxidation and ventricular rupture following acute myocardial infarction. *J Mol. Cell Cardiol* 50:426–432, 2011.

75. Chen SL, Fang WW, Ye F, et al: Effect on left ventricular function of intracoronary transplantation of autologous bone marrow mesenchymal stem cells in patients with acute myocardial infarction. *Am J Cardiol* 94:92–95, 2004.

76. Meyer GP, Wollert KC, Lotz J, et al: Intracoronary bone marrow cell transfer after myocardial infarction: eighteen months' follow-up data from the randomized controlled BOOST (BOne marrOw transfer to enhance ST-elevation infarct regeneration) trial. *Circulation* 113:1287–1294, 2006.

77. Lunde K, Solheim S, Aakhus S, et al: Intracoronary injection of mononuclear bone marrow cells in acute myocardial infarction. *N Engl J Med* 355:1199–1209, 2006.

78. Yousef M, Schannwell CM, Kostering M, et al: The BALANCE Study: clinical benefit and long-term outcome after intracoronary autologous bone marrow cell transplantation in patients with acute myocardial infarction. *J Am Coll Cardiol* 53:2262–2269, 2009.

79. Traverse JH, Henry TD, Vaughn DE, et al: Rationale and design for TIME: A phase II randomized double-blind placebo-controlled pilot trial evaluating the safety and effect of timing of administration of bone marrow mononuclear cells after acute myocardial infarction. *Am. Heart J* 158:356–363, 2009.

80. Cohen ED, Wang Z, Lepore JJ, et al: Wnt/beta-catenin signaling promotes expansion of Isl-1-positive cardiac progenitor cells through regulation of FGF signaling. *J Clin Invest* 117:1794–1804, 2007.

81. Tse HF, Kwong YL, Chan JK, et al: Angiogenesis in ischaemic myocardium by intramyocardial autologous bone marrow mononuclear cell implantation. *Lancet* 361:47–49, 2003.

82. Seiler C, Pohl T, Wustmann K, et al: Promotion of collateral growth by granulocyte-macrophage colony-stimulating factor in patients with coronary artery disease: a randomized double-blind placebo-controlled study. *Circulation* 104:2012–2017, 2001.

83. Assmus B, Honold J, Schachinger V, et al: Transcoronary transplantation of progenitor cells after myocardial infarction. *N Engl J Med* 355:1222–1232, 2006.

84. Perin EC, Dohmann HF, Borojevic R, et al: Transendocardial autologous bone marrow cell transplantation for severe chronic ischemic heart failure. *Circulation* 107:2294–2302, 2003.

85. Willerson JT, Perin EC, Ellis SG, et al: Intramyocardial injection of autologous bone marrow mononuclear cells for patients with chronic ischemic heart disease and left ventricular dysfunction (First Mononuclear Cells injected in the US [FOCUS]): Rationale and design. *Am Heart J* 160:215–223, 2010.

86. Kang HJ, Kim HS, Zhang SY, et al: Effects of intracoronary infusion of peripheral blood stem-cells mobilised with granulocyte-colony stimulating factor on left ventricular systolic function and restenosis after coronary stenting in myocardial infarction: the MAGIC cell randomised clinical trial. *Lancet* 363:751–756, 2004.

87. Valgimigli M, Rigolin GM, Cittanti C, et al: Use of granulocyte-colony stimulating factor during acute myocardial infarction to enhance bone marrow stem cell mobilization in humans: clinical and angiographic safety profile. *Eur Heart J* 26:1838–1845, 2005.

88. Ellis SG, Penn MS, Bolwell B, et al: Granulocyte colony stimulating factor in patients with large acute myocardial infarction: Results of a pilot dose-escalation randomized trial. *Am Heart J* 152:9–14, 2006.

89. Ripa RS, Jorgensen E, Wang Y, et al: Stem cell mobilization induced by subcutaneous granulocyte-colony stimulating factor to improve cardiac regeneration after acute ST-elevation myocardial infarction: result of the double-blind randomized placebo-controlled stem cells in myocardial infarction (STEMMI) trial. *Circulation* 113:1983–1992, 2006.

90. Zohlnhofer D, Ott I, Mehilli J, et al: Stem cell mobilization by granulocyte colony-stimulating factor in patients with acute myocardial infarction: a randomized controlled trial. *JAMA* 295:1003–1010, 2006.

91. Overgaard M, Ripa RS, Wang Y, et al: Timing of granulocyte-colony stimulating factor treatment after acute myocardial infarction and recovery of left ventricular function: results from the STEMMI trial. *Int. J Cardiol* 140:351–355, 2010.

Evaluation of Interventional Techniques

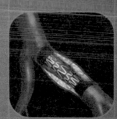

Qualitative and Quantitative Coronary Angiography

JEFFREY POPMA | ALEXANDRA ALMONACID | DAVID BURKE

KEY POINTS

- Although clinical outcomes after percutaneous coronary intervention have continued to improve over the past decade, precise assessment of coronary lesion complexity remains valuable in estimating early and late procedural risk. Aggregate scores that consider both the vessel patency and underlying lesion morphology provide the most predictive information for estimating outcome. A recent quantitative assessment of the extent of complexity of coronary artery disease, the SYNTAX score, has provided valuable insights into the selection of patients for multivessel percutaneous coronary intervention or coronary artery bypass surgery. Longer lesions, thrombus-containing lesions, degenerated saphenous vein grafts, severe tortuosity and angulation, and total coronary occlusions hold the highest risk for failure with percutaneous coronary intervention.

- Assessment of both myocardial blood flow and myocardial perfusion is useful in predicting prognosis in patients with ST-segment elevation myocardial infarction and may also be valuable in predicting events in patients with non-ST-segment elevation myocardial infarction as well. More quantitative indices are preferred over more qualitative ones in order to assess the value of new drugs and devices in patients with ST-segment elevation myocardial infarction.

- Interventional cardiologists remain firmly wedded to the coronary angiogram for the assessment of lesion severity before and after percutaneous coronary intervention, reserving the physiological assessment of intermediate (40%–70%) lesions to adjunct modalities, such as measurements of fractional flow reserve. More reliable and reproducible methods of severity assessment using quantitative angiography have provided important insights into the mechanism of benefit for new drugs and devices in patients undergoing coronary intervention. Use of novel quantitative programs has yielded three-dimensional imaging methods that may allow more precise characterization of total occlusions and bifurcation disease.

- Late clinical restenosis can be predicted by the quantitative measurement of percent diameter stenosis and late lumen loss on follow-up angiography in patients undergoing drug-eluting and bare metal stent placement, although controversy remains relating to their use as surrogate markers for clinical outcomes when assessing new generations of coronary stents. Nevertheless, quantitative angiographic methods remain extremely important for the assessment of outcome after new device and drug therapy in patients undergoing intervention for ischemic heart disease.

Introduction

Percutaneous coronary intervention (PCI) has evolved dramatically over the past 2 decades, fundamentally altering the management of ischemic coronary artery disease (CAD). Coronary stents and, more recently, drug-eluting coronary stents (DESs), are currently used in over 90% of PCI procedures. Coronary arteriography is a fundamental component of PCI, providing prognostic information about the baseline lesion morphology and severity, quantification of anterograde perfusion, and adequacy of the final angiographic result. Conventional "visual" angiography has formed the cornerstone of clinical decision making for patients undergoing cardiovascular intervention, but insights from more quantitative analysis of procedural and late angiograms have permitted a mechanistic understanding of the relative value of new devices and drugs developed for the treatment of ischemic cardiovascular disease. A better understanding of the factors predisposing to procedural complications, thrombosis, and restenosis has permitted more appropriate selection of patients for these procedures. The purposes of this chapter are threefold. First, the standard criteria used to stratify the baseline procedural risk in patients undergoing PCI are reviewed. These criteria have been modified since the availability of DESs, and a number of new predictive scores, such as the SYNTAX score, have provided useful tools for deciding between multivessel PCI and coronary artery bypass grafting (CABG) in patients with multivessel CAD. Second, newer methods to assess myocardial perfusion beyond coronary flow, which provide important prognostic information for patients with acute myocardial infarction (AMI), are discussed. Third, the quantitative angiographic methods used for evaluating early and late procedural outcomes after PCI are outlined, including the value of these indices as surrogates for clinical outcome in novel stent studies.

Qualitative Angiography

Assessment of procedural risk for PCI begins with accurate assessment of the complexity of the baseline coronary anatomy. Predictors for an adverse procedural outcome after balloon angioplasty were identified in early series, but a standardized approach to the assessment of lesion morphology in patients undergoing PCI was lacking until the late 1980s. Refinement of these criteria was necessary after the introduction of coronary stents in order to more appropriately estimate procedural risk, particularly with the continued availability of the alternative of CABG.

UPDATE ON THE ACC/AHA TASK FORCE ON LESION MORPHOLOGY

A joint task force of the American College of Cardiology (ACC) and American Heart Association (AHA) established criteria to estimate procedural success and complication rates after balloon angioplasty based on the presence or absence of specific high-risk lesion characteristics.[1] Although these criteria were developed based solely on the task force's clinical impressions (Table 56-1), their estimates of procedural success and complications were closely correlated with the procedural outcomes demonstrated in patients undergoing multivessel balloon angioplasty.[2] Chronic total occlusion, high-grade stenosis, stenosis on a bend of 60 degrees or more, and location in vessels with proximal tortuosity were associated with an adverse outcome.[2] The most complex lesion morphologies (i.e., "type C" lesions) were associated with less satisfactory procedural outcomes.[3,4] Definitions for these variables are provided (Table 56-2). With improved outcomes associated with the use of coronary stents, contemporary composite risk scores were proposed.[5,6] The Society for Cardiac Angiography and Interventions (SCAI) registry evaluated 61,926 patients (74.5% received stents) from the ACC National Cardiovascular Data Registry and classified their lesions into four groups: non-type C patent, type C patent, non-type C occluded, and type C occluded (Table 56-3).[5]

TABLE 56-1	ACC/AHA Characteristics of Type A, B, and C Coronary Lesions	
Type A lesions—high success (≈85%), low risk		
Discrete (<10 mm)	Little or no calcium	
Concentric	Less than totally occlusive	
Readily accessible	Not ostial in location	
Nonangulated segment (<45 degrees)	Smooth contour, no major side branch	
Absence of thrombus	No side branch involvement	
Type B lesions—moderate success (60%–85%), moderate risk		
Tubular (10- to 20-mm length)	Moderate to heavy calcification	
Eccentric	Total occlusion <3 months old	
Moderate tortuosity of proximal segment	Moderately angulated (45–90 degrees)	
Bifurcation lesion requiring double guidewire	Irregular contour	
Some thrombus present		
Type C low success (≈60%), high risk		
Diffuse (>20-mm length)	Total occlusion >3 months old	
Excessive tortuosity of proximal segment	Inability to protect major side branches	
Extremely angulated segment (>90 degrees)	Degenerated vein grafts with friable lesions	

Modified from Ryan TJ, Faxon DP, Gunnar RP, et al. Guidelines for percutaneous transluminal coronary angioplasty: a report of the American College of Cardiology/American Heart Association Task Force on Assessment of Diagnostic and Therapeutic Cardiovascular Procedures (Subcommittee on Percutaneous Transluminal Coronary Angioplasty). *J Am Coll Cardiol.* 1988;12:529–545.

These more simplified criteria provided better discrimination for success or complications than the ACC/AHA original classification, with a C statistic of 0.69 for success using the ACC/AHA original classification system, 0.71 using the modified ACC/AHA system, and 0.75 for the SCAI classification.[5] The Mayo Clinic risk score was constructed by adding integer scores for the presence of eight morphological variables and was compared with the ACC/AHA risk score in 5,064 patients undergoing PCI, of whom 183 (4%) experienced an adverse event (death, Q-wave myocardial infarction, stroke, emergency CABG).[6] The Mayo Clinic risk score offered significantly better risk stratification than the ACC/AHA lesion classification for the development of cardiovascular complications, whereas the ACC/AHA lesion classification was a better system for determining angiographic success.[6]

THE SYNTAX SCORE

The SYNTAX score was developed to incorporated both the complexity and extent of coronary artery disease in patients undergoing PCI or CABG.[7,8] A lesion is defined as significant when it causes a >50% reduction in luminal diameter by visual assessment in a vessel >1.5 mm in diameter.[8] A multiplication factor of 2 is used for nonocclusive lesions and 5 for occlusive lesions reflecting the difficulty of the percutaneous treatment.[8] Up to 12 lesions are identified within the coronary tree, and each is assessed for its severity, including the presence of a total occlusion (with appropriate characterization) and of side branches and their size.[8] Each lesion is also weighted by its contribution to the myocardial bed that it supplies.[8] In a right-dominant system, the right coronary artery (RCA) supplies approximately 16% and the left coronary artery (LCA) 84% of the flow to the left ventricle (LV), with 66% to the left anterior descending artery (LAD) and 33% to the left circumflex coronary artery (LCX). These factors are included in the weight given to each segment. Lesions are further graded by their complexity, including multiple tandem lesions, morphology of total occlusions, bifurcation and trifurcation involvement, aorto-ostial location, diffuse disease and small vessels, severe tortuosity, length >20 mm, heavy calcification, and thrombus.[8,9] The predictive value of the SYNTAX score in patients who had undergone PCI for three-vessel disease was evaluated for 1,292 lesions in 306 patients in the Arterial Revascularization Therapies Study Part II.[10] The rate of major adverse cardiac and cerebrovascular events at 370 days was 27.9% in the tertile

TABLE 56-2	Definitions of Preprocedural Lesion Morphology
Variable	*Definition*
Eccentricity	Stenosis that is noted to have one of its luminal edges in the outer quarter of the apparently normal lumen
Irregularity	Characterized by lesion ulceration, intimal flap, aneurysm, or "sawtooth" pattern
Ulceration	Lesion with a small crater consisting of a discrete luminal widening in the area of the stenosis provided that it does not extend beyond the normal arterial lumen
Aneurysmal dilation	Segment of arterial dilation larger than the dimensions of the normal arterial segment
Sawtooth pattern	Multiple sequential stenotic irregularities
Lesion length	Measured "shoulder-to-shoulder" in an unforeshortened view
Discrete	Lesion length <10 mm
Tubular	Lesion length 10–20 mm
Discrete	Lesion length >20 mm
Ostial location	Origin of the lesion within 3 mm of the vessel origin
Lesion angulation	Vessel angle formed by the center line through the lumen proximal to the stenosis and extending beyond it and a second center line in the straight portion of the artery distal to the stenosis
Moderate	Lesion angulation >45 to 90 degrees
Severe	Lesion angulation >90 degrees
Bifurcation	Present if a medium or large branch (>1.5 mm) originates within the stenosis and if the side branch is completely surrounded by stenotic portions of the lesion to be dilated
Lesion accessibility	
Moderate tortuosity	Lesion is distal to two bends <75 degrees
Severe tortuosity	Lesion is distal to three bends >75 degrees
Degenerated SVG	Graft characterized by luminal irregularities or ectasia comprising >50% of the graft length
Calcification	Readily apparent densities noted within the apparent vascular wall at the site of the stenosis
Moderate	Densities noted only with cardiac motion before contrast injection
Severe	Radiopacities noted without cardiac motion before contrast injection
Total occlusion	TIMI 0 or 1 flow
Thrombus	Discrete, intraluminal filling defect is noted with defined borders and is largely separated from the adjacent wall; contrast staining may or may not be present

SVG, saphenous vein graft; TIMI, Thrombolysis in Myocardial Infarction.

with the highest SYNTAX score and 8.7% in the tertile with the lowest SYNTAX score (hazard ratio [HR] 3.5, $P = 0.001$).[10] By multivariate analyses, SYNTAX score independently predicted outcome and the risk of major adverse cardiac and cerebrovascular events. Compared with the modified lesion classification scheme of the American Heart Association/American College of Cardiology, the SYNTAX score showed a greater discrimination ability and better goodness of fit.[10] The SYNTAX score has been used to predict outcomes in patients enrolled in studies of drug-eluting stents.[11,12] In an analysis of 819 patients with left main coronary artery disease who underwent revascularization in two Italian centers, the outcomes of patients undergoing PCI and CABG were studied. In patients with SYNTAX scores ≤ 34, the rates of 2-year mortality were similar between CABG and PCI (6.2% vs. 8.1%, respectively; $P = 0.461$).[11] Among patients with SYNTAX scores >34, those treated with CABG had lower rates of mortality than those treated with PCI (8.5% vs. 32.7%, respectively; $P < 0.001$).[11] A similar correlation with the SYNTAX score and surgical outcome was not found in patients undergoing CABG.[13,14] The SYNTAX score has also been incorporated into the recommendations by the European Society of Cardiology guidelines[15] and to evaluate patients as suitable candidates for CABG or PCI in clinical practice.[16] An improvement in the ability of the SYNTAX score to predict major

TABLE 56-3	SCAI Lesion Classification System: Class I to IV Lesions

Type I lesion (highest success expected, lowest risk)
(1) Does not meet ACC/AHA criteria for Type C lesion
(2) Patent
Type II lesion
(1) Meets any of the following criteria for Type C lesion
  Diffuse (>2 cm length)
  Excessive tortuosity of proximal segment
  Extremely angulated segments ≥ 90 degrees
  Inability to protect major side branches
  Degenerated vein grafts with friable lesions
(2) Patent
Type III lesion
(1) Does not meet ACC/AHA criteria for type C lesion
(2) Occluded
Type IV lesion
(1) Meets any of the following criteria for type C lesion
  Diffuse (>2 cm length)
  Excessive tortuosity of proximal segment
  Extremely angulated segments ≥90 degrees
  Inability to protect major side branches
  Degenerated vein grafts with friable lesions
(2) Occluded

Modified from Krone R, Shaw R, Klein L, et al. Evaluation of the American College of Cardiology/American Heart Association and the Society for Coronary Angiography and Interventions lesion classification system in the current "stent era" of coronary interventions (from the ACC National Cardiovascular Data Registry). *Am J Cardiol.* 2003;92:389–394.

adverse cardiovascular and cerebrovascular events (MACCE) and mortality can be achieved by combining the SYNTAX score with a simple clinical risk score incorporating age, ejection fraction, and creatinine clearance to produce the clinical SYNTAX score (CSS).[17] The CSS incorporates the SYNTAX score with a modified ACEF score ([age/ejection fraction] +1 for each 10 mL the creatinine clearance is <60 mL/min per 1.73 m[2]) to estimate major adverse cardiac events at 1 and 5 years after PCI.[17] At 1-year follow-up, rates of repeat revascularization and MACCE were significantly higher in the highest-tertile group.[17] At 5-year follow-up, those with high CSSs had a comparable rate of myocardial infarction, a trend toward a significantly higher rate of death, and significantly higher rates of repeat revascularization and overall MACCE compared with patients in the lower two tertiles.[17] The respective C statistics for the CSS, SYNTAX score, and ACEF score for 5-year mortality were 0.69, 0.62, and 0.65; for 5-year MACCE, they were 0.62, 0.59, and 0.57.

RISK ASSESSMENT USING SPECIFIC LESION MORPHOLOGICAL CRITERIA

Despite the value of risk scores in estimating aggregate procedural risk, there are several limitations of these criteria as applied to individual patients. Identification of lesion characteristics—such as eccentricity, irregularity, angulation, and tortuosity—is limited by substantial interobserver variability. Agreement with the ACC/AHA classification was noted in only 58% of lesions in one series, with disagreement by two classification grades noted in almost 10% of lesions.[2] Accordingly, rather than a composite score, description of individual morphological features may be more predictive of early and late outcome after PCI. Some ACC/AHA morphological features are associated with a complicated procedure (e.g., thrombus, saphenous vein graft [SVG] degeneration, angulated segments), whereas others are associated with an unsuccessful but uncomplicated procedure (e.g., chronic total occlusions, diffuse disease). The weighted kappa value for the interobserver reproducibility on the global score was 0.45, while the intraobserver weighted kappa value was 0.59.[9] The SYNTAX score is reproducible (Δ 2.1%–3.4%).[9,18] Other studies have also shown the importance of clinical variables in assessing early and late risk after PCI.[19–22] Individual morphological criteria may also have individual prognostic value in assessing outcomes.

Irregular Lesions

With the advent of coronary stents, the prognostic importance of irregular lesions has been diminished substantially, although identification of an irregular plaque at angiography suggests the presence of an acute coronary syndrome and intracoronary thrombus. Semiquantitative and quantitative measurements of lesion irregularity were developed in the early 1990s to better characterize lesion morphology in patients with acute coronary syndromes, but these methods have not found clinical utility independent of other clinical risk factors. A novel technique of identifying plaque rupture (PR) defined any irregular lesion with ulceration, flap, or aneurysm on a qualitative angiogram as suspicious for PR. Intravascular ultrasound (IVUS)-detected PR and non-PR lesions were compared with the corresponding angiograms.[23] A total of 224 distinct (ruptured or nonruptured) lesions were detected by IVUS in 65 patients; 49 of the 105 IVUS-detected nonculprit PRs were suspected on angiography.[23] The positive and negative predictive values for correct angiographic diagnosis of PR were 96% and 61%, respectively.[23] Proximal coronary location, wide cavity, and counter-flow rupture were strong predictors of correct angiographic diagnosis, enabling four specific angiographic patterns to be identified using three-dimensional IVUS PR reconstruction.[23]

Angulated Lesions

Vessel curvature at the site of maximal stenosis should be measured in the most unforeshortened projection using a length of curvature that approximates the balloon length used for coronary dilation. Balloon angioplasty of highly angulated lesions is associated with an increased risk of coronary dissection; however, in the era of coronary stenting, the greatest impediment of angulated lesions is inability to deliver the stent to the stenosis and straighten the arterial contour after stent placement, which may predispose to late stent fracture.

Lesion Calcification

Coronary artery calcium is an important marker for coronary atherosclerosis. Conventional coronary angiography has limited sensitivity for the detection of smaller amounts of calcium and is only moderately sensitive for the detection of extensive lesion calcium (60% and 85% sensitivity for three- and four-quadrant calcium, respectively).[24] The presence of coronary calcification reduces the compliance of the vessel and may predispose to dissection at the interface between calcified plaque and normal wall after balloon angioplasty.[25] The presence of coronary calcification also reduces the ability to cross chronic total occlusions; moreover, in severely calcified lesions, stent strut expansion is inversely correlated with the circumferential arc of calcium.[24] Higher target lesion revascularization rates have been shown in patients treated with sirolimus-eluting stents who had lesion calcification compared with those who did not.[26,27] Rotational atherectomy is the preferred pretreatment method in patients with severe lesion calcification, particularly ostial lesions; it facilitates the delivery and expansion of coronary stents by creating microdissection planes within the fibrocalcific plaque. Even with these contemporary methods, however, the presence of moderate or severe coronary calcification is associated with reduced procedural success and higher complication rates, including stent dislodgement. In less severely calcified lesions, no difference in restenosis rate was found after paclitaxel-eluting stent implantation in calcified versus noncalcified vessels.[28] Calcification noted within SVGs is usually within the reference vessel wall rather than within the lesion and is associated with older grafts, insulin-dependent diabetes, and history of smoking.[29] Calcified lesions were an independent predictor of stent thrombosis in one series.[30]

Degenerated Saphenous Vein Grafts

SVGs develop progressive degeneration over time, with 25% occluding within the first year after CABG[31] and 50% developing occlusion within 10 years after surgery. Although coronary stents and, more recently, DESs[11] reduce restenosis rates compared with balloon angioplasty, only embolic protection devices have reduced procedural complications.[32,33] One exception may be in patients treated for in-stent restenosis (ISR), where embolic protection may not be required. Self-expanding stents made with expanded polytetrafluoroethylene (ePTFE) provide no additional advantage over noncovered balloon-expandable stents on the development of early complications or late restenosis.[34] The risk for embolic complications appears to be related to both the degree of overall graft degeneration and the length of the lesion.[35] Using angiographic assessments of the extent of graft degeneration and estimated volume of plaque in the target lesion, independent correlates of an increased 30-day rate of major adverse cardiovascular events (MACE) were more extensive vein graft degeneration ($P < 0.0001$) and bulkier lesions (larger estimated plaque volume, $P < 0.0005$). SVG lesions have been associated with a worse late outcome after PCI than native vessel lesions.[4]

Thrombus

Conventional angiography is relatively insensitive for the detection of coronary thrombus. The presence of angiographic thrombus, usually identified by the appearance of discrete intraluminal filling defects within the arterial lumen, is also associated with a higher albeit widely variable (6% to 73%), incidence of ischemic complications after PCI. A large thrombus burden is an independent predictor of stent thrombosis in patients with ST-elevation myocardial infarction (STEMI) treated with DESs.[36] The primary complications related to PCI of thrombus-containing lesions are distal embolization and thrombotic occlusion, with the risk for complications with angiographic thrombus relating to the size of the coronary thrombus. Routine rheolytic thrombectomy provides no benefit in patients with AMI,[37] although it may be useful for patients with a large thrombus burden. A number of aspiration catheters have been used in patients with AMI and large thrombus burden, but large-scale studies are lacking. Traditionally, the extent of coronary thrombus has been determined using the semiquantitative TIMI thrombus grade (TTG). A novel method of assessing intracoronary thrombus burden uses the discrepancy between luminal areas assessed with edge detection (ED) and videodensitometry (VD) as measured with the Cardiovascular Angiography Analysis System II.[38] A good correlation between D-QCA and true occlusive volumes was found ($y = 9.21 + 0.99x$, correlation $r = 0.996$) with low intra- and interobserver variability.[38] TTG also decreased in an in vivo model, but in 9 (47%) patients in whom TTG remained unchanged, D-QCA detected a reduction in thrombus burden (pre: 148.17 ± 154.03 mm^3; post: 112.86 ± 117.82 mm^3; $P = 0.05$).[38] These results suggest that dual QCA appears to be a useful approach to the quantification of coronary thrombus volume, being more sensitive than the TTG in assessing changes in thrombus resulting from treatment strategies.[38] The presence of thrombus remains an important predictor of outcome after PCI.[3]

Ostial Location

Ostial lesions are defined as those that begin within 3 mm of the origin of the coronary artery; they are classified as aorto-ostial and non-aorto-ostial. Balloon angioplasty of ostial lesions is limited by suboptimal procedural outcome, primarily owing to technical factors such as difficulties with guide-catheter support, lesion inelasticity precluding maximal balloon expansion, and early vascular recoil limiting the acute angiographic result. Debulking techniques such as directional and rotational atherectomy improve the compliance of the aorto-ostial lesion but have had limited effect on preventing late restenosis. Ostial lesion of the RCA and left circumflex artery have been associated with higher rates of target lesion revascularization (TLR) after DES placement.[27] Coronary stenting, more recently with DESs, has become the default therapy for most aorto-ostial lesions. However, there are unique challenges of stent placement in the aorto-ostial location. These include protrusion of the stent into the aorta, thus precluding subsequent injection catheter engagement; compression;

and avulsion of the stent struts into the aorta when new techniques, such as cutting balloon angioplasty, are used to treat ISR. Isolated non-aorto-ostial stenoses of the left circumflex and LAD[39] and ostial side-branch bifurcation lesions are also effectively treated with DESs,[40] but they pose unique challenges regarding vessel wall geometry, adequate ostial branch coverage (particularly if there is a narrow angle with the adjacent branch), and plaque shifting, causing compromise of the parent or adjacent branch vessels. Whereas stent protrusion into the parent vessel of less than 1 mm is usually well tolerated, stent protrusion to greater degrees precludes treatment of the parent branches.[40] Stent fractures have been reported with more advanced stenting techniques used to treat the parent vessel and ostial side-branch stenoses.

Long Lesions

Lesion length may be estimated quantitatively as the "shoulder-to-shoulder" extent of atherosclerotic narrowing greater than 20%, although many clinicians estimate lesion length based on the identification of a "normal to normal" segment, which is usually longer than the length obtained with quantitative methods. Conventional balloon angioplasty of long lesions has been associated with reduced procedural success, particularly when the segment is diffusely diseased (i.e., <20 mm in length), primarily because of the more extensive plaque burden in long lesions. Stents improve late outcome compared with balloon angioplasty, but stent and lesion length remain the most important predictors of restenosis in the stent era.[41] Coronary stents have been used to treat suboptimal angiographic results ("spot stenting") and dissections after balloon angioplasty of longer lesions, although the "full metal jacket" stent approach to diffuse disease is associated with a higher recurrence rate in the absence of complete stent expansion, particularly in smaller vessels. Overlapping sirolimus-eluting stents provide safe and effective treatment for long coronary lesions.[42] In one series, longer stented lesions were associated with stent thrombosis.[30]

Bifurcation Lesions

The risk of side-branch occlusion in bifurcation lesions relates to the extent of atherosclerotic involvement of the side branch within its origin from the parent vessel, which ranges from 14% to 27% in side branches with ostial involvement. To accurately assess the risk of side-branch occlusion and avoid conflicting definitions of side-branch and ostial stenosis, a number of classification systems for bifurcation stenoses have been proposed (Fig. 56-1).[43–46] Bifurcation lesions are predictors of stent thrombosis.[47] One stent is preferable to stents in both the parent vessel and the side branch, because subacute thrombosis and restenosis remain higher in bifurcation disease treated with coronary stents in both branches.[48] If two stents are planned for the parent vessel and side branch, a number of stenting techniques are possible, including simultaneous kissing stents, crush, coulotte,[49] and T stenting. To date, the optimal technique has not been identified, although the use of DESs appears to reduce restenosis compared with bare metal stents. The origin of the side branch is the most common location of failure (recurrence) after bifurcation stenting.[50] A number of dedicated bifurcation stents have been developed to provide adequate vessel coverage[45] and side-branch access[51] during stent deployment. Common to all of these strategies is a final "kissing" balloon inflation in the parent vessel and side branch.[52] A specifically designed side-branch stent has also shown favorable initial results.[53] A new bifurcation software (QVA-CMS V. 6.0 with the Bifurcation Module, MEDIS, Leiden, The Netherlands) has been developed to assess the severity of stenosis in patients with bifurcation stenoses using an analysis system that will allow examination of the bifurcation in three separate segments.[54] A minimal cost algorithm is used to detect the contours of the proximal main vessel (PMV), distal main vessel (DMV), and sidebranch (SB) (QVA-CMS V. 6.0 with the Bifurcation Module, MEDIS, Leiden, The Netherlands). This new quantitative bifurcation analysis system can be consistently applied to the analysis of bifurcation lesions before and after angioplasty, with an intra- and interobserver reproducibility equal to

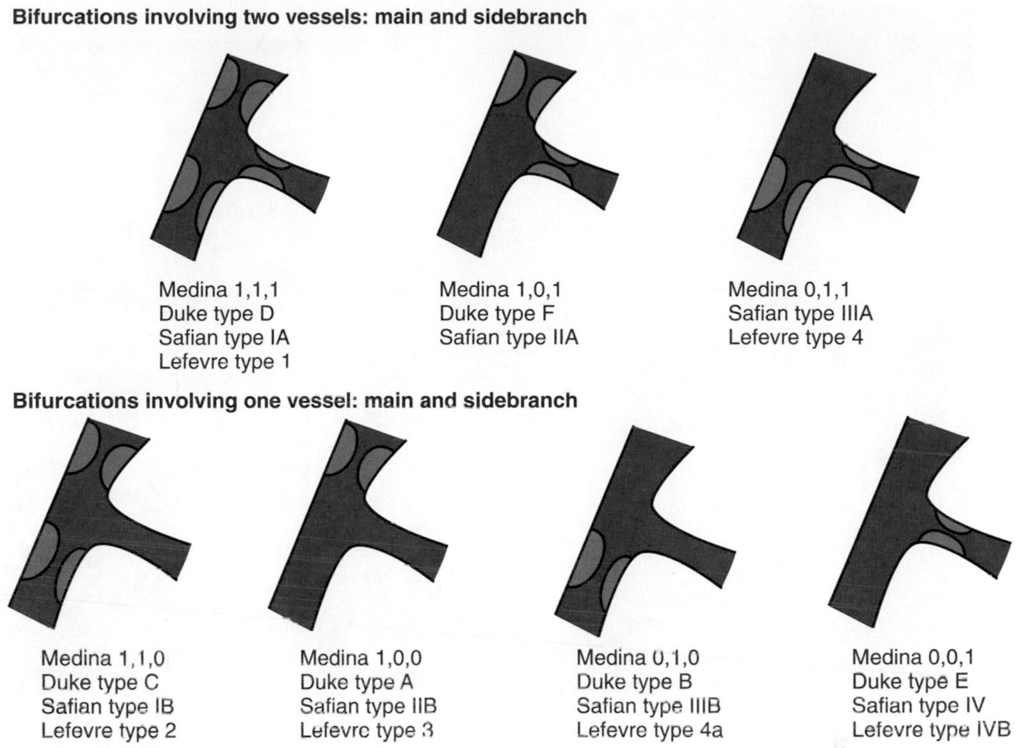

Bifurcations involving two vessels: main and sidebranch

Medina 1,1,1
Duke type D
Safian type IA
Lefevre type 1

Medina 1,0,1
Duke type F
Safian type IIA

Medina 0,1,1
Safian type IIIA
Lefevre type 4

Bifurcations involving one vessel: main and sidebranch

Medina 1,1,0
Duke type C
Safian type IB
Lefevre type 2

Medina 1,0,0
Duke type A
Safian type IIB
Lefevre type 3

Medina 0,1,0
Duke type B
Safian type IIIB
Lefevre type 4a

Medina 0,0,1
Duke type E
Safian type IV
Lefevre type IVB

Figure 56-1 Schematic classification system for types of bifurcation stenoses.

Total Occlusion

Coronary occlusion is identified as an abrupt termination of the epicardial vessel; anterograde and retrograde collaterals may be present and are helpful in quantifying the length of the totally occluded segment. Coronary occlusions are common findings[55] and often lead to the decision to perform CABG rather than PCI in the setting of multivessel disease.[56,57] The success rate for recanalization depends on the duration of the occlusion and on certain morphologic features of the lesion, such as bridging collaterals, occlusion length greater than 15 mm, and absence of a "nipple" to guide advancement of the wire. Although newer technologies and techniques have been used to recanalize refractory occlusions,[58,59] better guidewires and wire techniques have accounted for much of the improvement in crossing success over the years.[60] Simultaneous coronary injections are sometimes useful for identifying the length of the total occlusion (Fig. 56-2). Once the occlusion has been crossed, coronary stents, including DESs,[61,62] have been used to provide the best long-term outcomes. A key component to the assessment of total occlusion is definition of the collateral grades that provide blood flow to the jeopardized myocardium.[63] The Rentrop classification system includes Rentrop grade 0 (no filling), Rentrop grade 1 (small side branches filled), Rentrop grade 2 (partial epicardial filling of the occluded artery), and Rentrop grade 3 (complete epicardial filling of the occluded artery). Anatomical collaterals summarized by the 26 potential pathways were consolidated into four groups: septal, intra-arterial (bridging), epicardial with proximal takeoff (atrial branches), and epicardial with distal takeoff.[64] Finally, the size of the collateral connection can be quantified as group 0 (no continuous connection between donor and recipient artery), group 1 (continuous threadlike connection ≤0.3 mm), or group 2 (continuous small, branch-like collateral through its course ≥0.4 mm).[64] Three-dimensional (3D) imaging has been used for case planning in patients with chronic total occlusions.[65] The novel CardiOp-B system for 3D reconstruction of the coronary vessels has been used in 302

angiographic images from 58 consecutive patients undergoing interventional treatment for 61 chronic total occlusion (CTO).[65] The success rate of 3D reconstruction was 83%. When successful, these reconstructions led to a significant improvement in lesion analysis, especially at the stump area and/or missing segment. Importantly, in 92% of the successful 3D reconstructions, the artery path in the lesion area could be delineated. In most cases, 3D reconstruction of CTO can clearly image the stump area, delineate the lesion path, and provide enough information for the clinician to precisely calculate the severity of stenosis and lesion length. 3D reconstructions may serve as a useful tool for planning interventional procedures for CTO and improving their success rate.[65]

ANGIOGRAPHIC COMPLICATIONS AFTER PERCUTANEOUS CORONARY INTERVENTION

Although the frequency of angiographic complications during PCI has been reduced substantially with the use of coronary stents, untoward effects resulting from disruption of the atherosclerotic plaque and embolization of atherosclerotic debris, thrombus, and vasoactive mediators still occurs during 5% to 10% of PCI procedures (Table 56-4).

Coronary Dissection

Plaque fracture is an integral component of balloon angioplasty, although significant vessel wall disruption resulting in reduced anterograde flow and luminal compromise is a relatively uncommon occurrence (≈3%).[66] The National Heart, Lung and Blood Institute (NHLBI) coronary dissection criteria categorize the severity of coronary dissection after PCI (Table 56-4), with the prognostic implications of the coronary dissection depending on extension into the media and adventitia, axial length, presence of contrast staining, and effect on anterograde coronary perfusion. It is sometimes difficult to assess the angiographic residual lumen in the presence of coronary dissection because of the changes in frame-to-frame luminal diameter seen with two-dimensional imaging; in this setting, IVUS may provide a more accurate reflection of the true circumferential luminal dimensions.

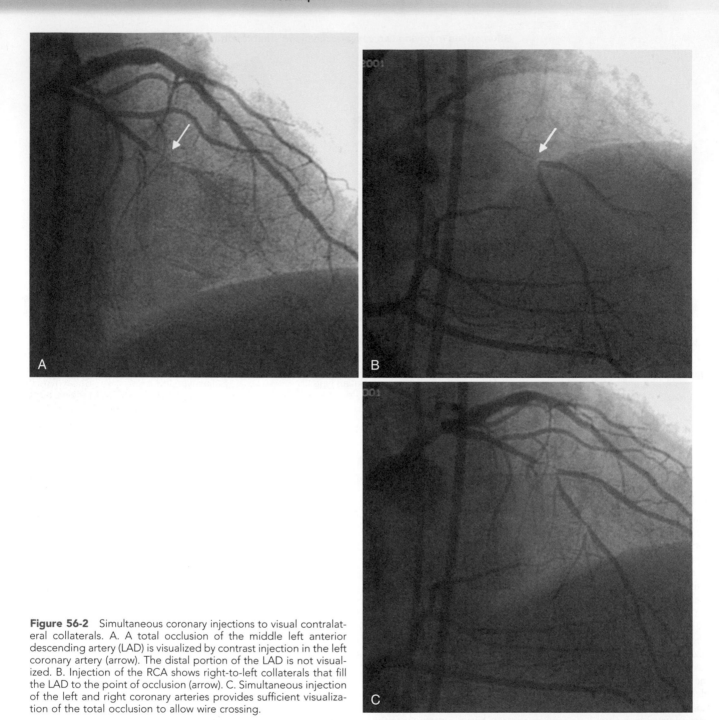

Figure 56-2 Simultaneous coronary injections to visual contralateral collaterals. A. A total occlusion of the middle left anterior descending artery (LAD) is visualized by contrast injection in the left coronary artery (arrow). The distal portion of the LAD is not visualized. B. Injection of the RCA shows right-to-left collaterals that fill the LAD to the point of occlusion (arrow). C. Simultaneous injection of the left and right coronary arteries provides sufficient visualization of the total occlusion to allow wire crossing.

Dissections resulting in a residual area of stenosis of 60% or greater by IVUS[67] and those extending more than 5 to 10 mm in axial length are associated with a worse prognosis. A residual coronary dissection is an independent predictor of stent thrombosis.[47]

"No-Reflow"

Reduced flow during PCI, also known as no-reflow, is defined as a reduction in anterograde flow despite a patent lumen at the site of PCI. It occurs during 1% to 5% of PCI procedures. No-reflow is a strong predictor of mortality after PCI.[68] It is more common (15%) during primary angioplasty for AMI.[69] Predictors of no-reflow include a higher plaque burden, thrombus, lipid pools by IVUS, a larger vessel cross-sectional area, preinfarction angina, and TIMI flow grade 0 on the initial coronary angiogram, among other factors.[70–72] Compared with aspirates obtained from patients without no-reflow, aspirates obtained from patients who developed no-reflow contained more atheromatous plaque and significantly more platelet and fibrin complex, macrophages, and cholesterol crystals.[73] The 30-day mortality rate was significantly higher (27.5%) in patients with combined slow-flow and no-reflow phenomena than in patients with normal coronary blood flow after PCI (5.3%; $P < 0.001$).[69] Intracoronary or intragraft nitroprusside,[74] adenosine,[75] verapamil,[76] and nicardipine[77] as well as the aspiration of atherosclerotic debris have each been used to correct the episode of no-reflow.

TABLE 56-4	Definition of Complications after Percutaneous Coronary Intervention
Variable	**Definition**
Abrupt closure	Obstruction of contrast flow (TIMI 0 or 1) in a dilated segment with previously documented anterograde flow
Ectasia	A lesion diameter greater than the reference diameter in one or more areas
Luminal irregularities	Arterial contour that has a "sawtooth pattern" consisting of opacification but not fulfilling the criteria for dissection or intracoronary thrombus
Intimal flap	A discrete filling defect in apparent continuity with the arterial wall
Thrombus	Discrete, mobile angiographic filling defect with or without contrast staining
Dissection*	
A	Small radiolucent area within the lumen of the vessel
B	Linear, nonpersisting extravasation of contrast
C	Extraluminal, persisting extravasation of contrast
D	Spiral-shaped filling defect
E	Persistent luminal defect with delayed anterograde flow
F	Filling defect accompanied by total coronary occlusion
Length	Measure end-to-end for type B through F dissections
Staining	Persistence of contrast within the dissection after washout of contrast from the remaining portion of the vessel
Perforation	
Localized	Extravasation of contrast confined to the pericardial space immediately surrounding the artery and not associated with clinical tamponade
Nonlocalized	Extravasation of contrast with a jet not localized to the pericardial space, potentially associated with clinical tamponade
Sidebranch loss	TIMI 0, 1, or 2 flow in a side branch >1.5 mm in diameter that previously had TIMI 3 flow
Coronary spasm	Transient or permanent narrowing >50% when a <25% stenosis was previously noted

TIMI, Thrombolysis in Myocardial Infarction

*National Heart, Lung, and Blood Institute classification system for coronary dissection.

Distal Embolization

Periprocedural myonecrosis provides clinical evidence of distal particulate embolization during PCI. Angiographic distal embolization is defined as the migration of a filling defect or thrombus to distally occlude the target vessel or one of its branches.[78] It occurs in approximately 10% of patients with an AMI undergoing PCI. Embolic complications occur more often in patients with AMI and in patients undergoing balloon angioplasty of SVG lesions, particularly those with recent occlusion.

Coronary Perforation

Coronary perforation is an uncommon (<1%) complication of PCI that is associated with significant morbidity and mortality.[79-83] Coronary perforations are infrequent in patients undergoing balloon angioplasty (0.1%) compared with those undergoing atheroablative therapy (1.3%; $P < 0.001$).[80] Perforation due to coronary guidewires may manifest late after the procedure. Initial management strategies include prolonged balloon inflation, reversal of anticoagulation, and, in refractory cases, use of PTFE-covered stents.[84-86] The prognosis after coronary perforation depends on the extent of extravasation into the pericardium.[80] A classification scheme has been developed based on the angiographic appearance of the perforation, with type I perforations including an extraluminal crater without extravasation, type II perforations containing pericardial or myocardial blushing, and type III perforations having a diameter equal to or greater than 1 mm with contrast streaming and cavity spilling.[80] Type I perforations were associated with no deaths, but cardiac tamponade occurred in 8% of patients; type II perforations were associated with no deaths, but cardiac tamponade occurred in 13% of patients; and type III perforations were associated with death in 19% and cardiac tamponade in 63% of patients.[80]

Coronary Spasm

Coronary spasm is defined as a transient or sustained reduction in the diameter of stenosis by more than 50% in an arterial segment with insignificant (<25%) baseline narrowing. Although coronary spasm may occur in approximately 5% of cases, its frequency has been reduced with the routine use of coronary vasodilators, such as nitroglycerin and calcium channel blockers. Wire straightening of the vessel can mimic coronary spasm.

Abrupt Closure

Abrupt closure during coronary intervention is defined as an abrupt cessation of coronary flow to TIMI 0 or 1; it occurs during 3% to 5% of balloon angioplasty procedures. Abrupt closure may be caused by coronary dissection, embolization, or thrombus formation within the vessel. Its incidence has been markedly reduced with the availability of coronary stents.[87]

Stent Thrombosis

With the addition of a thienopyridine derivative (i.e., ticlopidine or clopidogrel) to aspirin, the incidence of bare metal stent thrombosis within 30 days of the procedure is less than 1%. Predictive factors for stent thrombosis include persistent dissection of NHLBI grade B or higher after stenting, greater total stent length, and a smaller final minimal lumen diameter within the stent.[88] DESs administered with longer durations (3 to 6 months) of dual antiplatelet therapy have similar rates of stent thrombosis as those that occur with bare metal stents,[89,90] although premature discontinuation of dual antiplatelet therapy has been associated with higher (6% to 29%) rates of stent thrombosis.[91,92] In addition, diabetes, prior brachytherapy, bifurcation lesions with two stents, AMI, renal failure, lower EF, and longer stent length have been associated with stent thrombosis.[91,92] A recent concern is the occurrence of very late (>1 year) stent thrombosis with the use of DESs[93] due to inflammation from the stent.[94,95] The estimated incidence of very late stent thrombosis ranges from 0.2% to 0.6% per year up to 3 years after stent placement. Long-term dual antiplatelet therapy may not be completely sufficient to prevent stent thrombosis.[90] The Academic Research Consortium has proposed new criteria for the timing and definitions used to document stent thrombosis in clinical studies. Timing of stent thrombosis is defined as acute (<24 hours), subacute (24 hours to 30 days), late (30 days to 1 year), and very late (after 1 year).[96] The categories of definite, probable, and possible stent thrombosis have been proposed as a more inclusive and standardized way to characterize the occurrence of this event in patients undergoing stent implantation (Table 56-5).

Restenosis Pattern

When ISR occurs after bare metal stent implantation, the risk of recurrence can be predicted by the pattern of restenosis.[97,98] Using the Mehran classification system, pattern I includes focal (<10 mm in length) lesions, pattern II is defined as ISR greater than 10 mm within the stent, pattern III includes ISR greater than 10 mm extending outside the stent, and pattern IV is totally occluded ISR.[97] Pattern I can be classified further by the location of the restenosis: Ia, within the stent; Ib, at the edge of the stent; Ic, at the articulation or gap; or Id, multifocal.[97] The need for recurrent target lesion revascularization (TLR) increased with increasing ISR class, from 19% to 35%, 50%, and 83% in classes I through IV, respectively ($P < 0.001$).[97] Restenosis after DES implantation is generally more focal than after bare metal stent placement[99]; with the sirolimus-eluting stent, it is more commonly seen at the margin of the stent owing to balloon injury that is not covered with the stent.[100]

Late Aneurysm Formation

Late vessel wall expansion of greater than 20% after PCI has been termed a coronary artery aneurysm. Coronary artery aneurysms, or,

TABLE 56-5	Academic Research Consortium Stent Thrombosis Definitions
Event	**Definition**
Definite	
Angiographic Confirmation	TIMI flow grade 0 with occlusion originating in or within 5 mm of stent in the presence of a thrombus
	Or
	TIMI flow grade 1, 2, or 3 originating in or within 5 mm of stent in the presence of a thrombus
	AND at least one of the following criteria within the last 48 hours
	New acute onset of ischemic symptoms at rest (typical chest pain with duration >20 min)
	New ischemic ECG changes suggestive of acute ischemia
	Typical rise and fall in cardiac biomarkers
Pathologic Confirmation	Evidence of recent thrombus within the stent determined at autopsy or via examination of tissue retrieved after thrombectomy
Probable	Any unexplained death within the first 30 days Irrespective of the time after the index procedure, any MI that is related to documented acute ischemia in the territory of the implanted stent without angiographic confirmation of stent thrombosis and in the absence of any other cause.
Possible	Any unexplained death >30 days after intracoronary stenting

ECG, electrocardiographic; MI, myocardial infarction; TIMI, Thrombolysis in Myocardial Infarction.

TABLE 56-6	TIMI Flow Grade Classification
Grade	**Definition**
3 (complete reperfusion)	Anterograde flow into the terminal coronary artery segment through a stenosis is as prompt as anterograde flow into a comparable segment proximal to the stenosis. Contrast material clears as rapidly from the distal segment as from an uninvolved, more proximal segment.
2 (partial reperfusion)	Contrast material flows through the stenosis to opacify the terminal artery segment. However, contrast enters the terminal segment perceptibly more slowly than more proximal segments. Alternatively, contrast material clears from a segment distal to a stenosis noticeably more slowly than from a comparable segment not preceded by a significant stenosis.
1 (penetration with minimal perfusion)	A small amount of contrast flows through the stenosis but fails to fully opacify the artery beyond.
0 (no perfusion)	No contrast flow through the stenosis.

Modified from Sheehan FH, Braunwald E, Canner P, et al. The effect of intravenous thrombolytic therapy on left ventricular function: A report on tissue-type plasminogen activator and streptokinase from the Thrombolysis in Myocardial Infarction (TIMI) Phase I Trial. *Circulation.* 1987;72:817–829.

more precisely, pseudoaneurysms, are rare findings after balloon angioplasty, atheroablation, and coronary stenting. Coronary artery aneurysms most likely arise from tears or dissection and incomplete healing that compromises vessel wall integrity and results in vessel wall expansion. Coronary artery aneurysms are also rarely (<1%) seen after DES placement, although the pathological etiology of aneurysms in this setting may relate to the expansion of all three layers of the arterial wall owing to inflammation and the effects of cytostatic or cytotoxic drugs and malapposition of the stent struts.[101,102] Under rare circumstances, coronary artery aneurysms can become infected, requiring surgical intervention.[103,104]

CORONARY PERFUSION

Evaluation of pharmacological and mechanical methods of reperfusing coronary occlusions in patients with STEMI is supported by the development of a reproducible angiographic method to assess the degree of coronary recanalization achieved with these therapies. The classification scheme for TIMI flow grade characterizes the extent of coronary recanalization in patients with STEMI treated with systemic thrombolytic agents and in those presenting with non-STEMI and unstable angina (Table 56-6).[105] The TIMI frame count[106] and the TIMI myocardial perfusion grade were developed to further quantify anterograde flow and assess distal microvascular perfusion.[107]

Classification Scheme for TIMI Flow Grade

The TIMI flow grade system is a valuable tool for assessing the efficacy of reperfusion strategies in patients with STEMI and for identifying patients at higher risk for an adverse outcome with acute coronary syndromes or undergoing PCI. Several thrombolytic trials have identified an important relationship between 90-minute TIMI flow grade after thrombolysis and clinical outcome.[108] In the GUSTO (Global Utilization of Streptokinase and Tissue Plasminogen Activator for Occluded Coronary Arteries) angiographic substudy, the mortality rate for patients with TIMI 2 flow (7.4%) was similar to the mortality rate for those with TIMI 0 or 1 flow (8.9%). In contrast, the mortality rate was lowest (4.4%) in patients with TIMI 3 flow.[108] Despite these important associations, there are a number of limitations of the TIMI classification system. Substantial observer variability has been noted with the TIMI flow grade, with the best agreement between

the angiographic core laboratory and clinical centers occurring when the artery is graded as either open or closed (TIMI 0 or 1 flow; kappa value = 0.84).[106] Observer agreement is only moderate in assessing TIMI grade 3 flow (kappa value = 0.55) and is poor in the assessment of TIMI grade 2 flow (kappa value = 0.38). The lack of concordance for determining TIMI flow grade was also shown between experienced angiographic core laboratories. Another limitation of the TIMI flow grade is that it provides ordinal values rather than continuous ones, thus limiting its statistical power in clinical trials. Furthermore, although TIMI flow grade has classically compared flow in the infarct-related vessel to flow in the "normal" nonculprit artery, flow in the non-infarct-related artery in patients with STEMI is not truly normal compared with flow in patients without STEMI.[109] Difficulties in reproducibly assessing myocardial flow relative to flow in other vessels (e.g., the RCA, or in the setting of total occlusion of the contralateral vessel) led some investigators to modify the definition of "TIMI grade 3 flow" to include opacification of the distal coronary artery within three cardiac cycles.[110] The "three cardiac cycle" definition of TIMI 3 flow results in an absolute rate increase of approximately 10% compared with the original definition.[111] Accordingly, more quantitative measures of anterograde flow were developed.

TIMI Frame Count

The TIMI frame count (TFC) provides a quantitative assessment of the number of frames required for dye to reach standardized distal landmarks; it may provide a more objective and precise method of estimating coronary blood flow than the TIMI flow grade.[106] The first frame used for TIMI frame counting is defined as the cine frame, in which a column of dye touches both borders of the coronary artery and moves forward, and the last frame is characterized as the cine frame in which dye begins to enter (but does not necessarily fill) a standard distal landmark in the artery. The standard distal landmarks for epicardial vessels are the first branch of the posterolateral artery for the RCA; the most distal branch of the obtuse marginal branch in the dye path through the culprit lesion in the circumflex system; and the distal bifurcation—which is also known as the "moustache," "pitchfork," or "whale's tail"—in the LAD. These frame counts are corrected for the longer length of the LAD by dividing the TFC by 1.7 to arrive at the corrected TIMI frame count (CTFC). The CTFC provides a number of advantages over TIMI flow grades. The CTFC is quantitative rather than qualitative, objective rather than subjective, and a continuous rather than a categorical variable. Observer variability is also substantially less with TFC measurements compared with TIMI flow grades.[106] Furthermore, although it has traditionally been assumed that basal flow in nonculprit arteries in the setting of AMI after thrombolysis is "normal," it is now appreciated that basal flow in the uninvolved artery is abnormal using the CTFC.[109] The more objective CTFC has also been related to clinical outcomes.[107] Flow in the infarct-related artery in survivors of STEMI was significantly faster than in patients who died; mortality increased by 0.7% for every 10-frame rise in the CTFC ($P < 0.001$).[107] None of the patients in the TIMI studies who had a CTFC less than 14 (hyperemic or TIMI grade 4 flow) died within the first 30 days. In another series of patients undergoing PCI, none of the 376 patients with a CTFC less than 14 after angioplasty died, underscoring the fact that, within the subgroup of patients with "normal flow," there may be further subgroups with even better flow.

TIMI Myocardial Perfusion Grade

It is now apparent that epicardial flow does not necessarily imply tissue level or microvascular perfusion. These findings led to the development of the TIMI myocardial perfusion grade (TMPG) (Fig. 56-3; Table 56-7), which has been shown to be a multivariate predictor of mortality in AMI.[107] The TMPG permits risk stratification even within epicardial TIMI grade 3 flow. That is, despite achieving normal TIMI grade 3 flow after reperfusion therapy, patients with diminished microvasculature perfusion (TMPG 0 or 1) have a persistently elevated mortality rate of 5.4% compared with patients with both TIMI grade 3

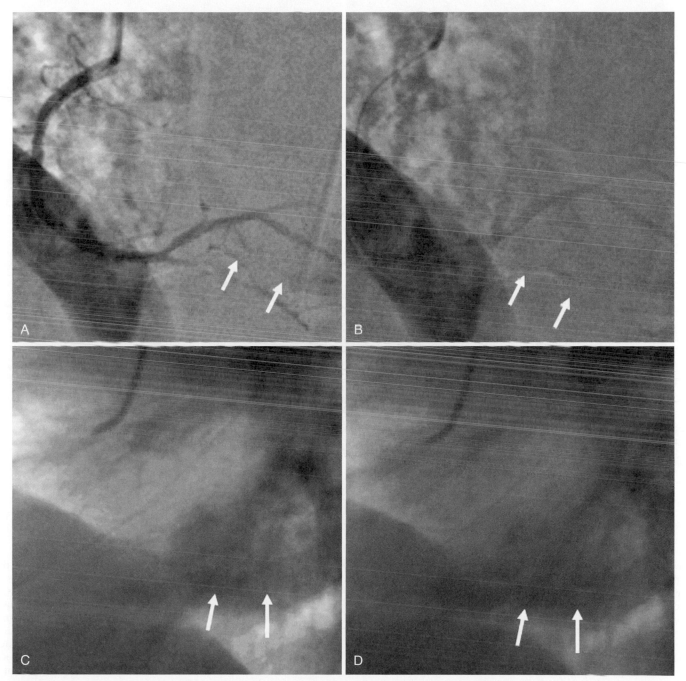

Figure 56-3 Thrombolysis in Myocardial Infarction (TIMI) myocardial perfusion grade using digital subtraction angiography. Perfusion grade 0 is characterized by the absence of the typical "ground-glass" filling of the distal vascular bed during coronary injection (A) and washout (B). Perfusion grade 1 is demonstrated by persistent contrast staining at the beginning (C) and end (D) of the coronary injection.

Continued

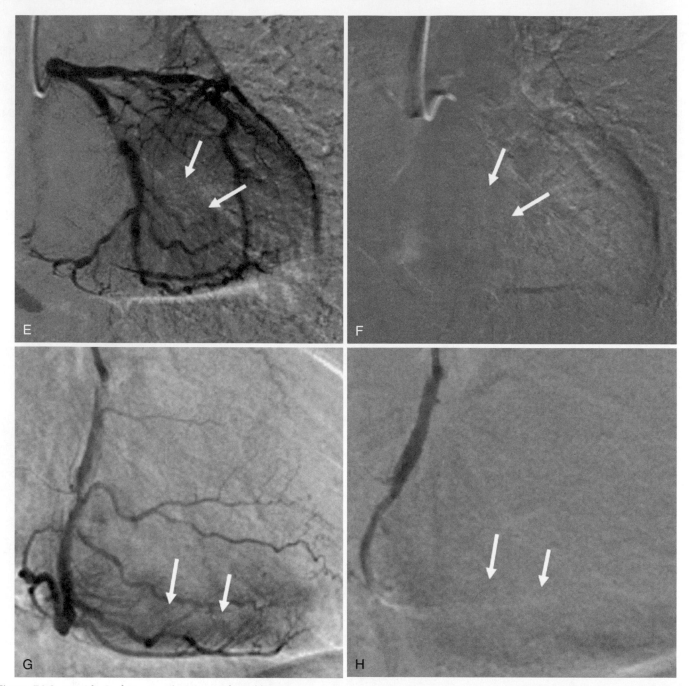

Figure 56-3, cont'd Perfusion grade 2 is manifested by a very prominent contrast appearance at the end of coronary injection (E) that washes out at the end of the contrast injection (F). Perfusion grade 3 is shown as a normal ground-glass appearance of the distal vascular bed at the end of the contrast injection (G) that washes out at the end of the injection (H).

flow and TMPG 3, who have a mortality rate less than 1%.[107] Accordingly, the TIMI flow grades and the TMPGs can be combined to identify a group of patients at "very low" or "very high" risk for mortality after STEMI. Those patients with both TIMI grade 3 flow and TMPG 3 flow had a mortality rate of 0.7%, whereas patients with both TIMI grade 0 or 1 and TMPG 0 or 1 flow had a mortality rate of 10.9%. Another approach to assess myocardial perfusion is to use digital subtraction angiography (DSA) to quantitatively characterize the kinetics of dye entering the myocardium during contrast angiography. DSA is performed at end-diastole by aligning cine frame images taken before dye fills the myocardium with those taken at the peak of myocardial filling to subtract spine, ribs, diaphragm, and epicardial artery. A representative region of the myocardium that is free of overlap by epicardial arterial branches is sampled to determine the increase in the gray-scale brightness of the myocardium when it first reached its peak intensity. The circumference of the myocardial blush is measured using a handheld planimeter. The number of frames required for the myocardium to first reach its peak brightness is converted into time (seconds) by dividing the frame count by 30 (for images acquired at 30 frames per second). The rate of rise in brightness (gray-scale change per second) and the rate of growth of blush in circumference (centimeters per second) can then be calculated. Using DSA, microvascular perfusion was reduced in AMI patients compared to normal patients, as demonstrated by a reduction in peak brightness (gray-scale peak), the rate of rise in brightness, the blush circumference, and the rate of growth of blush in circumference.[111]

TABLE 56-7	TIMI Myocardial Perfusion Grades
Grade	**Definition**
3	Normal entry and exit of dye from the microvasculature. There is a ground-glass appearance ("blush") or opacification of the myocardium in the distribution of the culprit lesion that clears normally and is either gone or mildly or moderately persistent at the end of the washout phase (approximately three cardiac cycles), similar to an uninvolved artery. Blush that is of only mild intensity throughout the washout phase but fades normally is also classified as grade 3.
2	Delayed entry and exit of dye from the microvasculature. There is a ground-glass appearance ("blush") or opacification of the myocardium in the distribution of the culprit lesion that is strongly persistent at the end of the washout phase (i.e., dye is strongly persistent after three cardiac cycles of the washout phase and either does not diminish or only minimally diminishes in intensity during washout).
1	Slow entry of dye into but failure to exit the microvasculature. There is a ground-glass appearance ("blush") or opacification of the myocardium in the distribution of the culprit lesion that fails to clear from the microvasculature, and dye staining is present on the next injection (approximately 30 seconds between injections).
0	Failure of the dye to enter the microvasculature. There is either minimal or no ground-glass appearance ("blush") or opacification of the myocardium in the distribution of the culprit artery, indicating lack of tissue-level perfusion.

CORONARY FLOW VELOCITY

Absolute flow velocity can be measured using PCI guidewire velocity.[112] With this technique, the guidewire tip is placed at the coronary landmark after PCI and a Kelly clamp is placed on the guidewire at the point at which it exits the Y adapter. The guidewire tip is then withdrawn to the catheter tip and a second Kelly clamp is placed on the wire where it exits the Y adapter. The distance between the two Kelly clamps outside the body is measured as the distance between the catheter tip and the anatomical landmark inside the body. Velocity (centimeters per second) may be calculated as this distance (centimeters) divided by the product of the TFC (frames) and the film frame speed (frames per second). Flow (milliliters per second) may be calculated by multiplying velocity and the mean cross-sectional lumen area (square centimeters) along the length of the artery to the TIMI landmark. In a series of 30 patients undergoing PCI, velocity increased from 13.9 ± 8.5 cm/sec before PCI to 22.8 ± 9.3 cm/sec after PCI ($P <$ 0.001). For all 30 patients, flow doubled from 0.6 ± 0.4 mL/sec before PCI to 1.2 ± 0.6 mL/sec after PCI ($P < 0.001$). In the 18 patients with TIMI grade 3 flow both before and after PCI, flow increased 86%, from 0.7 ± 0.3 to 1.3 ± 0.6 mL/sec ($P < 0.001$).

Quantitative Angiography

Quantitative coronary angiography (QCA) is most commonly performed using automated arterial contour detection, although videodensitometry and digital parametric imaging have also been tried with limited success. Whereas "online" QCA is somewhat cumbersome to use in the catheterization laboratory, "offline" QCA has proved to be valuable for research investigation in determining the effects of new drugs and devices on lumen dimensions early and late after PCI. Notably, for clinical decision making in intermediate lesions, neither trained visual estimates or online quantitative angiography is a substitute for precise physiological measurements of stenosis severity, such as fractional flow reserve or coronary Doppler measurements.[113]

NONQUANTITATIVE ESTIMATES OF LESION SEVERITY

Virtually every interventionalist uses an "eyeball" estimate to determine the severity of angiographic stenosis, although these visual estimations of lesion severity are of limited value for research studies because of substantial observer-to-observer variability. Blinded review of cineangiograms by experienced cardiologists found that the average visual diameter stenosis was 85% before PCI (vs. 68% using quantitative methods) and 30% after PCI (vs. 49% using quantitative methods); these differences correspond to a 200% error in the estimation of percent diameter stenosis.[114] Visual estimates of stenosis severity also result in some values (e.g., 90% to 99% diameter stenosis) that are physiologically untenable for antegrade flow. Inherent overestimation and underestimation of stenosis severity gauged visually can be overcome by retraining the clinician's eye. A more quantitative approach to the assessment of lesion severity uses handheld or digital calipers to estimate quantitative diameters and percent diameter stenosis. Angiographic images are magnified, and calibration is performed by measuring the known dimensions of the diagnostic or guiding catheter using digital calipers. The observer then visually identifies the lumen's border using the calipers, and a calibration factor is obtained to determine absolute coronary dimensions. Properly applied, this method appears to correlate weakly with automated edge-detection algorithms. If caliper measurements are obtained from nonmagnified images, the correlation with automated edge-detection algorithms is less accurate.

COMPUTER-ASSISTED QUANTITATIVE CORONARY ANGIOGRAPHY

QCA was initiated almost 30 years ago by Brown and colleagues, who magnified 35-mm cineangiograms obtained from orthogonal projections and hand-traced the arterial edges on a large screen. After computer-assisted correction for pincushion distortion, the tracings were digitized and the orthogonal projections were combined to form a 3D representation of the arterial segment, assuming an elliptical geometry. Although accuracy and precision were enhanced compared with visual methods, the time needed for image processing limited the clinical utility of this method. Several automated edge-detection algorithms were then developed and applied to directly acquired digital images or to 35-mm cine film digitized using a cine-video converter. Subsequent iterations of these first-generation devices used enhanced microprocessing speed and digital image acquisition to render the end-user interface more flexible and substantially shortened the time required for image analysis.

QCA is divided into several distinct processes, including film digitization (when applicable), image calibration, and arterial contour detection (Fig. 56-4). For processing 35-mm cine film, a cine-video converter is used to digitize images into a 512 by 512 (or larger) by 8-bit pixel matrix. Optical (preferably) or digital magnification results in an effective pixel matrix up to 2458 by 2458.[115] For estimation of absolute coronary dimensions, the diagnostic or guiding catheter usually serves as the scaling device. In general, a nontapered segment of the catheter is selected, and a center line through the catheter is drawn. Linear density profiles are then constructed perpendicular to the catheter center line and a weighted average of the first and second derivative functions is used to define the catheter edge points. Individual edge points are then connected using an automated algorithm, outliers are discarded, and the edges are smoothed. The diameter of the catheter is then used to obtain a calibration factor, expressed in millimeters per pixel. The dimensions of the injection catheter may be influenced by whether contrast or saline is imaged within the catheter tip and by the type of material used in catheter construction. As high-flow injection catheters have been developed, more quantitative angiographic systems have been using contrast-filled injection catheters for image calibration. The automated algorithm is then applied to a selected arterial segment: absolute coronary dimensions are obtained from the minimal lumen diameter (MLD) reference diameter, and, from these, the percent diameter stenoses are derived. For most angiographic systems, interobserver variabilities are 3.1% for diameter stenosis and 0.10 to 0.18 mm for MLD for cineangiographic readings; variabilities are slightly higher (<0.25 mm) for repeated analyses of the digital angiograms owing to the slightly lower resolution compared

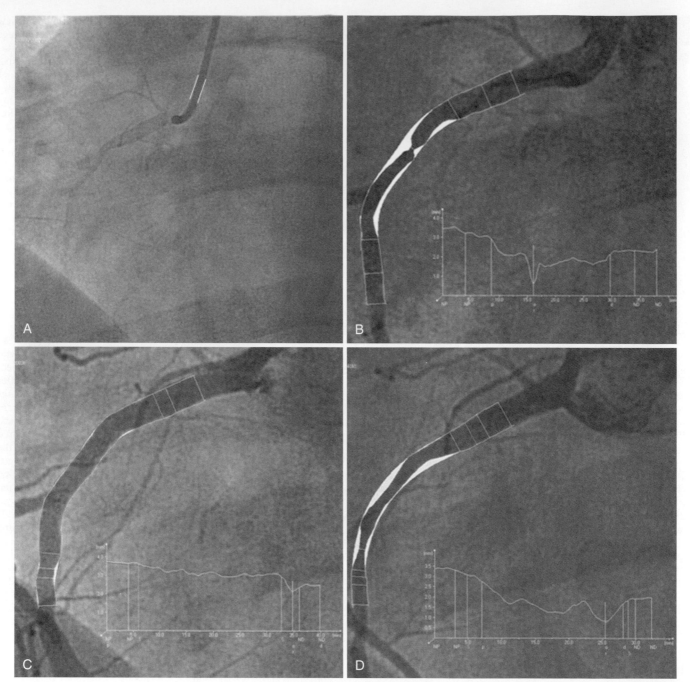

Figure 56-4 Quantitative coronary angiography. A. Image calibration is performed using the nontapered portion of the injection catheter as the calibration source. B. The automated edge detection algorithm (CMS, Leiden, The Netherlands) is applied to the arterial contour, and the minimal lumen diameter (MLD) is identified. A diameter function profile curve (insert) shows the diameters of the vessel along the length of the analysis segment. C. After coronary stent placement, the identical length of artery is analyzed to provide an assessment of the lumen improvement. D. At the time of angiographic follow-up, the location of late lumen loss along the length of the analysis segment is identified.

with cineangiography. The two most commonly used QCA systems are described.

Cardiovascular Angiography Analysis System

The Cardiovascular Angiography Analysis System (CAAS, Pie Data Medical B.V., Maastricht, The Netherlands) is a QCA system developed for offline cineangiographic analysis (Fig. 56-2). The edge-detection algorithm incorporates an optional correction for pincushion distortion; its edge detection uses a weighted (50%) sum of the first and second derivatives of the mean pixel density, and it applies minimal cost criteria for smoothing of the arterial edge contours. In addition

to reporting an interpolated reference diameter and an MLD, a subsegment analysis provides mean, minimal, and maximal subsegment diameters. Specific reporting algorithms have been developed for DESs, for patients undergoing radiation brachytherapy, and for those undergoing peripheral intervention.

Coronary Measurement System

Specific features of the Coronary Measurement System (CMS, MEDIS, Leiden, The Netherlands) include two-point user-defined center-line identification, arterial edge detection using a weighted (50%) sum of the first and second derivatives of the mean pixel density, arterial contour detection using a minimal cost matrix algorithm, and an "interpolated" reference vessel diameter. One limitation of the minimal cost algorithm used with the first-generation CMS system (as well as the CAAS-II system) has been its inability to precisely quantify arterial luminal contours characterized by abrupt changes. The CMS-Gradient Field Transformation (GFT) algorithm is not restricted in its search directions, incorporating multidirectional information about the arterial boundaries for construction of the arterial edge; it is suitable for the analysis of complex coronary artery lesions. Specific reporting algorithms have been developed for bifurcation lesions (Fig. 56-5), DESs (Fig. 56-6), patients undergoing radiation brachytherapy (Fig. 56-7), and those undergoing peripheral intervention.

FACTORS CONTRIBUTING TO VARIABILITY USING QUANTITATIVE CORONARY ANGIOGRAPHY

Variability associated with measurements of MLD and reference diameter is affected by a number of factors, including (1) the biological differences among luminal diameters (e.g., reference vessel size, vasomotor tone, thrombus); (2) inconsistencies in radiographic image acquisition parameters (e.g., quantum mottling, out-of-plane magnification, foreshortening); and (3) variability in angiographic measurement (e.g., frame selection, factors affecting the edge-detection algorithm) (Table 56-8). These factors should be controlled in order to improve the overall diagnostic accuracy of QCA.

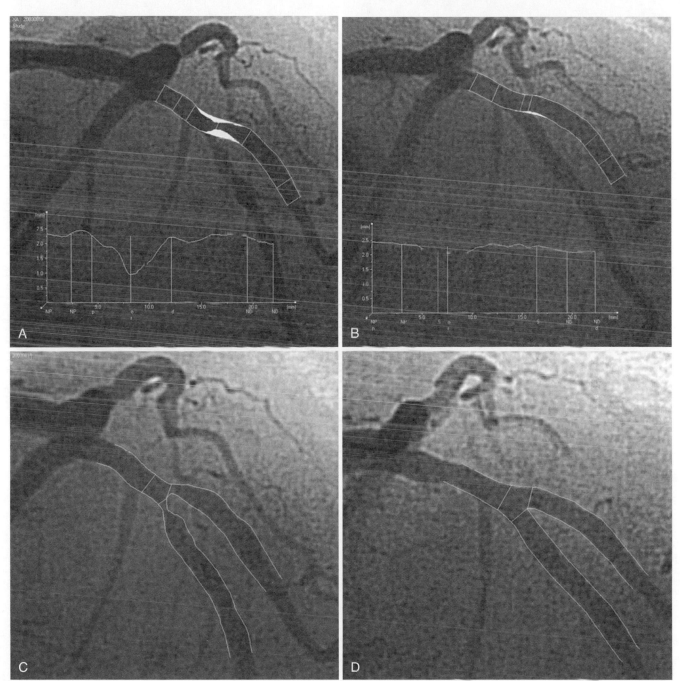

Figure 56-5 Bifurcation quantitative analysis. Quantitative angiographic analysis of bifurcation lesions is complicated by the difficulty in identifying minimal lumen diameter (MLD) at the site of vessel branching. Three methods of bifurcation analysis have been employed: conventional quantitative angiography separately applied to each branch (A. Before intervention. B. After intervention); application of the edge algorithm to both branches (C. Before intervention. D. After intervention); and beginning the analysis at the ostium of the branch (E. Before intervention. F. After intervention). *Continued*

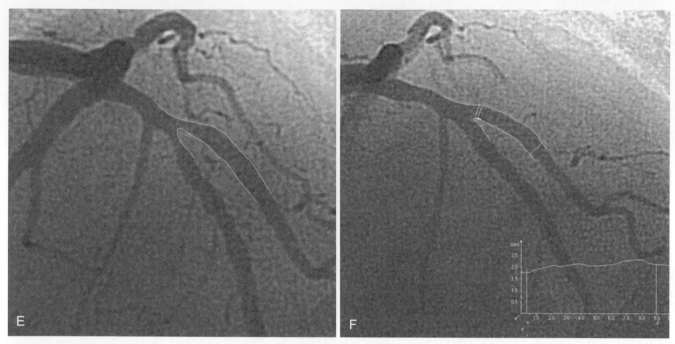

Figure 56-5, cont'd.

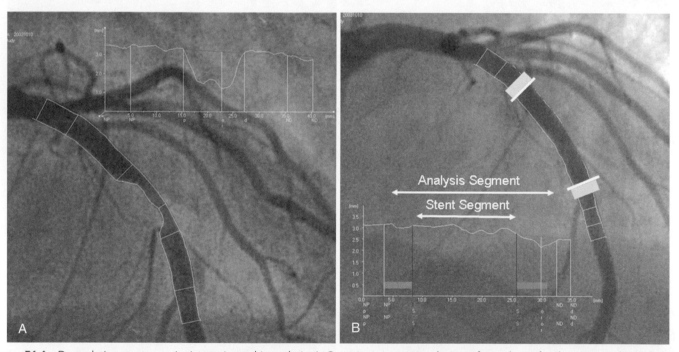

Figure 56-6 Drug-eluting stent quantitative angiographic analysis. A. Quantitative angiography is performed on a focal stenosis in the midportion of the left anterior descending coronary artery (LAD). B. After placement of a drug-eluting stent, the proximal and distal portions of the stent are identified (solid bars). A 5-mm proximal and distal edge is also analyzed (shaded boxes). From these measurements, the minimal lumen diameters within the stent ("stent" segment) and within the region of analysis ("analysis" segment) are identified.

Biological Variability

Studies that include a wide range of vessel sizes have more biological variability in vessel diameter (as reflected in the standard deviation of the measurements) than those that are more restrictive in their inclusion criteria. Vasomotor tone may also affect the size of the reference vessel, resulting in distal vasoconstriction and vasospasm that dynamically affect the arterial diameter in paired measurements. Transient maximum coronary vasodilation may be achieved with intracoronary

(50 to 200 mcg), intravenous (10 mcg/min), or sublingual (0.4 to 0.8 mg) nitroglycerin.

Acquisition Variability

Acquisition factors that affect variability include cardiac and respiratory motion artifact, vessel foreshortening, inadequate filling of the coronary artery ("streaming"), overfilling of the aortic cusp with contrast, and failure to separate overlapping branch vessels from the stenosis.[116] These factors may lead to either overestimation or

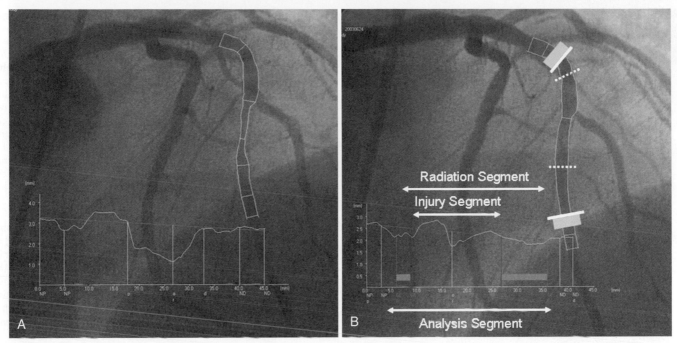

Figure 56-7 Brachytherapy analysis. A. Quantitative angiography is performed on a focal stenosis in the midportion of the left anterior descending coronary artery (LAD). B. After balloon angioplasty, the proximal and distal portions of the balloon injury are identified (dashed lines). After radiation brachytherapy, the proximal and distal portion of the radiation injury are identified (solid lines). A 5-mm proximal and distal edge of the radiation zone is also analyzed (shaded boxes) to identify the "edge effect." From these measurements, the minimal lumen diameters within the segment of balloon injury ("injury" segment), the segment of radiation injury ("radiation" segment), and within the region of analysis ("analysis" segment) are identified. The shaded portion in the diameter function profile curve (insert) represents the region of the artery that was treated with radiation but was not injured with the balloon.

underestimation of lesion severity. Out-of-plane magnification and pincushion distortion may also contribute to small errors in angiographic imaging. For sequential studies, use of the identical angiographic imaging laboratory allows replication of the x-ray generator, tube, and image intensifier parameters. With the introduction of digital imaging and archiving, image compression has raised potential problems with the quality of images for analysis. The standard Digital Imaging and Communications in Medicine (DICOM) 2.1 Joint Photographic Expert Group (JPEG) lossless compression has become the industry standard for image storage and transfer and requires approximately 500 megabytes of storage for each imaging study. The effect of image compression and decompression on image quality was evaluated by a joint task force of the American College of Cardiology and European Society of Cardiology using JPEG images at compression ratios of 1:1 (uncompressed), 6:1, 10:1, and 16:1.[117] The intraobserver analysis showed significant systematic and random errors in the calibration factor at JPEG compression ratios of 10:1 and higher; therefore these should not be used in QCA clinical research studies.[117] Similar issues exist for the analysis of S-VHS video tapes with substantial loss of image resolution. Flat-panel image acquisition does not affect the quality of QCA.[118]

Measurement Variability

Analysis of two or more orthogonal projections permits a more accurate assessment of the physiological significance of lesion severity, although a second, technically suitable projection is in many cases unavailable owing to vessel foreshortening, overlap, and poor image quality. If orthogonal projections are not available, analyses of the "worst view" projection may provide sufficiently accurate information for clinical studies. Herrington and colleagues[119] used a components-of-variance model to show that the process of acquiring and performing QCA on selected cine frames accounted for 57% of the total measurement variability, whereas day-to-day variations in the patient, procedure, and equipment accounted for 30% of total variability.

Frame selection accounted for the remaining 13% of total variability. When direct digital angiography is performed and random errors associated with noise in the cine video pathway are eliminated, frame selection may be a much more important contributor to overall measurement variability. Frame selection has been associated with substantial interobserver variability, and the frame demonstrating the sharpest and tightest view of the stenosis should be used. Angiographic core laboratory reproducibility of various angiographic parameters may affect sample size calculations for various studies.[120] In repeated (over 1 year) comparisons of five quantitative parameters (e.g., minimum lumen diameter [MLD], ejection fraction [EF], etc.) and six qualitative parameters (e.g., TIMI myocardial perfusion grade [TMPG] or TIMI thrombus grade [TTG], etc.), MLD and EF were the most reproducible, yielding the smallest sample size calculations, whereas percent diameter stenosis and center-line wall motion require substantially larger trials.[120] Of the qualitative parameters, all except TIMI flow grade gave reproducible characteristics, yielding sample sizes of many hundreds of patients. Reproducibility of TMPG and TTG was only moderately good both within and between core laboratories, underscoring an intrinsic difficulty in assessing these.[120] Automated QCA systems differ with respect to the preferred method of calibration, location of the arterial border, and construction of its contour; use of minimal-cost or "smoothing" algorithms; and selection of normal "reference" segments. Edge-detection algorithms that identify the arterial edge using a 50% weighted threshold of the first- and second-derivative extrema may produce systematically larger reference and obstruction diameters than those using a 75% weighted value (weighted toward the first-derivative extremum) or the first-derivative extremum itself. These systematic differences may also affect the accuracy and reproducibility of the absolute and relative angiographic measurements. Accordingly, each angiographic core laboratory should independently determine its own variabilities during the performance of QCA studies, potentially permitting standardization of techniques among different core laboratories.

TABLE 56-8	Correctable Sources of Imaging Error during Acquisition	
Source of Error	**Potential Corrections**
Biological variation in lumen diameter	
Vasomotor tone	Nitroglycerin, 100–200 mcg intracoronary every 10 minutes
Variations in image acquisition	
Single studies	
Vessel motion	
Cardiac	End-diastolic/end-systolic cineframe
Respiratory	Breath-holding
Vessel foreshortening	Obtain multiple angiographic projections
Insufficient contrast injection	Use 7- or 8-Fr large high-flow catheters
Branch vessel overlap	Obtain multiple angiographic projections
Pincushion distortion	Image objects in center of image
Sequential studies	
X-ray generator (pulse width/beam)	Repeat study in same imaging
X-ray tube (focal spot/shape/tube current)	As above
Image intensifier (magnification/resolution)	As above
Differences in angles and gantry height	Record gantry height/angle/skew on worksheet
Image calibration	Use measured catheter diameter
Errors in image analysis	
Electronic noise	Recursive digitization and frame averaging
Quantum noise	Spatial filtering of digital image data
Automated edge-detection algorithm	Minimize observer interaction
Selection of reference positions	Interpolated or averaged normal segment
Identification of lesion length	Use of side branches, other landmarks
Frame selection	End-diastolic frame showing "worst" view

QUANTITATIVE ANGIOGRAPHIC INDICES

Measurement of Plaque Regression

Although quantitative coronary angiography has generally been viewed as an insensitive tool to measure plaque regression after lipid-lowering therapy, particularly compared with intravascular ultrasound, one recent study has evaluated the effect of rosuvastatin on quantative angiographic regression.[121] In that study, which comprised 507 coronary disease patients treated with rosuvastatin 40 mg daily for 24 months, it was found that the percent diameter stenosis decreased from 37.3% ± 8.4% to 36.0% ± 10.1% ($P < 0.001$). The minimal lumen diameter increased from 1.65 ± 36 to 1.68 ± 0.38 mm ($P < 0.001$).[121]

Luminal Improvements after Percutaneous Coronary Intervention

Early and late angiographic results after PCI have been described using a number of QCA criteria. Coronary stents provide a superior residual lumen compared with balloon angioplasty, but they may result in higher amounts of late intimal hyperplasia (and late lumen loss) than is seen after balloon angioplasty. The net balance is that stents provide a net larger late angiographic result.

Angiographic Success

The change in MLD that occurs immediately after PCI is called the *acute gain* (in millimeters), and the loss of MLD that occurs during the follow-up period is defined as the *late loss* (in millimeters). Relative changes that occur in the percent diameter stenosis are provided by the following relationship: % diameter stenosis = (1 − [MLD/reference diameter]) × 100. Traditionally, angiographic success after PCI has

been defined as the achievement of a less than 50% residual diameter stenosis,[1] which is most often associated with at least 20% improvement from the baseline diameter stenosis as well as symptom improvement. With the advent of coronary stents and the determination that stent thrombosis was associated with a suboptimal initial angiographic result, a more contemporary definition of angiographic "stent success" was the attainment of a less than 20% residual diameter stenosis within the stent, although higher (up to 20% to 30%) "inflow" or "outflow" diameter stenosis may be present owing to residual plaque at the stent margins. Although the documented disparity between visual and quantitative estimates of angiographic success remains a challenge for self-reporting registries that describe procedural outcomes, there has been documented improvement in angiographic success rates over the past decade with the more widespread use of coronary stents.[122]

Binary Angiographic Restenosis

A number of binary criteria have been used to describe angiographic restenosis after PCI. Binary angiographic restenosis is best defined as a 50% or greater diameter stenosis at follow-up, although a number of other dichotomous criteria have been used (e.g., loss of <50% of the initial gain, loss in MLD of ≥0.72 mm). Binary angiographic restenosis after DES placement may occur within the stent ("in-stent" restenosis), within the 5-mm margins of the stent ("edge" restenosis), or within the segment between the proximal and distal reference segments ("in-segment" or "in-lesion" restenosis).

Late Luminal Loss

The long-term success of PCI can be measured by several other QCA parameters. Serial QCA studies have shown that there is an approximate 0.50-mm reduction in luminal diameter that develops within 3 to 6 months after balloon angioplasty, although angiography cannot differentiate whether this reduction is due to intimal hyperplasia or arterial remodeling (or constriction). Luminal loss after balloon angioplasty follows a near-gaussian distribution. Because there is little or no arterial remodeling after bare metal stent placement, late luminal loss after stent placement is primarily due to intimal hyperplasia, and angiographic estimates of volumetric percent volume obstruction have been well correlated with IVUS measurements of intimal hyperplasia.[123] A number of technical factors may compromise the ability of late luminal loss to characterize overall reductions in lumen diameters, including calibration errors at the time of postprocedural or follow-up assessments and the relocation of the MLD between the postprocedural and follow-up examinations.[124] The distribution of late luminal loss after placement of DESs is unlike the distribution of late luminal loss noted after bare metal stent placement, with a narrowing variance (i.e., standard deviation) due to the reduced tissue growth and a rightward skewing of the late-luminal-loss histogram,[125] suggesting an "all-or-none" response to the DES.[126] The patient-based relationship between late luminal loss and TLR was examined in 1,314 patients with de novo lesions who were treated with bare metal or paclitaxel-eluting stents.[127] In this analysis, the relationship between late luminal loss and TLR was monotonic and curvilinear,[98] with the likelihood of TLR not exceeding 5% until the late loss of the analysis segment was greater than 0.5 mm and not exceeding 10% until late loss was greater than 0.65 mm.[127] At lower magnitudes of late luminal loss, there was a very small incremental increase in the occurrence of TLR; with higher degrees of late luminal loss, the late loss-TLR relationship was steep and almost linear.[127] The rate of TLR was related not only to median late loss but also to measures of its statistical distribution. Specifically, TLR increased with lack of homogeneous biological response, manifested by greater variance (i.e., higher standard deviations) and greater rightward skewing of the late-luminal-loss histogram.[127] To correct for this skewing and to develop better predictive models of restenosis, an optimized power transformation was applied to data from patients enrolled in two trials of sirolimus-eluting stents to predict rates of binary angiographic restenosis and compare them with observed restenosis rates.[125] The mean in-stent late loss was 0.17 ± 0.45 mm after sirolimus-eluting stent placement and 1.00 ± 0.70 mm after bare metal stent placement. If a normal distribution was assumed, late loss accurately estimated in-stent binary angiographic restenosis for the bare metal stent (predicted 35.4% vs. observed 35.4%) but underestimated the binary restenosis rate in the sirolimus-eluting stent arm (predicted 0.6% vs. observed 3.2%). Power transformation improved the reliability of the estimate in the sirolimus arm (predicted 3.2% vs. observed 3.2%). In contrast, another study did not confirm the value of the power transformation as a predictor of binary angiographic restenosis.[128] To formally evaluate four potential angiographic surrogate markers for TLR by applying well-defined criteria of surrogacy to an extensive database of randomized DES trials, Pocock and colleagues analyzed 11 multicenter, prospective randomized stent trials comprising 5,381 patients, each with a single treated lesion and follow-up angiography.[129] Based on four surrogate criteria, late loss and percent diameter stenosis strongly predicted the risk of TLR, with in-segment percent diameter stenosis being the most highly predictive (C statistic = 0.95). Whereas late loss as a surrogate was dependent on vessel size, percent diameter stenosis was independent of vessel size. Differences in TLR rates for bare metal and drug-eluting stents were fully explained statistically by their differences in late loss and percent diameter stenosis. However, because of the curvilinearity of the logistic model, trials comparing two effective DESs can have significant differences in mean late losses and percent diameter stenosis but negligible expected differences in TLR risk. Others have suggested a stronger relationship between late loss and TLR for comparative DES trials,[130] but whether late luminal loss will serve as a meaningful surrogate endpoint in DES comparative trials remains controversial.

Three-Dimensional Imaging

A number of commercial software systems have developed 3D imaging software for quantifying coronary stenoses. In a phantom study that compared the two 3D QCA systems, the CardiOp-B and CAAS 5, the CardiOp-B system significantly underestimated the minimum luminal diameter MLD while both systems significantly overestimated the maximum luminal diameter at the minimal luminal area (MLA) over the phantom's true value.[131] The CAAS 5 system had a greater degree of accuracy and precision per millimeter than the CardiOp-B in assessing the minimal LD.[131] An increased precision per millimeter (SD =

0.01 vs. 0.29) and accuracy per millimeter (mean difference = 0.03 vs. 0.11) in the mean LD was observed with the CAAS 5. In comparing the MLA per millimeter (2), the CAAS 5 was more precise (SD = 0.14 vs. 0.55) and accurate (mean difference = 0.12 vs. 0.02) with regard to the true phantom MLA compared with the CardiOp-B system.[131]

Quantitative Coronary Angiography in Patients Undergoing Brachytherapy

New technologies, such as radiation brachytherapy, may cause injury at the margin of the treated segment, resulting in "edge" restenosis in regions that were not initially narrowed. Contemporary QCA analyses are performed to identify each of these regional changes in MLD to analyze the local biological effects of therapy. Radiation coverage may be inadequate in regions of balloon injury ("geographic miss"), or it may have an independent effect on the luminal diameter in regions that are not injured with a balloon catheter ("geographic extension").[132] These quantitative methods have led to the elucidation of the biological effects of radiation for the treatment of ISR.

LIMITATIONS OF QUANTITATIVE CORONARY ANGIOGRAPHY

The ability of QCA to accurately detect the presence and severity of coronary atherosclerosis is limited by several factors. Compensatory arterial dilation occurs during the early stages of coronary atherosclerosis, resulting in a preserved coronary lumen despite the presence of significant coronary atherosclerosis. Routine coronary angiography can accurately measure the arterial lumen but is relatively insensitive for the detection of arterial wall atherosclerosis, circumferential plaque distribution, vessel wall calcification, or luminal dimensions after stent implantation. Coronary angiography is limited to a lesser extent by radiographic factors, such as cardiac motion, pincushion distortion, and quantum mottling; most analysis systems have difficulty discriminating values less than 1.0 mm owing to limitations of radiographic imaging of small objects (e.g., veiling glare, point spread function). Newer methods incorporating adaptive simultaneous coronary border detection have been developed to more accurately assess the dimensions of smaller vessels.

REFERENCES

1. Smith S, Feldman T, Hirshfeld J, et al: ACC/AHA/SCAI 2005 Guideline Update for Percutaneous Coronary Intervention—summary article: a report of the American College of Cardiology/American Heart Association Task Force on Practice Guidelines (ACC/AHA/SCAI Writing Committee to Update the 2001 Guidelines for Percutaneous Coronary Intervention). *Circulation* 113(1):156–175, 2006.
2. Ellis SG, Roubin GS, King SB III, et al: Importance of stenosis morphology in the estimation of restenosis risk after elective percutaneous transluminal coronary angioplasty. *Am J Cardiol* 63:30–34, 1989.
3. Madan P, Elayda MA, Lee VV, et al: Predicting major adverse cardiac events after percutaneous coronary intervention: the Texas Heart Institute risk score. *Am Heart J* 155(6):1068–1074, 2008.
4. Waksman R, Buch AN, Torguson R, et al: Long-term clinical outcomes and thrombosis rates of sirolimus-eluting stents versus paclitaxel-eluting stents in an unselected population with coronary artery disease (REWARDS registry). *Am J Cardiol* 100(1):45–51, 2007.
5. Krone R, Shaw R, Klein L, et al: Evaluation of the American College of Cardiology/American Heart Association and the Society for Coronary Angiography and Interventions lesion classification system in the current "stent era" of coronary interventions (from the ACC-National Cardiovascular Data Registry). *Am J Cardiol* 92(4):389–394, 2003.
6. Singh M, Rihal CS, Lennon RJ, et al: Comparison of Mayo Clinic risk score and American College of Cardiology/American Heart Association lesion classification in the prediction of adverse cardiovascular outcome following percutaneous coronary interventions. *J Am Coll Cardiol* 44:357–361, 2004.
7. Serruys PW, Morice MC, Kappetein AP, et al: Percutaneous coronary intervention versus coronary-artery bypass grafting for severe coronary artery disease. *N Engl J Med* 360(10):961–972, 2009.

8. Sianos G, Morel MA, Kappetein AP, et al: The SYNTAX Score: an angiographic tool grading the complexity of coronary artery disease. *EuroIntervention* 1(2):219–227, 2005.
9. Serruys PW, Onuma Y, Garg S, et al: Assessment of the SYNTAX score in the Syntax study. *EuroIntervention* 5(1):50–56, 2009.
10. Valgimigli M, Serruys PW, Tsuchida K, et al: Cyphering the complexity of coronary artery disease using the syntax score to predict clinical outcome in patients with three-vessel lumen obstruction undergoing percutaneous coronary intervention. *Am J Cardiol* 99(8):1072–1081, 2007.
11. Capodanno D, Capranzano P, Di Salvo ME, et al: Usefulness of SYNTAX score to select patients with left main coronary artery disease to be treated with coronary artery bypass graft. *J Am Coll Cardiol Cardiovasc Interent* 2(8):731–738, 2009.
12. Wykrzykowska JJ, Garg S, Girasis C, et al: Value of the SYNTAX score for risk assessment in the all-comers population of the randomized multicenter LEADERS (Limus Eluted from A Durable versus ERodable Stent coating) trial. *J Am Coll Cardiol* 56(4):272–277, 2010.
13. Holzhey DM, Luduena MM, Rastan A, et al: Is the SYNTAX score a predictor of long-term outcome after coronary artery bypass surgery? *Heart Surg Forum* 13(3):E143–E148, 2010.
14. Lemesle G, Bonello L, de Labriolle A, et al: Prognostic value of the Syntax score in patients undergoing coronary artery bypass grafting for three-vessel coronary artery disease. *Catheter Cardiovasc Intervent* 73(5):612–617, 2009.
15. Wijns W, Kolh P, Danchin N, et al: Guidelines on myocardial revascularization: the Task Force on Myocardial Revascularization of the European Society of Cardiology (ESC) and the European Association for Cardio-Thoracic Surgery (EACTS). *Eur Heart J* 31(20):2501–2555, 2010.
16. Feldman T: The SYNTAX score in practice: an aid for patient selection for complex PCI. *Catheter Cardiovasc Intervent* 73(5):618–619, 2009.

17. Garg S, Sarno G, Garcia-Garcia HM, et al: A new tool for the risk stratification of patients with complex coronary artery disease: the Clinical SYNTAX Score. *Circ Cardiovasc Intervent* (4):317–326, 2010.
18. Garg S, Girasis C, Sarno G, et al: The SYNTAX score revisited: a reassessment of the SYNTAX score reproducibility. *Catheter Cardiovasc Intervent* 75(6):946–952, 2010.
19. Singh M, Peterson ED, Milford-Beland S, et al: Validation of the Mayo clinic risk score for in hospital mortality after percutaneous coronary interventions using the national cardiovascular data registry. *Circ Cardiovasc Intervent* 1(1):36–44, 2008.
20. Singh M, Gersh BJ, Li S, et al: Mayo Clinic Risk Score for percutaneous coronary intervention predicts in-hospital mortality in patients undergoing coronary artery bypass graft surgery. *Circulation* 117(3):356–362, 2008.
21. Lev EI, Kornowski R, Vaknin-Assa H, et al: Comparison of the predictive value of four different risk scores for outcomes of patients with ST-elevation acute myocardial infarction undergoing primary percutaneous coronary intervention. *Am J Cardiol* 102(1):6–11, 2008.
22. Negassa A, Monrad ES, Srinivas VS: A simple prognostic classification model for postprocedural complications after percutaneous coronary intervention for acute myocardial infarction (from the New York State percutaneous coronary intervention database). *Am J Cardiol* 103(7):937–942, 2009.
23. Gilard M, Rioufol G, Zeller M, et al: Reliability and limitations of angiography in the diagnosis of coronary plaque rupture: an intravascular ultrasound study. *Arch Cardiovasc Dis* 101(2):114–120, 2008.
24. Mintz GS, Popma JJ, Pichard AD, et al: Patterns of calcification in coronary artery disease. A statistical analysis of intravascular ultrasound and coronary angiography in 1155 lesions. *Circulation* 91(7):1959–1965, 1995.
25. Vavuranakis M, Toutouzas K, Stefanadis C, et al: Stent deployment in calcified lesions: can we overcome calcific restraint with

high-pressure balloon inflations? *Catheter Cardiovasc Intervent* 52:164–172, 2001.

26. Kawaguchi R, Tsurugaya H, Hoshizaki H, et al: Impact of lesion calcification on clinical and angiographic outcome after sirolimus-eluting stent implantation in real-world patients. *Cardiovasc Revasc Med* 9(1):2–8, 2008.

27. Mutoh M, Ishikawa T, Hasuda T, et al: Predictors of target lesion revascularization and documented stent thrombosis beyond 30 days after sirolimus-eluting stent implantation: retrospective analysis in consecutive 1070 angiographic follow-up lesions. *Circ J* 71(8):1328–1331, 2007.

28. Moussa I, Ellis SG, Jones M, et al: Impact of coronary culprit lesion calcium in patients undergoing paclitaxel-eluting stent implantation (a TAXUS-IV sub study). *Am J Cardiol* 96:1242–11247, 2005.

29. Castagna MT, Mintz GS, Ohlmann P, et al: Incidence location magnitude and clinical correlates of saphenous vein graft calcification: an intravascular ultrasound and angiographic study. *Circulation* 111:1148–1152, 2005.

30. Machecourt J, Danchin N, Lablanche JM, et al: Risk factors for stent thrombosis after implantation of sirolimus-eluting stents in diabetic and nondiabetic patients: the EVASTENT Matched-Cohort Registry. *J Am Coll Cardiol* 50(6):501–508, 2007.

31. Alexander JH, Hafley G, Harrington RA, et al: Efficacy and safety of edifoligide an E2F transcription factor decoy for prevention of vein graft failure following coronary artery bypass graft surgery: PREVENT IV: a randomized controlled trial. *JAMA* 294:2446–2454, 2005.

32. Baim D, Wahr D, George B, et al: Randomized trial of a distal embolic protection device during percutaneous intervention of saphenous vein aorto-coronary bypass grafts. *Circulation* 105(11):1285–1290, 2002.

33. Stone GW, Rogers C, Hermiller J, et al: Randomized comparison of distal protection with a filter-based catheter and a balloon occlusion and aspiration system during percutaneous intervention of diseased saphenous vein aorto-coronary bypass grafts. *Circulation* 108:548–553, 2003.

34. Turco MA, Buchbinder M, Popma JJ, et al: Pivotal randomized U.S. study of the Symbiottrade mark covered stent system in patients with saphenous vein graft disease: eight-month angiographic and clinical results from the Symbiot III trial. *Catheter Cardiovasc Intervent* 68:379–388, 2006.

35. Giugliano GR, Kuntz RE, Popma JJ, et al: Determinants of 30-day adverse events following saphenous vein graft intervention with and without a distal occlusion embolic protection device. *Am J Cardiol* 95:173–177, 2005.

36. Sianos G, Papafaklis MI, Daemen J, et al: Angiographic stent thrombosis after routine use of drug-eluting stents in ST-segment elevation myocardial infarction: the importance of thrombus burden. *J Am Coll Cardiol* 50(7):573–583, 2007.

37. Ali A, Cox D, Dib N, et al: Rheolytic thrombectomy with percutaneous coronary intervention for infarct size reduction in acute myocardial infarction: 30-day results from a multicenter randomized study. *J Am Coll Cardiol* 48:244–252, 2006.

38. Aleong G, Vaqueriza D, Del Valle R, et al: Dual quantitative coronary angiography: a novel approach to quantify intracoronary thrombotic burden. *EuroIntervention* 4(4):475–480, 2009.

39. Tsagalou E, Stancovic G, Iakovou I, et al: Early outcome of treatment of ostial de novo left anterior descending coronary artery lesions with drug-eluting stents. *Am J Cardiol* 97:187–191, 2006.

40. Kini AS, Moreno PR, Steinheimer AM, et al: Effectiveness of the stent pull-back technique for nonaorto-ostial coronary narrowings. *Am J Cardiol* 96:1123–1128, 2005.

41. Popma JJ, Leon MB, Moses JW, et al: Quantitative assessment of angiographic restenosis after sirolimus-eluting stent implantation in native coronary arteries. *Circulation* 110:3773–3780, 2004.

42. Kereiakes DJ, Wang H, Popma JJ, et al: Periprocedural and late consequences of overlapping Cypher sirolimus-eluting stents: pooled analysis of five clinical trials. *J Am Coll Cardiol* 48:21–31, 2006.

43. Gobeil F, Lefevre T, Guyon P, et al: Stenting of bifurcation lesions using the Bestent: a prospective dual-center study. *Catheter Cardiovasc Intervent* 55:427–433, 2002.

44. Medina A, de Lezo J: A new classification of coronary bifurcation lesions. *Rev Esp Cardiol* 59(2):183–184, 2006.

45. Lefevre T, Louvard Y, Morice MC, et al: Stenting of bifurcation lesions: classification treatments and results. *Catheter Cardiovasc Intervent* 49:274–283, 2000.

46. Movahed MR: Quantitative angiographic methods for bifurcation lesions: a consensus statement from the European Bifurcation Group. Shortcoming of the Medina classification as a preferred classification for coronary artery bifurcation lesions in comparison to the Movahed classification. *Catheter Cardiovasc Intervent* 74(5):817–818, 2009.

47. van Werkum JW, Heestermans AA, Zomer AC, et al: Predictors of coronary stent thrombosis: the Dutch Stent Thrombosis Registry. *J Am Coll Cardiol* 53(16):1399–1409, 2009.

48. Iakovou I, Schmidt T, Bonizzoni E, et al: Incidence predictors and outcome of thrombosis after successful implantation of drug-eluting stents. *JAMA* 293:2126–2130, 2005.

49. Adriaenssens T, Byrne RA, Dibra A, et al: Culotte stenting technique in coronary bifurcation disease: angiographic follow-up using dedicated quantitative coronary angiographic analysis and 12-month clinical outcomes. *Eur Heart J* 29(23):2868–2876, 2008.

50. Columbo A, Moses JW, Morice MC, et al: Randomized study to evaluate sirolimus-eluting stents implanted at coronary bifurcation lesions. *Circulation* 109:1244–1249, 2004.

51. Ikeno F, Kim YH, Luna J, et al: Acute and long-term outcomes of the novel side access (SLK-View) stent for bifurcation coronary lesions: a multicenter nonrandomized feasibility study. *Catheter Cardiovasc Intervent* 67:198–206, 2006.

52. Ge L, Airoldi F, Iakovou I, et al: Clinical and angiographic outcome after implantation of drug-eluting stents in bifurcation lesions with the crush stent technique: importance of final kissing balloon post-dilation. *J Am Coll Cardiol* 46:613–620, 2005.

53. Onuma Y, Muller R, Ramcharitar S, et al: Tryton I First-In-Man (FIM) study: six month clinical and angiographic outcome analysis with new quantitative coronary angiography dedicated for bifurcation lesions. *EuroIntervention* 3(5):546–552, 2008.

54. Goktekin O, Kaplan S, Dimopoulos K, et al: A new quantitative analysis system for the evaluation of coronary bifurcation lesions: comparison with current conventional methods. *Catheter Cardiovasc Intervent* 69(2):172–180, 2007.

55. Christofferson RD, Lehmann KG, Martin GV, et al: Effect of chronic total coronary occlusion on treatment strategy. *Am J Cardiol* 95:1088–1091, 2005.

56. Stone GW, Kandzari DE, Mehran R, et al: Percutaneous recanalization of chronically occluded coronary arteries: a consensus document: part I. *Circulation* 112:2364–2372, 2005.

57. Stone GW, Reifart NJ, Moussa I, et al: Percutaneous recanalization of chronically occluded coronary arteries: a consensus document: part II. *Circulation* 112:2530–2537, 2005.

58. Baim DS, Braden G, Heuser R, et al: Utility of the Safe-Cross-guided radiofrequency total occlusion crossing system in chronic coronary total occlusions (results from the Guided Radio Frequency Energy Ablation of Total Occlusions Registry Study). *Am J Cardiol* 94:853–858, 2004.

59. Orlic D, Stankovic G, Sangiorgi G, et al: Preliminary experience with the Frontrunner coronary catheter: novel device dedicated to mechanical revascularization of chronic total occlusions. *Catheter Cardiovasc Intervent* 64:146–152, 2005.

60. Saito S, Tanaka S, Hiroe Y, et al: Angioplasty for chronic total occlusion by using tapered-tip guidewires. *Catheter Cardiovasc Intervent* 59:305–311, 2003.

61. Rahel BM, Laarman GJ, Suttorp MJ: Primary stenting of occluded native coronary arteries II—rationale and design of the PRISON II study: a randomized comparison of bare metal stent implantation with sirolimus-eluting stent implantation for the treatment of chronic total coronary occlusions. *Am Heart J* 149:e1–e3, 2005.

62. Suttorp MJ, Laarman GJ, Rahel BM, et al: Primary Stenting of Totally Occluded Native Coronary Arteries II (PRISON II): a randomized comparison of bare metal stent implantation with sirolimus-eluting stent implantation for the treatment of total coronary occlusions. *Circulation* 114:921–928, 2006.

63. Seiler C: The human coronary collateral circulation. *Heart (England)* 89:1352–1357, 2003.

64. Werner GS, Ferrari M, Heinke S, et al: Angiographic assessment of collateral connections in comparison with invasively determined collateral function in chronic coronary occlusions. *Circulation* 107:1972–1977, 2003.

65. Dvir D, Assali A, Kornowski R: Percutaneous coronary intervention for chronic total occlusion: novel 3-dimensional imaging and quantitative analysis. *Catheter Cardiovasc Intervent* 71(6):784–789, 2008.

66. Laskey WK, Williams DO, Vlachos HA, et al: Changes in the practice of percutaneous coronary intervention: a comparison of enrollment waves in the National Heart Lung and Blood Institute (NHLBI) Dynamic Registry. *Am J Cardiol* 87:964–969; A3–A4, 2001.

67. Nishida T, Colombo A, Briguori C, et al: Outcome of nonobstructive residual dissections detected by intravascular ultrasound following percutaneous coronary intervention. *Am J Cardiol* 89:1257–1262, 2002.

68. Resnic FS, Wainstein M, Lee MK, et al: No-reflow is an independent predictor of death and myocardial infarction after percutaneous coronary intervention. *Am Heart J* 145:42–46, 2003.

69. Yip HK, Chen MC, Chang HW, et al: Angiographic morphologic features of infarct-related arteries and timely reperfusion in acute myocardial infarction: predictors of slow-flow and no-reflow phenomenon. *Chest* 122:1322–1332, 2002.

70. Iijima R, Shinji H, Ikeda N, et al: Comparison of coronary arterial finding by intravascular ultrasound in patients with "transient no-reflow" versus "reflow" during percutaneous coronary intervention in acute coronary syndrome. *Am J Cardiol* 97:29–33, 2006.

71. Iwakura K, Ito H, Kawano S, et al: Predictive factors for development of the no-reflow phenomenon in patients with reperfused anterior wall acute myocardial infarction. *J Am Coll Cardiol* 38:472–477, 2001.

72. Tanaka A, Kawarabayashi T, Nishibori Y, et al: No-reflow phenomenon and lesion morphology in patients with acute myocardial infarction. *Circulation* 105:2148–2152, 2002.

73. Kotani J, Nanto S, Mintz GS, et al: Plaque gruel of atheromatous coronary lesion may contribute to the no-reflow phenomenon in patients with acute coronary syndrome. *Circulation* 106:1672–1677, 2002.

74. Hillegass WB, Dean NA, Liao L, et al: Treatment of no-reflow and impaired flow with the nitric oxide donor nitroprusside following percutaneous coronary interventions: initial human clinical experience. *J Am Coll Cardiol* 37:1335–1343, 2001.

75. Barcin C, Denktas AE, Lennon RJ, et al: Comparison of combination therapy of adenosine and nitroprusside with adenosine alone in the treatment of angiographic no-reflow phenomenon. *Catheter Cardiovasc Intervent* 61:484–491, 2004.

76. Michaels AD, Appleby M, Otten MH, et al: Pretreatment with intragraft verapamil prior to percutaneous coronary intervention of saphenous vein graft lesions: results of the randomized controlled vasodilator prevention on no-reflow (VAPOR) trial. *J Invas Cardiol* 14:299–302, 2002.

77. Huang RI, Patel P, Walinsky P, et al: Efficacy of intracoronary nicardipine in the treatment of no-reflow during percutaneous coronary intervention [In Process Citation]. *Catheter Cardiovasc Intervent* 68:671–676, 2006.

78. Ishizaka N, Issiki T, Saeki F, et al: Angiographic follow-up after successful percutaneous coronary angioplasty for chronic total coronary occlusion: experience in 110 consecutive patients. *Am Heart J* 127(1):p8–p12, 1994.

79. Fasseas P, Orford JL, Panetta CJ, et al: Incidence correlates management and clinical outcome of coronary perforation: analysis of 16298 procedures. *Am Heart J* 147:140–145, 2004.

80. Ellis SG, Ajluni S, Arnold AZ, et al: Increased coronary perforation in the new device era. Incidence, classification, management, and outcome. *Circulation* 90:2725–2730, 1994.

81. Klein LW: Coronary artery perforation during interventional procedures. *Catheter Cardiovasc Intervent* 68:713–717, 2006.

82. Javaid A, Buch AN, Satler LF, et al: Management and outcomes of coronary artery perforation during percutaneous coronary intervention. *Am J Cardiol* 98:911–914, 2006.

83. Stankovic G, Orlic D, Corvaja N, et al: Incidence predictors in-hospital and late outcomes of coronary artery perforations. *Am J Cardiol* 93:213–216, 2004.

84. Ly H, Awaida JP, Lesperance J, et al: Angiographic and clinical outcomes of polytetrafluoroethylene-covered stent use in significant coronary perforations. *Am J Cardiol* 95:244–246, 2005.

85. Gercken U, Lansky AJ, Buellesfeld L, et al: Results of the Jostent coronary stent graft implantation in various clinical settings: procedural and follow-up results. *Catheter Cardiovasc Intervent* 56:353–360, 2002.

86. Lansky AJ, Yang YM, Khan Y, et al: Treatment of coronary artery perforations complicating percutaneous coronary intervention with a polytetrafluoroethylene-covered stent graft. *Am J Cardiol* 98:370–374, 2006.

87. Suh WW, Grill DE, Rihal CS, et al: Unrestricted availability of intracoronary stents is associated with decreased abrupt vascular closure rates and improved early clinical outcomes. *Catheter Cardiovasc Intervent* 55:294–302, 2002.

88. Cutlip D, Baim D, Ho K, et al: Stent thrombosis in the modern era: a pooled analysis of multicenter coronary stent clinical trials. *Circulation* 103(15):1967–1971, 2001.

89. Urban P, Gershlick AH, Guagliumi G, et al: Safety of coronary sirolimus-eluting stents in daily clinical practice: one-year follow-up of the e-Cypher registry. *Circulation* 113:1434–1441, 2006.

90. Moreno R, Fernandez C, Hernandez R, et al: Drug-eluting stent thrombosis: results from a pooled analysis including 10 randomized studies. *J Am Coll Cardiol* 45:954–959, 2005.

91. Park DW, Park SW, Park KH, et al: Frequency of and risk factors for stent thrombosis after drug-eluting stent implantation during long-term follow-up. *Am J Cardiol* 98:352–356, 2006.

92. Kuchulakanti PK, Chu WW, Torguson R, et al: Correlates and long-term outcomes of angiographically proven stent thrombosis with sirolimus- and paclitaxel-eluting stents. *Circulation* 113:1108–1113, 2006.

93. Ong AT, McFadden EP, Regar E, et al: Late angiographic stent thrombosis (LAST) events with drug-eluting stents. *J Am Coll Cardiol* 45:2088–2092, 2005.

94. Virmani R, Guagliumi G, Farb A, et al: Localized hypersensitivity and late coronary thrombosis secondary to a sirolimus-eluting stent: should we be cautious? *Circulation* 109:701–705, 2004.

95. Joner M, Finn AV, Farb A, et al: Pathology of drug-eluting stents in humans: delayed healing and late thrombotic risk. *J Am Coll Cardiol* 48:193–202, 2006.

96. Cutlip DE, Windecker S, Mehran R, et al: Clinical end points in coronary stent trials: a case for standardized definitions. *Circulation* 115(17):2344–2351, 2007.

97. Mehran R, Dangas G, Abizaid A, et al: Angiographic patterns of in-stent restenosis. Classification and implications for long-term outcome. *Circulation* 100:1872–1878, 1999.

98. Alfonso F, Cequier A, Angel J, et al: Value of the American College of Cardiology/American Heart Association angiographic classification of coronary lesion morphology in patients with in-stent restenosis. Insights from the Restenosis Intra-stent Balloon angioplasty versus elective Stenting (RIBS) randomized trial. *Am Heart J* 151(3):681–689, 2006.

99. Colombo A, Orlic D, Stankovic G, et al: Preliminary observations regarding angiographic pattern of restenosis after rapamycin-eluting stent implantation. *Circulation* 107(17):2178–2180, 2003.

100. Lemos PA, Saia F, Ligthart JM, et al: Coronary restenosis after sirolimus-eluting stent implantation: morphological description

and mechanistic analysis from a consecutive series of cases. *Circulation* 108:257–260, 2003.

101. Stabile E, Escolar E, Weigold G, et al: Marked malapposition and aneurysm formation after sirolimus-eluting coronary stent implantation. *Circulation* 110:e47–e48, 2004.

102. Gupta RK, Sapra R, Kaul U: Early aneurysm formation after drug-eluting stent implantation: an unusual life-threatening complication. *J Invas Cardiol* 18:E140–E142, 2006.

103. Alfonso F, Moreno R, Vergas J: Mycotic aneurysms after sirolimus-eluting coronary stenting. *Catheter Cardiovasc Intervent* 67:327–328, 2006.

104. Singh H, Singh C, Aggarwal N, et al: Mycotic aneurysm of left anterior descending artery after sirolimus-eluting stent implantation: a case report. *Catheter Cardiovasc Intervent* 65:282–285, 2005.

105. Group TS: The Thrombolysis in Myocardial Infarction (TIMI) trial. Phase I Findings. *N Engl J Med* 312:932–936, 1985.

106. Gibson CM, Cannon CP, Daley WL, et al: TIMI frame count: a quantitative method of assessing coronary artery flow. *Circulation* 93(5):879–888, 1996.

107. Gibson C, Cannon C, Murphy S, et al: Relationship of TIMI myocardial perfusion grade to mortality following thrombolytic administration. *Circulation* 101:125–130, 2000.

108. The GUSTO Angiographic Investigators: The effects of tissue plasminogen activator streptokinase or both on coronary artery patency ventricular function and survival after acute myocardial infarction. *N Engl J Med* 329:1615–1622, 1993.

109. Gibson C, Ryan K, Murphy S, et al: Impaired coronary blood flow in non-culprit arteries in the setting of acute myocardial infarction. *J Am Coll Cardiol* 34:974–982, 1999.

110. Stone GW, Brodie BR, Griffin JJ, et al: Prospective multicenter study of the safety and feasibility of primary stenting in acute myocardial infarction: in-hospital and 30-day results of the PAMI stent pilot trial. Primary Angioplasty in Myocardial Infarction Stent Pilot Trial Investigators. *J Am Coll Cardiol* 31(1):p23–p30, 1998.

111. Gibson CM, Cannon CP, Murphy SA, et al: Relationship of the TIMI myocardial perfusion grades flow grades frame count and percutaneous coronary intervention to long-term outcomes after thrombolytic administration in acute myocardial infarction. *Circulation* 105:1909–1913, 2002.

112. Gibson CM, Dodge JT, Goel M, et al: Angioplasty guidewire velocity: a new simple method to calculate absolute coronary blood velocity and flow. *Am J Cardiol* 80:1536–1539, 1997.

113. Fischer JJ, Samady H, McPherson JA, et al: Comparison between visual assessment and quantitative angiography versus fractional flow reserve for native coronary narrowings of moderate severity. *Am J Cardiol* 90:210–215, 2002.

114. Fleming RM, Kirkeeide RL, Smalling RW, et al: Patterns in visual interpretation of coronary arteriograms as detected by quantitative coronary arteriography. *J Am Coll Cardiol* 18(4):945–951, 1991.

115. Garrone P, Biondi-Zoccai G, et al: Quantitative coronary angiography in the current era: principles and applications. *J Intervent Cardiol* 22(6):527–536, 2009.

116. Garcia JA, Movassaghi B, Casserly IP, et al: Determination of optimal viewing regions for x-ray coronary angiography based on a quantitative analysis of 3D reconstructed models. *Int J Cardiovasc Imaging* 25(5):455–462, 2009.

117. Tuinenburg JC, Koning G, Hekking E, et al: American College of Cardiology/European Society of Cardiology International Study of Angiographic Data Compression Phase II: the effects of varying JPEG data compression levels on the quantitative assessment of the degree of stenosis in digital coronary angiography. Joint Photographic Experts Group. *J Am Coll Cardiol* 35:1380–1387, 2000.

118. Tuinenburg JC, Koning G, Seppenwoolde Y, et al: Is there an effect of flat-panel-based imaging systems on quantitative coronary and vascular angiography? *Catheter Cardiovasc Intervent* 68:561–566, 2006.

119. Herrington DM, Siebes M, Sokol DK, et al: Variability in measures of coronary lumen dimensions using quantitative coronary angiography. *J Am Coll Cardiol* 22(4):1068–1074, 1993.

120. Steigen TK, Claudio C, Abbott D, et al: Angiographic core laboratory reproducibility analyses: implications for planning clinical trials using coronary angiography and left ventriculography end-points. *Int J Cardiovasc Imaging* 24(5):453–462, 2008.

121. Ballantyne CM, Raichlen JS, Nicholls SJ, et al: Effect of rosuvastatin therapy on coronary artery stenoses assessed by quantitative coronary angiography: a study to evaluate the effect of rosuvastatin on intravascular ultrasound-derived coronary atheroma burden. *Circulation* 117(19):2458–2466, 2008;

122. Peterson ED, Lansky AJ, Anstrom KJ, et al: Evolving trends in interventional device use and outcomes: results from the National Cardiovascular Network Database. *Am Heart J* 139:198–207, 2000.

123. Tsuchida K, Garcia-Garcia HM, Ong AT, et al: Revisiting late loss and neointimal volumetric measurements in a drug-eluting stent trial: analysis from the SPIRIT FIRST trial. *Catheter Cardiovasc Intervent* 67:188–197, 2006.

124. Semeraro O, Agostoni P, Verheye S, et al: Re-examining minimal luminal diameter relocation and quantitative coronary angiography—intravascular ultrasound correlations in stented saphenous vein grafts: methodological insights from the randomised RRISC trial. *EuroIntervention* 4(5):633–640, 2009.

125. Mauri L, Orav EJ, O'Malley AJ, et al: Relationship of late loss in lumen diameter to coronary restenosis in sirolimus-eluting stents. *Circulation* 111:321–327, 2005.

126. Lemos PA, Mercado N, van Domburg RT, et al: Comparison of late luminal loss response pattern after sirolimus-eluting stent implantation or conventional stenting. *Circulation* 110:3199–3205, 2004.

127. Ellis SG, Popma JJ, Lasala JM, et al: Relationship between angiographic late loss and target lesion revascularization after coronary stent implantation: analysis from the TAXUS-IV trial. *J Am Coll Cardiol* 45:1193–1200, 2005.

128. Agostoni P, Valgimigli M, Abbate A, et al: Is late luminal loss an accurate predictor of the clinical effectiveness of drug-eluting stents in the coronary arteries? *Am J Cardiol* 97:603–605, 2006.

129. Pocock S, Lansky A, Mehran R, et al: Angiographic surrogate endpoints in drug-eluting stent trials: a systematic evaluation based on individual patient data from eleven randomized controlled trials. *J Am Coll Cardiol* 51:22–32, 2008.

130. Mauri L, Orav EJ, Candia SC, et al: Robustness of late lumen loss in discriminating drug-eluting stents across variable observational and randomized trials. *Circulation* 112:2833–2839, 2005.

131. Ramcharitar S, Daeman J, Patterson M, et al: First direct in vivo comparison of two commercially available three-dimensional quantitative coronary angiography systems. *Catheter Cardiovasc Intervent* 71(1):44–50, 2008.

132. Lansky AJ, Dangas G, Mehran R, et al: Quantitative angiographic methods for appropriate end-point analysis edge-effect evaluation and prediction of recurrent restenosis after coronary brachytherapy with gamma irradiation. *J Am Coll Cardiol* 39:274–280, 2002.

Intracoronary Pressure and Flow Measurement

MORTON J. KERN | MICHAEL J. LIM

KEY POINTS

- The physiologic consequences of a given coronary stenosis and its potential to produce myocardial ischemia are not always apparent from angiographic assessment alone. Intermediately severe stenoses can be assessed easily and reliably by sensor guidewire measurements in the catheterization laboratory (cath lab) facilitating appropriate clinical decision making.

- Fractional flow reserve (FFR) has been proven to be an accurate predictor of myocardial ischemia compared with noninvasive stress testing.

- Selective percutaneous coronary intervention (PCI) of only those lesions that are physiologically significant, as shown by FFR, has been prospectively demonstrated to be superior over angiographically guided PCI in patients with multi-vessel coronary artery disease (CAD).

- FFR is useful in that it can guide decision making within the cath lab with regard to common angiographic dilemmas, including side branch stenoses, left main coronary artery (LMCA) disease, or multi-vessel disease.

The goal of PCI is the relief of ischemia and restoration of coronary blood flow. The treatment of coronary stenosis with stenting improves exercise tolerance, reduces anti-ischemic medications, and improves survival in patients with ST elevation myocardial infarction (STEMI). However, stent placement is of no benefit to patients if the angiographic stenoses are not responsible for ischemia. It is common knowledge that the angiogram is limited in identifying flow-limiting stenoses because of the display of three-dimensional structures in only two dimensions.

It is of historical interest that Andreas Grüntzig understood this problem from the very first percutaneous transluminal coronary angioplasty (PTCA) performed in 1977. Because of the poor quality of angiography, he developed and used a 4 French (F) balloon dilation catheter with a double lumen, one for balloon inflation and one for distal lesion pressure recordings. The procedure was guided by a reduction in the trans-stenotic pressure gradient. With improvements in angiography and PCI equipment, especially drug-eluting stents (DESs) over the last three decades, many interventional cardiologists believe that angiographic information alone is sufficient for decision making regarding patient care and that lesion assessment by pressure and flow recordings can be reserved for research purposes. This erroneous "conventional wisdom" is no longer supported by substantial multi-center long-term clinical outcome studies of the benefits of physiologic lesion assessment. The rationale for physiologic lesion assessment is simple. The angiogram cannot be relied on exclusively to direct coronary revascularization.[1] Angiography cannot fully characterize the clinical or hemodynamic significance of many coronary stenoses. This fact is well recognized and documented repeatedly by intravascular ultrasound (IVUS) imaging, computed tomography angiography (CTA), and the ubiquitous necessity for stress testing to clarify lesions seen on coronary angiography. Moreover, even sophisticated imaging modalities such as densitometry, rotational angiography, and CTA with three-dimensional reconstruction do not reliably reflect the physiologic significance of a given lesion (Fig. 57-1).[2]

Coronary angiography produces two-dimensional luminograms, a silhouette image of the three-dimensional vascular lumen. It does not truly identify atherosclerosis, a disease within the vessel wall, but merely provides a "shadow" without any intraluminal details sufficient to characterize a plaque. The eccentric shapes of plaques do not permit the observer to determine whether such an opening is limiting coronary blood flow. The accurate identification of both "normal" and "diseased" vessel segments by angiography further complicates the determination of a lesion's significance in the setting of diffuse CAD, which cannot easily be seen on an angiogram. Angiographic artifacts, including contrast streaming, branch overlap, vessel foreshortening, calcifications, and ostial origins, further make the interpretation of some luminal narrowings unreliable. Despite numerous attempts to improve the angiographic imaging of complex anatomy, the angiographer is still confronted by a visual dilemma, in which no single view or multiple views can provide an answer. Hence, the use of the physiology to assess the coronary stenosis is required, either out of the cath lab via stress testing or by coronary pressure measurement.

Fundamental Concepts of Coronary Blood Flow

Coronary blood flow can increase from a resting level to a maximum, depending on increases in myocardial oxygen demand or in response to neurogenic or pharmacologic hyperemic stimuli. Normally, large epicardial vessel resistance to blood flow is trivial. Most of the regulation of coronary flow is by the myocardial precapillary arteriolar resistance vessels. In a normal adult artery supplying normal myocardium, coronary blood flow can increase more than threefold. However, several conditions, including left ventricular hypertrophy, myocardial ischemia, and diabetes, can affect the microcirculation, blunting the maximal absolute increase in coronary flow or increasing resting flow above the expected level for myocardial oxygen demand at rest. The regulation of coronary vasomotor tone and the influence of several mechanisms such as α-adrenoreceptor–mediated vasoconstriction have been extensively reviewed elsewhere and are beyond the scope of this chapter.[3] A significant atherosclerotic stenosis produces epicardial conduit resistance. In response to the loss of perfusion pressure and flow to the distal (poststenotic) vascular bed, the small resistance vessels dilate to maintain satisfactory basal flow appropriate for myocardial oxygen demand. Viscous friction, flow separation forces, and flow turbulence at the site of the stenosis produce energy loss at the stenosis (Fig. 57-2). Energy (heat) is extracted, reducing pressure distal to the stenosis, thereby producing a pressure gradient between the proximal and distal artery regions. The pressure loss or gradient increases with increasing coronary flow.[4] There exists an absolute poststenotic myocardial perfusion pressure threshold, below which myocardial ischemia may be easily induced.

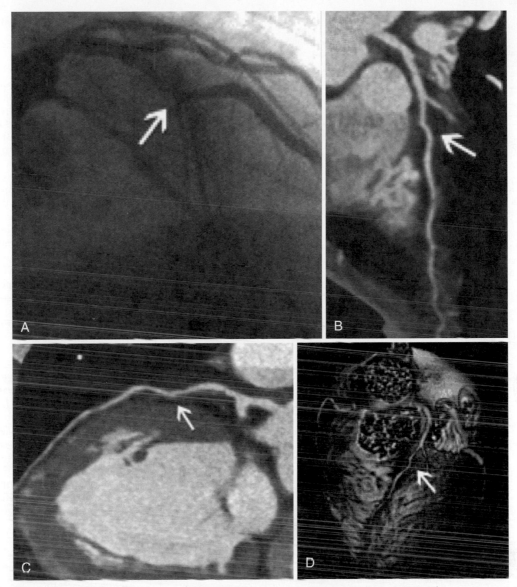

Figure 57-1 Multiple modality imaging of an intermediate coronary artery stenosis. **A,** Invasive angiographic assessment of a mid-LAD artery lesion visually appearing less than 50% in severity. **B and C,** Orthogonal curved multi-planar CT angiographic images depicting the same LAD lesion. **D,** Volume-rendered reconstructed CT angiographic image showing the same LAD lesion. Despite multiple projections and modalities, these images demonstrate the lack of ability of anatomic assessment to determine the LAD lesion's ability to produce anterior wall ischemia. *LAD,* left anterior descending; *CT,* computed tomography. (*From Meijboom WB, Van Mieghem CAG, van Pelt N, et al: Comprehensive assessment of coronary artery stenoses: Computed tomography coronary angiography versus conventional coronary angiography and correlation with fractional flow reserve in patients with stable angina, J Am Coll Cardiol 52:636–643, 2008.*)

CORONARY FLOW AND FLOW RESERVE

As the severity of stenosis increases, maximal coronary flow becomes attenuated, and coronary flow reserve (CFR) decreases. CFR is a combined measure of the capacity of the major resistance components (the epicardial coronary artery and the supplied vascular bed) to achieve maximal blood flow in response to hyperemic stimulation. A normal CFR implies that both epicardial and microvascular bed resistances are low (normal) (Fig. 57-3). However, if they are abnormal, CFR does not indicate which component is affected, a fact that limits the clinical applicability of this measurement. Although early studies in animals and humans indicated an absolute normal value for CFR of 3.5 to 5, the CFR in adult patients with chest pain syndromes and CAD risk factors undergoing cardiac catheterization with angiographically normal vessels was 2.7 ± 0.6, suggesting a degree of patient variability and microvascular disease. In patients with essential hypertension and normal coronary arteries and in those with aortic stenosis and normal coronary arteries, CFR may be reduced, in part related to myocardial hypertrophy and an abnormal microvasculature. Furthermore, CFR can be altered by changes in basal and hyperemic flows, which are influenced by hemodynamics, loading conditions, and contractility. For example, tachycardia increases basal flow and decreases hyperemic flow, thus reducing CFR by 10% for each 15-beat increase in heart rate. In clinical terms, CFR is best used to assess the microcirculation in the absence of epicardial artery narrowings. CFR should not be used to assess stenosis significance because of the influence of hemodynamics and the unknown impact of the microcirculation.

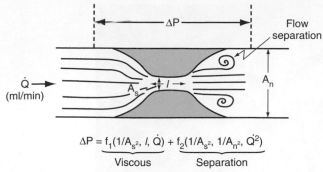

$$\Delta P = \underbrace{f_1(1/A_s{}^2,\, l,\, \dot{Q})}_{\text{Viscous}} + \underbrace{f_2(1/A_s{}^2,\, 1/A_n{}^2,\, \dot{Q}^2)}_{\text{Separation}}$$

Figure 57-2 Total pressure loss across a stenosis is derived from two sources: (1) frictional losses along the leading edge of the stenosis and (2) inertial losses stemming from the sudden expansion, which causes flow separation and eddies (exit losses). Frictional losses are linearly related to flow, $\dot{Q}$, by the law of Poiseuille, and exit losses increase with the square of the flow (law of Bernoulli). The total change in pressure gradient (ΔP) is the sum of the two: $\Delta P = f1 \times \dot{Q} + f2 \times \dot{Q}2$. The loss coefficients, $f1$ and $f2$, are functions of stenosis geometry and rheologic properties of blood (viscosity and density). The graphic representation of this equation results in a quadratic relationship, in which the curvilinear shape demonstrates the presence of nonlinear exit losses. If no stenosis is present, the second term is zero, and the curve becomes a straight line (with a positive slope that depends on the diameter of the vessel, based on the law of Poiseuille). A_n, area of the normal segment; A_s, area of the stenosis; L, length. (*Redrawn from Kern MJ: Coronary physiology revisited: Practical insights from the cardiac catheterization laboratory,* Circulation 101:1344–1351, 2000.)

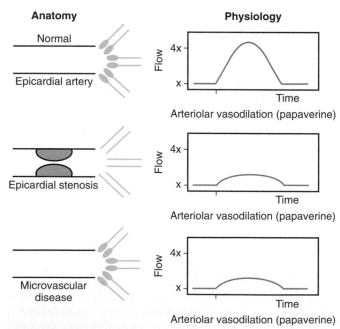

Figure 57-3 Schematic representation of coronary flow reserve findings. *Top panel,* A normal artery without any epicardial stenosis or microvascular disease demonstrates the ability to significantly increase coronary flow when a hyperemic agent is given. *Middle panel,* An artery with a significant epicardial stenosis that blunts the ability to increase flow over baseline. *Bottom panel,* The same finding of an artery unable to increase its flow rate. However, the reason in this case is not epicardial stenosis but severe microvascular disease. (*Redrawn from Wilson RF, Lascon DD: A clinician's guide to assessing the physiologic significance of arterial stenoses,* Cathet Cardiovasc Diagn 29:93–98, 1993.)

INTRACORONARY PRESSURE MEASUREMENTS AND FRACTIONAL FLOW RESERVE

As the limitations of invasive CFR were recognized, the development of pressure sensor guidewires yielded a new concept of lesion assessment. Pressure measurements, which were made across a lesion during maximal hyperemia, termed the *myocardial fractional flow reserve (FFRmyo),* were introduced.[5] When blood flows from the proximal to the distal part of the normal epicardial coronary artery, virtually no energy is lost; therefore, the pressure remains constant throughout the conduit. In the case of epicardial coronary narrowing, potential energy is transformed into kinetic energy and heat when blood traverses the lesion. The energy loss results in a pressure drop, which reflects the total loss of energy. To maintain resting myocardial perfusion at a constant level, a decrease in myocardial resistance compensates for any resistance of flow caused by the epicardial narrowing. The decrease in myocardial resistance reserve is proportional to the resistance that can be computed from the pressure gradient–flow relation; therefore, the pressure at constant maximal flow can represent an index of the physiologic consequences of a given coronary narrowing on the myocardium. The maximal myocardial blood flow in the presence of a stenosis is reduced relative to expected normal flow in the absence of a stenosis and can be expressed as a fraction of its normal expected value if there were no lesion. This value can be derived from pressure data alone for the myocardium (FFRmyo), the epicardial coronary artery (FFRcor), and the collateral supply (FFRcoll), based on several assumptions regarding trans-lesional pressure measured during maximal hyperemia.[5,6] The proposed equations have been derived from a theoretical model of the coronary circulation and have been validated experimentally in instrumented dogs, and later in humans, by comparison with myocardial flow measured by positron emission tomography (PET).[7] During maximal hyperemia (pharmacologic challenge with papaverine or adenosine), coronary resistance is at the lowest level and remains constant, so that flow is directly related to the measured pressure gradient. The total myocardial blood flow (Qn) in an area served by a coronary artery with a stenosis is the sum of the flow through the stenosis (QS) and the collateral flow (QC). FFRmyo is defined as the ratio of the measured flow (Qs) to the maximal flow that should be present without any stenosis (QN):

$$Qs = (Pd - Pv)/Rd$$

and

$$Qn = (Pa - Pv)/Ra$$

In practice, *Pv* is considered negligible relative to *Pa*, and hence:

$$FFR = Qs \div Qn = (Pd \div Rd) \div (Pa \div Ra)$$

where *Pa* = mean arterial pressure; *Pv* = mean venous pressure; *Pd* = mean pressure distal to the stenosis; and *R* = resistance of the myocardial vascular bed. Because this resistance is assumed to be constant and minimal at maximal hyperemia, *Rd* = *Ra*, and is canceled from the above equation.

FFRmyo can thus be estimated as the ratio of the mean distal coronary blood pressure (using ultra-thin pressure transducers) to the mean aortic blood pressure (measured by the guiding catheter). Because each myocardial territory serves as its own control, FFR is a lesion-specific index. Furthermore, it is independent of microcirculation, heart rate, blood pressure, and other hemodynamic variables and can be applied in multi-vessel disease.

FFRcoll and FFRcor are calculated with similar equations:

$$FFRcor = 1 - \Delta P/(Pa - Pw)$$

$$FFRcoll = FFRmyo - FFRcor$$

where *Pw* = the coronary wedge pressure measured distally when the PTCA balloon is inflated in the artery.

Unlike most other physiologic indexes, FFR has a normal value of 1.0 for every patient and every coronary artery. FFR has high

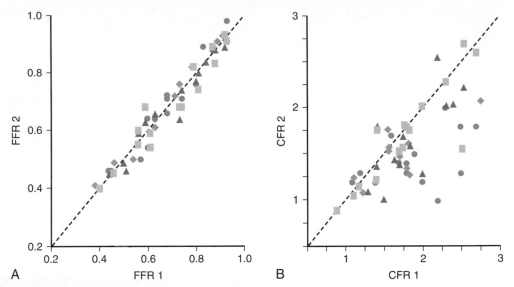

Figure 57-4 **A,** Reproducibility of fractional flow reserve (FFR) by serial measurements in a multi-center study of 325 patients in whom FFR was measured twice within a 10-minute interval. **B,** Reproducibility of coronary flow reserve (CFR) in the same patients. Blue boxes represent baseline conditions. Violet diamonds represent changes in blood pressure induced by infusion of nitroprusside. Blue triangles represent changes in heart rate induced by pacing. Pink circles represent changes in contractility induced by infusion of dobutamine. Despite variations in heart rate of 40%, blood pressure of 35%, and contractility of 50%, FFR but not CFR was unaffected by these changes. *(Data from De Bruyne B, Bartunek J, Sys SU, et al: Simultaneous coronary pressure and flow velocity measurements in humans: Feasibility, reproducibility and hemodynamic dependence of coronary flow velocity reserve, hyperemic flow versus pressure slope index and fractional flow reserve, Circulation 94:1842–1849, 1996.)*

reproducibility and low intra-individual variability (Fig. 57-4). Moreover, FFR, unlike CFR, is independent of gender or CAD risk factors such as hypertension and diabetes and has less variability with common doses of adenosine. De Bruyne and associates demonstrated that in humans, FFRmyo is independent of hemodynamic conditions. Changes in heart rate affected by pacing, in contractility by dobutamine infusion, and in blood pressure by nitroprusside infusion did not alter FFRmyo.[8] The coefficient of variation between two consecutive measurements was 4.2%, lower than the 17.7% for CFR measured with a Doppler wire.

Methodology of Coronary Pressure Measurement

GENERAL SETUP AND GUIDEWIRE MANIPULATION

The measurement of coronary pressure is similar to performing an angioplasty in that a sensor guidewire is passed through an angioplasty Y-connector attached to a guiding catheter, with anticoagulation (intravenous [IV] heparin) given beforehand. To minimize measurement variability caused by vessel spasm, intracoronary (IC) nitroglycerin (100 to 200 mcg) is given before the guidewire is advanced into the artery. For coronary pressure measurements, two pressure wire systems are available at this time: (1) the PressureWire (St. Jude Medical Inc., Minneapolis, MN) and (2) the PrimeWire (Volcano Therapeutics, Rancho Cardova, CA). Both can be used as angioplasty guidewires with mechanical properties close to standard "workhorse" guidewires. For both wires, a pressure sensor is located 3 cm from the tip, at the junction of the radiopaque and radiolucent portions of the wire, and the tip can be shaped to facilitate delivery to the distal vessel (Fig. 57-5). Before inserting the guidewire into the patient, the sensor-wire and guiding-catheter pressure signals are calibrated and set at zero. The sensor wire is then introduced and positioned at the tip of the guiding catheter, where the guiding catheter and wire pressures are equalized (assuming an accurate baseline before advancing down the artery). Next, the wire is advanced down the vessel and across the stenosis or to the most distal part of the coronary artery for assessment of serial lesions or diffuse disease. A pharmacologic hyperemic stimulus (e.g., adenosine, see below) is then administered through the guiding

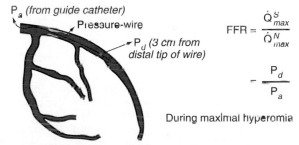

$$FFR = \frac{\dot{Q}^S_{max}}{\dot{Q}^N_{max}}$$

$$= \frac{P_d}{P_a}$$

During maximal hyperemia

Figure 57-5 Schematic representation showing how to measure fractional flow reserve (FFR) to assess the significance of stenosis of a proximal left anterior descending coronary artery. The proximal pressure (P_a) is the mean pressure taken from the guiding catheter during maximal hyperemia. The distal pressure (P_d) is measured by the guide wire sensor placed distal to the stenosis. FFR is calculated as P_d divided by P_a. $\dot{Q}^N_{max}$, maximal flow of normal vessel, $\dot{Q}^S_{max}$, maximal flow of stenotic vessel.

catheter or can be given by IV infusion. The mean and phasic pressure signals are continuously recorded, and at peak hyperemia (represented by the nadir, or lowest, distal pressure), the FFR is calculated as the ratio between the mean distal coronary pressure (measured by the pressure wire) and the mean aortic pressure (measured by the guiding catheter):

$$FFR = Pd \div Pa$$

To study the distribution of abnormalities along a diseased coronary artery (with serial lesions or diffuse disease), the pressure wire can be pulled back slowly during intravenously induced hyperemia. Simultaneously, observing the location of the wire and the pressure tracings indicates the location of hemodynamically significant atherosclerotic abnormalities. On pulling back the pressure wire, one can observe gradual pressure recovery because of diffuse atherosclerosis compared with a focal stenosis that is associated with an abrupt increase in pressure proximal to the lesion. By moving the sensor back and forth, the exact location of a pressure drop representing a focal obstruction to

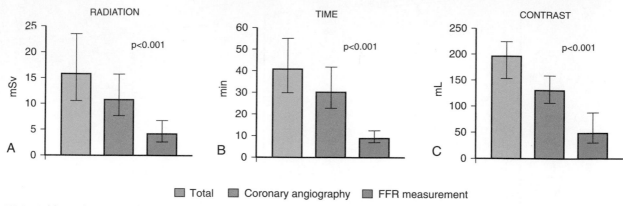

Figure 57-6 Additional amount of radiation, contrast, and procedure time to perform coronary angiography and fractional flow reserve (FFR) measurements. As can be seen in all three graphs, FFR measurement is associated with a small incremental increase in each variable. *(From Ntalianis A, Trana C, Muller O, et al: Effective radiation dose, time, and contrast medium to measure fractional flow reserve, J Am Coll Cardiol Interv 3:821–827.)*

TABLE 57-1	Pharmacologic Characteristics of Agents Used for Induction of Hyperemia				
Drug	*Dose*	*Plateau (seconds)*	*Half-life (minutes)*	*Side Effects*	*Comments*
Papaverine IC	15 mg LCA 10 mg RCA	30–60	2	Transient Q–T interval prolongation Torsades de pointes	
Adenosine IV	140 mcg/kg/min	60–120	1–2	Decreased blood pressure (10%–15%) chest burning	Avoid in patients with history of bronchospasm
Adenosine IC	>40 mcg LCA 24–36 mcg RCA	5–10	0.5–1	Transient AV block when injected into the dominant artery	Must repeat with escalating doses to ensure that maximal hyperemia is reached
Dobutamine IV	20–40 mcg/kg/min	60–120	3–5	Tachycardia, increase in blood pressure	
Nitroprusside IC	0.3–0.9 mcg/kg	20	1	Decreased blood pressure (20%)	

AV, atrioventricular; *IC*, intracoronary; *IV*, intravenous; *LCA*, left coronary artery; *RCA*, right coronary artery.

flow can be determined. After pressures are measured, the interface coupler can be disconnected and the pressure wire can be used as a "workhorse" guidewire to advance balloons or to deliver a stent. FFR is often measured using 6F guiding catheters but diagnostic catheters as small as 4F have been used. At the end of the procedure, the wire is withdrawn, and the guidewire pressure is verified in comparison with the guiding catheter pressure, thus ensuring that no pressure signal drift has occurred. A more complete description of the application and pitfalls of coronary pressure measurements can be found elsewhere.[9]

SAFETY OF INTRACORONARY SENSOR WIRE MEASUREMENTS

Qian and coworkers examined the safety of IC Doppler wire measurements in 906 patients.[10] Fifteen patients (1.7%) had severe transient bradycardia after administration of IC adenosine (14 in the right coronary artery [RCA] and 1 in the left coronary artery [LCA]). Nine patients (1%) had coronary spasm during passage of the Doppler guidewire (5 in the RCA and four in the left anterior descending [LAD] coronary artery). Two patients (0.2%) had ventricular fibrillation (VF) during the procedure. Hypotension with bradycardia and ventricular asystole occurred in one patient. Transplant recipients had more of these complications than did patients undergoing either diagnostic or interventional procedures. All complications were managed medically without long-term adverse consequences. These data support the safe clinical practice of sensor wire measurements with IC adenosine.

RADIATION, PROCEDURE TIME, CONTRAST USE FOR FRACTIONAL FLOW RESERVE

Performing FFR may increase the amounts of radiation dose, procedural time, and contrast medium after a diagnostic coronary angiogram. Ntalianis et al measured the amounts of radiation dose (mSv),

procedural time (min), and contrast medium (mL) in 200 patients (mean age 66 ± 10 years) undergoing diagnostic coronary angiography with FFR measured in at least one intermediate coronary artery stenosis.[11] In all, 296 stenoses (1.5 ± 0.7 stenoses per patient) were assessed after hyperemia was achieved by IC (n = 180) or IV (n = 20) adenosine. The additional amounts of mean radiation dose, procedural time, and contrast medium needed to obtain FFR as a percentage of the entire procedure were 30 ± 16% (median 4 mSv, range 2.4–6.7 mSv), 26 ± 13% (median 9 minutes, range 7–13 min), and 31 ± 16% (median 50 mL, range 30–90 mL), respectively. The additional procedural time was slightly longer with IV adenosine compared with IC adenosine (median 11 minutes vs. 9 minutes, P = 0.04), but there was no difference between IV and IC adenosine for radiation or contrast dosages (Fig. 57-6). There was no difference between IV and IC adenosine when FFR in radiation dose, procedural time, or contrast medium was measured in three or more lesions. The minimal increases in the amounts of radiation dose, procedural time, and contrast medium were low compared with IVUS or angioscopy. The clinical value of FFR measurements is worth the small additional amounts of radiation and procedure time involved.

PHARMACOLOGIC HYPEREMIC STIMULI

Maximal coronary hyperemia is required for in-lab coronary physiologic lesion assessment (Table 57-1). The most widely used maximal vasodilator agents are adenosine, adenosine triphosphate (ATP), and papaverine. Hyperosmolar ionic and low-osmolar nonionic contrast media do not produce maximal vasodilation. Nitrates increase volumetric flow, but because these agents also dilate the epicardial conductance vessels, the increase in coronary flow velocity is less than with adenosine or papaverine. IC nitroprusside has similar hyperemic effects compared with IC adenosine. Papaverine is no longer used for

IC hyperemic stimulation because of the occasional Q–T interval prolongation and associated ventricular tachycardia (VT) or VF.

Adenosine

Both IC adenosine and IV adenosine are the most commonly used hyperemic agents. Adenosine has a short half-life with a return to basal flow within 30 to 60 seconds after cessation of infusion. Adenosine is benign in appropriate dosages (20–30 mcg in the RCA or 40–60 mcg in the LCA, or infused IV at 140 mcg/kg/minute), although many have reported the use of much higher dosages with no adverse effects. Rarely, transient atrioventricular (AV) block and bradycardia may occur. IV administration tends to have a higher incidence of flushing, chest tightness, and AV block compared with IC dosing. Jeremias and colleagues examined differences in FFR between IC adenosine (15–20 mcg in the RCA or 18–24 mcg in the LCA) and IV adenosine (140 mcg/kg/minute) in 52 patients with 60 lesions.[12] There was a strong and linear relationship between IC and IV adenosine ($r = 0.978$ and $P < 0.001$). The mean measurement difference for FFR was 0.004 ± 0.03. A small random scatter in both directions of FFR was noted in 8.3% of stenoses, where the IC adenosine FFR value was 0.05 greater than the IV adenosine FFR value, suggesting a suboptimal IC hyperemic response. Changes in heart rate and blood pressure were significantly greater with IV adenosine. Two patients with IV adenosine but none with IC adenosine had side effects such as bronchospasm and nausea. These data indicated that IC adenosine is equivalent to IV infusion for determination of FFR in most patients. However, in a small percentage of cases, coronary hyperemia was suspected to be suboptimal with IC adenosine, suggesting that a repeated, higher IC adenosine dose may be helpful. IV adenosine also has the advantages of simplicity and weight-adjusted dosing and is required for the evaluation of ostial lesions or for the assessment of diffuse disease during pullback recordings.

Intracoronary Adenosine Triphosphate

Although it is unavailable in the United States, ATP may also be used to stimulate maximal hyperemia. Coronary flow velocity, hemodynamics, electrocardiography, and myocardial lactate metabolism before and after administration of 50 mcg of IC ATP and 10 mg of papaverine into the LCA were examined in 18 patients with normal coronary arteries. Dose responses were obtained with IC ATP doses of 0.5, 5, 15, 30, and 50 mcg and compared with the papaverine response in an additional 7 patients. ATP did not produce significant hemodynamic or electrocardiographic changes. The CFR was similar between ATP and papaverine. All 7 patients showed lactate production after papaverine; only 3 patients showed lactate production after ATP ($P < 0.001$). There was a significant correlation between CFR with ATP and with papaverine, indicating that maximal coronary vasodilation is safely obtained with IC ATP doses greater than 15 mcg.

Dobutamine Hyperemia

Bartunek and associates examined FFR in response to IC adenosine and IV dobutamine (10 to 40 mcg/kg/minute) in 22 patients with single-vessel CAD.[13] Peak dobutamine infusion produced similar distal coronary pressures and pressure ratios (Pd/Pa, 60 ± 18 and 59 ± 18 mm Hg; FFR, 0.68 ± 0.18 and 0.68 ± 0.17, respectively; all P = not significant [NS]). An additional bolus of IC adenosine given at peak dobutamine in 9 patients failed to change the FFR. As shown by angiography, high-dose IV dobutamine did not modify the area of the epicardial stenosis and, much like adenosine, fully exhausted myocardial resistance regardless of inducible left ventricular dysfunction.

Sodium Nitroprusside

IC nitroprusside may be an alternative to IC adenosine. Parham and associates examined coronary blood flow velocity, heart rate, and blood pressure in unobstructed LAD arteries in 21 patients at rest, after IC adenosine (boluses of 30–50 mcg), and after three serial doses of IC nitroprusside (boluses of 0.3, 0.6, and 0.9 mcg/kg).[14] IC nitroprusside produced equivalent coronary hyperemia with a longer duration

(about 25%) compared with IC adenosine. IC nitroprusside (0.9 mcg/kg) decreased systolic blood pressure by 20% with minimal change in heart rate, whereas IC adenosine had no effect on these parameters. FFR measurements with IC nitroprusside were identical to those obtained with IC adenosine ($r = 0.97$). IC nitroprusside, in doses commonly used for the treatment of the no-reflow phenomenon, can produce sustained coronary hyperemia without detrimental systemic hemodynamics. Sodium nitroprusside also appears to be a suitable hyperemic stimulus for coronary physiologic measurements.

Clinical Validation of Intracoronary Pressure Measurements

To define the threshold of FFRmyo below which inducible ischemia is present, Pijls et al and De Bruyne et al conducted independent but parallel and complementary investigations.[15,16] Pijls' group studied 60 patients accepted for single-vessel PTCA, who had a positive exercise test in the preceding 24 hours. FFRmyo was measured before and 15 minutes after PTCA, and the exercise test was repeated after 1 week. If the second exercise test had reverted to normal after PTCA, FFRmyo values were associated with inducible ischemia. All except two FFRmyo measurements greater than 0.74 were not associated with ischemia, and all FFRmyo measurements of 0.74 or less were related to inducible ischemia. In normal coronary arteries, FFRmyo was 0.98 ± 0.03. De Bruyne's group studied FFRmyo in 60 patients with one isolated lesion in one major coronary artery, who had a maximal exercise test 6 hours before catheterization. ST-segment depression was compared with FFRmyo, ΔP_{max}, and ΔP_{rest}. Intersections of sensitivity and specificity curves were at 87%, 83%, and 75%, respectively, for FFRmyo = 0.66, ΔP_{max} = 31 mm Hg, and ΔP_{rest} = 12 mm Hg. No abnormal test was present for FFRmyo greater than 0.72. FFRmyo has also been compared with the results of dobutamine echocardiography in 75 patients with normal left ventricular function and single-vessel CAD; the degree of dobutamine-induced dyssynergy correlated significantly with the quantitative coronary angiography (QCA) data, but the correlation was markedly better with FFRmyo. All but one patient with a FFRmyo greater than 0.75 had a normal stress test result. Among the most important reports of FFRmyo is that of Pijls and colleagues, who compared FFRmyo with the unique ischemic standard of common noninvasive testing modalities in 45 patients with moderate coronary stenoses and chest pain syndromes.[17] When the FFRmyo was lower than 0.75 (21 patients), reversible myocardial ischemia was demonstrated unequivocally on at least one noninvasive test (bicycle exercise testing, thallium scintigraphy, stress echocardiography with dobutamine), and all these positive test results were reversed after PTCA or coronary artery bypass grafting (CABG). In 21 of 24 patients with a FFRmyo greater than 0.75, all of the tests showed no demonstration of ischemia, and no revascularization procedure was performed. Importantly, no revascularization was required after 14 months of follow-up. The sensitivity of FFRmyo in the identification of reversible ischemia was 88%, the specificity was 100%, the positive predictive value was 100%, the negative predictive value was 88%, and the accuracy was 93%.

Intracoronary Pressure and Flow Measurements and Myocardial Perfusion Imaging

Strong correlations exist between myocardial stress testing and FFRmyo or CFR. An FFRmyo of less than 0.75 identifies physiologically significant stenoses associated with inducible myocardial ischemia with high sensitivity (88%), specificity (100%), positive predictive value (100%), and overall accuracy (93%). An abnormal CFR (<2) corresponds to reversible myocardial perfusion imaging defects with high sensitivity (86%–92%), specificity (89%–100%), predictive accuracy (89%–96%), and positive and negative predictive values (84%–100% and

TABLE 57-2	Summary of Correlation between Noninvasive Stress Test Results and Physiologic Measurements			
Index	Ischemic Test	N	BCV	Accuracy (%)
FFR	SPECT	763	0.74–0.78	75–95
	DSE	58	0.67–0.75	90
CFR	SPECT	704	1.7–2	75–92
	DSE	58	2	87–88
rCFR	SPECT	260	0.64–0.75	75–92
	DSE	28	0.75	81

BCV, best cut-off value (defined as the value with the highest sum of sensitivity and specificity); *CFR*, coronary flow reserve; *DSE*, dobutamine stress echocardiography; *FFR*, fractional flow reserve; *rCFR*, relative coronary flow reserve; *SPECT*, single photon emission tomography.

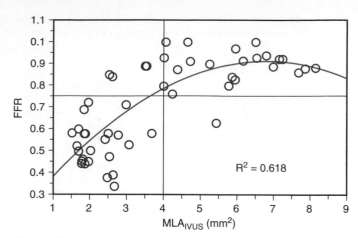

Figure 57-7 Correlation between fractional flow reserve (FFR) and quantified coronary angiography (QCA) and intravascular ultrasound (IVUS) measurements. *(From Takagi A, Tsurumi Y, Ishii Y, et al: Clinical potential of intravascular ultrasound for physiological assessment of coronary stenosis. Relationship between quantitative ultrasound tomography and pressure-derived fractional flow reserve, Circulation 100:250–255, 1999.)*

77%–95%, respectively). More recent studies have looked at the comparison of FFR with magnetic resonance myocardial perfusion imaging (MRMPI) to detect reversible myocardial ischemia. Previous studies have generally used quantitative coronary angiography as the standard to assess the accuracy of MRMPI despite the weak relationship that exists between stenosis severity and functional significance. To address this limitation of prior validation studies, Watkins et al studied 103 patients undergoing evaluation of angina with MRMPI using intravenous adenosine (140 mcg/kg-1/min), and first-pass 0.1 mmol/kg gadolinium bolus imaging technique to FFR performed within 1 week of MRMPI.[18] Perfusion defects were identified in 121 of 300 coronary artery segments (40%), of which 110 had an FFR less than 0.75; 168 of 179 normally perfused segments had an FFR greater than 0.75. The sensitivity and specificity of MRMPI for the detection of functionally significant coronary stenoses were 91% and 94%, respectively, with positive and negative predictive values of 91% and 94%. It appears that MRMPI can detect functionally significant CAD with high sensitivity, specificity, and positive and negative predictive values by using FFR as the standard.

Melikian et al reported on the correlation between ischemic myocardial perfusion imaging (MPI) with single-photon emission CT with FFR in patients with multi-vessel coronary disease.[19] Sixty-seven patients (201 vascular territories) with angiographic two-vessel or three-vessel coronary disease prospectively underwent MPI (rest or stress adenosine) and FFR in each vessel was measured within 2 weeks. In 42% of patients, MPI and FFR detected identical ischemic territories (mean number of territories 0.9 ± 0.8 for both; P = 1.00). In the remaining 36%, MPI underestimated (mean number of territories; MPI 0.46 ± 0.6; FFR 2.0 ± 0.6; P <0.001) and in 22% overestimated (mean number of territories; MPI 1.9 ± 0.8; FFR 0.5 ± 0.8; P <0.001) the number of ischemic territories in comparison with FFR. There was poor concordance to detect myocardial ischemia on both a per-patient (95% confidence interval [CI] −0.10–0.39, P = 0.14) and per-vessel (95% CI 0.15–0.42, P = 0.28) basis. In this study, there was poor concordance of MPI with FFR. MPI tends to underestimate or overestimate the functional significance of angiographic lesion severity compared with FFR in patients with multi-vessel disease. Table 57-2 summarizes the comparison between ischemic stress testing and coronary physiologic measurements.

Intracoronary Physiologic Measurements and Intravascular Ultrasound Measurements

IVUS offers a high degree of anatomic detail that can aid the operator in making clinical decisions and has been proposed as a surrogate measurement to determine the functional significance of a given stenosis. However, the two technologies are more complementary than similar, as FFR is designed for physiologic epicardial lesion assessment, whereas IVUS is designed to assess coronary lesion and vessel anatomy and morphology. IVUS is highly accurate for vessel sizing and confirming stent expansion and strut apposition. Given these differences, the clinician's first question should be: "Does this lesion limit blood flow and produce ischemia?" If the answer is yes, stenting is indicated. If the answer is no, then stenting is of no value and only results in introducing increased risk and cost, regardless of the IVUS images. A study comparing IVUS, QCA, and FFR in 42 patients with 51 stenoses also demonstrated that QCA alone was not accurate in determining physiologic lesion significance assessed by either IVUS or FFR.[20] There was a correlation of minimal lumen area (MLA) IVUS less than 3 mm² and cross-sectional area (CSA) IVUS stenosis greater than 60% with a measured FFR less than 0.75 (IVUS sensitivity 83%, specificity 92%). There are several IVUS studies comparing FFR to IVUS measurements, for example, MLA. Tagaki et al found that most MLA values less than 4 mm² were associated with FFR less than 0.75 (Fig. 57-7), although several patients had nonischemic FFR.[21] The reason for this variance is that resistance to flow is based on several different anatomic factors (entrance angle, length, MLA, eccentricity), of which MLA is only one. A 4-mm² MLA may limit flow in a large proximal vessel segment but will not impair flow in a smaller segment of the same artery. For assessment of the LMCA, unlike FFR, the IVUS threshold of "treat" or "not treat" changes. There are several different IVUS MLAs reported to be the cut-off value ranging from 5.9 to 7 mm² for treatment decisions.[22] Most IVUS thresholds are derived from clinical outcomes, with different areas from different studies. This variable IVUS "gold standard" can be understood on the basis of what we know about using only one dimension of a complex stenosis, including or not including the reference vessel segment dimensions. The loss of pressure across a stenosis can be computed from the simplified Bernouilli principle, which includes not only the stenosis area but also the length of the narrowing.

$$\Delta P = 1 \div As \times length \times V2$$

where *P* is the pressure drop across a stenosis, *As* is the minimal cross-sectional stenosis area (MCSa), and *V* is blood flow velocity through the tube. Moreover, unlike IVUS, FFR is not only lesion specific but also incorporates the variable myocardial blood flow across the stenosis supplying the specific myocardial bed. For example, a 70% stenosis in a vessel subtending a small diagonal or a previously infarcted mid-anterior descending territory will have less physiologic impact compared with an identical lesion in a mid-anterior descending territory subtending a normal anterior wall region because of the significantly higher flow requirements.

Usefulness of Fractional Flow Reserve in Daily Clinical Practice

DETERMINING THE NEED FOR REVASCULARIZATION IN SINGLE-VESSEL DISEASE WITH AN INTERMEDIATE STENOSIS

Determining the clinical significance of intermediate coronary stenoses on angiography frequently requires adjunctive noninvasive stress testing. Direct trans-lesional pressure measurements correlate well with myocardial perfusion imaging studies and may assist in clinical decision making. The clinical outcomes of deferring coronary intervention for intermediate stenoses with normal physiology are remarkably consistent, with clinical event rates of less than 10% over a 2-year follow-up period. No study has deferred treatment in symptomatic patients with abnormal trans-lesional physiology. Bech and colleagues recently reported the results of a large, randomized study (Deferral of PTCA versus performance of PTCA [DEFER]) of 325 patients for whom PTCA was planned who did not have documented ischemia.[23] The FFR of the stenosis was measured, and, if it was greater than 0.75, patients were randomly assigned to deferral of PTCA (deferral group; $n = 91$) or performance of PTCA (performance group; $n = 90$). If the FFR was less than 0.75, PTCA was performed as planned (reference group; $n = 144$). Clinical follow-up was obtained at 1, 3, 6, 12, and 24 months. Event-free survival was similar in the deferral and performance groups (92% vs. 89%, respectively, at 12 months; and 89% vs. 83% at 24 months) but was significantly lower in the reference group (80% at 12 months and 78% at 24 months) (Fig. 57-8). In addition, the percentage of patients free from angina was similar in the deferral

and performance groups (49% vs. 50% at 12 months; and 70% vs. 51% at 24 months) but was significantly higher in the reference group (67% at 12 months and 80% at 24 months). It was concluded that in patients with a coronary stenosis without evidence of ischemia, coronary pressure–derived FFR identifies those who will benefit from PTCA. Despite data showing durable safety of not treating lesions that are not physiologically significant, some patients with deferred procedures may still have recurrent angina, requiring continued medical therapy. Nonetheless, if they are physiologically normal, the functional and clinical impact of angiographically intermediate stenoses is associated with an excellent clinical outcome. Like other tests at a single point in time, in-lab trans-lesional hemodynamics may not reflect the episodic ischemia-producing conditions of daily life, particularly those related to vasomotor changes during exercise or emotional stress. Fortunately, most dynamic conditions are highly responsive to medical therapy. Physiologic thresholds validated by ischemic stress testing and clinical outcomes support decisions to defer intervention while continuing medical therapy for endothelial dysfunction, hypertension, hyperlipidemia, and episodic coronary vasoconstriction. Table 57-3 summarizes the results of studies deferring PCI for intermediate lesions on the basis of physiologic endpoints.

MULTI-VESSEL DISEASE

With the growing use of coronary stents in an increasingly complex patient population, a frequent application of physiologic assessment involves lesion selection in patients with multi-vessel disease. Accurate lesion selection is important because noninvasive studies have demonstrated that technetium 99m sestamibi single-photon emission computed tomography (MIBI-SPECT) failed to correctly indicate all ischemic areas in 90% of patients.[24] In 35% of such patients, no perfusion defect was present, possibly owing to balanced ischemia. Often, one ischemic area was masked by another, more severely underperfused area. Furthermore, when several stenoses or diffuse disease are present within one coronary artery, an abnormal MIBI-SPECT hypoperfusion image cannot discriminate among the different stenoses along the length of that vessel. In clinical practice, these observations highlight the fact that regions that may not appear responsible for ischemia can contain significant appearing narrowings, whereas other, more severe-appearing lesions may not be hemodynamically important. Coronary pressure measurements are particularly useful to localize regions of suspected ischemia. Tonino et al recently reported the results of the FAME (FFR versus Angiography for Multivessel Evaluation) trial.[25] This trial was designed to address the hypothesis that a physiologically guided PCI approach (FFR-PCI) was superior to

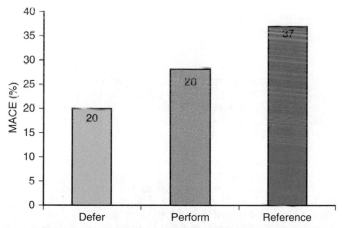

Figure 57-8 Graph showing the 5-year results from the Deferral of percutaneous transluminal coronary angioplasty (PTCA) versus performance of PTCA (DEFER) trial. The y-axis depicts the percentage of patients with major adverse cardiac events (MACEs): death, myocardial infarction, coronary artery bypass surgery, or percutaneous coronary intervention. The "DEFER" group ($n = 91$) consisted of those patients found to have an intermediate coronary stenosis in whom the measured FFR was greater than 0.75 and no angioplasty was performed (MACE = 20%). The "PERFORM" group ($n = 90$) consisted of those patients with an intermediate coronary stenosis with FFR values greater than 0.75 in whom angioplasty was performed (MACE = 28%). The "REFERENCE" group ($n = 144$) comprised patients whose lesions had measured FFR values of less than 0.75 in whom angioplasty was performed (MACE = 37%). (From Van Schaardenburgh P, Bech GJW, De Bruyne B, et al: Is it necessary to stent non-ischaemic stenoses? Five year follow-up of the DEFER study, Eur Heart J 26[Suppl 1]:3747, 2005.)

TABLE 57-3	Outcomes after Deferral of Coronary Intervention for Intermediate Coronary Artery Disease					
Index	**Author**	**Reference**	**N**	**Defer Value**	**MACE (%)**	**Follow-up (mo)**
FFR	Bech	17	100	0.75	8	18
	Bech	32	150	0.75	8	24
	Hernandez Garcia	54	43	0.75	12	11
	Bech*	21	24	0.75	21	29
	Rieber	55	47	0.75	13	12
	Chamuleau	56	92	0.75	9	12
	Rieber	57	24	0.75	8	12
	Lessar†	29	34	0.75	9	12
CFR	Kern	58	88	2.0	7	9
	Ferrari	59	22	2.0	9	15
	Chamuleau‡	60	143	2.0	6	12

*Patients with left main coronary artery disease.
†Patients with unstable angina.
‡Patients with multivessel disease.
CFR, coronary flow reserve; Defer Value, cut-off value used by study for decision making; FFR, fractional flow reserve; MACEs, major adverse cardiac events.

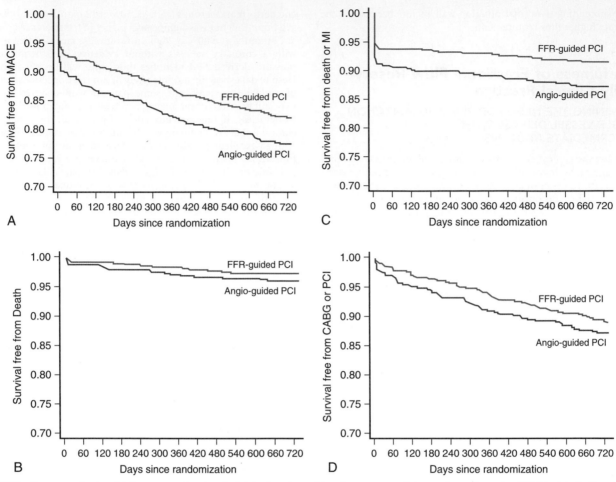

Figure 57-9 Two-year Kaplan–Meier curves showing individual and combined outcomes of the patients from the FAME trial. **A,** Freedom from major adverse cardiac events (MACEs). **B,** Overall survival. **C,** Freedom from death or myocardial infarction. **D,** Freedom from revascularization by percutaneous coronary intervention (PCI) or coronary artery bypass grafting (CABG). *(From Tonino PAL, De Bruyne B, Pijls, NHJ, et al: Fractional flow reserve versus angiography for guiding percutaneous coronary intervention, N Eng J Med 360:213–234, 2009.)*

conventional PCI (guided by angiographic findings) in patients with multi-vessel CAD. Twenty centers in Europe and the United States randomly assigned 1005 patients with multi-vessel CAD undergoing PCI with DESs to one of the two strategies. Following diagnostic angiography, operators selected lesions intended for stenting by visual angiographic appearance (approximately 50% diameter stenosis) before randomizing the patient. If the patient was randomized to the FFR-PCI strategy, FFR measurements were performed on all indicated lesions and the lesions were only stented if the FFR was 0.80 or less. Randomization to the angiographic strategy led to the treatment of all indicated lesions with a DES. The primary endpoints of death, MI, and repeat revascularization (CABG or PCI) were obtained at 1 year. Of the 1005 patients, 496 were assigned to the Angiography–PCI group, and 509 were assigned to the FFR-PCI group. Clinical characteristics and angiographic findings were similar in both groups. The Syntax (Synergy between PCI with Taxus and Cardiac Surgery) scores for gauging risk in multi-vessel disease involvement were identical at 14.5, indicating low- to intermediate-risk patients. Despite the number of lesions per patient being identical between the two groups, the FFR-PCI group used fewer stents per patient (1.9 ± 1.3 vs. 2.7 ± 1.2, $P <0.001$), less contrast (272 mL vs. 302 mL, $P <0.001$), had lower procedure cost ($5,332 vs. $6,007, $P <0.001$), and shorter hospital stay (3.4 days vs. 3.7 days, $P <0.05$). Even with fewer stents placed, patients in the FFR-PCI group had reductions in anginal symptoms equivalent to the angiographically guided group. The primary endpoint was strongly in favor of the FFR-PCI strategy, with lower MACE (13.2% vs. 18.4%, $P <0.02$).

There was also a lower combined incidence of death or MI (7.3% vs. 11%, $P <0.04$). These results remained durable for up to 2 years of follow-up (Fig. 57-9). When evaluating this large randomized study, it is obvious that the strategy of selectively using stent therapy to treat only the lesions that are responsible for ischemia provided patients with significant relief from angina, with concomitant reduction in follow-up MI rates. Many operators fear "leaving lesions uncovered" with stents because of concerns that these lesions will progress over time and require subsequent repeat catheterization and stenting or that the lesions will potentially rupture and cause MI. Over a 2-year follow-up, the FAME investigators showed that out of 513 deferred lesions in the FFR-PCI group, there were only 10 that showed clear progression and required stenting (target lesion revascularization [TLR] rate of 1.9%) and only 1 lesion that resulted in MI (0.2%). These data provide significant outcomes-based evidence that supports a strategy of only revascularizing ischemia-producing lesions when treating patients with multi-vessel disease.

FRACTIONAL FLOW RESERVE AND CORONARY ARTERY BYPASS GRAFTING

Several small, nonrandomized studies have reported the use of coronary physiology in multi-vessel disease. Recently, in patients with multi-vessel disease referred for CABG, patients who underwent selective PCI of hemodynamically significant stenoses, with medical therapy for all other nonsignificant lesions, had a prognosis similar to that of

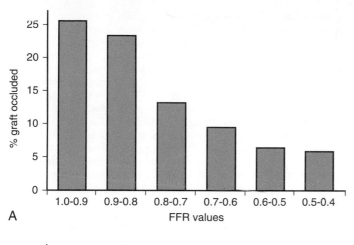

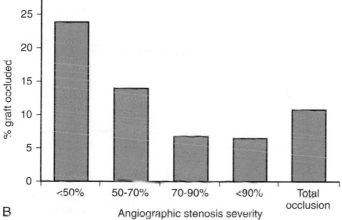

Figure 57-10 **A,** The relation between functional stenosis severity established by fractional flow reserve (FFR) measurements and graft failure at angiographic follow-up after 1 year. **B,** The relation between angiographic stenosis severity prior to bypass grafting and graft failure after angiographic follow-up at 1 year. (*From Botman CJ, Schonberger J, Koolen S, et al: Does stenosis severity of native vessels influence bypass graft patency? A prospective fractional flow reserve-guided study, Ann Thorac Surg 83:2093–2097, 2007.*)

patients who underwent CABG of all of the diseased vessels demonstrated by angiography.[26] In a similar study, 150 patients with multivessel disease referred for CABG had FFR performed.[27] If three vessels were significant (FFR < 0.75) or two vessels were significant with one being the proximal LAD artery, CABG was performed; otherwise, significant lesions were treated with stenting.[31] After a 2-year follow-up, there was no difference in event-free survival, including repeat revascularization, showing that an individually tailored approach to patients with multi-vessel disease can be accomplished by determining the hemodynamic significance of each lesion. In a group of 164 patients referred for bypass surgery on clinical grounds, preoperative FFR was performed with the surgeon blinded to the results.[28] Each patient returned for a repeat angiogram after 1 year, and the patency of the bypass grafts was compared with the preoperative angiographic stenosis and preoperative FFR. As shown in Figure 57-10, there was a higher percentage of occluded grafts at this early time when they were placed on vessels that had an FFR greater than 0.80. Although the highest percentage of occluded grafts was found in the group placed on vessels with less than 50% stenosis, there was still a high percentage of graft failure in the group with 50% to 70% stenosis. Thus, FFR-guided bypass is a reasonable strategy to predict bypass graft patency and has superiority over the strategy of grafting all vessels with lesions with 50% or more stenosis.

LEFT MAIN CORONARY ARTERY DISEASE

FFR can be used to assess narrowings of the LMCA with specific technical considerations with regard to the seating of the guiding catheter and the use of IV adenosine. Because of the potential for the guiding catheter obstructing blood flow across an ostial narrowing, FFR measurements should be performed with the guiding catheter disengaged from the coronary ostium and hyperemia induced with IV adenosine. Initially, the guiding catheter and wire pressures should be matched (equalized) before the guiding catheter is seated. Then, the guiding catheter is seated, and the pressure wire is advanced into the LAD artery or the left circumflex (LCx) artery. The guiding catheter is then disengaged, and IV adenosine infusion is initiated. After 1 to 2 minutes, the FFR is calculated, and thereafter the wire can be pulled back slowly to identify the exact location of the pressure drop. In case of a distal narrowing of the LMCA, this procedure may be performed twice, once with the pressure wire in the LAD artery and then again in the LCx artery. The use of FFR in LMCA stenosis was examined in 54 patients.[29] In 30 patients who had an FFR of less than 0.75, surgery was performed, and in 24 patients with an FFR of 0.75 or greater, medical therapy was chosen. After a follow-up of 3 years, there was no difference in event-free survival or functional class between the groups. No death or MI occurred in the patients in the medical group. Similar results were recently shown by Lindstaedt and colleagues, who monitored 51 patients with intermediate LMCA disease.[30] The decision to perform CABG was based on FFR measurement of the LMCA. In this patient population, 27 received CABG. After an average of 19 months of follow-up, there was no difference in event-free survival between those who underwent CABG and those who were treated medically. In a single-center retrospective evaluation, 274 consecutive patients with angiographically indeterminate LMCA stenosis underwent FFR evaluation to determine the need for revascularization similar to the prospective studies.[31] With 60 months follow-up, LMCA stenoses with FFR values of ≥0.80 had equivalent outcomes to those patients who underwent revascularization because of an FFR <0.80 (Fig. 57-11). With this patient series, there are now over 300 patients with published long-term outcomes demonstrating the ability of FFR to triage the use of revascularization for LMCA disease in a manner similar to that for single or multi-vessel coronary disease.

SERIAL (MULTIPLE) LESIONS IN A SINGLE VESSEL

If multiple stenoses are present in the same vessel, the hyperemic flow and pressure gradient through the first stenosis will be attenuated by the presence of the second one, and vice versa. Each stenosis will mask the true effect of its serial counterpart by limiting the achievable maximum hyperemia. This fluid dynamic interaction between two serial stenoses depends on the sequence, severity, and distance between the lesions as well as the flow rate. If the distance between two lesions is greater than six times the vessel diameter, the stenoses generally behave independently and the overall pressure gradient is the sum of the individual pressure losses at any given flow rate. When addressing two stenoses in series, equations have been derived to predict the FFR (FFRpred) of each stenosis separately (i.e., as if the other one were removed), using arterial pressure (Pa), pressure between the two stenoses (Pm), distal coronary pressure (Pd), and coronary occlusive pressure (Pw). FFRapp (ratio of the pressure just distal to that just proximal to each stenosis) and FFRtrue (ratio of the pressures distal and proximal to each stenosis but after removal of the other one) have been compared in instrumented dogs and in humans.[32,33] FFRtrue was more overestimated by FFRapp than by FFRpred. It was clearly demonstrated that the interaction between two stenoses is such that the FFR of each lesion cannot be calculated by the equation for isolated stenoses applied to each separately; however, the FFR for each lesion can be predicted by more complete equations that take into account Pa, Pm, Pd, and Pw. Although calculation of the exact FFR for each lesion separately is possible, it remains academic. In clinical practice, the use of the pressure pull-back recording is particularly well suited

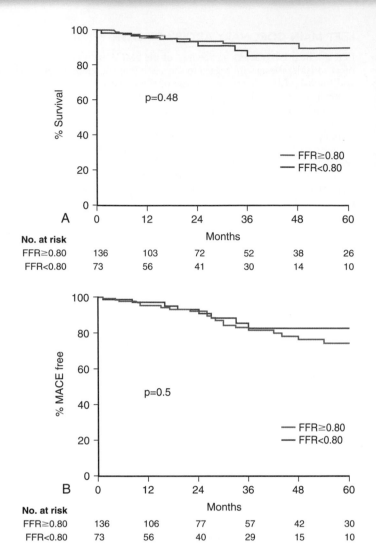

Figure 57-11 Outcomes in patients with intermediate left main coronary artery disease based on treatment guided by fractional flow reserve (FFR) assessment. **A,** Survival curves for patients with medical therapy (FFR >0.80) and coronary artery bypass grafting (CABG) (FFR<0.80) treated patients over 5 years. **B,** Major adverse cardiac events in patients treated with medical therapy (FFR >0.80) and CABG (FFR <0.80) over 5 years. *(From Hamilos M, Muller O, Cuisset T, et al: Long-term clinical outcome after fractional flow reserve–guided treatment in patients with angiographically equivocal left main coronary artery stenosis, Circulation 120:1505–1512, 2009.)*

to identify the several regions of a vessel with large pressure gradients that may benefit by treatment. The one stenosis with the largest gradient can be treated first, after which the FFR can be remeasured for the remaining stenoses to determine the need for further treatment (see case examples in Fig. 57-12 and 57-13).

DIFFUSE CORONARY DISEASE

A diffusely diseased atherosclerotic coronary artery can be viewed as a series of branching units diverting and gradually distributing flow along the longitudinally narrowing conduit length. The perfusion pressure gradually diminishes along this artery. CFR is reduced but is unassociated with a focal stenotic pressure loss. Therefore, mechanical therapy directed at a presumed "culprit" plaque to reverse such abnormal physiology would be ineffective in restoring normal coronary perfusion. With the use of FFRmyo during continuous-pressure wire pull-back from a distal location to a proximal location, the impact of

a specific area of angiographic narrowing can be examined, and the presence of diffuse atherosclerosis can be documented. Diffuse atherosclerosis, as opposed to a focal narrowing, is characterized by a continuous and gradual pressure recovery without localized abrupt increase in pressure related to an isolated region. De Bruyne and coworkers demonstrated the influence of diffuse atherosclerosis that often remains invisible at angiography.[34] FFRmyo measurements were obtained from 37 arteries in 10 individuals without atherosclerosis (group I) and from 106 nonstenotic arteries in 62 patients with arteriographic stenoses in another coronary artery (group II). In group I, the pressure gradient between the aorta and the distal coronary artery was minimal at rest (1 ± 1 mm Hg) and during maximal hyperemia (3 ± 3 mm Hg). Corresponding values were significantly larger in group II (5 ± 4 and 10 ± 8 mm Hg, respectively; both $P < 0.001$). The FFRmyo was near unity (0.97 ± 0.02; range, 0.92–1) in group I, indicating no resistance to flow in truly normal coronary arteries, but it was significantly lower (0.89 ± 0.08; range, 0.69–1) in group II, indicating a higher resistance to flow. This resistance to flow contributes to myocardial ischemia and has consequences for decision making during PCI. As for patients with several discrete stenoses within one coronary artery, similar considerations can be applied for patients with diffuse CAD or long lesions. The pressure pull-back recording at maximum hyperemia provides the necessary information to decide whether and where stent implantation may be useful. The location of a focal pressure drop superimposed on the diffuse disease can be identified as an appropriate location for treatment. In some cases, the gradual decline of pressure along the vessel occurs over a very long segment, such that interventional treatment is not possible (Fig. 57-14). Medical treatment (or CABG) can then be elected.

OSTIAL LESIONS AND "JAILED" SIDE BRANCHES

The ability to determine the physiologic significance of ostial lesions, particularly in side branch vessels, remains difficult with current angiographic techniques and equipment. This is particularly problematic after the side branch has been "jailed" by a stent in the parent vessel. Koo and coworkers examined the physiologic assessment of jailed side branches and compared the FFR with the QCA of stenosis severity.[35] Ninety-seven jailed side branch lesions in vessels larger than 2 mm with a percent stenosis greater than 50% by visual estimation after stent implantation had FFR performed, measuring the pressure 5 mm distal and proximal to the ostial side branch lesion. In 94 lesions, the mean FFR was 0.94 ± 0.04 at the main branch and 0.85 ± 0.11 at the jailed side branch. There was a negative correlation between percent stenosis and FFR ($r = 0.41$, $P < 0.001$). However, no lesion with less than 75% stenosis had an FFR less than 0.75. Among 73 lesions with greater than 75% stenosis, only 20 lesions were functionally significant (Fig. 57-15). The authors concluded that measurement of FFR in jailed side branch lesions is both safe and feasible and that as with other intermediate lesions, QCA is unreliable. Moreover, the measurement of FFR suggested that most of these lesions do not have functional significance and that intervention on these nonsignificant lesions may not be necessary (see example in Fig. 57-16). Similar findings have been reported for native ostial and branch lesions not "jailed" with intracoronary hardware that were found during routine coronary angiography.[36,37]

UNSTABLE ANGINA AND NON–ST SEGMENT ELEVATION MYOCARDIAL INFARCTION

After stabilization of patients with unstable angina or non–ST elevation myocardial infarction (NSTEMI), traditional management involves instituting maximal medical therapy and performing risk stratification by stress testing before coronary angiography and intervention based on the results. As an alternative approach, Leesar and colleagues used FFR to risk-stratify patients with acute coronary syndrome in the laboratory at the time of catheterization after medical stabilization.[38] Seventy patients were randomly assigned to either early

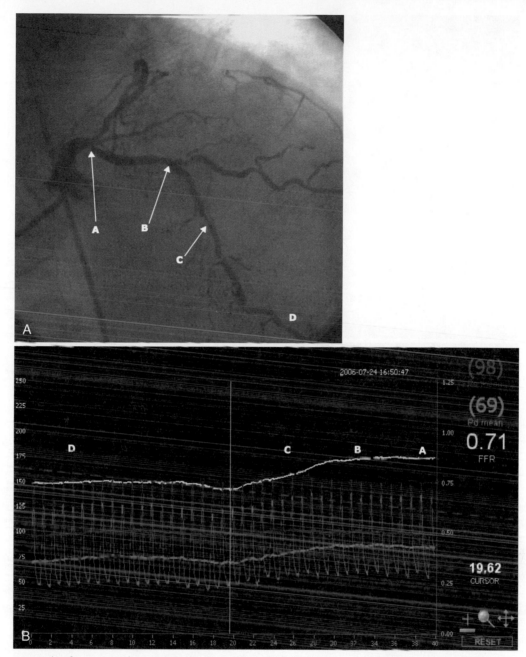

Figure 57-12 Case example of a patient who presented to the catheterization laboratory complaining of angina-like symptoms. **A,** Right anterior oblique (RAO) cranial angiogram shows multiple lesions (A through D) within the left anterior descending (LAD) coronary artery. **B,** A pull-back curve through the LAD during intravenous adenosine administration (points A through D represent the lesions identified in A).

in-hospital invasive evaluation ($n = 35$) with FFR or noninvasive evaluation by perfusion scintigraphy ($n = 35$). The decision to revascularize was based on abnormal FFR or MIBI-SPECT scans. The early invasive FFR-guided approach was as effective as the standard of care with noninvasive risk stratification. The rates of major adverse cardiac events (MACEs) at 1-year follow-up were similar between the groups. The FFR-guided approach was also associated with a shorter hospital stay and a significant decrease in total costs of the hospitalization. For patients who cannot be medically stabilized, current guidelines recommend urgent angiography with appropriate revascularization as indicated, without FFR. Nonetheless, FFR could be useful to assess other intermediately severe nonculprit lesions for consideration of complete revascularization.

RECENT ST ELEVATION MYOCARDIAL INFARCTION

After an acute MI, the predictive ability of FFR has some theoretic limitations, because the microvascular bed in the infarct zone does not necessarily have a uniform and constant resistance. However, DeBruyne and associates demonstrated that a threshold of 0.75 was also valid in 57 patients who had sustained an MI more than 6 days earlier.[39] Myocardial perfusion SPECT imaging and FFRmyo were obtained before and after angioplasty. The sensitivity and specificity of the 0.75 value of FFRmyo to detect flow maldistribution on SPECT imaging were 82% and 87%, respectively. The concordance between the FFR and SPECT imaging was 85% ($P < 0.001$). When only truly positive and truly negative SPECT imaging results were considered, the

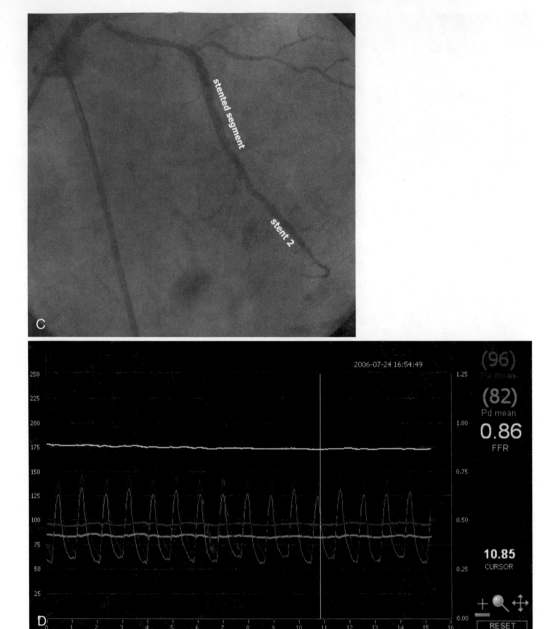

Figure 57-12, cont'd C, RAO cranial angiogram after treatment of lesions D and C with stents. **D,** Fractional flow reserve (FFR) of the LAD after stenting, with the wire distal to the last stent. The FFR of 0.86 reflects the fact that the ostial and middle lesions (A and B) did not need to be treated.

corresponding values were 87%, 100%, and 94% ($P < 0.001$). Patients with positive SPECT imaging before angioplasty had a significantly lower FFRmyo than did patients with negative SPECT imaging (0.52 ± 0.18 vs. 0.67 ± 0.16, $P < 0.0079$); they also had a significantly higher left ventricular ejection fraction (LVEF, 63% ± 10% vs. 52% ± 10%, $P < 0.0009$) despite a similar percent diameter stenosis (67% ± 13% vs. 68% ± 16%, $P = $ NS). A significant inverse correlation was found between LVEF and FFRmyo ($R = 0.29$, $P = 0.049$). It appears that, for a similar degree of stenosis, the value of FFRmyo depends on the mass of viable myocardium. The possibility of analyzing truly positive and negative SPECT imaging in this study confirmed the validity of the 0.75 threshold, which could not be derived from a study based only on angiographic parameters.[40]

Intracoronary Physiologic Measurements as a Research Tool

MICROVASCULAR DISEASE AND CHEST PAIN WITH NORMAL CORONARY ARTERIES

As part of the Women's Ischemic Syndrome Evaluation (WISE) study, Reis and associates examined 48 women with chest pain, normal coronary arteries, or minimal luminal irregularities with CFR.[41] Sixty percent of women with CFR of less than 2 had a hyperemic velocity 89% of baseline but no change in cross-sectional vessel area. Forty percent of women with normal microcirculation, with average CFR of 3.24, had associated increases in coronary flow velocity and CSA of 179% and 17%, respectively. A CFR of 2.2 provided a high sensitivity

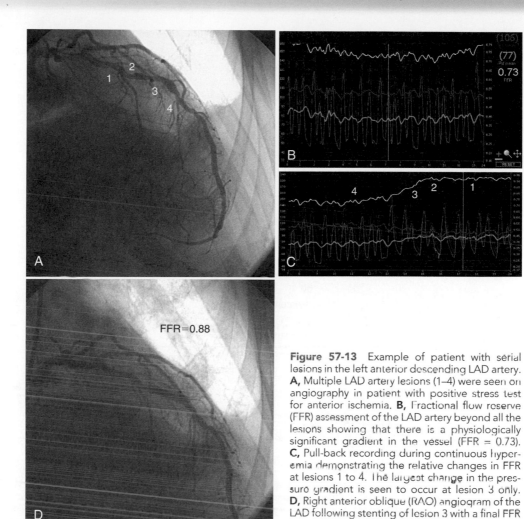

Figure 57-13 Example of patient with serial lesions in the left anterior descending LAD artery. **A,** Multiple LAD artery lesions (1–4) were seen on angiography in patient with positive stress test for anterior ischemia. **B,** Fractional flow reserve (FFR) assessment of the LAD artery beyond all the lesions showing that there is a physiologically significant gradient in the vessel (FFR = 0.73). **C,** Pull-back recording during continuous hyperemia demonstrating the relative changes in FFR at lesions 1 to 4. The largest change in the pressure gradient is seen to occur at lesion 3 only. **D,** Right anterior oblique (RAO) angiogram of the LAD following stenting of lesion 3 with a final FFR across all lesions of 0.88.

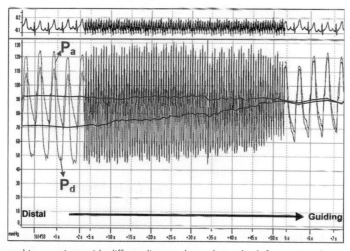

Figure 57-14 A pull-back curve created in a patient with diffuse disease throughout the left anterior descending (LAD) coronary artery. The fractional flow reserve (FFR) for this vessel is 0.67, reflecting ischemia-producing lesions. However, the gradual decrease in gradient from pressure distal to the stenosis (Pd) to arterial pressure (Pa) is reflective of severe, diffuse narrowing in the major portion of the vessel. This gradual change in the pressure curve shows that an extremely long segment is responsible for the ischemia and is most likely not best treated with multiple stents (i.e., "full metal jacket"). *(Courtesy of B. De Bruyne, Aalst, Belgium.)*

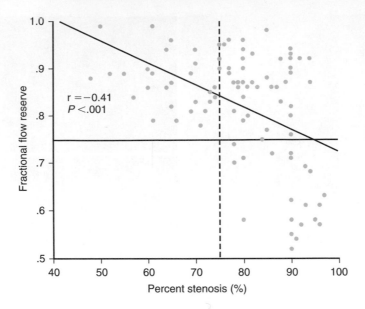

	% stenosis	
	≥50, <75	≥75
All lesions (*n* = 94)		
FFR <0.75	0	20 (27%)
FFR ≥0.75	20	53
Vessel size ≥2.5 mm (*n* = 28)		
FFR <0.75	0	8 (38%)
FFR ≥0.75	7	13

Figure 57-15 *Top,* Graph comparing percent diameter stenosis (by quantitative coronary angiography) to fractional flow reserve (FFR) across jailed side branches. Despite the statistical significance of the correlation, one should note the frequency of severely narrowed side branches without significant FFR values (*indicated by points in the upper right corner*). *Bottom,* Table showing the relationship between percent stenosis and FFR values across jailed side branches. *(From Koo BK, Kang HJ, Youn TJ, et al: Physiologic assessment of jailed side branch lesions using fractional flow reserve, J Am Coll Cardiol 46;633–637, 2005.)*

(90%) and specificity (89%) for the diagnosis of microvascular dysfunction. Failure of the epicardial coronary artery to dilate at least 9% was also a sensitive (79%) and specific (79%) surrogate marker of microvascular dysfunction. The attenuated epicardial coronary dilatory response likely represents significant microvascular dysfunction in women with chest pain and no obstructive CAD. Similar data were reported by Hasdai and colleagues in 203 patients with angiographically normal coronary arteries.[42] CFR and endothelial vasodilatory response to IC acetylcholine and adenosine were measured. Ninety-two percent of patients had at least one risk factor for atherosclerosis. Abnormal CFR was found in 59% of patients; 11% had impaired response to adenosine with CFR less than 2.5, and 29% had impaired response to acetylcholine with CFR less than 1.5; 18% had a combined abnormality. There was no correlation between endothelium-dependent and endothelium-independent flow response. The authors concluded that most patients with chest pain syndromes and nonobstructive CAD had risk factors for CAD with diverse abnormalities and endothelium-dependent and endothelium-independent function.

Simultaneous Measurement of Flow Velocity and Trans-Stenotic Pressure Gradient

Although the maximal flow and, consequently, the maximal trans-stenotic gradient is determined also by factors independent of the stenosis resistance, the pressure gradient–flow velocity relationship is intimately correlated with the stenosis hemodynamics. A method to assess the coronary vasculature that is easy to perform and currently poses the greatest clinical usefulness is the index of microcirculatory resistance (IMR). This index relies on using distal pressure and thermodilution flow, as assessed by the inverse of the arrival (transit) time of a room-temperature saline bolus to the distal coronary artery segment. By measuring the mean transit time at rest and comparing it with the mean transit time at peak hyperemia, a thermodilution CFR can be calculated. The ability to measure distal pressure and estimate flow using the thermodilution technique (example shown in Fig. 57-17) with a single wire also allows independent assessment of the microvasculature by calculating the index of microcirculatory resistance (IMR). Although principally a research tool, assessment of IMR permits a unique characterization of the microcirculation, and this has been shown to be prognostic in patients after STEMI.[43,44]

Conclusion

The technological advances in the field of interventional cardiology and the use of coronary physiology continue to provide valuable critical diagnostic assistance to the cath lab operator to make meaningful patient care decisions. Invasive assessment of coronary flow reserve is confined to research applications for the study of microvascular disease, but the use of FFR is increasingly being integrated into the daily practice in some laboratories. The physiologic assessment of intermediate stenoses in patients with complex CAD, including LMCA

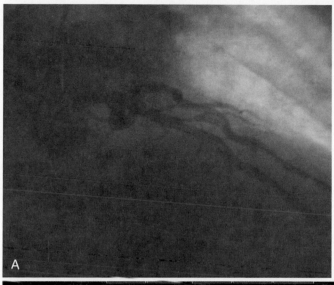

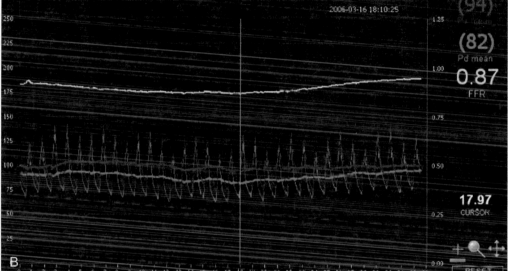

Figure 57-16 **A,** Right anterior oblique (RAO) cranial angiogram showing a left anterior descending (LAD) coronary artery without significant angiographic stenosis but a diagonal artery that appears to have a high-grade stenosis. **B,** Measurement of fractional flow rate (FFR) across the diseased ostial diagonal shows a value of 0.87, reflecting a nonsignificant ostial lesion despite its angiographic appearance.

Figure 57-17 Simultaneous measurement of pressure and flow (by thermodilution). The upper portion of the figure shows proximal (Pa) and distal (Pd) pressures at rest (left) and during hyperemia (right). The lower portion of the figure depicts the thermodilution curves at rest and during hyperemia with the associated average transit times at baseline and hyperemia circled. These values are used to calculate the coronary flow reserve (CFR) and the index of microcirculatory resistance (IMR), as seen on the right side of the panel. *FFR,* fractional flow reserve. *(From Martin KC, Yeung AC, Fearon WF: Invasive assessment of the coronary microcirculation,* Circulation *113:2054–2061, 2006.)*

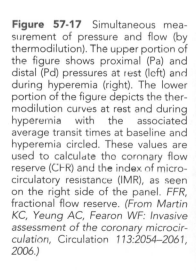

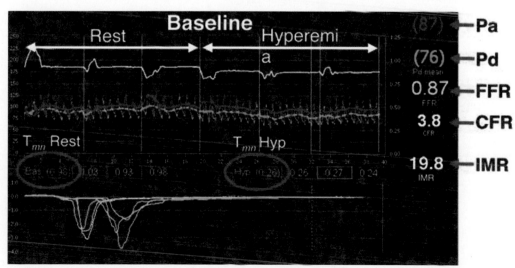

disease and multi-vessel disease, has improved the outcomes of patients with these complex anatomic subsets. FFR is especially useful with the replacement of surgical revascularization by percutaneous revascularization in recent years. FFR can help operators achieve complete resolution of coronary ischemia, similar to complete surgical revascularization. Future advances in coronary physiology will give practitioners the ability to evaluate the contribution of microvascular disease to a patient's symptoms, target therapies that can improve microvascular dysfunction, and evaluate endothelial dysfunction as a precursor to the atherosclerotic process. Conscientious operators employ FFR and IVUS for appropriate decision making and best outcomes in patients undergoing modern, complex PCI.

REFERENCES

1. Topol EJ, Nissen SE: Our preoccupation with coronary luminology. The dissociation between clinical and angiographic findings in ischemic heart disease. *Circulation* 92:2333–2342, 1995.
2. Meijboom WB, Van Mieghem CAG, van Pelt N, et al: Comprehensive assessment of coronary artery stenoses: Computed tomography coronary angiography versus conventional coronary angiography and correlation with fractional flow reserve in patients with stable angina. *J Am Coll Cardiol* 52:636–643, 2008.
3. Duncker DJ, Bache RJ: Regulation of coronary vasomotor tone under normal conditions and during acute myocardial hypoperfusion. *Pharmacol Ther* 86:87–110, 2000.
4. Gould KL, Kirkeeide RL, Buchi M: Coronary flow reserve as a physiologic measure of stenosis severity. *J Am Coll Cardiol* 15:459–474, 1990.
5. Pijls NHJ, van Son JAM, Kirkeeide RL, et al: Experimental basis of determining maximum coronary, myocardial, and collateral blood flow by pressure measurements for assessing functional stenosis severity before and after percutaneous transluminal coronary angioplasty. *Circulation* 86:1354–1367, 1993.
6. Pijls NHJ, Van Gelder B, Van der Voort P, et al: Fractional flow reserve: A useful index to evaluate the influence of an epicardial coronary stenosis on myocardial blood flow. *Circulation* 92:318–319, 1995.
7. De Bruyne B, Baudhuin T, Melin JA, et al: Coronary flow reserve calculated from pressure measurements in humans: Validation with positron emission tomography. *Circulation* 89:1013–1022, 1994.
8. De Bruyne B, Bartunek J, Sys SU, et al: Simultaneous coronary pressure and flow velocity measurements in humans: Feasibility, reproducibility and hemodynamic dependence of coronary flow velocity reserve, hyperemic flow versus pressure slope index and fractional flow reserve. *Circulation* 94:1842–1849, 1996.
9. Pijls NH, Kern MJ, Yock PG, et al: Practice and potential pitfalls of coronary pressure measurements. *Catheter Cardiovasc Interv* 49:1–16, 2000.
10. Qian J, Ge J, Baumgart D, et al: Safety of intracoronary Doppler flow measurement. *Am Heart J* 140:502–510, 2000.
11. Ntalianis A, Trana C, Muller O, et al: Effective radiation dose, time, and contrast medium to measure fractional flow reserve. *J Am Coll Cardiol Interv* 3:821–827, 2011.
12. Jeremias A, Whitbourn RJ, Filardo SD, et al: Adequacy of intracoronary versus intravenous adenosine-induced maximal coronary hyperemia for fractional flow reserve measurements. *Am Heart J* 140:651–657, 2000.
13. Bartunek J, Wijns W, Heyndrickx GR, et al: Effects of dobutamine on coronary stenosis physiology and morphology: Comparison with intracoronary adenosine. *Circulation* 100:243–249, 1999.
14. Parham WA, Bouhasin A, Ciaramita JP, et al: Coronary hyperemic dose responses to intracoronary sodium nitroprusside. *Circulation* 109:1236–1243, 2004.
15. Pijls NHJ, Van Gelder B, Van der Voort P, et al: Fractional flow reserve: A useful index to evaluate the influence of an epicardial coronary stenosis on myocardial blood flow. *Circulation* 92:3183–3193, 1995.
16. De Bruyne B, Bartunek J, Sys SU, et al: Relation between myocardial fractional flow reserve calculated from coronary pressure measurements and exercise-induced myocardial ischemia. *Circulation* 92:39–46, 1995.
17. Pijls NHJ, de Bruyne B, Peels K, et al: Measurement of fractional flow reserve to assess the functional severity of coronary-artery stenoses. *N Engl J Med* 334:1703–1708, 1996.
18. Watkins S, Chir B, McGeoch R, et al: Validation of magnetic resonance myocardial perfusion imaging with fractional flow reserve for the detection of significant coronary heart disease. *Circulation* 120:2207–2213, 2009.
19. Melikian N, De Bondt P, Tonino P, et al: Fractional flow reserve and myocardial perfusion imaging in patients with angiographic multivessel coronary artery disease. *J Am Coll Cardiol Interv* 3:307–314, 2010.
20. Abizaid A, Mint GS, Pichard AD, et al: Clinical, intravascular ultrasound, and quantitative angiographic determinants of the coronary flow reserve before and after percutaneous transluminal coronary angioplasty. *Am J Cardiol* 82:423–428, 1998.
21. Takagi A, Tsurumi Y, Ishii Y, et al: Clinical potential of intravascular ultrasound for physiological assessment of coronary stenosis. Relationship between quantitative ultrasound tomography and pressure-derived fractional flow reserve. *Circulation* 100:250–255, 1999.
22. Briguori C, Anzuini A, Airoldi F, et al: Intravascular ultrasound criteria for the assessment of the functional significance of intermediate coronary artery stenoses and comparison with fractional flow reserve. *Am J Cardiol* 87:136–141, 2001.
23. Bech GJ, De Bruyne B, Bonnier HJ, et al: Long-term follow-up after deferral of percutaneous transluminal coronary angioplasty of intermediate stenosis on the basis of coronary pressure measurement. *J Am Coll Cardiol* 31:841–847, 1998.
24. Lima RS, Watson DD, Goode AR, et al: Incremental value of combined perfusion and function over perfusion alone by gated SPECT myocardial perfusion imaging for detection of severe three-vessel coronary artery disease. *J Am Coll Cardiol* 42:64–70, 2003.
25. Tonino PAL, De Bruyne B, Pijls, NHJ, et al: Fractional flow reserve versus angiography for guiding percutaneous coronary intervention. *N Eng J Med* 360:213–234, 2009.
26. Berger A, Botman KJ, MacCarthy PA, et al: Long-term clinical outcome after fractional flow reserve-guided percutaneous coronary intervention in patients with multivessel disease. *J Am Coll Cardiol* 46:438–442, 2005.
27. Botman KJ, Pijls N, Bech JW, et al: Percutaneous coronary intervention or bypass surgery in multivessel disease? A tailored approach based on coronary pressure measurement. *Catheter Cardiovasc Interv* 63:184–191, 2004.
28. Botman CJ, Schonberger J, Koolen S, et al: Does stenosis severity of native vessels influence bypass graft patency? A prospective fractional flow reserve-guided study. *Ann Thorac Surg* 83:2093–2097, 2007.
29. Bech GJ, Drouste H, Pijls NH, et al: Value of fractional flow reserve in making decisions about bypass surgery for equivocal left main coronary artery disease. *Heart* 86:547–552, 2001.
30. Lindstaedt M, Yazar A, Germing A, et al: Clinical outcome in patients with intermediate or equivocal left main coronary artery disease after deferral of surgical revascularization on the basis of fractional flow reserve measurements. *Am Heart J* 152:156.e1–156.e9, 2006.
31. Hamilos M, Muller O, Cuisset T, et al: Long-term clinical outcome after fractional flow reserve–guided treatment in patients with angiographically equivocal left main coronary artery stenosis. *Circulation* 120:1505–1512, 2009.
32. De Bruyne B, Pijls NH, Heyndrickx GR, et al: Pressure-derived fractional flow reserve to assess serial epicardial stenoses: Theoretical basis and animal validation. *Circulation* 101:1840–1847, 2000.
33. Pijls NH, De Bruyne B, Bech GJ, et al: Coronary pressure measurement to assess the hemodynamic significance of serial stenoses within one coronary artery: Validation in humans. *Circulation* 102:2371–2377, 2000.
34. De Bruyne B, Hersbach F, Pijls NH, et al: Abnormal epicardial coronary resistance in patients with diffuse atherosclerosis but "normal" coronary angiography. *Circulation* 104:2401–2406, 2001.
35. Koo BK, Kang HJ, Youn TJ, et al: Physiologic assessment of jailed side branch lesions using fractional flow reserve. *J Am Coll Cardiol* 46;633–637, 2005.
36. Lim MJ, Kern MJ: Utility of coronary physiologic hemodynamics for bifurcation, aorto ostial and ostial branch stenoses to guide treatment decisions. *Catheter Cardiovasc Interv* 65:461–468, 2005.
37. Ziaee A, Parham WA, Herrmann SC, et al: Lack of relationship between imaging and physiology in ostial coronary artery narrowings. *Am J Cardiol* 93:1404–1407, 2004.
38. Leesar MA, Abdul-Baki T, Akkus NI, et al: Use of fractional flow reserve versus stress perfusion scintigraphy after unstable angina: Effect on duration of hospitalization, cost, procedural characteristics, and clinical outcome. *J Am Coll Cardiol* 44:1115–1121, 2003.
39. De Bruyne B, Pijls NH, Bartunek J, et al: Fractional flow reserve in patients with prior myocardial infarction. *Circulation* 104:157–162, 2001.
40. Caymaz O, Tezcan H, Fak AS, et al: Measurement of myocardial fractional flow reserve during coronary angioplasty in infarct-related and non-infarct related coronary artery lesions. *J Invasive Cardiol* 12:236–241, 2000.
41. Reis SE, Holubkov R, Lee JS, et al: Coronary flow velocity response to adenosine characterizes coronary microvascular function in women with chest pain and no obstructive coronary disease: Results from the pilot phase of the Women's Ischemia Syndrome Evaluation (WISE) study. *J Am Coll Cardiol* 33:1469–1475, 1999.
42. Hasdai D, Holmes DR, Jr., Higano ST, et al: Prevalence of coronary blood flow reserve abnormalities among patients with nonobstructive coronary artery disease and chest pain. *Mayo Clin Proc* 73:1133–1140, 1998.
43. Fearon WF, Balsam LB, Farouque HM, et al: Novel index for invasively assessing the coronary microcirculation. *Circulation* 107:3129–3132, 2003.
44. Fearon WF, Shah M, Ng M, et al: Predictive value of the index of microcirculatory resistance in patients with ST-Segment myocardial infarction. *J Am Coll Cardiol* 51:560–565, 2008.

58

Intravascular Ultrasound

YASUHIRO HONDA | PETER J. FITZGERALD | PAUL YOCK

KEY POINTS

- Intravascular ultrasound (IVUS) has evolved as the first clinical imaging method to directly visualize atherosclerosis and other pathologic conditions within the walls of blood vessels.

- Improvements in core IVUS technology have allowed for higher-resolution images and greater operator convenience.

- IVUS has provided significant insights into biologically mediated processes of the vasculature, such as the extent of plaque burden, vascular remodeling, and re-stenosis.

- IVUS has been established as a practically useful tool in clarifying situations in which angiography is equivocal or difficult to interpret, selecting the appropriate catheter-based intervention, and optimizing the results of coronary procedures.

- Advanced technical developments currently being explored may further enhance the usefulness of IVUS in both research and clinical arenas of future interventional cardiology, particularly with sophisticated therapeutic technologies to modify local vascular biology.

Intravascular ultrasound (IVUS) has evolved as the first clinical imaging method to directly visualize atherosclerosis and other pathologic conditions within the walls of blood vessels. Because the ultrasound signal is able to penetrate below the luminal surface, the entire cross-section of an artery—including the complete thickness of a plaque—can be imaged in real time. This offers the opportunity to gather diagnostic information about the process of atherosclerosis and to directly observe the effects of various interventions on the plaque and arterial wall. The first ultrasound imaging catheter system was developed by Bom and colleagues in Rotterdam in 1971 for intracardiac imaging of chambers and valves. In the early to mid-1980s, several groups began work on different catheter systems designed to image plaque and facilitate balloon angioplasty and other catheter-based interventions. The first images of human vessels were recorded by Yock and colleagues in 1988, with coronary images produced the next year by the same group and by Hodgson and colleagues.[1] The intervening period has seen rapid technical improvements of the systems, with significant enhancement in image quality and miniaturization of the imaging catheters.

Imaging Systems and Procedures

BASIC PRINCIPLES

IVUS imaging systems use reflected sound waves to visualize the vessel wall in a two-dimensional, tomographic format, analogous to a histologic cross-section. These systems use significantly higher frequencies than noninvasive echocardiography, achieving greater radial resolutions at the expense of limited beam penetration. The resolution, depth of penetration, and attenuation of the acoustic pulse by tissue are dependent on the geometric and frequency properties of the transducer. Current IVUS catheters used in the coronary arteries have center frequencies ranging from 20 to 45 megahertz (MHz), providing theoretical lower limits of resolution (calculated as half the wavelength) of 31 and 19 μm, respectively. In practice, the radial resolution is at least two to five times poorer (80 to 150 μm), determined by factors such

as the length of the emitted pulse and the position of the imaged structures relative to the transducer. There are two basic catheter designs, based on solid-state or mechanical approaches (Fig. 58-1). Both types of catheters generate a 360-degree, cross-sectional image plane that is perpendicular to the catheter tip.

Solid-State Dynamic Aperture System

In the solid-state approach, the individual elements of a circumferential array of transducer elements mounted near the tip of the catheter are activated with different time delays, to create an ultrasound beam that sweeps the circumference of the vessel. As the number of elements has increased, there have been progressive improvements in lateral resolution. Complex miniaturized integrated circuits in the catheter tip control the timing and integration of the transducer activation and route the resulting echocardiographic information to a computer, where cross-sectional images are reconstructed and displayed in real time. One of the technical advantages of the multi-element approach is the ability to manipulate the beam electronically—achieving, for example, the ability to focus at different depths. The current solid-state coronary catheter system (Volcano Corporation, Rancho Cordova, CA) has 64 transducer elements arranged around the catheter tip and uses a center frequency of 20 MHz. The latest coronary catheters in a rapid-exchange configuration are 3.5 French (F) in scanner diameter and thus compatible with a 5F guiding catheter. Larger peripheral imaging catheters are produced in both over-the-wire and rapid-exchange configurations. As an exception, a phased-array catheter (8F or 10F) for intracardiac imaging (Siemens Medical Solutions USA, Malvern, PA) uses a different technology, adapted from transesophageal echocardiography (TEE), which provides a sector ultrasound image with color and spectral Doppler capabilities. The catheter is compatible with multiple-frequency imaging (5 to 10 MHz) so that the operator can determine the desired trade-off between resolution and penetration (up to 15 cm).

Mechanically Rotating Single-Transducer System

In the mechanical approach, a single transducer element is rotated at 1800 revolutions per minute (rpm), inside a protective sheath at the distal tip of a catheter, via a flexible torque cable spun by an external motor drive unit attached to the proximal end of the catheter. Images from each angular position of the transducer are collected by a computerized image array processor, which synthesizes a cross-sectional ultrasound image of the vessel. The mechanical IVUS system is available commercially from two manufacturers in the United States and one in Japan. The imaging catheters use a 40-MHz or 45-MHz transducer with a distal crossing profile of 3.2F that is compatible with 6F (Boston Scientific Corporation, Natick, MA; Volcano Corporation) or 5F guiding catheters (Terumo Corporation, Tokyo, Japan). Larger catheters with lower center frequencies are also available for peripheral and intracardiac imaging. The catheters are advanced over a standard guidewire using a short rail section located distal to the protective sheath at the catheter tip. The fact that the guidewire runs outside the catheter, parallel to the imaging segment, results in a shadow artifact in the image (the so-called *guidewire artifact*).

Head-to-Head Comparisons

Mechanical systems have traditionally offered advantages in image quality compared with the solid-state systems because of the higher center frequencies and the larger effective aperture of a transducer element. Particularly, near-field resolution is excellent with mechanical catheters so that the digital subtraction of the ring-down artifact is not required. In addition, a stationary outer sheath of mechanical catheters allows the transducer to be moved through a segment of interest in a precise and controlled manner. Conversely, the longer rapid-exchange design of the solid-state catheter may track better than the short rail design of the mechanical systems in complex coronary anatomy. The distance of the transducer from the catheter tip is shorter than that of mechanical systems, which may also be beneficial in IVUS-guided intervention of chronic total occlusion (CTO) of lesions. The solid-state catheter includes no moving parts and, thus, is free from nonuniform rotational image distortion (NURD) (Fig. 58-2). This artifact can occur with mechanical systems when bending of the drive cable interferes with uniform transducer rotation, causing a wedge-shaped, smeared image to appear in one or more segments of the image. This may be corrected by straightening the catheter and motor drive assembly, lessening tension on the guiding catheter, or loosening the hemostatic valve of the Y-adapter.

Overall, however, in both systems, technical improvements are continuously being made, and good quality images can be achieved by either of them in the majority of cases. With both systems, serial cross-sectional images can be reconstructed into a longitudinal display mode, and both still frames and video images can be digitally archived on local storage memory or a remote server using Digital Imaging and Communications in Medicine (DICOM) Standard 3.0. Recently, both systems have begun installation directly into the cine-angiogram

system, enabling operators to quickly and easily incorporate IVUS interrogations into their interventional procedures. With this preinstalled IVUS system, IVUS is always on and ready, obviating the need for console transport between labs. Additionally, the system's tableside controller enables operator control of the device within the sterile field, facilitating direct investigation and exact location of a lesion of interest during the procedure.

IMAGING PROCEDURES

Before IVUS imaging, an intravenous injection of 5000 to 10,000 units of heparin or equivalent anticoagulation should be administered, as well as intracoronary (IC) nitroglycerine (100 to 300 mg), to reduce the risk for spasm. Mechanical catheters require a saline flush before insertion to eliminate any air in the protective sheath. Incomplete flushing can leave microbubbles adjacent to the transducer, resulting in poor image quality once the catheter is inserted (see Fig. 58-2). In either approach, image integrity should be checked before inserting the catheter. With a solid-state catheter, the catheter tip is first positioned in the aorta or a large proximal coronary vessel (not adjacent to any vessel wall) so that the ring-down artifact (a "halo" surrounding the catheter) can be electronically subtracted from the image before entering the coronary artery. If a significant ring-down artifact is observed with a mechanical catheter, microbubbles within the protective sheath may be suspected, requiring repeated saline flush procedures until the artifact is removed (see Fig. 58-2). The technique for delivering IVUS catheters is generally similar to that used for standard angioplasty or stent catheters. The imaging element is advanced distal to the area of interest, and the length of the target vessel is systemically scanned by withdrawal of the entire catheter (solid-state system) or by retracting the transducer within the protective sheath (mechanical system) over a standard 0.014-inch angioplasty guidewire. Automated pull-back devices withdraw the imaging element at a steady rate of 0.5 or 1.0 mm per second, which allows accurate axial registration of each cross-section for serial studies or precise longitudinal distance measurements.

◼ Safety

As with other interventional procedures, the risks of spasm, dissection, and thrombosis exist when intravascular imaging catheters are used. Early multi-center studies documented complication rates at 1% to 3%, including transient spasm as the most frequently reported event. Major complications, such as dissection, thrombosis, and abrupt closure with "certain relation" to IVUS, were identified in less than 0.5%. These studies were performed with first-generation catheters in

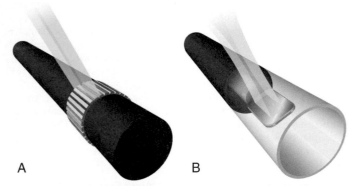

Figure 58-1 Diagrams of the two basic imaging catheter designs: solid-state (*A*) and mechanical (*B*).

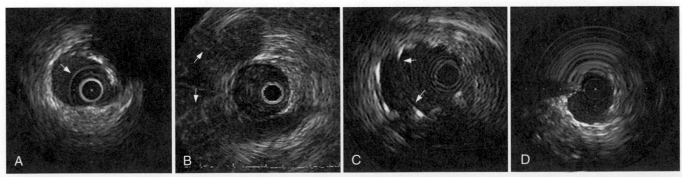

Figure 58-2 Common image artifacts. **A,** A "halo" or a series of bright rings immediately around the mechanical intravascular ultrasound (IVUS) catheter (*arrow*) is usually caused by air bubbles that need to be flushed out. **B,** Radiofrequency noise (*arrows*) appears as alternating radial spokes or random white dots in the far-field. The interference is usually caused by other electrical equipment in the cardiac catheterization laboratory. **C,** "White cap" artifacts caused by side lobe echoes (*arrows*) originate from a strong reflecting surface, such as metal stent struts or calcification. Smearing of the strut image can lead to the mistaken impression that the struts are protruding into the lumen, potentially interfering with area measurements and the assessment of apposition, dissection, and so on. **D,** Non-uniform rotational distortion (NURD) results in a wedge-shaped, smeared appearance in one or more segments of the image (between 9 and 4 o'clock in this example).

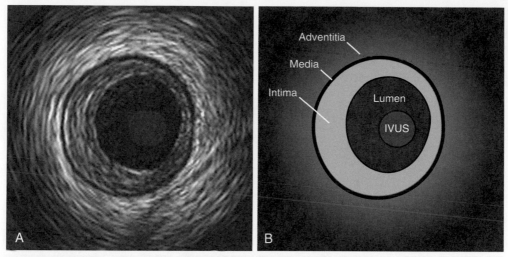

Figure 58-3 Intravascular ultrasound (IVUS) image (*A*) and schematic diagram (*B*) demonstrate the classic three-layered appearance of the intima (plaque), the media, and the adventitia. In many cases, the media can be difficult to resolve clearly in some portion of the image, but in this particular image, it stands out in all sectors. Note the speckled appearance of the blood within the lumen, particularly near the luminal border.

the early 1990s, and it is likely that the incidence of spasm and other complications is substantially lower with the current generation of catheters. No acceleration in the progression of atheroma or allograft vasculopathy of arteries previously imaged by IVUS has been reported compared with noninstrumented arteries.[2,3]

Image Interpretation

THREE-LAYERED APPEARANCE OF ARTERIAL WALL

The interpretation of IVUS images relies on the fact that the layers of a diseased arterial wall can be identified separately. Particularly in muscular arteries, such as the coronary tree, the media of the vessel stands out as a dark band compared with the intima and adventitia (Fig. 58-3). Media are less distinctly seen by IVUS in elastic arteries such as the aorta and the carotid, so differentiation of the layers in those vessels can be problematic. However, most of the vessels currently treated by catheter techniques are muscular or transitional, and identification of the medial layer is usually possible (this includes the coronary, ilio-femoral, renal, and popliteal systems).

The relative echolucency of the media compared with the intima and the adventitia gives rise to a three-layered appearance (bright–dark–bright) (see Fig. 58-3). The lower ultrasound reflectance of the media is caused by the presence of less collagen and elastin than in the neighboring layers. Because the intimal layer reflects ultrasound more strongly compared with the media, a spill-over effect, known as "blooming," is seen in the image. This results in a slight overestimation of the thickness of the intima and a corresponding underestimation of the medial thickness. Conversely, the media–adventitia border is accurately rendered because a step-up in echo reflectivity occurs at this boundary and no blooming appears. The adventitia and periadventitial tissues are similar enough in echo-reflectivity that a clear outer adventitial border cannot be defined.

Several deviations from the classic three-layered appearance are encountered in practice. In truly normal coronary arteries from young patients, echo-reflectivity of the intima and the internal lamina may not be sufficient to resolve a clear inner layer. This is particularly true when the media has a relatively high content of elastin. However, most adults seen in the cardiac catheterization laboratory (cath lab) have enough intimal thickening to show a three-layered appearance, even in angiographically normal segments. At the other end of the spectrum, patients with a significant plaque burden have thinning of the media underlying the plaque, often to the degree that the media is indistinct or undetectable in at least some part of the IVUS

cross-section. This problem is exacerbated by the blooming phenomenon. Even in these cases, however, the inner adventitial boundary (at the level of the external elastic lamina) is generally identifiable. For this reason, most IVUS studies measure and report the plaque-plus-media area as a surrogate measure for plaque area alone. Adding in the media represents only a tiny percentage increase of the total area of the plaque.

IMAGE ORIENTATION

Another important aspect of image interpretation is determining the position of the imaging plane within the artery. The IVUS beam penetrates beyond the artery, providing images of perivascular structures, including the cardiac veins, the myocardium, and the pericardium. These structures have a characteristic appearance when viewed from various positions within the arterial tree, so they provide useful landmarks with regard to the position of the imaging plane (Fig. 58-4). The branching patterns of the arteries are also distinctive and help identify the position of the transducer. In the left anterior descending (LAD) coronary artery system, for example, the septal perforators usually branch at a wider angle compared with the diagonals; on the IVUS scan, the septals appear to bud away from the LAD artery much more abruptly compared with the diagonals. The combination of perivascular landmarks and branching patterns allows the experienced operator to identify the vessel and the segment from the IVUS image alone. It is also important to understand that with the current systems, the rotational orientation of an IVUS image as presented on the screen is arbitrary and can vary between imaging runs. Here again, the branching pattern and perivascular landmarks, once understood, can provide a reference to the actual orientation of the image in space. Some operators prefer to have a standard rotational orientation for each imaging run and take the time to adjust the presentation on the screen by rotating it electronically so that the branches always appear in a uniform position.

QUANTITATIVE VESSEL MEASUREMENTS

Unlike coronary angiograms, IVUS has an intrinsic distance calibration, which is usually displayed as a grid on the image. Electronic caliper (diameter) and tracing (area) measurements can be performed at the tightest cross-section, as well as at reference segments located proximal and distal to the lesion.[4] In general, the reference segment is selected as the most normal-looking cross-section (i.e., largest lumen with smallest plaque burden) occurring within 10 mm of the lesion

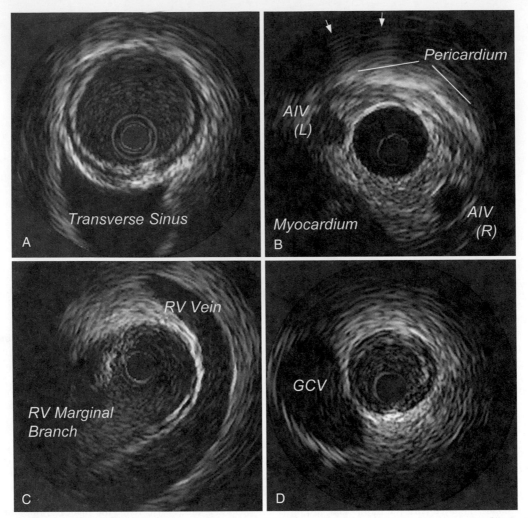

Figure 58-4 Perivascular landmarks. **A,** In the proximal portion of the left main coronary artery, a clear echo-free space filled with pericardial fluid, called the transverse sinus, is found adjacent to the artery, immediately outside of the left lateral aspect of the aortic root. **B,** In this distal cross-section from the left anterior descending (LAD) coronary artery, the right (R) and left (L) branches of the anterior interventricular vein (AIV) are seen to straddle the coronary artery. The pericardium appears as a typical bright stripe with rays emitting from it (arrows). **C,** At the level of the middle right coronary artery, the veins arc over the artery, typically at a position just adjacent to the right ventricular (RV) marginal branches. **D,** The great cardiac vein (GCV), running superiorly to the left circumflex (LCx) coronary artery appears as a large, low-echoic structure with fine blood speckle. Recurrent atrial branches emerge from the LCx artery in an orientation directed toward the GCV, whereas the obtuse marginal branches emerge opposite the GCV and course inferiorly to cover the lateral myocardial wall.

with no intervening major side branches. At lumen assessment, stagnant blood flow, the use of higher frequency IVUS, or both can increase the intensity of blood speckle, which may obscure the blood–tissue interface on a still image. A review of moving images can help identify the true lumen border. At procedure, saline can be injected through the guiding catheter to reduce blood speckle.

Vessel and lumen diameter measurements are important in everyday clinical practice, where accurate sizing of devices is needed. The maximum and minimum diameters (i.e., the major and minor axes of an elliptical cross-section) are the most widely used dimensions. The ratio of maximum diameter to minimum diameter defines a measure of symmetry. Area measurements are performed with computer planimetry. Lumen area is determined by tracing the leading edge of the blood–intima border, whereas the vessel (or external elastic membrane [EEM]) area is defined as the area enclosed by the outermost interface between the media and the adventitia. Plaque area (or plaque-plus-media area) is calculated as the difference between the vessel and lumen areas; the ratio of plaque to vessel area is termed *percent plaque area*, *plaque burden*, or *percent cross-sectional narrowing*. With the use of motorized pull-back, area measurements can be added to calculate volumes using Simpson's rule.

PLAQUE COMPOSITION ON GRAY-SCALE INTRAVASCULAR ULTRASOUND

The early changes of atherosclerotic disease, the so-called "fatty streaks," are too thin to be visualized with IVUS. As plaque continues to develop, it can be resolved on IVUS, with different acoustic properties, depending on the composition of the plaque. A plaque with *extensive lipid infiltration* has low echo-reflectivity (less than the adventitia) on IVUS. Plaques with predominantly *fibrous tissue* are more echogenic than fat-laden plaques and can cause signal attenuation to some degree. *Calcified plaque* is recognized by a bright interface that overlies a dark shadow extending radially outward (Fig. 58-5). This acoustic shadowing, often accompanied by "reverberations" (regularly spaced arcs deep to the initial bright interface), obscures the true thickness of the calcified plaque as well as any deeper tissue. Calcium is seen by IVUS in 60% to 80% of lesions undergoing intervention, only half of which are detected by fluoroscopy or angiography. A rough rule of thumb is that an arc of calcium must occupy two quadrants (180 degrees) on IVUS to be visible on fluoroscopy. Calcium on IVUS is seen more frequently with increasing age and in patients with stable (as opposed to unstable) angina, and correlates more with plaque

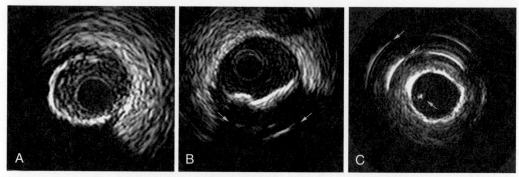

Figure 58-5 Examples of coronary calcification. **A,** A rim of calcium is seen between 5 and 10 o'clock positions, located beneath a fibro-fatty plaque that tightly surrounds the catheter. Note the shadowing beyond the calcium. **B,** Superficial calcium (between 3 and 7 o'clock positions) at the luminal surface. Speckles within the lumen are signals from blood. **C,** Circumferential, "napkin ring" calcification. Two arcs of reverberation are seen (*orange arrows*), and another pair of reverberations is seen to the right of the arrows. The small bright point adjacent to the catheter at 8:30 o'clock (*blue arrow*) is guidewire artifact from this mechanical catheter.

burden than lesion severity. One of the major limitations of IVUS in tissue identification is the difficulty in discriminating thrombus from soft plaque, which has a similar signal, or "texture," and brightness. IVUS clues to the presence of thrombus include (1) a nodular appearance or clefts in the tissue; (2) small channels within the mass; (3) scintillating appearance (reminiscent of amyloidosis on transthoracic echocardiography [TTE]); or (4) tissue that moves (wiggles) in response to motion of the vessel wall.[4]

ADVANCED TISSUE CHARACTERIZATION

To enhance the accuracy of in vivo plaque characterization by IVUS, several advanced signal analysis techniques have been developed and introduced into the research and clinical arenas. Current commercialized systems attempt to identify tissue components directly or the deformability of the tissue ("palpography") using computer-assisted analysis of raw radiofrequency (RF) signals in the reflected ultrasound beam.[5] This analysis is based on the fact that there is greater information contained in the backscattered ultrasound signal than is revealed by the conventional amplitude-based image presentation alone. One system simply uses integrated backscatter values, calculated as the average power of the backscattered ultrasound signal from a sample tissue volume, to differentiate tissue types (IB-IVUS, YD Co., Ltd.). Two other systems employ spectral RF analyses with a classification tree algorithm developed from ex vivo coronary datasets (Virtual Histology™, Volcano Corporation) or a pattern recognition technique based on the degree of spectral similarity between the backscattered signal and a reference library of spectra from known tissue types (iMap™, Boston Scientific Corporation).[6] All systems generate color-mapped images of the vessel wall, with a distinct color for each plaque component category (Fig. 58-6). When combined with automated pull-back and border detection techniques, these systems can provide a quantitative assessment of each tissue category over a three-dimensional coronary artery volume. Current technical limitations include limited spatial resolution (100 to 250 µm), no classifications for thrombus, blood, or intimal hyperplasia, and potential errors caused by poor ultrasound penetration through extensive calcification.

All systems have demonstrated a correlation of IVUS-determined plaque compositions with corresponding histopathology of coronary specimens.[5] Subsequent clinical studies showed that the IVUS-determined plaque vulnerability (large lipid or necrotic core) was related to unstable lesion characteristics or clinical presentations, but controversial results also exist (less necrotic core and more fibrous tissue in acute coronary syndromes). Among several multi-center studies initiated worldwide, PROSPECT (Providing Regional Observations to Study Predictors of Events in the Coronary Tree) is one of the largest natural history trials that prospectively employed three-vessel imaging with Virtual Histology and IVUS palpography in 700 patients with acute coronary syndrome (ACS). The interim 3-year results reported that a large necrotic core without a visible cap observed at baseline Virtual Histology was one of the strong independent predictors for future adverse cardiovascular events. Clinical follow-up to 5 years is ongoing, and the role of this technology in the detection of vulnerable plaque has yet to be established.

Diagnostic Applications: Insights into Plaque Formation and Distribution

The application of IVUS in clinical practice has given us several unique insights into the nature of coronary disease. For example, IVUS generally reveals a much larger plaque burden than that estimated by angiography. When a vessel appears to have a discrete stenosis by angiography, IVUS almost invariably shows that there is considerable atherosclerotic disease present through the entire length of the vessel. Even a reference that is normal or near-normal angiographically has, on average, plaque burden in 35% to 51% of the cross-sectional area. IVUS also gives a precise representation of the distribution of plaque within the vessel wall—specifically, the eccentricity or concentricity of atherosclerotic plaque—and the relationship of plaque volume to vessel wall area. Plaques that appear to be concentric by angiography are often eccentric by IVUS, and vice versa. Consistent with postmortem studies, IVUS has demonstrated that proximal LAD artery lesions are localized on the opposite wall from the flow divider between the LAD artery and the left circumflex (LCx) artery, supporting the theory that abnormally low shear forces contribute to plaque formation. Similarly, studies have shown that atherosclerotic plaque tends to form more on the inner curvature of the vessel arc (the wall opposite of pericardium when seen on IVUS).

Remodeling—localized expansion of the vessel wall in areas of high plaque burden as originally described by Glagov—occurs as if the vessel was stretching to accommodate the accumulation of plaque so as to avoid luminal encroachment. The remodeling response is, in fact, heterogeneous, with some segments showing the positive Glagov remodeling and others showing negative remodeling (shrinkage or constriction, that works in conjunction with plaque burden to accentuate luminal stenosis). The assessment of remodeling can be clinically important in determining optimal sizing for a therapeutic device. The degree of remodeling has also been shown to correlate with vulnerability to plaque rupture and with acute or long-term outcomes of intervention. The active lesions responsible for unstable angina or ACS have usually undergone extensive positive remodeling. Several studies have also shown that preinterventional positive remodeling predicts no-reflow phenomena, target lesion revascularization, and in-hospital

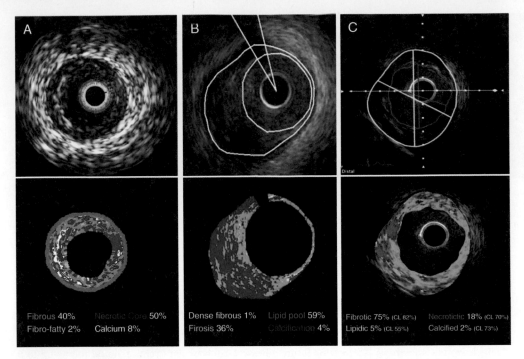

Figure 58-6 Examples of plaque characterization by radiofrequency intravascular ultrasound (IVUS) analysis. **A,** Virtual Histology™ (Volcano Corp.). Plaque components are determined using spectral radiofrequency signal analyses with a classification algorithm. *Dark green,* fibrous; *light green,* fibrofatty; *white,* calcium; *red,* necrotic core. **B,** A color-mapped presentation of integrated backscatter values (IB-IVUS. YD Co., Ltd.). *Blue,* lipid pool; *green,* fibrous; *yellow,* dense fibrous; *red,* calcification. **C,** iMap™ (Boston Scientific Corp.). Classification of tissue is made based on the degree of similarity between the sample and reference frequency spectrum. This method enables confidence level (CL) assessment of each plaque component along with a color-mapped presentation superimposed on the corresponding gray-scale image.

complications following coronary interventions. Although the predictive value in the context of stenting has not been established with certainty, cumulative evidence suggests that positively remodeled lesions are more biologically active than intermediate or negatively remodeled lesions.

Serial Monitoring of Disease Progression or Regression

The ability of IVUS to quantify arterial wall disease in a precise and reproducible manner allows serial evaluation of atherosclerotic plaque or transplant vasculopathy for the assessment of disease progression or regression. In serial studies for this purpose, the same IVUS system (in terms of catheter type, imaging console, and pull-back device) should be used for serial imaging procedures at baseline and follow-up in a given patient. The use of automated pull-back is mandatory for accurate axial registration of analysis segment. Some investigators recommend electrocardiogram (ECG)–gated image acquisition with a dedicated pull-back device, or software-based ECG-gated frame analysis of IVUS images obtained with a conventional pull-back device, although the exact impact of these approaches on the outcomes of clinical studies has not been documented. A certain length of untreated coronary segment (typically 30–50 mm) is preselected for serial analyses using anatomic landmarks such as major side branches. Volume data are often normalized by pull-back length (expressed as mean area) or vessel size (expressed as percent volume) for comparative analysis.

The change of the intima or the plaque volume measured by IVUS has been increasingly used as a surrogate endpoint in clinical trials of the natural history of atherosclerosis and transplant vasculopathy and in monitoring the results of pharmacologic interventions such as lipid lowering. Relying on angiographic assessment alone for accurate evaluation of disease progression or regression is extremely challenging, particularly with a diffuse extent of disease, a variable degree of arterial remodeling, or both. One pending question is whether disease progression or regression measured by IVUS would effectively reflect an increased or decreased risk of future cardiovascular events. Although several clinical trials suggest a significant association, a discrepancy between the imaging endpoint and clinical outcome has also been

implied in some studies.[7–10] Interestingly, recent clinical trials that employed IB-IVUS or Virtual Histology have demonstrated stabilization of plaque composition by anti-atherosclerotic agents, despite no change in total plaque volume observed by conventional IVUS measurement.[11,12] Advanced tissue characterization techniques may supplement the simple plaque quantification by gray-scale IVUS, thereby enhancing the usefulness of IVUS-defined endpoints in the evaluation of new pharmacologic therapies.

Interventional Applications

PREINTERVENTIONAL ASSESSMENT

Angiographic Lesion Ambiguity

Preinterventional IVUS has been used to clarify situations in which angiography is equivocal or difficult to interpret (especially in ostial lesions or tortuous segments in which the angiogram may not lay out the vessel well for interpretation). For intermediate lesions, the minimum lumen area (MLA) is the most commonly used IVUS parameter for deferring intervention. The ischemic MLA threshold is 3 to 4 mm^2 for major epicardial coronary arteries and 5.5 to 6 mm^2 for the left main coronary artery (LMCA), based on physiologic assessment with coronary flow reserve, fractional flow reserve, or stress scintigraphy. In practice, clinical and other lesion characteristics in a given patient should also be considered for final decision making.

In the assessment of LMCA disease, angulations, calcification, or spasm in this location can lead to poor catheter engagement and confounded angiographic interpretation (Fig. 58-7). Several investigators have demonstrated that high percentages of patients with angiographically normal LMCA are seen to have disease by IVUS. Conversely, a recent IVUS study demonstrated that less than half of the angiographically ambiguous LMCA lesions had significant stenosis.[13] This was especially true for ostial LMCA disease, where only 36% of the lesions had a significant stenosis, and 41% had plaque burden less than 50% as assessed by IVUS. Moreover, IVUS can also differentiate between true ostial and "pseudo-ostial" lesions. Thus, patients with LMCA disease merit IVUS or physiologic assessment before a blind decision about treatment strategy is made, since the result of detailed evaluation can dramatically alter management and prognosis.

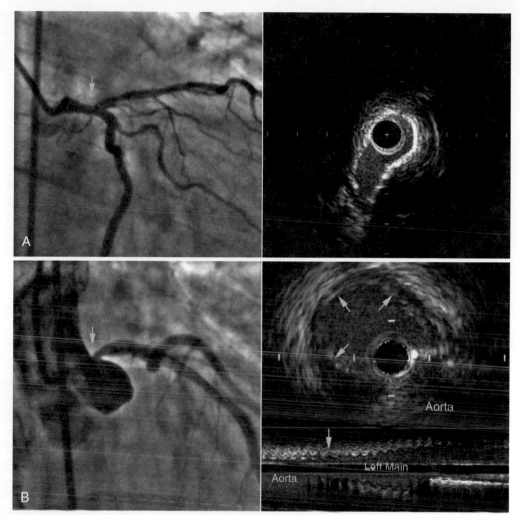

Figure 58-7 Two example cases of left main coronary artery (LMCA) assessment by intravascular ultrasound (IVUS). **A,** A moderate stenosis (*orange arrow*) is observed at the distal LMCA segment by angiography (*left*). IVUS reveals a significant lumen narrowing with napkin-ring superficial calcification at the corresponding segment (*right*). **B,** A significant stenosis (*orange arrow*) at the orifice of the LMCA is suspected by angiography (*left*). IVUS demonstrates reverse vessel tapering of the corresponding segment with only mild plaque accumulation (*blue arrows*) (*right*).

Strategic Plaque Assessment

Preinterventional IVUS imaging is useful in determining the appropriate catheter-based intervention strategy. With current IVUS catheters, most significant stenoses can be safely imaged before intervention, providing detailed information about circumferential and longitudinal extent of the plaque as well as the character of the tissue involved. When observed by IVUS, angiographically hazy lesions represent a spectrum of morphologies, including calcium, dissection, thrombus, and excessive plaque burden with extreme remodeling. In particular, the presence, location, and extent of calcium can significantly affect the results of intervention (see Fig. 58-5). Following balloon angioplasty, dissections are often observed at the junction of calcified and noncalcified plaque, where shear forces from dilation are high. For lesions with extensive superficial calcium, plaque modification through the use of rotational atherectomy may be required before balloon dilatation, stent implantation, or both. Conversely, lesions with deep calcium may be successfully treated by stand-alone stenting, even when severe calcification is seen on fluoroscopy. The amount and distribution of plaque can also be accurately determined, and precise measurements of lesion length and vessel size can guide the optimal sizing of devices to be employed.

Detailed assessment of target lesion anatomy in the coronary tree is also useful to prevent major side-branch encroachment by intervention. At bifurcation lesions, the extent of side-branch involvement can be difficult to assess with angiography alone, and the decision to pursue revascularization or protection of the side branch is often made based on ambiguous demonstration of these complex lesions.

The combination of plaque and carina shift following balloon dilatation or stenting may cause severe narrowing or occlusion of a side branch, particularly in the presence of a pre-existing ostial disease.[14] Such anatomic situations are responsible for the majority of creatine kinase elevations following stent implantation. Plaque deposition in the ostial lesion of a side branch can often be appreciated by looking across from the parent artery into the ostium of the branch, although accurate assessment requires direct imaging of the side branch.

In addition, evaluation of plaque composition by preinterventional IVUS may predict the occurrence of distal emboli during balloon dilatation or stenting that may result in the "slow-flow" or "no-reflow" phenomenon leading to peri-procedural myocardial infarction (MI). In gray-scale IVUS, predictive findings include large plaque burden with (non–calcium-related) signal attenuation, a large low-echoic region suggesting a lipid pool, and thrombus-containing plaque (Fig. 58-8).[15] Recent studies with IB-IVUS or Virtual Histology also demonstrated that the amount of lipid or necrotic core at preintervention was related to findings suggesting distal emboli.[16-19] Identification of high-risk plaques may help in selecting lesions suitable for distal protection devices.

RE-STENOTIC LESIONS

IVUS can accurately identify the primary mechanism of re-stenosis, which can significantly affect the treatment strategy in patients with re-stenotic lesions. In nonstent interventions, the majority of late

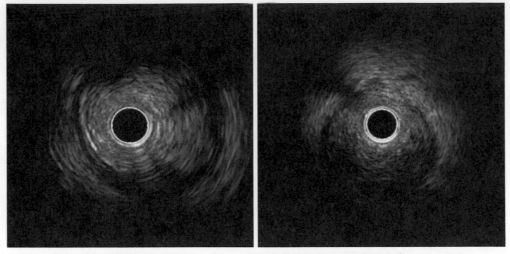

Figure 58-8 Lesions with large plaque burden and non–calcium-related signal attenuation. These characteristic appearances by gray-scale intravascular ultrasound are recognized as risk factors for occurrence of distal emboli during balloon dilatation or stenting.

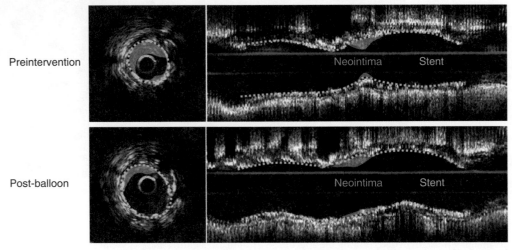

Preintervention

Post-balloon

Figure 58-9 Drug-eluting stent (DES) re-stenosis resulted primarily from stent underexpansion. Preinterventional intravascular ultrasound (*upper*) reveals significant stent underexpansion at the mid-segment with only a small amount of focal neointimal hyperplasia. This type of in-stent re-stenosis can be successfully treated with mechanical optimization by balloon dilatation and may not require additional DES implantation within the original re-stenotic stent.

lumen loss was caused by negative arterial remodeling (a decrease in vessel cross-sectional area), with only about a quarter of the late loss caused by tissue proliferation. In contrast, late loss in stented lesions is primarily caused by neointimal proliferation rather than by chronic stent recoil. It is important to note, however, that initial stent underexpansion can result in clinically significant lumen compromise, even with minimal neointimal hyperplasia (Fig. 58-9). Using preinterventional IVUS examination in 1090 consecutive in-stent re-stenosis (ISR) lesions, Castagna and colleagues showed that 20% of lesions had an MSA less than 5 mm^2 and that an additional 4.5% had other mechanical problems that contributed to re-stenosis.[20] In most of these cases, stent underexpansion or other mechanical problems were not suspected angiographically at the time of re-intervention. For this type of ISR, mechanical optimization is the first priority, and IVUS can be helpful to differentiate mechanical issues from exaggerated neointimal proliferation that may truly require drug-eluting stent (DES) implantation within the original re-stenotic stent.

BARE METAL STENTS

Insights into Mechanism of Action

Stent struts are easily visualized on IVUS examination as a collection of bright, distinct echoes, characteristic for each stent type. In contrast, the proliferative tissue within the stent struts has low echo-reflectivity, similar to thrombus, so that optimal instrument settings are required to visualize the re-stenotic material clearly. Stents essentially provide a rigid scaffold against the force of vessel recoil. During stent implantation, axial extrusion of noncalcified plaque into the adjacent reference zones can occur. Although a similar phenomenon can be observed in balloon angioplasty, the extrusion effect seen in stenting may be more prominent, commensurate with the increased ability of the stent to enlarge and hold open the treated segment. Extrusion of plaque may also contribute to the step-up or step-down appearance seen on angiography, as well as some of the side-branch encroachment after stent deployment.

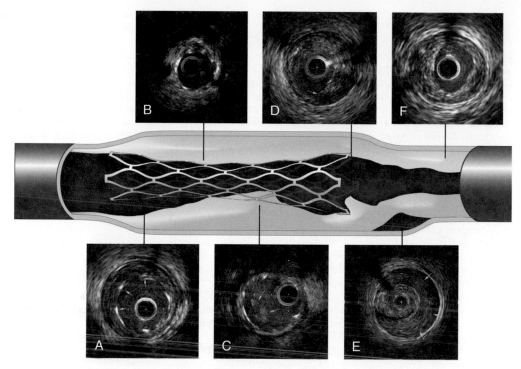

Figure 58-10 Problems with stent deployment detected by intravascular ultrasound (IVUS). The diagram indicates the cross-sections shown in the IVUS images. **A,** Incomplete apposition, in which there is a gap between a portion of the stent (*arrows*) and the vessel wall. **B,** Incomplete expansion relative to the ends of the stent and the reference segments. **C,** Tissue protrusion (plaque prolapse, thrombus, or both) (*arrows*) within the stent. **D,** An edge tear or "pocket flap" with a disruption of plaque (*arrow*) at the stent margin. **E,** Intramural hematoma detected as an accumulation of blood within the medial space (*arrows*) starting from the edge of the stent. **F,** Significant residual plaque burden at the segment uncovered by the stent.

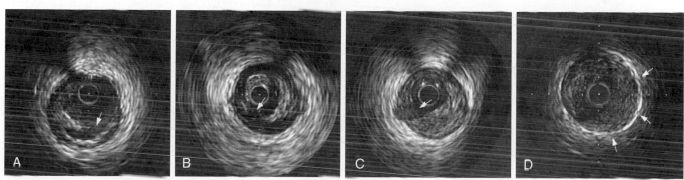

Figure 58-11 Four examples of dissections. **A,** A superficial (intimal) dissection starting at 6 o'clock and extending clockwise. The dissection flap does not extend far into the lumen. **B,** A deeper (medial) dissection with a flap extending into the lumen may compromise flow or precede abrupt closure. Injection of contrast in this setting can demonstrate free fluid flow behind the flap to better define the extent of tear. **C,** Eccentric plaque with a deep (adventitial) dissection at 8 o'clock that penetrates the external elastic lamina and extends into the adventitia. **D,** Intramural hematoma appears as an accumulation of blood within the medial space, displacing the internal elastic membrane inward and the external elastic membrane outward.

Common Stent Problems

IVUS has identified several stent deployment issues, including incomplete expansion and incomplete apposition (Fig. 58-10). Incomplete expansion occurs when a portion of the stent is inadequately expanded compared with the distal and proximal reference dimensions, as may occur where dense fibrocalcific plaque is present. Incomplete apposition occurs when part of the stent structure is not fully in contact with the vessel wall, possibly increasing local flow disturbances and the potential risk for subacute thrombosis in certain clinical settings. The collaborative work of Tobis and Colombo in the early 1990s demonstrated an unexpectedly high percentage of these stent deployment issues, leading to their development of the current high-pressure stent deployment techniques. After stent implantation, tears at the edge of the stent (marginal tears or pocket flaps) occur in 10% to 15% of cases (Fig. 58-11). These tears have been attributed to the shear forces created at the junction between the metal edge of the stent and the adjacent, more compliant tissue or to the effect of balloon expansion beyond the edge of the stent (the "dog–bone" phenomenon). Although minor non–flow-limiting edge dissections may not be associated with late angiographic ISR, significant residual dissections can lead to an increased risk of early major adverse cardiac events (MACEs). The current approach is to make a determination from the IVUS image as to whether the tear appears to be flow limiting (i.e., whether there is an extensive tissue arm projecting into the lumen). If this is the case, an additional stent is placed to cover this region. It is important to note, however, that an angiographic hazy appearance following stenting can represent a broad morphologic spectrum, including not only dissection but also calcium, thrombus, hematoma, tissue protrusion at the stent edge, and large residual plaque with positive vessel remodeling. These entities can be readily differentiated by direct visualization with post-stent IVUS, which is essential in determining the need and selection of appropriate adjunctive procedures.

Suboptimal Stenting and Subacute Thrombosis

Over the past decade, a number of studies have shown that IVUS-guided stent placement improves the clinical outcome of bare metal stents (BMSs). In the Multicenter Ultrasound-guided Stent Implantation in Coronaries (MUSIC) trial, IVUS-guided stenting required (1) complete apposition over the entire stent length; (2) in-stent minimum stent area (MSA) greater than or equal to 90% of the average of the reference areas or 100% of the smallest reference area; and (3) symmetric stent expansion with the minimum–maximum lumen diameter ratio greater than or equal to 0.7. Subacute thrombosis of less than 2% was believed to represent a reduction compared with non-IVUS guided deployment, although, with current anti-platelet regimens, similar results can usually be achieved with high-pressure postdilation without IVUS confirmation. Nevertheless, a number of studies have suggested a link between suboptimal stent implantation and stent thrombosis, including the Predictors and Outcomes of Stent Thrombosis (POST) registry, which demonstrated that 90% of thrombosis patients had suboptimal IVUS results (incomplete apposition, 47%; incomplete expansion, 52%; and evidence of thrombus, 24%), even though only 25% of patients had abnormalities on angiography.[21,22] These observations were replicated in a more recent study by Cheneau and colleagues, which suggested that mechanical factors continue to contribute to stent thrombosis, even in this modern stent era, with optimized anti-platelet regimens.[23] Although the use of IVUS in all patients for the sole purpose of reducing thrombosis is clearly not warranted from a cost standpoint, IVUS imaging should be considered in patients who are at particularly high risk for thrombosis (e.g., slow flow) or in whom the consequences of thrombosis would be severe (e.g., LMCA or equivalent).

Impact of Stent Expansion on Long-Term Outcomes

MSA, as measured by IVUS, is one of the strongest predictors for both angiographic and clinical re-stenosis after bare metal stenting. The predicted risk of re-stenosis decreases 19% for every 1-mm^2 increase in MSA, and stents with an MSA greater than 9 mm^2 have a greatly reduced risk of re-stenosis. In the Can Routine Ultrasound Improve Stent Expansion (CRUISE) trial, IVUS guidance by operator preferences increased MSA from 6.25 to 7.14 mm^2, leading to a 44% relative reduction in target vessel revascularization at 9 months compared with angiographic guidance alone.[24] In the Angiography versus IVUS-Directed stent placement (AVID) trial, IVUS-guided stent implantation resulted in larger acute dimensions compared with angiography alone (7.54 vs. 6.94 mm^2), with no increase in complications, and lower 12-month target lesion revascularization rates for vessels with angiographic reference diameter less than 3.25 mm, severe stenosis at preintervention (>70% angiographic diameter stenosis), and vein grafts.[25] However, controversial results were also reported in some IVUS-guided stent trials, presumably because of differing procedural endpoints for IVUS-guided stenting as well as various adjunctive treatment strategies that were used in these trials in response to suboptimal results (Table 58-1).[26,27] Overall, a meta-analysis of nine clinical studies (2972 patients) demonstrated that IVUS-guided stenting significantly lowers 6-month angiographic re-stenosis (odds ratio [OR] 0.75; 95% confidence interval [CI] 0.60–0.94, $P = 0.01$) and target vessel revascularizations (OR 0.62; 95% CI 0.49–0.78, $P = 0.00003$), with a neutral effect on death and nonfatal MI, compared with an angiographic optimization.[28]

DRUG-ELUTING STENTS

Mechanism of Action

IVUS observations from the clinical experience with anti-proliferative DESs have shown a striking inhibition of in-stent neointimal hyperplasia, whereas the mechanical performances of these new stents are similar to those of conventional BMSs.[29] Additionally, both statistical and geographic distributions of neointimal hyperplasia can be significantly different between the biologic (DES) and mechanical (BMS) stents. In general, neointimal volume (as a percentage of stent volume) within BMS follows a near-Gaussian or normal frequency distribution, with a mean value of 30% to 35%. The standard deviation of this statistical distribution represents biologic variability in vascular response to acute and chronic vessel injury by interventions. In contrast, biologic modifications by DES often result in a non-Gaussian frequency distribution, with variable degrees of the tail ends.[29] Because re-stenosis corresponds to the right tail end of the distribution curve, a discrepancy between mean neointimal volume and binary or clinical re-stenosis can occur in DES trials. Similarly, studies of the BMS have shown a wide individual variation in geographic distribution of neointima along the stented segment, whereas some types of DES demonstrated predilection of in-stent neointimal hyperplasia for specific locations (e.g., proximal stent edge).[29] In serial IVUS studies with multiple long-term follow-up, neointima within non–re-stenotic BMSs showed mild regression after 6 months. In contrast, both sirolimus-eluting and paclitaxel-eluting stents showed a slight but continuous increase in neointimal hyperplasia for up to 4 years.[29]

Intravascular Ultrasound Predictors of Failure of Drug-Eluting Stents

There is compelling clinical evidence that procedure-related factors are important contributors to the development of both re-stenosis and thrombosis after DES implantation. In particular, the most consistent risk factor is stent underexpansion, which has a reported incidence of 60% to 80% of DES failures. In a study of native coronary lesions treated with sirolimus-eluting stents, the only independent predictors of angiographic re-stenosis were postprocedural final MSA less than 5.5 mm^2 and IVUS-measured stent length greater than 40 mm (OR 0.586 and 1.029, respectively).[30] In a series of re-stenotic BMS lesions treated with sirolimus-eluting stents, 82% of recurrent lesions had an MSA less than 5 mm^2 versus 26% of nonrecurrent lesions ($P = 0.003$).[31] As previously discussed, the drugs on current DESs dramatically reduce the variability of the biologic response (neointimal proliferation) and, therefore, magnify the prognostic value of the MSA as a powerful predictor for ISR compared with that in the BMS era.[32]

Although published data on DES thrombosis are still limited, several small IVUS studies have suggested stent underexpansion and significant residual reference disease as risk factors of acute, subacute, or late DES thrombosis.[33-35] Some groups have also suggested baseline or late incomplete stent apposition (ISA) as another possible risk factor.[33-36] Notably, however, there is significant overlap in each risk factor between thrombosis and nonthrombosis cases, undoubtedly representing the multi-factorial process of this phenomenon. Nevertheless, the importance of procedural optimization cannot be overemphasized because these risk factors are the only variables that operators could alter in the cardiac cath lab.

Late-Acquired Incomplete Stent Apposition

ISA is characterized by IVUS as one or more struts clearly separated from the vessel wall, with evidence of blood speckle behind the strut in a segment not associated with any side branches. With serial IVUS performed immediately after the procedure and at follow-up ISA can be classified as baseline or late acquired (Fig. 58-12). At follow-up, baseline ISA may have resolved or may persist; therefore, ISA observed at follow-up could be either persistent baseline ISA (persistent ISA) or newly developed ISA in the segment where struts were completely apposed to the vessel wall at the baseline (late-acquired ISA).

Despite optimal angiographic results with high-pressure balloon dilatation, baseline ISA can be observed with IVUS in 8% to 30% of DES recipients. This morphologic abnormality primarily results from undersized stent selection, stent underexpansion, or insufficient stent conformability in calcified or complex-shaped lesions (the so-called *mechanical ISA*).

The incidence of late-acquired ISA appears to be dependent on treatment modality. This phenomenon was first brought into the spotlight in intracoronary brachytherapy trials (9.3% average incidence by IVUS). However, subsequent IVUS studies have revealed that this can

TABLE 58-1	Intravascular Ultrasound versus Angiographic Guidance of Bare Metal Stent Implantation						
	N	Population	Study Design	IVUS Criteria for Optimal Deployment	Criteria Fulfilled	Endpoints	Results
Albiero et al.	312	De novo Native	Multicenter Registry	Complete apposition, No ref disease, MSA ≥60% of average ref VA (early phase) or MSA ≥ distal ref LA (late phase)	NA	6-mo angiography	IVUS better (early phase)
Blasini, et al.	212	De novo & restenotic Native & SVG	Single center Registry	Complete apposition, No residual dissection, MSA >8 mm² and/or 90% of average ref LA	50%	6-mo angiography	IVUS better
Choi, et al.	278	De novo Native	Single center Registry	Complete apposition, No residual dissection, MSA ≥80% of distal ref LA	NA	Acute closure 6-mo MACE	IVUS better
Gaster, et al.	108	De novo & restenotic Native	Single center Randomized	MUSIC criteria	64%	6-mo angiography, CFR, FFR, TVR, 2.5-yr MACE	IVUS better
AVID	759	De novo Native & SVG	Multicenter Randomized	MUSIC criteria	NA	12-mo TLR	IVUS better (subset analysis)
CENIC	54526	De novo & restenotic Native & SVG	Multicenter Registry	Discretion of individual operator practice	—	In-hospital MACE	IVUS better
CRUISE	499	De novo & restenotic Native	Multicenter Nonrandomized	Discretion of individual operator practice	—	9-mo TVR	IVUS better
DIPOL	259	De novo Native	Multicenter Randomized	Complete apposition, MSA >7.5 mm³ or 80% of average ref LA	>90%	6-mo MACE	IVUS better
OPTICUS	550	De novo & restenotic Native	Multicenter Randomized	MUSIC criteria	56%	6-mo angiography, 12-mo MACE	No difference
PRESTO	9070	De novo & restenotic Native	Multicenter Nonrandomized	Discretion of individual operator practice	—	9-mo MACE	No difference
RESIST	155	De novo Native	Multicenter Randomized	MSA >80% of average ref LA	80%	6-mo angiography, 18-mo MACE	IVUS better (non-significant reduction)
SIPS	269	De novo & restenotic Native	Single center Randomized	MLA >65% of average ref LA	69%	6-mo angiography, 2-yr TLR	IVUS better
TULIP	144	Long lesions >20 mm	Single center Randomized	Complete apposition, MLD ≥80% of average ref diameter MSA ≥ distal ref LA	89%	6-mo angiography, 12-mo MACE	IVUS better

AVID, Angiography Versus IVUS-Directed stent placement trial; CENIC, Central Nacional de Intervenções Cardiovasculares; CFR, coronary flow reserve; CRUISE, Can Routine Ultrasound Influence Stent Expansion study; DIPOL, Direct Stenting versus Optimal Angioplasty; FFR, fractional flow reserve; IVUS, intravascular ultrasound; LA, lumen area; MACE, major adverse cardiac events; MLD, minimum lumen diameter; MSA, minimum stent area; MUSIC, Multicenter Ultrasound guided Stent Implantation in Coronaries; OPTICUS, OPTimization with ICUS to reduce stent restenosis; PRESTO, Prevention of REStenosis with Tranilast and its Outcomes trial; ref, reference vessel; RESIST, REStenosis after Intravascular ultrasound STenting; SIPS, Strategy for IVUS-guided PTCA and Stenting; SVG, saphenous vein graft; TLR, target lesion revascularization; TVR, target vessel revascularization; TULIP, Thrombocyte activity evaluation and effects of Ultrasound guidance in Long Intracoronary stent Placement; VA, vessel area.

also occur in up to 5% to 6% of balloon-expandable BMS recipients. In contrast the incidence of late acquired ISA related to DES significantly varies among different DES types and patient populations. In elective stenting, phosphorylcholine (PC)–coated zotarolimus-eluting stents have consistently shown extremely low incidences of late-acquired ISA (0.4% in ENDEAVOR-I to IV), compared to reports of 8–13% in patients treated with sirolimus- or paclitaxel-eluting stents.[37-39] Even higher incidences are observed in more complex studies enrolling patients with acute MI or CTO or those treated with atherectomy before stenting. Overall, a recent meta-analysis of seven randomized trials reported that the risk of late-acquired ISA in patients with DESs was four times higher compared with those with BMSs (OR 4.36, 95% CI 1.74–10.94, $P = 0.002$).[36] Late-acquired ISA primarily results from structural vessel wall changes that occur during the follow-up period (the so-called biological ISA). This is in contrast to the ISA seen with the initial deployment of either the BMS or the DES, which is a mechanical issue. The most commonly reported mechanisms for late ISA are (1) dissolution of thrombus present at the baseline and (2) regional positive vessel remodeling disproportional to peri-stent plaque area change.[39] Whereas thrombus dissolution can be seen in any type of stent in the treatment of thrombus-containing lesions, abnormal positive vessel remodeling is observed more frequently in patients who received DESs or brachytherapy. With regard to vessel remodeling, incompletely apposed struts are seen primarily in eccentric plaques, and the gaps develop mainly on the disease-free side of the vessel wall.[40] Thus, the combination of mechanical injury at stent implantation and biologic injury by DES components may predispose the vessel wall to chronic, pathologic dilatation in the setting of little underlying plaque.[41] At present, the clinical significance of late-acquired ISA is still being debated. The majority of clinical trials failed to show a direct association between late-acquired ISA and later thrombotic events at further follow-up. Conversely, IVUS examination of late DES thrombosis often shows significant ISA at the time of the event. This discrepancy may be partly caused by the number of late-acquired ISA in each study being too small to be powered to detect a causal relationship with rare thrombotic events. To overcome this issue, a literature-based meta-analysis was recently performed, suggesting a significantly higher risk of late or very late DES thrombosis in patients with late ISA (persistent or late-acquired) compared with those without late ISA (OR 6.51, 95% CI 1.34–34.91, $P = 0.02$).[36] However, careful interpretation of this association is still required because of the inherent limitations of literature-based analyses of heterogeneous studies. Another methodologic issue with respect to the clinical relevance of late-acquired ISA is lack of appropriate grading or classification. Reported late-acquired ISA is a spectrum ranging from tiny incomplete apposition to extensive aneurysm formation, and late-acquired ISA associated with thrombosis is often at the extreme end of this spectrum (Fig. 58-13). In addition, the mechanisms by which

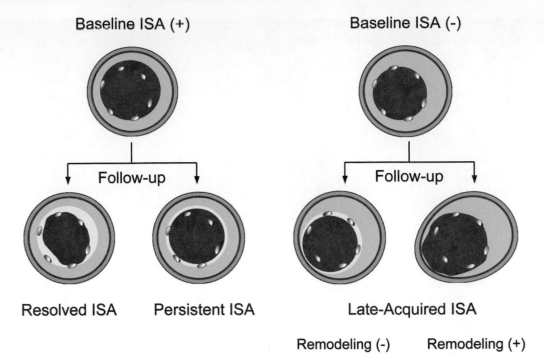

Figure 58-12 Classification of incomplete stent apposition (ISA). Baseline ISA can either be resolved (resolved ISA) or remain (persistent ISA) at follow-up. Late-acquired ISA without vessel expansion is typically seen in thrombus-containing lesions, whereas late-acquired ISA with focal, positive vessel remodeling is more characteristic with brachytherapy and drug-eluting stents.

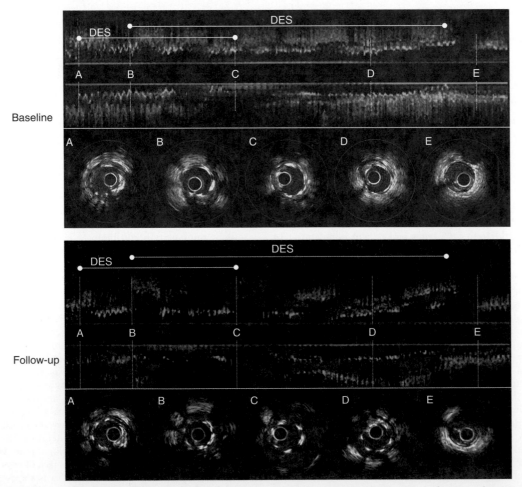

Figure 58-13 Extensive late-acquired incomplete stent apposition observed at follow-up after implantation of two overlapping drug-eluting stents (DESs). At follow-up, large gaps between the stent and the vessel wall (*red areas*) are detected throughout the stented segment, whereas the stent struts are well apposed to the vessel wall at baseline.

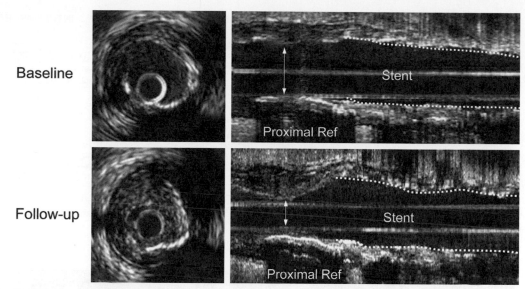

Figure 58-14 Proximal disease development 8 months after drug-eluting stent implantation. In this example, the new stenosis at the proximal stent margin is primarily caused by plaque proliferation despite minimal neointimal hyperplasia observed inside the stent. Baseline intravascular ultrasound reveals a significant residual plaque at the corresponding uncovered segment.

ISA may contribute to DES thrombosis appear to be multi-factorial. Long persistence of incompletely apposed DES struts (persistent baseline ISA or late acquired ISA) may be associated with delayed re-endothelialization allowing fibrin and platelet deposition. A significant gap or aneurysm formation may reduce local blood flow that promotes platelet adhesion and the coagulation cascade. Or the late development of ISA may simply represent a pathologic process within the arterial wall, such as chronic inflammation with endothelial dysfunction weakening the vessel structure, rather than serving as a direct cause of thrombosis.[41] To more accurately identify late acquired ISA posing a risk for future events across the spectrum, a better understanding of this phenomenon is essential.

Stent Edge Re-stenosis

Some early DES trials demonstrated a relatively high incidence of re-stenosis at the proximal edge segment compared with the distal edge, which led to an important clue for the optimal deployment of DES (Fig. 58-14). In our IVUS substudy of the SIRIUS trial, lesions with stent edge stenosis at 8 months had greater reference plaque burden (61% vs. 49%, $P = 0.03$) and a higher overexpansion index (maximum stent area/reference MLA: 1.8 vs. 1.5, $P = 0.03$) at baseline compared with those without edge stenosis.[42] More recently, the STLLR (The Impact of Stent Deployment Techniques on Clinical Outcomes of Patient Treated With the CYPHER® Stent) trial also demonstrated that geographic miss (defined as the length of injured or stenotic segment not fully covered by the DES) had a significant negative impact on both clinical efficacy and safety at 1 year following sirolimus-eluting stent implantation.[43] Therefore, complete coverage of the reference disease with less aggressive stent dilatation is currently recommended. Notably, however, longer stent length has been reported to be independently associated with DES thrombosis and re-stenosis.[30] Furthermore, significant underexpansion and incomplete strut apposition may also result in unfavorable outcomes. On-line IVUS guidance can facilitate both the determination of appropriate stent size and length as well as optimal procedural endpoint, achieving the goal of covering significant pathology with reasonable stent expansion, while anchoring the stent ends in relatively plaque-free vessel segments.[44]

For DES treatment of ISR, early clinical studies hypothesized that full DES coverage of an old BMS might be important for the prevention of recurrent re-stenosis. This aggressive optimization strategy, however, can be associated with several clinical issues and, thus, may not be feasible in every case of ISR. In a recent retrospective IVUS study

of patients with BMS re-stenosis treated with sirolimus-eluting stents, 77% of the uncovered BMS segments kept adequate lumen patency at follow-up.[45] Therefore, as long as the original BMS is well expanded and has a segment with sufficient lumen area, conservative coverage with a DES can be a clinical option. Another study from the TAXUS-IV, V, and VI trials evaluated 9-month IVUS results of patients who did not require revascularization at the time of 9-month angiography.[46] At 3 years, revascularization was required in 4.9% of paclitaxel-eluting stents and 6.7% of BMSs. Multivariate analysis identified minimum lumen area at 9 months as a significant predictor of late revascularization with the optimal thresholds to best predict subsequent revascularization-free survival of 4.2 mm^2 for paclitaxel-eluting stents and 4 mm^2 for BMSs.

Strut Fracture

Stent strut fracture is not a rare phenomenon in peripheral artery stenting (up to 65% in femoro-popliteal stenting) and can also occur following DES implantation in coronary lesions. By angiography, strut fracture is diagnosed as complete or partial separation of the stent at follow-up where there had been contiguity of the stent at the baseline. IVUS or optical coherence tomography (OCT) imaging can directly visualize stent struts, offering more detailed morphologic assessment and classifications. By IVUS, strut fracture is defined as longitudinal strut discontinuity and can be categorized on the basis of its morphologic characteristics: (1) strut separation, (2) strut subluxation, or (3) strut intussusception (Figs. 58-15 and 58-16).[29] Another recently proposed classification focuses on potential mechanisms of the strut fracture, categorizing them on the basis of the presence or absence of aneurysm at the fracture site (type I and II, respectively).[47] Angiographic or IVUS studies have reported the incidence of DES fracture as 0.8% to 7.7%, within which ISR or stent thrombosis occurred at 22% to 88%.[29] Theoretically, strut fracture of the DES can reduce the local drug dose delivered to the arterial wall, as well as affecting the mechanical scaffolding of the affected lesion segment. In addition, the irregular edge of the fractured struts may give chronic stimuli to the vessel wall under cardiac movement. Conversely, deployment of long and rigid stents in angulated lesions with hinge motion can lead to significant alteration of local physiology, and therefore, the strut fracture may help restore the original dynamic state in at least some cases. The exact incidence and clinical implications of strut fractures remain to be further investigated in large clinical studies.

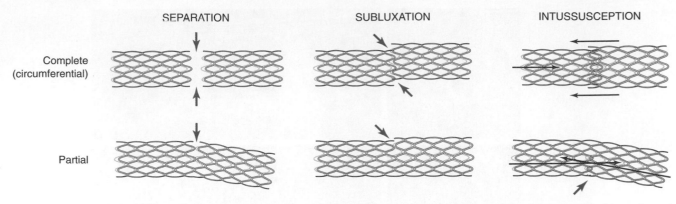

Figure 58-15 Stanford classification of stent strut fracture. By intravascular ultrasound, strut fracture is defined as longitudinal strut discontinuity and can be categorized on the basis of its morphologic characteristics.

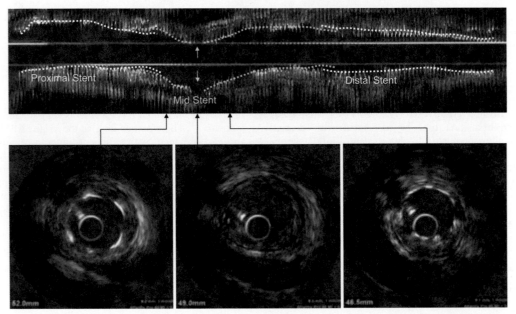

Figure 58-16 Stent strut discontinuity (fracture) observed 8 months after deployment of three overlapping drug-eluting stents. On the cross-sectional intravascular ultrasound (IVUS) image (*lower, middle*), an abnormal paucity of stent struts, not seen at baseline, is detected at a portion of the mid-stent. The longitudinal IVUS image (*upper*) shows an acute-angled bend at the corresponding segment (*arrows*). In this particular case, however, the stent fracture (complete separation type) is not associated with increased intimal hyperplasia.

IMPACT OF INTRAVASCULAR ULTRASOUND GUIDANCE ON THE OUTCOMES OF DRUG-ELUTING STENTS

To date, several large studies have assessed the impact of IVUS guidance during DES implantation on clinical outcomes (Table 58-2). In a single-center study of IVUS-guided DES implantation versus matched control population with angiographic guidance alone, a higher rate of definite stent thrombosis was seen in the angiography-guided group at both 30 days (0.5 vs. 1.4%, $P = 0.046$) and 12 months (0.7 vs. 2.0%, $P = 0.014$).[48] In addition, there was a trend in favor of IVUS guidance in 12-month target lesion revascularization (5.1 vs. 7.2%, $P = 0.07$). A multi-center registry, the MAIN-COMPARE (Revascularization for Unprotected Left MAIN Coronary Artery Stenosis: COMparison of Percutaneous coronary Angioplasty versus surgical REvascularization) study, enrolled patients with unprotected LMCA stenosis and demonstrated significantly lower 3-year mortality in the IVUS-guidance group compared with the conventional angiography-guidance group (4.7% vs. 16.0%, log-rank $P = 0.048$;

hazard ratio [HR] 0.39; 95% CI 0.15–1.02; Cox model $P = 0.055$) in patients treated with DESs.[49] Another single-center registry also reported that IVUS-guided DES implantation for the treatment of bifurcation lesions significantly reduced 4-year mortality compared with conventional angiography-guided stenting (HR 0.24; 95% CI 0.06–0.86; Cox model $P = 0.03$).[50] One small prospective multi-center randomized study (Angiography Versus IVUS Optimisation [AVIO]) has recently been conducted to investigate whether IVUS-guided DES implantation can improve acute outcomes in complex lesions.[51] This study used unique criteria for IVUS optimization, in which target MSA was determined according to the size of a postdilation, noncompliant balloon chosen on the basis of IVUS-measured media-to-media diameters at multiple sites within the stented segment. Post-procedure minimum lumen diameter, as the primary endpoint of this study, was significantly greater in the IVUS-guided group, particularly when optimal IVUS criteria were met, with no increased complications compared with the angiography-guided group (target IVUS criteria met: 2.86 mm, target IVUS criteria not met: 2.6 mm, angiography alone: 2.51 mm).

TABLE 58-2	Intravascular Ultrasound versus Angiographic Guidance of Drug-Eluting Stent Implantation						
	N	Population	Study Design	IVUS Criteria for Optimal Deployment	Criteria Fulfilled	Endpoints	Results
Costantini et al.	1350	De novo & restenotic Native	Single center Registry	Discretion of individual operator practice	—	3-yr MACE & stent thrombosis	IVUS better
Fujimoto, et al.	480	De novo Native & SVG	Single center Registry	Discretion of individual operator practice	—	8-mo angiography, MACE & TLR	No difference
Kim, et al.	758	De novo Native, Bifurcation (BMS + DES)	Single center Registry	Discretion of individual operator practice	—	4-yr MACE & stent thrombosis	IVUS better
Roy, et al.	1768	De novo & restenotic Native & SVG	Single center Registry	Discretion of individual operator practice	—	30-d &12-mo MACE & stent thrombosis	IVUS better
MAIN-COMPARE	975	De novo Native, Left main (BMS + DES)	Multicenter Registry	Discretion of individual operator practice	—	3-yr mortality	IVUS better
MATRIX	1504	De novo & restenotic Native & SVG	Multicenter Registry	Discretion of individual operator practice	—	2-yr TVF, MACE, stent thrombosis	IVUS better
AVIO	284	De novo Native	Multicenter Randomized	SA > "AOR" determined by the size of an optimal post-dilation balloon based on media-to-media diameter measurements	48%	Post-procedure MLD, 9-mo MACE	IVUS better (Post-procedure MLD)

AVIO, Angiography Versus IVUS Optimization; *AOR*, achievable optimal result; *IVUS*, intravascular ultrasound; *MAIN-COMPARE*, revascularization for unprotected left MAIN coronary artery stenosis: COMparison of Percutaneous coronary Angioplasty versus surgical REvascularization; *MACE*, major adverse cardiac events; *MLD*, minimum lumen diameter; *SA*, stent area; *ref*, reference vessel; *SVG*, saphenous vein graft; *TLR*, target lesion revascularization; *TVF*, target vessel failure.

Summary and Future Perspectives

Over the past two decades, IVUS has developed into an indispensable tool for research and clinical purposes. Although recent advances in noninvasive cardiovascular imaging now allow rapid and detailed visualization of cardiovascular structures, the demand for catheter-based imaging remains high because of its greater spatial resolution and practical usefulness for precise procedural guidance and real-time assessment of treatment effects. Current technical efforts in invasive imaging are aimed not only at further improvement of anatomic information but also at biologic or physiologic assessment of the target segment. These enhancements may allow a more comprehensive evaluation of the novel treatment device with both mechanical and biologic effects, and this could help achieve the ultimate goal to deliver the most effective treatment to patients with truly low rates of complications.

Acknowledgments

The authors acknowledge all the former and current coworkers at the Stanford Center for Cardiovascular Technology for their scientific contributions, as well as Heidi N. Bonneau, RN, MS, CCA, for her review and editing advice.

REFERENCES

1. Yock P, Linker D, Saether O, et al: Intravascular two-dimensional catheter ultrasound: Initial clinical studies. *Circulation* 78(4):II–21, 1988.
2. Ramasubbu K, Schoenhagen P, Balghith MA, et al: Repeated intravascular ultrasound imaging in cardiac transplant recipients does not accelerate transplant coronary artery disease. *J Am Coll Cardiol* 41(10):1739–1743, 2003.
3. Guedes A, Keller PF, L'Allier PL, et al: Long-term safety of intravascular ultrasound in nontransplant, nonintervened, atherosclerotic coronary arteries. *J Am Coll Cardiol* 45(4):559–564, 2005.
4. Mintz GS, Nissen SE, Anderson WD, et al: American College of Cardiology Clinical Expert Consensus Document on Standards for Acquisition, Measurement and Reporting of Intravascular Ultrasound Studies (IVUS). A report of the American College of Cardiology Task Force on Clinical Expert Consensus Documents. *J Am Coll Cardiol* 37(5):1478–1492, 2001.
5. Honda Y, Fitzgerald PJ: Frontiers in intravascular imaging technologies. *Circulation* 117(15):2024–2037, 2008.
6. Sathyanarayana S, Carlier S, Li W, et al: Characterisation of atherosclerotic plaque by spectral similarity of radiofrequency intravascular ultrasound signals. *EuroIntervention* 5(1):133–139, 2009.
7. Cannon CP, Braunwald E, McCabe CH, et al: Intensive versus moderate lipid lowering with statins after acute coronary syndromes. *N Engl J Med* 350(15):1495–1504, 2004.
8. von Birgelen C, Hartmann M, Mintz GS, et al: Relationship between cardiovascular risk as predicted by established risk scores versus plaque progression as measured by serial intravascular ultrasound in left main coronary arteries. *Circulation* 110(12):1579–1585, 2004.
9. Barter PJ, Caulfield M, Eriksson M, et al: Effects of torcetrapib in patients at high risk for coronary events. *N Engl J Med* 357(21):2109–2122, 2007.

10. Nissen SE, Tardif JC, Nicholls SJ, et al: Effect of torcetrapib on the progression of coronary atherosclerosis. *N Engl J Med* 356(13):1304–1316, 2007.
11. Kawasaki M, Sano K, Okubo M, et al: Volumetric quantitative analysis of tissue characteristics of coronary plaques after statin therapy using three-dimensional integrated backscatter intravascular ultrasound. *J Am Coll Cardiol* 45(12):1946–1953, 2005.
12. Serruys PW, Garcia-Garcia HM, Buszman P, et al: Effects of the direct lipoprotein-associated phospholipase A(2) inhibitor darapladib on human coronary atherosclerotic plaque. *Circulation* 118(11):1172–1182, 2008.
13. Sano K, Mintz GS, Carlier SG, et al: Assessing intermediate left main coronary lesions using intravascular ultrasound. *Am Heart J* 154(5):983–988, 2007.
14. Koo BK, Waseda K, Kang HJ, et al: Anatomic and functional evaluation of bifurcation lesions undergoing percutaneous coronary intervention. *Circ Cardiovasc Interv* 3(2):113–119, 2010.
15. Okura H, Taguchi H, Kubo T, et al: Atherosclerotic plaque with ultrasonic attenuation affects coronary reflow and infarct size in patients with acute coronary syndrome: An intravascular ultrasound study. *Circ J* 71(5):648–653, 2007.
16. Kawamoto T, Okura H, Koyama Y, et al: The relationship between coronary plaque characteristics and small embolic particles during coronary stent implantation. *J Am Coll Cardiol* 50(17):1635–1640, 2007.
17. Uetani T, Amano T, Ando H, et al: The correlation between lipid volume in the target lesion, measured by integrated backscatter intravascular ultrasound, and post-procedural myocardial infarction in patients with elective stent implantation. *Eur Heart J* 29(14):1714–1720, 2008.
18. Hong YJ, Jeong MH, Choi YH, et al: Impact of plaque components on no-reflow phenomenon after stent deployment in patients with acute coronary syndrome: A virtual histology-intravascular

ultrasound analysis. *Eur Heart J* 2009 Feb 19. [Epub ahead of print].
19. Wu X, Maehara A, Mintz GS, et al: Virtual histology intravascular ultrasound analysis of non-culprit attenuated plaques detected by grayscale intravascular ultrasound in patients with acute coronary syndromes. *Am J Cardiol* 105(1):48–53, 2010.
20. Castagna MT, Mintz GS, Leiboff BO, et al: The contribution of "mechanical" problems to in-stent restenosis: An intravascular ultrasonographic analysis of 1090 consecutive in-stent restenosis lesions. *Am Heart J* 142(6):970–974, 2001.
21. Honda Y, Fitzgerald PJ: Stent thrombosis: An issue revisited in a changing world. *Circulation* 108(1):2–5, 2003.
22. Uren NG, Schwaxzacher SP, Metz JA, et al: Predictors and outcomes on stent thrombosis: An intravascular ultrasound registry. *Eur Heart J* 23(2):124–132, 2001.
23. Cheneau E, Leborgne L, Mintz GS, et al: Predictors of subacute stent thrombosis: Results of a systematic intravascular ultrasound study. *Circulation* 108(1):43–47, 2003.
24. Fitzgerald PJ, Oshima A, Hayase M, et al: Final results of the Can Routine Ultrasound Influence Stent Expansion (CRUISE) study. *Circulation* 102(5):523–530, 2000.
25. Russo RJ, Silva PD, Teirstein PS, et al: A randomized controlled trial of angiography versus intravascular ultrasound-directed bare metal coronary stent placement (the AVID Trial). *Circ Cardiovasc Interv* 2(2):113–123, 2009.
26. Mudra H, di Mario C, de Jaegere P, et al: Randomized comparison of coronary stent implantation under ultrasound or angiographic guidance to reduce stent restenosis (OPTICUS Study). *Circulation* 104(12):1343–1349, 2001.
27. Orford JL, Denktas AE, Williams BA, et al: Routine intravascular ultrasound scanning guidance of coronary stenting is not associated with improved clinical outcomes. *Am Heart J* 148(3):501–506, 2004.

28. Casella G, Klauss V, Ottani F, et al: Impact of intravascular ultrasound-guided stenting on long-term clinical outcome: A meta-analysis of available studies comparing intravascular ultrasound-guided and angiographically guided stenting. *Catheter Cardiovasc Interv* 59(3):314–321, 2003.

29. Honda Y: Drug-eluting stents. Insights from invasive imaging technologies. *Circ J* 73(8):1371–1380, 2009.

30. Hong MK, Mintz GS, Lee CW, et al: Intravascular ultrasound predictors of angiographic restenosis after sirolimus-eluting stent implantation. *Eur Heart J* 27(11):1305–1310, 2006.

31. Fujii K, Mintz GS, Kobayashi Y, et al: Contribution of stent underexpansion to recurrence after sirolimus-eluting stent implantation for in-stent restenosis. *Circulation* 109(9):1085–1088, 2004.

32. Sonoda S, Morino Y, Ako J, et al: Impact of final stent dimensions on long-term results following sirolimus-eluting stent implantation: Serial intravascular ultrasound analysis from the SIRIUS trial. *J Am Coll Cardiol* 43(11):1959–1963, 2004.

33. Fujii K, Carlier SG, Mintz GS, et al: Stent underexpansion and residual reference segment stenosis are related to stent thrombosis after sirolimus-eluting stent implantation: An intravascular ultrasound study. *J Am Coll Cardiol* 45(7):995–998, 2005.

34. Alfonso F, Suarez A, Perez-Vizcayno MJ, et al: Intravascular ultrasound findings during episodes of drug-eluting stent thrombosis. *J Am Coll Cardiol* 50(21):2095–2097, 2007.

35. Okabe T, Mintz GS, Buch AN, et al: Intravascular ultrasound parameters associated with stent thrombosis after drug-eluting stent deployment. *Am J Cardiol* 100(4):615–620, 2007.

36. Hassan AK, Bergheanu SC, Stijnen T, et al: Late stent malapposition risk is higher after drug-eluting stent compared with bare-metal stent implantation and associates with late stent thrombosis. *Eur Heart J* 31(10):1172–1180, 2009.

37. Sakurai R, Bonneau HN, Honda Y, et al: Intravascular ultrasound findings in ENDEAVOR II and ENDEAVOR III. *Am J Cardiol* 100(8B):71M–76M, 2007.

38. Waseda K, Miyazawa A, Ako J, et al: Intravascular ultrasound results from the ENDEAVOR IV trial: Randomized comparison between zotarolimus- and paclitaxel-eluting stents in patients with coronary artery disease. *JACC Cardiovasc Interv* 2(8):779–784, 2009.

39. Hur SH, Ako J, Honda Y, et al: Late-acquired incomplete stent apposition: Morphologic characterization. *Cardiovasc Revasc Med* 10(4):236–246, 2009.

40. Ako J, Morino Y, Honda Y, et al:. Late incomplete stent apposition after sirolimus-eluting stent implantation: A serial intravascular ultrasound analysis. *J Am Coll Cardiol* 46(6):1002–1005, 2005.

41. Cook S, Ladich E, Nakazawa G, et al: Correlation of intravascular ultrasound findings with histopathological analysis of thrombus aspirates in patients with very late drug-eluting stent thrombosis. *Circulation* 120(5):391–399, 2009.

42. Sakurai R, Ako J, Morino Y, et al: Predictors of edge stenosis following sirolimus-eluting stent deployment (a quantitative intravascular ultrasound analysis from the SIRIUS trial). *Am J Cardiol* 96(9):1251–1253, 2005.

43. Costa MA, Angiolillo DJ, Tannenbaum M, et al: Impact of stent deployment procedural factors on long-term effectiveness and safety of sirolimus-eluting stents (final results of the multicenter prospective STLLR trial). *Am J Cardiol* 101(12):1704–1711, 2008.

44. Morino Y, Tamiya S, Masuda N, et al: Intravascular ultrasound criteria for determination of optimal longitudinal positioning of sirolimus-eluting stents. *Circ J* 74(8):1609–1616, 2010.

45. Sakurai R, Ako J, Hassan AH, et al: Neointimal progression and luminal narrowing in sirolimus-eluting stent treatment for bare metal in-stent restenosis: A quantitative intravascular ultrasound analysis. *Am Heart J* 154(2):361–365, 2007.

46. Doi H, Maehara A, Mintz GS, et al: Impact of in-stent minimal lumen area at 9 months poststent implantation on 3-year target lesion revascularization-free survival: A serial intravascular ultrasound analysis from the TAXUS IV, V, and VI trials. *Circ Cardiovasc Intervent* 1(2):111–118, 2008.

47. Doi H, Maehara A, Mintz GS, et al: Classification and potential mechanisms of intravascular ultrasound patterns of stent fracture. *Am J Cardiol* 103(6):818–823, 2009.

48. Roy P, Steinberg DH, Sushinsky SJ, et al: The potential clinical utility of intravascular ultrasound guidance in patients undergoing percutaneous coronary intervention with drug-eluting stents. *Eur Heart J* 29(15):1851–1857, 2008.

49. Park SJ, Kim YH, Park DW, et al: Impact of intravascular ultrasound guidance on long-term mortality in stenting for unprotected left main coronary artery stenosis. *Circ Cardiovasc Interv* 2(3):167–177, 2009.

50. Kim SH, Kim YH, Kang SJ, et al: Long-term outcomes of intravascular ultrasound-guided stenting in coronary bifurcation lesions. *Am J Cardiol* 106(5):612–618, 2010.

51. Colombo A, Caussin C, Presbitero P, et al: AVIO: a prospective, randomized trial of intravascular-ultrasound guided compared to angiography guided stent implantation in complex coronary lesions. *J Am Coll Cardiol* 56(13):xvii, 2010.

High-Risk Vulnerable Plaques: Definition, Diagnosis, and Treatment

PEDRO R. MORENO | CARLOS L. ALVIAR | JAVIER SANZ | VALENTIN FUSTER

KEY POINTS

- Plaque instability can now be detected through a number of invasive as well as noninvasive technologies.

- It is unclear at this time which of these technologies will emerge as the most pragmatic and useful.

- Validation of plaque instability imaging via clinical follow-up to determine natural history will be quite important.

Despite a steady decrease in the incidence of acute coronary events, cardiovascular disease (CVD) continues to be the major cause of death worldwide, with 16.7 million deaths per year, representing 29.2% of the total global deaths.[1-3] Coronary atherosclerosis is a condition that can be asymptomatic over decades. The transition from asymptomatic, nonobstructive disease to symptomatic, occlusive disease is related to acute coronary thrombosis. This condition, known as *atherothrombosis*, is mostly related to plaque rupture or erosion, which triggers a series of biochemical events ultimately leading to thrombus formation.[4,5] Atherosclerotic plaques at increased risk for rupture have been histologically characterized as thin cap fibroatheromas (TCFA), which can be properly identified by invasive imaging techniques.[6] As a result, the concept of early detection and treatment before clinical events has caused increased interest in the catheterization laboratory (cath lab). This chapter, divided into four sections, describes a systematic approach to high-risk vulnerable plaques (VPs). The first section is devoted to definition, incidence, risk factors, and anatomic location of plaque. The second section is devoted to plaque composition and to the pathophysiologic aspects of these lesions, setting up the foundations to understand the dynamics of plaque vulnerability. The third section summarizes the evolving field of invasive plaque imaging, with a brief comment on noninvasive imaging modalities. Finally, the fourth section is devoted to therapy, from conservative, pharmacologic options to aggressive percutaneous coronary intervention (PCI) alternatives.

Clinical Characteristics

DEFINITION AND CLINICAL EVIDENCE

A high-risk VP is a nonobstructive, silent coronary lesion that suddenly becomes obstructive and symptomatic (Fig. 59-1). The initial understanding of this process was described by Ambrose and Fuster in 1988 when they studied the baseline characteristics of nonobstructive lesions that evolved into acute myocardial infarction (AMI).[7] The investigators found that at baseline, the lesions evolving to complete occlusion had a mean diameter stenosis of 48%. Multiple investigators reproduced this finding using both angiographic and intravascular imaging modalities and supporting the concept that the majority of lesions responsible for AMI originate from nonobstructive disease.[8]

INCIDENCE

The number of nonobstructive, asymptomatic lesions that progress to obstructive, symptomatic lesions presenting as an acute event can give us the estimated incidence of this condition. Several studies have retrospectively addressed this issue. The first study included 1228 patients who underwent percutaneous coronary intervention (PCI) for symptomatic coronary artery disease (CAD). The incidence of nonobstructive, nonculprit lesions that required additional PCI was 12.4% in the first year and 5% to 7% per year from years 2 to 5 after the initial procedure (Fig. 59-2).[9] The second study included 3747 post-PCI patients from the National Heart Lung and Blood Institute (NHLBI) registry.[10] The incidence of nonobstructive, nonculprit lesions that required additional PCI was 6% in the first year, ranging from 4.4% to 12.8% according to the number of vessels involved (Fig. 59-3). A third study included a total of 1059 patients studied with computed tomographic angiography (CTA). VPs were classified according to the presence or absence of two variables: (1) positive remodeling, and (2) low attenuation ("soft") morphology on CT.[11] The incidence of acute coronary events was 11% in plaques with one variable and up to 22% in plaques with both variables. Notably, the absence of these two variables represented a strong negative predictive value, with an incidence of coronary events as low as 0.5%. Another study using intravascular modalities recently reported a 12% incidence of TCFAs by optical coherence tomography (OCT) in sites other than the culprit lesion responsible for the acute coronary syndrome (ACS).[12] Additionally, they found that the majority of TCFAs occurred in the proximal segments of the coronary vasculature. Despite this incidence of 11% to 22%, the actual area occupied by these plaques in the coronary circulation may not be as large. Cheruvu and Virmani performed detailed histopathology in the entire vasculature of 50 human hearts and demonstrated that only 1.1% to 1.6% of the coronary vessel area was occupied by TCFAs. Out of all the lesions studied, 10.8% corresponded to TCFA.[13] This is in agreement with a second study that identified a 11% incidence of TCFAs, with slightly higher incidence in patients with ACS, suggesting a more "unstable" profile of the coronary lesions in these subjects.[9,11] These retrospective and pathologic studies gave the foundation to design the first prospective natural-history study of VPs, also called the PROSPECT (Predictors of Response to CRT) Trial.[15] A total of 697 patients with ACS underwent three-vessel coronary angiography and gray-scale and radiofrequency (RF) intravascular ultrasound (IVUS) after multi-vessel coronary stenting. The incidence of nonculprit lesions developing major adverse cardiovascular events (MACEs) was 11.6% at 3.4 years. Most of these events were rehospitalization for progressive angina. Cardiac death or MI occurred in only 4.9% of the population. Three independent variables predicted these events and include (1) plaque burden of 70% or greater (hazard ratio [HR] 5.03; $P < 0.001$); (2) minimal lumen area (MLA) of 4 mm^2 or less (HR 3.21; $P = 0.001$); and (3) RF classification of TCFA (HR 3.35; $P < 0.001$). Of great interest, plaques exhibiting all three features had a higher HR, up to 11.05 ($P < 0.001$). Nevertheless, the prevalence of these high-risk plaques was only 4.2%. As a result, we now know that high-risk plaques are uncommon and are composed by a combination of anatomic features, which includes plaque burden and MLA, in addition to TCFA.

RISK FACTORS

Multiple regression analysis identified multi-vessel CAD at baseline (three- and two-vessel CAD), previous PCI, and age less than 65 years

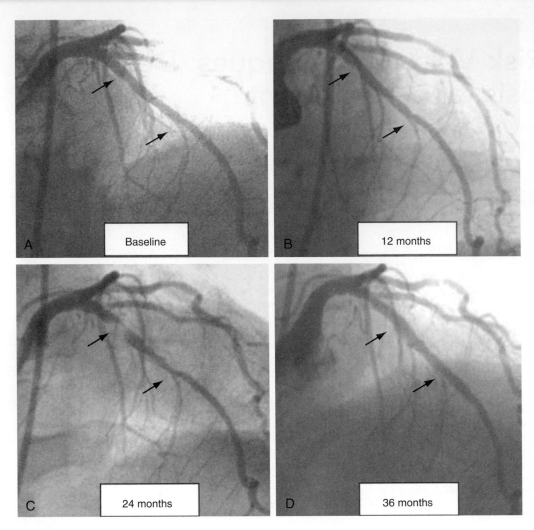

Figure 59-1 Sequential coronary angiograms of the left anterior descending coronary artery performed with 12-month intervals. Rapid progression from being nonobstructive and asymptomatic to being severely obstructive and symptomatic fulfills the clinical definition of vulnerable plaques. **A,** Completely normal vessel by angiography. **B,** Non-obstructive, asymptomatic coronary disease in the proximal segment (*black arrows*). **C,** Obstructive, symptomatic coronary disease presenting with acute coronary syndrome (*black arrows*). **D,** Stenosis is 10% to 20% in the segments 12 months after local therapy with stent (36 months after baseline angiogram). (*From the cardiac cath lab at Mount Sinai Medical Center, New York, NY.*)

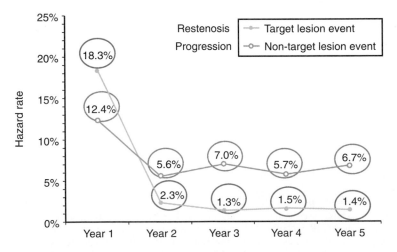

Figure 59-2 Hazard rates per year for target-lesion (*blue*) and nontarget-lesion (*red*) events derived from life table survival analysis. Target-lesion events include any repeat revascularization or other event (i.e., death, myocardial infarction [MI], acute coronary syndrome [ACS], or congestive heart failure [CHF]) attributed to the target lesion. Non–target-lesion events include all repeat revascularizations involving the target vessel outside the target lesion, any non–target vessel revascularization, and any death, MI, ACS, or CHF that was clearly not attributable to the target lesion. (*Adapted with permission from Cutlip DE, Chhabra AG, Baim DS, et al: Beyond restenosis: Five-year clinical outcomes from second-generation coronary stent trials, Circulation 110:1226–1230, 2004.*)

as independent predictors for VP. Of note, treatment with statins failed to protect patients within the first year.[10] IVUS studies also identified age, hypertension, diabetes mellitus (DM), heart failure, and dyslipidemia as predictors for IVUS-derived TCFA (ID-TCFA).[16] Diabetes is strongly associated with higher rates of ID-TCFA (21.6% vs. 13.1%, $P = 0.01$), and up to 54.4% in patients with a diagnosis of DM greater than 10 years.[17] The incidence of TCFA was also seven times higher in

males compared with females.[13] In terms of biomarkers and VP, serum myeloperoxidase is a new potential marker of plaque vulnerability.[18,19] Similarly, Lipoprotein-associated phospholipase (Lp-PLA2) may play a key role in necrotic core expansion as demonstrated by the Integrated Biomarkers and Imaging Study-2 (IBIS-2).[20] In isolated studies, highly sensitive cross-reactive protein (hs-CRP), white blood cell (WBC), interleukin (IL) 18, and tumor necrosis factor alpha (TNFα) inversely

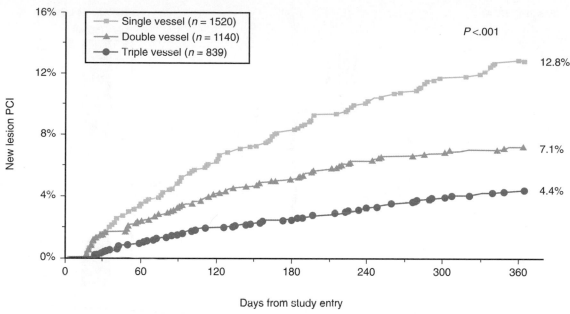

Figure 59-3   Kaplan–Meier analysis of nontarget lesion percutaneous coronary intervention (PCI) at 1 year, according to the initial degree of coronary artery disease. (*Adapted with permission from Glaser R, Selzer F, Faxon DP, et al: Clinical progression of incidental, asymptomatic lesions discovered during culprit vessel coronary intervention, Circulation 111:143–149, 2005.*)

correlated with fibrous cap thickness. However, hs-CRP appeared to be the only independent predictor by regression analysis.[21] Furthermore, hs-CRP has been postulated as a modulator of neovascularization.[22] Nevertheless, the clinical evidence for primary prevention of hs-CRP is rather limited and still subject to controversy, and further research is needed to completely elucidate the role of biomarkers to predict plaque rupture and coronary events.[23-25]

ANATOMIC DISTRIBUTION

The anatomic distribution of coronary lesions responsible for AMI is dominated by the proximal segment, which is responsible for 80% of MIs in all three major vessels.[26] These data were recently reproduced by OCT studies in vivo (Fig. 59-4).[12,27,28] When located in bifurcations, TCFAs are predominately located in the proximal rim of the bifurcation, as evaluated by OCT and IVUS.[29] After reviewing clinical characteristics, the next section provides the basis for understanding the pathophysiology of the disease. Most importantly, this section offers the foundation to critically evaluate novel imaging techniques that claim effectiveness in the diagnosis of high-risk VPs. For the interventionalist, the incidence of high-risk VPs evolving into clinical events is close to 13% in 3 years, in patients with ACS and multi-vessel disease. These lesions are positively remodeled, have large plaque burden, and are usually located in the proximal segment of the coronary arteries.

▉ Plaque Composition

Plaque rupture is, by far, the most common cause of atherothrombosis, responsible for 70% to 75% of all events and up to 85% in hypercholesterolemic white males. In plaque rupture, disease progresses through lipid core expansion and macrophage accumulation at the edges of the plaque, leading to fibrous cap disruption (Fig. 59-5). As a result, identifying plaques at risk for rupture offers the possibility of preventing the most common substrate for coronary thrombosis. The second cause of atherothrombosis is plaque erosion. Included initially as "other causes of coronary thrombosis," plaque erosion gained attention in the last decade as a significant substrate for coronary thrombosis and sudden cardiac death (SCD) in premenopausal females.[13] As

opposed to plaque rupture, erosion occurs in plaques with no specific features suitable for detection. Most of these plaques exhibit histologic patterns similar to plaques responsible for stable angina. They are characterized by a thick, smooth muscle cell–rich fibrous cap, reduced necrotic core areas, and a low degree of inflammation (Fig. 59-6). Plaque erosion is also associated with cigarette smoking, suggesting that thrombosis in these patients may be related to a systemic, prothrombogenic pathway rather than to a local, atherothrombotic mechanism. The characteristic lesion preceding plaque rupture is the TCFA, which is considered the hallmark of high-risk VPs (Fig. 59-7).[30] The classic histologic patterns of TCFA include, but are not limited to, (1) a thin fibrous cap with increased stress–strain relationship; (2) large necrotic core with increased free cholesterol–esterified cholesterol ratio; (3) increased plaque inflammation; (4) positive vascular remodeling; (5) increased vasa-vasorum neovascularization; and (6) intraplaque hemorrhage.[31]

THIN FIBROUS CAP WITH INCREASED STRESS–STRAIN RELATIONSHIP

Autopsy studies have shown that ruptured plaques are characterized by a very thin fibrous cap, measuring 23 ± 19 microns (μm) in thickness. Most importantly, 95% of ruptured caps measured 64 μm or less in the coronary and 60 μm or less in the aorta.[32] As a result, the first and probably most important histologic feature of TCFA is a fibrous cap 65 μm or more in thickness. These thin caps are unable to withstand the circumferential tensile stress applied by the oscillations of arterial blood pressure. The ratio of the circumferential tensile stress to the radial strain of the fibrous cap equals the stiffness of the tissue.[33] Hence, soft (fatty) tissue will be more strained than stiff (fibrous) tissue when equally stressed. Furthermore, as caps become thinner, the stress increases in an exponential pattern (Fig. 59-8). In addition, as lipid pools become larger, stress also increases. Therefore, the strength of a cap may be as important as the actual thickness of a fibrous cap. This stress–strain relationship in the fibrous cap is therefore considered a feature for plaque vulnerability.[34] Technology aiming to detect TCFA should have a radial resolution less than 65 μm and the ability to quantify the stress–strain relationship in the fibrous cap.

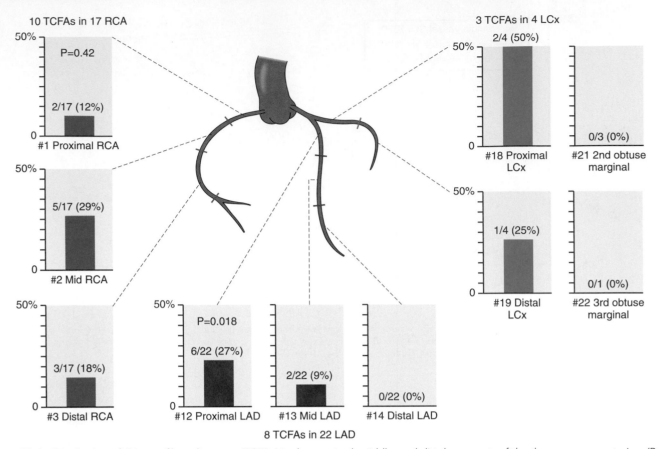

Figure 59-4 Distribution of thin cap fibroatheromas (TCFAs) in the proximal, middle, and distal segments of the three coronary arteries. *(Reproduced with permission from Tanaka A, Imanishi T, Kitabata H, et al: Distribution and frequency of thin-capped fibroatheromas and ruptured plaques in the entire culprit coronary artery in patients with acute coronary syndrome as determined by optical coherence tomography, Am J Cardiol 102:975–979, 2008.)*

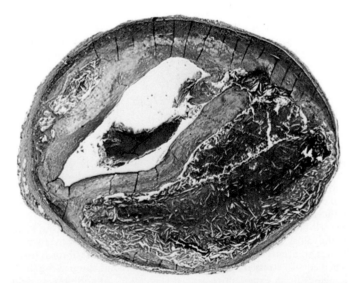

Figure 59-5 Cross-sectioned coronary artery containing a ruptured plaque at the shoulder of the fibrous cap with a nonocclusive thrombus superimposed. The large necrotic core can be identified by cholesterol crystals and extensive intra-plaque hemorrhage secondary to plaque rupture. Trichrome stain renders the thrombus red, the collagen blue, and the lipid colorless. *(Courtesy of Dr. K-Raman Purushothaman, Mount Sinai Hospital, New York, NY.)*

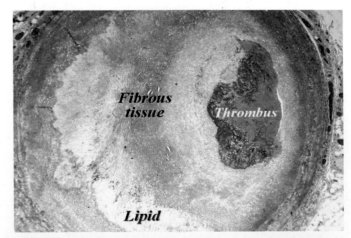

Figure 59-6 Plaque erosion. Cross-section of a coronary artery containing a stenotic atherosclerotic plaque with an occlusive thrombosis superimposed. The endothelium is missing at the plaque–thrombus interface, but the plaque surface is otherwise intact. Trichrome stain renders the thrombus red, the collagen blue, and the lipid colorless. *(Courtesy of Dr. Erling Falk, Aarhus, Denmark.)*

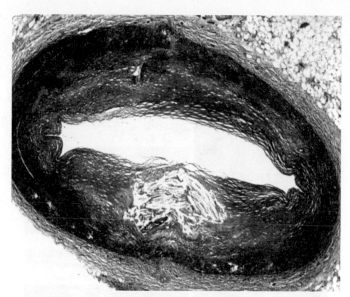

Figure 59-7 Thin cap fibroatheroma (TCFA), characterized by a very thin fibrous cap and a large necrotic core. Trichrome stain. *(Courtesy of Dr. K Raman Purushothaman, Mount Sinai Hospital, New York, NY.)*

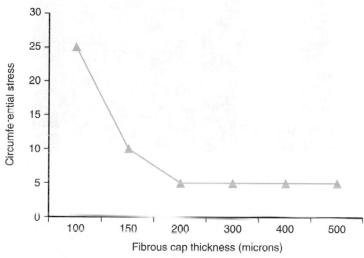

Figure 59-8 Relationship between circumferential stress (vertical axis) and fibrous cap thickness (horizontal axis). Note the exponential increase in circumferential stress when cap thickness is reduced to fewer than 200 microns. *(Adapted with permission from Loree HM, Kamm RD, Stringfellow RG, Lee RT: Effects of fibrous cap thickness on peak circumferential stress in model atherosclerotic vessels, Circ Res 71:850–858, 1992.)*

LARGE NECROTIC CORE WITH INCREASED FREE CHOLESTEROL TO ESTERIFIED CHOLESTEROL RATIO

Modified oxidized low-density lipoprotein (LDL) is avidly taken up by macrophages via scavenger receptors, leading to cytoplasm overload with lipid droplets. Continuous inflow of oxidized isoforms of LDL (oxLDL) leads to cell death with extracellular lipid accumulation within the matrix of the plaque. Preclinical experimentation has demonstrated how the oxLDL are associated with plaque vulnerability depending on the type of predominant molecule, mostly regulating apoptotic cell death.[35,36] This is the basic mechanism of the necrotic core, which is formed after death by necrosis, or apoptosis, of lipid-laden macrophages, foam cells, and erythrocytes. Active collagen

dissolution by metalloproteinases contributes to core expansion, which plays a major role in plaque vulnerability. In the aorta, TCFAs exhibit necrotic core areas of 40%, and ruptured plaques up to 50% of total plaque area.[37] However, other studies in coronary arteries show lower necrotic areas, down to 24% and 34% in TCFAs and ruptured plaques, respectively.[30] Core composition may influence the propensity for plaque rupture and thrombosis. An increased free cholesterol–esterified cholesterol ratio, with oxidized cholesterol, increases the likelihood of thrombosis by interacting with the oxLDL receptor-1 (LOX-1), and enhancing the expression of tissue factor.[38-40]

INCREASED PLAQUE INFLAMMATION

Macrophages and T cells are capable of degrading the extracellular matrix by secretion of proteolytic enzymes such as plasminogen activators and matrix metalloproteinases (MMPs), including collagenases, elastases, gelatinases, and stromelysins, weakening the already thin fibrous cap and predisposing it to rupture.[41] This has been recently confirmed by Suzuki et al, who found increased levels of MMP-1, MMP-13, and IL-6 in the coronary vessels of patients who had experienced MI, supporting the evidence behind the role of MMP in plaque rupture that leads to clinical events.[42] Among the multiple MMPs identified to have a role in atherosclerosis, two particular subtypes, MMP-7 and MMP-12, seem more selectively localized in specific subsets of macrophages; especially, those located in the necrotic core have low arginase-I expression and represent a marker of activation and enhanced inflammation.[43-45] The continuous entry, survival, and replication of monocytes or macrophages within plaques are aimed to remove oxLDL and reduce oxidation and reactive oxygen generation (ROS) products. In situations where the macrophage scavenger capacity is overloaded, cell death is activated by apoptosis, releasing MMPs and tissue factor.[46] This link among inflammation, apoptosis, and thrombosis was elegantly documented by Hutter et al in human and murine atherosclerotic lesions.[47] Therefore, plaque inflammation is a pivotal feature of plaque vulnerability.[4,48] Recent studies have reported two different subclasses of monocytes or macrophages inside the atheroma.[49] The first class of macrophages, classically known as activated macrophages, or M1, promote inflammation. The second subtype, identified as M2, appears to be anti-inflammatory. Therefore, the ratio between M1 and M2 macrophages has an impact on atherosclerosis progression, plaque regression, or both. It has been described that different factors shift this ratio toward an increased content of M2 cells, including increased T helper–secreted molecules, IL-4, IL-13, peroxisome proliferator activated receptor delta (PPAR δ) and the lipid sphingosin 1-phosphate (S1P).[50-52] These M2 macrophages are also responsible for efferocytosis, or the removal of short-lived apoptotic bodies from the atheroma. Defective efferocytosis leads to secondary necrosis, a process linked to advanced disease. The failure of macrophage efflux, prothrombotic factors, inflammatory chemokines, and collagenases increase the necrotic core, leading to plaque rupture and thrombosis.[53,54]

Technology aiming to detect TCFAs should have sufficient resolution to identify and quantify macrophages in the fibrous cap and shoulders of the atherosclerotic plaque.

DEGREE OF VASCULAR REMODELING

As a defense mechanism, the vessel wall can expand significantly to harbor large atheromas without obstructing the lumen (Fig. 59-9). Also known as *remodeling*, this process is linked to high-risk atherosclerosis. The mechanisms responsible for remodeling involve an inflammatory process at the base of the plaque, which leads to the digestion of the internal elastic lamina (IEL) and involves the deeper layers of the vessel wall, including the tunica media and the adventitia. Several studies have shown increased expression of MMPs within the intimo-medial interface of remodeled plaques.[55,56] Furthermore, disruption of the IEL is associated with medial and adventitial inflammation, and evidence suggests that MMP-10 plays a regulatory role in

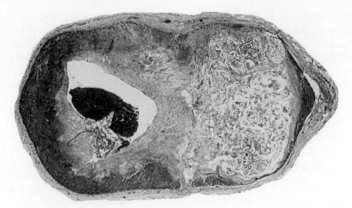

Figure 59-9 Large human thrombotic plaque in the left main coronary artery, with extensive remodeling containing a large necrotic core. (*Courtesy of Dr. K-Raman Purushothaman, Mount Sinai Hospital, New York, NY.*)

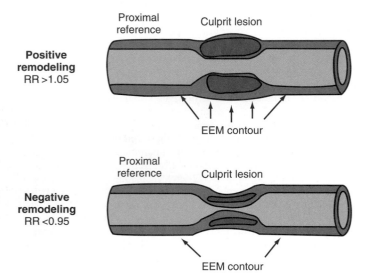

Remodeling ratio (RR) = EEM area lesion / EEM area proximal reference

Figure 59-10 Cartoon explaining the direction of positive and negative remodeling. (See text for details.) (*Adapted with permission from Schoenhagen P, Ziada KM, Kapadia SR, Crowe TD, Nissen SE, Tuzcu EM: Extent and direction of arterial remodeling in stable versus unstable coronary syndromes: An intravascular ultrasound study, Circulation 101:598–603, 2000.*)

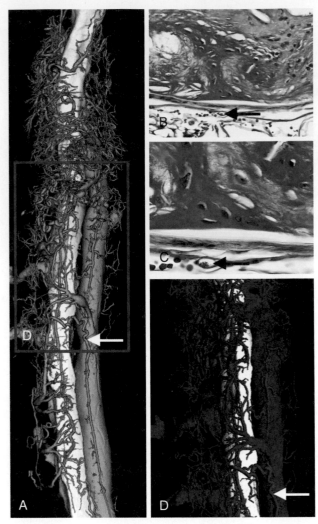

Figure 59-11 **A,** Volume-rendered high-resolution, three-dimensional micro-CT image of the descending aorta vasa vasorum. **B and C,** Corresponding histologic cross-sections demonstrate atherosclerotic lesions in the inferior vena cava (*black arrow*). **D,** Highlighted differentiated arterial (*red*) and venous (*blue*) vasa-vasorum. (Masson trichrome stain, bar 500 microns). (*Reproduced with permission from Langheinrich AC, Michniewicz A, Sedding DG, et al: Correlation of vasa vasorum neovascularization and plaque progression in aortas of apolipoprotein E(-/-)/low-density lipoprotein(-/-) double knockout mice, Arterioscler Thromb Vasc Biol 26:347–352, 2006.*)

atherosclerosis progression by influencing plaque inflammation and vascular remodeling.[32,57] Concordantly, Burke et al demonstrated that marked expansion of the IEL occurred also in plaque hemorrhage, with or without rupture.[58] The clinical relevance of remodeling was pioneered by Schoenhagen et al, who studied 85 patients with unstable coronary syndromes and 46 patients with stable coronary syndromes by using IVUS before PCI.[59] *Remodeling ratio (RR)* was defined as the area of the external elastic membrane at the lesion divided by the same area at the proximal reference site. Positive remodeling was defined as an RR greater than 1.05 and negative remodeling as an RR less than 0.95 (Fig. 59-10). The RR was higher at target lesions in patients with ACS than in patients with stable angina. As a result, positive remodeling was more frequent in ACS (51.8% vs. 19.6%), whereas negative remodeling was more frequent in stable angina (56.5% vs. 31.8%) ($P = 0.001$), confirming the histopathologic associations between plaque remodeling and vulnerability.[59] New technology aiming to detect TCFAs should provide exact measurements to quantify the degree of vascular remodeling. Of clinical relevance, Corti et al were

the first to document the same eccentric pattern for plaque regression after aggressive lipid therapy.[60] More recently, multiple studies have confirmed this observation (Figure 59-11).[61–63] Considering that lipid is the main plaque component that can be reversed with therapy, this eccentric pattern of plaque regression suggests an effective reverse lipid transport system through the deeper layers of the vessel wall, probably mediated by vasa-vasorum neovascularization.[4,64]

VASA-VASORUM NEOVASCULARIZATION

Atherosclerotic neovascularization evolves in early atherogenesis as a defense mechanism against hypoxia and oxLDL deposition within the tunica intima.[65,66] In advanced disease, neovessels may play a defensive role allowing for lipid removal from the plaque through the adventitia leading to plaque regression, as described above. The adventitial vasa-vasorum is the main source of neovascularization in atherosclerotic lesions (Fig. 59-12). Neovascularization, elegantly delineated by

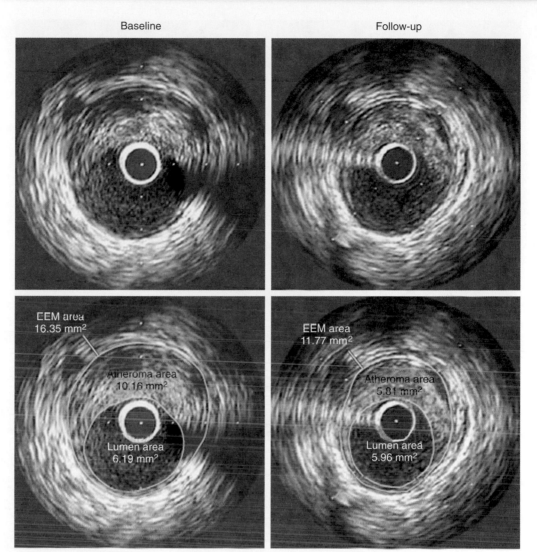

Figure 59-12 *Top panels,* The baseline and follow-up intravascular ultrasound (IVUS) images of a single coronary cross-section after 24 months of rosuvastatin treatment. *Bottom two panels,* Measurements superimposed on the same cross-sections, demonstrating the reduction in atheroma area. *EEM,* external elastic membrane. *(Reproduced with permission from Nissen SE, Nicholls SJ, Sipahi I, et al: Effect of very high-intensity statin therapy on regression of coronary atherosclerosis: The ASTEROID trial, JAMA 295:1556–1565, 2006.)*

Barger et al, who used cinematography (Fig. 59-13), is distributed from the epicardial fat to the plaque throughout vessel wall, although some can originate directly from the vessel lumen.[67] Nevertheless, neovessels from the adventitial vasa were 28 times more numerous (96.5%) compared with those from the luminal side (3.5%).[68] Neovessels from the adventitial vasa characterized severely stenotic lesions and correlated with the extent of inflammatory cell infiltration and lipid core size. Conversely, neovessels from a lumen origin were found in plaques with 40% to 50% stenosis and were associated more often with intra-plaque hemorrhage or hemosiderin deposits.[68] Neovessels may also serve as a pathway for leukocyte recruitment to high-risk areas of the plaque, including the cap and the shoulder. Expression of vascular cell adhesion protein 1 (VCAM-1), intercellular adhesion molecule 1 (ICAM-1), and E-selectin is twofold to threefold higher on neovessels compared with the arterial luminal endothelium, which confirms the pivotal role of neovessels as a pathway for leukocyte recruitment in human coronary plaques.[69] Angiogenesis is stimulated by inflammatory cells. For instance, apoptotic microvesicles at the submicron level, found in atherosclerosis plaques, are highly proangiogenic by regulating CD40L and are produced mostly from macrophages.[70,71] Histologic evidence for atherosclerotic neovascularization as a pathway for macrophage infiltration in advanced, lipid-rich plaques is also documented (Fig. 59-14).[72] Neovessel content was significantly increased in plaques with severe inflammation, associated with both increased macrophage and T lymphocyte infiltration.[73,74] Moreover, ruptured plaques exhibited the highest degree of neovascularization.[75] Further analysis of plaque

angiogenesis in diabetes documented a complex morphology, including sprouting, red blood cell (RBC) extravasation, and perivascular inflammation.[76] Lastly, neovascularization may increase calcification, as demonstrated by the close link between immature endothelial cells and osteoblasts in atherosclerotic plaques and in cellular tissue, expressing vascular calcification–associated factor (VCAF).[77] Using micro-CT imaging, recent studies have shown increased vasa-vasorum density, along with iron and glycophorin-A content in nonstenotic, noncalcified plaques. Moreover, calcium content was inversely proportional to neovessel content.[78] Technology detecting TCFAs should quantify vasa-vasorum neovascularization in the adventitia, in the tunica media, and within the atherosclerotic plaque.

In summary, plaque neovascularization, initially a defense mechanism to provide oxygen and to remove lipid from the plaque, may eventually fail leading to extravasation of RBCs, perivascular inflammation, and intra-plaque hemorrhage.

INTRA-PLAQUE HEMORRHAGE

Neovessel leakage leads to extravasation of plasma content and RBCs into the plaque, which is known as *intra plaque hemorrhage (IPH)*. The mechanisms by which IPH occurs involves the leakage of RBCs from immature neovessels, which is mediated by various growth factors and chemokines that are expressed more in VPs.[79] Compared with non-hemorrhagic atheromas, evidence has demonstrated lower levels of vascular endothelial growth factor (EGF), placental growth factor

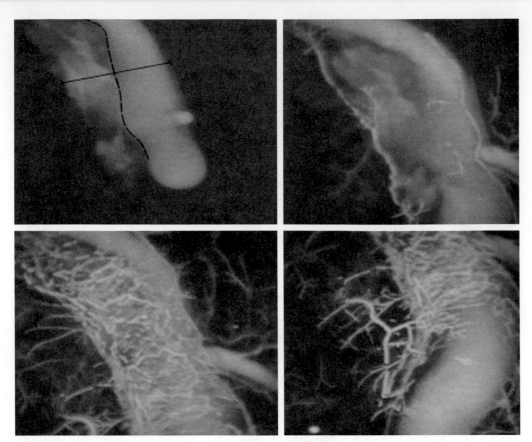

Figure 59-13 Color prints taken during the injection of silicone polymer into the coronary arteries of cleared hearts, demonstrating regions of vessels with abundant neovascularization. The positive regions are composed of networks of small-caliber vessels coming from the adventitia and penetrating the tunica media into the atherosclerotic plaque. *(Reproduced with permission from Barger AC, Beeuwkes R, 3rd, Lainey LL, Silverman KJ: Hypothesis: Vasa vasorum and neovascularization of human coronary arteries. A possible role in the pathophysiology of atherosclerosis, N Engl J Med 310:175–177, 1984.)*

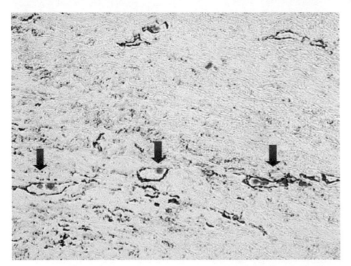

Figure 59-14 Histologic evidence of atherosclerotic neovascularization as a pathway for macrophage infiltration in human aortic plaques obtained at autopsy. Bicolor, contrasting immunohistochemical technique showing microvessels in cross-sections (*red arrows*) identified with the monoclonal endothelial cell marker CD34 linked to a blue chromogen and inflammatory cells identified with a combined macrophage–T cell marker CD68-CD3 linked to a red chromogen. *(Reproduced with permission from Fuster VM, Fayad PR, Corti ZA, Badimon RR: Atherothrombosis and high-risk plaque part I: Evolving concepts, J Am Coll Cardiol 46:937–954, 2005.)*

(PGF), and angiopoietin-1, in combination with an increased vascular endothelial growth factor (VEGF) expression, which are characteristic of hemorrhagic plaques.[80,81] Lysis of RBCs contributes to lipid deposition. In addition, extracorpuscular hemoglobin (Hb) can induce oxidative tissue damage by virtue of its heme iron, with subsequent production of reactive oxygen species.[79] The defense mechanism against free Hb is haptoglobin (Hp), which irreversibly binds to free Hb forming an Hp–Hb complex. Two classes of alleles (Hp-1 and Hp-2) characterize the human Hp locus at chromosome 16q22. The protein products of the two Hp alleles are structurally different, and the cardiovascular effects of this Hp polymorphism play a major role in patients with DM.[82–84] Multiple independent epidemiologic studies examining incident cardiovascular disease have demonstrated that individuals with DM and the Hp 2-2 (homozygous for the Hp 2 allele) genotype have the risk of cardiovascular events four to five times higher compared with individuals with the Hp 1-1 (homozygous for the Hp 1 allele) genotype. The mechanism by which this Hp 2-2 phenotype regulates inflammation and enhances plaque vulnerability is related to decreased Hp clearance in the Hp 2-2 phenotype. This is explained, in part, by a defective CD163 receptor in macrophages, which is the receptor in charge of removing the Hp–Hb complex from the atheroma.[85] Technology detecting TCFAs should identify intraplaque hemorrhage, iron deposition, RBC membranes, and hemosiderin deposits in macrophages. In patients with DM, Ha genotyping may offer additional prognostic value.

PLAQUE COMPOSITION: SUMMARY

Atherosclerotic plaques at high risk for rupture are composed of several features, including a large lipid core, a thin fibrous cap with increased shear stress, macrophage infiltration, positive remodeling, vasa-vasorum neovascularization, and increased intra-plaque hemorrhage. These concepts apply only to lesions at risk for plaque rupture and thrombosis (TCFAs). Of note, plaques at risk for erosion and thrombosis do not exhibit any specific morphologic feature that can be detected by any imaging technique at this point. This is a significant limitation of the individual, lesion-oriented approach to the high-risk VP hypothesis. Nevertheless, even by merely identifying and treating TCFAs, a significant reduction of clinical events can be achieved.

Plaque Imaging

INVASIVE TECHNIQUES

Coronary angiography has the ability to delineate the coronary lumen, but it does not provide any information about the vessel wall. Therefore, this technique is not appropriate for the detection of VPs. Thus multiple intracoronary imaging techniques have been proposed to identify TCFAs. Of pivotal importance, every imaging technique should have appropriate validation, with histology as the gold standard to identify key histo-morphologic components. Considering that the majority of atherosclerotic plaques (TCFAs and non-TCFAs) will have a certain degree of fibrous cap thickness, shear stress patterns, necrotic core area, macrophage area, positive remodeling, and vasa-vasorum neovascularization, the presence or absence of these features alone (sensitivity and specificity) is not enough. Proper histologic validation must include accurate assessment of the degree of these components, which involves linear regression analysis. This validation process should be confirmed in animal models of TCFA before being applied in human coronary arteries.[86] Then, the ultimate test should be a natural history study of all these techniques to determine if specific plaque components have any prognostic implications. Novel intracoronary techniques to detect TCFAs include (1) IVUS, (2) virtual histology (VH), (3) palpography, OCT, (4) IVUS elastography, or (5) intravascular magnetic resonance imaging (MRI), (6) angioscopy, (7) spectroscopy, and (8) thermography. A summary of these techniques, the component detected, and the resolution or accuracy is presented in Table 59-1. The first seven are already available for use in clinical practice or are under active evaluation in humans. With regard to thermography and the noninvasive modalities, an evidence-based approach for the understanding of their clinical usefulness will be presented. The interventionalist must develop a critical approach to evaluating these novel techniques, understanding their potential, and, most importantly, discerning their multiple limitations before considering them for clinical use.

Intravascular Ultrasound

Unlike angiography, IVUS allows proper visualization of the disease in the vessel wall and provides cross-sectional and longitudinal images of atherosclerotic plaques in vivo.[87] IVUS is based on transmitting and receiving high-frequency sound waves from tissue through a low-profile catheter (approximately 1 mm); reaching a radial resolution

between 100 to 250 µm. IVUS is safe, quick, and easy. Most importantly, IVUS allows identification of hemodynamically significant lesions that may be underestimated by angiography, particularly in nonocclusive plaques with positive remodeling. In addition, IVUS delineates the degree of calcification, plaque burden, and the degree of arterial remodeling. It uses the amplitude of the backscattered ultrasound signal to differentiate highly echogenic components such as calcium and dense fibrous tissue from echolucent tissue, including lipid and necrotic core. However, it cannot clearly differentiate between fibrous and fatty plaques.[88] As a consequence, it is accepted that grayscale IVUS, as an isolated technology, is not capable of distinguishing plaque types. Thus, the application of other imaging protocols and algorithms to IVUS, including integrated backscatter IVUS analysis and Virtual Histology (IVUS-VH), which is discussed below, may contribute to better identification of the different plaque components. Researchers have studied backscatter analysis that extracts frequency components of a signal buried in the original IVUS signal. The imaging signal from a small volume of tissue creates an integrated backscatter (IB) pattern.[89] Several studies have reported on the IVUS characteristics of culprit lesions and the presence of multiple ruptured plaques in patients with acute coronary events.[87,90] A recent study evaluated the long-term outcomes of VPs arbitrarily defined as plaques with rupture, lipid core, dissection, or thrombus by conventional IVUS during ACS both in culprit and nonculprit locations. Multiplicity of VPs in the nontarget vessels (HR 2.2, 95% confidence interval [CI] 1.4–3.4, $P = 0.001$) was the only independent predictor of long-term critical events. Finally, DM and ACS were significantly associated with the multiplicity of VP.[91]

The ability of IVUS to identify TCFAs can be summarized as follows:
1. *Fibrous cap thickness:* Considering that the resolution of IVUS is lower than that needed to detect TCFAs, efforts at quantifying cap thickness with IVUS will always overestimate the expected values provided by histology. With IVUS, ruptured plaques show thinner caps compared with nonruptured plaques (Fig. 59-15).[92] However, when ruptured plaques are evaluated with histology, the mean cap thickness is about 8 to 10 times lower than the resolution of IVUS, 23 ± 19 µm in the coronary, and 34 ± 16 µm in the aorta.[37] This significant overestimation of cap thickness by IVUS is related to its poor axial resolution, which makes it very unlikely for any IVUS-related technology to be able to detect TCFAs, the most common form of VP.[93]
2. *Necrotic core area:* The sensitivity of IVUS to detect the necrotic core has been reported to be 46%, with a specificity of 97%. Several studies have been performed trying to improve these results, using an integrated back scatter approach.[94,95] A prospective study demonstrated that 93% of the clinical events occurred in plaques with large echolucent areas, a surrogate of the necrotic core, suggesting a prognostic value for IVUS.[96] Similarly, recent studies propose the use of attenuation of the echo signal inside the plaque as being indicative of large necrotic cores, but no histologic validation has corroborated this finding.[97] We conclude that although IVUS provides useful information about plaque echogenicity, the exact sensitivity and accuracy to identify necrotic cores is unclear, and the resolution may not be sufficient to properly quantify this important feature of plaque vulnerability.[88]
3. *Plaque inflammation:* Detection of macrophages within the fibrous cap requires a resolution within 10 to 20 µm. Considering that the IVUS resolution is 10 to 20 times lower, it is impossible for IVUS to detect macrophages in atherosclerotic plaques.
4. *Degree of positive remodeling:* IVUS is an excellent tool for detecting remodeling, a major feature of plaque vulnerability, in contrast to detection of other features of plaque composition.[98] IVUS-derived arterial remodeling helped understand the actual paradox of lumen and plaque size in VP, as large plaques can appear as nonobstructive on angiography, leading to the realization that ruptured plaques are larger compared with nonruptured plaques.[37,90] No other imaging modality can show remodeling better than IVUS, so IVUS is considered the gold standard for this parameter in vivo.[99]

TABLE 59-1	Summary of Current Invasive Detection Technologies	
Technology	*Component Detected*	*Resolution/Accuracy*
Intravascular ultrasound (IVUS)	Remodeling, calcium	100–250 µm
IVUS–Virtual Histology	Necrotic core, calcium, collagen	480 µm
Optical coherence tomography	Necrotic core, fibrous cap thickness, macrophages	5–20 µm
IVUS–Elastography	Plaque strain	100–250 µm
Intravascular magnetic resonance imaging (MRI)	Necrotic core	250 µm
Angioscopy	Surface appearance of the plaque	N/A
Spectroscopy	Necrotic core	N/A
Thermography	Metabolic activity of the plaque	0.05° C accurate

N/A, not applicable.

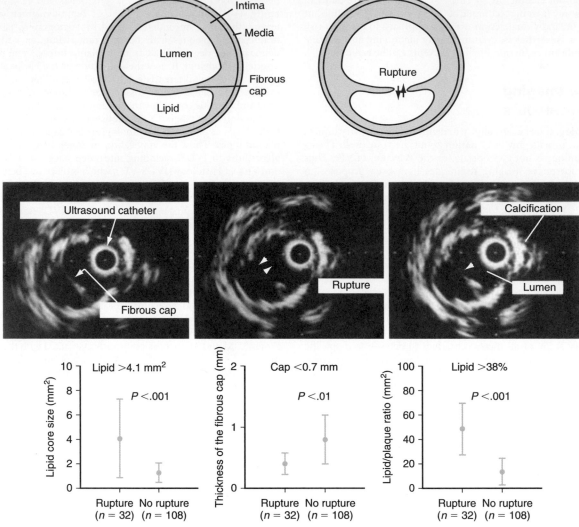

Figure 59-15 Intravascular ultrasound (IVUS) images of ruptured plaques, highlighting the fibrous cap and a large echolucent area under the cap suggestive of large necrotic cores (*upper panel*). Lipid area, cap thickness, and lipid percent area in ruptured (*red*) versus nonruptured (*black*) plaques (*lower panel*). (*Adapted with permission from Ge J, Chirillo F, Schwedtmann J, et al: Screening of ruptured plaques in patients with coronary artery disease by intravascular ultrasound, Heart 81:621–627, 1999.*)

5. *Plaque neovascularization:* IVUS has the potential to detect flow within the plaque and thus identify functional neovessels. While real-time IVUS is limited to evaluating plaque perfusion, recent developments with contrast agents have dramatically improved the quality of Doppler ultrasound. Intravascular injection of microbubbles (i.e., small encapsulated air or gas bubbles or albumin microspheres) can boost the Doppler signal from blood vessels. Microbubbles can help in visualizing flow in smaller vessels, even at the capillary level, as has been shown by contrast-enhanced echocardiography (CEE).[100] Direct visualization of atherosclerotic plaque microvessels using CEE was successfully done by Feinstein in carotid plaques; this has been also validated with histology in animal models and in humans.[101–103] In coronary arteries, IVUS-CEE has successfully identified plaque neovessels with spatiotemporal changes and enhancement–detection techniques (Fig. 59-16).[104] To improve resolution, an IVUS prototype using "harmonic" imaging, with transmission of ultrasound at 20 MHz (fundamental) and detection of contrast signals at 40 MHz (second harmonic), was developed with the aim to identify adventitial neovessels in rabbits models.[105,106] However, to date, vasa-vasorum detection of coronary atherosclerosis with IVUS imaging is still evolving for clinical use.

Virtual Histology

Considering the significant limitations of IVUS, Nair and Vince at Cleveland Clinic studied the ultrasound scattered reflection wave as a possible alternative to improve tissue characterization.[107] This backscattered reflection wave is received by the transducer, where it is converted into voltage. This voltage is known as *backscattered radiofrequency (RF)* data. Using a combination of previously identified spectral parameters of the backscattered ultrasound signal, a classification scheme was developed to construct an algorithm to test plaque composition ex vivo. Four major plaque components were tested, including fibrotic tissue (dark green), fibro-fatty tissue (yellow-green), calcific-necrotic core (red), and dense calcium (white). A color was assigned for each of these components and is displayed on the IVUS image (Fig. 59-17). The Movat-stained histologic images identified homogeneous regions representing each of the four plaque components (Fig. 59-18). The unit of analysis (also called *box*) was initially composed of 64 backscattered RF data samples in length (480 μm).[107] The algorithm developed was then validated ex vivo, with sensitivities and specificities between 79% and 93% for all four-plaque components.[107] The initial studies were performed in ex vivo human coronary specimens with a 30-MGz, 2.9F, mechanically rotating IVUS catheter (Boston Scientific Corp); the initial catheter approved by the U.S. Food and Drug

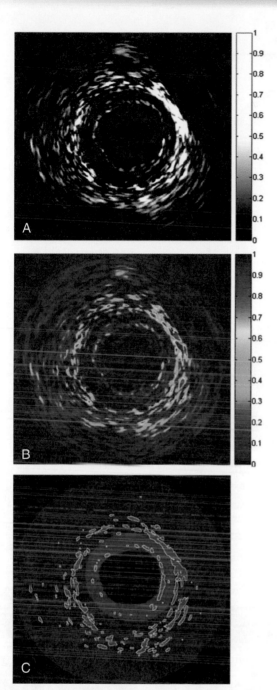

Figure 59-16 Differential intravascular ultrasound (IVUS) images to identify the vasa-vasorum, showing the subtracted post-injection signals from baseline signals. **A,** Black and white (signal intensity of Figure 59-1 A–C). **B,** Color-coded, panel A. **C,** Thresholded to show most significant areas of enhancement. *(Adapted with permission from Vavuranakis M, Kakadiaris IA, O'Malley SM, et al: Images in cardiovascular medicine. Detection of luminal-intimal border and coronary wall enhancement in intravascular ultrasound imaging after injection of microbubbles and simultaneous sonication with transthoracic echocardiography, Circulation 112:e1–e2, 2005.)*

Administration (FDA) was a 20-MHz (Eagle-Eye® Gold) device. Recently, the catheter was upgraded with a 45-MHz transducer that is currently available for clinical practice. In vivo validation studies have shown positive results.[108,109] Virtual histology gained significant attention with the PROSPECT Trial.[15] As previously discussed in this review, VH-derived TCFA was associated with increased events (HR 3.35, $P < 0.001$). Most importantly, the highest-risk lesions (HR 11.05,

$P < 0.001$) were a conglomerate of several features, including greater than 70% plaque burden, low MLA, and TCFA morphology. Therefore, isolating TCFA by using VH may not be enough to categorize a lesion as VP. The possibility of a PROSPECT II study randomizing patients with these lesions to aggressive medical therapy with or without stenting may be considered. However, the large number of patients needed and the increased costs may limit the ability to test this hypothesis.

The individual ability of VH to identify TCFAs can be described as follows:

1. *Fibrous cap thickness:* IVUS-VH is limited in cap thickness evaluation. This was elegantly addressed in the initial publication by Nair and Vince, in which they comment on the limitations: "The window size currently applied for selection of regions of interest and eventual tissue map reconstructions is 480 microns in the radial direction. Therefore, detection of thin fibrous caps (≤65 microns below the resolution of IVUS) would be compromised, restricting the detection of vulnerable atheromas".[107] As a result, lesions with fibrous cap thickness greater than 65 μm will be incorrectly classified as TCFAs and perhaps overestimated. Therefore, with its axial resolution of 250 μm, it is insufficient to determine fibrous cap thickness, and investigators have proposed a classification of "IVUS-VH–derived TCFA".[110] This has been defined as a plaque with a rich necrotic core (>10%), without evident overlying fibrous tissue, and with a percent plaque volume of 40% seen on at least three consecutive images. Such features are reflective of histologic TCFAs that are more prone to rupture. As also defined by histology, IVUS-VH–derived TCFAs cluster around the proximal segments of the arteries, are more often associated with positively remodeling, and are more frequently found in patients with ACS compared with those with stable angina.[111,112] Sawada et al evaluated the ability of both IVUS-VH and OCT to detect TCFAs in the same coronary lesions. IVUS-VH was very effective in detecting the absence of TCFA. However, IVUS-VH only diagnosed half of the TCFAs compared with OCT.[99,113] One of the initial concerns about the IVUS-VH–derived TCFA was its accuracy to serve as a surrogate for VPs and the actual prognostic value that this specific finding could provide. This question was mostly answered by the PROSPECT trial (described above), which highlighted the value of IVUS-VH–derived TCFA. In a similar way, this concept was reinforced by a recent publication by Kubo et al, which addressed the natural history of IVUS-VH-TCFA in 99 patients undergoing PCI, who were followed up for 12 months with serial evaluations of coronary vasculature with the use of IVUS-VH. They found that 75% of the 20 VH-TCFAs healed by either becoming TCFAs (65% of total) or by becoming fibrotic (10% of total), whereas only 25% of those remained unchanged. They also reported the occurrence of 12 new VH-TCFAs that developed during the follow-up period: 6 of them from pathologic intimal thickening and 6 from TCFAs identified at baseline. Notably, no acute coronary events occurred during the follow-up period from any of the initially identified or the newly formed VH-TCFAs.[114]

2. *Necrotic core area:* IVUS-VH was initially developed to identify calcific necrotic cores. However, the incidence and degree of calcification in necrotic cores is variable, and therefore necrotic cores without calcification may not be properly identified.[115] Most importantly, the majority of advanced atherosclerotic lesions will display a certain degree of necrotic core. As a result, when validating necrotic core using IVUS-VH, not only the presence or absence of the necrotic core is important (sensitivity/specificity) but also the area.[116] IVUS-VH routinely reports necrotic core area (mm²) and percent of total plaque area. A recent substudy from the PROSPECT cohort reported that plaques with large areas of attenuation by grayscale analysis are associated with large amount of VH-IVUS necrotic core and are markers of the presence of fibroatheromas (VH-TCFA or thick-capped fibroatheromas [VH-ThFA]).[117] However, despite the cumulative clinical evidence and proposed clinical applications of IVUS-VH, proper validation of these areas with histology using linear regression analysis have yet to be

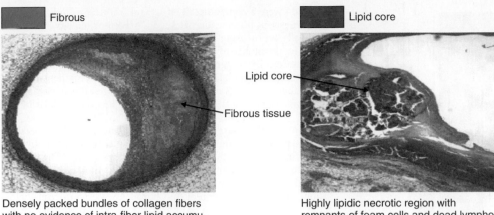

Fibrous

Fibrous tissue

Densely packed bundles of collagen fibers with no evidence of intra-fiber lipid accumulation. No evidence of macrophage infiltration. Appears dark yellow on Movat stained section.

Lipid core

Lipid core

Highly lipidic necrotic region with remnants of foam cells and dead lymphocytes present. No collagen fibers are visible and mechanical integrity is poor. Cholesterol clefts and micro calcifications are visible.

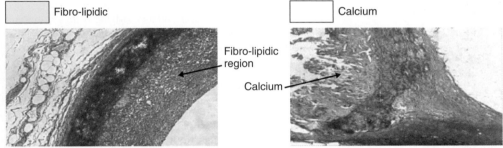

Fibro-lipidic

Fibro-lipidic region

Calcium

Loosely packed bundles of collagen fibers with regions of lipid deposition present. These areas are cellular and no cholesterol clefts or necrosis are present. Some macrophage infiltration. Increase in extracellular matrix. Appears turquoise on Movat stained section.

Calcium

Focal area of dense calcium. Appears purple on Movat. Usually falls out section, but calcium crystals are evident at borders

Figure 59-17 Color-coded reproduction of intravascular ultrasound Virtual Histology (IVUS-VH) plaque composition displayed in vivo in the cath lab.

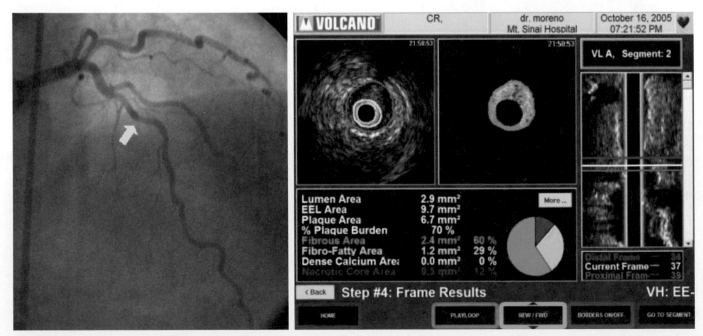

Figure 59-18 Definitions of the different plaque components obtained with intravascular ultrasound Virtual Histology (IVUS-VH). *(Reproduced with permission from Vince, DG, personal communication).*

performed in humans and probably never will be. Limited studies have attempted to identify the correlations between necrotic core areas by using IVUS-VH with histology; these were done in a porcine model, demonstrating that IVUS-VH is unreliable in terms of necrotic core assessment.[118,119] As discussed earlier in this review, multiple pathologic studies have established the concept that necrotic core areas from patients with ACS are larger compared with necrotic core areas from patients with chronic stable angina.[4,30] Conversely, fibrous plaque areas (collagen) have been found to be significantly smaller in patients with ACS.[38] Surmely et al concluded that data on plaque composition obtained by IVUS-VH contradict previously published histopathologic data.[120] However, Rodriguez-Granillo et al have identified larger necrotic areas in ruptured plaques and in nonculprit lesions from patients with ACS.[121,122] Validation with histology in carotid atherosclerosis shows diagnostic accuracy of 99.4% for TCFA, 96.1% for calcified TCFA, 85.9% for fibroatheroma, 85.5% for fibrocalcific atheroma, 83.4% for pathologic intimal thickening, and 72.4% for calcified fibroatheroma.[123] In a small prospective cohort, IVUS-VH analysis was correlated with coronary atherectomy specimens. The correlation coefficients ranged from 0.90 to 0.97 for plaque components.[124]

3. *Plaque inflammation:* Detection of macrophages within the fibrous cap requires a resolution within 10 to 20 μm. Considering that IVUS-VH resolution is at least 10 to 20 times lower, it is impossible for VH to detect macrophages in vivo.

4. *Degree of positive remodeling:* IVUS is an excellent tool to detect remodeling, and IVUS-VH should preserve this advantage. As reviewed earlier, positive remodeling is related to large necrotic core areas, more frequently seen in patients with ACS. Conversely, plaques with negative or constrictive remodeling are associated with smaller necrotic core areas, usually seen in patients with chronic

stable angina. Recent studies evaluated IVUS-VH–derived necrotic core areas in plaques with positive and negative remodeling and found smaller necrotic core areas in positively remodeled plaques.[90] Other investigators have confirmed these data.[125] However, some authors have demonstrated contradictory data with strong correlations between large IVUS-VH–derived necrotic core areas and positive remodeling.[117,126] Finally, vasa-vasorum neovascularization and IPH require highly sophisticated technology and cannot be identified with IVUS-VH. On the basis of the data presented above, it is difficult to reconcile these contradictory findings and, therefore, impossible to elucidate the real clinical value of IVUS-VH–derived plaque composition in clinical practice.

Elastography and Palpography

The mechanical stress induced by changes in blood pressure induces deformation on the fibrous cap (strain).[127] This stress–strain relationship in coronary lesions can be identified by using another IVUS-derived technique called *elastography* or *palpography*, which displays data in a color-coded scale (see Figure 59-18).[128] Purple indicates a low strain (hard, stiff), whereas yellow indicates a region of high strain (soft, deformable).[129] Palpography has high sensitivity and specificity to detect VP, with a deformation of more than 2% reflecting increased macrophage infiltration, reduced smooth muscle cell, and low collagen content (Fig. 59-19).[130] The Rotterdam Classification (ROC) divides strain into four subclasses; the worst is ROC IV, with a deformation greater than 1.2%.[129] Palpography shows correlations with CRP, and ST elevation myocardial infarction (STEMI). Aggressive treatment using statins can reduce, over a period of 6 months, the intensity and frequency of these high-strain spots. Recent improvements using reconstructive compounding by motion artifact correction are promising.[131,132] Nonetheless, palpography cannot detect fibrous cap thickness, necrotic core, degree of remodeling, neovascularization, or IPH,

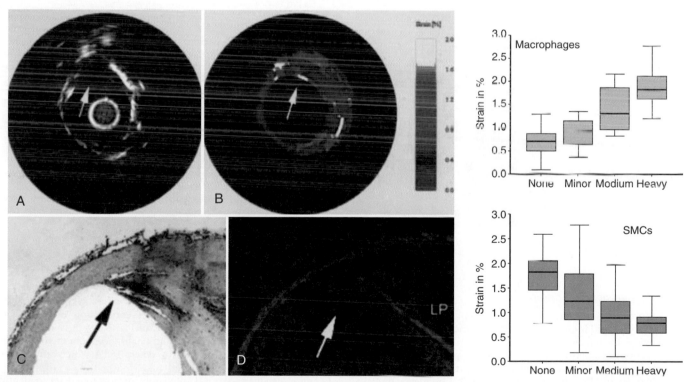

Figure 59-19 Vulnerable plaque marked in intravascular ultrasound (IVUS) (*A*), elastogram (*B*), macrophage staining (*C*), and collagen staining (*D*). In the elastogram, a vulnerable plaque is indicated by a high strain on the surface. In the corresponding histology, a high amount of macrophages (*C*) is visible with a thin cap (*D*) and a lipid pool (*LP*). See also box plots correlating the macrophage (*upper right*) and smooth muscle cell content (*lower right*) with the level of strain. High levels of strain are associated with significant increases in macrophage content and significant decreases in smooth muscle cell content. *SMCs,* smooth muscle cells. (*Adapted with permission from Schaar JA, De Korte CL, Mastik F, et al: Characterizing vulnerable plaque features with intravascular elastography,* Circulation *108:2636-2641, 2003.*)

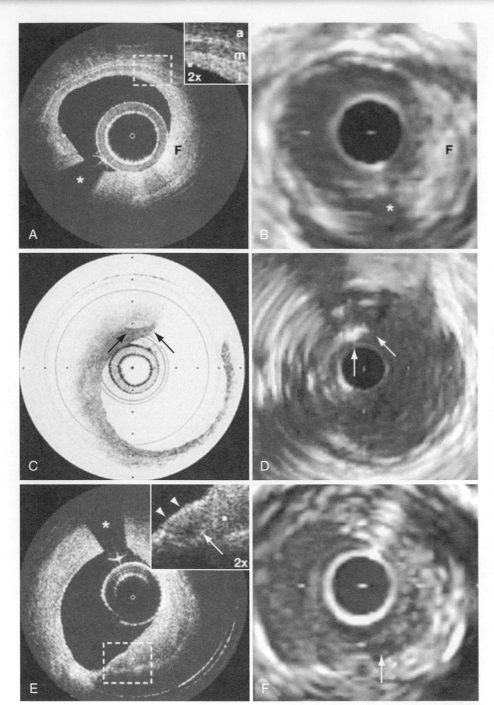

Figure 59-20 In vivo optical coherence tomography images of different coronary plaque types compared with intravascular ultrasonography of the corresponding sites. **A,** Fibrous plaque: from 9 o'clock to 2 o'clock, the three-layer structure of a typical intimal hyperplasia is shown and a magnified area is shown in the box. A homogeneous, signal-rich pattern indicates fibrous plaque (F), which is partly obscured by a guidewire artifact (*). **B,** Fibrous plaque: the intravascular ultrasound image corresponding to A. **C,** Calcific plaque: a signal-poor region surrounded by sharp borders represents calcific plaque, which is clearly delineated (arrows). **D,** Calcific plaque: on the corresponding intravascular ultrasound image calcium is easily identified but the strong signal obscures the structure in front of the calcium deposit and a back-shadow artifact obscures that behind the deposit. **E,** Lipid-rich plaque: a signal-poor region (arrow in inset) surrounded by diffuse borders and separated by a thin cap (arrow heads in inset) is consistent with thin cap fibroatheroma (TCFA). **F,** Lipid-rich plaque: the corresponding intravascular ultrasound image suggests a superficial echolucent region. a, adventitia; i, intima; m, media. (Adapted, with permission from Low AF, Tearney GJ, Bouma BE, Jang IK: Technology Insight: optical coherence tomography—current status and future development, Nat Clin Pract Cardiovasc Med 3:154–162; quiz 172, 2006.)

Optical Coherence Tomography

OCT is a novel high-resolution intravascular imaging technique that is currently approved for clinical use. Of all of the invasive modalities, OCT provides the highest resolution (5 to 20 μm).[133] Excellent sensitivity and specificity, between 92% and 100%, have been documented for all components of TCFA.[133] Superb resolution allows for improved images (Fig. 59-20). Recent advances using optical frequency domain imaging (OFDI) allow for high-speed comprehensive imaging, scanning up to 5 cm with one single saline flush (Fig. 59-21).[134] OCT is currently being used in clinical practice, providing significant information for the identification of plaque rupture, fibrous cap erosion, intracoronary thrombus, and TCFA location.[135,136] Similarly, OCT can

predict no-reflow phenomenon in patients with large lipid cores who undergo PCI during ACS.[137] A direct comparison of OCT with IVUS-VH to detect TCFAs is shown in Figure 59-22. With all these promising facts on OCT, the interventionalist needs objective information regarding the ability of OCT to detect TCFA, which can be summarized as follows:

1. *Fibrous cap thickness:* OCT is the only imaging tool that can identify plaques with cap thickness 65 μm or less. This was demonstrated with histologic studies using proper linear regression analysis (r = 0.89) (Fig. 59-23). In vivo studies showed that fibrous cap thickness was lowest in patients with AMI, intermediate in patients with unstable angina, and highest in patients with chronic stable angina

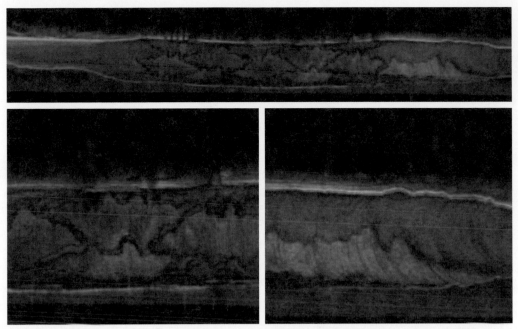

Figure 59-21 In vivo optical frequency-domain imaging (OFDI) of a coronary stent deployed in the porcine model. Normal endothelium is shown in red, dissections induced by the balloon during stent deployment are shown in white, and stent struts are shown in blue. *(Reproduced with permission from Bouma BE: New insights from OCT, polarization-sensitive OCT, and the emergence of OFDI. Presented at The Vulnerable Plaque Session: "Pathophysiology, detection, and therapeutic intervention," Transcatheter Therapeutic Intervention (TCT) Meeting, 2006, Washington, D.C.; 2006.)*

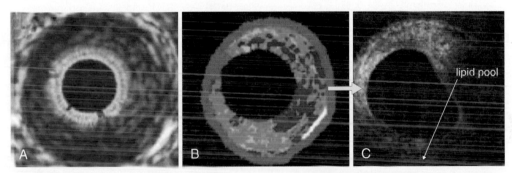

Figure 59-22 Definite thin cap fibroatheroma (TCFA) in vivo by three different invasive imaging modalities. *Panel A,* Conventional intravascular ultrasound (IVUS) imaging. *Panel B,* intravascular ultrasound–Virtual Histology (IVUS-VH). *Panel C,* Optical coherence tomography (OCT). *(Reproduced with permission from Sawada T, Shite J, Garcia-Garcia HM, et al: Feasibility of combined use of intravascular ultrasound radiofrequency data analysis and optical coherence tomography for detecting thin cap fibroatheroma, Eur Heart J 29:1136–1146, 2008.)*

(Fig. 59-24).[138] Using this analysis, OCT can estimate the incidence of TCFAs according to the clinical syndrome (see Fig. 59-23). The advantages of OCT extend not only to the ability to measure fibrous cap thickness but also to the identification of plaque rupture, fibrous cap erosion, and thrombosis more accurately compared with other imaging modalities, including IVUS and angioscopy. This was demonstrated by Kubo et al, who studied patients with ACS for the assessment of fibrous cap thickness after statin treatment.[136,139] For a comparison between different intracoronary imaging modalities assessing plaque rupture see Figure 59-25.

2. *Necrotic core area:* The lipid pool and the necrotic core are signal poor and therefore are diffusely delineated with respect to the surrounding tissue. The lipid-rich plaque can be recognized, therefore, by the presence of large areas of ill-defined, signal-poor regions that are evident to the naked eye (see Fig. 59-20, *C*). Conversely, when the cap is thick and the signal is strong, the operator can tell that

the signal is coming from a fibrous plaque mostly composed of collagen (see Figs. 59-20, *A*, 59-23, and 59-24). Thus, it is considered that OCT can still identify lipid-rich plaques according to the characteristics of the signal, as mentioned above. Such classification of the plaque moderately correlates with IVUS-VH for necrotic core identification.[113,136] Of note, linear correlations of human coronary plaque collagen were recently performed, showing regression plots between OCT and measured collagen, with a correlation value of 0.475 ($P < 0.002$), and the predictive values of collagen were between 89% and 93%.[140] Nevertheless, it is important to highlight that OCT does not validate necrotic core areas as effectively as it does cap thickness and collagen, and further experimentation is warranted to overcome this issue, particularly for necrotic and lipid tissue evaluation.[141] However, promising results from a recent study performed in the Thoraxcenter demonstrated how the different vessel wall components, including necrotic core and macrophages, can be

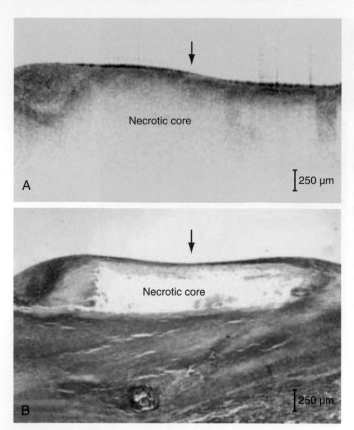

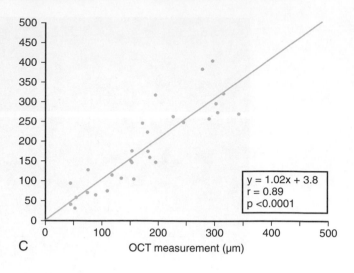

Figure 59-23 Optical coherence tomography evaluation of fibrous cap thickness. **A,** Minimal fibrous cap thickness measuring 44.1 microns by optical coherence tomography (OCT) (*black arrow*), obtained from plaque illustrated below. **B,** Minimal fibrous cap thickness measuring 40.4 microns by histology (*black arrow*). Necrotic core is visualized underneath the fibrous cap. **C,** Linear regression analysis showing an excellent correlation between OCT and histology measurements in 29 human atherosclerotic plaques. *(Reproduced with permission from Jang IK: Optical coherence tomography. Studies at MGH. Paper presented at Transcatheter Cardiovascular Therapeutics, TCT Conference, September 27, 2002.)*

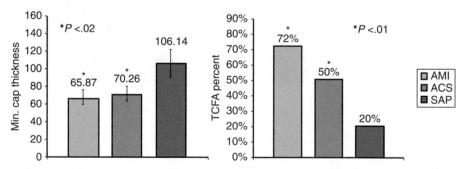

Figure 59-24 In vivo quantification of fibrous cap thickness by optical coherence tomography (OCT). Cap thickness was lowest in patients with acute myocardial infarction, intermediate in patients with acute coronary syndrome (ACS), and highest in patients with chronic stable angina. As a result, the incidence of thin cap fibroatheroma (TCFA) is highest in acute myocardial infarction and lowest in chronic stable angina. *(Reproduced with permission from Jang IK, Tearney GJ, MacNeill B, et al: In vivo characterization of coronary atherosclerotic plaque by use of optical coherence tomography, Circulation 111:1551–1555, 2005.)*

distinguished by their optical properties with has good histologic correlation.[142]

3. *Plaque inflammation:* As discussed for cap thickness, OCT resolution allows for proper identification of macrophages in atherosclerotic plaques.[133] The first correlation in vitro was performed by Tearney et al, who identified multiple strong back reflections from caps with abundant macrophage infiltration, resulting in a relatively high OCT signal variance.[143] This signal variance was then processed using logarithmic transformation (Fig. 59-26, *A* to *F*). Linear regression analysis showed correlations for raw and logarithmic OCT-derived and immunostained macrophages of 0.84 (*P* < 0.0001) and 0.47 (*P* < 0.05), respectively (see Figure 59-26). In vivo studies then showed increased macrophage density in ruptured plaques from patients with ACS (both in culprit and nonculprit lesions) compared with nonruptured plaques from patients with chronic stable angina (Fig. 59-27).[144] In addition to this, OCT has been able to assess the content of macrophages located in the fibrous cap and has correlated this macrophage density with peripheral white blood cell (WBC) count.[145]

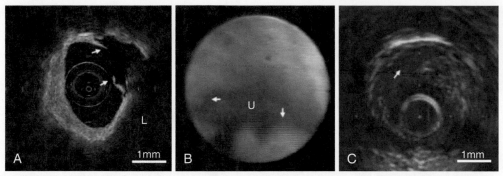

Figure 59-25   Fibrous cap rupture during acute coronary syndrome assessed by different invasive modalities. **A,** Optical coherence tomography (OCT) demonstrating a lipid-rich area (*L*) and fibrous cap discontinuation (*white arrows*) that protrudes into the lumen. **B,** Angioscopy with yellow lesion and cap disruption in white arrows and ulceration (*U*). **C,** Intravascular ultrasound (IVUS) showing an eccentric plaque rupture at the shoulder (*white arrow*). *(Reproduced with permission from Kubo T, Imanishi T, Takarada S, et al: Assessment of culprit lesion morphology in acute myocardial infarction: Ability of optical coherence tomography compared with intravascular ultrasound and coronary angioscopy, J Am Coll Cardiol 50:933–939, 2007.)*

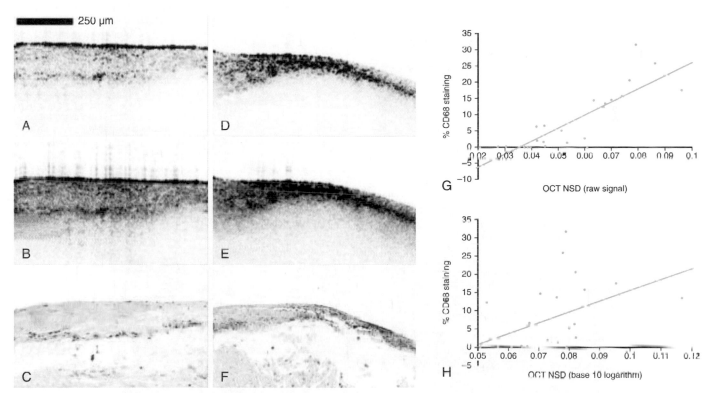

Figure 59-26   Raw (*A*) and logarithm base 10 (*B*) optical coherence tomography (OCT) images of a fibroatheroma with a low density of macrophages within the fibrous cap. **C,** Corresponding histology for A and B (CD68 immunoperoxidase; original magnification ×100). Raw (*D*) and logarithm base 10 (*E*) OCT images of a fibroatheroma with a high density of macrophages within the fibrous cap. **F,** Corresponding histology for D and E (CD68 immunoperoxidase; original magnification ×100). Correlation between the raw (*G*) and logarithm base 10 (*H*) OCT NSD and CD68 percent area staining (*diamonds,* NSD data; *solid line,* linear fit). *(Reproduced with permission from Tearney GJ, Yabushita H, Houser SL, et al: Quantification of macrophage content in atherosclerotic plaques by optical coherence tomography, Circulation 107:113–119, 2003.)*

4. *Degree of positive remodeling:* OCT has limited plaque penetration, and depth is reduced to 2 to 3 mm. Therefore, it is not possible to image beyond the internal elastic lamina. As a result, OCT cannot assess the actual diameter of the vessel to calculate the remodeling index. This is a significant limitation of OCT.

5. *Plaque neovascularization and intra-plaque hemorrhage:* OCT is the gold standard to quantify neovascularization and the effects of novel anti-angiogenic therapies in other common diseases such as age-related macular degeneration, extrafoveal choroid neo-vascularization, and proliferative diabetic retinopathy.[146] However, the number of studies specifically assessing atherosclerotic neovascularization or IPH is limited. An interesting study recently published by Kitabata et al proposed the use of OCT to identify intra-plaque structures that could probably represent neovessels. These were called "microchannels" and were defined as a no-signal tubulo-luminal structure without a connection to the vessel lumen on three consecutive cross-sectional OCT images (Fig. 59-28). These authors reported that plaques with microchannels displayed characteristics of vulnerability, including plaque rupture, positive remodeling, and thin fibrous caps compared with plaques without these structures. However, a histologic validation of these structures observed with in vivo OCT imaging has not yet been done.[147]

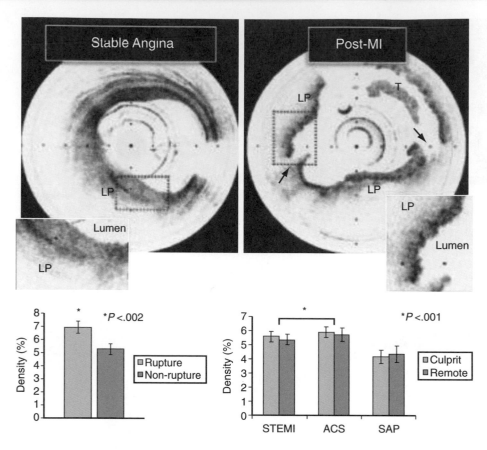

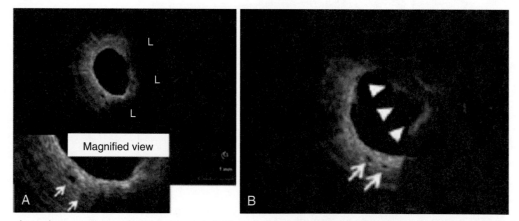

Figure 59-27 *Upper panel,* OCT images of plaques from patients with stable angina and after myocardial infarction. *LP,* lipid pool. See increased signal area at the fibrous cap in post-MI figure (detail) highlighting increased macrophage density areas. *Lower left panel,* Increased macrophage density in ruptured (*red bar*) compared with nonruptured (*blue bar*) plaques. *Lower right panel,* Macrophage density in culprit (*red bar*) and remote (*blue bar*) plaques from patients with ST elevation myocardial infarction (STEMI), acute coronary syndrome (ACS), and stable angina pectoris (SAP). Macrophage density is higher at both plaques (culprit and remote) in patients with STEMI and ACS compared with plaques from patients with SAP. *(Reproduced with permission from MacNeill BD, Jang IK, Bouma BE, et al: Focal and multi-focal plaque macrophage distributions in patients with acute and stable presentations of coronary artery disease, J Am Coll Cardiol 44:972–979, 2004.)*

Figure 59-28 Microchannels representing plaque neovascularization. **A,** Eccentric lipid rich plaque (*L*) with microchannels (*white arrows*). **B,** Intracoronary thrombus (*arrowheads*) and two additional microchannels. *(Adapted with permission from Kitabata H, Tanaka A, Kubo T, et al: Relation of microchannel structure identified by optical coherence tomography to plaque vulnerability in patients with coronary artery disease, Am J Cardiol 105:1673–1678, 2010.)*

Surface and Intravascular Magnetic Resonance Imaging

MRI is being increasingly recognized as a potential approach for the quantification of atherosclerotic plaque burden and lesion composition.[148] MRI allows for three-dimensional evaluation of vascular structures, with outstanding depiction of various components of the atherothrombotic plaque, including lipid, fibrous tissue, calcium, and thrombus formation.[149] In addition, combining MRI with cellular and molecular targeting is providing important data on the biologic activity of high-risk VPs, especially for carotid and aortic lesions.[150] However, MRI characterization of coronary plaques is considerably more difficult. The deep intra-thoracic position of coronary arteries

(4 to 10 cm from the surface), the smaller dimensions, and the tortuous and irregular course of these vessels under continuous movement further exacerbate the problem, resulting in a reduction in image quality.[151] To overcome some of these issues, MRI has been also applied to the intravascular imaging field given the low signal-to-noise ratio of surface MRI.[152] Whereas the conventional MRI resolution is approximately 460 μm, intravascular MRI (ivMRI) resolution is improved to 250 μm. As a result, ivMRI may provide valuable information in plaque characterization of coronary lesions. This technology is currently under aggressive clinical testing in the United States and Europe, with over 100 patients enrolled. To date, it is known that

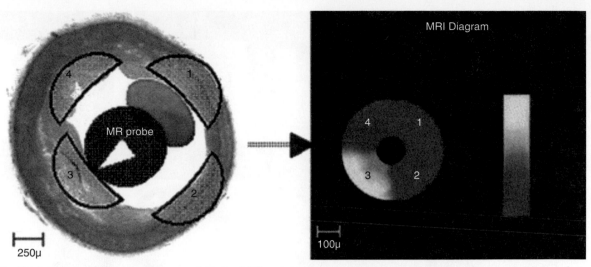

Figure 59-29   Depiction of the magnetic resonance imaging (MRI) catheter with imaging areas superimposed on a cross-section of a human coronary artery (*left*). Interrogation of the arterial wall is in four quadrants, each comprising a field of view. A single field of view is denoted by the white arrowhead. The MRI diagram (*right*) displays the lipid fraction in each quadrant assessed by the catheter. In this particular illustration, an increased lipid concentration is noted only in quadrant 3, as it displays yellow. Quadrants 1, 2, and 4 are shown in blue, indicating a low lipid content or increased fibrous content.

ivMRI has a safe profile at 30-day follow-up as evidenced in the first-in-human study published.[153] As a result, ivMRI requires careful attention regarding its ability to detect TCFAs, and it can be summarized as follows:

1. *Fibrous cap thickness and necrotic core:* As stated above, the resolution of ivMRI is higher than 65 μm, and thus it is a limited imaging modality for the identification of TCFAs. To overcome this limitation, the luminal surface of the plaque is simultaneously evaluated in two separate bands: a superficial, luminal 0–100-μm band, and a deeper 100-50-μmband.[154] TCFA was then defined as the presence of an increased lipid fraction within the superficial band (0–100 μm), which, in turn, denotes the presence of a thin fibrous cap, as well as increased lipid in the deep band, which indicates the presence of a necrotic core or an increased concentration of lipid-rich cells. Conversely, the absence of lipid within the superficial band may be indicative of a thick fibrous cap, which is associated with more stable lesions.[154] With the aid of a partially inflated balloon, the ivMRI catheter gets close to the vessel wall and obtains images in four quadrants (Fig. 59-29). Within each quadrant, the percentage of lipid is assessed in both the superficial and deep bands simultaneously, and the data are integrated to produce a circular color-coded display. Fibrous and fatty tissue could be differentiated according to their apparent water diffusion coefficients. Ex vivo experiments have shown a 95% sensitivity and 100% specificity for ivMRI probe to detect these components, with a penetration of about 250 μm.[154] The resulting image represents the sum of the four superficial and four deep bands from the four quadrants. However, this is not a real image but is more a chemical signature of the tissue generated by the computer. Validation studies were performed using a total of 34 human plaques (aortic and coronary) (see examples in Fig. 59-30). The results of histology, in addition to the aortic data, resulted in a sensitivity of 100% and a specificity of 89%.[154] The use of contrast agents for both ivMRI and surface MRI for plaque characterization is evolving. Among these, tyrosine polyethylene glycol micelles seem to accurately localize lipid-rich plaques in animal models, when combined with the ability of ivMRI to detect features of plaque stability.[155–157] Another promising contrast agent is gadofluorine M, which predominately detects extracellular matrix components but is not found in the lipid-rich areas, potentially allowing the identification of VPs.[158] Finally, novel markers such as P975 allow the identification of activated platelets in vivo by using

target-specific MRI, representing an accurate target for certain types of plaques during ACS.[159] However, these agents are still under development and, to date, their definitive role in plaque characterization is not completely known.

3. *Plaque inflammation:* With the advantage of molecular targeting, surface MRI can image macrophages using different pathways.[160] Several compounds, contrast agents, and nanoparticles are now available to target different molecules within macrophages.[161] The ultra-small super-paramagnetic particles of iron oxide compounds (USPIOs, SPIOs), also called *magnetic nanoparticles,* are internalized by macrophage receptors and can be properly imaged by MRI (Fig. 59-31). Similarly, lipid-based nanoparticles targeting scavenger receptor-B (CD36), as well as reconstituted high-density lipoprotein (rHDL) nanoparticles and monocrystalline iron-oxide nanoparticles (MION)-47, have also been used for macrophage identification in animal models.[162–164] In addition to macrophage receptor uptake, inflammatory cells can be imaged using targeting metabolic and proteolytic activities. The combination of MRI and 18Fluorodeoxyglucose positron emission tomography (PET) successfully images the metabolic activity of plaque macrophages in patients with symptomatic carotid atherosclerosis (Fig. 59-32).[165] Similarly, proteolytic activity by targeting cathepsin-B, MMPs, and myeloperoxidase, as well as inflammatory cell identification by targeting IL production, scavenger receptor, and apoptosis activation may also provide an estimation of the inflammatory component of the plaque.[161,166–171] Of note, macrophage imaging by MRI is only available as a noninvasive tool.

4. *Degree of positive remodeling:* The evaluation of remodeling requires perfect delineation of the external elastic lamina, both at the site of the plaque and at the reference segment. The current stage of ivMRI does not provide this degree of detail and therefore cannot quantify remodeling.

5. *Plaque neovascularization and intra-plaque hemorrhage:* As a general principle, molecular imaging for angiogenesis targets the endothelial cell.[172] Proliferating endothelial cells (ECs) respond to signaling by adhesion molecules, including integrins and cadherins, along with signals generated by secreted growth factors.[172] As a result, molecular imaging can target molecules such as the integrin αvβ3, which promotes angiogenesis by signaling basic fibroblast growth factor, or αvβ5, which promotes angiogenesis by signaling vascular endothelial growth factor. Winter et al evaluated atherosclerotic

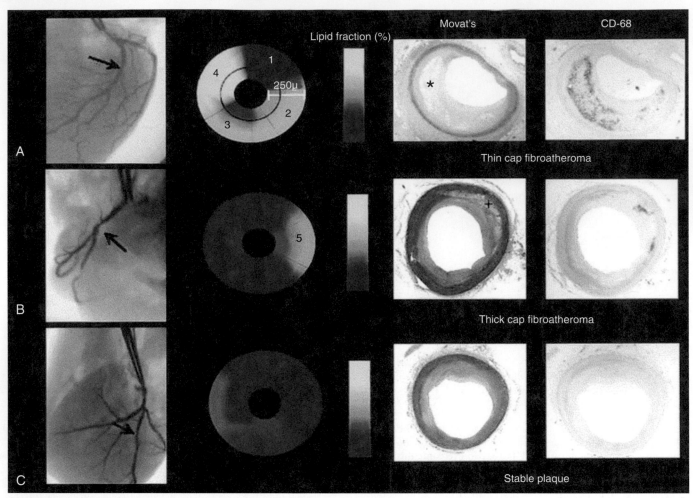

Figure 59-30 The magnetic resonance imaging (MRI) scan demonstrates excellent correlation with histology. Coronary angiography, MRI, and histologic cross-sections of three intermediate coronary lesions are shown. An arrow on the angiogram marks the site of interrogation. The corresponding MRI is shown in the second column, whereas corresponding histologic sections of the interrogated sections are shown in the third and fourth columns (Movat's pentachrome and anti-CD-68 antibody staining, respectively). **A,** Thin-cap fibroatheroma (*left to right*) in the proximal left anterior descending artery; the MRI display shows the presence of a high lipid content within three quadrants (2 to 4). Quadrant 1 has little lipid within the wall, as indicated by the lack of foam cells by Movat's staining or macrophages by CD-68 staining. Quadrant 2 has moderately increased lipid concentrations, as noted by an approximate lipid fractional index of 60%. Quadrant 3 has increased lipid only in the deep layer, whereas quadrant 4 has high lipid fractional indexes (± 100%) within the superficial and deep layers. Approximately 75% of the arterial circumference is lipid rich. The MRI display corresponds well with subsequent histology, as the Movat's section shows a large necrotic core (*) and a thin fibrous cap, and the adjoining immunohistochemical staining shows markedly positive staining for CD-68 in the area corresponding to quadrant 4 of the MRI display. **B,** Thick cap fibroatheroma in the right coronary artery. The MRI display shows no lipid content within the superficial layer (*blue*); however, a mild degree of increased lipid concentration is observed within the deep band >100 µm from the lumen in quadrant 5 only. The lipid fractional index is about 50%. The corresponding histologic section shows a thick cap fibroatheroma with a small, deep necrotic core (+), confirmed by the anti-CD-68 staining, corresponding with the MRI image. Because there is little to no lipid within the superficial layer, this lesion is considered a thick fibroatheroma. **C,** Stable lesion. A mild stenosis by angiography is seen in the intermediate branch of the left coronary artery. The MRI display of the lesion shows no increased lipid concentration in the shallow or the deep bands of any quadrant, indicating the presence of a fibrous lesion (hence, *blue* display). This diagnosis was confirmed by histology as adaptive intimal hyperplasia, and the corresponding anti-CD-68 staining was negative for foam cells or a necrotic core. (*Reproduced with permission from Schneiderman J, Wilensky RL, Weiss A, et al: Diagnosis of thin-cap fibroatheromas by a self-contained intravascular magnetic resonance imaging probe in ex vivo human aortas and in situ coronary arteries, J Am Coll Cardiol 45:1961–1969, 2005.*)

neovessels using αvβ3-targeted, paramagnetic nanoparticles in hypercholesterolemic rabbits (Fig. 59-33).[173] Other molecular targets have been successfully labeled for imaging atherosclerosis. Matter et al targeted a specific antibody against the fibronectin extra-domain B in ApoE-knockout mice.[174] Immunohistochemical studies revealed increased expression of extra-domain B not only in murine plaques but also in human plaques, predominantly around the vasa-vasorum.[174] Also, VCAM-1, a critical component of the leukocyte–endothelial adhesion cascade, was successfully targeted

using phage display–derived peptide sequences in ApoE-knockout mice, adding an additional method to interrogate angiogenesis in atherosclerotic plaques.[175] In recent years, delayed and dynamic contrast-enhanced MRI (CEMRI) has been employed to assess plaque neovascularization in animal models and in patients with atherosclerosis, providing an accurate quantification of the amount of neovessels in the plaque.[176] In the same way, we have recently demonstrated how gadofluorine M–enhanced MRI can accurately identify atherosclerotic neovascularization in an animal model of

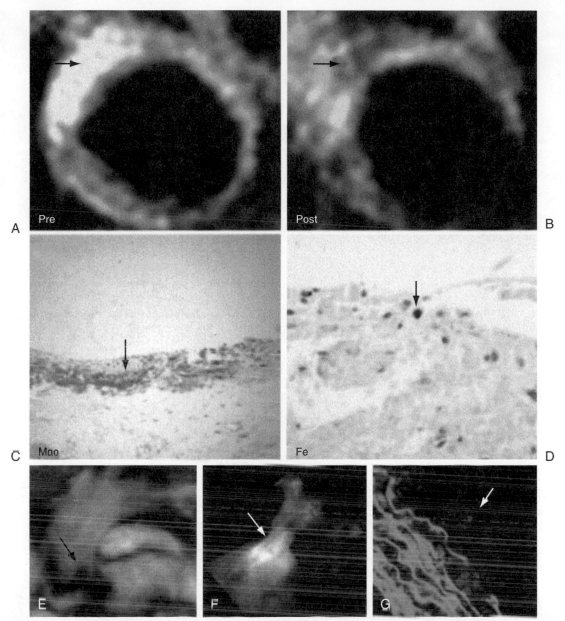

Figure 59-31   Cellular magnetic resonance image of macrophage (Mac) endocytosis in clinical and experimental atherosclerosis using magnetic nanoparticles. **A,** Dextranated magnetic nanoparticle injection (ferumoxtran, 2.6 mg/kg) produces focal signal loss within a carotid plaque of a neurologically symptomatic patient (*top*, "Pre" and "Post" images, *arrow*). Histologic examination of the carotid endarterectomy specimen demonstrates co-localization of macrophages. **B,** Multimodality magnetic resonance image and near infrared fluorescent imaging of murine atherosclerosis using a magneto-fluorescent nanoparticle. **C,** Anti-CD68 macrophage antibody (original magnification ×100) and iron (Fe). **D,** Pearls iron stain, neutral red counterstain (original magnification ×400). **E,** In vivo 9.4-T electrocardiogram-gated and respiratory-gated magnetic resonance image of an apolipoprotein E–/–-deficient mouse. Injection of a clinical-type near-infrared fluorescent dextranated magnetic nanoparticle (15 mg/kg of iron, 24-hour circulation time) produces focal signal loss (*arrow*) in the aortic root, a known site of atherosclerosis in the apo E–/– mouse. **F,** Fluorescence reflectance imaging of the resected aorta confirms a focal near-infrared fluorescent signal within the aortic root (*arrow*). **G,** On fluorescence microscopy, the near-infrared magneto-fluorescent nanoparticle accumulates in intimal macrophages (*red, arrow*) within aortic root plaque sections (original magnification ×200). In contrast, smooth muscle cells (stained here with a spectrally distinct α-actin fluorescent antibody, green) modestly co-localize with the magneto-fluorescent nanoparticle. *(Reproduced with permission from Jaffer FA, Libby P, Weissleder R: Molecular and cellular imaging of atherosclerosis: Emerging applications, J Am Coll Cardiol 47:1328–1338, 2006.)*

disease with adequate histologic validation.[177] However, some issues are still limiting the application of this technique in coronary atherosclerosis, mostly related to the small size of the plaque and to its proximity to the vessel wall, which adds noise to the imaging signal. Thus, despite promising results from this technique, further research should be performed with histologic validation before it is applied in clinical practice.

6. *Intra-plaque hemorrhage:* The evaluation of human carotid IPH with MRI was elegantly performed by Takaya et al (Fig. 59-34).[178] Of clinical relevance, IPH detected by MRI is associated with a significant increase in subsequent cerebrovascular events (HR 5.2, $P = 0.005$).[179] Other investigators have confirmed these findings, highlighting the value of MRI in detecting IPH in complex atherosclerosis.[154,180]

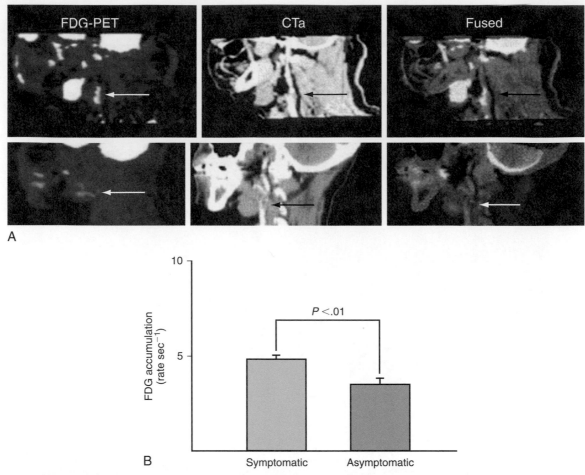

A

B

Figure 59-32 Positron emission tomography (PET) images from patients with unstable carotid disease after administration of fluorine-18–labeled deoxyglucose (FDG). **A,** FDG-PET (*left column*), computed tomographic angiography (CTA) (*middle column*), and fused images (*right column*) from patient with symptomatic carotid stenosis (*top row*) and contralateral asymptomatic carotid stenosis (*bottom row*). The yellow arrows highlight areas of FDG uptake corresponding to stenotic carotid plaque. **B,** A graph showing FDG accumulation rate in symptomatic versus asymptomatic carotid plaques. Note that the FDG uptake into symptomatic plaque was significantly higher. *(Reproduced with permission, from Davies JR, Rudd JH, Weissberg PL, Narula J: Radionuclide imaging for the detection of inflammation in vulnerable plaques, J Am Coll Cardiol 47:C57–C68, 2006.)*

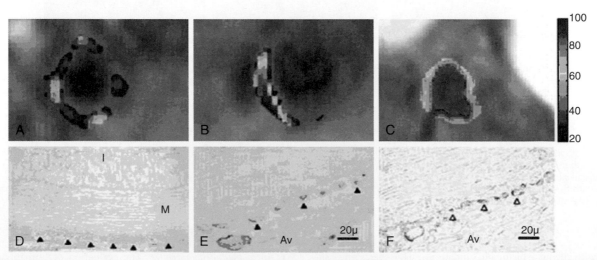

Figure 59-33 Molecular magnetic resonance imaging (MRI) of arterial neovessels in cholesterol-fed rabbits. Percent enhancement of adventitial signal (*false-colored from blue to red*) is shown in aortic segments at renal artery (A), mid-aorta (B), and diaphragm (C) 2 hours after αvß3-targeted Gd-loaded nanoparticles. Immunohistochemistry of αvß3-integrin (D) demonstrates thickened intima (I) and αvß3-integrin staining in adventitial neovessels (*black arrow heads*). Immunostaining in aorta from cholesterol-fed animal in A at 600× delineates neovascular αvß3-integrin (E, solid arrows) and platelet and endothelial cell adhesion molecule (F, open arrows) expression at the interface between media (M) and adventitia (Av). *(Reproduced with permission from Winter PM, Morawski AM, Caruthers SD, et al: Molecular imaging of angiogenesis in early-stage atherosclerosis with alpha(v)beta3-integrin-targeted nanoparticles, Circulation 108:2270–2274, 2003.)*

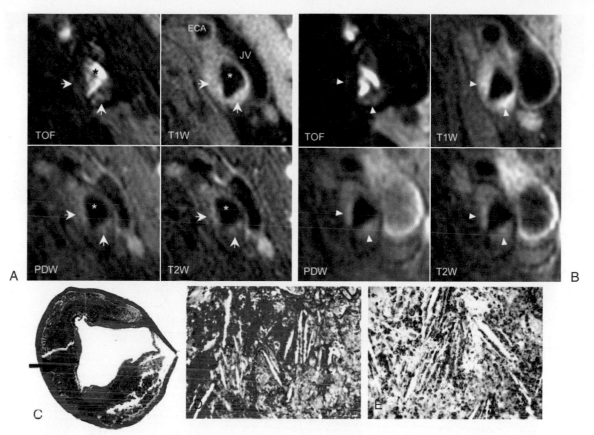

Figure 59-34 **A,** Signal intensity of type II hemorrhage at baseline examination. Type II hemorrhage is identified by hyperintense signals on TOF, T1W, PDW, and T2W images of left internal carotid artery (*arrow*). Asterisks show location of lumen. **B,** Images from 18 month follow-up scan showed a similar signal intensity pattern in the same regions (*arrowheads*). **C,** Matched Mallory's trichrome–stained section from excised CEA specimen. **D,** High power (×400) field taken from region (*arrow in C*) deep within necrotic core showing hemorrhagic debris and cholesterol clefts. **E,** Glycophorin A immunostaining of the same region (×400) in an adjacent section shows extensive staining of hemorrhagic debris indicating the presence of erythrocyte membranes. *JV,* jugular vein; *ECA,* external carotid artery. *(Reproduced with permission from Takaya N, Yuan C, Chu B, et al: Presence of intraplaque hemorrhage stimulates progression of carotid atherosclerotic plaques: Aa high-resolution magnetic resonance imaging study,* Circulation *111:2768–2775, 2005.)*

Angioscopy

Direct visualization of atherosclerotic plaques can provide information about plaque composition with the potential to identify specific components of the plaque.[181] Angioscopic classification of coronary lesions is performed according to the color of plaques in a bloodless field. White, yellow, and glistening yellow plaques have been quoted and studied in patients with CAD. Yellow plaques are associated with high concentrations of cholesterol-laden crystals with or without plaque degeneration, and intense yellow color indicates thin fibrous caps overlying a lipid core according to histologic studies. Uchida et el evaluated the clinical prospective value of these three different types of plaques in a prospective, three-vessel angioscopic study, which included 157 patients with chronic stable angina.[182] The incidence of ACS was evaluated 12 months later. The majority of patients (75%) had white plaques, which were associated with a low incidence of ACS (3.3%). The second group of patients (18%) had yellow plaques, which were associated with an intermediate incidence of ACS (7.6%). Finally, the third group of patients (8%) had glistening yellow plaques, which were associated with an impressive incidence of ACS (68%), including death in 22% of the cases.[182] These authors also evaluated the fibrous cap thickness of each of the three different plaques with autopsy specimens (Fig. 59-35). White plaques were associated with thick caps (400 μm), yellow plaques with thinner caps (80 μm), and glistening yellow with the thinnest caps (10–20 μm).[182] Other angioscopic studies in patients with ACS have shown a higher incidence of yellow plaques. Asakura

et al performed three-vessel angioscopy in patients 1 month after MI.[183] Yellow plaques were detected in 90% of 21 culprit lesions, and the number of these plaques was equally prevalent in the infarct-related and non–infarct-related coronary arteries (3.7 ± 1.6 vs. 3.4 + 1.8 plaques per artery), suggesting a diffuse, rather than a localized, process in patients with MI. To evaluate the predictive value of yellow plaques in clinical practice, Ohtani et al performed culprit vessel angioscopy in 552 patients with chronic stable angina, ACS, and AMI.[184] Yellow color intensity was also graded. The number of yellow plaques varied from 0 to 5 or more (Fig. 59-36). After 5 years, 7.1% of patients developed ACS. The mean number of yellow plaques was higher in the patients with an ACS event compared with those without the event (3.1 ± 1.8 vs. 2.2 ± 1.5, *P* = 0.008). However, the yellow color intensity scale was similar and did not lack any predictive value. In terms of in vivo evidence, a study that compared angioscopy with OCT demonstrated that yellow plaques identified by angioscopy had 98% and 96% sensitivity and specificity, respectively, for the identification of a fibrous cap measuring less than 110 μm by OCT. They also found that plaques with angioscopy yellow grade 3, had a mean fibrous cap thickness of 40 ± 14; however, these authors did not specify the sensitivity and the correlation coefficients for plaques with fibrous caps measuring less than 65 μm.[185] In the clinical arena, yellow plaques are seen more commonly at the site of culprit lesions, are more likely to rupture, and carry an increased risk of developing a subsequent coronary event. Similar to other imaging modalities mentioned above, angioscopy has also been used to demonstrate plaque stabilization with

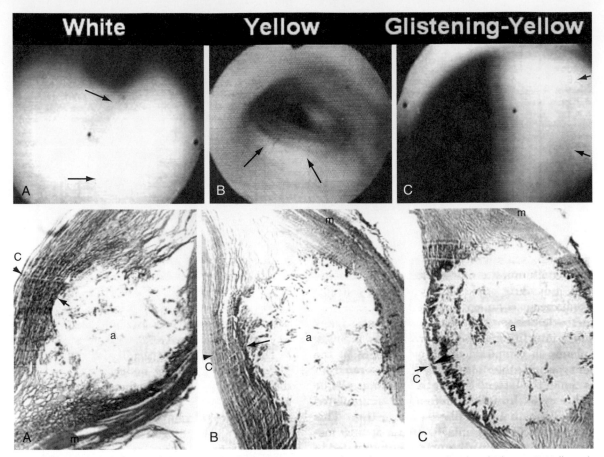

Figure 59-35 Angioscopic appearance of plaques at the time of autopsy. **A,** White plaque associated with a thick cap. **B,** Yellow plaque, associated with a thinner cap. **C,** Glistening yellow plaque, associated with the thinnest cap (see text for details). *(Reproduced with permission from Uchida Y, Nakamura F, Tomaru T, et al: Prediction of acute coronary syndromes by percutaneous coronary angioscopy in patients with stable angina, Am Heart J 130:195–203, 1995.)*

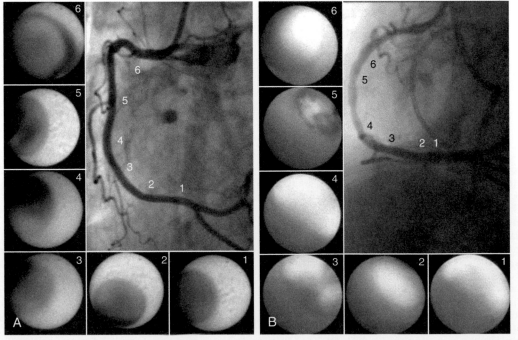

Figure 59-36 A representative case with no yellow plaque (*A*) and a representative case with multiple yellow plaques (*B*). **A,** No yellow plaque was detected in the right coronary artery: number of yellow plaques: 0, maximum color grade of yellow plaques: 0. **B,** Three yellow plaques were detected in the right coronary artery; maximum color grade of yellow plaques: 3. *(Reproduced with permission from Ohtani T, Ueda Y, Mizote I, et al: Number of yellow plaques detected in a coronary artery is associated with future risk of acute coronary syndrome: Detection of vulnerable patients by angioscopy, J Am Coll Cardiol 47:2194–2200, 2006.)*

statin therapy, as manifested by a decrease yellow intensity that correlates with plaque volume reduction shown by IVUS.[186] The main limitation of coronary angiography is the need for a blood-free environment to visualize the vessel wall, which requires proximal occlusion with a low pressure intracoronary balloon. The risk of ischemia and vessel injury is increased. Another option is to flush saline in a constant fashion before introducing the angioscope, which transiently displaces blood. Moreover, color interpretation is usually subjective and might be affected by the angulation of the catheter. To overcome these issues, a quantitative colorimetric method has been developed, as mentioned above. Ishibashi et al have proposed a more accurate grading system for coronary angioscopy interpretation that uses a quantitative colorimetric analysis based on the L*a*b* color space and brightness. Using this algorithm, plaque disruption was present in 79% of lesions with high yellow color intensity (defined as b* value >23) compared with 41% of lesions with b* values less than 23 ($P = 0.007$) in patients with ACS.[187] Finally, another limitation of angioscopy is that it is only a surface evaluation technique and does not provide direct information about plaque composition. As a result, fibrous cap thickness, inflammatory cell infiltration, necrotic core size, or remodeling are mostly considered surrogate parameters based on color-coding and correlation coefficients.

Spectroscopy

Spectroscopy is a nondestructive optical technology with the ability to analyze the chemical composition of plaque components.[188] After irradiation of tissue with a laser beam, scattered photons are acquired to identify specific features of plaque vulnerability.[188] Different plaque components such as calcium and cholesterol have specific absorption and reflectance patterns of light, producing a particular pattern, which is converted into an image. Two different modalities are currently under active evaluation for intravascular detection of high-risk VPs: Near-Infrared and Raman spectroscopy. Both techniques have good correlations with histologic analyses of coronary and aortic tissue.[189,190] However, the complexity of signal analysis may force investigators to focus on only one or two features of plaque vulnerability.

The physicochemical characteristics of lipid and calcium and their own Raman shift patterns make this modality highly sensitive for plaque detection. However, its main limitation is that only a small number of photons are recruited into the Raman shift, therefore providing poor tissue penetration and low signal-to-noise ratio. In a similar way backscattered noise can also decrease signal quality and imaging interpretation. However, new technologies have been shown to improve image quality by improving signal acquisition, including combination with IVUS.[191] The other spectroscopy modality, near-infrared spectroscopy (NIRS), measures diffuse reflectance signals with the use of near-infrared light. The spectrometer then emits light onto a substance and measures the light that is reflected back over a wide range of optical wavelengths, which are then processed as a spectrum, applied to an algorithm that predicts the probability of VPs, and displayed on a chemogram. The NIRS system was evaluated in 106 patients undergoing PCI in a multi-center study, with encouraging results.[192] They compared in vivo imaging with autopsy NIRS signals by using multivariate statistics. These authors found that NIRS appropriately identified lipid core-containing plaques in vivo. A main advantage of NIRS is that imaging can be performed without replacing the blood in the vessel, but it can only detect one characteristic of VP with no input on superficiality of lipid core or fibrous cap thickness. Catheters that combine NIRS with IVUS are currently being evaluated to test the ability of aggressive therapy to modify plaque composition. Multi-imaging technology has showed excellent correlation with events, as previously reported in the PROSPECT trial. A catheter providing IVUS for plaque burden and MLA and NIRS for necrotic core content will offer a more comprehensive assessment of the high risk lesion.[193] Although promising, clinical correlations with ACS are urgently needed. In the meantime, plaques with large lipid

core burden index (LCBI) by NIRS have demonstrated and increased risk for peri-procedural MI after PCI.[193,194] As a result, plaques with a very large LCBI may benefit from a protection device (filter) to prevent distal embolization and reduce the incidence of peri-procedural MI. This is the rationale of the CANARY trial. It will soon be known if spectroscopy will prove to be a useful clinical tool in the cath lab.

Thermography

Given the inflammatory nature of VP from macrophage and lymphocyte infiltration and from the release of inflammatory molecules from these cells, a local increase of temperature can occur in these areas of the vascular wall. This feature can be detected and measured by a catheter-based thermistor, which can differentiate changes of temperature of 0.05°C with a special discrimination of 0.5 mm. Thermography has been extensively evaluated in multiple settings with promising results.[195] In addition, thermography has been proposed as a useful tool for the identification of the culprit plaque, especially in cases of multi-vessel, complex disease.[196] Finally, like other imaging techniques, thermography can also be used for the assessment of plaque stabilization after statin therapy.[197] Toutouzas et al correlated thermography findings, expressed as changes in temperature, with plaque morphology by IVUS in 48 patients with ACS and 33 with stable angina. They found that change in temperature was an independent predictor of positive remodeling, plaque rupture, and ACS by multivariate analysis.[198] Nevertheless, despite all these efforts, the cooling effect of blood and other limitations significantly reduced the enthusiasm over thermography as a useful tool for intravascular detection of high-risk VPs. Furthermore, this technique is limited by two caveats. First, because this modality needs to be in direct contact with the vessel wall, the possibility of arterial injury is increased. Second, the diagnostic accuracy of thermography has several pitfalls related to confounding biases arising from temperature measurements generating artifacts from hemodynamic variations in blood pressure and blood flow within the vessels.[199]

NONINVASIVE IMAGING TECHNIQUES

Before completing the imaging section of this review, it is important to mention other noninvasive imaging techniques that have significantly evolved in the recent years in terms of VP assessment. These include MRI, CTA, and nuclear imaging. As noninvasive MRI has been already discussed, we will focus on briefly summarizing the other two modalities.

Coronary Computed Tomographic Angiography

In recent years, with the advancement of newer technologies in the field of CT and with the newer protocols and technologies allowing a more detailed examination of the vascular structures, coronary CTA has been proposed as a useful tool for the evaluation of coronary atherosclerotic plaques. A recent study reported that multi-detector CT (MDCT) could identify some differences in plaque morphologies when comparing TCFAs with non-TCFAs, highlighting the fact that a ring-like enhancement in MDCT could be a precursor lesion for plaque rupture.[200] Moreover, MDCT could provide prognostic information according to the type of plaque identified by this modality.[201] However, when compared with other imaging modalities with higher diagnostic accuracy to detect TCFAs, such as OCT or IVUS-VH, MDCT is only useful for the noninvasive evaluation of the calcified and fibro-fatty components of the plaque, but it cannot differentiate TCFA, which is one of the features of VP.[200,202–205]

Nuclear Imaging

Nuclear imaging using PET and CT technologies have been reported to provide useful information in patients with VPs.[206] They represent a feasible technique that addresses the molecular aspects of the atheroma and which, when used with dual gating protocols, can provide images with less motion artifact and image quality appropriate for clinical studies.[207] Also, specific tracers seem to be useful for the identification of different plaque components. Among the different tracers and markers of plaque vulnerability that have been studied with nuclear imaging 18F-Fluorodeoxyglucose (18F-FDG) is the most studied both in preclinical and clinical experiments, which have demonstrated that FDG uptake appropriately correlates with plaque macrophage density in animal models and human atherosclerosis and also predicts future cardiovascular events.[208,209] In the same way, it has been possible to detect MMP-rich plaques in preclinical studies with the use of radionuclear tracers, along with LDL receptor 1 with the use of 99mTc-LOX-1-mAb, apoptotic cells with annexin A5213, and neovascularization with alpha–beta₃ integrin-targeted PET.[210–216] Additionally, other promising contrast agents for noninvasive imaging modalities currently under development include HDL-based contrast and gold nanoparticles.[217,218] Figure 59-37 summarizes the potential targets in VP that are suitable for identification with nuclear imaging modalities. Unfortunately, despite these promising and encouraging results with noninvasive techniques, one of their main limitations is their inability to provide accurate plaque localization and anatomic evaluation of the

lesions. Further experimentation is required with appropriate histologic validation to identify the strengths and weakness of each of these technologies. The BioImage Study which includes a comprehensive assessment of cardiovascular risk factors, including noninvasive imaging for the identification of plaque vulnerability, will provide substantial data to establish the role of noninvasive modalities to address the vulnerability of the atherosclerotic plaque and will contribute to a better understanding of the natural history of such plaques, that will ultimately lead to a better therapeutic and preventive approach.[219]

PLAQUE IMAGING: SUMMARY

The development of new technologies for the purpose of detection of high-risk VPs is progressing rapidly. Although individual devices have reached a certain degree of technologic sophistication, a combination of these modalities may have a better future (i.e., OCT/backscattered IVUS; IVUS/Raman spectroscopy). The recently completed PROSPECT trial performed three-vessel coronary imaging in patients with ACS and has provided prognostic information related to invasive plaque imaging in CAD. If the event rate at follow-up is higher than expected with pharmacologic therapy, the scientific community will

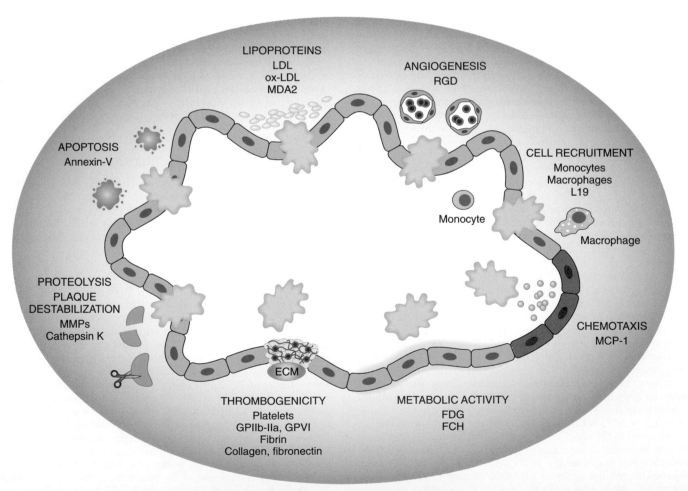

Figure 59-37 Potential targets in the pathophysiologic pathways of the atherosclerotic plaque that are susceptible for identification with nuclear imaging modalities. *FCM,* extracellular matrix; *FCH,* fluorocholine; *FDG,* fluorodeoxyglucose; *GP,* glycoprotein; *LDL,* low-density lipoprotein; *L19,* antibody against the extra-domain B of fibronectin; *MCP,* monocyte chemoattractant protein; *MDA2,* malondialdehyde epitope on oxidized low-density lipoprotein; *ox-LDL,* oxidized low-density lipoprotein; *RGD,* protein sequence "arginine-glycine-aspartic acid." *(Adapted with permission from Langer HF, Haubner R, Pichler BJ, Gawaz M: Radionuclide imaging: A molecular key to the atherosclerotic plaque, J Am Coll Cardiol 52:1–12, 2008.)*

need to consider additional therapeutic strategies. As a result, a comprehensive approach regarding invasive therapy is becoming mandatory for the interventionalist interested in the prevention of recurrent coronary events. Hence, as each currently available technology can provide information about different aspects of VP, an appropriate approach could be the combination of different technologies, including imaging, physiologic tests, and serum or genetic markers to enhance the detection of VP. The next section of this review will summarize current and future therapies for high-risk VPs.

Therapy

SYSTEMIC THERAPY

The treatment of high-risk VPs relies on aggressive medical therapy, which has been shown to reduce coronary events and improve survival. As a result, systemic therapy is the cornerstone of plaque stabilization, with documented reductions in lipid content, inflammation, and vasa-vasorum neovascularization.[220] Intensive statin therapy has demonstrated a significant decrease in coronary events in patients with stable disease (TNT and IDEAL trials), and in patients with ACS (A-to-Z and PROVE IT-TIMI-22 trials), not only in the incidence of coronary death or MI but also in the development of heart failure, independent of recurrent infarct.[221,222] Similarly, early intensive statin therapy for ACS was associated with clinical benefits that became evident after 4 to 12 months, including a decrease in serum VEGF levels, which probably represents an attenuation of plaque angiogenesis.[223,224] Most importantly, in the ASTEROID trial, aggressive therapy with rosuvastatin led to an absolute regression of atheroma volume (Fig. 59-38).[63] Another potent anti-atherogenic therapy involves increasing HDL. Studies using bezafibrate, a peroxisome proliferator-activated receptor (PPAR)-α agonist, and fenofibrate have demonstrated reduced events and plaque regression, respectively.[225,226] These beneficial effects may be caused not only by HDL augmentation and reverse cholesterol transport but also by recruitment of endothelial progenitor cells into the damaged endothelium.[227,228] As mentioned earlier, the beneficial effects of statin therapy on VP in terms of plaque regression and stabilization have been documented multiple times with different imaging techniques including OCT, angioscopy, MRI, and IVUS-VH.[60,139,229] In addition to high-dose statin therapy, angiotensin-converting enzyme (ACE) inhibitors, β-blockers, and aspirin have shown a reduction in the rates of death and MI and therefore are mandatory therapy to achieve stabilization of high-risk VPs.[220] Several interventions have been demonstrated to improve endothelial function by increasing endothelial progenitor cell (EPC) regeneration, mobilization, and release into the circulation, contributing to the passivation of the inflammatory environment. These modalities include exercise, statins, angiotensin receptor blockers (ARBs) and ACE inhibitors, and some peroxisome proliferator-activated receptor agonists.[230–232] Additionally n-3 fatty acids also have a stabilizing effect, and the mechanisms behind this beneficial effect involve the regulation of adhesion molecule expression, proinflammatory and proangiogenic growth factors by the endothelium, and the attenuation of the nuclear factor-κB system.[233] Another potential intervention for plaque stabilization is to impact the reverse cholesterol transport system. This has been proposed as a therapeutic alternative with the aim of promoting cholesterol efflux from macrophages, with the activation of ABCA1 and ABCG1 transporter systems. Further experimentation is ongoing.[66,234] In the search for other systemic therapies, substantial research is being performed. For instance, preclinical data have demonstrated that vaccination against TIE2, the angiopoetin receptor, promotes the formation of smaller atherosclerotic plaques with a more stable phenotype.[235] Similarly, both animal and human experiments have demonstrated that the selective inhibition of Lp-PLA2 reduces plasma Lp-PLA2 activity and is associated with decrease in the plaque area and the necrotic core area.[20,236] Despite the tremendous value of systemic therapy, patients still come back with recurrent events (22% recurrent event rate within 2 years) and therefore prove to be resistant to systemic therapy, as shown in the PROVE IT trial.[237] As a result, even the best combination of systemic therapies available today does not successfully prevent all episodes of plaque rupture and thrombosis. Therefore, new therapies are urgently needed as coadjuvants to systemic therapy in high-risk patients.

REGIONAL THERAPY

Regional therapy is defined as the intravascular treatment of coronary segments with therapeutic agents, including pharmacologic agents as well as physico-chemical therapies with the objective of stabilizing high-risk VPs. Regional therapies include photodynamic therapy (PDT), endoluminal phototherapy, and cryotherapy.[238–240] Of these, PDT has gained more attention in the recent years. It involves photosensitizing (light-sensitive) drugs, light, and tissue oxygen to treat targeted diseases, mostly in the field of oncology.[241] Photosensitizing agents (porphyrins) are administered locally or parenterally. They are selectively absorbed and retained within tissues for targeted therapy. This differential selectivity offers selective therapeutic effects when the target tissue is exposed to light at an appropriate wavelength; the surrounding normal tissue is then spared from therapeutic injury. Activation of the photosensitizer within tissue induces the production of free radicals leading to selective cytotoxic effects, mostly apoptosis (DNA fragmentation), or delayed necrosis. The application of PDT to atherosclerotic plaques was successfully performed in vivo by Waksman et al in hypercholesterolemic rabbits.[242] PDT induced a significant reduction (92% ± 6%) in the population of nuclei of all cell types in plaques relative to controls (P < 0.01). This effect was partly caused by reduction of smooth muscle cells (α-actin) and macrophages (RAM 11) (Fig. 59-39). These results suggest that PDT can almost eliminate macrophages from atherosclerotic plaques and may provide a therapeutic alternative for high-risk VPs refractory to aggressive systemic therapy. Two other therapies, endoluminal phototherapy and cryotherapy, are also under investigation, but experience with them is limited.

LOCAL THERAPY

Coronary stents offer the possibility of stabilizing high-risk VPs by thickening the fibrous cap through the formation of neointimal hyperplasia. As predicted by Peter Libby years ago, and then highlighted by Patrick Serruys in 2006, "If we could identify potentially unstable atheroma before they are evident, we might even contemplate angioplasty on non-significant stenosis to induce smooth muscle cell proliferation

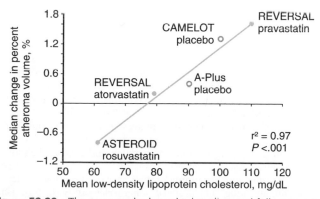

Figure 59-38 The top panels show the baseline and follow-up intravascular ultrasound (IVUS) images of a single coronary cross-section after 24 months of rosuvastatin treatment. The bottom two panels illustrate measurements superimposed on the same cross-sections, demonstrating the reduction in atheroma area. *EEM*, external elastic membrane. (*Reproduced with permission from Nissen SE, Nicholls SJ, Sipahi I, et al: Effect of very high-intensity statin therapy on regression of coronary atherosclerosis: The ASTEROID trial, JAMA 295:1556–1565, 2006.*)

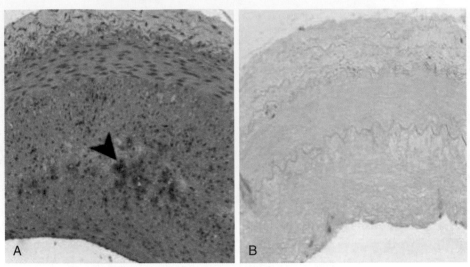

Figure 59-39 Histologic images of the effects of photodynamic therapy in atherosclerotic plaques from hypercholesterolemic rabbits. **A,** Control showing macrophages with black arrow. **B,** Seven days after photodynamic therapy. *(Reproduced with permission from Waksman R: Photodynamic therapy, New York and London, 2004, Taylor & Francis.)*

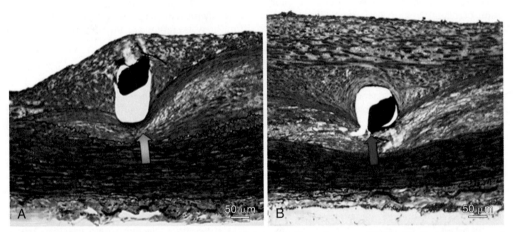

Figure 59-40 Histologic section illustrating different components of thin cap fibroatheroma (TCFA) 28 days after stent deployment. The strut compresses the old, thin fibrous cap (*yellow arrow*). A cellular neointimal layer has been laid down creating a new, thick fibrous cap (*red arrow*). Elastic-trichrome stain; 20× field.

and reinforce the plaque fibrous cap."[129,243] On the same subject, Michael Davies wrote in an editorial: "The time for prophylactic angioplasty has not come yet, but it may."[244] More recently, Eugene Brauwald also pinpointed this concept in his editorial entitled "Locking the Barn Door before the Horse Is Stolen": "The clinical application of VPs at risk of future rupture would require the development of measures for the prevention of plaque rupture that are more potent than those currently employed, in what we currently refer to as intensive prevention. Perhaps stenting or surgically bypassing these plaques could be considered in some patients."[6] However, considering the highly controversial concept of stenting VPs, the risk–benefit ratio must be evaluated in experimental animal models. To evaluate all these parameters, we developed an experimental animal model of spontaneous VPs in New Zealand hypercholesterolemic rabbits followed up for 4 years. These animals were randomized to metallic stents, drug-eluting stents (DESs), and controls ($n = 11$).[245] Only stent struts deployed into VPs were evaluated. Fibrous cap thickness, stent-induced fibrous cap rupture (Fig. 59-40), and peri-strut healing (Fig. 59-41), were evaluated, as well as peri-strut inflammation (see Fig. 59-41, *A*), fibrin deposition (see Fig. 59-41, *B*), hemorrhage (see Fig. 59-41, *C*), and strut

endothelialization (see Fig. 59-41, *D*). Metallic stents, β-estradiol-eluting stents, and everolimus-eluting stents increased fibrous cap thickness by 396%, 322%, and 270%, respectively ($P < 0.0001$ for all comparisons) (Table 59-2). Stent-induced fibrous cap rupture was present in 63% of stented lesions. Peri-strut inflammation, fibrin deposition, and hemorrhage increased, and endothelialization decreased in DESs compared with metallic stents ($P < 0.05$) (Table 59-3). These effects were obtained at the cost of increased cap damage and potentially iatrogenic, peri-strut healing patterns, including increased inflammation, fibrin deposition, hemorrhage, and decreased endothelialization. Similarly, new self-expanding devices with very thin struts and with low-pressure expanding profiles have been successfully tested in an animal model of localized atherosclerosis with promising results.[246,247] Other local delivery options are evolving, blocking proangiogenic factors.[248] Coated stents with the VEGF-specific antibody bevacizumab demonstrated encouraging results in terms of angiogenesis control in a small studies.[249,250] However, it is not known if local antiangiogenic therapy, with either stent-based or non–stent-based modalities, will require a single-dose or a multiple-dose approach. Evidence from experiments treating nonatherosclerotic angiogenesis

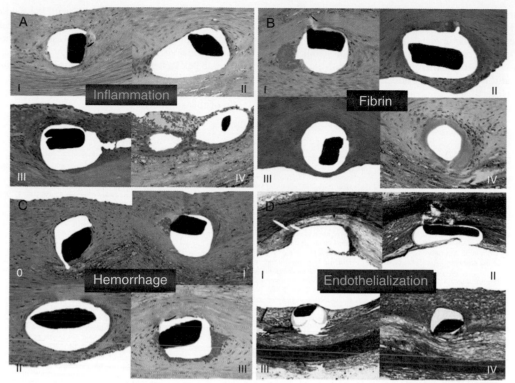

Figure 59-41 Composite of micrographs displaying examples of numerical scoring (scale I to IV) applied to four categories (A–D) of strut-related healing patterns at 28 days after stent deployment: **A,** Inflammation. **B,** Fibrin deposition. **C,** Hemorrhage. **D,** Endothelialization. Score criteria common to A, B, and C categories record the extent of the perimeter of each strut affected as follows: Score I: up to 1 quadrant around strut (or 25%); Score II: up to 2 quadrants (50%); Score III: up to 3 quadrants (75%); Score IV: up to 4 quadrants (100%). Endothelialization (category D) was recorded as Score I: up to 25% endothelial coverage; Score II: up to 75% endothelial coverage; Score III: up to 100% endothelial coverage; Score IV: Complete coverage with neointimal tissue.

TABLE 59-2	Planimetric Data Comparing Fibrous Cap Thickness in Stented and Nonstented Thin Cap Fibroatheromas			
Individual Strut Analysis	**Metallic** n = 127	**Beta-Estradiol** n = 46	**Everolimus** n = 41	**Control** n = 122
Old fibrous cap area (μm^2)	26 ± 3.9	24.4 ± 1.7	23 ± 1.9	27 ± 1.3
New fibrous cap area (μm^2)	107 ± 6.5*	87.6 ± 6.7*§	72.8 ± 3.9*§	27 ± 1.3

*$P < 0.0001$ in comparison with the Control group; §$P < 0.05$ in comparison with the Metallic stent group

TABLE 59-3	Planimetric Data Comparing Potential Iatrogenic Peri-Strut Healing Patterns after Metallic and Drug-Eluting Stents in Thin Cap Fibroatheromas		
Vascular Healing	**Metallic** n = 127	**Beta-Estradiol** n = 46	**Everolimus** n = 41
Inflammation score	0.9 ± 0.1	1.1 ± 0.1*	1.1 ± 0.1*
Fibrin score	0.6 ± 0.1	1.1 ± 0.1*	1.1 ± 0.2*
Hemorrhage score	0.1 ± 0.0	0.1 ± 0.0	0.2 ± 0.1*
Endothelization score	3.7 ± 0.1	3.2 ± 0.2*	3.6 ± 0.1

*$P < 0.05$ in comparison with Metallic stent group

favors repeated dosing. A controlled-release delivery system may ensure a sustained inhibitory effect on proangiogenic factors.[251] Finally, other local therapies, including blockage of molecular pathways or specific genes related to plaque vulnerability, have been tested.[252] However, further studies are still needed to elucidate the clinical applications of this approach.

Considering the diffuse pattern of the disease, local therapy to reinforce TCFA is subject to controversy. Furthermore, the risk of late stent thrombosis adds to the controversial application of coronary stents in VPs.[253] However, proponents of the stent hypothesis argue that the clinical event rate associated with high-risk TCFA (18% at 3 years in the PROSPECT trial) may be higher than the clinical event rate associated with stenting (4%–6% for the first year and about 1%–2% per year thereafter). Furthermore, new stent designs, including biodegradable materials, and self-expanding delivery systems may reduce the long-term risk of stent thrombosis, preserving the integrity of the fibrous cap with neointimal tissue.[254,255] The prediction of how we will treat high-risk TCFAs resistant to aggressive medical therapy is still a matter of great controversy as well as a promising opportunity for interventional cardiologists. Only prospective, randomized clinical trials will completely elucidate this issue.

Summary and Future Directions

Death and MI continue to result from high-risk lesions complicated by plaque rupture and thrombosis. The search for early diagnosis and treatment of these plaques offers the promise to prevent catastrophic consequences related to coronary thrombosis. Novel information has contributed to a better understanding of the complexity of this field. First, the established concept that VPs are responsible for a high number of future events has proved to be wrong. The incidence of death and MI in the PROSPECT trial was only 4.9% at 3.4 years, highlighting the excellent contemporary outcomes of aggressive medical therapy in secondary prevention. Second, a thin cap fibroatheroma, by itself, is not sufficient to fulfill the definition of VP. The new concept of the high-risk TCFA now includes large plaque burden and reduced lumen by IVUS. These three parameters consolidate the contemporary definition of VP.[5] The susceptibility of these plaques for stabilization, regression, or both with medical therapy, interventional therapy, or both is still unclear and may need to be addressed, especially for secondary prevention. Nevertheless, the real opportunity to make a difference is not in secondary prevention. The great majority of patients first present with SCD or MI. As a result, the field of VP must go into the community to identify patients with high-risk TCFAs and treat them accordingly. Therefore, noninvasive technology has a bright future in this regard. Regarding therapy, aggressive pharmacology has proved to be excellent in reducing future events. Interventional therapy may have an option for high-risk TCFAs refractory to medical therapy. Only randomized clinical trials will help to elucidate the risk–benefit ratio of this approach.

REFERENCES

1. Ford ES, Li C, Zhao G, et al: Trends in the prevalence of low risk factor burden for cardiovascular disease among United States adults. *Circulation* 120:1181–1188, 2009.
2. Yeh RW, Sidney S, Chandra M, et al: Population trends in the incidence and outcomes of acute myocardial infarction. *N Engl J Med* 362:2155–2165, 2010.
3. Lloyd-Jones D, Adams RJ, Brown TM, et al: Executive summary: Heart disease and stroke statistics—2010 update: A report from the American Heart Association. *Circulation* 121:948–954, 2010.
4. Fuster VM, Fayad PR, Corti ZA, et al: Atherothrombosis and high-risk plaque part I: Evolving concepts. *J Am Coll Cardiol* 46:937–954, 2005.
5. Moreno PR: The high-risk thin-cap fibroatheroma: A new kid on the block. *Circ Cardiovasc Interv* 2:500–502, 2009.
6. Braunwald E: Noninvasive detection of vulnerable coronary plaques: Locking the barn door before the horse is stolen. *J Am Coll Cardiol* 54:58–59, 2009.
7. Ambrose JA, Tannenbaum MA, Alexopoulos D, et al: Angiographic progression of coronary artery disease and the development of myocardial infarction. *J Am Coll Cardiol* 12:56–62, 1988.
8. Rdzanek A, Kochman J, Pietrasik A, et al: The prevalence of potentially unstable coronary lesions in patients with coronary artery disease—virtual histology study. *Kardiol Pol* 66:244–250, discussion 251–252, 2008.
9. Cutlip DE, Chhabra AG, Baim DS, et al: Beyond restenosis: Five-year clinical outcomes from second-generation coronary stent trials. *Circulation* 110:1226–1230, 2004.
10. Glaser R, Selzer F, Faxon DP, et al: Clinical progression of incidental, asymptomatic lesions discovered during culprit vessel coronary intervention. *Circulation* 111:143–149, 2005.
11. Motoyama S, Sarai M, Harigaya H, et al: Computed tomographic angiography characteristics of atherosclerotic plaques subsequently resulting in acute coronary syndrome. *J Am Coll Cardiol* 54:49–57, 2009.
12. Tanaka A, Imanishi T, Kitabata H, et al: Distribution and frequency of thin-capped fibroatheromas and ruptured plaques in the entire culprit coronary artery in patients with acute coronary syndrome as determined by optical coherence tomography. *Am J Cardiol* 102:975–979, 2008.
13. Cheruvu PK, Finn AV, Gardner C, et al: Frequency and distribution of thin-cap fibroatheroma and ruptured plaques in human coronary arteries: A pathologic study. *J Am Coll Cardiol* 50:940–949, 2007.
14. Lee WS, Kim SW, Ryu WS: Progression and observational frequency of atheromatous plaques in autopsied coronary arteries. *Korean Circ J* 39:399–407, 2009.
15. Stone GW, Maehara A, Lansky AJ, et al: A prospective natural-history study of coronary atherosclerosis. *N Engl J Med* 364:226–235, 2011.
16. Marso SP, House JA, Klauss V, et al: Diabetes mellitus is associated with plaque classified as thin cap fibroatheroma: an intravascular ultrasound study. *Diab Vasc Dis Res* 7:14–19, 2010.
17. Lindsey JB, House JA, Kennedy KF, et al: Diabetes duration is associated with increased thin-cap fibroatheroma detected by intravascular ultrasound with virtual histology. *Circ Cardiovasc Interv* 2:543–548, 2009.
18. Wong ND, Gransar H, Narula J, et al: Myeloperoxidase, subclinical atherosclerosis, and cardiovascular disease events. *JACC Cardiovasc Imaging* 2:1093–1099, 2009.
19. Meuwese MC, Stroes ES, Hazen SL, et al: Serum myeloperoxidase levels are associated with the future risk of coronary artery disease in apparently healthy individuals: The EPIC-Norfolk Prospective Population Study. *J Am Coll Cardiol* 50:159–165, 2007.
20. Serruys PW, Garcia-Garcia HM, Buszman P, et al: Effects of the direct lipoprotein-associated phospholipase A(2) inhibitor darapladib on human coronary atherosclerotic plaque. *Circulation* 118:1172–1182, 2008.
21. Li QX, Fu QQ, Shi SW, et al: Relationship between plasma inflammatory markers and plaque fibrous cap thickness determined by intravascular optical coherence tomography. *Heart* 96:196–201, 2010.
22. Turu MM, Slevin M, Matou S, et al: C-reactive protein exerts angiogenic effects on vascular endothelial cells and modulates associated signalling pathways and gene expression. *BMC Cell Biol* 9:47, 2008.
23. Wang TJ, Gona P, Larson MG, et al: Multiple biomarkers for the prediction of first major cardiovascular events and death. *N Engl J Med* 355:2631–2639, 2006.
24. Zethelius B, Berglund L, Sundstrom J, et al: Use of multiple biomarkers to improve the prediction of death from cardiovascular causes. *N Engl J Med* 358:2107–2116, 2008.
25. Koenig W, Khuseyinova N: Biomarkers of atherosclerotic plaque instability and rupture. *Arterioscler Thromb Vasc Biol* 27(1):15–26, 2006.
26. Wang JC, Normand SL, Mauri L, et al: Coronary artery spatial distribution of acute myocardial infarction occlusions. *Circulation* 110:278–284, 2004.
27. Valgimigli M, Rodriguez-Granillo GA, Garcia-Garcia HM, et al: Distance from the ostium as an independent determinant of coronary plaque composition in vivo: An intravascular ultrasound study based radiofrequency data analysis in humans. *Eur Heart J* 27:655–663, 2006.
28. Fujii K, Kawasaki D, Masutani M, et al: OCT assessment of thin-cap fibroatheroma distribution in native coronary arteries. *JACC Cardiovasc Imaging* 3:168–175, 2010.
29. Gonzalo N, Garcia-Garcia HM, Regar E, et al: In vivo assessment of high-risk coronary plaques at bifurcations with combined intravascular ultrasound and optical coherence tomography. *JACC Cardiovasc Imaging* 2:473–482, 2009.
30. Virmani R, Burke AP, Farb A, et al: Pathology of the vulnerable plaque. *J Am Coll Cardiol* 47:C13–C18, 2006.
31. Moreno PR: Vulnerable plaque: Definition, diagnosis, and treatment. *Cardiol Clin* 28:1–30, 2010.
32. Moreno PR, Purushothaman KR, Fuster V, et al: Intimomedial interface damage and adventitial inflammation is increased beneath disrupted atherosclerosis in the aorta: Implications for plaque vulnerability. *Circulation* 105:2504–2511, 2002.
33. Tang D, Teng Z, Canton G, et al: Local critical stress correlates better than global maximum stress with plaque morphological features linked to atherosclerotic plaque vulnerability: An in vivo multi-patient study. *Biomed Eng Online* 8:15, 2009.
34. Schaar JA, van der Steen AF, Mastik F, et al: Intravascular palpography for vulnerable plaque assessment. *J Am Coll Cardiol* 47:C86–C91, 2006.
35. Chen HH, Hosken BD, Huang M, et al: Electronegative LDLs from familial hypercholesterolemic patients are physicochemically heterogeneous but uniformly proapoptotic. *J Lipid Res* 48:177–184, 2007.
36. Shang YY, Wang ZH, Zhang LP, et al: TRB3, upregulated by ox-LDL, mediates human monocyte-derived macrophage apoptosis. *FEBS J* 276:2752–2761, 2009.
37. Moreno PR, Purushothaman KR, Fuster V, et al: Intimomedial interface damage and adventitial inflammation is increased beneath disrupted atherosclerosis in the aorta: Implications for plaque vulnerability. *Circulation* 105:2504–2511, 2002.
38. Moreno PR, Bernardi VH, Lopez-Cuellar J, et al: Macrophages, smooth muscle cells, and tissue factor in unstable angina. Implications for cell-mediated thrombogenicity in acute coronary syndromes. *Circulation* 94:3090–3097, 1996.
39. Kuge Y, Kume N, Ishino S, et al: Prominent lectin-like oxidized low density lipoprotein (LDL) receptor-1 (LOX-1) expression in atherosclerotic lesions is associated with tissue factor expression and apoptosis in hypercholesterolemic rabbits. *Biol Pharm Bull* 31:1475–1482, 2008.
40. Reininger AJ, Bernlochner I, Penz SM, et al: A 2-step mechanism of arterial thrombus formation induced by human atherosclerotic plaques. *J Am Coll Cardiol* 55:1147–1158, 2010.
41. Shah PK, Galis ZS: Matrix metalloproteinase hypothesis of plaque rupture: Players keep piling up but questions remain. *Circulation* 104:1878–1880, 2001.
42. Suzuki H, Kusuyama T, Sato R, et al: Elevation of matrix metalloproteinases and interleukin-6 in the culprit coronary artery of myocardial infarction. *Eur J Clin Invest* 38:166–173, 2008.
43. Newby AC: Metalloproteinases and vulnerable atherosclerotic plaques. *Trends Cardiovasc Med* 17:253–258, 2007.
44. Thomas AC, Sala-Newby GB, Ismail Y, et al: Genomics of foam cells and nonfoamy macrophages from rabbits identifies arginase-I as a differential regulator of nitric oxide production. *Arterioscler Thromb Vasc Biol* 27:571–577, 2007.
45. Newby AC, George SJ, Ismail Y, et al: Vulnerable atherosclerotic plaque metalloproteinases and foam cell phenotypes. *Thromb Haemost* 101:1006–1011, 2009.
46. Seshiah PN, Kereiakes DJ, Vasudevan SS, et al: Activated monocytes induce smooth muscle cell death: Role of macrophage colony-stimulating factor and cell contact. *Circulation* 105:174–180, 2002.
47. Hutter RV, Sauter C, Savontaus BV, et al: Caspase-3 and tissue factor expression in lipid-rich plaque macrophages: Evidence for apoptosis as link between inflammation and atherothrombosis. *Circulation* 109:2001–2008, 2004.
48. Libby P: Inflammation and cardiovascular disease mechanisms. *Am J Clin Nutr* 83:456S–460S, 2006.
49. Tabas I: Macrophage death and defective inflammation resolution in atherosclerosis. *Nat Rev Immunol* 10:36–46, 2010.
50. Odegaard JI, Ricardo-Gonzalez RR, Goforth MH, et al: Macrophage-specific PPARgamma controls alternative activation and improves insulin resistance. *Nature* 447:1116–1120, 2007.
51. Nofer JR, Bot M, Brodde M, et al: FTY720, a synthetic sphingosine 1 phosphate analogue, inhibits development of atherosclerosis in low-density lipoprotein receptor-deficient mice. *Circulation* 115:501–508, 2007.
52. Martinez FO, Helming L, Gordon S: Alternative activation of macrophages: an immunologic functional perspective. *Annu Rev Immunol* 27:451–483, 2009.
53. Tabas I: Consequences and therapeutic implications of macrophage apoptosis in atherosclerosis: The importance of lesion stage and phagocytic efficiency. *Arterioscler Thromb Vasc Biol* 25:2255–2264, 2005.
54. Schrijvers DM, De Meyer GR, Herman AG, et al: Phagocytosis in atherosclerosis: Molecular mechanisms and implications for plaque progression and stability. *Cardiovasc Res* 73:470–480, 2007.
55. Back M, Ketelhuth DF, Agewall S: Matrix metalloproteinases in atherothrombosis. *Prog Cardiovasc Dis* 52:410–428, 2010.
56. Page-McCaw A, Ewald AJ, Werb Z: Matrix metalloproteinases and the regulation of tissue remodelling. *Nat Rev Mol Cell Biol* 8:221–233, 2007.
57. Rodriguez JA, Orbe J, Martinez de Lizarrondo S, et al: Metalloproteinases and atherothrombosis: MMP-10 mediates vascular remodeling promoted by inflammatory stimuli. *Front Biosci* 13:2916–2921, 2008.
58. Burke AP, Kolodgie FD, Farb A, et al: Morphological predictors of arterial remodeling in coronary atherosclerosis. *Circulation* 105:297–303, 2002.
59. Schoenhagen P, Ziada KM, Kapadia SR, et al: Extent and direction of arterial remodeling in stable versus unstable coronary syndromes: An intravascular ultrasound study. *Circulation* 101:598–603, 2000.
60. Corti R, Fayad ZA, Fuster V, et al: Effects of lipid-lowering by simvastatin on human atherosclerotic lesions: A longitudinal study by high-resolution, noninvasive magnetic resonance imaging. *Circulation* 104:249–252, 2001.
61. Schoenhagen P, Tuzcu EM, Apperson-Hansen C, et al: Determinants of arterial wall remodeling during lipid-lowering therapy: Serial intravascular ultrasound observations from the Reversal of Atherosclerosis with Aggressive Lipid Lowering Therapy (REVERSAL) trial. *Circulation* 113:2826–2834, 2006.
62. Sipahi I, Nicholls SJ, Tuzcu EM, et al: Coronary atherosclerosis can regress with very intensive statin therapy. *Cleve Clin J Med* 73:937–944, 2006.
63. Nissen SE, Nicholls SJ, Sipahi I, et al: Effect of very high-intensity statin therapy on regression of coronary atherosclerosis: The ASTEROID trial. *JAMA* 295:1556–1565, 2006.
64. Moreno PR, Purushothaman KR, Zias E, et al: Neovascularization in human atherosclerosis. *Curr Mol Med* 6:457–477, 2006.
65. Moreno PR, Purushothaman KR, Sirol M, et al: Neovascularization in human atherosclerosis. *Circulation* 113:2245–2252, 2006.
66. Moreno PR, Sanz J, Fuster V: Promoting mechanisms of vascular health: Circulating progenitor cells, angiogenesis, and reverse cholesterol transport. *J Am Coll Cardiol* 53:2315–2323, 2009.
67. Barger AC, Beeuwkes R, 3rd, Lainey LL, et al: Hypothesis: Vasa vasorum and neovascularization of human coronary arteries. A possible role in the pathophysiology of atherosclerosis. *N Engl J Med* 310:175–177, 1984.
68. Kumamoto M, Nakashima Y, Sueishi K: Intimal neovascularization in human coronary atherosclerosis: its origin and pathophysiological significance. *Hum Pathol* 26:450–456, 1995.
69. O'Brien KD, McDonald TO, Chait A, et al: Neovascular expression of E-selectin, intercellular adhesion molecule-1, and vascular cell adhesion molecule-1 in human atherosclerosis and their relation to intimal leukocyte content. *Circulation* 93:672–682, 1996.
70. Leroyer AS, Isobe H, Leseche G, et al: Cellular origins and thrombogenic activity of microparticles isolated from human atherosclerotic plaques. *J Am Coll Cardiol* 49:772–777, 2007.
71. Leroyer AS, Rautou PE, Silvestre JS, et al: CD40 ligand+ microparticles from human atherosclerotic plaques stimulate endothelial proliferation and angiogenesis a potential mechanism for

intraplaque neovascularization. *J Am Coll Cardiol* 52:1302–1311, 2008.
72. Moreno PR, Fuster V: New aspects in the pathogenesis of diabetic atherothrombosis. *J Am Coll Cardiol* 44:2293–2300, 2004.
73. Purushothaman KR, Levy AP, Meeraranl P, et al: Atherosclerotic neovascularization in diabetes mellitus is related to plaque inflammation expressed as increased macrophage and T-cell lymphocyte infiltration. *Atherosclerosis* (8):P09–P259, 2007.
74. Purushothaman K-R, Fuster V, Sirol M, et al: Diabetic plaque inflammation and neovascularization are associated with increased reparative collagen content: Implication for plaque progression in diabetic atherosclerosis. *J Am Coll Cardiol* 47(Supp A):295A, 2006.
75. Moreno PR, Purushothaman KR, Fuster V, et al: Plaque neovascularization is increased in ruptured atherosclerotic lesions of human aorta: implications for plaque vulnerability. *Circulation* 110:2032–2038, 2004.
76. Moreno PR, O'Connor WN, Kini AS, et al: Microvessel sprouting, red blood cell extravasation, and peri-vascular inflammation is increased in plaques from patients with diabetes mellitus. *J Am Coll Cardiol* 45:430A, 2005.
77. Wilkinson FL, Liu Y, Rucka AK, et al: Contribution of VCAF-positive cells to neovascularization and calcification in atherosclerotic plaque development. *J Pathol* 211:362–369, 2007.
78. Gossl M, Versari D, Hildebrandt HA, et al: Segmental heterogeneity of vasa vasorum neovascularization in human coronary atherosclerosis. *JACC Cardiovasc Imaging* 3:32–40, 2010.
79. Hutter R SW, Fuster F, Moreno PR, et al: Pattern of angiogenesis regulators expressed in vulnerable coronary atheroma favors formation of immature and leaky neovessels: A role for VEGF and angiopoietin-1 in determining plaque stability. *J Am Coll Cardiol* 53:A457, 2009.
80. Le Dall J, Ho-Tin-Noe B, Louedec L, et al: Immaturity of microvessels in haemorrhagic plaques is associated with proteolytic degradation of angiogenic factors. *Cardiovasc Res* 85:184–193, 2010.
81. Post S, Peeters W, Busser E, et al: Balance between angiopoietin-1 and angiopoietin-2 is in favor of angiopoietin-2 in atherosclerotic plaques with high microvessel density. *J Vasc Res* 45:244–250, 2008.
82. Levy AP: Haptoglobin: A major susceptibility gene for diabetic cardiovascular disease. *Isr Med Assoc J* 6:308–310, 2004.
83. Asleh RG, Kalet-Litman J, Miller-Lotan S, et al: Haptoglobin genotype- and diabetes-dependent differences in iron-mediated oxidative stress in vitro and in vivo. *Circ Res* 96:435–441, 2005.
84. Levy AP, Roguin A, Hochberg I, et al: Haptoglobin phenotype and vascular complications in patients with diabetes. *N Engl J Med* 343:969–970, 2000.
85. Kalet-Litman S, Moreno PR, Levy AP: The haptoglobin 2-2 genotype is associated with increased redox active hemoglobin derived iron in the atherosclerotic plaque. *Atherosclerosis* 209:28–31, 2010.
86. Granada JF, Kaluza GL, Wilensky RL, et al: Porcine models of coronary atherosclerosis and vulnerable plaque for imaging and interventional research. *EuroIntervention* 5:140–148, 2009.
87. DeMaria AN, Narula J, Mahmud E, et al: Imaging vulnerable plaque by ultrasound. *J Am Coll Cardiol* 47:C32–C39, 2006.
88. Low AF, Kawase Y, Chan YH, et al: In vivo characterisation of coronary plaques with conventional grey-scale intravascular ultrasound: Correlation with optical coherence tomography. *EuroIntervention* 4:626–632, 2009.
89. Okubo M, Kawasaki M, Ishihara Y, et al: Tissue characterization of coronary plaques: Comparison of integrated backscatter intravascular ultrasound with virtual histology intravascular ultrasound. *Circ J* 72:1631–1639, 2008.
90. Fujii K, Mintz GS, Carlier SG, et al: Intravascular ultrasound profile analysis of ruptured coronary plaques. *Am J Cardiol* 98:429–435, 2006.
91. Kim SH, Hong MK, Park DW, et al: Impact of plaque characteristics analyzed by intravascular ultrasound on long-term clinical outcomes. *Am J Cardiol* 103:1221–1226, 2009.
92. Ge J, Chirillo F, Schwedtmann J, et al: Screening of ruptured plaques in patients with coronary artery disease by intravascular ultrasound. *Heart* 81:621–627, 1999.
93. Konig A, Bleie O, Rieber J, et al: Intravascular ultrasound radiofrequency analysis of the lesion segment profile in ACS patients. *Clin Res Cardiol* 99:83–91, 2010.
94. Komiyama N, Berry GJ, Kolz ML, et al: Tissue characterization of atherosclerotic plaques by intravascular ultrasound radiofrequency signal analysis: An in vitro study of human coronary arteries. *Am Heart J* 140:565–574, 2000.
95. Sano K, Kawasaki M, Ishihara Y, et al: Assessment of vulnerable plaques causing acute coronary syndrome using integrated backscatter intravascular ultrasound. *J Am Coll Cardiol* 47:734–741, 2006.
96. Yamagishi M, Terashima M, Awano K, et al: Morphology of vulnerable coronary plaque: insights from follow-up of patients examined by intravascular ultrasound before an acute coronary syndrome. *J Am Coll Cardiol* 35:106–111, 2000.
97. Bayturan O, Tuzcu EM, Nicholls SJ, et al: Attenuated plaque at nonculprit lesions in patients enrolled in intravascular ultrasound atherosclerosis progression trials. *JACC Cardiovasc Interv* 2:672–678, 2009.
98. Schoenhagen P, Nissen SE, Tuzcu EM: Coronary arterial remodeling: From bench to bedside. *Curr Atheroscler Rep* 5:150–154, 2003.
99. Raffel OC, Merchant FM, Tearney GJ, et al: In vivo association between positive coronary artery remodelling and coronary plaque characteristics assessed by intravascular optical coherence tomography. *Eur Heart J* 29:1721–1728, 2008.
100. Kaul S, Ito H. Microvasculature in acute myocardial ischemia: Part II: Evolving concepts in pathophysiology, diagnosis, and treatment. *Circulation* 109:310–315, 2004.
101. Staub D, Schinkel AF, Coll B, et al: Contrast-enhanced ultrasound imaging of the vasa vasorum: from early atherosclerosis to the identification of unstable plaques. *JACC Cardiovasc Imaging* 3:761–771, 2010.
102. Moguillansky D, Leng X, Carson A, et al: Quantification of plaque neovascularization using contrast ultrasound: A histologic validation. *Eur Heart J* 32(5):646–653, 2010.
103. Giannoni MF, Vicenzini E, Citone M, et al: Contrast carotid ultrasound for the detection of unstable plaques with neoangiogenesis: a pilot study. *Eur J Vasc Endovasc Surg* 37:722–727, 2009.
104. Carlier S, Kakadiaris IA, Dib N, et al: Vasa vasorum imaging: A new window to the clinical detection of vulnerable atherosclerotic plaques. *Curr Atheroscler Rep* 7:164–169, 2005.
105. Goertz DE, Frijlink ME, Tempel D, et al: Contrast harmonic intravascular ultrasound: A feasibility study for vasa vasorum imaging. *Invest Radiol* 41:631–638, 2006.
106. Vavuranakis M, Kakadiaris IA, O'Malley SM, et al: A new method for assessment of plaque vulnerability based on vasa vasorum imaging, by using contrast-enhanced intravascular ultrasound and differential image analysis. *Int J Cardiol* 130:23–29, 2008.
107. Nair A, Kuban BD, Tuzcu EM, et al: Coronary plaque classification with intravascular ultrasound radiofrequency data analysis. *Circulation* 106:2200–2206, 2002.
108. Van Herck J, De Meyer G, Ennekens G, et al: Validation of in vivo plaque characterisation by virtual histology in a rabbit model of atherosclerosis. *EuroIntervention* 5:149–156, 2009.
109. Hong MK, Park DW, Lee CW, et al: Effects of statin treatments on coronary plaques assessed by volumetric virtual histology intravascular ultrasound analysis. *JACC Cardiovasc Interv* 2:679–688, 2009.
110. Rodriguez-Granillo GA, Garcia-Garcia HM, Mc Fadden EP, et al: In vivo intravascular ultrasound-derived thin-cap fibroatheroma detection using ultrasound radiofrequency data analysis. *J Am Coll Cardiol* 46:2038–2042, 2005.
111. Hong MK, Mintz GS, Lee CW, et al: Comparison of virtual histology to intravascular ultrasound of culprit coronary lesions in acute coronary syndrome and target coronary lesions in stable angina pectoris. *Am J Cardiol* 100:953–959, 2007.
112. Nakamura T, Kubo N, Funayama H, et al: Plaque characteristics of the coronary segment proximal to the culprit lesion in stable and unstable patients. *Clin Cardiol* 32:E9–E12, 2009.
113. Sawada T, Shite J, Garcia-Garcia HM, et al: Feasibility of combined use of intravascular ultrasound radiofrequency data analysis and optical coherence tomography for detecting thin-cap fibroatheroma. *Eur Heart J* 29:1136–1146, 2008.
114. Kubo T, Maehara A, Mintz GS, et al: The dynamic nature of coronary artery lesion morphology assessed by serial virtual histology intravascular ultrasound tissue characterization. *J Am Coll Cardiol* 55:1590–1597, 2010.
115. Burke AP, Joner M, Virmani R: IVUS-VH: A predictor of plaque morphology? *Eur Heart J* 27:1889–1890, 2006.
116. Nasu K, Tsuchikane E, Katoh O, et al: Accuracy of in vivo coronary plaque morphology assessment: A validation study of in vivo virtual histology compared with in vitro histopathology. *J Am Coll Cardiol* 47:2405–2412, 2006.
117. Wu X, Maehara A, Mintz GS, et al: Virtual histology intravascular ultrasound analysis of non-culprit attenuated plaques detected by grayscale intravascular ultrasound in patients with acute coronary syndromes. *Am J Cardiol* 105:48–53, 2010.
118. Thim T, Hagensen MK, Wallace-Bradley D, et al: Unreliable assessment of necrotic core by virtual histology intravascular ultrasound in porcine coronary artery disease. *Circ Cardiovasc Imaging* 3:384–391, 2010.
119. Granada JF, Wallace-Bradley D, Win HK, et al: In vivo plaque characterization using intravascular ultrasound-virtual histology in a porcine model of complex coronary lesions. *Arterioscler Thromb Vasc Biol* 27:387–393, 2007.
120. Surmely JF, Nasu K, Fujita H, et al: Coronary plaque composition of culprit/target lesions according to the clinical presentation: A virtual histology intravascular ultrasound analysis. *Eur Heart J* 27(24):2939–2944, 2006.
121. Rodriguez-Granillo GA, Garcia-Garcia HM, Valgimigli M, et al: Global characterization of coronary plaque rupture phenotype using three-vessel intravascular ultrasound radiofrequency data analysis. *Eur Heart J* 27:1921–1927, 2006.
122. Rodriguez-Granillo GA, McFadden EP, Valgimigli M, et al: Coronary plaque composition of nonculprit lesions, assessed by in vivo intracoronary ultrasound radio frequency data analysis, is related to clinical presentation. *Am Heart J* 151:1020–1024, 2006.
123. Diethrich EB, Pauliina Margolis M, Reid DB, et al: Virtual histology intravascular ultrasound assessment of carotid artery disease: The Carotid Artery Plaque Virtual Histology Evaluation (CAPITAL) study. *J Endovasc Ther* 14:676–686, 2007.
124. Prasad A, Cipher DJ, Mohandas A, et al: Reproducibility of intravascular ultrasound virtual histology analysis. *Cardiovasc Revasc Med* 9:71–77, 2008.
125. Surmely JF, Nasu K, Fujita H, et al: Association of coronary plaque composition and arterial remodeling: A virtual histology intravascular ultrasound analysis. *Heart* 2006.
126. Rodriguez-Granillo GA, Serruys PW, Garcia-Garcia HM, et al: Coronary artery remodelling is related to plaque composition. *Heart* 92:388–391, 2006.
127. Gijsen FJ, Wentzel JJ, Thury A, et al: Strain distribution over plaques in human coronary arteries relates to shear stress. *Am J Physiol Heart Circ Physiol* 295:H1608–H1614, 2008.
128. Baldewsing RA, Schaar JA, Mastik F, et al: Local elasticity imaging of vulnerable atherosclerotic coronary plaques. *Adv Cardiol* 44:35–61, 2007.
129. Serruys PW: Fourth annual American College of Cardiology international lecture: A journey in the interventional field. *J Am Coll Cardiol* 47:1754–1768, 2006.
130. Schaar JA, De Korte CL, Mastik F, et al: Characterizing vulnerable plaque features with intravascular elastography. *Circulation* 108:2636–2641, 2003.
131. Liang Y, Zhu H, Gehrig T, et al: Measurement of the transverse strain tensor in the coronary arterial wall from clinical intravascular ultrasound images. *J Biomech* 41:2906–2911, 2008.
132. Danilouchkine MG, Mastik F, van der Steen AF: Reconstructive compounding for IVUS palpography. *IEEE Trans Ultrason Ferroelectr Freq Control* 56:2630–2642, 2009.
133. Low AF, Tearney GJ, Bouma BE, et al: Technology Insight: optical coherence tomography—current status and future development. *Nat Clin Pract Cardiovasc Med* 3:154–162; quiz 172, 2006.
134. Bouma BE: *New insights from OCT, polarization-sensitive OCT, and the emergence of OFDI. Presented at The Vulnerable Plaque Session: "Pathophysiology, detection, and therapeutic intervention,"* Washington, D.C., 2006, Transcatheter Therapeutic Intervention (TCT) Meeting, 2006.
135. Regar E, van Soest G, Bruining N, et al: Optical coherence tomography in patients with acute coronary syndrome. *EuroIntervention* 6(Suppl G):G154–G160, 2010.
136. Kubo T, Imanishi T, Takarada S, et al: Assessment of culprit lesion morphology in acute myocardial infarction: Ability of optical coherence tomography compared with intravascular ultrasound and coronary angioscopy. *J Am Coll Cardiol* 50:933–939, 2007.
137. Tanaka A, Imanishi T, Kitabata H, et al: Lipid-rich plaque and myocardial perfusion after successful stenting in patients with non-ST-segment elevation acute coronary syndrome: An optical coherence tomography study. *Eur Heart J* 30:1348–1355, 2009.
138. Jang IK, Tearney GJ, MacNeill B, et al: In vivo characterization of coronary atherosclerotic plaque by use of optical coherence tomography. *Circulation* 111:1551–1555, 2005.
139. Takarada S, Imanishi T, Kubo T, et al: Effect of statin therapy on coronary fibrous-cap thickness in patients with acute coronary syndrome: Assessment by optical coherence tomography study. *Atherosclerosis* 202:491–497, 2009.
140. Giattina SD, Courtney BK, Herz PR, et al: Assessment of coronary plaque collagen with polarization sensitive optical coherence tomography (PS-OCT). *Int J Cardiol* 107:400–409, 2006.
141. Manfrini O, Mont E, Leone O, et al: Sources of error and interpretation of plaque morphology by optical coherence tomography. *Am J Cardiol* 98:156–159, 2006.
142. van Soest G, Goderie T, Regar E, et al: Atherosclerotic tissue characterization in vivo by optical coherence tomography attenuation imaging. *J Biomed Opt* 15:011105, 2010.
143. Tearney GJ, Yabushita H, Houser SL, et al: Quantification of macrophage content in atherosclerotic plaques by optical coherence tomography. *Circulation* 107:113–119, 2003.
144. MacNeill BD, Jang IK, Bouma BE, et al: Focal and multi-focal plaque macrophage distributions in patients with acute and stable presentations of coronary artery disease. *J Am Coll Cardiol* 44:972–979, 2004.
145. Raffel OC, Tearney GJ, Gauthier DD, et al: Relationship between a systemic inflammatory marker, plaque inflammation, and plaque characteristics determined by intravascular optical coherence tomography. *Arterioscler Thromb Vasc Biol* 27:1820–1827, 2007.
146. Avery RL, Pieramici DJ, Rabena MD, et al: Intravitreal bevacizumab (Avastin) for neovascular age-related macular degeneration. *Ophthalmology* 113:363–372, e5, 2006.
147. Kitabata H, Tanaka A, Kubo T, et al: Relation of microchannel structure identified by optical coherence tomography to plaque vulnerability in patients with coronary artery disease. *Am J Cardiol* 105:1673–1678, 2010.
148. Fuster V, Fayad ZA, Moreno PR, et al: Atherothrombosis and high-risk plaque: Part II: Approaches by noninvasive computed tomographic/magnetic resonance imaging. *J Am Coll Cardiol* 46:1209–1218, 2005.
149. Fuster V, Corti R, Fayad ZA, et al: Integration of vascular biology and magnetic resonance imaging in the understanding of atherothrombosis and acute coronary syndromes. *J Thromb Haemost* 1:1410–1421, 2003.
150. Sirol M, Fuster V, Fayad ZA: Plaque imaging and characterization using magnetic resonance imaging: towards molecular assessment. *Curr Mol Med* 6:541–548, 2006.
151. Wilensky RL, Song HK, Ferrari VA: Role of magnetic resonance and intravascular magnetic resonance in the detection of vulnerable plaques. *J Am Coll Cardiol* 47:C48–C56, 2006.
152. Ferrari VA, Wilensky RL: Intravascular magnetic resonance imaging. *Top Magn Reson Imaging* 18:401–408, 2007.
153. Regar E, Hennen B, Grube E, et al: First-In-Man application of a miniature self-contained intracoronary magnetic resonance probe. A multi-centre safety and feasibility trial. *EuroIntervention* 2:77–83, 2006.

154. Schneiderman J, Wilensky RL, Weiss A, et al: Diagnosis of thin-cap fibroatheromas by a self contained intravascular magnetic resonance imaging probe in ex vivo human aortas and in situ coronary arteries. *J Am Coll Cardiol* 45:1961–1969, 2005.
155. Phinikaridou A, Ruberg FL, Hallock KJ, et al: In vivo detection of vulnerable atherosclerotic plaque by MRI in a rabbit model. *Circ Cardiovasc Imaging* 3:323–332, 2010.
156. Larose E, Kinlay S, Selwyn AP, et al: Improved characterization of atherosclerotic plaques by gadolinium contrast during intravascular magnetic resonance imaging of human arteries. *Atherosclerosis* 196:919–925, 2008.
157. Beilvert A, Cormode DP, Chaubet F, et al: Tyrosine polyethylene glycol (PEG)-micelle magnetic resonance contrast agent for the detection of lipid rich areas in atherosclerotic plaque. *Magn Reson Med* 62:1195–1201, 2009.
158. Meding J, Urich M, Licha K, et al: Magnetic resonance imaging of atherosclerosis by targeting extracellular matrix deposition with gadofluorine M. *Contrast Media Mol Imaging* 2:120–129, 2007.
159. Klink A, Lancelot E, Ballet S, et al: Magnetic resonance molecular imaging of thrombosis in an arachidonic acid mouse model using an activated platelet targeted probe. *Arterioscler Thromb Vasc Biol* 30:403–410, 2010.
160. Lipinski MJ, Frias JC, Fayad ZA: Advances in detection and characterization of atherosclerosis using contrast agents targeting the macrophage. *J Nucl Cardiol* 13:699–709, 2006.
161. Jaffer FA, Libby P, Weissleder R: Molecular and cellular imaging of atherosclerosis: Emerging applications. *J Am Coll Cardiol* 47:1328–1338, 2006.
162. Lipinski MJ, Frias JC, Amirbekian V, et al: Macrophage-specific lipid-based nanoparticles improve cardiac magnetic resonance detection and characterization of human atherosclerosis. *JACC Cardiovasc Imaging* 2:637–647, 2009.
163. Chen W, Vucic E, Leupold E, et al: Incorporation of an apoE-derived lipopeptide in high-density lipoprotein MRI contrast agents for enhanced imaging of macrophages in atherosclerosis. *Contrast Media Mol Imaging* 3:233–242, 2008.
164. Korosoglou G, Weiss RG, Kedziorek DA, et al: Noninvasive detection of macrophage-rich atherosclerotic plaque in hyperlipidemic rabbits using "positive contrast" magnetic resonance imaging. *J Am Coll Cardiol* 52:483–491, 2008.
165. Davies JR, Rudd JH, Weissberg PL, et al: Radionuclide imaging for the detection of inflammation in vulnerable plaques. *J Am Coll Cardiol* 47:C57–C68, 2006.
166. Lancelot E, Amirbekian V, Brigger I, et al: Evaluation of matrix metalloproteinases in atherosclerosis using a novel noninvasive imaging approach. *Arterioscler Thromb Vasc Biol* 28:425–432, 2008.
167. Lipinski MJ, Amirbekian V, Frias JC, et al: MRI to detect atherosclerosis with gadolinium-containing immunomicelles targeting the macrophage scavenger receptor. *Magn Reson Med* 56:601–610, 2006.
168. Fayad ZA, Amirbekian V, Toussaint JF, et al: Identification of interleukin-2 for imaging atherosclerotic inflammation. *Eur J Nucl Med Mol Imaging* 33:111–116, 2006.
169. Sosnovik DE, Schellenberger EA, Nahrendorf M, et al: Magnetic resonance imaging of cardiomyocyte apoptosis with a novel magneto-optical nanoparticle. *Magn Reson Med* 54:718–724, 2005.
170. Amirbekian V, Lipinski MJ, Briley-Saebo KC, et al: Detecting and assessing macrophages in vivo to evaluate atherosclerosis noninvasively using molecular MRI. *Proc Natl Acad Sci U S A* 104:961–966, 2007.
171. Burtea C, Laurent S, Lancelot E, et al: Peptidic targeting of phosphatidylserine for the MRI detection of apoptosis in atherosclerotic plaques. *Mol Pharm* 6:1903–1919, 2009.
172. Purushothaman KR, Sanz J, Zias E, et al: Atherosclerosis neovascularization and imaging. *Curr Mol Med* 6:549–556, 2006.
173. Winter PM, Morawski AM, Caruthers SD, et al: Molecular imaging of angiogenesis in early-stage atherosclerosis with alpha(v)beta3-integrin-targeted nanoparticles. *Circulation* 108:2270–2274, 2003.
174. Matter CM, Schuler PK, Alessi P, et al: Molecular imaging of atherosclerotic plaques using a human antibody against the extra-domain B of fibronectin. *Circ Res* 95:1225–1233, 2004.
175. Kelly KA, Allport JR, Tsourkas A, et al: Detection of vascular adhesion molecule-1 expression using a novel multimodal nanoparticle. *Circ Res* 96:327–336, 2005.
176. Calcagno C, Mani V, Ramachandran S, et al: Dynamic contrast enhanced (DCE) magnetic resonance imaging (MRI) of atherosclerotic plaque angiogenesis. *Angiogenesis* 13:87–99, 2010.
177. Sirol M, Moreno PR, Purushothaman KR, et al: Increased neovascularization in advanced lipid-rich atherosclerotic lesions detected by gadofluorine-M-enhanced MRI: Implications for plaque vulnerability. *Circ Cardiovasc Imaging* 2:391–396, 2009.
178. Takaya N, Yuan C, Chu B, et al: Presence of intraplaque hemorrhage stimulates progression of carotid atherosclerotic plaques: A high-resolution magnetic resonance imaging study. *Circulation* 111:2768–2775, 2005.
179. Takaya N, Yuan C, Chu B, et al: Association between carotid plaque characteristics and subsequent ischemic cerebrovascular events: A prospective assessment with MRI—initial results. *Stroke* 37:818–823, 2006.
180. Puppini G, Furlan F, Cirota N, et al: Characterisation of carotid atherosclerotic plaque: Comparison between magnetic resonance imaging and histology. *Radiol Med (Torino)* 111:921–930, 2006.
181. Uchida Y, Kawai S, Kanamaru R, et al: Detection of vulnerable coronary plaques by color fluorescent angioscopy. *JACC Cardiovasc Imaging* 3:398–408, 2010.
182. Uchida Y, Nakamura F, Tomaru T, et al: Prediction of acute coronary syndromes by percutaneous coronary angioscopy in patients with stable angina. *Am Heart J* 130:195–203, 1995.
183. Asakura M, Ueda Y, Yamaguchi O, et al: Extensive development of vulnerable plaques as a pan-coronary process in patients with myocardial infarction: An angioscopic study. *J Am Coll Cardiol* 37:1284–1288, 2001.
184. Ohtani T, Ueda Y, Mizote I, et al: Number of yellow plaques detected in a coronary artery is associated with future risk of acute coronary syndrome: Detection of vulnerable patients by angioscopy. *J Am Coll Cardiol* 47:2194–2200, 2006.
185. Takano M, Jang IK, Inami S, et al: In vivo comparison of optical coherence tomography and angioscopy for the evaluation of coronary plaque characteristics. *Am J Cardiol* 101:471–476, 2008.
186. Hirayama A, Saito S, Ueda Y, et al: Qualitative and quantitative changes in coronary plaque associated with atorvastatin therapy. *Circ J* 73:718–725, 2009.
187. Ishibashi F, Mizuno K, Kawamura A, et al: High yellow color intensity by angioscopy with quantitative colorimetry to identify high-risk features in culprit lesions of patients with acute coronary syndromes. *Am J Cardiol* 100:1207–1211, 2007.
188. Moreno PR, Muller JE: Detection of high-risk atherosclerotic coronary plaques by intravascular spectroscopy. *J Interv Cardiol* 16:243–252, 2003.
189. Moreno PR, Purushothaman KR, Charash WE, et al: Detection of lipid pool, thin fibrous cap, and inflammatory cells in human aortic atherosclerotic plaques by near-infrared spectroscopy. *Circulation* 105:923–927, 2002.
190. Gardner CM, Tan H, Hull EL, et al: Detection of lipid core coronary plaques in autopsy specimens with a novel catheter-based near-infrared spectroscopy system. *JACC Cardiovasc Imaging* 1:638–648, 2008.
191. Nazemi JH, Brennan JF: Lipid concentrations in human coronary artery determined with high wave number Raman shifted light. *J Biomed Opt* 14:034009, 2009.
192. Waxman S, Dixon SR, L'Allier P, et al: In vivo validation of a catheter-based near-infrared spectroscopy system for detection of lipid core coronary plaques: Initial results of the SPECTACL study. *JACC Cardiovasc Imaging* 2:858–868, 2009.
193. Fernandez-Friera L, Garcia-Alvarez A, Romero A, et al: Lipid-rich obstructive coronary lesions is plaque characterization any important? *JACC Cardiovasc Imaging* 3:893–895, 2010.
194. Goldstein JA, Grines C, Fischell T, et al: Coronary embolization following balloon dilation of lipid-core plaques. *JACC Cardiovasc Imaging* 2:1420–1424, 2009.
195. Madjid M, Willerson JT, Casscells SW: Intracoronary thermography for detection of high-risk vulnerable plaques. *J Am Coll Cardiol* 47:C80–C85, 2006.
196. Takumi T, Lee S, Hamasaki S, et al: Limitation of angiography to identify the culprit plaque in acute myocardial infarction with coronary total occlusion utility of coronary plaque temperature measurement to identify the culprit plaque. *J Am Coll Cardiol* 50:2197–2203, 2007.
197. Stefanadis C, Toutouzas K, Tsiamis E, et al: Relation between local temperature and C-reactive protein levels in patients with coronary artery disease: Effects of atorvastatin treatment. *Atherosclerosis* 192:396–400, 2007.
198. Toutouzas K, Synetos A, Stefanadi E, et al: Correlation between morphologic characteristics and local temperature differences in culprit lesions of patients with symptomatic coronary artery disease. *J Am Coll Cardiol* 49:2264–2271, 2007.
199. Cuisset T, Beauloye C, Melikian N, et al: In vitro and in vivo studies on thermistor-based intracoronary temperature measurements: Effect of pressure and flow. *Catheter Cardiovasc Interv* 73:224–230, 2009.
200. Kashiwagi M, Tanaka A, Kitabata H, et al: Feasibility of noninvasive assessment of thin-cap fibroatheroma by multidetector computed tomography. *JACC Cardiovasc Imaging* 2:1412–1419, 2009.
201. Rivera JJ, Nasir K, Cox PR, et al: Association of traditional cardiovascular risk factors with coronary plaque sub-types assessed by 64-slice computed tomography angiography in a large cohort of asymptomatic subjects. *Atherosclerosis* 206:451–457, 2009.
202. Narula J, Achenbach S: Napkin-ring necrotic cores: Defining circumferential extent of necrotic cores in unstable plaques. *JACC Cardiovasc Imaging* 2:1436–1438, 2009.
203. Sarno G, Vanhoenacker P, Decramer I, et al: Characterisation of the "vulnerable" coronary plaque by multi-detector computed tomography: A correlative study with intravascular ultrasound-derived radiofrequency analysis of plaque composition. *EuroIntervention* 4:318–323, 2008.
204. Kitagawa T, Yamamoto H, Horiguchi J, et al: Characterization of noncalcified coronary plaques and identification of culprit lesions in patients with acute coronary syndrome by 64-slice computed tomography. *JACC Cardiovasc Imaging* 2:153–160, 2009.
205. Pundziute G, Schuijf JD, Jukema JW, et al: Head-to-head comparison of coronary plaque evaluation between multislice computed tomography and intravascular ultrasound radiofrequency data analysis. *JACC Cardiovasc Interv* 1:176–182, 2008.
206. Langer HF, Haubner R, Pichler BJ, et al: Radionuclide imaging: A molecular key to the atherosclerotic plaque. *J Am Coll Cardiol* 52:1–12, 2008.
207. Teras M, Kokki T, Durand-Schaefer N, et al: Dual-gated cardiac PET-clinical feasibility study. *Eur J Nucl Med Mol Imaging* 37:505–516, 2010.
208. Wykrzykowska J, Lehman S, Williams G, et al: Imaging of inflamed and vulnerable plaque in coronary arteries with 18F-FDG PET/CT in patients with suppression of myocardial uptake using a low-carbohydrate, high-fat preparation. *J Nucl Med* 50:563–568, 2009.
209. Chen W, Dilsizian V: (18)F-fluorodeoxyglucose PET imaging of coronary atherosclerosis and plaque inflammation. *Curr Cardiol Rep* 12:179–184, 2010.
210. Schafers M, Schober O, Hermann S: Matrix-metalloproteinases as imaging targets for inflammatory activity in atherosclerotic plaques. *J Nucl Med* 51:663–666, 2010.
211. Ishino S, Mukai T, Kuge Y, et al: Targeting of lectinlike oxidized low-density lipoprotein receptor 1 (LOX-1) with 99mTc-labeled anti-LOX-1 antibody: Potential agent for imaging of vulnerable plaque. *J Nucl Med* 49:1677–1685, 2008.
212. Li D, Patel AR, Klibanov AL, et al: Molecular imaging of atherosclerotic plaques targeted to oxidized LDL receptor LOX-1 by SPECT/CT and magnetic resonance. *Circ Cardiovasc Imaging* 3:464–472, 2010.
213. Isobe S, Tsimikas S, Zhou J, et al: Noninvasive imaging of atherosclerotic lesions in apolipoprotein E-deficient and low-density-lipoprotein receptor-deficient mice with annexin A5. *J Nucl Med* 47:1497–1505, 2006.
214. Laufer EM, Winkens MH, Narula J, et al: Molecular imaging of macrophage cell death for the assessment of plaque vulnerability. *Arterioscler Thromb Vasc Biol* 29:1031–1038, 2009.
215. Laitinen I, Saraste A, Weidl E, et al: Evaluation of alphavbeta3 integrin-targeted positron emission tomography tracer 18F-galacto-RGD for imaging of vascular inflammation in atherosclerotic mice. *Circ Cardiovasc Imaging* 2:331–338, 2009.
216. Winter PM, Caruthers SD, Zhang H, et al: Antiangiogenic synergism of integrin-targeted fumagillin nanoparticles and atorvastatin in atherosclerosis. *JACC Cardiovasc Imaging* 1:624–634, 2008.
217. Skajaa T, Cormode DP, Falk E, et al: High-density lipoprotein-based contrast agents for multimodal imaging of atherosclerosis. *Arterioscler Thromb Vasc Biol* 30:169–176, 2010.
218. Cormode DP, Roessl E, Thran A, et al: Atherosclerotic plaque composition: Analysis with multicolor CT and targeted gold nanoparticles. *Radiology* 256(3):774–782, 2010.
219. Muntendam P, McCall C, Sanz J, et al: The BioImage Study: Novel approaches to risk assessment in the primary prevention of atherosclerotic cardiovascular disease—study design and objectives. *Am Heart J* 160:49–57, e1, 2010.
220. Ambrose JA, D'Agate DJ: Classification of systemic therapies for potential stabilization of the vulnerable plaque to prevent acute myocardial infarction. *Am J Cardiol* 95:379–382, 2005.
221. Cannon CP, Steinberg BA, Murphy SA, et al: Meta-analysis of cardiovascular outcomes trials comparing intensive versus moderate statin therapy. *J Am Coll Cardiol* 48:438–445, 2006.
222. Scirica BM, Morrow DA, Cannon CP, et al: Intensive statin therapy and the risk of hospitalization for heart failure after an acute coronary syndrome in the PROVE IT-TIMI 22 study. *J Am Coll Cardiol* 47:2326–2331, 2006.
223. Hulten E, Jackson JL, Douglas K, et al: The effect of early, intensive statin therapy on acute coronary syndrome: a meta-analysis of randomized controlled trials. *Arch Intern Med* 166:1814–1821, 2006.
224. Semenova AE, Sergienko IV, Masenko VP, et al: The influence of rosuvastatin therapy and percutaneous coronary intervention on angiogenic growth factors in coronary artery disease patients. *Acta Cardiol* 64:405–409, 2009.
225. Goldenberg I, Goldbourt U, Boyko V, et al: Relation between on-treatment increments in serum high-density lipoprotein cholesterol levels and cardiac mortality in patients with coronary heart disease (from the Bezafibrate Infarction Prevention trial). *Am J Cardiol* 97:466–471, 2006.
226. Corti R, Osende J, Hutter R, et al: Fenofibrate induces plaque regression in hypercholesterolemic atherosclerotic rabbits: In vivo demonstration by high-resolution MRI. *Atherosclerosis* 190(1):106–113, 2007.
227. Naik SU, Wang X, Da Silva JS, et al: Pharmacological activation of liver X receptors promotes reverse cholesterol transport in vivo. *Circulation* 113:90–97, 2006.
228. Tso C, Martinic G, Fan WH, et al: High-density lipoproteins enhance progenitor-mediated endothelium repair in mice. *Arterioscler Thromb Vasc Biol* 26:1144–1149, 2006.
229. Toi T, Taguchi I, Yoneda S, et al: Early effect of lipid-lowering therapy with pitavastatin on regression of coronary atherosclerotic plaque. Comparison with atorvastatin. *Circ J* 73:1466–1472, 2009.
230. Linke A, Erbs S, Hambrecht R: Effects of exercise training upon endothelial function in patients with cardiovascular disease. *Front Biosci* 13:424–432, 2008.
231. Deschaseaux F, Selmani Z, Falcoz PE, et al: Two types of circulating endothelial progenitor cells in patients receiving long term therapy by HMG-CoA reductase inhibitors. *Eur J Pharmacol* 562:111–118, 2007.
232. Werner C, Kamani CH, Gensch C, et al: The peroxisome proliferator-activated receptor-gamma agonist pioglitazone increases number and function of endothelial progenitor cells in patients with coronary artery disease and normal glucose tolerance. *Diabetes* 56:2609–2615, 2007.

233. Massaro M, Scoditti E, Carluccio MA, et al: Omega-3 fatty acids, inflammation and angiogenesis: basic mechanisms behind the cardioprotective effects of fish and fish oils. *Cell Mol Biol (Noisy-le-grand)* 56:59–82, 2010.

234. Petoumenos V, Nickenig G, Werner N: High-density lipoprotein exerts vasculoprotection via endothelial progenitor cells. *J Cell Mol Med* 13:4623–4635, 2009.

235. Hauer AD, Habets KL, van Wanrooij EJ, et al: Vaccination against TIE2 reduces atherosclerosis. *Atherosclerosis* 204:365–371, 2009.

236. Chauffe RJ, Wilensky RL, Mohler ER, 3rd.: Recent developments with lipoprotein-associated phospholipase A2 inhibitors. *Curr Atheroscler Rep* 12:43–47, 2010.

237. Cannon CP, Braunwald E, McCabe CH, et al: Intensive versus moderate lipid lowering with statins after acute coronary syndromes. *N Engl J Med* 350:1495–1504, 2004.

238. Waksman R, Leitch IM, Roessler J, et al: Intracoronary photodynamic therapy reduces neointimal growth without suppressing re-endothelialisation in a porcine model. *Heart* 92:1138–1144, 2006.

239. Magaraggia M, Marigo L, Pagnan A, et al: Porphyrin-photosensitized processes: Their applications in the prevention of arterial restenosis. *Cardiovasc Hematol Agents Med Chem* 5:278–288, 2007.

240. Dorval JF, Geoffroy P, Sirois MG, et al: Endovascular cryotherapy accentuates the accumulation of the fibrillar collagen types I and III after percutaneous transluminal angioplasty in pigs. *J Endovasc Ther* 13:104–110, 2006.

241. Triesscheijn M, Baas P, Schellens JH, et al: Photodynamic therapy in oncology. *Oncologist* 11:1034–1044, 2006.

242. Waksman R, et al. Novel photopoint photodynamic therapy for the treatment of atherosclerotic plaques [abstract]. *J Am Coll Cardiol* 41:259A, 2003.

243. Lafont A, Libby P: The smooth muscle cell: Sinner or saint in restenosis and the acute coronary syndromes? *J Am Coll Cardiol* 32:283–285, 1998.

244. Davies MJ: Detecting vulnerable coronary plaques. *Lancet* 347:1422–1423, 1996.

245. Echeverri DPK, Kilpatrick D, Moreno PR: Plaque stabilization by bare metal and drug-eluting stents in a rabbit model of of thin-cap fibroatheroma. *Brazilian J Interv Cardiol* 16:160–177, 2008.

246. Kaluza GL, Tellez A, Wallace-Bradley D, et al: First in-vivo experience with a novel low-pressure self-expanding intra-arterial shield: A one-month study comparing to balloon expandable stents in porcine coronary arteries. *Am J Cardiol* 100:(Suppl):2 31L, 2007.

247. Ramcharitar S, Gonzalo N, van Geuns RJ, et al: First case of stenting of a vulnerable plaque in the SECRITT I trial-the dawn of a new era? *Nat Rev Cardiol* 6:374–378, 2009.

248. Jain RK, Finn AV, Kolodgie FD, et al: Antiangiogenic therapy for normalization of atherosclerotic plaque vasculature: A potential strategy for plaque stabilization. *Nat Clin Pract Cardiovasc Med* 4:491–502, 2007.

249. Stefanadis C, Toutouzas K, Stefanadi E, et al: First experimental application of bevacizumab-eluting PC coated stent for inhibition of vasa vasorum of atherosclerotic plaque: Angiographic results in a rabbit atheromatic model. *Hellenic J Cardiol* 47:7–10, 2006.

250. Stefanadis C, Toutouzas K, Stefanadi E, et al: Inhibition of plaque neovascularization and intimal hyperplasia by specific targeting vascular endothelial growth factor with bevacizumab-eluting stent: An experimental study. *Atherosclerosis* 195:269–276, 2007.

251. Kolodgie FD, Narula J, Yuan C, et al: Elimination of neoangiogenesis for plaque stabilization: Is there a role for local drug therapy? *J Am Coll Cardiol* 49:2093–2101, 2007.

252. Roncal C, Buysschaert I, Gerdes N, et al: Short-term delivery of anti-PlGF antibody delays progression of atherosclerotic plaques to vulnerable lesions. *Cardiovasc Res* 86:29–36, 2010.

253. Serruys PW, Kukreja N: Late stent thrombosis in drug-eluting stents: Return of the "VB syndrome." *Nat Clin Pract Cardiovasc Med* 3:637, 2006.

254. Waksman R: Biodegradable stents: They do their job and disappear. *J Invasive Cardiol* 18:70–74, 2006.

255. Moreno P: First report of a vulnerable plaque specific stent capable of focal passivation without fibrous cap rupture. Paper presented in Transcatheter cardiovascular therapeutics, TCT Conference, Washington, D.C. 2006.

256. Loree HM, Kamm RD, Stringfellow RG, et al: Effects of fibrous cap thickness on peak circumferential stress in model atherosclerotic vessels. *Circ Res* 71:850–858, 1992.

257. Langheinrich AC, Michniewicz A, Sedding DG, et al: Correlation of vasa vasorum neovascularization and plaque progression in aortas of apolipoprotein E(-/-)/low-density lipoprotein(-/-) double knockout mice. *Arterioscler Thromb Vasc Biol* 26:347–352, 2006.

258. Vavuranakis M, Kakadiaris IA, O'Malley SM, et al: Images in cardiovascular medicine. Detection of luminal-intimal border and coronary wall enhancement in intravascular ultrasound imaging after injection of microbubbles and simultaneous sonication with transthoracic echocardiography. *Circulation* 112:e1–e2, 2005.

259. Jang IK: Optical coherence tomography. Studies at MGH. Paper presented at Transcatheter Cardiovascular Therapeutics, TCT Conference, September 27, 2002.

260. Waksman R: *Photodynamic therapy*, New York and London, 2004, Taylor & Francis.

Optical Coherence Tomography

GIULIO GUAGLIUMI | TAKASHI AKASAKA | VASILE SIRBU | TAKASHI KUBO

KEY POINTS

- *What is it?* Optical coherence tomography (OCT) is a new catheter-based imaging technology that uses light and fiberoptics to obtain unique details of vessels on a microscopic scale. OCT provides, with a high level of accuracy, real-time, full tomographic measurements of the tissue microstructure in living patients.

- *Why do we need it?* To assess the effectiveness of new devices and drug interventions, more quantitative indices are preferred. Because of its unrivaled high imaging axial resolution, OCT is able to overcome some of the limitations of angiography and intravascular ultrasound (IVUS) for assessing the significance of coronary stenoses and the results of stent procedures.

- *What can be obtained with OCT today?* OCT can reliably assess and quantify atherosclerotic plaque characteristics (thin fibrous cap, thrombus, neovessels, lipid pool, and possibly macrophages) and immediate and long-term vessel response to stent implantation (stent strut apposition and coverage). In complex interventional settings that hold a high risk of failure of percutaneous coronary intervention (PCI) (late stent thrombosis, in-stent re-stenosis, complex bifurcation), OCT can provide critical decision-making information. Currently, frequency-domain OCT (FD-OCT) systems allow a clear vision of very long segments of coronary arteries in few seconds, with a more complete picture of vessel involvement and easier image interpretation compared with standard methods.

- *What could be offered by OCT in the near future?* Three-dimensional reconstruction of OCT-images will automatically detect and quantify features of interest such as the shape of the lumen, the longitudinal position of the minimum lumen area (MLA), the site and amount of stent strut malapposition, and thrombus volume. The combination of FD-OCT with spectroscopic techniques will improve discrimination among tissue constituents in complex atherosclerotic lesions and allow for detailed analysis of the cellular and biochemical compositions of vulnerable plaques (VPs). Concurrent data collection from combined modalities will dramatically expand the structural and functional information available to the cardiologist and will hopefully guide the development and clinical use of novel cardiovascular therapies.

Optical coherence tomography (OCT) is an innovative real-time, tomographic imaging modality that can view microstructure in tissues. OCT delivers near-infrared light to the wall of the coronary artery through small-diameter optical fibers. The light that illuminates the vessel is absorbed and backscattered, or reflected, by the structures in tissue at different degrees, with an axial resolution of 1 to 10 microns (μm). Intravascular OCT imaging, based on advanced analysis of lesion morphology and accurate measurements, has the potential to overcome many of the limitations of conventional measures based on angiography and intravascular ultrasound (IVUS). The resolution of OCT is ideally suited for the measurement of tissue-level properties. Different tissue types have different optical properties. This makes OCT especially useful for studying the properties of tissues in ex vivo experimental models of various stages of atherosclerosis and for following plaque progression and regression and vascular response to coronary stent implantation in preclinical and clinical studies. Although its resolution is not sufficient to pick out individual cells (including regenerating endothelium), OCT is able to measure the density of

cellular aggregates and to provide some information about cellular composition. For example, it has been reported that some texture characteristics in OCT images of excised coronary arteries are correlated with macrophage cell density.[1] Also, fibrin deposition on stent struts, as detected by light and scanning electron microscopy (SEM), has specific attenuation characteristics in OCT.[2] Recent data support the concept that OCT imaging can be used to monitor cell culture progress and cellular transformation.[3] OCT provides excellent differentiation between the lumen and the arterial wall, with accurate measurements of the lumen areas and volumes as well as stent struts identification. Furthermore, quantitative measurements of the lumen, stent, and neointimal areas reveal highly reproducible results, driven by the unique resolution of this technology.[4] For OCT to be accepted by the medical community, ease of use and interpretation will be required. The new generation of frequency-doman OCT (FD-OCT) has significantly improved the signal-to-noise ratio, has a superior image quality, and enables faster acquisition. FD-OCT, which can grab the entire coronary artery in a few seconds (<5 seconds), will mostly be useful in the nonocclusive, high-volume contrast flushing method, without risk of major arrhythmias. On the basis of these properties, FD-OCT will probably permit a full scan of all major coronary vessels before and after coronary interventions. This represents a significant advantage for its use in PCIs, allowing quick evaluation of the entire vessel pathology (Fig. 60-1), identification of lesions to be treated, and assessment of landing zones for guiding stent implantation. Finally, FD-OCT can be combined with adjuvant techniques, including Doppler and IVUS, and can derive enormous advantage with miniaturization.[5]

Physical Principles of Optical Coherence Tomography Imaging

OCT's ability to create cross-sectional images of the vessel tissue is based on optical interference of near-infrared light.[6] Light is emitted and collected from the tip of a small-diameter optical fiber that rotates rapidly inside a transparent sheath. For longitudinal scanning of the vessel, a motor pulls back the fiber as it rotates within the sheath. The collected light carries information about the depth-resolved backscattering strength or reflectivity of the vascular tissue structures at the illuminated spot. Unlike ultrasound, where the depth information can be resolved by measuring the time-of-flight of acoustic reflections, light is too fast to resolve depth information by directly measuring photon time-of-flight. To overcome this, collected light is combined with a reference light beam, and lower-frequency optical interference signals are generated. These modulated interference signals can be measured with electronic components and digitally decoded to generate an optical backscattering profile (A-scan) of the tissue at the illuminated spot. Multiple backscattering profiles are collected as the catheter core rapidly rotates within the vessel. These profiles are then represented in a two-dimensional grayscale image, which is the OCT B-scan frame displayed to the user. OCT can be categorized into two approaches based on the scheme used for collecting and decoding the tissue backscattering profile from the collected light: time-domain OCT (TD-OCT) and FD-OCT (Fig. 60-2, Table 60-1). TD-OCT uses a broadband light source and a mechanically actuated sweep of the reference beam's optical path length (approximately 3–5 mm) to generate a temporal interference signal modulation. The modulated signal

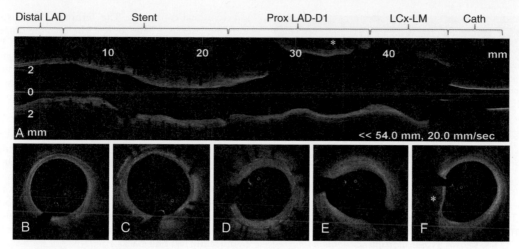

Figure 60-1 Frequency-domain optical coherence tomography (FD-OCT) scan of left anterior descending (LAD) coronary artery 6 months after drug eluting stent (DES) implantation **A,** Longitudinal view. **B,** Distal reference segment. **C,** Distal stented segment with homogeneous strut coverage. **D,** Proximal stented segment with homogeneous strut coverage but more neointimal tissue. **E,** Bifurcation LAD-D1. **F,** Ostial LAD with eccentric calcific plaque (*).

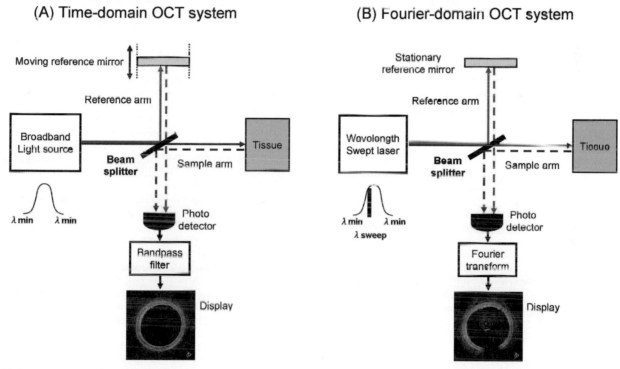

Figure 60-2 Main components of time-domain optical coherence tomography (TD-OCT) and FD-OCT. **A,** In TD-OCT, a broadband light source is divided by a beam splitter; part is sent to the tissue sample down the sample or measurement arm and the other down the reference arm to a moving mirror. The reflected signals are overlaid on a photodetector. The intensity of interference is detected and used to create images. **B,** In FD-OCT, the reference mirror does not move, and the light source is a laser that sweeps its output rapidly over a broad band of wavelengths. Fourier transformation of the interference signals stored during a single sweep reconstructs the amplitude profile of the reflections, analogous to a single A-line in an ultrasound scan. Lasers with narrow line widths and wide sweep ranges enable the acquisition of FD-OCT images with high resolution over a wide range of depths.

intensity is directly proportional to the tissue backscattering profile and is thus straightforward to extract. Unfortunately, the requirements for mechanical actuation limit the achievable A-scan repetition rate to a few kilohertz (kHz) and the B-scan frame rate to a few tens of hertz (Hz). This, in turn, limits the total intravascular region that can be safely visualized during a transient period of blood displacement by occlusion balloon or infusion of optically transparent fluid (saline or contrast media). In FD-OCT, interference signals generated by an interferometer at different wavelengths are processed mathematically by Fourier transformation to determine the amplitudes of reflections returning from different depths. As in magnetic resonance imaging (MRI), the frequency of the recorded signal encodes the position in the image. Although this makes FD-OCT more computationally intensive, A-scan repetition rates are typically 10 to 100 times higher than those of TD-OCT and therefore allow dramatically faster B-scan frame rates (hundreds of Hz). With its careful system and catheter designs,

TABLE 60-1	Performance of Frequency-Domain Optical Coherence Tomography System Compared with Time-Domain Optical Coherence Tomography System		
		TD-OCT	**FD-OCT**
Axial resolution (μm)		15–20	15–20
Lateral resolution (μm)		25–30	25–30
Scan diameter (mm)		6.8	8.3
Frame rate (frame/second)		15–20	100
Number of lines (/frame)		200–240	450
Maximum pullback speed (mm/second)		2–3	20
Coronary occlusion for imaging		Suggested	Not required

FD-OCT provides a far more comprehensive visualization of the intravascular region during the transient blood displacement period.

FD-OCT can be further subcategorized into two approaches: swept-source OCT (SS-OCT; also known as *optical frequency domain imaging [OFDI]*) and spectral-domain OCT (SD-OCT). SS-OCT uses a narrowband light source whose wavelength is tuned or "swept" through a broad spectral range as a function of time. The mechanical actuation necessary to sweep the source wavelength and create interference fringe modulation is on the nanometer scale and therefore can be accomplished rapidly and in compact Micro Electro Mechanical Systems (MEMS)-based packaging. SD-OCT uses a broadband light source similar to TD-OCT but avoids the need for mechanical actuation by dispersing the broadband spectral components in a spectrometer and by capturing modulated fringes using a parallel array of detectors such as a CCD (charge coupled device) camera. Commercial and research intravascular OCT imaging systems are usually the SS-OCT type, primarily because of instrumentation cost and the complexity advantages of SS-OCT in the 1250- to 1360-nm wavelength region that is appropriate for intravascular imaging. The C7XR OCT system, manufactured by LightLab Imaging, Inc. (Westford, MA), was introduced as the first commercially available FD-OCT imaging system for coronary imaging in the European Union in 2009 and in the United States in 2010. Employing a 2.7 French (F) intravascular catheter with a rapid-exchange monorail tip, the C7XR system has a spatial resolution of 15 μm and acquires 500 axial lines per frame at a rate of 100 frames per second. At the tip of the catheter is a 125-μm–diameter optical fiber assembly that consists of an integral side-looking fiber probe. The optical assembly is encapsulated in a hollow torque wire that translates motion from a drive motor located outside the patient's body. The C7XR system can volumetrically image a 5-cm vessel segment in approximately 3 seconds. High-speed data acquisition is a key feature of the C7XR system because it enables pull-back image acquisition during a low-volume injection of contrast medium or saline through the guiding catheter.[7] The current instructions for use of the C7XR system recommend an injection of a 14-mL bolus of contrast at a rate of 4 mL/second.

Three more FD-OCT systems are in advanced phases of development and testing. The Massachusetts General Hospital (MGH) optical frequency domain imaging (OFDI) system, developed by Bouma and Tearney's academic research group at the Wellman Center for Photomedicine, is the first of the second-generation intracoronary OCT systems to be used in vivo.[8] The light source of the MGH OFDI system is a high-speed wavelength swept laser that uses a polygon-mirror or grating filter to tune over a broad bandwidth of 120 nm, centered at 1320 nm. The high speed of this laser enables cross-sectional imaging at 100 frames per second with 512 A-lines per image. The axial resolution of the MGH OFDI system is 7 μm and the ranging depth is 4.6 mm in tissue (refractive index $n = 1.4$). MGH also fabricates its own OFDI catheters that use an asymmetric ball lens at the tip that is custom designed to correct for aberrations in the catheter sheath. The MGH OFDI system and catheter produce very-high-resolution images; the demonstration of two-dimensional and three-dimensional images obtained from this system paved the way for the development of current commercial FD-OCT systems that are now being adopted in interventional cardiology. The Terumo OFDI system uses a 1.3-μm scanning laser as a light source. The imaging range is 5 mm with an axial resolution of less than 20 μm in the water. The OFDI catheter (2.4F crossing profile) is a short monorail design for a 0.014-inch guidewire and contains the imaging core rotating within a sheath. The imaging core rotates at a speed of 9600 revolutions per minute (rpm) allowing imaging at 160 frames per second. Up to 150 mm pull-back in length is supported at the maximum pull-back speed of 40 mm per second.

The Volcano FD-OCT system and catheter were still under development at the time of this writing and final specifications were unavailable. Volcano (Rancho Cordova, CA) has demonstrated a prototype catheter with reduced profile and faster frame rate and pull-back compared with those currently available. The core technology that Volcano anticipates using enables the higher speeds and is based on a non-laser source of photons. This OCT system has been tested at breakthrough speeds of 200 kHz which will translate into ultra-fast imaging and significantly fast pull-backs.

IMAGE ACQUISITION

With TD-OCT, an occlusive technique is normally adopted to clear blood from the artery. An occlusion balloon (Helios Goodman, Advantec Vascular, Sunnyvale, CA) compatible with 6F guiding catheters (0.071-inch inner diameter) is advanced distal to the segment to be imaged over a conventional angioplasty guidewire. The guidewire is then replaced by the 0.019-inch OCT ImageWire (LightLab Imaging, Westford, MA). The occlusion balloon is repositioned proximal to the segment and inflated at low pressure (0.4–0.7 atmosphere [atm]), while flushing low volume (rate of 0.5–1.0 mL/second) of saline or Ringer's lactate solution through the distal lumen of the balloon. Images are acquired with an automated pull-back at a rate of 1 to 3 mm per second, generating 15 frames per second. Yamaguchi et al evaluated the safety and feasibility of OCT in 76 patients.[9] Procedural success rates were 97%, and no significant adverse events, including vessel dissection or fatal arrhythmia, were observed. Recently, a nonocclusive technique for OCT image acquisition has been developed as an alternative to the balloon-occlusion technique.[10] This nonocclusive technique, based on manual or injector infusion of contrast media or Dextran 40 and Ringer's lactate solution (Low Molecular Dextran L Injection®, Otsuka Pharmaceutical Factory, Tokushima, Japan) through the guiding catheter, simplifies the complex balloon-occlusion technique. Barlis et al reported data on 468 patients across six European medical centers, with occlusive and nonocclusive flushing techniques.[11] Transient chest pain and QRS widening or ST segment depression or elevation were observed in 48% and 46%, respectively. Major complications during OCT imaging included ventricular fibrillation (1.1%) caused by balloon occlusion, deep guiding catheter insertion, air embolism (0.6%), and vessel dissection (0.2%), or all. There was no major adverse cardiac event (MACE) within the 24 hours after OCT examination.

The imaging catheters of FD-OCT, which are designed for rapid-exchange delivery, have a 2.4F to 2.8F crossing profile and can be delivered over a 0.014-inch guidewire through a 6F or larger guiding catheter. Injecting saline, angiographic contrast media, or a mixture of contrast and saline through the guiding catheter (4–6 mL/second, 2–3 seconds) can achieve effective clearing of blood for FD-OCT imaging.[7] Because of its very high speed of pull-back, FD-OCT has the ability to scan longer segments of artery in a few seconds, without the need to occlude the vessel, showing minimal ischemic electrocardiogram (ECG) changes and no major arrhythmias during image acquisition.[12]

ARTIFACTS

Some artifacts are common in both OCT and IVUS, and others are unique to OCT imaging systems.[6] Residual blood attenuates the OCT signal. Nonuniform rotational distortion results in focal image loss or shape distortion. Sew-up artifact is the result of rapid artery or imaging wire movement in one frame's image formation, leading to single point misalignment of the lumen border. Saturation artifact occurs when light reflected from a highly specular surface such as stent struts produces signals with amplitudes that exceed the dynamic range of the data acquisition system. Fold-over artifact is more specific to the new generation of FD-OCT. It is the consequence of the "phase wrapping" or "alias" along the Fourier transformation when structure signals are reflected from outside the system's field of view. Bubble artifact occurs when small air bubbles are formed in the sheath of the ImageWire™ and it can attenuate the signal along a region of the vessel wall. Eccentricity of the ImageWire in the vessel lumen may result in the "sunflower effect" or the "merry-go-round artifact." Eccentric wire position can distort the image at the far site from ImageWire, leading to longer distance between A-lines and consequently decreasing the lateral resolution.

IMAGE INTERPRETATION

The high resolution of OCT allows us to identify the boundary of the intima and the media within the coronary arterial wall, which could not be distinguished by IVUS. In the OCT image, the intima is observed as a signal-rich layer nearest the lumen, and the media is visualized as a signal-poor middle layer (Table 60-2). The OCT measurement of intimal thickness is well correlated to histologic examination.[13] OCT has an ability to evaluate subtle intimal thickening in vivo, which is the early phase of coronary atherosclerosis. Several histologic examinations demonstrated that OCT is highly sensitive and specific for plaque characterization (Fig. 60-3 to 60-5).[14] Yabushita et al developed objective OCT image criteria for differentiating distinct components of atherosclerotic tissue.[15] In their histology-controlled OCT study with 357 autopsy segments from 90 cadavers, fibrous plaques were characterized by homogeneous signal-rich regions, fibrocalcific plaques by signal-poor regions with sharp borders, and lipid-rich plaques by signal-poor regions with diffuse borders (see Table 60-2). Validation tests revealed significant intra- and interobserver reliability ($\kappa = 0.83$–0.84) as well as excellent sensitivity and specificity—71% to 79% and 97% to 98% for fibrous plaques, 95% to 96% and 97% for fibrocalcific plaques, and 90% to 94%, and 90% to 92% for lipid-rich plaques, respectively. These definitions have formed the basis of plaque composition interpretation. Using these definitions, Kawasaki et al reported that OCT has a best potential for tissue characterization of coronary plaques compared with integrated backscatter IVUS and conventional IVUS (fibrous tissue: sensitivity—98% vs. 94% vs. 93%, specificity—94% vs. 84% vs. 61%; calcification: sensitivity—100% vs. 100% vs. 100%, specificity—100% vs. 99% vs. 99%; lipid pool: sensitivity—95% vs. 84% vs. 67%, specificity—98% vs. 97% vs. 95%, respectively).[16] OCT characteristics of coronary thrombi were studied by Kume et al in 108 coronary arterial segments at postmortem examination.[17] White thrombi were identified as signal-rich, low-backscattering protrusions in the OCT image, and red thrombi were identified as high-backscattering protrusions inside the lumen of the artery, with signal-free shadow (see Table 60-2)(Fig. 60-6 to 60-8). Using a measurement of the OCT signal attenuation within the thrombus, the authors demonstrated that a cut-off value of 250 μm in the half width of signal attenuation can differentiate white thrombi from red thrombi with a high sensitivity (90%) and specificity (88%). A further unique aspect of OCT is its ability to visualize the macrophages. Tearney et al proposed the potential of OCT to assess macrophage distribution within fibrous caps.[18] There was a high degree of positive correlation between OCT and histologic measurements of fibrous cap macrophage density ($r < 0.84$, $P < 0.0001$). A range of OCT signal standard deviation thresholds (6.15%–6.35%) yielded 100% sensitivity and specificity for identifying caps containing greater than 10% CD68 staining.

Current Clinical Applications

ASSESSMENT OF CORONARY ATHEROSCLEROSIS

Rupture of vulnerable plaque (VP) is responsible for acute coronary events. Morphologic features of VP include a large lipid core, a thin cap fibroatheroma (TCFA, fibrous cap thickness <65 μm), and an accumulation of macrophages localized in the fibrous cap. Since OCT has a near-histologic grade resolution, many in vitro and in vivo studies have been done to validate the capability of OCT to visualize these VP features (Fig. 60-9).[19,20] Kubo et al used OCT, IVUS, and angioscopy in patients with acute myocardial infarction (AMI) to assess the ability of each imaging method to detect the specific characteristics of vulnerable plaque.[21] OCT was superior in detecting plaque rupture (73% vs. 40% vs. 43%, $P = 0.021$), erosion (23% vs. 0% vs. 3%, $P = 0.003$), and thrombus (100% vs. 33% vs. 100%, $P < 0.001$) compared with IVUS and angioscopy. Intra- and interobserver variability of OCT yielded acceptable concordance for these characteristics ($\kappa = 0.61$–0.83). OCT might be the best tool available to detect

TABLE 60-2	Optical Coherence Tomography Image Characteristics
Histology	**OCT**
Intima	Signal-rich layer near lumen
Media	Signal-poor layer in middle of artery wall
Adventitia	Signal-rich outer layer of artery wall
Fibrotic tissue	Homogenous, high reflectivity, low attenuation
Calcification	Sharp edges, low reflectivity, low attenuation
Lipid	Diffuse edges, high reflectivity, high attenuation
Red thrombus	Medium reflectivity, high attenuation
White thrombus	Medium reflectivity, low attenuation

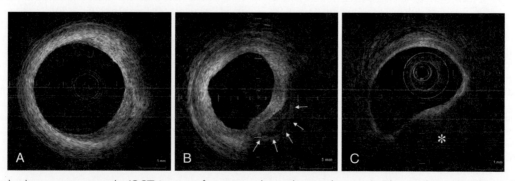

Figure 60-3 Optical coherence tomography (OCT) images of coronary atherosclerotic plaques. **A,** Fibrous plaque. **B,** Fibro-calcific plaque (calcify: arrows). **C,** Lipidic plaque (*).

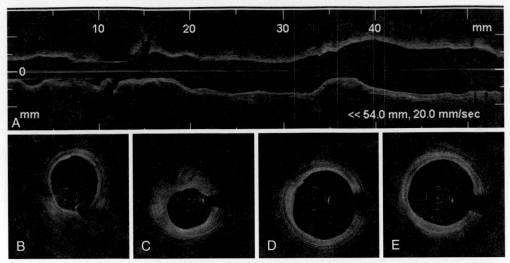

Figure 60-4 Frequency-domain optical coherence tomography (FD-OCT) scan of coronary artery with fibrous plaque. **A,** Longitudinal view. **B and E,** Normal coronary artery. OCT clearly demonstrates the appearance of a normal three-layered vessel wall. **C,** Eccentric fibrous plaque was imaged as a signal-rich region with diffuse border from the 9 o'clock to the 3 o'clock position. **D,** OCT shows fibrous intimal thickening at the 8 o'clock to the 11 o'clock position.

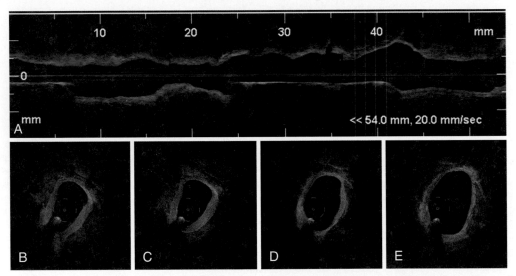

Figure 60-5 Frequency-domain optical coherence tomography (FD-OCT) scan of coronary artery with calcified plaque. Calcified plaque was imaged as a signal-poor region with sharp border extending to 320 to 360 degrees of the vessel circumference.

TCFAs.[22,23] Kume et al examined the reliability of OCT for measuring fibrous cap thickness.[24] In the examination of 35 lipid-rich plaques from 38 human cadavers, there was significant correlation in fibrous cap thickness between OCT and histologic examination ($r = 0.90$, $P < 0.001$). In the clinical setting, Sawada et al compared the feasibility for detecting TCFA between OCT and Virtual Histology IVUS (VH-IVUS).[25] Although the positive ratio of VH-IVUS for detecting TCFA was 45.9%, that of OCT was 77.8%. Jang et al analyzed OCT images from 57 patients who presented with stable angina pectoris (SAP), acute coronary syndrome (ACS), or AMI.[26] The AMI group was more likely than the ACS group (which was more likely than the SAP group) to have a thinner cap, more lipid, and a higher percentage of TCFA (72% vs. 50% vs. 20%, respectively, $P = 0.012$). Using OCT, Tanaka et al investigated the relationship between the culprit lesion morphology and the patient's activity at the onset of ACS.[20] TCFA was a lesion predisposed to rupture in both rest-onset and exertion-triggered ACS, and some plaque rupture occurred in fibrous caps greater than 65 μm thick, depending on exertion levels. Fujii et al performed a prospective

OCT analysis of all three major coronary arteries to evaluate the incidence and predictors of TCFAs in patients with AMI and SAP.[27] Multiple TCFAs were observed more frequently in patients with AMI than in SAP patients (69% vs. 10%, $P < 0.001$). In the entire cohort, multivariate analysis revealed that the only independent predictor of TCFA was AMI (odds ratio [OR] 4.12; 95% confidence interval [CI] 2.35–9.87, $P = 0.02$,). A recent OCT study conducted by Takarada et al[28] demonstrated that besides its reliability as a tool to measure fibrous cap thickness in vivo, lipid-lowering therapy with statin for 9 months follow-up significantly increased fibrous cap thickness in patients with hyperlipidemia (151 ± 110 to 280 ± 120 μm, $P < 0.01$). As therapies to prevent or make regression of atherosclerosis are developed, OCT can help assess treatment efficacy.

STENT ASSESSMENT

OCT can contribute to various stages of stent assessment, optimization of stent deployment techniques, quantification of the degree of stent

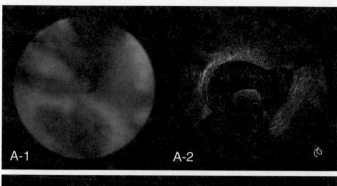

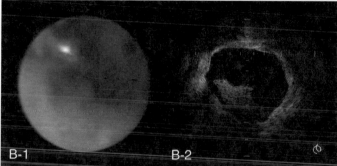

Figure 60-6 Red and white thrombus in the angioscopic images and the corresponding optical coherence tomography (OCT) images. Red thrombus identified by coronary angioscopy (A-1) was visualized as high-backscattering protrusions with signal-free shadowing in the OCT image (A-2). White thrombus (B-1) was characterized as signal-rich, low-backscattering projections in the OCT image (B-2).

coverage, and evaluation of the mechanisms of delayed healing and thrombus formation.[29] OCT provides complete visualization of the stent luminal surface in multiple cross-sections and allows accurate measurements at each strut level; it has similar ability to detect intraluminal thrombus (Fig. 60-10).[17,30] Malapposition, coverage, and abnormal intraluminal tissue formation can significantly vary among different stent segments as well as between struts in the same cross-section, an old pathologic notion recently highlighted in-vivo by OCT imaging obtained following drug-eluting stent (DES) deployment

(Fig. 60-11).[31] Vascular response to stent implantation cannot be fully appreciated by measuring only a few cross-sections of the stented segment. A more detailed analysis at the strut level is required, especially after DES implantation.[32] OCT provides clear high-resolution images of stent struts to perform a per-strut level analysis of apposition and coverage.

Optical Coherence Tomography Principles for Stent Analysis

Metallic stent struts are strong reflectors of light and appear as bright points along the circumference of the vessel. As light cannot penetrate the metallic strut, a nonsignal region (shadow) is generated behind the superficial strut. This can result in an excessive signal (blooming) at the strut surface and occasionally in saturation artifacts.[6] Therefore, light reflection from the luminal surface of the metal does not provide a direct measurement of strut thickness. Since the luminal surface of the strut is expected to be found in the middle of the blooming, half of the blooming value should be used as the standard for calculation. When a strut level analysis is performed, the center of the luminal surface of the strut blooming is determined for each strut, and its distance to the lumen contour of the vessel wall is automatically calculated. Magnification of stent struts is recommended to better assess strut apposition and tissue coverage.

Qualitative Stent Assessment

All cross-sectional images (frames) are initially screened for quality assessment and should be excluded from analysis if any portion of the image is out of the screen, a side branch occupies greater than 45 degrees of the cross-section, or the image has poor quality caused by residual blood, sew-up artifact, or reverberation.[33] Qualitative imaging assessment is normally performed in every frame to detect the presence of abnormal intraluminal tissue (AIT), defined as any irregular mass protruding beyond the stent strut into the lumen and further classified as related to uncovered or malapposed struts. Although OCT can accurately identify acute thrombus immediately after stent implantation, the distinction between fibrin clot and neointimal hyperplasia (NIH) is not always possible.[17,34] Thus, a more descriptive term of AIT to delineate intraluminal protruding masses can be adopted for qualitative assessment. AIT can be further classified into four categories according to its relationship with strut coverage, apposition, presence of underlining NIH, and location in a severely stenotic segment (Fig. 60-12). To avoid misclassification of small image artifacts, only AIT greater than 0.25 mm diameter should be included.

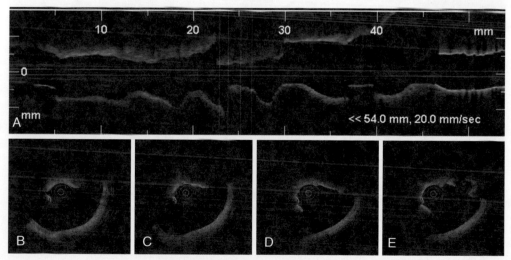

Figure 60-7 Frequency domain optical coherence tomography (FD-OCT) scan of coronary artery with red thrombus. Red thrombi were imaged as high-backscattering mass protruding into the vessel lumen of the artery with signal-free shadowing in the infarct-related lesion.

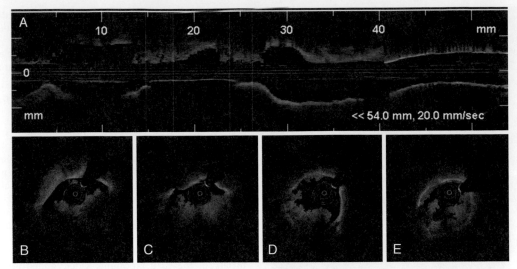

Figure 60-8 Frequency-domain optical coherence tomography (FD-OCT) scan of coronary artery with white thrombus. White thrombi were imaged as signal-rich, low-backscattering protrusions in the infarct-related lesion.

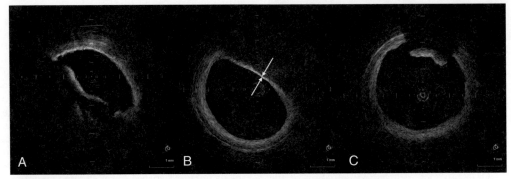

Figure 60-9 Optical coherence tomography (OCT) images of vulnerable plaques. **A,** Plaque rupture. **B,** Thin cap fibroatheroma (TCFA; fibrous-cap thickness = 60 μm: *arrows*). **C,** Intracoronary thrombus.

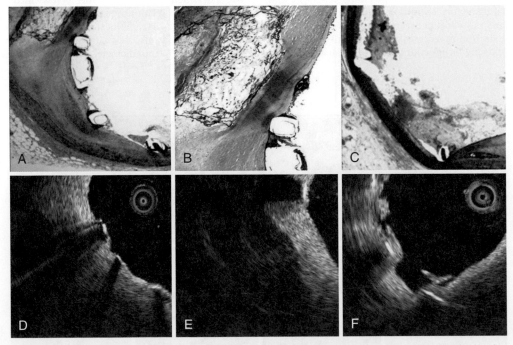

Figure 60-10 Correspondent postmortem pathology (*A to C*) and OCT cross-sections (*D to F*) in a patient who died 5 days after coronary stent implantation. High level of accuracy of optical coherence tomography (OCT) compared with pathology can be observed in: detection of uncovered struts (*A* versus *D*); identification of the cap thickness of a calcified plaque underlying stent struts (*B* versus *E*); peri-struts thrombus deposition (*C* versus *F*).

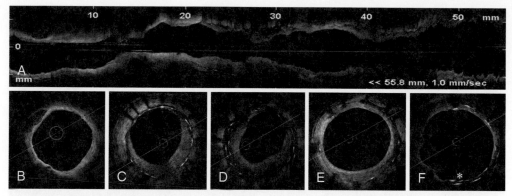

Figure 60-11   Intracoronary time-domain optical coherence tomography (TD-OCT) 6 months after multiple drug-eluting stent (DES) implantation with overlap. **A,** Longitudinal view of 5.5 cm of coronary artery with heterogeneity between segments in the amount of neointima and optical signal density. **B to F,** Multiple OCT cross-sections in different segments. **C and D,** Uneven and dark coverage in the same sections. **D,** overlapping struts. **E,** Homogeneous and bright tissue coverage. **F,** Combination of uncovered struts (6 o'clock) with signal attenuation (*).

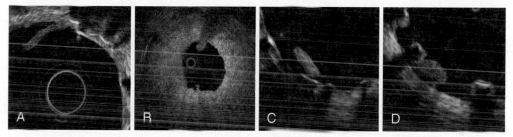

Figure 60-12   Abnormal intraluminal tissues (AIT) detected in coronary stents. AIT is classified into four categories. **A,** Intimal flap. **B,** Related to severely stenotic segment. **C,** Related to uncovered strut. **D,** Related to malapposed struts.

Quantitative Stent Assessment

Strut Apposition. To accurately evaluate stent apposition, the stent surface should be measured from the center of the stent reflection.[35] Two forms of strut apposition exist: (1) *protruding*, where the strut boundary is located above the level of the luminal surface; and (2) *embedded*, where the strut boundary is below the level of the luminal surface. *Incomplete stent apposition (ISA)*, synonymous with malapposition, is defined as separation of the strut from the lumen border by a distance greater than the width of the stent strut according to each stent specification plus a compensation factor of 20 μm to correct for strut blooming.[33] For DESs, strut malapposition is considered when the measured distance is greater than the sum of strut thickness plus the thickness of the abluminal polymer (Fig. 60-13). The cut-off value used to assess DES malapposition is somewhat arbitrary, given the possibility of polymer disruption during stent implantation. ISA can be addressed at a cross-section level and expressed as the number or length of consecutive cross-sections with ISA, or area or volume measurements, or expressed at the strut level as the maximum distance of ISA at each strut. Acute malapposition can be readily diagnosed by OCT immediately after stent deployment, whereas the detection of late malapposition requires the comparison of post intervention and follow-up images (Fig. 60-14).[33] Kubo et al showed that dissection (40 vs. 16%), tissue protrusion (58 vs. 20%), and ISA (47 vs. 18%) following stent deployment were observed more often by OCT compared with IVUS (Fig. 60-15).[36] By using serial OCT, Ozaki et al recently demonstrated that ISA observed at follow-up in sirolimus-eluting stents (SESs) is more frequently caused by acute ISA without neointimal growth, rather than by acquired ISA caused by vascular remodeling.[37] As a consequence, persistent ISA without strut coverage may be a substrate for DES late stent thrombosis (LST). Measurements for strut apposition and strut coverage are highly reproducible at the core laboratory.[4]

Strut Coverage. Histopathology results obtained from autopsy cases highlight delayed healing and incomplete endothelial coverage as predictors of LST after DES implantation. This pathologic phenomenon has not been reported in patients with bare metal stents (BMSs). Unlike BMSs, which develop circumferential coverage with an average thickness of 500 μm or more, easily measured by IVUS and angiography, the smaller amount of neointimal growth after DES implantation is largely under the limit of resolution of these imaging techniques (Fig. 60-16).[38] Preclinical studies demonstrated a close degree of correlation for coverage in DESs when OCT is compared with light and SEM.[2,30] All the struts that were completely covered by FD-OCT were also fully covered by SEM. Quantitative strut level analysis of coverage can be performed in vivo by OCT at different intervals along the stented segment, ranging approximately from 0.33 mm (every five frames) up to 1 mm intervals. Large intervals can produce a higher variability between consecutive sections.[39] Continuous assessment of every frame is not recommended because cardiac dynamics introduces forward and backward longitudinal displacement of the image wire, a phenomenon that can cause the "persistence" of the previous frame image in the current frame. Struts are normally classified on the basis of the coverage value of strut-intimal thickness (SIT): Struts covered by tissue have positive SIT values, and uncovered or malapposed struts have negative SIT values. Four types exist (Fig. 60-17): (1) struts covered by tissue where the strut boundary is below the luminal surface, defined as *embedded covered struts;* (2) those covered by tissue where the boundary is above the lumen, defined as *protruding covered struts;* (3) those not covered by tissue but abutting the vessel wall, classified as *uncovered apposed struts;* and (4) those not covered by tissue and not abutting the vessel wall, classified as *uncovered and malapposed struts.* The number of struts without coverage is counted for each frame analyzed, and the total number of frames with uncovered struts is recorded. The stent length lacking neointimal coverage is counted as

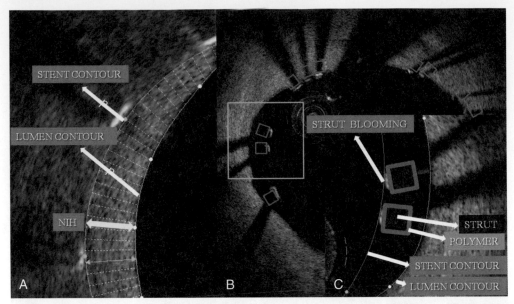

Figure 60-13   Automated contour detection algorithm for calculation of neointimal thickness and quantification of strut malapposition. **A,** Contour traces for measurements of lumen, stent and neointimal (stent-lumen) areas. **B and C,** Cross-section magnification and algorithm for calculation of strut malapposition; struts located from 7 to 9 o'clock are malapposed. Final malapposition distance (*red arrow*) obtained by considering strut thickness + polymer + half of the blooming (*arrow*).

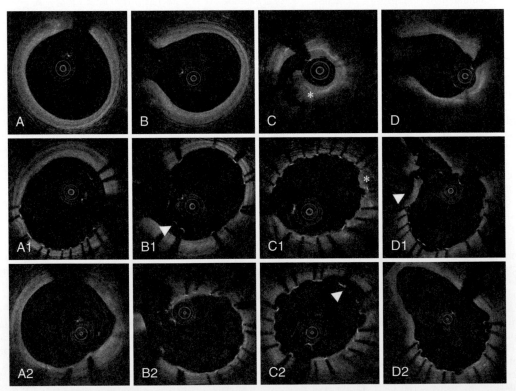

Figure 60-14   Frequency-domain optical coherence tomography (FD-OCT) assessment of the culprit lesion in acute myocardial infarction at pre-procedure (*A to D*), post-stent implantation (*A1 to D1*) and 6 months follow-up (*A2 to D2*). **A,** Regular contour and homogeneous optical characteristics of the distal reference segment; exit of the stent with small degree of strut malapposition (3 and 5 o'clock) (*A1*), resolved in follow-up (*A2*). **B,** Side branch (9 o'clock) patent after stent implantation (*B1*), with evidence of major strut malapposition (*arrowhead*), sealed in follow-up (*B2*). **C,** Infarct-related lesion with a large amount of white thrombus and plaque occluding the vessel (*); plaque protrusion through the stent struts (3 o'clock, *) (*C1*); late acquired stent malapposition (12 o'clock and 3 o'clock, arrowhead) caused by thrombus and plaque dissolution (*C2*). **D,** Fibro-fatty plaque proximally to the culprit lesion (9 o'clock and 11 o'clock) with residual post stent dissection (*D1, arrowhead*) normalized in follow-up (*D2*).

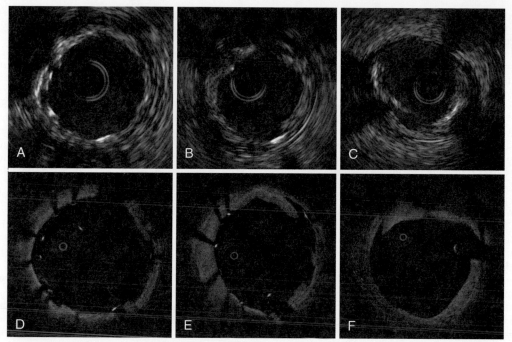

Figure 60-15 Intravascular ultrasound (IVUS) (*A to C*) and optical coherence tomography (OCT) correspondent cross-sections (*D to F*) obtained immediately after stent implantation; superiority of OCT in detecting: strut malapposition (*A versus D*), residual dissection inside (*B versus E*) and outside the stent (*C versus F*).

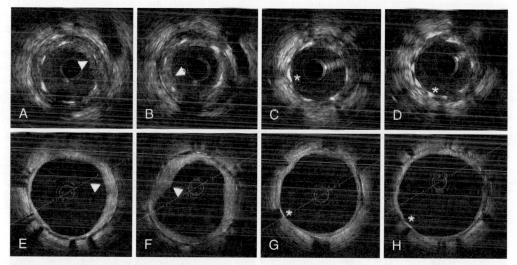

Figure 60-16 Intravascular ultrasound (IVUS) (*A to D*) and optical coherence tomography (OCT) (*E to H*) correspondent cross-sections obtained at the 6-month follow-up after stent implantation. Accuracy in detecting coverage in presence of different degree of neointima: moderate degree of neointima (*A, B versus E, F*) (*arrowheads*); lower degrees of neointima (*C, D versus G, H*) (***).

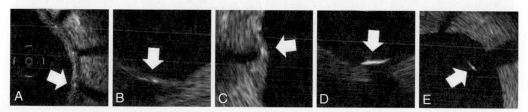

Figure 60-17 Stent strut coverage classification by optical coherence tomography (OCT). **A and B,** Covered embedded struts. **C,** Protruding covered strut. **D,** Protruding uncovered strut. **E,** Uncovered and malapposed strut. *(Reproduced with permission from Guagliumi G, Sirbu V: Optical coherence tomography: High resolution intravascular imaging to evaluate vascular healing after coronary stenting, Catheter Cardiovasc Interv 72:237–247, 2008.)*

maximum length (in consecutive frames) and total length (in cumulative frames). The time course of tissue coverage after stent implantation is different according to stent type. In BMSs, normal neointima was observed in all cross-sections 6 months after stent implantation. The proliferating tissue was recognized as a homogeneous OCT signal. In contrast, in a later phase, during an extended period (≥5 years), neointima transformed into various OCT signal patterns with intimal disruption, thrombus deposition, atherosclerotic progression, and neovascularization.[40] Conversely, OCT assessment of DESs at different time points demonstrated a significant rate of uncovered stent struts at early and late follow-up, ranging from 15% at 3 months to 5% at 2 years, and a high degree of heterogeneity. However, different DESs have completely different rates of coverage and uneven neointima responses, perhaps depending on the polymer characteristics and specific drug kinetics.[31] Even in patients with AMI, vascular responses can vary across DES types. While paclitaxel-eluting stents (PESs) implanted in ST elevated MI (STEMI) resulted in a significantly higher rate of uncovered and malapposed struts compared with BMSs, as detected by OCT at 13 months, similar strut coverage and vessel response were observed at 6 months follow-up in zotarolimus-eluting stents (ZESs) compared with identical BMSs.[33,41] Despite the fact that neointimal coverage in DESs may progress over time, previous long-term OCT studies have shown that uncovered stent struts decreased but did not disappear from 6 to 12 months.[42] The optimal time for assessing DES coverage remains to be defined. Early assessment of strut coverage can be faced with more difficult separation between fibrin and neointima tissues. Conversely, longer time intervals (6–13 months) might be more useful for measuring the advanced rate of strut coverage and the accelerated progression of underlying atherosclerotic lesions.[43] Strut coverage as assessed by OCT must be interpreted with caution, as OCT has not been established to detect the composition of the material covering stent struts (whether cellular or not cellular in nature), and, of course, it cannot determine endothelial functionality. Strut coverage observed by OCT does not exclude the possibility of LST (Fig. 60-18). No in vivo study has systematically determined DES coverage in patients with LST. Recently, optical density of stent strut coverage, measured with novel OFDI, revealed that fibrin-covered struts had lower signal density compared with neointimal tissue.[2] Densitometric analysis may be a promising method for the characterization of stent tissue coverage. The relationship between all these OCT morphometric findings and subsequent clinical events has to be determined in a larger number of stents or patients and with additional years of clinical follow-up.[41]

Bioabsorbable Stents and Polymers. Currently, stents coated with biodegradable polymer and fully absorbable stents are in advanced phase of development. New-generation DESs with biodegradable, only abluminal polymer, were recently tested for safety and effectiveness in prospective OCT studies, compared with DESs with permanent polymer.[44,45] Because of complete strut absorption, fully biodegradable stents can provide short-term vessel scaffolding of the coronary lesions without a permanent implantation, restoring normal vasomotion tone. Serial OCT data obtained after everolimus-eluting bioabsorbable stent implantation (Abbot Vascular, Santa Clara, CA) at up to 2 years of follow-up, revealed the rate of disappearance of struts over time and documented different degrees of bioabsorption of polymeric struts.[46] In summary, OCT is able to provide unique morphometric details across all stent types (metallic, permanent polymeric DESs, bioabsorbable DESs), setting the stage for a new possible standard of assessment in the early phase of development and clinical testing.[47]

Promising Clinical Applications in Stented Coronary Lesions. The use of OCT in PCI and stented patients has been demonstrated to be safe.[9,11] However, the benefit of OCT guidance in complex coronary interventions is not yet documented. At least three major clinical settings that hold the highest risk for failure with PCI can benefit from the use of OCT: (1) late and very late stent thrombosis (LST), (2) recurrence of re-stenosis in DES, and (3) complex bifurcation requiring advanced operative techniques.[48–50] In LST, OCT may detect and measure the rate and distribution of uncovered and malapposed struts, the heterogeneity of in-stent vascular response (Fig. 60-19), and eventually the formation of de novo atherosclerotic lesions within the stented segment (Fig. 60-20). In addition, OCT permits quantification of the completeness of thrombus removal after mechanical thrombus aspiration or the use of lytic agents.

Finally, OCT makes it possible to monitor whether strut coverage at sites of previously uncovered struts begins to grow or continues to persist even after re-treatment by balloon dilation or stent-in-stent implantation for LST. OCT, with small diameter hydrophilic-coated catheters, may easily reach and cross difficult lesions, including severe in-stent re-stenosis. Various OCT patterns of in-stent re-stenotic lesions after DES implantation have been observed, suggesting possible

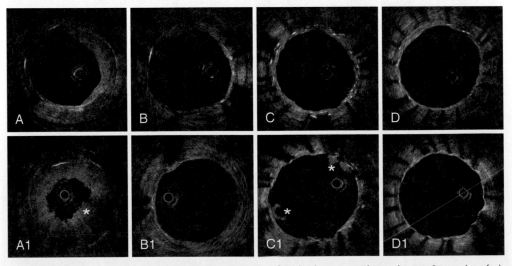

Figure 60-18 Paired optical coherence tomography (OCT) cross-sections of multiple stent with overlap, at 3 months of elective follow-up in an asymptomatic patient, and greater than 1 year later immediately after thrombus aspiration during very late stent thrombosis (VLST), 17 months after stent implantation. At 3 months, all struts were covered (*A* to *D*); irregular contour and inhomogeneous optical signal characteristics were observed at different cross-sections (*A* and *C*); during VLST, evidence of heterogeneous tissue responses at different cross-sections, with thrombus (*) deposition only at site levels of early irregular coverage (*A1* and *C1*).

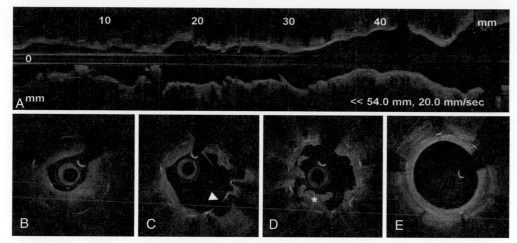

Figure 60-19 Frequency-domain optical coherence tomography (FD-OCT) scan during very late stent thrombosis (VLST), 36 months after drug-eluting stent (DES) implantation. **A,** longitudinal view. **B,** Severe neointimal proliferation in the distal segment. **C,** Largely uncovered and malapposed stent struts with residual thrombus over-imposed (*arrowhead*). **D,** White thrombus attached to the stent struts and protruding into the lumen (*). **E,** Uniform smooth and optimal coverage in the proximal stent segment.

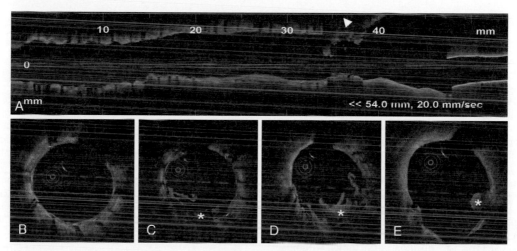

Figure 60-20 Frequency-domain optical coherence tomography (FD-OCT) during very late stent thrombosis (VLST) 2 years after drug-eluting stent (DES) implantation. Progression of atherosclerotic pathology with rupture of thin cap fibroatheroma (TCFA) at proximal stent border. **A,** Longitudinal view with evidence of thrombus formation at the stent entrance (*arrowhead*). **B,** Fully regular coverage inside the stent. **C and D,** Thrombus fragments attached to stent struts (*) at the entrance. **E,** ruptured TCFA with cavity and thrombus (*) immediately before the stent.

different tissue components.[49] In this context, OCT can be useful in assessing the immediate results of different mechanical interventions, pharmacologic interventions, or both. Bifurcation lesions and related stent procedures have been investigated with OCT, mainly to improve the accuracy of angiography in detecting complex anatomy at the branching points. OCT can provide unique data on the localization of plaque at a bifurcation lesion and a detailed assessment of apposition and coverage of new dedicated stents for bifurcation disease (Fig. 60-21). OCT has demonstrated the proximal rim of the side branch ostium as a region more likely to contain thin fibrous cap plaques as well as a variable pattern of strut coverage across DES technology.[51,52]

Use of Optical Coherence Tomography in Noncoronary Arteries

The ability of OCT to characterize the nature of atherosclerotic plaque can be expanded to assess carotid as well as peripheral vasculature. OCT is being assessed for its potential use in the identification of carotid stenosis and in distinguishing between stable and unstable atherosclerotic plaques.[53] Meissner et al studied the potential role of OCT in ex vivo peripheral vascular diseases, showing morphometric

findings comparable with those reported for coronary arteries.[54] Although evidences of safety and efficacy for in vivo application of OCT for carotid and peripheral arteries are lacking, this might represent a promising use of OCT for future vascular medicine.

Quantitative Measurements. Cross-sectional diameter and area measurements of coronary vessels provide interventional cardiologists with useful guidance for lesion assessment, stent sizing, and placement. Furthermore, optimization of the stent area is of critical importance for the prevention of in-stent re-stenosis. Frequency of OCT light is 10 million times faster than that of IVUS, with a much clearer delineation of intraluminal border, which allows the precise automated determination of lumen contour with fewer errors, an important feature for rapid intra-procedural image analysis. When OCT and IVUS measurements were carried out postmortem in perfusion-fixed samples, IVUS and OCT imaging modalities significantly overestimated the true lumen and stent dimensions compared with pathology.[55] However, histology measurements are not directly analogous to measurement in life and are subject to variable technical preparation and artifacts in the production of a histologic section.[56] The process of dehydration,

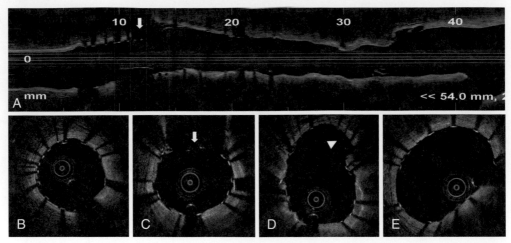

Figure 60-21 Use of frequency-domain optical coherence tomography (FD-OCT) in bifurcation lesion (Medina 1:1:1) treated with complex interventional techniques (drug-eluting stent [DES] implanted in the main vessel and dedicated stent for bifurcation implanted in the side branch). FD-OCT scan obtained after kissing balloon dilation. **A,** Longitudinal view. **B,** DES in the main vessel distally to the bifurcation. Apposition of all stent struts to the vessel wall. **C,** Level of bifurcation with largely patent side branch (*arrow*). **D,** presence of struts in the main and side branches (dedicated stent, *arrowhead*). **E,** Proximal DES segment: This product is not available for commercial use in the United States.

paraffin embedding, sectioning, and staining results in a reduction of the circumference by 19% ± 5% and wall thickness reduction by 18% ± 2%. Furthermore, backscattering of OCT signals caused by fixation of cross-link collagen may significantly enhance the delineation between lumen and vessel wall, compared with in vivo lumen measurements, with an artificial increase of reflectivity. The wide gap in lumen dimensions observed between OCT and histology in non stented coronary segments is less clear when the arteries are treated with metallic stents, demonstrating approximately 6% greater stent area and 10% greater lumen area as assessed by OCT across all stent types.[30] In measurements of lumen diameter and lumen area, there is a clear correlation between OCT and IVUS.[55] However, OCT systematically underestimates the lumen dimensions compared with IVUS.[9] Several factors may explain this difference, including the inadequate spatial resolution of IVUS, the stretch of small arteries by the IVUS catheter (Dotter effect), eccentric OCT wire position in the lumen with image border distortion, and reduction of intracoronary perfusion pressure during occlusive OCT image acquisition. A dedicated, semi-automated contour detection system is used for measurements. An important advantage of FD-OCT imaging is that it can precisely delineate three-dimensional contours of long segments of coronary arteries in a few seconds. A novel contour-finding algorithm that traces the lumen boundaries of OCT images automatically was recently developed. This software shows the cross-sectional areas calculated automatically for all frames in a pull-back sequence as a graph superimposed on the longitudinal (L)–mode image. OCT enables quick and precise comparison of minimal lumen areas (MLAs) with the reference areas over the entire length of the vessel scanned. A clear correlation ($r = 0.99$) between manual and quantitative, fully automated, three-dimensional lumen contour detection methods was recently demonstrated.[57]

Plaque Measurements. The following measures are normally performed:

- *Fibrous cap thickness in nonruptured plaque:* defined as the minimum distance from the coronary artery lumen to inner border of lipid pool, which is characterized by signal-poor region in OCT image.
- *TCFA:* defined as a plaque with a fibrous cap measuring less than 65 μm at the thinnest part. In the ruptured plaque, residual fibrous cap is identified as a flap between the lumen of coronary artery and the cavity of plaque, and its thickness is measured at the thinnest part.

- *Lipid core:* is semi-quantified as the number of involved quadrants on the cross-sectional OCT image. When lipid is present in two or more quadrants in any of the images within a plaque, it is considered a lipid-rich plaque.
- *Macrophage content:* to calculate macrophage content, the OCT data within a defined region of interest (ROI) are preprocessed using median filtering to remove background noise and reduce speckle. Within the ROI, the OCT signal is characterized by use of the normalized standard deviation (NSD): $NSD = \delta / (S_{max} - S_{min})$, where δ is the standard deviation of the OCT signal, S_{max} is the maximum OCT image value, and S_{min} is the minimum OCT image value. It has been demonstrated that the macrophage density, as determined by immunohistochemistry, correlated with the base 10 logarithm OCT NSD ($r = 0.47$, $P < 0.05$) and with the linear OCT NSD ($r = 0.84$, $P < 0.0001$).[1]

Stent Measurements. Lumen, stent, and NIH areas and volumes are usually determined at short intervals (0.6 mm). The following measurements at cross-sectional level are commonly reported with OCT in stented coronary arteries:

- *Stent MLA:* the area bounded by the stent border.
- *Minimum stent diameter:* the shortest diameter through the center of mass of the stent.
- *Stent expansion:* the minimum stent cross-sectional area (CSA) compared with the reference area, which can be the proximal, distal, largest, or average reference area.
- *Stent eccentricity:* (maximum stent diameter—minimum stent diameter) ÷ the maximum stent diameter.
- *NIH area:* the area bounded by the stent—the area bounded by the neointima.
- *Percent stent area obstruction:* (stent area—lumen area) ÷ stent area × 100.
- *Neointimal Unevenness Score (NUS):* the maximum neointimal thickness ÷ the average neointimal thickness in each analyzed frame. This index is expressing the heterogeneity of in stent strut coverage.[32]

Technologies Under Development

FD-OCT facilitates the acquisition of spectroscopic and polarization, Doppler and other imaging modes for plaque characterization.[58] Interpretation of current TD-OCT image is limited to the evaluation of

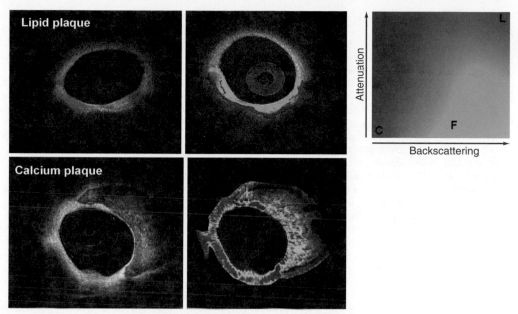

Figure 60-22 Examples of color-coded optical coherence tomography (OCT) images of lipidic plaque and calcified plaque. Using a postprocessing color-coding software-based algorithm on analysis of either spectral OCT backscattered data and attenuation data, lipid (*l*) was shown in blue, fibrous tissue (*F*) was shown in green, and calcium (*C*) was shown in red. (*Courtesy of LightLab Imaging, Westford, MA*)

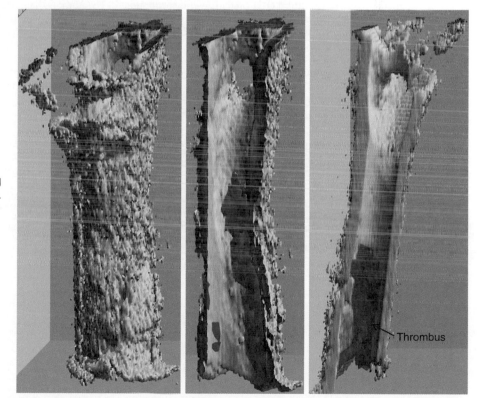

Figure 60-23 Examples of three dimensional optical coherence tomography (OCT) images. Intracoronary thrombus was shown in red. (*Courtesy of LightLab Imaging, Westford, MA.*)

grayscale image, and identification of individual plaque components by OCT requires experience. The application of a postprocessing, color-coding, software-based algorithm to the analysis of either spectral OCT backscattered data or other optical tissue properties should improve the characterization of atherosclerotic coronary plaques and provide a more objective assessment (Fig. 60-22). Moreover, Tearney et al reported that FD-OCT, called OFDI by the author's group, enables imaging of the three-dimensional microstructure of long segments of coronary arteries.[7] Three-dimensional reconstruction of OCT images improves the evaluation of lesion vulnerability, such as the distribution of necrotic core, thin fibrous cap, and intracoronary thrombus (Fig. 60-23). Also, OCT identification of plaque cellular components such as inflammatory cells is likely to be improved by three-dimensional visualization. When FD-OCT is fully exploited, it has the potential to dramatically change the way that physicians and researchers understand coronary artery disease to better diagnose and treat the disease.

Future of Optical Coherence Tomography

Some expected advances in intravascular OCT technology include improved imaging speed and usability, automated image classification, and enhanced visualization, incorporation of alternative optical contrast sources, and OCT-combination devices. Improvements in light source sweep rates will enable faster rotational rates and pull-back rates and provide physicians with the ability to capture a high-density scan of the entire coronary artery between consecutive heartbeats, thus minimizing motion artifacts and further reducing the volume of contrast injected to displace blood during image acquisition. Clinical usability of OCT systems will be improved by features such as robust catheter autocalibration, debris-insensitive connectors, self-synchronizing flush and acquisition, and integration with existing cath lab systems and networks. Advanced image processing algorithms will be developed to classify tissue types and automatically detect in three-dimensional display features of interest such as the shape of the vessel lumen, stent strut malapposition, and thrombi deposition. The longitudinal position between the reference and where the CSA is the smallest MLA will be found automatically. The algorithm will recognize and avoid residual blood, guidewire reflections, and other structures that may appear to be part of the vessel wall. Interpolation across side branches will be accomplished by imposing continuity of the inner surface of the vessel across neighboring frames. Volume co-registration with IVUS, angiography, CT, or previous OCT datasets will lead to better four-dimensional visualization of pathology and interventional guidance and feedback. To provide functional information and a wider range of classifiable tissue types, future OCT systems will incorporate alternative optical approaches such as polarization sensitivity, Doppler/phase sensitivity, and spectral sensitivity, to endogenous as well as exogenous sources of contrast (spectrally tunable optical nanoparticles). Other intravascular diagnostic devices that provide complementary information, such as ultrasound, absorption spectroscopy, fluorescence spectroscopy, and Raman spectroscopy, may be engineered to reside alongside OCT in the same catheter probe. IVUS and FD-OCT imaging with a single catheter may enable visualization of tissue microstructure in superficial layers of the artery wall at the same time as the deeper layers of the artery for evaluation of plaque burden and vessel remodeling. The combination of FD-OCT with near-infrared, Raman, or other spectroscopic techniques may improve discrimination among tissue constituents in complex atherosclerotic lesions and allow for detailed analysis of the cellular and biochemical composition of thin-capped lesions for vulnerable plaque detection.

Concurrent data collection from these modalities will dramatically expand the structural and functional information available to the cardiologist and will hopefully guide development and clinical use of novel cardiovascular therapies.

Conclusion

OCT enables real-time, full tomographic, in situ visualization of vessel microstructure with a unique high axial resolution. Previously unrevealed details on atherosclerotic plaque architecture and stent vascular response can be easily observed and quantified, and this would accelerate the understanding of the formation and treatment of coronary artery disease. Advances in the technology of FD-OCT improved the ease of use and broaden the application of OCT from a research diagnostic tool toward an established technique for guiding coronary procedures.

Acknowledgments

The Authors thank Hideyuki Ikejima, MD, and Hironori Kitabata, MD (Wakayama Medical University, Wakayama, Japan); Gary Tearney, MD, PhD, and Brett Bouma, PhD (Wellman Center for Photomedicine, Massachusetts General Hospital, MA); Joe Schmitt, PhD (LightLab Imaging, Westford, MA, a subsidiary of St Jude Medical); and Nate Kemp, PhD (Volcano Corporation, Billerica, MA) for assistance with the preparation of this chapter.

REFERENCES

1. Tanaka A, Tearney GJ, Bouma BE: Challenges on the frontier of intracoronary imaging: Atherosclerotic plaque macrophage measurement by optical coherence tomography. *J Biomed Opt* 15:011104, 2010.
2. Templin C, Meyer M, Müller MF, et al: Coronary optical frequency domain imaging (OFDI) for in vivo evaluation of stent healing: Comparison with light and electron microscopy. *Eur Heart J* 31:1792–1801, 2010.
3. Kull S, Celi S, Berti S, et al: Pre-implant evaluation of tissue engineered small diameter vascular grafts with optical coherence tomography: Preliminary results on bench-test. Proceedings ECCOMAS—International Conference on Tissue Engineering (ICTE), 2009; 301–308.
4. Gonzalo N, García-García HM, Serruys PW, et al: Reproducibility of quantitative optical coherence tomography for stent analysis. *EuroIntervention* 5:224–232, 2009.
5. Yin J, Yang HC, Li X, et al: Integrated intravascular optical coherence tomography ultrasound imaging system. *J Biomed Opt* 15:0105121–0105123, 2010.
6. Bezerra HG, Costa MA, Guagliumi G, et al: Intracoronary optical coherence tomography: A comprehensive review clinical and research applications. *JACC Cardiovasc Interv* 2:1035–1046, 2009.
7. Tearney GJ, Waxman S, Shishkov M, et al: Three-dimensional coronary artery microscopy by intracoronary optical frequency domain imaging. *JACC Cardiovasc Imaging* 1:752–761, 2008.
8. Yun SH, Tearney GJ, Vakoc BJ, et al: Comprehensive volumetric optical microscopy in vivo. *Nat Med* 12:1429–1433, 2006.
9. Yamaguchi T, Terashima M, Akasaka T, et al: Safety and feasibility of an intravascular optical coherence tomography image wire system in the clinical setting. *Am J Cardiol* 101:562–567, 2008.
10. Prati F, Cera F, Ramazzotti V, et al: Safety and feasibility of a new non-occlusive technique for facilitated intracoronary optical coherence tomography (OCT) acquisition in various clinical and anatomical scenarios. *EuroIntervention* 3:365–370, 2007.
11. Barlis P, Gonzalo N, Di Mario C, et al: A multicentre evaluation of the safety of intracoronary optical coherence tomography. *EuroIntervention* 5:90–95, 2009.
12. Takarada S, Imanishi T, Liu Y, et al: Advantage of next-generation frequency-domain optical coherence tomography compared with conventional time-domain system in the assessment of coronary lesion. *Catheter Cardiovasc Interv* 75:202–206, 2010.

13. Kume T, Akasaka T, Kawamoto T, et al: Assessment of coronary intima-media thickness by optical coherence tomography: Comparison with intravascular ultrasound. *Circ J* 69:903–907, 2005.
14. Kume T, Akasaka T, Kawamoto T, et al: Assessment of coronary arterial plaque by optical coherence tomography. *Am J Cardiol* 97:1172–1175, 2006.
15. Yabushita H, Bouma BE, Houser SL, et al: Characterization of human atherosclerosis by optical coherence tomography. *Circulation* 106:1640–1645, 2002.
16. Kawasaki M, Bouma BE, Bressner J, et al: Diagnostic accuracy of optical coherence tomography and integrated backscatter intravascular ultrasound images for tissue characterization of human coronary plaques. *J Am Coll Cardiol* 48:81–88, 2006.
17. Kume T, Akasaka T, Kawamoto T, et al: Assessment of coronary arterial thrombus by optical coherence tomography. *Am J Cardiol* 97:1713–1717, 2006.
18. Tearney GJ, Yabushita H, Houser SL, et al: Quantification of macrophage content in atherosclerotic plaques by optical coherence tomography. *Circulation* 107:113–119, 2003.
19. Kitabata H, Kubo T, Akasaka T: Identification of multiple plaque ruptures by optical coherence tomography in a patient with acute myocardial infarction: A three-vessel study. *Heart* 94:544, 2008.
20. Tanaka A, Imanishi T, Kitabata H, et al: Morphology of exertion-triggered plaque rupture in patients with acute coronary syndrome: An optical coherence tomography study. *Circulation* 118:2368–2373, 2008.
21. Kubo T, Imanishi T, Takarada S, et al: Assessment of culprit lesion morphology in acute myocardial infarction: Ability of optical coherence tomography compared with intravascular ultrasound and coronary angioscopy. *J Am Coll Cardiol* 50:933–939, 2007.
22. Kubo T, Imanishi T, Takarada S, et al: Implication of plaque color classification for assessing plaque vulnerability: A coronary angioscopy and optical coherence tomography investigation. *JACC Cardiovasc Interv* 1:74–80, 2008.
23. Tanaka A, Imanishi T, Kitabata H, et al: Distribution and frequency of thin-capped fibroatheromas and ruptured plaques in the entire culprit coronary artery in patients with acute coronary syndrome as determined by optical coherence tomography. *Am J Cardiol* 102:975–979, 2008.
24. Kume T, Akasaka T, Kawamoto T, et al: Measurement of the thickness of the fibrous cap by optical coherence tomography. *Am Heart J* 152:e1–e4, 2006.

25. Sawada T, Shite J, García-García HM, et al: Feasibility of combined use of intravascular ultrasound radiofrequency data analysis and optical coherence tomography for detecting thin-cap fibroatheroma. *Eur Heart J* 29:1136–1146, 2008.
26. Jang IK, Tearney GJ, MacNeill B, et al: In vivo characterization of coronary atherosclerotic plaque by use of optical coherence tomography. *Circulation* 111:1551–1555, 2005.
27. Fujii K, Masutani M, Okumura T, et al: Frequency and predictor of coronary thin-cap fibroatheroma in patients with acute myocardial infarction and stable angina pectoris a 3-vessel optical coherence tomography study. *J Am Coll Cardiol* 52:787–788, 2008.
28. Takarada S, Imanishi T, Kubo T, et al: Effect of statin therapy on coronary fibrous-cap thickness in patients with acute coronary syndrome: Assessment by optical coherence tomography study. *Atherosclerosis* 202:491–497, 2009.
29. Guagliumi G, Sirbu V: Optical coherence tomography: High resolution intravascular imaging to evaluate vascular healing after coronary stenting. *Catheter Cardiovasc Interv* 72:237–247, 2008.
30. Murata A, Wallace-Bradley D, Tellez A, et al: Accuracy of optical coherence tomography in the evaluation of neointimal coverage after stent implantation. *JACC Cardiovasc Imaging* 3:76–84, 2010.
31. Guagliumi G, Musumeci G, Sirbu V, et al: Optical coherence tomography assessment of in vivo vascular response after implantation of overlapping bare-metal and drug-eluting stents. *JACC Cardiovasc Interv* 3:531–539, 2010.
32. Otake H, Shite J, Ako J, et al: Local determinants of thrombus formation following sirolimus-eluting stent implantation assessed by optical coherence tomography. *JACC Cardiovasc Interv* 2:459–466, 2009.
33. Guagliumi G, Sirbu V, Bezerra H, et al: Strut coverage and vessel wall response to zotarolimus-eluting and bare-metal stents implanted in patients with ST-segment elevation myocardial infarction: The OCTAMI (Optical Coherence Tomography in Acute Myocardial Infarction) Study. *JACC Cardiovasc Interv* 3:680–687, 2010.
34. Kume T, Okura H, Kawamoto T, et al: Images in cardiovascular medicine. Fibrin clot visualized by optical coherence tomography. *Circulation* 118:426–427, 2008.
35. Sawada T, Shite J, Negi N, et al: Factors that influence measurements and accurate evaluation of stent apposition by optical coherence tomography assessment using a phantom model. *Circ J* 73:1841–1847, 2009.

36. Kubo T, Imanishi T, Kitabata H, et al: Comparison of vascular response after sirolimus-eluting stent implantation between patients with unstable and stable angina pectoris: A serial optical coherence tomography study. *JACC Cardiovasc Imaging* 1:475–484, 2008.

37. Ozaki Y, Okumura M, Ismail TF, et al: The fate of incomplete stent apposition with drug-eluting stents: An optical coherence tomography-based natural history study. *Eur Heart J* 31:1470–1476, 2010.

38. Matsumoto D, Shite J, Shinke T, et al: Neointimal coverage of sirolimus-eluting stents at 6-month follow-up: Evaluated by optical coherence tomography. *Eur Heart J* 28:918–919, 2007.

39. Bezerra HG, Guagliumi G, Kyono H, et al: Determining the optimal cross-sectional analysis interval for OCT assessment of coronary stenting. *Circulation* 120:S1000, 2009.

40. Takano M, Yamamoto M, Inami S, et al: Appearance of lipid-laden intima and neovascularization after implantation of bare-metal stents extended late-phase observation by intracoronary optical coherence tomography. *J Am Coll Cardiol* 55:26–32, 2010.

41. Guagliumi G, Costa MA, Sirbu V, et al: Strut coverage and late malapposition with paclitaxel-eluting stents compared with bare metal stens in acute myocardial infarction: optical coherence tomography substudy of the Harmonizing Outcomes with Revascularization and Stents in Acute Myocardial Infarction (HORIZONS-AMI) Trial. *Circulation* 123:274–281, 2008.

42. Katoh H, Shite J, Shinke T, et al: Delayed neointimalization on sirolimus-eluting stents: 6-month and 12-month follow up by optical coherence tomography. *Circ J* 73:1033–1037, 2009.

43. Nakazawa G, Vorpahl M, Finn AV, et al: One step forward and two steps back with drug-eluting-stents: From preventing restenosis to causing late thrombosis and nouveau atherosclerosis. *JACC Cardiovasc Imaging* 2:625–628, 2009.

44. Guagliumi G, Sirbu V, Musumeci M, et al: Strut coverage and vessel wall response to a new-generation paclitaxel-eluting stent with an ultrathin biodegradable abluminal polymer optical coherence tomography drug-eluting stent investigation (OCTDESI). *Circ Cardiovasc Interv* 3:367–375, 2010.

45. Windecker S, Serruys PW, Wandel S, et al. Biolimus-eluting stent with biodegradable polymer versus sirolimus-eluting stent with durable polymer for coronary revascularisation (LEADERS): A randomised non-inferiority trial. *Lancet* 372:1163–1173, 2008.

46. Serruys PW, Ormiston JA, Onuma Y, et al: A bioabsorbable everolimus-eluting coronary stent system (ABSORB): 2-year outcomes and results from multiple imaging methods. *Lancet* 373:897–910, 2009.

47. Daemen J, Simoons ML, Wijns W, et al: ESC forum on drug eluting stents European Heart House, Nice, 27–28 September 2007. *Eur Heart J* 30:152–161, 2009.

48. Sirbu V, Guagliumi G, Musumeci G: In-vivo mechanisms of late drug eluting stent thrombosis. Optical coherence tomography, intravascular ultrasound and thrombus aspirated findings [abstract]. *Eur Heart J* 29(Suppl):127, 2008.

49. Takano M, Xie Y, Murakami D, et al: Various optical coherence tomographic findings in restenotic lesions after sirolimus-eluting stent implantation. *Int J Cardiol* 134:263–265, 2009.

50. Ferrante G, Kaplan AV, Di Mario C: Assessment with optical coherence tomography of a new strategy for bifurcational lesion treatment: The Triton side-branch stent. *Catheter Cardiovasc Interv* 73:69–72, 2009.

51. Gonzalo N, García-García HM, Regar E, et al: In vivo assessment of high-risk coronary plaques at bifurcations with combined intravascular ultrasound and optical coherence tomography. *JACC Cardiovasc Imaging* 2:473–482, 2009.

52. Kyono H, Guagliumi G, Sirbu V, et al: Optical coherence tomography (OCT) strut-level analysis of drug-eluting stents (DES) in human coronary bifurcations. *EuroIntervention* 6:69–77, 2010.

53. Prabhudesai V, Phelan C, Yang Y, et al: The potential role of optical coherence tomography in the evaluation of vulnerable carotid atheromatous plaques: A pilot study. *Cardiovasc Intervent Radiol* 29:1039–1045, 2006.

54. Meissner OA, Rieber J, Babaryka G, et al: Intravascular optical coherence tomography: Comparison with histopathology in atherosclerotic peripheral artery specimens. *J Vasc Interv Radiol* 17:343–349, 2006.

55. Gonzalo N, Serruys PW, García-García HM, et al: Quantitative ex vivo and in vivo comparison of lumen dimensions measured by optical coherence tomography and intravascular ultrasound in human coronary arteries. *Rev Esp Cardiol* 62:615–624, 2009.

56. Siegel RJ, Swan K, Edwalds G, et al: Limitations of postmortem assessment of human coronary artery size and luminal narrowing: Differential effects of tissue fixation and processing on vessels with different degrees of atherosclerosis. *J Am Coll Cardiol* 5:342–346, 1985.

57. Sihan K, Botha C, Post F, et al: Fully automatic three-dimensional quantitative analysis of intracoronary optical coherence tomography: Method and validation. *Catheter Cardiovasc Interv* 74:1058–1065, 2009.

58. Nadkarni SK, Pierce MC, Park BH, et al: Measurement of collagen and smooth muscle cell content in atherosclerotic plaques using polarization-sensitive optical coherence tomography. *J Am Coll Cardiol* 49:1474–1481, 2007.

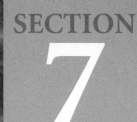

Outcome Effectiveness of Interventional Cardiology

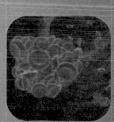

61

Medical Economics in Interventional Cardiology

DANIEL MARK

KEY POINTS

- The most influential determinant of an economic analysis is usually not the costs of the new therapy or strategy but, rather, the absolute magnitude of the clinical benefits being produced relative to the comparison therapy or strategy.

- An economic analysis should examine the full spectrum of incremental clinical and cost outcomes of the therapy or strategy being studied over a time horizon, typically the lifetime of the cohort, that reasonably reflects the long-term consequences of that technology for the patients being treated.

- Cost-effectiveness analysis assesses the extra or incremental costs for a new therapy or strategy that are incurred to produce an incremental or extra unit of health benefits, such as an extra life-year or quality-adjusted life-year (QALY). The focus is on the assessment of efficiency of a particular investment relative to alternative ways to spend health care dollars.

- Therapies with large upfront costs and delayed incremental clinical benefits, such as coronary artery bypass grafting (CABG), can be economically attractive over the long run, if applied to sufficiently high-risk populations.

- Infrequently, a new therapy or strategy is so effective at reducing complications that it fully offsets its cost (a therapy that offers better clinical outcomes with lower cost is referred to as a "dominant therapy"), but most new therapies that improve outcomes are also more costly in the long run, necessitating cost-effectiveness analysis.

According to recent American Heart Association (AHA) estimates, percutaneous coronary intervention (PCI) is performed in the United States about 1.18 million times each year.[1] Despite this astonishing level of its adoption into mainstream cardiovascular practice, controversies persist about the appropriate indications for PCI and about its value provided for money spent in different clinical contexts. The purpose of this chapter is to review what is known about this question of value for money. Rather than striving to be encyclopedic, this chapter will emphasize broad concepts and selected studies that best illustrate these concepts in different areas of interventional cardiology. The first part of the chapter provides an overview of important economic concepts and approaches. The second part reviews empirical research data on the economics of interventional cardiology.

Medical Economics: Concepts and Methods

MEDICAL COST DEFINITIONS AND TERMINOLOGY

To an economist, a "cost" is not the amount of money required to purchase a particular health care good or service but rather the consumption of societal resources required to produce that good or service, and deliver it to the consumer that could have been used for another purpose.[2] The term "opportunity cost" is used in the economics literature to indicate this particular meaning of cost. Society consumes resources to satisfy its wants, including those for food, housing, and recreation, as well as health care. However, because resources are ultimately finite, society cannot satisfy all wants and is obliged to choose from among the potential alternative uses of its resources. Economics provides a set of tools and approaches to assist with the decisions regarding what health care to produce, in what quantity, and for whom. The classic illustration of the constrained resources concept is the "guns-versus-butter" example from freshman economics. Resources expended in the production of weapons cannot also be applied to the production of food; therefore, in a world of limited resources, more weapons may mean less food. At the societal level, more health care may ultimately translate into less investment in education, transportation, housing, or other societal priorities.

Opportunity cost is a foundational concept but not a measurement tool. In most actual economic studies, accounting costs are measured as a surrogate for opportunity cost, in large part because the former are easier to measure. Accounting costs are the monetary prices we are more familiar with when we think about the concept of cost. In most businesses or industries, the market price of a product or service is equal to the cost of producing that item plus some amount of profit (typically reflecting a fair return on investment). In the U.S. medical sector, the discrepancy almost universally observed between *prices* (or charges) and *costs* (the true accounting cost of providing a given medical service) is largely attributable to "cost shifting," a set of accounting practices designed to shift costs from a variety of sources (Table 61-1) onto whichever group of payers is most willing and able to absorb them. The net effect of these cost-shifting practices is to distort the relationship between U.S. medical prices or charges and medical resource consumption. U.S. medical charges are, for that reason, never a good surrogate for medical costs, and their use in research and policy evaluations should be avoided.

The concepts of marginal and incremental costs are commonly used in medical economics. Strictly speaking, *marginal cost* is defined as the cost of producing *one* additional (or *one* less) unit of product, such as a PCI or bypass surgery procedure. Marginal cost excludes costs that do not vary as a direct function of production (termed *fixed costs*), such as the cost of the interventional laboratory or operating room facilities. Although the notion of one more or one less test or procedure is useful for some types of (usually theoretical) economic analyses, the more practical questions usually focus on examining the costs of shifting *groups* of patients from one diagnostic or therapeutic strategy to another. For this type of analysis, the term *incremental* is often substituted for *marginal*. (Unfortunately, some leading medical economics researchers use "marginal" and "incremental" synonymously, whereas others do not, leading to potential confusion for those outside the field.) Incremental cost analysis is an important component of cost-effectiveness analysis and is central to the economic notion of cost as a measure of alternative uses of scarce resources introduced at the beginning of this chapter. In the next section, we consider how incremental costs are actually measured and some of the problems involved in translating economic theory into practice.

Induced costs (or *savings*) are the costs of the tests or therapies added or averted as a consequence of some initial management decision, resource use, or both. A few examples will make the concept clear. The institution of an aggressive program of intravenous thrombolytic

TABLE 61-1	Major Components of Hospital Charges for Medical Services
1.	True costs to hospital of resources consumed (e.g., disposable supplies, personnel equipment allocated overhead)
2.	Cost-shifting accounting maneuvers
	Bad debts
	Free services (e.g., indigent care, employees)
	Disallowed costs by third party payers
3.	Replacement of existing equipment
4.	Acquisition of new technologies (e.g., magnetic resonance imaging)
5.	Budgeting for expansion of services (e.g., more inpatient beds, more outpatient clinics)

1, cost for given hospital service; *1–5*, Charge or price for given hospital service.
From Mark DB, Jollis J. Economic aspects of therapy for acute myocardial infarction. In: Bates ER, ed. *Adjunctive Therapy for Acute Myocardial Infarction.* New York: Marcel Dekker, Inc., 1991:471–496, with permission.

TABLE 61-2	Major Methodologic Issues in Medical Cost Studies

Measurement of cost:
Categories of cost items to be included:
- Disposable supplies
- Personnel (direct cost component)
- Department overhead (e.g., departmental administration, maintenance, equipment depreciation, utilities)
- Allocated hospital or clinic overhead (e.g., hospital administration, admissions, medical records)

Focus for cost analysis:
- Resources consumed/service provided ("bottom-up")
- Billed charges/fees ("top-down")
- Episode of care
- Historical data

Structural framework of this study:
- Randomized controlled trial
- Observational study
- Cost-effectiveness model

Possible perspectives of the cost analysis:
- Societal
- Medicare, managed care, other third-party payers
- Hospitals, clinics, physicians, other providers
- Patients

Time effects on medical costs:
- Inflation
- Discounting of future costs

Geographic effects on medical costs:
- Different practice settings
- Different geographic locations within a country

therapy in patients with acute myocardial infarction (AMI) by a given hospital or physician practice group may be accompanied by a rise in the number of patients with major disabling strokes who need long-term care. That latter cost is *induced* by the initial therapeutic decision. In the same way, performance of PCI induces the cost of repeat revascularization procedures to treat symptomatic restenosis or stent thrombosis. Use of statin therapy for secondary prevention induces a cost savings over the long term owing to reduced need for cardiac procedures and hospitalizations.

Finally, the term *indirect cost* is often used by health service researchers to discuss the societal costs associated with loss of employment or productivity caused by morbidity. Because of the potential for confusion with the accounting meaning of indirect cost, the alternative term *productivity cost* is currently preferred.

METHODOLOGIC ISSUES IN MEDICAL COST STUDIES

To perform a medical cost study, it is necessary to consider five major issues (Table 61-2): (1) the way cost is to be conceptualized and measured, (2) the type of study to be performed (the structural framework in which the cost analysis will be accomplished), (3) the perspectives of the analysis, (4) the importance of cost variations over time, and (5) the importance of cost variations caused by geographic and market factors.

Cost Measurement

In any clinical cost study, the investigators must decide at an early stage what categories of cost items they need to include in the analysis and at what level of detail they wish to focus (see Table 61-2). In practice, the types of detailed data required for marginal or incremental cost analysis are difficult to obtain unless the hospital or health system involved has a computerized cost-accounting system, and they are impractical (if not impossible) to obtain for all participants in the typical large cardiovascular multi-center trial. Therefore, rather than adding up the individual resources being consumed (which might be termed the *bottom-up approach*), most U.S. cost studies start with an aggregated measure of costs, such as can be obtained from hospital or physician bills (a *top-down analysis*). Although the top-down approach is much more practical for many cost studies, especially multi-center studies, it does reduce the ability of the investigator to control the factors that are included as costs in the analysis.

In an older, but still instructive, study examining the practical impact of using top-down versus bottom-up cost estimates, Hlatky and colleagues at Duke compared the magnitude of cost savings available by shifting from a more expensive treatment (i.e., coronary artery bypass grafting [CABG]) to a less expensive one (i.e., percutaneous transluminal coronary angioplasty [PTCA]) in 389 patients with coronary artery disease (CAD). Two bottom-up and three top-down cost estimates were examined (Table 61-3). Using only hospital charges (method 5), the cost savings was estimated at $10,000 per patient shifted to PTCA. However, if no hospital or departmental overhead were to be saved from this change in practice, then the true cost savings would be that estimated by method 1 or 2: 20% to 46% of the amount estimated from charges. Methods 3 and 4, which include varying amounts of overhead, overestimate the short-term cost savings from the CABG to PTCA shift; they are more correctly viewed as providing an estimate of the difference in *average* cost. Conversely, methods 1 and 2 indicate the *marginal* or *incremental* difference. Note that the difference between costs using the Medicare correction factors (method 4) and using charges (method 5) is attributed, at least in part, to the hospital's shifting of costs from nonpaying patients to the paying segment. This "surtax" would, of course, never be recoverable by changes in patient management. For this reason alone, charges represent a poor choice for evaluating the cost implications of different clinical strategies.

A true bottom-up cost analysis, sometimes referred to as a *microcosting analysis,* is a complex, time-consuming process that requires identification of all the inputs into a health care service and the assignment of an appropriate cost to each. This is easiest for a relatively simple service, such as the administration of an antibiotic, the performance of a radiograph, or a laboratory test. A more complex hospital laboratory procedure, such as a PCI, is a considerably greater challenge because of the large variability of inputs from one case to the next. Most complicated of all is an entire episode of care from admission to discharge because this requires detailed cost and resource-use data from virtually every major hospital department.

Of the top-down strategies for estimating costs, the most widely used in the United States involves converting hospital charges (taken from the hospital bill) to costs using the correction factors or *ratios of costs to charges (RCCs)* included in each hospital's annual Medicare Cost Report. Medicare RCCs are largely a holdover from the era before prospective payment, when Medicare reimbursed hospitals on the

TABLE 61-3	Five Estimates of the Cost Savings Available by Shifting Patients from CABG to PTCA				
	Cost Accounting Method*				
	1	2	3	4	5
Total Difference ($)†	1935	4593	5346	7837	10087
Room	283	2323	1939	3052	3277
Procedure	28	334	1014	876	1348
Blood Bank	342	390	466	532	749
Electrocardiography	3	16	33	47	70
Laboratory	65	146	368	1035	1392
Pharmacy	1061	1115	682	1076	1727
Respiratory	48	120	358	463	529
Supplies	68	68	93	135	271
Radiology	38	78	263	459	555

From Hlatky MA, Lipscomb J, Nelson C, et al. Resource use and cost of initial coronary revascularization. Coronary angioplasty versus coronary bypass surgery. *Circulation* 1990;82 (Suppl IV):IV-208-13, with permission.

†Cost differences are given in 1986 US dollars

Abbreviations: PTCA = coronary angioplasty; CABG = coronary artery bypass graft surgery; method 1 = disposable supplies only; method 2 = supplies plus personnel; method 3 = costs from charges using department level cost/charge ratios; method 4 = costs from charges using Medicare cost/charge ratios; method 5 = charges.

basis of costs incurred. To do so, Medicare developed a method of deciding how to reimburse hospitals for the reasonable and necessary costs of providing care to its beneficiaries (i.e., actual hospital cost), rather than paying the full charged amount. This method involved an elaborate reporting system that required each hospital to file with Centers for Medicare and Medicaid Services (CMS) each year. In this report, which is still required, the hospital details how expenses for direct patient care, overhead, capital equipment, and so forth relate to billed charges. To provide CMS with a means of converting charges to costs for its various ancillary services, each hospital includes in its report a set of ratios, the RCCs. Although not designed for research, the Medicare RCCs represent a moderately standardized means of estimating cost across all the hospitals in the United States that file a Medicare Cost Report. Although no longer used for reimbursement, the Medicare Cost Report still serves as the primary source of government data on hospital costs. In addition, costs calculated with the RCC method are used to recalibrate *diagnosis-related group (DRG)* weights. Therefore, this method provides a valuable tool for multi-center cost research.

There are three important limitations to the RCC method of cost estimation that should be noted. First, this approach does not separate out overhead and most other fixed costs and therefore provides an estimate of average rather than marginal cost; hence, it may overestimate potential cost savings. Second, Medicare Cost Reports have complex, detailed instructions for how they are to be filled out; as with the complex federal income tax reporting system, this means that hospitals may choose to interpret the instructions differently (just as different people choose to fill out their income tax forms differently). For this reason, the goal of uncovering a hospital's actual cost of providing care may be accomplished to a varying degree using this method. Finally, RCCs are themselves averages of all the cost–charge relationships within a large hospital revenue (ancillary) center such as the radiology, pharmacy, or laboratory departments. If an individual patient's resource consumption pattern in a given cost center is not "average," the Medicare RCCs may not be particularly accurate in converting those charges to costs. For the same reason, conversion of charges to costs for individual items on a detailed hospital bill may not be particularly accurate if the RCC for that item is not close to the average RCC of that cost center. By extension, the practice some have advocated of using one average RCC for an entire hospital may also be less accurate.

DRG reimbursement rates, which are available from CMS in the United States and are also used in some European countries, provide an alternative top-down cost estimation method. Once the patient's DRG assignment is known, it becomes a simple matter to calculate the "hospital costs." This system of cost estimation has a number of limitations, however. First, it is not sensitive to variations in

resource-use intensity within a DRG. Thus, DRG reimbursement rates are averages in the sense that they represent the "average cost" for a particular DRG among all (elderly) patients in that DRG. Second, if CMS decides not to increase reimbursement to cover the costs of new technology, which has been the case with many new, expensive drug therapies, the DRG reimbursement is insensitive to large differences in resource costs. To take a more complex example, a patient who is admitted for unstable angina and undergoes a diagnostic cardiac catheterization, a PCI, a repeat PCI for abrupt closure, and then CABG will likely be coded out as DRG 106 (CABG with catheterization); from CMS's point of view, the cost of the two PCIs is the hospital's problem. For all these reasons, DRG reimbursement is not a particularly good way of estimating costs in an economic analysis unless the analysis is being done from CMS's perspective.

The most approximate cost-estimation method used in clinical research involves counting only big-ticket items consumed (such as number of PCIs, cardiac catheterizations, or CABGs; days in the intensive care unit; and total hospital length of stay) and assigning unit prices to each item. The resulting linear formula:

$$\text{Total cost} = \sum \text{price} \times \text{quantity}$$

is simple and inexpensive to use (hence its appeal in clinical research), but it suffers from some important drawbacks. First, the source of cost weights is often external to the resource data being analyzed and, therefore, of uncertain relevance. Such cost weights are often chosen because they are conveniently available (e.g., published in some unrelated economic study) rather than because they are well suited to the problem at hand. Second, the appropriate set of big-ticket items necessary to estimate costs accurately using this method has never been rigorously defined. For example, days in the intensive care unit (ICU) is an important driver of hospital costs but is difficult to collect accurately in a multi-center study and may be omitted in favor of total length of stay. How much inaccuracy such a decision introduces into the costing and its effects on estimates of incremental costs are important, but often ignored, questions. Third, to preserve the desired simplicity, the method usually treats the big-ticket inputs as though they were homogeneous. For example, an uncomplicated single-vessel PCI would typically be assigned the same price as a complex three-vessel PCI procedure complicated by abrupt closure. The true costs of these two procedures may, in fact, differ substantially.

Assignment of costs to physician services in a cost analysis is usually done in one of two ways. In the past, physician fees (which are charges, analogous to hospital charges) have been used. Because most patients receive care from a variety of practitioners (each billing out of a separate office), collecting actual physician bills is several times more complicated than collecting hospital bills. Increasingly, however, physician fees have become a distorted measure of true resource inputs because physicians have been forced to employ the same types of cost shifting used by hospitals to cover unreimbursed and under-reimbursed services. Furthermore, it can be reasonably argued that physician fees in the "fee-for-service" era have never properly reflected a true market price for physician services. Unlike the situation for hospitals, however, Medicare has never required physicians to disclose their true costs in a cost report.

Because of these distortions, the Medicare Fee Schedule—based on the resource-based relative-value scale (RBRVS) of Hsiao and colleagues—has been adopted as a more appropriate method for assigning costs to physician services.[3] The basic concept of the RBRVS is that the price of a service should reflect the (long-term) cost of providing that service. Medicare fees are tied to the American Medical Association Physician's Current Procedural Terminology (CPT) classification system; therefore, to estimate physician costs from these fees, some map must be created between the CPT codes and the data available in the study database about physician services.

Although the Medicare Fee Schedule is not an ideal measure of the consumption of physician work in health care, it has the strong advantage of being more objective and consistent than charges or fees. Furthermore, the Medicare RBRVS payment schedule is now being used by many private insurers and managed care organizations, although with variations. Therefore, it represents the best available national measure of the economic value of physician work.

COST STUDY STRUCTURES

Medical cost studies generally fall into one of three categories: (1) randomized controlled trials (RCTs); (2) observational studies; and (3) cost-effectiveness models. *Cost-effectiveness models* are discussed in the next section. A cost study in a *randomized controlled trial* is usually ancillary to the primary objective of the trial. Typically, costs or resource consumption patterns are a secondary endpoint in a trial that has either a composite clinical or (preferably) a mortality primary endpoint. Some have argued that because RCTs are rarely performed with cost as a primary endpoint, the trials are usually not optimized to answer the economic questions of greatest interest, except insofar as these questions parallel the primary clinical ones. In addition, requirements of the clinical portion of the study may distort the economic substudy. For example, follow-up protocol angiography to define restenosis leads to repeat revascularization procedures that would not otherwise have been done. Even protocol-required clinic visits may lead to medical tests and therapies that would otherwise not have occurred.

Observational cost studies include both nonrandomized treatment comparisons and descriptive series without an intrinsic comparison group. Descriptive cost studies are useful in areas in which few empirical cost data have been published. Such data can be used to make sample size projections for RCTs or to inform cost-effectiveness and other health policy studies (in conjunction with appropriate sensitivity analyses). Little has been done, to date, with observational treatment comparisons involving cost data. As with observational comparisons of medical outcomes, statistical adjustment techniques to "level the playing field" are critical. However, because medical costs are subject to variations over time and over geographic location and practice settings, it is still uncertain what boundaries exist for defining when a nonrandomized cost comparison can provide useful, relatively unbiased information.

Importance of Perspective in Cost Analysis

Cost is always defined (either explicitly or implicitly) in terms of specific buyers and sellers (or consumers and producers). Table 61-2 lists the different perspectives that can be used for a medical cost analysis. Most commonly, economists and health policy analysts advocate the use of a societal perspective, in which total health expenditures (public and private) are examined as a function of the benefits produced and the opportunities forgone across the economy. Such an analysis ideally includes hospital costs, physician fees, outpatient testing, outpatient drug therapy costs, nonmedical direct expenses (e.g., transportation to the medical facility, child care, housekeeping), and the economic impact of lost productivity because of illness.

In contrast, analysis from the perspective of specific payers or providers typically includes only a portion of the costs listed for a societal analysis. For CMS, for example, hospital costs are defined by the payments specified by the relevant DRG regardless of the amount of services provided (or their cost to the provider). The Medicare Fee Schedule performs a similar function for physician services. For payers other than CMS, costs are the amount they are actually required to pay (or agree to reimburse providers) for health care services. Large insurance companies and managed care plans usually are able to obtain significant discounts off the list price, whereas the individual or the small company that is self-insured may be required to pay total charges. As a practical matter, perspectives other than societal and that of CMS or other national payers are infrequently used in cost studies in the medical literature.

Time Effects in Cost Analysis

Time effects are important to medical cost analyses for two major reasons (see Table 61-2). First, inflationary forces in the economy cause the value of money to diminish over time, so cost studies from different years should not be directly compared until differences caused solely by inflation are accounted for. Although there are several ways to make this adjustment (none of them ideal), perhaps the most widely used is the medical care component of the Producer Price Index (available at http://www.bls.gov/ppi/).

Independent of the effects of inflation, future medical expenditures are considered less costly than current ones because current expenditures take the money out of your pocket right away, whereas future expenditures allow you to hold onto your money for a period and invest it at the market rate of return. Assuming that the inflation-adjusted price for medical care does not change over time (i.e., no technological advances that increase or decrease true costs), one can buy more medical care with a given nominal sum of money in 5 or 10 years than is possible in the present. For this reason, cost studies using a long-term perspective employ a technique called *discounting* to account for the differences between the present value and the future value of money.

Geographic and Market Factors

Geographic and market economic factors also have important effects on medical care costs, although these have received little attention in empirical medical cost research. Different practice settings (e.g., within a particular region of the country) can affect the cost of providing a given type of care owing to variations in case mix, different practice patterns of the health care team (e.g., physicians, nurses, administrators), and different levels of efficiency within each setting. For example, for a given patient, care in an academic tertiary care center and care in a large private community hospital in the same city may be associated with quite different hospital costs. First, the teaching hospital must add at least part of the cost of its resident staff, and because an attending physician must supervise the residents, total physician time is usually increased per unit of care in a teaching hospital. Furthermore, residents typically order more tests per patient encounter. Other cost differences could arise from differing levels of nursing intensity at each stage in the hospitalization, differing use of intensive and intermediate care beds, and different typical lengths of stay for particular problems. In the second Thrombosis in Myocardial Infarction (TIMI II) trial, tertiary centers used more coronary angiography, coronary angioplasty, and CABG for initially admitted, medically equivalent patients compared with community hospitals.[4]

The costs of material and labor inputs to medical care can vary substantially from one part of the country to another, creating true differences in the cost of providing a given medical service according to geographic factors. Labor costs (e.g., nursing salaries) are probably the most important of the geographic determinants of health care cost variations. Thus, comparison of cost studies from different regions of the country or different practice settings should (but rarely do) include

		Effectiveness	Utility	QOL-Adjusted	
TABLE 61-4	**Cost Effectiveness, Cost Utility, and Cost Benefit: Sample Calculations***				
Strategy	Treatment Costs	Effectiveness (Life Expectancy)	Utility (Quality of Life)	QOL-Adjusted Life-Expectancy	Benefits[†]
Rx A	$20,000	4.5 Years	0.80	3.60 QALYs	$4000
Rx B	$10,000	3.5 Years	0.90	3.15 QALYs	$2000

Incremental Cost-effectiveness Ratio $= \dfrac{\$20,000 - \$10,000}{4.5\,years - 3.5\,years} = \$10,000$ per Life Year Saved

Incremental Cost-utility Ratio $= \dfrac{\$20,000 - \$10,000}{3.6\,QALYs - 3.15\,QALYs} = \$22,222$ per QALY Saved

Incremental Cost-benefit Ratio $= \dfrac{\$20,000 - \$10,000}{\$4000 - \$2000} = 5$

*From Detsky AS, Naglie IG. A clinician's guide to cost-effectiveness analysis. *Ann Intern Med* 1990;113:147–154, with permission.
[†]Shows health benefits valued in dollars

an adjustment for geographic cost differences. Several geographic adjustment indices are available, including the Medicare area wage index (for adjusting DRG reimbursement) and the Medicare Fee Schedule geographic adjustment factor.

COST-EFFECTIVENESS ANALYSIS

In clinical medicine, the term *cost-effective* is frequently used synonymously with *worthwhile* to indicate an intuitive, unspecified threshold between productive and wasteful medical expenditures. However, for economists the term *cost-effective* has a specific technical (and not particularly intuitive) meaning. Cost-effectiveness analysis involves the explicit comparison of one option or program with at least one alternative investment of dollars, and it never indicates whether a given expenditure is worthwhile in an absolute sense but, rather, how it stands relative to other potential expenditures. Therefore, it is incorrect to speak of any medical practice in isolation as cost-effective. The primary objective of cost-effectiveness analysis is to evaluate different health care expenditure options in common terms so that policy and other decision makers can choose the most efficient method of producing extra health benefits from among the alternative ways that health care dollars can be distributed.

The general term *cost-effectiveness analysis* actually refers to a family of methods for economic analysis (Table 61-4). For all methods, the final measure is expressed in ratio form, with incremental costs in the numerator and incremental health care benefits or outcomes in the denominator. The distinction among the methods derives primarily from how health benefits are measured. In cost-effectiveness analysis, the measure of incremental health effects chosen is typically the difference in life expectancy between the alternative strategies being evaluated (see Table 61-4). This is the most common type of economic health care analysis performed.

In *cost-utility analysis*, remaining survival is adjusted for less than full quality (quality-adjusted life-years [QALYs]). With both cost-effectiveness and cost-utility analysis, informal benchmarks are used to define results considered "economically attractive" [typically less than $50,000 per life-year or QALY] and "economically unattractive" [typically $100,000 per life-year or QALY or more]. The middle zone between these two benchmarks is considered of uncertain economic attractiveness.

Cost-benefit analysis is used much less often in medicine, probably because it requires measuring all health-related benefits of a program in monetary terms (see Table 61-4). The results of a cost–benefit analysis can either be expressed as a ratio of incremental monetary benefits to monetary costs or as a difference between the two. If the benefit: cost ratio exceeds 1 or the difference of benefits minus costs is positive, the assumed interpretation is that the treatment or program is worth doing, as it provides a net gain to the decision makers. Cost-benefit analysis has the useful feature of permitting comparison of medical care expenditures with societal expenditures on education, defense, transportation, and so forth, whereas cost-effectiveness analysis is

useful only in comparison of expenditures that produce the same type of outcome (e.g., QALYs). However, the difficulty of valuing health benefits in dollars in a valid and acceptable way has made this the least used method of efficiency analysis in medical economics.

Table 61-4 compares two hypothetical treatment strategies (A and B) for a particular disease and summarizes the calculations involved in the different analyses. Treatment A costs twice as much as treatment B but also improves average life expectancy by 1 year. Thus, the cost-effectiveness ratio for A relative to B is $10,000 per life-year saved. Whether switching from B to A is "worthwhile" depends on the alternative health care expenditures (aside from A) available for $10,000 or less. This is the most common sort of problem faced in cost-effectiveness analysis: whether to fund a new program that provides more health benefits than the standard therapy but at a substantially increased cost. (It is theoretically possible to go in the other direction—to give up health benefits to save substantial health care dollars—but this is rarely politically viable.)

QALYs allow us to factor in the *value* (to the decision maker, which may be the patient but could be someone else) of the extended survival offered by a new program or alternative therapy, as well as its quantity. In the example in Table 61-4, strategy A improves life expectancy relative to B, but the average quality of life for survivors is lower. This could come about in several ways. For example, with strategy B the sickest patients could die, leaving a relatively healthier group of survivors. In contrast, strategy A saves these sick patients from dying but cannot restore them to the same level of health as in the case of other patients with lower disease severity. These sicker surviving patients lower the average quality of life for the group. Alternatively, there could be something about strategy A that negatively affects quality of life, such as the need for chronic medication that is associated with significant side effects and that is not required with strategy B. In this example, moving from cost-effectiveness to cost-utility analysis more than doubles the cost of an additional unit of (quality-adjusted) survival with strategy A.

The underlying tenet of all these forms of economic analysis is that the analyst desires to determine the most efficient means of maximizing the net health benefits for a particular group or population under the constraint of limited resources (i.e., where it is not possible to provide every beneficial service to every potential recipient). Note that such economic analyses are neutral to the specific patients and diseases under study; the health benefits being maximized are abstractly conceptualized as belonging to a large group or population. In actual practice, however, political and other forces may play a large role in deciding where societal and other health care dollars are to be invested.

The ultimate problem in health care is that individual patients (and their physicians) wish to obtain all the health benefits that are available from modern medical technology. However, for the collection of all patients (i.e., society), the resources are not adequate to meet this need for every individual, which forces difficult and potentially divisive choices. The more we do for selected segments of the population (e.g., chronic renal failure patients receiving dialysis, patients with acquired

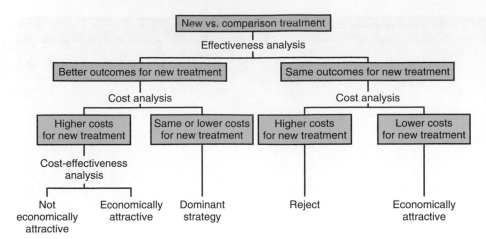

Figure 61-1 Schematic representation of patterns of outcome and cost differences that may result when a new therapy or strategy is compared with an existing standard. Effectiveness is always considered first because if the new therapy is less effective, its cost is rarely of concern. If effectiveness is better, or at least equivalent, then costs are examined. If the outcomes are better but the net costs are higher, cost-effectiveness analysis is then performed. If the costs are equivalent or lower, the therapy is said to be *dominant* (i.e., it becomes the preferred option). If outcomes are equivalent, cost analysis is used to select the more efficient, less costly option. This form of cost analysis is sometimes referred to as *cost minimization* or *cost-efficiency analysis.*

immune deficiency syndrome [AIDS], patients with AMI), the less we are able to do for the remainder. In the next section, we examine the costs of various interventional coronary disease therapies. We then return to the issue of cost-effectiveness at the end of this chapter and examine the ways in which this tool can be applied (and misapplied) in the analysis of these difficult choices.

Economics of Interventional Cardiology

GENERAL ISSUES

An economic analysis comparing a new drug, device, or strategy with "conventional" or "usual" care starts with an exploration of the ways in which the new approach will alter costs for the patients involved. At the most basic level, this involves understanding the resource consumption patterns and associated incremental costs of the new approach or technology. For a new interventional procedure, this includes the costs of the equipment and supplies used and the personnel changes required. A careful economic analysis also must determine what diagnostic or therapeutic procedures and what complications are added or averted, along with the cost effects of these changes in practice and outcome. Understanding these relationships is often difficult in practice, and one of the major advantages of empirical data collection over armchair models for cost studies is the frequency with which actual medical practices and outcomes diverge from the expected ideal.

In general, three major patterns of cost outcomes are possible when comparing alternative medical strategies or technologies (Fig. 61-1).
1. The new strategy or technology is associated with net higher costs but also provides additional clinical benefits. For example, CABG saves more lives than does medical therapy in patients with severe CAD, but it costs more money. In such cases, economic analysis attempts to define the relationship between incremental costs and incremental health benefits so that policy judgments can be made about adopting the new strategy. Cost-effectiveness analysis is the technique used to formalize this assessment. In some cases, the new strategy or technology may recoup some of its costs by reducing or preventing costly complications that occur with the comparison approach. For example, coronary stenting reduces the need for repeat revascularization procedures relative to conventional balloon angioplasty. These follow-up benefits provide at least a partial offset to the initially higher costs of stenting. However, because the total costs of the new strategy are often higher, cost-effectiveness analysis is still required to define its economic attractiveness.
2. The new strategy or technology produces better outcomes and has lower net costs. Use of enoxaparin in patients with acute coronary syndrome (ACS) in the Low Molecular Weight Heparin (Enoxaparin) in the Management of Unstable Angina (ESSENCE) trial is

an example. Such strategies are referred to by economists as *dominant.*
3. The new strategy or technology provides a less expensive, more efficient alternative to conventional therapy with the same benefits. For example, to the extent that PCI provides an equivalent revascularization option to CABG for some patients with CAD, it may substantially reduce costs.

CORONARY REVASCULARIZATION

In 2007, approximately 1.06 million diagnostic cardiac catheterizations, 1.18 million PCIs, and 408,000 CABGs were performed in the United States.[1] Because a hospitalization for PCI averages from $8000 to $15,000 and a hospitalization for CABG averages $30,000 or more, coronary revascularization costs in aggregate probably exceed $25 billion per year (Table 61-5). Although the procedures may be more efficient now than in the past owing to shortened hospital stays and lower complication rates, use in patients with more complex disease and advances in technology, especially for PCI, have tended to push costs back up. In this portion of the chapter, we review the available data addressing two key questions: First, what information do we have about how much these procedures cost? Second, what is the value of these procedures, where *value* refers to the balance between incremental costs and benefits? The literature on interventional cardiology tends to be divided into studies focused on the procedure, which may include both stable and unstable patients, and studies focused on a portion of the clinical spectrum of CAD, which typically examine strategies of care. Therefore, this section starts with a general review of economics of coronary revascularization.

Costs of Percutaneous Coronary Intervention

The costs of PCI have changed considerably over time, as have the clinical and technical aspects of the procedures. Stenting is now used in almost all PCI cases in the United States, and the use of drug-eluting stents (DESs) has varied from a high of over 90% of PCI cases to about 60% at present. Similar trends have been observed in Canada and Europe.

In an analysis of the cost of 335,000 Medicare beneficiaries undergoing PCIs in 2002, the average cost of hospitalization in patients who did not develop complications was $13,861 (mean length of hospital stay, 3 days), whereas patients undergoing PCI who developed complications had costs of $26,807 (mean length of hospital stay, 8 days).[5] Similar results were obtained in a Mayo Clinic analysis of PCI cases (1998–2003), with the cost of uncomplicated cases averaging $12,279 and the cost of complicated cases averaging $27,865.[6]

To understand what drives these costs, we must consider four major categories of determinants: (1) patient-specific, (2) treatment-specific, (3) hospital-specific, and (4) geographic–economic. Such costs include

TABLE 61-5	Cost of Initial Hospitalization for Revascularization			
Data source	Year(s)	# of Hospitalizations	Cost	Length of Stay
CABG				
Medicare Standard Analytic Files, 5% random sample of fee-for-service Medicare beneficiaries[1]	2001	4,664	$30,219 Mean	
PRIMO CABG trial[2]	1/2002–2/2003	2,102	$46,679 ± $37,946 for patients (pts) with MI by Day 4 post-op $33,051 ± $23,411 for pts with no MI by Day 4 post-op Means	13.9 ± 13.5 days for pts with MI by Day 4 post-op 9.4 ± 7.5 days for pts with no MI by Day 4 post-op Means
Perspective database, 164 hospitals in the U.S., mostly South[3]	10/2003–9/2005	81,289	$25,140 ($19,677–$33,121) Median	7 days (6–11) Median
Medicare Standard Analytic Files, 5% random sample of fee-for-service Medicare beneficiaries[1]	2004	4,056	$29,327 Mean	
Medicare Provider Analysis and Review file, Medicare beneficiaries[4]	10/2004–9/2005	114,233	$32,201 ± $23,059 Mean	9.9 ± 7.8 days Mean
Virginia state database, 99% of all isolated CABG cases in the Commonwealth of Virginia[5]	1/2004–12/2007	14,780	$30,654 Mean $24,414 Median	7.4 ± 5.8 days Mean
Maryland Health Services Cost Review Commission[6]	7/2005–6/2006	2,782	$27,580 ± $12,465 for people ages 40–50 To $42,115 ± $29,729 for people ages ≥80 Means	6.3 ± 3.3 days for people ages 40–50 To 10.4 ± 7.9 days for people ages ≥80 Means
PCI				
COURAGE trial[7]	1999–2004	1,149	$12,162 Mean	
Medicare Standard Analytic Files, 5% random sample of fee-for-service Medicare beneficiaries[1]	2001	9698	$14,067 Mean	
Medicare database[8]	10/2001–9/2002	335,477	$15,089 ± 13,063 Mean	3.5 ± 4.4 days Mean
TAXUS-IV trial[9]	2/2002–7/2002	1,314	$9,067 ± $3,387 for BMS group $11,096 ± $3,195 for PES group Means	1.9 ± 2.1 days for BMS group 2.0 ± 2.0 days for PES group Means
Medicare Standard Analytic Files, 5% random sample of fee-for-service Medicare beneficiaries[1]	2004	12,318	$14,639 Mean	
Hospital of the University of Pennsylvania and Pennsylvania Presbyterian Medical Center, patient-specific medical billing data[10]	9/2004–7/2006	39	$9,604 for early discharge PCI using femoral artery approach $10,565 for routine care PCI using femoral artery approach Means	
Maryland Health Services Cost Review Commission[6]	7/2005–6/2006	10,885	$13,230 ± $7,778 for people ages 40–50 To $14,412 ± $9,169 for people ages ≥80 Means	1.5 ± 1.6 for people ages 40–50 To 2.1 ± 2.7 for people ages ≥80 Means

CABG, coronary artery bypass graft surgery; MI, myocardial infarction; U.S., United States; PCI, percutaneous coronary intervention; BMS, bare metal stent; PES, paclitaxel-eluting stent.

[1]Ryan J, Linde-Zwirble W, Engelhart L, et al: Temporal changes in coronary revascularization procedures, outcomes, and costs in the bare-metal stent and drug-eluting stent eras: Results from the US Medicare program. *Circulation* 119:952–961, 2009.

[2]Chen JC, Kaul P, Levy JH, et al: Myocardial infarction following coronary artery bypass graft surgery increases healthcare resource utilization. *Crit Care Med* 35:1296–1301, 2007.

[3]Auerbach AD, Hilton JF, Maselli J, et al: Case volume, quality of care, and care efficiency in coronary artery bypass surgery. *Arch Intern Med* 170:1202–1208, 2010.

[4]Brown PP, Kugelmass AD, Cohen DJ, et al: The frequency and cost of complications associated with coronary artery bypass grafting surgery: Results from the United States Medicare program. *Ann Thorac Surg* 85:1980–1986, 2008.

[5]Speir AM, Kasirajan V, Barnett SD, et al: Additive costs of postoperative complications for isolated coronary artery bypass grafting patients in Virginia. *Ann Thorac Surg* 88:40–45, 2009.

[6]Agarwal S, Banerjee S, Tuzcu EM, et al: Influence of age on revascularization related costs of hospitalization among patients of stable coronary artery disease. *Am J Cardiol* 105:1549–1554, 2010.

[7]Weintraub WS, Spertus JA, Kolm P, et al: Effect of PCI on quality of life in patients with stable coronary disease. *N Engl J Med* 359:677–687, 2008.

[8]Kugelmass AD, Cohen DJ, Brown PP, et al: Hospital resources consumed in treating complications associated with percutaneous coronary interventions. *Am J Cardiol* 97:322–327, 2006.

[9]Bakhai A, Stone GW, Mahoney E, et al: Cost effectiveness of paclitaxel-eluting stents for patients undergoing percutaneous coronary revascularization. Results from the TAXUS-IV Trial. *J Am Coll Cardiol* 48:253–261, 2006.

[10]Glaser R, Gertz Z, Matthai WH, et al: Patient satisfaction is comparable to early discharge versus overnight observation after elective percutaneous coronary intervention. *J Invasive Cardiol* 21:464–467, 2009.

an entire episode of care, not simply the procedural costs in the catheterization laboratory (cath lab).

Patient-specific factors such as disease severity affect costs by influencing the type of procedure needed to treat the patient's CAD (e.g., number and type of stents, adjunctive procedures, medications), the associated likelihood of success, and the risks of short-term and long-term complications (e.g., abrupt closure, re-stenosis, stent thrombosis). Procedures in patients with complex lesions (e.g., chronic total occlusions) can be more costly, for example, because success rates are lower and long-term durability of successful dilations is reduced. The extent of CAD also has a modest effect on costs: Costs are lowest in single-vessel disease and highest in three-vessel disease. In addition, diabetes and older age have been associated with modestly higher costs.[7] Recently, patient insurance status has been shown to significantly influence the PCI procedure, with Medicaid and uninsured patients much less likely to receive a DES.[8,9]

Treatment-related factors include decisions made in the cath lab as well as management decisions before and after the procedures. In one large series, physician decision delay (i.e., delay between admission and diagnostic catheterization or between catheterization and revascularization) increased hospital costs by 86%, and weekend delay (procedure postponed because of an intervening weekend) increased costs by 61%.[7] Newer revascularization technologies are associated with significantly higher costs. In a sample of 4375 Medicare patients, use of DESs increased costs by $1882 at 30 days compared with bare metal stents (BMSs), although the difference was reduced to $647 by 1 year because of additional follow-up procedures required by patients receiving BMSs.[10] In addition, use of adjunctive pharmacotherapy also increases costs. In the Enhanced Suppression of the Platelet IIb/IIIa Receptor with Integrilin Therapy (ESPRIT) trial, use of eptifibatide added about $300 net to the hospital costs for PCI.[11] Use of a vascular closure device in one study lowered procedure costs by a very small amount ($44).[12] Same-day discharge after elective PCI in a small randomized study was associated with a savings of $1961 per patient.[13]

Less work has been done to define important hospital-specific or provider-related cost determinants. In a large-claims database, Topol and colleagues found that care at a teaching hospital resulted in lower charges.[14] In 250 patients treated at the University of California, San Francisco (UCSF), the physician operator was a major cost determinant, with the highest-cost physician averaging $4400 more than the lowest-cost physician.[15] This difference was attributed to a more resource-intensive style of practice and not to disease severity or procedure outcome differences. Another study found that high-volume operators (i.e., >50 cases per year) had slightly lower hospital costs than low-volume operators (approximately $300 difference, $P = 0.07$) despite performing more complex procedures on a higher-risk population.[16]

Finally, geographic factors have been infrequently studied but appear to explain modest differences in cost on a national level. In one study, costs in the West were the highest and costs in the Midwest were the lowest.[14]

Costs of Coronary Artery Bypass Grafting

In 2102, patients enrolled in 147 U.S. hospitals in the Pexelizumab for the Reduction of Infarction and Mortality in Coronary Artery Bypass Graft Surgery (PRIMO-CABG) trial, the hospital cost of a CABG (2002–2003) was almost $30,000, with an additional $4000 in physician fees.[17] In 114,233 Medicare patients treated with isolated CABG in 2005, the mean hospitalization cost was $32,201, with a mean length of hospital stay of 9.9 days.[18] As with the costs of PCI described in the previous section, the costs of CABG can be analyzed to identify their major determinants.

Patient characteristics typically account for 25% or less of the variance in hospital costs. In 12,807 patients in New York State who underwent CABG in 1992, patient characteristics accounted for 23% of the variance in log costs.[19] In a cohort of patients receiving their operation at Emory University, the major clinical correlates of higher costs included worse angina class, previous MI, older age, heart failure, and

more extensive CAD, with diabetes being a marginally significant predictor ($P = 0.07$).[20] In contrast, in the Bypass Angioplasty Revascularization Investigation (BARI) study, CABG in patients with diabetes had 5-year costs that were $15,000 higher compared with those in patients without diabetes.[21] In the New York state data referred to earlier, the major predictors of extremely high costs of CABG included older age, non-elective procedure, ejection fraction less than 50%, repeat heart surgery, diabetes, chronic obstructive pulmonary disease, hepatic failure, chronic renal insufficiency, and transfer from another acute care facility.

A retrospective study of 5,549,700 U.S. patients who underwent CABG between 1988 and 2005 found that the incidence of comorbidities increased significantly over the study period.[22] Chronic pulmonary disease went from 8.7% to 20.8%, diabetes from 16.7% to 33.9%, peripheral vascular disease from 4.5% to 10.7%, and cerebral vascular disease from 2.3% to 3.7%. Despite this increase in comorbidities, in-hospital mortality decreased from 4.6% to 2.5%, and length of stay decreased from 11 to 8 days.

Three major procedural factors increase CABG costs: (1) use of an internal mammary artery graft, (2) use of cardiopulmonary bypass, and (3) the need for additional procedures such as valvular repair or replacement.

In a trial conducted at a single academic medical center to assess clinical, economic, and quality-of-life outcomes, 200 patients were randomized to either elective off-pump CABG or to CABG with pulmonary bypass.[23] Follow-up out to 1 year showed similar graft patency; similar rates of death, MI, angina, stroke, and re-intervention procedures; and similar quality-of-life measures. Initial hospitalization costs were $2272 higher in the CABG with bypass arm, and 1-year costs in this arm were $1955 higher. In the Canadian Off-pump CABG Registry, involving 1657 consecutive off-pump patients and 1693 consecutive on-pump patients, the initial hospital costs for off-pump CABG were significantly lower ($11,744 vs. $13,720; $P < 0.01$).[24] These differences persisted out to 1 year.

The Randomized On/Off Bypass (ROOBY) trial assigned 2203 patients scheduled for urgent or elective CABG to either on-pump or off-pump procedures.[25] Patients assigned to off-pump procedures experienced worse graft patency and 1-year outcomes than did those randomized to on-pump procedures. No statistically significant differences were observed between the groups in measurements of resource use, including hours in the operating room, total hours on ventilator, postoperative length of stay in the surgical ICU, or total postoperative length of stay in the hospital.

Complications that occur after surgery (which may reflect a combination of patient-related, treatment-related, and provider-related factors) substantially increase costs. A retrospective study of Medicare beneficiaries undergoing CABG in fiscal year 2005 found the mean cost of the procedure ($32,201) increased by $15,468 and the mean length of hospital stay (9.9 days) increased by 5.3 days in the 14% of patients who experienced complications, including septicemia, postoperative infection, postoperative stroke, renal failure requiring hemodialysis, postoperative respiratory distress syndrome, reoperation, hemorrhage, or postoperative shock.[18]

Hospital-level provider-related factors explain about 40% of the variance in the initial costs of CABG.[19] In a Duke analysis, the attending surgeon was the most important determinant of cost among all factors examined.[26] The most expensive surgeon had a median cost that was $4200 higher than that of the least expensive surgeon. As with PCI costs, the explanation for this appears to lie in a more resource-intensive style of practice rather than in a difference in disease severity or in complication rates. An observational study of 81,289 patients who underwent CABG surgery between October 1, 2003, and September 1, 2005, at 164 hospitals in the United States found that low-volume hospitals and low-volume surgeons were both associated with higher costs.[27] In this same study, adherence to quality measures shortened the length of hospital stay and lowered costs.

A comparison of costs of CABG at five U.S. and four Canadian hospitals, using the same cost accounting software system, showed that

U.S. hospital costs were substantially higher ($20,673 vs. $10,373; $P < 0.001$).[28] These differences were not explained by clinical differences, and length of hospital stay in Canada was 17% longer.

Comparisons of Treatment Options for Coronary Artery Disease

Revascularization versus Medical Therapy in Stable Coronary Artery Disease. In one recent meta-analysis involving 61 trials and over 25,000 patients, PCI demonstrated no advantage over medical therapy in survival or MI risk.[29] A second meta-analysis compared medical therapy with PCI for angina relief. In 14 trials involving 7818 patients, PCI demonstrated an overall benefit in angina relief, but the effect was substantially smaller and not significant in trials performed between 2000 and 2009.[30]

Three contemporary trials have compared the costs of these two strategies. The Clinical Outcomes Utilizing Revascularization and Aggressive DruG Evaluation (COURAGE) trial randomized 2287 patients with evidence of ischemia and significant CAD to undergo either PCI with optimal medical therapy or optimal medical therapy alone. The patients were followed for a period of 2.5 to 7 years, with median follow-up of 4.6 years. In this cohort, the addition of PCI to optimal medical therapy did not reduce the risk of death, MI, or other major cardiovascular events.[31–33] However, the PCI group showed a statistically significant improvement in angina relief and quality of life at 1 month following randomization, with angina relief differences lasting through 24 months but disappearing by 36 months and quality of life differences lasting through 12 months but disappearing by 24 months.[34] The PCI strategy averaged $34,843 in costs per patient over the course of the study compared with $24,718 in the medical-therapy-alone group, with additional costs in the PCI group largely driven by initial procedural costs.[35] On the basis of these trial data, the lifetime incremental cost-effectiveness ratio for PCI was about $168,000 per QALY.

The Bypass Angioplasty Revascularization Investigation 2 Diabetes (BARI 2D) trial tested whether coronary revascularization added to state-of-the-art medical therapy in type 2 diabetics with stable CAD improved all-cause mortality.[36] At 5 years, there were no significant differences between PCI and medical therapy in the rate of death or in the composite endpoint of death, MI, or stroke. Cumulative 4-year costs in the PCI group were $5600 higher than in the medical therapy group ($73,400 for PCI vs. $67,800 for medical therapy, $P < 0.02$).[37] Over lifetime projections, medical therapy would incur minimally higher costs ($200 more than PCI) but have more life-years of survival (14.03 for medical therapy vs. 13.70 for PCI). Medical therapy would be economically attractive at $600 per life-year added compared with PCI in this cohort.

In a study of patients with an occluded infarct-related artery 3 to 28 days after MI, the Occluded Artery Trial (OAT) reported no significant difference between PCI and medical therapy in the composite of death, re-infarction, or hospitalization for New York Heart Association (NYHA) class IV heart failure.[38] An economic analysis was performed in the cohort of 469 U.S. patients enrolled in this trial.[39] The mean cost of hospitalization plus physician fees at 30 days was $22,859 for the PCI group and $12,683 for the medical therapy group. At 2 years, cumulative costs in the PCI group were $7,089 higher ($P < 0.001$) with no significantly different clinical benefit.

Percutaneous Coronary Intervention with Bare Metal Stents versus Coronary Artery Bypass Grafting in Stable Multi-vessel Disease. The most important early trials of PCI versus CABG are instructive but are limited because of significant changes in both procedures and in associated medical therapies relative to contemporary care. Of the trials comparing PTCA and CABG, the BARI trial was the largest, enrolling 1829 patients with multi-vessel CAD at 18 centers between 1988 and 1991. The BARI Substudy of Economics and Quality of Life (SEQOL) enrolled 934 of these patients at the seven largest enrolling sites.[21] Initial costs for the PTCA arm included $14,415 in hospital costs and $6698 in physician fees. For the CABG arm, initial hospital costs amounted to $21,534 and physician fees to $10,813. Total inpatient follow-up costs (hospital and physician fees) were $27,439 for PTCA and $19,529 for CABG. Outpatient follow-up care was equivalent in both arms. The cumulative 5-year cost for medications was higher in the PTCA arm ($4948 vs. $3670). Thus, at the end of 5 years, total discounted costs in the PTCA arm were 5% lower than in the CABG arm ($56,225 vs. $58,889). Five-year costs in patients with two-vessel disease were significantly lower with angioplasty ($52,390 vs. $58,498 for CABG), whereas in three-vessel disease, angioplasty was actually more expensive ($60,918 vs. $59,430). At 12 years of follow-up in the BARI SEQOL study, cumulative costs had narrowed to $120,750 for the PTCA arm versus $123,000 in the CABG arm, and the difference was no longer significant ($P = 0.55$). CABG yielded a cost-effectiveness ratio of $14,300 per life-year added compared with PTCA at 12 years.[40]

The British Randomized Intervention Treatment of Angina (RITA) trial compared the costs of PTCA and CABG (using U.K. costs) in 1011 patients and confirmed the results of the BARI trial.[41] Initial costs of PTCA were half those of CABG, but at the end of 2 years, PTCA costs had risen to 80% of CABG costs.

The Arterial Revascularization Therapies Study (ARTS) I compared PCI with BMS versus CABG in 1205 patients with multi-vessel disease.[42] By 1 year, the major difference between the two arms was a higher repeat revascularization rate in the stent arm (21.2% vs. 3.8% in the CABG arm), a difference that persisted at 3-year follow-up (26.7% vs. 6.6% in the CABG arm). One-year total costs were €11,117 for the stent group versus €13,896 for the CABG group, a difference of €2779. This difference in costs had narrowed to €1798 at the 3-year follow-up, with the stent group showing €14,302 in total costs versus €16,100 for the surgery group. These cost estimates, which were calculated from limited resource use data and European cost weights, appear to underestimate costs as typically seen in the United States. At 5 years, there was no difference in survival or freedom from death, MI, or stroke between the two strategies, but repeat revascularization remained higher in the PCI arm (30% vs. 9%; $P < 0.001$).[43] The diabetes subgroup (208 patients) showed a nonsignificant trend toward higher mortality with PCI (13.4% vs. 8.3%; $P = 0.27$).

Between 1996 and 1999, the Canadian/European Surgery or Stent (SoS) trial randomly assigned 988 patients with typical angina and multi-vessel disease to either PCI with BMS or CABG. In an economic analysis of this trial, initial hospitalizations costs were higher in the CABG arm, and follow-up costs were higher in the PCI arm, consistent with previous trials.[44] Total 1-year follow-up costs in the subgroup of patients with ACS were $6435 for the PCI arm and $8870 for the CABG arm. Total 1-year costs in the non-ACS subgroup were $5069 for the PCI arm and $7487 for the CABG arm. Patients with ACS had significantly higher initial costs and total 1-year costs.

Drug-Eluting Stents versus Bare Metal Stents. Meta-analyses of randomized trials have persuasively shown that use of DESs in PCI, compared with BMSs, has no effect on the rates of death or nonfatal MI.[45] The only endpoint consistently modified by DESs is the need for repeat target lesion revascularization. Further, data from Emory University showed that the occurrence of re-stenosis had no discernible effect on late survival.[46] Thus, the case for the cost-effectiveness of DESs expressed in terms of QALYs gained has rested primarily on the assumption that symptomatic re-stenosis and the need for repeat PCI is associated with a significant disutility. However, a recent study of this question using the time trade-off in 103 patients 2 weeks following PCI found that patients assigned these events a median disutility value of 0.[47] An earlier study of this question using a willingness-to-pay approach in 1642 patients in two PCI trials found that patients were willing to pay $1162 to avoid a 30% chance of re-stenosis and $366 to avoid a 20% chance of re-stenosis.[48] A second more recent analysis of the willingness to pay to eliminate restenosis in 270 patients who received PCIs found the median value of $2802, with higher-income patients willing to pay more.[49] These disparate results suggest that the questions surrounding the economic value of preventing re-stenosis remain unsettled.

In the Sirolimus-Eluting Balloon Expandable Stent in the Treatment of Patients With De Novo Native Coronary Artery Lesions (SIRIUS) trial, 1058 patients with complex coronary disease were randomized to receive either a sirolimus-eluting stent (SES) or a BMS. Cohen and colleagues performed a prospective economic analysis of this trial.[50] They found initial hospital costs per patient to be $2881 higher in the SES arm, but this additional cost had attenuated to $309 at 1 year as costs in the SES arm were reduced because of significant reductions in repeat revascularization rates. The incremental cost-effectiveness ratio for SES versus BMS was $1650 per repeat revascularization avoided. One important caveat about these results is that they were substantively influenced by the protocol of 8 month repeat coronary angiography, which led to a doubling in the rate of late repeat revascularization procedures in the BMS arm and a consequent narrowing in the cost difference between the two arms. If the extra procedures induced by the protocol angiograms are deleted from the calculations, the net cost of the DES strategy in this trial was $1300.

The cost-effectiveness of paclitaxel-eluting stents (PESs) was prospectively examined by Bakhai and colleagues in the TAXUS-IV trial.[51] In this study, 1314 patients undergoing PCIs were randomly assigned to either PESs or BMSs, with follow-up out to 1 year. Index hospitalization costs per patient for the PES arm were $2028 higher when compared with those for the BMS arm. Cost savings of $1456 per patient in the PES arm were realized at 1-year follow-up, primarily owing to reductions in repeat revascularization procedures. The incremental cost-effectiveness of the PES was $4678 per target vessel revascularization avoided and $47,798 per QALY gained.

In the Basel Stent Kasten Effekivitäts Trial (BASKET), 826 consecutive, unselected patients, reflecting "everyday practice," were randomized to DESs (both SESs and PESs were used) or BMSs.[52] After 6 months of follow-up, total costs in the DES arm were €10,544, compared with €9639 in the BMS arm (P < 0.0001). At 18 months, costs in the DES arm were €11,808 compared with €10,450 in the BMS arm.[53] The incremental cost-effectiveness ratio to avoid one major event (cardiac death, MI, or target vessel revascularization) was €64,732, and the cost per QALY gained with DES was €40,467.

Drug-Eluting Stents versus Coronary Artery Bypass Grafting. A meta-analysis of four trials comparing multi-vessel PCI with DES versus CABG (3895 patients) recently reported that major cardiac event rates (death, MI, stroke) were similar in the two arms but that target vessel revascularization was significantly higher in the PCI arm.[54] However, the Arterial Revascularization Therapy Study II (ARTS II) showed that complete revascularization was achieved in 61% of the PCI group versus 84% of the CABG group from ARTS I.[55] Whether such a difference should be expected to translate into measureable differences in long-term patient outcome, such as angina relief and quality of life, remains unclear.

The Synergy between Percutaneous Coronary Intervention with Taxus and Cardiac Surgery (SYNTAX) international trial randomly assigned 1800 patients with three-vessel or left main coronary artery (LMCA) disease to CABG or PCI with PESs.[56] At 12 months, rates of major cardiac or cerebrovascular events (death from any cause, stroke, MI, or repeat revascularization) were lower in the CABG group (12.4% vs. 17.8%, P = 0.002). Repeat revascularization rates were significantly higher in the PCI group, and rates of stroke were significantly higher in the CABG group. Index hospitalization costs were significantly higher in the CABG group ($33,254 vs. $27,560, P < 0.001) as were 12 months of follow-up costs ($39,581 vs. $35,991, P < 0.001).[57] Additional economic and quality-of-life results from this trial are expected.

REPERFUSION OF ACUTE ST ELEVATION MYOCARDIAL INFARCTION

In the United States, more than 200,000 patients each year get acute reperfusion therapy for ST elevation myocardial infarction (STEMI). In registry data from 420 U.S. hospitals involving 78,254 patients with AMI (2001 to 2006), 67% received reperfusion therapy.[58] These data also show that in the U.S., the use of thrombolytic therapy has substantially diminished in recent years in favor of primary PCI, which is now used in about 84% of acute reperfusion cases. Of the 16% of patients with AMI who received thrombolytic therapy, about half went on to subsequent rescue PCI.

Thrombolytic Therapy

The drug costs of thrombolytic therapy are now well known: the average wholesale price for 1.5 million units of streptokinase is about $590; for 100 mg of tissue plasminogen activator (t-PA), it is about $2800; and the same price is applied to both 30 mg of recombinant tissue plasminogen activator (rt-PA) and 50 mg of tenecteplase (TNK) (Fig. 61-2).[49] In the Global Use of Strategies to Open Occluded

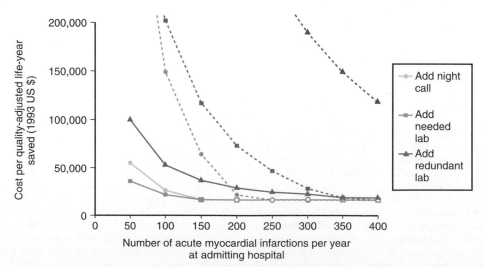

Figure 61-2   Cost per quality-adjusted life-year saved (1993 U.S. dollars) with different options to deliver primary percutaneous coronary intervention (PCI) for acute ST elevation myocardial infarction (STEMI). Solid symbols indicate comparison with thrombolysis. Open symbols indicate comparison with no reperfusion therapy (angioplasty dominant over thrombolysis at those points). Solid lines give three hospital scenarios, with most favorable assumption of efficacy based on pre-GUSTO IIb randomized trials. Dashed lines give three hospital scenarios using effectiveness data from community-based observational studies. *GUSTO IIb*, Global Use of Strategies To Open Occluded Arteries in Acute Coronary Syndromes trial IIb. (*From Lieu TA, Gurley J, Lundstrom RJ, et al: Projected cost-effectiveness of primary angioplasty for acute myocardial infarction, J Am Coll Cardiol 30:1741–1750, 1997. Reprinted with permission from the American College of Cardiology.*)

	Cost-effectiveness Ratios for t-PA as Compared with Streptokinase in the Primary Analysis and Selected Subgroups of Patients in GUSTO I		
TABLE 61-6			

Patient Groups	Increased Life Expectancy with t-PA (Years of Life Saved)		Cost Effectiveness ratio (Dollars per LY Saved)
	UNDISCOUNTED	DISCOUNTED	
Primary Analysis	0.14	0.09	32,678
Inferior MI ≤40	0.03	0.01	203,071
Inferior MI 41–60	0.07	0.04	74,816
Inferior MI 61–75	0.16	0.10	27,873
Inferior MI >75	0.26	0.17	16,246
Anterior MI ≤40	0.04	0.02	123,609
Anterior MI 41–60	0.10	0.06	49,877
Anterior MI 61–75	0.20	0.14	20,601
Anterior MI >75	0.29	0.21	13,410

LY = life year

Data from Mark DB, Hlatky MA, Califf RM, et al. Cost effectiveness of thrombolytic therapy with tissue plasminogen activator as compared with streptokinase for acute myocardial infarction. *N Engl J Med* 1995;332:1418–1424.

Coronary Arteries (GUSTO) I trial, t-PA (alteplase) was shown to save one extra life per 100 patients with AMI shifted from streptokinase and to produce a higher proportion of TIMI grade 3 coronary flow in the infarct vessel. In the prospective GUSTO I trial economic substudy, substitution of an accelerated t-PA regimen for intravenous streptokinase was economically attractive, with a cost-effectiveness ratio of $27,000 to $33,000, depending on the specific assumptions used in the calculations.[59] Subgroup analysis showed that t-PA was modestly more cost effective in anterior MIs but was considerably more effective in older patients (Table 61-6). These results were not substantially altered after taking into account the 1 per 1000 extra nonfatal disabling strokes produced by t PA. Tenecteplase is considered to be as effective as alteplase, has the same acquisition cost, and is preferred by many centers because of its ease of administration (single bolus versus bolus plus infusion).

Primary Percutaneous Coronary Reperfusion

Between 1990 and 2002, a total of 25 RCTs compared primary PCI with thrombolysis. Pooling of patient-level data from 22 of these trials revealed that primary PCI was associated with a 37% reduction in 30-day mortality rates.[60] This advantage was evident both in patients who presented early and in those who presented longer than 4 hours after symptom onset. The benefit of PCI was also sustained in trials with follow-up of 1 year or longer.[61] Angiographic comparisons showed a higher early reperfusion rate and a higher proportion of patients achieving TIMI grade 3 flow. In addition, two early RCTs suggested that direct PTCA might, in fact, be a less expensive reperfusion strategy than t-PA.[62]

The contemporary economic consequences of primary PCI versus thrombolysis have not been studied in the United States. The Stenting versus Thrombolysis in Acute Myocardial Infarction (STAT) trial, a small Canadian study of 123 patients, reported initial hospital costs (in 1999 U.S. dollars) of $6354 for primary PCI and $7893 for t-PA ($P < 0.01$).[63] The cost of t-PA in Canada at the time of the trial was about $1800, whereas the cost of the PCI using BMSs was approximately $2100. The study is difficult to interpret, both because it was unblinded and small and because 64% of the patients in the t-PA arm had an unscheduled coronary angiogram during the index hospitalization. An economic analysis of the Comparison of Angioplasty and Pre-hospital Thrombolysis in Acute Myocardial Infarction (CAPTIM) trial found no difference between the two reperfusion strategies in 1-year outcomes, but costs were lower for primary PCI.[64] The thrombolysis strategy in this trial included the use of rescue PCI, as needed. A small, 104-patient randomized trial in Sweden of primary PCI with enoxaparin and abciximab versus reteplase and enoxaparin found

higher initial treatment costs in the PCI arm, but lower hospitalization costs.[65] Total 1-year costs were similar: $25,313 for PCI versus $27,819 for thrombolysis. Early discharge of low-risk patients who received primary PCI is being explored as a method for reducing total costs of care for this subset of patients.[66]

Lieu and colleagues demonstrated that the costs of a primary PCI strategy vary importantly with the structural details of individual hospital programs.[67] Using a spreadsheet-based model and cost data obtained from a Kaiser Permanente Hospital, they showed that procedural costs varied from $1600 to $14,300, depending on extra costs for night call, annual procedural volume, and, particularly, the need to construct a new cath lab to handle the extra volume.

Using these data in a decision analytic model, along with effectiveness data from published clinical trials and other studies, Lieu and colleagues examined the cost-effectiveness of primary angioplasty.[68] In the base case analysis, they considered the case of a hospital with an existing cath lab with night and weekend coverage that admitted 200 patients with AMI each year. Under these assumptions, primary PCI was cost saving compared with thrombolysis (either t-PA or streptokinase regimens) and had a cost of $12,000 per QALY relative to no reperfusion therapy. In sensitivity analyses, the need to build a new cath lab, the need to add the costs of night call, and a diminution of laboratory volume all significantly increased the cost-effectiveness ratio. A recent analysis of this question found that transporting every patient in a defined cohort to an existing PCI facility was more effective and less costly than strategies involving building new PCI laboratories.[69]

Early Invasive Strategies versus Early Conservative Strategies in Patients with Acute Coronary Syndrome

In the United States, angiography is frequently performed after AMI. In the Acute Coronary Treatment and Intervention Outcomes Network (ACTION) Registry, 83% of 82,004 patients with AMI from 248 U.S. sites had a diagnostic catheterization during the index hospitalization.[70] In the subset with non–ST elevation acute MI (NSTEMI), 46% had PCI, whereas the rate of CABG was about 10%. The decision to refer for diagnostic catheterization in acute coronary disease (ACD) is at best modestly influenced by clinical factors but is substantially influenced by structural aspects of the practice environment, such as the availability of catheterization facilities at the admitting hospital, being admitted by a cardiologist rather than by a generalist, and having an attending cardiologist who performs invasive procedures.

Several major RCTs have compared early invasive management strategies with early conservative management strategies for non–ST elevation ACS. The Treat Angina with Aggrastat and Determine Cost of Therapy with an Invasive or Conservative Strategy (TACTICS-TIMI 18) trial reflects contemporary management, with coronary stents used in more than 80% of patients undergoing PCI and all patients receiving an intravenous glycoprotein (GP) IIb/IIIa inhibitor (tirofiban).[71] Diagnostic catheterization was performed in 51% of patients receiving early conservative management and in 97% of those receiving early invasive management. At 6 months, the early invasive arm had 2 per 1000 fewer deaths and 20 per 1000 fewer MIs. Economic analysis of this trial found that the early invasive arm had higher initial costs ($15,714 vs. $14,047) and lower follow-up costs out to 6 months ($6098 vs. $7180).[72] Cumulative 6-month costs were very similar. Cost per life-year added was estimated at $13,000.

The Fragmin and Revascularization during Instability in Coronary Artery Disease II (FRISC II) trial compared an invasive strategy (diagnostic catheterization rate, 96%) with a noninvasive strategy (diagnostic catheterization rate, 10%) in 2457 patients with ACS. At 1 year, the invasively treated group had a mortality rate of 2.2% compared with 3.9% in the noninvasive strategy group ($P = 0.016$); the corresponding rates for MI were 8.6% and 11.6%, respectively ($P = 0.015$).[73] The invasive strategy was also associated with a reduction in re-admissions (37% vs. 57%; $P < 0.001$) and (repeat) revascularization (7.5% vs. 31%; $P < 0.001$). An economic analysis of the Fast Revascularization During Instability in Coronary Artery Disease II (FRISC II) trial from the

Swedish perspective has been published. At the end of 1 year, cumulative costs in the invasive arm were SEK201,622 (U.S. $20,072) versus SEK177,746 (U.S. $16,939) for the noninvasive arm, leaving the invasive arm with a $3,133 cost at the end of 1 year. Five-year follow-up from this trial has recently been published.[74] Mortality was 9.7% in the invasive group and 10.1% in the noninvasive group (P = 0.69). Nonfatal MI rates were 12.9% in the invasive group and 17.7% in the noninvasive group (P = 0.002).

In contrast to the Treat angina with Aggrastat and determine Cost of Therapy with Invasive or Conservative Strategy (TACTICS)-TIMI 18 and FRISC II trials, the Invasive versus Conservative Treatment in Unstable Coronary Syndromes (ICTUS) trial of 1200 patients with ACS and elevated troponins failed to find any evidence of benefit from a reduction in hard cardiac events for the early invasive strategy.[75] A meta-analysis of seven trials involving 8375 patients and a mean follow-up of 2 years reported a 25% reduction in all-cause mortality and a 17% reduction in nonfatal MI for early invasive management.[76] However, these results did not take into account the heterogeneous varieties of "early invasive" management represented in the seven trials, with hospital angiography rates ranging from 10% to more than 50%. The more aggressive the "early conservative" arm, the more difficult it is to demonstrate any incremental benefit to routine early angiography. The most optimistic estimates of benefit for the early invasive strategy were seen in the smallest trial and in the trial with the most conservative version of the early conservative management strategy.

ANTI-PLATELET THERAPY

Use of intravenous GP IIb/IIIa blockers in ACS has now been extensively studied.[77] In pooled analyses, a short course of tirofiban or eptifibatide has reduced absolute 30-day death or MI rates by 1.5% (Platelet Glycoprotein IIb/IIIa in Unstable Angina: Receptor Suppression Using Integrilin Therapy [PURSUIT] trial) to 3.2% (Platelet Receptor Inhibition in Ischemic Syndrome Management in Patients Limited by Unstable Signs and Symptoms [PRISM PLUS] trial) with most of the effect on nonfatal MI. Two of the largest trials—Platelet Receptor Inhibition for Ischemic Syndrome Management (PRISM) and PRISM-PLUS—studied tirofiban, and PURSUIT used eptifibatide and GUSTO IV tested abciximab. Of these, only PURSUIT has published an economic analysis.[78] In the 3522 U.S. patients enrolled in the trial, there was no evidence that eptifibatide use altered resource use or costs through either a positive or a negative effect on clinical course. The absence of an effect on resource use despite reduced ischemic complications may be related to the very high (85%) rate of routine diagnostic catheterization in the U.S. cohort. The cost of the eptifibatide regimen was $1014, and the 3.5% absolute reduction in death or MI at 30 days in the U.S. cohort translated into an incremental life expectancy of 0.11 life-years per patient added by eptifibatide. The resulting cost-effectiveness ratio was $13,700 per added life-year.

In PCI populations, GP IIb/IIIa blockers reduced death, MI, or urgent revascularization by 33%.[79] Five trials with prospective economic analysis have been concluded, three with abciximab and one each with tirofiban and eptifibatide. The Evaluation of Platelet IIb/IIIa Inhibitor for Stenting (EPISTENT) trial extended the Evaluation of PTCA to Improve Long-term Outcome by c7E3 GP IIb/IIIa Receptor Blockade (EPILOG) trial results to the use of stenting. Patients were randomized to stenting with abciximab, stenting with placebo, or balloon angioplasty with abciximab. Prospective economic analysis in the 1438 U.S. patients showed that costs for the baseline hospitalization differed only in the costs of the stents and abciximab used: $13,228 for stent plus abciximab, $11,923 for stent plus placebo, and $11,357 for balloon plus abciximab.[80] Thus, stent plus abciximab therapy was $1300 more expensive than stent plus placebo and almost $1900 more expensive than balloon plus abciximab arm. In follow-up, the two stent groups had similar costs, whereas the balloon plus abciximab group exceeded these groups by more than $900. Therefore, at 1 year, the stent plus abciximab arm was $930 more expensive than balloon plus abciximab. At 1 year, 1% of the stent plus abciximab group had died,

compared with 2.4% of the stent plus placebo patients and 2.1% of balloon plus abciximab patients. Incremental life expectancy was projected from these data and used to calculate cost-effectiveness ratios. For stent plus abciximab relative to stent plus placebo, the cost to add a life-year was $6200; relative to balloon plus abciximab, the cost to add a life-year was $5300.

The European/Australasian Stroke Prevention in Reversible Ischaemia Trial (ESPRIT) (1999–2000) randomized 2064 patients undergoing PCI with stenting to either eptifibatide or placebo. The eptifibatide arm had reduced ischemic complications. The cost of the eptifibatide regimen was $495. Total hospital costs (including eptifibatide) were $10,721 for the eptifibatide arm versus $10,430 for placebo, an incremental cost of $291 per patient.[11] Follow-up costs out to 1 year were $2121 for eptifibatide versus $2254 for placebo. Therefore, the net 1-year costs of the eptifibatide strategy were $146. At 1 year, eptifibatide was associated with 6 per 1000 fewer deaths (P = 0.28) and 35 per 1000 fewer MIs (P = 0.004). This translated into 0.104 added life-years per patient (discounted at 3%) and a cost-effectiveness ratio of $1407 per added life-year.

Several studies have examined the economics of the use of oral adenosine diphosphate (ADP) receptor antagonist anti-platelet agents after PCI. In the PCI-CURE substudy of the Clopidogrel in Unstable angina to Prevent Recurrent Events (CURE) trial (1998–2000), 2658 patients were randomized to clopidogrel or placebo after PCI for a mean of 8 months. Clopidogrel reduced the rate of cardiovascular death or MI by 25% but had no effect on cardiovascular death alone. The cost per day of the clopidogrel therapy was $3.22, which was largely offset by reductions in complications, so at the end of 1 year, the net cost of the clopidogrel strategy was between $250 and $425.[81] Incremental cost-effectiveness was less than $5000 per life-year gained, making clopidogrel use in this setting highly economically attractive. The Clopidogrel for the Reduction of Events During Observation (CREDO) trial showed similar results for clopidogrel loading before PCI followed by 1 year of clopidogrel therapy, with incremental cost-effectiveness ratios (ICERs) ranging from $2929 to $4353 per life-year saved compared with placebo.[82] Two decision-model-based analyses of the use of clopidogrel for 1 year after PCI found slightly higher ICERs of $15,696 per life-year saved in the United States and €10,993 in Sweden.[83,84]

In the Trial to Assess Improvement in Therapeutic Outcomes by Optimizing Platelet Inhibition with Prasugrel Thrombolysis in Myocardial Infarction (TRITON-TIMI)-38, over 13,600 patients with moderate- to high-risk ACS scheduled for PCI were randomized to receive a loading dose of prasugrel or clopidogrel followed by a maintenance dose for 6 to 15 months. The prasugrel group experienced significantly fewer events in the combined endpoint of cardiovascular death, nonfatal MI, or nonfatal stroke (9.9% prasugrel vs. 12.1% clopidogrel, P < 0.001), as well as significantly fewer urgent target vessel revascularizations and stent thromboses. Patients receiving prasugrel had significantly higher rates of major bleeding (2.4% prasugrel vs. 1.8% clopidogrel, P < 0.03). An economic evaluation of this trial found average total costs over a median 14.7 months follow-up were $221 lower for those randomized to receive prasugrel.[85] Primarily because of the significantly lower rate of nonfatal MI, the prasugrel group showed a life expectancy gain of 0.102 year over the clopidogrel group rendering prasugrel the dominant therapy.

The Study of Platelet Inhibition and Patient Outcomes (PLATO) trial randomized 18,624 patients with ACS to receive ticagrelor (180 mg loading dose, 90 mg twice daily maintenance dose) or clopidogrel (300 to 600 mg loading dose, 75 mg daily maintenance dose).[86] The primary endpoint was a composite of death from vascular causes, MI, or stroke. At 12 months, the ticagrelor group reached significantly fewer primary endpoints (9.8% ticagrelor vs. 11.7% clopidogrel), and the rate of death from any cause was also significantly reduced with ticagrelor (4.5% ticagrelor vs. 5.9% clopidogrel). One of the complexities of this trial is the apparent lack of incremental efficacy of ticagrelor in the North American subset. A prospective economic analysis of this trial is expected to report results in 2012.

ANTI-THROMBIN THERAPY

On the basis of several small trials showing a reduction in death and nonfatal MI, heparin has been established as standard therapy for moderate-risk or high-risk patients with unstable angina. Several studies have been conducted with low-molecular-weight heparins (LMWHs) in patients with ACS. Enoxaparin was the first LMWH to be tested in a clinical trial that incorporated a prospective economic analysis. The Efficacy and Safety of Subcutaneous Enoxaparin in Non-Q Wave Coronary Events (ESSENCE) trial randomized 3171 patients with non-STEMI ACS in North and South America and Europe. At the end of 14 days, the enoxaparin therapy had resulted in a significant 15% lower rate of death, MI, or refractory angina (the primary endpoint) relative to standard unfractionated heparin (UH) therapy. Economic analysis of this trial, performed in the 923 patients randomized in the United States, showed that the enoxaparin regimen cost $75 more than standard heparin therapy. At the end of the initial hospitalization, the enoxaparin arm had not only recouped this cost difference but had also produced a cost savings of more than $700 owing to reduced invasive cardiac procedures and a small concurrent reduction in length of hospital stay. At 30 days, the cost advantage for the enoxaparin arm had risen to $1100.

The Superior Yield of the New Strategy of Enoxaparin Revascularization and Glycoprotein IIb/IIIa Inhibitors (SYNERGY) trial compared subcutaneous enoxaparin versus intravenous heparin in 10,027 patients with NSTEMI ACS (2001–2003).[87] No difference was observed in the primary endpoint of death or nonfatal MI. In addition, enoxaparin was associated with a moderate increase in major bleeding. Compared with earlier trials making this same comparison, the SYNERGY patients were older, and both the medical and interventional therapies were more aggressive. Whether these differences explain the lack of superiority for enoxaparin in SYNERGY remains unclear.

The Organization to Assess Strategies in Acute Ischemic Syndromes (OASIS-5) trial randomly assigned 20,078 NSTEMI ACS patients to fondaparinux or enoxaparin and reported no significant difference in the composite endpoint of death, MI, or refractory ischemia at 9 days.[88] However, fondaparinux did significantly reduce major bleeding events and death at 30 days and at 180 days. The cost analysis of this trial found using fondaparinux instead of clopidogrel would produce a cost saving of $547 per patient at 180 days, and long-term cost-effectiveness analysis found fondaparinux to be the dominant therapy.[89]

The FRISC II investigators prospectively examined the cost-effectiveness of extended treatment with dalteparin in 2267 patients with unstable CAD.[90] After a minimum of 5 days' open-label dalteparin treatment, patients were randomized to 3 months of subcutaneous dalteparin twice daily or to placebo. The dalteparin arm produced a significant reduction in death or MI at 1 month, at an additional cost of SEK849. The cost-effectiveness ratio was SEK30,300 per death or MI avoided. Despite these early gains, no significant difference was detected in death or MI between the two arms at 3 months.

Bivalirudin plus provisional GP IIb/IIIa inhibition was found to provide similar cardiac event rates out to 1 year while reducing the risk of severe bleeding events compared with routine GP IIb/IIIa inhibition plus heparin in the Randomized Evaluation in PCI Linking Angiomax to Reduced Clinical Events (REPLACE)-2 trial, a randomized, double-blind trial of 4651 U.S. patients undergoing non-emergent PCI.[91] Cohen and colleagues conducted a prospective economic evaluation of this study and found that bivalirudin produced a cost savings of $375 to $400 per patient at 30 days, primarily because of the reduction in bleeding episodes.[92]

PREVENTIVE THERAPIES

A number of secondary prevention programs have been shown to be effective in large-scale clinical trials and have also been shown to be economically attractive. These include statin therapy, smoking cessation interventions, aspirin therapy, β-blockers following MI, and angiotensin-converting enzyme (ACE) inhibitors for MI survivors with depressed left ventricular function. These data are reviewed elsewhere.[2]

Cost-Effectiveness and Health Policy

From 1994 to 1999, managed care had an almost unprecedented inhibitory effect on the growth of health care spending in the United States. During this period, the proportion of the gross domestic product (GDP) devoted to health care remained stable at 13% to 13.3%. The era of managed care acting as a restraining influence on health care spending is now history. Growth in annual medical spending has gone back up, and current estimates are that the United States is devoting 17.6% of its GDP to health care. Current projections are that medical costs will continue to grow into the foreseeable future, and this unrestrained growth is considered the number-one threat to the future fiscal health of the United States. The effect of the 2010 Patient Protection and Affordable Care Act on the national debt is currently very uncertain, as much depends on future decisions about spending in the Medicare program versus additional tax revenue for the federal government, both of which are heavily influenced by political pressures.

Any future health care reform that succeeds in restraining total annual U.S. medical care spending (public and private) will indirectly force patients to compete for health care resources and will directly force providers and policymakers to make more explicit decisions about which types of care are worthwhile.

As described in this chapter, defining the cost of medical care is an important first step. But when the overall goal is to choose the types of care to provide from among the available alternatives, cost must be explicitly tied to the health benefits produced, and the benefits must be valued in some uniform, comparable currency.

A host of controversial and complex allocation decisions will be required if providers can no longer count on payers to cover all the care they believe is appropriate for their patients. In the view of some, cost-effectiveness analysis provides the soundest and most logical method for making decisions about health care allocation. Canada, the United Kingdom, and other countries that seek to maximize health benefits within a fixed budget are much more receptive than the United States to the use of cost effectiveness as a decision aid. The Oregon Medicaid reform plan of the early 1990s attempted to make cost effectiveness the primary criterion for determining what to cover in the program. Although general conclusions from the Oregon experience were that current methodology and data were insufficient to permit a comprehensive cost-effectiveness ranking of all health care services and that ranking services by cost-effectiveness was also politically problematic, some aspects of the program remain in place and have guided coverage policy.[93]

Methodologic issues provide important challenges to the use of cost-effectiveness analysis as the primary tool for health care spending decisions. Principal among these is the absence of any uniform method for measuring either health care benefits or costs for use in cost-effectiveness analysis.

On the effectiveness side, several major problems face the analyst. Chief among these is the difficulty in accurately estimating the change in life expectancy attributable to a new therapeutic strategy. Unless the disease process under study is rapidly fatal, it is virtually impossible to obtain timely empirical life-expectancy data for use in cost-effectiveness calculations. Most commonly, analysts use survival or mortality rate measures at selected times, such as 30 days, 1 year, or 5 years, and attempt to project life expectancy from these figures with the aid of simple parametric survival modes. Examples include the Markov model and the Declining Exponential Approximation of Life Expectancy (DEALE) model. Other, more empirical, approaches have recently been developed.[78,94] Because currently there is no way to validate such projections and no gold standard to aid in choosing from among competing methods for making them, different analysts may come to substantially different conclusions about the effects on life expectancy of a given therapy.

Substantial additional difficulties arise if the analyst wishes to move from survival (cost-effectiveness analysis) to quality-adjusted survival (cost-utility analysis). No standard approach has been agreed on for quality adjustment of life expectancy figures, although QALYs have been used most often. One of the major assumptions of the QALY construct is that for a given person, it is possible to identify some point of indifference between living x years with some disease state or health impairment and living y years (where $y < x$) in full health. Another assumption is that improving the quality of life for one type of patient may provide more societal "value" than saving the life of another type of patient. Two main approaches have been used to derive the quality weights or utilities employed in calculating QALYs: (1) the standard reference gamble, and (2) the time trade-off technique. In each case, the resulting measure is presumed to reflect patient preferences in a way that would allow prediction of their future economic behavior (specifically, their purchase of future health care).

The advantage of the QALY for economic analysis is that it permits reduction of all survival, quality-of-life, and patient preference issues to a single measure. Whether such a reduction is valid or even appropriate continues to be vigorously debated among health policy investigators.

Critics of the QALY construct have pointed out that some of its major assumptions are probably invalid. For example, none of the current estimation methods take into account that good health is likely to be more highly valued at some stages in life (e.g., childrearing years) than at others. In addition, calculation of QALYs requires the assumption that patient preferences for different health states do not depend on the length of time spent in those states. Important technical issues relating to QALYs remain unsettled. For example, should ratings of disease states be obtained from patients who actually have the disease, from members of the general public asked to imagine that they have the disease, or from members of the medical profession familiar with the disease and its manifestations? Some data suggest that patient preferences (and consequently QALYs) may not be stable over time and that they are strongly influenced by the context of the assessment in which they are measured. Some have argued that QALYs and other utility scales are uniquely personal and cannot be averaged across a population, as is required in cost-effectiveness analysis. Furthermore, use of average utilities in cost-effectiveness analyses maximizes community preferences over those of the individual and raises important ethical questions. As might be expected, recent research has shown that different approaches to calculating quality-adjusted survival may yield significant differences in resulting cost-effectiveness ratios.

Finally, cost-effectiveness studies may differ substantially in the methodology used to estimate costs. Some use carefully measured data obtained from RCTs or observational studies, whereas others use expert opinions. As discussed earlier in the chapter, actually two factors must be estimated: (1) what resources were consumed in what quantities and (2) the associated unit costs. Often, none of the cost data used in cost-effectiveness models are derived from empirical research. In addition, substantial assumptions are required to project the lifetime health care costs of a cohort of patients. Although the importance of such assumptions can be examined through sensitivity analyses, as with life expectancy estimates, these data are rarely tested against empirical observations.

Thus, cost-effectiveness ratios are calculated by multiplying two imprecise measures—life expectancy gained and utilities of those years—and dividing the result into a third imprecise measure, the lifetime incremental costs. The resulting measure is necessarily imprecise. Despite these substantial limitations, which can severely limit the validity of comparing cost-effectiveness ratios from different studies, "league tables" providing such comparisons are common (Table 61-7). These figures, which are usually presented without any variability or distributional information, appear misleadingly precise and rigorous.

Several groups have proposed standards for cost-effectiveness analysis, thereby addressing some of the potential weaknesses described

TABLE 61-7	Cost-Effectiveness and Use of Selected Interventions in the Medicare Population*
Intervention	*Cost-Effectiveness (Cost/QALY)[†]*
Influenza vaccine	Cost saving
Pneumococcal vaccine	Cost saving
β-Blockers after myocardial infarction	<$10,000
Mammographic screening	$10,000–$25,000
Colon-cancer screening	$10,000–$25,000
Osteoporosis screening	$10,000–$25,000
Management of anti-depressants	Cost saving up to $30,000
Hypertension medication (DBP >105 mm Hg)	$10,000–$60,000
Cholesterol management, as secondary prevention	$10,000–$50,000
Implantable cardioverter defibrillator	$30,000–$85,000
Dialysis in end-stage renal disease	$50,000–$100,000
Lung-volume-reduction surgery	$100,000–$300,000
Left ventricular assist devices	$500,000–$1.4 million
Positron emission tomography in Alzheimer's disease	Dominated[‡]

*Ranges, rather than point estimates, are provided because the actual cost effectiveness will vary according to the target populations and the strategies used.

[†]Calculation based on 2002 U.S. dollars.

[‡]Benefits are lower and costs are higher compared with the use of the standard workup.

DBP, diastolic blood pressure; *QALY*, quality-adjusted life-year.

(Modified from Sanders GD, Hlatky MA, Owens DK: Cost-effectiveness of implantable cardioverter-defibrillators, *N Engl J Med* 353:1471–1480, 2005, with permission.)

earlier. The Panel on Cost Effectiveness in Health and Medicine convened by the U.S. Public Health Service, in particular, has generated a carefully researched monograph that should help to advance work in this area.[95] A number of commentators have noted that if cost-effectiveness assessment were an expensive new technology (which, in a sense, it is), health policy analysts would demand rigorous evaluations before it was unleashed on the public. In 2010, the Congress created a new Patient Centered Outcomes Research Institute to help support health reform and specifically prohibited it from using cost per QALYs thresholds for decision making.[96] Despite this apparent vote of no confidence, cost-effectiveness analysis is extremely useful when it focuses and informs professional and public debates, and much additional research is needed in this area.

Summary

The question of how much of societal resources to devote to health care is not one that can be settled by economic analysis. Rather, it is a political and ethical question that reflects, at least in part, the type of society we are (or purport to be) and our willingness to accept the necessity of trade-offs in a world of finite resources. In this context, the role of medical economic analysis is to define the relationship between dollars expended and benefits gained. Although the primary goal of economic analysis is theoretically to maximize efficient use of available health care resources, many pitfalls, both technical and ethical, separate theory from practice. Uncritical acceptance by medical professionals of the results of economic analyses does not serve the interests of patients any more than does uncritical acceptance of the dictates of any one RCT. However, uninformed skepticism applied uniformly to all economic analyses serves no useful purpose either. Much remains to be done to improve the empirical base and methodology of health care economic research. For this to happen, cost outcomes (with all their shortcomings) must become as much a routine part of clinical research as mortality and morbidity outcomes are now.

REFERENCES

1. Roger VL, Go AS, Lloyd-Jones DM, et al: Heart disease and stroke statistics—2011 update: A report from the American Heart Association. *Circulation* 123(4):e18–e209, 2010.
2. Mark DB: Medical economics in cardiovascular medicine. In Topol EJ, editor: *Textbook of cardiovascular medicine*, Philadelphia, 2006, Lippincott Williams & Wilkins.
3. Hsiao WC, Braun P, Dunn D, et al: Results and policy implications of the resource-based relative-value study. *N Engl J Med* 319:881–888, 1988.
4. Feit F, Mueller HS, Braunwald E, et al: Thrombolysis in Myocardial Infarction (TIMI) phase II trial: Outcome comparison of a "conservative strategy" in community versus tertiary hospitals. The TIMI Research Group. *J Am Coll Cardiol* 16:1529–1534, 1990.
5. Kugelmass AD, Cohen DJ, Brown PP, et al: Hospital resources consumed in treating complications associated with percutaneous coronary interventions. *Am J Cardiol* 97:322–327, 2006.
6. Jacobson KM, Hall LK, McMurtry EK, et al: The economic burden of complications during percutaneous coronary intervention. *Qual Saf Health Care* 16:154–159, 2007.
7. Ellis SG, Miller DP, Brown KJ, et al: In-hospital cost of percutaneous coronary revascularization. Critical determinants and implications. *Circulation* 92:741–747, 1995.
8. Gaglia MA, Jr, Torguson R, Xue Z, et al: Insurance type influences the use of drug-eluting stents. *JACC Cardiovasc Interv* 3:773–779, 2010.
9. Kao J, Vicuna R, House JA, et al: Disparity in drug-eluting stent utilization by insurance type. *Am Heart J* 156:1133–1140, 2008.
10. Groeneveld PW, Matta MA, Greenhut AP, et al: The costs of drug-eluting coronary stents among Medicare beneficiaries. *Am Heart J* 155:1097–1105, 2008.
11. Cohen DJ, O'Shea JC, Pacchiana CM, et al: In-hospital costs of coronary stent implantation with and without eptifibatide (the ESPRIT Trial). Enhanced suppression of the platelet IIb/IIIa receptor with integrilin. *Am J Cardiol* 89:61–64, 2002.
12. Resnic FS, Arora N, Matheny M, et al: A cost-minimization analysis of the angio-seal vascular closure device following percutaneous coronary intervention. *Am J Cardiol* 99:766–770, 2007.
13. Glaser R, Gertz Z, Matthai WH, et al: Patient satisfaction is comparable to early discharge versus overnight observation after elective percutaneous coronary intervention. *J Invasive Cardiol* 21:464–467, 2009.
14. Topol EJ, Ellis SG, Cosgrove DM, et al: Analysis of coronary angioplasty practice in the United States with an insurance-claims data base. *Circulation* 87:1489–1497, 1993.
15. Heidenreich PA, Chou TM, Amidon TM, et al: Impact of the operating physician on costs of percutaneous transluminal coronary angioplasty. *Am J Cardiol* 77:1169–1173, 1996.
16. Shook TL, Sun GW, Burstein S, et al. Comparison of percutaneous transluminal coronary angioplasty outcome and hospital costs for low-volume and high volume operators. *Am J Cardiol* 77:331–336, 1996.
17. Chen JC, Kaul P, Levy JH, et al: Myocardial infarction following coronary artery bypass graft surgery increases healthcare resource utilization. *Crit Care Med* 35:1296–1301, 2007
18. Brown PP, Kugelmass AD, Cohen DJ, et al: The frequency and cost of complications associated with coronary artery bypass grafting surgery: Results from the United States Medicare program. *Ann Thorac Surg* 85:1980–1986, 2008.
19. Cowper PA, DeLong ER, Peterson ED, et al: Variability in cost of coronary bypass surgery in New York State: Potential for cost savings. *Am Heart J* 143:130–139, 2002.
20. Mauldin PD, Becker ER, Phillips VL, et al. Hospital resource utilization during coronary artery bypass surgery. *J Interv Cardiol* 7:379–384, 1994.
21. Hlatky MA, Rogers WJ, Johnstone I, et al: Medical care costs and quality of life after randomization to coronary angioplasty or coronary bypass surgery. Bypass Angioplasty Revascularization Investigation (BARI) Investigators. *N Engl J Med* 336:92–99, 1997.
22. Song HK, Diggs BS, Slater MS, et al: Improved quality and cost-effectiveness of coronary artery bypass grafting in the United States from 1988 to 2005. *J Thorac Cardiovasc Surg* 137:65–69, 2009.
23. Puskas JD, Williams WH, Mahoney EM, et al: Off-pump vs conventional coronary artery bypass grafting: Early and 1-year graft patency, cost, and quality-of-life outcomes: a randomized trial. *JAMA* 291:1841–1849, 2004.
24. Lamy A, Wang X, Farrokhyar F, et al: A cost comparison of off-pump CABG versus on-pump CABG at one-year: The Canadian off-pump CABG registry. *Can J Cardiol* 22:699–704, 2006.
25. Shroyer AL, Grover FL, Hattler B, et al: On-pump versus off-pump coronary-artery bypass surgery. *N Engl J Med* 361:1827–1837, 2009.
26. Smith LR, Milano CA, Molter BS, et al: Preoperative determinants of postoperative costs associated with coronary artery bypass graft surgery. *Circulation* 90:II124–II128, 1994.
27. Auerbach AD, Hilton JF, Maselli J, et al: Case volume, quality of care, and care efficiency in coronary artery bypass surgery. *Arch Intern Med* 170:1202–1208, 2010.
28. Eisenberg MJ, Filion KB, Azoulay A, et al: Outcomes and cost of coronary artery bypass graft surgery in the United States and Canada. *Arch Intern Med* 165:1506–1513, 2005.
29. Trikalinos TA, sheikh-Ali AA, Tatsioni A, et al: Percutaneous coronary interventions for non-acute coronary artery disease: A quantitative 20-year synopsis and a network meta-analysis. *Lancet* 373:911–918, 2009.
30. Wijeysundera HC, Nallamothu BK, Krumholz HM, et al: Meta-analysis: Effects of percutaneous coronary intervention versus medical therapy on angina relief. *Ann Intern Med* 152:370–379, 2010.
31. Boden WE, O'Rourke RA, Teo KK, et al: Design and rationale of the Clinical Outcomes Utilizing Revascularization and Aggressive DruG Evaluation (COURAGE) trial Veterans Affairs Cooperative Studies Program no. 424. *Am Heart J* 151:1173–1179, 2006.
32. Weintraub WS, Barnett P, Chen S, et al: Economics methods in the Clinical Outcomes Utilizing percutaneous coronary Revascularization and Aggressive Guideline-driven drug Evaluation (COURAGE) trial. *Am Heart J* 151:1180–1185, 2006.
33. Boden WE, O'Rourke RA, Teo KK, et al: Optimal medical therapy with or without PCI for stable coronary disease. *N Engl J Med* 356:1503–1516, 2007.
34. Weintraub WS, Spertus JA, Kolm P, et al: Effect of PCI on quality of life in patients with stable coronary disease. *N Engl J Med* 359:677–687, 2008.
35. Weintraub WS, Boden WE, Zhang Z, et al: Cost-effectiveness of percutaneous coronary intervention in optimally treated stable coronary patients. *Circ Cardiovasc Qual Outcomes* 1:12–20, 2008.
36. Frye RL, August P, Brooks MM, et al: A randomized trial of therapies for type 2 diabetes and coronary artery disease. *N Engl J Med* 360:2503–2515, 2009.
37. Hlatky MA, Boothroyd DB, Melsop KA, et al: Economic outcomes of treatment strategies for type 2 diabetes mellitus and coronary artery disease in the Bypass Angioplasty Revascularization Investigation 2 Diabetes trial. *Circulation* 120:2550–2558, 2009.
38. Hochman JS, Lamas GA, Buller CE, et al: Coronary intervention for persistent occlusion after myocardial infarction. *N Engl J Med* 355:2395–2407, 2006.
39. Mark DB, Pan W, Clapp-Channing NE, et al: Quality of life after late invasive therapy for occluded arteries. *N Engl J Med* 360:774–783, 2009.
40. Hlatky MA, Boothroyd DB, Melsop KA, et al: Medical costs and quality of life 10 to 12 years after randomization to angioplasty or bypass surgery for multivessel coronary artery disease. *Circulation* 110:1960–1966, 2004.
41. Sculpher MJ, Seed P, Henderson RA, et al: Health service costs of coronary angioplasty and coronary artery bypass surgery: The Randomised Intervention Treatment of Angina (RITA) trial. *Lancet* 344:927–930, 1994.
42. Legrand VM, Serruys PW, Unger F, et al: Three-year outcome after coronary stenting versus bypass surgery for the treatment of multivessel disease. *Circulation* 109:1114–1120, 2004.
43. Serruys PW, Ong AT, van Herwerden LA, et al: Five-year outcomes after coronary stenting versus bypass surgery for the treatment of multivessel disease: The final analysis of the Arterial Revascularization Therapies Study (ARTS) randomized trial. *J Am Coll Cardiol* 46:575–581, 2005.
44. Zhang Z, Spertus JA, Mahoney EM, et al: The impact of acute coronary syndrome on clinical, economic, and cardiac-specific health status after coronary artery bypass surgery versus stent-assisted percutaneous coronary intervention: 1-year results from the stent or surgery (SoS) trial. *Am Heart J* 150:175–181 2005,.
45. Roiron C, Sanchez P, Bouzamondo A, et al: Drug eluting stents: An updated meta analysis of randomised controlled trials. *Heart* 92:641–649, 2006.
46. Weintraub WS, Ghazzal ZM, Douglas JS, Jr, et al: Long-term clinical follow-up in patients with angiographic restudy after successful angioplasty. *Circulation* 87:831–840, 1993.
47. Ploegmakers MM, Viscaal AM, Finch L, et al: The disutility of restenosis—the impact of repeat percutaneous coronary intervention on quality of life. *Can J Cardiol* 26:197–200, 2010.
48. Greenberg D, Bakhai A, Neumann PJ, et al: Willingness to pay for avoiding coronary restenosis and repeat revascularization: Results from a contingent valuation study. *Health Policy* 70:207–216, 2004.
49. Guertin JR, Liu A, Abrahamowicz M, et al: Willingness to pay to eliminate the risk of restenosis following percutaneous coronary intervention: A contingent valuation. *Circ Cardiovasc Qual Outcomes* 4(1):46–52, 2011.
50. Cohen DJ, van Hout B, Juliard JMJ, et al: Economic Outcomes After Coronary Stenting or Balloon Angioplasty in the BENESTENT II Trial: The US perspective. *Circulation* 96:455A, 1997.
51. Bakhai A, Stone GW, Mahoney E, et al: Cost effectiveness of paclitaxel-eluting stents for patients undergoing percutaneous coronary revascularization: Results from the TAXUS-IV Trial. *J Am Coll Cardiol* 48:253–261, 2006.
52. Kaiser C, Brunner-La Rocca HP, Buser PT, et al: Incremental cost-effectiveness of drug-eluting stents compared with a third-generation bare-metal stent in a real-world setting: Randomised Basel Stent Kosten Effektivitats Trial (BASKET). *Lancet* 366:921–929, 2005.
53. Brunner-La Rocca HP, Kaiser C, Bernheim A, et al: Cost-effectiveness of drug-eluting stents in patients at high or low risk of major cardiac events in the Basel Stent Kosten Effektivitats Trial (BASKET): An 18-month analysis. *Lancet* 370:1552–1559, 2007.
54. From AM, Al Badarin FJ, Cha SS, et al: Percutaneous coronary intervention with drug-eluting stents versus coronary artery bypass surgery for multivessel coronary artery disease: A meta-analysis of data from the ARTS II, CARDia, ERACI III, and SYNTAX studies and systematic review of observational data. *EuroIntervention* 6:269–276, 2010.
55. Sarno G, Garg S, Onuma Y, et al: Impact of completeness of revascularization on the five-year outcome in percutaneous coronary intervention and coronary artery bypass graft patients (from the ARTS-II study). *Am J Cardiol* 106:1369–1375, 2010.
56. Serruys PW, Morice MC, Kappetein AP, et al: Percutaneous coronary intervention versus coronary-artery bypass grafting for severe coronary artery disease. *N Engl J Med* 360:961–972, 2009.
57. Cohen DJ, Lavelle TA, Serruys PW, et al: Health related quality of life and U.S. based economic outcomes of PCI with drug-eluting stents vs. bypass surgery for patients with 3-vessel and left main coronary artery disease: 1-year results from the SYNTAX trial, American College of Cardiology 2009 Scientific Sessions.
58. Jneid H, Fonarow GC, Cannon CP, et al: Sex differences in medical care and early death after acute myocardial infarction. *Circulation* 118:2803–2810, 2008.
59. Mark DB, Hlatky MA, Califf RM, et al: Cost effectiveness of thrombolytic therapy with tissue plasminogen activator as compared with streptokinase for acute myocardial infarction. *N Engl J Med* 332:1418–1424, 1995.
60. Boersma E: Does time matter? A pooled analysis of randomized clinical trials comparing primary percutaneous coronary intervention and in-hospital fibrinolysis in acute myocardial infarction patients. *Eur Heart J* 27:779–788, 2006.
61. Huynh T, Perron S, O'Loughlin J, et al: Comparison of primary percutaneous coronary intervention and fibrinolytic therapy in ST-segment-elevation myocardial infarction: Bayesian hierarchical meta-analyses of randomized controlled trials and observational studies. *Circulation* 119:3101–3109, 2009.
62. Grines CL, Browne KF, Marco J, et al: A comparison of immediate angioplasty with thrombolytic therapy for acute myocardial infarction. The Primary Angioplasty in Myocardial Infarction Study Group. *N Engl J Med* 328:673–679, 1993.
63. Le May MR, Davies RF, Labinaz M, et al: Hospitalization costs of primary stenting versus thrombolysis in acute myocardial infarction: Cost analysis of the Canadian STAT Study. *Circulation* 108:2624–2630, 2003.
64. Machecourt J, Bonnefoy E, Vanzetto G, et al: Primary angioplasty is cost-minimizing compared with pre-hospital thrombolysis for patients within 60 min of a percutaneous coronary intervention center: The Comparison of Angioplasty and Pre-hospital Thrombolysis in Acute Myocardial Infarction (CAPTIM) cost-efficacy sub-study. *J Am Coll Cardiol* 45:515–524, 2005.
65. Aasa M, Henriksson M, Dellborg M, et al: Cost and health outcome of primary percutaneous coronary intervention versus thrombolysis in acute ST-segment elevation myocardial infarction—results of the Swedish Early Decision reperfusion Study (SWEDES) trial. *Am Heart J* 160:322–328, 2010.
66. Kotowycz MA, Cosman TL, Tartaglia C, et al: Safety and feasibility of early hospital discharge in ST-segment elevation myocardial infarction—a prospective and randomized trial in low-risk primary percutaneous coronary intervention patients (the Safe-Depart Trial). *Am Heart J* 159:117–e1-6, 2010.
67. Lieu TA, Lundstrom RJ, Ray GT, et al: Initial cost of primary angioplasty for acute myocardial infarction. *J Am Coll Cardiol* 28:882–889, 1996.
68. Lieu TA, Gurley RJ, Lundstrom RJ, et al: Projected cost-effectiveness of primary angioplasty for acute myocardial infarction. *J Am Coll Cardiol* 30:1741–1750, 1997.
69. Concannon TW, Kent DM, Normand SL, et al: Comparative effectiveness of ST-segment-elevation myocardial infarction regionalization strategies. *Circ Cardiovasc Qual Outcomes* 3:506–513, 2010.
70. Chin CT, Chen AY, Wang TY, et al: Risk adjustment for in-hospital mortality of contemporary patients with acute myocardial infarction: The Acute Coronary Treatment and Intervention Outcomes Network (ACTION) Registry((R))-Get With The Guidelines (GWTG) acute myocardial infarction mortality model and risk score. *Am Heart J* 161:113–122, 2011.
71. Cannon CP, Weintraub WS, Demopoulos LA, et al: Comparison of early invasive and conservative strategies in patients with unstable coronary syndromes treated with the glycoprotein IIb/IIIa inhibitor tirofiban. *N Engl J Med* 344:1879–1887, 2001.
72. Mahoney EM, Jurkovitz CT, Chu H, et al: Cost and cost-effectiveness of an early invasive vs conservative strategy for the treatment of unstable angina and non-ST-segment elevation myocardial infarction. *JAMA* 288:1851–1858, 2002.
73. Wallentin L, Lagerqvist B, Husted S, et al: Outcome at 1 year after an invasive compared with a non-invasive strategy in unstable coronary-artery disease: The FRISC II invasive randomised trial. FRISC II Investigators. Fast Revascularisation during Instability in Coronary artery disease. *Lancet* 356:9–16, 2000.
74. Lagerqvist B, Husted S, Kontny F, et al: 5-year outcomes in the FRISC-II randomised trial of an invasive versus a non-invasive strategy in non-ST-elevation acute coronary syndrome: A follow-up study. *Lancet* 368:998–1004, 2006.

75. de Winter RJ, Windhausen F, Cornel JH, et al: Early invasive versus selectively invasive management for acute coronary syndromes. *N Engl J Med* 353:1095–1104, 2005.

76. Bavry AA, Kumbhani DJ, Rassi AN, et al: Benefit of early invasive therapy in acute coronary syndromes: A meta-analysis of contemporary randomized clinical trials. *J Am Coll Cardiol* 48:1319–1325, 2006.

77. Lincoff AM, Califf RM, Topol EJ: Platelet glycoprotein IIb/IIIa receptor blockade in coronary artery disease. *J Am Coll Cardiol* 35:1103–1115, 2000.

78. Mark DB, Harrington RA, Lincoff AM, et al: Cost-effectiveness of platelet glycoprotein IIb/IIIa inhibition with eptifibatide in patients with non-ST-elevation acute coronary syndromes. *Circulation* 101:366–371, 2000.

79. Sabatine MS, Jang IK: The use of glycoprotein IIb/IIIa inhibitors in patients with coronary artery disease. *Am J Med* 109:224–237, 2000.

80. Topol EJ, Mark DB, Lincoff AM, et al: Outcomes at 1 year and economic implications of platelet glycoprotein IIb/IIIa blockade in patients undergoing coronary stenting: Results from a multicentre randomised trial. EPISTENT Investigators. Evaluation of Platelet IIb/IIIa Inhibitor for Stenting. *Lancet* 354:2019–2024, 1999.

81. Mahoney EM, Mehta S, Yuan Y, et al: Long-term cost-effectiveness of early and sustained clopidogrel therapy for up to 1 year in patients undergoing percutaneous coronary intervention after presenting with acute coronary syndromes without ST-segment elevation. *Am Heart J* 151:219–227, 2006.

82. Beinart SC, Kolm P, Veledar E, et al: Long-term cost effectiveness of early and sustained dual oral antiplatelet therapy with clopidogrel given for up to one year after percutaneous coronary intervention results: From the Clopidogrel for the Reduction of Events During Observation (CREDO) trial. *J Am Coll Cardiol* 46:761–769, 2005.

83. Lindgren P, Stenestrand U, Malmberg K, et al: The long-term cost-effectiveness of clopidogrel plus aspirin in patients undergoing percutaneous coronary intervention in Sweden. *Clin Ther* 27:100–110, 2005.

84. Cowper PA, Udayakumar K, Sketch MH, Jr, et al: Economic effects of prolonged clopidogrel therapy after percutaneous coronary intervention. *J Am Coll Cardiol* 45:369–376, 2005.

85. Mahoney EM, Wang K, Arnold SV, et al: Cost-effectiveness of prasugrel versus clopidogrel in patients with acute coronary syndromes and planned percutaneous coronary intervention: Results from the trial to assess improvement in therapeutic outcomes by optimizing platelet inhibition with Prasugrel-Thrombolysis in Myocardial Infarction TRITON-TIMI 38. *Circulation* 121:71–79, 2010.

86. Wallentin L, Becker RC, Budaj A, et al: Ticagrelor versus clopidogrel in patients with acute coronary syndromes. *N Engl J Med* 361:1045–1057, 2009.

87. Ferguson JJ, Califf RM, Antman EM, et al: Enoxaparin vs unfractionated heparin in high-risk patients with non-ST-segment elevation acute coronary syndromes managed with an intended early invasive strategy: Primary results of the SYNERGY randomized trial. *JAMA* 292:45–54, 2004.

88. Yusuf S, Mehta SR, Chrolavicius S, et al: Comparison of fondaparinux and enoxaparin in acute coronary syndromes. *N Engl J Med* 354:1464–1476, 2006.

89. Sculpher MJ, Lozano-Ortega G, Sambrook J, et al: Fondaparinux versus enoxaparin in non-ST-elevation acute coronary syndromes: Short-term cost and long-term cost-effectiveness using data from the Fifth Organization to Assess Strategies in Acute Ischemic Syndromes Investigators (OASIS-5) trial. *Am Heart J* 157:845–852, 2009.

90. Janzon M, Levin LA, Swahn E: Cost effectiveness of extended treatment with low molecular weight heparin (dalteparin) in unstable coronary artery disease: Results from the FRISC II trial. *Heart* 89:287–292, 2003.

91. Lincoff AM, Bittl JA, Harrington RA, et al: Bivalirudin and provisional glycoprotein IIb/IIIa blockade compared with heparin and planned glycoprotein IIb/IIIa blockade during percutaneous coronary intervention: REPLACE-2 randomized trial. *JAMA* 289:853–863, 2003.

92. Cohen DJ, Lincoff AM, Lavelle TA, et al: Economic evaluation of bivalirudin with provisional glycoprotein IIB/IIIA inhibition versus heparin with routine glycoprotein IIB/IIIA inhibition for percutaneous coronary intervention: Results from the REPLACE-2 trial. *J Am Coll Cardiol* 44:1792–1800, 2004.

93. Saha S, Coffman DD, Smits AK: Giving teeth to comparative-effectiveness research–the Oregon experience. *N Engl J Med* 362:e18, 2010.

94. Mark DB, Nelson CL, Anstrom KJ, et al: Cost-effectiveness of defibrillator therapy or amiodarone in chronic stable heart failure: Results from the Sudden Cardiac Death in Heart Failure Trial (SCD-HeFT). *Circulation* 114:135–142, 2006.

95. Weinstein MC, Siegel JE, Gold MR, et al: Recommendations of the Panel on Cost-effectiveness in Health and Medicine. *JAMA* 276:1253–1258, 1996.

96. Neumann PJ, Weinstein MC: Legislating against use of cost-effectiveness information. *N Engl J Med* 363:1495–1497, 2010.

62

Quality of Care in Interventional Cardiology

GREGORY J. DEHMER | RALPH G. BRINDIS

KEY POINTS

- In the present era of increasing state and federal regulations, consumer demands for quality, and pressures from payers for cost-efficiency, quality in the cardiac catheterization laboratory (cath lab) is being examined closely.

- Efforts to improve the quality of medical care in the United States started over 150 years ago and new initiatives including public reporting which have been incorporated into the *Patient Protection and Affordable Care Act (PPAHA-Public Law 111-148)* of 2010.

- Donabedian's triad consists of three domains (structure, process, and outcomes), which provide a conceptual framework for evaluating the quality of medical care.

- The key building blocks of quality include clinical practice guidelines, data standards, performance measures, outcome measures, and appropriate use criteria, all of which can contribute to continuous quality improvement projects.

- Continuous quality improvement (CQI) is an organized scientific process for evaluating, planning, improving, and controlling quality and has been demonstrated to reduce variation and improve overall performance in the cardiac cath lab.

- Clinical registries such as the CathPCI Registry of the National Cardiovascular Data Registry provide a cornerstone for benchmarking patient outcomes and are superior to simple volume standards or administrative databases.

- Public reporting increases transparency and is part of the proposed mechanisms to tie reimbursement to quality, but the substantial challenge is to ensure that public reporting occurs in a fair, accurate, and meaningful way that benefits patients yet minimizes the possibilities of negative unintended consequences.

"Quality is everyone's responsibility."

W. Edwards Deming[1]

Interventional cardiology has grown rapidly since its inception about 30 years ago. Invasive cardiovascular procedures have become a cornerstone for the evaluation and management of many cardiovascular diseases, especially coronary artery disease (CAD). Since these procedures are widely used, easily identified with claims data, and expensive, considerable attention has been focused on the cardiac cath lab. This attention has intensified in the present era because of increasing state and federal regulations, more frequent requests for the public reporting of hospital and physician data, consumer pressures for care of the highest quality, and increasing pressure from payers for care to be cost efficient with an increasing focus on ensuring the appropriate use of cardiac catheterization and percutaneous coronary interventions (PCIs). At the same time, there is a growing awareness that the quality of health care is compromised by several factors, including (1) preventable medical errors, (2) the absence of evidence-based standards in many areas, (3) a lack of emphasis on disease prevention, (4) inadequate personal responsibility for maintaining health, and (5)

disparities in health care delivery related to race, gender, income, and insurance status. The desire to improve the quality of cardiovascular care was growing even before these recent trends in the health care marketplace and the focus on health care reform. Numerous government and private agencies in the United States have been involved in the development of quality measures and the dissemination of data for several years (Table 62-1). Statewide "report cards" on cardiac surgeries and PCIs for hospitals and individual physicians exist in some states.[2,3] Interest in such reports on quality continues to increase as data have emerged showing that patients fail to receive up to 45% of the tests and treatments recommended by evidence-based guidelines.[4] In an attempt to promote quality and improve outcomes, programs generally referred to as "pay-for-performance," in which providers receive financial incentives for achieving certain benchmark goals in patient care, have been developed.[5]

Although there are no formal national standards to judge the quality of cardiac cath labs, some states have used clinical practice guidelines and expert consensus documents published by the American College of Cardiology Foundation (ACCF), the American Heart Association (AHA), and the Society for Cardiovascular Angiography and Interventions (SCAI) to develop quality standards.[6-8] Although these documents were never intended to serve as state or national standards, they have often become the de facto basis for licensure regulations imposed by state health departments in an attempt to improve quality. To more completely understand the current status of quality efforts in the cardiac cath lab, it is helpful to examine some of the major events that form the history of quality efforts in U.S. health care.

A Brief History of Quality Efforts in U.S. Medicine

Despite the many concerns about the state of American medicine today, there have been profound improvements during the past 150 years. The American Medical Association (AMA) was founded in 1847, in part, to address the disorganized and poor quality of health care in the United States. As a forerunner of efforts to come, in 1917, the American College of Surgeons established the Hospital Standardization Program promoting five minimal patient care standards and began surveying health care organizations to determine their acceptability for accreditation. On the basis of these early efforts, in 1952, several other organizations collaborated with the American College of Surgeons to form the Joint Commission on Accreditation of Hospitals.[9] The U.S. concepts of quality in health care were advanced by Avedis Donabedian in 1966 with the publication of his classic article that provided a broad definition of quality and recommended evaluations in three areas: *structure*, *process*, and *outcome*.[10] This format was widely adapted and is still in use today. During this early period, quality was often assessed by random chart audits or outcome-oriented chart surveys to evaluate metrics such as the use of blood products in surgical cases. Audit requirements were later minimized in favor of hospital-wide quality assurance programs designed to detect care that was felt to be outside acceptable standards. Physician profiles reflecting the number of procedures performed, indications, and complications were compared with grouped data from similar physicians to identify

TABLE 62-1	Organizations Involved in the Assessment of Quality Care	
Organization	*Mission / Goals / Focus*	*Web Site*
Agency for Healthcare Research and Quality (AHRQ)	Lead Federal agency charged with improving the quality, safety, efficiency, and effectiveness of health care for all Americans	www.ahrq.gov
National Guideline Clearinghouse (NGC)	An initiative of AHRQ that is a public resource for evidence-based clinical practice guidelines	www.guideline.gov
Centers for Medicare & Medicaid Services (CMS)	Host site for Hospital Compare (www.hospitalcompare.hss.gov), a Web site that reports process of care, risk-adjusted outcome, and patient satisfaction measures for all hospitals in the United States	www.medicare.gov
Department of Health and Human Services (DHHS)	Provides links to hundreds of sites on the Internet that contain reliable health care information and links to many government and nongovernment sources of information on healthcare quality	www.healthfinder.gov
The Joint Commission	Provides accreditation to hospital and other health care facilities; provides quality care and hospital quality measures for public reporting through the ORYX reporting program	www.jointcommission.org
National Committee for Quality Assurance (NCQA)	A private, 501(c)(3) not-for-profit organization dedicated to improving health care quality. Operate the Healthcare Effectiveness Data and Information Set (HEDIS), a tool used by more than 90 percent of America's health plans to measure performance on important dimensions of care and service	www.ncqa.org
The American Health Quality Association (AHQA)	An educational, not-for-profit national membership association dedicated to health care quality through community-based, independent quality evaluation and improvement programs	www.ahqa.org
National Quality Forum (NQF)	Sets national priorities and goals for performance improvement and endorses national consensus standards for measuring and publicly reporting on performance	www.qualityforum.org
American Medical Association (AMA)	Sponsored by the AMA, the Physician Consortium for Performance Improvement (PCPI) is committed to enhancing quality of care and patient safety by taking the lead in the development, testing, and maintenance of evidence-based clinical performance measures and measurement resources for physicians	www.ama-assn.org/
American College of Cardiology Foundation (ACCF)	In collaboration with other professional organizations develops clinical practice guidelines, expert consensus documents, and other quality programs including: Guidelines Applied in Practice (GAP) to provide assistance with guideline application in clinical practice and Hospital to Home (H2H), an effort to improve the transition from inpatient to outpatient status for individuals hospitalized with cardiovascular disease	www.cardiosource.org
American Heart Association (AHA)	In collaboration with other professional organizations develops clinical practice guidelines, expert consensus documents, and other quality programs including: Get With The Guidelines, a hospital-based quality improvement program designed to ensure that every patient is consistently treated according to the most recent evidence-based guidelines and Mission: Lifeline, a national, community-based initiative to improve systems of care for patients with ST elevation myocardial infarction (STEMI)	www.my.americanheart.org
The Leapfrog Group	A voluntary program organized by large employers to promote big leaps in healthcare safety, quality, and customer value.	www.leapfroggroup.org

"outliers" with the hope that they might be induced to change their practice habits by colleagues, the hospital, or other agencies.[11] Around 1990, a technique developed primarily for industry, called *continuous quality improvement (CQI)*, was advocated by the Joint Commission. Compared with quality assurance programs, this approach tries to improve the performance of the entire group, rather than simply identifying poor performers.[12–14] As quality efforts by the medical profession were maturing, state and federal agencies were also becoming interested in regulating health care, developing standards, and promoting high-quality medical care. By the late 1800s, many states required physician licensure and mandated educational standards for physicians. The National Board of Medical Examiners was founded in 1915 to provide a nationwide examination that licensing authorities could accept and use to judge candidates for licensure. As the medical field expanded and specialty training became available, it was recognized that some type of certification process for specialists was necessary. To establish a uniform system, the American Board of Medical Specialties was formed in 1933. There are now 24 specialty boards that certify physicians, and this process has evolved to one of continuous professional development and life-long learning through a Maintenance of Certification process requiring ongoing measurement of six core competencies.[15] One of the first federal initiatives was the formation of the U.S. Food and Drug Administration (FDA) in 1906. With the enactment of Social Security in 1935, followed by Medicare in 1965, the Federal government became more involved in setting requirements for the delivery of health care funded by federal dollars. To monitor the care of Medicare patients, Congress enacted rules called *Conditions of Participation*, which required hospitals to provide certain services and conduct utilization reviews to determine the appropriateness of hospital admissions. In 1972, amendments to the *Social Security Act* created the Professional Standards Review Organization program to promote hospital efficiency and eliminate unnecessary hospital use. This program failed to meet expectations and was unpopular, as many felt it emphasized cost containment rather than quality.[11] It was abandoned but was replaced by other peer review organizations (PROs).[16] As this was evolving, substantial changes in hospital reimbursement occurred with a shift to a cost-per-case system based on assignment to a diagnosis-related group (DRG). The PROs were responsible for validating correct assignment to a DRG and also for monitoring hospital admissions, re-admissions, surgical procedures, complications, and hospital deaths. PROs emphasized quality but focused more on outcomes metrics rather than on structure and process metrics and so were not without their critics.[17] Not surprisingly, as the amount of Medicare spending increased, the federal government became increasingly involved in monitoring and controlling payments to physicians and hospitals. Before 1989, physician payments for services within the Medicare program were based on usual and customary charges for services by similar physicians in the previous year. Substantial changes in Medicare payments to physicians occurred as a result of the *Budget Reconciliation Act* of 1989, which redirected payments based on costs rather than charges. Costs were determined for the actual work involved, the overhead required to provide the service, and malpractice costs, with all three elements further adjusted for geographic differences in cost. This caused major changes in practice patterns, which had both positive and negative effects on the quality of care. Additional federal funding led to the formation of the Agency for Health Care

Policy and Research, which had a turbulent history and narrowly escaped being eliminated in 1995, only to be reauthorized in 1999 with a new mandate and name as the Agency for Healthcare Research and Quality (AHRQ). Many other quality initiatives and programs were developed by professional organizations and government agencies over the next 10 years with variable degrees of success. Now, several more are proposed as part of the Patient Protection and Affordable Care Act (PPAHA-Public Law 111-148) of 2010. In addition to the sweeping changes in the delivery of health care, there are several provisions in this legislation specifically targeting the quality of health care. These include (1) establishment of a Patient-Centered Outcomes Research Institute, (2) formation of a Medicare Innovation Center with $10 billion to fund payment reform and quality improvement pilots, and (3) development of new systems linking payment to quality outcomes. These PPAHA and other progressive initiatives are aimed at ushering in substantial transformation of the American health care delivery system through the re-alignment of payment incentives rewarding quality rather than quantity of care.

Quality in Interventional Cardiology

"But even though Quality cannot be defined, you know what Quality is."

Robert M. Persig[18]

Quality is something everyone wants in health care, but it is not easily defined. Patients, physicians, payers, and government all have different perspectives on the elements that contribute to high-quality health care. Patients frequently place greater emphasis on the interaction and the time they have with their physician rather than on a strict focus on issues such as adherence to practice guidelines. In contrast, payers and government agencies are likely to place more emphasis on adherence to performance measures and on reduction in unnecessary procedures and costs.

The potential to deliver high-quality care in the cardiac cath lab centers on the core values promoted by the Institute of Medicine (IOM). In its report titled *"Crossing the Quality Chasm,"* quality is defined as "the degree to which health care systems, services, and supplies for individuals and populations increase the likelihood for desired health outcomes in a manner consistent with current professional knowledge."[19] The IOM further states that health care should be safe, effective, evidence based, timely, equitable, and patient centered. Several different definitions of *quality* have been proposed, reflecting the complexity of the health care system and its heterogeneous

stakeholders. The Rand Institute defines quality care as "providing patients with appropriate services in a technically competent manner, with good communications, shared decision making, and cultural sensitivity."[20] An increasingly popular operational definition of *quality* is based on error reduction and the recognition that there are three major types of errors in health care: (1) underuse, (2) overuse, and (3) misuse.[21] *Underuse* is defined as failure to provide a medical intervention when it is likely to produce a favorable outcome for a patient, such as the failure to prescribe lipid-lowering therapy for secondary prevention following a myocardial infarction (MI) in a patient with hyperlipidemia. *Overuse* is defined as the use of a test or therapy, even though its benefits do not justify the potential harm or costs, such as performance of a PCI in an asymptomatic patient with a stenosis of intermediate severity without first documenting the presence of important ischemia. *Misuse* occurs when a preventable complication eliminates the benefit of a therapy such as stent thrombosis because platelet inhibitors were not prescribed after placement of a coronary stent or when a stent is inadequately deployed in an artery and thus is not opposed to the vessel wall. Whatever definition of *quality* is used, there are several key elements that contribute to the development of quality health care.

Building Blocks of Quality in Health Care

Fundamental to the development of a quality health care environment is the assurance that the patient is receiving the correct treatment for his or her condition. Obviously, if the patient receives flawless and efficient delivery of the wrong treatment for his or her condition, quality cannot exist. A model for the integration of quality into the cycle of therapeutic development has been proposed (Fig. 62-1).[22] This starts with a hypothesis derived from the basic sciences, animal research, or other observations, progresses into early clinical research with small nonrandomized and unblinded case series, and eventually leads to a large randomized, blinded, and well-designed clinical trial. After one or more well-performed clinical trials provide clear information about a clinical question, the substrate is established for a clinical practice guideline.

CLINICAL PRACTICE GUIDELINES

The IOM defines *guidelines* as "systematically developed statements to assist practitioner and patient decisions about appropriate health care for specific clinical circumstances."[23] For nearly 20 years, the AHA and

Figure 62-1 A model for the integration of quality into the therapeutic development cycle. Concepts from the basic laboratory eventually lead to clinical studies. After well-conducted clinical studies are completed, clinical practice guidelines are developed, leading to quality indicators and then performance measures intended to elevate the level of care and improve outcomes. *(From Califf RM, Peterson ED, Gibbons RJ, et al: Integrating quality into the cycle of therapeutic development, J Am Coll Cardiol 40(11):1895–1901, 2002.)*

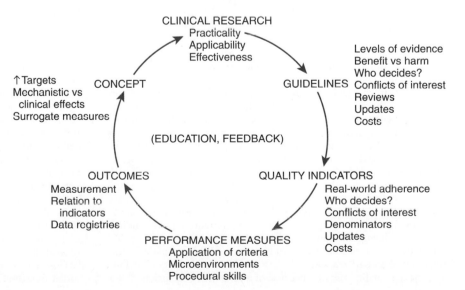

SIZE OF TREATMENT EFFECT ⟶

	CLASS I *Benefit > > > Risk* Procedure/Treatment SHOULD be performed/ administered	CLASS IIa *Benefit > > Risk* *Additional studies with* *focused objectives needed* IT IS REASONABLE to perform procedure/administer treatment	CLASS IIb *Benefit ≥ Risk* *Additional studies with broad* *objectives needed; additional* *registry data would be helpful* Procedure/Treatment MAY BE CONSIDERED	CLASS III *Risk ≥ Benefit* Procedure/Treatment should NOT be performed/administered SINCE IT IS NOT HELPFUL AND MAY BE HARMFUL
LEVEL A Multiple populations evaluated* Data derived from multiple randomized clinical trials or meta-analyses	• Recommendation that procedure or treatment is useful/effective • Sufficient evidence from multiple randomized trials or meta-analyses	• Recommendation in favor of treatment or procedure being useful/effective • Some conflicting evidence from multiple randomized trials or meta-analyses	• Recommendation's usefulness/efficacy less well established • Greater conflicting evidence from multiple randomized trials or meta-analyses	• Recommendation that procedure or treament is not useful/effective and may be harmful • Sufficient evidence from multiple randomized trials or meta-analyses
LEVEL B Limited populations evaluated* Data derived from a single randomized trial or nonrandomized studies	• Recommendation that procedure or treatment is useful/effective • Evidence from single randomized trial or nonrandomized studies	• Recommendation in favor of treatment or procedure being useful/effective • Some conflicting evidence from single randomized trial or nonrandomized studies	• Recommendation's usefulness/efficacy less well established • Greater conflicting evidence from single randomized trial or nonrandomized studies	• Recommendation that procedure or treament is not useful/effective and may be harmful • Evidence from single randomized trial or nonrandomized studies
LEVEL C Very limited populations evaluated* Only consensus opinion of experts, case studies, or standard of care	• Recommendation that procedure or treatment is useful/effective • Only expert opinion, case studies, or standard of care	• Recommendation in favor of treatment or procedure being useful/effective • Only diverging expert opinion, case studies, or standard of care	• Recommendation's usefulness/efficacy less well established • Only diverging expert opinion, case studies, or standard of care	• Recommendation that procedure or treament is not useful/effective and may be harmful • Only expert opinion, case studies, or standard care
Suggested phrases for writing recommendations†	should is recommended is indicated is useful/effective/beneficial	is reasonable can be useful/effective/beneficial is probably recommended or indicated	may/might be considered may/might be reasonable usefulness/effectiveness is unknown/unclear/uncertain or not well established	is not recommended is not indicated should not is not useful/effective/beneficial may be harmful

(left axis label) ESTIMATE OF CERTAINTY (PRECISION) OF TREATMENT EFFECT

Figure 62-2 Classification of recommendations and level of evidence used in the American College of Cardiology Foundation (ACCF)/the American Heart Association (AHA) clinical practice guidelines. The current definitions for treatment recommendations and level of evidence are shown. (*From* http://assets.cardiosource.com/Methodology_Manual_for_ACC_AHA_Writing_Committees.pdf: *Accessed August 10, 2010.*)

the ACCF, in conjunction with subspecialty organizations, where appropriate, have collaborated to develop clinical practice guidelines in cardiology. Guidelines have the potential to improve the quality of cardiovascular care and enhance the appropriateness of clinical practice, which, in turn, should lead to better patient outcomes, improved cost-effectiveness, and the identification of knowledge gaps that require further research. After a thorough review of all relevant evidence, guideline recommendations are developed with a level of evidence in a structured format (Fig. 62-2). To remain relevant and be embraced by clinicians, clinical practice guidelines must incorporate new evidence in a timely fashion; therefore, more focused guideline updates are now produced as new and important data are published. Recommendations contained within a guideline can be synthesized into algorithms, which then can be used to develop quality indicators, specifying the clinical circumstances under which a technology or treatment should or should not be used. In general, class I and III guideline recommendations with a level of evidence A identify recommendations that can be considered for the development of a quality measure. Unfortunately, the process is not as straightforward as it seems because of the many treatment considerations for which reasonable uncertainty exists. A challenging issue in the development of quality indicators occurs during the attempt to define which patients actually qualify for a particular indicator. In one study involving Medicare patients, less than half of all patients with an acute MI (AMI) actually qualified for a particular quality measure because of a long list of exclusions.[24] If a

large number of patients are excluded from a particular quality measure, the measure may not be a meaningful reflection of a physician's or a facility's care. Determining how well a provider or an institution meets specified quality indicators is one potential way to gauge the quality of the health care delivered.

DATA STANDARDS

A critical step for the success and application of quality standards is to have standardized data elements and corresponding definitions so that there is consistency in what is reported. For comparisons to be meaningful, there must be a common lexicon for describing the process and outcomes of clinical care, whether in randomized trials, observational studies, registries, or quality improvement initiatives. Particularly for quality performance measurement initiatives in which comparison of facilities or providers is proposed, common data standards and definitions must be clearly understood, consistently used, and properly interpreted by a broader audience for the entire process to be meaningful. To that end, the ACC/AHA Task Force on Clinical Data Standards has undertaken the job of developing and publishing clinical data standards, data elements, and corresponding definitions that can be used in the assessment of patient management and outcomes and for research and epidemiologic assessments.[25] Data standards have been developed for acute coronary syndromes (ACS), atrial fibrillation (AF), cardiac imaging, congestive heart failure (CHF), peripheral arterial

TABLE 62-2	American College of Cardiology/American Heart Association (ACC/AHA) Attributes for Satisfactory Performance Measures
Useful in improving patient outcomes	
Evidence-based	
Interpretable	
Actionable	
Measure design	
Denominator precisely defined	
Numerator precisely defined	
Validity	
Face validity	
Content validity	
Construct validity	
Reliability	
Measure implementation	
Feasibility	
Reasonable effort	
Reasonable cost	
Reasonable time period for collection	

(Adapted from Spertus JA, Eagle KA, Krumholtz HM, et al: American College of Cardiology and American Heart Association methodology for the selection and creation of performance measures for quantifying and quality of cardiovascular care, *J Am Coll Cardiol* 45(7):1147–1156, 2005.)

TABLE 62-3	Current and Planned American College of Cardiology Foundation/American Heart Association Performance Measure Sets	
Topic	*Publication Date*	*Partnering Organizations*
Chronic heart failure	2005	ACC/AHA: Inpatient measures ACC/AHA/PCPI Outpatient measures
Chronic stable coronary artery disease	2005	ACC/AHA/PCPI
Hypertension	2005	ACC/AHA/PCPI
ST and non-ST myocardial infarction	2006	ACC/AHA
Cardiac rehabilitation	2007	AACVPR/ACC/AHA
Atrial fibrillation	2008	ACC/AHA/PCPI
Primary prevention of cardiovascular disease	2009	ACCF/AHA
Peripheral artery disease	2010	ACCF/AHA/ACR/SCAI/SIR/ SVM/SVN/SVS
Cardiac diagnostic imaging	2011	Planned
Percutaneous coronary intervention	2011	Planned

ACC(F), American College of Cardiology (Foundation); *AHA*, American Heart Association; *PCPI*, American Medical Association—Physician Consortium for Performance Improvement; *AACVPR*, American Association of Cardiovascular and Pulmonary Rehabilitation; *ACR*, American College of Radiology; *SCAI*, Society for Cardiovascular Angiography and Interventions; *SIR*, Society for Interventional Radiology; *SVM*, Society for Vascular Medicine; *SVN*, Society for Vascular Nursing; *SVS*, Society for Vascular Surgery.

disease (PAD), and electrophysiologic studies and are planned for several other topics.[26] Cardiovascular data standards and their corresponding definitions then become the source for the data elements used in cardiovascular registries.

PERFORMANCE MEASURES

A quality indicator is simply a variable (e.g., primary PCI performed in patients with ST elevation MI [STEMI] within 90 minutes, if PCI is immediately available). In contrast, performance measures must have a well-defined numerator and denominator and appropriate and specified reasons to exclude patients from the tabulation within the measure. Without this structure, data for the measure cannot be collected in a reliable way. Using the above example, the corresponding performance measure would then be the proportion of eligible patients with STEMI who arrive at a PCI-capable hospital and receive primary PCI within 90 minutes of arrival. Guideline recommendations that clearly specify the patient population appropriate for a specified treatment or the optimal timing of a treatment are ideal for translation into performance measures.

Selecting performance measures involves evaluating the strength of evidence supporting the performance measure, defining the importance of the outcome most likely to be achieved by adherence to the performance measure, and assessing the association between adherence to the performance measure and a clinically important outcome. A detailed description of the methodology for the selection and creation of ACC/AHA performance measures has been published.[27] Similar to quality measures, class I guideline recommendations identify potential patient care decisions that could be considered for a performance measure. Performance measures, in general, represent "must do" elements of clinical care, whereas failure to adhere to a performance measure represents inadequate or inferior care. Other important attributes to consider in the development of a performance measure are the cost associated with implementing the measure, availability of reimbursement for the therapy or intervention, and the cost of collecting data required for the measure (Table 62-2).

Performance measures also require that a threshold for acceptable performance be developed. This leads to questions regarding who determines the threshold and how the threshold level of performance is determined, as it is unlikely that 100% compliance will be achieved for every performance measure. One proposed method to define thresholds is to establish achievable benchmarks of care.[28] Adherence

TABLE 62-4	Individual Measures and Domains Included in the Society of Thoracic Surgeons Composite Score
Operative care domain	
Use of at least one internal mammary artery graft	
Perioperative medical care domain	
Preoperative β-blockers	
Discharge β blockers	
Discharge anti-platelet medication	
Discharge anti-lipid medication	
Risk-adjusted mortality domain	
Operative mortality	
Risk-adjusted major morbidity domain	
Prolonged ventilation (>24 hours)	
Deep sternal wound infection	
Permanent stroke	
Renal insufficiency	
Reoperation	

(From O'Brien SM, Shahian DM, DeLong ER, et al: Quality measurement in adult cardiac surgery: Part 2—Statistical considerations in composite measure scoring and provider rating, *Ann Thorac Surg* 83(4 Suppl):S13–S26, 2007.)

to a performance measure is determined in a large sample and then the rate of adherence in the top 10% of facilities or physicians is set as the achievable benchmark. Using this method avoids establishing unreasonable goals which could paradoxically lead to inappropriate actions to achieve the established goal. Table 62-3 lists current performance measures related to cardiology and some additional measures under development. More recently, there has been interest in developing composite performance measures.[29] A composite performance measure is the combination of two or more measures into a single index. Such composite measures reduce the information burden by distilling the available indicators into a simple summary that can examine multiple dimensions of provider performance and facilitate comparisons. The Society of Thoracic Surgeons has developed and validated a composite measure for coronary artery bypass grafting (CABG) consisting of five process measures and six outcome measures, all of which are endorsed by the National Quality Forum[30,31] (Table 62-4). However, there are challenges to this approach. Details of an important individual measure can be diluted in the overall composite; methods for deriving the composite must be transparent to prevent it from being perceived as a black box.

OUTCOME MEASURES

The ultimate goal of performance measures is to identify patient care opportunities that are likely to improve outcomes for patients and thereby the quality of care. Among interventional cardiologists, there is general agreement regarding the outcomes measures of importance, and these have been used in many trials. Mortality, freedom from major adverse cardiac events (MACEs) such as MI, stroke, bleeding, and target lesion or vessel revascularization are all important, are relatively easy to quantify, and have been used in many trials. Improvements in symptoms and quality of life also are important but are more subjective and challenging to quantify; and collecting these data also involve additional cost and effort. Many outcome measures require risk adjustment to compare outcomes at the provider level in a fair manner, but adjusting for the effects of comorbid medical conditions, severity of the underlying disease, and socioeconomic status is not uniformly easy. This challenge is particularly huge when analyses are restricted to administrative claims data, which often have inferior data quality and lack the necessary clinical covariables for risk adjustment. Because of the challenges in measuring outcomes, especially some long-term outcomes at the provider level, it is often easier to assess quality by adhering to performance measures as surrogates of actual quality on the assumption that a high level of adherence to performance measures will result in better outcomes.

REAL-WORLD IMPACT OF PERFORMANCE MEASURES AND GUIDELINES

With the goal to improve outcomes for patients with cardiovascular disease at the forefront of all the efforts described above, it is important to note that some studies do show a positive relationship between adherence to performance measures and clinical outcomes.[32] However, this relationship is not necessarily strong and does not completely explain all of the variations. In one study using the National Registry of Myocardial Infarction (NRMI) database, only 6% of the hospital-level variations in 30-day mortality after AMI could be attributed to differences in the use of performance measures.[33] Relatively few studies have been performed to assess the extent to which guidelines are applied by clinicians in daily practice. Using data from the National Cardiovascular Data Registry (NCDR) collected between 2001 and 2004, it was shown that 64% of patients undergoing PCI had a class I indication, and 21% were class IIa, 7% were class IIb, and 8% were class III.[34] The clinical success of a PCI was directly related to the class of indication. *Clinical success*, defined as less than 25% residual stenosis without MI, same-admission bypass surgery, or death, occurred in 92.8% of patients with a class I indication, 91.7% of those with class IIa indications, 89% of those with class IIb indications, and 85.5% of those with a class III indication. Unfortunately, other studies have evaluated the extent to which guidelines are followed in clinical practice with disappointing results. For example, Lopes et al examined a large cohort of patients from three randomized double-blind clinical trials to determine if patients with AF were being treated with antithrombotic therapy in accordance with accepted guidelines.[35] Only 13.5% of the patients in these trials were receiving indicated prophylactic anti-thrombotic therapy with warfarin. Similarly, data from the Worcester Heart Attack Study and the Global Registry of Acute Coronary Events (GRACE) show an increase in the use of guideline-recommended medications (β-blockers, angiotensin-converting enzyme [ACE] inhibitors, aspirin, and lipid-lowering agents) over time, but still only about 60% of patients are receiving these medications.[36,37] These findings are not unusual as other studies have documented that guideline recommendations are followed for a disappointingly small portion of inpatients and outpatients.[38] Several reasons have been postulated to explain why care providers are not

using guidelines to a greater extent in daily practice.[39] These include (1) the sheer number of guidelines and their length, (2) the desire of clinicians to use "tried and true" approaches to managing disease entities, which are comfortable patterns for the physician, (3) the desire to avoid standardized and rigid order sets which may not apply to every patient and are perceived as "cookbook" medical therapy, and (4) the fact that in many cases, there are limitations to the guidelines such that there are no specific recommendations available or, when available, are based more on expert consensus than on data from multiple randomized trials. This latter point was highlighted by Tricoci et al, who evaluated the 16 most current ACC/AHA guideline documents.[40] Out of 2711 separate guideline recommendations, a median of 11% was level of evidence A compared with a median of 48% that was level of evidence C, and only 19% of class I recommendations were based on level of evidence A. Expert consensus was used more frequently in relation to imaging recommendations, whereas recommendations related to revascularization procedures were more commonly based on level A or level B of evidence. These limitations exist not only in the United States but also in other countries. The Reassessing European Attitudes about Cardiovascular Treatment (REACT) survey obtained responses from 754 physicians, each with more than 10 years' experience, from five European countries (France, Germany, Italy, Sweden, and the United Kingdom) to assess whether physicians' perceptions of coronary heart disease management matched their treatment practices and whether their perceptions of patients' awareness was an accurate reflection of their patients' understanding.[41] In the REACT survey, physicians were asked to specify what the most common barriers were that prevented them from implementing guideline recommendations. The most common barrier, cited by 38% of the respondents, was lack of time (Fig. 62-3). The potential effect of decision-maker bias regarding the recommendation for coronary artery revascularization has also been examined.[42] Using the New York State database, the treatment decision (CABG surgery, PCI, medical therapy, or no treatment) made by the cardiologist performing the cardiac catheterization was compared with the recommendations of the relevant ACC/AHA guideline document. Among the patients included in the study, guideline-supported indications for CABG occurred in 13% of patients, guideline-supported indications for PCI in 59% of patients, and guideline-supported indications for either CABG or PCI in 17% of patients. Of the patients who were indicated for CABG, the cardiologist recommended CABG in 53% and PCI in 34%. Of the patients indicated for PCI, 94% were recommended for PCI. For patients who had indications for either CABG or PCI, 93% were recommended for PCI and 5% for CABG. Treatment recommendations also varied, depending on whether the cath lab offered PCI or not. These findings show the potential effect of decision bias on the application of guideline recommendations for coronary revascularization. Considerable geographic variation in the use of PCI within the Medicare population has been noted in other large surveys (Fig. 62-4).[43] Variation in cardiologists' propensity to make treatment recommendations is also affected by several nonclinical factors.[44] In a survey of 598 cardiologists, several nonclinical reasons to recommend cardiac catheterization, including protection from malpractice litigation, were identified (Table 62-5).

APPROPRIATE USE CRITERIA

Although clinical practice guidelines provide a foundation for summarizing evidence-based cardiovascular care, there are many gaps in current knowledge and thus wide variation in practice patterns as noted above. This marked variability exists in the use of cardiovascular procedures, raising questions of overuse or underuse. Realizing that clinical practice guidelines do not cover all possible clinical situations, Appropriate Use Criteria (AUC) have been developed for both cardiovascular imaging procedures and coronary revascularization.[45] AUC should serve as a supplement to ACC/AHA clinical practice guideline documents. They are designed to examine the use of diagnostic and therapeutic procedures to support efficient use of medical resources during the provision of quality medical care. AUC provide

REASONS FOR NON-ADHERENCE TO GUIDELINES

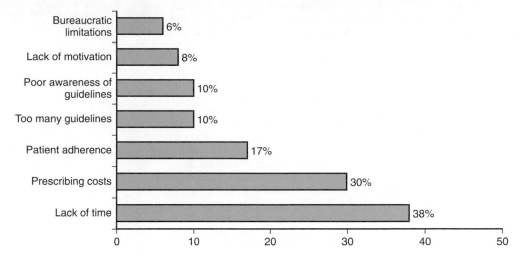

Figure 62-3 Barriers cited by physicians that prevent guideline implementation. *(Adapted from Hobbs FD, Erhardt L: Acceptance of guideline recommendations and perceived implementation of coronary heart disease prevention among primary care physicians in five European countries: The Reassessing European Attitudes about Cardiovascular Treatment (REACT) survey, Fam Pract 19(6):596–604, 2002.)*

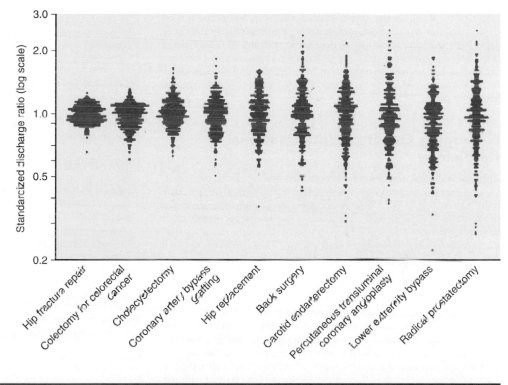

Figure 62-4 Profile of variation for 10 common surgical procedures. Each dot represents the ratio of the actual number of procedures performed compared with the average number in each of the 306 hospital referral regions in the United States. Little variation is seen per region for hip fracture repair *(far left of the graph)*. However, there is considerable and largely unexplained regional variation in the use of percutaneous transluminal coronary angioplasty. *(From Dartmouth Atlas Cardiovascular Report: Available at http://www.dartmouthatlas.org/downloads/reports/Cardiac_report_2005.pdf: Accessed August 3, 2010.)*

TABLE 62-5	Nonclinical Reasons for Recommending Cardiac Catheterization				
	Frequently	*Sometimes*	*Rarely*	*Never*	*Association with Cardiac Intensity Score (P Trend)*
The patient expected to undergo the procedure	9 (1.5%)	91 (15.6%)	271 (46.4%)	213 (36.5%)	
Mean Cardiac Intensity Score	51.5	49.7	49.8	49.9	0.99
Your colleagues would do so in the same situation	22 (3.8%)	134 (23.3%)	240 (41.7%)	180 (31.3%)	
Mean Cardiac Intensity Score	52.7	50.1	50.2	48.7	0.02
You wanted to satisfy the expectations of the referring physician	11 (1.9%)	156 (26.9%)	257 (44.2%)	157 (27%)	
Mean Cardiac Intensity Score	52.6	50.0	49.3	50.3	0.90
You wanted to protect against a possible malpractice suit	16 (2.7%)	123 (21.1%)	245 (42.0%)	200 (34.3%)	
Mean Cardiac Intensity Score	51.8	50.5	50.1	48.8	0.02
Doing so would enhance the financial stability of your practice	2 (0.3%)	3 (0.5%)	46 (7.9%)	532 (91.3%)	
Mean Cardiac Intensity Score	49.7	55.9	51.1	49.7	0.22

We would like you to think about your own cardiac catheterization recommendations. Sometimes, a cardiologist will recommend cardiac catheterization for other than purely clinical reasons. During the past 12 months, how often, if ever, has each of the above led you to recommend cardiac catheterization for a patient?

(From Lucas FL, Sirovich BE, Gallagher PM, et al: Variation in cardiologists' propensity to test and treat. Is it associated with regional variation in utilization? *Circ Cardiovasc Qual Outcomes* 3(3):253–260, 2010.)

practical tools to measure variations in care and examine use patterns. The process of AUC development has been well defined.[46] First, the AUC writing group combines specific clinical characteristics to create prototypical patient scenarios. Second, a technical panel is created from panelist nominations by relevant professional societies and provider-led organizations as well as from health policy and payer communities. The scenarios are then provided to the technical panel for appropriateness rating, and the technical panel is provided with summaries of the relevant evidence from the medical literature and practice guidelines. To preserve objectivity, the technical panels do not include a majority of individuals whose livelihood is tied to the technology under study. Third, members of the technical panel assess, individually and then collectively, the benefits and risks of the test or procedure in the context of the potential benefits to patients' outcomes, with an implicit understanding of the associated resource use and costs. At several steps in this process, a numerical score is assigned to each scenario with a score of 7 to 9 indicating appropriateness, 4 to 6 indicating uncertainty, and 1 to 3 indicating inappropriateness to perform that test or procedure. After the ranking process, the final appropriateness ratings are summarized by using an established rigorous methodology.[47]

AUC are intended to assist patients and clinicians but are not intended to diminish the acknowledged difficulty or uncertainty of clinical decision making and cannot act as substitutes for sound clinical judgment and practice experience. Rather, the aim of these criteria is to allow assessment of use patterns for a test or procedure. Comparing use patterns across a large subset of provider's patients can allow for an assessment of a provider's management strategies with those of his or her peers.

■ Judging Quality in Interventional Cardiology

Although there are many methods by which quality can be evaluated, Donabedian's triad provides a conceptual framework that has been used extensively.[10] This framework has three domains, *structure, process*, and *outcomes*, each identifying a major area of health care, containing metrics that should be assessed to determine the programmatic features needed to achieve quality.[48]

STRUCTURE

Structure refers to the physical components of health care delivery. For PCIs, structural measures include factors such as the training, experience, and board certification of physicians performing PCIs; the adequacy of diagnostic and therapeutic equipment; the presence of educational opportunities for the staff; the presence of a functioning peer-review process; and the presence of internal methods used for tracking procedural data so they can be compared with state or national data (Table 62-6). To assess the knowledge base of interventional cardiologists, the American Board of Internal Medicine (ABIM) has administered an additional qualification examination for board certification in interventional cardiology. The first such examination was held in 1999. Maintenance of certification is required after 10 years. Maintenance of certification not only involves another examination but also maintenance of a valid certification in internal medicine and cardiovascular disease, documentation of adequate procedure volumes (150 cases in the 2 years before expiration of the certificate), evidence of participation in a quality improvement project, and completion of self-evaluation modules for medical knowledge and practice performance. As of April 2010, there are 5108 ABIM-certified interventional cardiologists in the United States.[49] A requirement for board certification is more frequently being adopted by hospitals and payers, but there are no data to prove that board-certified physicians provide a higher quality of care than those who are not board certified. For other laboratory personnel, structural measures could include requirements for all technologists to be Registered Cardiovascular Invasive

TABLE 62-6	Examples of Structure, Process, and Outcome Measures in the Cardiac Catheterization Laboratory
Structural indicators	
Personnel indicators	
Credentialing (training and certification) of physicians and staff	
Re-appointment criteria for physicians	
Presence of a functioning peer-review process for operators	
Staff development and continuing education	
Equipment Indicators	
Fluoroscopic image quality	
Quality of stored images and stability of image archive	
Maintenance schedule for equipment	
Evaluation of new equipment and disposables	
Laboratory time lost or rescheduling because of equipment failure or problems	
Electrical safety systems	
Organizational Indicators	
Presence of internal methods for tracking and comparing procedural data	
Laboratory use (hours per day; procedures per lab per day; lab time per procedure)	
Total full time equivalents (FTEs) per procedure	
Disposable equipment costs per procedure; total costs per procedure and per operator	
Personnel costs per procedure	
Delay time between procedures	
Adherence to Occupational Safety and Health Administration (OSHA) guidelines	
Procedure fluoroscopy and cine-angiography times	
Radiation dosage to personnel	
Radiation protection practices	
Radiographic contrast use per case	
In-hospital delays for procedures	
Outpatient waiting times for procedures	
Outpatient waiting times for procedure starts	
Process indicators	
Indications for procedures or adherence to appropriateness use criteria	
Indications for hospital admissions	
Length of stay after procedures (total for lab and per physician)	
Quality of angiographic studies	
Quality (correctness) of study interpretation	
Precautions for patients with renal insufficiency, contrast allergy, latex allergy, etc.	
Outcome indicators	
Success rates for percutaneous coronary interventions (PCIs)	
Risk-adjusted outcomes, especially mortality, emergency bypass surgery, coronary perforation	
Satisfaction surveys (patient, family, referring physician)	
Frequency of coronary angiograms showing no significant disease	

(Adapted from Heupler FA, Al-Hani AJ, Dear WE, et al: Guidelines for continuous quality improvement in the cardiac catheterization laboratory, *Cathet Cardiovasc Diagn* 30(3):191–200, 1993.)

Specialists (RCIS) and to maintain certification in Advanced Cardiac Life Support (ACLS).

Education in the form of cardiac catheterization conferences, which provide a forum to discuss difficult management issues, and morbidity and mortality reviews as part of a peer review quality improvement program are important structural components.[50] To be effective, these programs must emphasize improvement of performance rather than simply punishing individual physicians as potential one-time outliers. Collection of laboratory data with benchmarking against state or national data is an important structural element to accurately assess clinical outcomes. Examples of such programs include the National Cardiovascular Data Registry's (NCDR), Cath PCI Registry, and ACTION-GWTG Registry of Myocardial Infarction.[51] Participation in such programs provides caregivers with standardized tools for data collection, including relevant data elements and definitions, and also validated risk-adjustment of patient outcomes, such as mortality-based on relevant individual patient clinical factors. In addition to tracking outcomes, these data reports are helpful to assess adherence to guidelines and performance measure recommendations and can serve as a focus for quality improvements within an institution. Such feedback systems, typically offered in a benchmarked format against one's peers, are known to be a critical element in quality improvement (see Fig. 62-1).[52]

PROCESS

In simple terms, *process* measures assess how the system works and how health care is delivered (see Table 62-6). A relevant example in interventional cardiology is the door-to-balloon (D2B) time metric for patients with STEMI. The actions which are necessary to achieve an optimal D2B time are complex, with many individual steps that cut across several hospital departments and services. For example, the emergency department must quickly recognize and triage a patient with a possible STEMI, and an electrocardiogram (ECG) must be obtained rapidly to confirm the diagnosis. Then appropriate treatment must be started, and there must be a process to quickly alert the interventional team. There should be separate processes to ready the cardiac cath lab, transport the patient to the laboratory, and finally open the culprit artery.[53] A flaw in any of these multiple steps will lead to a poor D2B time and contribute to a process failure within the system. Realizing that D2B times were suboptimal in many facilities, the Door-to-Balloon Alliance was launched in late 2006 with a goal of achieving a D2B time of 90 minutes or less in at least 75% of nontransferred patients.[54] Adoption of several process measures, all of which were found to improve D2B times, was tracked and increased during this effort, resulting in a significant improvement in national D2B times (Fig. 62-5).[55] Another example of a process measure is the appropriateness of performing a PCI. Proper patient selection for PCIs is receiving increasing scrutiny by all health care stakeholders, as there is wide variation in the use of PCIs (see Fig. 62-4).[43] Assessing the appropriateness of a PCI involves understanding the patient's history and clinical presentation, physical findings, noninvasive testing to determine the presence and severity of ischemia, knowledge of the left ventricular function, anatomic findings as determined by coronary angiography, and the accuracy of the interpretation of the angiographic findings. Appropriate use criteria for coronary artery revascularization have

recently been developed to determine whether coronary revascularization is a "reasonable" approach for a given clinical circumstance (Fig. 62-6).[56] Although acceptable indications outside of the AUC exist, measuring the degree of adherence to the clinical situations covered by such criteria is valuable for assessing the quality of patient selection. Application and assessment of appropriateness of care requires accurate collection of the relevant patient clinical variables.

Outcomes

The final component of Donabedian's triad is *outcome*, which is simply the final product or result. Outcomes are tangible measures such as procedure mortality rates and other related adverse outcomes such as vascular complications, bleeding, stroke, contrast nephropathy, cardiac tamponade, peri-procedural MI, or the rate of emergency CABG (see Table 62-6). The attraction to measuring outcomes as quality indicators relates to the implied association between the outcome measure and hospital or physician performance. However, these associations can be tenuous at the hospital or physician level, creating challenges for the accurate assessment of outcomes. For example, there is debate not only regarding the definition of a peri-procedural MI (i.e., any troponin rise versus three times baseline or five times baseline) but also the clinical significance of increased biomarkers in the peri-procedural period. In addition, besides the absence of a standardized biomarker collection protocol during the postprocedural period, additional challenges include interpretation of biomarker elevations in patients in the middle of an ACS event. Clinical data standards and definitions as well as standards for statistical models have been developed to help ensure consistency, but important issues remain.[57]

Many PCI-related adverse events such as mortality or emergency CABG are infrequent, especially when assessed at the operator level, where total procedures annually are modest. For example, the 95% confidence interval (CI) around a 2% mortality rate for 100 PCI procedures is 0% to 7%. This is a wide range for judging whether the operator has a low or a high mortality rate. Therefore, quarter-to-quarter or year-to-year outcome measures can often vary widely when measured at the single center or operator level. Another critical issue is risk adjustment. Multiple factors beyond the operator and the facility must be accounted for so that outcome comparisons are meaningful. The acuity of the patient, certain demographic features, and the presence of many comorbid conditions all have substantial roles

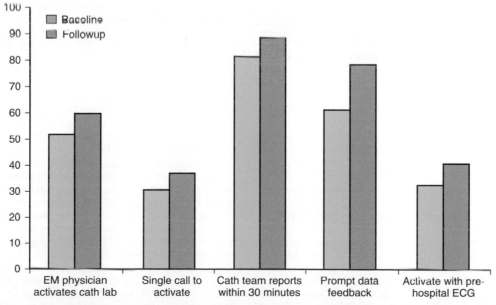

Figure 62-5 Percentage of Door-2-Balloon Alliance hospitals reporting use of recommended strategies at baseline and follow-up surveys. *cath,* catheterization; *ECG,* electrocardiogram; *EM,* emergency medicine. *(From Bradley EH, Nallamothu BK, Herrin J, et al: National efforts to improve door-to-balloon time results from the Door-to-Balloon Alliance, J Am Coll Cardiol 54(25):2423–2439, 2009.)*

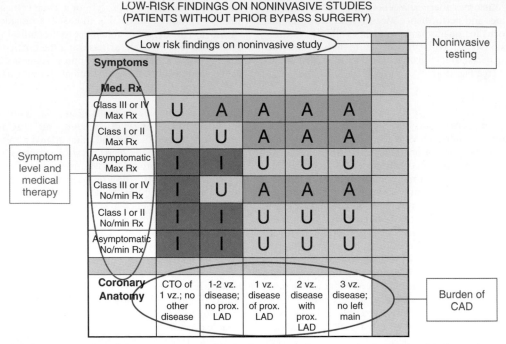

REVASCULARIZATION APPROPRIATENESS FOR PATIENTS WITH LOW-RISK FINDINGS ON NONINVASIVE STUDIES (PATIENTS WITHOUT PRIOR BYPASS SURGERY)

Figure 62-6 Format for the presentation of the coronary revascularization appropriate use criteria (AUC): table for patients with low risk findings on noninvasive studies. The burden of coronary artery disease is shown on the bottom of the table. The symptom class and degree of medical therapy is shown on the vertical axis. *A*, appropriate; *I*, inappropriate; *U*, uncertain; *CTO*, chronic total occlusion; *vd*, vessel disease; *LAD*, left anterior descending coronary artery; *Prox*, proximal; *Max*, maximal; *Med. Rx*, medical therapy *(From Patel MR, Dehmer GJ, Hirshfeld JW, et al: ACCF/SCAI/STS/AATS/AHA/ASNC 2009 Appropriateness Criteria for Coronary Revascularization: a report by the American College of Cardiology Foundation Appropriateness Criteria Task Force, Society for Cardiovascular Angiography and Interventions, Society of Thoracic Surgeons, American Association for Thoracic Surgery, American Heart Association, and the American Society of Nuclear Cardiology Endorsed by the American Society of Echocardiography, the Heart Failure Society of America, and the Society of Cardiovascular Computed Tomography, J Am Coll Cardiol 53(6):530–553, 2009.)*

in determining patient outcome, independent of the quality of care actually provided. To accomplish risk adjustment for key clinical outcomes, accurate and detailed clinical data are necessary, coupled with a rigorous risk adjustment methodology to truly and accurately describe provider outcome measurements.

To help health care provider groups and institutions respond to increasing requirements to document their processes and outcomes of care in the cardiac cath lab, the NCDR was started in 1997. Today, the NCDR is the most comprehensive, outcomes-based data repository program in the United States, with five hospital-based registries and one practice-based registry. More than 2200 hospitals nationwide participate in the NCDR, which has amassed over 11 million patient records.[58] Participation in some of the NCDR registries is now required by several states and several payers. Moreover, the Center for Medicare and Medicaid Services (CMS) requires participation in the NCDR's Implantable Cardioverter Defibrillator (ICD) Registry to receive reimbursement for ICD implantation for primary prevention of sudden cardiac death (SCD). The NCDR's CathPCI Registry now contains almost 10 million patient records and receives data from over 1300 facilities. Comprehensive data from the Cath PCI Registry are provided back to member institutions for use in their internal quality assessment and improvement. In addition, the development and validation of the most recent NCDR risk adjustment results have been published (Table 62-7).[59] In 2011, Chan et al, reported on appropriateness of over 500,000 PCI procedures from the NCDR and documented that nearly all acute PCIs were appropriate, while ~12% of elective PCIs, comprising only 30% of the overall database, were deemed "inappropriate."[59a] Outcomes assessment often overlaps with and represents the aggregate effect of the other two components of the triad, namely, structure and process. Thus, improving the end product is the ultimate measure of the overall success of medical care. Ideal outcomes assessment would not only examine an isolated episode of care (i.e., single PCI

procedure) but also include a longitudinal follow-up assessment of the PCI. This could include the impact of care on indirect health-related measures, such as patient satisfaction related to the overall care process itself, along with quantification of the actual cost of the care delivery, including cost-effectiveness and cost-efficiency calculations.

QUALITY ASSURANCE VERSUS CONTINUOUS QUALITY IMPROVEMENT

Quality assurance is a process that is based largely on the retrospective review of selected outcomes to determine the presence of discrepancies between actual practice and recommended standards of care.[60] In simple terms, it can be likened to inspecting the final product as it comes off the assembly line. Criteria are established to identify an "acceptable product," and items not meeting these criteria are judged as flawed or damaged and rejected before leaving the factory. By this process, a certain level of product quality is maintained, with only "acceptable products" reaching the market. Applied to the clinical environment, quality assurance seeks to identify outliers in some aspect of clinical care. Once identified, outliers are often provided an opportunity to improve, but if that fails, they can be denied further participation in clinical care (Fig. 62-7, *A*). As structured, the quality assurance process promotes a level of defensiveness among physicians, as the process is often focused at determining who is at fault if something goes wrong—the so called "bad apple" concept.[61] In contrast, the CQI process provides an alternative approach whereby specific problems are first identified, which is followed by the formulation of a solution by various stakeholders; this is validated by re-evaluation of the process once the solution is implemented (see Fig. 62-7, *B*). For example, a facility may have an excessive number of cases of hematomas following PCIs performed through the femoral artery access. Although hematomas do not occur in most patients, which is "acceptable," patients with

TABLE 62-7	National Cardiovascular Data Registry (NCDR) CathPCI Risk Score System					
Variable	**Scoring Response Categories (years)**				*Total Points*	*Risk of In-Patient Mortality*
AGE	<60	≥60, <70	≥70, <80	≥80		
	0	4	8	14	5	0.1%
Cardiogenic shock	No	Yes	–	–	10	0.1%
	0	25	–	–	15	0.2%
Prior CHF	No	Yes	–	–	20	0.3%
	0	5	–	–	25	0.6%
Peripheral vascular disease	No	Yes	–	–	30	1.1%
	0	5	–	–	35	2.0%
Chronic lung disease	No	Yes	–	–	40	3.6%
	0	4	–	–	45	6.3%
GFR	<30	30–60	60–90	>90	50	10.9%
	18	10	6	0	55	18.3%
NYHA functional class IV	No	Yes	–	–	60	29.0%
	0	4	–	–	65	42.7%
PCI status (STEMI)	Elective	Urgent	Emergent	Salvage	70	57.6%
	12	15	20	38	75	71.2%
PCI status (no STEMI)	Elective	Urgent	Emergent	Salvage	80	81%
	0	8	20	42	85	89.2%
					90	93.8%
					95	96.5%
					100	98.0%

National Cardiovascular Data Registry (NCDR) risk prediction model for percutaneous coronary intervention mortality. Points are assigned for the different variables and the total number of points used to predict the risk of in-patient mortality.

(From Peterson ED, Dai D, DeLong ER, et al: Contemporary mortality risk prediction for percutaneous coronary intervention: Results from 588,398 procedures in the National Cardiovascular Data Registry, *J Am Coll Cardiol* 55(18):1923–1932, 2010.)

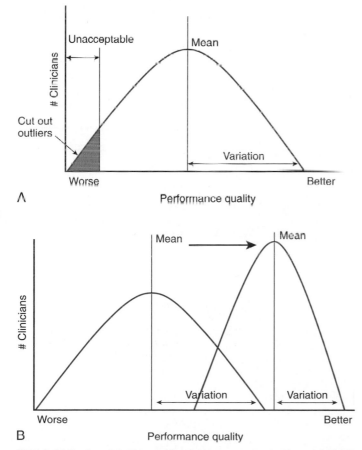

Figure 62-7 *Panel A,* The quality assurance approach. The goal of this process is to identify outliers that are unacceptable and excluded. *Panel B,* The continuous quality improvement approach. The goal of this process is to identify opportunities for practice improvement and develop methods to respond to these opportunities and improve overall practice.

hematomas are unhappy, have a prolonged hospitalization, and cost the facility more in resources. A CQI project could be initiated to reduce the number of cases of hematomas. This would require participation of all of the individuals involved, including physicians, cath lab personnel, nursing staff in the recovery area, and others who interact with the patient. Each step in the process is carefully examined, opportunities for improvement are identified, and appropriate steps are taken to address any defects in the process. The new process is initiated, and then the results are measured in this case by determining if the number of cases of hematomas has been reduced. The CQI process has now become a vital and expected component of a quality cardiovascular program with the goal of reducing variation and improving overall performance.[62] Several models for CQI exist. One model frequently used is the Plan-Do-Study-Act (PDSA) model and an alternative is the Focus-Analyze-Develop-Execute (FADE) model (Figs. 62-8 and 62-9).

The core actions of these models and most CQI programs include the following:

- The collection of data containing relevant patient variables that allows assessment of clinical processes, performance, and outcomes
- Feedback of this performance and outcomes to the clinicians, with risk adjustment, if necessary, and benchmarking of the data
- Implementation of appropriate interventions to promote reduction in wasteful and inefficient variation of care and simultaneously improving performance

Despite the emphasis on the importance of CQI efforts, relatively few studies have formally examined the results or improvements in patient outcomes related to CQI. Ferguson et al examined the effect of CQI interventions to improve preoperative β-blocker use in all patients and the use of the internal mammary artery as a bypass conduit in older patients in a large cohort undergoing CABG.[63] Compared with the control arm, the CQI interventions lead to an increase in the use of both β-blockers and the internal mammary artery, especially at centers with lower surgical volumes. Moscucci et al reported the results of a statewide CQI PCI initiative in Michigan.[64] This involved the use of a wide range of CQI strategies, which particularly relied on quarterly feedback reports to clinicians on their adherence to process and

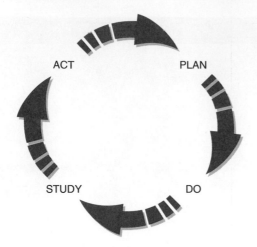

PLAN: Plan a change or test of how something works
DO: Carry out the plan
STUDY: Look at the results. What did you find out?
ACT: Decide what actions should be taken to improve

Figure 62-8 The Plan-Do-Study-Act (PDSA) model.

performance measures, along with reports of crude and risk-adjusted outcomes. The program resulted in a demonstrable decrease in bleeding, transfusion requirements, vascular complications, and contrast use, leading to a trend in the reduction of contrast nephropathy. In a temporal observational study at the Mayo Clinic, Rihal et al also identified the benefit of CQI intervention for PCI delivery, showing improvements in both clinical and economic outcomes.[65] Unfortunately, there are several barriers to the implementation of CQI programs. Lack of hospital administrative and financial supports, the time and expense of internal data collection, and the lack of physician leadership frequently hamper CQI efforts.[66]

Developing a Quality Culture in Interventional Cardiology

ORGANIZATIONAL CULTURE

Amid the escalating demands for quality health care, it is increasingly important to encourage an organizational "culture of quality" in the cardiac cath lab. *Organizational culture* is the term used to describe the shared beliefs, perceptions, and expectations of individuals in organizations. Because of its shared nature, organizational culture can have a dramatic effect on efforts to change specific procedures or processes.

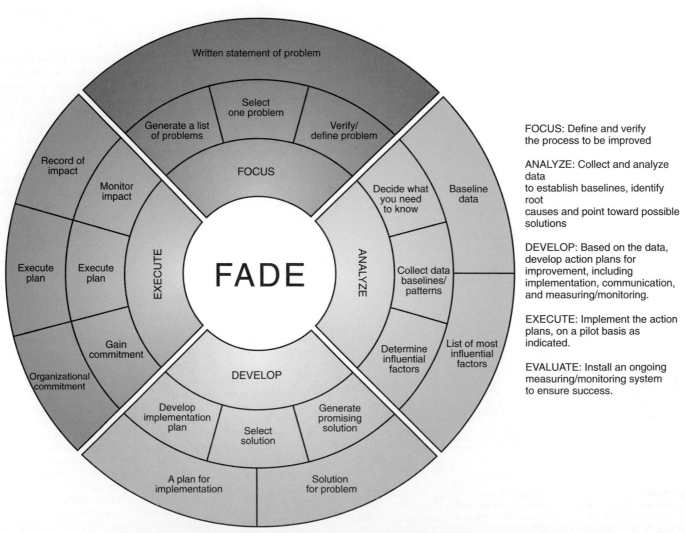

FOCUS: Define and verify the process to be improved

ANALYZE: Collect and analyze data to establish baselines, identify root causes and point toward possible solutions

DEVELOP: Based on the data, develop action plans for improvement, including implementation, communication, and measuring/monitoring.

EXECUTE: Implement the action plans, on a pilot basis as indicated.

EVALUATE: Install an ongoing measuring/monitoring system to ensure success.

Figure 62-9 The Focus-Analyze-Develop-Execute and Evaluate (FADE*) model. (***The FADE Model**, Organizational Dynamics Institute, Wakefield, MA.)*

For better or worse, organizational culture affects any effort to implement change. Characteristics of organizational culture have also been linked to various aspects of organizational performance such as financial performance, customer and employee satisfaction, and innovation. In the health care environment, organizational culture has been associated with several elements that contribute to quality, such as nursing care, job satisfaction, and patient safety.[67,68] A supportive organizational culture is often cited as a key component of successful quality improvement initiatives in a variety of industries, including health care. Measures of organizational culture are related to an organization's ability to adapt to rapidly changing health care demands, to remain competitive, and to sustain high levels of performance. Successful organizations portray organizational culture as being central to the operation and function of the organization, providing a shared vision that can serve as an effective guide to appropriate and goal-directed social and individual behaviors. However, some aspects of organizational culture can have an opposite effect that unfortunately undermines any efforts for positive change. Many quality initiatives fail because of resistance to change, ingrained attitudes, lack of understanding, and poor communication. For success, the high-level leaders of an organization must focus on the mission and vision of the organization. Mission is seen as a fundamental unit of culture, and as such, the failure to fulfill the organization's mission impedes quality improvement efforts. By focusing on the mission and the vision, leaders may facilitate the dissemination of quality-oriented values throughout an organization. Once the leadership embraces the role of advancing a quality culture through the organization's mission and vision, these can be disseminated through the multiple levels of the organization. Four levels of intervention have been proposed to influence organizational culture: (1) individual, (2) team or microsystem, (3) organizational, and (4) environmental.[69] In its landmark publication *Crossing the Quality Chasm*, the Institute of Medicine asserts that all interventions must address these four dimensions.[19]

PHYSICIAN-CHAMPIONS

Key in the development of a quality culture in interventional cardiology is the role of the physician-champion. A physician-champion should be an opinion leader, a change agent, and a physician who influences colleagues and friends. A physician-champion is a respected individual who provides expert education, champions a cause or a product, or gives support to staff for the diffusion and implementation of clinical practice guidelines, protocols, or research evidence. In all cases, the physician-champion is perceived as a credible individual who has the ability to persuade others. Often, the physician-champion is able to influence other physicians to adopt or implement a new or revised process or guideline for quality improvement or to become physician-champions themselves. The champion's role can be an invaluable tool for change within a health care organization. However, when the chosen physician is unable or unwilling to engage in the variety of tasks required to be an effective physician-champion, the role is not clearly defined, or the prospective champion only has a narrow sphere of influence and lacks the required institutional support, the physician-champion will not be able to fulfill the expectations of the organization, and change may not be thoroughly implemented or sustainable.

BENCHMARKING

An additional essential element for a quality culture is the process of *benchmarking*. Simply put, a *benchmark* is a standard by which something can be measured or judged. Only by the collection of data can clinicians or hospitals compare, or benchmark, their care and outcomes with those of their peers and with national standards. Major strides in quality improvement require this process, coupled with changes in the systems of care and the engagement of local clinical leaders and administrative support.[70] The process must be iterative so that the effectiveness of the changes can be assessed. Therefore, quality improvement is a process that mandates answers to the questions "How am I doing compared with others?" and "Am I getting better?"

As noted earlier, the NCDR was developed to assist facilities in the collection of data for use in benchmarking and quality improvement. Specifically, the NCDR-CathPCI Registry and the ACTION-GWTG Registry provide data for benchmarking key outcome metrics for the cath lab and in patients with ACS, respectively. These reports include both regional benchmarking (to "like" hospitals) and national benchmarking against all participating facilities. Sample sections of such a benchmark report from the CathPCI and ACTION-GWTG Registries are shown in Figures 62-10 and 62-11. The intention is that this feedback with benchmarking be used by hospitals and practices to target areas for improvement. For example, a hospital participating in the CathPCI Registry may find that it has a high vascular complication rate compared with "like hospitals" or with the national standard. This should lead to the development of a CQI team that includes all stakeholders to examine the cases, identify possible causes, develop an action plan to correct the identified problems, implement the plan, and then evaluate whether the plan has been effective.

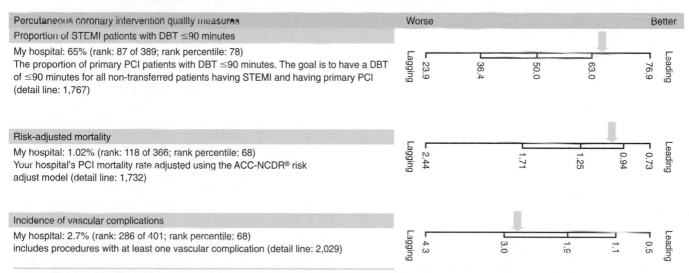

ACC-NCDR® = American College of Cardiology National Cardiovascular Data Registry; DBT = door to balloon time; PCI = percutaneous coronary intervention; STEMI = ST-elevation myocardial infarction.

Figure 62-10 Sample from the executive summary of a report from the NCDR CathPCI Registry.

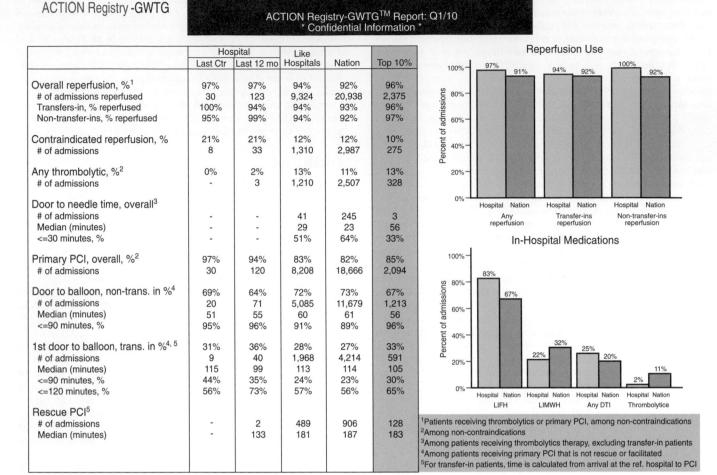

Figure 62-11 Sample page from a report from the ACTION-GWTG Registry.

Public Reporting—the New Frontier

Although many superb aspects of the U.S. health care system exist, its shortcomings, including unacceptable gaps in care and concerns over quality issues, are increasingly becoming more apparent to all stakeholders. Employers have seen an increasing portion of their revenue being consumed in providing health care for their employees, as has the federal government for Medicare beneficiaries. This increasing financial burden has pressured payers, who, in turn, have pressured providers to accelerate quality improvement efforts. Public reporting of physician, health plan, and institutional performances is increasingly being used in an attempt to steer patients to the best performing providers and facilities on the assumption that patients will receive better and more cost-effective care. Patients are also becoming more engaged in this process and are increasingly interested in public performance reports on providers and facilities. The public release of performance data has been proposed as a mechanism for improving the quality of care by providing more transparency and greater accountability of health care providers.[71] Public reporting is not particularly new in the cardiovascular arena, especially in the case of cardiac surgeons. Beginning in the mid-1990s, New York and Pennsylvania publicly reported cardiac surgery outcomes; Massachusetts started a program (Mass-DAC) in 2002, and California in 2003.[2,3,72,73] After its early years of operation, the New York program reported a reduction in risk-adjusted mortality from 4.17% to 2.45%, with smaller yearly improvements thereafter.[74] The Pennsylvania CABG public reporting program has documented a similar trend.[75] In evaluating public reporting programs, it is important to understand the source of the data and the distinction between administrative (claims) data and clinical data sources. For example, the Mass-DAC cardiac surgery reporting program uses clinical data from the Society of Thoracic Surgery database. In an important comparative study, the cardiac surgery performance results based on clinical data were compared with performance results derived from administrative data during the same period. Considerable disparities in the results between these two data sets were found, which led to the conclusion that report cards using administrative data are problematic compared with those derived from audited and validated clinical data.[76] This same comparison was made within the New York cardiac surgery reporting program with similar conclusions.[77] The use of pure administrative data was inferior to clinical data in identifying outliers and assessing surgical outcomes. At the national level, in collaboration with the Hospital Quality Alliance, the CMS issues a Web-based public report.[78] The following are reported: (1) several process of care measures for patients with acute MI, CHF, other selected medical conditions, and some surgical procedures; (2) outcomes of care measures, including 30-day risk-adjusted mortality and re-admission rates for MI, heart failure, and pneumonia; (3) patients' hospital experiences, using data collected from the Hospital Consumer Assessment of Healthcare Providers and Systems (HCAHPS) Survey; (4) the number of Medicare patients treated (volume) for certain illnesses or diagnoses; and (5) Medicare inpatient hospital payment information. Up to this point, large-scale public reporting efforts in cardiology and interventional cardiology have primarily focused on events such as acute MI and CHF or on procedures such as CABG or PCIs. Although some state programs report physician-level metrics, the CIs around any point estimate are necessarily wide because of the small sample size for any single physician. Therefore, the majority of public reporting has been at the facility level, as greater statistical validity exists with larger denominators. The more meaningful programs rely on clinical data sources to avoid the pitfalls of administrative data and allow for a more robust risk adjustment of outcomes. Although more public reporting is coming in the future, concern has been expressed that such programs may lead to unintended consequences that could offset their benefits.[79,80]

THE UNINTENDED CONSEQUENCES OF PUBLIC REPORTING

Although the early reduction in risk-adjusted mortality from CABG in the New York experience was deemed a success, another perspective subsequently emerged. Omoigui et al reviewed 9442 isolated CABG operations performed from 1989 through 1993 at the Cleveland Clinic to assess referral patterns, case-mix, and outcomes.[81] Patients referred to Cleveland from New York had a higher frequency of prior open heart surgery and were more likely to be NYHA functional class III or IV compared with patients from Ohio, other states, and even other countries. Accordingly, their expected mortality rate was higher than among other referral cohorts. The observed 5.2% mortality rate among patients referred from New York was significantly greater than any of the other referral sources, leading the authors to speculate that the public reporting of outcomes data in New York may have provoked the increased referral of high-risk patients out of state, explaining the reduction of CABG mortality in New York.

Schneider and Epstein surveyed cardiologists and cardiac surgeons to determine whether they were aware of the Pennsylvania Consumer Guide to Cardiac Surgery and, if so, to determine their views on its usefulness, limitations, and influence on providers.[82] Only 10% reported that the published mortality rates were "very important" in assessing the performance of a cardiothoracic surgeon. Less than 10% reported discussing the guide with more than 10% of their patients before CABG. Among cardiologists, 87% reported that the guide had minimal or no influence on their referral recommendations. When the limitations of the guide were assessed, 78% cited the absence of indicators of quality other than mortality, 79% cited inadequate risk adjustment methods, and 53% cited the unreliability of data provided by hospitals and surgeons. Importantly, 59% of cardiologists reported increased difficulty in finding surgeons willing to perform CABG in severely ill patients who required it, and 63% of cardiac surgeons reported that they were reluctant to operate on such patients. In a subsequent publication, awareness and use of the consumer guide was assessed among patients undergoing CABG in the prior year.[83] Only 12% of patients were aware of the guide before surgery, and less than 1% knew the correct rating of their surgeon or hospital and reported that it had a moderate or major impact on their selection of provider. These studies, however, are roughly 10 years old, and now the general public, especially the informed patient, seems more keenly aware of these issues.

Currently, there are several Web sites where patients can report their individual experiences with physicians, both good and bad, in an unregulated and nonscientific manner. This, in turn, has resulted in some physicians requiring patients to agree to not participate in such activities before any treatment is provided.[84] The public reporting of PCI data has a shorter history compared with that of cardiac surgery, but similar observations are now being made. Moscucci et al compared the demographics, indications, and outcomes of 11,374 patients undergoing PCIs in Michigan, where no public reporting is present, with 69,048 patients from New York, where public reporting exists.[85] Patients in Michigan more frequently underwent PCIs for acute MI (14.4% vs. 8.7%, $P < 0.0001$) and cardiogenic shock (2.56% vs. 0.38%, $P < 0.0001$) compared with those in New York and had a higher prevalence of CHF and extracardiac vascular disease. The unadjusted in-hospital mortality rate was lower in New York than in Michigan, but after adjustment

for comorbidities, there was no significant difference in mortality between the two groups. The authors concluded that a propensity in New York toward nonintervention in the case of higher risk patients may be related to the fear of public reporting of high mortality rates. This was confirmed in a separate retrospective study of the SHOCK (Should We Emergently Revascularize Occluded Coronaries for Cardiogenic Shock?) registry comparing the outcomes of patients from New York with those from other states.[86] Patients from New York State presenting with cardiogenic shock were less likely to receive angiography, PCI, or CABG; in-hospital mortality among these patients was 1.5 times higher in New York, possibly indicating that life-saving treatments were being withheld to avoid the reporting of adverse outcomes. Survey data from New York physicians confirmed this, with 83% of practitioners agreeing that patients who were at high risk were denied PCI because of fear of public reporting and 79% confirming that their own decisions on performing PCIs on individual patients had been influenced by fear of public reporting.[87] Similar concerns have been raised about the public reporting of PCI data in Massachusetts.[88] To minimize this unintended consequence, some reporting efforts now specifically exclude extremely high-risk and salvage patients. In addition to concerns that the risk adjustment methods currently available are suboptimal and do not include all relevant variables, there has been a suggestion that mortalities be adjudicated to determine if they were procedure related or not procedure related. About 80% of the mortalities at one Massachusetts hospital were felt, after further blinded review, to not be directly related to the procedure and more related to the natural history of disease in the patient.[88]

Payers have been more focused on cost profiling physicians, but the accuracy of these methods have also been questioned.[89] Fung and colleagues conducted a systematic review of the evidence that public reporting leads to an improvement in the quality of care.[90] They concluded that there is minimal evidence about public reporting of individual provider data and practices and that a rigorous evaluation of many major public reporting systems is lacking. They found some evidence suggesting that public release of performance data stimulates quality improvement activity at the hospital level, but the overall effect of public reporting on effectiveness, safety, and patient-centeredness remains uncertain.

The most compelling justification for the public reporting of clinical outcomes is the public's right to know about the care that they are likely to receive from hospitals and physicians. Such transparency of information should allow patients to make better informed decisions about their health care choices, but the reporting process must be accurate and fair. Realizing the importance of public reporting, the ACC published six principles of public reporting as a possible roadmap for the future (Table 62-8).[91] There is also a growing interest in changing reimbursement models to be based on the quality of care, rather

TABLE 62-8	**2008 American College of Cardiology Foundation Principles for Public Reporting of Physician Performance Data**

- The driving force behind physician performance measurement and reporting systems should be to promote quality improvement.
- Public reporting programs should be based on performance measures with scientific validity
- Public reporting programs should be developed in partnership with physicians.
- Every effort should be made to use standardized data elements to assess and report performance and to make the submission process uniform across all public reporting programs
- Performance reporting should occur at the appropriate level of accountability.
- All public reporting programs should include a formal process for evaluating the impact of the program on the quality and cost of health care, including an assessment of unintended consequences.

(From Drozda JP Jr., Hagan EP, Mirro MJ, et al: ACCF 2008 health policy statement on principles for public reporting of physician performance data: A report of the American College of Cardiology Foundation Writing Committee to Develop Principles for Public Reporting of Physician Performance Data, *J Am Coll Cardiol* 51(20):1993–2001, 2008.)

than quantity of care, and on the development of more quality measures approved by the National Quality Forum.

Conclusion

There is no doubt that all people, if asked, would say they want the highest quality medical care for themselves and their loved ones.

Moving forward, it is important to recognize that current efforts to achieve this goal have fallen short in certain areas and that important gaps exist in the ability to always provide the highest quality of care to all patients. Improving the quality of care in interventional cardiology is a lofty, but achievable, goal if physicians and other members of the interventional care delivery team make this effort a part of their daily practice.

REFERENCES

1. Deming WE: The W. Edwards Deming Institute: Available at www.deming.org: Accessed July 12, 2010.
2. New York State Department of Health: *Cardiovascular disease: Data and statistics:* Available at http://www.nyhealth.gov/statistics/diseases/cardiovascular/: Accessed July 8, 2010.
3. Pennsylvania Health Care Cost Containment Council: *Cardiac surgery in Pennsylvania:* Available at http://www.phc4.org/reports/cabg/: Accessed July 8, 2010.
4. McGlynn EA, Asch SM, Adams J, et al: The quality of health care delivered to adults in the United States. *N Engl J Med* 348(26):2635–2645, 2003.
5. Dehmer GJ, Powell W: Pay for quality—what every interventional cardiologist needs to know: Part I. *Catheter Cardiovasc Interv* 68(1):169–172, 2006.
6. Smith SC, Jr, Feldman TE, Hirshfeld JW, Jr, et al: ACC/AHA/SCAI 2005 guideline update for percutaneous coronary intervention: A report of the American College of Cardiology/American Heart Association Task Force on Practice Guidelines (ACC/AHA/SCAI Writing Committee to Update the 2001 Guidelines for Percutaneous Coronary Intervention). *J Am Coll Cardiol* 47(1):216–235, 2006.
7. Bashore TM, Bates ER, Berger PB, et al: Cardiac catheterization laboratory standards: A report of the American College of Cardiology Task Force on Clinical Expert Consensus Documents (ACC/SCA&I Committee to Develop an Expert Consensus Document on Catheterization Laboratory Standards). *J Am Coll Cardiol* 37(8):2170–2214, 2001.
8. Dehmer GJ, Blankenship J, Wharton TP, Jr, et al: The current status and future direction of percutaneous coronary intervention without on-site surgical backup: An expert consensus document from the Society for Cardiovascular Angiography and Interventions. *Catheter Cardiovasc Interv* 69(4):471–478, 2007.
9. Roberts J, Coale J, Redman R: A history of the Joint Commission on Accreditation of Hospitals. *JAMA* 258(7):936–940, 1987.
10. Donabedian A: Evaluating the quality of medical care. *Milbank Mem Fund Q* 44(3 Suppl):166–206, 1966.
11. Luce JM, Bindman AB, Lee PR: A brief history of health care quality assessment and improvement in the United States. *West J Med* 160(3):263–268, 1994.
12. Laffel G, Blumenthal D: The case for using industrial quality management science in health care organizations. *JAMA* 262(20):2869–2873, 1989.
13. Berwick D: Continuous improvement as an ideal in health care. *N Engl J Med* 320(1):53–56, 1989.
14. Kritchevsky S, Simmons B: Continuous quality improvement: Concepts and applications for physician care. *JAMA* 266(13):1817–1823, 1991.
15. The American Board of Medical Specialties: Available at www.abms.org: Accessed April 7, 2010.
16. Dans P, Weiner J, Otter S: Peer review organizations: Promises and potential pitfalls. *N Engl J Med* 313(18):1131–1137, 1985.
17. Rubin HR, Rogers WH, Kahn KL, et al: Watching the doctor-watchers: How well do peer review organization methods detect hospital care quality problems? *JAMA* 267(17):2349–2354, 1992.
18. Persig RM: *Zen and the art of motorcycle maintenance: An inquiry into values,* New York, 1974, William Morrow Company, Inc..
19. Committee on Quality of Health Care in America, Institute of Medicine: *Crossing the quality chasm: A new health system for the 21st century,* Washington D.C., 2001, National Academy Press.
20. Schuster MA, McGlynn EA, Brook RH: How good is the quality of health care in the United States? *Milbank Q* 76(4):517–563, 1998.
21. Lee TH: A broader concept of medical errors. *N Engl J Med* 347(24):1965–1967, 2002.
22. Califf RM, Peterson ED, Gibbons RJ, et al: Integrating quality into the cycle of therapeutic development. *J Am Coll Cardiol* 40(11):1895–1901, 2002.
23. Field MJ, Lohr KN, editors: *Guidelines for clinical practice: From development to use,* Washington, D.C., 1992, National Academy Press.
24. Marciniak TA, Ellerbeck EF, Radford MJ, et al: Improving the quality of care for Medicare patients with acute myocardial infarction: Results from the Cooperative Cardiovascular Project. *JAMA* 279(1):1351–1357, 1998.
25. Radford MJ, Heidenreich PA, Bailey SR, et al: ACC/AHA 2007 methodology for the development of clinical data standards: A Report of the American College of Cardiology/American Heart Association Task Force on Clinical Data Standards. *J Am Coll Cardiol* 49(7):830–837, 2007.
26. American College of Cardiology Cardiosource: Available at http://www.cardiosource.org/Science-And-Quality/Practice-Guidelines-and-Quality-Standards.aspx?type=KXaIWJdFFUW5Txwigr32qg: Accessed July 8, 2010.

27. Spertus JA, Eagle KA, Krumholtz HM, et al: American College of Cardiology and American Heart Association methodology for the selection and creation of performance measures for quantifying and quality of cardiovascular care. *J Am Coll Cardiol* 45(7):1147–1156, 2005.
28. Kiefe CI, Allison JJ, Williams OD, et al: Improving quality improvement using achievable benchmarks for physician feedback: A randomized controlled trial. *JAMA* 285(22):2871–2879, 2001.
29. Peterson ED, DeLong ER, Masoudi FA, et al: ACCF/AHA 2010 position statement on composite measures for healthcare performance assessment. *J Am Coll Cardiol* 55(16):1755–1766, 2010.
30. O'Brien SM, Shahian DM, DeLong ER, et al: Quality measurement in adult cardiac surgery: part 2—Statistical considerations in composite measure scoring and provider rating. *Ann Thorac Surg* 83(4 Suppl):S13–S26, 2007.
31. Shahian DM, O'Brien SM, Normand ST, et al: Association of hospital coronary artery bypass volume with processes of care, mortality, morbidity, and the Society of Thoracic Surgeons composite quality score. *J Thorac Cardiovasc Surg* 139(2):273–282, 2010.
32. Mehta RH, Peterson ED, Califf RM: Performance measures have a major effect on cardiovascular outcomes: A review. *Am J Med* 120(5):398–402, 2007.
33. Bradley EH, Herrin J, Elbel B, et al: Hospital quality for acute myocardial infarction: Correlation among process measures and relationship with short-term mortality. *JAMA* 296(1):72–78, 2006.
34. Anderson HV, Shaw RE, Brindis RG, et al: Relationship between procedure indications and outcomes of percutaneous coronary interventions by American College of Cardiology/American Heart Association Task Force Guidelines. *Circulation* 112(18):2786–2791, 2005.
35. Lopes RD, Starr A, Pieper CF, et al: Warfarin use and outcomes in patients with atrial fibrillation complicating acute coronary syndromes. *Am J Med* 123(2):134–140, 2010.
36. Goldberg RJ, Spencer FA, Steg PE, et al, for the Global Registry of Acute Coronary Events Investigators: Increasing use of single and combination medical therapy in patients hospitalized for acute myocardial infarction in the 21st century. *Arch Intern Med* 167(16):1766–1773, 2007.
37. Fornasini M, Yarzebski J, Chirboga D, et al: Contemporary trends in evidence-based treatment for acute myocardial infarction. *Am J Med* 123(2):166–172, 2010.
38. Cabana MD, Rand CS, Powe NR, et al: Why don't physicians follow clinical practice guidelines? A framework for improvement. *JAMA.* 282(15):1458–1465, 1999.
39. Alpert JS: Why are we ignoring guideline recommendations? *Am J Med* 123(2):97–98, 2010.
40. Tricoci P, Allen JM, Kramer JM, et al: Scientific evidence underlying the ACC/AHA clinical practice guidelines. *JAMA* 301(8):831–841, 2009.
41. Hobbs FD, Erhardt L: Acceptance of guideline recommendations and perceived implementation of coronary heart disease prevention among primary care physicians in five European countries: The Reassessing European Attitudes about Cardiovascular Treatment (REACT) survey. *Fam Pract* 19(6):596–604, 2002.
42. Hannan EL, Racz MJ, Gold J, et al: Adherence of catheterization laboratory cardiologists to American Collage of Cardiology/American Heart Association guidelines for percutaneous coronary interventions and coronary artery bypass graft surgery. What happens in actual practice? *Circulation* 121(2):267–275, 2010.
43. Dartmouth Atlas Cardiovascular Report: Available at http://www.dartmouthatlas.org/downloads/reports/Cardiac_report_2005.pdf: Accessed August 3, 2010.
44. Lucas FL, Sirovich BE, Gallagher PM, et al: Variation in cardiologists' propensity to test and treat. Is it associated with regional variation in utilization? *Circ Cardiovasc Qual Outcomes* 3(3):253–260, 2010.
45. American College of Cardiology Cardiosource: Available at http://www.cardiosource.org/Science-And-Quality/Practice-Guidelines-and-Quality-Standards.aspx?type=KkmZefu5Ikel7rdhS3uegw: Accessed August 11, 2010.
46. Patel MR, Spertus JA, Brindis RG, et al: ACCF proposed method for evaluating the appropriateness of cardiovascular imaging. *J Am Coll Cardiol* 46(8):1606–1613, 2005.
47. Fitch K, Bernstein SJ, Aguilar MD, et al: *The RAND/UCLA appropriateness method user's manual,* Arlington, VA, 2001, RAND.
48. Heupler FA, Al-Hani AJ, Dear WE, et al: Guidelines for continuous quality improvement in the cardiac catheterization laboratory. *Cathet Cardiovasc Diagn* 30(3) 191–200, 1993.

49. American Board of Internal Medicine: Available at http://www.abim.org/pdf/data-candidates-certified/all-candidates.pdf: Accessed July 3, 2010.
50. Heupler FA, Chambers CE, Dear WE, et al: Guidelines for internal peer review in the cardiac catheterization laboratory. *Cathet Cardiovasc Diagn* 4(1):21–32, 1997.
51. Brindis RG, Fitzgerald S, Anderson HV, et al: The American College of Cardiology-National Cardiovascular Data Registry (ACC-NCDR(r)): Building a national clinical data repository. *J Am Coll Cardiol* 37(8):2240–2245, 2001.
52. Eagle KA, Montoye CK, Riba AL, et al: American College of Cardiology's Guidelines Applied in Practice (GAP) Projects in Michigan; American College of Cardiology Foundation Guidelines Applied in Practice Steering committee. Guideline-based standardized care is associated with substantially lower mortality in Medicare patients with acute myocardial infarction. *J Am Coll Cardiol* 46(7):1242–1248, 2005.
53. Bradley EH, Curry LA, Webster TR, et al: Achieving rapid door-to-balloon times: How top hospitals improve complex clinical systems. *Circulation* 113(8):1079–1085, 2006.
54. Krumholz HM, Bradley EH, Nallamothu BK, et al: A campaign to improve the timeliness of primary percutaneous coronary intervention: Door-to-Balloon: An Alliance for Quality. *JACC Cardiovasc Interv* 1(1):97–104, 2008.
55. Bradley EH, Nallamothu BK, Herrin J, et al: National efforts to improve door-to-balloon time results from the Door-to-Balloon Alliance. *J Am Coll Cardiol* 54(25):2423–2429, 2009.
56. Patel MR, Dehmer GJ, Hirshfeld JW, et al: ACCF/SCAI/STS/AATS/AHA/ASNC 2009 Appropriateness Criteria for Coronary Revascularization: A Report of the American College of Cardiology Foundation Appropriateness Criteria Task Force, Society for Cardiovascular Angiography and Interventions, Society of Thoracic Surgeons, American Association for Thoracic Surgery, American Heart Association, and the American Society of Nuclear Cardiology. *J Am Coll Cardiol* 53(6):530–553, 2009.
57. Krumholz HM, Brindis RG, Brush JE, et al; American Heart Association; Quality of Care and Outcomes Research Interdisciplinary Writing Group; Council on Epidemiology and Prevention; Stroke Council; American College of Cardiology Foundation: Standards for statistical models used for public reporting of health outcomes: An American Heart Association Scientific Statement from the Quality of Care and Outcomes Research Interdisciplinary Writing Group: Cosponsored by the Council on Epidemiology and Prevention and the Stroke Council. Endorsed by the American College of Cardiology Foundation. *Circulation* 113(3):456–462, 2006.
58. National Cardiovascular Data Registry: Available at www.NCDR.com: Accessed July 5, 2010.
59. Peterson ED, Dai D, DeLong ER, et al: Contemporary mortality risk prediction for percutaneous coronary intervention: Results from 588,398 procedures in the National Cardiovascular Data Registry. *J Am Coll Cardiol* 55(18):1923–1932, 2010.
59a. Chan PS, Patel MR, Klein LW, et al: Appropriateness of percutaneous coronary intervention. *JAMA* 306:53–61, 2011.
60. Colton D: Quality improvement in health care—Conceptual and historical foundation. *Eval Health Prof* 23(1):7–42, 2000.
61. Hammermeister KE: Participatory continuous improvement. *Ann Thorac Surg* 58(6):1815–1821, 1994.
62. Jencks SF, Wilensky GR: The health care quality improvement initiative. A new approach to quality assurance in Medicare. *JAMA* 268(7):900–903, 1992.
63. Ferguson TB, Peterson ED, Coombs LP, et al: Use of continuous quality improvement to increase use of process measures in patients undergoing coronary artery bypass graft surgery. A randomized controlled trial. *JAMA* 290(1):49–56, 2003.
64. Moscucci M, Rogers EK, Montoye C, et al: Association of a continuous quality improvement initiative with practice and outcomes variations of contemporary percutaneous coronary interventions. *Circulation* 113(6):814–822, 2006.
65. Rihal CS, Kamath CC, Holmes DR, et al: Economic and clinical outcomes of a physician-led continuous quality improvement intervention in the delivery of percutaneous coronary intervention. *Am J Manag Care* 12(8):445–452, 2006.
66. Brindis RG, Dehmer GJ: Continuous quality improvement in the cardiac catheterization laboratory: Are the benefits worth the cost and effort? *Circulation* 113(6):767–770, 2006.
67. Aiken LH, Clarke SP, Sloane DM, et al: Hospital nurse staffing and patient mortality, nurse burnout, and job dissatisfaction. *JAMA* 288(16):1987–1993, 2002.
68. Aiken LH, Sochalski J, Lake ET: Studying outcomes of organizational change in health services. *Med Care* 35(11 Suppl):NS6–N18, 1997.

69. Ferlie E, Shortell SM: Improving the quality of health care in the United Kingdom and the United States: A framework for change. *Milbank Quarterly* 79(2):281–315, 2001.

70. Majumdar SR, McAlister FA, Furberg CD: From knowledge to practice in chronic cardiovascular disease: A long and winding road. *J Am Coll Cardiol* 43(10):1738–1742, 2004.

71. Lansky D: Improving quality through public disclosure of performance information. *Health Aff* 21(4):52–62, 2002.

72. Department of Health Care Policy, Massachusetts Data Analysis Center (Mass-DAC): Available at http://www.massdac.org/reports/surgery.html: Accessed July 8, 2010.

73. Li Z, Carlile DM, Marcin JP, et al: Impact of public reporting on access to coronary artery bypass surgery: The California Outcomes Reporting Program. *Ann Thorac Surg* 89(4);1131–1138, 2010.

74. Hannan EL, Kumar D, Racz M, et al: New York State's Cardiac Surgery Reporting System: Four years later. *Ann Thorac Surg* 58(6):1852–1857, 1994.

75. Bentley JM, Nash DB: How Pennsylvania hospitals have responded to publicly released reports on coronary artery bypass graft surgery. *Jt Comm J Qual Improv* 24(1):40–49, 1998.

76. Shahian DM, Silverstein T, Lovett AF, et al: Comparison of clinical and administrative data sources for hospital coronary artery bypass graft surgery report cards. *Circulation* 115(12):1518–1527, 2007.

77. Hannan EL, Racz MJ, Jollis JG, et al: Using Medicare claims data to assess provider quality for CABG surgery: Does it work well enough? *Health Serv Res* 31(6):659–678, 1997.

78. Centers for Medicare and Medicaid Services: *Hospital quality initiatives: Hospital compare*: Available at http://www.hospitalcompare.hhs.gov/: Accessed July 8, 2010.

79. Werner RM, Asch DA: The unintended consequences of publicly reporting quality information. *JAMA* 293(10):1239–1244, 2005.

80. Marshall MN, Shekelle PG, Leatherman S, et al: The public release of performance data: what do we expect to gain? A review of the evidence. *JAMA* 283(14):1866–1874, 2000.

81. Omoigui NA, Miller DP, Brown KJ, et al: Outmigration for coronary bypass surgery in an era of public dissemination of clinical outcomes. *Circulation* 93(1):27–33, 1996.

82. Schneider EC, Epstein AM: Influence of cardiac-surgery performance reports on referral practices and access to care. A survey of cardiovascular specialists. *N Engl J Med* 335(4):251–256, 1996.

83. Schneider EC, Epstein AM: Use of public performance reports: A survey of patients undergoing cardiac surgery. *JAMA* 279(20): 1638–1642, 1998.

84. Pesce NL: *New York Daily News*, January 14, 2010: Available at http://www.nydailynews.com/lifestyle/health/2010/01/14/2010-01 14_some_doctors_requiring_gag_orders_to_keep_patients_from_posting_unflattering_int.html: Accessed August 12, 2010.

85. Moscucci M, Eagle KA, Share D, et al: Public reporting and case selection for percutaneous coronary interventions: An analysis from two large multicenter percutaneous coronary intervention databases. *J Am Coll Cardiol* 45(11):1759–1765, 2005.

86. Apolito RA, Greenberg MA, Menegus MA, et al: Impact of the New York State Cardiac Surgery and Percutaneous Coronary Intervention Reporting System on the management of patients with acute myocardial infarction complicated by cardiogenic shock. *Am Heart J* 155(2):267–273, 2008.

87. Narins CR, Dozier AM, Ling FS, et al: The influence of public reporting of outcome data on medical decision making by physicians. *Arch Intern Med* 165(1):83–87, 2005.

88. Resnic FS, Welt FG: The public health hazards of risk avoidance associated with public reporting of risk-adjusted outcomes in coronary intervention. *J Am Coll Cardiol* 53(10):825–830, 2009.

89. Adams JL, Mehrotra A, Thomas JW, et al: Physician cost profiling—reliability and risk of misclassification. *N Engl J Med* 362(11):1014–1021, 2010.

90. Fung CH, Lim Y-W, Mattke S, et al: Systematic review: Evidence that publishing patient care performance data improves quality of care. *Ann Intern Med* 148(2):111–123, 2008.

91. Drozda JP, Jr, Hagan EP, Mirro MJ, et al: ACCF 2008 health policy statement on principles for public reporting of physician performance data: A report of the American College of Cardiology Foundation Writing Committee to Develop Principles for Public Reporting of Physician Performance Data. *J Am Coll Cardiol* 51(20):1993–2001, 2008.

Volume and Outcome

JAMES G. JOLLIS

A series of studies over 30 years have repeatedly identified a relationship between increased procedural volume and lower mortality, particularly for higher-risk procedures or patients.[1-11] The finding of better outcomes with increased experience seems rather obvious and, in isolation, should not engender much controversy. When the volume–outcome relationship is applied to health policy in a manner that suggests that patients should avoid low-volume hospitals or physicians, passionate debate ensues. Fueled by intense policy interests, papers that support or refute volume standards continue to be published in the medical and health services research literature. This chapter will examine the volume–outcome relationship for PCIs in depth according to the strength of the evidence and the underlying reasons why study conclusions may vary despite the consistency of the relationship. On the basis of this review, a practical framework for public policy will be proposed. To provide some perspective on the issue, one must first understand that the proposed volume thresholds represent very low numbers and impact relatively few patients. The relationship between worse outcome and low volume is most apparent among the very-low-volume operators. In the case of interventional cardiologist volume, an overall PCI volume of 75 cases per year requires performance of fewer than two procedures per week, and a primary PCI volume of 12 involves treatment of one ST elevation myocardial infarction (STEMI) per month. A hospital must perform 4 cases per week to reach a threshold of 200 elective PCI cases, and 3 cases per month to reach a primary PCI threshold of 36 cases. With such low thresholds, low-volume providers treat relatively few patients. A reasonable gauge of the relative proportion of patients treated in low-volume institutions can be obtained from the National Inpatient Sample (NIS), a nationally representative cohort of patients of all ages treated at 20% of the U.S. hospitals.[1] Data from the NIS indicate that only 4% of patients undergoing PCI are treated in hospitals with volumes below 200 cases per year, yet the low-volume institutions treating these relatively few patients represent 27% of hospitals (Fig. 63-1). Similarly, extrapolating physician volumes from the New York State Coronary Angioplasty

Reporting System, 7% of patients are treated by physicians who perform fewer than 75 cases per year, and these operators represent 30% of all physicians performing PCI.

Evidence for a Volume–Outcome Relationship

The origins of the volume–outcome relationship date back to 1979 when Luft, Bunker, and Enthoven of Stanford University identified higher mortality at lower-volume hospitals for a number of surgical procedures, including open heart and vascular surgeries.[2] Of 12 surgeries, the relationship was most evident among the higher-risk procedures, and their initial data identified a threshold of approximately 200 surgical procedures above which procedural mortality decreased by 25% to 41%. In their initial work, the authors suggested that the observed relationships supported the regionalization of higher-risk procedures. Since the initial work, the volume–outcome relationship has repeatedly been demonstrated for a number of procedures and conditions, most recently by Ross et al.[12] Examining over three million Medicare patients hospitalized at 4679 hospitals between 2004 and 2006 for acute myocardial infarction (AMI), congestive heart failure (CHF), or pneumonia, those treated at lower-volume hospitals had significantly higher 30-day mortality rates. For AMI, the upper volume threshold was 610 cases, beyond which significant differences in mortality were no longer observed.

Volume standards for PCI were first introduced in the 1988 American College of Cardiology/American Heart Association (ACC/AHA) guidelines.[13] Lacking empirical evidence for coronary angioplasty volume, the task force selected the threshold volume of 50 cases based on the rationale that one must golf about once per week to remain proficient and that such an experiential relationship likely extended to PCIs. The publication of this standard unleashed a flood of concerns from approximately half the cardiologists performing angioplasty at the time who did not meet the one-case-per-week standard. Providers opposed to volume standards were concerned about restrictions to practice in the absence of empirical evidence of a volume–outcome relationship for PCI. They were also concerned that such standards may impede high-quality but low-volume physicians and that annual volume standards did not take into account aggregate experience over a number of years.

Empirical evidence supporting a volume–outcome relationship for PCI began to emerge in the 1990's. In a study of Medicare procedures, Jollis et al found in-hospital mortality increasing from 2.5% for high-volume hospitals to 3.9% for those treated at low-volume hospitals.[3] Among the 217,836 patients studied, the relationship between volume and outcome appeared "J" shaped, with the highest mortality for hospital volumes at below 100 Medicare procedures per year (Fig. 63-2). As Medicare primarily involves patients over age 65 years, a Medicare case volume of 100 represents an overall hospital volume of roughly 200 cases per year. For 19,594 patients undergoing elective PCI in 48 hospitals in the Society for Cardiac Angiography and Interventions registry, Kimmel found significantly higher mortality, emergency bypass, and major complications for patients treated at hospitals with volumes below 400 cases per year.[4] In the New York State Coronary Angioplasty Reporting System, Hannan et al identified significantly higher risk-adjusted mortality for patients treated at hospitals with annual volumes below 600.[5] Following the widespread adoption of

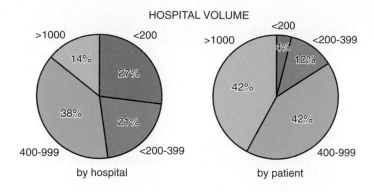

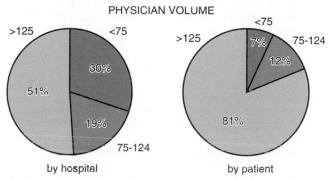

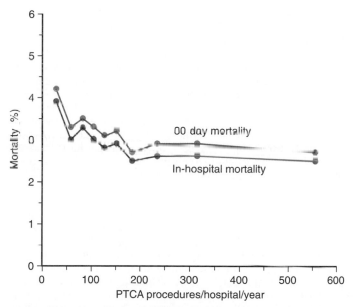

Figure 63-1 Distribution of percutaneous coronary intervention (PCI) volume by hospitals, physicians, and patients. (Adapted from Epstein, Hannan 2005)[1,10]

Figure 63-2 Mortality for Medicare beneficiaries according to hospital volume. (Data from Jollis JG, Peterson ED, DeLong ER, et al: The relation between the volume of coronary angioplasty procedures at hospitals treating Medicare beneficiaries and short-term mortality, N Engl J Med 331:1625–1629, 1994.)

coronary stents, repeat analyses of Medicare data by McGrath et al continued to identify higher mortality for low-volume hospitals.

Evidence for a relationship between physician volume and outcome also emerged in related analyses, with both Jollis and Hannan identifying higher in-hospital mortality for physician volumes below 75 cases per year.[5,6] Thus, with substantial compelling evidence, the PCI

guidelines revised the minimum volume standards upward to 75 cases per year for physicians and 200 cases per year for hospitals.[14] Since the original evidence was incorporated into the updated guidelines, the volume–outcome relationship continues to be examined in contemporary studies. With improved technology and lower event rates, the question remains whether this relationship should continue to guide policy regarding hospital and operator volumes. To understand empirical evidence concerning the volume–outcome relationship, one must keep in perspective three basic concepts of observational research: (1) frequency of the endpoint, (2) representativeness of the sample, and (3) regression analyses techniques. Considering more recent evidence in light of these concepts, the relationship continues to be observed in higher-risk populations and samples with an adequate representation of low-volume providers.

The first consideration when evaluating empirical evidence is whether the study involves an adequate number of endpoints to observe a volume–outcome relationship. The relationship is most apparent in high-risk patients who are more likely to experience complications and death. In the first study of volume and outcome for PCIs, the greatest differences in mortality by volume were seen in the subset of patients with AMI, with mortality for low-, medium-, and high-volume hospitals of 8.1%, 7.1%, and 6.4%, respectively, compared with 1.3%, 1.2%, and 1.0% mortality for patients without MI treated at low-, medium-, and high-volume hospitals.[3] This finding follows the clinical intuition that experience is likely to be most important in managing complications and high-risk situations.

Contemporary studies of patients with AMI that include the universe of low-volume operators continue to provide persuasive evidence of a volume–outcome relationship. Srinivas et al examined in-hospital mortality in 7321 patients receiving primary PCI in New York State at 41 hospitals (volume range 1 to 172 primary PCIs per year) from 266 physicians (volume range 1 to 55 primary PCIs per year).[8] Risk-adjusted mortality was substantially lower for higher-volume hospitals at a volume threshold of 50 cases per year (≤50, >50 primary PCIs per year mortality 5.4%, 3.4%; odds ratio [OR] 0.58; 95% confidence interval [CI] 0.38–0.88) and for physicians at 20 cases per year (≤20, >20 primary PCIs per year mortality 4.2%, 2.9%; OR 0.63; 95% CI 0.44–0.91) (Fig. 63-3). Stratifying risk-adjusted mortality by hospital and physician volume, the highest mortality of 7.9% (P = 0.01) was seen for patients treated by low-volume physicians (<20 primary PCIs per year) practicing in low-volume hospitals (<50 primary PCIs/year), and, conversely, the lowest mortality of 2.8% was seen among patients treated by high-volume physicians (>20 primary PCIs/year) at high-volume hospitals (>50 primary PCIs/year). The stratified analysis showing an interaction between physician and hospital volumes suggests that both physician and staff experience contribute to better outcomes. Conversely, when adverse outcomes decline, the volume–outcome relationship is mitigated. Following the introduction of coronary stents, abrupt coronary artery closure and the need for urgent bypass surgery markedly decreased from 3.8% to 1.9% in Medicare patients.[3,7] Repeat analyses by McGrath et al found that the inverse relationship between volume and surgery was no longer apparent following the adoption of coronary stents. By combining endpoints, the ability of an observational study to observe a volume–outcome relationship increases. Moscucci et al examined the composite endpoint of death, bypass surgery, stroke or transient ischemic attack, MI, and repeat PCI for 18,504 patients treated at 14 Michigan hospitals while participating in a quality improvement initiative.[9] Although individual complications were more common for low-volume physicians, the relationships did not reach statistical significance until combined as a composite endpoint (Fig. 63-4).

To understand empirical evidence, a second important consideration is whether the study population includes a representative sample of low-volume operators. Studies that include the universe of low-volume operators according to mandatory registries or hospital claims, such as the New York Coronary Angioplasty Reporting System or the National Inpatient Sample (NIS), consistently identify volume–outcome relationships, whereas those that rely on voluntary

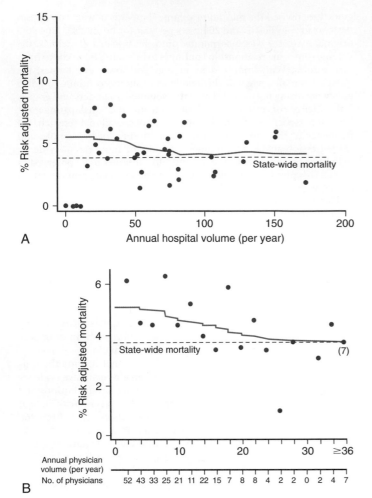

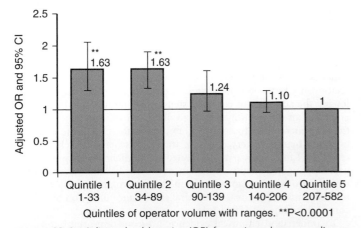

Figure 63-3 Volume–outcome relationships for hospitals (*A*) and physicians (*B*) for primary percutaneous coronary interventions in New York State. (*Adapted from Srinivas VS, Hailpern SM, Koss E, Monrad ES, Alderman MH: Effect of physician volume on the relationship between hospital volume and mortality during primary angioplasty, J Am Coll Cardiol 53:574–579, 2009.*)

Figure 63-4 Adjusted odds ratios (OR) for major adverse cardiovascular events with generalized estimating equations clustering modeling. ** *P* < 0.0001. (*Adapted from Moscucci M, Share D, Smith D, et al: Relationship between operator volume and adverse outcome in contemporary percutaneous coronary intervention practice: An analysis of a quality-controlled multicenter percutaneous coronary intervention clinical database, J Am Coll Cardiol 46:625–632, 2005.*)

participation by hospitals focused on quality improvement are less likely to include an adequate sample of low-volume providers sufficient to characterize the volume–outcome relationship. The most representative cohort of PCI patients involves the NIS cited above, involving discharge records for a random sample of acute care hospitals that approximates a 20% stratified sample of U.S. community hospitals.[15] The NIS includes all payers and thus includes patients under age 65 years. Examining 362,748 patients treated at 457 hospitals, including 122 hospitals with volumes below 200 cases per year, Epstein et al found a stepwise increase for in-hospital mortality according to volume categories (<200: 2.6%, 200–399: 1.8%, 400–999: 1.6%, 1000+: 1.4%; *P* < 0.001).[1] The greatest mortality differences were seen among high-risk patients, including those over age 75 years (<200: 5.8%, 1000+: 3.0%, *P* < 0.001) and with AMI (<200: 4.5%, 1000+: 3.4%, *P* < 0.001). A related consideration involves the prevalence of low-volume PCI programs as a function of state regulation. Historically, New York has been highly regulated, resulting in relatively few low-volume institutions, whereas the regulatory environment in California has been conducive to low-volume hospitals. Comparing the statewide PCI data from New York and California, Carey et al found New York hospital volume to be substantially higher (PCI cases per hospital per year, New York 1007, California 376).[16] This difference in hospital volume was associated with almost double the rate of in-hospital mortality for California (New York 0.76%, California 1.43%) for corresponding years. Although patient descriptors cannot be directly compared between New York registry data and California claims data, population-based rates of PCI were similar between these states making patient selection an unlikely explanation for the higher mortality in California. The study by Carey also attributed 33% higher bypass surgery mortality in California to a predominance of low-volume surgery programs in the state. The New York and California comparison indicates that studies that include regions with a predominance of low-volume operators are more likely to identify a volume–outcome relationship.

Careful consideration of regression models represents a third important element of volume–outcome relationship studies. Regression analyses simply examine the mathematical relationship between two variables according to a set of data points. As regression techniques become more complex, their presentation in papers must be abbreviated to meet editorial requirements. Thus, elaborate regression procedures have evolved into "black box" approaches to balancing comparisons. Without detailed presentations, readers are unable to assess whether regression techniques have overcome critical obstacles that limit their ability to reliably identify relationships of interest, namely, confounding, multi-co-linearity, unmeasured risk, and model fit. Even the most sophisticated modeling techniques are limited by sample size and the potential for type II errors, incorrectly accepting the null hypothesis of no difference when a significant difference exists. Mortality differences by volume that are apparent in unadjusted data may lose their statistical significance in regression models as statistical thresholds are raised to satisfy probability assumptions. For example, Kumbhani et al examined primary PCI volume and outcome for 29,513 patients directly presenting to 116 hospitals while participating in the Get With The Guidelines (GWTG) registry.[17] Stratified by annual hospital primary PCI volume, there was a trend toward higher mortality for lower-volume institutions (<36 procedures: 3.9%, 36–70 procedures: 3.2%, and >70 procedures: 3.0%) These differences were present despite the exclusion of patients treated in hospitals that submitted fewer than 30 patients and irrespective of the select nature of GWTG hospitals. Following adjustment in regression models, the mortality difference did not reach statistical significance (low volume vs. high volume, adjusted OR 1.3, *P* = 0.15). The study used generalized estimating equations, a technique that has become widespread over the past decade. This conservative approach accounts for the lack of independence of patients treated within the same hospital but requires larger samples or absolute differences to identify statistically significant findings compared with regression analyses that ignore "within-hospital" clustering.

Generalized estimating equations raise the threshold for statistical significance, increasing the likelihood of a type II error. In viewing negative findings from regression adjusted analyses such as the Kumbhani study, one must not confuse the "absence of proof" with "proof of absence."

Public Policy Implications

As noted above, those who argue against volume standards cite concerns about restricting high-quality but low-volume providers. Participation in national registries has been put forth as an alternative to minimal procedural volumes such that quality can be measured and ensured. Another advantage of this approach is that low-volume providers are motivated to avoid high-risk patients, the patients for whom the volume–outcome relationship is most apparent. Unfortunately, registries lack statistical power to reliably identify quality low-volume providers because of insufficient sample size. Low-volume hospitals and physicians have worse outcomes, on average, and policies that broadly apply volume standards should avert procedural complications and deaths. Although national guidelines have incorporated volume standards, the majority of decisions regarding physician and hospital practice occur at the local or state level irrespective of these guidelines.[18] Interventional cardiologists are granted privileges at the hospital level, and hospitals have significant incentives to encourage all physicians to perform procedures in their facilities regardless of volume standards. The ability of hospitals to open and operate interventional cardiology programs is regulated by states, and standards vary widely. In many regions of the country, low-volume PCI programs are common and increasing in number despite national standards and empirical evidence. Coronary intervention represents a profitable activity from the hospitals' perspective, and hospitals have successfully lobbied many state governments to allow the expansion of low-volume facilities. With national declines in cardiac catheterization procedures since 2000, the need for the continued expansion of PCI facilities becomes even more questionable.[19] The necessity of additional hospitals and operators varies according to the elective or urgent nature of the procedure. Elective PCI procedures are relatively low risk and less subject to the volume–outcome relationship. However, the very nature of elective procedures allows for diversion of patients to higher-volume facilities, obviating the need for more PCI facilities. Whether volume standards should be strictly applied for primary PCI procedures represents a more challenging and uncertain policy question. The time-dependent relationship between device activation and patient survival, coupled with extraordinarily long "first hospital door-to-device" times for patients requiring hospital transfer for acute intervention, favor a broadening of the availability of primary PCI.[20,21] Particularly for patients presenting to rural hospital emergency departments, where transport times to PCI facilities are longer than 30 to 40 minutes, a case can be made for expanding PCI facilities to rural areas. High-risk patients including those with AMI have the worst outcomes with low-volume providers, however, and a better strategy may involve reperfusion with fibrinolysis at the rural hospital, followed by transfer to a regional PCI facility.

Conclusion

A relationship between lower volume and worse outcomes has been established by sizeable and compelling empirical evidence over the past 30 years. This association is most apparent among high-risk patients and procedures. The strength of supporting evidence varies as a function of representation by low-volume providers, sample size, the number of outcomes of interest, and regression techniques. Although procedural volume represents only one facet of quality cardiovascular care, the supporting evidence and concern for patients compels the medical community to foster experienced interventional operators and facilities to the extent possible.

REFERENCES

1. Epstein AJ, Rathore SS, Volpp KG, et al: Hospital percutaneous coronary intervention volume and patient mortality, 1998 to 2000. *J Am Coll Cardiol* 43:1755–1762, 2004.
2. Luft HS, Bunker JP, Enthoven AC: Should operations be regionalized? The empirical relation between surgical volume and mortality. *N Engl J Med* 301:1364–1369, 1979.
3. Jollis JG, Peterson ED, DeLong ER, et al: The relation between the volume of coronary angioplasty procedures at hospitals treating Medicare beneficiaries and short-term mortality. *N Engl J Med* 331:1625–1629, 1994.
4. Kimmel SE, Berlin JA, Laskey WK: The relationship between coronary angioplasty procedure volume and major complications. *JAMA* 274:1137–1142, 1995.
5. Hannan EL, Racz M, Ryan TJ, et al: Coronary angioplasty volume outcome relationships for hospitals and cardiologists. *JAMA* 279:892–898, 1997.
6. Jollis JG, Peterson ED, Nelson CL, et al: Relationship between physician and hospital coronary angioplasty volume and outcome in elderly patients. *Circulation* 95:2485–2491, 1997.
7. McGrath PD, Wennberg DE, Malenka DJ, et al: Operator volume and outcomes in 12,988 percutaneous coronary interventions. *J Am Coll Cardiol* 31:570–576, 1998.
8. Srinivas VS, Hailpern SM, Koss E, et al: Effect of physician volume on the relationship between hospital volume and mortality during primary angioplasty. *J Am Coll Cardiol* 53:574–579, 2009.
9. Moscucci M, Share D, Smith D, et al: Relationship between operator volume and adverse outcome in contemporary percutaneous coronary intervention practice: An analysis of a quality-controlled multicenter percutaneous coronary intervention clinical database. *J Am Coll Cardiol* 46:625–632, 2005.
10. Hannan EL, Wu C, Walford G, et al: Volume-outcome relationships for percutaneous coronary interventions in the stent era. *Circulation* 112:1171–1179, 2005.
11. Vakili BA, Kaplan R, Brown DL: Volume-outcome relation for physicians and hospitals performing angioplasty for acute myocardial infarction in New York State. *Circulation* 104:2171–2176, 2001.
12. Ross JS, Normand SLT, Wang Y, et al: Hospital volume and 30 day mortality for three common medical conditions. *N Engl J Med* 362:1110–1118, 2010.
13. Ryan TJ, Faxon DP, Gunnar RM, et al: Guidelines for percutaneous transluminal coronary angioplasty: A report of the American College of Cardiology/American Heart Association Task Force on Assessment of Diagnostic and Therapeutic Cardiovascular Procedures. *Circulation* 78:486–502, 1988.
14. Ryan TJ, Bauman WB, Kennedy JW, et al: Guidelines for percutaneous transluminal coronary angioplasty. A report of the American Heart Association/American College of Cardiology Task Force on Assessment of Diagnostic and Therapeutic Cardiovascular Procedures (Committee on Percutaneous Transluminal Coronary Angioplasty). *Circulation* 88:2987–3007, 1993.
15. http://www.hcup-us.ahrq.gov/nisoverview.jsp: Accessed December 23, 2010.
16. Carey JS, Danielsen B, Gold JP, et al: Procedure rates and outcomes of coronary revascularization procedures in California and New York. *J Thorac Cardiovasc Surg* 129:1276–1282, 2005.
17. Kumbhani DJ, CP Cannon, GC Fonarow, et al: Association of hospital primary angioplasty volume in ST-segment elevation myocardial infarction with quality and outcomes. *JAMA* 302:2207–2213, 2009.
18. Smith SC, Jr, Feldman TE, Hirshfeld JW, Jr, et al: ACC/AHA/SCAI 2005 guideline update for percutaneous coronary intervention: A report of the American College of Cardiology/American Heart Association Task Force on Practice Guidelines (ACC/AHA/SCAI Writing Committee to Update the 2001 Guidelines for Percutaneous Coronary Intervention). *J Am Coll Cardiol* 47:1–121, 2006.
19. Lloyd Jones D, Adams RJ, Brown TM, et al; on behalf of the American Heart Association Statistics Committee and Stroke Statistics Subcommittee: Heart disease and stroke statistics— 2010 update: A report from the American Heart Association. *Circulation* 121:e46–e215, 2010.
20. Boersma E, The Primary Coronary Angioplasty vs. Thrombolysis (PCAT)-2 Trialists' Collaborative Group: Does time matter? A pooled analysis of randomized clinical trials comparing primary percutaneous coronary intervention and in-hospital fibrinolysis in acute myocardial infarction patients. *Eur Heart J* 27:779–788, 2006.
21. Jollis JG, Roettig ML, Aluko AO, et al: Implementation of a statewide system for coronary reperfusion for ST-segment elevation myocardial infarction. *JAMA* 298:2371–2380, 2007.